CANCER
OF THE HEAD AND NECK

CANCER
OF THE HEAD AND NECK

FOURTH EDITION

Eugene N. Myers, MD

Professor and Eye & Ear Foundation Chair
Department of Otolaryngology University of Pittsburgh School of Medicine
Professor Department of Oral and Maxillofacial Surgery University of Pittsburgh School
of Dental Medicine Pittsburgh, Pennsylvania

James Y. Suen, MD

Professor and Chairman
Department of Otolaryngology–Head and Neck Surgery
University of Arkansas for Medical Sciences Director, Arkansas Cancer Research Center
Professor and Chairman Department of Otolaryngology–Head and Neck Surgery
Arkansas Children's Hospital Little Rock, Arkansas

Jeffrey N. Myers, MD, PhD

Assistant Professor of Surgery
Department of Head and Neck Surgery
University of Texas M.D. Anderson Cancer Center
Houston, Texas

Ehab Y. N. Hanna, MD

Professor and Vice-Chairman Director of Head and Neck Oncology and Skull Base
Surgery, Department of Otolaryngology–Head and Neck Surgery
University of Arkansas for Medical Sciences, Little Rock, Arkansas

SAUNDERS
An Imprint of Elsevier

BS

SAUNDERS
An Imprint of Elsevier

The Curtis Center
Independence Square West
Philadelphia, Pennsylvania 19106

CANCER OF THE HEAD AND NECK   ISBN 0-7216-9480-2
Copyright © 2003, 1996, 1989, Elsevier Science (USA). All Rights Reserved
Copyright © 1987, Mosby, Inc. All Rights Reserved

Notice

Otolaryngology is an ever-changing field. Standard safety precautions must be followed but as new research and clinical experience broaden our knowledge, changes in treatment and drug therapy may become necessary or appropriate. Readers are advised to check the most current product information provided by the manufacturer of each drug to be administered to verify the recommended dose, the method and duration of administration, and contraindications. It is the responsibility of the treating physician, relying on experience and knowledge of the patient, to determine dosages and the best treatment for each individual patient. Neither the Publisher nor the author assumes any liability for any injury and/or damage to persons or property arising from this publication.

The Publisher

Library of Congress Cataloging-in-Publication Data

Cancer of the head and neck / [edited by] Eugene N. Myers... [et al.].—4th ed.
    p. cm.
 Includes bibliographical references and index.
 ISBN 0-7216-9480-2
 1. Head–Cancer. 2. Neck–Cancer.   I. Myers, Eugene N.

 RC280.H4 C35 2003
 616.99′491–dc21   2002042704

Acquisitions Editor: Rebecca Schmidt
Project Manager: Amy Norwitz
Cover Designer: Ellen Zanolle

CE/MVY

Printed in the United States of America

Last digit is the print number: 9   8   7   6   5   4   3   2   1

12/12/04

This book is dedicated to

My wife, Barbara,
Our children, Marjorie Myers Fulbright and Jeffrey Nicholas Myers, MD, PhD;
Our grandchildren, Alex and Chip Fulbright and Keith, Brett, and Blake Myers,
who are a constant source of joy and inspiration;
My parents, the late Dr. David Myers and Mrs. Rosalind Myers,
whose dedication to patient care was a way of life;
and Dr. John Conley, with whom I learned the principles of head and neck surgery

EUGENE N. MYERS, MD

In memory of
My parents, brothers, Carol Anne, and my patients
all have inspired me;
and to
My family, Karen, Brad, Brennan, Brent, Agnieszka, and Tiffany:
my love to them;
My staff, office staff, and nurses:
thanks for all that you do
Eugene N. Myers, my partner and friend,
for a wonderful sojourn

JAMES Y. SUEN, MD

Lisa, Keith, Brett, and Blake Myers,
who are constant sources of love, pride, and inspiration for me,
and to
My parents, Barbara and Eugene Myers,
for giving me the "right stuff"
I would also like to thank Dr. Helmuth Goepfert
for giving me the opportunity to pursue my dream of being a surgeon-scientist
at a very special institution

JEFFREY N. MYERS, MD, PHD

My wife, Sylvie,
for her patience, sacrifice, and support while I was working on "the book";
Our daughters, Gabrielle Grace (Gigi) Hanna and Camille Lauren Hanna,
for the joy and blessing they bring to our lives;
My parents
who encouraged me to follow my dreams,
The senior editors, Dr. Eugene N. Myers and Dr. James Y. Suen,
for giving me the opportunity and the honor to be part of this work;
My residents and students
who continue to teach me;
And my patients
whose endurance, resilience, and faith continue to amaze me.

EHAB Y. N. HANNA, MD

Contributors

K. Kian Ang, MD, PhD
Professor of Radiation Oncology, Professor and Deputy
Chairman, University of Texas M.D. Anderson Cancer
Center, Houston, Texas
    Chapter 14: *Cancer of the Oropharynx*
    Chapter 31: *General Principles of Radiation Therapy
        for Cancer of the Head and Neck*

Jenny L. Badley, BSN, RNP
Registered Nurse Practitioner, Department of
Otolaryngology, University of Arkansas for
Medical Sciences, Little Rock, Arkansas
    Chapter 30: *Nursing Care*

Leon Barnes, MD
Professor of Pathology and Otolaryngology,
University of Pittsburgh School of Medicine;
Chief, Division of Head and Neck Pathology,
University of Pittsburgh Medical Center, Presbyterian
Shadyside Hospital; Professor and Chairman, Department
of Oral Medicine and Pathology,
University of Pittsburgh School of Dental Medicine,
Pittsburgh, Pennsylvania
    Chapter 3: *Pathology of the Head and Neck: Basic
        Considerations and New Concepts*

Keith E. Blackwell, MD
Associate Professor, David Geffen School of Medicine at
the University of California Los Angeles, Los Angeles,
California
    Chapter 28: *Reconstruction of Major Defects in the
        Head and Neck Following Cancer Surgery*

Donald L. Bodenner, MD
Assistant Professor, Department of Geriatrics; Chief,
Endocrine Oncology, Arkansas Cancer Research Center,
University of Arkansas for Medical Sciences,
Little Rock, Arkansas
    Chapter 19: *Cancer of the Thyroid*

Randall L. Breau, MD
Associate Professor, Department of Otolaryngology,
University of Arkansas for Medical Sciences,
Little Rock, Arkansas
    Chapter 19: *Cancer of the Thyroid*
    Chapter 23: *Cancer of the Ear and Temporal Bone*

Eduardo D. Bruera, MD
Professor and Chair, Department of Palliative Care and
Rehabilitative Medicine, University of Texas
M.D. Anderson Cancer Center, Houston, Texas
    Chapter 36: *Supportive and Palliative Care*

Ricardo L. Carrau, MD
Associate Professor of Otolaryngology; Medical Director,
UPMC Swallowing Disorders Center;
Assistant Professor of Oral and Maxillofacial Surgery;
University of Pittsburgh School of Medicine,
Pittsburgh, Pennsylvania
    Chapter 10: *Surgery of the Anterior and Lateral
        Skull Base*
    Chapter 35: *Rehabilitation of Swallowing and Speech in
        Head and Neck Surgery*

Mark S. Chambers, DMD
Associate Professor, Section of Oncologic Dentistry and
Prosthodontics, Department of Head and Neck Surgery,
University of Texas M.D. Anderson Cancer Center,
Houston, Texas
    Chapter 29: *Oral Rehabilitation of Patients With
        Head and Neck Cancer*

Dominique Chevalier, MD
Professor, Ear Nose Throat/Head and Neck Surgery,
Medical School, Lille University II; Hospital Huriez
C.H.R.U., Lille Cedex, France
    Chapter 16: *Cancer of the Hypopharynx and Cervical
        Esophagus*

Gary L. Clayman, MD, DDS
Professor and Director, Head and Neck Cancer Program;
Alando J. Ballantyne Distinguished Chair of Head and
Neck Surgery, University of Texas M.D. Anderson Cancer
Center, Houston, Texas
    Chapter 14: *Cancer of the Oropharynx*

Bernard Coche-Dequeant, MD
Radiation Oncologist, Centre Oscar Lambret, Lille, France
    Chapter 16: *Cancer of the Hypopharynx and Cervical
        Esophagus*

Michael J. Cunningham, MD
Associate Professor of Otology and Laryngology,
Harvard Medical School; Surgeon, Department of
Otolaryngology, Massachusetts Eye & Ear Infirmary,
Boston, Massachusetts
    Chapter 24: *Cancer of the Head and Neck in the
        Pediatric Population*

Hugh D. Curtin, MD
Professor of Radiology, Harvard Medical School; Chief of
Radiology, Massachusetts Eye & Ear Infirmary, Boston,
Massachusetts
    Chapter 5: *Radiologic Evaluation of Cancer of the
        Head and Neck*
    Chapter 22: *Tumors of the Parapharyngeal Space*

Frederic F. W.-B. Deleyiannis, MD, MPhil, MPH
Assistant Professor, Division of Plastic Surgery,
Department of Surgery, University of Pittsburgh School
of Medicine, Pittsburgh, Pennsylvania
    Chapter 37: *Quality of Life in Patients With
         Head and Neck Cancer*

John L. Dornhoffer, MD
Associate Professor, Department of Otolaryngology,
University of Arkansas for Medical Sciences,
Little Rock, Arkansas
    Chapter 23: *Cancer of the Ear and Temporal Bone*

Thomas B. Dougherty, MD, PhD
Professor of Anesthesiology, University of Texas
M.D. Anderson Cancer Center, Houston, Texas
    Chapter 6: *Anesthetic Considerations*

Ahmed Elsayem, MD
Assistant Professor, Department of Palliative Care and
Rehabilitation Medicine, University of Texas
M.D. Anderson Cancer Center, Houston, Texas
    Chapter 36: *Supportive and Palliative Care*

Cathy Eng, MD
Assistant Professor, GI Medical Oncology,
University of Texas M.D. Anderson Cancer Center,
Houston, Texas
    Chapter 33: *Chemotherapy in the Treatment of Cancer
         of the Head and Neck*

Chun-Yang Fan, MD, PhD
Assistant Professor of Pathology and Otolaryngology,
University of Arkansas for Medical Sciences,
Little Rock, Arkansas
    Chapter 3: *Pathology of the Head and Neck: Basic
         Considerations and New Concepts*

Melanie B. Fukui, MD
Director of Neuroradiology, Allegheny General Hospital,
Pittsburgh, Pennsylvania
    Chapter 5: *Radiologic Evaluation of Cancer of the
         Head and Neck*

Adam S. Garden, MD
Associate Professor, Department of Radiation Oncology,
University of Texas M.D. Anderson Cancer Center,
Houston, Texas
    Chapter 29: *Oral Rehabilitation of Patients With
         Head and Neck Cancer*

Javier Gavilán, MD
Professor of Otolaryngology, Universidad Autonoma;
Chairman, La Paz University Hospital, Madrid, Spain
    Chapter 18: *Cancer of the Neck*

Eric M. Genden, MD
Assistant Professor, Mount Sinai School of Medicine,
New York, New York
    Chapter 28: *Reconstruction of Major Defects in the
         Head and Neck Following Cancer Surgery*

Hermes C. Grillo, MD
Emeritus Professor of Surgery, Harvard Medical School;
Visiting Surgeon, Emeritus Chief of General Thoracic
Surgery, Massachusetts General Hospital, Boston,
Massachusetts
    Chapter 17: *Tumors of the Cervical Trachea*

Zane T. Hammoud, MD
Chief Resident, Cardiothoracic Surgery; Massachusetts
General Hospital, Boston, Massachusetts
    Chapter 17: *Tumors of the Cervical Trachea*

Ehab Y. N. Hanna, MD
Professor and Vice-Chairman, Director of Head and Neck
Oncology and Skull Base Surgery, Department of
Otolaryngology–Head and Neck Surgery,
University of Arkansas for Medical Sciences,
Little Rock, Arkansas
    Chapter 9: *Cancer of the Nasal Cavity,
         Paranasal Sinuses, and Orbit*
    Chapter 21: *Malignant Tumors of the Salivary Glands*

Jeffrey R. Harris, MD
Assistant Professor, Division of Otolaryngology–Head and
Neck Surgery, University of Alberta Faculty of Medicine
and Dentistry, Edmonton, Alberta, Canada
    Chapter 28: *Reconstruction of Major Defects in the
         Head and Neck Following Cancer Surgery*

Jesús J. Herranz-Gonzalez, MD
Chief of Section, Juan Canalejo Hospital, La Caruña,
Spain
    Chapter 18: *Cancer of the Neck*

Waun Ki Hong, MD
Professor of Medicine; Head, Division of Cancer
Medicine; Chairman, Thoracic/Head and Neck Medical
Oncology Department, University of Texas
M.D. Anderson Cancer Center, Houston, Texas
    Chapter 32: *Chemoprevention*

Mary Ann Horn, BSN, RNP
Otolaryngology Nurse Practitioner, Department of
Otolaryngology, University of Arkansas for Medical
Sciences, Little Rock, Arkansas
    Chapter 30: *Nursing Care*

Carla M. Huff, MD
Resident-Chief, Washington University School of
Medicine, Saint Louis, Missouri
    Chapter 4: *Evaluation, Classification, and Staging*

Jonas T. Johnson, MD
Professor, Departments of Otolaryngology and Radiation
Oncology, University of Pittsburgh School of Medicine;
Professor, Department of Oral and Maxillofacial Surgery,
University of Pittsburgh School of Dental Medicine; Vice
Chairman, Department of Otolaryngology; Director,
Otolaryngology Residency Training Program, Eye & Ear
Institute, Pittsburgh, Pennsylvania
    Chapter 22: *Tumors of the Parapharyngeal Space*

Ashutosh Kacker, MD
Assistant Professor of Otorhinolaryngology, Weill College
of Medicine of Cornell University; Assistant Attending,
New York Presbyterian Hospital–Cornell Campus,
New York, New York
    Chapter 15: *Cancer of the Larynx*
    Chapter 25: *Cancer of the Head and Neck in*
        HIV-Infected Patients

Erik S. Kass, MD
Senior Research Investigator, Laboratory of Tumor
Immunology and Biology, National Cancer
Institute/National Institutes for Health; Staff physician,
Warren Grant Magnusen Clinical Center, Bethesda,
Maryland
    Chapter 34: *Immunotherapy of Cancer of the*
        Head and Neck

Merrill S. Kies, MD
Professor of Medicine, Department of Otolaryngology,
University of Texas M.D. Anderson Cancer Center,
Houston, Texas
    Chapter 14: *Cancer of the Oropharynx*

Dennis H. Kraus, MD
Associate Attending, Head and Neck Service; Director,
Speech, Hearing, and Rehabilitation Center, Department
of Surgery, Memorial Sloan-Kettering Cancer Center,
New York, New York
    Chapter 15: *Cancer of the Larynx*

Stephen Y. Lai, MD, PhD
Head and Neck Surgical Oncology Fellow, Department
of Otolaryngology, University of Pittsburgh School of
Medicine, Pittsburgh, Pennsylvania
    Chapter 7: *Nonmelanoma Skin Cancer of the*
        Head and Neck

James C. Lemon, DDS
Professor, Department of Head and Neck Surgery,
Section of Oncologic Dentistry and Prosthodontics,
University of Texas M.D. Anderson Cancer Center,
Houston, Texas
    Chapter 29: *Oral Rehabilitation of Patients With*
        Head and Neck Cancer

Eric J. Lentsch, MD
Assistant Professor, Department of Otolaryngology–Head
and Neck Surgery, University of Louisville, Louisville,
Kentucky
    Chapter 2: *Pathogenesis and Progression of Squamous*
        Cell Carcinoma of the Head and Neck
    Chapter 8: *Melanoma of the Head and Neck*
    Chapter 18: *Cancer of the Neck*

Jean-Louis Lefebvre, MD
Professor, ENT/Head and Neck Surgery, Medical School,
Lille University II; Chief, Head and Neck Surgery
Department, Centre Oscar Lambret, Lille, France
    Chapter 16: *Cancer of the Hypopharynx and Cervical*
        Esophagus

Jack W. Martin, DDS
Professor and Chief, Section of Oncologic Dentistry,
Department of Head and Neck Surgery,
University of Texas M.D. Anderson Cancer Center,
Houston, Texas
    Chapter 29: *Oral Rehabilitation of Patients With*
        Head and Neck Cancer

Douglas J. Mathisen, MD
Professor or Surgery, Harvard Medical School; Visiting
Surgeon, Chief, General Thoracic Surgery, Massachusetts
General Hospital, Boston, Massachusetts
    Chapter 17: *Tumors of the Cervical Trachea*

Christina A. Meyers, PhD
Professor of Neuropsychology, Department of
Neuro-Oncology, University of Texas M.D. Anderson
Cancer Center, Houston, Texas
    Chapter 36: *Supportive and Palliative Care*

Luka Milas, MD, PhD
Professor and Gilbert H. Fletcher Chair in Radiation
Oncology, University of Texas M.D. Anderson Cancer
Center, Houston, Texas
    Chapter 31: *General Principles of Radiation Therapy*
        for Cancer of the Head and Neck

Thomas Murry, PhD
Professor of Speech Pathology, Department of
Otolaryngology; Clinical Director, The Voice and
Swallowing Center, Columbia University College of
Physicians & Surgeons, New York, New York
    Chapter 35: *Rehabilitation of Swallowing and Speech in*
        Head and Neck Surgery

Eugene N. Myers, MD
Professor and Eye & Ear Foundation Chair,
Department of Otolaryngology, University of Pittsburgh
School of Medicine; Professor, Department of Oral and
Maxillofacial Surgery, University of Pittsburgh
School of Dental Medicine, Pittsburgh, Pennsylvania
    Chapter 1: *Perspectives in Head and Neck Cancer*
    Chapter 13: *Cancer of the Oral Cavity*
    Chapter 22: *Tumors of the Parapharyngeal Space*

Jeffrey N. Myers, MD, PhD
Assistant Professor of Surgery, Department of Head and
Neck Surgery, University of Texas M.D. Anderson Cancer
Center, Houston, Texas
    Chapter 2: *Pathogenesis and Progression of Squamous*
        Cell Carcinoma of the Head and Neck
    Chapter 8: *Melanoma of the Head and Neck*

Daniel W. Nuss, MD
Professor and Chairman, Department of
Otolaryngology–Head and Neck Surgery;
Professor, Department of Neurosurgery, Louisiana State
University Health Sciences Center, New Orleans,
Louisiana
    Chapter 10: *Surgery of the Anterior and Lateral*
        Skull Base

Vassiliki A. Papadimitrakopoulou, MD
Assistant Professor of Medicine, Department of
Thoracic/Head and Neck Medical Oncology, University of
Texas M.D. Anderson Cancer Center, Houston, Texas
   Chapter 32: *Chemoprevention*

David G. Pfister, MD
Associate Attending, Department of Medicine, Memorial
Sloan-Kettering Cancer Center, New York, New York
   Chapter 15: *Cancer of the Larynx*

Jay F. Piccirillo, MD
Course Master, Clinical Epidemiology, Washington
University School of Medicine; Attending Physician,
Barnes-Jewish Hospital, St. Louis, Missouri
   Chapter 4: *Evaluation, Classification, and Staging*

Frederic A. Pugliano, MD
St. Joseph's Hospital/Active Staff, St. Mary's Health
Center/Active Staff, St. Louis, Missouri
   Chapter 4: *Evaluation, Classification, and Staging*

Gregory J. Renner, MD
Associate Professor of Surgery, Division of
Otolaryngology–Head and Neck Surgery, University of
Missouri-Columbia School of Medicine, Columbia, Missouri
   Chapter 12: *Cancer of the Lip*

Maria A. Rodriguez, MD
Associate Professor, Ad-Interim Chair, Department of
Lymphoma/Myeloma, University of Texas
M.D. Anderson Cancer Center, Houston, Texas
   Chapter 26: *Lymphomas Presenting in the Head and
      Neck: Current Issues in Diagnosis and
      Management*

Duane A. Sewell, MD
Assistant Professor, Department of Otorhinolaryngology,
University of Pennsylvania School of Medicine,
Philadelphia, Pennsylvania
   Chapter 7: *Nonmelanoma Skin Cancer of the
      Head and Neck*

Ashok R. Shaha, MD
Professor of Surgery, Cornell University College of
Physicians and Surgeons; Attending Surgeon, Head and
Neck Service, Memorial Sloan-Kettering Cancer Center,
New York, New York
   Chapter 20: *Tumors of the Parathyroid Glands*

Jonathan Shun Tong Sham, MD
Professor, Department of Clinical Oncology, University of
Hong Kong, Hong Kong
   Chapter 11: *Cancer of the Nasopharynx*

Almon S. Shiu, MD, PhD
Associate Professor and Director of Stereotactic Service,
University of Texas M.D. Anderson Cancer Center,
Houston, Texas
   Chapter 31: *General Principles of Radiation Therapy
      for Cancer of the Head and Neck*

Alfred A. Simental, Jr., MD
Assistant Professor, Division of Otolaryngology–Head and
Neck Surgery, Department of Surgery, Loma Linda
University School of Medicine, Loma Linda,
California
   Chapter 13: *Cancer of the Oral Cavity*

Bhuvanesh Singh, MD
Assistant Professor, Weill Medical College of Cornell
University; Director, Laboratory of Epithelial Cancer
Biology, Assistant Attending Surgeon, Memorial
Sloan-Kettering Cancer Center, New York, New York
   Chapter 25: *Cancer of the Head and Neck in
      HIV-Infected Patients*

Steven H. Sloan, MD
Assistant Clinical Professor, Department of
Otolaryngology, University of California, San Francisco,
San Francisco, California
   Chapter 28: *Reconstruction of Major Defects in the
      Head and Neck Following Cancer Surgery*

Carl H. Snyderman, MD
Associate Professor of Otolaryngology; Co-Director for
Cranial Base Surgery, University of Pittsburgh School of
Medicine, Pittsburgh, Pennsylvania
   Chapter 10: *Surgery of the Anterior and Lateral
      Skull Base*

James Y. Suen, MD
Professor and Chairman, Department of
Otolaryngology–Head and Neck Surgery,
University of Arkansas for Medical Sciences;
Director, Arkansas Cancer Research Center;
Professor and Chairman, Department of
Otolaryngology–Head and Neck Surgery, Arkansas
Children's Hospital, Little Rock, Arkansas
   Chapter 1: *Perspectives in Head and Neck Cancer*
   Chapter 19: *Cancer of the Thyroid*
   Chapter 21: *Malignant Tumors of the Salivary Glands*
   Chapter 27: *Unusual Tumors*

Daniel E. Supkis, MD
Associate Professor of Anesthesiology, University of Texas
M.D. Anderson Cancer Center, Houston, Texas
   Chapter 6: *Anesthetic Considerations*

Béla B. Toth, MD, DDS
Professor, Department of Head and Neck Surgery,
University of Texas M.D. Anderson Cancer Center,
Houston, Texas
   Chapter 29: *Oral Rehabilitation of Patients With
      Head and Neck Cancer*

Mark L. Urken, MD
Professor and Chairman, Department of Otolaryngology,
Mount Sinai School of Medicine; Attending,
Derald Ruttenberg Cancer Center, New York,
New York
   Chapter 28: *Reconstruction of Major Defects in the
      Head and Neck Following Cancer Surgery*

Carter Van Waes, MD, PhD
Investigator, Tumor Biology Section, Head and Neck
Surgery Branch, National Institute on Deafness and Other
Communication Disorders, Bethesda, Maryland
> Chapter 34: *Immunotherapy of Cancer of the
> Head and Neck*

Everett E. Vokes, MD
John E. Ultmann Professor of Medicine and Radiation and
Cellular Oncology, Pritzker School of Medicine; Director,
Section of Hematology/Oncology, University of Chicago,
Chicago, Illinois
> Chapter 33: *Chemotherapy in the Treatment of Cancer
> of the Head and Neck*

Emre A. Vural, MD
Assistant Professor, Department of Otolaryngology–Head
and Neck Surgery, University of Arkansas for Medical
Sciences, Little Rock, Arkansas
> Chapter 27: *Unusual Tumors*

Milton Waner, MD
Professor, Department of Otolaryngology–Head and Neck
Surgery, University of Arkansas for Medical Sciences;
Director of the Vascular Anomalies Center of Excellence,
Arkansas Children's Hospital, Little Rock,
Arkansas
> Chapter 27: *Unusual Tumors*

Tamara Wasserman, MS
Coordinator, Swallowing Disorders Center, University of
Pittsburgh Medical Center, Pittsburgh, Pennsylvania
> Chapter 35: *Rehabilitation of Swallowing and Speech in
> Head and Neck Surgery*

Randal S. Weber, MD
Gabriel Tucker Professor and Vice-Chair, Department of
Otorhinolaryngology–Head and Neck Surgery;
Director, Center for Head and Neck Cancer,
University of Pennsylvania Health System,
Philadelphia, Pennsylvania
> Chapter 7: *Nonmelanoma Skin Cancer of the
> Head and Neck*

William Ignace Wei, FRCS, FRCSE
W. Mong Professor of Otorhinolaryngology,
Department of Surgery, University of Hong Kong,
Hong Kong
> Chapter 11: *Cancer of the Nasopharynx*

Jane L. Weissman, MD
Professor of Radiology and Otolaryngology; Director of
Head and Neck Imaging, Oregon Health and Science
University, Portland, Oregon
> Chapter 5: *Radiologic Evaluation of Cancer of the
> Head and Neck*

Christopher T. Westfall, MD
Professor of Ophthalmology, University of Arkansas for
Medical Sciences, Little Rock, Arkansas
> Chapter 9: *Cancer of the Nasal Cavity, Paranasal
> Sinuses, and Orbit*

Ernest A. Weymuller, Jr., MD
Professor and Chairman, Department of
Otolaryngology–Head and Neck Surgery, University of
Washington School of Medicine, Seattle, Washington
> Chapter 37: *Quality of Life in Patients With
> Head and Neck Cancer*

Kenneth R. Whittemore, Jr., MD
Resident, Department of Otolaryngology, Massachusetts
Eye & Ear Infirmary, Boston, Massachusetts
> Chapter 24: *Cancer of the Head and Neck in the
> Pediatric Population*

Suzanne Wolden, MD
Assistant Attending, Department of Radiation Oncology,
Memorial Sloan-Kettering Cancer Center, New York,
New York
> Chapter 15: *Cancer of the Larynx*

Bevan Yueh, MD, MPH
Associate Professor, Department of Otolaryngology–Head
and Neck Surgery, University of Washington; Staff Surgeon
and Research Associate, VA Puget Sound, Seattle,
Washington
> Chapter 37: *Quality of Life in Patients With
> Head and Neck Cancer*

Robert P. Zitsch III, MD
Associate Professor and Interim Chief, Division of
Otolaryngology, Department of Surgery, University of
Missouri-Columbia School of Medicine, Columbia,
Missouri
> Chapter 12: *Cancer of the Lip*

Preface

The management of cancer of the head and neck is the best example we know in medicine of a multidisciplinary team approach to a disease entity. It incorporates surgeons, medical specialists, anesthesiologists, radiation oncologists, radiologists, pathologists, and oral, maxillofacial, and plastic surgeons, to name a few. These team members do not necessarily work in the same office or clinic or inpatient unit, but all make a tremendous contribution to the care of this group of patients who have very challenging diseases.

Because most head and neck patients are first referred to a head and neck surgeon, that surgeon must be the leader of the team. However, as the concept of organ preservation has become pervasive in our field, it appears that, at least in the community practice, chemotherapy and radiation therapy have become the first line of treatment for many patients, even though their efficacy in certain anatomic sites has not been proven. This approach decreases the number of patients available for resident training and may decrease the need for fellowship training in head and neck oncologic surgery.

Cancer of the Head and Neck is written primarily for surgeons but also emphasizes all of the specialists who are involved as members of the health care team. In this fourth edition we have have consolidated all of the information given in the previous edition and included additional information in fewer chapters. We have incorporated into the site-specific chapters items previously dealt with in individual chapters, such as the use of antibiotics in head and neck surgery, management of complications of head and neck surgery, and others. We have given more emphasis to reconstruction and rehabilitation of the patient by such chapters as "Oral Rehabilitation of Patients With Head and Neck Cancer" by Mark Chambers and the group from M.D. Anderson; "Rehabilitation of Swallowing and Speech in Head and Neck Surgery" by Thomas Murry, Tamara Wasserman, and Ricardo L. Carrau; and "Supportive and Palliative Care" by Ahmed Elsayem and colleagues from M.D. Anderson. The major change has not been so much in new chapters as in new authors, and we have searched for colleagues both in the United States and abroad to contribute to the book to make it contemporary and not to overlook any item that would contribute to the understanding and management of this disease.

We would like to welcome Jeffrey N. Myers, MD, PhD, and Ehab Y. N. Hanna, MD, as coeditors of this fourth edition, and we are hoping that their contribution in the future as editors of the book will provide a seamless transition and uphold the quality of *Cancer of the Head and Neck*.

EUGENE N. MYERS

JAMES Y. SUEN

Acknowledgments

We are very happy to have the fourth edition of *Cancer of the Head and Neck* published by Elsevier. The medical editors of Elsevier, Stephanie Smith Donley, Hilarie Surrena, and Rebecca Schmidt, have shown great dedication and have been supportive to us since the fourth edition was being created.

We are grateful to our contributors for their time and effort. We know it was a sacrifice for them.

Once again, we owe a great debt to Mary Jo Tutchko, who has been the editorial assistant for the last two editions of our book. She has been the point person from the beginning to the last detail of each book and has devoted herself to making certain that the book was completed despite her otherwise incredibly heavy workload.

Contents

CHAPTER 1

Perspectives in Head and Neck Cancer

Eugene N. Myers
James Y. Suen

In this chapter, we offer our perspectives as editors of the three previous editions of *Cancer of the Head and Neck*; having practiced the specialty of head and neck cancer for more than 30 years, we have participated in an exciting evolution in our field.

In the first edition, the evaluation of the patient with head and neck cancer was fairly simple and consisted primarily of a careful examination of the head and neck, a biopsy, a computed tomography (CT) scan of the head and neck, and a chest radiograph. Now, in addition to CT scans, we have magnetic resonance imaging (MRI), magnetic resonance angiography (MRA), and positron emission tomography (PET) scans to choose from, all of which are expensive and have driven costs even higher, although they provide important information. Today, biopsied specimens frequently undergo immunohistochemical studies, genetic evaluation, and tests for molecular markers, in addition to routine histopathologic examination. Marked improvements in staining techniques have added greater precision to the histopathologic diagnosis of a variety of tumors (see Chapter 3). Enhancements in molecular biologic diagnoses, such as p53 evaluation of surgical margins, are not widely used but certainly can be performed in laboratories with the resources and expertise required to carry out these techniques.[1]

Treatment has become more complex as well. Thirty years ago, the choice was surgery, radiation therapy, or combined therapy. Surgical resections can now be more radical because of the availability of microvascular free-tissue flaps for reconstruction. Radiation treatments can be hyperfractionated or hypofractionated. Three-dimensional conformal planning is commonly used. Neutron or proton beam therapy, intensity-modulated radiation therapy (IMRT), and tomotherapy are available at specialized centers, some causing greater tissue damage and others minimizing tissue damage.

The most significant change in our specialty is the new role of chemotherapy. It has gone from being used for palliation only to a more major role in combination with radiation therapy (organ-sparing therapies) to obviate the need for surgery. A number of studies indicate that chemoradiation is equivalent to surgery–radiation therapy.[2–4] Even though chemoradiation can prevent surgery in many instances, the function of the organ afterward is not always ensured. Most head and neck surgeons believe that patients treated with chemoradiation should be included in protocols so that they can be carefully evaluated and so that the best role for this therapy can be established. Other preliminary data support the use of chemotherapy alone for the treatment of early laryngeal cancer.

◨ TRAINING OF THE HEAD AND NECK SURGEON

The specialty of head and neck surgery was founded by Dr. Hayes Martin, who became Chief of Head and Neck Surgery at Memorial Sloan-Kettering Hospital in 1934. At that time, head and neck surgery was a subspecialty of general surgery, requiring general surgery training followed by a surgical oncology fellowship. It was in the 1950s that a few otolaryngologists with advanced training in oncology established themselves as head and neck surgeons. This created conflicts between the specialties, and as a result, two different societies were formed. In 1956, general and plastic surgeons formed the Society of Head and Neck Surgeons. In 1958, six otolaryngologists—Franklin Keim, William Trible, Edwin Cocke, John S. Lewis, John M. Loré, and George A. Sisson, Sr.—founded the American Society for Head and Neck Surgeons.[5]

In the 1960s, subspecialty training fellowships in head and neck oncologic surgery, which were 1 year in duration, were offered following the completion of general otolaryngology training. By the 1970s, both of the head and neck societies began to admit into their own membership members of the other society. In an effort to make training more uniform, the Joint Council on Advanced Training in Head and Neck Oncologic Surgery was formed in 1977 and was initially chaired by Dr. John Loré. Fellowship programs approved by this joint council had to show commitment, resources, and the ability to train fellows in oncology (including radiotherapy, rehabilitation, and research). A residency in general surgery, otolaryngology, or plastic surgery was a prerequisite for participation in a fellowship program. Fellowships could be 1 or 2 years in duration. In 1992, the Joint Council on Advanced Training in Head and Neck Oncologic Surgery changed the duration of the fellowships to a minimum of 2 years because new technologies were developing, and such a change was compatible with its goal of producing clinician-scientists who would be the leaders of our specialty. When this 2-year minimum was initiated, the number of applicants decreased significantly and many fellowships went unfilled, and non-approved 1-year fellowships became more popular. As a result of these events, in 2000, the Joint Council on Advanced Training in Head and Neck Oncologic Surgery changed the duration of head and neck fellowships back to a 1-year minimum. At present, there are 16 approved fellowship programs, and several applications are pending.

As mentioned, two separate head and neck societies had their beginnings during the 1950s. Many years passed before the barriers between the two societies began to fall. One of the most significant breakthroughs was the establishment of joint scientific meetings and joint international conferences (held every 4 years). Because of the decreased numbers of general surgeons and plastic surgeons applying for fellowships and specializing in head and neck surgery, the two societies made the decision to merge in 1999; in the year 2000, the American Head and Neck Society was formed, with Dr. Jesus Medina as its first president—a development that fulfilled the dream of many past presidents of the two societies.

■ ROLE OF THE SURGEON

In times past, the surgeon was the person who was in charge of the head and neck cancer patient's care—making the diagnosis, deciding the treatment, performing the surgery, prescribing the rehabilitation, and taking care of the patient whose treatment failed until his or her death. Now, because of the active roles of the medical oncologist and the radiation oncologist, the surgeon is part of a multidisciplinary team that makes treatment decisions, although he or she is usually still the leader. In addition, the expanded roles of maxillofacial prosthodontists, speech pathologists, and physical therapists, working with the help of surgeons, have benefited patients in achieving maximal functional outcomes.

Once, the head and neck surgeon did the extirpative surgery and the reconstruction; it is now commonplace for a separate reconstructive surgeon to do the reconstruction, especially when a microvascular free-tissue transfer is indicated. Because free-tissue flaps can cover large defects, the head and neck surgeon can take larger margins, a practice that provides better opportunity for local control.

Because of organ-sparing protocols, many patients in whom initial treatment has failed undergo major salvage surgery. Salvage surgery has a high risk of complications and generally should be performed by a surgeon with significant oncologic experience. Cancer involving the cranial base has evolved into a specialty in itself that combines the work of cranial base surgeons and neurosurgeons.

As a response to the concept of organ preservation by chemoradiation, there are those who have adopted the idea of organ preservation by surgery. Dr. Gregory Weinstein's recent book entitled *Organ Preservation Surgery for Laryngeal Cancer* has particularly emphasized the use of supracricoid laryngectomy in patients with various cancers of the larynx who previously would have had total laryngectomy.[6] Dr. Wolfgang Steiner from Germany has also emphasized the use of microsurgical laser techniques in the management of cancers of the supraglottic larynx.[7]

With the evolution of health care economics, head and neck cancer surgery is being performed less often in the community. Poor reimbursement by third party carriers, higher-risk patient populations, and lack of trained head and neck nurses are the primary reasons. Patients commonly are referred to academic health centers for their cancer care.

A greater number of surgical procedures are being done with the use of endoscopes. Although the morbidity and the healing time may be reduced with these procedures, one must be mindful that when dealing with cancer, adequate margins are important. It is better to have a scar and a live patient than to have no scars and a dead patient.

Certainly, given all of these developments, one has to consider the potentially changing role of the surgeon in the management of cancer of the head and neck. Those of us who have spent most of our careers in the management of surgery of the head and neck recognize that no longer will everybody be treated surgically, as they have been in the past. This reduced need for head and neck surgery will, of course, have an effect on the teaching of head and neck surgery in both residency and fellowship training programs.

■ ECONOMIC CHANGES

The cost of health care continues to spiral out of control because of more advanced technology and the higher costs of doing business, especially malpractice costs. A major move is under way to develop guidelines for treatment based on evidence-based data; such guidelines could change the way head and neck cancer patients are treated, from an individualized treatment approach to algorithm-specified (flow-diagram) therapies.

■ QUALITY OF LIFE ISSUES

A great deal of attention is now being focused on outcomes research and quality of life issues. These have become very important to patients and surgeons alike. The work of Piccirillo (see Chapter 4) and Weymuller (see Chapter 37) has greatly influenced the thinking on how to apply various management plans in the treatment of cancer of the head and neck. Piccirillo's work, which pointed out to us the importance of comorbidities in the outcome of treatment for patients with cancer of the head and neck, has made us all think twice before operating not only on patients with advanced-stage disease, but also on those with earlier-stage disease who have severe comorbidities.

Weymuller and his colleagues have studied the issue of quality of life and have focused their attention on the fact that we need to consider this important issue before prescribing treatment programs for patients. Most of us who are involved in head and neck surgery certainly now think about the oncologic outcome, along with issues of quality of life; both of these are taken very seriously. The surgeon's attention to these matters helps the patient in choosing the proper treatment program—one that will be sound oncologically and will also consider appearance and functionality.

RESEARCH CHANGES

Major advances in research have occurred over the past 10 years. These are discussed in the chapters by Myers (see Chapter 2) and van Waes (see Chapter 34). Genetic abnormalities associated with malignant transformation of cells and control of apoptosis are being elucidated, which will allow new methods of prevention and treatment to be developed very soon.

The identification of genetic abnormalities in some cancers, such as medullary carcinoma of the thyroid, allows us to screen family members so that premalignant lesions can be identified and treated before they become malignant (see Chapter 19). The ability to find specific tumor markers in some cancers will enable molecular targeting of drugs specific for individual tumors, in the way that Gleevec (imatinib mesylate) has been developed for the treatment of chronic myelocytic leukemia.[8]

The old saying that "research cures cancer" will certainly be the case for the treatment of head and neck cancer.

THE FUTURE

It is always risky and interesting to predict the future. Some things seem obvious and are predictable. It is impressive to see the caliber of the students who have been choosing otolaryngology over the past 10 or more years. Overall, they are intelligent and innovative, which, it is hoped, will result in improved research in the areas of head and neck cancer.

Today, the staging of head and neck cancer is a clinical one, with radiologic considerations. Molecular staging should complement clinical staging and improve its accuracy, as more information is obtained regarding genetic and molecular abnormalities that lead to malignancies.

The surgical role of the head and neck surgeon in treating cancer of the head and neck will diminish as new methods of chemoprevention are developed with acceptable morbidity and as new therapies are discovered, such as gene therapy and molecular targeting of drugs. New technology, such as the use of endoscopes in surgery, may make possible minimally invasive surgery in neck dissection; its efficacy has already been noted in thyroid and parathyroid surgery.

We feel confident that despite all of the progress that has been made (as described here), the head and neck surgeon will continue to play a major role in health care, and we strongly encourage those interested in this field not to put away their scalpels. Even the radiation oncologist needs to be aware that today's "standard radiotherapy" will probably be obsolete in 10 or more years.

Because the computer has become such a powerful information tool, we predict that textbooks such as this one will be unnecessary in the future. This is an exciting time in medicine because technology is so advanced and available. It will take lots of research dollars combined with the bright young minds our specialty has attracted, but it will be only a matter of time before cures for head and neck cancer are found, hopefully within our lifetime.

On the other hand, it is sad to see the careers of most of the "giants" in our specialty coming to an end and to mourn those who have died. We are indebted to many, among them John Conley, George Sisson, John M. Loré, John S. Lewis, Edwin Cocke, Richard Jesse, William McComb, Alondo J. Ballantyne, Joseph Ogura, Hugh Biller, Robert Byers, and Helmuth Goepfert.

REFERENCES

1. Brennan JA, Mao L, Hruban RH, et al: Molecular assessment of histopathological staging in squamous cell carcinoma of the head and neck. N Engl J Med 332:429–435, 1995.
2. Wolf GT, Hong WK, Urba S, et al: Induction chemotherapy plus radiation compared with surgery plus radiation in patients with advanced laryngeal cancer. N Engl J Med 324:1685–1690, 1991.
3. Adelstein DJ, Saxton JP, Lavertu P, et al: Maximizing local control and organ preservation in advanced squamous cell head and neck cancer (SCHNC) with hyperfractionated and concurrent chemotherapy. Proc Am Ann Meet Soc Clin Oncol 20:A893, 2001.
4. Calais G, Alfonsi M, Bardet E: Radiation alone (RT) versus RT with concomitant chemotherapy (CT) in stage III or IV oropharynx carcinoma. Final results of the 94–01 GORTEC randomized study. Int J Radiat Oncol Biol Phys 51:A2, 2001.
5. Sisson GA Sr: The Head and Neck Story. Chicago, Kascot Media, 1983.
6. Weinstein GS, Laccourreye O, Brasnu D, Laccourreye H (eds): Organ Preservation Surgery for Laryngeal Cancer. San Diego, Singular Thomson Learning, 2000.
7. Steiner W, Ambrosch P: Endoscopic Laser Surgery of the Upper Aerodigestive Tract. New York, Thieme Stuttgart, 2000.
8. Druker BJ, Talpaz M, Resta DJ, et al: Efficacy and safety of a specific inhibitor of the Bcr-Abl tyrosine kinase in chronic myeloid leukemia. N Engl J Med 344:1031–1037, 2001.

Pathogenesis and Progression of Squamous Cell Carcinoma of the Head and Neck

Eric J. Lentsch
Jeffrey N. Myers

◾ INTRODUCTION

Recent developments in molecular medicine have led us to understand that neoplastic cell growth results from disruption of normal mechanisms that regulate cellular proliferation, differentiation, and death. With the advent of newer molecular techniques, we are now better able to comprehend the genetic changes a cell undergoes during carcinogenesis. As we acquire greater knowledge of tumor biology and develop new molecular technology, it is increasingly important for oncologists to understand the molecular mechanisms underlying neoplastic diseases of the head and neck so that new therapies may be rationally applied.

This chapter presents a useful conceptual framework for organizing information and theories of cancer. Specific steps in the development and progression of neoplasia are discussed within this context, and recent data relevant to head and neck tumors are presented. Finally, the potential use of biologic therapeutics to target molecules that play a role in the development and maintenance of the malignant phenotype is examined.

Basic Concepts of Tumor Biology

Clonal Evolution

The dominant theory of tumor development over the past 30 years has been the clonal evolution theory, first proposed in 1976 by Nowell.[1] This model is built on the theory of natural selection and posits that cancer cells develop strategies to survive a hostile host environment (e.g., tissue barriers, the immune system, induction of programmed cell death) and use host resources (e.g., oxygen, nutrients) to grow and proliferate. In this model, repeated carcinogenic insults, or "events," occur within a cell, usually at the genetic or epigenetic level. When enough events occur, a selective growth advantage is conferred on the affected cell. As this cell proliferates, mutant progeny arise as a result of further insults and genomic instability. Most of the offspring do not

survive because of immunologic surveillance, apoptosis, or metabolic derangement. Eventually, however, a dominant clonal population of cells is produced that not only survives, but flourishes. As evolution occurs within this clonal population, new clones are produced with acquired additional characteristics, such as the capacity for invasion, that define cancer (Fig. 2–1). Thus, within the resulting malignancy, a vast majority of cells have developed from a single clone; they therefore are genotypically similar, or clonal.

Molecular Progression Models

Nowell's model is now well accepted and has led to the understanding that most malignancies arise from a multistep process of accumulated genetic events. Epidemiologic analysis indicates that six to ten independent events are required for the development of most tumors, including squamous cell carcinoma of the head and neck (SCCHN).[2] Over the past decade, investigators have attempted to dissect these events and better understand the pathways that tumor cells take in their development into cancer. The molecular progression model represents the sum of these events. The first, and still most comprehensive, molecular progression model is that of Fearon and Vogelstein, who developed a multistep model of colon carcinogenesis.[3] Colon carcinoma is well suited to this type of modeling because the disease has a continuum ranging from normal mucosa, to benign adenomatous growth, to carcinoma in situ, to invasive carcinoma. In this model, specific molecular events, including oncogene activation and inactivation of tumor suppressor genes, lead to progression from normal cell growth to frank neoplasia and tumor formation. It is the accumulation of events, rather than their ordered occurrence, that leads to cancer. This model fits well with epidemiologic data that have shown an increased prevalence of colon carcinoma among the elderly and in families in which specific gene defects are found in the germline.[4]

As is the case with colon carcinogenesis, head and neck carcinogenesis proceeds through distinct phenotypic and genotypic steps. It has been shown that a histologic progression occurs from normal mucosa to dysplastic mucosa to carcinoma in situ to frank invasive carcinoma.[5] Over the past 20 years, investigators have identified a number of acquired alterations in oncogenes and tumor suppressor genes and

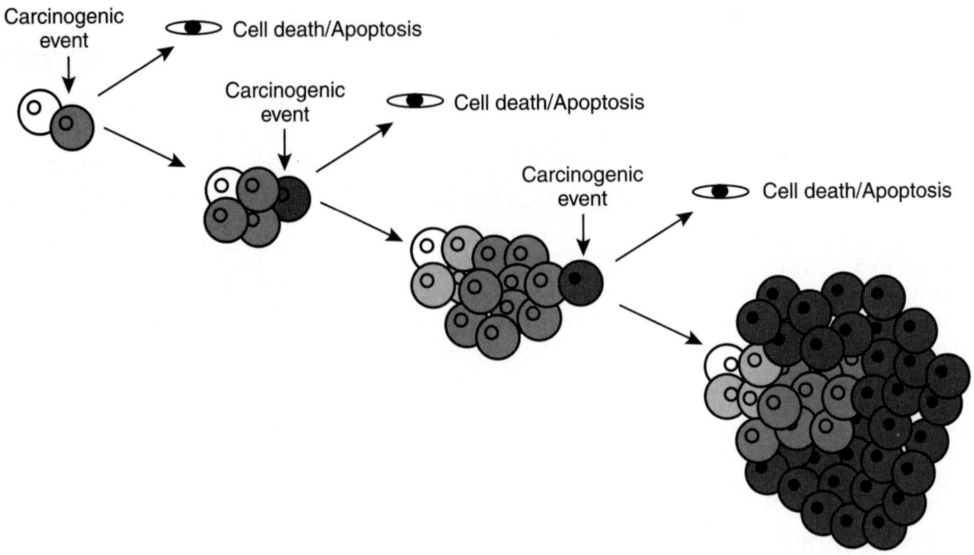

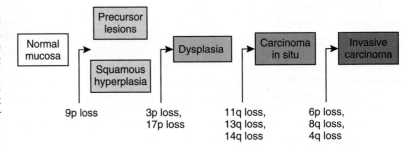

FIGURE 2–1 Clonal evolution. Cells undergo genetic or epigenetic events that lead to either cell death or a selective growth advantage for the cell and its progeny. As successive events occur, a clonal population of tumor cells that are genotypically similar is produced.

have tried to coordinate these genotypic changes with the phenotypic changes seen clinically. Initial work by van der Riet and coworkers[6, 7] has assembled these genetic events, whether they result from cytogenetic alterations, interaction with viral products, or damage from radiation or chemical carcinogens, into an "allelotype" for head and neck carcinoma. This has led to the development of a molecular progression model for head and neck cancer (Fig. 2–2).[8] Again, it is the accumulation of genetic events and not the specific ordering of the events that appears to be associated with phenotypic progression. This model is important not only for understanding the pathogenesis of head and neck cancer but also for developing new diagnostic, staging, and therapeutic techniques.

Field Carcinogenesis

Clear evidence exists that exposure to the carcinogens in tobacco is responsible for the vast majority of SCCHN.[9] These carcinogens can induce molecular changes throughout the entire upper aerodigestive tract. Slaughter[10] first described these changes, originating the concept of field carcinogenesis or "condemned mucosa" in 1953. Slaughter hypothesized that because of constant carcinogenic pressure, the entire upper aerodigestive tract is at increased risk of developing multiple primary tumors. The original

hypothesis was that multiple genetic events occurred throughout the involved mucosa, allowing the development of multiple molecularly distinct lesions (Fig. 2–3).

Recently however, an alternative hypothesis has been postulated to explain field carcinogenesis. In it, a single lesion is thought to form multiple upper aerodigestive tract lesions through the process of intraepithelial migration (see Fig. 2–3). That is, rather than several molecularly distinct lesions that arise independently, a single group of molecularly similar transformed progenitor cells migrates to distant sites, thus explaining the appearance of multiple primary lesions, second primary lesions, and recurrent lesions.

Evidence exists for both hypotheses. For instance, van Oijen and associates[11] analyzed metachronous primaries from nine patients with SCCHN and found that in all patients studied, distinct *TP53* (formerly *p53*) mutations were noted and different patterns of loss of heterozygosity were identified. This has been corroborated by other studies.[12, 13] In addition, a recent study has demonstrated molecular evidence for genetically altered fields surrounding the primary tumor and has also shown that these fields vary in size and consist of genetically different subclones within each field.[14] Taken together, these data argue for the Slaughter hypothesis of field cancerization. On the other hand, Bedi and colleagues[15] studied patterns of X-chromosome inactivation in head and neck patients with multiple primaries.

FIGURE 2–2 Molecular progression model. Multiple mutations are involved in the progression from normal mucosa to dysplasia to carcinoma in situ to invasive carcinoma. It is not the specific order of events, but rather the accumulation of events, that is important. (Derived from Califano J, van der Riet P, Westra W, et al: Genetic progression model for head and neck cancer: Implications for field cancerization. Cancer Res 56:2488–2492, 1996.)

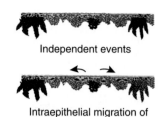

Independent events

Intraepithelial migration of progenitor cells

FIGURE 2–3 Theories of field carcinogenesis. Theories of field carcinogenesis include Slaughter's original description of condemned mucosa with independent events causing the formation of genotypically dissimilar multiple primaries *(top)*, and a competing theory that hypothesizes the migration of cells submucosally to form genotypically similar multiple primaries *(bottom)*. (Used with permission from van Oijen MG, Slootweg PJ: Oral field cancerization: Carcinogen-induced independent events or micrometastatic deposits. Cancer Epidemiol Biomarkers Prev 9:249–256, 2000.)

In four evaluable patients, they showed that the same X chromosome was inactivated in each of the primary tumors. In the same study, analysis of loss of heterozygosity revealed similar findings in several tumor pairs. These data lend credence to the hypothesis of migrating clones.

Currently, it seems likely that both hypotheses may help explain the concept of field carcinogenesis. It is easy to conceptualize that second primary and metachronous tumors that lie near each other may, in many cases, be a result of the migrating clone theory; however, second primary and metachronous tumors separated by long distances are more likely to occur as a result of independent molecular events. Evidence for this was recently put forth by Jang and coworkers,[16] who found, in a series of 26 patients, that the majority of multiple primary tumors developed from clonally independent cells affected by field carcinogenesis, and that a small but significant percentage were clonally related and may have formed by submucosal spread.

Squamous Cell Carcinoma Arising in Nonsmokers

Though SCCHN has been strongly linked to tobacco, a disturbing trend has been observed recently—an increase in incidence among nonsmokers. In 1975, Byers[17] brought attention to a small subgroup of patients with oral tongue cancer who had none of the traditional risk factors. Since that time, several studies have echoed Byers' initial findings, demonstrating that this subgroup tended to be young (usually younger than 40 years) women with cancer of the oral cavity, and the clinical impression was that survival was worse in this subgroup.[18] In addition, several studies have indicated that the incidence of SCCHN in this subgroup is increasing.[19, 20] The reason for this is unclear at this time.

In the absence of carcinogenic pressure from tobacco, several causative agents have been theorized to play a role in the pathogenesis of these cancers. These include the consumption of alcohol, human papilloma virus (HPV) infection, exposure to secondhand smoke, immunosuppression, and genetic susceptibility. The consumption of alcohol has long been believed to be a contributing factor in the development of SCCHN, although it has been difficult to separate its effects from those of tobacco. In a recent study of 864 nonsmokers, however, consumption of alcohol was found to be the major risk factor for cancer of the oral cavity and pharynx.[21] Despite this and other epidemiologic evidence associating the use of alcohol with SCCHN, no evidence points to a direct role for alcohol in the pathogenesis of SCCHN.

A second possible etiologic agent is HPV infection. The HPV family of viruses comprises more than 70 subtypes. They are double-stranded DNA viruses that integrate into the host genome after infection. HPVs are believed to contribute to carcinogenesis by producing viral oncoproteins E6 and E7, which can inactivate tumor suppressor genes such as *TP53* and *RB*. High-risk HPV subtypes 16 and 18 have long been known to cause other epithelial malignancies, especially cancer of the cervix in women. However, the most common subtypes found in the head and neck, HPV-6 and HPV-11, are considered to be low-risk subtypes. Early data were inconsistent, but more recent reports have strengthened the hypothesis that HPV infection is a risk factor in the development of SCCHN.[22, 23] The data appear to be especially strong for HPV as a causal agent for a small proportion of cancers of the oropharynx. In one study,[24] HPV positivity was associated with the oropharyngeal site, and the causal subtype was almost always HPV-16. These tumors were less likely to occur among moderate to heavy smokers, and they had a lower rate of *TP53* mutation than did HPV-negative tumors. In addition, patients with HPV-positive tumors had improved disease-specific survival compared with patients with HPV-negative tumors. These data support an etiologic role for specific HPV subtypes in a subgroup of patients with SCCHN.

Finally, increased susceptibility to DNA damage from environmental factors has been implicated as a causative factor in nonsmokers with SCCHN. Genetic susceptibility to carcinogens has been quantitated by counting the number of chromosome breaks induced by the exposure of peripheral blood lymphocytes in culture to carcinogens and comparing the results of cases with those of matched control groups. The initial studies of mutagen sensitivity in SCCHN were performed using bleomycin. These studies found that nonsmokers with SCCHN are more sensitive to chromosomal damage than are control subjects without evidence of SCCHN.[25] These findings have been confirmed recently with the more relevant tobacco carcinogen benzo[a]pyrenediol epoxide, or BPDE.[26] It has been postulated that increased mutagen sensitivity is the result of variations in carcinogen metabolism, deficiencies in DNA repair, or both. To date, studies of young patients with SCCHN have identified abnormalities in carcinogen-metabolizing genes (e.g., *glutathione-S-transferase*),[27] DNA repair genes (e.g., *XRCC1*),[28] and tumor suppressor genes (e.g., *TP53*).[29]

Genetic Basis of Cancer

It is currently understood that cancer is a genetic disease in which genes normally involved in essential cellular functions undergo mutation or alteration, causing the phenotypic changes seen in cancer. These genes have traditionally been classified as either oncogenes or tumor suppressor genes. Oncogenes are genes that when activated or "turned on" may lead to the malignant phenotype. Conversely, tumor suppressor genes are those genes that when deactivated or "turned off" may lead to unchecked proliferation. As our understanding of the molecular mechanisms of cancer has advanced, we have come to appreciate that other types of genes participate in the process of tumor progression, including those involved in angiogenesis, apoptosis, invasion, and metastasis, some of which do not fit neatly into the oncogene–tumor suppressor gene paradigm.

Oncogenes

Oncogenes are genes that when "activated" are responsible for tumorigenesis. Prior to activation, these genes are termed *proto-oncogenes,* and they have been shown to be important in normal intracellular signaling pathways. Typically, activation of oncogenes results in a gain of function that may be *quantitative* (e.g., an increase in the production of an unaltered product) or *qualitative* (e.g., the production of an altered product). As a result of such alterations, activated oncogenes induce cellular proliferation and therefore tumor development. A vast majority of oncogenes have some function related to cellular growth and/or differentiation; however, they may play various roles in cellular function.

The prototypic oncogene is the *RAS* oncogene. The *RAS* gene and its protein product are involved in a complex cascade of signals from the cell surface to the nucleus that activate cellular growth. Various receptors, such as the receptor tyrosine kinases, activate RAS proteins. The activated guanosine triphosphate (GTP)-bound form of RAS exerts its effects through various target proteins, such as the mitogen-activated protein kinase and phosphatidylinositol-3-kinase cascades, which are important in the activation of gene transcription and cell proliferation.[30] When growth signals are no longer needed, RAS proteins return to their deactivated guanosine diphosphate (GDP)-bound form, effectively "turning off" the cell's growth machinery. Thus, by acting as a "molecular switch," *RAS* exerts an important effect on the cell's growth and differentiation pathways. Mutated forms of *RAS* commonly cause the protein to be constitutively activated, thus turning on the cell's growth machinery and allowing uncontrolled proliferation and survival, two of the hallmarks of cancer. Since its discovery, *RAS* has served as a paradigm for oncogenic activation of normal cells to neoplastic cells.

Some of the known oncogenes, their cellular functions, and the cancers they are associated with are listed in Table 2–1.

Tumor Suppressor Genes

We now understand that certain genes play a vital role in preventing normal cells from becoming neoplastic. The past three decades have brought heightened understanding of the role of these tumor suppressor genes in the development of human cancer. In general, tumor suppressor genes act as molecular "brakes," or as Lane[31] phrased them, "guardians of the genome,"—preventing cells from undergoing uncontrolled growth and division. In their normal state, most tumor suppressor genes act on cell-cycle control, transcriptional regulation, or apoptosis, acting as checkpoints to control entry into active proliferative states or causing apoptosis. When these genes are deactivated, through mutation or other events, the cell loses this negative control and is free to undergo uncontrolled growth and division.

TABLE 2-1 Oncogenes

Oncogenes	Associated Neoplasms
Growth Factors	
V-*sis*	Glioma/fibrosarcoma
Int2	Mammary carcinoma
KS3	Kaposi's sarcoma
HST	Stomach carcinoma
Growth Factor Receptors	
EGF-R	Squamous cell carcinoma
v-*fms*	Sarcoma
v-*kit*	Sarcoma
v-*ros*	Sarcoma
MET	MNNG-treated human osteocarcinoma cell line
TRK	Colon/thyroid carcinomas
NEU	Neuroblastoma/breast carcinoma
RET	Carcinomas of thyroid MEN-2A, MEN-2B
Mas	Epidermoid carcinoma
Signal Transducers	
SRC	Colon carcinoma
v-*yes*	Sarcoma
v-*fgr*	Sarcoma
v-*fes*	Sarcoma
ABL	CML
H-RAS	Colon, lung, pancreas carcinomas
K-RAS	AML, thyroid carcinoma, melanoma
N-RAS	Carcinoma, melanoma
Gsp	Adenomas of thyroid
Gip	Ovary, adrenal carcinoma
Dbl	Diffuse B-cell lymphoma
Vav	Hematopoietic cells
v-*mos*	Sarcoma
v-*raf*	Sarcoma
Pim-1	T-cell lymphoma
v-*crk*	
Transcription Factors	
v-*myc*	Carcinoma myelocytomatosis
N-MYC	Neuroblastoma: lung carcinoma
L-MYC	Carcinoma of the lung
v-*myb*	Myeloblastosis
v-*fos*	Osteosarcoma
v-*jun*	Sarcoma
v-*ski*	Carcinoma
v-*rel*	Lymphatic leukemia
v-*ets-1*	Erythroblastosis

AML, acute myelogenous leukemia; CML, chronic myelogenous leukemia; MEN, multiple endocrine neoplasia; MNNG, N-methyl-N′-nitro-N-nitrosoguanidine.

The prototypic tumor suppressor gene is the retinoblastoma (*RB*) gene. It was originally described by Knudson,[32] who, while studying children with retinoblastoma, noted a consistent region of loss on chromosome 13 in all patients. Knudson postulated that two genetic "hits" must occur at a specific locus for a retinoblastoma to develop. In familial cases, one allele of this gene must already be mutated or deleted in the germline; then an acquired mutation in the normal remaining allele leads to development of retinoblastoma.[32] In sporadic cases, however, both alleles must be mutated; the relatively low probability of the occurrence of this event accounts for the infrequency of this tumor in the general population and the enhanced peak of incidence of sporadic forms of the disease in older patients.

TABLE 2-2 Tumor Suppressor Genes

Tumor Suppressor Genes	Associated Neoplasms
RB1	Familial retinoblastoma, retinoblastoma, osteosarcoma, SCLC, breast, prostate, bladder, pancreas, esophageal, others
TP53	Li-Fraumeni syndrome; approx. 50% of all cancers (rare in some types, such as prostate carcinoma and neuroblastoma)
*INK4–p16	Familial melanoma, familial pancreatic carcinoma, approx. 25%–30% of many different cancer types (e.g., breast, lung, pancreatic, bladder)
*INK4–p19^{ARF}	Familial melanoma?, approx. 15% of many different types of cancer
APC	Familial adenomatous polyposis coli, Gardner's syndrome, Turcot's syndrome, colorectal, desmoid tumors
BRCA1	Inherited breast and ovarian cancer, ovarian (~10%), rare in breast cancer
BRCA2	Inherited breast (both female and male), pancreatic cancer, ?others?; rare mutations in pancreatic, ?others?
WT-1	WAGR, Denys-Drash syndrome, Wilms' tumor
NF-1	Neurofibromatosis type 1, melanoma, neuroblastoma
NF-2	Neurofibromatosis type 2, schwannoma, meningioma, ependymoma
VHL	von Hippel-Lindau syndrome, renal (clear cell type), hemangioblastoma
MEN-1	Multiple endocrine neoplasia type 1, parathyroid adenoma, pituitary adenoma, endocrine tumors of the pancreas
PTCH	Gorlin's syndrome, hereditary basal cell carcinoma syndrome, basal cell skin carcinoma, medulloblastoma
PTEN/MMAC1	Cowden's syndrome; sporadic cases of juvenile polyposis syndrome, glioma, breast, prostate, follicular thyroid carcinoma, head and neck squamous carcinoma
DPC4	Familial juvenile polyposis syndrome, pancreatic (~50%), approx. 10%–15% of colorectal cancers, rare in others
E-CAD	Familial diffuse-type gastric cancer; lobular breast cancer, gastric (diffuse type), lobular breast carcinoma, rare in other types (e.g., ovarian)
LKB1/STK1	Peutz-Jeghers syndrome, rare in colorectal, not known in others
SNF5/INI1	Rhabdoid predisposition syndrome (renal; or extrarenal malignant rhabdoid tumors), choroid plexus carcinoma medulloblastoma; central primitive neuroectodermal tumors, rare in rhabdoid tumors, choroid plexus carcinoma, medulloblastoma
EXT1	Hereditary multiple exostoses, not known
EXT2	Hereditary multiple exostoses, not known
TSC1	Tuberous sclerosis, not known
TSC2	Tuberous sclerosis, not known
MSH2, MLH'1, PMS1, PMS2, MSH6	Hereditary nonpolyposis colorectal cancer, colorectal, gastric, endometrial
TGF-B type IIR	RER+ colorectal and gastric cancer, head and neck, lung, and esophageal squamous cell carcinoma
BAX	RER+ colorectal
FHIT	Lung, cervical, renal, others
α-CAT	Some prostate and lung, ?others?
DCC	Some colorectal, neuroblastoma, male germ cell cancer, gliomas, ?others?
MADR2/SMAD2	Some colorectal
CDX2	Rare mutations in colorectal
MKK4	Rare mutations in pancreas, lung, breast, and colorectal; ?others?
PP2RIB	Lung, colorectal
MCC	Rare mutations in colorectal

RER+, replication error positive; SCLC, small cell lung cancer; WAGR, Wilms' tumor, aniridia, genitourinary malformations, and mental retardation (syndrome).

Knudson's dominant negative model has served as a useful paradigm for the identification of a growing number of tumor suppressor genes that are important in the development of a variety of tumor types.

Since the identification of the RB gene, several other tumor suppressor genes have been identified, many of which play a role in SCCHN (Table 2–2).

◼ HALLMARKS OF CANCER

Over the past several decades, remarkable advances in multiple fields of cancer research have allowed for better understanding of the molecular and cellular pathogenesis and progression of cancer. Nowell's theory of clonal evolution[1] and Fearon and Vogelstein's[3] multistep model of carcinogenesis have unified observations from different fields of cancer research into a coherent conceptual framework. In Nowell's model,[1] tumors are viewed as heterogeneous collections of cancer cells. Successful cancer cells are those that have acquired characteristics that confer a selective growth advantage over their neighbors. The work of Fearon and Vogelstein[3] has led to the identification of discrete genetic events that occur in the progression of colon cancers from precancerous polyps to invasive tumors. Although the precise order and number of events required for tumorigenesis remain unknown, a recent series of experiments performed by Hahn and colleagues demonstrated six important steps that are believed to be necessary for a cancer to develop.[33, 34] These steps include the following: (1) acquisition of autonomous proliferative signaling, (2) inhibition of growth inhibitory signals, (3) evasion of programmed cell death (apoptosis), (4) immortalization, (5) acquisition of a nutrient blood supply (angiogenesis), and (6) tissue invasion and metastasis (Fig. 2–4). Herein, we review some developments in the study of SCCHN in the context of this conceptual framework.

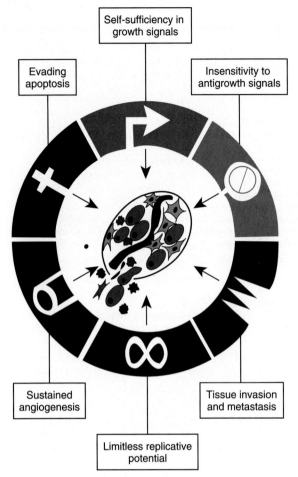

FIGURE 2–4 Hallmarks of cancer. Hanahan and Weinberg described six important steps that are believed to be necessary for a cancer to develop. (Used with permission from Hanahan D, Weinberg RA: The hallmarks of cancer. Cell 100:57–70, 2000.)

Acquisition of Autonomous Proliferative Signaling

All normal cells require growth signals for proliferation. Growth signals can be provided in a variety of ways, such as diffusible molecules (growth factors), extracellular matrix components, or cell-to-cell interactions, to name a few. In general, growth signals are transmitted from the cell surface to the nucleus through various intracellular signaling pathways (Fig. 2–5). A distinct characteristic of neoplastic cells is their ability to acquire autonomy from exogenous growth signaling. The work of a number of investigators has shown that aberrant expression of growth factors and growth factor receptors may play a role in the pathogenesis of SCCHN.[35] In addition, other aspects of intracellular signaling may be altered in neoplastic cells, helping to provide this autonomy of growth.

Epidermal Growth Factor Axis

Cohen originally purified epidermal growth factor (EGF) from mouse submandibular glands in 1962.[36] The isolation and characterization of EGF and its receptor (EGF-R) have furthered our understanding of the regulation of normal cell proliferation and the loss of this regulation that occurs in neoplastic cell growth. Investigators have begun to study the role of EGF, the EGF-R, and transforming growth factor-α (TGF-α; another ligand for the EGF-R) in the development of SCCHN.[17]

Most studies of EGF and the EGF-R in SCCHN have involved quantitation of expression at the DNA, RNA, or protein level in cell lines or fresh tissues, and the correlation of these findings to clinical parameters. Although conflicting data have been obtained, some general trends have been noted. Specifically, it appears that the EGF axis is upregulated in a large proportion of cases of SCCHN; however, the clinical significance of this upregulation is uncertain at this time. For instance, in an immunohistochemical analysis of squamous cell carcinoma (SCC) of the base of the tongue, the EGF-R and TGF-α were routinely seen in normal squamous mucosa adjacent to the tumors, with overexpression of the EGF-R and TGF-α seen in 60% and 35% of tumors, respectively.[37] However, overexpression appeared to have no effect on survival. Similar results were seen in an analysis of tumors of the nasal cavity and paranasal sinuses.[38] Conversely, in a study of 103 laryngeal tumors, EGF-R expression was elevated, particularly in tumors that were poorly differentiated when compared with normal mucosa.[39] In this study, however, the 2-year survival of patients with EGF-R–positive tumors was 58%, compared with 82% for patients with EGF-R–negative lesions.

To further investigate the role that TGF-α and EGF-R expression may play in the pathogenesis of SCCHN, Grandis and Tweardy[40] systematically evaluated the level of mRNA encoding these two proteins in tumors and normal mucosa from patients with SCCHN, as well as in normal mucosa from patients without a history of tobacco or alcohol consumption. In their analysis, TGF-α mRNA was elevated in 95% of histologically normal samples in patients with SCCHN, and in 87.5% of patients with SCCHN when compared with normal mucosa from individuals without cancer. The mRNA for the EGF-R was found to be elevated in 91% of histologically normal tissue from tumor-bearing patients and in 92% of tumors, when compared with normal mucosa from tumor-free control subjects. The high levels of both the ligand and the receptor in tumors and normal mucosa from patients with cancer of the head and neck suggest that environmental influences, such as tobacco and alcohol consumption, lead to upregulation of growth factor production and receptor expression, which may play a role in tumor development. Correlations between growth factor and receptor levels and clinical data have begun to yield clinically meaningful results. In a detailed analysis of 91 patients, levels of EGF-R and TGF-α were quantified via immunohistochemical staining, and increased levels of both were found to be independent predictors of decreased disease-free survival.[41] Several subsequent studies corroborate these data.[42, 43]

Some functional data to support this hypothesis have come from a study of two SCCHN cell lines that were examined for levels of EGF-R expression by means of immunoprecipitation of metabolically labeled cells with specific anti–EGF-R antibodies.[44] In this study, the cell line that grew more efficiently in plating assays was found to have fivefold higher levels of EGF-R. The immunoprecipitated receptors were also

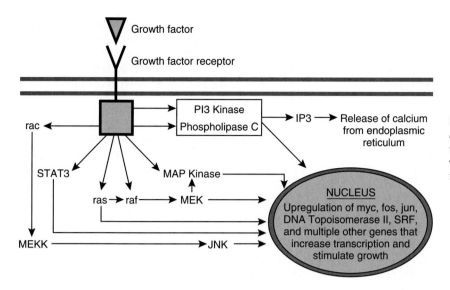

FIGURE 2–5 Growth factor pathways. An example of a growth factor pathway that involves the binding of a growth factor to its receptor, which then may result in the activation of multiple downstream pathways.

analyzed for intrinsic tyrosine kinase activity, an enzymatic activity that is indispensable for EGF-R signal transduction; the more rapidly proliferating cell line was found to possess greater kinase activity. Furthermore, kinase activity was increased in immunoprecipitates from both cell lines by the addition of exogenous EGF.

More recently, EGF-R and its ligands have been studied in invasion and metastasis. Increasing evidence suggests an association between an upregulated EGF axis and activation of matrix metalloproteinases (MMPs) in SCCHN cell lines.[45] In this study, upregulation of MMP-9 was demonstrated by exposing cells to EGF-R ligands; in addition, monoclonal antibodies against EGF-R inhibited MMP-9 upregulation and impeded tumor cell invasion. A second study upheld these findings and also showed an upregulation of urokinase-type plasminogen activator (uPA).[46] These data suggest a role for the EGF axis in the regulation of invasion and metastasis of SCCHN.

Signal Transducers and Activators of Transcription Proteins

Signal transducers and activators of transcription (STATs) are a family of cytoplasmic proteins responsible for transmitting signals from cell-surface receptors to the nucleus, where they act as transcription factors. STATs have been implicated as playing a role in the development of several types of tumors, including SCCHN.[47] In SCCHN, STAT proteins, specifically STAT3, have been shown to play an important role in EGF/TGF-mediated cell growth.[48] Activation of the EGF/TGF pathway results in constitutive expression of STAT3. This association has been strengthened by experiments in which abrogation of STAT3 function (via mutant constructs or antisense oligonucleotides) resulted in significant growth inhibition of SCCHN cells.[49] In addition, further studies using antisense oligonucleotides have showed that STAT3 activation causes a significant decrease in apoptosis. This downregulation appears to be due to elevated levels of the antiapoptotic protein BCL-X_L.[50] Further studies of this downstream signaling molecule are being actively pursued.

Nuclear Factor-Kappa B

Nuclear factor-kappa B (NF-κB) is a well-established transcription factor that acts to regulate genes that drive immune and inflammatory responses. In normal cells, NF-κB remains largely in the cytoplasm, complexed to inhibitor proteins (IκBs), and therefore remains transcriptionally inactive until a cell receives an appropriate stimulus. In response to a stimulus, IκB proteins become phosphorylated and ubiquitinated, and undergo rapid proteolysis by the 26S proteasome. This degradation of the IκB proteins results in the liberation of NF-κB, allowing this transcription factor to accumulate in the nucleus, where it activates the expression of specific genes involved in immune and inflammatory responses and in cell growth control.[51]

Recently, NF-κB has been connected with the acquisition of multiple hallmarks of cancer development and progression. Through the increased transcription of genes important for mediating increased cell proliferation (cyclin D1), apoptosis evasion (c-IAP-2, XIAP), invasion (matrix metalloproteinase [MMP-9]), and angiogenesis (interleukin-8 [IL-8]), NF-κB has been found to promote tumor progression in multiple ways. Evidence for the role of NF-κB in human oncogenesis was first seen in Hodgkin's lymphoma.[52] Other cancer types have been investigated as well.[53] Duffey and associates studied NF-κB function in a murine keratinocyte tumor progression model and in human SCCHN cell lines and showed that enhanced NF-κB activity is positively associated with local tumor growth and metastatic potential in animal models.[54] More recent studies using cDNA microarrays indicate that NF-κB may activate proliferation via upregulation of cyclin D1 and other cell-cycle regulators.[55]

Fibroblast Growth Factors

Investigators studying cell lines as well as primary tumors have shown that the expression of fibroblast growth factors (FGFs) FGF-1 and FGF-2 is elevated compared with the level of those in normal mucosa.[56] Interestingly, treatment of an SCC cell line expressing FGF-1, with FGF antisense oligonucleotides or anti-FGF antibody, led to significant inhibition of cell growth.[57] Because biochemical studies also confirmed that this cell line expresses the receptor for this ligand on its cell surface, it has been postulated that an autocrine growth pathway involving FGF-1 may play a role in SCCHN progression.

Hepatocyte Growth Factor Axis

Hepatocyte growth factor/scatter factor (HGF/SF) has remarkably diverse biologic functions in different tissues and has been implicated in mitogenic responses, cell motility, and angiogenesis.[58] This growth factor may have a critical role in a variety of biologic processes, including normal development, wound healing, and carcinogenesis. The HGF/SF receptor (HGF-R) is coded by the c-met proto-oncogene.[59] The c-met–encoded receptor belongs to the family of transmembrane growth factor receptors with tyrosine kinase activity.

Recent evidence has implicated both HGF and c-met in invasion and metastasis of oral cavity cancer cell lines.[60, 61] It appears that this increase in invasiveness may be the result of HGF's ability to upregulate both MMP-1 and MMP-9.[62] In addition, Dong and colleagues[63] have shown that HGF may play a role in angiogenesis in SCCHN via upregulation of proangiogenic cytokine IL-8 and vascular endothelial growth factor (VEGF). Thus, HGF and c-met appear to play diverse and important roles in the pathogenesis of SCCHN.

Inhibition of Growth Inhibitory Signals

In the normal cell, growth and differentiation are tightly controlled. Although constitutive stimulation of cell proliferation through normal growth factors is necessary for tumor development, it is insufficient in itself to cause oncogenic transformation of normal cells. Another important and related step in tumorigenesis is the loss of normal antigrowth signals. Extensive study in this field has delineated a complex interplay of factors, resulting in regulation of a cell's progression through the "cell cycle" (Fig. 2–6). The cell cycle is the process by which each cell replicates its DNA and divides. It consists of several phases—G1 (growth phase 1), S (DNA synthesis), G2 (growth phase 2), and M (mitosis)—each of which is tightly controlled. Central to the control of the cell cycle is a group of molecules called cyclins and their regulators—cyclin-dependent kinases (CDKs) and cyclin-dependent kinase inhibitors (CDKIs). Any molecule that affects or regulates cyclins, CDKs, or CDKIs will have a profound effect on cell growth and is a potential carcinogenic mediator. Several of these molecules are discussed in the following sections as they relate to SCCHN.

Retinoblastoma Gene

The retinoblastoma (*RB*) gene and its protein product (pRB) have been referred to as the gateway to the cell cycle. In its active form, pRB prevents progression through the cell cycle by binding to and inactivating the transcription factor E2F, which is vital to the expression of other genes required for DNA synthesis. Various cyclin/CDK combinations are able to respond to mitogenic stimuli and inactivate pRB via the process of phosphorylation. When it is phosphorylated, pRB releases E2F, leading to the transcription of genes critical for progression of cells from the G1 to the S-phase of the cell cycle. This then initiates the DNA synthesis phase of the cell cycle.

Because of its critical role in cell-cycle initiation, *RB* has been intensively studied in various tumor types, including SCCHN. Examination of 60 SCCHN tumor specimens revealed loss of heterozygosity of the *RB* region of chromosome 13 in 52% of patients. However, a decreased level of pRB expression could be detected in only 19.4% of these specimens by immunochemistry.[64] Other studies have also demonstrated low rates of pRB alterations in SCCHN.[65] These findings suggest that *RB* inactivation is an uncommon event in the development of SCCHN, and that other mechanisms of cell cycle inhibition are at work. Because several signaling molecules reside upstream of pRB, any alterations to this pathway that lead to increased phosphorylation of pRB can lead to the loss of negative growth control. Some of these molecules are discussed here.

TP53 Gene

The most intensely studied gene involved in carcinogenesis is a tumor suppressor gene called *TP53*. The *TP53* locus is the most commonly mutated locus in human cancers. Located on the short arm of chromosome 17, TP53 is a 393-amino-acid protein that is evolutionarily well conserved and is expressed in all tissues of the body. Although the overall sequence of this protein in humans is nearly 82% homologous with murine TP53, five regions of approximately 20 amino acids each within the protein are nearly identical across species lines.[66] Mutagenesis and x-ray crystallographic studies

FIGURE 2–6 Cell cycle control. Each step of the cell cycle is tightly controlled by cyclin and CDK interactions and is further regulated by a variety of intracellular molecules, including the INK4 and the p21 protein families, as well as oncogenes such as RB and tumor suppressor genes such as *TP53*. (Used with permission from Gillet CE, Barnes DM: Demystified ... cell cycle. Mol Pathol 51: 310–316, 1998.)

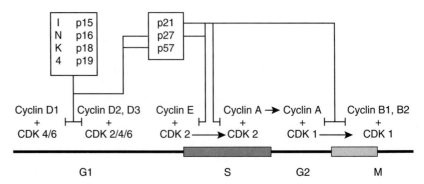

have localized specific functions to these regions. The first 75 amino acids of TP53 are involved in the activation of transcription of specific genes, whereas amino acids 120 to 290 are involved in the specific recognition of DNA sequences.[67] The carboxyl terminus is believed to be important for nuclear localization and oligomerization of TP53 into tetramers.[68]

Although the mechanism of action of TP53 is through the positive or negative regulation of gene transcription, its biologic role is to protect cells from DNA damage caused by radiation, chemical carcinogens, or other mechanisms. TP53 does this either by arresting the cell cycle so that DNA repair can occur or by inducing programmed cell death (apoptosis).[69-71] Analysis of extensive data on sites of mutation of the *TP53* gene in human cancers has revealed certain "hot spots" for mutations at sites that are believed to be important in carrying out these functions.[72] The majority of these (more than 92%) are found in the five "conserved regions" of the gene. Mutations within these regions impair a cell's ability to repair its DNA, which leads to genomic instability of the cancer cell and additional alterations in oncogene and tumor suppressor gene products. Mutations of *TP53* also prevent apoptosis in response to DNA damage, which may make tumor cells resistant to treatment with irradiation or chemotherapeutic agents that act by damaging cellular DNA and triggering apoptosis. The role of this gene in the pathogenesis of SCCHN has been extensively studied; some of this work is outlined in the following paragraphs.

Somers and colleagues[73] analyzed TP53 in SCCHN using immunohistochemical studies and demonstrated TP53 overexpression in 13 of 13 SCCHN cell lines and in 10 of 13 fresh tissue specimens. DNA sequencing of the *TP53* gene revealed G to T transversions that resulted in single amino acid substitutions. Because G to T transversions can result from the interaction of DNA with benzopyrene, a component of cigarette smoke, the results of this study suggest a mechanism by which smoking may play a role in the pathogenesis of tobacco-associated malignancy.

Numerous studies have documented overexpression and point mutations in *TP53* genes from both SCCHN cell lines and fresh tumors from sites within the head and neck. As is the case with other cancer types, mutation of the *TP53* gene is one of the most common abnormalities in SCCHN, with a frequency of approximately 50%.[74] It seems clear that TP53 plays an important functional role in the progression of SCCHN. Early evidence for this was revealed by Boyle and coworkers,[75] who found that 19% of premalignant lesions and 43% of malignant lesions had *TP53* mutations. Similar results have been seen in immunohistochemical studies performed by other groups.[76, 77] Experiments carried out by investigators at the University of Texas M.D. Anderson Cancer Center[78] have shown a steady increase in *TP53* abnormalities during progression of head and neck tumors, with 19% of normal epithelium, 29% of hyperplastic lesions, 45% of dysplastic lesions, and 58% of invasive cancers demonstrating TP53 overexpression. These researchers also demonstrated a significant association between TP53 expression and genomic instability, suggesting that *TP53* alterations may lead to the accumulation of genetic events during head and neck tumorigenesis.

Although *TP53* can be altered through mutations, there are several other mechanisms by which *TP53* function is altered that are believed to play a role in tumorigenesis. As was discussed previously, the HPV proteins E6 and E7 can bind to TP53 and inactivate its function.[79] Another example is the cellular protein mdm-2, which binds to the transcriptional activation domain of TP53, effectively blocking its ability to regulate target genes and exert its antiproliferative or apoptotic effects.[80] In addition, mdm-2 appears to play a major role in TP53 degradation, thus providing a new mechanism for ensuring effective termination of the TP53 signal.[81] To date, few studies of mdm-2 in SCCHN have been performed, and the data are unclear at this point; however, one study of TP53 inactivation revealed that in 95% of patients, TP53 was inactivated by mutation, HPV infection, or mdm-2 overexpression.[82]

INK4 Gene Family

The *INK4* (*IN*hibitors of CD*K4*) family of genes consists of several proteins—p15[INK4B], p16[INK4A], p18[INK4C], p19[INK4D]— that appear to act mainly on the G1 phase in the cell cycle. By far, the most studied of this gene family is *p16*. Independent studies of the *9p21-22* region in human cancers revealed that a gene, encoding a protein known as p16, was important in inhibiting cells from entering the cell cycle.[83] Serrano and colleagues[84] demonstrated that p16 binds to and inhibits the enzyme CDK4, which is important in enabling cells to pass through the cell cycle. The p16/cyclin story is complex, but the promotion of cell proliferation through the inactivation of a cell-cycle inhibitor or the overexpression of a cell-cycle activator demonstrates how quantitative and qualitative alterations in the expression of oncogenes and tumor suppressor genes contribute to tumorigenesis.

Alterations in *p16* have been shown to be important in a variety of human cancers. Early studies on SCCHN indicated that *p16* alterations were among the most common abnormalities found. Reed and associates[85] showed that p16 activity was lost in 83% of primary tumors. Various distinct mechanisms appear to be responsible, including homozygous deletion, point mutation, and promoter methylation.

More recently, researchers have attempted to identify whether *p16* is affected early or late in the carcinogenic pathway. Studies of premalignant and malignant oral cavity lesions have also shown frequent alterations of the coding region of the *p16* gene.[86-88] The frequent finding of *p16* gene mutations or loss of its expression in dysplastic as well as neoplastic oral lesions indicates that this may be an early step in oral carcinogenesis.[86] Because *p16* is so widely altered in head and neck cancer, it is an attractive target for newer molecular therapeutic techniques. A recent study showed that gene therapy directed toward the p16 protein might have potential benefit; using an adenoviral gene therapy approach, Rocco and coworkers[89] demonstrated inhibition of cell growth in human SCCHN cell lines. The same vector also showed stabilization or reduction in tumor volumes in a nude mouse model. This work has the potential to lead to new therapies for treatment of SCCHN.

Cyclin D1

The cyclin family of cellular proteins, along with their partners, the CDKs, are responsible for driving the cell through the cell cycle. As would be expected, proteins involved in driving the cell cycle, including cyclins, are frequently overexpressed in primary tumors.[90] Of the many cell-cycle regulators implicated in the development of cancers, cyclin D1 is among the most prevalent.[91]

Cyclin D1 amplification has been identified in as many as 64% of cases of SCCHN.[92] Overexpression of cyclin D1 has been studied in various head and neck subsites. For instance, in oral cavity cancer, Bova and associates[93] analyzed 148 tongue cancers immunohistochemically for the expression of cyclin D1 and found it was overexpressed in 68%. This finding correlated with reduced disease-free and overall survival in a statistically significant fashion. A recent study confirmed these results and correlated high expression of cyclin D1 with lymph node metastases.[94] Likewise, in a study of squamous cell carcinomas of the larynx, amplification of cyclin D1 was identified in 37% of neoplasms, which correlated with local invasion, locoregional recurrence, and pathologic stage.[95] A high correlation of cyclin D1 mRNA overexpression with gene amplification supports a role for this protein in the pathogenesis of SCCHN. Also, in studies of hypopharyngeal sites, cyclin D1 gene amplification and protein overexpression not only were correlated with prognosis but were also useful in identifying optimum treatment regimens[96]; cyclin D1–negative tumors responded particularly well to multimodality treatment.

Overexpression of cyclin D1 protein in SCCHN was found to be an independent prognostic indicator of recurrence,[97] a finding that was confirmed in another study.[98] Further confirmation of the importance of cyclin D1 in SCCHN was provided recently by Nakashima and Clayman,[99] who showed that transfection of antisense cyclin D1 into head and neck cancer cell lines caused decreased in vitro growth rates and decreased tumorigenicity in a nude mouse model. This finding leads to the possibility of new gene therapy approaches to SCCHN.

p21 Family

The p21 family consists of p21, p27, and p57. p21 was one of the first CDK inhibitors identified.[100] It was found by several different laboratories and thus has multiple names, including WAF1, CIP1, SDI1, and mda-6. p27 and p57 are also known as KIP1 and KIP2. This family is known to have a wide variety of inhibitory effects on CDKs. Currently, data concerning the role of the p21 family of proteins in the development of head and neck cancer are limited. One study evaluated p21 protein levels in tumors and found that overexpression of p21, as evaluated immunohistochemically, correlated with increasing recurrence rates and shortened disease-free and overall survival times.[101] A more recent study, evaluating p27 levels in patients with oral tongue SCC, found that patients with low p27 levels, as evaluated by immunohistochemical and Western blotting techniques, had higher-stage disease and lower rates of overall survival.[102] A similar study by the same group in patients with hypopharyngeal SCC also showed poorer survival rates in patients with low expression of p27.[103] Further corroborative studies are needed to fully elucidate the role of this family of proteins in the pathogenesis of SCCHN.

Evasion of Programmed Cell Death (Apoptosis)

Programmed cell death, or apoptosis, is a critical step in cell differentiation and turnover and in tissue homeostasis. Intensive study in this area over the past decade has led to a greater understanding of the initiation and regulation of apoptosis. It is now clear that one of the requisites for cancer cells to prosper is the development of resistance to apoptosis, shifting the balance between cell division and cell death.

The biochemical process of apoptosis is one of the most studied aspects of cell biology. It has been found to be a precisely orchestrated series of steps triggered by physiologic stimuli that lead to membrane dissolution, breakdown of the nuclear and cytosolic skeletons, chromosomal degradation, and fragmentation of the nucleus (Fig. 2–7). Currently, apoptosis is thought of as a three-step process. The first step of this process is the initiation, or signal step. In general, a signal, either extracellular or intracellular, triggers the apoptotic machinery. The second step is the execution, or actual "program," of cell death. Within this phase, multiple effector molecules act on the signal event to cause the release of caspases, the ultimate destroyers of the cell. The third step involves the morphologic changes seen in the dying cell and the responses of the surrounding cells to its death. As would be expected for such a complex process, multiple regulatory and effector molecules are needed for the successful initiation and completion of this process. Mutations of any of the genes encoding these apoptotic proteins or any changes in their levels of expression can lead to increased cell survival, a critical step in tumorigenesis.

Apoptosis can be initiated by extracellular or intracellular pathways. Extracellular initiators of the apoptotic machinery include ligands that bind cell-surface receptors such as Fas, tumor necrosis factor receptor, TRAMP, TRAIL-R1, TRAIL-R2, and DR-6. These have been called "death receptors." The best studied of these is the Fas/Fas ligand complex, which serves as a model for all other death receptors. The signal in this pathway is the binding of Fas ligand to Fas, which causes clustering of Fas complexes and the subsequent intracellular binding of Fas-associated death domain (FADD). This in turn causes the recruitment of an initiator caspase, caspase 8, which initiates apoptosis by cleavage of downstream effector caspases 3, 6, and 7. Although this pathway has been well defined and studied in other cancers, little is known of its role in SCCHN.

Intracellular molecules can also act as initiators of apoptosis. By far, the best studied example is the *TP53* gene. This gene and its protein product have multiple functions, as described earlier, including the induction of apoptosis in response to DNA damage. This induction of apoptosis appears to occur through a downstream effector molecule known as BAX—a potent proapoptotic molecule. Mutations in the *TP53* gene can result in loss of this function, which can lead to survival of cells with damaged DNA. This in turn can lead to genomic instability with the development of multiple genetic abnormalities that can foster tumor progression. Evidence for this phenomenon in SCCHN was demonstrated by Ravi and colleagues,[104] who showed that the presence of mutant TP53 protein has an inverse correlation to the extent of apoptosis in oral cavity cancer. Significant correlation was also evident between the

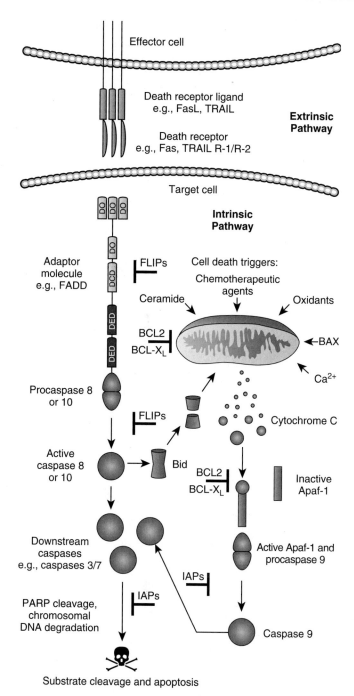

FIGURE 2–7 Apoptosis. Intracellular and extracellular pathways are involved in the orchestrated series of steps leading to cell death. Initiator and effector caspases are depicted, as are regulatory molecules such as BCL2 and BCL-X$_L$. (Used with permission from Gastman BR: Apoptosis and its clinical impact. Head Neck 23:409–425, 2001.)

BAX/BCL2 ratio and cyclin D1 levels and apoptosis. These results suggest that apoptosis decreases as histologic abnormality increases, apparently because of alterations in the levels of apoptotic regulatory proteins.

More data that support a role for TP53 in the induction of apoptosis come from gene transfer studies by Clayman and coworkers[105] and Liu and associates.[106] Using adenoviral vectors to restore wild-type *TP53* to human SCCHN cell lines with *TP53* alterations, these investigators were able to demonstrate a loss of tumorigenesis in nude mice and induction of apoptosis in the wild-type *TP53*–transduced tumors. As well as shedding new light on the role of *TP53* mutations in the pathogenesis of SCCHN, these data have served as the basis for phase I and II trials of adenovirus *TP53* in patients with advanced or refractory SCCHN, which have established the safety of this type of gene therapy.[107] The efficacy of this type of treatment alone or in combination with other modalities remains to be established.

Regardless of whether the apoptotic cascade is initiated by cell-surface receptors or intracellular initiators, the cellular effectors of apoptosis are the caspase family of proteases. This family includes at least 13 proteins and is classically divided into three groups: *nonapoptotic caspases* (caspases 1, 4, 5, 11, 12, and 13), which appear to have no role in apoptosis; *initiator caspases* (caspases 8, 9, and 10), which function to begin and amplify the caspase cascade; and *effector caspases* (caspases 2, 3, 6, and 7), which appear to be the ultimate effectors of apoptosis. Thus, the initial step in the apoptotic cascade is the activation of a cellular receptor or intracellular initiator, which in turn activates one or more initiator caspases. This step is also the major regulatory step and is controlled by many proapoptotic and antiapoptotic proteins, which are discussed later. Once activated, the initiator caspases process and activate one or more effector caspases. These, then, cleave cellular proteins, organelles, and chromosomes and provide the final mechanism for apoptosis.

It has become clear over the past decade that various chemotherapeutic agents exert their antitumor effects by inducing apoptosis, and several of these do so by specifically upregulating caspases. For instance, 5-fluorouracil has been shown to specifically upregulate caspases 1, 3, and 8.[108] Moreover, inhibitors of these caspases consistently blocked apoptosis. Likewise, in head and neck cancer cell lines, cisplatin administration selectively upregulated caspases 3, 8, and 9.[109] Further experiments have shown that inhibitors of caspase 9 completely block apoptosis, whereas inhibitors of caspases 3 and 8 partially block apoptosis. Other chemotherapeutic agents, such as 9-cis-retinoic acid[110] and arsenic trioxide,[111] also act by upregulating various caspases.

Various regulatory molecules play a role in the apoptotic pathway. Perhaps the best studied is the BCL2 family of molecules, which is responsible for regulating the release of cytochrome C from the mitochondria. This family consists of pro-apoptotic molecules (e.g., BAX, BAK, and BID) and antiapoptotic molecules (e.g., BCL2, BCL-X$_L$, and BFL-1). Complex (and as yet not fully understood) interactions between these regulators control the release of cytochrome C from mitochondria and the subsequent activation of the apoptotic machinery. The best studied molecules in SCCHN are BCL2 and BAX, but the findings have varied. For instance, BCL2 overexpression has been associated with both worse[112] and better[113] overall survival rates in patients with SCCHN. Data from one study suggest that in carcinoma of the tongue, overexpression of BCL2 and loss of BAX expression, quantitated as the BCL2/BAX ratio, is significantly associated with poor prognosis.[114] Further studies are necessary to elucidate the role of these regulatory proteins in the pathogenesis of SCCHN.

The transcription factor NF-κB has also been shown to enhance cell survival in a variety of tumor types, including SCCHN.[115] The suppression of apoptosis by NF-κB may occur through transcriptional modulation of the expression of multiple apoptosis inhibitory proteins, including c-FLIP, TRAF1, TRAF2, c-IAP-1, c-IAP-2, A1/BFL-1, BCL-X$_L$, IEX-1, and XIAP.[116] In addition, activation of NF-κB appears to decrease TP53-dependent apoptosis.[117] In SCCHN, overexpression of NF-κB has been shown to decrease tumor necrosis factor-α (TNF-α)–mediated apoptosis, which is reversed by NF-κB inhibitors.[118] These data indicate that inhibitors of NF-κB signaling have great therapeutic potential alone or in combination with apoptosis-inducing chemotherapeutic agents or radiotherapy.

Immortalization

Normal cells can replicate themselves a finite number of times before they become senescent, enter a "crisis" state, and ultimately die.[119] Tumor cells, in contrast, acquire the ability to overcome this process, allowing them to replicate indefinitely. This is termed *immortalization*. Mechanisms by which tumors achieve immortalization are currently under investigation. Over the past decade, it has become apparent that the DNA at the ends of chromosomes, the so-called telomeric DNA (or telomeres), has been found to play an important role in cell senescence.[34] These telomeres appear to act as "protective caps" at the ends of chromosomes,

preventing destruction of the chromosomes. It is now known that with each replicative cycle, a small amount of telomeric DNA is lost. Over the life of the organism, therefore, the telomeres become shorter and shorter. Once enough telomeric DNA has been lost, the chromosomal ends are no longer protected, leading to the fusion of chromosomes and karyotypic abnormalities that eventually precipitate cell death. Nearly all tumor cells have acquired one or another mechanism to maintain their telomeric length.[17] The best studied of these mechanisms is the expression of the enzyme telomerase, which extends the length of telomeres (Fig. 2–8).

Several groups have investigated telomerase activity in SCCHN. In an analysis of 16 SCCHN cell lines and 29 tumor specimens, telomerase activity was found in 100% of cell lines and 90% of invasive cancers but was not detected in any normal tissues.[120] These findings are supported by those in other published reports.[121, 122] At least one study has demonstrated that telomerase activity has a relationship with the degree of tumor differentiation and treatment response[123]; another study showed that advanced cancers (e.g., stage T4) had significantly higher telomerase levels than did early cancers (e.g., stage T1/T2).[124] In studies of premalignant lesions, telomerase appears to be activated as well.[125] These early data indicate that telomerase is important in the pathogenesis of SCCHN, that it has prognostic value, and that it appears to be activated early in the development of head and neck cancers.

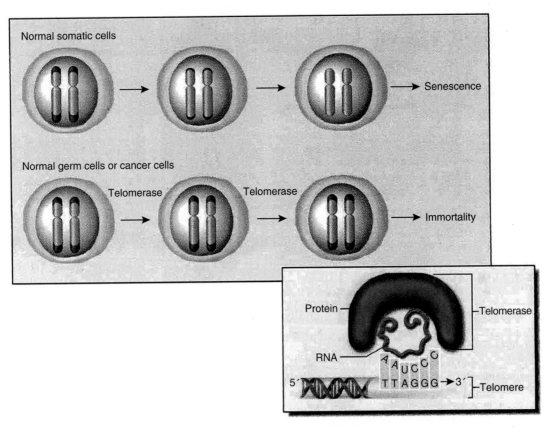

FIGURE 2–8 Immortalization. The enzyme telomerase is critical for the maintenance of telomeric DNA, allowing indefinite cellular replication. (Used with permission from Haber DA: Telomeres, cancer, and immortality. N Engl J Med 332:955–956, 1995.)

Acquisition of a Nutrient Blood Supply (Angiogenesis)

As tumors grow, invade, and metastasize, formation of new blood vessels is critical. Although many tumor cells have metabolic derangements, they still require essential nutrients and gas exchange for survival. Without adequate vascularization, tumors larger than 1 mm^3 may undergo necrosis. Not surprisingly, most tumors are able to overcome this impediment by stimulating endothelial cell proliferation and new blood vessel formation. This process of neovascularization, or angiogenesis, is itself a multistep process that appears to be regulated by both stimulatory and inhibitory factors.[34] Steps critical to successful neovascularization include degradation of the extracellular matrix, endothelial cell proliferation, migration, and assembly into higher-order structures (Fig. 2–9). Molecules that regulate angiogenesis may affect one or more of these steps.

Microvessel Density

Initial studies attempted to quantitate tumor angiogenesis through the staining of blood vessels with endothelial cell markers such as factor VIII, CD31, and CD34 and the subsequent measurement of "microvessel density." This measurement has been found to be an independent prognostic indicator for patients with breast, ovarian, prostatic, and gastric carcinomas.[126] Several studies[127–130] have looked at microvessel density in relation to the clinical outcome of patients with SCCHN, but these studies have yielded conflicting results. One study of 25 patients with stage T1 lesions of the oral cavity showed a correlation between elevated microvessel density, as determined by factor VIII staining, and the development of cervical metastases.[127] Another study found that patients who had SCCHN with increased microvessel density had a better prognosis, with a median survival of 69 months, than did patients with low microvessel density, with a median survival of 10 months.[128] Two additional studies, of 106 patients and 19 patients, showed no correlation between microvessel density and clinical outcomes.[129, 130]

Regulators of Angiogenesis

A number of significant advances have been made in recent years to further our understanding of tumor angiogenesis, including the isolation and characterization in several tumor systems of specific angiogenic factors and their inhibitors.[131] The complex interplay of both positive and negative regulators of the angiogenic process determines the degree of new blood vessel formation in and around a tumor.[126] Studies of these molecules in the pathogenesis of SCCHN have been limited, but they indicate that angiogenesis is important for SCCHN biology, may be clinically important for prognostic information, and may be a target for biologic therapy in the future. A few of these molecules and their purported roles in the angiogenic pathway, with special reference to SCCHN, are discussed in the next sections.

POSITIVE REGULATORS OF ANGIOGENESIS

Vascular Endothelial Cell Growth Factor (VEGF). VEGF has pleiotropic angiogenic effects. Not only is VEGF a potent endothelial cell mitogen, but it also promotes cell survival, cell motility, and endothelial cell organization, as well as permeability across endothelial cell monolayers.[126] Studies have attempted to correlate VEGF overexpression with various clinical endpoints such as cervical nodal metastases, tumor microvessel counts, and overall survival.[132, 133] Thus far, the results of studies of VEGF in SCCHN are conflicting. In one study of 77 patients with oral or oropharyngeal carcinoma, VEGF was found to be present in 41% of tumors and was identified as the most significant predictor of poor prognosis.[134] Similar findings have been reported in other subsites.[135] In addition, in vitro studies have demonstrated that downregulation of VEGF by transfection of antisense VEGF in head and neck cancer cell lines reduced endothelial cell migration by 50%.[136] However, no decrease in tumorigenicity in these cell lines was noted. This supports other data that have shown no prognostic relationship between VEGF levels and tumor stage, invasiveness, or survival parameters.[137, 138] Thus, currently no consensus exists about the role of VEGF in the pathogenesis of SCCHN.

Basic Fibroblast Growth Factor (bFGF). bFGF has been found to be among the most potent of the endothelial cell mitogens.[126] This molecule promotes endothelial cell motility and survival as well as the organization of endothelial cells into tubules, when grown in vitro in the presence of extracellular matrix components. bFGF also upregulates the production of the tissue proteases, MMP-1 and uPA.

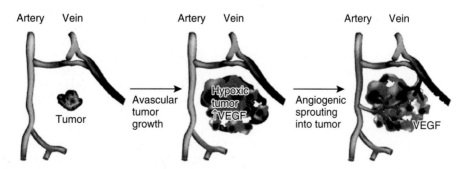

FIGURE 2–9 Angiogenesis. As tumors are established, they require new blood vessel formation to allow continued growth. A complex interplay of molecular events, including regulation by pro-angiogenic (such as VEGF) and anti-angiogenic molecules, is required for this to occur. (Used with permission from Yancopoulos GD, Davis S, Gale NW, et al: Vascular-specific growth factors and blood vessel formation. Nature 407:242–248, 2000.)

Expression of bFGF and its receptor FGF-2 has been identified in normal oral keratinocytes as well as in oral cancers.[139] A study performed at the M.D. Anderson Cancer Center on 11 head and neck cancer specimens showed high levels of bFGF in well-differentiated tumor specimens but an absence of expression in poorly differentiated tumors.[140] Furthermore, the levels of bFGF found in these tumors were similar to or lower than those found in the adjacent normal mucosa. In addition, several groups have reported elevated levels of bFGF in the serum and urine of patients with SCCHN and have correlated this with poor prognosis.[141, 142]

Platelet-Derived Endothelial Cell Growth Factor (PD-ECGF). PD-ECGF is an endothelial cell mitogen with in vivo angiogenic activity that also displays thymidine phosphorylase activity. PD-ECGF expression was studied in 58 patients with oral or oropharyngeal cancers; PD-ECGF was found to be overexpressed in a high percentage of tumor cells.[143] Those patients with higher percentages of tumor cells expressing PD-ECGF had higher rates of relapse and death from their disease than did those with a lesser degree of staining. However, there was no correlation between microvessel density and PD-ECGF staining.

Interleukin 8 (IL-8). Several lines of evidence indicate that IL-8 is a cytokine with angiogenic activity.[126] Homogenates of nine fresh SSCHN tumor specimens were found to contain IL-8 by radioimmunoassay.[144] Further evaluation of these tumors by immunohistochemical techniques showed that this cytokine was localized within the tumor cells. In addition, stimulation of cultures of SCCHN cells and established tumor cell lines with interleukin 1 or tumor necrosis factor increased IL-8 expression by the tumor cells. A follow-up study by the same research group showed that in a high percentage of SCCHN tumors, the IL-8 receptors could be detected on both cancer cells and endothelial cells within the tumor.[145]

NEGATIVE REGULATORS OF ANGIOGENESIS

Interferons. Studies of the interferons (IFNs) have shown that the members of this family of cytokines have potent antiangiogenic activity. IFN-α and IFN-β have been particularly well studied in this regard. Both have been found to inhibit endothelial cell proliferation and migration.[126] In addition, decreased IFN-β expression has been inversely correlated with microvessel density and new blood vessel formation and has been shown to downregulate the expression of IL-8, bFGF, and MMPs.[146, 147] Although the role of IFNs in the pathogenesis of SCCHN is largely unknown at this time, they have shown promise as a potential therapeutic strategy in mouse models either by direct replacement[148] or through upregulation by other cytokines.[149]

Thrombospondins. Thrombospondins (TSPs) are a multigene family of five secreted glycoproteins that are involved in the regulation of cell proliferation, adhesion, and migration. Two members of the TSP family—TSP-1 and TSP-2—are also naturally occurring inhibitors of angiogenesis.[150] Evidence shows that TSP-1 inhibits angiogenesis by inducing endothelial cell apoptosis[151]; this was achieved by increased expression of BAX, decreased expression of BCL2, and activation of caspase 3. As yet, little is known of the role of TSPs in the pathogenesis of SCCHN.

Others. Recently, data that also implicate nitric oxide[152] and the PTEN gene[153] as angiogenesis inhibitors have been produced. However, these molecules have not yet been studied in SCCHN.

Tissue Invasion and Metastasis

The subsequent phases of tumor progression include tissue invasion and metastasis. The specific events that must take place for invasion and metastasis to occur have been identified, and a number of proteins that facilitate these events have been isolated and characterized in SCCHN, as well as in other tumor types (Fig. 2–10).[154] Invasion of adjacent normal tissue is one of the pathologic criteria central to the diagnosis of malignancy; the three steps critical to epithelial tumor cell invasion are the attachment of tumor cells to the basement membrane, proteolysis of the extracellular matrix, and migration of the tumor cell.[155] Some of the specific molecules involved in these steps have been studied in many tumor types, including SCCHN.

Attachment to the Basement Membrane

The basement membrane underlying squamous epithelium serves as a natural barrier to tumor cell invasion and has been biochemically characterized using a variety of methods. Collagen type IV, laminin, collagen type VII, and heparan sulfate proteoglycans have all been found in epithelial basement membranes.[156, 157] However, loss of the basement membrane has not been correlated with invasive behavior in SCCHN, as it is in other tumor types.[158, 159]

INTEGRINS

Both normal and neoplastic squamous cell epithelia have been found to have specific receptors for basement membrane constituents through which cells adhere to the extracellular matrix. By raising monoclonal antibodies to human SCCHN cells, van Waes and Carey[160] isolated a tumor-expressed antigen known as A9, which was subsequently shown to be identical to the α6β4 integrin. Integrins are a family of cell adhesion molecules, and the α6β4 integrin is known to bind specifically to laminin. Immunohistochemical studies of normal squamous epithelium and SCCHN specimens have shown a polarized pattern of expression of the α6β4 integrin on the basal pole of normal skin or mucosal keratinocytes, which are adjacent to the basement membrane, and a more diffuse staining pattern in tumors.[161] When A9 antigen expression was correlated with clinical parameters, increased levels of α6β4 integrin expression were correlated with early recurrence and metastasis.[162] Another integrin that has been studied in SCCHN is αvβ5 integrin. Unlike α6β4 integrins, αvβ5 integrin has reduced expression in SCCHN.[163] In vitro studies suggest that this integrin may be important in oral neoplasia because αvβ5-negative cell lines show a malignant phenotype that can be reversed by transfection of the missing integrin.[164] Thus, it appears that integrins have important but widely varied roles in the progression of SCCHN.

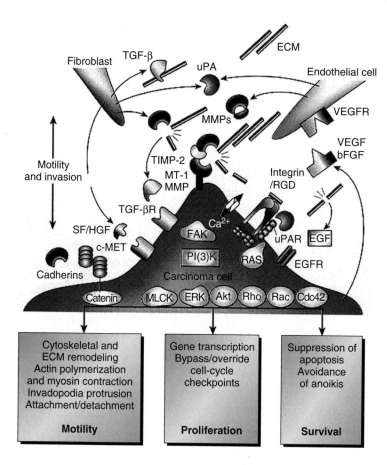

FIGURE 2–10 Invasion and metastasis. A variety of molecular regulators are required for tissue invasion and the formation of metastasis. Some of the more common regulators, including MMPs, uPa, cadherins, and catenins, are pictured above. (Used with permission from Liotta LA, Kohn EC: The microenvironment of the tumour-host interface. Nature 411:375–379, 2001.)

E-CADHERIN

E-cadherin is another cell-surface receptor molecule that plays a role in maintaining cell-cell contacts, an important feature of epithelial cells. With the use of immunohistochemical methods, E-cadherin levels have been associated with differentiation in squamous cell carcinomas[165]; that is, well-differentiated tumors express high levels of E-cadherin, whereas poorly differentiated tumors have significantly lower levels of expression.[165] E-cadherin expression has also been examined in relation to clinical outcome in patients with SCCHN.[166] Although E-cadherin expression was not related to tumor size or stage, patients with increased tumor levels of E-cadherin appeared to have a more favorable survival rate. This finding was corroborated in a recent study in which patients with strong E-cadherin staining in tumors had a 5-year survival rate of 85%, compared with 53% for those with weak staining.[167] Decreased levels of E-cadherin have also been associated with the metastatic phenotype in SCCHN cell lines.[168] This relationship has been shown in tumor specimens as well,[169] indicating that loss of E-cadherin may be an important step in the development of metastasis in SCCHN.

CATENINS

More recently, a group of cytoplasmic proteins called catenins, which form complexes with cadherins, have been shown to assist in the maintenance of cell-cell contacts. Studies in oral cavity cancers have revealed that as with E-cadherin, catenin levels show an inverse relationship with degree of tumor differentiation.[170] Further studies are ongoing to assess whether catenins may play a complementary role with cadherins in invasion and metastasis.

Proteolysis and Migration

Proteolysis of the extracellular matrix is thought to be a critical step for tissue invasion by tumors.[171] A wide variety of proteases have been evaluated in many tumor types, and there is an expanding body of literature regarding the potential role of several specific proteolytic enzymes and their specific inhibitors in the development of tissue invasion and regional metastases of human SCCHN.

MATRIX METALLOPROTEINASES

The MMPs are a diverse group of proteinases that require metal ions for their activity, hence their name. They have been found to be important mediators of invasion and metastasis in many tumor types, including breast, colon, and prostate. In SCCHN, several individual MMPs have been studied. Using a combination of immunohistochemical, in situ hybridization, and zymographic methods, Sutinen and colleagues[172] found relatively increased expression of MMP-2 in oral cancer specimens, compared with oral dysplastic lesions. These data have been corroborated in other studies.[173, 174] The expression of this enzyme, also known as 72-kD type IV collagenase, has been correlated with the development of cervical lymph node metastases and lymphatic and vascular invasion in patients with oral cavity tumors.[175]

MMP-3, also known as stromelysin-1, has also been shown to be upregulated in approximately 50% of head and neck cancers.[176] This MMP degrades laminin, fibronectin, and type IV collagen. With the use of in situ hybridization, MMP-3 was identified in tumor cells in 23 of 26 SCCHN samples studied, suggesting a role for MMPs in stromal invasion by SCCHN.[177] These data were further substantiated in a study of 107 SCCHN samples using Northern blot analysis, in which several MMPs, including MMP-3, were found to be overexpressed.[178] Further analysis by immunohistochemical staining indicates that expression of this MMP appears to be concentrated at the advancing or invasive front of the tumor.[179] These studies have also demonstrated that MMP-3 is associated with higher T stage and advanced nodal status.

Another MMP implicated in the development of SCCHN is MMP-9, also known as the 92-kD type IV collagenase. Initial investigations showed that SCCHN cell lines expressed MMP-9,[180] and subsequent analysis of fresh SCCHN biopsy specimens with antibodies to MMP-9 confirmed the presence of this protease in invasive SCCHN.[181] Several studies have verified this.[182] The presence of increased MMP-9 activity has been associated with invasiveness in oral cavity cancer.[174] In addition, suppression of MMP-9 activity has been shown to decrease tumor cell invasiveness in tongue cancer cells.[183] More recent evidence points toward a new role for MMP-9 in invasion and metastasis of SCCHN. Riedel and coworkers[184] found that MMP-9 staining was correlated with increased microvessel density and upregulation of VEGF, indicating that MMP-9 and VEGF may cooperate in the process of angiogenesis in SCCHN. This presents an exciting avenue for the application of MMP inhibitors that might block invasion and attenuate angiogenesis.

It has recently become evident that MMPs are regulated within the cell by various molecules, the most important of which are a group of inhibitors called tissue inhibitors of metalloproteinases (TIMPs). TIMPs participate actively in the dynamic regulation of proteolysis, and they are usually produced by surrounding stromal cells in an attempt to block the proteolytic effects of MMPs.[172] Only recently has this area of research been examined with respect to SCCHN. One of the few studies available suggests that both high levels of MMPs and low levels of TIMPs may be required for metastasis to occur.[174] Many additional questions regarding the interaction of SCCHN with the extracellular matrix still need to be answered, and it is likely that important information about the biology of these tumors as well as clinical applications will arise from studies in this area.

UROKINASE-TYPE PLASMINOGEN ACTIVATOR

The uPA system is also believed to play a role in invasion and metastasis. uPA is known to bind to a specific receptor, urokinase-type plasminogen activator receptor (uPAR), and uPA activity can be inhibited by a specific inhibitor, plasminogen activator inhibitor (PAI).[185] The uPA system has been well studied in several tumor models, including SCCHN. Early work indicated that uPA levels were significantly elevated in SCCHN cell lines, compared with those in fibroblasts.[186] In addition, uPAR has been shown to be upregulated in SCCHN.[187] Another recent study of 34 primary oral cavity cancers showed that uPA and uPAR are expressed in 23.5% and 29.4% of tumors, respectively, and that coexpression of these two molecules is associated with highly invasive tumors and lymph node metastases.[188] Clayman and associates[189] were able to show that inhibition of uPA by a specific anti-uPA antibody abrogated the ability of SCC cell lines to invade. Likewise, evidence indicates that blocking the uPAR molecule abrogates tumor metastasis.[190] These data suggest that the uPA system plays an important role in the ability of SCCHN to invade and metastasize.

SERPINS

The serpin family of proteins is a group of protease inhibitors just coming to prominence for their role in carcinogenesis. Several recent studies have highlighted their importance in SCCHN.[191–193] Spring and colleagues identified and cloned a serpin member they named "headpin," which maps to chromosome 18q, a site of frequent loss of heterozygosity in SCCHN.[191] They found headpin to be expressed in normal oral mucosa but underexpressed in oral cavity SCC. This downregulation appears to occur at the transcriptional level in SCCHN cell lines studied by the same group.[192]

Another serpin family member, maspin, is also located on chromosome 18q and is also known to have tumor suppressor functions. Using immunohistochemical techniques, Xia and colleagues[193] showed that patients with oral SCC tumors that had high maspin expression had lower rates of regional metastases and better overall survival rates. Further studies are necessary to delineate the role of the serpin family of proteins in the pathogenesis of SCCHN.

■ MOLECULAR TARGETS FOR CANCER THERAPY

As our understanding of the basic molecular pathways responsible for the pathogenesis of SCCHN has improved, more rational approaches to cancer therapy have been developed. Molecular medicine holds tremendous promise and potential for the treatment of head and neck cancer. Gene therapy, antibody-toxin conjugates, antisense molecules, and small molecule inhibitors are all being studied, at both basic science and clinical levels. It is clear that molecular therapy for cancer will become increasingly important in the next millennium.

Conventional treatments for cancer, such as surgery, radiotherapy, and chemotherapy, all have untoward side effects on normal tissue as a consequence of tumor killing. Since the time of Erlich, who described the so-called magic bullet, scientists have striven to find more specific cancer therapies that can target cancer cells without damaging normal cells. The promise of molecular medicine is that as we learn more about what makes cancer cells different, we can better use that knowledge to target specific components of tumor cells not found in normal cells, thus mimicking the "magic bullet." From the results of initial trials, it has become clear that not all molecules (regardless of how vital they are to the carcinogenic pathway) are good targets for molecular therapies. The ideal target should be commonly found on cancer cells, should be specific to cancer cells, and should also be involved in several aspects of carcinogenesis. Thus, a molecule that plays a role in proliferative signaling, apoptosis, invasion, and angiogenesis, such as NF-κB, is theoretically a better target than a molecule that plays only one role in the carcinogenic pathway. In the next sections, we outline a few of the best studied and most promising molecular targets for the treatment of SCCHN.

Molecular Targets

NF-κB

As was previously discussed, the NF-κb transcription factor can enhance tumor progression by increasing the expression of cellular regulatory proteins that inhibit apoptosis, increase proliferative signaling, and enhance invasion and angiogenesis.[194] This makes NF-κB an ideal target for molecular therapies.

Initial attempts at inhibiting NF-κB activation used specific IκBs, usually IκBα or IκBβ. These are repressors that bind to and sequester NF-κB in the cytoplasm, inhibiting its nuclear translocation and transcriptional activation.[195] In several model systems, IκBα inhibition of NF-κB has been found to enhance tumor cell apoptosis. In fibrosarcoma cell lines, IκBα sensitizes cells to apoptosis induced by either ionizing radiation or chemotherapeutic agents.[196] Wang and coworkers[197] have shown that IκBα reduces the tumorigenicity of human SCCHN cells in mice with severe combined immunodeficiency disease. Therefore, IκBα may have potential benefit as a sensitizing agent for radiotherapy or chemotherapy in patients with SCCHN.

Another potential method for downmodulating the NF-κB pathway is the inhibition of IκB degradation by the 26 S proteasome. Several proteasome inhibitors have been studied, including peptide aldehydes (e.g., MG101, MG132, MG115), acylating agents (e.g., lactacystin), and boronic acid peptides (e.g., PS341). These inhibitors block proteasome function, thus allowing IκB levels in the cell to remain high, effectively decreasing the activity of NF-κB. In SCCHN cell lines, PS341 in particular has been found to be a potent inhibitor of NF-κB activation, causing reductions in tumor cell survival, tumor growth, and angiogenesis.[198] In addition, PS341 appears to enhance the effects of chemotherapeutic agents, as demonstrated by Cusack and associates,[199] who found a significant reduction in tumor size and an increase in apoptosis in colon cancer cell lines treated with PS341 plus irinotecan when compared with cells treated with irinotecan alone. A similar study showed enhancement of radiosensitivity as well.[200]

Other interesting potential agents of NF-κB inhibition are the nonsteroidal anti-inflammatory drugs (NSAIDs), which include aspirin, sulfasalazine, sulindac, and cyclooxygenase-2 (COX-2) inhibitors. These agents have been shown to decrease NF-κB activity in vitro and in vivo; however, the mechanism of action is not as yet understood.[201] The role of NSAIDs in the prevention of colon cancer is well documented.[202] Likewise, several dietary compounds, including flavonoids, curcumin, and resveratrol, appear to block NF-κB activation and may be potential adjunctive treatments or preventive therapies.[201]

RAS

Another potential target for molecular therapy is the *RAS* oncogene. As was discussed earlier, *RAS* is the prototypic oncogene and has varied roles in carcinogenesis, including cell survival, cell proliferation, and apoptosis. Although *RAS* is mutated in most human cancers, studies in SCCHN have shown a relatively low frequency of *RAS* mutations.[203] Because of its importance in the overall development of many cancers, attempts to inhibit *RAS* have led to the development of farnesyltranferase inhibitors (FTIs). These molecules act by inhibiting farnesylation, a critical post-translational modification of the RAS protein required for its function. FTIs have shown great potential in phase I and II trials and appear to affect only cancer cell physiology, without affecting normal cellular functions.[204] It is interesting that although FTIs were developed to inhibit RAS, a major portion of their mechanism of action appears to be secondary to the blockade of farnesylation of several non-RAS proteins, especially RhoB.[205]

The current generation of FTIs appears to act specifically on cancer cells, having shown few if any side effects in clinical trials. In one trial of 42 tumor cell lines, more than 70% of cell lines lost anchorage-independent growth when treated with FTIs.[206] This effect was independent of *RAS* mutational status. In vitro studies have shown FTIs to act synergistically with chemotherapeutic agents and radiotherapy.[207, 208] Several phase I and II trials with FTIs have been completed,[209] and these have shown minimal side effects when used in the treatment of advanced tumors.

Epidermal Growth Factor Receptor

Probably the best studied molecular target is the EGF-R. As has been described previously, EGF-R activation occurs in a large percentage of human cancers and has been reported in 80% to 90% of SCCHN specimens. As with other targets, the EGF-R seems to play multiple roles in carcinogenesis, including cell growth and apoptosis. Several methods of blocking EGF-R–mediated pathways have been described and are outlined in the following section.

Multiple ligands for EGF-R, including EGF, TGF-α, betacellulin, heparin-binding EGF, amphiregulin, Cripto, and epiregulin, have been identified.[210] By conjugating these ligands to bacterially derived toxins (e.g., diphtheria or *Pseudomonas* toxins), Azemar and colleagues[211] were able to show antitumor effects in SCCHN cell lines. However, although it was initially promising, severe side effects, including hepatotoxicity, appear to limit the usefulness of this approach.[212]

Monoclonal antibodies engineered to block EGF-R activation appear to be much better tolerated than bacterially derived toxins and have fewer side effects. The humanized monoclonal antibody C225 has shown promise in the treatment of SCCHN. Early work found that C225 inhibited growth of SCCHN in vitro.[213] Furthermore, when used in conjunction with chemotherapeutic agents or radiotherapy,

C225 has been shown to enhance tumor cell kill.[214, 215] In phase I and II trials in humans, impressive responses have been elicited in patients with SCCHN.[216] Currently, multi-institutional, randomized phase III trials are under way to determine whether synergistic effects can be demonstrated when C225 is added to either radiotherapy or chemotherapy regimens.

Several other methods of inhibiting EGF-R have recently been developed. A series of small molecule inhibitors that block the tyrosine kinase activity of the EGF-R has been developed. The best studied of these, ZD1839 (Iressa), has shown promise when used in combination with chemotherapeutic agents.[217] Currently, phase III trials of ZD1839 are under way in non–small cell lung cancer and other tumor types.[218] Lastly, antisense strategies, designed to inhibit the translation of the EGF-R protein, have shown promise in in vitro and in vivo models and have entered phase I trials.[219]

TP53

As has been described earlier, the *TP53* gene plays a major role in the pathogenesis of SCCHN. Evidence demonstrates that it helps regulate cell-cycle progression and apoptosis. When *TP53* is mutated or abnormally expressed, as it is in more than 50% of cases of SCCHN, these cellular functions are affected, allowing tumor formation and progression. For this reason, the *TP53* gene is a logical target for molecular therapies.

Most attempts to restore *TP53* function to tumors have involved gene therapy techniques. Gene therapy uses vectors, usually adenoviral or retroviral, to deliver a functionally normal gene to replace a mutated gene within a tumor. In most cases, the *TP53* vector is delivered to the tumor via intratumoral injection. Pioneering work by Roth and colleagues at the M.D. Anderson Cancer Center[220, 221] showed that by restoring *TP53* function via gene therapy, tumor regression was observed; the mechanism appears to be increased apoptosis in cancer cells. Phase I and II human trials conducted by this group showed that *TP53* gene therapy was feasible and safe and induced tumor regression in patients with lung cancer. Clayman and his group[97, 222] initiated *TP53* gene therapy for SCCHN and showed similar preclinical results, further demonstrating its feasibility and safety in human trials including SCCHN patients. Currently, randomized phase III trials are under way to determine the efficacy of this technique both as a surgical adjuvant and in combination with chemotherapeutic agents.[99]

A second method of affecting the *TP53* gene in tumor cells involves the use of an adenovirus, ONYX-015, that is genetically engineered to delete the 55-kD *E1B* gene.[223] This deletion renders it replication selective; that is, it can replicate only in cells that are TP53 null. Thus, this virus will replicate in and eventually lyse TP53 null cells while leaving TP53 competent cells unaffected; this virus, then, has exciting potential to selectively kill tumor cells. Preclinical studies demonstrated selective killing both in vitro and in vivo.[224] Phase I and II trials in more than 200 cancer patients to date have shown the treatments to be generally well tolerated, with no maximally tolerated doses identified. Viral replication

was tumor selective, and replication was generally transient.[225] Clinical trials have also demonstrated synergism with chemotherapeutic agents[226] and radiotherapy,[227] suggesting that ONYX-015 may be a useful adjunctive treatment in SCCHN. Studies are under way to determine its potential efficacy.

Identification of Novel Targets for Molecular Therapy

Identification of the genes that cause carcinogenesis is the central aim of cancer research. The logical extension of this aim is to use those identified genes to develop novel therapeutic modalities. Recent improvements in molecular biologic techniques and genomics have resulted in an explosion of information and a huge increase in the number of genes and proteins known to be involved in carcinogenesis. This in turn leads to a great increase in potential molecular targets.

Human Genome Project

The Human Genome Project was spawned in the mid-1980s when the National Research Council recognized the need for the creation of genetic, physical, and sequential maps of the human genome. With the advent of newer sequencing techniques, these goals were recently realized with the publication of the initial sequencing and analysis of the human genome in 2001.[228] In this report, it is estimated that the human genome contains 30,000 to 40,000 genes, far fewer than was first suspected (and only twice as many as the recently sequenced worm genome contains). However, the complexity of these genes is greater, and the number of subsequently produced protein products is also much greater.

The importance of the Human Genome Project to oncology is difficult to overemphasize. Future work in identifying genes important in carcinogenesis could lead to new and unique genetic tests that could help in the identification of patients at risk for developing cancer. In addition, improvements in the identification and classification of tumors will allow clinicians to make better diagnostic and therapeutic decisions. And, perhaps more importantly, a huge number of potential targets for pharmaceutical and molecular therapies have been identified. The effect of the Human Genome Project in oncology is so important that the National Cancer Institute recently developed a program called the Cancer Genome Anatomy Project, in an effort to compile a comprehensive record of all the genes involved in human cancer.

Microarray Technology

Another revolution in the way scientists are able to study cancer at the molecular level is the development of microarray technology, which provides researchers with a powerful new tool for observing patterns of gene expression in cells and allows comparison of tumor tissue with normal tissue. The most commonly used microarrays—DNA microarrays or gene chips—usually comprise micron-range–sized spots of genomic DNA, cDNA, or oligonucleotides arrayed on a glass slide. When cDNA samples obtained from tumor samples and normal tissue are placed on this slide, differences in gene expression between the tissue types can be observed. Advanced computing techniques can then catalog these differences, providing the researcher with a list of differentially expressed genes.

Microarray technology has been used for a wide scope of applications, including sequencing, detection of mutations or polymorphisms, and differential gene expression. The power of this technology is its ability to generate a genome-wide expression profile of thousands of genes in one experiment. An example of its use in SCCHN was provided by Villaret and coworkers,[229] who identified 13 differentially expressed genes in SCCHN using DNA microarrays. Four of these were genes not previously described; identification of these genes is currently under way. In addition, Hanna and associates have used microarray technology to identify tumor-related genes that can be used as predictors of radiation response of SCCHN.[230] It is therefore easy to see how microarrays can be used for diagnostic and predictive purposes, as well as for helping to identify novel targets for molecular therapies.

Proteomics

With the accumulation of vast numbers of DNA sequences in data bases, and indeed the entire sequence of the human genome, researchers are realizing that having only genetic information is not sufficient for elucidating biologic function. Instead, it will become important to understand the relationship between genes and the protein complement or "proteome" of a cell. Proteomics, the study of the proteome, includes not only the identification of proteins but also the determination of their localization, modifications, interactions, activities, and ultimately, function. As in the case of genomics, there has been an explosion in growth of the field of proteomics, fueled by discoveries of the Human Genome Project and the development of powerful protein technologies such as mass spectrometry, two-hybrid techniques, and protein arrays.

Because the proteome is much more complex than the genome, progress in proteomics has been slower. However, it is expected that a wealth of information about the protein makeup of tumor cells will become available over the next decade as a result of proteomics. Because proteins are one step closer to function than genes are, these studies are expected to lead directly to biologic discoveries, especially in cancer research, where additional insight into how cancer cells are "functionally" different from normal cells is needed. Combined, this information will then be available to assist in the development of new diagnostic, prognostic, and therapeutic strategies for clinical oncologists to use.

◼ SUMMARY

The past decade has brought about an explosion of information about the pathogenesis of cancer in general, and SCCHN specifically. We are now better able to understand the molecular events underlying carcinogenesis. The clonal evolution theory and molecular progression models have given researchers a better framework from which to explore the specifics of carcinogenesis. For instance, we now understand that SCCHN arises from the accumulation of multiple genetic alterations, sometimes inherited, but usually acquired somatically from exposure to environmental agents, including tobacco, alcohol, and viruses. Each of these genetic events provides cells with a selective growth advantage, leading to the production of a dominant clonal population. Further genetic events lead to the development of cancer cells that can overcome normal growth controls and host defenses and establish a tumor. The accumulation of subsequent molecular events leads to abnormalities in proliferation, cell-cycle control, apoptosis, immortalization, angiogenesis, invasion, and metastasis, all of which factor into the pathogenesis and progression of SCCHN.

Certainly, as we improve our understanding of the steps responsible for cancer formation, we will be better able to diagnose and treat this disease. The lexicon of alterations that are important in the pathogenesis of SCCHN is being expanded at a rapid pace through the use of powerful new molecular methods. As more studies correlating clinical outcomes with specific molecular aberrations are completed, molecular diagnosis will play an increasingly important role in determining the prognosis and need for specific treatments for patients with SCCHN. Perhaps even more important is the prospect of targeting molecules critical in the pathogenesis of SCCHN with specific biologically based therapies. Novel therapeutic approaches using antisense technology, gene therapy, and immunoconjugates have yielded exciting results in preclinical models, some of which have led to the initiation of clinical protocols. These provide the promise and excitement of developing molecular therapies to combat this disease. Thus, as we learn more about the molecular pathogenesis of SCCHN, and as our ability to target specific molecules increases, the potential for rationally treating SCCHN by targeting specific molecular defects critical to the biology of this tumor should become a reality and will have a tremendous impact on the way we diagnose and treat SCCHN in the future.

REFERENCES

1. Nowell PC: The clonal evolution of tumor cell populations. Science 194:23–28, 1976.
2. Renan MJ: How many mutations are required for tumorigenesis? Implications from human cancer data. Mol Carcinog 7:139–146, 1993.
3. Fearon ER, Vogelstein B: A genetic model for colorectal tumorigenesis. Cell 61:759–767, 1990.
4. Vogelstein B, Kinzler KW: The multistep nature of cancer. Trends Genet 9:138–141, 1993.
5. Batsakis JG: Tumors of the Head and Neck, ed 2. Baltimore, Williams & Wilkins, 1979, pp 121–129.
6. Nawroz H, van der Reit P, Hruban RH, et al: Allelotype of head and neck squamous cell carcinoma. Cancer Res 54:1152–1155, 1994.
7. van der Riet P, Nawroz H, Hruban RH, et al: Frequent loss of chromosome 9p21-22 early in head and neck cancer progression. Cancer Res 54:1156–1158, 1994.
8. Califano J, van der Riet P, Westra W, et al: Genetic progression model for head and neck cancer: Implications for field cancerization. Cancer Res 56:2488–2492, 1996.
9. Vokes EE, Weichselbaum RR, Lippman SM, et al: Head and neck cancer. N Engl J Med 328:184–194, 1993.
10. Slaughter DP, Southwick HW, Smejkal W: Field cancerization in oral stratified squamous epithelium: Clinical implications of multicentric origin. Cancer 6:963–968, 1953.

11. van Oijen MG, Leppers Vd, Straat FG, Tilanus MG, et al: The origins of multiple squamous cell carcinomas in the aerodigestive tract. Cancer 88:884–893, 2000.

12. Chung KY, Mukhopadhyay T, Kim J, et al: Discordant p53 gene mutations in primary head and neck cancers and corresponding second primary cancers of the upper aerodigestive tract. Cancer Res 53:1676–1683, 1993.

13. Partridge M, Emilion G, Pateromichelakis S, et al. Field cancerisation of the oral cavity: Comparison of the spectrum of molecular alterations in cases presenting with both dysplastic and malignant lesions. Oral Oncol 33:332–337, 1997.

14. Tabor MP, Brakenhoff RH, van Houten VMM, et al: Persistence of genetically altered fields in head and neck cancer patients: Biological and clinical implications. Clin Cancer Res 7:1523–1532, 2001.

15. Bedi GC, Westra WH, Gabrielson E, et al: Multiple head and neck tumors: Evidence for a common clonal origin. Cancer Res 56:2484–2487, 1996.

16. Jang SJ, Chiba I, Hirai A, et al: Multiple oral squamous epithelial lesions: Are they genetically related? Oncogene 20:2235–2242, 2001.

17. Byers RM: Squamous cell carcinoma of the oral tongue in patients less than thirty years of age. Am J Surg 130:475–478, 1975.

18. Cusumano RJ, Persky MS: Squamous cell carcinoma of the oral cavity and oropharynx in young adults. Head Neck 10:229–234, 1988.

19. Atula S, Grenman R, Laippala P, et al: Cancer of the tongue in patients younger than 40 years. A distinct entity? Arch Otolaryngol Head Neck Surg 122:1313–1319, 1996.

20. Myers JN, Elkins T, Roberts D, et al: Squamous cell carcinoma of the tongue in young adults: Increasing incidence and factors that predict treatment outcomes. Otolaryngol Head Neck Surg 122:44–51, 2000.

21. Fioretti F, Bosetti C, Tavani A, et al: Risk factors for oral and pharyngeal cancer in never smokers. Oral Oncol 35:375–378, 1999.

22. Gillison ML, Koch WM, Shah KV: Human papillomavirus in head and neck squamous cell carcinoma: Are some head and neck cancers a sexually transmitted disease? Curr Opin Oncol 11:191–199, 1999.

23. Franceschi S, Munoz N, Bosch XF, et al: Human papillomavirus and cancers of the upper aerodigestive tract: A review of epidemiological and experimental evidence. Cancer Epidemiol Biomarkers Prev 5:567–575, 1996.

24. Gillison ML, Koch WM, Capone RB, et al: Evidence for a causal association between human papillomavirus and a subset of head and neck cancers. J Natl Cancer Inst 92:709–720, 2000.

25. Schantz SP, Hsu TC, Ainslie N, et al: Young adults with head and neck cancer express increased susceptibility to mutagen-induced chromosome damage. JAMA 262:3313–3315, 1989.

26. Wang LE, Sturgis EM, Eicher SA, et al: Mutagen sensitivity to benzo(a)pyrene diol epoxide and the risk of squamous cell carcinoma of the head and neck. Clin Cancer Res 4:1773–1778, 1998.

27. Cheng L, Sturgis EM, Eicher SA, et al: Glutathione-S-transferase polymorphisms and risk of squamous-cell carcinoma of the head and neck. Int J Cancer 84:220–224, 1999.

28. Sturgis EM, Castillo EJ, Li L, et al: Polymorphisms of DNA repair gene XRCC1 in squamous cell carcinoma of the head and neck. Carcinogenesis 20:2125–2129, 1999.

29. Lingen MW, Chang KW, McMurray SJ, et al: Overexpression of p53 in squamous cell carcinoma of the tongue in young patients with no known risk factors is not associated with mutations in exons 5–9. Head Neck 22:328–335, 2000.

30. Hernandez-Alcoceba R, del Peso L, Lacal JC: The Ras family of GTPases in cancer cell invasion. Cell Mol Life Sci 57:65–76, 2000.

31. Lane D: p53, guardian of the genome. Nature 358:15–16, 1992.

32. Knudson AG: Mutation and cancer: Statistical study of retinoblastoma. Proc Natl Acad Sci USA 68:820–823, 1971.

33. Hahn WC, Counter CM, Lundberg AS, et al: Creation of human tumour cells with defined genetic elements. Nature 400:464–468, 1999.

34. Hanahan D, Weinberg RA: The hallmarks of cancer. Cell 100:57–70, 2000.

35. Grandis JR, Tweardy DJ: The role of peptide growth factors in head and neck carcinoma. Otolaryngol Clin North Am 25:1105–1115, 1992.

36. Cohen S: Isolation of a mouse submaxillary gland protein accelerating incisor eruption and eyelid opening in the newborn animal. J Biol Chem 237:1555, 1962.

37. Sauter ER, Ridge JA, Gordon J, et al: p53 overexpression correlates with increased survival in patients with squamous carcinoma of the tongue base. Am J Surg 164:651–653, 1992.

38. Furata Y, Takasu T, Asai T, et al: Clinical significance of the epidermal growth factor receptor gene in squamous cell carcinomas of the nasal cavities and paranasal sinuses. Cancer 69:358–362, 1992.

39. Maurizi M, Scambia G, Benedetti Panici P, et al: EGF receptor expression in primary laryngeal cancer: Correlation with clinico-pathological features and prognostic significance. Int J Cancer 52:862–866, 1992.

40. Grandis JR, Tweardy D: Elevated levels of transforming growth factor alpha and epidermal growth factor receptor messenger RNA are early markers of carcinogenesis in head and neck cancer. Cancer Res 53:3579–3584, 1993.

41. Grandis JR, Melhem MF, Gooding WE, et al: Levels of TGF-alpha and EGFR protein in head and neck squamous cell carcinoma and patient survival. J Natl Cancer Inst 90:824–832, 1998.

42. Dassonville O, Formento JL, Francoual M, et al: Expression of epidermal growth factor receptor survival in upper aerodigestive tract cancer. J Clin Oncol 11:1873–1878, 1993.

43. Formento JL, Francoual M, Ramaioli A, et al: EGF receptor, a prognostic factor in epidermoid cancers of the upper aerodigestive tracts. Bull Cancer 81:610–615, 1994.

44. Maxwell SA, Sacks PG, Gutterman JU, et al: Epidermal growth factor receptor protein-tyrosine kinase activity in human cell lines established from squamous carcinomas of the head and neck. Cancer Res 49:1130–1137, 1989.

45. O-charoenrat P, Modjtahedi H, Rhys-Evans P, et al: Epidermal growth factor–like ligands differentially up-regulate matrix metalloproteinase 9 in head and neck squamous carcinoma cells. Cancer Res 60:1121–1128, 2000.

46. Shibata T, Kawano T, Nagayasu H, et al: Enhancing effects of epidermal growth factor on human squamous cell carcinoma motility and matrix degradation but not growth. Tumour Biol 17:168–175, 1996.

47. Turkson J, Jove R: STAT proteins: Novel molecular targets for cancer drug discovery. Oncogene 19:6613–6626, 2000.

48. Grandis JR, Chakraborty A, Zeng Q, et al: Downmodulation of TGF-alpha protein expression with antisense oligonucleotides inhibits proliferation of head and neck squamous carcinoma but not normal mucosal epithelial cells. J Cell Biochem 69:55–62, 1998.

49. Grandis JR, Drenning SD, Chakraborty A, et al: Requirement of Stat3 but not Stat1 activation for epidermal growth factor receptor–mediated cell growth in vitro. J Clin Invest 102:1385–1392, 1998.

50. Grandis JR, Drenning SD, Zeng Q, et al: Constitutive activation of Stat3 signaling abrogates apoptosis in squamous cell carcinogenesis in vivo. Proc Natl Acad Sci USA 97:4227–4232, 2000.

51. Ghosh S, May M, Kopp E: NF-κB and Rel proteins: Evolutionarily conserved mediators of immune respones. Annu Rev Immunol 16:225–260, 1998.

52. Bargou RC, Emmerich F, Krappmann D, et al: Constitutive nuclear factor-κB-RelA activation is required for proliferation and survival of Hodgkin's disease tumor cells. J Clin Invest 100: 2961–2969, 1997.

53. Sovak M, Bellas RE, Kim DW, et al: Aberrant NF-κB/Rel expression and pathogenesis of breast cancer. J Clin Invest 100:2952–2960, 1997.

54. Duffey D, Chen Z, Dong G, et al: Expression of a dominant negative mutant inhibitor of NF-κB in human head and neck squamous cell carcinoma inhibits survival, proinflammatory cytokine expression and tumor growth in vivo. Cancer Res 59:3468–3474, 1999.

55. Guttridge DC, Albanese C, Reuther JY, et al: NFκB controls cell growth and differentiation through transcriptional regulation of cyclin D1. Mol Cell Biol 19:5923–5929, 1999.

56. Myoken Y, Myoken Y, Okamoto T, et al: Immunocytochemical localization of fibroblast growth factor-1 (FGF-1) and FGF-2 in oral squamous cell carcinoma (SCC). J Oral Pathol Med 23:451–456, 1994.

57. Myoken Y, Myoken Y, Okamoto T, et al: Release of fibroblast growth factor-1 by human squamous cell carcinoma correlates with autocrine cell growth. In vitro cell. Dev Biol 30:790–795, 1994.

58. Jiang W, Hiscox S, Matsumoto K, et al: Hepatocyte growth factor/scatter factor, its molecular, cellular and clinical implications in cancer. Crit Rev Oncol Hematol 29:209–248, 1999.

59. Bottaro DP, Rubin JS, Faletto DL, et al: Identification of the hepatocyte growth factor receptor as the c-met proto-oncogene product. Science 251: 802–805, 1991.

60. Uchida D, Kawamata H, Omotehara F, et al: Role of HGF/c-met system in invasion and metastasis of oral squamous cell carcinoma cells in vitro and its clinical significance. Int J Cancer 93:489–496, 2001.

61. Hasina R, Matsumoto K, Matsumoto-Taniura N, et al: Autocrine and paracrine motility factors and their involvement in invasiveness in a human oral carcinoma cell line. Br J Cancer 80:1708–1717, 1999.

62. Hanzawa M, Shindoh M, Higashino F, et al: Hepatocyte growth factor upregulates E1AF that induces oral squamous cell carcinoma cell invasion by activating matrix metalloproteinase genes. Carcinogenesis 21:1079–1085, 2000.

63. Dong G, Chen Z, Li ZY, et al: Hepatocyte growth factor/scatter factor–induced activation of MEK and PI3K signal pathways contributes to expression of proangiogenic cytokines interleukin-8 and vascular endothelial growth factor in head and neck squamous cell carcinoma. Cancer Res 61:5911–5918, 2001.

64. Yoo GH, Xu HJ, Brennan JA, et al: Infrequent inactivation of the retinoblastoma gene despite frequent loss of chromosome 13q in head and neck squamous cell carcinoma. Cancer Res 54:4603–4606, 1994.

65. Xu J, Gimenez-Conti IB, Cunningham JE, et al: Alterations of p53, cyclin D1, Rb, and H-ras in human oral carcinomas related to tobacco use. Cancer 83:204–212, 1998.

66. Levine AJ, Chang A, Dittmer D, et al: The p53 tumor suppressor gene. J Lab Clin Med 123:817–822, 1994.

67. Farmer GE, Bargonetti J, Shu H, et al: Wild-type p53 activates transcription in vitro. Nature 358:82–86, 1992.

68. Levine AJ: The p53 tumor-suppressor gene. N Engl J Med 326:1350–1352, 1992.

69. Kastan MB, Onyekere O, Sidransky D, et al: Participation of p53 protein in the cellular response to DNA damage. Cancer Res 51:6304–6311, 1991.

70. Yin Y, Tainsky MA, Bischoff FZ, et al: Wild-type p53 restores cell cycle control and inhibits gene amplification in cells with mutant p53 alleles. Cell 70:937–948, 1992.

71. Yonish-Rouach E, Resnitzky D, Lotem J, et al: Wild-type p53 induces apoptosis of myeloid leukaemic cells that are inhibited by interleukin-6. Nature 352:345–347, 1991.

72. Chang A, Levine AJ, Silver A, et al: The Princeton University database of p53 mutations. Princeton, NJ, Princeton University, 1994.

73. Somers KD, Merrick MA, Lopez ME, et al: Frequent p53 mutations in head and neck cancer. Cancer Res 52:5997–6000, 1992.

74. Sakai E, Tsuchida N: Most human squamous cell carcinomas in the oral cavity contain mutated p53 tumor-suppressor genes. Oncogene 7:927–933, 1992.

75. Boyle JO, Hakim J, Koch W, et al: The incidence of p53 mutations increases with progression of head and neck cancer. Cancer Res 53:4477–4480, 1993.

76. Shin DM, Kim J, Ro JY, et al: Activation of p53 gene expression in premalignant lesions during head and neck tumorigenesis. Cancer Res 54:321–326, 1994.

77. Zhang L, Rosin M, Priddy R, et al: p53 expression during multistage human oral carcinogenesis. Int J Oncol 3:735–739, 1993.

78. Shin DM, Charuruks N, Lippman SM, et al: p53 protein accumulation and genomic instability in head and neck multistep tumorigenesis. Cancer Epidemiol Biomarkers Prev 10:603–609, 2001.

79. Syrjanen SM, Syrjanen KJ: New concepts on the role of human papillomavirus in cell cycle regulation. Ann Med 31:175–187, 1999.

80. Oliner JD, Pietenpol JA, Thiagalingam S, et al: Oncoprotein MDM2 conceals the activation domain of tumour suppressor p53. Nature 362:857–860,1993.

81. Haupt Y, Maya R, Kazaz A, et al: Mdm2 promotes the rapid degradation of p53. Nature 387:296–299, 1997.

82. Ganly I, Soutar DS, Brown R, et al: p53 alterations in recurrent squamous cell cancer of the head and neck refractory to radiotherapy. B J Cancer 82:392–398, 2000.

83. Kamb A, Gruis NA, Weaver-Feldhaus J, et al: A cell cycle regulator potentially involved in genesis of many tumor types. Science 264:436–440, 1994.

84. Serrano M, Hannon GJ, Beach D: A new regulatory motif in cell-cycle control causing specific inhibition of cyclin D/CDK4. Nature 366:704–707, 1993.

85. Reed AL, Califano J, Cairns P, et al: High frequency of p16 (CDKN2/MTS-1/INK4A) inactivation in head and neck squamous cell carcinoma. Cancer Res 56:3630–3633, 1996.

86. Papadimitrakopoulou V, Izzo J, Lippman SM, et al: Frequent inactivation of p16ink4a in oral premalignant lesions. Oncogene 14:1799–1803, 1997.

87. El-Naggar A, Lai S, Clayman GL, et al: Expression of p16, Rb, and cyclin D1 gene products in oral and laryngeal squamous carcinoma: Biological and clinical implications. Hum Pathol 30:1013–1018, 1999.

88. Mao L, Lee JS, Fan YH, et al: Frequent microsatellite alterations at chromosomes 9p21 and 3p14 in oral premalignant lesions and their value in cancer risk assessment. Nat Med 2:682–685, 1996.

89. Rocco JW, Li D, Liggett WH Jr, et al: p16INK4A adenovirus–mediated gene therapy for human head and neck squamous cell cancer. Clin Cancer Res 4:1697–1704, 1998.

90. Cordon-Cardo C: Mutations of cell cycle regulators: Biological and clinical implications for human neoplasia. Am J Pathol 147:545–560, 1995.

91. Peters G: The D-type cyclins and their role in tumorigenesis. J Cell Sci 18:89–96, 1994.

92. Bartkova J, Lukas J, Muller H, et al: Abnormal patterns of D-type cyclin expression and G1 regulation in human head and neck cancer. Cancer Res 55:949–956, 1995.

93. Bova RJ, Quinn DI, Nankervis JS, et al: Cyclin D1 and p16INK4A expression predict reduced survival in carcinoma of the anterior tongue. Clin Cancer Res 5:2810–2819, 1999.

94. Mineta H, Miura K, Takebayashi S, et al: Cyclin D1 overexpression correlates with poor prognosis in patients with tongue squamous cell carcinoma. Oral Oncol 36:194–198, 2000.

95. Jares P, Fernandez PL, Campo E, et al: PRAD-1/Cyclin D1 gene amplification correlates with messenger RNA overexpression and tumor progression in human laryngeal carcinomas. Cancer Res 54:4813–4817, 1994.

96. Masuda M, Hirakawa N, Nakashima T, et al: Cyclin D1 overexpression in primary hypopharyngeal carcinomas. Cancer 78:390–395, 1996.

97. Michalides RJ, van Veelen NM, Kristel PM, et al: Overexpression of cyclin D1 indicates a poor prognosis in squamous cell carcinoma of the head and neck. Arch Otolaryngol Head Neck Surg 123:497–502, 1997.

98. Akervall JA, Michalides RJ, Mineta H, et al: Amplification of cyclin D1 in squamous cell carcinoma of the head and neck and the prognostic value of chromosomal abnormalities and cyclin D1 overexpression. Cancer 79:380–389, 1997.

99. Nakashima T, Clayman GL: Antisense inhibition of cyclin D1 in human head and neck squamous cell carcinoma. Arch Otolaryngol Head Neck Surg 126:957–961, 2000.

100. El Deiry WS, Tokino T, Velculeccu VE, et al: WAF1, a potential mediator of p53 tumor suppression. Cell 75:817–825, 1993.

101. Erber R, Klein W, Andl T, et al: Aberrant p21(CIP1/WAF1) protein accumulation in head-and-neck cancer. Int J Cancer 74:383–389, 1997.

102. Mineta H, Miura K, Suzuki I, et al: Low p27 expression correlates with poor prognosis for patients with oral tongue squamous cell carcinoma. Cancer 85:1011–1017, 1999.

103. Mineta H, Miura K, Suzuki I, et al: p27 expression correlates with prognosis in patients with hypopharyngeal cancer. Anticancer Res 19:4407–4412, 1999.

104. Ravi D, Ramadas K, Matthew BS, et al: De novo programmed cell death in oral cancer. Histopathology 34:241–249, 1999.

105. Clayman GL, El-Naggar AK, Roth JA, et al: In vivo molecular therapy with p53 adenovirus for microscopic residual head and neck squamous carcinoma. Cancer Res 55:1–6, 1995.

106. Liu T-J, Zhang W-W, Taylor DL, et al: Growth suppression of human head and neck cancer cells by the introduction of a wild-type p53 gene via a recombinant adenovirus. Cancer Res 54:3662–3667, 1994.

107. Clayman GL: The current status of gene therapy. Semin Oncol 27:39–43, 2000.

108. Ohtani T, Hatori M, Ito H, et al: Involvement of caspases in 5-FU induced apoptosis in an oral cancer cell line. Anticancer Res 20:3117–3121, 2000.

109. Kuwahara D, Tsutsumi K, Kobayashi T, et al: Caspase-9 regulates cisplatin-induced apoptosis in human head and neck squamous cell carcinoma cells. Cancer Lett 148:65–71, 2000.

110. Hayashi K, Yokozaki H, Naka K, et al: Overexpression of retinoic acid receptor beta induces growth arrest and apoptosis in oral cancer cell lines. Jpn J Cancer Res 92:42–50, 2001.

111. Seol JG, Park WH, Kim ES, et al: Potential role of caspase-3 and -9 in arsenic trioxide–mediated apoptosis in PCI-1 head and neck cancer cells. Int J Oncol 18:249–255, 2001.

112. Gallo O, Chiarelli I, Boddi V, et al: Cumulative prognostic value of p53 mutations and bcl-2 protein expression in head-and-neck cancer treated by radiotherapy. Int J Cancer 84:573–579, 1999.

113. Pena JC, Thompson CB, Recant W, et al: Bcl-xL and Bcl-2 expression in squamous cell carcinoma of the head and neck. Cancer 85:164–170, 1999.

114. Xie X, Clausen OP, De Angelis P, et al: The prognostic value of spontaneous apoptosis, Bax, Bcl-2, and p53 in oral squamous cell carcinoma of the tongue. Cancer 86:913–920, 1999.

115. Barkett M, Gilmore T: Control of apoptosis by Rel/NF-κB transcription factors. Oncogene 18:6910–6924, 1999.

116. Baldwin AS: Control of oncogenesis and cancer therapy resistance by the transcription factor NF-κB. J Clin Invest 107:241–246, 2001.

117. Webster G, Perkins N: Transcriptional cross-talk between NF-κB and p53. Mol Cell Biol 19:3485–3495, 1999.

118. Duffey DC, Crowl-Bancroft CV, Chen Z, et al: Inhibition of transcription factor nuclear factor-kappa B by a mutant inhibitor-kappa B alpha attenuates resistance of human head and neck squamous cell carcinoma to TNF-alpha caspase-mediated cell death. Br J Cancer 83:1367–1374, 2000.

119. Counter CM, Hahn WC, Wei W, et al: Dissociation among in vitro telomerase activity, telomere maintenance, and cellular immortalization. Proc Natl Acad Sci USA 95:14723–14728, 1998.

120. Mao L, El-Naggar AK, Fan YH, et al: Telomerase activity in head and neck squamous cell carcinoma and adjacent tissues. Cancer Res 56:5600–5604, 1996.

121. Patel MM, Patel DD, Parekh LJ, et al: Evaluation of telomerase activation in head and neck cancer. Oral Oncol 35:510–515, 1999.

122. Sumida T, Sogawa K, Hamakawa H, et al: Detection of telomerase activity in oral lesions. J Oral Pathol Med 27:111–115, 1998.

123. Mutirangura A, Supiyaphun P, Trirekapan S, et al: Telomerase activity in oral leukoplakia and head and neck squamous cell carcinoma. Cancer Res 56:3530–3533, 1996.

124. Curran AJ, St. Denis K, Irish J, et al: Telomerase activity in oral squamous cell carcinoma. Arch Otolaryngol Head Neck Surg 124:784–788, 1998.

125. Kannan S, Tahara H, Yokozaki H, et al: Telomerase activity in premalignant and malignant lesions of human oral mucosa. Cancer Epidemiol Biomarkers Prev 6:413–420, 1997.

126. Fidler IJ, Kumar R, Bielenberg DR, et al: Molecular determinants of angiogenesis in cancer metastasis. Cancer J 4:S58–S66. 1998.

127. Shpitzer T, Chaimaoff M, Gal R, et al: Tumor angiogenesis as a prognostic factor in early oral tongue cancer. Arch Otolaryngol Head Neck Surg 122:865–868, 1996.

128. Zatterstrom K, Brun E, Willen R, et al: Tumor angiogenesis and prognosis in squamous cell carcinoma of the head and neck. Head Neck 17:312–318, 1995.

129. Dray TG, Hardin NJ, Sofferman RA: Angiogenesis as a prognostic marker in early head and neck cancer. Ann Otol Rhinol Laryngol 104:724–729, 1995.

130. Gleich LL, Biddinger PW, Pavelic ZP, et al: Tumor angiogenesis in T1 oral cavity squamous cell carcinoma: Role in predicting tumor aggressiveness. Head Neck 18:343–346, 1996.

131. Folkman J: Angiogenesis and breast cancer. J Clin Oncol 12:441–443, 1994.

132. Denhart BC, Guidi AJ, Tognazzi K, et al: Vascular permeability factor/vascular endothelial growth factor and its receptors in oral and laryngeal squamous cell carcinoma and dysplasia. Lab Invest 77:659–664, 1997.

133. Salven P, Heikkila P, Anttonen A, et al: Vascular endothelial growth factor in squamous cell head and neck carcinoma: Expression and prognostic significance. Mod Pathol 10:1128–1133, 1997.

134. Smith BD, Smith GL, Carter D, et al: Prognostic significance of vascular endothelial growth factor protein levels in oral and oropharyngeal squamous cell carcinoma. J Clin Oncol 18:2046–2052, 2000.

135. Mineta H, Miura K, Ogino T, et al: Prognostic value of vascular endothelial growth factor (VEGF) in head and neck squamous cell carcinomas. Br J Cancer 83:775–781, 2000.

136. Nakashima T, Hudson JM, Clayman GL: Antisense inhibition of vascular endothelial growth factor in human head and neck squamous cell carcinoma. Head Neck 22:483–488, 2000.

137. Tae K, El-Naggar AK, Yoo E, et al: Expression of vascular endothelial growth factor and microvessel density in head and neck tumorigenesis. Clin Cancer Res 6:2821–2828, 2000.

138. Burian M, Quint C, Neuchrist C: Angiogenic factors in laryngeal carcinomas: Do they have prognostic relevance? Acta Otolaryngol 119:289–292, 1999.

139. Myoken Y, Okamoto T, Sato JD, et al: Immunocytochemical localization of fibroblast growth factor-1 (FGF-1) and FGF-2 in oral squamous cell carcinoma (SCC). J Oral Pathol Med 23:451–456, 1994.

140. Janot F, El-Naggar AK, Morrison RS, et al: Expression of basic fibroblast growth factor in squamous cell carcinoma of the head and neck is associated with degree of histologic differentiation. Int J Cancer 64:117–123, 1995.

141. Dietz A, Rudat V, Conradt C, et al: Prognostic relevance of serum levels of the angiogenic peptide bFGF in advanced carcinoma of the head and neck treated by primary radiochemotherapy. Head Neck 22:666–673, 2000.

142. Leunig A, Tauber S, Spaett R, et al: Basic fibroblast growth factor in serum and urine of patients with head and neck cancer. Oncol Rep 5:955–958, 1998.

143. Fujieda S, Sunaga H, Tsuzuki H, et al: Expression of platelet-derived endothelial cell growth factor in oral and oropharyngeal carcinoma. Clin Cancer Res 4:1583–1590, 1998.

144. Cohen RF, Contrino J, Spiro JD, et al: Interleukin-8 expression by head and neck squamous cell carcinoma. Arch Otolaryngol Head Neck Surg 121:202–209, 1995.

145. Richards BL, Eisma RJ, Spiro JD, et al: Coexpression of interleukin-8 receptors in head and neck squamous cell carcinoma. Am J Surg 174:507–512, 1997.

146. Riedel F, Gotte K, Bergler W, et al: Expression of basic fibroblast growth factor protein and its down-regulation by interferons in head and neck cancer. Head Neck 22:183–189, 2000.

147. Slaton JW, Perrotte P, Inoue K, et al: Interferon-alpha-mediated down-regulation of angiogenesis-related genes and therapy of bladder cancer are dependent on optimization of biological dose and schedule. Clin Cancer Res 5:2726–2734, 1999.

148. Li S, Zhang X, Xia X, et al: Intramuscular electroporation delivery of IFN-alpha gene therapy for inhibition of tumor growth located at distant site. Gene Ther 8:400–407, 2001.

149. Hanna E, Zhang X, Woodlis J, et al: Intramuscular electrophoration delivery of IL-12 gene for treatment of squamous cell carcinoma located at distant site. Cancer Gene Ther 8:151–157, 2001.

150. Lawler J: The functions of thrombospondin-1 and -2. Curr Opin Cell Biol 12:634–640, 2000.

151. Nor JE, Mitra RS, Sutorik MM, et al: Thrombospondin-1 induces endothelial cell apoptosis and inhibits angiogenesis by activating the caspase death pathway. J Vasc Res 37:209–218, 2000.

152. Norrby K: Constitutively synthesized nitric oxide is a physiological negative regulator of mammalian angiogenesis mediated by basic fibroblast growth factor. Int J Exp Pathol 81:423–427, 2000.

153. Giri D, Ittmann M: Inactivation of the PTEN tumor suppressor gene is associated with increased angiogenesis in clinically localized prostate carcinoma. Hum Pathol 30:419–424, 1999.

154. Stetler-Stevenson WG, Asnavoorian S, Liotta LA: Tumor cell interactions with the extracellular matrix during invasion and metastasis. Annu Rev Cell Biol 9:541–573, 1993.

155. Liotta L: Tumor invasion and metastasis: Role of the extracellular matrix. Cancer Res 46:1–7, 1986.

156. Wetzels RHW, van der Velden L-A, Schaafsm HE, et al: Immunohistochemical localization of basement membrane type VII collagen and laminin in neoplasms of the head and neck. Histopathology 21:459–464, 1992.

157. Sakr WA, Zarbo RJ, Jacobs JR, et al: Distribution of basement membrane in squamous cell carcinoma of the head and neck. Hum Pathol 18:1043–1050, 1987.

158. Carter RL, Burman JF, Barr L, et al: Immunohistochemical localization of basement membrane type IV collagen in invasive and metastatic squamous carcinomas of the head and neck. J Pathol 147:159–164, 1985.

159. Visser R, Beek JMH, Havenith MG, et al: Immunocytochemical detection of basement membrane antigens in the histopathological evaluation of laryngeal dysplasis and neoplasia. Histopathology 10:171–180, 1986.

160. van Waes C, Carey TE: Overexpression of the A9 antigen/α6β4 integrin in head and neck cancer. Otalaryngol Clin North Am 25:1117–1139, 1992.

161. Carey TE, Nair TS, Chern C, et al: Blood group antigens and integrins as biomarkers in head and neck cancer: Is aberrant tyrosine

phosphorylation the cause of altered α6β4 integrin expression? J Cell Biochem (Suppl) 17F:223–232, 1993.

162. Wolf GT, Carey TE: Tumor antigen phenotype, biologic staging, and prognosis in head and neck squamous carcinoma. J Natl Cancer Inst Monogr 13:67–74, 1992.

163. Thomas GJ, Jones J, Speight PM: Integrins and oral cancer. Oral Oncol 33:381–388, 1997.

164. Jones J, Sugiyama M, Speight PM, et al: Restoration of alpha v beta 5 integrin expression in neoplastic keratinocytes results in increased capacity for terminal differentiation and suppression of anchorage-independent growth. Oncogene 12:119–126, 1996.

165. Wu H, Lotan R, Menter D, et al: Expression of E-cadherin is associated with squamous differentiation in squamous cell carcinomas. Anticancer Res 20:1385–1390, 2000.

166. Mattijssen V, Peters HM, Schalkwijk L, et al: E-cadherin expression in head and neck squamous cell carcinoma is associated with clinical outcome. Int J Cancer 55:580–585, 1993.

167. Chow V, Yuen AP, Lam KY, et al: A comparative study of the clinicopathological significance of E-cadherin and catenin (alpha, beta, gamma) expression in the surgical management of oral tongue carcinoma. J Cancer Res Clin Oncol 127:59–63, 2001.

168. Nakayama S, Sasaki A, Mese H, et al: Establishment of high and low metastasis cell lines derived from a human tongue squamous cell carcinoma. Invasion Metastasis 18:219–228, 1999.

169. Schipper JH, Unger A, Jahnke K: E-cadherin as a functional marker of the differentiation and invasiveness of squamous cell carcinoma of the head and neck. Clin Otolaryngol Allied Sci 19:381–384, 1994.

170. Lo Muzio L, Staibano S, Pannone G, et al: Beta- and gamma-catenin expression in oral squamous cell carcinomas. Anticancer Res 19:3817–3826, 1999.

171. Liotta L: Tumor invasion and metastasis. Role of the extracellular matrix. Cancer Res 46:1–7, 1986.

172. Sutinen M, Kainulainen T, Hurskainen T, et al: Expression of matrix metalloproteinases (MMP-1 and -2) and their inhibitors (TIMP-1, -2 and -3) in oral lichen planus, dysplasia, squamous cell carcinoma and lymph node metastasis. Br J Cancer 12:2239–2245, 1998.

173. Tokumaru Y, Fujii M, Otani Y, et al: Activation of matrix metalloproteinase-2 in head and neck squamous cell carcinoma: Studies of clinical samples and in vitro cell lines co-cultured with fibroblasts. Cancer Lett 150:15–21, 2000.

174. Ikebe T, Shinohara M, Takeuchi H, et al: Gelatinolytic activity of matrix metalloproteinase in tumor tissues correlates with the invasiveness of oral cancer. Clin Exp Metastasis 17:315–323, 1999.

175. Kusukawa J, Sasaguri Y, Shima I, et al: Expression of matrix metalloproteinase-2 related to lymph node metastasis of oral squamous cell carcinoma. A clinicopathologic study. Am J Clin Pathol 99:18–23, 1993.

176. Kusukawa J, Harada H, Shima I, et al: The significance of epidermal growth factor receptor and matrix metalloproteinase-3 in squamous cell carcinoma of the oral cavity. Eur J Cancer (Part B), Oral Oncol 32B:217–221, 1996.

177. Polette M, Clavel C, Muller D, et al: Detection of mRNAs encoding collagenase I and stromelysin 2 in carcinomas of the head and neck by in situ hybridization. Invasion Metastasis 11:76–83, 1991.

178. Muller D, Breathnach R, Engelmann A, et al: Expression of collagenase-related metalloproteinase genes in human lung or head and neck tumours. Int J Cancer 48:550–556, 1991.

179. Kusukawa J, Sasaguri Y, Morimatsu M, et al: Expression of matrix metalloproteinase-3 in stage I and II squamous cell carcinoma of the oral cavity. J Oral Maxillofac Surg 53:530–534, 1995.

180. Charous SJ, Stricklin GP, Nanney LB, et al: Expression of matrix metalloproteinases and tissue inhibitor of metalloproteinases in head and neck squamous cell carcinoma. Ann Otol Rhinol Laryngol 106:271–278, 1997.

181. Juarez J, Clayman G, Nakajima M, et al: Role and regulation of expression of 92-kDa type-IV collagenase (MMP-9) in 2 invasive squamous-cell-carcinoma cell lines of the oral cavity. Int J Cancer 55:10–18, 1993.

182. Pickett KL, Harber GJ, DeCarlo AA, et al: 92K-GL (MMP-9) and 72K-GL (MMP-2) are produced in vivo by human oral squamous cell carcinomas and can enhance FIB-CL (MMP-1) activity in vitro. J Dent Res 78:1354–1361, 1999.

183. Baba Y, Tsukuda M, Mochimatsu I, et al: Inostamycin, an inhibitor of cytidine 5′-diphosphate 1,2-diacyl-sn-glycerol (CDP-DG): Inositol

184. transferase suppresses invasion ability by reducing productions of matrix metalloproteinase-2 and -9 and cell motility in HSC-4 tongue carcinoma cell line. Clin Exp Metastasis 18:273–279, 2000.

184. Riedel F, Gotte K, Schwalb J, et al: Expression of 92-kDa type IV collagenase correlates with angiogenic markers and poor survival in head and neck squamous cell carcinoma. Int J Oncol 17:1099–1105, 2000.

185. Andreasen PA, Egelund R, Petersen HH: The plasminogen activation system in tumor growth, invasion, and metastasis. Cell Mol Life Sci 57:25–40, 2000.

186. Petruzzelli GJ, Snyderman CH, Johnson JT: In vitro urokinase type plasminogen activator levels and total plasminogen activator activity in squamous cell carcinomas of the head and neck. Arch Otolaryngol Head Neck Surg 120:989–992, 1994.

187. Schmidt M, Schler G, Gruensfelder P, et al: Urokinase receptor up-regulation in head and neck squamous cell carcinoma. Head Neck 22:498–504, 2000.

188. Nozaki S, Endo Y, Kawashiri S, et al: Immunohistochemical localization of a urokinase-type plasminogen activator system in squamous cell carcinoma of the oral cavity: Association with mode of invasion and lymph node metastasis. Oral Oncol 34:58–62, 1998.

189. Clayman G, Wang SW, Nicolson GL, et al: Regulation of urokinase-type plasminogen activator expression in squamous-cell carcinoma of the oral cavity. Int J Cancer 54:73–80, 1993.

190. Ignar DM, Andrews JL, Witherspoon SM, et al: Inhibition of establishment of primary and micrometastatic tumors by a urokinase plasminogen activator receptor antagonist. Clin Exp Metastasis 16:9–20, 1998.

191. Spring P, Nakashima T, Frederick M, et al: Identification and cDNA cloning of headpin, a novel differentially expressed serpin that maps to chromosome 18q. Biochem Biophys Res Commun 264:299–304, 1999.

192. Nakashima T, Pak SC, Silverman GA, et al: Genomic cloning, mapping, structure and promoter analysis of HEADPIN, a serpin which is down-regulated in head and neck cancer cells. Biochim Biophys Acta 1492:441–446, 2000.

193. Xia W, Lau YK, Hu MC, et al: High tumoral maspin expression is associated with improved survival of patients with oral squamous cell carcinoma. Oncogene 19:2398–2403, 2000.

194. Baldwin AS: Control of oncogenesis and cancer therapy resistance by the transcription factor NF-kappa B. J Clin Invest 107:241–246, 2001.

195. Baldwin AS: The NF-kappa B and I kappa B proteins: New discoveries and insights. Annu Rev Immunol 14:649–683, 1996.

196. Wang CY, Mayo MW, Baldwin AS Jr: TNF- and cancer therapy-induced apoptosis: Potentiation by inhibition of NF-kappaB. Science 274:784–787, 1996.

197. Wang CY, Cusack JC Jr, Liu R, et al: Control of inducible chemoresistance: enhanced anti-tumor therapy through increased apoptosis by inhibition of NF-kappaB. Nat Med 5:412–417, 1999.

198. Sunwoo JB, Chen Z, Dong G, et al: Novel proteasome inhibitor PS-341 inhibits activation of nuclear factor-kappa B, cell survival, tumor growth, and angiogenesis in squamous cell carcinoma. Clin Cancer Res 7:1419–1428, 2001.

199. Cusack JC Jr, Liu R, Houston M, et al: Enhanced chemosensitivity to CPT-11 with proteasome inhibitor PS-341: Implications for systemic nuclear factor-kappaB inhibition. Cancer Res 61:3535–3540, 2001.

200. Russo SM, Tepper JE, Baldwin AS Jr, et al: Enhancement of radiosensitivity by proteasome inhibition: Implications for a role of NF-kappaB. Int J Radiat Oncol Biol Phys 50:183–193, 2001.

201. Yamamoto Y, Gaynor RB: Therapeutic potential of inhibition of the NF-kappaB pathway in the treatment of inflammation and cancer. J Clin Invest 107:135–142, 2001.

202. Fournier DB, Gordon GB: COX-2 and colon cancer: Potential targets for chemoprevention. J Cell Biochem (Suppl) 34:97–102, 2000.

203. Kiaris H, Spandidos DA, Jones AS, et al: Mutations, expression and genomic instability of the H-ras proto-oncogene in squamous cell carcinomas of the head and neck. Br J Cancer 72:123–128, 1995.

204. Sebti SM, Hamilton AD: Farnesyltransferase and geranylgeranyltransferase I inhibitors and cancer therapy: Lessons from mechanism and bench-to-bedside translational studies. Oncogene 19:6584–6593, 2000.

205. Prendergast GC: Farnesyltransferase inhibitors define a role for RhoB in controlling neoplastic pathophysiology Histol Histopathol 16:269–275, 2001.

206. Sepp-Lorenzino L, Ma Z, Rands E, et al: A peptidomimetic inhibitor of farnesyl:protein transferase blocks the anchorage-dependent and -independent growth of human tumor cell lines. Cancer Res 55:5302–5309, 1995.

207. Moasser MM, Sepp-Lorenzino L, Kohl NE, et al: Farnesyl transferase inhibitors cause enhanced mitotic sensitivity to taxol and epothilones. Proc Natl Acad Sci USA 95:1369–1374, 1998.

208. Bernhard EJ, McKenna WG, Hamilton AD, et al: Inhibiting Ras prenylation increases the radiosensitivity of human tumor cell lines with activating mutations of ras oncogenes. Cancer Res 58: 1754–1761, 1998.

209. Sebti SM, Hamilton AD: Farnesyltransferase and geranylgeranyltransferase I inhibitors and cancer therapy: Lessons from mechanism and bench-to-bedside translational studies. Oncogene 19:6584–6593, 2000.

210. Lango MN, Shin DM, Grandis JR: Targeting growth factor receptors: Integration of novel therapeutics in the management of head and neck cancer. Curr Opin Oncol 13:168–175, 2001.

211. Azemar M, Schmidt M, Arlt F, et al: Recombinant antibody toxins specific for ErbB2 and EGF receptor inhibit the in vitro growth of human head and neck cancer cells and cause rapid tumor regression in vivo. Int J Cancer 86:269–275, 2000.

212. Schumann J, Angermuller S, Bang R, et al: Acute hepatotoxicity of *Pseudomonas aeruginosa* exotoxin A in mice depends on T cells and TNF. J Immunol 161:5745–5754, 1998.

213. Goldstein NI, Prewett M, Zuklys K, et al: Biological efficacy of a chimeric antibody to the epidermal growth factor receptor in a human tumor xenograft model. Clin Cancer Res 1:1311–1318, 1995.

214. Hoffmann T, Hafner D, Ballo H, et al: Antitumor activity of anti-epidermal growth factor receptor monoclonal antibodies and cisplatin in ten human head and neck squamous cell carcinoma lines. Anticancer Res 17:4419–4425, 1997.

215. Milas L, Mason K, Hunter N, et al: In vivo enhancement of tumor radioresponse by C225 antiepidermal growth factor receptor antibody. Clin Cancer Res 6:701–708, 2000.

216. Mendelsohn J, Baselga J: The EGF receptor family as targets for cancer therapy. Oncogene 19:6550–6565, 2000.

217. Ciardiello F, Caputo R, Bianco R, et al: Antitumor effect and potentiation of cytotoxic drug activity in human cancer cells by ZD-1839 (Iressa), an epidermal growth factor receptor-selective tyrosine kinase inhibitor. Clin Cancer Res 6:2053–2063, 2000.

218. Baselga J, Averbuch SD: ZD1839 ("Iressa") as an anticancer agent. Drugs 60:33–40, 2000.

219. He Y, Zeng Q, Drenning SD, et al: Inhibition of human squamous cell carcinoma growth in vivo by epidermal growth factor receptor antisense RNA transcribed from the U6 promoter. J Natl Cancer Inst 90:1080–1087, 1998.

220. Roth JA, Nguyen D, Lawrence DD, et al: Retrovirus-mediated wild-type p53 gene transfer to tumors of patients with lung cancer. Nat Med 2:985–991, 1996.

221. Roth JA: Clinical protocol: Modification of tumor suppressor gene expression and induction of apoptosis in non-small cell lung cancer (NSCLC) with an adenovirus vector expressing wildtype p53 and cisplatin. Hum Gene Ther 7:1013–1030, 1996.

222. Clayman GL, El-Naggar AK, Lippman SM, et al: Adenovirus-mediated p53 gene transfer in patients with advanced recurrent head and neck squamous cell carcinoma. J Clin Oncol 16: 2221–2232, 1998.

223. Bischoff JR, Kirn DH, Williams A, et al: An adenovirus mutant that replicates selectively in p53-deficient human tumor cells. Science 274:373–376, 1996.

224. Heise C, Sampson-Johannes A, Williams A, et al: ONYX-015, an E1B gene-attenuated adenovirus, causes tumor-specific cytolysis and antitumoral efficacy that can be augmented by standard chemotherapeutic agents. Nat Med 3:639–645, 1997.

225. Kirn D: Clinical research results with dl1520 (Onyx-015), a replication-selective adenovirus for the treatment of cancer: What have we learned? Gene Ther 8:89–98, 2001.

226. Khuri FR, Nemunaitis J, Ganly I, et al: A controlled trial of intratumoral ONYX-015, a selectively-replicating adenovirus, in combination with cisplatin and 5-fluorouracil in patients with recurrent head and neck cancer. Nat Med 6:879–885, 2000.

227. Rogulski KR, Freytag SO, Zhang K, et al: In vivo antitumor activity of ONYX-015 is influenced by p53 status and is augmented by radiotherapy. Cancer Res 60:1193–1196, 2000.

228. Lander ES, Linton LM, Birren B, et al: International Human Genome Sequencing Consortium. Initial sequencing and analysis of the human genome. Nature 409:860–921, 2001.

229. Villaret DB, Wang T, Dillon D, et al: Identification of genes overexpressed in head and neck squamous cell carcinoma using a combination of complementary DNA subtraction and microarray analysis. Laryngoscope 110:374–381, 2000.

230. Hanna E, Shrieve DC, Ratanatharathorn V, et al: A novel alternative approach for prediction of radiation response of squamous cell carcinoma of head and neck. Cancer Res 61:2376–2380, 2001.

Pathology of the Head and Neck: Basic Considerations and New Concepts

Leon Barnes

Chun-Yang Fan

Tumors of the head and neck are a heterogeneous group of neoplasms that display a wide range of biologic behaviors. Excluding those found in the skin, central nervous system, eye, thyroid, and lymph nodes, they account for 3% of the total cancer burden in the United States, and of these, 80% to 90% are squamous cell carcinomas. Each year, approximately 40,000 new cases of cancer of the head and neck are diagnosed in this country, resulting in 11,700 deaths.[1]

Successful management of patients with cancer of the head and neck requires a close collaborative relationship between the surgeon, medical oncologist, radiation oncologist, and pathologist. This is especially so in the head and neck because the anatomy is complex, biopsies are often small, and tumors are among the most complex found in the human body.

The traditional role of the pathologist is to provide precise information with respect to tumor type and grade, the presence or absence of angiolymphatic and perineural invasion, the adequacy of resection margins, and the assessment of regional lymph nodes that assists clinicians in the care of their patients. This traditional role, however, is rapidly changing with the emergence of innovative technologies that greatly improve our understanding of basic biology and our ability to detect malignant cells at the molecular and genetic levels.

With the advent of these modern procedures, more challenging questions are being asked of pathologists, such as

1. Do second primary cancers arise from the same genetically altered progenitor cell as the first primary cancer, or do they arise independently from a different clone?
2. Is a microscopically "negative or clear" surgical resection margin also negative at the genetic level? If not, what is the impact of the genetically altered cells on local recurrence and patient survival?
3. Can we make use of this new technology to detect genetically altered cells before they become morphologically malignant?
4. Can we predict the potential for malignant progression (invasion) in head and neck premalignant lesions?
5. Are microscopically negative lymph nodes truly negative at the genetic level?
6. In a clinically negative neck (N0), can we predict the likelihood that a primary tumor will spread to cervical lymph nodes?

To address the "old" and "new" pathology, this chapter is divided into two sections: (1) general histologic and cytologic considerations and (2) molecular pathology.

GENERAL HISTOLOGIC AND CYTOLOGIC CONSIDERATIONS

The Surgical Pathology Report

The surgical pathologist serves as a consultant to the surgeon. The consultation and the surgical pathology report represent a "distillation of [the pathologist's] experience, knowledge, and wisdom" about a specific disease.[2]

The generation of an accurate and informative surgical pathology report, however, is a dual responsibility. It begins in the operating room with the surgeon, who must provide on the tissue requisition form a brief but pertinent clinical history, state the operative procedure, and indicate the diagnosis. Information regarding details such as whether a patient has received any prior treatment, especially irradiation or chemotherapy, or whether a given lesion is clinically suspicious of a verrucous carcinoma can be of immense value to the pathologist.

A surgeon who submits a tumor to a pathologist for evaluation is usually seeking the answers to four questions: (1) What is the diagnosis? (2) How extensive is the disease (i.e., which structures are involved, are positive lymph nodes present)? (3) Are the surgical margins of resection free of disease? (4) Are there any other histologic features that influence the prognosis, such as the presence or absence of extranodal spread of tumor or perineural invasion? If the pathology report contains the answers to these four questions, then the pathologist has done the job well.

Because the pathology report becomes a part of the patient's permanent medical records and may even be used as a legal document, it is imperative that it be accurate not only anatomically and pathologically but also grammatically. It should also be concise.

The Tissue Specimen

Once the decision has been made to perform a biopsy, the surgeon must assume the responsibility for obtaining tissue that is representative, placing it in the appropriate fixative (or, in some instances, submitting it in the fresh state), and properly labeling it. Pathologically, the ideal biopsy is one that is large enough to include both normal and abnormal tissue and is free of extraneous artifacts. Necrotic and ulcerative areas should be avoided if possible. If this cannot be done, the necrotic ulcerated tissue or crust should be removed and the remaining tumor biopsied. If a verrucous carcinoma is suspected, it is essential that the biopsy be deep enough to include the tumor-stroma interface, or the biopsy will most likely be nondiagnostic. If the differential diagnosis includes a malignant lymphoma and a lymph node is to be removed, the largest, not the most accessible, lymph node should be removed. It must be removed intact, free of crush artifact, and must be delivered immediately to the pathologist in an unfixed state so that fresh tissue for T- and B-cell markers and for other studies can be obtained. If a previous biopsy of a tumor revealed only a "malignant tumor of undetermined type," the surgeon should anticipate the need for electron microscopy or other diagnostic procedures; above all, the surgeon should communicate with the pathologist before proceeding with a second biopsy.

If the resected specimen is complex, it may be appropriate to call the pathologist to the operating room for orientation, or it may be helpful for the surgeon to go to the pathology laboratory to describe the specimen.

Histologic Features

Type of Tumor

The accurate classification of neoplasms is one of the most basic tasks of the diagnostic pathologist and is the fundamental principle on which effective tumor therapy is based. Although most malignant neoplasms are carcinomas, sarcomas, or lymphomas, such generic designations are too vague for intelligent patient management. Each tumor has its own peculiarities. For instance, papillary carcinoma of the thyroid metastasizes primarily to cervical lymph nodes, whereas follicular carcinoma of the thyroid generally spreads through blood vessels to the lungs and bones, and only rarely metastasizes to lymph nodes. Adenoid cystic carcinoma of salivary origin, in turn, has an unexplained neurotropism that must be taken into account. Squamous cell carcinoma can exist in several forms (e.g., verrucous, conventional, and spindle cell), each of which has its own clinicopathologic features with varying degrees of malignancy and variable response to radiotherapy.

In regard to sarcomas, there is a growing dogma that histologic grade may be more important than histologic type. We do not agree. Although grade is significant, histologic type is equally important. For example, some sarcomas (e.g., angiosarcoma, embryonal and alveolar rhabdomyosarcoma) are especially prone to metastasize to lymph nodes, whereas others (e.g., Kaposi's sarcoma and epithelioid sarcoma) tend to be multifocal; a few may even involve and spread along the course of nerves (e.g., malignant schwannoma). Some are only locally aggressive and rarely metastasize (e.g., dermatofibrosarcoma protuberans), whereas

others may disseminate widely (malignant fibrous histiocytoma). Highly effective treatment protocols have been developed for a few sarcomas (e.g., triple therapy for embryonal rhabdomyosarcoma).

The division of malignant lymphomas into two broad categories—Hodgkin's and non-Hodgkin's—has proved useful. Patients with Hodgkin's disease tend to be younger and to present with localized disease that spreads in a predictable pattern; the disease is often curable in these patients. In contrast, patients with non-Hodgkin's lymphoma are usually older, present with multifocal or disseminated disease, and suffer from other health problems; the disease in these patients is therefore more difficult to treat and/or cure.

Location of Tumor

The importance of the site of origin of a neoplasm cannot be overstated. Tumors that arise in sites that are highly visible to the patient, do not involve vital structures, and can be easily approached surgically with minimal disruption of function or form often have a good prognosis. Likewise, those that compromise function early and arise in areas relatively devoid of lymphatics, such as the true vocal cord, are potentially curable as compared with those that arise in clinically silent, lymphatic-rich areas, such as the supraglottic larynx, base of the tongue, and hypopharynx. However, neoplasms originating in highly innervated sites can be a mixed blessing. They may present early because of pain or functional disturbances but display prominent perineural invasion; even if they are small, sacrificing a major nerve may be necessary in order to accomplish complete removal.

Size of Tumor

The dictum "the larger the tumor, the worse the prognosis" is generally valid; indeed, it forms one of the three components (T, or tumor) of the TNM (tumor, nodes, metastasis) system of cancer staging.[3] There are exceptions, however. Some carcinomas, particularly those of the floor of the mouth, may have a large surface component but show only superficial invasion of the lamina propria. Such tumors are less likely to disseminate to regional lymph nodes and tend to have a better prognosis than those that are smaller but more deeply invasive.[4-6] Still other tumors, although small, may demonstrate a propensity for early vascular invasion. This is especially so for small cell (oat cell) carcinoma of the larynx.[7]

Tumor Thickness

Breslow[8] has clearly shown that prognosis in cutaneous malignant melanoma correlates with the thickness of the tumor. The same principle is now being applied to squamous cell carcinoma of the head and neck to target patients with clinically negative necks (N0) who are at risk of developing nodal metastasis and might therefore benefit from elective neck dissection.

Mohit-Tabatabai and associates[9] retrospectively studied 84 patients with stage I and II squamous cell carcinoma of the floor of the mouth and concluded that any patient with an N0 floor of the mouth lesion measuring more than 1.5 mm in thickness should have an elective neck dissection, whereas those with lesions smaller than 1.5 mm could be followed with no further therapy. The incidence of cervical node metastasis in this study (with a mean follow-up of 69 months) was 1.8% for lesions less than 1.5 mm thick, and 48% for those thicker than 1.5 mm. Spiro and colleagues[10] also evaluated the predictive value of tumor thickness in a retrospective study of 105 patients with T1, T2, and T3N0 squamous cell carcinoma of the oral tongue and floor of the mouth. They concluded that elective neck dissection was indicated for any patient with a tumor that exceeded 2 mm in thickness. In this study (with a minimum follow-up of 2 years), the incidence of cervical lymph node metastasis was 7.5% for tumors 2 mm or less in thickness, compared with 38% for those exceeding 2 mm.

Frierson and Cooper[11] studied 187 squamous cell carcinomas of the lower lip and observed that 75% of those measuring 6 mm or more in thickness metastasized, primarily to cervical lymph nodes. This strongly suggests the need for elective neck dissection in any patient with a squamous cell carcinoma of the lip that is 6 mm or greater in thickness.

Differentiation of Tumor

There is a relationship to some extent between tumor grade (differentiation) and the site of the primary lesion, the stage of the disease, lymph node involvement, and prognosis.[12–15] Anaplastic tumors in general tend to have a more rapid doubling time, usually contain an aneuploid chromosome population, and metastasize earlier than neoplasms that are more differentiated.

Pattern of Tumor Invasion

The mode in which a malignant tumor invades the stroma of the host has prognostic significance.[15–17] Tumors composed of large cohesive masses of cells with pushing borders are less likely to metastasize. In contrast, neoplasms that invade in a noncohesive pattern of single and small aggregates of cells have a greater incidence of regional lymph node and distant metastases.

Inflammatory Response to Tumor

It is apparent that some patients with squamous cell carcinoma of the head and neck can mount an immunologic response to the tumor, and that the greater the inflammatory reaction, the better the prognosis.[9, 18–20] The vast majority of inflammatory cells are T-lymphocytes of both helper-inducer and suppressor-cytotoxic subsets. B-lymphocytes are distinctly uncommon.

Reichert and coworkers[21] have also shown that the number of S-100 protein–positive dendritic cells in a tumor and the level of epsilon-chain expression in tumor-infiltrating lymphocytes are significant predictors of survival in patients with squamous cell carcinoma of the oral cavity. The greater the number and expression, the better the survival.

Perineural Invasion

Perineural invasion by squamous cell carcinoma is more common than was previously thought and is an ominous sign that correlates with an increased incidence of local recurrence, regional lymph node metastasis, and decreased survival.[10, 22–27] The frequency of this finding varies according to the institution and patient referral patterns, the number of histologic sections examined, and the diligence of the pathologist (Table 3–1).

Patients with perineural invasion may or may not manifest neurologic abnormalities. In some instances, the degree of involvement is so extensive that it results in enlargement of the nerve with subsequent erosion of osseous foramina and obliteration of tissue planes, all of which may be apparent on radiologic evaluation.[28, 29] Histologically, perineural invasion may have no effect on the nerve, or the tumor can expand, invade, or interfere with blood supply of the nerve, resulting in local edema, demyelinization, or segmental infarction (Fig. 3–1).

Once cancer enters the perineural space, it may spread proximally or distally and compromise an otherwise adequate margin of resection. Although the tumor can extend for long distances along the course of the nerve (i.e., 6 cm or more), autopsy studies by Soo and others[26] and Carter and associates[30] indicate that perineural tumor tends to remain localized to the terminal 1 or 2 cm of the nerve, and that skip lesions are not found. It is important to note in these studies, however, that most patients were treated with radiotherapy, which may have induced fibrosis in the nerve and prevented more extensive tumor spread, or it may have destroyed malignant cells that had previously propagated more distantly along the nerve.

TABLE 3–1 Perineural Invasion in Squamous Cell Carcinoma of the Head and Neck

Reference	Site	Total No. of Patients	Incidence of Perineural Invasion (%)	Incidence of Cervical Node Metastasis in Patients With Perineural Invasion (%)
Frierson & Cooper[11]	Lower lip	185	11	60
Byers et al[23]	Lower lip	1308	2	80
Cottel[24]	Skin of head and neck		5	0
Goepfert et al[25]	Skin of head and neck	520	14	35
Soo et al[26]	Mucosal, primarily oral cavity, larynx, and pharynx	239	27	70
Fagan et al[27]	Mucosal, primarily oral cavity, tongue, and pharynx	142	52	73

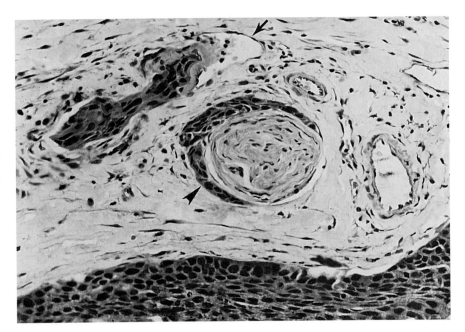

FIGURE 3–1 Squamous cell carcinoma showing both perineural invasion *(arrowhead)* and lymphatic invasion *(arrow)* (hematoxylin-eosin, ×315).

Perineural invasion is a histologic sign of biologic aggressiveness and, in the case of mucosal squamous cell carcinoma, appears to be independent of tumor size.[26] Once identified, postoperative radiotherapy to the site of the primary tumor and the neck, even if the neck is clinically negative, may be warranted, according to some investigators.[25, 26]

There is evidence to suggest that the nerve cell adhesion molecule (N-CAM) may play a role in perineural spread in a variety of tumors, especially adenoid cystic carcinoma.[31–33] Tumors that express N-CAM by immunohistochemistry are more likely to involve nerves than are those that lack this marker.

Blood Vessel Invasion

Surprisingly few clinical studies address the significance of blood vessel invasion in cancers of the head and neck. The issue is further clouded by investigators who use the term "vascular invasion" in a generic sense, to denote both blood vessel and lymphatic invasion. Such generic usage, however, is not unreasonable because venolymphatic communications occur, and histologically it is often difficult to distinguish with confidence between lymphatics and small blood vessels (Fig. 3–2).

Access of cancer cells to blood vessels and the subsequent development of metastases is dose-dependent and involves a

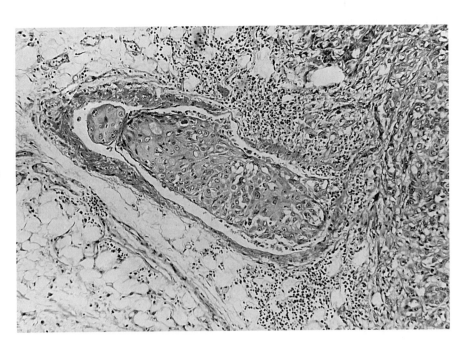

FIGURE 3–2 Venous invasion by squamous cell carcinoma (hematoxylin-eosin, ×125).

clonal selection of cells that are able to overcome mechanical and immunologic barriers.[34] Hence, although it is a worrisome sign, the mere presence of tumor emboli within blood vessels cannot always be equated with dissemination. With this background information, it is interesting to note that Poleksic and Kalwaic[35] and Close and associates[36] have observed a statistical correlation between blood vessel invasion and lymph node metastasis in patients with squamous cell carcinoma of the oral cavity and pharynx. In a study of 30 consecutive untreated T2 or greater squamous cell carcinomas of the oral cavity and oropharynx, Close and associates noted that the absence of blood vessel invasion predicted negative regional lymph nodes in 7 of 8 cases, and the presence of vascular invasion predicted lymph node metastases in 19 of 22 cases. This is in contrast to the study of McGavran and coworkers,[22] who found no relationship between venous invasion and lymph node metastasis in patients with squamous cell carcinoma of the larynx.

Djalilian and associates[37] reviewed 4300 radical neck dissections and found invasion of the lumen of the jugular vein in 48 cases (1.1%). The primary tumor was a squamous cell carcinoma located in the larynx (30), mouth (6), tongue (4), pharynx (4), ear (1), or cheek (1); the site was unknown in 2. Forty-four of the patients died (72% within the first 2 years of neck dissection), and of these, 13 had evidence of pulmonary metastasis. The overall 5-year survival rate of these 48 patients with jugular vein invasion was 10.4%. The authors concluded that invasion of the jugular vein tended to be a late phenomenon associated with massive, often matted, cervical lymph nodes, and it was usually grossly obvious.

Bone and Cartilage Invasion

It is generally accepted in squamous carcinoma of the oral cavity that the extent of osseous invasion correlates with the size of the lesion but not with its histologic grade.[38–40] Although neoplastic cells gain access to bone by direct extension or along neural pathways, the actual destruction of bone is mediated primarily through host cells (osteoclasts) that are stimulated by local tumor-derived products.[41]

Sessions[42] and Pittam and Carter[43] have observed that carcinomas of the larynx that invade the cartilaginous framework are associated with a high incidence of cervical lymph node metastasis. Likewise, patients with squamous cell carcinoma of the external ear whose tumors extend into the auricular cartilage and invade the stroma over a broad front are more prone to develop nodal metastasis than when these features are absent.[44]

Margins of Resection

According to Lee,[45] 15% of all oral cavity, 9% of oropharyngeal, 4% of laryngeal, and 3% of hypopharyngeal carcinomas are inadequately excised. Just how widely should head and neck carcinomas be excised? What is the significance of a microscopically positive margin? And does a pathologically free margin ensure that local disease has been adequately controlled? These are questions that have perplexed clinicians and pathologists for years.

Categorically, there is no "magic number" that applies to the amount of normal tissue that should be removed in excising head and neck cancers. The amount depends to a large extent on the anatomic site. In the larynx, a margin of a few millimeters may suffice, whereas in the hypopharynx–cervical esophagus, where submucosal spread is so common, a margin of 1 cm or more is desirable. For partial glossectomies, Harrison[46] advocates a 1-cm cuff of normal tissue and indicates that it probably should be extended to 2 cm. Questionable margins, however, should always be monitored with frozen sections.

With the possible exception of the larynx (see following discussion), most studies of mucosal squamous cell carcinoma indicate that 50% to 80% of patients with positive surgical margins will either develop local recurrences or demonstrate residual tumor on reexcision.[45, 47–50] Presumably, in those instances in which the lesion has been reexcised and no residual tumor has been found, one of the following occurred: (1) the tumor extended only to and not beyond the original plane of excision, (2) the residual tumor was subsequently destroyed in the ensuing reparative process, or (3) the report of a positive margin was a false-positive finding.

Conversely, 15% to 30% of patients with margins that are judged to be pathologically "adequate or free" develop recurrence.[45, 47–50] These false-negative findings can result from the following: (1) small, remote satellite tumor nodules that were not removed at the time of the original procedure; (2) subclinical multicentric lesions ("field cancerization," in situ carcinoma); or (3) unrecognized lymphatic or blood vessel tumor emboli or perineural invasion.[51]

Bauer and associates[52] studied 111 consecutive hemilaryngectomy specimens to determine the significance of a positive margin. Of 39 patients who had a positive margin, only 7 (18%) subsequently developed a biopsy-proved local recurrence. Four of 72 patients (6%) with negative margins also developed recurrence.

Zieske and colleagues[53] reviewed 349 patients with advanced squamous cell carcinoma of the head and neck and identified 31 (8.8%) who had positive margins on permanent histologic sections. Of these 31 individuals, 29 had stage III or IV disease, primarily of the pharynx, larynx, or oral cavity. Postoperative radiotherapy was administered to 25; of these, locoregional control was not achieved in 60%, and 84% eventually died. The authors concluded that the presence of a positive margin carries a grave prognosis for patients with stage III or IV squamous cell carcinoma of the head and neck, and that when additional surgical free margins cannot be obtained owing to anatomic limitations or other patient factors, postoperative external beam radiation is inadequate for locoregional control.

Scholl and coworkers[50] evaluated 268 patients with squamous cell carcinoma of the tongue treated by glossectomy with and without radiotherapy. Fifty-four (20%) had positive margins on initial frozen section evaluation. They observed that patients who had positive margins on initial frozen section examination that were subsequently rendered negative at the completion of the procedure and were treated by surgery alone had a significantly increased local recurrence rate and decreased survival compared with patients similarly treated with initially negative margins. The use of immediate postoperative irradiation appeared to improve local control in this instance. They noted that positive mucosal margins were more often seen in T1 or T2 tumors, whereas positive soft tissue margins were more common in T3 and T4 lesions.

Lymph Nodes

The status of the regional lymph nodes is one of the most important parameters that determines prognosis in patients with head and neck cancers. The presence of even a single positive node decreases survival by as much as 50%.

Whether the absolute number of positive lymph nodes correlates with survival is controversial. For instance, Schuller and associates,[54] in a study of 242 patients with squamous cell carcinoma of various sites in the head and neck whose treatment included a radical neck dissection, concluded that the number of positive lymph nodes failed to demonstrate any consistent prognostic value. Johnson and colleagues[55] came to a similar conclusion in a study of 177 radical neck specimens. Sessions[42] also noted that multiplicity of positive lymph nodes does not correlate with the survival of patients with supraglottic and glottic cancers, but that more than one positive lymph node in a patient with cancer of the inferior hypopharynx results in a statistically significant decrease in survival. However, Kalnins and coworkers,[56] in a review of 340 patients with squamous cell carcinoma of the oral cavity, observed the 5-year determinant survival to be 75% when cervical lymph nodes were negative, 49% when one lymph node was positive, 30% when two lymph nodes were positive, and 13% when three or more lymph nodes were positive. Most other investigators have also found that the number of positive lymph nodes correlates to some extent with prognosis: As the number increases, survival decreases proportionately.[18, 57–60] Patients with bilateral lymph node metastases have a worse prognosis than do those with unilateral neck disease.[57]

The level (site) of cervical lymph node involvement is also important. Patients with positive lymph nodes in the lower level of the neck tend to do poorly.[56, 57, 61, 62] This is not unexpected, because the next echelon of lymph node involvement might be the mediastinal lymph nodes. Moreover, patients often have additional diseased lymph nodes at high levels in the neck. If one is aware of the lymphatic drainage of various anatomic regions of the head and neck, the level of the positive lymph node may allow the clinician to predict the most likely primary site in a patient who presents with a tumor of unknown origin.

The spread of tumor beyond the capsule of a lymph node into the perinodal soft tissue (extracapsular spread [ECS]) is an ominous finding that is associated statistically with an increased incidence of neck recurrence and decreased survival; when found, this spread warrants the use of postoperative radiation and/or chemotherapy[63] (Figs. 3–3 and 3–4). The reported incidence of extracapsular spread ranges from 24% to 85% and varies, to some extent, with the size of the lymph node.[56, 59, 60, 64, 65] Studies indicate that extracapsular spread occurs in 15% to 25% of lymph nodes up to 1 cm in size and in 75% of those in excess of 3 cm.[55, 59, 60] Distinction should be made between extracapsular spread that is microscopic versus macroscopic, because the macroscopic type is associated with a 10-fold greater risk of neck recurrence than the microscopic type.[64]

Whether the immunomorphology of regional lymph nodes in patients with cancer of the head and neck has prognostic significance remains controversial; this is especially so if the patient has received preoperative radiation. Berlinger and associates[66] reported the 5-year survival rate for 84 patients with squamous cell carcinoma of various sites in the head and neck to be 85% when the cervical lymph nodes showed a predominant germinal center pattern, 80% for a lymphocytic pattern, 44% for an unstimulated pattern, and 0% for a lymphocyte-depleted pattern. Gilmore and colleagues,[67] however, found no strong correlation between cervical lymph node immunomorphology and survival or metastases. It is generally agreed that sinus histiocytosis has no prognostic influence in head and neck cancers.[18, 68]

Sentinel Lymph Nodes

Depending on the site and size of the tumor, about 30% of patients with a squamous cell carcinoma of the upper

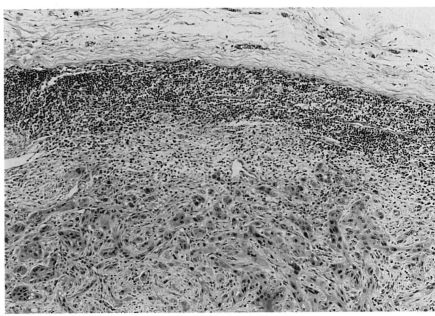

FIGURE 3–3 Metastatic squamous cell carcinoma in a cervical lymph node. In this instance, the tumor is confined to the node (hematoxylin-eosin, ×125).

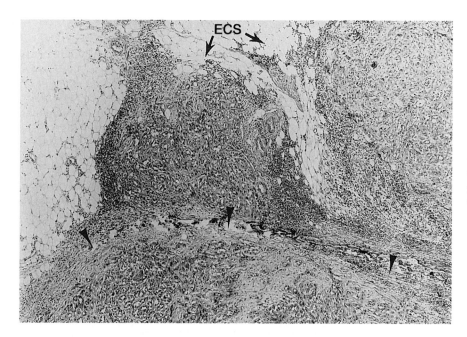

FIGURE 3–4 Metastatic squamous cell carcinoma in a cervical lymph node with extracapsular spread (ECS) into adjacent adipose tissue. *Arrowheads* show capsule of lymph node (hematoxylin-eosin, ×50).

aerodigestive tract and a clinically negative neck (N0) will harbor occult metastasis on elective neck dissection.[69, 70] To triage these patients into operative and nonoperative groups, sentinal lymph node mapping, as applied in breast and melanoma protocols, is now being used in some medical centers, with varying degrees of success.[71–76]

The concept of a sentinel lymph node is based on the premise that metastasis from a primary tumor follows an orderly progression and will first involve the most proximal draining (sentinel) lymph node before spreading to other lymph nodes. Accordingly, if the sentinel lymph node is free of tumor, it is assumed that the remaining cervical lymph nodes are free as well, and a neck dissection will not be done. If, on the other hand, the sentinel lymph node is positive, a neck dissection is warranted.

The sentinel node is identified by injecting the primary tumor site with a radioactive tracer and excising the "hot" (sentinel) lymph node for pathologic evaluation. Such lymph nodes need special processing by the pathologist because, in many instances, the tumor deposits are very small, consisting of only a cluster of two or more cells that may be easily overlooked on routine evaluation. The lymph node should be totally submitted for microscopic study, and multiple sections obtained at different levels should be examined; these analyses should be augmented with immunohistochemical stains for cytokeratin.

Distant Metastases

The frequency with which squamous cell carcinoma of the head and neck spreads below the clavicles varies according to whether the results are derived from clinical or autopsy data. Studies based on clinical data report an incidence of 10% to 30%,[77, 78] whereas autopsy series report distant metastases in 30% to 50%.[78–81] The lungs, liver, and bones (especially the vertebrae, ribs, and skull) are the most common sites.

About half of all distant metastases are detected clinically within 9 months of treatment, and 80% within 2 years.[77] Their presence is an ominous sign because almost 90% of patients are dead within 2 years of detection of the first metastasis.[82]

The probability of developing distant metastases is related to some extent to the site and stage of the primary cancer. Tumors of the hypopharynx, nasopharynx, supraglottic larynx, and oropharynx are more likely to disseminate than are those of the oral cavity, sinuses, middle ear, and glottis. Although the incidence varies with both the T and N stages, Merino and associates[77] indicate that the N stage has the greater influence. Leemans and colleagues[83] indicate that patients with three or more positive lymph nodes and extranodal spread are at increased risk of developing metastases below the clavicles and may benefit from adjuvant systemic therapy when such metastases are observed.

Distant metastases are often preceded by locoregional recurrence. In fact, only 10% to 20% of patients develop distant spread without first experiencing locoregional recurrence.[77, 78, 84]

Multiple Primary Cancers

Ten percent to 20% of patients with head and neck cancers either have or will develop additional primary malignancies during their lifetime.[85–89] Most of these are found in other head and neck sites, in the lungs, or in the esophagus. It is important to recognize this phenomenon because the discovery of a second primary may alter the initial therapeutic approach to the index tumor; represent a more aggressive, life-threatening neoplasm; or compromise previously successful treatment.

Multiple primary cancers are classified according to their temporal sequence as synchronous or metachronous. There is confusion, however, in the usage of these terms. Some authors define synchronous cancers as those that are diagnosed at the same time as or within 6 months of identification of the primary lesion; metachronous neoplasms are defined as those that develop longer than 6 months after the index tumor. Others apply the term "synchronous carcinoma" only to neoplasms that are identified during initial evaluation of the index tumor.

Prospective endoscopic studies of head and neck cancer patients indicate that during workup of the index tumor, additional simultaneous primaries will be found in 10% to 20% of cases.[87, 88] Gluckman and associates[87] observed that in metachronous carcinomas (defined as those appearing 6 months or longer after the index tumor), the average interval between the diagnoses of the first and the second carcinoma was 26 months, with a range of 8 months to 6 years.

Exfoliative and Imprint Cytology

Exfoliative Cytology

Although it still has some staunch advocates, exfoliative cytology for the detection of mucosal cancers of the head and neck (excluding the esophagus) is not widely employed for several reasons. First, most head and neck cancers can be visualized either grossly or through endoscopes and are therefore amenable to direct biopsy. Second, physicians today are better trained in the detection of premalignant/early malignant lesions of the mucous membranes. Third, even if the cytologic findings are positive, a confirmatory biopsy is still desirable.

The accuracy of exfoliative cytology in biopsy-proven cancer of the oral cavity is 75% to 95%; stated otherwise, cytologic findings are false-negative in 5% to 25% of all oral malignancies.[90–92] In the larynx, accuracy is about 85%.[93] Tumors that are heavily keratinized, well differentiated, inflamed, necrotic, or crusted or that have been previously irradiated are more often associated with false-negative smears.

It is well known that patients with head and neck cancer have a high incidence of second primary cancer, and that bronchogenic carcinoma is one of the most frequently encountered second primaries in this population. The value of cytologic examination of sputum and bronchial washings for the detection of lung cancer is unquestionable. However, what is the significance of positive bronchial cytologic findings in a patient with a known primary malignancy in the upper aerodigestive tract? Can cancer cells desquamated from a primary cancer in the upper aerodigestive tract be recovered in the tracheobronchial tree and be mistaken for an occult pulmonary carcinoma? Johnson and coworkers[94] addressed this issue in a prospective study of 100 consecutive untreated patients who had squamous cell carcinoma of the upper aerodigestive tract and a normal chest radiograph. Each individual had panendoscopy and bronchial washings obtained for cytologic evaluation. Only one patient (1%) had positive bronchial cytologic findings, probably from the shedding of tumor cells from an upper aerodigestive source. The authors concluded that cancers of the upper aerodigestive tract rarely desquamate identifiable tumor cells into the tracheobronchial tree, and that when such cells are found in bronchial washings, every effort should be made to localize a second primary cancer in the lung.

It has been known for many years that cytologic examinations of washings obtained from operative wounds of cancer patients are positive for malignant cells in 10% to 25% of cases.[95, 96] This is especially so if the cancer is ulcerated and extends to the surgical margins. Follow-up of such patients, however, indicates that this type of "wound seeding" has no significant prognostic value. Patients with washings that are cytologically positive are no more prone to develop local recurrences or metastases than are those with negative washings.

Imprint Cytology

Tumor imprints are easy to prepare and can be of immense value to the surgical pathologist. They are obtained by simply pressing a microscopic slide against the cut surface of the tumor, followed by immediate fixation and staining.

Imprints are indispensable in the classification of hematologic malignancies, and in the case of biopsies that are crushed or distorted, they may be the only source of material that is diagnostic. They are especially useful as an adjunct in the frozen section evaluation of small biopsies, such as those from the central nervous system,[97] or as a supplement in the intraoperative evaluation of thyroid lesions.

Histochemical and immunoperoxidase stains can also be done on tumor imprints. In fact, if the substance being stained for is labile, it is better to perform the stain on the imprint than on formalin-fixed, paraffin-embedded tissue.

Fine-Needle Aspiration

Fine-needle aspiration (FNA) is a safe, rapid, inexpensive method of evaluating neoplastic and non-neoplastic lesions throughout the body. In the hands of experienced personnel, it is quite accurate in the evaluation of the salivary glands and thyroid, of masses in the neck, and of orbital lesions. The procedure has several advantages. First, it allows for better presurgical planning and patient counseling, especially with respect to the possible need for a neck dissection or sacrifice of the facial nerve. Second, in patients who are thought to have benign tumors or are poor operative risks, a benign FNA would allow the patient to be followed with more confidence. Third, it provides an alternative to the danger of open neck biopsy and the inaccuracies of relying on clinical judgment alone. Fourth, it can be used to verify suspected recurrences or metastases in patients with a known primary cancer. Our own bias, however, is that radical surgery should never be performed on the basis of an FNA alone; the diagnosis should be confirmed by frozen section or by permanent histologic sections.

The procedure is simple, requires little equipment, and can be performed easily in the physician's office. The skin over the mass is sterilized and a local anesthetic is injected. A 22-gauge, 1- to 3-in. needle attached to a 10- to 20-mL disposable syringe held in a metal syringe holder is used for aspiration. The mass is immobilized between the fingers, and the needle is introduced. Once the needle is through the skin, negative pressure is applied to the syringe, and the needle is moved back and forth within the tumor in several different planes. The pressure is then released and the syringe is withdrawn. The aspirated cells are spread on a microscopic slide and are immediately fixed and stained; a cover slip is placed and the specimen examined (Fig. 3–5).

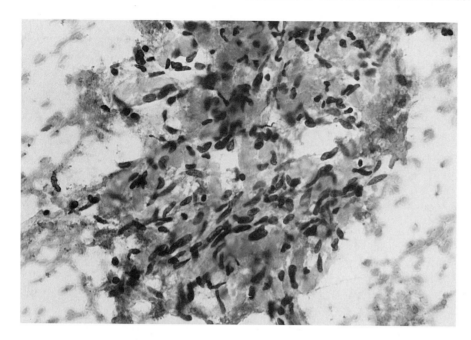

FIGURE 3–5 Fine-needle aspiration biopsy of a pleomorphic adenoma of the parotid gland, composed primarily of spindle cells with a few admixed epithelial cells lying in a myxoid background (Papanicolaou stain, ×500).

Occasionally, small bits of tissue or fluid may also be aspirated. This specimen can be submitted as a "cell block" for routine tissue processing and may supplement, or even be more diagnostic than, the aspirate (Fig. 3–6).

Some head and neck surgeons have been reluctant to use FNA for fear of seeding the needle tract with tumor cells, damaging the facial or recurrent laryngeal nerve, or inducing a salivary fistula. Experience has shown, however, that these complications are practically nonexistent. Engzell and coworkers[98] studied 157 patients with a pleomorphic adenoma of the major salivary glands who had undergone FNA prior to surgical excision. None of these developed tumor seeding of the needle tract during a 10-year follow-up. Smith[99] reviewed 63,108 FNAs and found only three examples of

needle tract seeding, an incidence of only 0.005%. These three tumors occurred in the pancreas, uterine cervix, and kidney. Although dissemination of tumor cells through punctured vascular channels is a potential danger, experiments in rabbits indicate that puncturing the tumor with a needle rarely results in release of malignant cells into lymphatics or blood vessels, and even when it does, the volume of cells is too small for a successful "take."[99] Hematoma is the most common complication of FNA, followed by infection.

Salivary Glands

The accuracy of FNA of the major salivary glands is shown in Table 3–2.[100–104] According to Cohen and associates[103] and

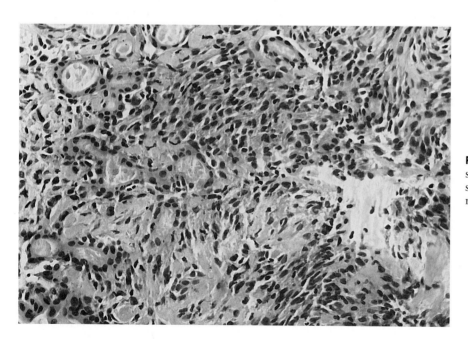

FIGURE 3–6 Cell block of needle aspirate shown in Figure 3–5, exhibiting diagnostic salivary ducts, spindle cells, and focal myxoid matrix (hematoxylin-eosin, ×315).

TABLE 3-2 Accuracy of Fine-Needle Aspiration of the Salivary Glands

Reference	No. of Aspirations With Histology	Overall Accuracy (%)		Accuracy for Benign Lesions %		Accuracy for Malignant Lesions (%)		False-Negatives (%)	False-Positives (%)
		According to Histology	Benign vs. Malignant	According to Histology	Benign Only	According to Histology	Malignant Only		
Sismanis et al[100]	44	74	91	87	96	60	85	4	5
Qizilbash et al[101]	101	87	98	90	100	79	88	12	0
O'Dwyer et al[102]	341	70	90	83	94	27	73	27	6
Cohen et al[103]	40	88	—	91	—	71	—	—	—
Layfield et al[104]	171	77	92	82	95	74	—	4.7	3.5
Average	—	79	93	87	96	62	82	12	3.6

Layfield and colleagues,[104] the diagnosis of salivary gland tumors by FNA is as accurate as frozen section at surgery (compare Tables 3–2 and 3–3). A majority of diagnostic errors involve cellular pleomorphic adenoma, mucoepidermoid carcinoma, sialoadenitis, and lymphoma.

Cervical Lymph Nodes–Neck Masses

FNA is especially useful in the evaluation of patients with enlarged cervical lymph nodes and a mass in the neck because the results, when coupled with the clinical findings, can be used to determine whether additional time-consuming and expensive evaluation is indicated. In experienced hands, it is 87% to 100% sensitive for the presence of tumor and 88% to 98% specific for the absence of tumor.[105, 106] It has also been shown that FNA generally does not interfere with subsequent histologic evaluation, should the lymph node require excision for further pathologic study.[107]

Lymphadenopathy is most often caused by reactive hyperplasia, infection, metastatic cancer, or lymphoma. Although the recognition of metastatic cancer is relatively easy, the distinction between hyperplasia-lymphadenitis and lymphoma with FNA may be difficult, if not impossible. Even if the smear is positive for lymphoma, excision of a lymph node for confirmation of a primary diagnosis and tissue staging of lymphoma is essential. The excised node also offers valuable prognostic information as to whether the lymphoma is nodular or diffuse, and it can be used as an additional source for cell markers.

In performing needle biopsy of a mass in the neck, one should always be aware of tumors near the bifurcation of the common carotid artery, which might be a carotid body paraganglioma. Listen for a bruit; if one is heard, an FNA is contraindicated for fear of inducing hemorrhage, carotid artery thrombosis, or even a cerebrovascular accident. Clinicians and cytopathologists must also be aware of cervical lesions that appear to be cystic because some of these will prove to be metastases that have undergone cystic degeneration.

Thyroid

Solitary cold nodules of the thyroid are common, and about 20% are malignant. FNA is a potentially useful tool for distinguishing those patients with solitary nodules who are in need of immediate surgery from those who can be followed safely.[108, 109] In published series, the sensitivity and specificity values of thyroid FNAs vary from 65% to 98% and from 73% to 100%, respectively.[108, 109] The overall accuracy of FNA, as far as the thyroid is concerned, compares quite favorably with the coarse (Tru-Cut) needle biopsy and with frozen section diagnosis.[110–114]

The most difficult areas of differential diagnosis in thyroid aspirations include distinguishing an adenoma from low-grade follicular carcinoma (which is virtually impossible short of tissue evaluation) and distinguishing some atypical Hürthle cell changes in Hashimoto's thyroiditis from malignant cells. Although fine-needle aspiration may release thyroglobulin into the circulation, antithyroglobulin antibodies apparently do not form.[115]

Orbit

The use of FNA in the evaluation of a mass in the orbit is becoming increasingly more common. It is used primarily to identify nonresectable deep orbital lesions that would otherwise require extensive surgery for diagnosis. Of 156 orbital FNAs reported by Kennerdell and colleagues,[116] 80% were positive or diagnostically helpful, 18% were inadequate, and 2% were false-positive or false-negative findings. Metastatic carcinomas, inflammatory lesions, and lymphoid tumors were most often encountered. Because of difficulty in aspiration, soft tissue tumors were responsible for most inadequate smears.

As might be expected, complications are not uncommon and are sometimes serious. These include hemorrhage, globe perforation, and transient or permanent blindness.

Frozen Sections

Frozen sections, or operating room consultations (as some prefer to call them because the tissue is not always frozen for microscopic examination), are indispensable to the head and neck surgeon. They offer a quick, usually definitive, diagnosis so that an appropriate therapeutic decision can be made while the patient is still on the operating table.

Large retrospective studies of frozen sections in general surgery have shown the procedure to be 95% to 98% accurate, with false-negative findings ranging from 0.9% to 1.7% and false-positive findings from 0.15% to 0.4%.[117–120] Fewer than 4% of cases have to be deferred for permanent histologic sections. Similar reviews of frozen sections limited to the head and neck region have shown identical results.[121–123] This method of diagnosis, however, always achieves its highest degree of accuracy when "there is cooperation between an experienced surgeon with an interest in pathology and a pathologist with a clinical viewpoint."[117]

Errors in diagnoses are most often due to misinterpretation of the biopsy, inadequate sampling, technical problems, or lack of communication between the surgeon and pathologist.[118, 120] To reduce errors, we strongly endorse the policy whereby the pathologist personally goes into the operating room, rather than communicating with the surgeon indirectly over an intercom or through a messenger. This allows the pathologist to acquire firsthand the pertinent clinical history, receive information about specimen orientation, see the surgical wound, or review the patient's clinical records and radiographs.

The pathologist must always be aware of the clinical implication of the diagnosis because few diagnostic procedures can have as immediate and serious treatment consequences as a frozen section. Likewise, the surgeon must not fall into a sense of complacency about frozen sections. Errors, though rare, do occur, and the results can be disastrous not only for the patient but also medicolegally for the surgeon and the pathologist.

As with any diagnostic procedure, indications for its use should be specific; frozen sections are not excluded from this rule. Indications for frozen sections include the following:

1. To determine if a tumor is benign or malignant; if it is malignant, a more extensive operation might be done.
2. To determine if the surgical margins of resection are adequate; if not, the frozen section should be repeated on additional margins.
3. To determine if a biopsy is representative or diagnostic. Occasionally, a biopsy of a suspected tumor may reveal only necrotic debris with no viable cells. A frozen section would indicate whether excision of more tissue is required.
4. To verify or confirm the identity of tissue removed. For example, in a parathyroidectomy, it can be difficult to distinguish a parathyroid gland from a lymph node. This is a simple task with frozen section.
5. To hasten the identification of microorganisms. Certain microorganisms, such as *Aspergillus* species and *Mucor* species, can often be recognized in tissue sections. Specific therapy can be employed immediately, rather than waiting days for the results of cultures.
6. To determine if a lesion needs special handling, such as estrogen receptors for breast carcinomas or cultures for inflammatory processes.
7. To assess the presence or absence of rejection in organ transplant patients, so that antirejection therapy, if needed, can be started immediately.

Frozen sections should not be requested in the following situations:

1. When the results would not alter the operation.
2. If the tissue is heavily calcified or ossified.
3. If the biopsy specimen is exceedingly small and no additional tissue will be obtained for permanent histologic studies. The freezing and thawing of tissue results in artifacts that might interfere with subsequent histologic evaluation.
4. For certain lesions, such as small cutaneous growths suspected of being malignant melanomas; melanocytic lesions are difficult enough to characterize on permanent sections, let alone on frozen section.

A majority of frozen sections of the head and neck are concerned with assessing margins of excision, benign versus malignant salivary gland tumors, lymph node and neck masses, and disorders of the thyroid and parathyroid glands. In a review of 1146 consecutive frozen sections of head and neck lesions, Remsen and others[122] singled out the nasopharynx and the oropharynx as the areas in which frozen sections were the least accurate.

There is a prevailing opinion among surgeons that frozen section evaluation of salivary gland tumors is unreliable. This, in part, stems from a bygone era in which (1) the classification and behavior of salivary gland neoplasms were unknown, unsettled, or evolving; (2) the quality of frozen sections was far inferior to the quality of those currently available with the cryostat; and (3) the policy of incisional rather than excisional biopsy was practiced, often yielding a limited or nonrepresentative portion of the neoplasm for pathologic evaluation. Even so, in some large teaching centers, frozen section accuracy may be less than desirable. This relates to a variety of factors: (1) The responsibility for frozen sections, in some instances, is delegated to senior pathology residents or fellows who are less experienced; (2) large pathology departments rotate the responsibility of frozen sections among all staff pathologists, who have varying interests and expertise in head and neck pathology; and (3) surgeons from a variety of technical and philosophical backgrounds (general, maxillofacial, and head and neck) are involved in the removal of these tumors. Table 3–3 summarizes studies pertaining to the accuracy of frozen section evaluation of the salivary glands.[123–129]

Common pitfalls in frozen section evaluation of salivary gland neoplasms include mistakenly identifying (1) monomorphic adenomas and cellular pleomorphic adenomas (mixed tumors) as malignant, (2) malignant lymphomas as inflammatory lesions or anaplastic carcinomas, (3) acinic cell carcinomas as adenomas, (4) low-grade mucoepidermoid carcinomas as benign, or (5) benign lymphoepithelial lesions as anaplastic carcinomas. If the tumor does not conform to the "usual" histologic pattern of a salivary gland tumor, the possibility of metastasis should always be considered.

Frozen section evaluation of the thyroid continues to be a problem for most pathologists. In a review of 363 thyroidectomies examined by frozen section, Montone and Livolsi observed that in only 50% of cases could an accurate diagnosis of benign or malignant be made during surgery.[130] In the remaining 50%, the diagnosis had to be deferred until permanent sections were available. Of the deferred cases, 78% were eventually found to be benign and 22% malignant. Distinguishing adenomas from encapsulated follicular carcinomas, recognizing the follicular variant of papillary carcinoma, and evaluating Hürthle cell lesions are the circumstances responsible for most deferred diagnoses.[130–132]

Because the accuracy of FNA of the thyroid is equivalent to that of the frozen section and because up to half of all frozen sections of the thyroid are deferred, many medical centers have started to experience a decline in requests for frozen sections.[130, 133]

Immunohistochemistry

Few procedures have had such an enormous impact on anatomic pathology as immunoperoxidase stains. The stains

TABLE 3-3 Accuracy of Frozen Section Diagnosis of Salivary Glands

Reference	No. of Cases	Overall Accuracy (%)		Accuracy for Benign Lesions (%)		Accuracy for Malignant Lesions (%)		Deferred (%)	False-Negatives (%)	False-Positives (%)
		According to Histology	Benign vs. Malignant	According to Histology	Benign Only	According to Histology	Malignant Only			
Miller et al[123]	132	83	88	93	94	36	60	8	24	0
Hillel & Fee[124]	75	84	95	93	95	43	71	9	5	0
Wheelis & Yarington[125]	256	86	96	88	98	77	88	0	12	2
Dindzans & Van Nostrand[126]	110	94	97	97	—	80	—	2	3	0
Granick et al[127]	462	96	—	97	—	86	—	—	14	2
Rigual et al[128]	100	92	96	96/100*	—	77/67*	—	0	9	3
Gnepp et al[129]	301	—	96	—	98	—	89	2	6	0.9
Average	—	89	95	94	96	66	77	4	10	1

*Separate figures given for parotid and submandibular glands, respectively.

are antigen-antibody reactions that rely on the binding of an antibody to a specific cellular component. A chromogen is then used to locate and visualize the immune reaction in tissue.[134]

The number of antibodies that can be developed against specific antigens appears to be unlimited. Antibodies can be developed not only against tumor antigens but also against immunoglobulins, hormones, infectious agents (e.g., herpes, cytomegalovirus), and various cytoplasmic components (e.g., intermediate filaments, neurosecretory granules). A few of the more common immunoperoxidase stains and their diagnostic applications are shown in Table 3-4.

Immunoperoxidase stains are especially useful in evaluating tumors that are categorized as "anaplastic" or "undifferentiated" on routine histologic section.[135–137] Although they are highly accurate, only a few of these stains are actually tumor-specific. Most allow only a general categorization of a tumor as carcinoma, sarcoma, or lymphoma. However, this information, when coupled with hematoxylin-eosin–stained sections, histochemical stains, and clinical information, generally allows the pathologist to make a specific diagnosis.

The value of immunoperoxidase stains can be appreciated by the following case report.

A 55-year-old man presented with an enlarged right superior jugular lymph node in level II of the right neck and a history of having had a Clark's level III, 0.85-mm-thick, superficial spreading malignant melanoma removed from his right temple 3 years previously. Metastasis was suspected and the lymph node was removed for verification. The pathologist confirmed the presence of a "malignant tumor," but, on hematoxylin-eosin section, it was uncertain whether it was metastatic melanoma, carcinoma, or lymphoma (Fig. 3–7A). Immunoperoxidase stains for S-100 protein, keratin, and common leukocyte antigen were requested. The common leukocyte antigen stain was strongly positive, whereas both the S-100 protein and keratin stains were negative (Fig. 3–7B). The results clearly indicated that the patient had another primary tumor (a malignant lymphoma) and not metastatic melanoma, as had been clinically suspected. Inappropriate therapy was therefore avoided.

Immunoperoxidase stains are time-consuming and expensive. The need for them depends entirely on the histologic appearance of the tumor on hematoxylin-eosin section, the differential diagnosis formulated by the pathologist, and the clinical information provided. The stains, on average, take 1 to 2 days to perform. Immunohistochemistry offers several advantages over electron microscopy for tumor diagnosis.

TABLE 3-4 Diagnostic Application of Immunoperoxidase Stains

Marker	Diagnostic Application
Keratin	Distinguishes epithelial tumors from lymphomas and most sarcomas; also found in synovial sarcomas, epithelioid sarcomas, and mesotheliomas
Carcinoembryonic antigen	Distinguishes epithelial tumors (especially adenocarcinomas) from lymphomas, sarcomas, and mesotheliomas; also found in medullary carcinoma of thyroid
Common leukocyte antigen	Distinguishes lymphomas and leukemias from carcinomas and sarcomas
Myoglobin	Identifies neoplasms of skeletal muscle origin only; not found in smooth muscle tumors
Desmin	Identifies tumors of both smooth muscle and skeletal muscle origin
Factor VIII–related antigen	Identifies tumors of endothelial origin
S-100 protein	Identifies neural tumors (including granular cell tumor), malignant melanomas, histiocytosis X, lipomas, cartilaginous tumors, and myoepithelial cells
Calcitonin	Medullary carcinoma of the thyroid
Chromogranin	Neuroendocrine tumors
Prostatic specific antigen	Prostatic carcinoma

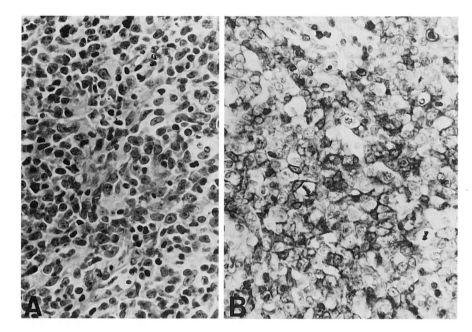

FIGURE 3–7 *A*, Hematoxylin-eosin–stained section of cervical lymph node composed of malignant cells with poorly defined cytoplasmic borders and round-to-reniform nuclei with prominent nucleoli (×500). *B*, Immunoperoxidase stain for common leukocyte antigen with typical brown-black staining of tumor cells shown in *A* (×500).

First, in contrast to electron microscopy, which requires forethought of need and specific fixation for optimal results, immunoperoxidase stains can be done on archival, formalin-fixed, paraffin-embedded tissue. Second, immunoperoxidase stains do not require expensive equipment, as electron microscopy does. And third, many different tissue blocks can be examined, as opposed to the minute fragments of tissue that are examined with the electron microscope. Thus, sampling errors are less of a problem.

Electron Microscopy

Transmission electron microscopy has reached a plateau in tumor pathology and, for reasons mentioned previously, has largely been supplanted by immunoperoxidase stains. There are occasions, however, when specific antibodies are not available, or when immunoperoxidase stains are inconclusive or do not support the light microscopic impression. In these instances, electron microscopy may be of help. The recent application of immunohistochemical techniques at the ultrastructural level, however, offers a new vista and perhaps a resurgence of this instrument's use in investigative pathology.

Flow Cytometry

The light microscopic evaluation of tumors is subjective and at best semiquantitative; yet it has been, and continues to be, the basis on which neoplasms are diagnosed and prognosis predicted. The application of flow cytometry to the field of surgical pathology initially offered some hope for a more objective and quantitative means of assessing biologic parameters and tumor virulence at a cellular level. Indeed, this has occurred in some instances, whereas, in others, the data generated from flow cytometric studies have been confusing, controversial, or even contradictory.

Flow cytometry can be carried out on body fluids, needle aspirates, and fresh and formalin-fixed paraffin-embedded tissue. Although the instrumentation is complex, the principle is simple. A suspension of cells or cell nuclei is allowed to pass singly through a laser light source. The cells or nuclei scatter the light, which is picked up by sensors that convert the scattered light into electrical impulses. The electrical signals are then digitized and stored in a computer, which then analyzes the data and produces a histogram.

Although flow cytometry has been used extensively for determining cell markers in patients with leukemias, lymphomas, and immunologic disorders, it can also be used to quantify DNA and to determine the ploidy of solid tumors. Data from flow cytometric analysis of solid tumors from various body sites allow some generalizations. First, cancers may be either diploid or aneuploid.[138–140] Second, aneuploidy per se is not an absolute criterion of malignancy.[141] Third, although aneuploid cancers tend to be more aggressive than those that are diploid, notable exceptions exist. For instance, Goldsmith and colleagues[140] observed that in squamous cell carcinoma of the larynx, aneuploid tumors have a better prognosis than do diploid tumors. In direct contrast, they noted that squamous cell carcinomas of the oral cavity that were aneuploid or tetraploid tended to have a poor response to treatment compared with those that were diploid.

The significance of aneuploidy in lesions judged to be benign by conventional light microscopy is uncertain. Joensuu and coworkers[142] studied 67 follicular adenomas of the thyroid and found 18 (27%) that were aneuploid. Although it is well known that pathologists occasionally have difficulty in distinguishing between follicular adenomas and encapsulated, well-differentiated follicular carcinomas, these investigators could find no evidence of blood vessel or capsular invasion on subserial sectioning of the aneuploid adenomas. Moreover, 12 of the patients were followed for 5 years or longer, and none developed distant metastases. Aneuploidy has also been identified in a few adenomatous goiters.[141] Whether such lesions are actually premalignant or are extremely well differentiated carcinomas beyond recognition at the light microscopic level is unknown. Certainly such patients need to be followed more closely.

Data derived from flow cytometric evaluation must be interpreted and used cautiously because studies of similar tumors have occasionally produced disparate conclusions. This, in part, may be related to tumor heterogeneity and inadequate sampling, or to flawed statistical analysis of noncomparable groups of patients.[143]

MOLECULAR PATHOLOGY

It is well recognized that the development of squamous cell carcinoma of the head and neck (SCCHN) is a multistep process with progressive accumulation of adverse chromosomal or genetic aberrations resulting in activation of oncogenes and/or inactivation of tumor suppressor genes, ultimately leading to selective growth advantage over normal cells and tumor formation.[144] Chromosomal abnormalities have been shown to be valuable markers for the diagnosis and prognosis of cancers and provide a chromosomal basis for the location of some common genetic defects.[145] Cytogenetic studies have revealed that the structural chromosomal alterations most commonly seen in SCCHN are losses of 3p, 5q, 8p, 9p, and 18q (found in 40% to 60% of tumors), followed by gains of 3q, 5q, 7p, 8q, and 11q (found in 30% to 40% of tumors).[146, 147] Allelic imbalance (AI) or loss of heterozygosity (LOH) studies have been used extensively to identify regions on chromosomes that may harbor tumor suppressor genes.[148] Regions that frequently show LOH are on chromosomal arms 9p, 3p, 11q, 13q, 17p, and 18q, and less frequently on 6p, 8p, 8q, 17q, and 19q.[149, 150]

Characterization of chromosomal aberrations (karyotype)[146, 147] and allelic imbalance (allelotype)[149, 150] allows investigators to locate important oncogenes or tumor suppressor genes that may play crucial roles in head and neck carcinogenesis. For example, chromosomal gains on 7p12 and 11q13 are frequently seen in SCCHN, and these correspond to the increased gene copy number and gene expression of epidermal growth factor receptor (EGF-R) and cyclin D1, respectively.[147] Allelic losses on 9p21, 11q13, and 17p13 are also very common in SCCHN, and these regions contain p16, a cyclin-dependent kinase inhibitor; cyclin D1, a proto-oncogene; and *TP53*, a tumor suppressor gene, respectively.[150, 151] Apparent allelic loss at 11q13 actually represents amplification of cyclin D1, which has been confirmed by fluorescence in situ hybridization.[152] Among the genetic alterations associated with corresponding gene functions and products identified, overexpression of EGF-R and cyclin D1, and inactivation of *TP53* and *p16* are most commonly and consistently seen in SCCHN.[153, 154]

Tumor karyotype and allelotype analyses in combination with characterization of *TP53* gene mutations help clinicians to identify some chromosomal and genetic markers that are associated with certain important processes in the carcinogenesis of SCCHN, such as field cancerization[155–160] and the genetic basis of tumor progression (from hyperplasia to dysplasia to carcinoma in situ to invasive carcinoma).[151, 161, 162]

The remaining portion of this chapter focuses on the roles of molecular and genetic technologies and resultant new concepts in the practice of head and neck pathology. The following issues are discussed: (1) field cancerization, (2) early detection of cancer, (3) surgical resection margin, (4) second primary cancers, and (5) cervical lymph nodes.

Field Cancerization

Field cancerization is perhaps the most basic and important concept in head and neck squamous carcinogenesis. This concept has been intimately linked to local recurrences and second primary cancers, which together are responsible for most treatment failures in patients with SCCHN. In 1953, Slaughter and associates proposed the concept of field cancerization in patients with oral cancers.[163] They hypothesized that the entire epithelial surface of the upper aerodigestive tract is "condemned" or "preconditioned" and thereby has an increased risk of developing premalignant or malignant lesions due to prolonged exposure primarily to tobacco carcinogens. They based their field cancerization theory on their observation of 783 oral cancer patients with the following supportive features: (1) high rate of local recurrence, (2) high incidence of second primary cancers, (3) multiple independent lesions within the sample specimen, and (4) presence of abnormal mucosa at surgical resection margins.

With the development of sophisticated molecular technologies, the original, morphology-based field cancerization theory has gained increasing support at the genetic and molecular levels. The genetic or molecular alterations that have key roles in head and neck carcinogenesis are demonstrated in both histologically normal and dysplastic upper aerodigestive tract mucosa. These genetic "field changes" include, but are not limited to, the following: (1) allelic imbalance (AI) or loss of heterozygosity (LOH) at the chromosomal arms of 3p, 9p, 17p, 4q, 6p, 8p, 11q, 13q, and 14q that are frequently seen in SCCHN[151, 155, 158, 161, 164–167]; (2) *TP53* gene mutations[155, 162, 168, 169] or *TP53* gene overexpression[170, 171]; (3) cyclin D1 gene amplification[172] and overexpression[173, 174]; (4) epidermal growth factor receptor (EGF-R) gene overexpression[175]; and (5) proto-oncogene eukaryotic initiation factor 4E (eIF4E) amplification and overexpression.[176, 177]

In general, the genetic "field changes" have the following features: (1) The changes can be detected in microscopically "benign" mucosa[151, 155, 164, 166, 168, 169]; (2) the accumulation of genetic alterations (genetic progression) parallels the histopathologic progression from hyperplasia to dysplasia to carcinoma in situ to invasive carcinoma[151, 161, 165, 166]; (3) the number of genetic events sufficient for a malignant phenotype can be acquired in a preinvasive epithelial lesion long before the clinical appearance of malignancy[161]; and (4) multiple preinvasive and invasive lesions within the same field frequently share the same genetic changes, supporting the notion that the process of field cancerization is derived from the expansion and migration of clonally related preneoplastic cells, at least in a significant number of cases.[151, 155, 158–161, 178]

Early Detection of Cancer

Failure to detect head and neck cancer early is one of the most important factors contributing to poor outcome for SCCHN patients. For example, patients with tumors arising in the lip and true vocal cords have an excellent prognosis, with an overall 5-year survival approaching 80%[179, 180]; this may be largely due to the fact that tumors of these two locations can be detected early because of the ease of self-inspection for cancer of the lip and the change in voice quality (hoarseness) for cancer of the vocal cords. By contrast, cancer of the hypopharynx behaves the worst, with an overall 5-year survival of 20% to 40%. Because this is a relatively silent area that is not amenable to self-inspection, tumors arising from this area are quite large when first detected; most are T3 or T4 lesions. It is fair to say that many SCCHN patients die because of delayed diagnosis, leading to advanced stages of their disease. The development of early detection technologies at the genetic level would be an important step toward improved survival for SCCHN patients.

Currently, a few encouraging studies have applied microsatellite analysis in detecting occult cancer cells in saliva from SCCHN patients[181] to predict the potential for malignant progression in oral preinvasive lesions.[165, 166, 182, 183]

In a feasibility test involving 44 patients with known head and neck cancer and 43 healthy control subjects, Spafford and coworkers successfully detected specific genetic alterations in exfoliated oral mucosal cells in saliva samples from 35 of 38 SCCHN patients, compared with none in 43 saliva samples obtained from healthy control subjects, demonstrating a very high sensitivity of 92% and specificity of 100% for the test.[181] It has also been previously documented that tumor-associated microsatellite alterations can be detected in morphologically benign oral mucosa in patients with early cancer.[151, 155, 164, 166, 168, 169] Thus, with further validation and refinement, this microsatellite analysis–based saliva test could be used as a screening tool to detect occult cancer among high-risk populations.

Traditionally, the likelihood for malignant progression in oral preinvasive lesions has been judged by the degree of epithelial dysplasia. Such assessment is subjective, however, and does not always correctly predict the final outcome of preinvasive lesions. Using microsatellite analysis, several groups of investigators have independently proved that cumulative allelic loss of two or more of the chromosomal regions at 3p, 8p, 9p, 17p, 4q, 5q, 11q, 13q, and 18q can accurately predict the potential for malignant progression in oral preinvasive lesions.[165, 166, 182, 183] On the basis of these findings, Partridge and colleagues advocate complete excision of all suspicious areas that show allelic loss at two or more key loci, regardless of the degree of dysplasia.[165]

By using a much simpler immunohistochemical approach, Cruz and coworkers have shown that the distribution of TP53-positive cells in squamous mucosa, rather than the percentage of TP53-positive cells, can predict the likelihood for malignant progression.[171] In their study involving 35 oral preinvasive lesions, they found that suprabasal expression of TP53 protein, in combination with the presence of moderate to severe dysplasia, had a very high sensitivity for identifying lesions that later progressed to invasive carcinoma (91%). Interestingly, they also found that suprabasal TP53 protein expression was present in three oral lesions with no or mild dysplasia, and all three later progressed to invasive carcinoma.[171] With further validation of a larger series, this immunohistochemical method could become an invaluable and practical tool in pathology because of its cost-effectiveness and relative simplicity.

Currently, no molecular or genetic test can replace the traditional role of an experienced otolaryngologist and pathologist in cancer detection and diagnosis. These tests are still evolving and should be regarded only as supplementary to more standard practices of thorough examination and biopsy.

Surgical Resection Margins

With surgical resection being the mainstay of therapy for patients with SCCHN, histologic assessment of resection margins is essential to ensure complete removal of a tumor. This method, however, may not always detect minute foci of cancer cells that can lead to local recurrence.

Tumor-specific genetic alterations have been frequently detected in microscopically "benign" surgical resection margins both by *TP53* gene mutational analysis[155, 168, 169] and by microsatellite analysis.[155, 165] Thus, persistence of a small number of cancer cells at the margin that are beyond the limit of the light microscope may represent a major factor contributing to frequent local recurrence (15%–30%) and subsequent treatment failure in those patients with margins that are judged to be microscopically "negative, or free."[184–187]

Currently, investigators have succeeded in detecting residual cancer cells at histopathologically "negative" resection margins and have shown that patients with positive margins at the genetic levels experience recurrence much more frequently than those with negative genetic margins.[168, 169]

Amplification and overexpression of the eukaryotic initiation factor *4E* (*eIF4E*) gene have been demonstrated in SCCHN and adjacent normal-appearing mucosa.[176] Using immunohistochemistry, Nathan and associates have demonstrated that overexpression of the *eIF4E* gene at surgical resection margins that are histopathologically "negative" is associated with increased local recurrence.[177] With further prospective documentation, this procedure could become very useful in extending the ability of pathologists to assess surgical resection margins.

Second Primary Cancers

A second primary cancer is defined as a cancer that is geographically separate and distinct, and not connected by neoplastic epithelial changes with the original primary cancer.[188] Clinically, these new cancers develop either simultaneously with the primary tumor (synchronous) or after a period of time (metachronous). Second primary cancers have a negative impact on long-term survival of patients and are often the cause of treatment failure and death.[189–191] The frequency of second primary cancers is estimated to be 3% to 5% per year, with 5-year cumulative incidence ranging from 15% to 40%.[188, 192–194]

Second primary cancers are related to Slaughter's field cancerization concept[163] and have long been considered to be genetically unrelated, independent lesions, arising in upper aerodigestive tract mucosa that has accumulated multiple independent genetic alterations as a result of continued exposure to environmental carcinogens. This traditional view on the origin of multiple SCCHNs has been challenged during the 1990s with the advent of modern molecular technologies.

Currently, there are two different theories on the genesis of multiple SCCHNs: (1) a monoclonal theory, in which a single cell is transformed and through clonal expansion gives rise to one large extended premalignant field, from which multiple genetically related tumors develop[155, 159, 160, 178, 195, 196]; and

(2) a polyclonal theory, in which multiple transforming events lead to genetically unrelated tumors.[156, 157, 197, 198]

The monoclonal theory appears to be gaining support for the following reasons: (1) Neoplastic transformation is an extremely rare event, even in individuals with hereditary predispositions to cancer[159]; and (2) identical genetic alterations, such as specific types of *TP53* mutations,[155, 196] patterns of X-chromosome inactivation and allelic loss,[160, 178] and chromosomal aberrations[195] between primary and second primary cancers, provide compelling supportive evidence for a monoclonal origin of multiple primary tumors.

Conversely, a number of studies have shown discordant genetic alterations between the primary and second primary cancers using *TP53* gene mutational and allelic loss analyses, respectively.[156, 197, 198] However, these features are not conclusive evidence in support of an independent origin of multiple head and neck cancers. It has been shown that progression of neoplasms is related to the accumulation of a number of genetic events but not necessarily to the exact order of these events.[199] Thus, in tumors displaying different patterns of genetic alteration, the genetic alterations being analyzed in these studies may have occurred after clonal expansion. An unidentified earlier genetic event may still be shared by these cancers.[159, 160]

The genesis of multiple primary cancers may have important therapeutic implications. For example, if multiple primary cancers develop from genetically independent clones, we should focus more on prevention and early detection. On the other hand, if multiple primary tumors are monoclonal in origin, then our effort should focus on the prevention of local spread and metastasis and on early use of systemic therapy.[159] It has been demonstrated that certain chemopreventive agents, such as isotretinoid, can reduce the incidence of second primary cancers.[193, 194]

Currently, very few studies have applied genetic and molecular techniques in predicting the occurrence of second primary cancers. In one such study involving 105 SCCHN patients, Homann and colleagues observed that overexpression of the TP53 protein in tumor-distant mucosa (at least 4 cm from the resection margin of the primary tumor), but not in the primary tumor, is associated with an increased incidence of secondary primary cancer.[170]

Cervical Lymph Nodes

The status of the cervical lymph nodes is one of the most important prognostic factors in patients with SCCHN. The presence of metastatic squamous cell carcinoma in cervical lymph nodes is an adverse event associated with decreased survival.[187, 200–203] Nodal metastases, however, must be of a certain size to allow successful detection by clinical palpation or modern imaging techniques. Microscopic metastatic deposits can escape clinical detection, and evaluation of cervical lymph node metastases by computed tomography (CT) and magnetic resonance imaging (MRI) has a specificity of only 70% to 85%.[204, 205] Consequently, the management of the clinically negative (N0) neck is controversial.[206–208] The identification of genetic and molecular markers for prediction of neck lymph node metastases would be most helpful in the surgical management of SCCHN patients.

Several investigators have used immunohistochemical procedures to predict metastasis to cervical lymph nodes.[209, 210] In these studies, overexpression of cyclin D1 and retinoblastoma (*RB*) tumor suppressor genes, loss of expression of epithelial cell adhesion molecule (Ep-CAM), and the absence of inflammatory reaction and eosinophilic infiltration in the primary tumor are molecular and histopathologic changes associated with increased risk of nodal metastasis.[209, 210] With these markers, the detection of nodal metastases appears highly accurate, with a sensitivity of 100% and specificity of 79%.[209]

Molecular and genetic technologies have also allowed more accurate assessment of lymph nodes in neck dissection specimens. Conventional morphologic examination often fails to detect small foci of metastatic disease (micrometastases) in lymph nodes,[211, 212] resulting in errors in tumor staging. Using *TP53* gene mutation analysis, two groups of investigators have detected cancer cells in 2 of 2 (100%) and 6 of 28 (21%) lymph nodes that were initially judged to be negative by histopathologic assessment.[168, 169]

◨ CONCLUSION

The pace of modern molecular and genetic evolution and the knowledge derived from these events may have tremendous impact on the future management of patients with SCCHN. The polymerase chain reaction (PCR) technique has revolutionized biomedical science and is perhaps the single most dominant technique responsible for advances in molecular biology and genetics. Allelic loss and microsatellite instability analyses, DNA sequencing, and mutation analysis all are PCR-based assays that are sensitive enough to detect specific genetic alterations derived from DNA of just a few cancer cells. Automation using a PCR-based microcapillary array technology for microsatellite-based cancer detection allows cancer detection simultaneously in a large volume of samples.[213] Most processes related to cancer development, progression, and responsiveness to chemo- and radiation therapies are regulated by multiple genetic events that coordinate with one another. The arrival of Serial Analysis of Gene Expression (SAGE), cDNA microarrays, and proteomic technology now allows the pursuit of gene and protein expression profiling achieved through simultaneous analysis of thousands of genes.[214] In head and neck cancer, gene expression profiling for the development of malignant phenotypes[215, 216] and for the assessment of tumor responsiveness to radiation[217] has been tentatively created.

Although the light microscope continues to be the gold standard by which tumors are diagnosed, we are at the dawn of a new era in which molecular-genetic studies may become the new standard of care for patients with cancer of the head and neck.

REFERENCES

1. Greenlee RT, Hill-Harmon MB, Murray T, Than M: Cancer statistics, 2001. CA Cancer J Clin 51:15–36, 2001.
2. Wagner BM: The surgical pathology report. Hum Pathol 15:1, 1984.
3. Fleming T, Cooper JS, Henson DE, et al (eds): AJCC Cancer Staging Manual, 5th ed. Philadelphia, Lippincott-Raven, 1997.
4. Crissman JD, Gluckman J, Whitely J, et al: Squamous cell carcinoma of the floor of the mouth. Head Neck Surg 3:2, 1986.

5. Schramm VL Jr, Myers EN, Sigler BA: Surgical management of early epidermoid carcinoma of the anterior floor of the mouth. Laryngoscope 90:207, 1980.

6. Moore C, Flynn MB, Greenberg RA: Evaluation of size in prognosis of oral cancer. Cancer 58:158, 1986.

7. Gnepp DR, Ferlito A, Hyams V: Primary anaplastic small cell (oat cell) carcinoma of the larynx: Review of the literature and report of 18 cases. Cancer 51:1731, 1983.

8. Breslow A: Thickness, cross-sectional areas and depth of invasion in the prognosis of cutaneous melanoma. Ann Surg 172:902–908, 1970.

9. Mohit-Tabatabai MA, Sobel HJ, Rush BF, et al: Relationship of thickness of floor of mouth stage I and II cancer to regional metastasis. Am J Surg 152:351, 1986.

10. Spiro RH, Huvos AG, Wong GV, et al: Predictive value of tumor thickness in squamous carcinoma confined to the tongue and floor of the mouth. Am J Surg 153:345, 1986.

11. Frierson HF Jr, Cooper PH: Prognostic factors in squamous cell carcinoma of the lower lip. Hum Pathol 17:346, 1986.

12. Arthur K, Farr HW: Prognostic significance of histologic grade in epidermoid carcinoma of the mouth and pharynx. Am J Surg 124:489, 1972.

13. Jakobsson PA: Histologic grading of malignancy and prognosis in glottic carcinoma of the larynx. In Albert PW, Bryce DE (eds): The Centennial Conference on Laryngeal Carcinoma. New York, Appleton-Century-Crofts, 1974, p 847.

14. Chung CK, Styker JA, Abt AB, et al: Histologic grading in the clinical evaluation of laryngeal carcinoma. Arch Otolaryngol 106:623, 1980.

15. Crissman JD: Tumor-host interactions as prognostic factors in the histologic assessment of carcinomas. In Sommers SC, Rosen PP, Fechner RE (eds): Pathology Annual, vol 21, part 1. Norwalk, Conn, Appleton-Century-Crofts, 1986, p 29.

16. Crissman JD, Liu WY, Gluckman JL, et al: Prognostic value of histopathologic parameters in squamous cell carcinoma of the oropharynx. Cancer 54:2995, 1984.

17. Yamaoto E, Miyakawa A, Kohama G: Mode of invasion and lymph node metastasis in squamous cell carcinoma of the oral cavity. Head Neck Surg 6:938, 1984.

18. Noone RB, Booner H Jr, Raymond S, et al: Lymph node metastases in oral cancer: A correlation of histopathology with survival. Plast Reconstr Surg 53:158, 1974.

19. Hiratsuka H, Imamura H, Ishii Y, et al: Immunohistologic detection of lymphocyte subpopulations infiltrating in human oral cancer with special reference to its clinical significance. Cancer 53:2456, 1984.

20. Guo M, Rabin BS, Johnson JJ, et al: Lymphocyte phenotypes at tumor margins in patients with head and neck cancer. Head Neck Surg 9:265, 1987.

21. Reichert TE, Scheuer C, Day R, et al: The number of intratumoral dendritic cells and epsilon-chain expression in T cells as prognostic and survival biomarkers in patients with oral carcinoma. Cancer 91:2136, 2001.

22. McGavran MH, Bauer WC, Ogura JH: The incidence of cervical lymph node metastases from epidermoid carcinoma of the larynx and their relationship to certain characteristics of the primary tumor: A study based on the clinical and pathological findings for 96 patients treated by en bloc laryngectomy and radical neck dissection. Cancer 14:55, 1961.

23. Byers RM, O'Brien J, Waxier J: The therapeutic and prognostic implications of nerve invasion in cancer of the lower lip. Int J Radiat Oncol Biol Phys 4:215, 1978.

24. Cottel WI: Perineural invasion by squamous-cell carcinoma. J Dermatol Surg Oncol 8:589, 1982.

25. Goepfert H, Dichtel WJ, Medina JE, et al: Perineural invasion in squamous cell skin carcinoma of the head and neck. Am J Surg 148:542, 1984.

26. Soo K, Carter RL, O'Brien CJ, et al: Prognostic implications of perineural spread in squamous carcinomas of the head and neck. Laryngoscope 96:1145, 1986.

27. Fagan JJ, Collins B, Barnes L, et al: Perineural invasion in squamous cell carcinoma of the head and neck. Arch Otolaryngol Head Neck Surg 124:637, 1998.

28. Dodd GD, Dolan PA, Ballantyne AJ, et al: The dissemination of tumors of the head and neck via the cranial nerves. Radiol Clin North Am 8:445, 1970.

29. Curtin HD, Williams R, Johnson J: CT of perineural tumor extension: Pterygopalatine fossa. Am J Roentgenol 144:163, 1985.

30. Carter RL, Pittam MR, Tanner NSB: Pain and dysphagia in patients with squamous carcinomas of the head and neck: The role of perineural spread. J R Soc Med 75:598, 1982.

31. Gandour-Edwards R, Kapadia SB, Barnes L, et al: Neural cell adhesion molecule in adenoid cystic carcinoma invading the skull base. Otolaryngol Head Neck Surg 117:453, 1997.

32. McLaughlin RB Jr, Montone KT, Wall SJ, et al: Nerve cell adhesion molecule expression in squamous cell carcinoma of the head and neck: A predictor of propensity toward perineural spread. Laryngoscope 109:821, 1999.

33. Vural E, Hutcheson J, Karourian S, et al: Correlation of neural cell adhesion molecules with perineural spread of squamous cell carcinoma of the head and neck. Otolaryngol Head Neck Surg 122:717, 2000.

34. Sugarbaker EV: Cancer metastasis: A product of tumor-host interactions. Curr Probl Cancer 3:3, 1979.

35. Poleksic S, Kalwaic HJ: Prognostic value of vascular invasion in squamous cell carcinoma of the head and neck. Plast Reconstr Surg 61:234, 1978.

36. Close LG, Burns DK, Reisch J, et al: Microvascular invasion of intraoral carcinoma. Presented at the Society for Head and Neck Surgery, April 28, 1987, Denver, Colorado.

37. Djalilian M, Weiland LH, Devine KD, et al: Significance of jugular vein invasion by metastatic carcinoma in radical neck dissection. Am J Surg 126:566, 1973.

38. Cady B, Catlin D: Epidermoid carcinoma of the gum: A 20-year survey. Cancer 23:551, 1969.

39. Platz H, Fries R, Hudec NI, et al: The prognostic relevance of various factors at the time of the first admission of the patient: Retrospective DOSAK study on carcinoma of the oral cavity. J Maxillofac Surg 11:3, 1983.

40. O'Brien CJ, Carter RL, Soo K, et al: Invasion of the mandible by squamous carcinoma of the oral cavity and oropharynx. Head Neck Surg 8:247, 1986.

41. Carter RL, Tanner NSB, Clifford P, et al: Direct bone invasion in squamous carcinoma of the head and neck: Pathological and clinical implications. Clin Otolaryngol 5:107, 1980.

42. Sessions DG: Surgical pathology of the larynx and hypopharynx. Laryngoscope 86:814, 1976.

43. Pittam MR, Carter RL: Framework invasion by laryngeal carcinomas. Head Neck Surg 4:200, 1982.

44. Afzelius LE, Gunnarsson M, Nordgren H: Guidelines for prophylactic radical lymph node dissection in cases of carcinoma of the external ear. Head Neck Surg 2:361, 1980.

45. Lee JG: Detection of residual carcinoma of the oral cavity, oropharynx, hypopharynx, and larynx: A study of surgical margins. Trans Am Acad Ophthalmol Otolaryngol 78:49, 1974.

46. Harrison D: The questionable value of total glossectomy. Head Neck Surg 6:632, 1983.

47. Byers RM, Bland KI, Borlase B, et al: The prognostic and therapeutic value of frozen section determinations in the surgical treatment of squamous carcinoma of the head and neck. Am J Surg 136:525, 1978.

48. Looser KG, Shah JP, Strong EW: The significance of "positive" margins in surgically resected epidermoid carcinomas. Head Neck Surg 1:107, 1978.

49. Chen TY, Emrich U, Driscoll DL: The clinical significance of pathological findings in surgically resected margins of the primary tumor in head and neck carcinoma. Int J Radiat Oncol Biol Phys 13:833, 1987.

50. Scholl P, Byers RM, Batsakis JG, et al: Microscopic cut-through of cancer in the surgical treatment of squamous carcinoma of the tongue: Prognostic and therapeutic implications. Am J Surg 152:354, 1986.

51. Barnes L, Johnson JT: Pathologic and clinical considerations in the evaluation of major head and neck specimens resected for cancer. In Sommers SC, Rosen PP, Fechner RE (eds): Pathology Annual, vol 21, part 1. Norwalk, Conn, Appleton-Century-Crofts, 1986, p 173.

52. Bauer WC, Lesinski SG, Ogura JH: The significance of positive margins in hemilaryngectomy specimens. Laryngoscope 85:1, 1975.

53. Zieske LA, Johnson JT, Myers EN, et al: Squamous cell carcinoma with positive margins. Arch Otolaryngol Head Neck Surg 112:863, 1986.

54. Schuller DE, McGuirt WF, McCabe BF, et al: The prognostic significance of metastatic cervical lymph nodes. Laryngoscope 90:557, 1980.

55. Johnson JT, Barnes EL, Myers EN, et al: The extracapsular spread of tumors in cervical node metastasis. Arch Otolaryngol 107:725, 1981.

56. Kalnins IK, Leonard AG, Sako K, et al: Correlation between prognosis and degree of lymph node involvement in carcinoma of the oral cavity. Am J Surg 134:450, 1977.

57. Spiro RH, Alfonso AE, Farr HW, et al: Cervical lymph node metastasis from epidermoid carcinoma of the oral cavity and oropharynx: A critical assessment of current staging. Am J Surg 128:562, 1974.

58. Rollo J, Rozenbom CV, Thawley S, et al: Squamous carcinoma of the base of the tongue: A clinicopathologic study of 81 cases. Cancer 47:333, 1981.

59. Snow GB, Annyas AA, Van Slooten EA: Prognostic factors of neck node metastasis. Clin Otolaryngol 7:185, 1982.

60. Richard JM, Sancho-Garnier H, Micheau C, et al: Prognostic factors in cervical lymph node metastasis in upper respiratory and digestive tract carcinomas: Study of 1,713 cases during a 15-year period. Laryngoscope 97:97, 1987.

61. Grandi C, Alloisio M, Moglia D, et al: Prognostic significance of lymphatic spread in head and neck carcinomas: Therapeutic implications. Head Neck Surg 8:67, 1985.

62. Stell PM, Morton RR, Singh SD: Cervical lymph node metastases: The significance of the level of the lymph node. Clin Oncol 9:101, 1983.

63. Johnson JT, Myers EN, Srodes CH, et al: Maintenance chemotherapy for high-risk patients: A preliminary report. Arch Otolaryngol 111:727, 1985.

64. Carter RL, Bliss JM, Soo KC, et al: Radical neck dissections for squamous carcinomas: Pathological findings and their clinical implications with particular reference to transcapsular spread. Int J Radiat Oncol Biol Phys 13:825, 1987.

65. Johnson JT, Myers EN, Bedetti CD, et al: Cervical lymph node metastases: Incidence and implications of extracapsular carcinoma. Arch Otolaryngol 111:534, 1985.

66. Berlinger NT, Tsakraklides V, Pollak K, et al: Immunologic assessment of regional lymph node history in relation to survival in head and neck carcinoma. Cancer 37:697, 1976.

67. Gilmore BB, Repola D, Batsakis JG: Carcinoma of the larynx: Lymph node reaction patterns. Laryngoscope 88:1333, 1978.

68. Zoller M, Goodman ML, Cummings CW: Guidelines for prognosis in head and neck cancer with nodal metastases. Laryngoscope 88:135, 1978.

69. Snow GB, Patel P, Leemans CR, et al: Management of cervical lymph nodes in patients with head and neck cancer. Eur Arch Otorhinolaryngol 249:187, 1992.

70. Don DM, Anzai Y, Lufkin RB, et al: Evaluation of cervical lymph node metastases in squamous cell carcinoma of the head and neck. Laryngoscope 105:669, 1995.

71. Pitman KT, Johnson JT, Edington H, et al: Lymphatic mapping with isosulfan blue dye in squamous cell carcinoma of the head and neck. Arch Otolaryngol Head Neck Surg 124:790, 1998.

72. Alex JC, Sasaki LT, Krag DN, et al: Sentinel lymph node radiolocalization in head and neck squamous cell carcinoma. Laryngoscope 110:198, 2000.

73. Zitsch RP III, Todd DW, Renner GJ, et al: Intraoperative radiolymphoscintigraphy for detection of occult nodal metastasis in patients with head and neck squamous cell carcinoma. Otolaryngol Head Neck Surg 122:662, 2000.

74. Taylor RJ, Wahl RL, Sharma PK, et al: Sentinel node localization in oral cavity and oropharynx squamous cell carcinoma. Arch Otolaryngol Head Neck Surg 127:970, 2001.

75. Stoeckli SJ, Steinert H, Pfaltz M, et al: Sentinel lymph node evaluation in squamous cell carcinoma of the head and neck. Otolaryngol Head Neck Surg 125:221, 2001.

76. Shoaib T, Soutar DS, McDonald DG, et al: The accuracy of head and neck carcinoma sentinel lymph node biopsy in the clinically N0 neck. Cancer 91:2077, 2001.

77. Merino OR, Lindberg RD, Fletcher GH: An analysis of distant metastases from squamous cell carcinoma of the upper respiratory and digestive tracts. Cancer 40:145, 1977.

78. Zbaren P, Lehmann W: Frequency and sites of distant metastases in head and neck squamous cell carcinoma: An analysis of 101 cases at autopsy. Arch Otolaryngol Head Neck Surg 113:762, 1987.

79. O'Brien PH, Carlson R, Steubner EA Jr, et al: Distant metastases in epidermoid cell carcinoma of the head and neck. Cancer 27:304, 1971.

80. Dennington ML, Carter DR, Meyers AD: Distant metastases in head and neck epidermoid carcinoma. Laryngoscope 90:196, 1980.

81. Chung TS, Stefani S: Distant metastases of carcinoma of tonsillar region: A study of 475 patients. J Surg Oncol 14:5, 1980.

82. Probert JC, Thompson RW, Bagshaw MA: Patterns of spread of distant metastases in head and neck cancer. Cancer 33:127, 1974.

83. Leemans CR, Tiwari R, Nautz JJP, et al: Regional lymph node involvement and its significance in the development of distant metastases in head and neck carcinoma. Cancer 71:452, 1993.

84. Papac RJ: Distant metastases from head and neck cancer. Cancer 53:342, 1984.

85. Vrabec DP: Multiple primary malignancies associated with index cancers of the oral, pharyngeal and laryngeal areas. Trans Pa Acad Ophthalmol Otolaryngol 32:177, 1979.

86. Shapshay SM, Hong WK, Fried MP, et al: Simultaneous carcinomas of the esophagus and upper aerodigestive tract. Otolaryngol Head Neck Surg 88:373, 1980.

87. Gluckman JL, Crissman JD, Donegan JO: Multicentric squamous-cell carcinoma of the upper aerodigestive tract. Head Neck Surg 3:90, 1980.

88. McGuirt WF, Matthews B, Koufman JA: Multiple simultaneous tumors in patients with head and neck cancer: A prospective, sequential panendoscopic study. Cancer 50:1195, 1982.

89. Vikram B, Strong EW, Shah JP, et al: Second malignant neoplasms in patients successfully treated with multimodality treatment for advanced head and neck cancer. Head Neck Surg 6:734, 1984.

90. King OH Jr, Coleman SA: Analysis of oral exfoliative cytologic accuracy by control biopsy technique. Acta Cytol 9:351, 1965.

91. Rovin S: An assessment of the negative oral cytologic diagnosis. Am Dent Assoc 74:759, 1967.

92. Shklar G, Meyer I, Cataldo E, et al: Correlated study of oral cytology and histopathology: Report on 2,052 oral lesions. Oral Surg 25:61, 1968.

93. Lundgren J, Olofsson J, Hellquist HB, et al: Exfoliative cytology in laryngology: Comparison of cytologic and histologic diagnoses in 350 microlaryngoscopic examinations—a prospective study. Cancer 47:1336, 1981.

94. Johnson JT, Turner J, Dekker A, et al: Significance of positive bronchial cytology in presence of squamous cell carcinoma of upper aerodigestive tract. Ann Otol Rhinol Laryngol 90:454, 1981.

95. Harris AH, Smith RR: Operative wound seeding with tumor cells:Its role in recurrences of head and neck cancer. Ann Surg 151:330, 1960.

96. Fisher JC, Ketcham AS, Hume RB, et al: Significance of cancer cells in operative wounds. Am J Surg 114:514, 1967.

97. Burger PC: Use of cytological preparations in the frozen section diagnosis of central nervous system neoplasia. Am J Surg Pathol 9:344, 1985.

98. Engzell U, Esposti PL, Rubio C, et al: Investigation on tumor spread in connection with aspiration biopsy. Acta Radiol Ther Stockh 10:385, 1971.

99. Smith EH: The hazards of fine-needle aspiration biopsy. Ultrasound Med Biol 10:629, 1984.

100. Sismanis A, Merrian JM, Kline TS, et al: Diagnosis of salivary gland tumors by fine needle aspiration biopsy. Head Neck Surg 3:482, 1981.

101. Qizilbash AH, Sianos J, Young JEM, et al: Fine needle aspiration biopsy cytology of major salivary glands. Acta Cytol 29:503, 1985.

102. O'Dwyer P, Farrar WB, James A, et al: Needle aspiration biopsy of major salivary gland tumors: Its value. Cancer 57:554, 1986.

103. Cohen MB, Liung BME, Boles R: Salivary gland tumors: Fine-needle aspiration vs frozen-section diagnosis. Arch Otolaryngol Head Neck Surg 112:867, 1986.

104. Layfield U, Tan P, Glasgow BJ: Fine-needle aspiration of salivary gland lesions: Comparison with frozen sections and histologic findings. Arch Pathol Lab Med 111:346, 1987.

105. Frable WJ: Thin-needle aspiration biopsy. In Major Problems in Pathology, vol 14. Philadelphia, WB Saunders, 1983.

106. Shaha A, Webber C, Marti J: Fine-needle aspiration in the diagnosis of cervical lymphadenopathy. Am J Surg 152:420, 1986.

107. Behm FG, O'Dowd GJ, Frable WJ: Fine-needle aspiration effects on benign lymph node histology. Am J Clin Pathol 82:195, 1984.

108. Ravetto C, Colombo L, Dottorini ME. Usefulness of fine-needle aspiration in the diagnosis of thyroid carcinoma. A retrospective study in 37,895 patients. Cancer (Cancer Cytopathol) 90:357, 2000.

109. Amrikachi M, Ramzy I, Rubenfeld S, et al: Accuracy of fine-needle aspiration of thyroid. A review of 6226 cases and correlation with surgical or clinical outcome. Arch Pathol Lab Med 125:484, 2001.

110. Miller JM, Hamburger JI, Kini S: Diagnosis of thyroid nodules: Use of fine-needle aspiration and needle biopsy. JAMA 241:481, 1979.

111. Lo Gerfo P, Colacchio T, Caushaj F, et al: Comparison of fine-needle and coarse-needle biopsies in evaluating thyroid nodules. Surgery 92:835, 1982.

112. Hamburger JL, Hamburger SW: Declining role of frozen section in surgical planning for thyroid nodules. Surgery 98:307, 1985.

113. Bugis SP, Young EM, Archibald SD, et al: Diagnostic accuracy of fine-needle aspiraton biopsy versus frozen section in solitary thyroid nodules. Am J Surg 152:411, 1986.

114. Mandell DS, Genden EM, Mechanick JI, et al: Diagnostic accuracy of fine-needle aspiration and frozen section in nodular thyroid disease. Otolaryngol Head Neck Surg 124:531, 2001.

115. Catania A, Cantalamessa L, Gasparmni P: Circulating thyroglobulin and anti-thyroglobulin antibodies after fine-needle aspiration of thyroid nodules. Horm Metab Res 17:49, 1985.

116. Kennerdell JS, Slamovits TL, Dekker A, et al: Orbital fine-needle aspiraton biopsy. Am J Ophthalmol 99:547, 1985.

117. Ackerman LV, Ramirez GA: The indications and limitations of frozen section diagnosis: A review of 1269 consecutive frozen section diagnoses. Br J Surg 46:336, 1959.

118. Saltzstein SL, Nahum AM: Frozen section diagnosis: Accuracy and errors; uses and abuses. Laryngoscope 83:1128, 1973.

119. Holaday WJ, Assor D: Ten thousand consecutive frozen sections: A retrospective study focusing on accuracy and quality control. Am J Clin Pathol 61:769, 1974.

120. Rogers C, Klatt EC, Chandrasoma P: Accuracy of frozen-section diagnosis in a teaching hospital. Arch Pathol Lab Med 11:514, 1987.

121. Bauer WC: The use of frozen sections in otolaryngology. Trans Am Acad Ophthalmol Otolaryngol 78:88, 1974.

122. Remsen KA, Lucente FE, Biller HF: Reliability of frozen section diagnosis in head and neck neoplasms. Laryngoscope 94:519, 1984.

123. Miller RH, Calcaterra TC, Paglia DE: Accuracy of frozen section diagnosis of parotid lesions. Ann Otol Rhinol Laryngol 88:573, 1979.

124. Hillel AD, Fee WE Jr: Evaluation of frozen section in parotid gland surgery. Arch Otolaryngol 109:230, 1983.

125. Wheelis RF, Yarington CT Jr: Tumors of the salivary glands: Comparison of frozen-section diagnosis with final pathologic diagnosis. Arch Otolaryngol 110:76, 1984.

126. Dindzans LI, Van Nostrand AWP: The accuracy of frozen section diagnosis of parotid lesions. J Otolaryngol 13:382, 1984.

127. Granick MS, Erickson ER, Hanna DC: Accuracy of frozen-section diagnosis in salivary gland lesions. Head Neck Surg 7:465, 1985.

128. Rigual NR, Milley P, Lore JM Jr, et al: Accuracy of frozen section diagnosis in salivary gland neoplasms. Head Neck Surg 8:442, 1986.

129. Gnepp DR, Rader WR, Cramer SF, et al: Accuracy of frozen section diagnosis of the salivary gland. Otolaryngol Head Neck Surg 96: 325, 1987.

130. Montone KT, Livolsi VA: Frozen section analysis of thyroidectomy specimens: Experience over a 12-year period. Pathol Case Rev 2:241, 1997.

131. Rosen Y, Rosenblatt P, Saltzman E: Intraoperative pathologic diagnosis of thyroid neoplasms. Report on experience with 504 specimens. Cancer 66:2001, 1990.

132. Leteurtre E, Leroy X, Pattou F, et al: Why do frozen sections have limited value in encapsulated or minimally invasive follicular carcinoma of the thyroid? Am J Clin Pathol 115:370, 2001.

133. DeMay RM: Frozen section of thyroid? Just say no. Am J Clin Pathol 110:423, 1998.

134. Taylor CR: Immunoperoxidase technique: Theory and applicability to surgical pathology. In Barnes L (ed): Surgical Pathology of the Head and Neck. New York, Marcel Dekker, 1985, p 23.

135. Mackay B, Ordonez NG: The role of the pathologist in the evaluation of poorly differentiated tumors. Semin Oncol 9:396, 1982.

136. Goodwin WJ Jr, Nadji NI: Immunoperoxidase staining in the diagnosis of malignant tumors of the head and neck. Otolaryngol Head Neck Surg 93:259, 1985.

137. Abemayor E, Kessler DJ, Ward PH, et al: Evaluation of poorly differentiated head and neck neoplasms. Immunocytochemistry techniques. Arch Otolaryngol Head Neck Surg 113:506, 1987.

138. Lovett EL III, Schnitzer B, Keren DF, et al: Application of flow cytometry to diagnostic pathology. Lab Invest 50:115, 1984.

139. Friedlander ML, Whedley DW, Taylor LW: Clinical and biological significance of aneuploidy in human tumors. J Clin Pathol 37:961, 1984.

140. Goldsmith MM, Cresson DH, Arnold LA, et al: DNA flow cytometry as a diagnostic indicator in head and neck cancer: Part 1. Otolaryngol Head Neck Surg 96:307, 1987.

141. Joensuu H, Klemi PJ, Eerola E: Diagnostic value of flow cytometric DNA determination combined with fine needle aspiration biopsy in thyroid tumors. Anal Quant Cytol Histol 9:328, 1987.

142. Joensuu H, Klemi PJ, Eerola E: DNA aneuploidy in follicular adenomas of the thyroid gland. Am J Pathol 124:373, 1986.

143. Carter R: Pathology of squamous cell carcinomas of the head and neck. Curr Opin Oncol 4:485, 1992.

144. Weinberg RA: How cancer arises. Sci Am 275:62–70, 1996.

145. Solomon E, Borrow J, Goddard AD: Chromosome aberrations and cancer. Science 254:1153–1160, 1991.

146. Carey TE, Worsham MJ, Van Dyke DL: Chromosomal biomarkers in the clonal evolution of head and neck squamous neoplasia. J Cell Biochem Suppl 17F:213–222, 1993.

147. Gollin SM: Chromosomal alterations in squamous cell carcinoma of the head and neck: Window to the biology of disease. Head Neck 23:238–253, 2001.

148. Lasko D, Cavenee W, Nordenskjold M: Loss of constitutional heterozygosity in human cancer. Ann Rev Genet 25:281–314, 1991.

149. Nawroz H, van der Riet P, Hruban RH, et al: Allelotype of head and neck squamous cell carcinoma. Cancer Res 54:1152–1155, 1994.

150. Field JK: Genomic instability in squamous cell carcinoma of the head and neck. Anticancer Res 16:2421–2432, 1996.

151. Califano J, van der Riet P, Westra W, et al: Genetic progression model for head and neck cancer: Implications for field cancerization. Cancer Res 56:2488–2492, 1996.

152. Lee CM, Rossie KM, Appel BN, et al: Visualization of Int2 and Hst1 amplification in oral squamous cell carcinomas. Genes Chromosomes Cancer 12:288–295, 1995.

153. Reed AL, Califano J, Cairns P, et al: High frequency of p16 (CDKN2/MTS-1/INK4A) inactivation in head and neck squamous cell carcinoma. Cancer Res 56:3630–3633, 1996.

154. Quon H, Liu FF, Cummings BJ: Potential molecular prognostic markers in head and neck squamous cell carcinomas. Head Neck 23:147–159, 2001.

155. Tabor MP, Brakenhoff RH, van Houten VMM, et al: Persistence of genetically altered fields in head and neck cancer patients: Biological and clinical implications. Clin Cancer Res 7:1523–1532, 2001.

156. Jang SJ, Chiba I, Hirai A, et al: Multiple oral squamous epithelial lesions: Are they genetically related? Oncogene 20:2235–2242, 2001.

157. van Qijen MGCT, Slootweg PJ: Oral field cancerization: Carcinogen-induced independent events or micrometastatic deposits? Cancer Epidemiol Biomarkers Prev 9:249–256, 2000.

158. Lydiatt WM, Anderson PE, Bazzana T, et al: Molecular support for field cancerization in the head and neck. Cancer 82:1376–1380, 1998.

159. Carey TE: Field cancerization: Are multiple primary cancers monoclonal or polyclonal? Ann Med 28:183–188, 1996.

160. Bedi GC, Westra WH, Gabrielson E, et al: Multiple head and neck tumors: Evidence for a common clonal origin. Cancer Res 56: 2484–2487, 1996.

161. Califano J, Westra WH, Meininger G, et al: Genetic progression and clonal relationship of recurrent premalignant head and neck lesions. Clin Cancer Res 6:347–352, 2000.

162. Boyle JO, Hakim J, Koch W, et al: The incidence of p53 mutations increases with progression of head and neck cancer. Cancer Res 53:4477–4480, 1993.

163. Slaughter DP, Southwick HW, Smejkal W: "Field cancerization" in oral stratified squamous epithelium: Clinical implications of multicentric origin. Cancer 6:963–968, 1953.

164. Guo ZM, Yamaguchi K, Sanchez-Cespedes M, et al: Allelic losses in OralTest-directed biopsies of patients with prior upper aerodigestive tract malignancy. Clin Cancer Res 7:1963–1968, 2001.

165. Partridge M, Pateromichelakis S, Phillips E, et al: A case-control study confirms that microsatellite assay can identify patients at risk of developing oral squamous cell carcinoma within a field of cancerization. Cancer Res 60:3893–3898, 2000.

166. Rosin MP, Cheng X, Poh C, et al: Use of allelic loss to predict malignant risk for low-grade oral epithelial dysplasia. Clin Cancer Res 6:357–362, 2000.

167. van der Riet P, Nawroz H, Hruban RH, et al: Frequent loss of chromosome 9p21-22 early in head and neck cancer progression. Cancer Res 54:1156–1158, 1994.

168. Partridge M, Li SR, Pateromichelakis S, et al: Detection of minimal residual cancer to investigate why oral tumors recur despite seemingly adequate treatment. Clin Cancer Res 6:2718–2725, 2000.

169. Brennan JA, Mao L, Hruban RH, et al: Molecular assessment of histopathological staging in squamous-cell carcinoma of the head and neck. N Engl J Med 332:429–435, 1995.

170. Homann N, Nees M, Conradt C, et al: Overexpression of p53 in tumor-distant epithelia of head and neck cancer patients is associated with increased incidence of second primary carcinoma. Clin Cancer Res 7:290–296, 2001.

171. Cruz IB, Snijders PJF, Meijer CJ, et al: p53 expression above the basal cell layer in oral mucosa is an early event of malignant transformation and has predictive value for developing oral squamous cell carcinoma. J Pathol 184:360–368, 1998.

172. Roh HJ, Shin DM, Lee JS, et al: Visualization of the timing of gene amplification during multistep head and neck tumorigenesis. Cancer Res 60:6496–6502, 2000.

173. Izzo JG, Papadimitrakopoulou VA, Li XQ, et al: Dysregulated cyclin D1 expression early in head and neck tumorigenesis: In vivo evidence for an association with subsequent gene amplification. Oncogene 17: 2313–2322, 1998.

174. Bartkova J, Lukas J, Muller H, et al: Abnormal pattern of D-type cyclin expression and G1 regulation in human head and neck cancer. Cancer Res 55:949–956, 1995.

175. Shin DM, Ro JY, Hong WK, Hittelman WN: Dysregulation of epidermal growth factor receptor expression in premalignant lesions during head and neck tumorigenesis. Cancer Res 54:3153–3159, 1994.

176. Sorrells D, Ghali GE, De Benedetti A, et al: Progressive amplification and overexpression of the eukaryotic initiation factor 4E gene in different zones of head and neck cancers. J Oral Maxillofac Surg 57: 294–299, 1999.

177. Nathan CO, Liu L, Li BDL, et al: Detection of the proto-oncogene eIF4E in surgical margins may predict recurrence in head and neck cancer. Oncogene 15:579–584, 1997.

178. Califano J, Leong PL, Koch WM, et al: Second esophageal tumors in patients with head and neck squamous cell carcinoma: an assessment of clonal relationships. Clin Cancer Res 5:1862–1867, 1999.

179. Sinard RJ, Netterville JL, Garrett CG, Ossoff RH: Cancer of the larynx. In Suen JY, Myers EN (eds): Cancer of the Head and Neck, 3rd ed. New York, Churchill Livingstone, 1996, pp 381–421.

180. Renner GJ, Zitsch RB III: Cancer of the lip. In Suen JY, Myers EN (eds): Cancer of the Head and Neck, 3rd ed. New York, Churchill Livingstone, 1996, pp 294–320.

181. Spafford MF, Koch WM, Reed AL, et al: Detection of head and neck squamous cell carcinoma among exfoliated oral mucosal cells by microsatellite analysis. Clin Cancer Res 7:607–612, 2001.

182. Partridge M, Emilion GG, Pateromichelakis S, et al: Allelic imbalance at chromosomal loci implicated in the pathogenesis of oral precancer; cumulative loss and its relationship with progression to cancer. Eur J Cancer Oral Oncol 34:77–83, 1998.

183. Mao L, Lee JS, Fan YH, et al: Frequent microsatellite alterations at chromosome 9p21 and 3p14 in oral premalignant lesions and their value in cancer risk assessment. Nat Med 2:682–685, 1996.

184. Rubin P: A unified classification of cancers: An oncotaxonomy with symbols. Cancer 31:963, 1973.

185. Jones E, Lund VJ, Howard DJ, et al: Quality of life of patients treated surgically for head and neck cancer. J Laryngol Otol 106:238–242, 1992.

186. de Visscher AVM, Manni JJ: Routine long-term follow-up in patients treated with curative intent for squamous cell carcinoma of the larynx, pharynx, and oral cavity. Does it make sense? Arch Otolaryngol Head Neck Surg 120:934–939, 1994.

187. Leemans CR, Tiwari R, Nauta JJP, et al: Recurrence at the primary site in head and neck lymph node metastasis as a prognostic factor. Cancer 73:187–190, 1994.

188. Moore C: Cigarette smoking and cancer of the mouth, pharynx and larynx. JAMA 218:553–560, 1971.

189. Jones AS, Morar P, Phillips DE, et al: Second primary tumors in patients with head and neck squamous cell carcinoma. Cancer 75:1343–1353, 1995.

190. Schwartz LH, Ozsahin M, Zhang GN, et al: Synchronous and metachronous head and neck carcinomas. Cancer 74:1933–1938, 1994.

191. Lippman SM, Hong WK: Second malignant tumors in head and neck squamous cell carcinoma: The overshadowing threat for patients with early-stage disease. Int J Radiat Oncol Biol Phys 17: 691–694, 1989.

192. Wynder EL, Mushinski MH, Spivak JC: Tobacco and alcohol consumption in relation to the development of multiple primary cancers. Cancer 40:1872–1878, 1997.

193. Hong WK, Lippman SM, Itri LM, et al: Prevention of second primary tumors with isotretinoin in squamous-cell carcinoma of the head and neck. N Engl J Med 323:795–801, 1990.

194. Benner SE, Pajak TF, Lippman SM, et al: Prevention of second primary tumors with isotretinoin in patients with squamous cell carcinoma of the head and neck: Long-term follow-up. J Natl Cancer Inst 86:140–141, 1994.

195. Worsham MJ, Wolman SR, Carey TE, et al: Common clonal origin of synchronous primary head and neck squamous cell carcinomas: Analysis by tumor karyotypes and fluorescence in situ hybridization. Hum Pathol 26:251–261, 1995.

196. Koch WM, Boyle JO, Mao L, et al: p53 gene mutations as markers of tumor spread in synchronous oral cancers. Arch Otolaryngol Head Neck Surg 120:943–947, 1994.

197. van Oijen MG, Leppers Vd Straat FG, Tilanus MG, Slootweg PJ: The origins of multiple squamous cell carcinomas in the aerodigestive tract. Cancer 88:884–893, 2000.

198. Chung KY, Mukhopadhyay T, Kim J, et al: Discordant p53 gene mutations in primary head and neck cancers and corresponding second primary cancers of the upper aerodigestive tract. Cancer Res 53:1676–1683, 1993.

199. Fearon ER, Vogelstein B: A genetic model for colorectal tumorigenesis. Cell 61:759–767, 1990.

200. Alvi A, Johnson JT: Extracapsular spread in the clinically negative neck (N0): Implications and outcome. Otolaryngol Head Neck Surg 114:65–70, 1996.

201. Don DM, Anzai Y, Lufkin RB, et al: Evaluation of cervical lymph node metastases in squamous cell carcinoma of the head and neck. Laryngoscope 105:669–674, 1995.

202. Kowalski LP, Magrin J, Waksman G, et al: Supraomohyoid neck dissection in the treatment of head and neck tumors. Survival results in 212 cases. Arch Otolaryngol Head Neck Surg 119:958–963, 1993.

203. Johnson JT, Barnes EL, Myers EN, et al: The extracapsular spread of tumors in cervical node metastasis. Arch Otolaryngol 107: 725–729, 1981.

204. Close LG, Merkel M, Vuitch MF, et al: Computed tomographic evaluation of regional lymph node involvement in cancer of the oral cavity and oropharynx. Head Neck 11:309–317, 1989.

205. van den Brekel MW, Castelijns JA, Croll GA, et al: Magnetic resonance imaging vs palpation of cervical lymph node metastasis. Arch Otolaryngol Head Neck Surg 117:663–673, 1991.

206. Pitman KT, Johnson JT, Myers EN: Effectiveness of selective neck dissection for management of the clinically negative neck. Arch Otolaryngol Head Neck Surg 123:917–922, 1997.

207. Friedman M, Mafee MF, Pacella BLJ, et al: Rationale for elective neck dissection in 1990. Laryngoscope 100:54–59, 1999.

208. Martin H: The case for prophylactic neck dissection. CA Cancer J Clin 40:245–251, 1990.

209. Takes RP, Baatenburg de Jong RJ, Schuuring E, et al: Markers for assessment of nodal metastasis in laryngeal carcinoma. Arch Otolaryngol Head Neck Surg 123:412–419, 1997.

210. Capaccio P, Pruneri G, Carboni N, et al: Cyclin D1 expression is predictive of occult metastases in head and neck cancer patients with clinically negative cervical lymph nodes. Head Neck 22:234–240, 2000.

211. Fielding LP, Fenoglio-Preiser CM, Freedman LS: The future of prognostic factors in outcome prediction for patients with cancer. Cancer 70:2367–2377, 1992.

212. Feinmesser R, Freeman JL, Feinmesser M, et al: Role of modern imaging in decision-making for elective neck dissection. Head Neck 14:173–176, 1992.

213. Wang Y, Hung SC, Linn JF, et al: Microsatellite-based cancer detection using capillary array electrophoresis and energy-transfer fluorescent primers. Electrophoresis 18:1742–1748, 1997.

214. Duggan DJ, Bittner M, Chen Y, et al: Expression profiling using cDNA microarrays. Nat Genet 21:10–14, 1999.

215. Villaret DB, Wang T, Dillon D, et al: Identification of genes overexpressed in head and neck squamous cell carcinoma using a combination of complementary DNA subtraction and microarray analysis. Laryngoscope 110:374–381, 2000.

216. Leethanakul C, Patel V, Gillespie J, et al: Distinct pattern of expression of differentiation and growth-related genes in squamous cell carcinomas of the head and neck revealed by the use of laser capture microdissection and cDNA arrays. Oncogene 19:3220–3224, 2000.

217. Hanna E, Shrieve DC, Ratanatharathorn V, et al: A novel alternative approach for prediction of radiation response of squamous cell carcinoma of head and neck. Cancer Res 61:2376–2380, 2001.

CHAPTER 4

Evaluation, Classification, and Staging

Jay F. Piccirillo
Carla M. Huff
Frederic A. Pugliano

■ INTRODUCTION

Every patient with cancer of the head and neck requires a comprehensive evaluation by a multidisciplinary team. This chapter addresses general principles applicable to the broad topic of evaluation, classification, and staging. A combined approach, including the head and neck surgeon, radiation oncologist, medical oncologist, speech pathologist, nutritionist, social worker, and clinical nurse specialist, provides each patient with a thorough and organized diagnostic evaluation and treatment plan. The standard collection of patient, tumor, treatment, and outcome information allows for outcome and quality of care assessment.

■ EVALUATION

The history and physical examination at the initial consultation establish a foundation for subsequent laboratory and radiographic evaluation and treatment planning. Psychosocial and nutritional assessments, followed by intervention when indicated, are vital to achieving optimal outcomes. Treatment should not begin until the patient and physician have a clear understanding of the goals of treatment.

Regular post-treatment follow-up visits provide an opportunity for the patient and physician to achieve the goals of treatment, typically, eradication of tumor and rehabilitation of function. Although the primary function of follow-up is to provide surveillance for new or recurrent disease, the physician also provides guidance and reassurance and can provide access to resources that can improve the patient's quality of life and functional capacity.

History

Although many patients present with an established diagnosis, a careful history generates a complete differential diagnosis, ensuring that all diagnostic possibilities are considered prior to establishment of a definitive diagnosis. Symptoms related to the tumor often suggest a specific anatomic site. For example, hoarseness indicates probable laryngeal involvement. The presence of risk factors for the development of cancer of the head and neck, such as the use of tobacco products, alcohol abuse, and environmental exposure to wood dust or heavy metals, increases the likelihood of cancer.

The history also provides estimates of prognosis and aids in the selection of proper treatment. The severity of the disease is determined by the duration, type, and rate of progression of symptoms and the functional impairment experienced by the patient. Symptoms of systemic disease, such as bone pain, jaundice, or hemoptysis, necessitate a complete metastatic evaluation.

Medical comorbidities significantly affect the patient's treatment planning and prognosis. Review of the past medical history helps in identification of specific comorbidities. The severity of a patient's comorbidities is determined by functional and objective criteria. Communication with the primary care physician may provide insights into the patient's general health. The clinician is well advised to seek medical consultation for patients who have newly diagnosed or inadequately treated complex medical problems.

Physical Examination

The examiner must correlate physical findings with the patient's history. The specifics of the examination of the head and neck are beyond the scope of this chapter. In general, careful inspection and palpation of the surfaces and cavities of the head and neck enable the clinician to localize and characterize the pathologic changes that are causing the patient's symptoms. For example, the gloved finger may detect a firm mass in the base of the tongue that is responsible for a patient's ankyloglossia. The examiner should give special attention to abnormalities in the texture and color of the mucosal linings of the upper aerodigestive tract. Areas of ulceration or leukoplakia are suspicious for malignancy, as is a mass that is abnormally firm or fixed to adjacent structures. Clinical assessment of the neck is based on determination of the size, number, and consistency of palpable lymph nodes. The examination of the head and neck confirms the location of the tumor and along with radiographic evaluation forms the basis for the tumor, node, and metastasis (TNM) staging system.[1]

The introduction of fiberoptic technology into the office setting has greatly enhanced the clinician's ability to examine the upper aerodigestive tract.[2] Videolaryngoscopy produces a permanent record of the examination that allows for subsequent review and also may be used in patient education.[3]

Medical Evaluation

Medical comorbidities are identified by history; review of the medical records, including the results of laboratory tests; and communication with the patient's primary care physician. The severity of comorbidities is determined by the subjective complaints of the patient and objective findings from examination and diagnostic testing. For example, the severity of a patient's congestive heart failure can be revealed by the presence of orthopnea or paroxysmal nocturnal dyspnea, and an echocardiogram provides an objective measurement of cardiac function. The American Society of Anesthesiologists (ASA) scoring guide estimates a patient's anesthetic risk based on age, medical comorbidities, anatomic abnormalities, and prior anesthetic experience.[4] The ASA score gives an objective assessment of a patient's ability to tolerate a planned surgical procedure. Appropriate preoperative testing should be based on age, sex, concomitant medical disease, and type of surgery to be performed. Preoperative testing performed on a routine basis without careful consideration has been shown to be neither clinically useful nor cost-effective.[5]

Assessment of performance status is important in the medical evaluation of the patient with cancer of the head and neck. Performance status is a global assessment of a patient's ability to perform activities of daily living and has been shown to be an important prognostic factor in a wide variety of cancers.[6] Poor performance status as established by the Specific Activities Scale has proved to be one of the strongest predictors of postoperative medical complications.[7] A number of tools have been developed to provide reliable data on performance status. A patient's performance status should be followed from the pretreatment phase through recovery. Changes in performance status enable the clinician to evaluate the impact of interventions on the patient's overall health. In addition to performance status, measurements of health-related quality of life should be recorded as an integral part of the pretreatment and posttreatment assessment.

Metastatic Workup

Cancer of the head and neck is generally considered a regional disease owing to the tendency of metastatic spread to be restricted to the lymph nodes in many histologic cell types. However, the possibility of systemic metastasis should not be overlooked, particularly in patients with a large primary tumor mass or bulky neck disease. In squamous cell carcinoma, the lungs are the most common sites of metastasis (83%), followed by the skeletal system (31%) and liver (6%).[8, 9]

A chest radiograph is adequate for routine screening; however, the additional sensitivity of computed tomography (CT) can be invaluable in ruling pulmonary metastasis in or out. In patients with abnormal liver function studies, CT scan of the abdomen is useful in ruling out metastasis to the liver. Although positron emission tomography (PET) scanning in the patient with advanced-stage disease may demonstrate distant metastasis, the utility of bone scanning in the asymptomatic patient must be questioned.[10, 11] Although metastatic disease has a profound impact on treatment and outcome, restricting the use of adjunctive testing to patients with suspicious symptoms or abnormal laboratory findings results in a more cost-effective and appropriate evaluation.

Nutritional Assessment

Patients with cancer of the head and neck often present with nutritional depletion from disruption of the normal anatomic pathways for dietary intake. Frequently, these patients are known abusers of alcohol and tobacco, which results in further nutritional depletion. Malnutrition can compromise immunologic function, inhibit wound healing, and increase susceptibility to infection. Regardless of the chosen course of treatment, patients with nutritional deficiencies will benefit from nutritional support.

Choosing the appropriate form of support requires a thorough baseline nutritional assessment. Although a registered dietician is indispensable in generating accurate baseline measures, the physician can quickly identify the high-risk patient based on readily available data. A patient who experiences a 10% decrease in his or her usual weight and is found to have a serum albumin less than 3.2 mg/dL or a total lymphocyte count less than 1500 cells/mL is considered malnourished and will benefit from nutritional supplementation.[12] Additional data may be obtained to more clearly define the patient's specific nutritional needs. The nature of the patient's malignancy, type of therapy, and duration of need for support are considered so that the safest, most cost-effective form of nutritional support can be administered to the individual patient.

The prognostic nutritional index (PNI) has been studied as an indicator of postoperative complications in patients with head and neck cancer.[13] Combining anthropometric data, laboratory evaluation, and measurements of immune function, the PNI accurately gauges a patient's nutritional status. The triceps skinfold (TSF) thickness, the serum albumin (ALB) and transferrin (TFN) levels, and the number of positive responses to delayed hypersensitivity (DH) skin testing are combined using the following formula:

$$PNI = 158\% - 0.78\,(TSF) - 16.6\,(ALB) - 0.2\,(TFN) - 5.8\,(DH)$$

Patients with advanced-stage head and neck cancer and a PNI greater than 20% have been shown to be at increased risk for a major complication following surgery for head and neck cancer.[13]

The goals of nutritional support must be established prior to supplementation. In most cases, the primary goal of nutritional support is the reversal of the catabolic state seen in many cancer patients. Increases in serum transferrin and prealbumin provide the earliest evidence of anabolic metabolism.[14] Increase in lean body mass has been suggested as a goal for pretreatment supplementation. However, owing to the metabolic demands of the tumor, attempts to build lean body mass are usually unsuccessful. Optimization of nutritional status must be balanced with prompt therapy of the malignancy. A low threshold for initiating nutritional supplementation should be maintained because of the high complication rate associated with malnutrition.[15]

Once the need for nutritional support has been established, the route of supplementation is selected. Whenever possible, nutritional support is provided through the natural alimentary tract. The implementation of tube feedings has been shown to be more effective than ad libitum oral supplementation.[16] Preoperatively, anorexia, lethargy, and tumor bulk may compromise the effectiveness of oral supplementation, and postoperatively, structural alterations affecting deglutition and ability to protect the airway may continue to impair oral intake.

Traditionally, the nasogastric tube has been used for supplementation in these situations. However, technical improvement in the fluoroscopic and endoscopic placement of gastrostomy tubes has provided an alternative in patients requiring long-term tube feedings. In our experience, patient satisfaction is greater with the gastrostomy than with the nasogastric tube. Although it is apparently more invasive and costly, one study has shown a decrease in postoperative complications and length of hospital stay with the use of gastrostomy.[17] The use of total parenteral nutrition (TPN) in patients with cancer of the head and neck may be necessary for patients who cannot tolerate enteral feeding. TPN should be implemented in a timely fashion to achieve optimal results.

Psychosocial Assessment

Patients are more psychologically invested in the head and neck than in other parts of the body.[18] Patients with head and neck cancer suffer the burden of a life-threatening illness, yet unlike many cancer patients, they are unable to conceal their affliction from public view. Treatments that result in dysfunction or disfigurement of the structures of the head and neck can have great psychological impact on the patient and may lead to social isolation. Each tumor site in the head and neck presents unique challenges that must be met if quality of life issues are considered in treatment. It is the physician who must recognize the differences and provide the patient with options to overcome these challenges.[19] Patients with advanced-stage cancer tend to have a greater number of quality of life issues than do those with limited disease; younger patients and female patients tend to have worse emotional and social adjustment to their disease. The presence of comorbidities and a lack of social support may also have a negative impact on the patient's quality of life.[19] Other factors to consider when treating patients with cancer of the head and neck include coping skills, personality disorders, and a history of psychiatric illness or substance abuse. Preoperative psychosocial evaluation can identify patients at risk for developing psychiatric problems during the course of the disease.[20]

Patients who undergo treatment for head and neck cancer frequently have problems with self-esteem due to a change in self-image.[21] These effects are greatest after major disfiguring surgery. Emotional maturity and ability to cope with changes in body image directly affect patients' psychological health during the postoperative period. Reactive anxiety and depression are the most common psychiatric problems seen in cancer patients.[22] Patients with preexisting anxiety or depressive disorders are at risk for developing major psychiatric problems as a result of oncologic therapy. Suicidal ideation is not uncommon.

Alcohol and tobacco abuse are noted in many patients with cancer of the head and neck. Alcohol abuse can create many medical and psychological problems during treatment.

Patients actively abusing alcohol should undergo detoxification to avoid withdrawal reaction during therapy. Nicotine withdrawal can lead to anxiety, sleep disturbances, and headache. Withdrawal can be avoided by the judicious use of transdermal or oral nicotine supplements. A history of abuse of certain analgesics or mood elevators should be sought because withdrawal from these medications can be as severe as alcohol withdrawal.

Preoperative counseling can reduce uncertainty and restore a feeling of self-control in the head and neck cancer patient. An understanding of the treatment plan, which is developed with patient input, reduces the patient's anxiety during the preoperative period. Meeting with speech therapists, support groups, and former patients helps patients understand the post-treatment changes and provides tangible proof that patients can survive the cancer and its treatment. The clinician should provide appropriate pretreatment counseling and encourage patient participation in support groups.

Radiologic Evaluation

CT and magnetic resonance imaging (MRI) are useful in the assessment of the deep tissue extensions of tumors of the head and neck.[23] CT effectively demonstrates bone changes such as erosive lesions at the skull base or mandible. MRI has multiplanar imaging capability and can show subtle variations in soft tissue, distinguishing inflammatory changes from fibrosis or recurrent tumor.[24] Each modality has its advantages, even within anatomic subsites. For example, a CT scan shows early erosion of the bone of the cranial base, whereas MRI can show intracranial extension through the foramen ovale or pterygoid canal. The decision to use MRI versus CT is based on the information needed in a particular case. The sensitivity for these modalities in finding disease ranges from 80% to 90%.[25]

PET using ^{18}F fluorodeoxyglucose ([18]FDG) is a newer imaging modality that has been evaluated at various institutions for a variety of indications in patients with cancer of the head and neck. Compared with CT and MRI, PET has lower spatial resolution, rendering it less suitable for accurate anatomic assessment of tumor extent. However, because [18]FDG-PET is able to assess tissue metabolic activity, it has shown promise in distinguishing recurrent tumor from post-treatment fibrosis. Currently, the high cost of PET prohibits its widespread use; therefore, it is usually reserved for selected cases of head and neck cancer for which more specific information is needed than CT or MRI can provide.[25] Machines that combine PET with CT are currently being evaluated and will, no doubt, prove to be useful in certain situations.

Accurate evaluation of the extent of local tumor involvement and regional metastasis is critical in treatment planning for cancer of the head and neck. Radiologic criteria for cervical lymph node metastasis have been correlated with pathologic specimens in several studies. Lymph nodes larger than 1 cm and the presence of central necrosis have been shown to be the most reliable radiographic criteria.[26] CT has been shown to alter the clinical description of neck metastasis in 20% to 30% of cases, with most cases being upstaged from the physical examination.[27] The presence of extensive local or regional metastasis noted on CT affects treatment planning.

Patients with metastasis to the cervical lymph nodes and an unknown primary lesion present a challenging diagnostic problem. When the primary lesion is too small to be detected or is located in an area inaccessible to endoscopic evaluation, metastatic cancer may be detected before the primary lesion. Diagnostic imaging is used to locate the occult primary cancer or to identify suspicious areas for tissue biopsy and/or fine-needle aspiration. CT and ultrasound guidance are used to increase the accuracy of such biopsies.[28]

Future developments in radiographic techniques may prove beneficial to the evaluation of the patient with head and neck cancer. Magnetic resonance angiography (MRA) has shown promise for assessing flow in the carotid artery and for determining the presence of invasive tumor within the lumen.[29] MRA may also prove useful in evaluation of both donor and recipient vascular beds when free-flap reconstruction is planned.

Cytology

In patients with a known primary tumor and clinically positive cervical metastasis, fine-needle aspiration biopsy (FNAB) adds little to the diagnostic evaluation. However, in the patient with a neck mass of unknown cause, FNAB can save the time and expense of extensive evaluation for malignant disease and can avoid the potential complications of open biopsy. Several studies have shown the excellent diagnostic accuracy of FNAB.[30, 31] To achieve this high degree of diagnostic accuracy, the cytopathologist must be well trained in the interpretation of head and neck aspiration cytology. As in other areas of medicine, if the findings of FNAB do not correlate with the clinical picture, the clinician should pursue further diagnostic evaluation until he or she is confident about the findings.

Endoscopy

Preoperative evaluation of the patient with squamous cell carcinoma of the head and neck includes panendoscopy to detect the presence of synchronous secondary primary cancers. This is typically performed in the operating room when the patient is undergoing biopsy of the primary lesion. In the interest of reducing costs, clinicians have attempted to reduce the use of operating room time. Many biopsies can be performed in the office setting, and fiberoptic technology has helped improve the effectiveness of this practice.[32] In addition, many clinicians have supplanted esophagoscopy and bronchoscopy with barium swallow esophagrams and chest radiographs.

In one study, in which patients were selected for endoscopy based on having one or more risk factors for a second primary cancer, panendoscopy revealed a synchronous lesion in less than 2% of cases.[33] The cost-effectiveness of routine panendoscopy was prospectively evaluated in 100 patients.[34] Results of the study showed a one-third savings in total cost and a reduction in unnecessary procedures if bronchoscopy and esophagoscopy were reserved for symptomatic patients. It should be noted that Japanese investigators have been able to increase the yield of esophagoscopy with the addition of Lugol's solution to endoscopic evaluation.[35]

A recent study,[36] which evaluated 358 patients who underwent panendoscopy for primary tumor, showed an incidence of 6.4% synchronous primary tumors; 3% of these were found on panendoscopy. The remainder were seen on outpatient examination or chest radiograph. The location of the synchronous lesion varied depending on primary site. Patients with cancer of the oral cavity and oropharynx had tumors throughout the entire aerodigestive tract. Patients with hypopharyngeal cancer primaries tended to have synchronous tumors in the esophagus. Patients with laryngeal tumors most often had second primary cancer in the lung. Owing to the varied locations of the synchronous lesions, a chest radiograph alone was believed to be insufficient for diagnosing these tumors. These studies demonstrate the controversy surrounding the role of panendoscopy in the diagnosis of head and neck cancer.

Future Directions

Incorporation of the findings of molecular biology into the clinical practice of head and neck oncology has yet to become a reality. However, Bradford and associates[37] studied the prognostic utility of several specific tumor markers and biologic factors in patients with advanced-disease laryngeal cancer. Traditional tumor staging information was recorded before treatment, and biopsy specimens were analyzed for histologic characteristics, proliferating cell nuclear antigen (PCNA), and *TP53* expression. Multivariable analysis identified extranodal extension as the only factor predictive of overall survival; extranodal extension and aggressive growth pattern were predictive of decreased disease-free survival. Extent of primary tumor (T class) was the only factor predictive of chemotherapy response; T class, *TP53* overexpression, and elevated PCNA index were predictive of successful organ preservation. It is likely that molecular biologic techniques, as they become more widely used and their prognostic value is validated, will be incorporated into clinical practice.

Post-treatment Follow-up

Follow-up of patients treated for cancer of the head and neck currently focuses on surveillance for new or recurrent disease. A recent review of nationwide practices shows that a majority of clinicians see patients monthly during the first post-treatment year.[38] Sixty percent of respondents recommend an annual chest radiograph, whereas other testing is reserved for symptomatic patients. A majority of second malignant tumors arise in the lung, which explains the current practice of using the annual chest radiograph as a screening tool.[39] In a meta-analysis of 40,287 head and neck cancer patients, Haughey and coworkers[40] found a 14.2% prevalence of second malignant tumors, with the majority presenting as metachronous lesions. Based on these results, the authors emphasized aggressive follow-up monitoring. Recent studies have suggested a role for [18]FDG-PET in detecting recurrent cancer in the irradiated patient.[41]

Surveillance for recurrent disease in the postoperative period is essential. A prospective study of 428 head and neck cancer patients showed improved survival when recurrence was detected on routine follow-up rather than on self-referral (58 vs. 32 months, $P < .05$).[42]

In addition to recognition of recurrent disease, recent literature has increasingly stressed the importance of measuring and improving functional status and quality of life. Cancer of the head and neck and its treatment can have tremendous impact on these. Clinicians have long recognized the importance of survival, pain control, and impairment of speech and swallowing. Studies have also shown the importance of body image, social acceptance, and sexual function on patient satisfaction postoperatively.[43, 44] Patient-based questionnaires can provide much information about the impact of various treatment regimens on health status and quality of life. These data can reveal important problems in a patient's life that may not have been evident to the physician and other members of the health care team. The clinician can then direct treatment and counseling efforts to the specific areas identified. In addition, this information can be used to evaluate the effectiveness of treatment and to improve patient care in the future.

CLASSIFICATION OF TUMORS

Historical Perspective on Classification of Cancer

The problem of the classification of cancers has occupied the attention of physicians and other scientists for decades.[45] Denoix and Schwartz[46] originally described the TNM system of cancer classification in 1948. This system was incorporated in 1953 by the Union International Contre le Cancer (UICC) and the International Congress of Radiology into a formal classification system for cancer.[47] The TNM system was adopted in the United States in 1959, when the American College of Surgeons, the American College of Radiology, the College of American Pathologists, the American College of Physicians, the American Cancer Society, and the National Cancer Institute sponsored the formation of the American Joint Committee on Cancer (AJCC) Staging and End-Results Reporting.[1] The stated purpose of the AJCC was "to develop systems for the clinical classification of cancer, which would be of value to practicing American physicians."[48] During the past 30 years, the AJCC has worked to develop TNM definitions and stage classifications for all anatomic sites and subsites, to revise definitions and classifications from results of clinical studies, and to educate physicians and other health care professionals about the TNM classification system. In 1988, the AJCC reached agreement with the UICC for a common TNM and stage classification system, thereby resolving many minor differences that had previously prevented the creation of a single tumor classification system. In 1992, Public Law 102-515[49] authorized $30 million annually for 5 years to establish a national cancer registry. Managed by the Centers for Disease Control and Prevention (CDC), the registry allows individual states to collect comprehensive, consistent information on the incidence of cancer by type, severity, and patient background.[49]

Reasons for Classification

A series of rules for classifying cancers has evolved to describe the extent of the cancer. Difficulties arise because different cancers may be classified by a variety of methods. Without standard definitions for the reporting of cancers and cancer patients, confusion arises in cancer statistics, including the reporting of results and evaluation of treatment. The standardization of cancer classification provides uniform collection and reporting of cancer-related information in cancer registries. The objectives of cancer classification have been stated by the UICC and AJCC and include the following: (1) to aid the clinician in planning treatment,

(2) to give an indication of prognosis, (3) to assist in the evaluation of end results, (4) to facilitate the exchange of information between treatment centers, and (5) to assist in the continuing investigation of cancer.

To investigate the reasons for and value of cancer classification, one of us (J.F.P.) surveyed by mailed questionnaire 101 physicians specializing in the care of patients with cancer of the head and neck.[50] Of the five stated purposes of cancer staging, *to assist in the evaluation of end results* was rated most important overall. However, a considerable degree of variation existed among the respondents in the relative importance of the five purposes.

Rules for Morphologic Classification

Morphologic classification is an attempt to establish standard measures of the physical extent of neoplasms across different anatomic sites. Differences in clinical presentation are due to differences in the location of the cancer, the function of the affected structure, the clinical biology of the cancer, and the health status of the host. The clinical evaluation varies by the accessibility of the tumor to physical examination and radiographic study. The criteria for classification do not change from site to site, nor are negative inferences made simply because of an inability to fully evaluate the disease process.[47] Owing to the variability in clinical presentation, tumors from all sites are classified in general terms according to the anatomic extent of primary tumor (T), the degree of regional lymph node involvement (N), and the presence or absence of distant metastatic disease (M). Classification must be distinguished from staging, which is the grouping of cancers with similar crude survival rates.

Classification of Microscopic Morphology

The histologic type is determined qualitatively by comparing the cancer with the most closely related tissue or cell type.[1] The predominant histologic type of cancer in the head and neck is squamous cell carcinoma. The histologic type can be further classified according to the degree of differentiation of the tumor, as follows: GX, grade cannot be assessed; G1, well differentiated; G2, moderately well differentiated; G3, poorly differentiated; and G4, undifferentiated.

Other tumors of the head and neck may originate from tissues of glandular, odontogenic, lymphoid, bony, or cartilaginous origin. Only tumors of squamous cell origin are included in the AJCC TNM cancer staging system.[1]

Classification of Gross Morphology

The TNM system classifies a cancer's gross morphology or macroscopic spread from primary to distant sites according to the following three dimensions:

T = extent of primary tumor, described in five T categories: T in situ, T1, T2, T3, and T4

N = extent of regional lymph node spread, described in four N categories: N0, N1, N2, and N3

M = presence of distant metastases, dichotomized as M0 or M1

T Categories. The general criteria for categorizing cancer of the head and neck are extent of surface spread and size of the tumor. Vocal cord function is used for classifying laryngeal cancers. Depth of invasion has been shown to be prognostically important for cancers of the oral cavity[51] but is not used for tumor classification. Size of the tumor is related to the number of cells and may also be related to the age of the tumor. However, assumptions about the age of the tumor (i.e., "early" or "late") based on its size are fraught with hazard because rate of growth, cell removal or loss, and host resistance factors all affect the size of the tumor.[47] The use of the term "early cancer" should therefore be discouraged.

N Categories. The general criteria for the classification of regional lymph node metastasis are based on size, number, distribution, and level of involvement.

Size is one of the most important criteria in node classification. However, size may be difficult to determine clinically. A superficial node that is greater than 0.5 cm in diameter is usually palpable, whereas a more deeply situated node must reach 1 cm in diameter before it becomes palpable.[52] Level of lymph node involvement is generally discussed in terms of *echelon*[53] or station. Station refers to a regular stopping place in a stage of progression. The first station is the cluster of lymph nodes receiving direct drainage of a specific site or organ. The second station refers to those nodes that commonly receive lymph drainage from other lymph nodes rather than directly from the site or organ. Level of lymph node involvement has been shown to be of prognostic importance[54, 55] but is not included in the N classification.

M Categories. Metastasis is classified as present or absent, that is, M0 or M1. When a metastatic workup has not been completed and the probability of metastasis is low, the designation MX should be used.

◐ STAGING

TNM System for Unified Stage Grouping

The Venn diagram[45] (Fig. 4–1) illustrates the possible spread of cancer. For each cancer, the individual T, N, and M category ratings are combined to form expressions such as T2N1M0 or T3N2M1. Because five categories of T, four categories of N, and two categories of M create 40 possible combinations for the TNM expressions, the combinations were combined into stage groupings to ease statistical analyses (*stages I, II, III,* and *IV*).[1,56] The various combinations were selected based on the observation that patients with localized tumors had higher survival rates than patients with widespread tumors. When there is no nodal involvement, the stage is determined by the extent of primary tumor. Thus, T1 = stage I; T2 = stage II; T3 = stage III; and T4 = stage IV. With nodal involvement, stage is essentially determined by assessment of extent of nodal involvement. Thus, N1 is classified as stage III for T1 to T3 and stage IV when T = 4. When N is greater than N1, the stage is stage IV (Table 4–1).

The terms "localized" and "widespread" are often interchanged with "early" and "late," implying some regular progression with time. This implication erroneously led to the thought that stage I progressed to stage II, then to stage III. Denoix and Schwartz[46] recognized that orderly progression was not observed at all times, a point that has been restated by the AJCC: "Actually the stage of disease at the time of diagnosis may be a reflection of the neoplasm but also of the type of tumor and of the tumor-host relationship."[1]

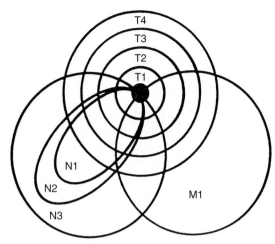

FIGURE 4–1 Venn diagram of cancer spread illustrates the lack of an orderly, predictable progression. The black central focus represents subclinical disease, and each large circle illustrates the different tumor (T), node (N), and metastasis (M) categories. The potential for spread exists in any of these directions. (From Rubin P: A unified classification of cancers: An oncotaxonomy with symbols. Cancer 31:963, 1973.)

In the AJCC *Manual for Staging of Cancer,*[1] the following head and neck sites are included: the oral cavity, the pharynx (nasopharynx, oropharynx, and hypopharynx), the larynx, and the paranasal sinuses. The various subsites and exact anatomic boundaries are discussed in detail in the *Manual* and elsewhere in this text. The T and N definitions for the various major head and neck subsites are shown in Table 4–2 and Table 4–3.

Cancer Statistics

Definition of Starting Time

A definition of the starting time or "zero" time[57,58] forms the basis for the calculation of survival and other outcomes measures. Various starting times are commonly used: (1) date of diagnosis, (2) date of first visit to physician or clinic, (3) date of hospital admission, and (4) date of treatment initiation.[1] If the time to recurrence of a cancer after apparent complete remission is being studied, the starting time is the date of apparent complete remission.

TABLE 4–1 Stage Grouping for All Head and Neck Sites (Except for Salivary Glands and Thyroid Gland) According to UICC and AJCC

Stage I	T1N0M0
Stage II	T2N0M0
Stage III	T3N0M0
	T1 or T2 or T3N1M0
Stage IV	T4N0 or N1M0
	any T N2 or N3M0
	any T any N M1

From Snow GB, Balm AJ, Arendse JE, et al: Prognostic factors in neck node metastasis. In Larson DL, Ballantyne AJ, Guillamondegui OM (eds): Cancer in the Neck: Evaluation and Treatment. New York, Macmillan, 1986, p 53.

TABLE 4-2 Definition of TNM for Cancer of the Nasopharynx, Oropharynx, and Hypopharynx

Primary Tumor (T)
TX Primary tumor cannot be assessed
T0 No evidence of primary tumor
Tis Carcinoma in situ

Nasopharynx
T1 Tumor confined to the nasopharynx
T2 Tumor extends to soft tissues
    T2a Tumor extends to the oropharynx and/or nasal cavity without parapharyngeal extension°
    T2b Any tumor with parapharyngeal extension°
T3 Tumor involves bony structures and/or paranasal sinuses
T4 Tumor with intracranial extension and/or involvement of cranial nerves, infratemporal fossa, hypopharynx, orbit, or masticator space

°Note: Parapharyngeal extension denotes posterolateral infiltration of tumor beyond the pharyngobasilar fascia.

Oropharynx
T1 Tumor 2 cm or less in greatest dimension
T2 Tumor more than 2 cm but not more than 4 cm in greatest dimension
T3 Tumor more than 4 cm in greatest dimension
T4a Tumor invades the larynx, deep/extrinsic muscle of tongue, medial pterygoid, hard palate, or mandible
T4b Tumor invades lateral pterygoid muscle, pterygoid plates, lateral nasopharynx, or skull base or encases carotid artery

Hypopharynx
T1 Tumor limited to one subsite of hypopharynx and 2 cm or less in greatest dimension
T2 Tumor invades more than one subsite of hypopharynx or an adjacent site, or measures more than 2 cm but not more than 4 cm in greatest diameter without fixation of hemilarynx
T3 Tumor more than 4 cm in greatest dimension or with fixation of hemilarynx
T4a Tumor invades thyroid/cricoid cartilage, hyoid bone, thyroid gland, esophagus, or central compartment soft tissue°
T4b Tumor invades prevertebral fascia, encases carotid artery, or involves mediastinal structures

°Note: Central compartment soft tissue includes prelaryngeal strap muscles and subcutaneous fat.

Regional Lymph Nodes (N)

Nasopharynx
The distribution and the prognostic impact of regional lymph node spread from nasopharynx cancer, particularly of the undifferentiated type, are different from those of other head and neck mucosal cancers and justify the use of a different N classification scheme.

NX Regional lymph nodes cannot be assessed
N0 No regional lymph node metastasis
N1 Unilateral metastasis in lymph node(s), 6 cm or less in greatest dimension, above the supraclavicular fossa°
N2 Bilateral metastasis in lymph node(s), 6 cm or less in greatest dimension, above the supraclavicular fossa°
N3 Metastasis in a lymph node(s)°>6 cm and/or to supraclavicular fossa
    N3a Greater than 6 cm in dimension
    N3b Extension to the supraclavicular fossa°°

°Note: Midline nodes are considered ipsilateral nodes.
*°°*Supraclavicular zone or fossa is relevant to the staging of nasopharyngeal carcinoma and is the triangular region originally described by Ho. It is defined by three points: (1) the superior margin of the sternal end of the clavicle, (2) the superior margin of the lateral end of the clavicle, (3) the point where the neck meets the shoulder. Note that this would include caudal portions of Levels IV and V. All cases with lymph nodes (whole or part) in the fossa are considered N3b.

Oropharynx and Hypopharynx
NX Regional lymph nodes cannot be assessed
N0 No regional lymph node metastasis
N1 Metastasis in a single ipsilateral lymph node, 3 cm or less in greatest dimension
N2 Metastasis in a single ipsilateral lymph node, more than 3 cm but not more than 6 cm in greatest dimension, or in multiple ipsilateral lymph nodes, none more than 6 cm in greatest dimension, or in bilateral or contralateral lymph nodes, none more than 6 cm in greatest dimension
    N2a Metastasis in a single ipsilateral lymph node more than 3 cm but not more than 6 cm in greatest dimension
    N2b Metastasis in multiple ipsilateral lymph nodes, none more than 6 cm in greatest dimension
    N2c Metastasis in bilateral or contralateral lymph nodes, none more than 6 cm in greatest dimension
N3 Metastasis in a lymph node more than 6 cm in greatest dimension

Distant Metastasis (M)
MX Distant metastasis cannot be assessed
M0 No distant metastasis
M1 Distant metastasis

TABLE 4-3 Definition of TNM for Cancer of the Supraglottis, Glottis, and Subglottis

Primary Tumor (T)
TX Primary tumor cannot be assessed
T0 No evidence of primary tumor
Tis Carcinoma in situ

Supraglottis
T1 Tumor limited to one subsite of supraglottis with normal vocal cord mobility
T2 Tumor invades mucosa of more than one adjacent subsite of supraglottis or glottis or region outside the supraglottis (e.g., mucosa of base of tongue, vallecula, medial wall of pyriform sinus) without fixation of the larynx
T3 Tumor limited to larynx with vocal cord fixation and/or invades any of the following: postcricoid area, pre-epiglottic tissues, paraglottic space, and/or minor thyroid cartilage erosion (e.g., inner cortex)
T4a Tumor invades through the thyroid cartilage and/or invades tissues beyond the larynx (e.g., trachea, soft tissues of neck including deep extrinsic muscle of the tongue, strap muscles, thyroid, or esophagus)
T4b Tumor invades prevertebral space, encases carotid artery, or invades mediastinal structures

Glottis
T1 Tumor limited to the vocal cord(s) (may involve anterior or posterior commissure) with normal mobility
T1a Tumor limited to one vocal cord
T1b Tumor involves both vocal cords
T2 Tumor extends to supraglottis and/or subglottis, and/or with impaired vocal cord mobility
T3 Tumor limited to the larynx with vocal cord fixation and/or invades paraglottic space, and/or minor thyroid cartilage erosion (e.g., inner cortex)
T4a Tumor invades through the thyroid cartilage and/or invades tissues beyond the larynx (e.g., trachea, soft tissues of neck including deep extrinsic muscle of the tongue, strap muscles, thyroid, or esophagus)

T4b Tumor invades prevertebral space, encases carotid artery, or invades mediastinal structures.

Subglottis
T1 Tumor limited to the subglottis
T2 Tumor extends to vocal cord(s) with normal or impaired mobility
T3 Tumor limited to larynx with vocal cord fixation
T4a Tumor invades cricoid or thyroid cartilage and/or invades tissues beyond the larynx (e.g., trachea, soft tissues of neck including deep extrinsic muscles of the tongue, strap muscles, thyroid, or esophagus)
T4b Tumor invades prevertebral space, encases carotid artery, or invades mediastinal structures

Regional Lymph Nodes (N)
NX Regional lymph nodes cannot be assessed
N0 No regional lymph node metastasis
N1 Metastasis in a single ipsilateral lymph node, 3 cm or less in greatest dimension
N2 Metastasis in a single lpsilateral lymph node, more than 3 cm but not more than 6 cm in greatest dimension, or in multiple ipsilateral lymph nodes, none more than 6 cm in greatest dimension, or in bilateral or contralateral lymph nodes, none more than 6 cm in greatest dimension
N2a Metastasis in a single ipsilateral lymph node, more than 3 cm but not more than 6 cm in greatest dimension
N2b Metastasis in multiple ipsilateral lymph nodes, none more than 6 cm in greatest dimension
N2c Metastasis in bilateral or contralateral lymph nodes, none more than 6 cm in greatest dimension
N3 Metastasis in a lymph node, more than 6 cm in greatest dimension

Distant Metastasis (M)
MX Distant metastasis cannot be assessed
M0 No distant metastasis
M1 Distant metastasis

The most convenient starting time for treatment effectiveness studies is the date of first antineoplastic therapy. For untreated patients, the most comparable date is the time at which it was decided that no cancer-directed treatment would be given. For both treated and untreated patients, the times from which survival rates are calculated usually coincide with the date of the initial staging of cancer.

Classifications of Treatment

The classification of treatment is based on the type, timing, and sequence of treatment. The extraction of these data from the medical record has been carefully and completely described elsewhere.[57,59-61] Treatment types include surgery, radiotherapy, and chemotherapy. Within each treatment type, subtypes can be easily defined (e.g., supraglottic laryngectomy is a specific type of surgical treatment). Treatment sequence can be defined as either initial or subsequent, and treatments can be used singly or in combination. Initial treatment refers to the first course of antineoplastic therapy, which can be given as a single modality or as combination therapy. Subsequent treatment is any treatment used after initial treatment and initiated as a result of persistence, recurrence, or some clinical change in the tumor. According to this classification, therapy that included surgery and postoperative radiotherapy could be classified as either initial combination therapy or initial surgery and subsequent radiotherapy, depending on the clinical scenario. In the first scenario, surgery and postoperative radiotherapy is classified as initial combination therapy when the decision to use radiotherapy was made prior to surgery. In the second scenario, postoperative radiotherapy is classified as subsequent therapy when the decision to use radiotherapy was made *after* surgery and as a result of findings at surgery (e.g., tumor too extensive for complete removal or extracapsular spread of tumor in a lymph node).

Classification of Staging Times

The following rules for classification are recommended by the AJCC. Four classification times are described for each site.

Clinical Classification (cTNM or TNM). This classification is based on evidence acquired before treatment. Such evidence arises from physical examination, imaging, endoscopy, biopsy, and other relevant findings. The use of diagnostic imaging technology can affect the way patients are staged. The impact that diagnostic imaging has on cancer staging and statistics is referred to as "stage migration."[62]

Pathologic Classification (pTNM). Pathologic classification is based on evidence acquired before treatment, supplemented or modified by additional evidence acquired from pathologic examination of a resected specimen.

Retreatment Classification (rTNM). Retreatment classification is used after a disease-free interval and when further definitive treatment is planned. All information available at the time of retreatment should be used in determining the stage of the recurrent tumor.

Autopsy Classification (aTNM). If classification of a cancer is done after the death of a patient and a postmortem examination has been done, all pathologic information should be used.

Description of Outcome

Vital Status. The post–zero time vital status for each patient can be classified as alive, dead, or unknown (i.e., lost to follow-up). Survival time is the time from the starting point to the terminal event to the end of the study or to the date of last observation. Completeness of follow-up is crucial in any study of survival time. Vital status at survival time can be further classified as follows:

Alive; tumor-free; no recurrence
Alive; tumor-free; after recurrence
Alive; with persistent, recurrent, or metastatic disease
Alive; with primary tumor
Dead; tumor-free
Dead; with cancer (primary, recurrent, or metastatic disease)
Dead; post operation
Unknown; lost to follow-up

Health Status and Health-Related Quality of Life. Although survival rate is the standard outcome measure in oncology, it does not capture fully the essence of clinical practice and human illness.[63, 64] Important information collected in daily practice includes patient-based measures of symptoms, functional capacity, social and emotional consequences of disease and its treatment, and satisfaction with care.[65] An expanded definition of patient outcome has been described by Fries and Spitz.[66] Patient outcome is described in a hierarchical fashion,[67] with mortality and morbidity forming the first two levels of outcome. The next level of patient outcome is described by the health status of the patient. Health status can be described by the physical, functional, and emotional limitations experienced by a patient.[68,69] Health-related quality of life (HRQOL) represents the fourth level of patient outcome. A definition of HRQOL on which all patients, physicians, and researchers can agree may be impossible to obtain. However, during the past decade, sufficient research has been conducted over a wide range of conditions and by a large number of investigators that a common core description of HRQOL may now be possible.[70,71] Health-related quality of life includes a suitable description of the health status of the patient and the value, importance, or utility placed on that condition by the patient.[72] Patient satisfaction with medical care is viewed as the final level or feature of patient outcome. Patient outcomes may also be described in terms of the resources used or monies spent to obtain a certain health outcome state.[73] The three general types of economic analyses are cost-identification, cost-effectiveness, and cost-benefit.[74]

Calculation of Survival Rates

The calculation of survival rates is the primary outcome measurement in cancer statistics. The basic concept is simple: Of a given number of patients, what percentage will be alive at the end of a specified interval, such as 5 years? There are several ways to measure survival rates.[75]

Direct Method. The simplest procedure for summarizing patient survival is to calculate the percentage of patients alive at the end of a specified interval, such as 5 years.

Actuarial or Life-table Method. This method provides a means for using all follow-up information accumulated up to the closing date of the study. This approach also provides information on the pattern of survival or the manner in which the patient group was depleted during the total period of observation.

Observed Survival Rate. The observed survival rate accounts for all deaths, regardless of cause, and is a true reflection of total mortality.

Adjusted Survival Rate. The adjusted survival rate is the proportion of the initial patient group that escaped death due to cancer if all other causes of death were not operant. The use of adjusted survival rate is particularly important in comparing patient groups that may differ with respect to factors such as sex, age, race, and socioeconomic status.

Relative Survival Rate. The relative survival rate is the ratio of the observed survival rate to the expected rate for a group of people in the general population similar with respect to sex, age, race, and the calendar period of observation.

Problems With the Present Classification System for Cancer

Many problems and weaknesses of current cancer staging practices have been identified.[50,54] These problems can be related directly to the current TNM system or can be relevant to cancer staging overall. Proposals for improvements for each of these problems are suggested in the following paragraphs.

PROBLEMS WITH THE CURRENT TNM SYSTEM

Definition Criteria. The most important problems with the current system arise from ambiguity and variability of the actual definitions for the various T, N, and M categories. More explicit definitions and criteria are required to reduce ambiguity. A reduction in ambiguity will allow for the standardized collection of tumor information. For clinical staging, improvements are needed in definitions for vocal cord function and in T definitions for the supraglottis, glottis, and pyriform sinus. For patients with clinically positive cervical lymph node metastasis, criteria for the classification of clinical nodal disease should include size of largest node, consistency of nodal metastasis (e.g., soft, mobile, firm, immobile, matted), and level of the metastatic lymph node farthest from the primary tumor. The five-level nodal classification system described by Suen and Goepfert[76] and used at Memorial Sloan-Kettering Cancer Center[77] could be used for this purpose. In 1997, a Strategic Planning Conference was convened to help standardize and clarify the reporting of the pathologic stage of head and neck cancer. Conference participants recommended including information such as adjacent structures involved, adequacy of margins, complications during the operation, surgical approach, and type of neck dissection. This information could be entered into a data base via a menu-driven user interface.[78] New definitions with explicit criteria should be created for other morphologic characteristics, such as *exophytic* and *endophytic, depth of invasion,* and *microscopic characteristics of the tumor border* for excised tumors. Microscopic pathologic examination of nodal disease should also report status of the node capsule (e.g., intact or extracapsular spread).

Stage Groupings. The grouping together of the various T, N, and M combinations into stages was thought by many of the respondents in the previously described survey[50] to be inconsistent and biologically inaccurate. The original and current stage groupings were created based on *presumed* prognosis.[1] No prospective, multivariate analysis was performed to create the four stage groupings from the various combinations of T, N, and M. New stage groupings, based on multivariate studies of the relative impact of the T, N, and M categories, should be undertaken.

Observer Variability. Observer variability and measurement error create significant problems with the use of the staging system. For instance, in a retrospective review of outcomes for 193 patients with laryngeal carcinoma, one of us (J.F.P.) identified 44 examples of two or more physicians staging the same patient differently.[79] Through education and establishment of "validated TNM physician" programs, observer variability could be reduced. These educational training sessions could use videotapes to demonstrate cancers in various head and neck sites and demonstration neck mannequins to aid in examination and estimation of the size and character of various regional nodal presentations.

Inclusion of CT and MRI Scans. The proper role and criteria for sophisticated radiographic and other imaging techniques in the staging of patients are not clear, and this ambiguity creates another problem with the current system. Clinical studies should be conducted to examine the relative prognostic impact of these studies and the impact of their results on therapeutic decisions.

Stage Migration. Stage migration can occur whenever new diagnostic technology is used to assign disease stages.[62] This situation most commonly arises when advances in diagnostic technology are applied only to relatively recent groups of patients. Because the sensitive new methods can identify "silent" or "subclinical" advanced lesions that would have previously been undetected, the new technological data allow recently diagnosed patients with silent spread to "migrate" or "shift" from localized stages with generally good prognoses (i.e., TNM stages I and II) into advanced stages with generally worse prognoses (i.e., TNM stages III and IV).[80] The result is that the survival rates within each stage increase, while the overall survival for all patients remains the same. A recent study[81] showed that 17% of patients with laryngeal cancer were reclassified after receiving CT scan information and, as a result, stage-specific survival rates improved in three of the four TNM stages.

One solution to the stage migration problem is to stage patients in ways that are not sensitive to technological advances. For example, a simple, universally applicable staging system could be created based on clinical features, such as symptom severity, medical comorbidity, and morphologic extent of tumor as defined by history and simple physical examination alone. A secondary or advanced staging system based on new diagnostic technology could also be used. The adoption of a stable staging system would eliminate the problems that result from comparing patients based on different staging modalities.

PROBLEMS RELEVANT TO OVERALL CANCER STAGING

The current system fails to address other areas important to cancer description, prognosis, and treatment evaluation. These areas include host- and patient-based prognostic variables.

Exclusion of Host Factors. Despite providing an excellent description of the size of the cancer and its extent of anatomic spread, the TNM system does not account for the clinical biology of the cancer,[82,83] which is manifested by both the *structural form* of the tumor and its *physiologic function* in the patient. Human cancers do not necessarily or always spread in an orderly fashion. Thus, the clinical biology of the tumor cannot be fully described by assessment of the extent or size of the tumor alone.

The tumor's morphologic structure can be reported for gross anatomy (TNM categories), microscopic forms (e.g., cell type, degree of differentiation), and biomolecular attributes (e.g., tumor markers, ploidy). The functional effects of the tumor can be described by the severity of illness created in the patient. These functional effects are manifested by the type, duration, and severity of cancer symptoms (e.g., weight loss, fatigue,[84-86] and the performance or functional status of the host).[87,88] Another important aspect of clinical biology is the comorbidity of the patient who is the "setting" in which the cancer occurs. Although unrelated to the cancer itself, the patient's concomitant disease can affect the clinical course of the cancer, as well as the choice of treatment and the prognosis.[89-93] Each aspect of the clinical features of cancer is discussed in the paragraphs that follow.

Symptoms as an Index of Biologic Behavior. Cancer symptoms (and certain physical signs) provide important prognostic information[84] because they reflect the tumor's biologic behavior. Although a patient's symptoms are regularly noted in medical student histories, presented at tumor boards, and used in the "clinical judgment" of experienced clinicians, the patient's presenting symptoms are generally not cited, categorized, or analyzed in the evaluation of prognosis and therapy. One main reason for the neglect of symptoms has been their variability.[65] Because cancer with similar morphologic properties can be accompanied by different symptoms, physicians have often concluded that symptoms are too subjective to merit scientific consideration. A second reason for the scientific exclusion of symptoms has been the assumed absence of a suitable taxonomy for classifying the symptoms into appropriate subgroups. This assumption is incorrect, however, because several taxonomies have been created to classify symptoms, as is illustrated in the following examples of the prognostic importance of symptoms.

When patients with carcinoma of the nasopharynx were classified based on the number and duration of symptoms at initial presentation, a significant difference in survival rates was found.[86] For example, 97 of 166 patients (58%) with fewer than seven symptoms survived 5 years, whereas only 4 of 16 patients (25%) with seven or more symptoms survived 5 years (*P* < .001). These differences remained statistically significant even after other prognostic variables (such as extent of tumor and antibody-dependent cellular cytotoxicity) were controlled.

In 1966, Feinstein[84] proposed a taxonomic system based on type, duration, and severity of symptoms and physical signs. Symptoms and physical signs are classified as primary, systemic, or distant based on their presumed mechanism. Primary symptoms are related to a tumor at its primary site. For example, in cancer of the larynx, symptoms such as hoarseness and voice change are classified as primary symptoms. Systemic symptoms are due to effects of the tumor away from the primary site. Constitutional symptoms, such as weight loss and fatigue, are examples of systemic symptoms. Distant symptoms, when accompanied by appropriate

supporting documentation of distant spread, imply that the cancer has extended beyond its primary locus. Distant symptoms in cancer of the larynx include bone pain from distant metastasis, or visual changes from invasion of the base of the skull.

In a hierarchical arrangement that resembles the TNM system, cancer in patients with distant symptoms is classified as *distant*, regardless of the presence of primary or systemic symptoms. In patients with systemic symptoms but no distant symptoms, the cancer is classified as *systemic*, regardless of the presence or absence of primary symptoms. In patients with primary symptoms alone, the cancer is classified as *primary*. In patients without any pertinent symptoms, the cancer is classified as *asymptomatic*.

This taxonomy has been used to show the prognostic importance of symptoms in a variety of cancers.[94-96] In one study of 192 patients with cancer of the larynx,[97] the total 5-year survival was 50% (96/192), but the rates ranged from 77% (37/48) in the *primary* symptom stage, to 56% (38/68) in the *systemic* symptom stage, to 28% (21/76) in the *distant* symptom stage. In a later study of cancer of the larynx,[79] the total 5-year survival rate was 66% (127/193), with rates ranging from 79% (91/115), to 48% (30/62), to 38% (6/16), respectively, in the *primary, systemic,* and *distant* stages (Table 4–4). In each of these cancers, the prognostic gradients described by symptoms were statistically significant, even when other known prognostic variables were controlled for with multivariate analysis. A recent study of 1010 patients with cancer of the head and neck evaluated 23 symptoms related to the site of the lesion to determine their prognostic impact on survival.[98] Four symptoms–dysphagia, otalgia, mass in the neck, and weight loss—had a negative impact on overall survival. The cancer was classified based on symptom severity, where *None* was designated if 0 of the 4 symptoms were present, *Mild* if 1 was present, *Moderate* if 2 were present, and *Severe* if 3 or 4 were present. Overall survival was strongly related to the symptom severity stage, and this association was independent of TNM stage, comorbidity, age, and alcohol use. Similar results have been shown for oral cavity and oropharyngeal cancer.[99-101]

Performance Status. Performance status can be viewed as measurable outcomes that affect quality of life.[102] At the time of diagnosis, a patient can have not only symptoms but other functional effects that are manifested in overall performance status or physical capacity. The Karnofsky Performance Status (KPS) Scale,[103] the Spitzer Quality of Life Index,[104] the Eastern Cooperative Oncology Group Scale,[105] and the Host (AJCC)1 Scale are examples of rating scales that have been used in oncology to assess a patient's functional capacity for

TABLE 4–4 Five-Year Survival Rates in Larynx Cancer According to Symptom Stage

Symptom Stage	Feinstein et al[97] (1977)		Piccirillo et al[79] (1994)	
	Total Patients	Survival Rate	Total Patients	Survival Rate
Primary	37/48	77	91/115	79
Systemic	38/68	56	30/62	48
Distant	21/76	28	6/16	38
Total	96/192	50	127/193	66

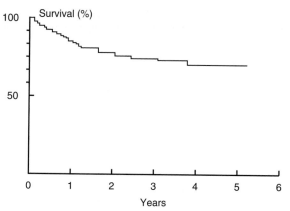

FIGURE 4–2 Survival results for 763 patients with previously untreated cancer of the larynx. (Adapted from Stell PM: Prognosis in laryngeal carcinoma: Host factors. Clin Otolaryngol 13:399–409, 1989.)

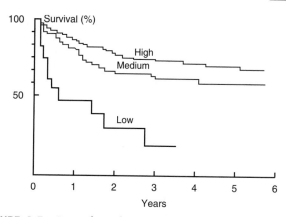

FIGURE 4–3 Survival results according to performance status. (Adapted from Stell PM: Prognosis in laryngeal carcinoma: Host factors. Clin Otolaryngol 13:399–409, 1989.)

work and for daily activities of self-care. However, these scales are not specific to head and neck cancer patients.[102] Several tumor-specific instruments are being tested, such as the European Organization for Research and Treatment of Cancer Quality of Life Questionnaire—Head and Neck,[106] the University of Washington Quality of Life Questionnaire,[107] and the Functional Assessment of Cancer Therapy–Head and Neck Scale.[108]

Prognosis for cancer patients is much better if they have ample functional capacity and can perform activities of self-care than if function and activities are impaired. The patient's performance status can affect not only prognosis but also the choice of treatments. Patients with decreased functional capacity may be deemed "too sick" for one treatment (e.g., surgery) and may receive an alternative therapy (e.g., irradiation). The prognostic impact of the KPS scale can be illustrated by the observed survival results for 763 patients with previously untreated larynx cancer (Fig. 4–2).[87]

The results reveal major prognostic differences when the patients are divided according to their high, medium, or low KPS ratings (Fig. 4–3). The results led Stell to comment: "Performance status is a very important prognostic factor—more significant in fact than T status. Furthermore, assessment of performance status requires no technology."[87]

Comorbidity. Although not a feature of the cancer itself, comorbidity is an important attribute of the patient. Concomitant disease(s) can strongly affect the patient's survival as well as the choices of treatment for the cancer. The cancers for which comorbidity is particularly important are cancers that are not rapidly fatal and that affect middle-aged or older people. The cancers in which comorbidity has been

shown to be important or could be expected to be important based on the previous statement include cancers of the oral cavity,[99,109] pharynx, larynx,[79,97,110] breast,[92,93] prostate,[90,94] bladder, ovary, and endometrium,[89] and non-Hodgkin's lymphoma. Based on recent cancer incidence rates,[111] these cancers represent approximately 61% of all cancers for men and 65% of those for women. Several comorbidity instruments have been validated and are available for use. These include the Charlson Comorbidity Index[112] and the Kaplan-Feinstein Comorbidity Index.[113]

The Kaplan-Feinstein Comorbidity Index[113] was developed from a study of the impact of comorbidity on outcomes for patients with diabetes mellitus. Although it is not specific for head and neck cancer, it is frequently used to measure comorbidity. Specific diseases and conditions were classified, according to their severity of organ decompensation, as mild, moderate, or severe. Severe comorbidity is also referred to as *prognostic* comorbidity because it is likely to affect prognosis. Examples of severe or prognostic comorbidity include malignant hypertension; congestive heart failure, myocardial infarction, or significant arrhythmias within the past 6 months; and marked pulmonary insufficiency. Examples of moderate comorbidity include congestive heart failure more than 6 months ago; old stroke, with residua; and recurrent asthmatic attacks with chronic obstructive pulmonary disease. Examples of mild comorbidity include myocardial infarction more than 6 months ago; old stroke without residua; and chronic lung disease manifested only on radiologic or pulmonary function tests. Table 4–5 shows the impact of comorbidity alone on 5-year survival rates, regardless of the TNM stage of the tumor, for five different cancers.

TABLE 4–5 Impact of Prognostic Comorbidity on 5-Year Survival Rates°

Prognostic Comorbidity	Rectum Cancer[95]	Larynx Cancer[97]	Endometrial Cancer[89]	Prostate Cancer[94]	Larynx Cancer[79]
Absent	85/264 (32%)	93/172 (54%)	102/131 (78%)	137/229 (60%)	123/166 (74%)
Present	6/54 (11%)	3/20 (15%)	3/11 (27%)	6/38 (16%)	4/27 (15%)
Total	91/318 (29%)	96/192 (50%)	105/142 (74%)	143/267 (54%)	127/193 (66%)
χ^2	9.76	10.94	3.54	25.41	36.27
P value	.0018	.0009	.0599	<.0001	<.0001

°Denominators, number of patients in each category; numerators, corresponding number of 5-year survivors.

TABLE 4-6 Impact of Comorbidity on 5-Year Survival Rates Within TNM Stages°

Prognostic Comorbidity	TNM Stages				
	I	II	III	IV	Total
Absent	59/71 (83%)	31/41 (76%)	25/38 (66%)	8/16 (50%)	123/166 (74%)
Present	1/6 (17%)	1/7 (14%)	2/7 (28%)	0/7 (0%)	4/27 (15%)
Total	60/77 (78%)	32/48 (67%)	27/45 (60%)	8/23 (35%)	127/193 (66%)

°Denominators, number of patients in each category; numerators, corresponding number of 5-year survivors.

In each of the five case series in Table 4–5, the 5-year survival rates were reduced when prognostic comorbidity was present and were elevated when it was absent. For each series except endometrial cancer, the impact of prognostic comorbidity remained significant, even when other prognostic factors were controlled. For instance, in cancer of the larynx,[79] survival rates were not only significantly different based on comorbidity but were also significantly different *within* TNM stages based on comorbidity (Table 4–6).

A modified version of the Kaplan-Feinstein Comorbidity Index was used by Piccirillo to assess the independent impact of comorbidity on head and neck cancer survival and treatment.[114] This prospective cohort study of 3378 cancer patients included 341 head and neck cancer patients. When compared with other cancer sites, a significant percentage (21%) of patients with head and neck cancer had comorbidities scored as *moderate* or *severe*. Comorbidity was significantly associated with 2-year survival.

The Charlson Comorbidity Index[112] was created from studies of 1-year mortality rates for patients admitted to a medical unit of a teaching hospital (Table 4–7). The Charlson Comorbidity Index is a weighted index that takes into account the number and seriousness of comorbid diseases. The scoring system for this instrument assigns weights of 1, 2, 3, and 6 for each of the existing comorbid diseases present at initial assessment and derives from that a total score that determines the patient's overall prognostic status.

Although useful in predicting survival, these indices are not cancer-specific. Recently, the Adult Comorbidity Evaluation-27 (ACE-27) was developed and validated.[114] It is the only comorbidity index designed specifically for cancer patients.

TABLE 4-7 Weighted Index of Comorbidity

Assigned Weights For Diseases°	Disease
1	Myocardial infarct
	Congestive heart failure
	Peripheral vascular disease
	Cerebrovascular disease
	Dementia
	Chronic pulmonary disease
	Connective tissue disease
	Ulcer disease
	Mild liver disease
	Diabetes
2	Hemiplegia
	Moderate or severe renal disease
	Diabetes with end-organ damage
	Any tumor
	Leukemia
	Lymphoma
3	Moderate or severe liver disease
6	Metastatic solid tumor
	Acquired immunodeficiency syndrome (AIDS)

°Assigned weights for each condition that a patient has. The total equals the score. Example: chronic pulmonary (1) and lymphoma (2) = total score (3).
From Charlson ME, Pompei P, Ales HL, et al: A new method of classifying prognostic comorbidity in longitudinal studies: Development and validation. J Chronic Dis 40:373, 1987.

Aside from direct effects on survival, severe comorbidity can also have a prognostic impact by altering therapy. A patient who is "too sick" to tolerate a preferred treatment may be given a less aggressive treatment or even palliative treatment. The ASA[4] has devised a system for the collection and tabulation of statistical data to classify preoperative conditions. The ASA scale uses a five-category rating process ranging from class 1—"healthy normal patient"—to class 5—"moribund patient who is not expected to survive for 24 hours with or without operation."

The ASA scale was strictly limited to a definition of preoperative physical status and did not express total operative risk.[115] Total operative risk depends not only on the physical status of the patient but also on the proposed surgery and the skill of the surgeon. Vacanti and coworkers[116] found that operative mortality (deaths within the first 48 postoperative hours) was significantly associated with ASA physical status category (Table 4–8). Marx and colleagues[117] also found that operative mortality (deaths within the first 7 postoperative days) was significantly related to ASA score (see Table 4–8).

TABLE 4-8 Mortality Rates According to American Society of Anesthesiologists (ASA)

Physical Status Class	Vacanti et al[116]		Marx et al[117]	
	Deaths/Anesthetic Procedures	Mortality Rate (%)	Deaths/Anesthetic Procedures	Mortality Rate (%)
I	43/50,703	0.08	11/18,320	0.06
II	34/12,601	0.27	50/10,609	0.47
III	66/3,626	1.82	168/3,820	4.40
IV	66/850	7.76	252/1,073	23.48
V	57/608	9.38	164/323	50.77
Total	266/68,388	0.39	645/34,145	1.89

As has been demonstrated earlier, the presence of comorbidity, rather than the extent of tumor, may sometimes determine the selection of treatment and the patient's eventual outcome. Nevertheless, comorbidity data are not currently collected or included in cancer statistics. As was demonstrated in Table 4–5 and in the reports previously cited, this omission continues to render the classification of patients imprecise, and it affects the subsequent interpretation of both 5-year survival rates and therapeutic effectiveness.

Reasons for the Exclusion of Host Factors. Despite the numerous examples of the importance of patient factors to prognosis and evaluation of treatment effectiveness, these variables continue to be excluded from the standard system for cancer classification. There are multiple reasons for the exclusion of these important patient-based variables: (1) belief in the exclusive importance of morphology, (2) desire to avoid soft data, (3) previous lack of a taxonomy for patient-based variables, (4) desire to avoid multiple variables and components, and (5) desire to keep the system simple for clinical practice.[50, 118]

Incorporation of Additional Prognostic Variables Into Cancer Staging Systems. The incorporation of additional variables into a cancer staging system, even if prognostically important, has been regarded as a cumbersome and time-consuming activity that could impair the physician's documentation of the patient's pretherapeutic condition. Many tumor registry technicians would probably agree with the reply received from an otolaryngology professor who was asked if he thought performance status should be included in a cancer staging system: "It is difficult enough just to get TNM reported on all patients by all physicians."[119] The unwillingness of clinicians to obtain and include important clinical information is a peculiar inexplicability in an era when they have been willing to order a plethora of additional laboratory and imaging tests.

In addition to presenting problems in data collection, the inclusion of additional prognostic variables presents problems in data analysis. The TNM system is based on a "bin" model[56] in which the number of bins increases rapidly as additional prognostic variables are added. For example, if the presence or absence of prognostic comorbidity was directly added to the TNM staging system, the number of bins would increase from 40 to 80 [$2 \times (5 \times 4 \times 2)$]. The inclusion of new factors in the TNM system was therefore deemed not to be practical. Furthermore, before the advent of computers and appropriate statistical programs, the analysis of multiple variables and the identification of independent prognostic variables were difficult. Limiting the staging system to one component—anatomic extent of tumor—was therefore a practical necessity.

Multivariable regression analyses, such as Cox's proportional hazard method,[120] however, can now be easily done with microcomputers, and independent prognostic variables can readily be identified. Independent prognostic variables are those variables that significantly contribute to predictions of prognosis even after other known prognostic variables are controlled. In addition to identifying important prognostic variables, the "output" from these analyses quantifies the relative impact (or "weight") of each of the prognostic variables.[121] Interactions between variables can also be examined.

These outputs can be used to construct clinical prediction models to estimate prognosis.[122, 123] The operational rules for the clinical prediction models can then be stored in microcomputers, and the myriad of important individual data can be entered to produce a prognostic estimate.[124] This multivariable regression process has obvious analytic appeal, but it may not seem appealing to clinicians because of its reliance on microcomputers and "black-box" mathematics.[125]

A different form of multivariate analysis, generally referred to as conjunctive consolidation[96] or targeted-cluster analysis, can be used to incorporate the additional prognostic variables without reliance on cryptic mathematical equations or additional bins. In this form of analysis, a staging system is created through the combination of multiple prognostic variables, based on biologic sensibility and statistical criteria. One of the most important characteristics of this type of analysis is that a staging system can include a greater number of prognostic variables (e.g., including symptom severity and prognostic comorbidity into the TNM system) yet maintain a discrete number of stages (usually three or four). A second important characteristic is that conjunctive consolidation is an uncomplicated analytic technique that is generally more relevant and meaningful to clinicians than are the results of regression equations. The use of conjunctive consolidation to create the clinical severity (CS) staging system for cancer of the larynx[79] is demonstrated in the following section.

The goal of the CS staging system project was twofold: (1) to demonstrate the prognostic importance of symptom severity and comorbidity and (2) to demonstrate that a composite CS staging system, created by the addition of symptom severity and comorbidity to the TNM system, could substantially improve the prognostic precision of cancer staging. The first step in the creation of the CS system was the creation of a functional severity (FS) system through the conjunction of symptom severity and comorbidity. As can be seen in Table 4–9, in each category of symptom stage, survival rates were substantially lowered when prognostic comorbidity was present.

Because both symptom severity and prognostic comorbidity stages were distinctively important, the categories were combined using conjunctive consolidation techniques. Thus, the eight symptom comorbidity groups were consolidated into three composite stages, labeled as alpha, beta, and gamma. Next, the prognostic impact of FS was examined

TABLE 4–9 Five-Year Survival Rates in Conjunctive Consolidation of Symptom Severity and Prognostic Comorbidity Stages

Symptom Stage		Prognostic Comorbidity Stage		
		Absent	Present	Total
1	Alpha	64/76 (84%)	Gamma 1/5 (20%)	65/81 (80%)
2		25/31 (81%)	1/3 (33%)	26/34 (76%)
3	Beta	28/47 (60%)	2/15 (13%)	30/62 (48%)
4		6/12 (50%)	0/4 (0%)	6/16 (38%)
Total		123/166 (74%)	4/27 (15%)	127/193 (66%)

From Piccirillo JF, Wells CK, Sasaki CT, et al: New clinical severity staging system for cancer of the larynx. Five-year survival rates. Ann Otol Rhinol Laryngol 103:83, 1994.

TABLE 4-10 Five-Year Survival Rates in Conjunction With Functional Severity and TNM Anatomic Stages

Functional Severity Stage	TNM Anatomic Stage				
	I	II	III	IV	Total
Alpha	53/60 (88%)	24/30 (80%)	9/13 (69%)	3/4 (75%)	89/107 (83%)
Beta	6/11 (55%)	7/11 (64%)	16/25 (64%)	5/12 (42%)	34/59 (58%)
Gamma	1/6 (17%)	1/7 (14%)	2/7 (28%)	0/7 (0%)	4/27 (15%)
Total	60/77 (78%)	32/48 (67%)	27/45 (60%)	8/23 (35%)	127/193 (66%)

From Piccirillo JF, Wells CK, Sasaki CT, et al: New clinical severity staging system for cancer of the larynx. Five-year survival rates. Ann Otol Rhinol Laryngol 103:83, 1994.

within each TNM stage. As is shown in Table 4–10, within each vertical column of TNM anatomic stage, the FS staging system defined an important and consistent prognostic gradient.

The gradients in 5-year survival rates extend from 88% to 17% in TNM stage I, from 80% to 14% in stage II, from 69% to 28% in stage III, and from 75% to 0% in stage IV. These results demonstrate the profound prognostic heterogeneity that can exist among patients who are in the same TNM stage. The 12 FS-TNM anatomic stage categories were then consolidated into four composite stages, as is shown in Table 4–11. The survival rate was 88% (53/60) in stage A, 80% (24/30) in stage B, 63% (38/60) in stage C, and 28% (12/43) in stage D. This survival gradient was highly significant ($\chi^2 = 30.47$, $P < .0001$).

The CS staging system contains the same number of stages as the TNM system (four) but incorporates two additional prognostic variables and produces a larger range of overall survival gradient (60% vs. 43%) and a larger χ^2 linear trend value (30.47 vs. 15.55). The main advantage of conjunctive consolidation is that the additional prognostic variables (i.e., symptom severity and comorbidity) can be added to the existing TNM staging system without the need to increase the number of bins exponentially. As stated by Burke and Henson,[56] ". . . to increase our prognostic accuracy, the current system must be enhanced by the creation of a system that contains the TNM variables as well as the new predictive variables."

Evaluation of Staging Systems

The purpose of staging is to divide a large, usually heterogeneous group into a number of smaller subgroups that are

TABLE 4-11 Pattern of Consolidation of Functional Severity and TNM Anatomic Stages to Form Composite Clinical Severity Staging System

Functional Severity Stage	TNM Anatomic Stage			
	I	II	III	IV
Alpha	A	B	C	D
Beta	C	C	C	D
Gamma	D	D	D	D

From Piccirillo JF, Wells CK, Sasaki CT, et al: New clinical severity staging system for cancer of the larynx. Five-year survival rates. Ann Otol Rhinol Laryngol 103:83, 1994.

internally homogeneous and externally disparate. The qualitative comparison of different staging systems is best done with "face validity" or "common sense"[126]; statistical scores and tests are used for the quantitative evaluation of each system's mathematical accomplishments. Some of the quantitative scores and tests used for dichotomous outcomes (i.e., survival) are described in the paragraphs that follow. It must be always kept in mind that when different staging systems or the same staging system in different populations is evaluated, the level of "performance" of the staging system will largely depend on the variance of the predictor variables and the rate of development of the outcome event in each of the study populations. Several excellent sources exist for those who are interested in reading more about the quantitative evaluations of staging systems.[127–132]

Monotonicity of Survival Gradient. The survival gradient is monotonic if each of the successive subgroups has a consistently lower (or higher) survival rate than the preceding group.

Range of Survival Gradient. The range of survival gradient is the difference between the highest and lowest survival rates in the staging system. A wide range is obviously desirable.

Sensitivity and Specificity. These indices can be calculated from a standard 2×2 table of predicted alive/dead versus actual alive/dead. *Sensitivity* is defined as the proportion of dead patients who were predicted to die, and *specificity* is the proportion of live patients who were predicted to survive. The perfect staging system would have a sensitivity and specificity of 1. Few staging systems reach this measure of perfection; there is usually a trade-off between sensitivity and specificity. The more sensitive the staging system (i.e., the fewer false-negatives), the less specific (i.e., the more false-positives) it becomes. This reciprocal relationship between sensitivity and specificity is represented by the test's receiver operating characteristics (ROC) curve.

Proportionate Reduction in Predictive Errors. A prognostic staging system divides a population into unique prognostic strata. When the outcome of interest is a dichotomous event, all the members of a stratum are "predicted" to have attained or not attained the target event, depending on whether the stratum rate is above or below 50%. The total improvement in congruent fit can be expressed as the proportionate reduction in predictive errors. Thus, if E is the number of predictive errors in the total unstratified data, the proportionate reduction in error is $(E - \Sigma e_i)/E$, where e_i is the number of errors in each

TABLE 4-12 Quantitative Evaluation of Staging Systems

Category of Evaluation	Staging System		
	TNM Anatomic (1988)	Functional Severity	Clinical Severity
Monotonicity of survival gradient	Yes	Yes	Yes
Range of overall survival gradient	43%	68%	60%
Proportionate reduction in predictive errors	11%	29%	29%
Proportionate reduction in variance	0.094	0.240	0.219
χ^2 for linear trend	15.55	47.30	30.47

From Piccirillo JF, Wells CK, Sasaki CT, et al: New clinical severity staging system for cancer of the larynx. Five-year survival rates. Ann Otol Rhinol Laryngol 103:83, 1994.

stratum. The larger the proportionate reduction in predictive error, the better the staging system.

Proportionate Reduction in Variance. This is the proportion of group variance in the original population that was later reduced by the division into stages. The score ranges from 0 to 1, and higher values represent better achievements for staging systems having the same number of categories.

χ^2 **for Linear Trend (lt).** This score represents a test of the linear monotonicity of the survival rates within ordered categories. It is not equivalent to the standard χ^2. For comparative purposes, the higher the value of χ^2_{lt}, the better. For nonparametric data, the Mann-Whitney U-test should be used.

c-Statistic. The c-statistic is derived from measures of sensitivity and specificity and is equal to the area under the ROC curve. The larger the number, the better the staging system.

R^2. When the outcome event is a continuous variable, the appropriate type of multivariate analysis is a linear regression, and the R^2 is the standard summary measure. R^2 represents the fraction of total variance in the outcome explained by or attributed to differences in baseline or predictor variables. When the outcome event is a dichotomous variable, logistic regression should be used, and an analogue of R^2 can be used as a summary measure.

Several of these quantitative evaluation principles were applied to three staging systems for the 193 patients with laryngeal cancer[79]: the standard 1988 AJCC TNM criteria, the FS system, and the CS system. As is shown in Table 4–12, all three systems had a monotonic survival gradient. In every other feature, however, the FS and CS systems were quantitatively superior to the TNM system.

Evaluation of Treatment Effectiveness

As stated earlier in this chapter, the evaluation of treatment effectiveness is one of the most important functions of cancer staging. If the staging system is not accurate, precise, and reliable, then inexact assessments of treatment effectiveness result. To illustrate the importance of staging to the evaluation of treatment effectiveness, unpublished data from the cancer of the larynx[79] project are presented here.

The three main forms of initial treatment (radiation, surgery, or combined radiation and surgery) for patients with cancer of the larynx are compared in Tables 4–13 and 4–14. The overall 5-year survival rate, regardless of treatment, was 67% (124/184), and for the three forms of initial treatment, the survival rates were 73% (74/101), 67% (28/42), and 54% (22/41). These differences were not statistically different.

By looking at Table 4–13 and examining rates within TNM stages, it can be seen that survival rates within stages are not dramatically different between treatments. However, survival rates for patients in stages II and III are highest with radiation treatment, and in stages I and IV they are highest with surgical treatment. Comparisons of treatment effectiveness within CS stages are presented in Table 4–14. For patients in

TABLE 4-13 Five-Year Survival Rates Within TNM Stages as a Function of Initial Treatment*

TNM Stage	Radiation	Surgery	Combined	Total
I	45/56 (80%)	9/11 (82%)	6/8 (75%)	60/75 (80%)
II	22/32 (69%)	7/11 (64%)	3/5 (60%)	32/48 (67%)
III	6/9 (67%)	11/18 (61%)	9/17 (53%)	26/44 (59%)
IV	1/4 (25%)	1/2 (50%)	4/11 (36%)	6/17 (35%)
Total	74/101 (73%)	28/42 (67%)	22/41 (54%)	124/184 (67%)

*Denominators, number of patients in each category; numerators, corresponding number of 5-year survivors.

TABLE 4-14 Five-Year Survival Rates Within Clinical Severity Stages as a Function of Initial Treatment*

Clinical Severity Stage	Radiation	Surgery	Combined	Total
I	42/47 (89%)	6/6 (100%)	5/5 (100%)	53/58 (91%)
II	24/33 (73%)	9/13 (69%)	4/6 (67%)	37/52 (71%)
III	7/17 (41%)	12/21 (57%)	9/19 (47%)	28/57 (49%)
IV	1/4 (25%)	1/2 (50%)	4/11 (36%)	6/17 (35%)
Total	74/101 (73%)	28/42 (67%)	22/41 (54%)	124/184 (67%)

*Denominators, number of patients in each category; numerators, corresponding number of 5-year survivors.

CS stages I, III, and IV, surgical treatment has provided the highest survival rates, whereas survival rates for patients in CS stage II were highest with radiation treatment.

Although the differences in survival overall and within TNM and CS stages as a result of different treatments are not statistically significant, it is interesting to see what impact the different staging systems have had on the evaluation of treatment effectiveness.

For example, consider the patient with a T2N0 carcinoma of the glottis. Based on the TNM staging system and according to Table 4–13, radiation therapy has a slightly higher 5-year survival rate than does surgery or combined treatment (69% vs. 64% vs. 60%). Now consider that this patient has respiratory difficulty, cough, and malaise at the time of presentation but does not have severe comorbidity. Based on these clinical factors and the TNM stage, this patient would be classified into CS stage III. By referring to Table 4–14, it can be seen that surgery—not radiation therapy—produces the highest 5-year survival rate (57% vs. 41%). This example illustrates how using different staging systems can lead to different inferences about treatment effectiveness.

The conclusions about which treatment is most effective are based not only on the type of staging system used but also on the outcome of interest. In the previous examples, the outcome measure was 5-year survival. Quantity of survival is very important but is not the only outcome of interest to physicians and patients.[61] Many other outcomes, such as cancer recurrence, health status, quality of life, and cost of care, are also important. Similar treatment effectiveness analyses can be performed with these other important outcomes. To incorporate both quantity and quality of survival requires the use of quality-adjusted life-years and other utility calculations.[133, 134]

Finally, because these treatments were not selected randomly, definitive conclusions about treatment effectiveness are not possible. The results of observational (i.e., noncontrolled) studies can be helpful in the care of patients and the design of future randomized clinical trials. However, only the results of randomized trials can be used to make definitive conclusions about treatment effectiveness.

◼ CONCLUSION

Patients with cancer of the head and neck present a significant challenge to health care professionals. Because of the anatomic complexity of the head and neck, the various treatment options available, and the functional limitations resulting from treatment, the initial evaluation, treatment, and follow-up of the patient with head and neck cancer require a multidisciplinary team approach. When excellence in delivery of treatment is coupled with complete and valid assessments of the extent of disease, the severity of illness, the psychosocial situation, and patient preference, successful outcomes can often be achieved. The AJCC TNM system is an excellent method for the classification of extent of tumor. Nevertheless, other notable features of the patient with cancer are important for prognosis, treatment selection, and evaluation of therapeutic effectiveness. Improvements in the care of patients with head and neck cancer will result from improvements in its evaluation, classification, and treatment.

REFERENCES

1. American Joint Committee on Cancer: AJCC Cancer Staging Manual, 6th ed. New York, Springer-Verlag, 2002.
2. Lancer JM, Moir AA: The flexible fibreoptic rhinolaryngoscope. J Laryngol Otol 99:767, 1985.
3. Gates GA, Painter C: Objective assessment of laryngeal function. In Cummings CW, Fredrickson JM, Krause CJ, et al (eds): Otolaryngology: Head and Neck Surgery. Update II. St. Louis, Mosby–Year Book, 1990, pp 3–9.
4. Saklad M: Grading of patients for surgical procedures. Anesthesiology 2:281, 1941.
5. Velanovich V: Preoperative laboratory screening based on age, gender, and concomitant medical diseases. Surgery 115:56, 1994.
6. Orr ST, Aisner J: Performance status assessment among oncology patients: A review. Cancer Treat Rep 70:1423, 1986.
7. Pelczar BT, Weed HG, Schuller DE, et al: Identifying high-risk patients before head and neck oncologic surgery. Arch Otolaryngol Head Neck Surg 119:861, 1993.
8. Snow GB, Balm AJ, Arendse JW, et al: Prognostic factors in neck node metastasis. In Larson DL, Ballantyne AJ, Guillamondegui OM (eds): Cancer in the Neck: Evaluation and Treatment. New York, Macmillan, 1986, p 53.
9. Calhoun KH, Fulmer P, Weiss R, Hokanson JA: Distant metastases from head and neck squamous cell carcinomas. Laryngoscope 104:199, 1994.
10. Sham JS, Tong CM, Choy D, Yeung DW: Role of bone scanning in detection of subclinical bone metastasis in nasopharyngeal carcinoma. Clin Nucl Med 16:27, 1991.
11. van Veen SA, Balm AJ, Valdes Olmos RA, et al: Occult primary tumors of the head and neck: Accuracy of thallium 201 single-photon emission computed tomography and computed tomography and/or magnetic resonance imaging. Arch Otolaryngol Head Neck Surg 127:406, 2001.
12. Dudrick SJ, O'Donnell JJ, Weinmann-Winkler S: Nutritional management of head and neck tumor patients. In Thawley SE, Panje WR (eds): Comprehensive Management of Head and Neck Tumors. Philadelphia, WB Saunders, 1987, p 14.
13. Hooley R, Levine H, Flores TC, et al: Predicting postoperative head and neck complications using nutritional assessment. The prognostic nutritional index. Arch Otolaryngol 109:83, 1983.
14. Fletcher JP, Little JM, Guest PK: A comparison of serum transferrin and serum prealbumin as nutritional parameters. J Parenteral Enteral Nutr 11:144, 1987.
15. Flynn MB, Leightty FF: Preoperative outpatient nutritional support of patients with squamous cancer of the upper aerodigestive tract. Am J Surg 154:359, 1987.
16. Meguid MM, Campos AC, Hammond WG: Nutritional support in surgical practice: Part 1. Am J Surg 159:345, 1990.
17. Gibson S, Wenig BL: Percutaneous endoscopic gastrostomy in the management of head and neck carcinoma. Laryngoscope 102:977, 1992.
18. Breitbart W, Holland J: Psychosocial aspects of head and neck cancer. Semin Oncol 15:61, 1988.
19. Hammerlid E, Bjordal K, Ahlner-Elmqvist M, et al: A prospective study of quality of life in head and neck cancer patients. Part I: At diagnosis. Laryngoscope 111:669, 2001.
20. Lucente FE, Strain JJ, Wyatt DA: Psychological problems of the patient with head and neck cancer. In Thawley SE, Panje WR (eds): Comprehensive Management of Head and Neck Tumors. Philadelphia, WB Saunders, 1987, p 69.
21. Gamba A, Romano M, Grosso IM, et al: Psychosocial adjustment of patients surgically treated for head and neck cancer. Head Neck 14:218, 1992.
22. Derogatis LR, Morrow GR, Fetting J, et al: The prevalence of psychiatric disorders among cancer patients. JAMA 249:751, 1983.
23. Dillon WP, Harnsberger HR: The impact of radiologic imaging on staging of cancer of the head and neck. Semin Oncol 18:64, 1991.
24. Piollet H, Lufkin RB, Hanafee W: Magnetic resonance imaging of tumors of the upper aerodigestive tract. Oncology 3:93, 1989.
25. Di Martino E, Nowak B, Hassan HA, et al: Diagnosis and staging of head and neck cancer: A comparison of modern imaging modalities (positron emission tomography, computed tomography, color-coded duplex sonography) with panendoscopic and histopathologic findings. Arch Otolaryngol Head Neck Surg 126:1457, 2000.

26. van den Brekel MW, Stel HV, Castelijns JA, et al: Cervical lymph node metastasis: Assessment of radiologic criteria. Radiology 177:379, 1990.

27. Stevens MH, Harnsberger HR, Mancuso AA, et al: Computed tomography of cervical lymph nodes. Staging and management of head and neck cancer. Arch Otolaryngol 111:735, 1985.

28. Knappe M, Louw M, Gregor RT: Ultrasonography-guided fine-needle aspiration for the assessment of cervical metastases. Arch Otolaryngol Head Neck Surg 126:1091, 2000.

29. Langman AW, Kaplan MJ, Dillon WP, Gooding GA: Radiologic assessment of tumor and the carotid artery: Correlation of magnetic resonance imaging, ultrasound, and computed tomography with surgical findings. Head Neck 11:443, 1989.

30. Shaha A, Webber C, Marti J: Fine-needle aspiration in the diagnosis of cervical lymphadenopathy. Am J Surg 152:420, 1986.

31. Karayianis SL, Francisco GJ, Schumann GB: Clinical utility of head and neck aspiration cytology. Diagn Cytopathol 4:187, 1988.

32. Bastian RW, Collins SL, Kaniff T, Matz GJ: Indirect videolaryngoscopy versus direct endoscopy for larynx and pharynx cancer staging. Toward elimination of preliminary direct laryngoscopy. Ann Otol Rhinol Laryngol 98:693, 1989.

33. Hordijk GJ, Bruggink T, Ravasz LA: Panendoscopy: A valuable procedure? Otolaryngol Head Neck Surg 101:426, 1989.

34. Benninger MS, Enrique RR, Nichols RD: Symptom-directed selective endoscopy and cost containment for evaluation of head and neck cancer. Head Neck 15:532, 1993.

35. Ina H, Shibuya H, Ohashi I, Kitagawa M: The frequency of a concomitant early esophageal cancer in male patients with oral and oropharyngeal cancer. Screening results using Lugol dye endoscopy. Cancer 73:2038, 1994.

36. Stoeckli SJ, Zimmermann R, Schmid S: Role of routine panendoscopy in cancer of the upper aerodigestive tract. Otolaryngol Head Neck Surg 124:208, 2001.

37. Bradford CR, Wolf GT, Carey TE, et al: Predictive markers for response to chemotherapy, organ preservation, and survival in patients with advanced laryngeal carcinoma. Otolaryngol Head Neck Surg 121:534, 1999.

38. Marchant FE, Lowry LD, Moffitt JJ, Sabbagh R: Current national trends in the posttreatment follow-up of patients with squamous cell carcinoma of the head and neck. Am J Otolaryngol 14:88, 1993.

39. McDonald S, Haie C, Rubin P, et al: Second malignant tumors in patients with laryngeal carcinoma: Diagnosis, treatment, and prevention. Int J Radiat Oncol Biol Phys 17:457, 1989.

40. Haughey BH, Gates GA, Arfken CL, Harvey J: Meta-analysis of second malignant tumors in head and neck cancer: The case for an endoscopic screening protocol. Ann Otol Rhinol Laryngol 101:105, 1992.

41. Stokkel MP, Draisma A, Pauwels EK: Positron emission tomography with 2-[18F]-fluoro-2-deoxy-D-glucose in oncology. Part IIIb: Therapy response monitoring in colorectal and lung tumours, head and neck cancer, hepatocellular carcinoma and sarcoma. J Cancer Res Clin Oncol 127:278, 2001.

42. de Visschar AV, Manni JJ: Routine long-term follow-up in patients treated with curative intent for squamous cell carcinoma of the larynx, pharynx, and oral cavity. Does it make sense? Arch Otolaryngol Head Neck Surg 120:934, 1994.

43. Hess M, Kugler J, Kalveram KT, Vosteen KH: The effect of functional impairments and autonomic symptoms on the quality of life after the therapy of tumors in the ENT area. Laryngorhinootologie 69:647, 1990.

44. Jones E, Lund VJ, Howard DJ, et al: Quality of life of patients treated surgically for head and neck cancer. J Laryngol Otol 106:238, 1992.

45. Rubin P: A unified classification of cancers: An oncotaxonomy with symbols. Cancer 31:963, 1973.

46. Denoix PF, Schwartz D: Regeles generales de classification des cancers et de presentation des resultats therapeutics. Acad Chir (Paris) 85:415, 1959.

47. International Union Against Cancer: TNM Classification of Malignant Tumours, 4th ed. Berlin, Springer-Verlag, 1987, p 1.

48. Copeland MM: Clinical staging of cancer for end result reporting. In Clark RL, Cumley RW (eds): Yearbook of Cancer. Chicago, Ill, Yearbook, 1960, p 498.

49. Cancer Registries Amendment Act of 1992. 42 USC 280e, 1994.

50. Piccirillo JF: Purposes, problems, and proposals for progress in cancer staging. Arch Otolaryngol Head Neck Surg 121:145, 1995.

51. Spiro RH, Huvos AG, Wong GY, et al: Predictive value of tumor thickness in squamous carcinoma confined to the tongue and floor of the mouth. Am J Surg 152:345, 1986.

52. Sako K, Pradier RM, Marchetta FC, Pickren JW: Fallibility of palpation in the diagnosis of metastases to cervical nodes. Surg Gynecol Obstet 118:989, 1964.

53. Rouviere H: Anatomy of the Human Lymphatic System. Ann Arbor, Mich, Edwards, 1938.

54. Spiro RH, Alfonso AE, Farr HW, Strong EW: Cervical node metastasis from epidermoid carcinoma of the oral cavity and oropharynx. A critical assessment of current staging. Am J Surg 128:562, 1974.

55. Stell PM, Morton RP, Singh SD: Cervical lymph node metastases: The significance of the level of the lymph node. Clin Oncol 9:101, 1983.

56. Burke HB, Henson DE: Criteria for prognostic factors and for an enhanced prognostic system. Cancer 72:3131, 1993.

57. Feinstein AR, Pritchett JA, Schimpff CR: The epidemiology of cancer therapy. II. The clinical course: data, decisions, and temporal demarcations. Arch Intern Med 123:323, 1969.

58. Feinstein AR: Clinical Judgment. Melbourne, Fla, Krieger, 1974.

59. Feinstein AR, Spitz H: The epidemiology of cancer therapy. I. Clinical problems of statistical surveys. Arch Intern Med 123:171, 1969.

60. Feinstein AR, Pritchett JA, Schimpff CR: The epidemiology of cancer therapy. III. The management of imperfect data. Arch Intern Med 123:448, 1969.

61. Feinstein AR, Pritchett JA, Schimpff CR: The epidemiology of cancer therapy. IV. The extraction of data from medical records. Arch Intern Med 123:571, 1969.

62. Feinstein AR, Sosin DM, Wells CK: The Will Rogers phenomenon. Stage migration and new diagnostic techniques as a source of misleading statistics for survival in cancer. N Engl J Med 312:1604, 1985.

63. McNeil BJ, Weichselbaum R, Pauker SG: Speech and survival: Tradeoffs between quality and quantity of life in laryngeal cancer. N Engl J Med 305:982, 1981.

64. McNeil BJ, Weichselbaum R, Pauker SG: Fallacy of the five-year survival in lung cancer. N Engl J Med 299:1397, 1978.

65. Feinstein AR: Clinical biostatistics. XLI. Hard science, soft data, and the challenges of choosing clinical variables in research. Clin Pharmacol Ther 22:485, 1977.

66. Fries JF, Spitz PW: The hierarchy of patient outcome. In Spilker B (ed): Quality of Life Assessments in Clinical Trials. New York, Raven Press, 1990, p 25.

67. Piccirillo JF: Outcomes research and otolaryngology. Otolaryngol Head Neck Surg 111:764, 1994.

68. Institute of Medicine: Disability in America. Toward a National Agenda for Prevention. Washington, DC, National Academy Press, 1991.

69. U.S. Department of Health and Human Services: Healthy People 2000 (Publication DHHS 91-50212). Washington, DC, U.S. Department of Health and Human Services, 1991.

70. The Portugal Conference: Measuring quality of life and functional status in clinical and epidemiological research. Proc J Chron Dis 40:459, 1987.

71. Guyatt G, Feeny D, Patrick D: Issues in quality of life measurement in clinical trials. Control Clin Trials 12:81S, 1991.

72. de Haes JCJM, van Knippenberg FCE: Quality of life of cancer patients: Review of the literature. In Aaronson NK, Beckmann J (eds): The Quality of Life of Cancer Patients. New York, Raven Press, 1987, p 167.

73. Torrance GW: Measurement of health state utilities for economic appraisal. A review. J Health Econ 5:1, 1986.

74. Eisenberg JM: Clinical economics. A guide to the economic analysis of clinical practices. JAMA 262:2879, 1989.

75. Entrom JE, Austin DF: Interpreting cancer survival rates. Science 195:847, 1977.

76. Suen JY, Goepfert H: Standardization of neck dissection nomenclature. Head Neck Surg 10:75, 1987.

77. Shah JP, Strong E, Spiro RH, Vikram B: Surgical grand rounds. Neck dissection: Current status and future possibilities. Clin Bull 11:25, 1981.

78. Weymuller EA Jr: Clinical staging and operative reporting for multi-institutional trials in head and neck squamous cell carcinoma. Head Neck 19:650, 1997.

79. Piccirillo JF, Wells CK, Sasaki CT, Feinstein AR: New clinical severity staging system for cancer of the larynx. Five-year survival rates. Ann Otol Rhinol Laryngol 103:83, 1994.

80. Pfister DG, Wells CK, Chan CK, Feinstein AR: Classifying clinical severity to help solve problems of stage migration in nonconcurrent comparisons of lung cancer therapy. Cancer Res 50:4664, 1990.

81. Champion GA, Piccirillo JF: The impact of computer tomography on pretherapeutic staging of patients with laryngeal cancer: Demonstration of the Will Rogers phenomenon. Presented at the Annual Meeting of the American Academy of Otolaryngology Head and Neck Surgery, Dever, CO, Septemeber 10, 2001. [Submitted for publication.]

82. Feinstein AR: On classifying cancers while treating patients [editorial]. Arch Intern Med 145:1789, 1985.

83. Barr LC, Baum M: Time to abandon TNM staging of breast cancer? Lancet 339:915, 1992.

84. Feinstein AR: Symptoms as an index of biological behaviour and prognosis in human cancer. Nature 209:241, 1966.

85. Feinstein AR, Bondy PK: A new staging system for cancer, and a reappraisal of "early" treatment and "cure" by radical surgery. Trans Assoc Am Physicians 80:111, 1967.

86. Neel HB, Taylor WF, Pearson GR: Prognostic determinants and a new view of staging for patients with nasopharyngeal carcinoma. Ann Otol Rhinol Laryngol 94:529, 1985.

87. Stell PM: Prognosis in laryngeal carcinoma: Host factors. Clin Otolaryngol 15:111, 1990.

88. Zelen M: Keynote address on biostatistics and data retrieval. Cancer Chemother Rep 4:31, 1973.

89. Wells CK, Stoller JK, Feinstein AR, Horwitz RI: Comorbid and clinical determinants of prognosis in endometrial cancer. Arch Intern Med 144:2004, 1984.

90. Concato J, Horwitz RI, Feinstein AR, et al: Problems of comorbidity in mortality after prostatectomy. JAMA 267:1077, 1992.

91. Greenfield S, Aronow HU, Elashoff RM, Watanbe D: Flaws in mortality data. The hazards of ignoring comorbid disease. JAMA 260:2253, 1988.

92. Satariano WA: Comorbidity and functional status in older women with breast cancer: Implications for screening, treatment, and prognosis. J Gerontol 47:24, 1992.

93. Satariano WA, Ragland DR: The effect of comorbidity on 3-year survival of women with primary breast cancer. Ann Intern Med 120:104, 1994.

94. Clemens JD, Feinstein AR, Holabird N, Cartwright S: A new clinical-anatomic staging system for evaluating prognosis and treatment of prostatic cancer. J Chron Dis 39:913, 1986.

95. Feinstein AR, Schimpff CR, Hull EW: A reappraisal of staging and therapy for patients with cancer of the rectum. I. Development of two new systems of staging. Arch Intern Med 135:1441, 1975.

96. Feinstein AR, Wells CK: A clinical-severity staging system for patients with lung cancer. Medicine 69:1, 1990.

97. Feinstein AR, Schimpff CR, Andrews JFJ, Wells CK: Cancer of the larynx: A new staging system and a re-appraisal of prognosis and treatment. J Chron Dis 30:277, 1977.

98. Pugliano FA, Piccirillo JF, Zequeira MR, et al: Symptoms as an index of biologic behavior in head and neck cancer. Otolaryngol Head Neck Surg 120:380, 1999.

99. Ribeiro KC, Kowalski LP, Latorre MR: Impact of comorbidity, symptoms and patient's characteristics on the prognosis of oral carcinomas. Arch Otolaryngol Head Neck Surg 126:1079, 2000.

100. Pugliano FA, Piccirillo JF, Zequeira MR, et al: Clinical-severity staging system for oral cavity cancer: Five-year survival rates. Otolaryngol Head Neck Surg 120:38, 1999.

101. Pugliano FA, Piccirillo JF, Zequeira MR, et al: Clinical-severity staging system for oropharyngeal cancer: Five-year survival rates. Arch Otolaryngol Head Neck Surg 123:1118, 1997.

102. de Boer MF, McCormick LK, Pruyn JF, et al: Physical and psychosocial correlates of head and neck cancer: A review of the literature. Otolaryngol Head Neck Surg 120:427, 1999.

103. Karnofsky DA, Abelmann WH, Craver LF, Burchenal JH: The use of the nitrogen mustards in the palliative treatment of carcinoma. Cancer 1:634, 1948.

104. Spitzer WO, Dobson AJ, Hall J, et al: Measuring the quality of life of cancer patients: A concise QL index for use by physicians. J Chron Dis 34:585, 1981.

105. Zubrod CG, Schneiderman M, Frei E: Appraisal of methods for the study of chemotherapy of cancer in man: Comparative therapeutic trial of nitrogen mustards and triethylene thiophosphoramide. J Chron Dis 11:7, 1960.

106. Bjordal K, Ahlner-Elmqvist M, Tollesson E, et al: Development of a European Organization for Research and Treatment of Cancer (EORTC) questionnaire module to be used in quality of life assessments in head and neck cancer patients. EORTC Quality of Life Study Group. Acta Oncol 33:879, 1994.

107. Hassan SJ, Weymuller EA Jr: Assessment of quality of life in head and neck cancer patients. Head Neck 15:485, 1993.

108. Cella DF TDBA: The functional assessment of cancer therapy (FACT) scales: Incorporating disease-specificity and subjectivity into quality of life assessment. Proc Annu Meet Am Soc Oncol 9:325, 1990.

109. Piccirillo JF: Impact of comorbidity and symptoms on the prognosis of patients with oral carcinoma. Arch Otolaryngol Head Neck Surg 126:1086, 2000.

110. Chen AY, Matson LK, Roberts D, Goepfert H: The significance of comorbidity in advanced laryngeal cancer. Head Neck 23:566.

111. Boring CC, Squires TS, Tong T, Montgomery S: Cancer statistics, 1994. Cancer J Clin 44:7, 1994.

112. Charlson ME, Pompei P, Ales KL, MacKenzie CR: A new method of classifying prognostic comorbidity in longitudinal studies: Development and validation. J Chron Dis 40:373, 1987.

113. Kaplan MH, Feinstein AR: The importance of classifying initial comorbidity in evaluating the outcome of diabetes mellitus. J Chron Dis 27:387, 1974.

114. Piccirillo JF: Importance of comorbidity in head and neck cancer. Laryngoscope 110:593, 2000.

115. Ross, Tinker: Anesthesia risk. In Miller RD (ed): Anesthesia. New York, Churchill Livingstone, 1995, p 723.

116. Vacanti CJ, Van Houten RJ, Hill RC: A statistical analysis of the relationship of physical status to postoperative mortality in 68,388 cases. Anesth Analg 49:564, 1970.

117. Marx GF, Mateo CV, Orkin LR: Computer analysis of postanesthetic deaths. Anesthesiology 39:54, 1973.

118. Piccirillo JF: Problems in the American Joint Committee System for Staging Cancer. Presented at the RWJ National Clinical Scholars Meeting, Fort Lauderdale, FL, November, 1991.

119. Stell PM: Letter to author (JFP). March 1992.

120. Cox DR: Regression methods and life tables (with discussion). J Royal Stat Soc, B34:187–220, 1972.

121. Harrell FEJ, Lee KL, Matchar DB, Reichert TA: Regression models for prognostic prediction: Advantages, problems, and suggested solutions. Cancer Treat Rep 69:1071, 1985.

122. Concato J, Feinstein AR, Holford TR: The risk of determining risk with multivariable models. Ann Intern Med 118:201, 1993.

123. Sox HC Jr, Blatt M, Higgins MC, Marton KI: Medical Decision Making. London, Butterworths, 1987.

124. Feinstein AR, Rubinstein JF, Ramshaw WA: Estimating prognosis with the aid of a conversational-mode computer program. Ann Intern Med 76:911, 1972.

125. Piccirillo JF, Feinstein AR: Black-box mathematics and medical practice. Arch Otolaryngol Head Neck Surg 119:147, 1993.

126. Feinstein AR: Clinimetrics. New Haven, Conn, Yale University Press, 1987.

127. Feinstein AR: Clinical biostatistics. XIV. The purposes of prognostic stratification. Clin Pharmacol Ther 13:285, 1972.

128. Feinstein AR: Clinical biostatistics. XV. The process of prognostic stratification. Part 1. Clin Pharmacol Ther 13:442, 1972.

129. Feinstein AR: Clinical biostatistics. XVI. The process of prognostic stratification. Part 2. Clin Pharmacol Ther 13:609, 1972.

130. Ash AS, Shwartz M: Evaluating the performance of risk adjustment methods: Dichotomous measures. In Iezzoni LI (ed): Risk Adjustment for Measuring Health Care Outcomes. Ann Arbor, Mich, Health Administration Press, 1994, p 313.

131. Kramer MS: Clinical Epidemiology and Biostatistics. New York, Springer-Verlag, 1988.

132. Harrell FEJ, Lee KL, Califf RM, et al: Regression modeling strategies for improved prognostic prediction. Stat Med 3:143, 1984.

133. Llewellyn-Thomas H, Sutherland HJ, Tibshirani R, et al: Describing health states. Methodologic issues in obtaining values for health states. Med Care 22:543, 1984.

134. Lane DA: Utility, decision, and quality of life. J Chron Dis 40:585, 1987.

CHAPTER 5

Radiologic Evaluation of Cancer of the Head and Neck

Melanie B. Fukui

Hugh D. Curtin

Jane L. Weissman

Imaging technology continues to develop.[1, 2] Many of the initial problems associated with magnetic resonance imaging (MRI) have been addressed, and superb images of the head and neck are the routine rather than the exception. Computed tomography (CT) is faster, so patient motion is not as much of a limitation as with MRI.

The basic principles of head and neck cancer imaging have not changed. Some progress has been made in functional imaging, in which the examination reflects metabolism as well as anatomy. Usually, though, the task of the radiologist is to define the margin of abnormal anatomy and the location and the extent of disease.

The radiologist is rarely the first to diagnose the presence of a tumor. Tumors are almost always detected clinically by palpation or by direct visualization. The role of the radiologist is to define the depth of extension of a lesion and the relationship of the tumor to various structures, which are key determinants of surgical approach and potential resectability. The first section of this chapter describes some of the more commonly used imaging modalities, in addition to newer imaging techniques. Later, modes of tumor extension are described and discussed in relation to the different regions of the head and neck.

■ IMAGING METHODS

Plain Films and Fluoroscopy

The density of tissue determines the number of x-rays stopped by a tissue and thus the number of x-rays reaching a film. This principle is the basis of plain film radiography, fluoroscopy, tomography, and CT.

Plain films offer excellent spatial resolution (the ability to separate small objects that are close together) if the density differences are great enough. The spatial resolution of a plain film is greater than that of CT. Plain films can be used when air abuts a soft tissue or when soft tissue is against bone because density differences are high and one tissue can be "contrasted" against another. Plain radiographs provide little information about the soft tissues because the densities of the various components of soft tissue are similar.

Some materials, such as metal, absorb even more x-rays than are absorbed by bone and so can easily be seen on plain films or by fluoroscopy. Barium and iodinated contrast media can be used as contrast agents to outline an area in which the natural contrast is not high enough to allow adequate visualization (Fig. 5–1). Fluoroscopy is a dynamic study that enables evaluation of motion or of position over time.

Plain films of the head and neck are rarely used to evaluate head and neck cancer if CT and MRI are available. However, the radiologist may discover a tumor on a plain film taken to investigate sinusitis. Plain films of the chest are still the routine survey examination. Fluoroscopy is used during an esophagram so that long segments can be evaluated quickly. The dynamic capability of the fluoroscopy is important because distensibility and pliability of the esophagus are important parts of the examination.

Computed Tomography

CT is based on the same physical principles as for plain film radiography, but detectors are used instead of films, and a computer uses complicated algorithms to calculate the relative electron density at each point on a plane, called the *image slice*. The image does not have the resolution of a plain film, but the ability to differentiate the various soft tissues and to see structures unobscured by superimposed bone more than compensates for this slight disadvantage. CT separates muscle from fat and gives an excellent image of bone. Tumor can be identified by its effect on the fat planes, which become important landmarks throughout the head and neck.

Indeed, the ability of CT to distinguish tumor from fat is one of the most useful attributes of this modality in the evaluation of tumors of the head and neck. Separation of tumor from muscle is more difficult in that the densities can be the same (Figs. 5–2 and 5–3). Similarly, determining the relationship of tumor to blood vessels is very important but difficult because tumor and vessels have very similar densities. The use of intravenous contrast helps to resolve these problems.

Iodine has a high electron density and stops many x-rays in much the same way as does bone. Thus, iodine can easily be differentiated from almost all nonenhancing soft tissue. Compounds of iodine can be injected intravenously and are harmlessly excreted through the kidneys. With contrast agent in a vessel or in the soft tissue, the structure is more

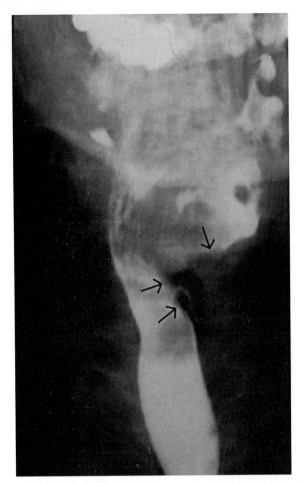

FIGURE 5–1 Frontal view of a barium swallow showing a bulky tumor of the left pyriform sinus (*arrows*).

dense or more opaque to x-rays. Its white appearance is similar to that of bone. Because different tissues enhance to different degrees, tumor can be differentiated from vessels and usually from muscle. The tumor may enhance more than does muscle, so the interface between tumor and muscle is appreciated.

The rapidity with which an image can be generated has a direct bearing on the quality of the image. The longer it takes to collect the data for a particular image, the more likely it is that patient motion (e.g., swallowing, breathing, even pulsation of vessels) will occur and degrade an image. Shorter image times allow less time for possible movement and therefore characteristically result in better images. When CT was first used in the 1970s, a single slice required 10 seconds for data collection. Modern scanners can do a complete study through the entire neck in almost the same time. Spiral or helical technology continuously collects data as the scanner "spirals" down the neck, rather than going slice by slice.

Data are still collected in one primary plane, which is in the plane of the gantry or perpendicular to the axis of the "bore" of the scanner. In obtaining a direct coronal image, the patient must be positioned so that the body part to be examined is in the appropriate orientation relative to the

CT gantry. Direct coronal images of the sinus can usually be achieved, although with some patient discomfort. Direct coronal images of the neck are impossible.

Reformatted images are computer manipulations of the data. Data points from many slices are stacked and cut so that an approximation of a coronal image can be obtained (Fig. 5–4). With rapid acquisition of a complete data set through the neck by means of helical scanning, the reformatted images approach the quality of direct scans. Certainly, reformatted images now are better than the direct scans of the not too distant past.

The next step in image manipulation is development of a three-dimensional image (Fig. 5–5) by image stacking and data remanipulation. Although these images do not provide information beyond that already available on the axial scan, they provide an additional perspective that can be very helpful in communicating the extent of a lesion.

Once a data set is collected, various algorithms can be applied to the data (see Figs. 5–2A and B). An algorithm is simply a computer software program that can accentuate a certain characteristic of the image. For instance, the *bone algorithm* accentuates or sharpens margins that have a great difference in density. Bone–soft tissue interfaces are made more obvious by the large differences between bone and soft tissue. Margins between air and soft tissue also benefit from such programs. The detail within the soft tissues is poor; separation of muscle and fat, for instance, is not obvious. However, bone detail (cortex, medullary cavity) is superb. The data can be reworked with soft tissue algorithms without reimaging (i.e., reexposing) the patient.

Magnetic Resonance Imaging

MRI uses radio waves rather than x-rays to create an image. The dangers associated with ionizing radiation are not a factor in MRI. Imaging times are still longer than those for CT, but considerable progress has been made toward addressing this problem. Resolution rivaling that of CT can now be achieved by MRI. The thinnest slice available with the most modern MRI unit is actually slightly smaller than the thinnest available with CT. However, the thinnest slices with the highest resolution often require a significant investment of scanner time if a pleasing image is to be produced. Each year brings faster and better MRI, and this is likely to continue for some time.

The key advantage of MRI is its ability to differentiate soft tissues more easily than they can be differentiated on CT (see Figs. 5–2 and 5–3). In addition, images can be made in any slice orientation without the need for repositioning the patient. Sagittal, coronal, and even oblique images can be produced as easily as axial images.

MRI produces an image by using magnets and radio waves. A complete description of the process is beyond the scope of this chapter, but many good descriptions are available.[3] Some brief comments are in order.

Certain nuclei have magnetic properties and thus react with any other magnetic field in the vicinity. Radio waves can stimulate these nuclei to move to a higher energy level. When the stimulating radiofrequency is turned off, the nuclei tend to return to the lower energy level, giving off a radiofrequency wave in the process. If, by using a very complex system of coils, the magnetic field is varied, the radiofrequency that emanates from any point can be defined and an image produced.

Several terms and ideas are necessary for an understanding of MRI.

1. Almost all imaging currently is done by stimulating hydrogen nuclei.

2. The amount of radiofrequency coming from a region is called *signal intensity* and is usually shown as brightness or whiteness on the image. Lack of signal (no radiofrequency from an area) is dark or black (signal void).

3. *T1-weighting* is a function of how quickly the stimulated nuclei return to their base state after the stimulating radiofrequency is turned off. T1-weighted

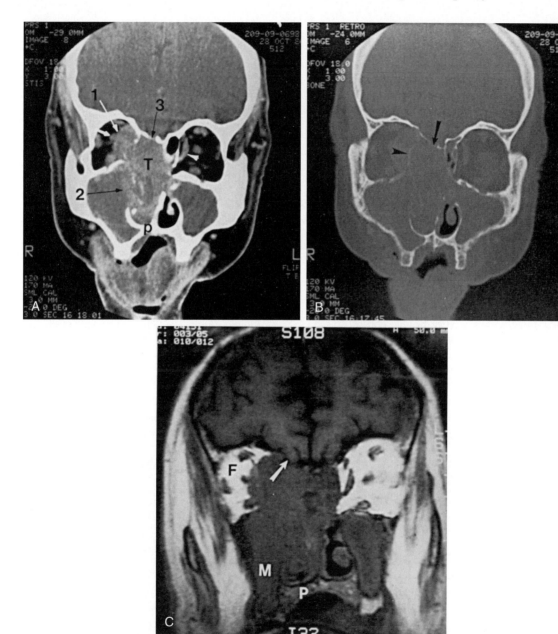

FIGURE 5–2   Carcinoma of the nasal cavity, ethmoid sinus, and orbit. *A*, Coronal CT scan (soft tissue algorithm) shows the tumor (T) in the nasal cavity, extending through the lamina papyracea into the right orbit (1), close to the optic nerve *(unlabeled arrow)*. The medial rectus muscle is inseparable from the tumor; the left medial rectus muscle is normal *(arrowhead)*. The tumor margin (2) is seen against the low-density obstructed secretions in the maxillary sinus. The tumor erodes the cribriform plate (3) and extends down to the hard palate (P). *B*, Coronal CT scan (bone algorithm) shows the erosion of the cribriform plate *(arrowhead)* much more clearly than in *A*. Bone algorithms do not distinguish tumor from orbital fat *(arrowhead)* or from brain or obstructed secretions. *C*, Coronal T1-weighted MR image shows intermediate-signal tumor against the normal white orbital fat (F). Cribriform plate is not seen well, but tumor is separated from brain *(arrow)* by low-signal CSF. M, maxillary antrum; P, hard palate.

Continued

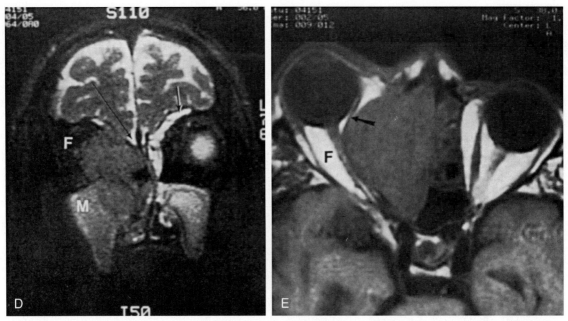

FIGURE 5–2, Cont'd *D*, Coronal T2-weighted MR image shows normal white CSF *(long arrow)* between tumor and brain. Fat (F) is darker than tumor on this T2-weighted image, and the obstructed secretions in the maxillary sinus (M) and the left ethmoid sinus *(short arrow)* are brighter than tumor. *E*, Axial T1-weighted MR image shows the tumor bowing the medial rectus muscle *(arrow)* laterally. The margin of tumor is easily seen against the bright orbital fat (F).

images have relatively short imaging times and produce clear images. Fat is very bright, cerebrospinal fluid (CSF) is dark, and muscle is of moderate signal intensity (see Figs. 5–2C and E and 5–3B).

4. *T2-weighting* relates to the loss of phase coherence of the nuclei after the stimulating sequence is turned off.

This is a more difficult property to measure. Conventional T2-weighted images take longer to produce and tend to be less sharp than T1-weighted images of comparable image time (see Fig. 5–2D). T2-weighted images are worth having because their ability to contrast one tissue with another is enhanced

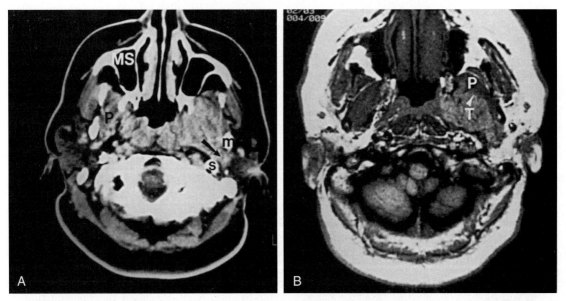

FIGURE 5–3 Thyroid carcinoma metastatic to the parapharyngeal space. *A*, Axial CT image shows tumor in the left parapharyngeal space, inseparable from the lateral pterygoid muscles, extending through the stylomandibular tunnel *(arrow)*, between the mandible (m) and the styloid process (s). M, maxillary sinus. *B*, Axial T1-weighted MR image of the same patient shows the tumor (T) inseparable from the pterygoid muscle (P), with an irregular interface *(arrowhead)* suggesting invasion. Tumor and muscle have very different signal intensities.

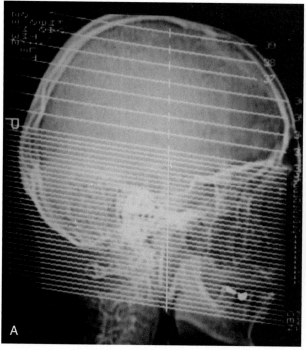

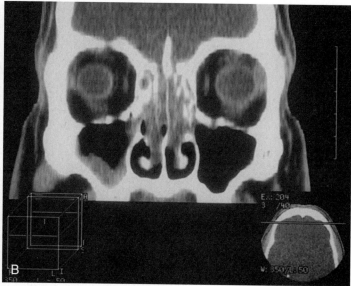

FIGURE 5–4 *A,* Scout view from a CT study posted with lines indicating the locations of axial images. *B,* Reformatted coronal CT image, which was created by the computer software from axial images such as those shown in *A.*

in certain situations. The CSF is bright, and fat tends to darken with stronger T2-weighting.

5. *Pulse sequence* refers to the number and the timing of radiofrequency pulses directed into the patient.

6. Regions giving no signal (signal void) are black on the MRI image. Examples of this phenomenon are cortical bone and air. Rapidly flowing blood gives a signal void in most routine pulse sequences (Fig. 5–6). The blood that was stimulated by the radiofrequency has moved

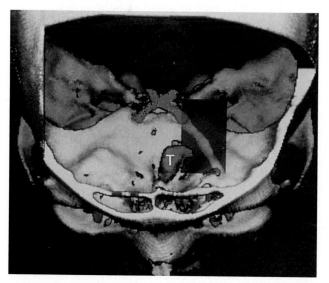

FIGURE 5–5 Three-dimensional (3-D) reconstruction of axial CT. A small tumor (T) is seen in the cribriform plate area. The position relative to the optic nerves can be judged on the 3-D image.

out of the region and has been replaced by nonstimulated blood. Sequences have been developed that actually cause a bright signal from flowing blood. These are used to create magnetic resonance angiograms.

7. Surface coils are small antennas that when placed close to an area are efficient at picking up a signal. These are good for examining areas close to the surface, but they lose their advantage with increasing depth.

MRI can distinguish between tissues that may be of similar densities on CT. For instance, tumors tend to have the same CT appearance as muscle and be indistinguishable. MRI can often define the margin of the tumor (see Fig. 5–6). As tumor extends intracranially, the relationship of a tumor to the brain can usually be better defined with MRI than with CT (see Fig. 5–6). The CSF is more clearly imaged by MRI than by CT because the signal difference between CSF and soft tissue (brain) is greater than are the CT density differences.

Intravenous iodinated contrast medium (with its potential allergic complications) is not a factor in MRI. Paramagnetic intravenous agents (gadolinium) are used to improve the signal from some tissues and are considered to be safer than CT contrast agents.

The use of MRI offers some advantages. Although imaging times with MRI are fairly long, allowing patient motion (e.g., swallowing, breathing) to interfere, recent advances in technology have decreased the imaging time and motion artifacts. A technique called *fast spin-echo imaging* (Fig. 5–7) allows the MRI machine to acquire more than one image in the same time interval. Thus, anatomic regions can be imaged with a much shorter sequence than was previously required. The time saved can be used to produce a sharper

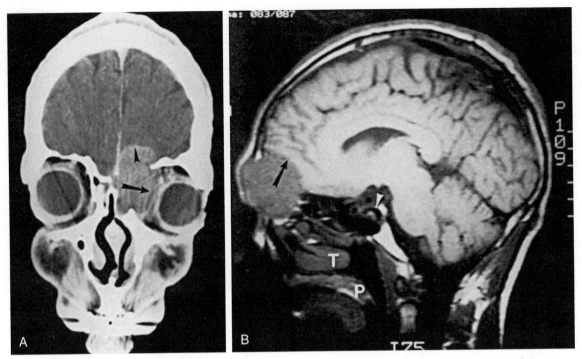

FIGURE 5–6 Lymphoma of the ethmoid sinus and orbit. *A,* Coronal CT image shows tumor eroding through left lamina papyracea into orbit *(arrow)* and extending intracranially through cribriform plate and fovea ethmoidalis *(arrowhead). B,* Sagittal T1-weighted MR image shows the intracranial extent of the tumor *(arrow),* which has a different signal intensity from the frontal lobe displaced by the tumor. The signal void of rapidly flowing blood in the carotid artery *(arrowhead)* is the same as the signal void of air in the adjacent sphenoid sinus. T, inferior turbinate; P, soft palate.

image. This concept is particularly true with the T2-weighted sequence. The fast spin-echo T2-weighted image is much sharper and is achieved in much less time.

The tissue characteristics of a fast spin-echo sequence are almost the same as those of a conventional spin-echo sequence. On the fast spin-echo T2-weighted image, fluid is bright but the fat is not dark. This can lead to problems. Normally, the "darkening" on T2-weighted sequences can be helpful in differentiating fat from some other substances, such as hemorrhage. A second technologic development can be used to address this problem.

Fat suppression is a technique that allows the signal coming from fat to be obliterated (see Fig. 5–7A). The hydrogen nuclei in fat and those in water have slightly different characteristic frequencies. The frequencies are close enough that both fat and water contribute to the final image, but electronic manipulations allow separation and obliteration of signals coming either from fat or from water. In the case of the T2-weighted fast spin-echo image, the signal from fat can be "suppressed" so that the final result has the appearance of the more familiar conventional spin-echo image: fluid is bright and fat is dark.

Fat suppression is also useful on T1-weighted images obtained after gadolinium administration. After gadolinium, a tissue that "enhances" is bright and so is very clearly seen against a tissue that is dark. If, however, the enhancement abuts fat, both the enhancing tissue and the fat are bright and the interface is lost. Selective fat suppression is used to turn the fat dark so that the enhancing tissues can be easily differentiated.

Another problem with MRI is the difficulty in evaluating structures that provide little or no signal. Imaging of bone can be a problem; cortical bone gives no signal. This has not been a major problem in tumor imaging because as tumor destroys a cortical surface, signal (from the tumor) is seen where there should be none. The medullary portions of bone have a high enough fat content that a bright signal is seen on a T1-weighted image. As tumor invades such an area, the relatively high signal medullary cavity is replaced by tumor with a less intense signal. Nonetheless, the thin slice and bone algorithm of CT do provide an advantage for the imaging of cortical margins.

The use of MRI presents more of a problem in the middle ear and mastoid. The mastoid and ossicles are predominantly cortical bone. Here, the bone is adjacent to air, with almost no intervening soft tissue. Neither cortical bone nor air gives signal, so the ossicles and the mastoid septations are invisible on MRI. If, however, tumor invades the middle ear or mastoid, the air is replaced; signal is seen where there should be none, and the tumor can be visualized.

Metals can cause artifacts with MRI but tend to be less of a problem than with CT. Metals distort the magnetic field and interfere with signal near the metal, but the "spray" artifact seen from the teeth on CT is not encountered on MRI.

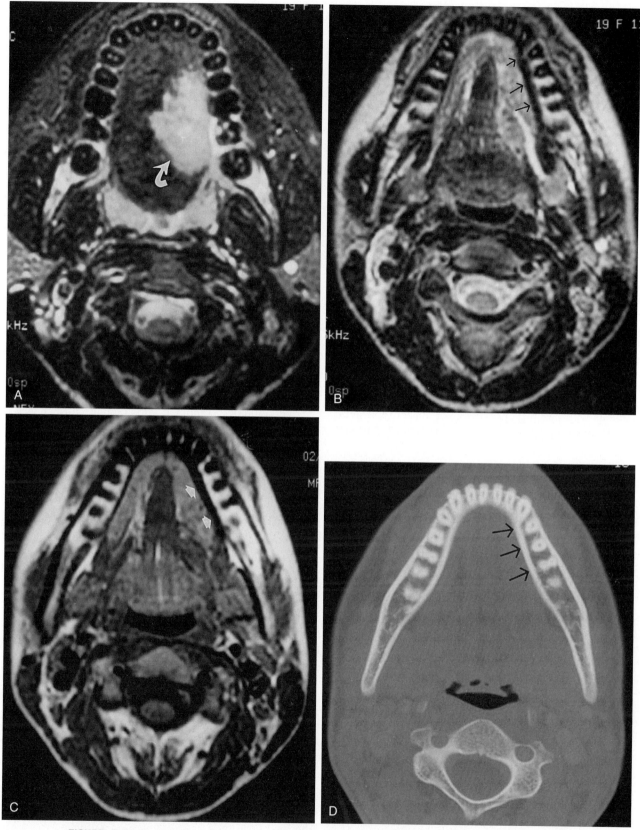

FIGURE 5–7 Tongue carcinoma. *A*, T2-weighted fast spin-echo image with fat suppression. The outline of the tumor is clearly seen *(arrow)*, and its medial margin can be assessed relative to midline. *B*, Slightly lower slice shows an intact black line *(arrows)*, which represents an intact cortex of the mandible. *C*, T1-weighted image shows the intact cortex *(arrows)*. *D*, High-resolution CT scan bone algorithm shows an intact white line, which represents the cortex *(arrows)*.

Iron Oxide Particle (Combidex) MRI

Iron oxide particles (Combidex) are a contrast agent for identifying lymph node involvement with tumor.[4, 5] The principle underlying iron oxide imaging is that lymph nodes replaced by tumor do not concentrate the agent, whereas normal lymph nodes do take up the particles. Because iron produces low signal on MRI, normal lymph nodes appear dark (Fig. 5–8); lymph nodes harboring tumor are brighter than normal nodes (Fig. 5–9). This technique is limited by the inability of MRI to resolve small lymph nodes.[5]

Proton Magnetic Resonance Spectroscopy

Proton magnetic resonance spectroscopy measures specific metabolites that may be elevated in neoplasia and other disease processes. Spectroscopy has been used extensively in the brain to distinguish recurrent tumor from radiation necrosis. In many neoplasms, the metabolite choline is elevated with respect to creatine (an increased choline/creatine ratio). In vitro studies confirm an elevated choline/creatine ratio in squamous cell carcinoma of the head and neck.[6] Although this application is highly desirable in the head and neck, magnetic resonance spectroscopy in vivo is made challenging by air-filled structures that impede the homogeneous magnetic field needed for reliable spectroscopy data to be acquired. In the future, magnetic resonance scanners able to obtain smaller voxels than current scanners may overcome this obstacle.

Patients with pacemakers or with certain ferromagnetic aneurysm clips, implants, or foreign bodies cannot be placed in the magnet because the effect of the magnet on these metals can be dangerous to the patient.

Ultrasound

Ultrasound is of limited usefulness in the head and neck because bone does not transmit sound. If the mass is approachable by an ultrasound probe, an examination can determine whether a lesion is cystic or solid. Ultrasound is used extensively in thyroid-parathyroid evaluation and is occasionally used in assessment of the salivary glands. Some investigators have tried to evaluate possible tumor invasion of the carotid artery, with variable success.

Carcinoma of the tongue has been reported to give fewer echoes than the muscles of the tongue. Therefore, the relationship of a tumor to midline can be determined. This methodology has not been widely accepted.

Neck nodes can be easily seen with the use of ultrasound. The margin of the node reflects the sound waves to a much greater extent than does the surrounding fat, making them obvious on the image monitor. Size can be determined, and if the node is larger than normal, an aspiration biopsy can be done using ultrasound as a guide. Several reports have found this to be an excellent method for evaluating neck nodes.[7]

Nuclear Medicine

Radioisotopes combined with certain carriers that are injected or ingested will concentrate in certain soft tissues.

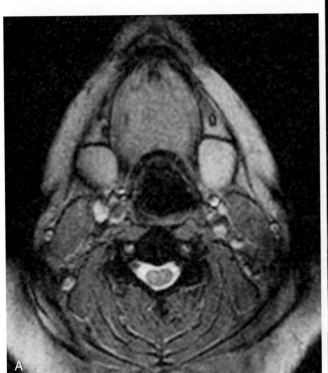
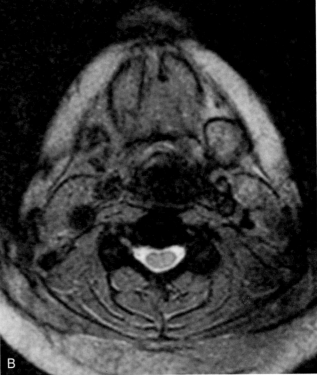

FIGURE 5–8 Iron oxide particle (Combidex) MRI of normal lymph nodes. *A,* Axial T2-weighted MR imaging before Combidex injection. The normal level II lymph nodes are slightly bright on the precontrast image. *B,* After contrast, normal lymph nodes become low in signal as their functioning histiocytes concentrate iron oxide particles. (Courtesy of Yoshimi Anzai.)

Once the isotope is in the soft tissues, images can be made by defining the degree to which the isotope has been taken up by that tissue. Nuclear medicine is frequently used to evaluate thyroid function and pathology. Parathyroid imaging is done in search of functioning tissue in patients with hyperparathyroidism.

Another helpful nuclear medicine examination that is used for evaluation of head and neck cancer is the bone scan using Tc99m-labeled phosphate compounds. This examination is more sensitive than are plain films or other radiographic techniques for detecting metastatic deposits to bone.

Lymphoscintigraphy uses the injection of a primary tumor with Tc99m-labeled phosphate compounds and subsequent imaging (Fig. 5–10) to provide a map of lymphatic drainage of the tumor. The objective of this technique is to direct lymph node dissection. This method has been used in combination with intraoperative sentinel node mapping and biopsy in head and neck melanoma, and its role in the management of upper aerodigestive tract tumors is currently being evaluated.

Positron emission tomography (PET) has been used to differentiate malignancy from normal tissue. ^{18}F fluorodeoxyglucose (FDG) is an imaging isotope that detects tissue with increased metabolism. Preliminary work attempted to detect unknown primary lesions and to differentiate postoperative changes resulting from recurrent or residual tumor.[8, 9] Although ^{18}FDG-PET is expensive, its efficacy has prompted insurance reimbursement for oncologic imaging and in turn has stimulated wider availability.

^{18}FDG-PET has proved superior to either CT or MRI in detecting recurrence and distinguishing tumor from postirradiation effects and scar in extracranial head and neck cancer.[10] Greven and associates[10] reported a sensitivity and specificity of 80% and 81%, respectively, for PET in the identification of postirradiation recurrence compared with a sensitivity of 58% and a specificity of 100% for CT. The success of ^{18}FDG-PET in detecting tumor depends on several factors, including ^{18}FDG-avid tumor, lesion size, differentiation of tumor from physiologic metabolic activity, and accurate localization of abnormal ^{18}FDG uptake. Certain tumors are variable in their ^{18}FDG uptake, especially tumors of salivary gland origin; therefore, ^{18}FDG-PET is unreliable both in tumor detection and in distinguishing benign from malignant tumors of salivary origin. A malignant lesion of at least 1 cm should be detectable on current PET scanners if the tumor takes up ^{18}FDG. The standardized uptake value (SUV) is a measure of ^{18}FDG uptake that takes into account the injected dose of ^{18}FDG and the patient's body weight. SUVs higher than 3 are considered suspicious for malignancy. Physiologic ^{18}FDG uptake, however, may be quite intense, especially in muscles, and may confound diagnosis. PET alone suffers from limited anatomic localization and spatial resolution, particularly in the head and neck region, which are crucial in treatment planning. The ability to distinguish abnormal from physiologic ^{18}FDG uptake and accurate

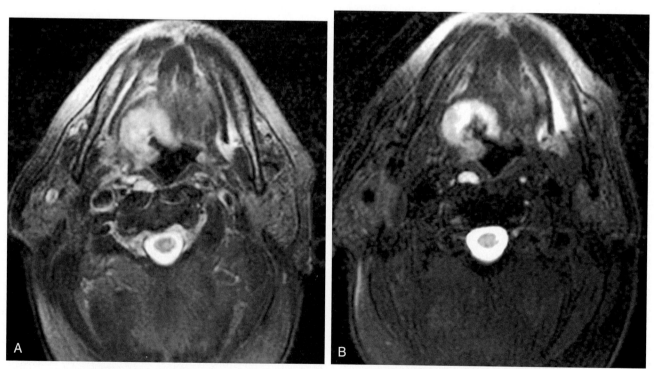

FIGURE 5–9 Iron oxide particle (Combidex) MRI of metastatic squamous cell carcinoma of the base of the tongue. *A*, Axial T2-weighted MR imaging before Combidex injection. The abnormal right retropharyngeal lymph node is hyperintense on the precontrast image, representing a metastasis from the large mass in the right tongue base. *B*, After contrast, the abnormal right retropharyngeal lymph node remains bright in signal, unable to take up iron oxide particles because its reticuloendothelial cells are replaced by metastatic carcinoma. (Courtesy of Yoshimi Anzai.)

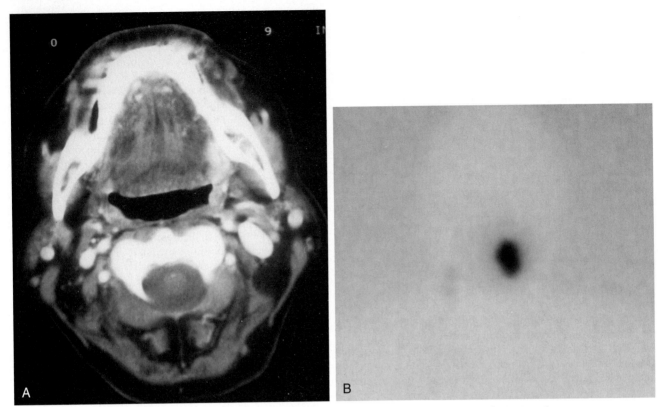

FIGURE 5–10 Sentinal lymph node mapping. *A,* Axial contrast-enhanced CT scan shows an enhancing soft tissue mass at the left tongue base. *B,* An anterior view obtained after injection of the left tongue base squamous cell carcinoma with ^{99m}Tc sulfur colloid demonstrates intense tracer uptake in the tongue base in addition to faint uptake in the right neck, contralateral to the primary focus. This case illustrates the variability in lymphatic drainage of the oropharynx.

tumor localization, however, has been greatly improved with the development of the combined PET/CT scanner.

Although the combination of separately acquired CT and PET images using retrospective or prospective registration methods[11] is more accurate (89% to 97%) than CT alone (69% to 75%),[12, 13] this approach is limited by patient movement and by imprecise localization of points between CT and PET. Computer algorithms to coregister functional and anatomic images are less successful in the diagnosis of head and neck tumors, where the anatomic orientation can change between scans, than in anatomically fixed organs such as the brain.[14, 15] The most reliable solution to this problem is to obtain both functional and anatomic images sequentially in the same scanner, without moving the patient between acquisitions. Such a device, a combined PET and CT scanner, has been designed and built by collaboration between the University of Pittsburgh and CTI Molecular Imaging, Incorporated (Knoxville, Tenn); it allows functional and anatomic images to be acquired at the same imaging session. PET/CT scanners have recently become commercially available. Our initial experience in evaluating cancer of the head and neck suggests greatly improved interpretability of ^{18}FDG-PET scans when coregistered CT data are used. The combination of ^{18}FDG-PET and CT offers the potential for improved detection and localization of cancer of the head and neck, with one tool to guide surgery, external beam irradiation, brachytherapy, or needle biopsy.

Initial experience with the prototype combined PET/CT at the University of Pittsburgh has demonstrated its benefit in detecting tumor recurrence in the treated patient with cancer of the head and neck, detecting the primary cancer site in patients who have a mass in the neck with an occult primary lesion (Fig. 5–11), detecting recurrent tumors of the cranial base, and detecting recurrent cancer of the thyroid in patients with elevated thyroglobulin levels and negative radioactive iodine (^{131}I) studies (Fig. 5–12). Of those who underwent ^{18}FDG-PET/CT scanning for suspected recurrent tumor of the cranial base, seven of eight patients had foci of increased ^{18}FDG uptake (SUV ≥ 3.0) in the region of clinically suspected tumor.[16] In one case with histologically proven invasion of the second and third divisions of the trigeminal nerve, PET/CT did not demonstrate the perineural invasion seen on MRI but showed unsuspected recurrence in the right masticator space. In one case of squamous cell carcinoma, PET/CT predicted the site of next recurrence in the clivus. Thus, PET/CT has already demonstrated the potential to help in patient management. Differentiation of residual or recurrent tumor from scar tissue is extremely difficult using static CT or MRI alone. Serial imaging with CT or MRI to determine tumor growth results in lost treatment time.

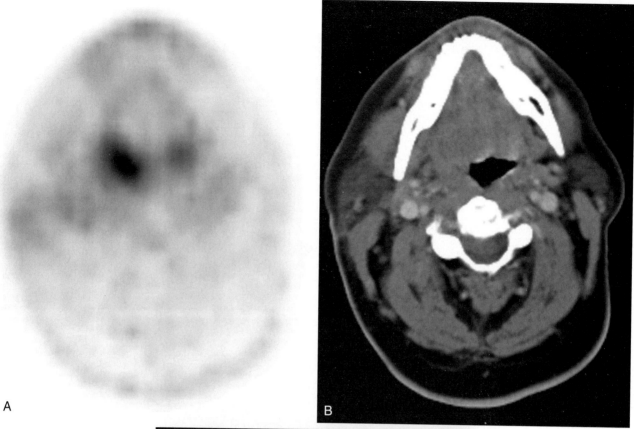

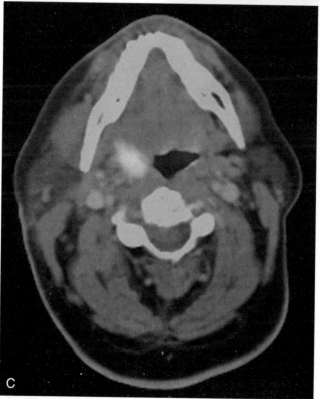

FIGURE 5–11 Combined FDG PET/CT imaging of an undiscovered primary cancer. The patient had undergone a series of five biopsies of Waldeyer's ring before PET/CT without evidence of a primary lesion. *A*, Axial FDG PET image at the level of the tonsils shows intensely elevated FDG uptake on the right (SUV = 4). *B*, Axial contrast-enhanced CT scan at the same level shows fullness in the right tonsil. *C*, Combined FDG PET/CT image localizes the increased FDG uptake to the right tonsil. Six additional biopsies of the tongue base and tonsil, directed by PET/CT, were obtained before the right tonsil squamous cell carcinoma could be proven on histology.

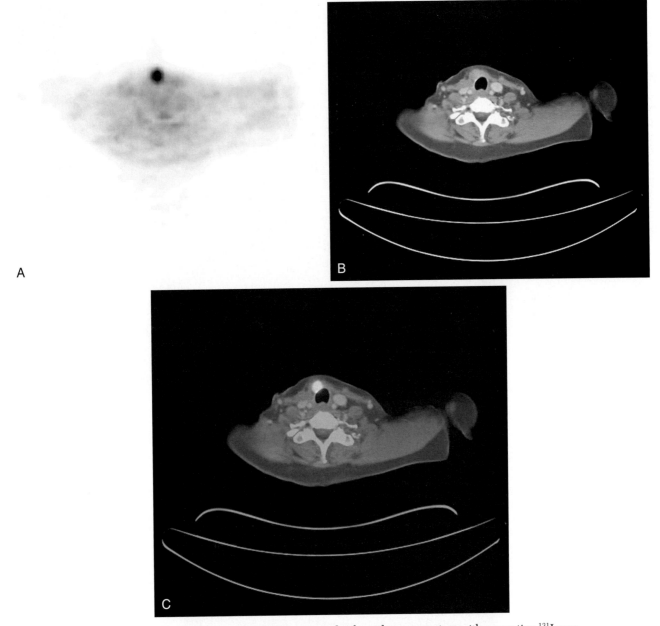

FIGURE 5–12 Combined FDG PET/CT imaging of a thyroid cancer patient with a negative ^{131}I scan and elevated thyroglobulin. *A*, Axial FDG PET image at the level of the thyroid bed shows intensely elevated FDG uptake slightly to the right of midline. *B*, Axial contrast-enhanced CT scan at the same level shows right paratracheal soft tissue prominence. *C*, Combined FDG PET/CT image localizes the increased FDG uptake to the right thyroid bed. Resection proved recurrent papillary carcinoma.

Combined anatomic images (CT) and functional images (PET) may also provide a more powerful approach for monitoring or targeting therapy than is offered by PET or CT images obtained separately. Changes in [18]FDG uptake appear to coincide with a decline in the number of viable tumor cells.[17] Importantly, metabolic response to therapy may precede changes in tumor volume.[17–19] Minn and colleagues[19] demonstrated that patients who ultimately had a good response to radiation therapy had a marked reduction in [18]FDG uptake from baseline level during the course of radiotherapy. Lowe and coworkers[20] evaluated [18]FDG-PET in assessing the response to chemotherapy of patients with stage III/IV head and neck cancer. They hypothesized that a

reduction in tumor metabolism, as evidence by decreased standardized uptake values (SUVs), would correlate with tumor response to chemotherapy.[20] They determined the sensitivity and specificity of PET for residual disease to be 90% and 83%, respectively.[20] These findings suggest that [18]FDG-PET may be useful in assessing response of the tumor to chemotherapy. The SUV, a relative measure of FDG uptake, is a prognostic indicator in cancer of the head and neck and has also been linked with clinical gauges of prognosis in pancreatic cancer.[21] Although the precise SUV that allows a significant threshold for diagnosis varies among laboratories, the SUV has been correlated with clinical measures of prognosis in several types of cancer.[20, 22] In a study by Minn and associates,[22] cancer of the head and neck with an SUV greater than 9.0 was associated with advanced disease and had a 3-year survival of 22%, compared with 73% in patients with SUVs of less than 9.0.

Combined PET/CT imaging allows accurate localization of increased metabolic activity. In the future, studies may address the efficacy of PET/CT-guided targeting for external beam irradiation and brachytherapy. Ultimately, the ability to focus therapy on the most metabolically active portion of the tumor may both improve treatment response and decrease morbidity. Combined anatomic images (CT) and functional images (PET) may also provide a more powerful approach for monitoring therapy than is possible with the use of PET or CT images obtained separately.

Angiography

Contrast medium is injected into the arteries to determine the vascularity of a tumor as well as to delineate the blood supply. When a patient has a tumor close to the carotid artery, the arteriogram may be combined with temporary balloon occlusion and xenon blood flow study (CT) of the brain to determine the risk of resecting the artery.

Xenon Flow Study

Xenon-enhanced CT is used to determine the relative perfusion of different areas of the brain.[23, 24] It is useful in the evaluation of tumors for which adequate resection would necessitate sacrifice of the internal carotid artery. Although stable xenon gas is currently not available because its use for this indication was "off label," it will likely return to clinical use in the future.

Xenon has a high enough electron density to be visualized on CT. Unlike iodinated contrast agents, xenon readily crosses the blood-brain barrier. Accumulation of xenon in the brain is therefore related to blood flow. A stable form of xenon is inhaled by the patient and diffuses from the lung into the bloodstream. The amount of xenon that actually enters the patient is determined by analyzing the amount of xenon inhaled versus the amount exhaled. The concentration in the tissues is then calculated.

At each of several predetermined locations in the brain, axial CT slices are acquired rapidly. Because several slices are imaged at the same level over a set interval, the rate of change in density resulting from the xenon can be plotted. This calculation corresponds to the blood flow at that location.

During an arteriogram, a balloon can be temporarily inflated to occlude the carotid artery. The patient inhales xenon, and the effect of the carotid occlusion on cerebral blood flow to the ipsilateral hemisphere is measured. This is, of course, done under continuous neurologic monitoring. This examination has proved useful in predicting which patients can tolerate resection of the carotid artery.

☐ EVALUATION OF TUMORS

In imaging tumors of the head and neck, the radiologist is usually trying to define the extent of a tumor rather than to

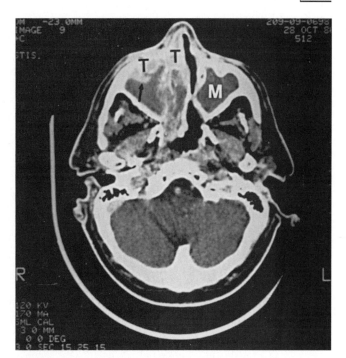

FIGURE 5–13 Axial contrast-enhanced CT image of a tumor (T) of the right nasal cavity and anterior maxillary sinus. Both left (M) and right maxillary sinuses contain obstructed low-density secretions, which can be differentiated from the enhancing tumor.

establish a diagnosis. CT and MRI are the primary tools used to make this determination. Tumors can spread by direct tumor encroachment or by a lymphatic, perineural, or hematogenous route.

Direct Encroachment by Tumor

As a tumor grows, it can invade bone or infiltrate normal soft tissue structures. This direct extension can be detected on CT or MRI by visualization of the bulk of the tumor replacing the normal structures. The muscle groups of the head and neck are well defined by intervening fat planes. Fat is an ideal subject for CT or MRI. Bone involvement can be detected on CT or MRI (see Fig. 5–7). The relationship of tumor to muscle is better determined by MRI because the density of muscle is often identical to that of tumor on CT (see Fig. 5–3). The interface between tumor and sinuses can frequently be visualized on CT (Fig. 5–13) but is more consistently delineated by MRI (see Fig. 5–2).

Lymphatic Spread

CT has become very useful in the detection of metastasis of cancer into the lymph node (Fig. 5–14).[25–27] It is especially helpful in visualizing nodes that may not be accessible to palpation (see Fig. 5–14B).

When squamous cell carcinoma replaces a node, the node may have a lower attenuation number or density (see Fig. 5–14). On CT, the central portion is dark with a definable rim. This low-density center is thought to represent necrosis (see Fig. 5–9). Nodes larger than 1 cm, even without a low-density center, are considered to be suspicious. In

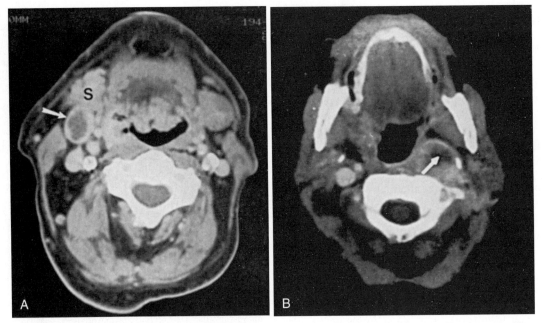

FIGURE 5–14 Metastatic lymphadenopathy: CT images. *A*, Axial CT image shows a necrotic zone II node with a low-density center and a thick, enhancing rim *(arrow)*. S, submandibular gland. *B*, Axial CT image shows a necrotic left retropharyngeal node of Rouvière *(arrow)* with a low-density center.

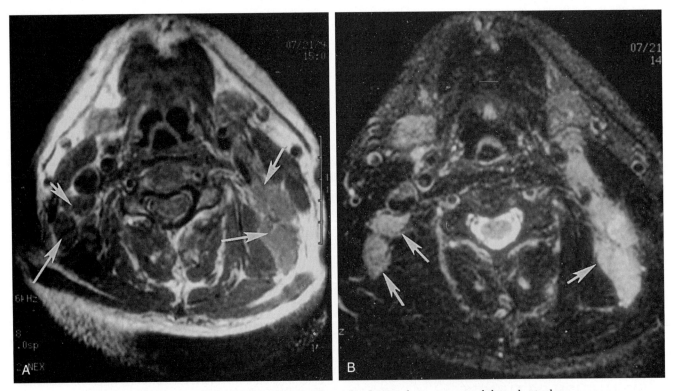

FIGURE 5–15 Cervical adenopathy: MRI. *A*, T1-weighted MRI shows extensive bilateral spinal accessory adenopathy *(arrows)* in a patient with lymphoma. The nodes are homogeneous. *B*, T2-wighted image of the same patient shows that the nodes *(arrows)* are hyperintense *(white)*, whereas the surrounding fat is less hyperintense. *Continued*

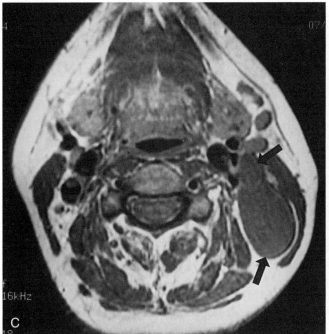

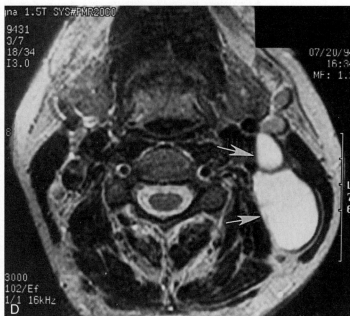

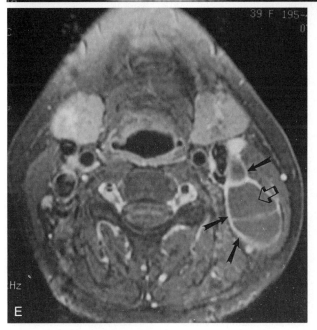

FIGURE 5–15, Cont'd *C,* Axial T1-weighted MRI of another patient shows a large cystic, bi-lobed mass *(arrows)* in the posterior left side of the neck. This was initially believed to be a cystic hygroma, but excisional biopsy revealed metastatic squamous cell cancer. *D,* On a T2-weighted sequence, the necrotic (cystic) adenopathy is hyperintense *(arrows)*. *E,* After gadolinium, a T1-weighted image shows enhancement of the periphery of the node *(black arrows)* but not of the necrotic material in the center *(open arrow)*. Fat suppression makes the surrounding fat less white, so the enhancing mass is more conspicuous.

the upper jugular–jugulodigastric area, a 1.5-cm size limit is used. If a node of borderline size is round instead of oval (which is normal), suspicion is increased.[27] Clustering of multiple lymph nodes may be indicative of metastases.

Occasionally, a node is replaced by fat and so has a low-density center. However, the density reading is much lower than that of a necrotic node, which enables the radiologist to make a determination.

Superficial nodes are easily palpated by the clinician. The usefulness of CT increases with the depth of the nodes. The radiologist may find clinically undetected nodes in the jugular chain or in the spinal accessory chain deep to the sternocleidomastoid. The retropharyngeal nodes (nodes of Rouvière)

are usually undetectable clinically, and CT is very sensitive in their evaluation. These nodes are found at the oropharyngeal-nasopharyngeal level just medial to the carotid artery (see Fig. 5–14*B*). Submental, submandibular, parotid, and other superficial nodes can be found on CT, but these are usually palpable by the clinician.

Nodes are also easily detected on MRI (Fig. 5–15). Because they are surrounded by fat, nodes are easily seen and measured on a T1-weighted image. Evaluation of the internal architecture based on the MRI signal has potential usefulness, but it is an extrapolation of the CT findings. If the center of the node does not enhance with gadolinium, tumor or necrosis is suspected. MRI is more expensive than CT and

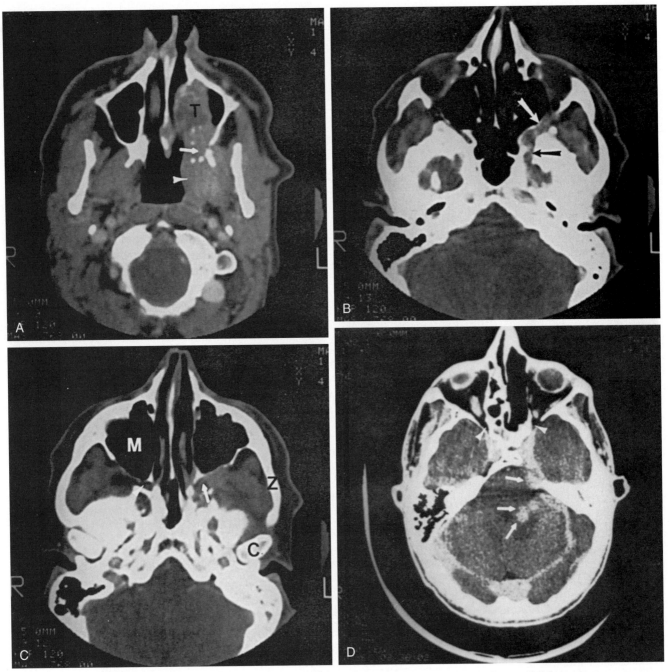

FIGURE 5–16 Perineural tumor: CT scans. *A*, Tumor from the left maxillary sinus has eroded bone in the expected location of the greater and lesser palatine foramina *(arrow)*, giving tumor access to the palatine nerves, branches of V2. Tumor also infiltrates the lateral wall of the nasopharynx *(arrowhead)*. *B*, There is a tumor at the junction of the superior portion of pterygopalatine fossa with an inferior orbital fissure *(white arrow)*. Tumor extends back along foramen rotundum *(black arrow)*, which is also enlarged. *C*, The left pterygopalatine fossa is widened *(arrow)* and contains soft tissue, which replaces the normal fat seen on the right side *(arrowhead)*. M, maxillary sinus; Z, zygomatic arch; C, mandibular condyle. *D*, Tumor has extended intracranially from Meckel's cave along the trigeminal nerve *(arrows)*. Fat in the superior orbital fissures is intact *(arrowheads)*. (From HD Curtin, R Williams, J Johnson: CT of perineural tumor extension: Pterygopalatine fossa. AJNR 5:731–737, fig 2A, 2B, 2C, 1984. by Amercian Society of Neuroradiology www.ajnr.org.)

is more complicated to perform. However, if MRI is done for evaluation of a primary lesion, information regarding node status can be obtained during the same examination.

Ultrasound is used frequently, especially by practitioners in Europe, to evaluate nodal status. The technique is very effective for examination of the main nodal beds. However, ultrasound has limitations in some areas. Because the sound frequencies that are used cannot penetrate bone, evaluation of the retropharyngeal nodes is impossible. Data regarding primary lesions of the mucosal surface are also limited.

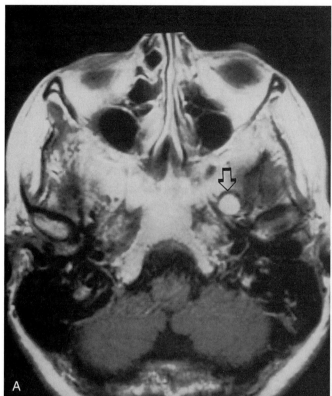

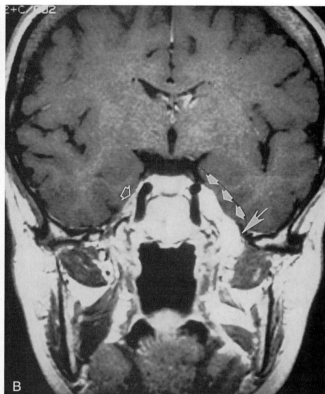

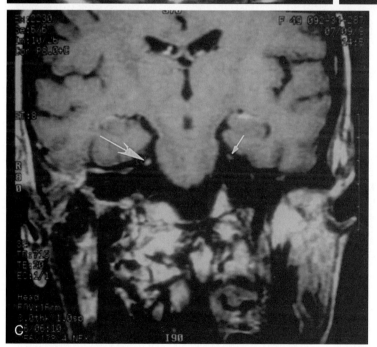

FIGURE 5–17 Perineural tumor: MRI studies. *A,* The enlarged, enhancing cranial nerve V3 is quite conspicuous as it passes through the foramen ovale *(arrow)* on this contrast-enhanced axial T1-weighted image. *B,* The enlarged V3 passes through an enlarged foramen ovale *(long white arrow)* on this enhanced T1-weighted coronal image. The cavernous sinus on the left *(short white arrows)* is wider than that on the right *(open arrow),* which suggests the presence of tumor here as well. *C,* Another patient's coronal T1-weighted image after contrast shows enhancement of the cisternal portion of the right trigeminal nerve *(large arrow).* The left trigeminal nerve *(small arrow)* is normal.

Perineural Extension

Many tumors of the head and neck can escape the limits of a proposed resection by following the nerves. This perineural spread is especially common in adenoid cystic carcinoma but can also occur in other tumors, such as squamous cell carcinoma. The tumor can follow the nerve through a neural foramen to an intracranial site.

CT (Fig. 5–16) or MRI (Figs. 5–17 and 5–18) can detect this tumor extension.[28] A nerve enlarged by perineural tumor often expands or erodes the bony canal through which the nerve passes. More importantly, as the cranial nerves approach the skull base, almost all pass through small regions that contain fat. As the tumor extends through the area, fat is replaced. As stated, fat is the ideal medium for either CT or MRI because tumor infiltrating fat can be readily detected. Key areas, depending on the origin of a tumor, are the superior orbital fissure, the pterygopalatine fossa, and the stylomastoid foramen.[28, 29] The amount of fat around the jugular vein and

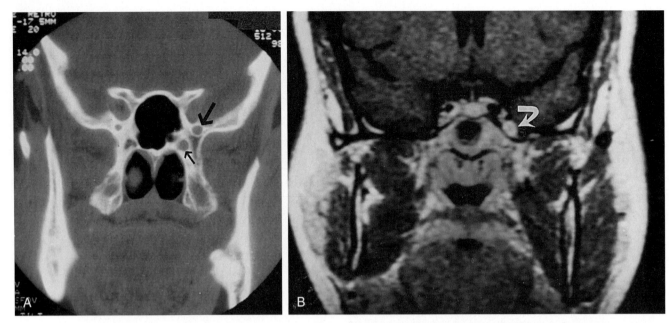

FIGURE 5–18 Adenoid cystic carcinoma involving foramen rotundum. *A,* Coronal CT scan shows enlargement of foramen rotundum *(large arrow)* and vidian canal *(small arrow). B,* Postcontrast MRI shows enhancement *(arrow),* which indicates tumor extension through the foramen rotundum.

carotid artery is sufficient for an enlarged nerve to be detectable. Cranial nerve V3 also passes through fat in the masticator space while exiting the skull base.

Tumors extending through the neural fascia can be visualized when they are contrasted against the CSF spaces. If perineural tumor reaches the cavernous sinus, the lesion may blend with the enhancing cavernous sinus on CT, but the cavernous sinus usually appears to be enlarged. MRI appears to be better able to demonstrate tumor involvement in the cavernous sinus.

The presence of a normal-sized nerve does not absolutely exclude perineural extension. The possibility remains that microscopic spread would not enlarge a nerve and fat would not be obliterated. MRI is considered to be more sensitive than CT for detecting tumor within a normal-sized nerve (see Fig. 5–18). For instance, if the nerve (V2) within the foramen rotundum enhances, tumor is considered to be present even if the foramina are not involved. The preganglionic segment of the trigeminal nerve may also enhance, even though it might not be enlarged (see Fig. 5–17).

Hematogenous Spread

Local recurrence is the rule for head and neck primary tumors, but distant metastases do occur. Chest radiographs are the initial studies used to search for pulmonary metastases, but a CT scan is more sensitive. CT is also used to evaluate possible metastases to the abdomen or head. MRI can be used to evaluate the head. Bone scans with Tc99m phosphate compounds can be used to search for bone metastases. In the absence of obvious lung metastases in cancer of the head and neck, the likelihood of bone metastasis is extremely low, and a bone scan is not usually indicated unless there is a high suspicion of involvement. PET scanning is also very sensitive in diagnosing cancer in the lungs.

Second Primary Tumors

Patients with cancer of the head and neck often have second primary cancers. These synchronous or metachronous cancers are found in the mouth, larynx, lungs, and esophagus and, more rarely, in the stomach.

At the University of Pittsburgh, chest radiographs and barium swallow are performed before endoscopy is undertaken. On barium swallow, the radiologist searches for obvious cancers and for areas of the esophagus that lack pliability or distensibility.

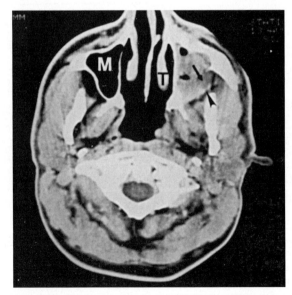

FIGURE 5–19 CT image of a tumor in the left maxillary sinus that extends through the posterolateral wall of the sinus *(arrow)* and into the fat of the infratemporal fossa *(arrowhead).* On the right, there is normal fat in this location. M, normal right maxillary sinus; T, turbinate.

If the radiologist can state that the walls are pliable and distensible throughout the esophagus, the examination is very accurate. If there is an area of apparent lack of pliability or even minor irregularity, this should be reported to the endoscopist as an area that cannot be cleared and should be visualized directly.

The postcricoid region almost always has a slight irregularity. Even this area is usually pliable when the barium column is watched fluoroscopically as it passes throughout the postcricoid-cricopharyngeal area.

◼ REGIONAL EXAMINATION AND LANDMARKS

Paranasal Sinuses, Nasal Cavity, Orbit, and Anterior Skull Base

Axial and coronal scans are often needed to stage a cancer in this area. The anterior and posterior walls of the maxillary sinuses are seen in axial slices (Fig. 5–19). Many landmarks crucial to staging are better seen in the coronal plane. The palate, orbital floor, maxilloethmoid plate, roof of the ethmoid, cribriform plate, and floor of the anterior cranial fossa are all horizontally positioned and are best seen in the coronal plane (see Figs. 5–2 and 5–6). The lamina papyracea and ethmoid air cells are seen well on either axial or coronal images.

Direct encroachment usually occurs through the bony walls of a sinus. Detection depends on demonstration of the bony defect and of the tumor in the tissue on the opposite side of the wall. Bone erosion can be seen on either CT or MRI. CT offers a slight advantage with bone algorithms and thin slices. MRI can often visualize a bone defect as a signal intensity replacing the normal signal void of cortical bone (i.e., a defect in a cortical line).

Obliteration of fat along the outer surface of the posterolateral wall of the maxillary sinus is a very sensitive sign of tumor extension (see Fig. 5–19). CT and MRI are equally useful in this area. Further tumor progression brings a tumor into contact with muscles such as the pterygoids, and here MRI is better at demonstrating the tumor-muscle interface.

At the roof of the ethmoid and cribriform plate, CT shows small bony erosions, but MRI has an advantage in showing the relationship of tumor to the inferior surface of the frontal lobe (see Fig. 5–6B). Sagittal images that can be obtained directly with MRI or reconstructed for CT are useful in showing the junction of the floor and the anterior wall of the anterior cranial fossa (see Fig. 5–6B).

Once outside a sinus, a tumor can spread through fissures to reach other anatomic areas. The pterygopalatine fossa and the inferior orbital fissure are the most important because they connect the infratemporal fossa, the nasal cavity, and the orbit, as well as give access to the foramen rotundum and the middle cranial fossa. Fat is abundant, so both CT and MRI are excellent techniques.

As a tumor grows within a sinus, the air is replaced with soft tissue. Tumors can also obstruct the outflow of mucus from the sinus. Often the mucus retained in the sinus can be differentiated from the tumor. On CT, the retained mucus has a low density (see Fig. 5–13). Most tumors are dense and so can be contrasted against mucus of lower density. If the sinus is filled with low-density material reaching the bony walls, one can be confident that this represents obstruction. Rarely, portions of a tumor can be low enough in density to mimic the appearance of mucus retention, so the density within the sinus should always be compared with that of the bulk of the tumor. In addition, most tumors enhance after intravenous contrast. Secretions do not enhance.

The low-density obstruction phenomenon is usually most obvious in large sinuses, such as the maxillary sinus. Even small amounts of mucosal thickening can completely occlude a small ethmoid air cell. Because the mucosa enhances slightly, the appearance can be the same as that of tumor. In this instance, visualization of the small ethmoid septations can be helpful. If these septations are intact, one leans toward a diagnosis of obstruction rather than of tumor; however, this finding is not absolute, and it may be impossible to determine the exact margin of a lesion.

MRI has a distinct advantage in differentiating tumor from obstruction.[30–32] With the use of multiple sequences (Fig. 5–20), this determination can almost always be made. An obstructed sinus fills with mucus. Initially, the retained secretions are very watery and have a low protein content (see Figs. 5–20A and D). The MRI signal at this stage reflects the watery consistency with low signal on T1-weighted images and high signal on T2-weighted images. With chronic obstruction, protein concentration increases, which changes the signal characteristics (see Fig. 5–20A). The T1-weighted image is brighter (higher signal) and the T2-weighted image remains bright. With continued obstruction, higher protein concentration and desiccation of secretions eventually lead to a drop in signal intensity on both sequences. The sinus becomes "darker." The final stage of obstruction reveals a dense, dry material that is low in signal intensity. At this stage, a completely obstructed sinus can be represented on MRI by a signal void and thus can have the same appearance as an aerated normal sinus (see Figs. 5–20B and C).

Even though an obstructed sinus can have almost any appearance, it is rare that tumor and obstruction cannot be differentiated on some sequence. Most tumors are relatively dark on T1-weighted image and brighter than muscle, but they are not as bright as fluid on T2-weighted image. Rarely, some adenocarcinomas and some neural lesions can be quite bright on T2-weighted image. Very rarely is the signal of the tumor exactly the same as that of obstructed secretions.

The use of gadolinium can be helpful. Tumors, unless completely necrotic, cystic, or avascular, enhance to some degree. Secretions in a sinus destroyed by cancer do not enhance at all. The signal is the same before and after gadolinium injection. Contrast does not reach the lumen of the sinus. The mucosa of an obstructed sinus does enhance. Indeed, the sinonasal mucosa usually enhances to a much greater degree than does the moderately enhancing tumor. The enhancing wall of the obstructed sinus can be a very useful sign in differentiating tumor from obstructed secretions (see Fig. 5–20A).[33]

Perineural extension can play a significant role in the area of the paranasal sinus (see Figs. 5–16 through 5–18). The major nerves supplying this region are the first two divisions of the trigeminal nerve. The second branch (maxillary division) of the trigeminal nerve is most likely to be involved. Tumor may reach the infraorbital nerve or superior alveolar nerve by invasion of the roof of the maxillary sinus and posterolateral

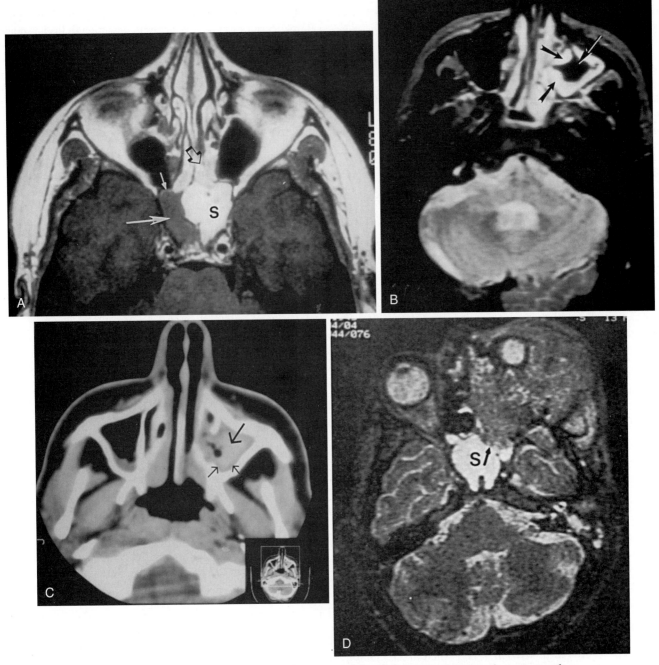

FIGURE 5–20 Obstructed sinuses. *A,* Axial contrast-enhanced T1-weighted image of a patient with an esthesioneuroblastoma shows enhancing tumor *(open arrow)* in the nasal cavity. High-signal material in the left sphenoid air cell (S) was also bright before contrast and therefore represents proteinaceous secretions in an obstructed sinus. Lower-signal, more watery obstructed secretions fill the right sphenoid air cell *(long white arrow).* The thin, normal mucosa enhances *(short white arrow). B,* Axial T2-weighted MRI of another patient shows thick mucosa *(black arrows)* lining the left maxillary sinus, and low signal *(highlighted arrow)* in the lumen of the sinus, which suggests residual aeration. *C,* Axial CT image obtained the same day reveals that the maxillary lumen is, in fact, filled with hyperdense material *(large arrow).* This appearance on CT and MRI is characteristic of proteinaceous, desiccated secretions. The lower-density edematous mucosa *(small arrows)* is less conspicuous than on MRI. *D,* Axial T2-weighted image of another patient shows a large tumor filling the left ethmoid sinus and orbit. The watery obstructed secretions in the sphenoid sinus (S) are white, and the interface with tumor *(arrow)* is easily seen.

wall, respectively. The superior alveolar nerves extend through the posterolateral wall and so can be accessed directly through the sinus mucosa. Direct perineural invasion from the skin and superficial soft tissues of the face gives access to the infraorbital nerve, and invasion of the palatal mucosa can reach the palatine nerves. All these neural pathways converge on the pterygopalatine fossa, making this a key structure (see Fig. 5–16A). The pterygopalatine fossa is filled with fat, which lends itself to evaluation by CT or MRI. Either modality seems exquisitely sensitive for detection of tumors in the pterygopalatine fossa. From the pterygopalatine fossa,

the foramen rotundum carries tumor to Meckel's cave and the middle cranial fossa. These regions must be examined closely, especially if the fat in the pterygopalatine fossa is obliterated. In the foramen rotundum and in the region of Meckel's cave, gadolinium-enhanced MRI is considered more sensitive. The involved nerve is thought to enhance even if it is still of normal size. In most cases, either CT or MRI can detect this extension because the nerve and the foramen are enlarged.

Once reaching the pterygopalatine fossa by perineural extension, tumor can extend directly through (1) the

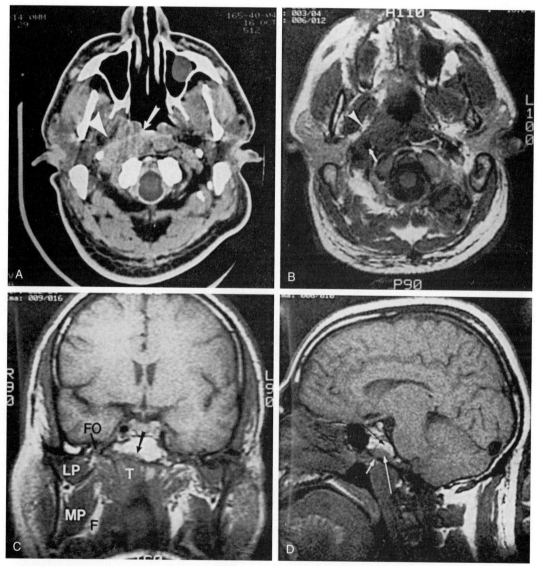

FIGURE 5–21 Nasopharyngeal tumor. *A*, Axial CT image shows a tumor in the right fossa of Rosenmüller (*arrow*) that extends through the deglutitional ring toward the spine and narrows the fat of the parapharyngeal space (*arrowhead*). The relationship of tumor to carotid artery is difficult to determine. *B*, Axial T1-weighted MRI of the same patient shows the tumor surrounding the signal void of the carotid artery and jugular vein (*arrow*). Parapharyngeal fat is compressed by tumor (*arrowhead*). *C*, Coronal T1-weighted image shows the tumor (T) eroding into the clivus (*arrow*), replacing normal white clivus marrow. LP, lateral pterygoid muscle; MP, medial pterygoid muscle; FO, foramen ovale; F, parapharyngeal fat. *D*, Sagittal T1-weighted image shows interruption of the signal void of cortical bone (*short white arrow*) and replacement of normal clivus (*black arrow*) marrow by lower-signal tumor (*long white arrow*).

pterygomaxillary fissure to the infratemporal fossa, (2) the sphenopalatine foramen to the nasal cavity, or (3) the inferior orbital fissure to the orbit. Again, the pterygopalatine fossa can serve as an ominous crossroad for tumor extension.

Tumors of the superficial orbit and eyelid can access the first division of the trigeminal nerve and follow this nerve through the superior orbital fissure to the cavernous sinus. Here a small amount of fat situated in the superior orbital fissure becomes the sentinel point. The tumor obliterates the fat en route to the cavernous sinus.

The number of cases of perineural extension in the radiology literature is small. More experience is necessary before a confident determination can be made about the sensitivity of CT or MRI in finding perineural spread. Microscopic extension is theoretically possible without abnormality at imaging.

Perineural spread of cancer can be antegrade as well as retrograde. Tumor reaching a branch point can spread in either direction. For instance, tumor reaching the pterygopalatine fossa from the palatine nerves can spread anteriorly along the infraorbital nerve, can pass through the foramen rotundum to the middle cranial fossa, or pass in both directions at once.

MRI can detect both enhancement and enlargement of a nerve (see Figs. 5–17A and B). Perineural cancer may cause enhancement of a nerve without enlargement (see Fig. 5–17C). For this reason, MRI is probably more sensitive than CT in the diagnosis of perineural tumor.

The lymph nodes most at risk for metastases depend on the site of origin of the primary cancer. Cancers originating in the anterior part of the face and nasal cavity spread to submental or submandibular nodes as well as to lateral nodal groups such as the parotid nodes. Cancers originating more posteriorly spread to the jugular and retropharyngeal chains. The key nodal groups should be included in the area imaged, especially if the primary sites of lymphatic drainage extend into deeper chains, such as occurs with the posterior nasal cavity and sinus.

Nasopharynx

Direct extension of a cancer of the nasopharynx is determined by the osseous borders and limiting fascial planes.[34–36] The roof of the nasopharynx is made up of bone covered by mucosa. Laterally and posteriorly, the pharyngobasilar fascia forms a strong barrier that at least initially limits extension. There is a gap between the superior margin of the pharyngobasilar fascia and the skull base. This gap is called the hiatus of Morgagni, and through this gap pass the levator veli palatini muscle and the eustachian tube.

Aggressive cancer can spread through the pharyngobasilar fascia to reach the parapharyngeal spaces (which are filled with fat). Tumor encroaches on this fat and is therefore detectable. An axial slice can enable visualization of the torus tubarius, the fossa of Rosenmüller, and the eustachian tube orifice. Initially, the cancer can obliterate these structures and fill the airway so that the soft tissue on one side of the airway is wider than that on the other side (Fig. 5–21A). This soft tissue at the nasopharyngeal level is normally made up of the pharyngobasilar fascia and the levator veli palatini and is analogous to the ring formed by the constrictor muscle at lower levels. At either level, one can use the term

"deglutitional ring," although the ring is much thicker at lower levels. Asymmetry is the key finding. As tumor spreads beyond the pharyngobasilar fascia, the deglutitional ring and tumor impinge on the fat of the parapharyngeal space, causing apparent narrowing of the fat. This effect can be seen on CT (see Fig. 5–21A) or MRI (Fig. 5–21B).

The cancer may pass between the pharyngobasilar fascia and bone and extend along the course of the eustachian tube.[34–35] This gives the cancer access to the carotid canal, middle ear, and thin portions of the floor of the middle cranial fossa.

Along the roof of the nasopharynx, bone is the barrier. The cancer may seek the path of least resistance, such as the petro-occipital fissure or the foramen lacerum, but the cancer can also erode directly into bone (Figs. 5–22 and 5–23; see also Fig. 5–21). Early erosion can be seen by using the bone algorithm on CT (see Fig. 5–23D). MRI becomes very sensitive as tumor growing into marrow obliterates the normal high signal (fat in the medullary spaces) on T1-weighted images (see Fig. 5–23C). Coronal scans (either MRI or CT) are very helpful in evaluating the roof of the nasopharynx. Sagittal scans give a good slice through the roof and posterior wall of the nasopharynx (see Fig. 5–23E).

After the cancer passes through the bone or fissures, it impinges on the air of the sphenoid sinus, the cavernous sinus, or the CSF spaces. Air spaces can be evaluated by CT or MRI. Both the CSF spaces and the cavernous sinus can be evaluated by CT or MRI but are probably best evaluated by MRI.

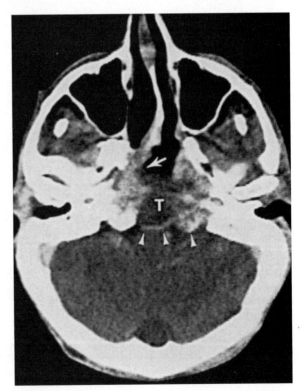

FIGURE 5–22 Axial CT scan shows an aggressive nasopharyngeal cancer (T) that extends from the nasopharynx *(arrow)*, erodes the clivus, and extends intracranially. Enhancing dura are indicated by *arrowheads*.

If the cancer is located in the anterior part of the nasopharynx, spread can also occur laterally through the sphenopalatine foramen into the pterygopalatine fossa. Here the cancer reaches neural structures and can pass along the maxillary division of the trigeminal nerve to reach the cavernous sinus. The vidian canal is just lateral to the sphenopalatine foramen and so can become a potential pathway of spread (see Fig. 5–23D).

Nodal involvement can include the nodes of Rouvière (lateral retropharyngeal) and the upper jugular nodes. However, special attention must be given to a careful search for posterior triangle nodes because of their high frequency of involvement.

Infratemporal Fossa, Parapharyngeal, Masticator, and Parotid Regions

Lateral to the muscles of deglutition lies an area that has been divided and subdivided into a multitude of spaces based on various interpretations of fascial layers. Radiologically, some advantages can be gained by attempting to place a lesion in one space or another, in that the differential diag-

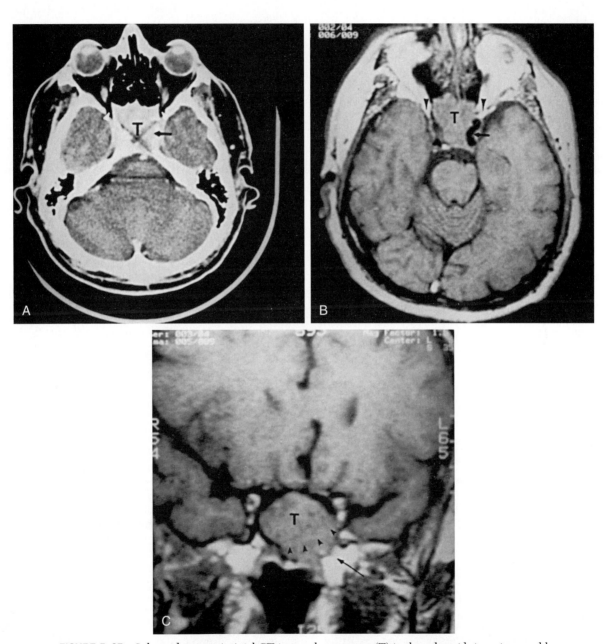

FIGURE 5–23 Sphenoid tumor. *A,* Axial CT image shows tumor (T) in the sphenoid sinus, inseparable from the cavernous carotid artery *(arrow). B,* Axial T1-weighted MRI shows the tumor (T) and the signal void of the cavernous carotid artery *(arrow).* Normal fat is seen in the superior orbital fissures *(arrowheads). C,* Coronal T1-weighted image shows tumor (T) in the sphenoid sinus, eroding through the floor of the sinus with loss of the signal void of normal cortex *(arrowheads)* and infiltration of the normal white marrow fat *(arrow).*

Continued

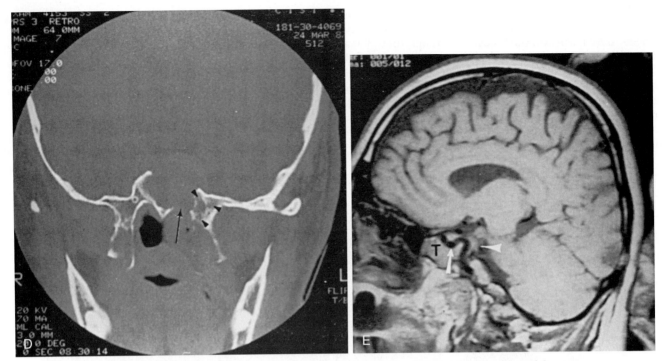

FIGURE 5–23, Cont'd *D,* Coronal CT (bone algorithm) shows the destruction of the floor of the sinus *(arrow)* and tumor infiltrating the medullary bone *(arrowheads)* around the vidian canal. The vidian canal on the right is normal. *E,* Sagittal T1-weighted MRI shows the curvilinear signal void of carotid artery *(arrow)* passing through the tumor (T, *arrowhead*).

nosis can be restricted to a few possibilities.[37–40] One system divides the area into four basic compartments: poststyloid parapharyngeal space, prestyloid parapharyngeal space, masticator space, and parotid compartments.[39] These are based on compartmentalization caused by thicker layers of fascia. The parotid space communicates with the prestyloid para-

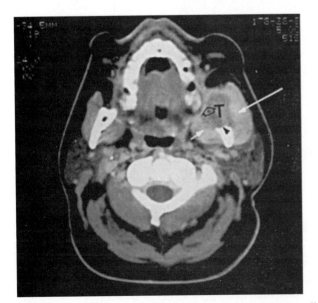

FIGURE 5–24 Contrast-enchanced CT image of a squamous cell cancer (T) of the retromolar trigone *(open arrow)* shows the tumor invading and displacing the medial pterygoid muscle *(short arrow),* eroding the ramus of the mandible *(arrowhead),* and invading the masseter muscle *(long arrow).*

pharyngeal space with no significant intervening fascial layers. A small portion of the parotid gland passes through the stylomandibular tunnel to reach the prestyloid compartment. Indeed, the prestyloid compartment contains little else other than this small portion of the parotid gland and fat. The poststyloid parapharyngeal space contains the carotid artery, jugular vein, and cranial nerves IX, X, XI, and XII and is separated from the prestyloid space by fascia stretching from the styloid muscles to the tensor veli palatini muscle. The masticator space contains the pterygoid, temporalis, and masseter muscles, cranial nerve V3, the mandibular ramus, and the terminal branches of the external carotid artery (internal maxillary artery) that pass through the space en route to the pterygopalatine fossa. The masticator space is separated from the prestyloid space by the medial fascial covering of the medial pterygoid muscle and the interpterygoid fascia. The medial pterygoid fascia fuses with the interpterygoid fascia, and together this fused fascial layer continues to the base of the skull, forming the medial wall of the masticator compartment. The fascial covering of the medial pterygoid fuses to the posterior margin of the mandible before continuing along the outside (lateral) surface of the masseter muscle.

Most lesions arising in the parapharyngeal-masticator-parotid area are benign, but several points relating to malignancy are appropriate in this chapter. Most malignancies involving this area arise elsewhere and extend into the region. Squamous cell carcinomas of the oropharynx, nasopharynx, tonsillar pillar, or retromolar trigone extend directly into these spaces and are visualized as the cancer invades or distorts fat (Fig. 5–24). When a tumor involves muscle, MRI appears to have an advantage (see Figs. 5–2 and 5–7).

A malignancy in the parotid gland can have the same appearance as a benign lesion. If a tumor has an irregular margin, and especially if the lesion extends into another fascial compartment, malignancy should be strongly suspected.

Perineural extension is a factor in the parotid, poststyloid, and masticator spaces. Cancer of the parotid gland can extend along the facial nerve, and adenocystic carcinoma is the most frequent example. As the cancer extends toward the temporal bone, a small fat pad must be crossed before the stylomastoid foramen is reached. This fat can be obliterated by cancer, which can be detected easily by MRI or CT. Tumor extending along the intratemporal facial nerve can expand the bony canal of the facial nerve and so can be detected by either MRI or CT. The bony canal of the facial nerve has soft tissue within, which gives an MRI signal, unlike the air or cortical bone of the mastoid. Enlargement on CT or MRI indicates tumor extension following the nerve. Enhancement of a normal-sized nerve on MRI is considered suspicious as well.

The masticator space contains the third division of the trigeminal nerve; malignancies of the masticator space

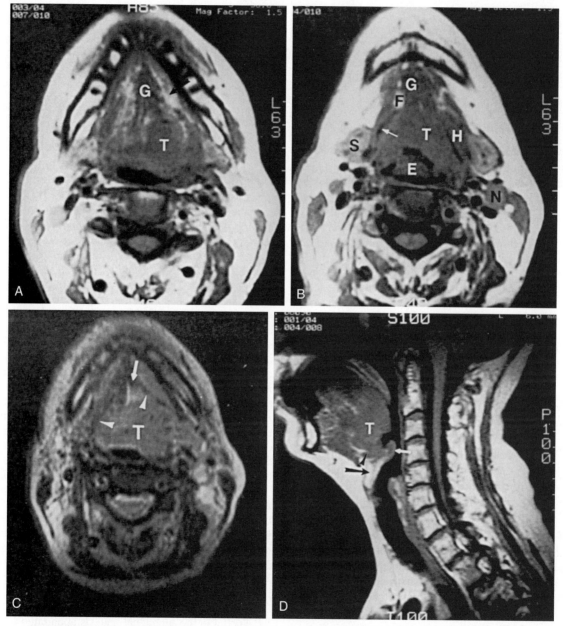

FIGURE 5–25 Carcinoma of the tongue: MRI studies. *A,* Axial T1-weighted image shows tumor (T) at the base of tongue, displacing the genioglossus muscle (G) but sparing the sublingual fat *(arrowhead). B,* Axial T1-weighted image in lower plane shows the relationship of the left-sided tumor (T) to the genioglossus (G) and the hyoglossus (H) muscles. The tumor crosses the midline and approaches the right lingual artery *(arrow).* S, submandibular gland; F, submental fat; E, epiglottis. One enlarged left lymph node (N) is seen. *C,* Axial T2-weighted image shows that tumor (T, *arrowheads)* is hyperintense with respect to muscle *(arrow). D,* Sagittal T1-weighted MRI shows the tumor (T)—specifically the inferior extent of tumor *(arrowhead)*—with respect to pre-epiglottic fat *(black arrow)* and epiglottis *(white arrow).*

Continued

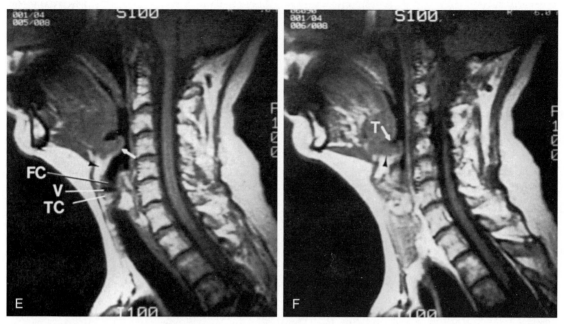

FIGURE 5–25, Cont'd *E*, Plane lateral to that shown in *D*. The tumor abuts the epiglottis *(arrow)*. FC, false vocal cords; TC, true vocal cords; V, laryngeal ventricle. *F*, Plane lateral to that shown in *E*. Tumor (T) fills the vallecula *(arrowhead)*.

therefore have access to this nerve and can pass through the skull base via the foramen ovale. Most malignancies arising outside the masticator space must violate the fascial boundaries before reaching the nerve. The lingual nerve can carry tumor through the masticator space from the floor of the mouth or the submandibular gland. Cancer of the parotid gland can follow the auriculotemporal branch of the trigeminal nerve (V3) through a small gap in the fascia and thus reach the masticator space and foramen ovale.

The poststyloid parapharyngeal space is also a potential route of transit as cancers of the tongue or pharynx pass along the cranial nerves found in this space. A nonenhancing soft tissue mass extending along the great vessels toward the skull base should be viewed with suspicion. The intracranial end of the hypoglossal canal and the jugular foramen should be inspected closely.

No discussion of the parapharyngeal spaces would be complete without a brief mention of the retropharyngeal nodes, the so-called nodes of Rouvière. These nodes technically are not in the poststyloid parapharyngeal space. Most anatomists place the nodes in the retropharyngeal spaces, separated from the poststyloid parapharyngeal space by a separate fascial layer extending from the pharyngobasilar fascia to the prevertebral fascia. However, as nodes enlarge, the resultant mass is seen as a poststyloid tumor (see Fig. 5–14*B*) that is usually medial to the carotid artery.[27] The low-density center of a node, however, indicates its identity.

Oral Cavity/Oropharynx

Carcinoma of the tongue can be difficult to visualize on CT because the tumor and the muscles of the tongue can have the same density, which makes the precise margin difficult to pinpoint.[41] Bolus contrast enhancement has improved the abilities of CT in addressing this problem. MRI can usually generate different signals for tumor and tongue muscles and so can define the margins of the tumor more precisely; it is therefore considered the most accurate imaging study for this purpose (Fig. 5–25; see also Fig. 5–7).[42, 43]

Cancer from the tongue can cross the glossopharyngeal sulcus and spread up the tonsillar pillar to the free margin of the soft palate (Figs. 5–26 and 5–27). Submucosal spread can continue to the level of the nasopharynx.[44] As tumor spreads here, the ring of deglutition is widened. This can be difficult to assess in the area of the tonsil because the size of the tonsil may vary. Superior to the tonsil, especially at the level of the nasopharynx, the widening is a more sensitive sign for the presence of tumor.

Cancer arising in the tonsillar region can grow down into the tongue or up into the nasopharynx as well as extend directly laterally into the region of the nasopharynx. The same principle for detection holds as for tumor arising in the tongue and extending superiorly to reach the tonsillar pillar.

A cancer at the base of the tongue may infiltrate the tongue musculature or spread onto the epiglottis. Here the irregular tumor alters the usual thin appearance of the epiglottis. This extension is usually obvious to the clinician. The radiologist, however, must carefully examine the pre-epiglottic space to exclude further inferior and deep extension. The pre-epiglottic space is filled with fat, so either CT or MRI is very sensitive in tumor detection (see Fig. 5–25).

The floor of the mouth includes several regions that contain fat. The fat in the sublingual space is obliterated by tumor. As tumor infiltrates the geniohyoid and genioglossus, enough fat usually borders the muscles to allow evaluation. Evaluating involvement of the mylohyoid muscle can be difficult (see Fig. 5–25). Tumor bordering the muscle often has the same CT density as the muscle, so the radiologist cannot always tell whether the tumor is abutting or growing into the muscle. If the tumor grows through the muscle, the fat on the external

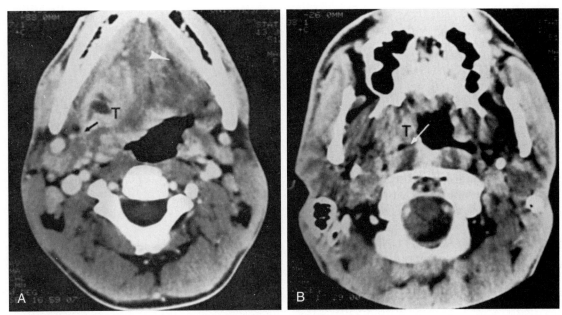

FIGURE 5–26 Tongue tumor invading tonsillar pillar: CT studies. *A,* Carcinoma from the lateral margin of the tongue (T, *arrow*) obliterates fascial planes in the right floor of mouth. Normal left sublingual fat is seen (*arrowhead*). *B,* In a higher plane, the lateral nasopharyngeal wall is widened by tumor (T), which extends submucosally. The fossa of Rosenmüller (*arrow*) is compressed by tumor.

surface is obliterated and the tumor becomes detectable again. A more reliable determination can be made by MRI.

Involvement of bone is particularly important in surgical planning. Cancer of the floor of the mouth can invade the lingual surface of the mandible or grow over the alveolar process and involve its superior surface. In the roof of the mouth, the hard palate and the alveolar processes can be eroded. In the region of the retromolar trigone, the ramus of the mandible and the maxillary buttress are at risk.

In each of these areas, the same principles apply as are used for evaluation of the nasopharynx and the sinuses. CT is still more sensitive for evaluation of the cortex of the bone, whereas MRI can demonstrate involvement of a marrow cavity. Recent reports have indicated that an intact cortical line at MRI is a very accurate indication that the cortex is not involved. However, an irregular cortex and even an abnormal marrow cavity can be seen in many benign conditions, such as chronic infection and dental abnormality. In addition, edema from nearby tumor may be indistinguishable from tumor itself. Plain dental radiography, including panorex and dental occlusal views, can also provide useful information regarding bony involvement of the mandible or maxilla by tumor.

Perineural extension may occur along branches of the trigeminal (V3), hypoglossal, or glossopharyngeal nerves. The masticator space and the poststyloid parapharyngeal space regions should be carefully inspected for an unexplained soft tissue mass.

Cancer arising from the mucosa of the posterior hard palate can spread along the palatine nerves and through the palatine foramina to reach the pterygopalatine fossa. This is of particular importance because many cancers of the posterior hard palate arise from the minor salivary glands that are abundant there. Adenoid cystic carcinoma frequently arises in this location.

Identification of lymph nodes should be attempted in the submandibular, submental, and jugular chains. Cancer of the lateral border of the oral tongue eventually drains to the omohyoid nodes (level 4), which are slightly inferior to the jugulodigastric nodes. Again, perhaps the most important nodal group to the radiologist is the lateral retropharyngeal nodes. These nodes are often readily defined by CT or MRI and may be undetectable by the clinician (see Fig. 5–9B and 5–14B).

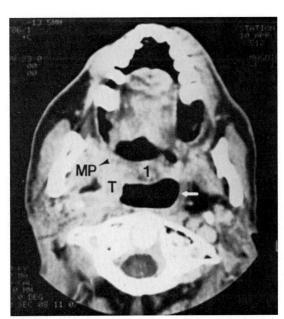

FIGURE 5–27 CT study of a tongue cancer that has extended submucosally up the tonsillar pillar (T) and into the soft palate (1). Tumor probably invades medial pterygoid muscle (MP, *arrowhead*). Normal deglutitional ring is seen on the left (*arrow*).

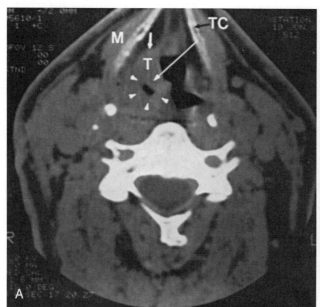

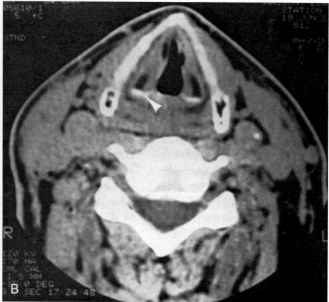

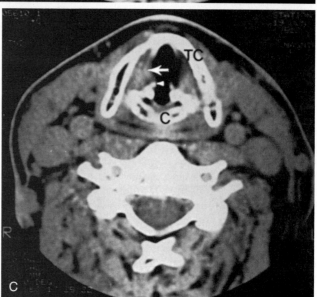

FIGURE 5–28 Supraglottic tumor: CT studies. *A,* Image through the hypopharynx shows tumor (T) invading fat *(arrow)* and concentrically narrowing the right pyriform sinus *(arrowheads).* Thyroid cartilage (TC) is irregularly mineralized; this is normal. M, strap muscles. *B,* Lower-plane image through the false vocal cords at the level of the upper arytenoid cartilage *(arrowhead).* No tumor is present. *C,* Lower-plane image through the true vocal cords shows the thyroarytenoid muscle *(arrow)* and vocal process of the arytenoid *(arrowhead)* and the thyroid (TC) and cricoid (C) cartilage.

Submandibular Gland

The question that is usually asked in regard to a tumor of the submandibular gland is whether tumor is within the gland or arises outside the gland, and is therefore more likely to involve a lymph node. The radiologist can usually make the decision as to whether the gland is actually involved because as with the parotid gland, the submandibular gland has a characteristic density that is intermediate (between those of muscle and fat) (see Fig. 5–14A).

Larynx and Hypopharynx

Imaging of the larynx is one of the greatest challenges to the radiologist.[45] As in other anatomic areas, the mucosal surface remains the domain of the clinician, whereas the radiologist attempts to determine deep extension. Identification of

fat planes is of great importance in this anatomic site. Accurate imaging influences the choice of organ-sparing surgery.

The pre-epiglottic space contains fat and is readily evaluated by CT or MRI. One of the areas for which the radiologist can provide the most help is the paraglottic space, which lies between the mucosal surface and the inner lamina of the thyroid cartilage (Fig. 5–28). At the level of the false cord (see Fig. 5–28B), most of the paraglottic space is made up of fat. At the level of the cord, however, the thyroarytenoid muscle occupies most of the paraglottic region (see Fig. 5–28C). Axial imaging has been the mainstay of evaluation. Coronal imaging (Figs. 5–29 and 5–30) can be very helpful, especially in determining the vertical limit of a tumor.

The cartilages are also used as landmarks for determination of location. The vocal process of the arytenoid cartilage pinpoints the level of the true vocal cord. The upper arytenoid is seen at the level of the false cord. The definition of

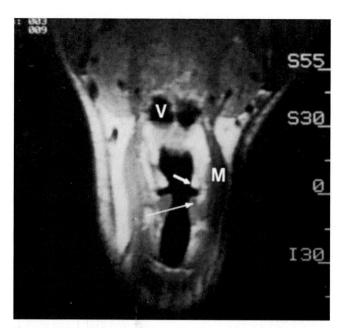

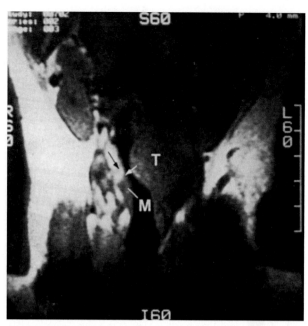

FIGURE 5–29 Coronal MRI of the larynx. The false vocal cord *(short arrow)* contains fat and is therefore white; the true vocal cord *(long arrow)* is mostly thyroarytenoid muscle, and is less white. The ventricle is visible between false and true cords. V, vallecula; M, strap muscles.

FIGURE 5–30 Left supraglottic tumor (T) extends into false vocal cord, and from there passes through paraglottic space into true vocal cord. The right false *(arrows)* and true (M) vocal cords are normal.

the inferior extent of a glottic-subglottic lesion relies on position relative to the cricoid.

Cartilage

Involvement of laryngeal cartilage is best appreciated on axial views and can be seen with CT or MRI. One must be cautious in stating that there is involvement of cartilage on the basis of a defect in the calcification of a cartilage because the variability in calcification makes this finding unreliable (Fig. 5–31). The most definite sign is demonstration of tumor beyond the external surface of the cartilage (Fig. 5–32).

MRI is considered to be more sensitive than other modalities for detection of cartilage invasion (Fig. 5–33).

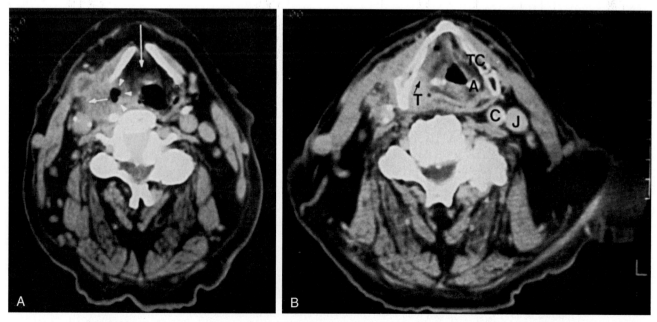

FIGURE 5–31 Pyriform sinus tumor: CT images. *A,* The right pyriform sinus tumor *(arrowheads)* extends into the strap muscles and soft tissues of the neck *(short arrow).* The pre-epiglottic fat is spared *(long arrow). B,* In a lower plane, tumor (T) extends between thyroid and arytenoid cartilage *(arrow).* A, normal left arytenoid; C, common carotid artery; J, internal jugular vein; TC, thyroid cartilage.

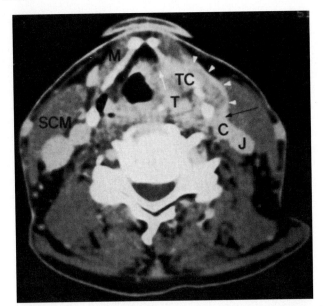

FIGURE 5–32 Pyriform sinus tumor (T) erodes through thyroid cartilage (TC) and into overlying strap muscles *(arrowheads)*; it extends posteriorly *(arrow)* to contact common carotid artery (C) but not internal jugular vein (J). M, normal right strap muscle; SCM, sternocleidomastoid.

The normal MRI appearance of cartilage is unlike that of cancer.[46] Cancer is intermediate in intensity on T1-weighted image and relatively brighter than muscle on T2-weighted image. The normal components of the thyroid and cricoid cartilages are cortex, fatty medullary space, and nonossified cartilage. The cortex is a signal void, and the medullary fat is bright on T1-weighted image. Nonossified cartilage can look like cancer on T1-weighted image, but it is relatively dark on T2-weighted image. Therefore, a normal-appearing cartilage on MRI is an accurate indicator that the cartilage is normal. An abnormal appearance of cartilage is a good indicator that cancer is present, but some findings are falsely positive. Squamous cell carcinoma can cause an inflammatory response that gives an appearance quite similar to that of tumor. The findings at MRI cannot be considered entirely specific.

Tumor can extend into the extralaryngeal soft tissues by passing through the cartilage. Another frequent route of egress is through the cricothyroid membrane into the anterior soft tissues. Small fat planes close to the cricothyroid membrane and beneath the strap muscles make imaging a very sensitive method of evaluation. This is another important finding to the surgeon in choosing a voice-sparing procedure or total laryngectomy.

Supraglottis

The ventricle is one of the most important landmarks in the larynx. A laryngeal lesion that crosses the ventricle may require a different treatment plan than a lesion confined to the glottis or supraglottis. On axial images, the level of the ventricle can be difficult to determine because of the horizontal orientation of the slitlike structure. As the cancer approaches the ventricle through the paraglottic space, the fat is obliterated. If a section can be found below the tumor where the paraglottic fat is not obliterated, then one can be confident that the lesion is supraglottic. If the cancer reaches the ventricle, involvement of the cord can be suggested by comparing the width of one cord with that of the other by using the vocal process to determine the cord level. This determination is less reliable than is evaluation of

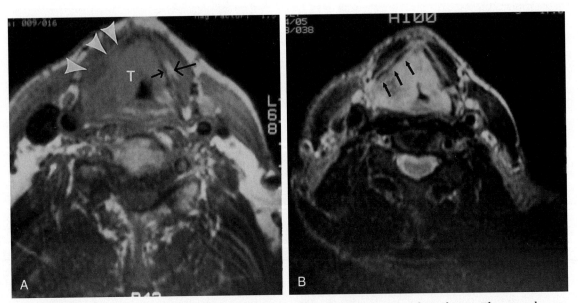

FIGURE 5–33 *A,* T1-weighted axial image. A tumor (T) is seen in the supraglottic larynx. The normal cartilage on the left has high-signal fat *(large arrow)* and a low-signal bony cortex *(small arrow)*. On the opposite side *(arrowheads)*, the cartilage has an intermediate signal intensity. *B,* T2-weighted image shows high signal in the cartilage, which indicates tumor involvement. The key finding is that the abnormality is intermediate to low signal on T1-weighted image and to high signal on T2-weighted image.

tumor in the paraglottic fat. If, however, the lesion continues below the cord into the subglottic region, the airway is distorted and tumor is easily detected. Unfortunately, the area in which one would prefer to have the greatest reliability can be the most difficult to visualize. If the cord is normal and the fat of the paraglottic space is obliterated on the next-higher slice, the lesion can be just above the ventricle, at the ventricle, or slightly into the true cord.

Coronal images can help provide answers about extent of tumor into the ventricle. MRI provides excellent coronal images as well as axial images (see Figs. 5–29 and 5–30). On coronal images, the ventricle may be invisible. The thyroarytenoid muscle again becomes the landmark. The upper margin of the muscle is at the level of the ventricle. Ideally, the precise inferior margin of a tumor will be reliably defined with respect to the relationship of the tumor to the muscle (see Fig. 5–30).

Glottis/Subglottis

The inferior extent of a carcinoma of the vocal cord is very important. Less extension is allowed posteriorly than anteriorly because of the shape of the cricoid cartilage. The cricoid cartilage is easily seen on CT or MRI, and so the position of the tumor relative to the cricoid is readily defined.

Pyriform Sinus/Postcricoid Region

Cancer of the hypopharynx should be described relative to anatomic structures in the larynx as well as in the pharynx itself. The pharynx and particularly the pyriform sinus have an intimate association with the larynx.

The thyroarytenoid gap is a radiologic landmark seen on either CT or MRI (see Fig. 5–31). This is the point at which the posterior paraglottic fat meets the pyriform sinus, which invaginates slightly between the two cartilages. Obliteration of fat in the landmark can be helpful in determining passage of tumor in one direction or the other. Cancer of the pyriform sinus can invade the larynx, usually by passing through the thyroarytenoid gap to reach the false cord and the paraglottic space.

Of equal importance is the lateral extension. Lateral extension of the cancer brings the lesion into the immediate vicinity of the carotid (see Figs. 5–31 and 5–32). CT or MRI can demonstrate the gross relationship of tumor to vessel. MRI has the advantage of clearly showing the vessel as a signal void because of the rapidly flowing blood.

Barium studies can be helpful in evaluating the pyriform apex. A thick barium is used to coat the pyriform sinus mucosa, and plain films are taken while the patient puffs out the cheeks. The lower extent of the mucosal irregularity is identified.

The pyriform apex is usually evaluated with cross-sectional imaging. Similarly, the inferior extent of a cancer of the hypopharynx can be predicted at imaging because the cancer causes a thickening of the wall of the pharynx. The inferior extent is estimated relative to the position of the cricopharyngeus muscle. The position of the inferior edge of this muscle is the point at which the shape of the food passage, in axial image, changes from linear (oval) to round, signifying the change from pharynx to esophagus.

The relationship of the inferior margin of the cancer relative to the cricopharyngeus can also be determined by barium swallow. The irregularity caused by the cancer is described relative to the indentation of the cricopharyngeus muscle. The barium study is also useful in judging the fixation of the tumor to the prevertebral fascia and musculature. If the tumor slides easily relative to the spine as the patient swallows, then the tumor is not fixed to the prevertebral structures. If the tumor and pharynx do not move up and down with swallowing, then the lesion is presumed to have invaded these structures. This study is much more accurate than CT/MRI in determining involvement of vertebral fascia.

Nodes

Nodal involvement depends on the level of a tumor. In supraglottic tumors, images should be taken of the upper nodal groups, whereas the subglottic lesion must be evaluated through the lower neck for paratracheal and upper mediastinal involvement to be detected.

Thyroid

The evaluation of thyroid disease is complex, and there are many and varied indications for thyroid imaging. In the context of this chapter, the primary concern is differentiation between benign and malignant tumors. Ultrasound and radionuclide imaging are used to evaluate the thyroid gland.[47, 48] A solitary thyroid nodule is the most common management problem for the clinician.

The initial step in the workup of a solitary nodule is often fine-needle aspiration. The differentiation between benign and malignant tumors can be made in more than 90% of cases by a skilled cytologist. If a benign diagnosis is established, the nodule may often be observed clinically. If malignant cells are obtained, surgery is indicated. If the cytologic findings reveal atypical benign cells, radionuclide imaging will give functional information about the nodule.

The anatomy of the thyroid area is well demonstrated on CT or MRI. The location of a mass relative to the thyroid gland and surrounding tissues can be accurately assessed. A smooth margin of the gland is reassuring. As tumor extends beyond the confines of the gland and invades the contiguous soft tissue, the fat planes are obliterated.

Nodal spread from thyroid carcinoma can have a wide variety of appearances. Metastatic nodes can enhance, can be cystic, or can be inhomogeneous. Metastatic papillary cancer may contain calcifications. Posterior cervical triangle nodes are commonly involved.

One must be cautious in the use of iodine contrast CT for the evaluation of differentiated thyroid cancers if radioiodine ablation is contemplated. Therefore, ultrasound or MRI is often more useful in this setting.

Temporal Bone

Determination of the extent of a tumor of the temporal bone (Fig. 5–34A) relies on definition of involvement of bony and soft tissue structures. A lesion of the external auditory

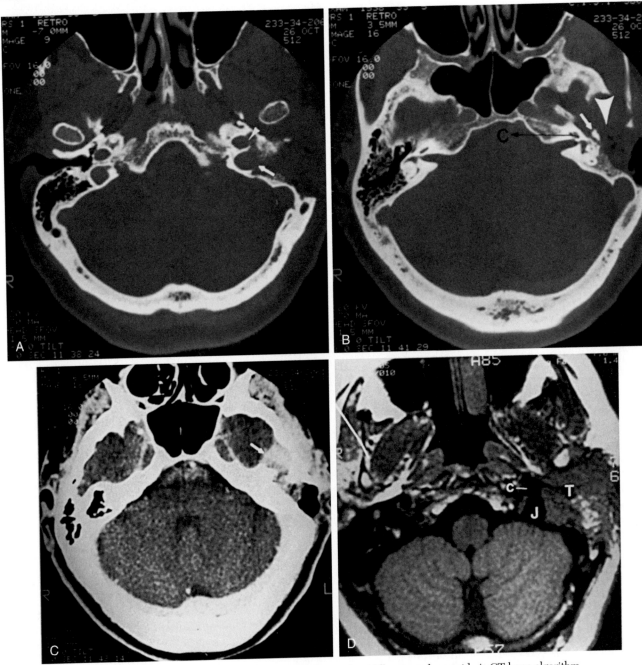

FIGURE 5–34 Carcinoma of the external auditory canal, middle ear, and mastoid. *A,* CT bone algorithm shows erosion of the mastoid extending into the lateral wall of the jugular fossa *(arrow)* and petrous carotid canal *(arrowhead). B,* CT bone algorithm in a higher plane shows the mass eroding the mastoid and middle ear *(arrowhead)* but sparing the malleus and incus *(arrow). C,* CT soft tissue algorithm shows the tumor eroding through the petrous bone into the middle cranial fossa *(arrow). D,* T1-weighted MR image shows the tumor (T) in the mastoid. The signal void of internal carotid artery (C) and internal jugular vein (J) indicates that these vessels are patent, but the signal void of cortical bone cannot be distinguished from the vessel. CT is a better means to assess erosion of the bone in this location.

canal may erode the cortical margins of the canal (see Fig. 5–34*A*) and proceed in any direction. Cancer extending superiorly or posteriorly will distort the normally aerated mastoid cells (see Fig. 5–34*B*). Intracranial extension is apparent on CT and MRI (see Fig. 5–34*C*). Inferior and anterior extension obliterates the fat planes that are beneath the temporal bone and in the temporomandibular joint region (see Fig. 5–34*D*). Extension into the middle ear through the tympanic membrane obliterates the air in the middle ear. In the middle ear and mastoid, it can be difficult to distinguish tumor from obstruction. Cancer reaching the medial wall of the middle ear can erode into the jugular or carotid canal (see Fig. 5–34*B*). Currently, erosion of bone is best evaluated on CT.

The CT findings in carcinoma of the external auditory canal can be indistinguishable from necrotizing external otitis.[49] Often this malignant external otitis can extend inferiorly, obliterating the fat planes inferior to the temporal bone.

More aggressive approaches to the skull base have increased the importance of evaluation of the internal carotid artery as it approaches and travels within the cavernous sinus. CT has the advantage of thinner cuts, which emphasize bone. MRI has the advantages of easy definition of the artery and cavernous sinus and of availability of a multiplicity of slice orientations.

◼ CONCLUSION

Evaluation of head and neck tumors requires many different imaging modalities. The radiologist must be cognizant of the usual route of spread if the extreme boundaries of a lesion are to be defined.

REFERENCES

1. Bergeron RT, Som PM (eds): Head and Neck Imaging Excluding the Brain, 2nd ed. St Louis, CV Mosby, 1984.
2. Valvassori GE, Mafee MF (eds): Diagnostic imaging. Otolaryngol Clin North Am 21:(entire issue), 1988.
3. Brant-Zawadzki M, Norman D (eds): Magnetic Resonance Imaging of the Central Nervous System. New York, Raven, 1987.
4. Anzai Y, McLachlan S, Morris M, et al: Dextran-coated superparamagnetic iron oxide: The first human use of a new contrast agent for assessing lymph nodes in the head and neck. Am J Neuroradiol 15:87, 1994.
5. Hoffman HT, Quets J, Toshiaki T, et al: Functional magnetic resonance imaging using iron oxide particles in characterizing head and neck adenopathy. Laryngoscope 110:1425, 2000.
6. Maheshwari SR, Mukherji SK, Neelon B, et al: The choline/creatine ratio in five benign neoplasms: Comparison with squamous cell carcinoma by use of in vitro MR spectroscopy. Am J Neuroradiol 21:1930, 2000.
7. Van den Brekel MW, Stel HV, Castelijno JA, et al: Lymph node staging in patients with clinically negative neck examination by ultrasound and ultrasound guided aspiration cytology. Am J Surg 162:362, 1991.
8. Rege S, Maass A, Chaiken L, et al: Use of positron emission tomography with fluoro-deoxyglucose in patients with extracranial head and neck cancers. Cancer 73:3047, 1994.
9. Rege SD, Chaiken L, Hoh CK, et al: Change induced by radiation therapy in FDG uptake in normal and malignant structures of the head and neck: Quantitation with PET. Radiology 189:807, 1993.
10. Greven KM, Williams DW 3rd, Keyes JW Jr, et al: Can positron emission tomography distinguish tumor recurrence from irradiation sequelae in patients treated for larynx cancer? Cancer J Sci Am 3:333, 1997.
11. Wahl RL, Quint LE, Cieslak RD, et al: "Anatometabolic" tumor imaging: Fusion of FDG PET with CT or MRI to localize foci of increased activity. J Nucl Med 34:1190, 1993.
12. Wong WL, Hussain K, Chevretton E, et al: Validation and clinical application of computer-combined computed tomography and positron emission tomography with 2-[18F]fluoro-2-deoxy-D-glucose head and neck images. Am J Surg 172:628, 1996.
13. Magnani A, Rizzo G, Fazio F: FDG/PET and spiral CT image fusion for mediastinal lymph node assessment of non-small cell lung cancer patients. J Cardiovasc Surg 40:741, 1999.
14. Sercarz J, Bailet JW, Abemayor E, et al: Computer coregistration of positron emission tomography and magnetic resonance images in head and neck cancer. Am J Otolaryngol 19:130, 1998.
15. Woods R, Cherry S, Mazziotta J: Rapid automated algorithm for aligning and reslicing PET images. J Comput Assist Tomogr 16:620, 1992.
16. Fukui M, Meltzer CC, Snyderman CH: Combined PET/CT evaluation of recurrent skull base neoplasm: A new tool. Skull Base 11:17, 2001.
17. Abe Y, Matsuzawa T, Fujiwara T, et al: Assessment of radiotherapeutic effects on experimental tumors using 18F-2-fluoro-2-deoxy-D-glucose. Eur J Nucl Med 12:325, 1986.
18. Ichiya Y, Kuwabara Y, Otsuka M, et al: Assessment of response to cancer therapy using fluorine-18-fluorodeoxyglucose and positron emission tomography. J Nucl Med 32:1655, 1991.
19. Minn H, Paul R, Ahonen A: Evaluation of treatment response to radiotherapy in head and neck cancer with fluorine-18 fluorodeoxyglucose. J Nucl Med 29:1521, 1988.
20. Lowe V, Dunphy FR, Varvares M, et al: Evaluation of chemotherapy response in patients with advanced head and neck cancer using [F-18] fluorodeoxyglucose positron emission tomography. Head Neck 19:666, 1997.
21. Stollfuss J, Glatting G, Friess H, et al: 2-(Fluorine-18)-fluoro-2-deoxy-D-glucose PET in detection of pancreatic cancer: Value of quantitative image interpretation. Radiology 195:339, 1995.
22. Minn H, Lapela M, Klemi PJ, et al: Prediction of survival with fluorine-18-fluoro-deoxyglucose and PET in head and neck cancer. J Nucl Med 38:1907, 1997.
23. Erba SM, Horton JA, Latchaw RE, et al: Balloon test occlusion of the internal carotid artery with xenon CT. AJNR Am J Neuroradiol 9:533, 1988.
24. Barker DW, Jungreis CA, Horton JA, et al: Balloon test occlusion of the internal carotid artery: Change in stump pressure over 15 minutes and its correlation with xenon CT cerebral blood flow. AJNR Am J Neuroradiol 14:587, 1993.
25. Som PM: Lymph nodes of the neck. Radiology 165:593, 1987.
26. Mancusco AA, Maceri D, Rice D, et al: CT of cervical lymph node cancer. AJR Am J Roentgenol 136:381, 1981.
27. Mancusco AA, Harnsberger HR, Muraki AS, et al: Computed tomography of cervical and retropharyngeal lymph nodes: Normal anatomy, variants of normal, and applications in staging head and neck cancer: I. Normal anatomy. Radiology 148:709, 1983.
28. Curtin HD, Williams R, Johnson J: CT of perineural tumor extension: Pterygopalatine fossa. AJR Am J Roentgenol 144:163, 1984 and AJNR Am J Neuroradiol 5:731, 1984.
29. Curtin HD, Wolfe P, Snyderman N: The facial nerve between the stylomastoid foramen and the parotid: Computed tomographic imaging. Radiology 149:165, 1983.
30. Som PM, Dillon WP, Curtin HD, et al: Hypointense paranasal sinus foci: Differential diagnosis with MR imaging and relation to CT findings. Radiology 176:777, 1990.
31. Dillon WP, Som PM, Fullerton GD: Hypointense MR signal in chronically inspissated sinonasal secretions. Radiology 174:73, 1990.
32. Som PM, Dillon WP, Fullerton GD, et al: Chronically obstructed sinonasal secretions: Observations on T1 and T2 shortening. Radiology 172:515, 1989.
33. Lanzieri CF, Shah M, Krauss D, et al: Use of gadolinium-enhanced MR imaging for differentiating mucoceles from neoplasms in the paranasal sinuses. Radiology 178:425, 1991.
34. Teresi LM, Lufkin RB, Vinuela F, et al: MR imaging of the nasopharynx and floor of the middle cranial fossa: I. Normal anatomy. Radiology 164:811, 1987.
35. Teresi LM, Lufkin RB, Vinuela F, et al: MR imaging of the nasopharynx and floor of the middle cranial fossa: II. Malignant tumors. Radiology 164:817, 1987.
36. Curtin HD, Tabor EK: Nose, paranasal sinuses, and facial bones. In Latchaw RE (ed): MR and CT Imaging of the Head, Neck, and Spine, 2nd ed. St Louis, Mosby–Year Book, 1991, p 947.
37. Som PM, Biller HF, Lawson W: Tumors of the parapharyngeal space: Preoperative evaluation, diagnosis and surgical approaches. Ann Otol Rhinol Laryngol 90(suppl):3, 1985.
38. Som PM, Biller HF, Lawson W, et al: Parapharyngeal space masses: An updated protocol based upon 104 cases. Radiology 153:149, 1984.
39. Curtin HD: Separation of the masticator space from the parapharyngeal space. Radiology 163:195, 1987.
40. Som PM, Braun IF, Shapiro MD, et al: Tumors of the parapharyngeal space and upper neck: MR imaging characteristics. Radiology 164:823, 1987.
41. Mukari AS, Mancusco AA, Harnsberger HR, et al: CT of the oropharynx, tongue base, and floor of the mouth: Normal anatomy and range of variations, and application in staging carcinoma. Radiology 148:725, 1983.
42. Lufkin RB, Wortham DG, Dietrich RB, et al: Tongue and oropharynx: Findings on MR imaging. Radiology 161:69, 1986.

43. Shaefer SK, Maravilla R, Suss RA, et al: Magnetic resonance imaging versus computed tomography: Comparison in imaging oral cavity and pharyngeal carcinomas. Radiology 160:860, 1986.

44. Mancusco AA, Hanafee WN: Elusive head and neck cancers beneath intact mucosa. Laryngoscope 93:133, 1983.

45. Curtin HD: Imaging of the larynx: Current concepts. Radiology 173:1, 1989.

46. Castelijns JA, Gerritsen AJ, Kauser MC, et al: Invasion of laryngeal cartilage by cancer: Comparison of CT and MR imaging. Radiology 167:199, 1988.

47. James EM, Charboneau JW: High-frequency (10 MHz) thyroid ultrasonography. Semin Ultrasound CT MR 6:294, 1985.

48. Atkins HL: The thyroid. In Freeman LM (ed): Freeman and Johnson's Clinical Radionuclide Imaging, 3rd ed, vol 2. Orlando, Fla, Grune & Stratton, 1984, p 1275.

49. Curtin HD, Wolfe P, May M: Malignant external otitis: CT evaluation. Radiology 145:383, 1982.

CHAPTER 6

Anesthetic Considerations

Daniel E. Supkis
Thomas B. Dougherty

A variety of problems unique to patients undergoing head and neck oncologic surgery are of concern to the anesthesiologist. Many of these patients have a history of chronic cigarette smoking and alcohol use.[1, 2] They usually have multiple medical problems, including, in particular, coronary artery disease and chronic obstructive pulmonary disease. These systemic problems impact significantly on the anesthetic plan. Such patients often present to the operating room with conditions that make mask ventilation and tracheal intubation potentially difficult during and following the induction of general anesthesia. Frequently, the surgical procedures, especially those involving plastic reconstruction of a large defect, are lengthy. The surgical team usually requires complete and easy access to one or more operative sites, including either the airway itself or an area near it,[3] and the anesthesiologist is often unable to be positioned near the patient's head.[4] The timely establishment of general anesthesia in the patient, a quiet operative field free of bulky equipment, and the patient's smooth emergence from anesthesia at the conclusion of the operation are expected.[3]

This chapter addresses these unique concerns by describing a concise and safe approach to the anesthetic management of patients undergoing surgical therapy for cancer of the head and neck. The approach is based on current airway management principles and techniques and emphasizes the prevention of airway problems associated with this type of surgery.[5]

PREOPERATIVE EVALUATION

Of all the phases in the surgical treatment of the head and neck oncologic patient, the assessment of his or her general state of health and the condition of the upper airway before undertaking the operative procedure ranks among the most important.[6] The anesthesiologist's preoperative clinical evaluation includes pertinent information from the patient's history, physical examination, previous anesthetic records, laboratory and special studies, and surgical plan.[7] A good evaluation not only provides a reasonable assessment of the patient's perioperative risk but allows the anesthesiologist to plan in advance the techniques of airway and anesthetic management that will be used.

History

The medical history should focus on the patient's disease state and current medications, a review of organ systems, and information on allergies. Particular emphasis is placed on the upper airway and on the cardiovascular, respiratory, and renal systems. Patients with cancer of the head and neck often have a history of tobacco and alcohol abuse and may have evidence of bronchitis, chronic obstructive pulmonary disease, hypertension, coronary artery disease, or alcohol withdrawal.[3, 4] These systemic problems greatly increase the complexity of anesthetic requirements and demand special attention to proper management of the airway.[8] For example, provision of supplemental oxygen to the patient or prevention of increased sympathetic nervous system activity may be necessary.[8] The patient may be taking one or more drugs for control of hypertension, angina, bronchospasm, an endocrine disorder, pain, or a psychological disturbance.[6] The anesthesiologist should be familiar with the classes of drugs involved, the anticipated adverse effects, and any possible interactions between the drugs and planned anesthetics. With few exceptions, the patient's usual medications, especially cardiovascular, pulmonary, and pain medications, should be administered up to and including the day of surgery. Exceptions to this are aspirin, which is usually stopped at least 5 to 7 days beforehand, and warfarin (Coumadin). Because angiotensin-converting enzyme (ACE) inhibitors and ACE receptor–blocking agents can be associated with severe hypotension during standard anesthetic induction techniques,[9] these two classes of antihypertensive drugs should be discontinued preoperatively.[10]

Information should be obtained about previous operations and recent anesthetic procedures, including whether airway management or tracheal intubations were difficult.[3] The difficult airway can be viewed as a clinical situation in which a conventionally trained anesthesiologist experiences difficulty with mask ventilation, tracheal intubation, or both, following the induction of general anesthesia.[11] A difficult intubation is one in which correct insertion of the tracheal tube with conventional (rigid) laryngoscopy requires multiple attempts or takes longer than 10 minutes.[11]

The degree of difficulty can range from extremely easy to impossible. Between these extremes, several well-defined degrees of difficulty are encountered,[12] depending on how much of the glottis is seen during laryngoscopy. Cormack and Lehane define four grades of view.[13] In grade I, most of the glottis, including anterior and posterior commissures, is visible. In grade II, the posterior portion of the glottis is visible, but the anterior commissure is not seen. In grade III, only the epiglottis is visible (the glottis cannot be seen). In grade IV, only the soft palate is visible (the epiglottis and glottis cannot be seen). The patient with a grade I or II view is easily intubated most of the time, whereas a patient with a grade III or IV view can be very difficult to intubate. In particular, the presence of tumor, together with associated anatomic changes and/or bleeding, can create a potentially difficult airway in the patient. A past history of an easy intubation 1 to 2 years earlier is no assurance that the patient remains easy to intubate. The tumor may have progressed, or concurrent problems such as cervical arthritis or arthritis of the temporomandibular joint may have worsened. Even if a large tumor of the head and neck region resolves somewhat with chemotherapy and radiation treatments, the patient is still at risk of having a difficult airway because of post-treatment fibrosis that limits the compliance of the submandibular space and the ability to extend the neck.

The detection of upper airway obstructive signs and symptoms is particularly important. The patient should be asked about problems with shortness of breath, dyspnea (especially when lying down), exercise intolerance, handling of secretions, and hoarseness.[7] If any airway obstruction is present, the patient has a compromised airway, which can be a difficult one.[3] Changes in the character of the patient's voice may suggest the site of the tumor as well as the progression of disease.[14] A coarse, scratchy-sounding voice suggests a glottic tumor, whereas a muffled voice is characteristic of a tumor of the supraglottis, base of the tongue, or pharynx.[14, 15] The patient with obstructive sleep apnea without an obvious anatomic abnormality may have a hidden problem such as a mass in the vallecula.[14] This condition can hinder mask ventilation and tracheal intubation following the induction of general anesthesia.[16] The patient who has difficulty breathing in the supine position but not in the lateral or prone position may have a mass in the pharynx, neck, or anterior mediastinum. Anesthetizing such a patient in the supine position without first securing the airway with an awake intubation can lead to severe airway obstruction.[3, 14]

If tumor has interfered with fluid intake and eating, dehydration, electrolyte imbalance, weight loss, malnutrition, and anemia may be significant.[17] The seriously malnourished or dehydrated patient has reduced cardiopulmonary reserve and will demonstrate poor tolerance to general anesthesia, immunocompromise, and impaired wound healing.[18]

Physical Examination

In addition to the patient's chest and heart, the upper airway should be evaluated systematically and thoroughly.

TABLE 6-1 General Physical Indicators of a Difficult Airway or Intubation in Patients

Short neck with a full set of teeth
Small mouth or limited mouth opening
Obesity
Receding lower jaw (micrognathia)
Protruding upper incisors (overbite)
Large tongue (e.g., caused by myxedema, acromegaly, hemangioma)
Enlarged thyroid (goiter) displacing or impinging on the airway
Limited mobility of cervical spine

From Dougherty TB, Nguyen DT: Anesthetic management of the patient scheduled for head and neck cancer surgery. J Clin Anesth 6:74, 1994.

Procedures for the physical examination of the upper airway are described in detail elsewhere,[8, 14, 19] and only pertinent features are discussed here. It is good practice to consider the patient scheduled for head and neck oncologic surgery as representing a potentially difficult tracheal intubation involving problems in airway management.[17] The preoperative airway evaluation will nearly always identify the patient who may be more safely managed by securing a patent airway before the induction of general anesthesia.

The patient's head and neck should be inspected in the frontal plane and in profile so that micrognathia, retrognathia, prognathia, and overbite can be detected.[14] Congenital or acquired factors other than head and neck tumors that suggest that the patient could develop a difficult airway following the induction of general anesthesia are listed in Table 6–1. The following three maneuvers described by Benumof[8] when considered together yield information about the possibility of visualizing the patient's vocal cords with conventional (rigid) laryngoscopy.

1. Can the patient assume the "sniffing" position by extending the head at the atlanto-occipital joint and moving the lower jaw forward by flexing the neck at the shoulders? This indicates the degree to which the anesthesiologist will be able to align the oral, pharyngeal, and laryngeal axes in the straightest line possible during rigid laryngoscopy. The presence of an obstructive tumor or a history of previous surgery or radiation fibrosis may limit mobility of the neck and hinder mask ventilation or rigid laryngoscopy.[3] Moreover, preoperative irradiation may lead to glottic edema, trismus, and an immobile epiglottis and larynx.[7]

2. When the patient's mouth is opened as widely as possible, and the tongue protrudes maximally, can the soft palate, uvula, and tonsillar pillars be visualized? The ability to do so embodies the Mallampati test and has been correlated with ease of rigid laryngoscopy and intubation.[19, 20] Although this test provides valuable information about the size of the tongue relative to the oral cavity space and is a useful predictor of tracheal intubation difficulty, it has been associated with both false-positive[21] and false-negative results.[22] The Mallampati test should not be considered conclusive when used by itself. Despite the limitations of the test, if only the soft palate is seen, visualization of the glottis with rigid laryngoscopy is expected to be difficult.[19] In an adult, the distance between the upper and lower incisors should be at least 4 to 6 cm (2.5–3 fingerbreadths) to successfully permit placement of a rigid laryngoscope in the oral cavity and the endotracheal tube beside it.[14]

3. Can at least 2 fingerbreadths be placed on the patient's neck between the lower border of the mandible and the larynx (thyromental distance)? A variation of this maneuver is to have the patient extend the head fully. If the distance between the mental prominence of the mandible and the thyroid notch is less than 6 cm in the adult, visualization of the vocal cords by rigid laryngoscopy may be extremely difficult.[23] The submandibular space should be palpated to determine its compliance or the presence of tumor, abscess, or hematoma. The compliance of this space can be greatly

reduced by scar tissue formation from previous surgery or fibrosis from radiation therapy. During conventional rigid laryngoscopy, the tongue is displaced into the submandibular space. If that space is noncompliant or is occupied by a mass lesion, displacement of the tongue will be insufficient to allow adequate visualization of the vocal cords.

In addition to the information obtained from the previously listed maneuvers, answers to the following questions should be sought during the airway evaluation.[6]

1. What is the condition of the patient's teeth? The presence of dental appliances or protruding, loose, or diseased teeth may contribute to a difficult intubation.[3, 14]

2. Is the patient's tongue protruding, swollen, or fixed in position? A tongue that is large relative to the size of the oral cavity will interfere with adequate mask ventilation and tracheal intubation.[8] A tongue fixed in position, regardless of its size, can prevent a successful laryngoscopy.[14]

3. Does the patient exhibit stridor during either inspiration or expiration, or both, on auscultation of the larynx or trachea? Stridor is caused by increased turbulence and rate of air flow through a narrowed passage, which suggests partial obstruction.[3, 24] A tumor at or above the vocal cords may be associated with inspiratory stridor, whereas a bronchial obstruction is indicated by expiratory stridor.[15] A subglottic or tracheal lesion is suggested by a biphasic stridor occurring during both inspiration and expiration.[15]

Finally, tumors and any accompanying edema of the oral cavity, pharynx, and hypopharynx, together with previous surgery on the patient's airway, can greatly limit the open space of the upper airway or distort its anatomy.[3] All of these factors can interfere with mask application, maintenance of an adequate airway, and tracheal intubation.[25] Dysfunction of the ninth, tenth, or twelfth cranial nerve, whether the result of injury from previous surgery or tumor invasion (e.g., glomus tumor), can predispose the patient to aspiration or obstruction.[26] Table 6–2 summarizes the common causes of a problematic airway unique to head and neck oncologic patients.

Laboratory and Special Studies

Information from the patient's history and physical examination guides the selection of laboratory tests and special studies.[3, 6] For many of our patients, a hemoglobin or

TABLE 6–2 Common Causes of a Difficult Airway or Intubation in Head and Neck Cancer Patients

Limited head and neck mobility and position
Limited mouth opening
Limited upper airway open space, resulting from tumor, edema, or previous surgery
Distorted anatomy of the airway by tumor expansion or previous surgery
Fixation of tissues of head and neck, oral cavity, pharynx, or larynx by tumor, surgical scars, or radiation fibrosis

From Dougherty TB, Nguyen DT: Anesthetic management of the patient scheduled for head and neck cancer surgery. J Clin Anesth 6:74, 1994.

hematocrit level, coagulation profile, platelet count, 12-lead electrocardiogram (ECG), chest radiograph, and room air arterial oxygen saturation value are obtained.[3] In the patient with significant functional limitations secondary to chronic obstructive pulmonary disease, baseline arterial blood gas analysis allows an assessment of the acid-base status and the degree of hypoventilation and hypoxemia.[14] If partial airway obstruction is present, flow-volume loop studies are helpful in distinguishing the location of the obstruction and in determining whether it is fixed or variable.[14] Frequently, the cardiac status of the patient with symptomatic heart disease has to be evaluated further by consultation with a cardiologist and additional testing.[3] Determination of electrolyte, glucose, blood urea nitrogen, and creatinine levels is suggested for the patient who has a known or suspected metabolic disease, is malnourished, or is receiving drug therapy such as diuretics or digoxin.[18] In addition, plasma drug levels should be checked to ensure that the maximum benefit of medications such as theophylline or digoxin is being attained. Liver function tests are obtained in patients suspected of alcohol abuse.

Radiographic studies are becoming increasingly important in the airway evaluation of the surgical patient with cancer of the head and neck.[27] Computed tomography images are especially helpful in determining the location, size, and extent of lesions and in detecting any erosion of bony or cartilaginous structures.[28] Magnetic resonance imaging offers multiplanar views of cartilage and soft tissue and is useful in the evaluation of tumor extension. The results of these studies may be helpful in evaluating the degree of airway obstruction, as well as in selecting which technique of tracheal intubation should be used.

Communication With the Surgeon

Preoperative communication and cooperation between the anesthesiologist and the surgeon are essential in determining special surgical requirements and unique consequences of various head and neck procedures. The nature of the patient's significant medical problems and airway management options should be discussed with the surgeon before induction of general anesthesia or intubation is attempted.[3, 7] In this manner, last-minute, impulsive decisions are prevented and the patient is provided with a smooth, safe anesthetic. Moreover, the surgeon, using information from indirect or flexible fiberoptic laryngoscopy, should be able to predict whether the airway or tracheal intubation will be difficult.[29]

Before being brought to the operating room, the patient should be in the best possible medical condition, keeping in mind the status of the tumor and the time available for preoperative medical treatment of significant problems.[3] If time allows, for example, hypertension and myocardial ischemia should be adequately controlled before surgery is performed. The patient with bronchitis and chronic obstructive lung disease might benefit from preoperative treatment with antibiotics and bronchodilators.

Patients with vascular tumors of the head and neck require special attention. They have the potential to lose massive quantities of blood in a short period of time. This is usually technically difficult surgery. This information should be related to the anesthesia care team during preoperative communication. If massive transfusion is likely necessary, the blood bank should be informed several days to a week before the procedure to ensure that an adequate supply of blood is on hand for the patient. A type and screen should be sent once the decision for surgery has been made. A call should be made to blood bank personnel to inform them of the potential need for large quantities of blood products. Intraoperative management of the patient requires that multiple large-bore intravenous lines be established. Invasive arterial pressure monitoring is useful in these patients for beat-to-beat monitoring of the blood pressure and to ensure that blood samples can be obtained for determination of hemoglobin, hematocrit, and coagulation factors. Central venous pressure/pulmonary artery monitoring is helpful for determination of volume status. Use of intraoperative cell saver techniques has not been well established for these types of procedures. Basically, the cell saver or intraoperative autologous blood salvage devices work best for cardiovascular procedures (mainly aneurysm and open heart surgery) and for orthopedic procedures. It is best to use the cell saver in procedures where blood will pool into dependent areas. The surface skimming of shed blood can result in a postoperative coagulopathy.[30, 31] In addition, cell saver use mandates that the blood be provided from a non-contaminated source. Surgical fields that connect with the oral-pharyngeal cavity are unacceptable for the use of cell saver technology because of potential bacterial contamination.

ANESTHETIC MANAGEMENT

One of the most effective methods of reducing anxiety in the patient facing head and neck oncologic surgery is to give him or her a thorough description of the anesthetic events about to take place and the rationale behind them.[6, 32, 33] This includes placement of invasive monitors and, especially, performance of an awake fiberoptic-guided intubation following sedation and topical analgesia. If premedication is still necessary to allay anxiety, administration of small doses of midazolam is acceptable in the patient who has no upper airway obstruction. If evidence of some airway compromise is present, premedication should be deferred until the patient is near the operating room and can be monitored appropriately. If airway obstruction is severe, premedication is best avoided.[3, 7]

Airway Management and Induction of Anesthesia

Statistical studies of anesthesia-related adverse respiratory events suggest that one third of severe perioperative complications are the result of inability to establish and maintain an adequate upper airway following the induction of general anesthesia.[34, 35] In few other situations is the problem of airway management greater and more challenging than in surgery for head and neck cancer. With only slight modification, the American Society of Anesthesiologists (ASA) algorithm for the difficult airway[11] is useful for managing the airway in patients undergoing surgery for cancer of the head and neck (Fig. 6–1).

Choice of Tracheal Intubation Method. If the patient has no evidence of a difficult airway or airway compromise, general anesthesia is usually safely induced before the airway is secured with tracheal intubation. Although sodium thiopental and propofol are commonly used induction agents, etomidate is preferable when myocardial depression is to be avoided. Addition of a potent inhalational agent (e.g., isoflurane, desflurane, or sevoflurane) by mask, plus moderate doses of an intravenous narcotic (e.g., fentanyl or sufentanil), greatly reduces the sympathetic response that results from rigid laryngoscopy and intubation. Early administration of a muscle relaxant during anesthetic induction facilitates mask ventilation and intubation.

If the airway or intubation is potentially difficult, we apply a topical anesthetic to the upper airway, carefully sedate the patient, and proceed with direct examination of the airway with rigid laryngoscopy while the patient is awake.[5] During preparation of the patient for this examination, as outlined in Table 6–3, it should be remembered that in some patients, airway obstruction may actually occur or worsen as a result of topical application of local anesthetic to the larynx.[3] Also, translaryngeal instillation of local anesthetic or percutaneous blocks of the glossopharyngeal and superior laryngeal nerves, although effective in promoting analgesia of the upper airway, are generally avoided because these procedures are frequently contraindicated by the presence of tumor.[3] In fact, Sitzman and coworkers[37] demonstrated that glossopharyngeal nerve blocks are no more effective than topical application of lidocaine as a route of local anesthetic administration for awake laryngoscopy.[25]

Direct upper airway evaluation performed while the patient is awake allows the selection of the safest technique for securing the airway. If, during the examination, the patient's vocal cords can be visualized, it is appropriate to proceed with induction of general anesthesia before intubation, the technique of which is determined by the patient's medical condition.[25] After the patient loses consciousness and ventilation is established, the short-acting muscle relaxant succinylcholine is administered intravenously to facilitate laryngoscopy and intubation. Sivarajan and associates[38, 39] caution that the ability to visualize the glottis in the awake patient with a potentially difficult airway does not guarantee the same ability following induction of general anesthesia. The induction of anesthesia and paralysis results in an anterior displacement of the larynx, which can hinder visualization of the vocal cords.

Fiberoptic-Guided Intubation in the Awake Patient. If a difficult airway or intubation is certain based on the findings of the preoperative airway evaluation or of an awake examination of the airway, and if the patient does not have a large, friable supraglottic tumor, the airway is secured by an awake tracheal intubation technique. Our preference is to proceed with an awake fiberoptic-guided intubation, which is generally well tolerated by the properly prepared, spontaneously breathing patient. Adequate sedation and topical analgesia of the upper airway are achieved as described in Table 6–3. If the patient has undergone a previous reconstructive procedure of the head and neck and is returning for a second surgery, it is wise to consider performing an elective fiberoptic intubation and to avoid rigid conventional laryngoscopy, which might damage the reconstructed area. An

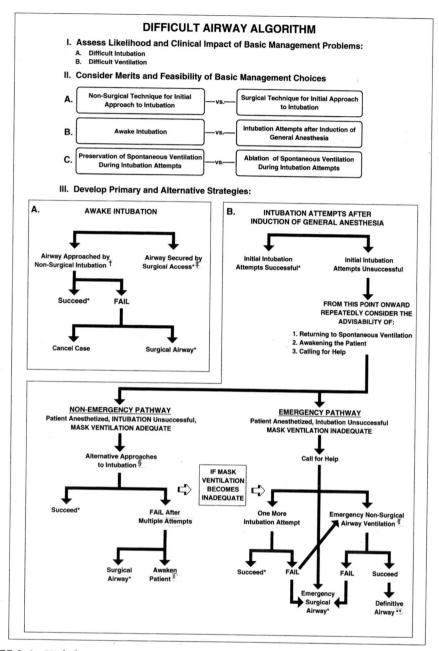

FIGURE 6–1 With few exceptions, the American Society of Anesthesiologists' algorithm for managing the difficult airway or intubation is applicable to the patient undergoing head and neck cancer surgery. *Confirm intubation with exhaled carbon dioxide. †Awake nonsurgical intubation includes oral or nasal fiberoptic intubation at our institution. ‡Awake surgically secured airway is indicated in the patient with a bulky, friable intraoral, pharyngeal, or other large supraglottic tumor. §Alternative approaches to difficult intubation include (but are not limited to) use of different laryngoscope blades, oral or nasal fiberoptic guidance, laryngeal mask airway (LMA), intubating stylet or tube changer, or surgically created airway access. ‖See Awake Intubation. ¶At the present time, emergency nonsurgical airway is limited to LMA or transtracheal jet ventilation in our patient population. **If endotracheal intubation through an LMA is unsuccessful, the definitive airway is usually established by a tracheotomy in the head and neck cancer patient. (Adapted from American Society of Anesthesiologists: Practice guidelines for management of the difficult airway. A report by the American Society of Anesthesiologists' task force on management of the difficult airway. Anesthesiology 78:597, 1993.)

awake fiberoptic intubation also may be preferable if a difficult airway is even a possibility in the patient who has ischemic heart disease.[3] This procedure should produce less sympathetic stimulation than is produced by an awake, direct laryngoscopy or a difficult intubation after induction of general anesthesia. The route of intubation, either nasal or oral, is determined by the planned surgical procedure and the patient's physical condition.[40] Detailed instructions for

TABLE 6-3 Topical Anesthesia for Awake Instrumentation of the Upper Airway

1. Give the patient an adequate explanation of the events that are about to occur.
2. Administer an anticholinergic, such as glycopyrrolate, early in the sedation process to dry the patient's secretions and provide a clear field for laryngoscopy.
3. Supply supplemental oxygen to the patient at the start of sedation. Use of a pulse oximeter, electrocardiogram, and automatic blood pressure cuff to monitor the patient is mandatory.
4. Sedate the patient with a combination of a benzodiazepine and narcotic. We use midazolam (0.25–0.5 mg increments) and sufentanil (0.1–0.2 µg/kg). Because patient response to these doses can vary greatly, they are titrated to effect while meaningful contact is maintained with the patient.°
5. To achieve topical analgesia of the upper airway, apply 4% lidocaine with a high-flow atomizer, which creates a fine, dense, deeply penetrating spray. For adequate anesthesia of the larynx itself, the patient breathes vigorously while the pharyngeal region behind the base of the tongue is sprayed. Limit the total dose of lidocaine to 3–4 mg/kg to prevent central nervous system toxicity from excessive absorption of the drug from the oral and laryngeal mucous membranes.[36]

°"Meaningful contact" means the patient remains rational and appropriately follows commands.[8]
Modified from Dougherty TB, Nguyen DT: Anesthetic management of the patient scheduled for head and neck cancer surgery. J Clin Anesth 6:74, 1994.

performing fiberoptic intubations are beyond the scope of this chapter and are described elsewhere.[8, 14, 41] Certain key features of these intubations, however, are mentioned here.

The nasal route is particularly useful in patients with a large tongue, a receding lower jaw, limited mouth opening, or tracheal deviation. For this route, the patient's nostrils are anesthetized topically, as described in Table 6–4. After the selected nostril is dilated with soft, progressively larger nasal airways, a well-lubricated nasotracheal tube is loaded proximally onto a fiberoptic laryngoscope before the tip of the laryngoscope is inserted into the nostril. While performing the laryngoscopy, one can insufflate oxygen through the suction port of the laryngoscope. This effectively supplements the patient's respirations with oxygen and has the added benefit of blowing secretions away from the tip of the scope, which reduces fogging of the lens.[42] When the laryngoscope enters the trachea, the nasotracheal tube is advanced gently over the laryngoscope through the nose and into the trachea. The fiberoptic scope is removed only after the correct tracheal position of the tube above the carina is verified. Tracheal tubes constructed of a soft, flexible material, such as polyvinylchloride or reinforced silicone, pass more easily through the vocal cords and cause less damage. The size difference between the endotracheal tube and the fiberoptic scope should be minimal. If the space is too great, the tube may catch on the vocal cords during attempts to pass the tube through the glottic opening.[8] General anesthesia is induced in the patient only after the breathing circuit is attached to the tracheal tube and the presence of end-tidal carbon dioxide is confirmed. Suggestions for a successful fiberoptic-guided intubation are summarized in Table 6–5.

Fiberoptic-guided intubation by the oral route is greatly facilitated by inserting an airway intubator bite-block such as the Ovassapian[43, 44] or Williams[43] airway behind the patient's tongue in the midline of the mouth. The airway not only keeps the fiberoptic scope in the midline during laryngoscopy but also displaces the tongue anteriorly away from the soft palate, enabling the fiberoptic scope to pass more easily between the tongue and the soft palate.

The latest generation of fiberoptic scope has a video chip at the tip of the scope. This allows for increased image resolution without the matrix pattern that is obtained by viewing through a fiberoptic bundle. It now is possible to have the surgical team examine the airway as the anesthesia care team performs a fiberoptic intubation. The surgical team can help guide the anesthesia care team if the airway anatomy is severely distorted.

Other Awake Intubation Techniques. When an attempted fiberoptic intubation in the awake patient is unsuccessful or when excessive blood and secretions are present in the airway, a retrograde endotracheal intubation technique can be used to secure the airway.[45–48] Sanchez and Pallares[49] describe various modifications of this approach in detail. Their suggested technique using the retrograde kit supplied by Cook Incorporated (Bloomington, Ind) is summarized as follows.[25] The patient is placed ideally in the supine sniffing position with the neck hyperextended. The skin is prepared, and anesthesia of the airway is achieved if not already carried out in the awake patient. Translaryngeal analgesia, if not contraindicated, facilitates performance of the technique. The kit's 18-gauge angio-catheter is advanced initially into the larynx through the

TABLE 6-4 Preparation of the Nose for Fiberoptic–Guided Intubation

1. Spray the nostrils initially with 0.05% oxymetazoline hydrochloride (e.g., Afrin Nasal Spray), or 0.5% phenylephrine hydrochloride to shrink the nasal mucosa to gain more space and to reduce the risk of bleeding.
2. Spray the nostrils with 4% lidocaine using an atomizer connected to a high-flow oxygen source while the patient inhales through the nose and exhales through the mouth.
3. Dilate the nostril selected for intubation by gently inserting soft, progressively larger nasal airways coated with 2% lidocaine gel.

Modified from Dougherty TB, Nguyen DT: Anesthetic management of the patient scheduled for head and neck cancer surgery. J Clin Anesth 6:74, 1994.

TABLE 6-5 Suggestions for a Successful Fiberoptic Intubation

Work with a well-sedated, well-oxygenated patient who remains cooperative, breathes adequately, and has a dry oral cavity.
Allow sufficient time to achieve adequate topical analgesia of the airway. If the analgesia begins to wear off, apply additional local anesthetic between intubation attempts.
Keep the operating room table at its lowest position, and work from a high position. Use a standing stool, if necessary.
Use a 7.5-mm or smaller endotracheal tube. Too much space between the fiberoptic laryngoscope and a larger tube may interfere with passage of the tube through the glottic opening.

From Dougherty TB, Nguyen DT: Anesthetic management of the patient scheduled for head and neck cancer surgery. J Clin Anesth 6:74, 1994.

cricothyroid membrane and is angled so that the sheath of the angiocatheter is advanced cephalad. After the needle is removed, the J-tipped guide wire is advanced through the angiocatheter sheath and the tip is retrieved from the patient's mouth. The angiocatheter is removed, and a hemostat is clamped on the guide wire flush with the skin of the neck. The tapered tip of the Teflon guide catheter is then passed over the guide wire into the mouth and is advanced through the vocal cords to the cricothyroid membrane. A 6.0-mm endotracheal tube is advanced over the entire structure through the vocal cords until the cricothyroid membrane is reached. The wire and the guide catheter are removed together. Use of the guide catheter reduces the discrepancy between the external diameter of the guide and the internal diameter of the endotracheal tube, thereby allowing greater success with this technique.

Combinations of conventional, fiberoptic, and retrograde techniques may be helpful in achieving successful intubation in some situations.[8] For example, a fiberoptic laryngoscope can be used as an antegrade guide when a retrograde wire is passed through the suction port. Direct laryngoscopy can occasionally facilitate placement of the tip of a fiberoptic scope near the patient's glottic opening.

Tracheotomy With Local Anesthesia. If the patient presenting for surgery is experiencing acute respiratory distress because of upper airway obstruction, a tracheotomy performed by the head and neck surgeon with local anesthesia is indicated to secure the airway before the induction of general anesthesia. Intravenous sedation should be administered with extreme caution, if it is used at all.[3] In the patient with severe airway obstruction, the tracheotomy may need to be performed with the patient in the sitting position. A tracheotomy in the awake patient is also indicated if the patient has a bulky, friable laryngeal cancer. The performance of rigid or fiberoptic laryngoscopy and the passage of an endotracheal tube in such a patient greatly increase the risk of uncontrolled hemorrhage, aspiration of tumor, and airway obstruction.[16] The airway can be secured with an endotracheal tube or a tracheotomy tube. The choice would depend on the proposed procedure. If the surgical procedure is supraglottic, a tracheotomy tube is preferable. If the proposed procedure is a tracheal/laryngeal surgery, the endotracheal tube would be appropriate. After the airway is secured with the tracheotomy, general anesthesia is carefully induced in the patient.

Unanticipated Difficult or Failed Intubation. An unexpectedly difficult airway or failed intubation following the induction of general anesthesia is not uncommon in head and neck cancer patients, and the anesthesiologist must have a clear plan of action formulated beforehand to manage this eventuality. Fortunately, as one gains experience in airway assessment and management, the likelihood of such difficulty or failure decreases. Suggestions to minimize the incidence of an unanticipated difficult or failed intubation are outlined in Table 6–6. If, after induction of anesthesia, the patient's trachea cannot be intubated with rigid laryngoscopy after a reasonable number of attempts using varying neck positions and different laryngoscope blades, the subsequent course of action depends on the ability to ventilate the patient by mask (see Fig. 6–1).[3]

Fiberoptic-Guided Intubation of the Anesthetized Patient. If mask ventilation of the patient is adequate,

TABLE 6–6 Minimizing the Frequency of Unanticipated Difficult or Failed Intubation

Always keep the patient's safety as the first priority.
Be aware that a note in the patient's chart concerning his or her airway status 2 weeks ago may not be accurate if the tumor has progressed or the patient has received radiation therapy in the interim.
If the status of the airway is in doubt, intubate the patient while he or she is awake.
Resist the temptation to rush, and maintain good communication with other members of the operating team.
Know your limits, and do not hesitate to seek help from a more experienced endoscopist.

From Dougherty TB, Nguyen DT: Anesthetic management of the patient scheduled for head and neck cancer surgery. J Clin Anesth 6:74, 1994.

anesthesia is continued with a potent inhalational agent (e.g., isoflurane, desflurane, or sevoflurane), and attempts are made to secure the patient's airway with either a nasal or oral fiberoptic-guided intubation. If the nasotracheal route is selected, a self-sealing bronchoscopy swivel adapter is connected to the end of the tracheal tube. The tube is well lubricated and is carefully passed through one of the patient's nostrils to the 15-cm mark.[8] An assistant occludes the patient's mouth and opposite nostril to allow ventilation through the bronchoscope adapter as the fiberoptic laryngoscope is advanced through the tube into the trachea (Fig. 6–2). If the oral route is chosen, an intubator biteblock[43, 44] is inserted into the midline of the mouth as before. The regular anesthesia face mask is replaced with one containing a diaphragm-covered endoscopy port (e.g., the

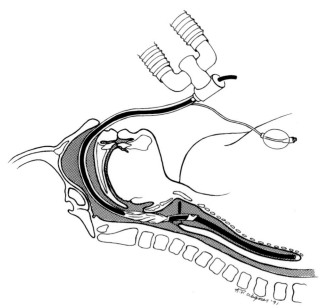

FIGURE 6–2 Nasal fiberoptic intubation in an anesthetized patient. The nasotracheal tube is passed through a nostril to the 15-cm mark. The patient can be ventilated through the swivel adapter attached to the tube. The fiberoptic laryngoscope is passed through the nasotracheal tube into the trachea, and the nasotracheal tube is advanced over the laryngoscope. (From Dougherty TB, Nguyen DT: Anesthetic management of the patient scheduled for head and neck cancer surgery. J Clin Anesth 6:74, 1994.)

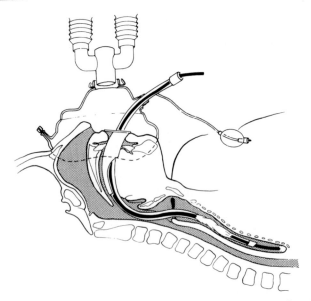

FIGURE 6–3 Use of anesthesia mask with diaphragm and oral airway intubator as aids to oral fiberoptic endotracheal intubation in the anesthetized patient. The fiberoptic laryngoscope and endotracheal tube have been introduced through the mask's diaphragm. After the endotracheal tube is in place and the laryngoscope has been withdrawn, the mask is removed over the endotracheal tube. Removal of the oral airway is optional. (From Dougherty TB, Nguyen DT: Anesthetic management of the patient scheduled for head and neck cancer surgery. J Clin Anesth 6:74, 1994.)

Patil-Syracuse endoscopy mask [Keomed Incorporated, Minnetonka, Minn]).[50, 51] This mask allows the patient to be ventilated by an assistant while the anesthesiologist accomplishes the fiberoptic intubation through the self-sealing diaphragm, as shown in Figure 6–3. If a Patil-Syracuse endoscopy mask is not available, a regular anesthesia face mask can still be used to accomplish an oral intubation. In this case, the breathing circuit is removed from the mask's connector and is reattached to a self-sealing bronchoscopy swivel adapter connected to the proximal (anesthesia machine) end of the endotracheal tube. The cuff of the tube is placed in the mask's connector and is inflated to allow ventilation of the patient through the bronchoscope adapter. The fiberoptic laryngoscope is passed through the airway intubator and into the trachea. The cuff of the endotracheal tube is deflated as the tube is advanced over the fiberoptic scope in the trachea. After the fiberoptic scope is withdrawn, the mask is cautiously removed over the endotracheal tube. This technique is useful for the nasal route as well.

Laryngeal Mask Airway. The ease and speed of its insertion without the use of rigid laryngoscopy have prompted an increasing number of anesthesiologists to use the laryngeal mask airway (LMA)[52] as an important aid for management of the difficult airway or failed intubation.[53, 54] The LMA (Fig. 6–4) was originally conceived in 1981 by Brain,[55] and in that same year, commercial production of the LMA began. The LMA was approved for use in the United States in 1991.

The LMA is a major advance in two areas. The first is as an alternative to tracheal intubation. This is especially

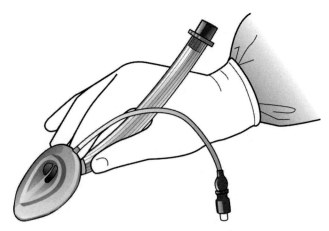

FIGURE 6–4 Classic laryngeal mask airway.

useful for ambulatory surgery cases. There are indications that patients who undergo ambulatory surgery, including that of the head and neck, recover faster and may be discharged from the hospital more quickly, resulting in lower costs.[56, 57]

The second area is in the management of the difficult airway. In 1993, the LMA was listed in the ASA Algorithm for the Difficult Airway.[11] The indications for the LMA were expanded in the second revision of the Difficult Airway Algorithm in 1996.[58]

The LMA is an effective ventilatory device in most patients,[59, 60] and it has been advocated as a conduit for intubation in the anesthetized patient.[61, 62] An endotracheal tube can be passed with or without fiberoptic guidance through the LMA.[63, 64] Because the opening of the LMA is positioned close to the glottis, tracheal intubation can be accomplished more quickly than with other airway devices. After the LMA has been inserted and adequate ventilation through it has been confirmed (Fig. 6–5), a well-lubricated 4-mm fiberoptic laryngoscope is loaded with a 6.5-mm endotracheal tube, and the scope is advanced through a size 4 or 5 LMA.[58, 63] The endotracheal tube is advanced over the

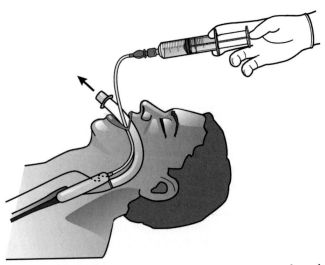

FIGURE 6–5 Correct positioning of the classic laryngeal mask airway.

fiberoptic scope into the trachea. After the cuff of the endotracheal tube has been inflated, the fiberoptic scope is removed. If a larger endotracheal tube is desired, the LMA is deflated and is carefully removed from the oral cavity over the 6.5-mm tube, which is then changed to a larger endotracheal tube with the aid of a tube exchanger.[40]

The recently introduced LMA-Fastrach (The Laryngeal Mask Company Ltd., San Diego, Calif) is specifically designed to facilitate tracheal intubation with an endotracheal tube.[64] The LMA-Fastrach differs from the regular LMA in that it has a rigid handle to facilitate oral insertion, an epiglottis-elevating bar, and a rigid, anatomically curved airway tube that can accommodate up to an 8.0-mm endotracheal tube. The LMA-Fastrach requires use of a flexible, wire-reinforced, silicone tube to accomplish tracheal intubation successfully. Although experience with the LMA and the LMA-Fastrach in patients with difficult or failed intubations is increasing, use of these devices in the surgical patient with head and neck cancer and distorted upper airway anatomy is at best controversial and may not be practical.[25]

If all attempts at intubation, including LMA and fiberoptic techniques, continue to be unsuccessful, anesthesia is discontinued and the airway is supported as the patient is allowed to awaken. The anesthesiologist then proceeds with an awake fiberoptic intubation, which generally results in a successful tracheal intubation more often than in the anesthetized patient.

Mask Ventilation Inadequate. If, during management of the unanticipated difficult airway in the anesthetized patient, mask ventilation becomes inadequate, the emergency limb of the ASA difficult airway algorithm should be followed, because securing the airway now becomes critical. Most head and neck patients who have received standard doses of opioids, benzodiazepines, intravenous induction agents, and muscle relaxants are unlikely to reestablish spontaneous respiration before they become hypoxemic, with subsequent bradycardia and cardiac arrest. Additional help should be requested to improve ventilation techniques and to aid in application of specialized airway techniques.[64] For example, two-person mask ventilation (i.e., one person managing the anesthesia mask and the other person squeezing the bag) usually improves ventilation by creating a better mask seal and jaw thrust than are associated with conventional one-person mask ventilation. Use of a large oral or nasal airway should be considered. If mask ventilation remains inadequate despite optimal technique, the anesthesiologist should insert an LMA.[58, 64] Successful ventilation is usually achieved with the LMA, and as has been described previously, it can be used as a conduit for placement of an endotracheal tube.

If placement of an LMA fails to establish adequate ventilation, initiation of transtracheal jet ventilation (TTJV) can be life saving. The assembly and use of TTJV are described in detail by Benumof and Scheller.[65] The technique includes inserting a 14-gauge intravenous catheter percutaneously through the cricothyroid membrane into the airway in a caudal direction and connecting the hub of the catheter to a jet ventilating system. Our system consists of a hand-controlled jet injector (blowgun) powered by oxygen at a pressure that can be regulated up to 50 psi.[3, 65] During TTJV, the chest is observed to rise and fall with each activation of the jet injector.

Attempts to maintain the patient's own airway must continue, to allow passive exhalation of the injected oxygen. Finally, the operator of TTJV must maintain a firm grip on the injection catheter at all times. Without such a grip, activation of the jet injector can eject the catheter out of the trachea and into the surrounding subcutaneous tissue. Subsequent jet ventilation through the displaced catheter causes massive subcutaneous emphysema, making subsequent attempts at securing the airway nearly impossible. Once the patient has been stabilized with TTJV, an assistant can accomplish endotracheal intubation in a more leisurely fashion by using conventional laryngoscopy, fiberoptic laryngoscopy, or a retrograde technique. As an alternative, the surgical team may elect to perform a tracheotomy to secure the airway.

Rigid Ventilating Bronchoscopy. In circumstances of subglottic obstructive or potentially obstructive processes, rigid ventilation bronchoscopy may be the most appropriate means of rapidly obtaining and maintaining the airway.[25] Examples include airway-compromising tracheal pathology, such as direct thyroid cancer invasion, and extraluminal compression of the trachea, usually from mediastinal or paratracheal lymph nodes.

Airway management in the situation of subglottic obstruction requires a team approach involving the surgeon, anesthesiologist, and nursing personnel.[25] Communication and preparedness are essential for successful implementation of rigid bronchoscopy. The patient is usually examined with the bronchoscope while under general anesthesia following a slow and careful inhalational induction with the patient breathing spontaneously. At other times, topical analgesia supplemented with carefully titrated sedation may be employed. In the emergent obstructive circumstance, awake, nonanesthetized passage of the rigid ventilating bronchoscope may be the only means of establishing an airway. Rapid debulking of obstructing tracheal pathology may be necessary if the bronchoscope cannot pass the intratracheal lesion. Once the bronchoscope has passed the obstruction, attachments allowing ventilation through the scope can be connected. End-tidal carbon dioxide is monitored, and general anesthesia is induced.

The rigid ventilating bronchoscope can be passed beyond most tumors, even those causing nearly total obstruction.[25] Often during placement of the bronchoscope, nearly-obstructing tumors can be "cored out" with the tip of the scope. Once the status of the distal airway has been evaluated, the tumor can be removed partially with forceps. If bleeding occurs because of the tumor's vascularity, distal placement of the bronchoscope can provide ventilation while the shaft of the bronchoscope tamponades the tumor. If indicated, a laser can be used for further tumor debulking and homeostasis.

Rigid endoscopy is a technical procedure that requires expertise for successful implementation. As flexible fiberoptic bronchoscopy has become the standard method for the intraluminal evaluation of pulmonary disease, experience with the rigid bronchoscope among head and neck surgeons has diminished. Therefore, in instances in which rigid bronchoscopy is planned, a skilled team should be present in the operating suite. In an organized, controlled, well-communicated environment, this often highly tense situation can become a safe and effective airway management process.

Maintenance of General Anesthesia

Monitors During Anesthesia. During the time the airway is secured and anesthesia is induced, the patient's cardiovascular and pulmonary status is monitored with at least an automatic noninvasive blood pressure cuff, a continuous ECG (leads II and V_5), a pulse oximeter, and an end-tidal capnograph. If the surgical procedure will be lengthy or considerable blood loss is expected, urine output should be monitored with an indwelling urinary catheter to guide intraoperative fluid management. Adequacy of fluid management is indicated by a urine output of 0.5 to 1.0 mL/kg/hour. An indwelling catheter also prevents overdistention of the bladder and its associated problems of hypertension, pain, and urinary retention.[18] Careful attention to monitoring intraoperative blood loss provides an additional guide to fluid and blood replacement. One or two large-bore peripheral intravenous lines should be established to provide a low-resistance portal for rapid infusion of fluids or blood should this become necessary.[18] A radial arterial line involves minimal risk and is convenient in patients requiring close control of blood pressure and periodic blood sampling for laboratory tests.[3] Depending on the predicted blood loss, the expected fluid requirements, and the patient's cardiac, pulmonary, or renal function, placement of a central venous or pulmonary arterial catheter may be indicated. These catheters can be placed via antecubital or femoral veins if the subclavian or neck veins cannot be used because of their involvement in the operative field.

Patient Positioning. Because the patient's head is often draped and the anesthesiologist's access to the airway is frequently restricted, the endotracheal tube and connectors must be nonkinking, of low profile, and secured to minimize pressure on the nasal ala or buccal commissure.[3] Whenever possible, the breathing circuit connected to the endotracheal tube should be secured to the patient's head to enable the surgeon to reposition the head, if necessary, without causing an accidental extubation. For certain surgical procedures, an oral tracheal tube must be secured at the buccal commissure and directed laterally away from the patient. Operative field requirements may dictate that any tape used for securing the tube cannot extend more than 1 or 2 cm toward the opposite side of the patient's face. Constant vigilance is needed to prevent the breathing circuit from pulling downward on the tube's adapter. If this occurs, the commissure can act as a fulcrum, and the distal end of the tube can work its way out of the trachea.[16] Many operations for cancer of the head and neck are of long duration, and special attention must be paid to body positioning and padding of pressure points to prevent pressure sores and nerve injury.[18] Extreme extension or lateral rotation of the head is avoided to prevent arterial or venous occlusion at the neck, leading to cerebral ischemia. It is important to protect the patient's eyes by lubrication, closure with tape, or tarsorrhaphy in certain cases, and padding.

For superficial operations involving the head or neck with the patient under monitored anesthesia care, surgical draping needs to be performed in a manner that avoids trapping any supplemental oxygen that the patient may be receiving. The drapes should be made of fire-resistant material and should be positioned well away from the surgical site to minimize any risk of ignition by electrocautery or laser. The surgeon should notify the anesthesia personnel long before electrocautery will be used so that the oxygen can be turned off. Although supplemental oxygen may be helpful in older individuals, its use in young, healthy patients is debatable.

Anesthetic Agents. Techniques using a combination of intravenous opioids and potent inhalational agents maintain general anesthesia satisfactorily in most patients undergoing head and neck cancer operations. The opioid sufentanil, administered as a constant infusion (0.1–0.5 µg/kg/hour) plus supplementation with isoflurane, sevoflurane, or desflurane (0.5–1.0 minimal alveolar concentration [MAC]) has proved particularly safe in our often debilitated patient population. A muscle relaxant such as rocuronium, also administered as a constant infusion (3–7 µg/kg/min), is relied on to provide a motionless field, especially during operations near large vascular structures (e.g., the internal jugular vein and the carotid artery). If, on the other hand, the surgical team needs to monitor motor nerve function (e.g., facial nerve function) during the procedure, a muscle relaxant is generally avoided.[3] In this situation, smaller doses of opioids are used and more reliance is placed on inhalational agents to prevent patient movement. If the patient's blood pressure cannot tolerate the concentrations of inhalational agents required to prevent movement, low doses of a muscle relaxant can be titrated to provide a motionless field without interfering with adequate motor nerve response to stimulation. This condition is usually met when the patient demonstrates a three-out-of-four twitch ratio during peripheral nerve stimulation. A vasodilating agent may be required to aid in the aggressive control of hypertension to prevent unnecessary blood loss throughout the procedure.

Tracheotomy Under General Anesthesia. Tracheotomy performed after induction of general anesthesia and endotracheal intubation is a common procedure and approach for many major head and neck surgeons. Often 100% oxygen is administered before the actual tracheotomy is performed, to provide the patient with some oxygen reserve and prevent hypoxemia should loss of control of the airway occur.[66] However, a word of caution is important here. Electrocautery is commonly used around the tracheotomy to control bleeding after the trachea has been opened. The combination of electrocautery, oxygen escaping around the endotracheal tube cuff, and a flammable tube can be a major fire hazard. In this situation, the tube can ignite and produce a blowtorch effect, resulting in third-degree burns to the trachea and bronchi. The surgeon and anesthesiologist should always be aware of this potential complication. When the surgeon reaches the anterior tracheal wall, the anesthesiologist and surgeon should communicate the anticipated entry into the trachea itself. If electrocautery is being used to control bleeding, reduction in the oxygen concentration is mandatory to avoid an airway fire. Because nitrous oxide supports combustion, it should not be used to lower the oxygen concentration. As the trachea is transected, the nasal or oral endotracheal tube should be carefully pulled from the surgeon's field so that the tip of the endotracheal tube is at the cephalic margin of the tracheal incision (which allows rapid reinsertion should there be a false passage of the tracheotomy tube).[16]

Following creation of the tracheotomy, the surgeon usually places a sterile, flexible, reinforced, cuffed tracheal tube through the stoma into the trachea. A short length of flexible tubing and an adapter are attached to this tube and passed under the surgical drapes for connection to the awaiting breathing circuit. The anesthesiologist must be thoroughly familiar with this maneuver before transection of the patient's trachea is performed, to avoid unnecessary delay in providing ventilation to the patient. Correct placement of the tracheal tube must be verified by the presence of breath sounds on auscultation and by the appearance of an end-tidal carbon dioxide waveform. The endotracheal tube should be secured by suturing it to the skin of the neck or chest.

Special Intraoperative Concerns. Two important aspects of neck dissection are of concern to the anesthesiologist. First, venous air embolism can occur during the procedure from entrainment of air by open neck veins. Diagnosis is suggested by an acute decrease in end-tidal carbon dioxide, followed by a decrease in blood pressure.[4] Treatment consists of placing the head down, giving the patient 100% oxygen, and covering the wound with fluid.[4] Using positive pressure ventilation and minimally elevating the patient's head during the operation greatly reduces the likelihood of air embolism. Second, bradycardia, which can be profound or can even result in asystole, is sometimes seen during neck dissection when pressure is inadvertently placed on the carotid sinus.[18] Effective treatment includes elimination of the inciting stimulus, which is usually pressure applied to the carotid sinus, and administration of intravenous atropine for persistent bradycardia. If the bradycardia is recurrent during the dissection, the surgeon should infiltrate the area around the carotid sinus with lidocaine to block the reflex.[18]

Any procedure involving free-flap reconstruction with microsurgical techniques for vascular anastomoses is usually lengthy. Every effort must be made to maintain adequate blood flow to the flap at all times.[3] In general, we administer fluids or blood to ensure an adequate blood volume, blood pressure, and flap perfusion pressure and avoid, if possible, the use of vasoconstrictors. Elevation of the operating room temperature plus a warming blanket, breathing circuit humidifier, and fluid warmer are used to prevent hypothermia and accompanying vasoconstriction in the patient.

Laser Surgery of the Upper Airway

The carbon dioxide (CO_2) and neodymium:yttrium-aluminum-garnet (Nd:YAG) lasers are most commonly used for microsurgery of the upper airway and trachea.[17] Important advantages of laser surgery include increased precision of dissection, preservation of normal tissues, ability to coagulate small vessels, less tissue edema and bleeding, and maintenance of sterile conditions. The CO_2 laser emits light in the far-infrared range, and the beam is almost entirely absorbed by the surface of the target tissue, which is destroyed by vaporization of cellular water.[4] The CO_2 laser beam must be aimed directly at the target and is more useful for lesions of the upper airway. The Nd:YAG laser beam can be transmitted by fiberoptics and is therefore well suited to tumor debulking in the lower airway. The physics and medical uses of lasers, including safety and implications for anesthetic management, have been reviewed in depth by Sosis,[67] Van Der Spek and coworkers,[68] and Hermens and associates.[69] Only major considerations of laser airway surgery are presented here.

TABLE 6–7 Precautions Taken to Prevent Eye Damage From Laser Surgery

The operating room should have a warning sign posted outside indicating that a laser is in use.
All operating room personnel must wear goggles specific for absorbing the wavelength of light produced by the laser.
The patient's eyes should be protected with opaque, moistened gauze.
Instruments with a nonreflective (matte) finish should be used to help disperse the beam.
The laser should be in standby mode when not in use.

From Joseph MM: Anesthesia for ear, nose, and throat surgery. In Longnecker DE, Tinker JH, Morgan GE, Jr (eds): Principles and Practice of Anesthesiology, 2nd ed, vol 2. St Louis, Mosby–Year Book, 1998, p 2200.

Reflected or misdirected laser beams can harm other tissues, especially the eyes of the patient and other operating room personnel. Precautions taken to prevent damage to the eye are listed in Table 6–7. In addition, the patient's skin and tissues adjacent to the field should be protected with moistened sponges or towels to dissipate heat.[69, 70] A major anesthetic consideration for laser surgery is maintaining complete immobility of the patient to prevent laser damage to adjacent healthy tissue. This is accomplished by the use of an adequate depth of anesthesia and a muscle relaxant.

The most ominous hazard of laser surgery is creation of a fire in the upper airway itself, with the greatest risk being ignition of the endotracheal tube.[71–73] Once the endotracheal tube becomes ignited, a "blowtorch" flame can be produced within the tube because everything needed for a fire is present—a combustible material, heat, and oxygen to support combustion.[4] General precautions to reduce the risk of fire are outlined in Table 6–8. Although an endotracheal tube fire can be avoided altogether by ventilating the patient's lungs with jet or Venturi ventilation,[75, 76] these techniques can result in smoke inhalation and instillation of debris or tumor into the patient's trachea.

When choosing an endotracheal tube to manage ventilation during laser surgery, it is important to remember that all endotracheal tubes not made of metal are capable of eventual combustion if exposed to a laser beam for a sufficient time. Methods of trying to protect polyvinylchloride or red rubber tubes with metallic tape are not entirely satisfactory either. Some types of tape are penetrated by the laser beam or have a flammable backing.[77] Also, gaps between tape wraps leave portions of the tube unprotected, rough tape edges can

TABLE 6–8 General Precautions to Reduce the Risk of Fire in Laser Airway Surgery

Use the lowest possible F_{IO_2} because oxygen supports combustion.
Note that N_2O also supports combustion.
Keep paper drapes away from the operative field.
Use laser on lowest effective power setting. Use intermittent mode to avoid heat buildup.[74]
Use water-soluble ointments because oil-based ointments are flammable.[68]

From Joseph MM: Anesthesia of ear, nose, and throat surgery. In Longnecker DE, Tinker JH, Morgan GE, Jr (eds): Principles and Practice of Anesthesiology, 2nd ed, vol 2. St Louis, Mosby–Year Book, 1998, p 2200.

damage mucosal surfaces, and pieces of tape broken off can be aspirated.[69]

In an effort to overcome the drawbacks of taping tubes, various special purpose endotracheal tubes have been developed specifically for CO_2 laser surgery of the airway. Laser-resistant tubes should be manufactured and labeled according to specifications of the American Society for Testing and Materials (ASTM). The ASTM uses a standard method of determining laser resistance, thereby allowing the practitioner to judge which laser-resistant tube is appropriate for the type of laser used during surgery. Of these tubes, the authors have found the Laser-Flex (Mallinckrodt, Inc., St. Louis) to be the most satisfactory. The shaft of this tube is constructed entirely of flexible stainless steel. The two cuffs, although made of polyvinylchloride, still maintain a seal even if one cuff becomes deflated after being struck by a laser beam. The cuffs of the endotracheal tube should be filled with saline. This fluid will act as a heat sink should either cuff be struck by a laser.[78] If the cuff is penetrated, the leaking fluid may help extinguish any resulting fire. A solution of dilute methylene blue is often added to the proximal cuff so that the appearance of any dye in the airway will warn the surgeon of penetration of the cuff by the laser beam.[66] Further protection is provided by packing the cuff area with wet gauze or pledgets. Frequent irrigation of any packing is mandatory because adsorption by the CO_2 laser can quickly dry it out, causing a fire.

Unfortunately, at the time of publication, no endotracheal tube, not even the various specialized laser tubes, can be used safely with the Nd:YAG laser. The laser is most often delivered to the surgical site via a fiberoptic guide inserted through either a rigid or a flexible bronchoscope. If a flexible bronchoscope is employed, a polyvinylchloride tube is usually used for ventilation because the laser fiber will be at a point below the end of the endotracheal tube.[66] No part of the endotracheal tube should be below the tip of the laser fiber, and the lowest possible fractional inspired oxygen concentration should be used. Nitrous oxide should be avoided during laser surgery because it supports combustion. High fresh gas flow rates from the anesthesia machine will facilitate removal of smoke and improve the surgical field.

All anesthetic techniques for laser airway surgery are associated with some risk of fire; therefore, knowledge of how to manage an airway fire is critical.[4] It is particularly important to remember that these fires can occur suddenly and without warning. Table 6–9 describes the appropriate steps to take in the event of an airway fire. Management of an airway fire is the sole responsibility of the surgeon and the anesthesiologist. Because these fires are devastating to the patient's airway, the surgeon should first disconnect oxygen flow through the endotracheal tube, then extubate the trachea immediately at the first indication of a fire.

Extubation of the Trachea

The patient should remain anesthetized until the operation is completed. Premature emergence from anesthesia before all dressings are applied should be avoided to prevent the patient from straining and coughing on the endotracheal tube, which elevates the patient's blood pressure and may increase the risk of postoperative bleeding.[3] The patient should not be stimulated vigorously at the end of the procedure to hasten awakening, particularly if the patient's muscle paralysis is not yet fully reversed. Enough time should be allowed for the patient's smooth emergence. All patients receive supplemental oxygen therapy following emergence from general anesthesia because transient hypoxemia immediately postoperatively is a common problem.[18, 79, 80]

Following those procedures in which no tracheotomy is established, eventual extubation of the patient's trachea is desirable. The timing depends both on the length of the procedure and on the degree of edema or distortion of the upper airway produced by the operation. Often, the anesthesia and surgical teams need to be involved jointly in the decision to extubate. Some patients (e.g., those after superficial procedures) can usually be extubated in the operating room or in the postanesthesia care unit when fully awake. Based on the severity of their medical problems or the level of observation required to prevent postoperative complications (e.g., hematoma, airway compromise), these patients are either sent to a dedicated head and neck nursing floor or kept overnight in the postanesthesia care unit.[3] Patients undergoing lengthy procedures, including free-flap reconstruction, usually remain intubated overnight in the surgical intensive care unit. Sedation and, if necessary, muscle paralysis are continued to enhance flap survival by preventing the patient from moving and coughing during this period. These patients are maintained in a 30-degree head-up position to minimize edema.

If extubation of the patient is contemplated, the following conditions must be met to accomplish this safely.[3] The

TABLE 6–9 Response Algorithm for Management of an Airway Fire

	Steps	Measures
Immediate	First	Immediately disconnect oxygen source from the endotracheal tube, and remove burning objects from the patient's airway.
	Second	Irrigate the site with saline if the fire is still smoldering.
	Third	Ventilate the patient by mask, reintubate with an endotracheal or rigid bronchoscope, and ventilate with as low an FIO_2 as possible.
Secondary	Fourth	Evaluate the extent of injury by bronchoscopy and laryngoscopy, and remove debris.
	Fifth	The surgeon should perform a tracheotomy if indicated.
	Sixth	Monitor the patient with oximetry, arterial blood gas analysis, and serial chest radiographs.
	Seventh	Use ventilatory support, steroids, and antibiotics as needed.

From Joseph MM: Anesthesia for ear, nose and throat surgery. In Longnecker DE, Tinker JH, Morgan GE, Jr (eds): Principles and Practice of Anesthesiology, 2nd ed, vol 2. St. Louis, Mosby–Year Book, 1998, p 2200.

patient has to be easily arousable and able to follow simple commands such as squeezing the anesthesiologist's hand. The patient should have no residual muscle paralysis following administration of an appropriate dose of a reversal agent. Adequate recovery from muscle paralysis is indicated by a train-of-four response to neuromuscular stimulation in which the fourth twitch height is at least 70% of the first twitch height. The patient's pulmonary mechanics must be suitable for extubation. Commonly used criteria include, for example, a vital capacity of 10 mL/kg or greater and a negative inspiratory force of at least –20 cm H_2O.[81] Finally, the equipment used for securing the airway at the induction of anesthesia must be immediately available at extubation.

In most patients, particularly in those whose airway was easily managed during induction or without airway edema postoperatively, extubation will be simple and straightforward. In others, however, it may be even more of a challenge than the original intubation.[3] Airway edema, nasal packing, and surgical changes in the patient's anatomy may prevent adequate mask ventilation, should the patient develop acute airway obstruction following extubation. The use of nasal or oral airways may be contraindicated by the risk of disrupting surgical repair or reconstruction in the nasopharynx or oropharynx. If some doubt exists as to whether the patient can maintain an adequate airway following extubation, even after surgically caused upper airway edema is allowed to subside, the trachea should be extubated over a fiberoptic laryngoscope using the following suggested technique.[3] The patient is given supplemental oxygen and placed in a semisitting position. Lidocaine (4%) is sprayed topically in the oropharynx, around the glottic area, and through the endotracheal tube. If necessary, the patient may be carefully and lightly sedated. Then the fiberoptic laryngoscope is inserted through the endotracheal tube, and the tip is positioned near the carina. After the cuff of the endotracheal tube is deflated, the tube is slowly backed out of the trachea and larynx while the fiberoptic scope is maintained in the trachea. If the patient can breathe adequately for 15 to 30 minutes, the laryngoscope and endotracheal tube are removed from the airway. If, however, the patient cannot maintain an adequate airway during this time, the endotracheal tube can be advanced back into the trachea over the fiberoptic scope, and extubation can be attempted later.

Alternatively, the patient can be extubated over a jet stylet.[8, 82] A jet stylet is a hollow tube exchanger with a small external diameter that is passed through the endotracheal tube into the trachea. The tracheal tube is withdrawn over the stylet following the same approach as that described for the fiberoptic laryngoscope. The stylet affords the added advantage, though, of allowing immediate jet ventilation of the patient should hypoxemia develop before replacement of the endotracheal tube has been completed.

◖ SUMMARY

A critical phase in the surgical treatment of the head and neck oncologic patient is the anesthesiologist's preoperative clinical evaluation of the patient. This involves obtaining pertinent information from the patient's medical history, physical examination, previous medical records, laboratory studies, and special tests. In particular, emphasis is placed on the patient's upper airway and cardiovascular, pulmonary, and renal systems. Before the patient is brought to the operating room, any serious medical problems should be identified and treated as much as possible, keeping in mind the status of the tumor and the urgency of the surgery.

Communication and cooperation between the anesthesiologist and head and neck surgeon are essential, not only to determine the specific surgical requirements and unique consequences of the proposed operation but also to select the best approach for managing the patient's airway. If the patient has no evidence of a difficult airway, general anesthesia is usually safely induced before the airway is secured with tracheal intubation. If the airway or intubation is potentially difficult, the patient may require an awake, direct examination of the airway with sedation and topical analgesia to determine the best intubation technique before induction of general anesthesia. If a difficult airway or intubation is certain, our preference is to secure the patient's airway with an awake fiberoptic-guided intubation. An initial tracheotomy performed by the surgeon under local anesthesia is generally indicated before anesthesia is induced in the patient who is experiencing acute upper airway obstruction or who has a bulky, friable tumor of the larynx or base of the tongue.

The anesthesiologist must always have a clear plan of action formulated beforehand in the event an unexpectedly difficult airway is encountered and the patient cannot be intubated with rigid laryngoscopy after general anesthesia has been induced.[3] Should mask ventilation become inadequate during intubation attempts, use of the LMA or, if necessary, initiation of TTJV can be life saving until an airway can be established by other means.

Techniques that employ a combination of intravenous opioids and potent inhalational agents maintain general anesthesia satisfactorily in most patients undergoing head and neck operations. Because many of these procedures are lengthy, careful attention must be paid to correct positioning of the patient, sufficient cardiopulmonary monitoring, and adequate intraoperative fluid management. During laser surgery on the airway, efforts are made to prevent accidental laser beam injury to the patient and other operating room personnel and to minimize the risk of airway fire. The timing of extubation of the patient's trachea after surgery depends both on the length of the procedure and on the degree of edema or distortion of the upper airway produced by the operation. Frequently, extubation can be more of a challenge than the original intubation and requires a joint decision by the anesthesia and surgical teams.

REFERENCES

1. Merletti F, Boffetta P, Ciccone G, et al: Role of tobacco and alcohol beverages in the etiology of cancer of the oral cavity/oropharynx in Torino, Italy. Cancer Res 49:4919, 1989.
2. Binnie WH: Etiology. In Smith C, Pindborg JJ, Binnie WH (eds): Oral Cancer, Epidemiology, Etiology, and Pathology. New York, Hemisphere, 1990, p 17.
3. Dougherty TB, Nguyen DT: Anesthetic management of the patient scheduled for head and neck cancer surgery. J Clin Anesth 6:74, 1994.
4. Joseph MM: Anesthesia for ear, nose, and throat surgery. In Longnecker DE, Tinker JH, Morgan GE Jr (eds): Principles and Practice of Anesthesiology, 2nd ed, vol 2. St Louis, Mosby–Year Book, 1998, p 2200.

5. Supkis DE Jr, Dougherty TB, Nguyen DT, et al: Anesthetic management of the patient undergoing head and neck cancer surgery. Cancer Bull 47:19, 1995.
6. Scamman FL: Anesthesia for surgery of head and neck tumors. In Thawley SE, Panje WR (eds): Comprehensive Management of Head and Neck Tumors. Philadelphia, WB Saunders, 1987, p 25.
7. Donlon JV Jr: Anesthesia for eye, ear, nose, and throat surgery. In Miller RD (ed): Anesthesia, 2nd ed, vol 3. New York, Churchill Livingstone, 1986, p 1837.
8. Benumof JL: Management of the difficult adult airway with special emphasis on awake tracheal intubation. Anesthesiology 75:1087, 1991.
9. Coriat P, Richer C, Douraki T, et al: Influence of chronic angiotensin-converting enzyme inhibition on anesthetic induction. Anesthesiology 81:299, 1994.
10. Roizen MF: Anesthetic implications of concurrent diseases. In Miller RD (ed): Anesthesia, 5th ed, vol 1. Philadelphia, Churchill Livingstone, 2000, p 903.
11. American Society of Anesthesiologists: Practice guidelines for management of the difficult airway. A report by the American Society of Anesthesiologists' task force on management of the difficult airway. Anesthesiology 78:597, 1993.
12. Benumof JL: Definition and incidence of the difficult airway. In Benumof JL (ed): Airway Management Principles and Practice. St Louis, Mosby, 1996, p 121.
13. Cormack RS, Lehane J: Difficult tracheal intubation in obstetrics. Anaesthesia 39:1105, 1984.
14. Ovassapian A: Management of the difficult airway. In Ovassapian A (ed): Fiberoptic Endoscopy and the Difficult Airway, 2nd ed. Philadelphia, Lippincott-Raven, 1996, p 201.
15. Barratt GE, Coulthard SW: Upper airway obstruction: Diagnosis and management options. In Brown BR (ed): Contemporary Anesthesia Practice. Philadelphia, FA Davis, 1987, p 73.
16. Dougherty TB: The difficult airway in conventional head and neck surgery. In Benumof JL (ed): Airway Management Principles and Practice. St Louis, Mosby, 1996, p 686.
17. Donlon JV Jr: Anesthesia for eye, ear, nose, and throat surgery. In Miller RD (ed): Anesthesia, 5th ed, vol 2. Philadelphia, Churchill Livingstone, 2000, p 2173.
18. Golden KJ: Anesthetic considerations. In Myers EN, Suen JY (eds): Cancer of the Head and Neck, 2nd ed. New York, Churchill Livingstone, 1989, p 145.
19. Mallampati SR: Recognition of the difficult airway. In Benumof JL (ed): Airway Management Principles and Practice. St Louis, Mosby, 1996, p 126.
20. Mallampati SR, Gatt SP, Gugino LD, et al: A clinical sign to predict difficult tracheal intubation: A prospective study. Can Anaesth Soc J 32:429, 1985.
21. Wilson ME, John R: Problems with the Mallampati sign. Anaesthesia 45:486, 1990.
22. Charters P, Perera S, Horton WA: Visibility of pharyngeal structures as a predictor of difficult intubation. Anaesthesia 42:1115, 1987.
23. Patil VU, Stehling LC, Zauder HL: Predicting the difficulty of intubation utilizing an intubation guide. Anesthesiol Rev 10:32, 1983.
24. Prust RS, Calkins JM: Considerations for managing the airway in the ENT patient. In Brown BR (ed): Contemporary Anesthesia Practice. Philadelphia, FA Davis, 1987, p 49.
25. Dougherty TB, Clayman GL: Airway management of surgical patients with head and neck malignancies. Anesth Clin North Am 16:547, 1998.
26. Jensen NF: Glomus tumors of the head and neck: Anesthetic considerations. Anesth Analg 78:112, 1994.
27. Londy F, Norton ML: Radiologic techniques for evaluation and management of the difficult airway. In Norton ML, Brown ACD (eds): Atlas of the Difficult Airway. St Louis, Mosby–Year Book, 1991, p 62.
28. Jensen NF, Benumof J: The difficult airway in head and neck tumor surgery. Anesth Clin North Am 11:475, 1993.
29. Yamamoto K, Tsubokawa T, Shibata K, et al: Predicting difficult intubation with indirect laryngoscopy. Anesthesiology 86:316, 1997.
30. Bull BS, Bull MH: The salvaged blood syndrome: A sequel to mechanochemical activation of platelets and leukocytes? Blood Cells 16(1):5–20, 1990; discussion 20–3.
31. Tawes RL Jr, Duvall TB: Is the "salvaged-cell syndrome" myth or reality? Am J Surg 172(2):172–174, 1996.
32. Egbert LD, Battit GE, Turndorf H, et al: The value of the preoperative visit by an anesthetist. JAMA 185:553, 1963.
33. Leigh JM, Walker J, Janaganathan P: Effect of preoperative anaesthetic visit on anxiety. BMJ 2:987, 1977.
34. Caplan RA, Posner KL, Ward RJ, et al: Adverse respiratory events in anesthesia: A closed claims analysis. Anesthesiology 72:828, 1990.
35. Keenan RL, Boyan CP: Cardiac arrest due to anesthesia. A study of incidence and causes. JAMA 253:2373, 1985.
36. Ovassapian A: Topical anesthesia of the airway. In Ovassapian A (ed): Fiberoptic Endoscopy and the Difficult Airway, 2nd ed. Philadelphia, Lippincott-Raven Publishers, 1996, p 47.
37. Sitzman BT, Rich GF, Rockwell JJ, et al: Local anesthetic administration for awake direct laryngoscopy. Anesthesiology 86:34, 1997.
38. Sivarajan M, Fink BR: The position and the state of the larynx during general anesthesia and muscle paralysis. Anesthesiology 72:439, 1990.
39. Sivarajan M, Joy JV: Effects of general anesthesia and paralysis on upper airway changes due to head position in humans. Anesthesiology 85:787, 1996.
40. Ovassapian A: Fiberoptic-assisted management of the airway. In 1990 Annual Refresher Course Lectures, No. 254. Park Ridge, Ill, American Society of Anesthesiologists, 1990.
41. Ovassapian A, Wheeler M: Fiberoptic endoscopy-aided techniques. In Benumof JL (ed): Airway Management Principles and Practice. St Louis, Mosby, 1996, p 282.
42. Benumof JL: Management of the difficult or impossible airway. In 1990 Annual Refresher Course Lectures, No. 163. Park Ridge, Ill, American Society of Anesthesiologists, 1990.
43. Ovassapian A, Dykes MHM: The role of fiberoptic endoscopy in airway management. Semin Anesth 6:93, 1987.
44. Williams RT, Harrison RE: Prone tracheal intubation simplified using an airway intubator. Can Anaesth Soc J 28:288, 1981.
45. Waters DJ: Guided blind endotracheal intubation for patients with deformities of the upper airway. Anaesthesia 18:158, 1963.
46. Butler FS, Cirillo AA: Retrograde tracheal intubation. Anesth Analg 39:333, 1960.
47. Barriot P, Riou B: Retrograde technique for tracheal intubation in trauma patients. Crit Care Med 16:712, 1988.
48. Purcell T: Retrograde tracheal intubation. In Dailey RH, Simon B, Young GP, et al (eds): The Airway: Emergency Management. St Louis, Mosby–Year Book, 1992, p 135.
49. Sanchez A, Pallares V: Retrograde intubation technique. In Benumof JL (ed): Airway Management Principles and Practice. St Louis, Mosby, 1996, p 320.
50. Rogers SN, Benumof JL: New and easy techniques for fiberoptic endoscopy-aided tracheal intubation. Anesthesiology 59:569, 1983.
51. Patil V, Stehling LC, Zauder HL, et al: Mechanical aids for fiberoptic endoscopy. Anesthesiology 57:69, 1982.
52. Brain AIJ: The laryngeal mask—a new concept in airway management. Br J Anaesth 55:801, 1983.
53. Calder I, Ordman AJ, Jackowski A, et al: The brain laryngeal mask airway: An alternative to emergency tracheal intubation. Anaesthesia 45:137, 1990.
54. Pennant JH, White PF: The laryngeal mask airway: Its uses in anesthesiology. Anesthesiology 79:144, 1993.
55. Brain AIJ. The development of the laryngeal mask—a brief history of the invention, early clinical studies and experimental work from which the laryngeal mask evolved. Eur J Anaesthesiol 4:5, 1991.
56. Todd DW: A comparison of endotracheal intubation and use of the laryngeal mask airway for ambulatory oral surgery patients [Journal Article]. J Oral Maxillofac Surg 60:2, 2002; discussion 4–5.
57. Joshi GP, Inagaki Y, White PF, et al: Use of the laryngeal mask airway as an alternative to the tracheal tube during ambulatory anesthesia [see comments]. Anesth Analg 85:573, 1997.
58. Benumof J: The laryngeal mask airway and the ASA difficult airway algorithm. Anesthesiology 84:686, 1996.
59. Smith I, White PF: Use of the laryngeal mask airway as an alternative to a face mask during outpatient arthroscopy. Anesthesiology 77:850, 1992.
60. Verghese C, Brimacombe JR: Survey of laryngeal mask airway usage in 11,910 patients: Safety and efficacy for conventional and non-conventional usage. Anesth Analg 82:129, 1996.
61. Heath ML, Allagain J: Intubation through the laryngeal mask: A technique for unexpected difficult intubation. Anaesthesia 46:545, 1991.
62. Crosby ET, Cooper RM, Douglas JM, et al: The unanticipated difficult airway with recommendations for management. Can J Anaesth 45:757, 1998.
63. Benumof JL: Use of the laryngeal mask airway to facilitate fiberscope-aided tracheal intubation. Anesth Analg 74:313, 1992.

64. Domino KB: Management of the patient with a difficult airway: An update. Clin Anesth Updates 8:2, 1999.

65. Benumof JL, Scheller MS: The importance of transtracheal jet ventilation in the management of the difficult airway. Anesthesiology 71:769, 1989.

66. Feinstein R, Owens WD: Anesthesia for ear, nose, and throat surgery. In Barash PG, Cullen BF, Stoelting RK (eds): Clinical Anesthesia, 2nd ed. Philadelphia, JB Lippincott, 1992, p 1113.

67. Sosis MB: Anesthesia for laser airway surgery. In Benumof JL (ed): Airway Management Principles and Practice. St Louis, Mosby, 1996, p 698.

68. Van Der Spek AFL, Spargo PM, Norton ML: The physics of lasers and implication for their use during airway surgery. Br J Anaesth 60:709, 1988.

69. Hermens JM, Bennett MJ, Hirshman CA: Anesthesia for laser surgery. Anesth Analg 62:218, 1983.

70. Pashayan AG: Anesthesia for laser surgery. In ASA Refresher Courses in Anesthesiology. Philadelphia, JB Lippincott, 1995, p 276.

71. Snow JC, Norton ML, Saluja TS, et al: Fire hazard during CO_2 laser microsurgery on the larynx and trachea. Anesth Analg 55:146, 1976.

72. Burgess GE, LeJeune FE: Endotracheal tube ignition during laser surgery of the larynx. Arch Otolaryngol 105:561, 1979.

73. Cozine K, Rosenbaum LM, Askanazi J, et al: Laser-induced endotracheal tube fire. Anesthesiology 55:583, 1981.

74. Patel KF, Hicks JN: Prevention of fire hazards associated with the use of carbon dioxide lasers. Anesth Analg 60:885, 1981.

75. Ruder CB, Rapheal NL, Abramson AL: Anesthesia for carbon dioxide laser microsurgery of the larynx. Otolaryngol Head Neck Surg 89:732, 1981.

76. Gussack GS, Evans RF, Tacchi EJ: Intravenous anesthesia and jet ventilation for laser microlaryngeal surgery. Ann Otol Rhinol Laryngol 96:29, 1987.

77. Sosis MB: Evaluation of five metallic tapes for protection of endotracheal tubes during CO_2 laser surgery. Anesth Analg 68:392, 1989.

78. LeJeune FE, Guice C, Letard F, et al: Heat sink protection against lasering endotracheal cuffs. Ann Otol Rhinol Laryngol 91:606, 1982.

79. Bay J, Nunn JF, Prys-Roberts C: Factors influencing arterial PO_2 during recovery from anesthesia. Br J Anaesth 40:398, 1968.

80. Marshall BE, Wyche MQ: Hypoxemia during and after anesthesia. Anesthesiology 37:178, 1972.

81. Moon RE, Camporesi EM: Respiratory monitoring. In Miller RD (ed): Anesthesia, 3rd ed, vol 1. New York, Churchill Livingstone, 1990, p 1129.

82. Bedger RC, Chang JL: A jet stylet catheter for difficult airway management. Anesthesiology 66:221, 1987.

CHAPTER 7

Nonmelanoma Skin Cancer of the Head and Neck

Duane A. Sewell

Stephen Y. Lai

Randal S. Weber

INTRODUCTION

Skin cancer is the most common malignancy in the United States, with an estimated one million new cases diagnosed annually.[1-3] In fact, it is estimated that one in six Americans will develop a skin cancer at some time in their life.[1] Among these malignancies, squamous cell carcinoma (SCC) and basal cell carcinoma (BCC) are by far the most frequent pathologic types, and the incidence of these cancers continues to rise.[4] Because of the effects of direct ultraviolet radiation, these cancers disproportionately affect the sun-exposed areas of the skin of the head and neck. In this chapter, we review the causes, clinical assessment, histopathology, and treatment modalities of nonmelanoma skin cancer (NMSC).

ETIOLOGY AND RISK FACTORS

Studies have shown that the most important causative factor for the development of skin cancer is the cumulative amount of ultraviolet radiation (UVR) exposure.[5, 6] UVR occupies the portion of the light spectrum from 200 to 400 nm (Fig. 7–1). This portion is divided into three segments—UV A, UV B, and UV C. UV B (290 to 320 nm) is the most harmful of these wavelengths. Light within the UV B spectrum can cause genetic mutations by promoting the formation of pyrimidine dimers at the DNA level. This leads to the inactivation of tumor suppressor genes such as $p53$, which are seen to be altered in almost 60% of NMSC cases.[7, 8] In addition, it has been shown that UVR alters the detection and elimination of malignant cells by inducing suppressor T-cell activity and by decreasing the number of epidermal Langerhans antigen-presenting cells.[9]

The incidence of NMSC can be directly correlated with cumulative amount of UVR exposure. For instance, it has been demonstrated that the incidence of NMSC increases in the United States as latitude decreases.[10] In addition, UVR exposure and NMSC incidence increase with the ongoing depletion of the ozone layer.[11-13] Studies have shown that for each 1% decrease in ozone, there is a corresponding 2%

increase in the incidence of NMSC,[14] and the ozone layer has been depleted by 10% to 40% over recent decades because of industrial by-products.[10, 12, 15, 16] Other environmental factors that may lead to NMSC include exposure to ionizing radiation, coal tar, and asphalt and the oral consumption of arsenic. Also, there are rare genetic syndromes that carry a high risk of development of skin cancer, such as xeroderma pigmentosum and nevoid basal cell syndrome. The former syndrome is an autosomal recessive disorder that causes defects in DNA excision-repair and synthesis; the latter is an autosomal dominant disorder associated with mandibular cysts and multiple BCCs.[17]

The risk of developing NMSC varies greatly with ethnicity. This is most likely due to differences in melanin content in the skin; melanin has been shown to protect the cutaneous cells from the harmful effects of UV B radiation. It is estimated that five times the amount of UV B radiation reaches the dermis in those with lighter skin than in those with dark skin.[18] Thus, populations with lighter skin pigmentation, such as those from northern Europe, have a far greater risk of NMSC.[19, 20] Another confounding variable in the assessment of the risk of developing skin cancer is the individual's ability to tan. When skin reaction to UVR has been calculated in terms of the tendency to freckle or sunburn, it was shown that people who tan rather than freckle or burn with UVR exposure have a lower incidence of NMSC despite a fair complexion. Thus, Irish, Scottish, and Welsh populations have a higher propensity toward development of NMSC than do southern Europeans, who tan more readily.[21]

PREMALIGNANT LESIONS

Many skin cancers arise from known precancerous lesions. Common precursor lesions for both SCC and BCC include actinic, or solar, keratoses (AK). Controversy exists regarding these lesions. Some clinicians believe that they represent an intraepidermal form of SCC instead of a precursor.[22, 23] This is based on the similar histologic characteristics of the two lesions. Nonetheless, there is consensus that once these lesions invade the dermis, there is potential for local spread and distant metastasis. Upon review of several studies, it was estimated that the approximate risk of development of invasive SCC from AK is 8% to 10%. The prevalence of this disease process in populations with lighter complexions is very high, ranging from 11% to 26%.[24]

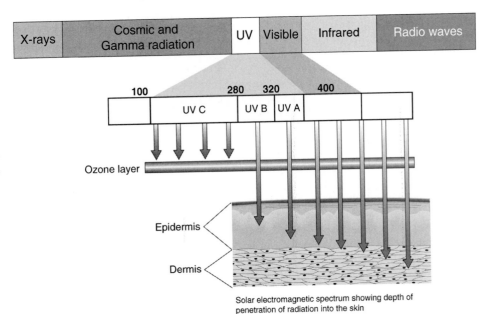

FIGURE 7–1 Penetration of ultraviolet and visible-spectrum radiation into the skin.

These lesions are usually erythematous and scaly, appearing on sun-exposed areas of the head and neck. Sometimes, the lesion is palpable as a rough scale before it is visible. Clinical variants exist, including a cutaneous horn in which a hyperkeratotic lesion protrudes from the skin, and actinic cheilitis wherein the lesion forms on the vermilion of the lips. The diagnosis can be made only by biopsy, and treatment should include excision of the lesion, given the previously mentioned possibility of invasion.

Bowen's disease is another pathologic entity that is thought to represent in situ SCC of the skin (Fig. 7–2). Clinically, it presents as a red, scaling plaque or nodule that is commonly misdiagnosed as eczema or psoriasis. On mucous membranes of the mouth and genital areas, the lesions are known as erythoplasia of Queyrat.[25] Bowen's disease is estimated to become invasive in 3% to 5% of patients, and approximately 13% of those patients will develop metastases.[26] Therefore, it should be treated aggressively with excision, cryotherapy, or radiation.[27]

Unlike AK and Bowen's disease, keratoacanthoma (KA) is a cutaneous lesion that is histologically similar to SCC and is considered by many experts to have malignant potential. This common tumor presents most often on sun-exposed skin as a rapidly enlarging nodule with central ulceration and is thought to arise from the hair follicle. Within a few weeks, it can grow to 2 cm or larger. Although these lesions usually regress spontaneously, biopsy and treatment should be undertaken to definitively rule out SCC and to prevent impingement on surrounding structures.[28] The treatment of choice is surgical excision.

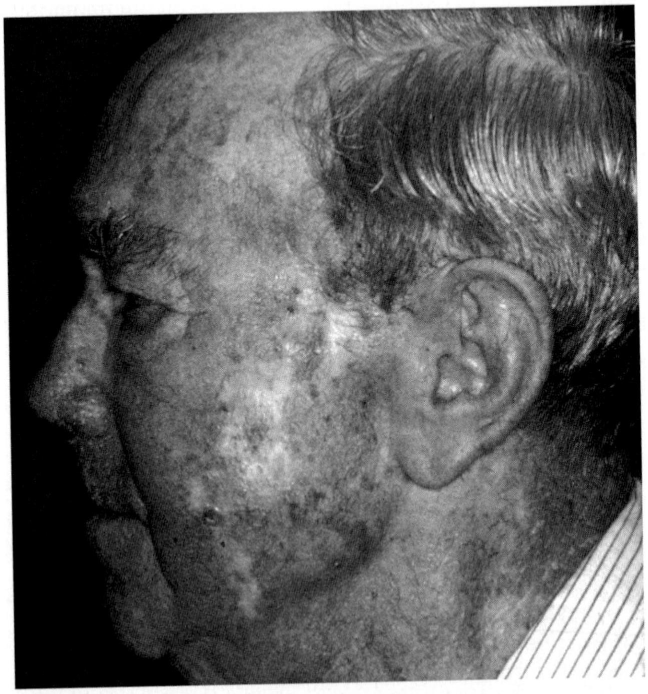

EPITHELIAL SKIN CANCERS

Basal Cell Carcinoma

It is well documented that BCC is the most common skin cancer, but this presupposes that AKs are premalignant lesions and not SCCs in situ.[29] BCC accounts for 70% of cutaneous malignancies.[1] Histologically, several key features lead to the diagnosis of BCC. Most commonly seen are epithelial cells with large nuclei, ill-defined borders, and a lack of intracellular bridges. Fixation artifact includes the separation of the stroma from the tumor cells, or *clefting*.

FIGURE 7–2 Bowen's disease presents as a red, geographic plaque with irregular borders. (Reprinted with permission from Weber RS: Clinical assessment and staging. In Weber RS, Miller MJ, Goepfert H [eds]: Basal and Squamous Cell Skin Cancers of the Head and Neck. Philadelphia, Williams & Wilkins, 1996.)

The stroma is composed of collagen fibers and mucin. Mucin shrinks with fixation, causing the retraction of the stroma from the tumor islands.

Clinically, several distinct histomorphologic growth patterns of BCC have been noted. Three are mentioned with the greatest frequency—nodular, morpheaform, and superficial. *Nodular* lesions are the most common and often present as raised, pearly, well-circumscribed lesions with overlying telangiectases. Also known as noduloulcerative, this form of BCC can, if neglected, ulcerate in the manner of a SCC. Seventy-five percent of BCCs are of this type.[2]

The *superficial* type of BCC was formerly incorrectly labeled "superficial multifocal" because of its propensity for clefting upon fixation. This type accounts for 10% of BCCs and affects the trunk and extremities more often than the head and neck. It is usually a red, scaly plaque that can be difficult to distinguish from Bowen's disease. These increase in size through peripheral extension.[29, 30]

Morpheaform, or sclerosing, type is the most aggressive form of BCC. Examination shows a fibrotic yellowish plaque with indistinct borders. These tumors tend to be deeply invasive and often extend peripherally beyond the apparent clinical margin. Histologically, morpheaform differs from the other types of BCC in that the stroma contains little mucin, and therefore separation artifact is uncommon. At the periphery, fingerlike projections of tumor extend into the surrounding dermis, leading to a high recurrence rate after treatment. A desmoplastic reaction of the surrounding tissues is common.[2, 30]

Infrequently encountered BCCs include keratotic BCC, which is also known as metatypical or basosquamous carcinoma. This intermediate lesion has characteristics of both BCC and SCC and has a higher metastatic potential than do other forms of BCC.[31] Another variant is the fibroepithelioma, first described by Pinkus in 1953,[31a] which usually presents on the trunk as a firm, pedunculated lesion. Pigmented BCC resembles the nodular type of BCC except for its brown color secondary to dendritic melanocytes. It can be confused with malignant melanoma on clinical inspection alone.

Metastasis from BCC is very rare. The reported rate is less than 0.1% of all lesions.[9, 32] Most patients with metastatic disease have the morpheaform variant, as well as perineural invasion and multiple local recurrences.[32] Nonetheless, the overall 5-year survival rate for patients diagnosed with BCC is more than 95%.[2]

Squamous Cell Carcinoma

The second most common skin cancer is SCC, which arises from the keratinocytes of the spinous layer of the epidermis. Nests of atypical squamous cells infiltrate the dermis with a surrounding inflammatory infiltrate. The four most common histopathologic patterns are conventional, acantholytic, spindle cell, and verrucous carcinoma. *Conventional* SCC can be subdivided into well-differentiated, moderately differentiated, or poorly differentiated. In general, the more poorly differentiated the tumor, the fewer keratin pearls are apparent, the higher the nuclear-cytoplasmic ratio, and the more striking the nuclear atypia.

The other types are less common. *Acantholytic* SCC, also mentioned in the literature as adenoid type, is characterized histologically by a pseudoglandular appearance. *Spindle cell* SCC is often associated with extensive UVR exposure or chronic burns.[33] *Verrucous* carcinoma is a well-differentiated, papillomatous variant of SCC.

The classic appearance of SCC is a shallow ulcer with elevated, indistinct borders on a sun-exposed area of the body, especially near the ears, nose, and lips. A plaque often covers the lesion. Although usually preceded by actinic changes in sun-exposed areas, SCC can also arise in skin damaged by ionizing radiation, thermal injury, or a previous scar (Marjolin's ulcer). Tumors that arise from these causes, as opposed to those caused by sun exposure, are generally more aggressive and metastasize more frequently.

Approximately 2% to 14% of SCCs demonstrate spread along cutaneous nerves in the head and neck (Fig. 7–3).[34] Although most patients with SCC who have perineural invasion are asymptomatic, some patients present with pain, paresthesias, facial paralysis, or diplopia as the different cranial nerves of the head and face are affected.[35] Neurotropism can involve both small peripheral nerves and major nerve trunks, and tumors of the midface and forehead have a higher propensity for this type of invasion. Although the molecular mechanisms for perineural invasion remain poorly understood, recent studies have demonstrated the potential importance of laminin-5 isoforms and of the nerve-cell adhesion molecule (N-CAM).[36, 37] Perineural extension of SCC is associated with a high incidence of regional lymph node metastasis (35%) and a 5-year survival rate of less than 30%.[34]

Cutaneous SCC can metastasize to regional lymph nodes. One large meta-analysis estimated the rate to be 5.2% for all lesions on sun-exposed areas of the skin, excluding the lip and external ear.[38] This study identified several clinical factors that increased the risk of regional metastasis. Size greater than 2 cm was identified as a risk factor for metastasis. Sites that are associated with higher rates include the external ear and the lip.[39] Tumors that arise in a previous scar have a metastatic rate of 38%; those with perineural invasion metastasize

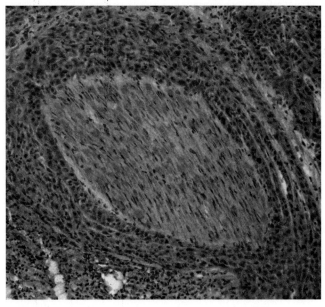

FIGURE 7–3 Microscopic view of perineural infiltration of a peripheral nerve with squamous cell carcinoma.

at a rate of 47%. As would be expected, patients with lymph node metastasis have a decreased survival rate; it has been estimated at between 28% and 45%.[38] Because of early detection, however, the overall 5-year survival rate for SCC is still greater than 90%.[40]

NONEPITHELIAL SKIN CANCERS

Ninety-five percent of NMSCs are either BCC or SCC. The remaining 5% include a diverse mix of tumors arising from skin appendages, neuroendocrine cells, mesenchymal cells, or vascular structures. The same principles of biopsy-confirmed diagnosis and treatment that applied to BCC and SCC also apply to most of these lesions.

Merkel cell carcinoma is a rare malignancy that is one of the more aggressive nonmelanoma skin cancers. First described in 1972 as trabecular carcinoma of the skin, it is now named for its presumed cell of origin.[41] The Merkel cell is located near the basal layer of the epidermis and is thought to be neuroendocrine in origin.[42] Merkel cell carcinoma typically appears as a red, shiny dermal nodule on sun-exposed areas of elderly patients. It affects the skin of the head and neck approximately 50% of the time.[42, 43] The tumors are often smaller than 2 cm and can mimic basal or SCC in clinical presentation, which can cause a delay in diagnosis.

Histologically, Merkel cell carcinoma is similar to other tumors of neuroendocrine origin. It is characterized by small blue cell tumors with a high nuclear-cytoplasmic ratio and hyperchromatic nuclei.[44] These tumors can be further differentiated from more common skin cancers by means of neuron-specific enolase and electron microscopy, the latter of which usually shows dense neurosecretory granules.[44]

Treatment for these lesions must be aggressive. Local recurrence after resection has been reported in as many as 44% of patients.[42, 45] Regional nodal metastases are reported in 31% to 80% of cases,[45, 46] and distant metastases occur in up to one third of patients.[30] Thus, wide surgical margins of 2 to 3 cm are recommended in most studies.[45–47] Because of the high rate of lymph node metastasis, treatment of the regional lymphatics is indicated, with surgical neck dissection, postoperative radiation therapy, or both. Many studies can be cited that show the efficacy of either modality.[43, 48–50] Survival rates based on small sample sizes have been reported as 72% at 2 years,[51] but 21% at 5 years.[43] Adjuvant chemotherapy is indicated for the treatment of distant metastases, although several reports have revealed inconsistent improvement in overall survival.[52–54]

Dermatofibrosarcoma protuberans (DFSP) is a sarcoma of the dermal fibroblasts. It usually occurs in patients between the ages of 20 and 50 and is found in the head and neck in 10% to 15% of cases.[55, 56] It rarely metastasizes, but it is often locally aggressive. It presents as an indurated, violaceous plaque but can progress to a multicentric lesion that spreads well beyond its apparent borders. Because of its dermal origin and tentacle-like projections of tumor cells beneath normal-appearing skin, recurrence rates of up to 60% have been reported.[56, 57] Several recent studies have concluded that wide surgical margins are necessary if this tumor is to be treated adequately. These studies also suggest that Mohs' micrographic surgery is the procedure of choice

for this particular tumor.[57–59] The prognosis after surgical resection with negative margins is very good, with 5-year survival rates greater than 80%.[60]

Atypical fibroxanthoma is a low-grade malignant lesion of mesenchymal origin.[61] Elderly patients typically present with these nodular lesions involving sun-exposed areas of the head and neck. Histologically, these lesions comprise pleomorphic cells with irregular, hyperchromatic nuclei and atypical giant cells, with demonstrated aggressive infiltration into the subcutaneous fat.[62] Careful pathologic analysis is necessary to distinguish this lesion from dermatofibrosarcoma or malignant fibrous histiocytoma. Treatment is usually surgical with wide local excision.

Sebaceous gland carcinoma is a very uncommon lesion that accounts for approximately 0.2% of all skin cancers.[63] Seventy-five percent of these tumors arise from malignant changes in the meibomian glands of the eyelid, although they can also appear elsewhere on the skin of the head and neck.[30] This lesion may appear as a verrucous, nodular growth with ulcerations. Histologically, sebaceous gland carcinoma has irregular lobules with undifferentiated cells and distinct sebaceous cells containing the foamy cytoplasm. An early biopsy may distinguish sebaceous cell carcinoma from benign processes such as keratoconjunctivitis or a chalazion and from more common cutaneous malignancies.

Ocular sebaceous gland carcinoma is an aggressive lesion. The rate of metastatic disease is 14% to 25%,[64] and the overall mortality rate is 22%.[65] Treatment requires wide surgical excision with removal of involved regional lymph nodes. Radiation therapy is indicated for metastatic disease or unresectable tumors.[30, 44] Chemotherapy may be used to treat distant metastasis.[64]

Carcinoma of the eccrine sweat glands and apocrine glands is extremely rare, and no common clinical features have been described.[66] Diagnosis typically requires pathologic interpretation following excision or biopsy of a suspicious lesion. Both of these lesions tend to be locally invasive, and regional/distal metastasis is unusual.[67, 68] Lesions of the head and neck that represent primary lesions may be difficult to distinguish from metastatic disease from other sites. Extramammary Paget's disease can manifest as a variation of apocrine carcinoma involving the external auditory canal or orbital skin. Treatment of these lesions involves wide local excision and treatment of regional lymph nodes if they are involved.

STAGING

The tumor, node, metastasis (TNM) staging system for NMSC recommended by the American Joint Committee on Cancer Staging is based on retrospective data and uses the endpoints of recurrence and survival (Table 7–1). A T1 tumor is 2 cm or smaller, T2 tumors are larger than 2 cm but not larger than 5 cm, and T3 lesions are those larger than 5 cm. T4 tumors are characterized by invasion of adjacent structures such as cartilage, nerve, muscle, or bone. Only two categories are used to classify regional lymph node metastasis: N0 for no metastasis and N1 for any positive lymph node regardless of size. If upon pathologic evaluation the stage changes, the new stage is denoted with a "p" as a prefix, for example, "pT4."[69]

TABLE 7-1 Definition of TNM for Nonmelanoma Skin Cancer

Definitions for clinical (cTNM) and pathologic (pTNM) classifications are the same.

Primary Tumor (T)

TX	Primary tumor cannot be assessed
T0	No evidence of primary tumor
Tis	Carcinoma in situ
T1	Tumor 2 cm or less in greatest dimension
T2	Tumor more than 2 cm, but not more than 5 cm, in greatest dimension
T3	Tumor more than 5 cm in greatest dimension
T4	Tumor invades deep extradermal structures (i.e., cartilage, skeletal muscle, or bone)

Note: In case of multiple simultaneous tumors, the tumor with the highest T category will be classified and the number of separate tumors will be indicated in parentheses, e.g., T2 (5).

Regional Lymph Nodes (N)

NX	Regional lymph nodes cannot be assessed
N0	No regional lymph node metastasis
N1	Regional lymph node metastasis

Distant Metastasis (M)

MX	Distant metastasis cannot be assessed
M0	No distant metastasis
M1	Distant metastasis

Stage Grouping

Stage 0	Tis	N0	M0
Stage I	T1	N0	M0
Stage II	T2	N0	M0
	T3	N0	M0
Stage III	T4	N0	M0
	Any T	N1	M0
Stage IV	Any T	Any N	M1

Used with the permission of the American Joint Committee on Cancer (AJCC), Chicago, Illinois. The original source for this material is the *AJCC Cancer Staging Manual, Sixth Edition* (2002) published by Springer-Verlag New York, www.springer-ny.com.

◾ CLINICAL ASSESSMENT

As with any disease process, the initial step in treating a patient with a cutaneous malignancy is to obtain a complete history and physical examination. With regard to the history, a patient should be asked about any previous history of skin cancer, as well as any family history of skin cancer. The degree of lifetime sun exposure and any history of previous therapeutic radiation should be elicited. The presence of pain, paresthesias, or diplopia should also be ascertained.

The physical examination should include a complete evaluation of the head and neck. Particular characteristics of skin lesions should be noted and compared with the characteristics previously described in this chapter. The location and size of the tumor determine the cosmetic and functional deficits that may result from surgical resection. Additional reconstructive planning should be undertaken with tumors near the eyes, ears, skull, or dura. Many of these patients will also require a whole body examination by a dermatologist owing to the high rate of multiple primary tumors in high-risk populations.

The neurologic examination should include assessment of extraocular function and facial movement. The facial skin should be examined for perception of light touch and pinprick. Any history of abnormalities in cranial nerve VII function should be elicited and a careful examination performed. Clinical signs and symptoms of perineural invasion include pain, paresthesia, anesthesia, facial twitching/spasms, and facial paralysis. However, a majority of patients with perineural invasion are asymptomatic at initial presentation.[34]

Finally, the presence or absence of regional adenopathy is very important to assess. The nodes in the parotid, postauricular, upper cervical, and submandibular regions merit special consideration. Metastasis from primary skin cancer sites to the cervical nodes often follows predictable drainage routes (Fig. 7–4). Fine-needle aspiration may be indicated for enlarged nodes.

Although the physical examination is typically sufficient for a well-localized lesion, certain patients with skin cancer require diagnostic imaging for the purpose of assessing the full extent of primary disease and possible metastasis. The extent of deeply invasive or recurrent skin cancers may be impossible to assess clinically. These tumors, as well as those in high-risk areas like the preauricular region, may require either a computed tomographic (CT) scan or a magnetic resonance imaging (MRI) scan before treatment is initiated.

A contrast-enhanced CT scan should be obtained for the determination of bone invasion and lymph node metastasis from a skin lesion. The possibility of bone involvement should be entertained with any bulky or fixed lesion in the head and neck. Lymph nodes seen on CT scan that are greater than 1.5 cm in diameter or that demonstrate central hypodensity are indicative of possible metastasis. Extracapsular spread of metastatic tumor is suggested by the loss of adjacent fat planes on CT imaging.

For lesions at risk for intracranial extension, the MRI scan is the imaging modality of choice. A BCC in the medial canthal region would require assessment of the orbit as well as of the anterior cranial fossa. The MRI scan is available and provides for accurate evaluation of both intracranial and periorbital invasion and of involvement of cranial nerves by tumor.

Before treatment is begun, the histologic diagnosis is confirmed by biopsy. For smaller lesions, an excisional biopsy is appropriate; for larger tumors, an incisional or punch biopsy is usually sufficient for diagnosis. In either case, a full-thickness biopsy that includes the epidermis, dermis, and a portion of subcutaneous tissue is required.

◾ TREATMENT

Surgical Treatment

Surgical resection is the most common method of treatment for skin cancer of the head and neck.

Surgical Options

Surgical options include cryosurgery, electrodesiccation and curettage, Mohs' micrographic surgery, and standard excision. The choice of which modality to use depends on the type and size of the tumor, the suitability of the patient for surgery, and the availability and experience of the practitioners of each of these techniques. As long as the modality used

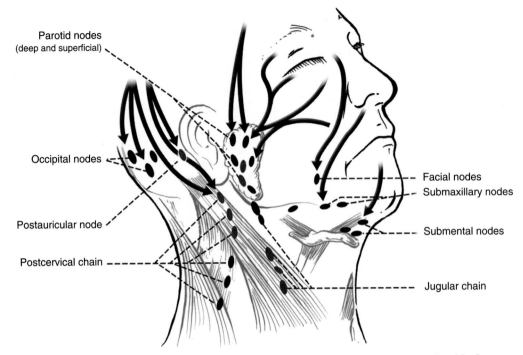

FIGURE 7–4 Regional metastasis from the primary skin cancer site tends to follow predictable drainage pathways to the cervical nodal groups.

is appropriate for the lesion and for the patient, comparable cure rates can be achieved in most cases.

Cryosurgery and Electrodesiccation. Cryosurgery and electrodesiccation are two treatment modalities with similar indications and limitations. Cryosurgery is the use of freezing temperatures to selectively destroy skin cancers. Liquid nitrogen is the most commonly used cryogen and is applied via spray or metal probe. Conversely, electrodesiccation and curettage uses heat to kill residual tumor cells left after sharp curettage. The advantages of both these modalities include low cost, ease of treatment in the office, and comparable cure rates of 94% to 99%.[2] Because they do not allow for pathologic control of margins, these treatments should be limited to nonmalignant lesions. True malignancies are more definitively treated with other therapies.

Mohs' Micrographic Surgery. For NMSC in areas that demand maximal preservation of normal tissue, Mohs' micrographic surgery is a favorable treatment option. Frederic E. Mohs developed the procedure when he was a medical student in the 1930s. His original technique involved the preoperative application of zinc chloride paste in order to "fix" the specimen in vivo. Currently, a fresh tissue technique is employed. The Mohs' surgeon, who serves as his or her own pathologist, first outlines the tumor with 1- to 3-mm margins. After appropriate anesthesia has been administered, the tumor is debulked of gross disease. Then, a scalpel angled at 45 degrees is used to excise the lesion along with 1 to 3 mm of the surrounding tissue in the shape of a saucer. Before the tumor has been completely excised, small nicks are made on the specimen and on the remaining wound edge for orientation purposes. Once the specimen has been excised, it is divided and a map is created with the use of color and numeric coding. Horizontal frozen sections are prepared so that the entire tumor margin is examined histologically. After reference has been made to the tumor map, any area of residual tumor is removed from the defect. This cycle of resection and pathologic examination is repeated until the margins are tumor-free.[2, 70]

Because the entire tumor is examined (not just representative samples of the margin), this technique has a high cure rate for NMSC.[2, 71, 72] However, in cases of large or aggressive SCC, en bloc surgical resection with the patient under general anesthesia is preferable. Wide surgical margins are required in these cases owing to the possibility of deep infiltration into subcutaneous tissues, muscle, and peripheral nerves. As with treatment of tumors of the upper aerodigestive tract, an attempt should be made to remove the entire tumor with clear margins. Mohs' micrographic surgery is best suited for smaller, less aggressive lesions.

Standard Surgical Excision. Standard surgical excision is the most common method used by the head and neck surgeon to treat skin cancer. Cure rates are quoted at 90% to 95% for primary tumors.[72] In areas in which there is elasticity of the tissues, excisional surgery is ideal.[38] For early lesions, excision may be performed in the outpatient setting. Local anesthesia is often sufficient for patient comfort; depending on the patient's cardiac status, epinephrine may be added for vasoconstriction. The specimen is oriented with a suture before removal and is subjected to permanent histologic analysis. For lesions of intermediate size, an ambulatory surgery center where sedation can be administered safely is an appropriate venue for the procedure. For large and/or aggressive tumors treated with surgical excision, en bloc surgical resection with the patient under general anesthesia is recommended.

Other Considerations

The most important principle in the management of these lesions is complete tumor excision. Wentzell and Robinson have suggested that surgeons frequently underestimate the depth of invasion of aggressive NMSC and that the potential cosmetic and functional consequences of surgical resection may lead to less aggressive excision of these tumors.[73] Despite their importance, cosmetic and functional concerns must remain secondary. Depending on the size and location of the tumor, proper surgical resection may require resection of surrounding structures and the use of rotational flaps or free flaps for reconstruction. Careful preoperative assessment, including diagnostic imaging and consultation with an experienced reconstructive surgeon, is essential in these cases.

Adequate margins of resection are of primary importance in the ultimate success of surgical treatment. Inadequate margins can lead to local recurrence and uncontrollable disease. The amount of normal skin that should be excised along with the tumor ultimately depends on the histologic and clinical behavior of the individual tumor. However, there are general principles with which the head and neck surgeon should be familiar. For tumors that are smaller than 2 cm, it has been shown that 4-mm margins are sufficient for local control in the vast majority of both BCC and SCC cases.[74, 75]

Aggressive lesions require wider surgical resection and additional clinical suspicion for potential regional metastasis and/or perineural invasion. Rowe and associates identified several common features of aggressive NMSC (Table 7–2).[38] These lesions grow rapidly, are often 2 cm or larger, may be recurrent, and may present with regional metastases. Histologic features include poorly differentiated lesions, spindle cell SCC, and basosquamous or morpheaform BCC. These lesions frequently occur in the "H-zone," encompassing the central midface and the lateral face from the temporal fossa to the mandibular angle (Fig. 7–5).[76] Clinical judgment should be used in each case; margins of up to 2 cm may be advisable when possible. As stated earlier, highly aggressive Merkel cell or DFSP tumors may require extensive resection.[45]

TABLE 7-2 Characteristics of Aggressive Nonmelanoma Skin Cancer

Large lesion (>2 cm)
Rapid growth
Recurrent disease
Regional metastasis
Perineural invasion
Pathologic findings
   Poorly differentiated
   Spindle cell squamous cell carcinoma
   Basosquamous or morpheaform basal cell carcinoma
Involvement of the midface H-zone
Invasion of bone, cartilage, and/or muscle

Care must also be taken to acquire appropriate deep margins. For superficial lesions, the deep margin should include a substantial amount of subcutaneous tissue. For more invasive tumors, a deep margin of the underlying fascia or muscle is included. Resection of muscle or bone may be necessary, depending on the extent of the tumor. Preoperative diagnostic imaging and intraoperative palpation should assist the surgeon in determining the appropriate deep margin to include with the resection.

After the specimen has been excised, intraoperative frozen section margin assessment should be performed. The surgeon should orient the specimen, preferably in the presence of the surgical pathologist (Fig. 7–6). Peripheral margins should be obtained around the entire circumference of the specimen, as well as in the entire deep margin. The surgeon and pathologist should create a specimen map so that if a positive margin is found, the location of the residual tumor can be precisely identified and additional resection performed.

Local and regional metastasis must be evaluated and treated appropriately when present. Although it has been commonly employed in the treatment of melanoma, sentinel node excision is not routinely practiced for NMSC.[77] Elective neck dissections are also not indicated for NMSC.

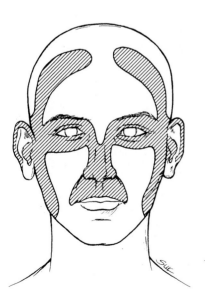
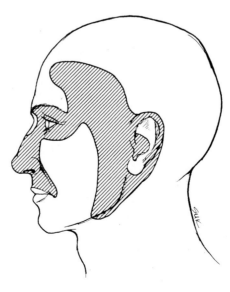

FIGURE 7–5 The H-zone encompasses the midface, extending from the lower eyelids horizontally to the preauricular region. The region spans the temple to the level of the angle of the mandible and includes the ear, postauricular sulcus, upper lip, nose, and medial canthus. (Reprinted with permission from Weber RS: Clinical assessment and staging. In Weber RS, Miller MJ, Goepfert H [eds]: Basal and Squamous Cell Skin Cancers of the Head and Neck. Philadelphia, Williams & Wilkins, 1996.)

SPECIMEN A: RESECTION POSTAURICULAR
MORPHEAFORM BASAL CELL CARCINOMA

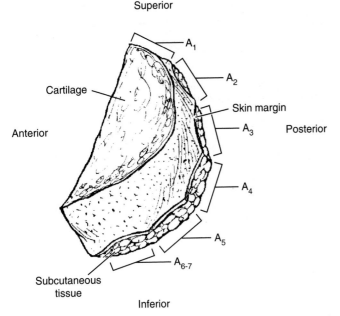

FIGURE 7–6 The head and neck surgeon and pathologist should collaborate in creating a tumor map that carefully describes the surgical specimen and the structures resected. The margin is carefully delineated so that sections submitted for frozen section analysis can be correlated with the original en bloc specimen. Positive margins can be precisely localized if additional margins must be obtained. (Reprinted with permission from Weber RS: Surgical principles. In Weber RS, Miller MJ, Goepfert H [eds]: Basal and Squamous Cell Skin Cancers of the Head and Neck. Philadelphia, Williams & Wilkins, 1996.)

When cervical metastatic disease is present, a regional neck dissection is performed in conjunction with resection of the primary tumor.

Metastasis to the parotid gland must also be carefully evaluated (Fig. 7–7). Parotidectomy in the treatment of skin cancer should be considered when intraparotid metastasis is present, the lesion has invaded the parotid capsule, facial nerve invasion has occurred, or the temporal bone is involved.[78, 79] Postoperative radiation therapy is indicated in these cases. Taylor and colleagues demonstrated the value of this combined approach. Ultimate control of disease in patients with parotid metastases from head and neck skin cancers was 62.5% with surgical treatment and 46% with radiation therapy, but it improved to 89% when both forms of treatment were used.[80]

Reconstruction of the defect can take many forms. For smaller lesions, primary closure and healing by secondary intention are appropriate options. Intermediate defects may warrant a skin graft or local advancement of a rotational flap for adequate closure. For large defects, regional or distant pedicled flaps or free flaps are used. The reconstructive options depend not only on the size of the defect but also on the nature of the tumor excised. In general, the use of flaps that will cover areas with close or indistinct margins should be avoided so that recurrence may be more quickly diagnosed.

Site-Specific Management of Nonmelanoma Skin Cancer

The management of NMSC requires special considerations in particular subsites of the head and neck. Of particular concern are aggressive lesions that are larger than 2 cm, those that invade underlying structures, and those that present with regional metastases or that require the surgical removal of cosmetic and/or functional units. Treatment of these lesions requires proper assessment of tumor extent and an understanding of factors that influence tumor resection and facial reconstruction.

Forehead and Scalp

The skin of the forehead and scalp includes the temporal, supra-eyebrow, and glabellar regions. The skin of the forehead and scalp is thick and contains abundant vascular subcutaneous tissue; however, the temporal skin is quite thin, and facial nerve branches are directly under the surface. Lesions of the forehead and scalp may have "silent" microscopic extensions that require interdisciplinary management.[81, 82]

A majority of nodular and nodular-ulcerative types of BCC can be controlled even when the lesions are quite large. Although the more aggressive morpheaform type of BCC represents 10% of all BCC lesions, 32% of forehead and temple lesions are of this type.[83] BCC lesions rarely metastasize; aggressive lesions of the ear and scalp that are deeply invasive or larger than 3 cm are more likely to metastasize than are lesions located in other head and neck sites. These lesions spread along lymphatics within the parotid gland and the cervical chain or to distant sites, including lung, bone, and skin.[84] Both aggressive BCC and SCC lesions of the scalp and forehead have an increased likelihood of parotid gland involvement, and the prognosis of these patients is worse, especially if the facial nerve is involved.[78, 79]

SCC lesions are typically well differentiated in the forehead and scalp. Aggressive lesions tend to occur in areas of previous radiation therapy, thermal injury, and chemical burn. These malignancies tend to be more invasive and are more likely to metastasize locally.[85] Additionally, there is increased concern about perineural invasion by SCC in this area. In one study, 14% of lesions in the forehead and scalp demonstrated invasion into one or more major cranial nerve branches.[34] Lesions in the frontozgomatic region have an increased frequency of perineural invasion, especially to the supraorbital nerves. Most often, the facial and trigeminal nerves were involved, and in 60% of cases, no signs or symptoms were noted at initial presentation. Although treatment can provide local cancer control, survival of patients with perineural invasion by SCC of the skin is quite poor; 5-year survival rates for patients treated with radiation therapy alone or with surgery and postoperative radiation therapy are about 30%.

Local invasion of the underlying bone by SCC in the forehead and scalp region can compromise excision and tumor control. Risks for involvement of the calvarium include large lesions, tumor fixation, CNS symptoms, and a history of previous radiation therapy. The physical examination and a contrast-enhanced CT scan are the primary means of determining the presence and extent of bone

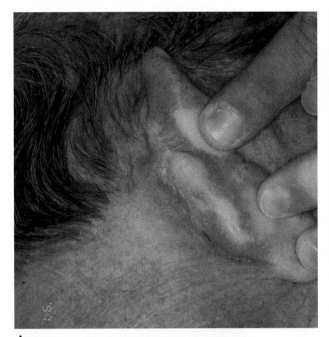

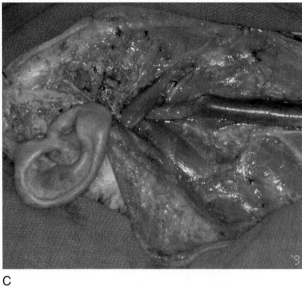

C

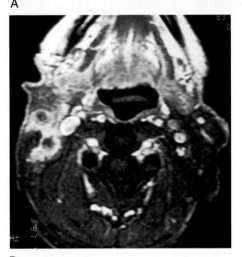

A

B

FIGURE 7–7 *A*, A postauricular squamous cell carcinoma was initially controlled by local excision. *B*, Delayed neck and parotid metastases were detected 6 months later. Axial magnetic resonance image demonstrates regional metastasis. *C*, Surgical treatment included superficial parotidectomy and cervical lymphadenectomy.

involvement. MRI studies can demonstrate intracranial tumor extent. The head and neck surgeon must be prepared to remove the outer table or full thickness of calvarium if invasion is present at time of resection. Neurosurgical involvement is required when the tumor involves the full thickness of the skull. Full-thickness craniectomy is recommended owing to the possibility of bone invasion or extension of tumor along venous channels. Tumor involving the inner cortex of the cranium may require resection of the underlying dura. Violation of the inner dura may require coagulation and resection of adjacent brain tissue at the site of involvement. However, the likelihood of cure for patients with transdural involvement of cutaneous SCC is exceedingly low.

Following standard wide local excision or Mohs' surgery, numerous options for reconstruction are available. Depending on size and location, options include healing by secondary intention, primary closure, or skin graft placement. Larger defects may require the use of tissue expanders, closure with local rotational flaps or regional myocutaneous/muscle flaps, or free-tissue transfer (Fig. 7–8). Resection of bone might require reconstruction with split calvarium, split rib, or prosthetic implants. The details of these reconstructive options are discussed more fully in Chapter 28.

Periauricular Region

Lesions of the ear and periauricular region account for 5% to 8% of all skin cancers of the head and neck.[86] Given the various embryologic origins of structures in this area, routes of tumor extension depend on the location of origin. Cancer arising in the preauricular skin tends to spread to the helix and tragus, rather than to the external auditory canal. Helical lesions spread toward adjacent areas of the external ear. Tumors may extend along the plane between the parotid gland and the external auditory canal to involve the superficial temporal vessels and spread toward the stylomastoid foramen. Tumors arising in the postauricular skin spread along

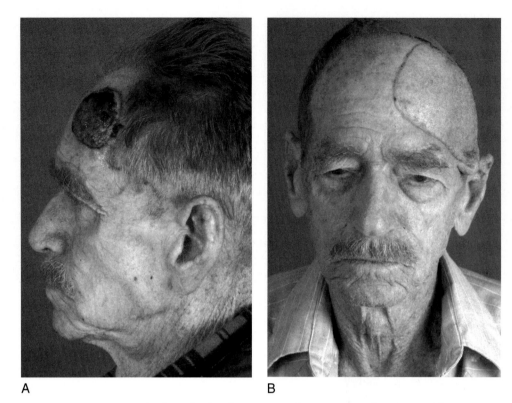

A   B

FIGURE 7–8 *A*, Patient with a large forehead squamous cell carcinoma with invasion of the periosteum but no bone involvement. *B*, Following a full-thickness excision, a split-thickness skin graft was inappropriate for coverage of the calvarium. The surgical defect was reconstructed with a rotational scalp flap.

the postauricular sulcus, and deep lesions in this area can involve the mastoid periosteum and the posteroinferior portion of the parotid gland. Tumors of the external auditory canal (EAC) may spread directly to the parotid gland or along the cranial base through the cartilaginous fissures of Santorini or the bony dehiscence in the medial canal floor (Huschke's foramen).

Patients with SCC in this region are especially at risk for regional metastasis and perineural invasion.[79] The head and neck surgeon should carefully evaluate the preauricular, parotid, retroauricular, and superior deep jugular lymph nodes for metastasis. Metastasis from the pinna to the parotid and superior deep jugular nodes occurs in 12% to 18% of patients.[87, 88] Perineural invasion most often occurs in BCC and SCC lesions of the malar and preauricular areas.[89] In the study by Niazi and coworkers of 4376 cases,[89] all of the tumors with perineural spread were recurrent lesions. Although many patients may be asymptomatic, clinicians encountering skin cancers in the periauricular region must carefully examine the patient for paresthesias and hypoesthesias in this region and must completely evaluate cranial nerve function.

Cancer of the skin of the periauricular region should be carefully evaluated for potential deep extension, especially in cases of recurrent cancer. CT scans are the preferred imaging modality for this region, given the closely related bone and cartilaginous structures. The lesions should be evaluated for potential involvement of the EAC and the tympanic bone. The mastoid cortex, air cell complex, and middle ear should be closely examined. The temporomandibular joint (TMJ), the ascending ramus of the mandible, and the transverse process of the second cervical vertebra should also be carefully assessed. Asymmetrical enlargement or bony erosion in the stylomastoid foramen or the foramen ovale may indicate potential perineural invasion. MRI studies help to define the potential involvement of the infratemporal fossa or parapharyngeal space. In cases of intracranial extension, MRI studies aid the clinician in determining involvement of the dura, brain, and internal carotid artery. Finally, subtle changes and thickening of cranial nerves may indicate perineural invasion.[90]

Surgical excision is the primary modality used in the periauricular region, especially given the potential for deep tumor invasion. Small tumors along the helix can be treated with a wedge resection. Tumors within the concha are likely to invade the auricular cartilage and do require a partial or total auriculectomy. Tumors arising in the skin of the conchal bowl and the lateral aspect of the external EAC may require an auriculectomy and sleeve resection.

Management of tumors in this region requires the careful consideration of several adjacent structures. Involvement of the parotid gland requires at least a superficial parotidectomy (Fig. 7–9). Although dermatologic surgeons occasionally resect a portion of the parotid gland during Mohs' micrographic surgery, only formal identification of the facial nerve during a parotidectomy can safely ensure facial nerve function. Deep involvement of the parotid gland or perineural invasion of the facial nerve may require a radical parotidectomy with

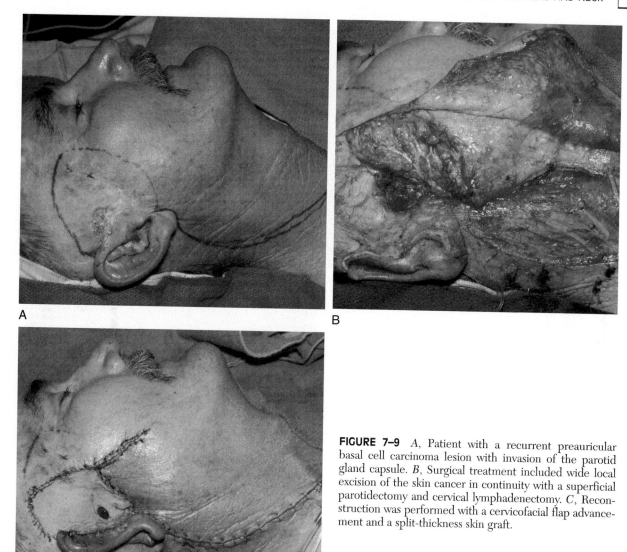

FIGURE 7–9 *A*, Patient with a recurrent preauricular basal cell carcinoma lesion with invasion of the parotid gland capsule. *B*, Surgical treatment included wide local excision of the skin cancer in continuity with a superficial parotidectomy and cervical lymphadenectomy. *C*, Reconstruction was performed with a cervicofacial flap advancement and a split-thickness skin graft.

excision of the facial nerve and immediate reconstruction of the nerve when possible.

Cancers of the skin that involve the mandible and TMJ require more radical surgical resection. Extension of tumor into the infratemporal fossa and the parapharyngeal space may require resection of the ascending ramus, the condyle, or both. A lateral temporal bone resection may require excision of the condyle, the TMJ, and the capsule of the joint. Extensive involvement of the joint may further require resection of the medial aspect of the glenoid fossa, potentially requiring exposure of the carotid artery through the temporal bone to permit bony dissection.

Lateral temporal bone resection may be indicated when a tumor involves the skin and cartilage of the pinna and the EAC, or when a tumor involves or is contiguous with the tympanic bone or the mastoid cortex.[91, 92] There must be no evidence of tumor invasion of the middle ear or the mastoid air cell complex. Otherwise, more extensive involvement of the temporal bone will require more radical resection. In all cases, an audiogram should be obtained and the patient should be counseled regarding the effects of surgical treatment on hearing and the vestibular system. Finally, the need for postsurgical radiation therapy depends on findings at surgery, the histology of the lesion, and the extent of nodal involvement.

Midface (Nose and Upper Lip)

Within the midface, the H-zone describes an area that encompasses the glabella, medial canthus, nasolabial sulcus, columellolabial junction, alar rim, and posterolateral nares.[38] Nonmelanoma skin lesions in this H-zone have a higher incidence of recurrence and are more difficult to treat surgically. These tumors tend to grow vertically, rather than laterally in a superficial plane, perhaps owing to the presence of facial embryologic fusion planes in this region

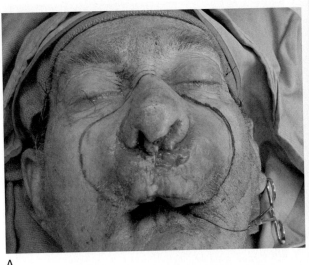

A

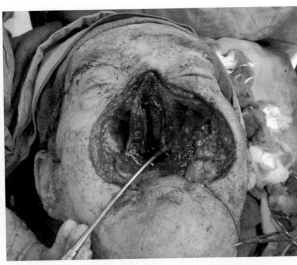

B

C

FIGURE 7–10 *A,* Patient with a squamous cell carcinoma lesion involving the upper lip and columella with extension into the maxillary sinuses. *B,* Surgical excision required a total rhinectomy and bilateral maxillectomies. *C,* Anterior view of the resected surgical specimen.

(Fig. 7–10).[93] Care must be exercised with the use of Mohs' micrographic treatment in these regions, especially with recurrent lesions or tumors that may demonstrate perineural invasion.

The portion of the H-zone encompassing the nose and upper lip represents a challenging area for tumor resection and subsequent reconstruction to preserve cosmetic and functional attributes. Tumors adherent to underlying nasal cartilage or bone will require at least a partial rhinectomy. Intraoperative frozen section assessment of surgical margins is necessary to ensure complete tumor resection. Reconstruction often requires the collaborative efforts of a multidisciplinary team. The head and neck surgeon manages the cancer treatment, the dental oncologist creates necessary oral/nasal prostheses, and the facial plastic surgeon oversees the reconstructive effort (Fig. 7–11).

The goal of reconstruction is to provide as normal an appearance as possible and to preserve function through maintaining patency of the nasal airway and competence of the oral sphincter. In the review of reconstruction strategies, the patient's general health and prognosis should be considered. Additionally, the surgeon should assess the willingness of the patient to have a staged reconstruction. For some

patients who are older or who are not good surgical candidates, a prosthesis may be the best choice. However, these are expensive; they also may be difficult to create and will require continued maintenance and periodic replacement.

Partial-thickness nasal defects should be reconstructed as early as possible once excision of the tumor has been verified. This may be an issue with recurrent lesions or with deeply invasive tumors such as morpheaform BCC. Skin grafts are the best choice if there is any concern regarding excision. The skin graft is relatively simple to place and to remove if necessary. Additionally, the skin graft facilitates close observation of the tumor site for recurrence. Better cosmetic results can be achieved with locoregional flaps that match skin texture and color. Options include nasolabial, nasal dorsal, and glabellar flaps.

Full-thickness defects require reconstruction of the nasal mucosal surface and the external skin. Potential sources for nasal mucosal surface reconstruction include septal mucosa and local flaps such as the nasolabial flap or other skin turnover flaps.[94] Flaps from the forehead provide good color and texture match and remain the best choice for subtotal or total nasal reconstruction. If necessary, forehead flaps may be employed in a delayed reconstruction and in conjunction

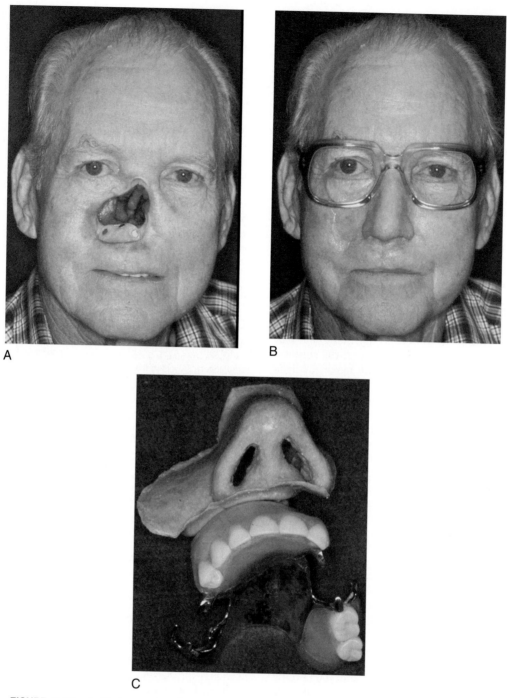

FIGURE 7–11 *A,* Patient with a large defect following partial rhinectomy and maxillectomy for a squamous cell carcinoma lesion. *B,* Same patient with his prosthetic device in position. *C,* The prosthetic device that was designed to accommodate the patient's surgical defect.

with tissue expanders for additional coverage.[95] Excision of skeletal support requires reconstruction with cartilage or bone grafts. Autologous donor material includes auricular cartilage and rib bone/cartilage grafts. Reconstruction of the skeletal support should occur during the initial repair of the external skin. Local flaps are less pliable and do not mold as well to the bone/cartilage grafts if they are introduced at a later procedure. This can result in increased seromas, infections, and graft failures.

Reconstruction of the lip depends on the size of the lip defect. Any remnant of the lip should be employed in the reconstruction when possible so that lip function is maintained along with oral competence. Small defects involving one fourth of the upper lip or one third of the lower lip can be closed primarily. A layered closure approximating the mucosa, muscle, and skin ensures proper lip function. Defects of moderate size will benefit from local flaps that employ lip remnants and the opposite lip in the reconstruction. These well-described flaps include the Karapandzic flap and the Abbé-Estlander flap.

When lip defects involve more than three quarters of the lip, repair can be adequately achieved only with distant flaps. Unlike local lip flaps, distant flaps do not contain the appropriate musculature to reproduce lip function and are more abnormal in appearance. Cheek flaps may be employed in the Bernard or Webster technique for reconstruction. Often, complex, staged reconstructions may be necessary, especially if remaining portions of the lip are incorporated into the reconstruction. Following the reconstruction of large defects of the lip, the patient will often have varying degrees of microstomia that can be improved by a later commissureplasty and scar revision.

Radiation Therapy

Although less than 10% of NMSC cases are treated with primary radiation therapy, it is estimated that 90% of lesions 2 cm or smaller can be controlled with radiation therapy.[31, 96] In cases in which surgical excision would cause functional or cosmetic deficits, primary radiotherapy is an important treatment option. Lesions of the eyelid, lip, nose, and ear should be considered for radiation treatment if the surgical morbidity is deemed too high. Patients with major medical comorbidities who are not surgical candidates may also benefit from primary radiation instead of surgical ablation.

Radiotherapy is an important adjunct to surgical ablation in the treatment of aggressive cutaneous malignancies. Indications for postoperative radiation therapy include large or recurrent primary lesions, close or positive tumor margins, and/or perineural invasion. Tumors that are poorly differentiated and spindle cell SCC may also benefit from radiotherapy. Lesions that are located in the embryologic fusion planes of the perinasal and periauricular regions can spread deeply and should also be considered for treatment with adjunctive radiation.[93] Additionally, postoperative radiation therapy may improve regional control in patients with lymph node metastases at multiple neck levels and in those with extracapsular spread. As was previously mentioned, Merkel cell carcinoma is an aggressive neuroendocrine tumor that is radiosensitive and should be treated with surgery, radiation, and chemotherapy.[97, 98]

Dosages are carefully determined to minimize damage to surrounding tissues. Typical regimens range from 4000 cGy in 8 fractions to 6000 cGy in 30 fractions, depending on the size and characteristics of the tumor.[96] Despite the care taken to affect only the tumor, morbidity can occur with radiation. Erythema, skin necrosis, alopecia, and hypopigmentation can occur within the radiation field.[99] If the tumor is near an important radiosensitive organ, such as the eye, the organ can be shielded so that it will suffer minimal damage. Radiation therapy is relatively contraindicated in patients with basal cell nevus syndrome, who have a propensity to develop tumors within previously irradiated skin.[2]

Additional Treatment Options

Other modalities of particular interest include topical chemotherapy, CO_2 laser ablation, and photodynamic therapy. Topical 5-FU and laser treatments are indicated in superficial lesions, and photodynamic therapy has been shown to be effective in large, aggressive head and neck tumors in elderly patients.[100]

CONCLUSION

NMSC of the head and neck is quite common. BCCs are the most common form and are curable in a great majority of patients. A variety of surgical and nonsurgical options are available for the treatment of NMSC. Aggressive skin lesions tend to invade more deeply, spread to regional lymphatics in the parotid and the neck, and present with perineural invasion. The management of these lesions is much more difficult and may require radical surgery with postoperative radiation. Reconstruction of defects following the resection of aggressive lesions is very challenging as surgeons attempt to restore both cosmetic appearance and normal function.

REFERENCES

1. Miller DL, Weinstock MA: Nonmelanoma skin cancer in the United States: Incidence. J Am Acad Dermatol 30:774, 1994.
2. Padgett JK, Hendrix JD Jr: Cutaneous malignancies and their management. Otolaryngol Clin North Am 34:523, 2001.
3. Strom SS, Yamamura Y: Epidemiology of nonmelanoma skin cancer. Clin Plast Surg 24:627, 1997.
4. Kaldor J, Shugg D, Young B, et al: Non-melanoma skin cancer: Ten years of cancer-registry-based surveillance. Int J Cancer 53:886, 1993.
5. Leffell DJ: The scientific basis of skin cancer. J Am Acad Dermatol 42:18, 2000.
6. Preston DS, Stern RS: Nonmelanoma cancers of the skin. N Engl J Med 327:1649, 1992.
7. Ananthaswamy HN, Pierceall WE: Molecular mechanisms of ultraviolet radiation carcinogenesis. Photochem Photobiol 52:1119, 1990.
8. Buzzell RA: Carcinogenesis of cutaneous malignancies. Dermatol Surg 22:209, 1996.
9. Buzzell RA: Effects of solar radiation on the skin. Otolaryngol Clin North Am 26:1, 1993.
10. Johnson TM, Rowe DE, Nelson BR, et al: Squamous cell carcinoma of the skin (excluding lip and oral mucosa). J Am Acad Dermatol 26:467, 1992.
11. Kelfkens G, de Gruijl FR, van der Leun JC: Ozone depletion and increase in annual carcinogenic ultraviolet dose. Photochem Photobiol 52:819, 1990.
12. Coldiron BM: Ozone depletion update. Dermatol Surg 22:296, 1996.
13. Madronich S, McKenzie RL, Bjorn LO, et al: Changes in biologically active ultraviolet radiation reaching the Earth's surface. J Photochem Photobiol B 46:5, 1998.
14. Urbach F: Ultraviolet radiation and skin cancer of humans. J Photochem Photobiol B 40:3, 1997.
15. Oikarinen A, Raitio A: Melanoma and other skin cancers in circumpolar areas. Int J Circumpolar Health 59:52, 2000.
16. Slaper H, Velders GJ, Daniel JS, et al: Estimates of ozone depletion and skin cancer incidence to examine the Vienna Convention achievements. Nature 384:256, 1996.
17. Shumrick KA, Coldiron B: Genetic syndromes associated with skin cancer. Otolaryngol Clin North Am 26:117, 1993.
18. Kaidbey KH, Agin PP, Sayre RM, et al: Photoprotection by melanin—a comparison of black and Caucasian skin. J Am Acad Dermatol 1:249, 1979.
19. Hogan DJ, Lane PR, Gran L, et al: Risk factors for squamous cell carcinoma of the skin in Saskatchewan, Canada. J Dermatol Sci 1:97, 1990.
20. Hunter DJ, Colditz GA, Stampfer MJ, et al: Risk factors for basal cell carcinoma in a prospective cohort of women. Ann Epidemiol 1:13, 1990.

21. Magnus K: The Nordic profile of skin cancer incidence. A comparative epidemiological study of the three main types of skin cancer. Int J Cancer 47:12, 1991.
22. Lober BA, Lober CW, Accola J: Actinic keratosis is squamous cell carcinoma. J Am Acad Dermatol 43:881, 2000.
23. Cockerell CJ: Histopathology of incipient intraepidermal squamous cell carcinoma ("actinic keratosis"). J Am Acad Dermatol 42:11, 2000.
24. Salasche SJ: Epidemiology of actinic keratoses and squamous cell carcinoma. J Am Acad Dermatol 42:4, 2000.
25. Petter G, Haustein UF: Histologic subtyping and malignancy assessment of cutaneous squamous cell carcinoma. Dermatol Surg 26:521, 2000.
26. Kao GF: Carcinoma arising in Bowen's disease. Arch Dermatol 122:1124, 1986.
27. Dupree MT, Kiteley RA, Weismantle K, et al: Radiation therapy for Bowen's disease: Lessons for lesions of the lower extremity. J Am Acad Dermatol 45:401, 2001.
28. Pagani WA, Lorenzi G, Lorusso D: Surgical treatment for aggressive giant keratoacanthoma of the face. J Dermatol Surg Oncol 12:282, 1986.
29. Brand D, Ackerman AB: Squamous cell carcinoma, not basal cell carcinoma, is the most common cancer in humans. J Am Acad Dermatol 42:523, 2000.
30. Skidmore RA Jr, Flowers FP: Nonmelanoma skin cancer. Med Clin North Am 82:1309, 1998.
31. Goldberg LH: Basal cell carcinoma. Lancet 347:663, 1996.
31a. Pinkus H: Premalignant fibroepithelial tumors of the skin. Arch Dermatol Syph 67:598, 1953.
32. Lo JS, Snow SN, Reizner GT, et al: Metastatic basal cell carcinoma: Report of twelve cases with a review of the literature. J Am Acad Dermatol 24:715, 1991.
33. Emmett AJ: Surgical analysis and biological behaviour of 2277 basal cell carcinomas. Aust N Z J Surg 60:855, 1990.
34. Goepfert H, Dichtel WJ, Medina JE, et al: Perineural invasion in squamous cell skin carcinoma of the head and neck. Am J Surg 148:542, 1984.
35. Dodd GD, Dolan PA, Ballantyne AJ, et al: The dissemination of tumors of the head and neck via the cranial nerves. Radiol Clin North Am 8:445, 1970.
36. Anderson TD, Feldman M, Weber RS, et al: Tumor deposition of laminin-5 and the relationship with perineural invasion. Laryngoscope 111:2140, 2001.
37. McLaughlin RB Jr, Montone KT, Wall SJ, et al: Nerve cell adhesion molecule expression in squamous cell carcinoma of the head and neck: a predictor of propensity toward perineural spread. Laryngoscope 109:821, 1999.
38. Rowe DE, Carroll RJ, Day CL Jr: Prognostic factors for local recurrence, metastasis, and survival rates in squamous cell carcinoma of the skin, ear, and lip. Implications for treatment modality selection. J Am Acad Dermatol 26:976, 1992.
39. Byers R, Kesler K, Redmon B, et al: Squamous carcinoma of the external ear. Am J Surg 146:447, 1983.
40. Gloster HM Jr, Brodland DG: The epidemiology of skin cancer. Dermatol Surg 22:217, 1996.
41. Toker C: Trabecular carcinoma of the skin. Arch Dermatol 105:107, 1972.
42. Haag ML, Glass LF, Fenske NA: Merkel cell carcinoma. Diagnosis and treatment. Dermatol Surg 21:669, 1995.
43. Goepfert H, Remmler D, Silva E, et al: Merkel cell carcinoma (endocrine carcinoma of the skin) of the head and neck. Arch Otolaryngol 110:707, 1984.
44. Brown MD: Recognition and management of unusual cutaneous tumors. Dermatol Clin 18:543, 2000.
45. Lawenda BD, Thiringer JK, Foss RD, et al: Merkel cell carcinoma arising in the head and neck: Optimizing therapy. Am J Clin Oncol 24:35, 2001.
46. Ott MJ, Tanabe KK, Gadd MA, et al: Multimodality management of Merkel cell carcinoma. Arch Surg 134:388, 1999.
47. Yiengpruksawan A, Coit DG, Thaler HT, et al: Merkel cell carcinoma. Prognosis and management. Arch Surg 126:1514, 1991.
48. Kokoska ER, Kokoska MS, Collins BT, et al: Early aggressive treatment for Merkel cell carcinoma improves outcome. Am J Surg 174:688, 1997.
49. Allen PJ, Zhang ZF, Coit DG: Surgical management of Merkel cell carcinoma. Ann Surg 229:97, 1999.
50. Eich HT, Eich D, Staar S, et al: Role of postoperative radiotherapy in the management of Merkel cell carcinoma. Am J Clin Oncol 25:50, 2002.
51. Hitchcock CL, Bland KI, Laney RG III, et al: Neuroendocrine (Merkel cell) carcinoma of the skin. Its natural history, diagnosis, and treatment. Ann Surg 207:201, 1988.
52. Redmond J III, Perry J, Sowray P, et al: Chemotherapy of disseminated Merkel-cell carcinoma. Am J Clin Oncol 14:305, 1991.
53. Feun LG, Savaraj N, Legha SS, et al: Chemotherapy for metastatic Merkel cell carcinoma. Review of the M.D. Anderson Hospital's experience. Cancer 62:683, 1988.
54. Poulsen M, Harvey J: Is there a diminishing role for surgery for Merkel cell carcinoma of the skin? A review of current management. Aust N Z J Surg 72:142, 2002.
55. Mark RJ, Bailet JW, Tran LM, et al: Dermatofibrosarcoma protuberans of the head and neck. A report of 16 cases. Arch Otolaryngol Head Neck Surg 119:891, 1993.
56. Gloster HM Jr: Dermatofibrosarcoma protuberans. J Am Acad Dermatol 35:355, 1996.
57. Ratner D, Thomas CO, Johnson TM, et al: Mohs micrographic surgery for the treatment of dermatofibrosarcoma protuberans. Results of a multiinstitutional series with an analysis of the extent of microscopic spread. J Am Acad Dermatol 37:600, 1997.
58. Gloster HM Jr, Harris KR, Roenigk RK: A comparison between Mohs micrographic surgery and wide surgical excision for the treatment of dermatofibrosarcoma protuberans. J Am Acad Dermatol 35:82, 1996.
59. Parker TL, Zitelli JA: Surgical margins for excision of dermatofibrosarcoma protuberans. J Am Acad Dermatol 32:233, 1995.
60. Bowne WB, Antonescu CR, Leung DH, et al: Dermatofibrosarcoma protuberans: A clinicopathologic analysis of patients treated and followed at a single institution. Cancer 88:2711, 2000.
61. Hakim I: Atypical fibroxanthoma. Ann Otol Rhinol Laryngol 110:985, 2001.
62. Ma CK, Zarbo RJ, Gown AM: Immunohistochemical characterization of atypical fibroxanthoma and dermatofibrosarcoma protuberans. Am J Clin Pathol 97:478, 1992.
63. Marenda SA, Otto RA: Adnexal carcinomas of the skin. Otolaryngol Clin North Am 26:87, 1993.
64. Nelson BR, Hamlet KR, Gillard M, et al: Sebaceous carcinoma. J Am Acad Dermatol 33:1, 1995.
65. Rao NA, Hidayat AA, McLean IW, et al: Sebaceous carcinomas of the ocular adnexa: A clinicopathologic study of 104 cases, with five-year follow-up data. Hum Pathol 13:113, 1982.
66. Gupta A, Flowers FP, Lessner AM: Asymptomatic eyelid papule in a 57-year-old healthy man. Arch Dermatol 136:1409, 2000.
67. Snow SN, Reizner GT: Mucinous eccrine carcinoma of the eyelid. Cancer 70:2099, 1992.
68. Thomson SJ, Tanner NS: Carcinoma of the apocrine glands at the base of eyelashes: A case report and discussion of histological diagnostic criteria. Br J Plast Surg 42:598, 1989.
69. Beahrs OH, American Joint Committee on Cancer, American Cancer Society, National Cancer Institute: Manual for Staging of Cancer, 4th ed. Philadelphia, Lippincott, 1992.
70. Shriner DL, McCoy DK, Goldberg DJ, et al: Mohs micrographic surgery. J Am Acad Dermatol 39:79, 1998.
71. Nelson BR, Railan D, Cohen S: Mohs' micrographic surgery for nonmelanoma skin cancers. Clin Plast Surg 24:705, 1997.
72. Rowe DE, Carroll RJ, Day CL Jr: Long-term recurrence rates in previously untreated (primary) basal cell carcinoma: Implications for patient follow-up. J Dermatol Surg Oncol 15:315, 1989.
73. Wentzell JM, Robinson JK: Embryologic fusion planes and the spread of cutaneous carcinoma: A review and reassessment. J Dermatol Surg Oncol 16:1000, 1990.
74. Wolf DJ, Zitelli JA: Surgical margins for basal cell carcinoma. Arch Dermatol 123:340, 1987.
75. Brodland DG, Zitelli JA: Surgical margins for excision of primary cutaneous squamous cell carcinoma. J Am Acad Dermatol 27:241, 1992.
76. Baker SR, Swanson NA, Grekin RC: Moh's surgical treatment and reconstruction of cutaneous malignancies of the nose. Fac Plast Surg 5:29, 1987.
77. Chao C, McMasters KM: Update on the use of sentinel node biopsy in patients with melanoma: Who and how. Curr Opin Oncol 14:217, 2002.
78. Jackson GL, Ballantyne AJ: Role of parotidectomy for skin cancer of the head and neck. Am J Surg 142:464, 1981.

79. Lai SY, Weinstein GS, Chalian AA, et al: Parotidecomy in the treatment of aggressive cutaneous malignancies. Arch Otol Head Neck Surg 128:521, 2002.

80. Taylor BW Jr, Brant TA, Mendenhall NP, et al: Carcinoma of the skin metastatic to parotid area lymph nodes. Head Neck 13:427, 1991.

81. Mohs FE, Zitelli JA: Microscopically controlled surgery in the treatment of carcinoma of the scalp. Arch Dermatol 117:764, 1981.

82. Hanke CW, Weisberger EC, Lingeman RE: Cancer of the scalp. Dermatol Clin 7:797, 1989.

83. Grekin RC, Schaler RE, Crumley RL: Cancer of the forehead and temple regions. Dermatol Clin 7:699, 1989.

84. Snow SN, Sahl W, Lo JS, et al: Metastatic basal cell carcinoma. Report of five cases. Cancer 73:328, 1994.

85. Stern HS, Haertsch P: Local recurrence and intracerebral spread of squamous cell carcinoma of the scalp. Plast Reconstr Surg 85:284, 1990.

86. Bailin PL, Levine HL, Wood BG, et al: Cutaneous carcinoma of the auricular and periauricular region. Arch Otolaryngol 106:692, 1980.

87. Cassisi NJ, Dickerson DR, Million RR: Squamous cell carcinoma of the skin metastatic to parotid nodes. J Fla Med Assoc 65:760, 1978.

88. Afzelius LE, Gunnarsson M, Nordgren H: Guidelines for prophylactic radical lymph node dissection in cases of carcinoma of the external ear. Head Neck Surg 2:361, 1980.

89. Niazi ZB, Lamberty BG: Perineural infiltration in basal cell carcinomas. Br J Plast Surg 46:156, 1993.

90. Medina JE, Pavlovich A, Wilson DA: Magnetic resonance imaging in the diagnosis of intracranial spread of carcinoma via the trigeminal nerve. Otolaryngol Head Neck Surg 102:416, 1990.

91. Kinney SE, Wood BG: Malignancies of the external ear canal and temporal bone: Surgical techniques and results. Laryngoscope 97:158, 1987.

92. Arena S, Keen M: Carcinoma of the middle ear and temporal bone. Am J Otol 9:351, 1988.

93. Panje WR, Ceilley RI: The influence of embryology of the midface on the spread of epithelial malignancies. Laryngoscope 89:1914, 1979.

94. Burget GC, Menick FJ: The subunit principle in nasal reconstruction. Plast Reconstr Surg 76:239, 1985.

95. Kroll SS: Forehead flap nasal reconstruction with tissue expansion and delayed pedicle separation. Laryngoscope 99:448, 1989.

96. Morrison WH, Garden AS, Ang KK: Radiation therapy for nonmelanoma skin carcinomas. Clin Plast Surg 24:719, 1997.

97. Meeuwissen JA, Bourne RG, Kearsley JH: The importance of postoperative radiation therapy in the treatment of Merkel cell carcinoma. Int J Radiat Oncol Biol Phys 31:325, 1995.

98. Pacella J, Ashby M, Ainslie J, et al: The role of radiotherapy in the management of primary cutaneous neuroendocrine tumors (Merkel cell or trabecular carcinoma): Experience at the Peter MacCallum Cancer Institute (Melbourne, Australia). Int J Radiat Oncol Biol Phys 14:1077, 1988.

99. Halpern JN: Radiation therapy in skin cancer. A historical perspective and current applications. Dermatol Surg 23:1089, 1997.

100. Gayl SV: Photofrin-mediated photodynamic therapy for treatment of aggressive head and neck nonmelanomatous skin tumors in elderly patients. Laryngoscope 111:1091, 2001.

CHAPTER 8

Melanoma of the Head and Neck

Eric J. Lentsch

Jeffrey N. Myers

INTRODUCTION

Cutaneous malignant melanoma (CMM) is an aggressive neoplasm known for its capricious nature that arises from melanocytes. First described by Rene Laennec in 1806,[1] melanoma has rightfully garnered a reputation as a dreaded disease. Although it is less common than basal cell and squamous cell carcinomas, the mortality rates associated with CMM far outstrip those of its less aggressive counterparts. When CMM is detected early, the chance of cure is very high, but advanced-stage melanoma has a dismal prognosis. Because as many as one third of CMMs arise in the head and neck, it is important for head and neck surgeons to have a thorough working knowledge of the disease, including an understanding of its natural history, diagnosis, staging, and treatment. In addition, it is important for clinicians to be aware of certain rare types of melanoma, such as mucosal melanoma and desmoplastic melanoma, because these may occur in the head and neck.

EPIDEMIOLOGY

Incidence

In the year 2002, it is estimated that 53,600 new cases of CMM, and between 20,000 and 40,000 new cases of melanoma in situ, were diagnosed.[2] The overall incidence of CMM is increasing at the disturbing rate of 5% per year. In 1935, the estimated lifetime risk of developing CMM was 1 in 1500; in 2001, estimates were that 1 in 75 Americans will develop CMM.[3] This increase is greater than the increase in any other cancer among men and is second only to the increase in lung cancer among women (Fig. 8–1).[2]

Primary melanoma of the head and neck accounts for approximately 25% to 30% of all melanomas, despite the fact that the head and neck represents only 9% of the total surface area of the body.[4] This predilection for the head and neck can be attributed to multiple factors, including sun exposure and regional variations in the distribution of melanocytes in the skin: The melanocytic content in the head and neck is two to three times higher than it is in other anatomic sites.[5]

Mortality

The number of deaths from melanoma continues to increase as well, with an estimated 7400 persons dying from CMM in the United States in 2002.[2] This represents approximately a 2% annual increase in mortality since 1960. This increase, however, appears to be due in large part to the overall increase in incidence of the disease. Examination of the survival rates over the past few decades reveals that the survival of patients diagnosed with CMM is improving. The 5-year cancer-related survival rates have increased by nearly 10% over the past 20 years—from 80% to 88%[2]—largely owing to earlier detection, resulting in the treatment of earlier-stage disease. Unfortunately, despite advances made in the management of this disease, survival rates with more advanced disease have not improved.

ETIOLOGY AND RISK FACTORS

Sun Exposure

The most important predisposing factor in the development of melanoma is exposure to sunlight. Evidence for this comes from site-specific incidence rates for melanoma. Investigators have shown that incidence rates are higher for exposed body parts, such as the face, neck, and upper back, than they are for nonexposed body parts.[6] In addition, epidemiologic studies have indicated that excessive lifetime exposure to sunlight, intermittent exposure to sunlight, and a history of sunburn are risk factors for the development of CMM. Many investigators currently believe that intermittent acute exposure is more damaging than cumulative exposure and that early exposures during childhood or adolescence, including blistering sunburn, may be particularly important.[7]

Ultraviolet B radiation (UV B; 280–320 nm) has long been thought to be the most critical element of sunlight in the formation of CMM. However, recent evidence indicates that ultraviolet A (UV A; 320–400 nm) and even visible-light radiation may also play a role.[8] At this time, no good evidence exists to pinpoint the effective UV wavelength responsible for the initiation and promotion of CMM.

Because of the role played by sunlight exposure in the development of CMM, much interest has centered on prevention strategies using sunscreens. Epidemiologic evidence has shown that sunscreens can be effective in the prevention of CMM.[9] However, there is also compelling evidence that they are not. Results from a European case-control study[10] and

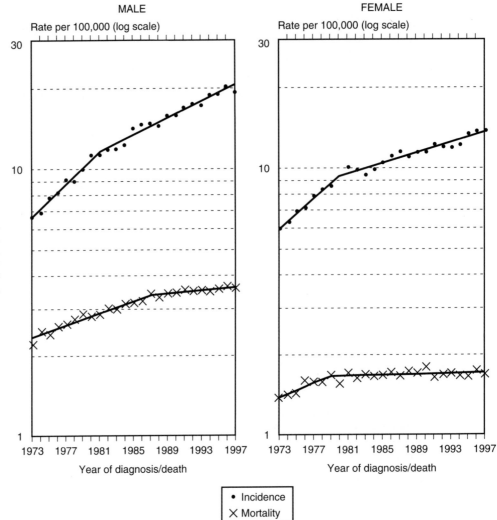

FIGURE 8–1 Incidence and mortality rates, by sex. (From The Surveillance, Epidemiology, and End Results (SEER) Program of the National Cancer Institute, Cancer Statistics Review 1973–1997.)

from one animal study[11] suggest that sunscreens may not protect against CMM. There are several explanations for this counterintuitive finding. First, sunscreens were developed to prevent (or at least delay) the development of sunburn, the body's alarm against overexposure. In doing so, they may be promoting a "safe" feeling among users, resulting in longer exposure to sunlight. Second, most sunscreens are effective in reducing UV B but not UV A or visible-spectrum radiation. As has been noted previously, exposure to these forms of radiation is now believed to be important in the development of CMM.

Despite these equivocal data, sun protection measures in the form of sunscreens, protective clothing and hats, and a general decrease in daily exposure, especially between the hours of 10 AM and 2 PM, are generally felt to be effectively preventive. In fact, the experience in Australia has shown that through education to promote public awareness, the incidence of CMM can decrease and melanomas that do develop can be diagnosed earlier.[12]

Precursor Lesions

A majority of patients with head and neck melanoma have a history of a preexisting pigmented lesion. In an early report,

one third of melanomas were found to have arisen in congenital nevi, one third in nevi present longer than 5 years, and one third in newly acquired nevi (nevi present <5 years).[13] A more recent report has shown that 81% of patients with CMM noticed a change in a preexisting lesion.[14]

At least three types of lesions are known to be precursors to CMM (Fig. 8–2). *Congenital nevi* are present at birth. Patients with large congenital nevi (i.e., >20 cm) have a lifetime risk of developing CMM of between 5% and 20%.[15] *Dysplastic nevi* may occur sporadically or as part of a familial syndrome (dysplastic nevus syndrome [DNS]). The lifetime risk of CMM in those with the sporadic form is unknown, but the risk in those with DNS is felt to be nearly 100%.[15] *Lentigo maligna* lesions are considered a preinvasive phase of lentigo maligna melanoma that frequently occurs on the face or neck. The rate of progression of lentigo maligna to melanoma is between 5% and 33%.[16]

Several pigmented cutaneous lesions have been associated with CMM, either because they were previously thought to be precursor lesions or because they mimic CMM in appearance (Fig. 8–3). *Acquired melanocytic nevi* typically are small (<1 cm) and relatively evenly colored. These benign lesions are most commonly tan to brown, but

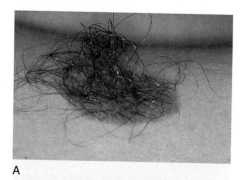

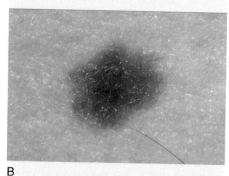

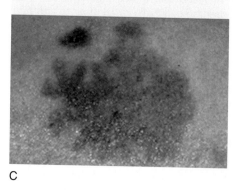

FIGURE 8-2 Precursor lesions. Known precursor lesions to CMM include congenital nevi (*A*), dysplastic nevi (*B*), and lentigo maligna (*C*). (Images courtesy of Department of Dermatology, University of Erlangen, Erlangen, Germany. Used with permission.)

coloration can be quite variable. *Spitz nevi* represent a distinctive variant of melanocytic nevus that is also benign. Many exhibit considerable vascular ectasia and thus may mimic hemangiomas. *Blue nevi* are a form of melanocytic nevi that are often heavily pigmented. They often appear to be nodular and therefore arouse considerable suspicion despite being benign. *Seborrheic keratoses* typically appear as light brown areas on the skin that appear to be "stuck on." As they mature, they often become darkly pigmented; however, they are benign and require no treatment. *Pigmented basal cell carcinoma* often has the color and contour of CMM; however, it does not display the aggressive characteristics of the lesion it mimics. Although these lesions are usually diagnosed clinically, biopsy of any suspicious lesion is recommended, to rule out CMM.

Patient Characteristics

Indirect evidence exists that certain phenotypic characteristics increase the risk that a patient will develop CMM. These include blue or green eyes, blond or red hair, a fair complexion, a freckling pattern, and an inability to tan.[17] Rigel[18] used multivariate analysis to identify six independent risk factors for CMM, including family history, blond or red hair, freckling of the upper back, history of three or more blistering sunburns before age 20 years, history of 3 or more years at an outdoor job as a teenager, and the presence of actinic keratoses. Persons with one or two of these risk factors had a 3.5-fold increased risk of developing CMM, whereas those with three or more factors had a 20-fold increased risk.[18]

Genetics

Familial Melanoma/Dysplastic Nevus Syndrome (FM/DNS)

The familial clustering of melanoma in association with clinically atypical moles was independently reported by Clark and associates[19] as the B-K mole syndrome, and by Lynch and colleagues[20] as the familial atypical multiple mole and melanoma (FAMMM) syndrome in 1978. Further studies by Clark and coworkers demonstrated that members of FM/DNS families have a lifetime risk of developing melanoma that approaches 100%.[21]

Several groups have performed linkage analyses in patients with FM/DNS. An early unconfirmed study that demonstrated a linkage of familial melanoma to chromosome 1p36 was followed by multiple studies that demonstrated a linkage to chromosome 9p21.[22–25] Subsequent investigations demonstrated that the relevant gene at the 9p21 locus was the previously described *p16* gene (also known as *CDKN2A* or *INK4A*). This gene appears to be involved in the development of familial melanoma; studies are exploring its role in the development of sporadic melanoma.

Xeroderma Pigmentosum

Another hereditary syndrome that predisposes to skin cancer is xeroderma pigmentosum (XP). This rare autosomal recessive disease leads to a risk of skin cancer that is approximately 1000 times that of the general population.[25] Clinical features of XP include the early onset of freckling (usually by age 2 years) and multiple skin cancers, including basal cell carcinoma, squamous cell carcinoma, and melanoma. Skin cancer in these patients often occurs before the age of 10 years.[26]

Patients with XP are hypersensitive to the sun, and skin cells from these patients exhibit both increased mutagenesis and decreased survival after exposure to UV radiation. We now know that most cases of XP are the result of a heterogeneous group of defects in nucleotide excision repair.[27] The high incidence of cutaneous cancers in XP patients supports an important role for UV-induced DNA damage in the pathogenesis of all three types of skin cancer.

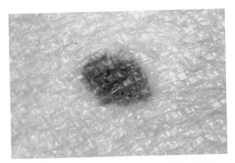

A

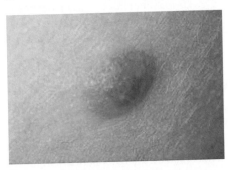

B

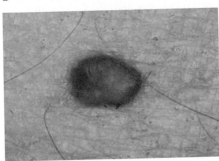

C

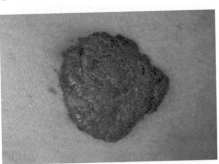

D

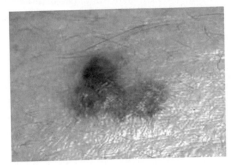

E

FIGURE 8–3 Lesions that may mimic melanoma. Lesions that have the same general appearance as CMM include melanocytic nevi (*A*), Spitz nevi (*B*), blue nevi (*C*), seborrheic keratoses (*D*), and pigmented basal cell carcinoma (*E*). (Images courtesy of Department of Dermatology, University of Erlangen, Erlangen, Germany. Used with permission.)

Sporadic Melanoma

As with most cancers, CMM is caused by a complex interplay of environmental factors (e.g., sun exposure) and genetic events (e.g., mutations, deletions) that either causes or allows the development of melanoma. Some of the molecular events involved in the pathogenesis and progression of melanoma are now coming to light and are discussed in the following paragraphs.

***INK4* Gene Family.** The *INK4* (INhibitors of CDK4) family of genes consists of several proteins—$p15^{INK4B}$, $p16^{INK4A}$, $p18^{INK4C}$, and $p19^{INK4D}$—that appear to act mainly on the G1 phase in the cell cycle. By far, the most studied of this gene family is *CDKN2A*. Independent studies of *CDKN2A* revealed that it was important in inhibiting cells from entering the cell cycle by binding to and inhibiting the enzyme cyclin-dependent kinase 4 (CDK4), which is important in enabling cells to pass through the cell cycle.[28, 29] Alterations in *CDKN2A* have been shown to be important in the pathogenesis of melanoma, with up to 61% of melanoma cell lines and 28% of melanoma tissue samples showing *CDKN2A* inactivation.[30] Various mechanisms of *CDKN2A* inactivation appear to be responsible, including homozygous deletion, point mutation, and promoter methylation. In addition, further studies have indicated that *CDKN2A* is affected early in the development of CMM[31] and that melanoma patients with *CDKN2A* alterations appear to have a worse prognosis than those without *CDKN2A* alterations.[32]

p21. The *CDKN2A* family consists of *p21, p27,* and *p57. p21* was one of the first CDK inhibitors identified.[33] It was found by several different laboratories and thus has multiple names, including WAF1, CIP1, SDI1, and mda-6. *p27* and *p57* are also known as KIP1 and KIP2. This family is known to have a wide variety of inhibitory effects on cyclin-dependent kinases (CDKs). Cells with *p21* alterations can evade cell-cycle arrest in response to DNA damage. In melanoma, *p21* appears to be infrequently affected; however, *p27* alterations appear in 72% of thick melanomas when compared with noninvasive lesions.[34] In addition, in cell culture experiments, *p27* levels are inversely related to anchorage-dependent growth, suggesting a role in melanoma invasion and metastasis.[35]

Retinoblastoma Pathway. The retinoblastoma (*RB*) gene and its protein product (pRB) have been called the gateway to the cell cycle. In its active form, pRB prevents progression through the cell cycle by binding to and inactivating the transcription factor E2F, which is vital to the expression of other genes required for DNA synthesis.[36] Various cyclin/CDK combinations are able to inactivate pRB via the process of phosphorylation. When it is phosphorylated, pRB releases E2F, leading to the transcription of genes critical for progression of cells from the G1 to the

S-phase of the cell cycle.[36] This sequence of events initiates the DNA synthesis phase of the cell cycle.

Because of the critical role it plays in cell-cycle initiation, *RB* has been intensively studied in various tumor types, including melanoma. Interestingly, the *RB* gene is rarely mutated in melanoma; however, it is frequently inactivated through phosphorylation, allowing release of E2F.[37, 38] This allows constitutive upregulation of E2F activity and subsequent deregulated cellular proliferation.

***TP53* Gene.** The most intensely studied gene involved in carcinogenesis is a tumor suppressor gene called *TP53* (formerly *p53*). The *TP53* locus is the most commonly mutated locus in human cancers.[39] Although the mechanism of action of *TP53* occurs through the regulation of gene transcription, its biologic role is to protect cells from DNA damage caused by radiation, chemical carcinogens, or other mechanisms. *TP53* does this by arresting the cell cycle so that DNA repair can occur, or by inducing apoptosis.[40, 41]

The role of *TP53* in the development of melanoma is controversial. Less than 25% of melanomas harbor mutations in the *TP53* gene[42]; however, overexpression of TP53 protein is common in melanoma.[43] Melanomas in which TP53 is overexpressed appear to be associated with a more aggressive phenotype.[44]

***PTEN* Gene.** The phosphatase and tensin homologue (*PTEN*) gene is a protein phosphatase that is important in the development of Cowden disease and hamartomas. It acts as an intracellular phosphatase that regulates the G1 cell-cycle checkpoint by blocking the phosphatidylinositol-3-kinase (PI3-K) pathway.[45] *PTEN* has been found to be mutated in up to 44% of primary melanomas and 58% of metastatic melanomas.[46] In addition, a recent study has shown that overexpression of *PTEN* inhibited the tumorigenicity of B16F10 melanoma cells in culture and also inhibited the ability of these cells to metastasize in an animal model.[47] These results suggest that mutation and deletion of *PTEN/MMAC1* may contribute to the development and progression of malignant melanoma.

RAS. The prototypic oncogene is the *RAS* oncogene. The *RAS* gene and its protein product are involved in a complex cascade of signals from the cell surface to the nucleus that activate cellular growth. *RAS* exerts its effects through various target proteins, such as the mitogen-activated protein kinase and phosphatidylinositol-3-kinase cascades, which are important in the activation of gene transcription and cell proliferation.[48] Mutated forms of *RAS* commonly cause constitutive activation of the protein, thus turning on the cell's growth machinery and allowing uncontrolled proliferation and survival.

Activating *RAS* mutations have been shown to lead to enhanced proliferation, survival, and migration of melanoma cells.[49] In addition, in vitro animal models have shown that *RAS* is vital for the development and progression of melanoma and that downregulation of *RAS* resulted in the regression of primary and explanted tumors.[50] These data indicate an important role for *RAS* in the pathogenesis of melanoma.

PTKs. Tyrosine phosphorylation is an important component of intracellular pathways that has diverse and crucial functions, including proliferation, survival, death, differentiation, migration, and attachment.[51] Protein phosphorylation is regulated by the balance between the activities of protein tyrosine kinases (PTKs) and protein tyrosine phosphatases. A number of PTKs are encoded by oncogenes and are thus strongly implicated in cancer. In melanoma cells, PTKs are overexpressed up to 90% of the time.[52] Therefore, PTKs are likely to play a role in melanoma genesis and progression; however, their precise function has yet to be defined.

Several other genes have been implicated in the ability of melanoma cells to invade and metastasize. These include integrins, *Nm-23*, fibroblast growth factor, and transforming growth factor-β_2 (TGF-β_2); however, a detailed discussion of these genes is beyond the scope of this chapter.

PATHOLOGY

Lentigo Maligna Melanoma

Lentigo maligna melanoma is the least common subtype of melanoma, accounting for 5% to 10% of all cases (Fig. 8–4). Its defining feature is a prolonged radial growth phase that may last for decades. These tumors are therefore very slow to invade. The neoplastic melanocytes tend to remain at the dermo-epidermal junction, and intraepithelial growth extends along hair follicles and ducts of the sweat glands. Invasion into the papillary dermis is required for differentiation of lentigo maligna melanoma from lentigo maligna.

Superficial Spreading Melanoma

Superficial spreading melanoma is the most common subtype of melanoma, accounting for 75% of cases (see Fig. 8–4). It is characterized by an initial radial growth phase; however, a vertical growth phase eventually develops, often heralded by ulceration and bleeding. The melanoma cells are uniform and form aggregates in all levels of the epidermis. The distinctive feature of this form of melanoma is that the tumor cells, although atypical, have a very uniform appearance.

Nodular Melanoma

Approximately 10% to 15% of patients with melanoma have the nodular subtype (see Fig. 8–4). This is characterized by a complete lack of radial growth and an early vertical growth phase. These melanomas are invasive almost from their onset.

Acral Lentiginous Melanoma

Acral lentiginous melanoma is found predominantly on the palms and soles. Uniformly large neoplastic cells, located in the basal layer, that have heavily pigmented dendritic processes characterize this subtype.

Desmoplastic Melanoma

Desmoplastic melanomas are characterized by a dermal population of spindle cells among a fibrous stroma, a pattern that has been likened to "schools of fish." These lesions often are not pigmented; they often infiltrate and expand nerves and may show neuron-like differentiation. In these instances, the term *neurotropic melanoma* is often used.

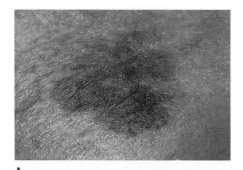

A

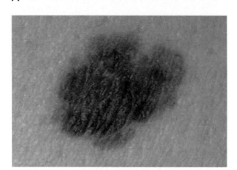

B

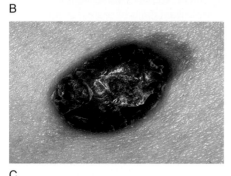

C

FIGURE 8–4 Pathologic types of melanoma found in the head and neck. Types of melanoma found in the head and neck include lentigo maligna melanoma (*A*), superficial spreading melanoma (*B*), and nodular melanoma (*C*). (Images courtesy of Department of Dermatology, University of Erlangen, Erlangen, Germany. Used with permission.)

This propensity to spread perineurally must be considered during the evaluation and treatment of these lesions.[53]

◘ DIAGNOSTIC EVALUATION

History

Early recognition and diagnosis are the keys to effective treatment of malignant melanoma. Most melanomas are detected by the patient or by a family member, with only 25% being detected by physicians.[54] The most common presenting signs are growth or change in color of a preexisting lesion. Other signs include bleeding, itching, ulceration, and pain. Unfortunately, these are usually late signs of CMM,

occurring much more frequently in thick melanomas than in thin ones. It is important to ask patients about a family history of melanoma, about overall sun exposure, and about their history of sunburn.

Physical Examination

An assessment of the total number and types of pigmented moles present is important. Specifically, one should search for congenital nevi, dysplastic nevi, and lentigo malignas. When examining lesions, one should use a bright light and a magnifying glass to assess their size, color, border, and surface characteristics. Hallmarks of melanoma include (1) variation in color, (2) an irregular raised surface, (3) an irregular border, and (4) ulceration. These features are usually distinct from those seen in benign nevi.

ABCD Checklist

The ABCD checklist has been used by clinicians to identify lesions that could potentially be malignant.[55] This checklist takes into account the following clinical factors:

Asymmetry—Uneven growth rates cause asymmetrical growth patterns.

Border irregularities—Lesions exhibiting border irregularities are more likely to be melanomas.

Color variegation—Differential coloring and shading is indicative of malignant potential.

Diameter—Any increase in the diameter of a lesion, or a diameter > 6 mm should raise suspicion.

Each of these factors has been shown to predict malignant lesions, but the strongest of them is border irregularity.[56] Any lesion believed to be suspicious according to these criteria should be investigated by biopsy.

Biopsy

All suspicious cutaneous lesions should undergo biopsy by a method that will confirm the diagnosis and provide accurate staging criteria and will not interfere with subsequent resection and reconstructive efforts should they be required. Several methods of biopsy are available to clinicians, and most have at least some role in the diagnosis of CMM.

If the lesion is small and the location is amenable, we recommend performing an *excisional biopsy* with 1- to 2-mm margins. This allows optimal pathologic evaluation of the entire lesion without the worry of a misdiagnosis secondary to nonrepresentative tissue. In addition, evidence suggests that patients who have had an excisional biopsy, as opposed to other types of biopsy, have a better overall survival rate.[57] It does not appear that excisional biopsy affects subsequent staging procedures such as lymphoscintigraphy. However, it must be kept in mind that the wide local excision (WLE) of lesions before lymphoscintigraphy is performed may alter lymphatic drainage patterns, thus making it difficult for the clinician to accurately identify sentinel nodes and drainage basins.[58]

If the lesion is large or is located in an area that would not permit excisional biopsy without significant disfigurement, we recommend an *incisional biopsy* through the thickest part of the tumor. *Punch biopsies*, if they encompass the entire

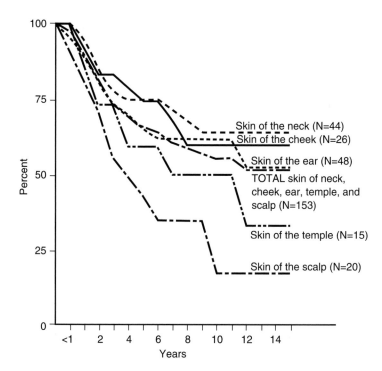

FIGURE 8–5 Actuarial survival rates for melanoma of the head and neck by primary site. (Reprinted from Am J Surg. v. 132: Ames FC, Sugarbaker EJ, Ballantyne AJ: Analysis of survival and disease control in stage I melanoma of the head and neck, pp 484–489, 1976, with permission from "Excerpta Medica, Inc".)

thickness of the lesion, are often sufficient and can easily be performed in the clinic or office. *Needle* and *shave biopsies* of primary lesions are discouraged because they do not adequately assess thickness, which is critical to proper treatment planning. Needle biopsies, however, may be useful for assessment of suspicious lymph nodes or distant metastasis

STAGING

Anatomic Location of the Primary Tumor

Multiple studies have reported the prognostic significance of anatomic site of the primary for survival rates. In general, patients with a primary melanoma in the head and neck are thought to have a worse prognosis than patients with tumors on the extremities.[59] Several studies have reported that tumors arising in the so-called BANS region (upper *b*ack, upper *a*rm, posterior *n*eck, and *s*calp) have worse survival rates than those in non-BANS regions, although this remains controversial.[60, 61]

A review from the M.D. Anderson Cancer Center showed that patients with a lesion located on the scalp do significantly worse than patients with a lesion on the ear, face, or neck (Fig. 8–5).[62] This finding has been corroborated by other investigators.[63, 64]

Depth of Invasion

The first significant attempts at staging of melanoma made no attempt to classify tumors according to depth of invasion, which is the criterion now believed to be the most important prognostic factor in stage I and II tumors. During the 1960s, several groups began to discover the importance of depth of invasion, culminating in the landmark histologic

staging system of Clark,[65] who defined levels of invasion, and Breslow,[66] who demonstrated the importance of tumor thickness (Table 8–1). It is currently believed that Breslow thickness represents a more powerful prognostic factor than do Clark levels; however, both remain widely used in the literature and in clinical practice.

American Joint Council on Cancer (AJCC) Staging

The AJCC staging system for CMM was first published in 1978 and has undergone several changes since that time in attempts to incorporate current knowledge into each iteration. It is based on the tumor, node, metastasis (TNM) classification and incorporates Breslow thickness and Clark levels into the primary tumor stages.

TABLE 8–1 Histopathologic Staging Systems— Clark Levels and Breslow Thickness

Clark Levels

Level I:	Lesions involving only the epidermis (in situ melanoma); not an invasive lesion
Level II:	Invasion of the papillary dermis but does not reach the papillary-reticular dermal interface
Level III:	Invasion fills and expands the papillary dermis but does not penetrate the reticular dermis
Level IV:	Invasion into the reticular dermis but not into the subcutaneous tissue
Level V:	Invasion through the reticular dermis into the subcutaneous tissue

Breslow Thickness

Stage I:	0.75 mm or less
Stage II:	0.76 mm to 1.50 mm
Stage III:	1.51 mm to 4.0 mm
Stage IV:	4.1 mm or greater

TABLE 8-2 Definition of TNM for Melanoma

Primary Tumor (T)

TX	Primary tumor cannot be assessed (e.g., shave biopsy or regressed melanoma)
T0	No evidence of primary tumor
Tis	Melanoma in situ
T1	Melanoma ≤ 1.0 mm in thickness with or without ulceration
T1a	Melanoma ≤ 1.0 mm in thickness and level II or III, no ulceration
T1b	Melanoma ≤ 1.0 mm in thickness and level IV or V or with ulceration
T2	Melanoma 1.01–2.0 mm in thickness with or without ulceration
T2a	Melanoma 1.01–2.0 mm in thickness, no ulceration
T2b	Melanoma 1.01–2.0 mm in thickness, with ulceration
T3	Melanoma 2.01–4.0 mm in thickness, with or without ulceration
T3a	Melanoma 2.01–4.0 mm in thickness, no ulceration
T3b	Melanoma 2.01–4.0 mm in thickness, with ulceration
T4	Melanoma greaterthan 4.0 mm in thickness with or without ulceration
T4a	Melanoma > 4.0 mm in thickness, no ulceration
T4b	Melanoma > 4.0 mm in thickness, with ulceration

Regional Lymph Nodes (N)

NX	Regional lymph nodes cannot be assessed
N0	No regional lymph node metastasis
N1	Metastasis in one lymph node
N1a	Clinically occult (microscopic) metastasis
N1b	Clinically apparent (macroscopic) metastasis
N2	Metastasis in two to three regional nodes or intra-lymphatic regional metastasis without nodal metastases
N2a	Clinically occult (microscopic) metastasis
N2b	Clinically apparent (macroscopic) metastasis
N2c	Satellite or in-transit metastasis *without* nodal metastasis
N3	Metastasis in four or more regional nodes, or matted metastatic nodes, or in-transit metastasis or satellite(s) *with* metastasis in regional node(s)

Distant Metastasis (M)

MX	Distant metastasis cannot be assessed
M0	No distant metastasis
M1	Distant metastasis
M1a	Metastasis to skin, subcutaneous tissues or distant lymph nodes
M1b	Metastasis to lung
M1c	Metastasis to all other visceral sites or distant metastasis at any site associated with an elevated serum lactic dehydrogenase (LDH)

Clinical Stage Grouping

Stage 0	Tis	N0	M0
Stage IA	T1a	N0	M0
Stage IB	T1b	N0	M0
	T2a	N0	M0
Stage IIA	T2b	N0	M0
	T3a	N0	M0
Stage IIB	T3b	N0	M0
	T4a	N0	M0
Stage IIC	T4b	N0	M0
Stage III	Any T	N1	M0
	Any T	N2	M0
	Any T	N3	M0
Stage IV	Any T	Any N	M1

Note: Clinical staging includes microstaging of the primary melanoma and clinical/radiological evaluation for metastases. By convention, it should be used after complete excision of the primary melanoma with clinical assessment for regional and distant metastases.

Pathologic Stage Grouping

Stage 0	Tis	N0	M0
Stage IA	T1a	N0	M0
Stage IB	T1b	N0	M0
	T2a	N0	M0
Stage IIA	T2b	N0	M0
	T3a	N0	M0
Stage IIB	T3b	N0	M0
	T4a	N0	M0
Stage IIC	T4b	N0	M0
Stage IIIA	T1–4a	N1a	M0
	T1–4a	N2a	M0
Stage IIIB	T1–4b	N1a	M0
	T1–4b	N2a	M0
	T1–4a	N1b	M0
	T1–4a	N2b	M0
	T1–4a/b	N2c	M0
Stage IIIC	T1–4b	N1b	M0
	T1–4b	N2b	M0
	Any T	N3	M0
Stage IV	Any T	Any N	M1

Note: Pathologic staging includes mirostaging of the primary melanoma and pathologic information about the regional lymph nodes after partial or complete lymphadenectomy. Pathologic Stage 0 or Stage IA patients are the exception; they do not require pathologic evaluation of their lymph nodes.

Used with the permission of the American Joint Committee on Cancer (AJCC), Chicago, Illinois. The original source for this material is the *AJCC Cancer Staging Manual, Sixth Edition* (2002) published by Springer-Verlag New York, *www.springer-ny.com.*

The staging system was revised in 1997 (Table 8–2)[67]; however, research into melanoma continued and new areas of controversy surfaced, prompting investigators at the M.D. Anderson Cancer Center to call for a reappraisal of the 1997 staging system.[68] First, the 1997 system was not using the optimal cut-offs for tumor thickness. Second, multiple studies have shown that ulceration is a powerful prognostic indicator, yet it is not employed in the 1997 system. Third, satellites, in-transit metastases, and local recurrences are afforded different levels of importance in the 1997 staging system yet probably have similar outcomes. Fourth, it is clear that the number of positive nodes is much more important than the size of the nodes involved.

Therefore, on the basis of these considerations, Buzaid and associates suggested several changes in the 1997 staging system.[68] These include the following:

1. Cut-offs for tumor thickness should be 1.0, 2.0, and 4.0 mm. These provide a simpler and more statistically powerful separation than do the currently used cut-offs.
2. Tumor ulceration should be incorporated into the staging system because it is a powerful independent prognostic factor.
3. Patients with nodal, in-transit, and satellite metastases and local recurrences have similar prognoses and should be grouped together for staging purposes in a new category called "regional skin/subcutaneous metastases."
4. The number of positive nodes should replace nodal size in the staging system.

In addition, within the new staging system, the sites of distant metastases and the presence of elevated serum lactic dehydrogenase (LDH) are used in the M category. Also, a new convention for defining clinical and pathologic staging has been added to take into account the staging information gained from intraoperative lymphatic mapping and sentinel node biopsy.[69] Table 8–2 shows the official 2002 AJCC staging system and highlights some of the changes that have been instituted. It is hoped that this updated staging classification will allow better stratification of patients and will provide better treatment guidelines and that it will assist in the development of useful experimental protocols.

Pretreatment Evaluation by Stage

In the absence of clinical evidence of any regional metastasis, further workup will depend on the stage of the primary tumor, which is best determined by the depth of invasion. Each patient should be evaluated individually. Table 8–3 presents the general guidelines followed at the M.D. Anderson Cancer Center. (*Note:* These diagnostic and treatment algorithms are available at www.mdanderson.org. Similar guidelines are available from the National Comprehensive Cancer Network at www.nccn.org and the National Cancer Institute at www.nci.nih.gov.)

In situ/Clark level I lesions require no further workup and are effectively treated with WLE. In the asymptomatic patient with *stage I or II melanoma,* a metastatic screen in the form of an ultrasound (US) of the neck, LDH, and a chest radiograph (CXR) is performed. For lesions of intermediate thickness, for thin lesions that are ulcerated, or for lesions that extend into Clark's level IV, consideration should be given to preoperative lymphoscintigraphy, especially if elective lymph node dissection is part of the treatment plan. This is based on data that reveal a 37% discordancy rate between the suspected site of drainage and the site identified by lymphoscintigraphy.[70] Thick lesions (>4 mm) or those that are locally recurrent are considered to be at high risk for distant metastasis; for these, therefore, consideration should be given to a metastatic imaging workup (i.e., computed tomography [CT] of the chest, abdomen, and pelvis, and magnetic resonance imaging [MRI] of the brain). All patients with clinically evident *regional disease (stage III)* require imaging of the cervical lymphatics as well as metastatic screening. Most will undergo a CT or ultrasound of the head and neck, CXR, and LDH. Selective metastatic imaging should be performed for patients with signs or symptoms of metastatic disease. Finally, all patients with known *systemic disease (stage IV)* require a full metastatic workup, including CXR; LDH; CT or ultrasound of the head and neck; CT of the chest, abdomen, and pelvis; and MRI of the brain.

Several newer modalities are currently being evaluated for use in melanoma patients, with the most studied technique being positron emission tomography (PET). Although there is hope that PET may be effective in detecting regional and metastatic lesions, its current role in the evaluation and follow-up of melanoma patients remains controversial. A meta-analysis revealed a sensitivity and specificity of 79% and 86%, respectively, when PET was used to evaluate regional and distant metastasis in melanoma patients.[71] With respect to detection of occult *regional* metastatic disease, current data suggest that PET is inferior to sentinel lymph node biopsy. This is best illustrated by Acland and colleagues,[72] who showed that PET was unable to detect any regional metastases in 14 patients with regional metastases verified by sentinel node biopsy. Wagner and colleagues[73] corroborated these data by showing that PET detected only 16% of patients with regional nodal metastasis verified by sentinel node biopsy. However, PET does appear to have a role in the detection of *distant* metastatic disease and may be superior to current modalities such as CT, MRI, and ultrasonography.[74–76] Thus, currently we feel that PET has a limited role in the initial evaluation of patients with early-stage disease, but it may have an increasing role in the evaluation of patients with advanced-stage disease.

◩ MANAGEMENT

General Treatment Options

Surgery

SURGERY FOR PRIMARY DISEASE

Surgery is generally accepted as the primary treatment modality for CMM. In almost every patient, complete surgical excision of the primary tumor is mandatory. The size of the margins that should be taken around the primary tumor has been debated for most of the past century. Recent studies have indicated that for melanomas of intermediate thickness, 2-cm margins are sufficient; for thinner melanomas, 1-cm margins result in equivalent local control and survival.[77, 78] These findings have been corroborated after long-term follow-up, with the additional finding that ulceration at the primary site is a risk factor for local recurrence, indicating that greater care should be taken when these lesions are excised.[79]

Surgeons must understand, however, that these recommendations are derived from studies of truncal and extremity melanoma, and that in the head and neck, one does not always have the luxury of being able to take 1- to 2-cm margins without imposing significant functional disability and/or cosmetic deformity. In addition, the surgeon must think in three dimensions, that is, how to best obtain a deep margin as well as lateral margins. This issue is largely site specific. In the scalp, WLE is usually taken down to the periosteum, unless the deep portion of the tumor encroaches on this, in which case resection of the periosteum, resection of the outer table of the cranium, or even resection of the full thickness of the cranial bone may be necessary. On the face, WLE is usually taken to the depth of the facial mimetic musculature, but

TABLE 8–3 Recommendations for Workup, on the Basis of Stage

Stage	Workup
Melanoma in situ	None
Stage I or II	CXR, LDH
Stage I or II with ulceration or T3	CXR, LDH Consider lymphoscintigraphy
T4 or recurrent primary	CXR, LDH Consider metastatic imaging
Stage III	CXR, LDH, CT, or ultrasound of the neck Consider metastatic imaging
Stage IV	CXR, LDH, metastatic imaging

CT, computed tomography; CXR, chest radiography; LDH, lactate dehydrogenase.

again resection of muscle and facial bones may be required as needed for adequate margins. Over the parotid, WLE is usually taken to the level of the parotid-masseteric fascia. If deeper resections are required, formal parotidectomy with facial nerve dissection or sacrifice of the nerve is required. On the ear, superficial tumors may be amenable to WLE taken to the level of the perichondrium; however, owing to the thin nature of the skin over the ear, partial or total auriculectomy is often required. If the external auditory canal is involved, more complex procedures such as lateral temporal bone resection may be required to ensure adequate margins of resection.

When tissue conservation is important, intraoperative frozen section analysis may be helpful; however, this is a controversial topic even among pathologists. In the hands of experienced pathologists, frozen section analysis of margins appears to have adequate sensitivity and specificity[80]; however, the risk of a false-negative report is very real, and such an event can be catastrophic. Thus, frozen section analysis should be used judiciously and only by surgeons and pathologists who are experienced and comfortable with it.

Lastly, the use of Mohs' micrographic surgery in the treatment of CMM has been reported[81]; however, its efficacy has not been widely tested, and we cannot recommend this modality at this time.

SURGERY FOR REGIONAL DISEASE

The parotid and cervical lymphatics are the most common sites of spread for CMM of the head and neck. It is well accepted that the clinically positive neck requires treatment. It is important to remember that in these patients, all intervening lymphatics between the primary site and the node(s) must be addressed. Thus, if a patient presents with a primary melanoma on the temple, anterior scalp, or face, along with a clinically positive node in level II, a parotidectomy must be performed along with the neck dissection. For primary sites on the chin or neck, a parotidectomy is probably not required. For posterior scalp lesions, it is important that the postauricular and suboccipital nodes be addressed. The type of neck dissection must be tailored to the disease; however, a modified radical neck dissection or a selective neck dissection is usually sufficient.[82]

What should be done with the clinically N0 neck is less clear. Patients with stage I disease have a relatively low rate of occult metastasis; however, a substantial percentage of patients with stage II disease will harbor occult regional metastasis. Thus, elective treatment of the neck is often considered in this population. Currently, prospective data do not support the use of any type of elective neck treatment for improving either locoregional control or overall survival.

The most commonly employed elective treatment of the neck is *elective neck dissection (END)*. If END is undertaken, it should be based on a sound knowledge of the pathways of lymphatic spread (Fig. 8–6). In general, tumors arising on the scalp and forehead anterior to a line drawn through the external auditory canal most commonly spread to the parotid/periparotid lymph nodes and upper jugular lymph nodes; therefore, a parotidectomy and lateral neck dissection is recommended. Tumors arising on the scalp and occiput posterior to a line drawn through the external auditory canal most commonly spread to the postauricular, suboccipital, and posterior triangle lymph nodes; therefore, a posterolateral neck dissection is recommended.[83] Tumors located anteriorly on the face and neck generally spread

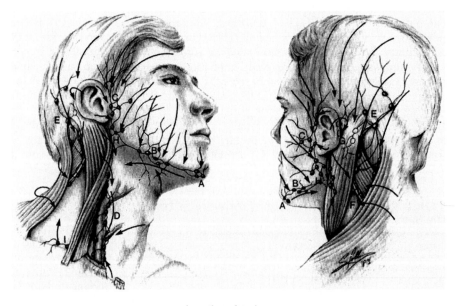

FIGURE 8–6 Predicted patterns of lymphatic drainage from primary sites in the head and neck. (Used with permission from Byers RM: Cervical and parotid node dissection. *In* Balch CM, Houghton AN, Milton GW, et al [eds]: Cutaneous Melanoma, 2nd ed. Philadelphia, JB Lippincott, 1992.)

Location of nodes

A. Submental
B. Submandibular
C. Preauricular
D. Jugular Chain
E. Occipital
F. Posterior Cervical
G. Retroauricular
H. Jugulodigastric
I. Supraclavicular

to the facial, submental, submandibular, and deep cervical nodes; therefore, a supraomohyoid neck dissection is recommended.

A newer option for elective treatment of the neck is *sentinel lymph node biopsy (SLNB)*. The theoretical basis for SLNB is as follows: The first stop along the route of lymphatic drainage from a primary tumor is a limited set of regional lymph nodes. With the use of dyes, radiographic contrast agents, or radioactive tracers, these "sentinel" lymph nodes can be identified and removed. It is thought that close examination of these nodes enables a better decision as to whether more extensive lymphadenectomy should be performed and/or systemic adjuvant therapy offered.

SLNB is a well-accepted procedure in the treatment of truncal and extremity melanoma. It provides clinically useful information for both treatment and prognosis. The results of a multi-institutional study that used lymphatic mapping for patients with stage I and II disease showed that the status of the sentinel nodes was the strongest predictor of disease-free survival[84] (Fig. 8–7). Additional work by this

group of investigators has shown that one of the benefits of this method is that it can focus the pathologist's attention on fewer lymph nodes than are found in an elective neck dissection. This enables a more thorough search for metastases through serial sectioning of lymph nodes or application of molecular methods, thus increasing the sensitivity of detection of metastases.[85, 86] Lastly, SLNB offers clinicians the means of saving a significant proportion of patients the potential morbidity of an elective neck dissection.

Despite its promise, the role of SLNB in the management of CMM of the head and neck has not yet been fully defined. The complexity of lymphatic drainage patterns and the frequent need for removal of sentinel lymph nodes from the parotid gland, thus placing the facial nerve at risk, have made head and neck surgical oncologists slow to adopt this method. Currently, the data from studies of head and neck sites are conflicting. Most studies have shown that sentinel nodes can be identified in about 95% of patients and that the rates of false-negative results are low.[86, 87] However, other studies have found disturbingly high rates of regional

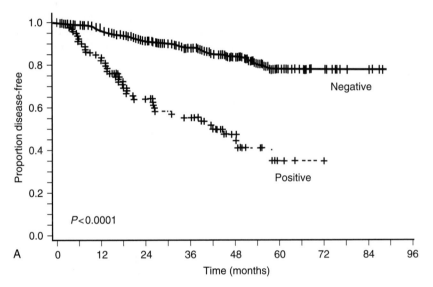

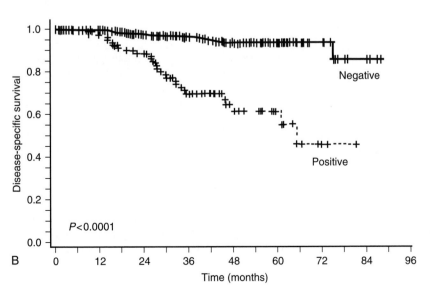

FIGURE 8–7 Disease-free survival and disease-specific survival according to sentinel lymph node status. Kaplan-Meier survival for patients undergoing sentinel lymph node biopsy. *A,* Disease-free survival. *B,* Disease-specific survival. (Used with permission from Gershenwald JE, Thompson W, Mansfield PF, et al: Multi-institutional melanoma lymphatic mapping experience: The prognostic value of sentinel lymph node status in 612 stage I or II melanoma patients. J Clin Oncol 17:976–983, 1999.)

TABLE 8-4 Sentinel Lymph Node Biopsy in Cutaneous Malignant Melanoma of the Head and Neck

Study/Year	Institution	Patients	SLN Identified (%)	Positve SLN (%)	False-Negatives (%)
Morton DL et al/1993[89]	John Wayne Cancer Institute	72	90	15	0
O'Brien CJ et al/1995[88]	Sydney Melanoma Unit	20	96	20	25
Bostick P et al/1995[90]	John Wayne Cancer Institute	117	96	12	0
Wells KE et al/1997[86]	University of South Florida	58	95	11	?
Alex JC et al/1998[91]	University of Vermont	23	96	14	5
Wells KE et al/1999[92]	University of South Florida	28	86	17	7
Jansen L et al/2000[93]	Netherlands Cancer Institute	30	90	28	6
Carlson GW et al/2000[94]	Emory University	58	96	18	21
Maffioli L et al/2000[95]	UO Medicina Nucleare, Milan	17	88	24	0
Wagner JD et al/2000[96]	Indiana University	70	99	17	2
Eicher SA et al/2002[98]	M.D. Anderson Cancer Center	43	98	21	0

SLN, sentinel lymph node.

recurrence in patients with negative results on sentinel node biopsy.[88] In addition, a steep learning curve is associated with the technique, as are potential risks to the facial nerve and other cranial nerves during the biopsy procedure.

Despite these potential shortcomings, many centers have adopted SLNB for CMM of the head and neck and are reporting its efficacy. A summary of recent large trials is presented in Table 8–4.[86, 88–97] The three largest studies, those reported by Bostick and colleagues,[90] Wagner and coworkers,[98] and Wells and associates,[97] have shown that SLNB can be performed 96% to 99% of the time with a combination of blue dye and radiocolloid detection methods. In addition, the percentage of positive SLN ranged from 12% to 17%, and complications rates were low. In all of these studies, false-negative rates had to be inferred from rates of regional recurrence after negative SLNB. Because of differences in follow-up and use of adjuvant treatments, the inferred false-negative rates reported in these studies are somewhat varied, ranging from 0% to 25%. It is unclear from the available studies what the true false-negative rate is with SLNB in the head and neck.

To help answer this question, a prospective trial was performed at the M.D. Anderson Cancer Center to evaluate the efficacy of SLNB in the setting of a comprehensive elective node dissection.[98] In this trial, sentinel nodes are identified, then lymphadenectomy is performed, to evaluate all of the regional nodes with respect to the status of the sentinel node. Current data from the trial indicate, as do other studies, that sentinel lymph nodes can be identified reliably—98% of the time in this study—using intraoperative lymphatic mapping. In addition, in no patients who had negative sentinel nodes was a positive nonsentinel node found in the neck dissection specimen—more evidence that SLNB is associated with a low false-negative rate. However, this technique appears to be complicated by the large number of sentinel lymph nodes found in individual patients (3.6 SLNs per patient), their frequent location in the parotid gland (44% of patients), and their frequent location in multiple levels of the neck (2.2 basins per patient). The authors concluded that these difficulties, which are largely peculiar to the head and neck, might preclude sentinel lymph node biopsy in many patients. In addition, they advocated selective removal of the entire sentinel node basin(s), rather than individual nodes, thus allowing histologic staging of the sentinel node basin with the least morbidity.

The difficulties with multiple sentinel nodes and multiple levels may be largely dependent on the technique and timing of lymphoscintigraphy. A recent study on SLNB in squamous cell carcinoma of the head and neck[99] highlighted the need to apply lymphoscintigraphy in a *dynamic* rather than a *static* mode. The authors emphasize that after accumulation in the SLN, the radiotracer moves to the next lymph node station in a considerable number of patients, giving the impression of more than one SLN in static imaging. Observing the dynamics of lymphoscintigraphy in real time allows the accurate identification of the first echelon node, which by definition is the SLN. This may limit the number and anatomic location of lymph nodes identified as "sentinel." Multiple trials are ongoing; these are required to define the true role of sentinel lymph node biopsy in the treatment of CMM of the head and neck.

SURGERY FOR METASTATIC DISEASE

Surgery for a solitary distant metastasis is sometimes recommended but is beyond the scope of this chapter.

Radiotherapy

Historically, melanoma was considered a radioresistant tumor. However, experience over the past 20 years has clearly shown that different dosimetry and fractionation schemes are required to treat CMM than are used to treat other tumors. With the advent of large dose fractions, significant improvements in locoregional control have been noted with the use of adjuvant radiotherapy.[100]

Data from the M.D. Anderson Cancer Center reveal that 88% locoregional control is possible in patients with stage II and III disease when postoperative radiotherapy is used at a dose of 30 Gy given in five fractions.[101] Specifically, three groups of patients were studied: (1) those who had undergone excision of a stage II primary tumor, (2) those with palpable lymphadenopathy who had undergone WLE and neck dissection, and (3) those with nodal relapse who had undergone neck dissection. In all three groups, the locoregional control rates were higher than in historical controls. In addition, the overall survival rate in patients with

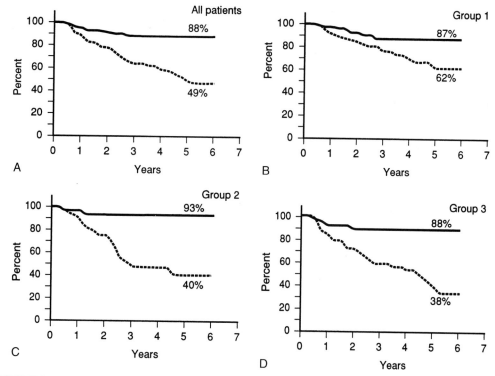

FIGURE 8–8 Locoregional control and survival rates of patients treated with elective or adjuvant radiotherapy. *A*, All patients. *B*, Group 1 = elective irradiation. *C*, Group 2 = adjuvant irradiation after wide local excision plus neck dissection. *D*, Group 3 = irradiation after nodal recurrence. In all cases, the *upper curve* indicates survival with radiation, and the *lower curve* indicates survival of historical controls without radiation. (Redrawn from Ang KK, Peters LH, Webers RS, et al: Postoperative radiotherapy for cutaneous melanoma of the head and neck region. Int J Radiat Oncol Biol Phys 30:795–798, 1994.)

stage II lesions was better than that in historic controls (Fig. 8–8).

Reports have indicated that adjuvant radiotherapy may not be beneficial (one study showed only a 14% regional recurrence rate after neck dissection alone was performed for patients with stage III disease).[102] However, a majority of reports have shown much higher recurrence rates (24%–47%) for patients treated with surgery alone.[103, 104] Therefore, at the M.D. Anderson Cancer Center, postoperative radiotherapy is recommended for all patients with stage II lesions in whom the regional lymphatics are not treated surgically, as well as for patients with pathologically proven nodal disease or nodal recurrence, after the appropriate nodal dissection has been performed. It should be understood, however, that this dosimetry is harmful to nervous tissue and thus cannot be used for lesions near the eye or central nervous system.

Chemotherapy

Chemotherapy traditionally has had two major uses—as adjuvant therapy in high-risk patients and as palliative therapy in patients with stage IV disease. To date, no prospective randomized trials have supported the use of chemotherapy as adjuvant treatment for CMM. Three major randomized trials have been performed using adjuvant chemotherapy after surgical resection.[105–107] Two of them found no difference in disease-free interval or overall survival rate,[106, 107] and the third found a worse overall survival rate with chemotherapy.[107] More commonly, chemotherapy is used to treat patients with metastatic or recurrent disease. In this case, the most active single agent is dacarbazine, which remains the only single agent approved for the treatment of advanced melanoma. Response rates to dacarbazine alone are 10% to 20%. Small, nonsignificant improvements in response rates can be achieved using combination chemotherapy.

Immunotherapy

Because melanoma is the most immunogenic type of solid tumor, it has served as the primary model for immunotherapy, both in the laboratory and in the clinic. Several approaches to enhancing the body's immune system have been examined in patients with CMM, including biologic response modifiers (e.g., interleukins and interferons), immunostimulants, and vaccines. Each of these approaches has shown some promise, but all remain investigational. As is the case with chemotherapy, the main clinical use for these therapies is as adjuvant therapy for high-risk patients and for patients with metastatic or recurrent disease.

Biologic response modifiers have been studied extensively, with interferon-α 2b (IFNα-2b) being the most promising. The results of at least one prospective randomized trial[108] revealed significant improvement in relapse-free and overall survival rates in patients treated with high-dose IFNα-2b as a postoperative adjuvant. A more recent trial, the Eastern Cooperative Oncology Group (ECOG) trial 1690, was performed to verify these results and to assess the efficacy of *low-dose* IFNα-2b.[109] Results showed that *low-dose* IFNα-2b had no efficacy, although as in the first study, an improvement in relapse-free survival was demonstrated in those patients given *high-dose* IFNα-2b. However, unlike in the previous study, no significant difference in overall survival rate was found in ECOG 1690. An interesting note is that this lack of difference in the overall survival rate was due to a significant increase in the survival rate of the observation group in the trial. The authors speculated that this could have been a result of the use of IFNα-2b as salvage therapy in patients who experienced a relapse in this arm of the study.

Other studies have appeared to validate the use of IFNα-2b in high-risk melanoma patients. Specifically, ECOG trial 1694 compared *high-dose* IFNα-2b therapy versus a GM2 ganglioside vaccine. This trial was closed because of the clear superiority of IFNα-2b therapy in terms of both disease-free and overall survival compared with the vaccine arm.[110] Two studies of *low-dose* IFNα-2b in high-risk patients have shown conflicting results. One, a prospective randomized trial conducted by the French Cooperative Group on Melanoma, demonstrated an increased disease-free survival rate and a trend toward better overall survival when *low-dose* IFNα-2b was used after resection of melanomas thicker than 1.5 mm in patients without clinically detectable node metastases.[111] However, the second trial, a multicenter randomized trial conducted by the WHO Melanoma Programme, showed no increase in either disease-free or overall survival in stage III patients treated with *low-dose* IFNα-2b after resection of regional nodes.[112] Thus, at this time, adjuvant IFNα-2b when given in *high doses* appears to improve disease-free survival, but its effect on the overall survival rate of patients with melanoma remains to be elucidated. The role of *low-dose* IFNα-2b therapy is unclear at this time.

The use of immunostimulants such as bacillus Calmette-Guérin, *Corynebacterium parvum,* and levamisole has yielded either conflicting or negative results. It is currently believed that these agents do not play a role in the treatment of CMM.[113]

Melanoma vaccines are among the most widely touted cancer treatments, and dramatic anecdotal responses are frequently described in the lay press. Indeed, many advances in the field of melanoma vaccination have been made during the past decade. As a result, many clinical trials of melanoma vaccines are now under way, including studies on peptide-based vaccines, DNA vaccines, carbohydrate-based vaccines, and antibody-based vaccines. Although the results of several phase II trials have shown feasibility and have suggested efficacy, no phase III trial has yet shown improvement in disease-free survival or overall survival rates in vaccinated patients.[114]

The efficacy of gene therapy is also being studied in melanoma patients. The most promising preliminary results have come from a multi-institutional study using allovectin-7,[115] which is a plasmid that enhances HLA-B7 expression of melanoma, thus making it more susceptible to antitumor immune responses. This study demonstrated that intratumoral administration of allovectin-7 in metastatic melanoma produces responses both in injected lesions and in overall disease.

Biochemotherapy

Because response rates achieved with chemotherapy or immunotherapy alone have been disappointing, attempts have been made to combine the two modalities to achieve higher response and survival rates. Many different combinations have been evaluated. At the M.D. Anderson Cancer Center, trials have usually combined cisplatin, vinblastine, and dacarbazine with interleukin 2 and IFNα-2b. The few prospective randomized trials that have been conducted have documented higher response rates, similar survival rates, and increased toxicity with biochemotherapy, compared with chemotherapy or immunotherapy alone.[116, 117] Several large ongoing trials are further evaluating the potential role of biochemotherapy, both as a postoperative adjuvant treatment and as treatment for systemic disease.

Treatment by Stage

The management of CMM must address the primary tumor, the regional lymphatics, and distant metastasis (if any). As head and neck surgeons, we are able to provide an acceptably high rate of locoregional control; however, many patients, particularly those with stage II disease and higher, will eventually die of distant disease. The treatment guidelines presented in this section are summarized in Table 8–5.

Melanoma In Situ

The recommended treatment for melanoma in situ is surgical excision. Conservative margins (0.5–1.0 cm) are acceptable. No regional or metastatic treatment is required because the risk of metastasis is essentially zero.

TABLE 8–5 Recommendations for Treatment, on the Basis of Stage

Stage	Treatment
I	Primary tumor—WLE
II	Primary tumor—WLE
	Regional lymphatics—Observation vs. END vs. SLNB vs. ENI
III	Primary tumor—WLE
	Regional lymphatics—Neck dissection +/– parotidectomy
	Consider postoperative radiotherapy
	Consider systemic adjuvant therapy trials
IV	Primary tumor—WLE
	Regional lymphatics—Neck dissection +/– parotidectomy if N+
	Metastasis—Site-directed surgery or radiotherapy
	Consider systemic adjuvant therapy trials
	Supportive care

END, elective neck dissection; ENI, elective neck irradiation; N+, node positive; SLNB, sentinel lymph node biopsy; WLE, wide local excision.

Stage I

In patients with stage I melanoma, the primary tumor is treated by wide local excision.[118] As has previously been described, margins of 1 cm are acceptable. The defect can be closed primarily or reconstructed with the use of local flaps or skin grafts. No regional or metastatic treatment is required because the risk of metastasis is very low.

Stage II

In patients with stage II melanoma, the primary tumor is treated by wide local excision. If possible, 2-cm margins are obtained. If 1-cm or smaller margins are obtained, adjuvant radiotherapy should be considered. The defect can be closed primarily or reconstructed with local flaps or skin grafts.

Because a substantial percentage of patients with stage II disease will harbor occult regional metastasis, elective treatment of the neck is often considered in this population. It bears repeating that prospective data do not support the use of any type of elective neck treatment to improve either locoregional control or overall survival rates. However, should elective treatment of the neck be performed, several options are available.

Elective neck dissection (END) is the most widely used treatment option. Generally, the dissection should include all nodal groups considered to be at risk, as mentioned earlier. One important advantage to END is the prognostic information it provides. Patients whose nodes contain occult metastases can be upstaged and are eligible for consideration for adjuvant radiotherapy and systemic treatment in the form of immunotherapy or biochemotherapy.

A second option is *elective neck irradiation*. In patients with stage II disease who were given irradiation to the primary site after WLE and to the undissected draining lymphatics, locoregional control is achieved in 85% of patients[101]—a rate that compares quite favorably with historical controls. However, data from prospective trials are not available to corroborate this finding.

Lastly, *sentinel lymph node biopsy (SLNB)* is undergoing investigation in the treatment of stage II patients (Fig. 8–9). The rationale for this modality and clinical experiences with its use in head and neck melanoma have been outlined previously. It is likely that in the future, this method will have a role in enhancing the sensitivity of regional nodal dissection.

In patients with stage II disease, no metastatic treatment is required because the risk of metastasis remains low.

Stage III

In patients with stage III melanoma, the primary tumor is treated by wide local excision. If possible, 2-cm margins are obtained. The defect can be closed primarily or reconstructed with the use of local flaps or skin grafts.

Regional disease is addressed by incorporating the appropriate neck dissection into the treatment plan (Fig. 8–10). If the disease is limited, a selective or modified radical neck dissection should be performed rather than a classical radical neck dissection. As has already been described, the addition of postoperative radiotherapy appears to improve locoregional control.[101] In-transit metastasis and/or satellitosis poses a particularly difficult problem (Fig. 8–11). Surgical extirpation may be attempted, but often these metastases are inoperable and nonsurgical therapy must be used.

Systemic therapy, in the form of chemotherapy, immunotherapy, or biochemotherapy, should be considered in all stage III patients because of the high risk for distant metastasis. Should systemic treatment be chosen, participation in a prospective clinical trial is recommended.

Stage IV

Treatment for metastatic melanoma must be individualized and is usually best undertaken by an experienced medical oncologist in the context of a clinical trial. Although the prognosis is extremely poor for patients with stage IV disease, attaining locoregional control remains important because of the devastating effects of uncontrolled locoregional disease. Palliative care is also of importance in these patients.

Recurrent Disease

Recurrent disease is an ominous finding that indicates a poor prognosis. Recurrences can be local, regional, or distant. Local and regional recurrences are usually addressed by reexcision, when possible, which has been shown to render up to 27% of patients disease free.[119] Adjuvant radiotherapy should be considered if it has not already been given. If surgery is not possible, radiation therapy and systemic treatment are secondary options, but they are usually only palliative options. Distant metastases that are amenable to surgical resection should be considered for aggressive treatment because, in rare instances, a cure or a long-term progression-free interval may be possible. Pulmonary metastases have a better prognosis than do brain or liver metastases, which are associated with an expected survival of only 2 to 4 months. Again, radiotherapy and systemic therapy are options for palliative treatment of recurrent disease. Occasionally, isolated distant metastases may be left in place initially to "monitor" the response to systemic treatment; then, depending on response, they are excised at a later time. It is important to remember that although the vast majority of patients with recurrence will die of their disease, locoregional control remains an important goal, if only to improve quality of life.

◼ SPECIAL ISSUES IN MELANOMA

Mucosal Melanoma

Mucosal melanoma of the head and neck is rare, accounting for 1% to 2% of melanomas. The most common sites of its occurrence in the head and neck are the nose, paranasal sinuses, oral cavity, and nasopharynx. Patients with sinonasal melanoma generally present with symptoms of nasal obstruction, epistaxis, pain, facial deformity, or visual disturbance. Oral lesions may cause dysphagia but more commonly present as asymptomatic masses. These indolent symptoms commonly result in a delay in presentation. In addition, several nonmalignant melanotic processes such as

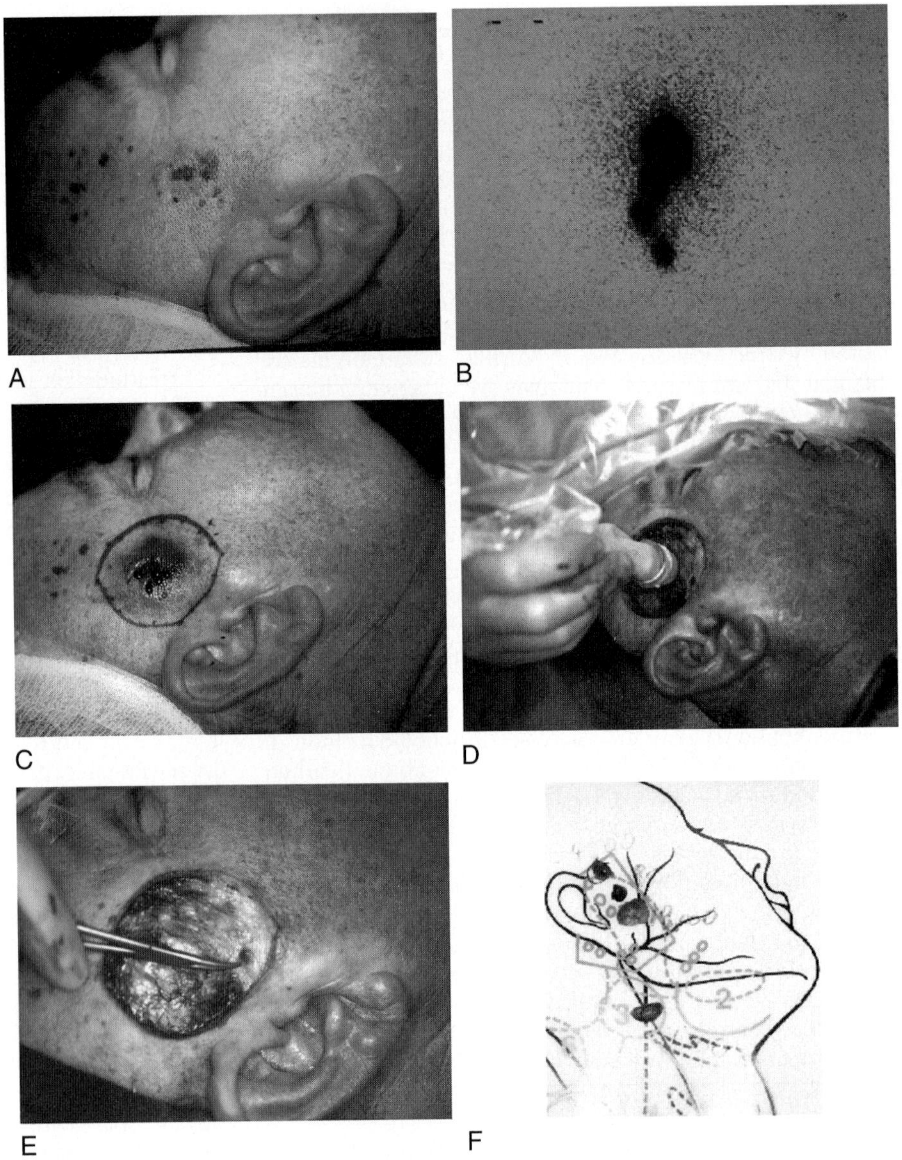

FIGURE 8–9 Sentinel node biopsy for CMM of the head and neck. Fifty-year-old patient with a 2.7-mm Clark level IV melanoma of the right cheek. *A,* Primary lesion. *B,* Preoperative lymphoscintigraphy. *C,* Intraoperative blue dye injection. *D,* Intraoperative localization of a sentinel node with handheld gamma probe. *E,* Intraoperative blue dye localization. *F,* Identification of four sentinel lymph nodes, one of which was positive for nodal metastasis.

pigmented nevi and mucosal melanotic macules may simulate oral mucosal melanomas. Because these are more common than mucosal melanoma, they are often observed rather than biopsied, again causing a delay in diagnosis.[120]

From a histopathologic standpoint, diagnosing mucosal melanoma may be difficult because these tumors often lack melanin. The anatomic site of the primary lesion appears to affect prognosis; 5-year survival rates are 30.9% for lesions in the nasal cavity, 12.3% for those in the oral cavity, and 0% for those located in the paranasal sinuses.[121] Moreover, most of the criteria used to determine the stage of CMM, including depth of invasion and regional lymphadenopathy, have not been shown to be important predictors of prognosis in mucosal melanoma.

As a group, mucosal melanomas are highly aggressive and lethal. Because of their rarity and their uniformly low survival rate, determination of the ideal treatment is difficult. Radical surgery is the most common primary treatment.

Adjuvant radiotherapy appears to improve local control rates but probably does not affect the overall survival rate because of the high rate of distant metastases.[120] Overall, 5-year survival rates are usually reported to be 15% to 20%, although rates as high as 40% have been reported as well.[121, 122] Death usually results from distant metastatic spread, and this is the limiting factor for long-term survival.[123]

Desmoplastic Melanoma

First described by Conley and colleagues in 1971, desmoplastic melanoma is a rare spindle cell variant of melanoma.[53] Frequently, this tumor arises from a benign-appearing lesion, often nonpigmented, and evolves into an aggressive neoplasm. It may be confused with other, less aggressive tumors, frequently causing a delay in proper therapy. These lesions tend to occur in older patients than do other forms of CMM, are more frequent in men, and are most common in the head and neck region.

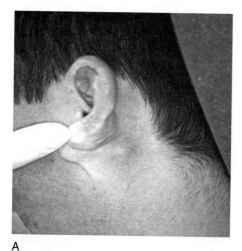

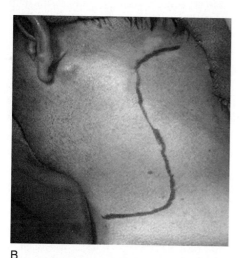

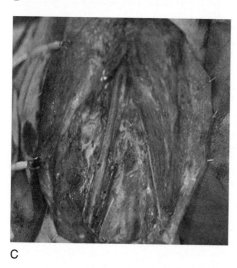

C

At diagnosis, these lesions tend to be thicker than other melanomas; however, thickness may not be as predictive of prognosis as in other types of melanoma. One of the hallmarks of this subtype of melanoma is its propensity for perineural spread. This trait is especially important in the head and neck because even small desmoplastic melanomas can gain access to cranial nerves, leading to palsies or intracranial spread. This propensity to spread perineurally has also been implicated in the particularly high rate of local recurrence seen with these tumors. For this reason, WLE with a careful analysis of the specimen for evidence of perineural invasion is especially important. Adjuvant radiotherapy is usually recommended. An interesting note is that the rate of regional lymph node metastasis from desmoplastic melanomas seems to be lower than for other forms of CMM,[124] regardless of the tumor's thickness. Overall, survival rates appear to be similar to those for other forms of CMM.[125]

Metastatic Melanoma of Unknown Origin

Rarely, melanoma is identified in cervical or parotid lymph nodes without any evidence of a primary tumor. It is suspected that a vast majority of such tumors represent metastases from primary tumors that have undergone spontaneous regression. In cases like this, unusual mucosal or ocular sites of the primary tumor should also be considered.

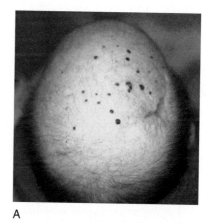

A

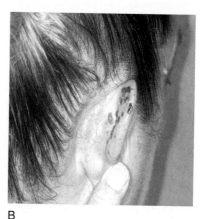

B

FIGURE 8–10 Regional treatment of CMM of the head and neck. Twenty-four-year-old patient with a regressed pigmented lesion of the vertex scalp. *A,* He presented with a clinically apparent left postauricular lymph node, which was pathologically positive for melanoma. *B* and *C,* He was treated with a posterolateral neck dissection.

FIGURE 8–11 In-transit/satellite metastases in the head and neck. Two patients with stage III cutaneous involvement manifested as in-transit (*A*) and/or satellite (*B*) lesions.

TABLE 8-6 Recommendations for Follow-up, on the Basis of Stage

Stage	Physical Examination	Radiology	Laboratory Tests
Melanoma in situ	Every 6 months × 4 years, then annually	None	None
Stage I or II (no ulceration, thickness < 1.0 mm)	Every 6 months × 4 years, then annually	CXR	LDH
Stage I or II (with ulceration, or thickness > 1.0 mm)	Every 4 months × 2 years, then every 6 months × 2 years, then annually	CXR	LDH
Stage III, or recurrent primary	Every 3 months × 2 years, then every 6 months × 3 years, then annually	CXR	LDH, CBC
Stage IV	Individualize	Individualize	Individualize

CBC, complete blood count; CXR, chest x-ray; LDH, lactate dehydrogenase.

Patients with this type of melanoma should be treated with an appropriate lymphadenectomy and postoperative radiotherapy. As with any stage III disease, these patients should be considered for trials of adjuvant systemic therapy. The prognosis for these patients does not appear to be worse than that for patients with known primary tumors; it may, in fact, be better.[126]

FOLLOW-UP

Because CMM remains a disease of younger people (average age, 45 years), the clinical and financial considerations of patient follow-up are significant. One report demonstrated that intensive follow-up in the post-treatment phase (5 years) resulted in a mean cost of $421,000 for laboratory tests alone.[127] Obviously, a balance must be struck between adequate surveillance and fiscal responsibility. It is estimated that 28% to 56% of recurrences are detected by physicians,[128, 129] indicating that routine examinations are an important part of follow-up. Most researchers agree that physical examinations should be supplemented by periodic laboratory testing and radiologic assessment. The optimal frequency and extent of these examinations, however, are undetermined.

At the M.D. Anderson Cancer Center, follow-up depends on the stage of the disease at diagnosis. For in situ lesions, physical examination is performed every 6 months for 4 years, then annually. Table 8–6 summarizes the follow-up we recommend for various stages of disease.

CONCLUSION

At the beginning of the 20th century, the diagnosis of melanoma spelled certain death. Over the past century, however, as our understanding of the natural history of the disease—including the causes and major risk factors—has improved, so has our ability to diagnose and treat it. As we begin the new millennium, we are able to cure as many as 80% of early melanomas and achieve high locoregional control rates for advanced tumors. Still, CMM remains a difficult challenge for practitioners and a significant health hazard for the entire population. It is hoped that patient education and measures to prevent the steady rise in the incidence of melanoma will help curtail the increasing mortality rates associated with this disease. Early diagnosis by physicians and prompt referral to qualified oncologists are key to improvement of cure rates. New developments in diagnostic and treatment strategies hold promise for further improvements in control and survival rates for those afflicted with this disease.

REFERENCES

1. Laennec RTH: Sur les melanoses. Bull Soc Med Paris 1:1–24, 1806.
2. Jemal A, Thomas A, Murray T, Thun M: Cancer statistics, 2000. CA Cancer J Clin 52:23–47, 2002.
3. Wingo PA, Ries LA, Giovino GA, et al: Annual report to the nation on the status of cancer, 1973–1996, with a special section on lung cancer and tobacco smoking. J Natl Cancer Inst 91:675–690, 1999.
4. Goldsmith HS: Melanoma: An overview. Cancer 29:194–197, 1979.
5. Batsakis JG: Tumors of the Head and Neck. Clinical and Pathological Considerations, 2nd ed. Baltimore, Williams & Wilkins, 1979.
6. Buettner PG, Raasch BA: Incidence rates of skin cancer in Townsville, Australia. Int J Cancer 78:587–593, 1998.
7. Koh HK: Cutaneous melanoma. N Engl J Med 325:171–182, 1991.
8. Setlow RB, Grist E, Thompson K, et al: Wavelengths effective in induction of malignant melanoma. Proc Natl Acad Sci USA 90:6666–6670, 1993.
9. Rodenas JM, Delgado-Rodriguez M, Herranz MT, et al: Sun exposure, pigmentary traits, and risk of cutaneous malignant melanoma: A case-control study in a Mediterranean population. Cancer Causes Control 7:275–283, 1996.
10. Autier P, Dore JF, Schifflers E, et al: Melanoma and use of sunscreens: An EORTC case-control study in Germany, Belgium and France. Int J Cancer 61:749–755, 1995.
11. Wolf P, Donawho CK, Kripke ML: Effect of sunscreens on UV radiation-induced enhancement of melanoma growth in mice. J Natl Cancer Inst 86:99–105, 1994.
12. Marks R: Two decades of the public health approach to skin cancer control in Australia: Why, how and where are we now? Australas J Dermatol 40:1–5, 1999.
13. McNeer G, Das Gupta TK: Prognosis in malignant melanoma. Surgery 56:512–515, 1964.
14. Balch CM, Karakousis C, Mettlin C: Management of cutaneous melanoma in the United States. Surg Gynecol Obstet 18:311–315, 1984.
15. Kaplan EN: The risk of malignancy in large congenital nevi. Plast Reconstr Surg 53:421–425, 1974.
16. Consensus Conference: Precursors to malignant melanoma. JAMA 251:1864–1867, 1984.
17. Evans RD, Kopf AW, Lew RA, et al: Risk factors for the development of malignant melanoma—I: Review of the case-control studies. J Dermatol Surg Oncol 14:393–408, 1988.
18. Rigel DS: Epidemiology and prognostic factors in malignant melanoma. Ann Plast Surg 28:7–8, 1992.
19. Clark WH Jr, Reimer RR, Greene M, et al: Origin of familial malignant melanomas from heritable melanocytic lesions. The B-K syndrome. Arch Dermatol 114:732–738, 1978.
20. Lynch HT, Frichot BC III, Lynch JF: Familial atypical multiple mole-melanoma syndrome. J Med Genet 15:352–356, 1978.

21. Greene MH, Clark WH Jr, Tucker M, et al: High risk of malignant melanoma in melanoma-prone families with dysplastic nevi. Ann Intern Med 102:458–465, 1985.

22. Bale SJ, Dracopoli NC, Tucker MA, et al: Mapping the gene for hereditary cutaneous malignant melanoma-dysplastic nevus to chromosome 1p. N Engl J Med 320:1367–1372, 1989.

23. Goldstein AM, Dracopoli NC, Engelstein M, et al: Linkage of cutaneous malignant melanoma/dysplastic nevi to chromosome 9p, and evidence for genetic heterogeneity. Am J Hum Genet 54:489–496, 1994.

24. Cannon-Albright LA, Goldgar DE, Meyer LJ, et al: Assignment of a locus for familial melanoma, MLM, to chromosome 9p13-p22. Science 258:1148–1152, 1992.

25. Gruis NA, Sandkuijl LA, Weber JL, et al: Linkage analysis in Dutch familial atypical multiple mole-melanoma (FAMMM) syndrome families. Effect of naevus count. Melanoma Res 3:271–277, 1993.

26. Kraemer KH, Levy DD, Parris CN, et al: Xeroderma pigmentosum and related disorders: Examining the linkage between defective DNA repair and cancer. J Invest Dermatol 103:96S–101S, 1994.

27. Cleaver JE: Defective repair replication of DNA in xeroderma pigmentosum. Nature 218:652–656, 1968.

28. Kamb A, Gruis NA, Weaver-Feldhaus J, et al: A cell cycle regulator potentially involved in genesis of many tumor types. Science 264:436–440, 1994.

29. Serrano M, Hannon GJ, Beach D: A new regulatory motif in cell-cycle control causing specific inhibition of cyclin D/CDK4. Nature 366:704–707, 1993.

30. Flores JF, Walker GJ, Glendening JM, et al: Loss of the p16INK4a and p15INK4b genes, as well as neighboring 9p21 markers, in sporadic melanoma. Cancer Res 56:5023–5032, 1996.

31. Reed JA, Loganzo F, Shea CR, et al: Loss of expression of the p16/cyclin-dependent kinase inhibitor 2 tumor suppressor gene in melanocytic lesions correlates with invasive stage of tumor progression. Cancer Res 55:2713–2718, 1995.

32. Straume O, Sviland L, Akslen LA: Loss of nuclear p16 protein expression correlates with increased tumor cell proliferation (Ki-67) and poor prognosis in patients with vertical growth phase melanoma. Clin Cancer Res 6:1845–1853, 2000.

33. El Deiry WS, Tokino T, Velculescu VE, et al: WAF1, a potential mediator of p53 tumor suppression. Cell 75:817–825, 1993.

34. Bales ES, Dietrich C, Bandyopadhyay D, et al: High levels of expression of p27KIP1 and cyclin E in invasive primary malignant melanomas. J Invest Derm 113:1039–1046, 1999.

35. Kawada M, Uehara Y, Mizuno S, et al: Up-regulation of p27Kip1 correlates inversely with anchorage-independent growth of human cancer cell lines. Jpn J Cancer Res 89:110–115, 1998.

36. Nevins JR: The Rb/E2F pathway and cancer. Hum Mol Gen 10:699–703, 2001.

37. Halaban R, Cheng E, Smicun Y, et al: Deregulated E2F transcriptional activity in autonomously growing melanoma cells. J Exp Med 191:1005–1016, 2000.

38. Halaban R: Melanoma cell autonomous growth: The Rb/E2F pathway. Cancer Metastasis Rev 18:333–343, 1999.

39. Kastan MB, Onyekere O, Sidransky D, et al: Participation of p53 protein in the cellular response to DNA damage. Cancer Res 51:6304–6311, 1991.

40. Yin Y, Tainsky MA, Bischoff FZ, et al: Wild-type p53 restores cell cycle control and inhibits gene amplification in cells with mutant p53 alleles. Cell 70:937–948, 1992.

41. Yonish-Rouach E, Resnitzky D, Lotem J, et al: Wild-type p53 induces apoptosis of myeloid leukaemic cells that are inhibited by interleukin-6. Nature 352:345–347, 1991.

42. Albino AP, Vidal MJ, McNutt NS, et al: Mutation and expression of the p53 gene in human malignant melanoma. Melanoma Res 4:35–45, 1994.

43. Weiss J, Heine M, Arden KC, et al: Mutation and expression of TP53 in malignant melanomas. Recent Results Cancer Res 139:137–154, 1995.

44. Staibano S, Lo Muzio L, Pannone G, et al: P53 and hMSH2 expression in basal cell carcinomas and malignant melanomas from photoexposed areas of head and neck region. Int J Oncol 19:551–559, 2001.

45. Myers MP, Pass I, Batty Ih, et al: The lipid phosphatase activity of PTEN is critical for its tumor suppressor function. Proc Natl Acad Sci USA 95:13513–13518, 1998.

46. Birck A, Ahrenkiel V, Zeuthen J, et al: Mutation and allelic loss of the PTEN/MMAC1 gene in primary and metastatic melanoma biopsies. J Invest Dermatol 114:277–280, 2000.

47. Hwang PH, Yi HK, Kim DS, et al: Suppression of tumorigenicity and metastasis in B16F10 cells by PTEN/MMAC1/TEP1 gene. Cancer Lett 172:83–91, 2001.

48. Hernandez-Acoceba R, del Peso L, Lacal JC: The Ras family of GTPases in cancer cell invasion. Cell Mol Life Sci 57:65–76, 2000.

49. Fujita M, Norris DA, Yagi H, et al: Overexpression of mutant ras in human melanoma increases invasiveness, proliferation and anchorage-independent growth in vitro and induces tumour formation and cachexia in vivo. Melanoma Res 9:279–291, 1999.

50. Chin L, Tam A, Pomerantz J, et al: Essential role for oncogenic Ras in tumour maintenance. Nature 400:468–472, 1999.

51. Hunter T: Protein kinases and phosphatases: The yin and yang of protein phosphorylation and signaling. Cell 80:225–236, 1995.

52. Easty DJ, Bennett DC: Protein tyrosine kinases in malignant melanoma. Melanoma Res 10:401–411, 2000.

53. Conley J, Lattes R, Orr W: Desmoplastic malignant melanoma (a rare variant of spindle cell melanoma). Cancer 28:914–936, 1971.

54. Koh HK, Miller DR, Geller AC, et al: Who discovers melanoma? Patterns from a population-based survey. J Am Acad Dermatol 26:914–919, 1992.

55. Friedman RJ, Rigel DS, Kopf AW: Early detection of malignant melanoma: The role of physician examination and self-examination of the skin. CA Cancer J Clin 35:130–151, 1985.

56. Mackie RM: Illustrated Guide to Recognition of Early Malignant Melanoma. Edinburgh, Blackwood Pillans and Wilson Ltd, 1986.

57. Austin JR, Byers RM, Brown WD, et al: Influence of biopsy on the prognosis of cutaneous melanoma of the head and neck. Head Neck 18:107–117, 1996.

58. Morton DL, Giuliano AE, Reintgen DS, et al: Symposium: Lymphatic mapping and sentinel node biopsy in patients with breast cancer and melanoma, part 2. Contemp Surg 53:353–358, 1993.

59. Balch CM, Soong S, Shaw HM, et al: An analysis of prognostic factors in 8,500 patients with cutaneous melanoma. In Balch CM, Houghton AN, Milton GW, et al (eds): Cutaneous Melanoma, 2nd ed. Philadelphia, JB Lippincott, 1992.

60. Wong JH, Wanek L, Chang LJ, et al: The importance of anatomic site in prognosis in patients with cutaneous melanoma. Arch Surg 126:486–489, 1991.

61. Garbe C, Buttner P, Bertz J, et al: Primary cutaneous melanoma. Prognostic classification of anatomic location. Cancer 75:2492–2498, 1995.

62. Ballantyne AJ: Malignant melanoma of the skin of the head and neck. An analysis of 405 cases. Am J Surg 120:425–431, 1970.

63. Close LG, Goepfert H, Ballantyne AJ, et al: Malignant melanoma of the scalp. Laryngoscope 89:1189–1196, 1979.

64. Loree TR, Spiro RH: Cutaneous melanoma of the head and neck. Am J Surg 158:388–391, 1989.

65. Clark WH Jr, From L, Bernardino EA, et al: The histogenesis and biologic behavior of primary human malignant melanomas of the skin. Cancer Res 29:705–727, 1969.

66. Breslow A: Thickness, cross-sectional areas and depth of invasion in the prognosis of cutaneous melanoma. Ann Surg 172:902–908, 1970.

67. American Joint Committee on Cancer: Malignant melanoma of the skin. In Fleming ID, Cooper JS, Henson DE, et al (eds): AJCC Cancer Staging Manual, 5th ed. Philadelphia, Lippincott Williams & Wilkins, 1997, pp 163–170.

68. Buzaid AC, Ross MI, Balch CM, et al: Critical analysis of the current American Joint Committee on Cancer staging system for cutaneous melanoma and proposal of a new staging system. J Clin Oncol 15:1039–1051, 1997.

69. Balch CM, Buzaid AC, Soong SJ, et al: Final version of the American Joint Committee on Cancer staging system for cutaneous melanoma. J Clin Oncol 19:3635–3648, 2001.

70. Leong SP, Achtem TA, Habib FA, et al: Discordancy between clinical predictions vs lymphoscintigraphic and intraoperative mapping of sentinel lymph node drainage of primary melanoma. Arch Dermatol 135:1472–1476, 1999.

71. Mijnhout GS, Hoekstra OS, van Tulder MW, et al: Systematic review of the diagnostic accuracy of (18)F-fluorodeoxyglucose positron emission tomography in melanoma patients. Cancer 91:1530–1542, 2001.

72. Acland KM, Healy C, Calonje E, et al: Comparison of positron emission tomography scanning and sentinel node biopsy in the detection of micrometastases of primary cutaneous malignant melanoma. J Clin Oncol 19:2674–2678, 2001.

73. Wagner JD, Schauwecker D, Davidson D, et al: Prospective study of fluorodeoxyglucose-positron emission tomography imaging of lymph node basins in melanoma patients undergoing sentinel node biopsy. J Clin Oncol 17:1508–1515, 1999.

74. Boni R, Boni RA, Steinert H, et al: Staging of metastatic melanoma by whole-body positron emission tomography using 2-fluorine-18-fluoro-2-deoxy-d-glucose. Br J Dermatol 132:556–562, 1995.

75. Blessing C, Feine U, Geiger L, et al: Positron emission tomography and ultrasonography. A comparative study assessing the diagnostic validity in lymph node metastasis of malignant melanoma. Arch Dermatol 131:1394–1398, 1995.

76. Damian DL, Fulham MJ, Thompson E, Thompson JF. Positron emission tomography in the detection and management of metastatic melanoma. Melanoma Res 6:325–329, 1996.

77. Balch CM, Urist MM, Karakousis CP, et al: Efficacy of 2-cm surgical margins for intermediate thickness melanomas (1-4 mm). Ann Surg 218:262–269, 1993.

78. Veronesi U, Cascinelli N, Adamus J, et al: Thin stage I primary cutaneous malignant melanoma: Comparison of excision with margins of 1 or 3 cm. N Engl J Med 318:1159–1162, 1988.

79. Balch CM, Soong SJ, Smith T, et al: Long-term results of a prospective surgical trial comparing 2 cm vs. 4 cm excision margins for 740 patients with 1–4 mm melanomas. Ann Surg Oncol 8:101–108, 2001.

80. Zitelli JA, Moy RL, Abell E: The reliability of frozen sections in the evaluation of surgical margins for melanoma. J Am Acad Dermatol 24:102–106, 1991.

81. Zalla MJ, Lim KK, Dicaudo DJ, et al: Mohs micrographic excision of melanoma using immunostains. Dermatol Surg 26:771–784, 2000.

82. Byers RM: The role of modified neck dissection in the treatment of cutaneous melanoma of the head and neck. Arch Surg 121:1338–1341, 1986.

83. Goepfert H, Jesse RH, Ballantyne AJ: Posterolateral neck dissection. Arch Otolaryngol 106:618–620, 1980.

84. Gershenwald JE, Thompson W, Mansfield PF, et al: Multi-institutional melanoma lymphatic mapping experience: The prognostic value of sentinel lymph node status in 612 stage I or II melanoma patients. J Clin Oncol 17:976–983, 1999.

85. Gershenwald JE, Colome MI, Lee JE, et al: Patterns of recurrence following a negative sentinel lymph node biopsy in 243 patients with stage I or II melanoma. J Clin Oncol 16:2253–2260, 1998.

86. Wells KE, Rapaport DP, Cruse CW, et al: Sentinel lymph node biopsy in melanoma of the head and neck. Plast Reconstr Surg 100:591–594, 1997.

87. Alex JC, Krag DN, Harlow SP, et al: Localization of regional lymph nodes in melanomas of the head and neck. Arch Otolaryngol Head Neck Surg 124:135–140, 1998.

88. O'Brien CJ, Uren RF, Thompson JF, et al: Prediction of potential metastatic sites in cutaneous head and neck melanoma using lymphoscintigraphy. Am J Surg 170:461–466, 1995.

89. Morton DL, Wen DR, Foshag LJ, et al: Intraoperative lymphatic mapping and selective cervical lymphadenectomy for early-stage melanomas of the head and neck J Clin Oncol 11:1751–1756, 1993.

90. Bostick P, Essner R, Sarantou T, et al: Intraoperative lymphatic mapping for early-stage melanoma of the head and neck. Am J Surg 174:536–539, 1995.

91. Alex JC, Krag DN, Harlow SP, et al: Localization of regional lymph nodes in melanomas of the head and neck. Arch Otolaryngol Head Neck Surg 124:135–140, 1998.

92. Wells KE, Stadelmann WK, Rapaport DP, et al: Parotid selective lymphadenectomy in malignant melanoma. Ann Plast Surg 43:1–6, 1999.

93. Jansen L, Koops HS, Nieweg OE, et al: Sentinel node biopsy for melanoma in the head and neck region. Head Neck 22:27–33, 2000.

94. Carlson GW, Murray DR, Greenlee R, et al: Management of malignant melanoma of the head and neck using dynamic lymphoscintigraphy and gamma probe-guided sentinel lymph node biopsy. Arch Otolaryngol Head Neck Surg 126:433–437, 2000.

95. Maffioli L, Belli F, Gallino G, et al: Sentinel node biopsy in patients with cutaneous melanoma of the head and neck. Tumori 86:341–342, 2000.

96. Wagner JD, Park HM, Coleman JJ 3rd, et al: Cervical sentinel lymph node biopsy for melanomas of the head and neck and upper thorax. Arch Otolaryngol Head Neck Surg 126:313–321, 2000.

97. Wells KE, Rapaport DP, Cruse CW, et al: Sentinel lymph node biopsy in melanoma of the head and neck. Plast Reconstr Surg 100:591–594, 1997.

98. Eicher SA, Clayman GL, Myers JN, et al: A prospective study of intraoperative lymphatic mapping for head and neck cutaneous melanoma. Arch Otolaryngol Head Neck Surg 128:241–245, 2002.

99. Stoeckli SJ, Steinert H, Pfaltz M, et al: Sentinel lymph node evaluation in squamous cell carcinoma of the head and neck. Otolaryngol Head Neck Surg 125:221–226, 2001.

100. Ang KK, Byers RM, Peters LJ, et al: Regional radiotherapy as adjuvant treatment for head and neck melanoma. Preliminary results. Arch Otolaryngol Head Neck Surg 116:169–172, 1990.

101. Ang KK, Peters LH, Weber RS, et al: Postoperative radiotherapy for cutaneous melanoma of the head and neck region. Int J Radiat Oncol Biol Phys 30:795–798, 1994.

102. Shen P, Wanek LA, Morton DL: Is adjuvant radiotherapy necessary after positive lymph node dissection in head and neck melanomas? Ann Surg Oncol 7:554–559, 2000.

103. O'Brien CJ, Petersen-Schaefer K, Ruark D, et al: Radical, modified, and selective neck dissection for cutaneous malignant melanoma. Head Neck 17:232–241, 1995.

104. Lee RJ, Gibbs JF, Proulx GM, et al: Nodal basin recurrence following lymph node dissection for melanoma: Implications for adjuvant radiotherapy. Int J Radiat Oncol Biol Phys 46:467–474, 2000.

105. Lejeune FJ, Lienard D, Leyvraz S, et al: Regional therapy of melanoma. Eur J Cancer 29A:606–612, 1993.

106. Veronesi U, Adamus J, Aubert C, et al: A randomized trial of adjuvant chemotherapy and immunotherapy in cutaneous melanoma. N Engl J Med 307:913–916, 1982.

107. Hill GJ, Moss SE, Golomb FM, et al: DTIC and combination therapy for melanoma: III. DTIC (NSC 45388) Surgical Adjuvant Study COG PROTOCOL 7040. Cancer 47:2556–2562, 1981.

108. Kirkwood JM, Strawderman MH, Ernstoff MS, et al: Interferon-alfa-2b adjuvant therapy of high risk resected cutaneous melanoma: The Eastern Cooperative Oncology Group Trial EST 1684. J Clin Oncol 14:7–17, 1996.

109. Kirkwood JM, Ibrahim JG, Sondak VK, et al: High- and low-dose interferon alfa-2b in high-risk melanoma: First analysis of intergroup trial E1690/S9111/C9190. J Clin Oncol 18:2444–2458, 2000.

110. Kirkwood JM, Ibrahim J, Sondak VK, et al: Relapse-free and overall survival are significantly prolonged by high-dose IFN[alpha]2b (HDFI) compared to vaccine GM2-KLH with QS21 (GMK, Progenics) for high-risk resected stage I/B-III melanoma: Results of the Intergroup Phase III Study E1694/S9512/C509801. Paper presented at the European Society of Medical Oncologists Annual Meeting, October 2000, Hamburg, Germany.

111. Grob JJ, Dreno B, de la Salmoniere P, et al: Randomised trial of interferon alpha-2a as adjuvant therapy in resected primary melanoma thicker than 1.5 mm without clinically detectable node metastases. French Cooperative Group on Melanoma. Lancet 351:1905–1910, 1998.

112. Cascinelli N, Belli F, MacKie RM, et al. Effect of long-term adjuvant therapy with interferon alpha-2a in patients with regional node metastases from cutaneous melanoma: A randomised trial. Lancet 358:866–869, 2001.

113. Sondak VK, Wolfe JA: Adjuvant therapy for melanoma. Curr Opin Oncol 9:189–204, 1997.

114. Ollila DW, Kelley MC, Gammon G, et al: Overview of melanoma vaccines: Active specific immunotherapy for melanoma patients. Semin Surg Oncol 14:328–336, 1998.

115. Stopeck AT, Jones A, Hersh EM, et al: Phase II study of direct intralesional gene transfer of allovectin-7, an HLA-B7/beta2-microglobulin DNA-liposome complex, in patients with metastatic melanoma. Clin Cancer Res 7:2285–2291, 2001.

116. Rosenberg SA, Yang JC, Schwartzentruber DJ, et al: Prospective randomized trial of the treatment of patients with metastatic melanoma using chemotherapy with cisplatin, dacarbazine, and tamoxifen alone or in combination with interleukin-2 and interferon alfa-2b. J Clin Oncol 17:968–975, 1999.

117. Keilholz U, Goey SH, Punt CJ, et al: Interferon alfa-2a and interleukin-2 with or without cisplatin in metastatic melanoma: A randomized trial of the European Organization for Research and Treatment of Cancer Melanoma Cooperative Group. J Clin Oncol 15:2579–2588, 1997.

118. Ames FC, Sugarbaker EJ, Ballantyne AJ: Analysis of survival and disease control in stage I melanoma of the head and neck. Am J Surg 132:484–489, 1976.

119. Zitsch RP, Roberts GD, Smith RB: Recurrent cutaneous melanoma of the head and neck. Otolaryngol Head Neck Surg 120:391–393, 1999.

120. Hicks MJ, Flaitz CM: Oral mucosal melanoma: Epidemiology and pathobiology. Oral Oncol 36:152–169, 2000.

121. Manolidis S, Donald PJ: Malignant mucosal melanoma of the head and neck: Review of the literature and report of 14 patients. Cancer 80:1373–1386, 1997.

122. Stern SJ, Guillamondegui OM: Mucosal melanoma of the head and neck. Head Neck 13:22–27, 1991.

123. Loree TR, Mullins AP, Spellman J, et al: Head and neck mucosal melanoma: A 32-year review. Ear Nose Throat J 78:372–375, 1999.

124. Beenken S, Byers R, Smith JL, et al: Desmoplastic melanoma. Histologic correlation with behavior and treatment. Arch Otolaryngol Head Neck Surg 115:374–379, 1989.

125. Quinn MJ, Crotty KA, Thompson JF, et al: Desmoplastic and desmoplastic neurotropic melanoma: Experience with 280 patients. Cancer 83:1128–1135, 1998.

126. Santini H, Byers RM, Wolf PF: Melanoma metastatic to cervical and parotid nodes from an unknown primary site. Am J Surg 150:510–512, 1985.

127. Weiss M, Loprinzi CL, Greagan ET, et al: Utility of follow-up tests for detecting recurrent disease in patients with malignant melanoma. JAMA 274:1703–1707, 1995.

128. Baughan CA, Hall VL, Leppard BJ, et al: Follow-up in stage I cutaneous malignant melanoma: An audit. Clin Oncol (R Coll Radiol) 5:174–180, 1993.

129. Poo-Hwu WJ, Ariyan S, Lamb L, et al: Follow-up recommendations for patients with American Joint Committee on Cancer stages I–III malignant melanoma. Cancer 86:2252–2258, 1999.

Cancer of the Nasal Cavity, Paranasal Sinuses, and Orbit

Ehab Y. N. Hanna
Christopher T. Westfall

INTRODUCTION

Over the past two decades, significant advances have been made in both the diagnosis and management of cancer of the nasal cavity and paranasal sinuses. The most significant advances in diagnosis are office endoscopy and high-resolution imaging. These diagnostic tools have allowed more accurate delineation of the extent of sinonasal tumors, and hence improved treatment planning. Significant advances in treatment include progress made in cranial base surgery that allows for safe excision of tumors involving the cranial base. In addition, the development of microvascular free-tissue transfer has made possible the effective reconstruction of more extensive surgical defects. Advances have also been made in both planning and delivery of radiotherapy, such as 3-D conformal radiation therapy (3-D CRT) and intensity-modulated radiation therapy (IMRT). Both modalities allow the administration of optimal radiation dosimetry to the tumor while sparing normal surrounding tissue. Various new combinations of effective cytotoxic chemotherapeutic agents are also being increasingly incorporated into the overall management of patients with sinonasal cancer.

Recent advances in the diagnosis and treatment of patients with sinonasal cancer have had a clear impact on our ability to control the disease and improve survival. Survival rates have improved from 25% to 40% in the 1960s, to 65% to 75% in most recently reported series.[1] Despite these improvements, a significant number of patients die of their disease. The rarity of these tumors and the similarity of their presenting symptoms to those of more common benign conditions, coupled with their propensity for early spread and involvement of surrounding critical structures, are reflected in the fact that most patients still present with advanced-stage disease. This has clearly hampered attempts to further improve prognosis. In this chapter, we present the current trends in diagnosis, classification, staging, and treatment of patients with cancers of the nasal cavity, paranasal sinuses, and orbit. We also discuss some strategies for improving outcome in these patients.

ANATOMY

Nasal Cavity

The nasal cavity is bounded by the bony pyriform aperture and the external framework of the nose. The nasal cavity opens anteriorly through the skin-lined nasal vestibule into the nares, and it communicates posteriorly through the choanae with the nasopharynx. The nasal cavity is divided in the midline by the *nasal septum,* which includes both cartilaginous and bony components (Fig. 9–1). The cartilage of the septum is somewhat quadrilateral in form and is thicker at its margins than at its center. Its anterior margin is connected to the nasal bones and is continuous with the anterior margins of the lateral cartilages; below, it is connected to the medial crura of the greater alar cartilages by fibrous tissue. Its posterior margin is connected to the perpendicular plate of the ethmoid; its inferior margin to the vomer and the palatine process of the maxilla.

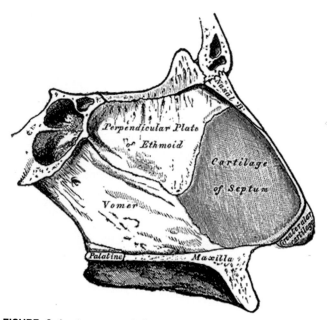

FIGURE 9–1 Anatomy of the nasal septum. (From Gray H: Anatomy of the Human Body, 20th ed. Edited by WH Lewis. New York, Bartelby, 2000.)

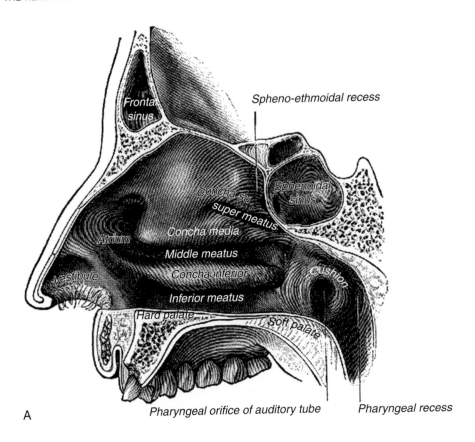

A

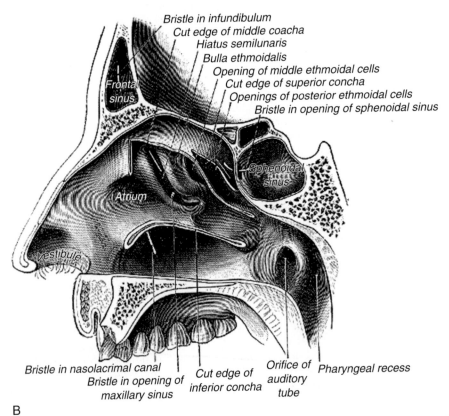

B

FIGURE 9–2 *A*, Anatomy of the lateral nasal wall. *B*, Removal of the middle turbinate reveals the anatomy of the middle meatus. (From Gray H: Anatomy of the Human Body, 20th ed. Edited by WH Lewis. New York, Bartelby, 2000.)

On the *lateral nasal wall* are the superior, middle, and inferior nasal turbinates; below and lateral to each turbinate (concha) is the corresponding nasal passage or meatus (Fig. 9–2A). Above the superior turbinate is a narrow recess—the sphenoethmoid recess—into which the sphenoid sinus opens. The superior meatus is a short oblique passage extending about halfway along the upper border of the middle turbinate; the posterior ethmoid cells open into the front part of this meatus. The middle meatus is below and lateral to the middle turbinate. The anatomy of the middle meatus is fully displayed by removal of the middle turbinate (Fig. 9–2B). The bulla ethmoidalis is the most prominent anterior ethmoid air cell. The hiatus semilunaris is a curved cleft lying below and in front of the bulla ethmoidalis. It is bounded inferiorly by the sharp concave margin of the uncinate process of the ethmoid bone; it leads into a curved channel—the infundibulum—bounded above by the bulla ethmoidalis and below by the lateral surface of the uncinate process of the ethmoid. The anterior ethmoid air cells open into the front part of the infundibulum. The frontal sinus drains through the nasofrontal duct, which in approximately 50% of subjects also drains into the infundibulum; however, when the anterior end of the uncinate process fuses with the front part of the bulla, this continuity is interrupted and the frontonasal duct then opens directly into the anterior end of the middle meatus. Below the bulla ethmoidalis, and partially hidden by the inferior end of the uncinate process, is the ostium of the maxillary sinus. An accessory ostium from the maxillary sinus is frequently present below the posterior end of the middle nasal concha. The inferior meatus is below and lateral to the inferior nasal turbinate. The nasolacrimal duct opens into the inferior meatus under cover of the anterior part of the inferior turbinate.

The *roof* of the nasal cavity is narrow from side to side and slopes downward (at about a 30-degree angle) from front to back. The cribriform plate, which transmits the filaments of the olfactory nerve, forms the roof of the nasal cavity medial to the superior attachment of the middle turbinate. Lateral to the middle turbinate, the fovea ethmoidalis forms the roof of the ethmoid sinuses. Careful assessment of the anatomy of the nasal roof, especially the relationship of the cribriform plate to the fovea ethmoidalis, is critical in avoiding a cerebrospinal fluid (CSF) leak during surgery in this region. The cribriform plate is usually at a slightly lower horizontal plane than is the fovea ethmoidalis, forming a shallow olfactory groove. This configuration is described as Keros type I (Fig. 9–3).[2, 3] However, the cribriform plate may be moderately or significantly lower than the fovea ethmoidalis, resulting in a medium (Keros type II) or deep (Keros type III) olfactory groove. The topography of the roof may also be asymmetrical (see Fig. 9–3).

The *floor* of the nasal cavity is concave from side to side and almost horizontal anteroposteriorly. The palatine process of the maxilla forms the anterior three fourths, and the horizontal process of the palatine bone forms the posterior fourth of the nasal floor.

The majority of the nasal cavity is lined by pseudostratified ciliated columnar epithelium, which contains mucous and serous glands (respiratory epithelium). Specialized olfactory epithelium lines the most superior portion of the

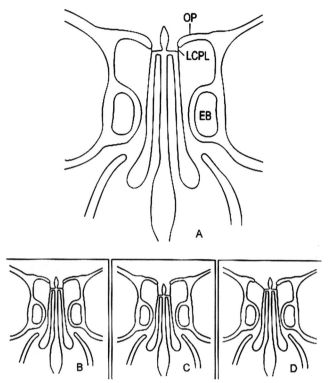

FIGURE 9–3 Anatomy of the ethmoid roof and lateral lamella of the cribriform plate. *A*, Keros type I. *B*, Keros type II. *C*, Keros type III. *D*, Asymmetrical ethmoid roof. Note that the right lateral lamella of the cribriform plate is very thin and long and is obliquely oriented, as is much of the right ethmoid roof. *OP*, Orbital plate of frontal bone; *LCPL*, lateral cribriform plate lamella; *EB*, ethmoid bulla.

nasal cavity and has direct connections with the olfactory tracts through openings in the cribriform plate.

The *arteries* of the nasal cavities are the anterior and posterior ethmoid branches of the ophthalmic artery, which supply the ethmoid and frontal sinuses, as well as the roof of the nose. The sphenopalatine artery supplies the mucous membrane covering the lateral nasal wall. The septal branch of the superior labial artery supplies the anterior inferior septum. The *veins* form a close cavernous plexus beneath the mucous membrane. This plexus is especially well marked over the lower part of the septum and over the middle and inferior turbinates. Venous drainage follows a pattern similar to arterial supply. The *lymphatic drainage* from the anterior part of the nasal cavity, similar to that from the external nose, goes to the submandibular group of lymph nodes (level I). Lymphatics from the posterior two thirds of the nasal cavities and from the paranasal sinuses drain to the upper jugular (level II) and retropharyngeal lymph nodes.

The sensory *nerves* of the nasal cavity transmit either somato-autonomic or olfactory sensation. *Somato-autonomic* nerves include the nasociliary branch of the ophthalmic, which supplies the anterior septum and lateral wall. The anterior alveolar nerve, a branch of the maxillary (V2), supplies the inferior meatus and the inferior turbinate. The nasopalatine nerve supplies the middle of the septum. The anterior palatine nerve supplies the lower nasal branches to the middle and inferior turbinates. The nerve of the

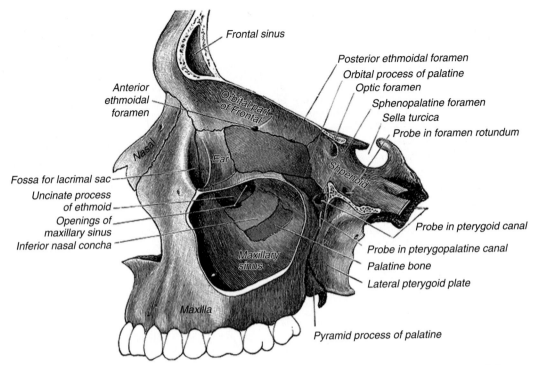

FIGURE 9–4   Anatomy of the maxillary sinus (lateral wall removed). (From Gray H: Anatomy of the Human Body, 20th ed. Edited by WH Lewis. New York, Bartelby, 2000.)

pterygoid canal (vidian) and the nasal branches from the sphenopalatine ganglion supply the upper and posterior septa, along with the superior turbinate. The *olfactory nerve* fibers arise from the bipolar olfactory cells and unite in fasciculi, which form a plexus beneath the mucous membrane and then ascend, passing into the skull through the foramina in the cribriform plate. Intracranially, olfactory nerve fibers enter the undersurface of the olfactory bulb, in which they ramify and form synapses with the dendrites of the mitral cells of the olfactory tract.

Maxillary Sinus

The maxillary sinus *(the antrum of Highmore),* the largest of the accessory sinuses of the nose, is a pyramidal cavity in the body of the maxilla (Fig. 9–4). Its base is formed by the lateral wall of the nasal cavity, and its apex extends into the zygomatic process. Its roof or orbital wall is frequently ridged by the infraorbital canal; its floor is formed by the alveolar process of the maxilla and is usually 1 to 10 mm below the level of the floor of the nose. Projecting into the floor are several conical elevations that correspond with the roots of the first and second molars; in some cases, the floor is perforated by one or more of these roots. The natural ostium of the maxillary sinus is partially covered by the uncinate process and communicates with the lower part of the hiatus semilunaris of the lateral nasal wall (see Figs. 9–2 and 9–4). An accessory ostium is frequently seen in, or immediately behind, the hiatus. The maxillary sinus appears as a shallow groove on the medial surface of the bone during about the fourth month of fetal life, but it does not reach its full size until after eruption of the second dentition.

Ethmoid Sinus

The ethmoid air cells consist of numerous thin-walled cavities situated in the ethmoid labyrinth and bounded by the frontal, maxillary, lacrimal, sphenoid, and palatine bones. They lie in the upper part of the nasal cavity between the orbits. The ethmoid sinuses are separated from the orbital cavity by a thin bony plate, the lamina papyracea. On each side, they are arranged in three groups—*anterior, middle,* and *posterior.* The anterior and middle groups open into the middle meatus of the nose, the former by way of the infundibulum, the latter on or above the bulla ethmoidalis (see Figs. 9–2 and 9–3). The posterior cells open into the superior meatus under cover of the superior nasal concha. Sometimes one or more ethmoid air cells extend over the orbital cavity (supraorbital ethmoid cells) or the optic nerve (Onodi cell). The ethmoid cells begin to develop during fetal life.

Frontal Sinus

The paired frontal sinuses appear to be outgrowths of the most anterior ethmoid air cells. They are located behind the superciliary arches and are rarely symmetrical, and the septum between them frequently deviates to one or the other side of the middle line. Absent at birth, the frontal sinuses are generally fairly well developed between the seventh and eighth years, but they reach their full size only after puberty. The frontal sinus is lined with respiratory epithelium and drains into the anterior part of the corresponding middle meatus of the nose through the frontonasal duct, which traverses the anterior part of the labyrinth of the ethmoid. The soft tissues of the forehead are located anteriorly, the orbits are located inferiorly, and the anterior cranial fossa is located posteriorly (see Figs. 9–2 and 9–4). Blood and neural supply is from the supraorbital and supratrochlear neurovascular bundles.

Sphenoid Sinus

The sphenoid sinus begins at the most posterior and superior portion of the nasal cavity (see Fig. 9–2). This midline structure, which is contained within the body of the sphenoid bone, is irregular and often has an eccentrically located intersinus septum. When exceptionally large, the sphenoid sinus may extend into the roots of the pterygoid processes or great wings, and it may pneumatize the basilar part of the occipital bone. The sphenoid sinus ostium is located on the anterior wall of the sinus and communicates directly with the sphenoethmoid recess above and medial to the superior turbinate (see Fig. 9–2). The sphenoid sinuses are present as minute cavities at birth, but their main development takes place after puberty. The posterior superior wall of the sphenoid sinus displays the forward convexity caused by the floor of the sella turcica, which contains the pituitary gland. The optic nerve and the internal carotid artery are closely related to the superior lateral wall of the sphenoid sinus, and their bony canals may be dehiscent within the sinus cavity (Fig. 9–5). Vascular and neural supplies come from the sphenopalatine and posterior ethmoid arteries and the branches of the sphenopalatine ganglion, respectively.

Infratemporal Fossa

The infratemporal fossa is an irregularly shaped cavity, located below and medial to the *zygomatic arch*. It is bounded anteriorly by the posterior surface of the maxilla; superiorly by the greater wing of the sphenoid and by the undersurface of the squamous portion of the temporal bone; medially by the lateral pterygoid plate; and laterally by the ramus of the mandible (Fig. 9–6A). It contains the inferior aspect of the temporalis muscle, along with the medial and lateral pterygoid muscles. It also contains branches of the internal maxillary vessels, and the mandibular (V3) and maxillary nerves (V2). The *foramen ovale* and the *foramen spinosum* open on its roof, and the *alveolar canals* on its anterior wall. The *inferior orbital* and *pterygomaxillary fissures* communicate with and may act as routes of spread of cancer to the infratemporal fossa (Fig. 9–6A and B).

Pterygopalatine Fossa

The pterygopalatine fossa is a small, triangular space located behind the maxillary sinus, in front of the pterygoid plates, and beneath the apex of the orbit. This fossa communicates with the orbit by the inferior orbital fissure, with the nasal cavity by the sphenopalatine foramen, and with the infratemporal fossa by the pterygomaxillary fissure (see Fig. 9–6). Five foramina open into it. Of these, the

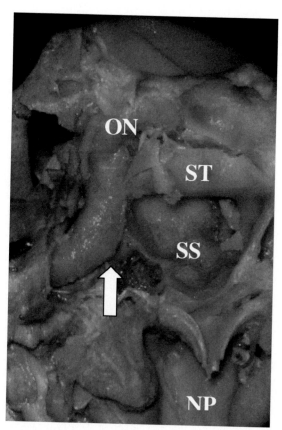

FIGURE 9–5 Cadaver dissection of the sphenoid sinus (SS). The sinus is located in the midline superior to the nasopharynx (NP). The sella turcica (ST) forms a convexity in the posterior superior wall. The internal carotid artery *(arrow)* courses through the lateral wall of the sinus and is related superiorly to the optic nerve (ON).

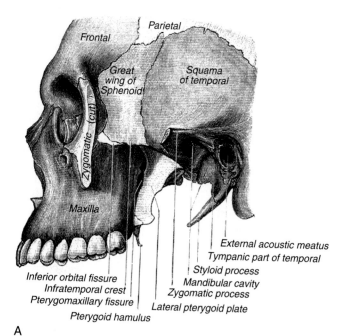

A

FIGURE 9–6 *A,* Lateral view of the skull showing the boundaries of the infratemporal fossa. The pterygomaxillary fissure is located between the maxilla anteriorly and the pterygoid plates posteriorly. It allows communication between the pterygopalatine fossa and the infratemporal fossa.

Continued

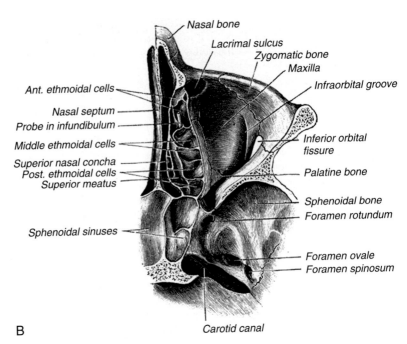

FIGURE 9–6, Cont'd *B,* Inferior view of the infratemporal fossa showing its relations to the foramina ovale, rotundum, and spinosum. (From Gray H: Anatomy of the Human Body, 20th ed. Edited by WH Lewis. New York, Bartelby.com, 2000, fig. 190.)

B

three on the posterior wall, including the *foramen rotundum,* the *pterygoid canal,* and the *pharyngeal canal,* are located in this order downward and medial. On the medial wall is the *sphenopalatine foramen,* and below is the superior orifice of the *pterygopalatine canal* (see Figs. 9–4 and 9–6). The fossa contains the maxillary nerve, the sphenopalatine ganglion, and the terminal part of the internal maxillary artery. The fissures and foramina of the pterygopalatine fossa serve as "highways" for spread of cancer from the sinonasal region to the orbit, infratemporal fossa, and cranial base.

Anterior Cranial Fossa

The floor of the anterior fossa is formed by the orbital plates of the frontal bone, the cribriform plate of the ethmoid, and the lesser wings and front part of the body of the sphenoid. In the midline, it presents, from anterior to posterior, the *frontal crest* for the attachment of the falx cerebri; the *foramen cecum,* which usually transmits a small vein from the nasal cavity to the superior sagittal sinus; and the *crista galli,* the free margin of which affords attachment to the falx cerebri (Fig. 9–7). On each side of the crista galli is the *olfactory groove* formed by the cribriform plate, which supports the olfactory bulb and presents foramina for transmission of the olfactory nerves. Lateral to each olfactory groove are the internal openings of the anterior and posterior ethmoid foramina—the anterior, located at about the middle of the lateral margin of the olfactory groove, transmits the anterior ethmoid vessels and the nasociliary nerve, which runs in a groove along the lateral edge of the cribriform plate; the posterior ethmoid foramen opens at the back part of this margin under cover of the projecting lamina of the sphenoid and transmits the posterior ethmoid vessels and nerve. More laterally, the cranial floor forms the orbital roof and supports the frontal lobes of the cerebrum. Farther back in the middle is the planum sphenoidale, which forms the roof of the sphenoid sinus, and the anterior margin of

the chiasmatic groove, which runs laterally on each side to the upper margin of the optic foramen (see Fig. 9–7).

Orbit

The orbits are two quadrilateral pyramidal cavities; their bases are directed forward and laterally, and their apices backward and medially, so that their long axes diverge at a 45-degree angle and if continued backward, would meet over the body of the sphenoid. The orbit is anatomically defined by seven bones (Fig. 9–8)—frontal, zygomatic, maxillary, lacrimal, ethmoid, sphenoid, and palatine—and by the orbital septum, which originates at the arcus marginalis and fuses with the levator aponeurosis above and the capsulopalpebral fascia below. It is bounded by the ethmoid and sphenoid sinuses at its medial aspect, the frontal sinus superomedially, the cranial vault superiorly and posteriorly, the temporal fossa laterally, and the maxillary sinus inferiorly. Each orbital cavity has a *roof,* a *floor,* a *medial* and a *lateral wall,* a *base,* and an *apex.*

The roof is formed anteriorly by the orbital plate of the frontal bone, and posteriorly by the lesser wing of the sphenoid. It presents medially the *trochlear fovea* for the attachment of the cartilaginous pulley of the superior oblique muscle, and laterally the *lacrimal fossa* for the lacrimal gland.

The floor is formed mainly by the orbital surface of the maxilla—anteriorly and laterally, by the orbital process of the zygomatic bone, and posteriorly and medially, to a small extent, by the orbital process of the palatine bone. At its medial angle is the superior opening of the nasolacrimal canal, immediately to the lateral side of which is a depression for the origin of the inferior oblique muscle. Running anteriorly near the middle of the floor is the infraorbital canal, which ends anterior to the maxilla in the infraorbital foramen and transmits the infraorbital nerve and vessels.

The medial wall is formed anteriorly to posteriorly by the frontal process of the maxilla, the lacrimal bone, the lamina

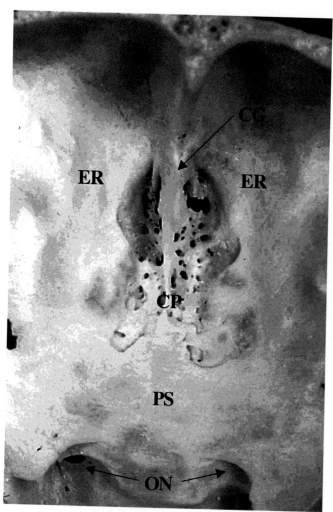

FIGURE 9–7 The floor of the anterior cranial fossa. The cribriform plate (CP) is characterized by the presence of foramina for the olfactory nerves on each side of the crista galli (CG), which is seen in the midline. Lateral to the CP is the ethmoidal roof, and even more lateral is the roof of the orbit. Posterior to the CP is the planum sphenoidale (PS). The optic nerves (ON) form the optic chiasm behind the PS.

papyracea of the ethmoid, and a small part of the body of the sphenoid anterior to the optic foramen. Anteroinferiorly, the lacrimal sac is located between the anterior and posterior lacrimal crests at the junction between the medial wall and the floor. The lacrimal part of the orbicularis oculi arises from the posterior lacrimal crest. At the junction of the medial wall and the roof, the frontoethmoid suture presents the *anterior* and *posterior ethmoid foramina*, the former transmitting the nasociliary nerve and anterior ethmoid vessels, the latter the posterior ethmoid nerve and vessels. These foramina indicate the level of the cranial base within the orbit.

The lateral wall is formed by the orbital process of the zygomatic and orbital surfaces of the greater wing of the sphenoid. On the orbital process of the zygomatic bone are the orbital tubercle (Whitnall's) and the orifices of one or two canals, which transmit the branches of the zygomatic

nerve. Between the roof and the lateral wall, near the apex of the orbit, is the *superior orbital fissure*. Through this fissure, the oculomotor, the trochlear, the ophthalmic division of the trigeminal (V1), and the abducent nerves enter the orbital cavity, as do some filaments from the cavernous plexus of the sympathetic and the orbital branches of the middle meningeal artery. Passing posteriorly through the fissure are the ophthalmic vein and the recurrent branch from the lacrimal artery to the dura mater. The lateral wall and the floor are separated posteriorly by the *inferior orbital fissure,* which transmits the maxillary nerve (V2) and its zygomatic branch, the infraorbital vessels, and the ascending branches from the sphenopalatine ganglion.

The base of the orbit (orbital rim), quadrilateral in shape, is formed superiorly by the supraorbital arch of the frontal bone, in which is located the *supraorbital notch* or *foramen* for passage of the supraorbital vessels and nerve; inferiorly by the zygomatic bone and maxilla, united by the zygomaticomaxillary suture; laterally by the zygomatic bone and the zygomatic process of the frontal joined by the zygomaticofrontal suture; and medially by the frontal bone and the frontal process of the maxilla united by the frontomaxillary suture.

The apex is located in the posterior aspect of the orbit. The optic foramen is a short, cylindrical canal, through which pass the optic nerve and ophthalmic artery.

The extraocular muscles—four rectus muscles and two obliques—enable movement of the eye. The third cranial nerve innervates all but the lateral rectus and the superior oblique muscles, which are innervated by the fourth and sixth cranial nerves, respectively. The rectus muscles originate at the annulus of Zinn and insert on the globe, forming a muscle cone, which is the central anatomic space in the orbit.

The *lacrimal system* comprises secretory and drainage systems. Secretory glands—the glands of Moll, Krause, and Wolfring—may be found along the margin of the eyelid. The lacrimal gland with its palpebral and orbital lobes is located in the superotemporal orbit. The lacrimal drainage system, located in the inferonasal orbit, is represented by the puncta, canaliculi, lacrimal sac, and nasolacrimal duct. Tumor involvement of the lacrimal system may present with epiphora.

The skin of the eyelid is continuous with the palpebral and bulbar conjunctivae, which are, in turn, contiguous with the globe. Each of these epithelial surfaces represents a potential site of origin for cancer.

◘ ETIOLOGY

The cause of sinonasal neoplasms is unknown. There is some epidemiologic evidence, however, to support an occupational risk for developing cancer of the sinonasal tract (SNT). Occupational exposure to inhalation of certain metal dusts or aerosols can cause loss of olfactory acuity, atrophy of the nasal mucosa, mucosal ulcers, perforated nasal septum, dysplasia of the nasal mucosa, or sinonasal cancer. Cancer of the nose and paranasal sinuses has been reported to be more frequent in workers exposed to nickel compounds in nickel refining, cutlery factories, and alkaline

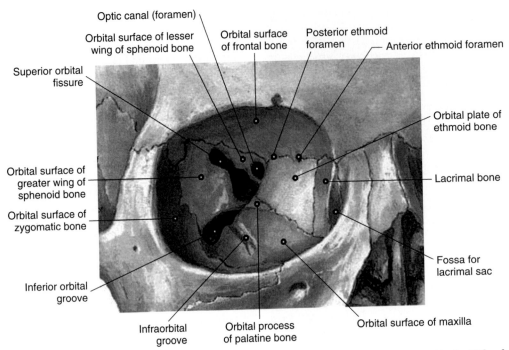

Optic canal (foramen)
Orbital surface of lesser wing of sphenoid bone
Orbital surface of frontal bone
Posterior ethmoid foramen
Anterior ethmoid foramen
Superior orbital fissure
Orbital plate of ethmoid bone
Orbital surface of greater wing of sphenoid bone
Lacrimal bone
Orbital surface of zygomatic bone
Fossa for lacrimal sac
Inferior orbital groove
Infraorbital groove
Orbital process of palatine bone
Orbital surface of maxilla

FIGURE 9–8 Bony anatomy of the right orbit. (From Gray H: Anatomy of the Human Body, 20th ed. Edited by WH Lewis. New York, Bartelby, 2000.)

battery manufacture, or to chromium in chromate production and chrome plating.[4] In a report on the risk of developing sinonasal cancer in Scandinavian countries, nickel workers involved with electrolytic work for longer than 15 years were found to have a 250-fold increased incidence of cancer of the sinus. In the same study, random biopsy of the middle turbinate showed evidence of dysplasia in 21% of workers. These changes were independent of their smoking history. All workers had been employed for at least 10 years, and there was an average latent period of 18 to 36 years before the development of carcinomas, most of which were squamous cell or anaplastic.[5] Similarly, in a Swedish cohort of workers (n = 6454) from seven aluminum foundries and three secondary aluminum (scrap) smelters, significantly elevated risk estimates for sinonasal cancer were observed.[6]

In animals, several heavy metals (e.g., Al, Cd, Co, Hg, Mn, Ni, Zn) have been shown to pass via olfactory receptor neurons from the nasal lumen through the cribriform plate to the olfactory bulb. Some metals (e.g., Mn, Ni, Zn) can even cross synapses in the olfactory bulb and migrate via secondary olfactory neurons to distant nuclei of the brain. The olfactory bulb tends to accumulate certain metals (e.g., Al, Bi, Cu, Mn, Zn) with greater avidity than do other regions of the brain. The molecular mechanisms responsible for metal translocation in olfactory neurons and deposition in the olfactory bulb are unclear, but chelation by metal-binding molecules such as carnosine (beta-alanyl-L-histidine) may be involved.[4]

Other occupational exposures may also increase the risk that cancer of the sinonasal tract will develop. A recent European case-control study revealed that exposure to leather and wood dust was associated with an excess risk of sinonasal cancer.[7] Both wood and leather dusts were associated more with adenocarcinoma than with squamous

cell carcinoma. In these European populations, occupation was associated with about 11% of all sinonasal cancers in women and 39% in men. A meta-analysis of 12 large case-control studies estimated that male woodworkers had a summary odds ratio of sinonasal cancer of 2.6 (95% confidence interval = 2.1–3.3).[8] The risk, which was greatest among men who had been employed in jobs with the highest wood dust exposure, increased with duration of exposure.[9, 10] Employment in the boot and shoe industry has also been associated with adenocarcinoma of the nasal cavity in England and Italy.[11] Data from a case-control study conducted at 27 hospitals in France showed that exposure to textile dust was associated with an elevated risk of squamous cell carcinoma and adenocarcinoma of the sinonasal tract, and that the risk increased with the duration and level of exposure.[12]

Although epidemiologic studies have not addressed the relationship between outdoor air pollution and sinonasal malignant neoplasms, a recent report on the incidence of sinonasal cancer in urban polluted cities suggests such a correlation.[13] Both primary and environmental (secondary) tobacco smoke also appear to be related to an increased incidence of sinonasal cancer, particularly squamous cell carcinoma.[7, 14, 15]

◻ PATHOLOGY

Cancer of the Nasal Cavity and Paranasal Sinuses

The mucosal lining of the nose—*the schneiderian membrane*—is derived from ectoderm. This is uniquely different from the mucosa of the rest of the upper respiratory tract, which is derived from endoderm. Olfactory neuroepithelium lines the superior portion of the nasal cavity and the roof of the nose. The sinonasal epithelium also has mucinous and minor salivary glands. The unique histology of this region is reflected in the histogenesis of a complex variety of epithelial and nonepithelial tumors (Table 9–1). These tumors have a wide range of biologic behavior, and a few (e.g., inverted papilloma, olfactory neuroblastoma) arise only in the sinonasal tract. However, the most common epithelial neoplasms of the sinonasal tract are those arising from "metaplastic" (squamous) epithelium and those originating from the seromucinous glands of the mucosal lining. Nonepithelial tumors are similar to those in other regions in the head and neck (see Table 9–1).

Sinonasal cancer accounts for about 1% of all malignancies and approximately 3% of cancers of the head and neck.[16, 17] There is a male predominance and a strong predilection for whites. A majority of patients are older than 50 years of age at the time of diagnosis. The most common malignant tumor of the nasal cavity and paranasal sinuses is squamous cell carcinoma, followed in frequency by adenocarcinoma (Fig. 9–9A).[18, 19] The maxillary sinus is the most common site of origin, followed in frequency by the lateral nasal wall and ethmoid sinuses. Primary carcinoma of the frontal sinus is uncommon,[20] and those arising in the sphenoid sinus are rare (Fig. 9–9B).[16]

Schneiderian Papillomas

Schneiderian papillomas are relatively uncommon, representing 0.4% to 4.7% of all sinonasal tumors. Their cause is unknown, but recent investigations have suggested that human papilloma virus (HPV) is involved in the development of sinonasal papilloma.[21–23]

There are three distinct types of schneiderian papillomas—fungiform, inverted, and cylindrical cell papilloma. The fungiform variety, which constitutes 50% of all schneiderian papillomas, arises almost invariably from the nasal septum, usually the anterior portion. The other two varieties originate primarily from the lateral nasal wall. Fungiform papillomas are multifocal in 25% of cases, are not considered premalignant, and have a relatively low incidence of associated invasive squamous cell carcinoma (3.5%). They must be distinguished from the more common keratinizing papillomas that originate from the hair-bearing skin of the nasal vestibule. The treatment of choice for fungiform papilloma is complete surgical excision. Inadequate excision accounts for the 22% to 50% incidence of local recurrence.[17]

Inverted papilloma accounts for 47% of sinonasal papillomas. They are more common among men and occur mostly in the 40- to 70-year-old age group. They usually originate from the lateral nasal wall in the region of the middle turbinate and ethmoid sinuses. Less common sites of origin, such as the nasopharynx, oropharynx, middle ear, nasal septum, lacrimal system, and frontal and sphenoid sinuses, have been described.[24–27] Although histologically "benign," inverted papillomas of the nose are locally aggressive and invade the paranasal sinuses, the nasopharynx, and occasionally the orbit and even the brain.[26, 28] Inverted papilloma is frequently multicentric, and there is a 3% to 24% (average 13%) incidence of coexisting carcinoma, mostly squamous cell.[17]

Because inverted papilloma is locally aggressive and may harbor coexisting carcinoma in a significant number of patients, the main goal of treatment should be complete surgical excision. This minimizes the risk of recurrence and allows comprehensive evaluation of the specimen for the presence of any coexisting malignancy. The recurrence rates quoted in the literature vary from less than 5% to as high as 75%, possibly depending on the surgical approach and the completeness of the surgical excision. Although

---

TABLE 9–1 Tumors of the Sinonasal Tract

Benign
Epithelial
  Papilloma
  Adenoma
  Dermoid
Nonepithelial
  Fibroma
  Chondroma
  Osteoma
  Neurofibroma
  Hemangioma
  Lymphangioma
  Nasal glioma
Intermediate
Schneiderian papilloma
  Inverted
  Fungiform
  Cylindrical
Angiofibroma
Ameloblastoma
Fibrous dysplasia
Ossifying fibroma
Giant cell tumor
Malignant
Epithelial
  Squamous cell carcinoma
    Differentiated (well, moderately, poorly)
    Basaloid squamous
    Adenosquamous
  Non-squamous cell carcinoma
    Adenoid cystic carcinoma
    Mucoepidermoid carcinoma
    Adenocarcinoma
    Neuroendocrine carcinoma
    Hyalinizing clear cell carcinoma
  Melanoma
  Olfactory neuroblastoma
  Sinonasal undifferentiated carcinoma (SNUC)
Nonepithelial
  Chondrosarcoma
  Osteogenic sarcoma
  Chordoma
  Soft tissue sarcoma
    Fibrosarcoma
    Malignant fibrous histiocytoma
    Hemangiopericytoma
    Angiosarcoma
    Kaposi's sarcoma
    Rhabdomyosarcoma
  Lymphoproliferative
    Lymphoma
    Polymorphic reticulosis
    Plasmacytoma
Metastatic
  Renal
  Lung
  Breast
  Ovary

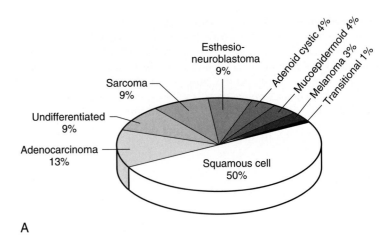

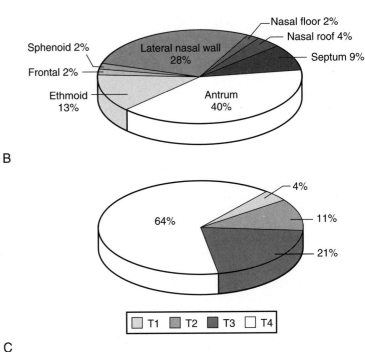

FIGURE 9–9 Data of 86 consecutive patients with sinonasal malignancy treated at the University of Arkansas for Medical Sciences between 1988 and 1998. Patients are classified according to (A) histopathologic diagnosis, (B) site of tumor origin, and (C) T-stage. (From Hanna E, Vural E, Teo C, et al: Sinonasal tumors: The Arkansas experience. Skull Base Surg 8[suppl]:15, 1998.)

multicentricity of the tumor has been suggested to be responsible for the high rate of recurrence, inadequate removal of the tumor during the initial resection seems to be the most important predictive factor of local recurrence.[29] This is supported by the correlation of low recurrence rates with more definitive procedures that permit adequate exposure and resection, such as lateral rhinotomy and medial maxillectomy.[30] Conservative surgical approaches, such as transnasal or transantral excision, have 27% to 78% recurrence rates; more definitive procedures, such as medial maxillectomy with lateral rhinotomy or with facial degloving approaches, have 0% to 29% recurrence rates.[29–31] In the University of Pittsburgh experience, recurrence rates following lateral rhinotomy with medial maxillectomy and meticulous removal of all additional mucosa from the ipsilateral maxillary, ethmoid, and sphenoid sinuses were lower than 5%.[30] Several recent reports described good results with endoscopic resection of inverted papilloma.[32–35] Although endoscopic resection may be adequate for small inverted papilloma limited to the lateral nasal wall,

more extensive lesions should probably be removed via an open approach.[36, 37]

Rarely, inverted papilloma invades the cranium, the meninges, and even the brain. A report from the University of Arkansas reviewed 21 cases of inverted papilloma with intracranial extension.[26] Coexisting squamous cell carcinoma was identified in almost half of patients. Of the 12 patients with "pure" inverted papilloma and intracranial extension, a majority (83%) had recurrent disease after initial treatment of inverted papilloma confined to the nose and sinuses. Patients with extradural disease had a survival rate of 86% with an average follow-up of 4.4 years. Eighty-six percent of these survivors were treated with craniofacial resection. In contrast, 75% of patients with intradural inverted papilloma were dead of disease within an average of 9 months regardless of the treatment modality. This review demonstrates that intracranial extension of inverted papilloma is most often associated with recurrent and incompletely excised tumors. Although intracranial *extradural* inverted papilloma can be effectively controlled with craniofacial resection, *intradural* disease has a poor prognosis regardless of treatment. Aggressive initial treatment of intranasal inverted papilloma may be the most important factor in preventing intracranial extension.[26]

Squamous Cell Carcinoma

SQUAMOUS CELL CARCINOMA OF THE NASAL CAVITY

Primary squamous cell carcinoma (SCC) of the nasal cavity is an uncommon malignancy. Most reported series include it with cancer of the paranasal sinuses.[38] The lateral nasal wall is the most common site of origin, followed by the nasal septum (see Fig. 9–9B).[18] About three fourths of cases of cancer of the septum arise anteriorly at or near the mucocutaneous junction, and the majority are of low grade. Prognosis is more closely related to size and location than to histologic grade. The nasal vestibule is lined by hair-bearing skin, and some consider it part of the integument rather than the nasal cavity proper. However, SCC of the nasal vestibule is more capricious than is cutaneous SCC found elsewhere on the face. Extension of these tumors into the base of the columella, nasal floor, or upper lip indicates aggressive behavior and is often associated with nodal metastasis.[17]

Treatment of SCC of the nasal cavity depends on the stage of disease. In general, early lesions (T1–T2) can be effectively managed by either surgery or radiation therapy (external or implant). Advanced cancer (T3–T4) is best approached with a combination of these two modalities. Regional lymph node metastasis occurs in 10% to 20% of cases. Elective treatment of the neck, therefore, may be considered in these cases. Local recurrence is common, occurring in 30% to 40% of cases. It is most often due to underestimation of the extent of disease, or to attempts at less radical treatment to preserve function and avoid the risk of complications. Systemic metastasis occurs in 10% of patients; another 15% have or will develop a second primary malignancy, about half of which occur in the head and neck. The 3-year and 5-year survival rates reported for patients with SCC of the nasal cavity were 86% and 69%, respectively[39]; the main cause of death is uncontrolled or recurrent disease at the primary site. Signs of poor prognosis include involvement of more than one area within the nasal cavity, extension outside of the nose, invasion of bone, metastasis to cervical lymph nodes, and large size of the primary lesion.

SQUAMOUS CELL CARCINOMA OF THE PARANASAL SINUSES

The majority of SCC of the paranasal sinuses is keratinizing but tends to be only moderately differentiated. Nonkeratinizing and undifferentiated carcinomas are less common, and undifferentiated carcinomas show a more rapid course of growth. Sinonasal basaloid SCC is a histologically distinct variant with pathologic features and a more aggressive biologic behavior, similar to basaloid SCC in other locations in the head and neck.[40] Verrucous carcinoma is another distinct variant of SCC that is well differentiated and has less tendency for deeper invasion. Its occurrence in the maxillary antrum is rare.[41] However, the extent of disease rather than the degree of differentiation is the most important determinant of prognosis. Because of the advanced stage of most paranasal sinus carcinomas at the time of presentation, the disease remains highly lethal despite aggressive treatment. Most recent reports show that the majority of patients (85%) still present with advanced-stage (T3–T4) cancer (Fig. 9–9C).[18, 19, 42, 43]

Another important factor responsible for the poor prognosis of SCC of the paranasal sinuses is early invasion of the cranial base. This is most common in superiorly or posteriorly located cancer. Perhaps this is the reason for the poorer prognosis for "suprastructure" carcinomas arising above or behind Ohngren's line (vide infra). Their relatively early extension to the cranial base is directly related to the close proximity of the paranasal sinuses to many of the foramina and fissures that transmit neurovascular structures through the cranial base. This, in addition to direct bony invasion of the cranial floor, provides yet another route of cranial base extension.

Although the reported incidence of clinically evident lymph node metastasis presentation is around 10% to 15%, the overall risk of nodal involvement from SCC of the paranasal sinuses is closer to 30%.[44] Regional spread to the lymph nodes is uncommon in cancer confined within the sinus walls. Once invasion into the overlying soft tissue and adjacent structures occurs (e.g., in the oral cavity), nodal involvement and even dissemination to distant sites are noted more frequently.[45]

Optimal treatment strategies for SCC of the paranasal sinuses remain to be defined, but there is almost universal agreement that advanced-stage disease is best treated with multimodal therapy.[1, 42, 43, 46] The most commonly employed treatment is radical en bloc surgical resection followed by postoperative radiation therapy. The 5-year survival rates associated with this approach range from 55% to 70%.[1, 18, 43, 46] Other treatment options, such as preoperative radiotherapy and chemotherapy followed by surgical salvage,[42] or the incorporation of conservative surgery with radiotherapy and regional chemotherapy,[47–49] have resulted in similar survival rates, but with less frequent need for radical resection.

Sinonasal Undifferentiated Carcinoma

In 1987, Levine and coworkers first described the clinical and pathologic findings of an undifferentiated carcinoma with distinct features arising in the nasal cavity and paranasal sinuses.[50] Clinically, sinonasal undifferentiated carcinoma (SNUC) is characterized by extensive tissue destruction and frequent involvement of the orbit and anterior cranial fossa (Fig. 9–10A).[51] Curiously, these tumors exhibit a paucity of significant symptoms relative to the extent of disease at the time of diagnosis. Histologically, SNUC is composed of pleomorphic cells with a high nuclear-cytoplasmic ratio, arranged in nests, sheets, and trabeculae. The differential diagnosis includes esthesioneuroblastoma (see under Olfactory Neuroblastoma), lymphoma, rhabdomyosarcoma, melanoma, and lymphoepithelioma. Light microscopy can usually distinguish SNUC from these neoplasms, but occasionally immunohistochemistry or electron microscopy is required.[52–54]

The distinction between SNUC and esthesioneuroblastoma is important because the behavior, prognosis, and

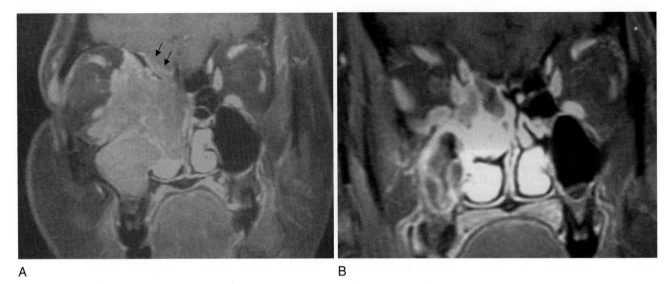

A   B

FIGURE 9–10 A 37-year-old woman presented with right-sided proptosis and diplopia. On ophthalmologic examination, she had limitation of ocular motility and an afferent pupillary defect, indicating involvement of the extraocular muscles and optic nerve, respectively. Biopsy was consistent with sinonasal undifferentiated carcinoma (SNUC). *A,* T1-weighted coronal MRI with gadolinium showed a right sinonasal tumor involving the nasal cavity, maxillary antrum, and ethmoid sinus, with significant extension and invasion into the right orbit. Contrast enhancement along the cribriform plate and the dura of the anterior cranial fossa *(arrows)* suggests intracranial extension. *B,* T1-weighted coronal MRI with gadolinium after two cycles of induction chemotherapy consisting of cisplatinum and 5-FU. Note the remarkable response in the tumor. The nasal cavity shows the normal enhancement of the turbinates, and the signal characteristics in the maxillary and ethmoid sinuses suggest inflammatory changes and no evidence of residual tumor. The extraocular muscles and optic nerve, which were indistinguishable from tumor on the pretreatment MRI, are now clearly visible. There is no further contrast enhancement along the cribriform plate or dura. The patient was subsequently treated with concurrent chemotherapy and intensity-modulated radiation therapy (IMRT). She had a complete tumor response to treatment and was spared a maxillectomy, craniofacial resection, and probable orbital exenteration. AT 2 years follow-up, she remained without evidence of disease.

treatment for these differ. Whereas esthesioneuroblastoma is usually slow growing and has a relatively better prognosis, SNUC is a tumor that progresses more rapidly, resulting in an extremely poor prognosis. In a recent report of 25 patients with SNUC, the median survival was 18 months.[53]

Distinguishing SNUC from esthesioneuroblastoma is not always easy. SNUC exhibits a greater number of mitotic figures, more abundant nuclear pleomorphism, extensive necrosis, and vascular invasion. On the other hand, esthesioneuroblastoma typically consists of small uniform cells with neurofibrillary processes and rosette formation.[53, 54] In a recent report, almost 95% of SNUC showed a diffuse positive immunoreaction for AE1/AE3 cytokeratins, whereas neither olfactory neuroblastoma nor malignant melanoma revealed positive immunostaining to these markers. Also, 80% of SNUC showed positive immunostaining for LMP-1, an Epstein-Barr virus (EBV)-related protein, whereas none of the olfactory neuroblastomas were LMP-1 positive.[55] The role of EBV infection in the pathogenesis of SNUC is, however, still under debate.[53]

There has been no consensus yet on the best therapeutic approach to SNUC. Deutsch and coworkers reported an improved outcome in patients with SNUC who were treated with preoperative combination chemotherapy (cyclophosphamide, doxorubicin, and vincristine) and radiation therapy.[56] This regimen is followed by definitive surgical resection in patients without extensive intracranial involvement and without distant metastasis. This regimen was compared with the results from an earlier report by the same authors wherein radiation therapy alone or in combination with chemotherapy was used in a similar group of patients. The data from this study and others suggest that patients without intracranial or metastatic disease may have improved survival with this multimodal approach.[51, 53–56] Induction chemotherapy may also limit the extent of resection or may enhance the chances of orbital preservation in patients with extensive SNUC (see Fig. 9–10).

Non–Squamous Cell Carcinoma

Nonepidermoid epithelial malignant neoplasms of the sinonasal tract can arise either from the surface epithelium or from the salivary glandular elements of the mucosa. There are numerous ways to classify such tumors, but perhaps the easiest classification divides them into salivary and nonsalivary histologic types.[17] A review of 106 patients with non–squamous cell cancer of the nasal cavity and paranasal sinuses treated at the Memorial Sloan-Kettering Cancer Center revealed the following histologic types: salivary-type carcinoma (33 patients); sarcoma (25 patients); melanoma (18 patients); esthesioneuroblastoma (11 patients); lymphoma (11 patients); and anaplastic cancer

(9 patients).[57] Most tumors arose in the nasal cavity (50%), followed by the antrum (39%), ethmoid sinus (9%), and frontal sinus (2%). Determinate 5-year and 10-year cure rates were as follows, respectively: esthesioneuroblastoma, 70% and 50%; lymphoma, 45% and 30%; anaplastic, 33% and 25%; salivary, 31% and 18%; sarcoma, 25% and 21%; and melanoma, 19% and 0%.[57]

ADENOID CYSTIC CARCINOMA

Adenoid cystic carcinoma (ACC) accounts for approximately 10% of all nonsquamous carcinomas in the head and neck and 15% of all cancers of the salivary glands.[58, 59] It is the second most common cancer of salivary glands, after mucoepidermoid carcinoma. ACC arises more commonly in the minor salivary glands than in all the major glands combined. It accounts for more than 35% of all tumors involving the minor salivary glands.[17] The oral cavity, including the palate, and the sinonasal tract are the most common sites, representing 50% and 18% of all ACC in the minor salivary glands, respectively. ACC represents 3% to 15% of malignant tumors arising in the paranasal sinuses (see Fig. 9–9A).[18] It is slightly more common among women, and approximately 90% of patients are between 30 and 70 years of age, with a peak incidence in the fifth and sixth decades of life.

Adenoid cystic carcinoma exhibits three histologic subtypes based on tumor architecture: cribriform, tubular, and solid. The *cribriform* pattern, which is the most common subtype, has the classic "Swiss cheese" appearance in which the cells are arranged in nests separated by round or oval spaces (Fig. 9–11). This characteristic stromal architecture of ACC, represented by stromal pseudocysts, may be due to the ability of ACC cells to synthesize, secrete, and degrade basement membrane proteins such as fibronectin[60] and heparan sulfate proteoglycan.[61] The biosynthesis and secretion of these basement membrane proteins are regulated by the rate of cell growth and may reflect the correlation between histologic appearance and biologic behavior of ACC.[62, 63] The *tubular* (or trabecular) pattern has a more

glandular architecture, and the *solid* (or basaloid) pattern shows sheets of cells with little or no luminal spaces. The tubular variety has the best prognosis, the solid variety has the worst prognosis, and the cribriform pattern has an intermediate prognosis.[64, 65] Most ACCs exhibit a mixed architecture of more than one pattern; their classification in such cases depends on the predominant histologic subtype.[66]

Adenoid cystic carcinoma exhibits a slow-growing, locally aggressive, relentless progression of disease. Patients may have symptoms from 10 weeks to 15 years before diagnosis, with an average of 5 years. Recurrence can occur 10 to 20 years after the initial treatment, and 5-year "survival" rates may give an erroneous indication of absolute survival.[67] Perineural spread—the hallmark of adenoid cystic carcinoma—is usually evident and provides avenues of spread to the cranial base and the central nervous system.[68, 69] The maxillary, mandibular, and vidian nerves are the most frequently involved; they allow perineural spread of sinonasal ACC through the foramina rotundum and ovale and the vidian canal (Fig. 9–12). Retrograde spread intracranially, or alternatively, antegrade spread from the Gasserian ganglion to the nerve branches in the infratemporal and pterygopalatine fossae, can then occur. Achievement of negative surgical margins in such cases is difficult.[58] Perhaps this is one of the reasons why ACC of the sinonasal tract has the worst prognosis of all sites in the head and neck.[67] The mechanism of perineural spread of cancer is poorly understood. Recently, investigators from the University of Arkansas have shown that neural cell adhesion molecules (NCAMs) may have a role in the pathogenesis of perineural spread of malignant tumors, including ACC and squamous cell carcinoma.[68, 70]

Lymphatic spread of ACC is uncommon. The incidence of lymph node metastasis from ACC detected at presentation or developing later in the course of the disease ranges from 10% to 30%.[71, 72] Metastasis to the regional lymphatics is more common in tumors originating from the parotid glands than the minor salivary glands, and in those with a solid rather than a cribriform or tubular histopathologic pattern.[71] The development of lymph node metastasis was associated with poor outcome despite aggressive therapy.[64, 72–75]

Distant hematogenous dissemination is considerably more frequent than lymphatic metastasis, with an average incidence of 40%. The incidence of distant metastasis correlates highly with the stage of disease (i.e., size of the primary tumor and status of the lymph nodes) on presentation. The lungs and bones are the sites most frequently involved in systemic metastasis. Although distant metastases usually indicate poor prognosis, more than 20% of patients with metastatic adenoid cystic carcinoma of the minor salivary glands live 5 years or longer after developing metastases.[76]

Surgical excision of ACC remains the most commonly used method of treatment. Obtaining tumor-free margins is very difficult in most cases because of perineural spread.[58, 77] Craniofacial surgery has facilitated the gross total excision of advanced lesions that were deemed inoperable in the past. In a recent report from the University of Pittsburgh of 35 patients with ACC of the sinonasal tract treated with craniofacial resection and postoperative radiation, the local

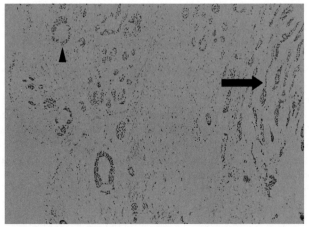

FIGURE 9–11 The classic "Swiss cheese" appearance of the cribriform variety of adenoid cystic carcinoma. Note the presence of perineural (*arrowhead*) and intraneural (*arrow*) tumor.

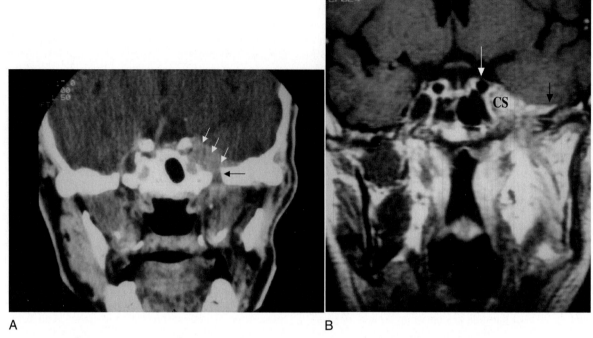

A   B

FIGURE 9–12 Imaging studies in a patient with perineural spread of adenoid cystic carcinoma along the third division of the trigeminal nerve (V3), involving the cavernous sinus and the dura of the middle cranial fossa. *A,* A coronal CT with IV contrast showing widening of the left foramen ovale *(black arrow),* compared with the one on the right. There is also enhancement and thickening along the left Meckel's cave *(white arrows).* *B,* A coronal T1-weighted MRI with gadolinium showing marked thickening and enhancement of V3, trigeminal ganglion, and the lateral cavernous sinus (CS). The tumor abuts the cavernous carotid artery *(white arrow).* There is enhancement of the dura along the floor of the middle cranial fossa *(black arrow).* This "dural tail" is usually a sign of involvement of the dura with tumor.

control rate was 64%.[78] This high rate of local disease control, however, did not translate to an improvement in disease-free survival (46% at median follow-up of 40 months), probably because of the high incidence of distant metastasis (20%).

Postoperative radiation is used to achieve better local control, especially if there is microscopic evidence of disease at or close to the resection margin. In a recent report of patients with ACC of the maxillary sinus, patients who were treated with combined surgery and radiation achieved a much lower local recurrence rate than those treated with either modality alone.[67] Postoperative radiation therapy may also improve survival. In the University of Michigan experience with patients with ACC of the sinonasal tract, the 6-year survival for patients treated with surgery and radiation was 73% compared with 50% for those treated with radiation only.[77] In another recent study, preoperative radiation was thought to decrease the incidence of distant metastasis.[79] However, owing to the increased rate of postoperative complications associated with preoperative radiation, most surgeons still recommend the use of adjuvant radiation after surgery.

Over the past decade, there has been growing evidence that fast-neutron radiation therapy provides higher rates of locoregional control of unresectable or recurrent ACC compared with photon or electron radiation therapy, and perhaps should be considered the initial treatment of choice in some cases.[80, 81] In one study of patients treated with fast-neutron radiation for gross inoperable, residual unresectable,

or recurrent disease, the 5-year locoregional control rates were 92% for patients treated definitively (without a previous surgical procedure), 63% for those treated postoperatively for gross residual disease, and 51% for those treated for recurrent disease after a surgical procedure.[82] This study suggested that neutron irradiation alone may be the therapy of choice in the treatment of some patients with unresectable advanced-stage ACC, and that surgery should be limited to those patients in whom disease-free margins can be obtained. A potentially morbid "debulking" surgical procedure before neutron irradiation is not warranted because no improvement in locoregional control can be demonstrated over that achievable with neutron therapy alone.[82]

A recent study of 75 patients with inoperable, recurrent, or incompletely resected ACC showed that fast neutron radiotherapy provides higher local control rates than a mixed beam and photons. This advantage for neutrons in local control, however, was not transferred to significant differences in survival because of a high incidence of distant metastasis, which occurred in 40% of these patients.[81] In another recent study of 72 patients with recurrent or gross residual ACC after surgery treated with fast neutron therapy, the recurrence-free survival rates were 83% after 1 year, 71% after 2 years, and 45% after 5 years.[80] These impressive results are encouraging; however, the use of fast-neutron radiation therapy is hampered by the lack of its widespread availability. Currently, only a few facilities are equipped with the technology and expertise of delivering fast-neutron radiation therapy. It is hoped, therefore, that fast-neutron therapy will become more widely available for patients with unresectable ACC.

Currently, the use of chemotherapy in the treatment of ACC is investigational.[83, 84] Generally, combination therapy is more effective than single-drug treatment.[85] The most effective drug regimens include cisplatin, paclitaxel, doxorubicin (Adriamycin), 5-fluorouracil, and epirubicin in different combinations.[86] Locally recurrent disease is best treated with repeated resection followed by radiation therapy, if it was not used in the initial treatment. Because the median survival after the appearance of distant metastases exceeds 6 years, aggressive local therapy may be indicated even in patients with metastatic disease.

Similar to patients with ACC in other sites, the reported outcome of patients with ACC of the sinonasal tract depends on the length of follow-up. Unlike in squamous cell carcinoma, survival curves of patients with ACC do not show a plateau at 5 years, and survival continues to decline even after 20 years.[58] For patients with ACC of the nasal cavity and paranasal sinuses, the 10-year overall and disease-specific survival rates range from 40% to 60%.[67, 79] Series with longer follow-up show these rates to decline to 20% by 30 years.[87]

Overall, the prognosis of patients with ACC of the nasal cavity and paranasal sinuses is worse than for those with ACC originating from other sites.[58, 67, 79, 88] Other adverse prognostic factors for patients with sinonasal ACC include advanced stage of disease, solid and high-grade histology, positive surgical margins, perineural spread along major nerves, locoregional failure, and systemic metastasis. Detailed discussion of these clinical factors, as well as newly described biologic and molecular markers that affect prognosis of patients with ACC, is presented in Chapter 21, Malignant Tumors of the Salivary Glands.

ADENOCARCINOMA

Adenocarcinoma is the second most common malignant tumor of the sinonasal tract after squamous cell carcinoma. It accounts for approximately 15% of all sinonasal cancers (see Fig. 9–9A).[18] Adenocarcinoma can arise from any site in the sinonasal tract, but the ethmoid sinuses are most frequently involved. Adenocarcinoma exhibits a striking male predominance (75%–90%), with a peak age incidence between 55 and 60 years. As was mentioned earlier, there is a higher incidence of these tumors in persons involved in wood, leather, textile, and furniture industries (see under Etiology).[7-12] These are generally adult male occupations, which may at least partially explain the sex and age predominance.

Adenocarcinoma of the sinonasal tract may originate from the surface epithelium, the minor salivary glands, or both. There are three basic growth forms: papillary, sessile, and alveolar-mucoid. The papillary type arises primarily from the surface epithelium and is characterized by a delicate fibrovascular core covered by malignant cells. The sessile type probably arises from the minor salivary glands and goblet cells, and it resembles adenocarcinoma of the gastrointestinal tract. The alveolar-mucoid type arises from the mucoserous glands and is confined to the lamina propria. It is characterized by signet ring cells, multiple goblet cells, and clusters of tumor cells floating in lakes of mucin.[17] A combination of the three patterns may occur in any given tumor, or one pattern may predominate. It seems that the papillary type may have a better prognosis.

Immunohistochemical stains showed that a number of sinonasal adenocarcinomas demonstrate the presence of secretory granules containing gastrin, glucagon, somatostatin, serotonin, and other neurosecretory amines. Whether the presence of neuroendocrine granules in adenocarcinoma is associated with a different biologic behavior is unknown. The incidence of a "true" neuroendocrine carcinoma in the paranasal sinuses is extremely rare, and its presentation as part of multiple endocrine neoplasia type 1 (MEN 1) has been described.[89] Other biologic markers have been recently reported to have prognostic significance in patients with adenocarcinoma of the sinonasal tract. Overexpression of c-erbB-2 was associated with a high incidence of local recurrence, reduced overall and disease-specific survival, and overall poor prognosis in patients with adenocarcinoma of the ethmoid sinuses.[90] Other recent studies demonstrated that the presence of H-RAS point mutations defines a subgroup of patients with ethmoid sinus adenocarcinomas for whom the prognosis is very poor.[91]

Because most adenocarcinomas of the sinonasal tract originate from the ethmoid sinuses, surgical excision frequently involves a craniofacial resection. In 2002, a report from Bordeaux, France, described the outcome of 76 patients with adenocarcinoma of the ethmoid sinuses treated with radical surgery.[9] Approximately 60% of these patients were staged as T3N0M0. Fifty percent of the patients were treated with craniofacial resection, and approximately 60% received postoperative radiation therapy. Local recurrence developed in 23% of patients, and 10% experienced cervical node and systemic metastasis. Survival rates were 82% at 3 years, 80% at 5 years, and 72% at 10 years. The prognosis was significantly correlated with local control. Local recurrence was more likely in patients with involvement of the dura, brain, and sphenoid sinus.[9]

One year earlier, another report from Rotterdam, the Netherlands, challenged the concept of radical surgery and reported results with surgical debulking and topical chemotherapy in a similar number of patients (70) with adenocarcinoma of the ethmoid sinuses.[92] Surgical debulking was done via an extended anterior maxillary antrostomy followed by a combination of repeated topical chemotherapy (fluorouracil) and frequent debridement of necrotic tumor. Radiotherapy was given for local recurrence, which occurred in 13% of patients. Adjusted disease-free survival at 2, 5, and 10 years was 96%, 87%, and 74%, respectively. The authors concluded that in patients with adenocarcinoma of the ethmoid sinuses, a combination of surgical debulking and repeated topical chemotherapy results in disease control and survival rates that are not different from those obtained by craniofacial resection and postoperative radiation therapy.[92] These contrasting reports illustrate that the optimal treatment for adenocarcinomas of the sinonasal tract remains unclear.

Melanoma

Melanoma of the sinonasal tract is rare. It accounts for approximately 3% of sinonasal cancers (see Fig. 9–9A).[18]

The nasal cavity is more commonly affected than the paranasal sinuses, and the maxillary antrum is more frequently involved than the ethmoid sinuses. The peak age incidence is between the fifth and eighth decades.[93] Presenting symptoms of melanoma are the same as those of other sinonasal neoplasms. On examination, the diagnosis may be obvious if a heavily pigmented polypoid or fleshy mass is seen within the nasal cavity. Some melanomas, however, are amelanotic and may appear pink-tan in color. Also, darkly pigmented people may have normal pigmentation of the mucosa within the nasal cavity.

The histologic appearance of sinonasal melanoma could be as varied as that of its cutaneous counterpart. Several histologic subtypes are described, including, in descending order, amelanotic small blue cell, pleomorphic, epithelioid, spindle cell, and myxoid. High mitotic rate and vascular invasion, absence of tumor-infiltrating lymphocytes, and regression are features shared by all sinonasal melanomas.[94] In the absence of identifiable melanin, the differential diagnosis includes anaplastic carcinoma, lymphoma, rhabdomyosarcoma, esthesioneuroblastoma, and other small round cell malignancies. Special stains and electron microscopy are used to establish the diagnosis. Negative staining of B- and T-cell markers and leukocyte common antigen (LCA) differentiate melanoma from lymphoma. Neuroendocrine markers such as neuron-specific enolase (NSE), chromogranin, and synaptophysin are usually expressed in esthesioneuroblastoma but not in melanoma. Cytokeratin differentiates melanoma from undifferentiated carcinoma. S-100 protein is usually expressed in mucosal melanomas, but variable staining intensity is demonstrated, with areas of complete negativity. HMB45 is strongly and uniformly (>80%) expressed in all undifferentiated small blue cell sinonasal melanomas. Some pigmented sinonasal melanomas, however, are predominantly HMB45-negative. The stronger HMB45 staining in amelanotic small blue cell mucosal melanomas is explained by the reaction of HMB45 antibody with an oncofetal antigen found in immature melanosomes. In poorly differentiated amelanotic malignant melanomas, antibody to HMB45 has proved to be a superb diagnostic marker.[94]

In general, mucosal melanomas of the head and neck, as a group, are rapidly lethal neoplasms. They are preponderantly thick melanomas and as a consequence can present with cervical lymph node metastasis with or without distant spread. Long-term survival is unusual to rare; 5-year survival is poor, and 10-year survival is dismal.[93] In a recent report of 72 patients with sinonasal mucosal melanoma treated with radical surgery with and without adjuvant radiation therapy, overall 5-year actuarial survival was 28%, and overall 10-year actuarial survival was 20%, with a median survival of 21 months.[95] A majority of disease-related deaths occurred within the first 36 months owing to local and/or systemic disease, irrespective of the treatment modality. There was no statistical difference in local control or survival between patients receiving surgery alone and those receiving surgery and radiotherapy. The addition of chemotherapy had no impact on survival, nor did the site of the tumor, the surgical procedure, the presence of lymph node metastases, or the age of the patient.[95] These data illustrate the need for new, more effective therapy for sinonasal mucosal melanoma. Several new biologic and immunomodulatory treatments are currently being investigated for use in patients with mucosal melanoma; the results of such treatment approaches are eagerly awaited.

Olfactory Neuroblastoma

Olfactory neuroblastoma, also known as esthesioneuroblastoma, is a tumor of neural crest origin. It arises almost exclusively from the olfactory epithelium of the nasal cavity and paranasal sinuses. Olfactory neuroblastoma represents 7% to 10% of sinonasal malignancy (see Fig. 9–9A).[18] It occurs with equal frequency in men and women. There is a bimodal age distribution, with one peak occurring in the group 11 to 20 years old and the second in the group 51 to 60 years old.

Microscopically, the tumor is composed of round cells larger than lymphocytes, with round nuclei, dense chromatin, and inconspicuous cytoplasm. The hallmark of this tumor is the arrangement of these cells into rosettes, pseudorosettes, or sheets and clusters.[17] In the absence of rosettes and pseudorosettes, the differential diagnosis includes anaplastic carcinoma, malignant lymphoma, malignant melanoma, plasmacytoma, embryonal rhabdomyosarcoma, and metastatic small cell carcinoma. Electron microscopy and special stains for neurofibrils are needed to establish the diagnosis. Esthesioneuroblastoma usually expresses a variety of neuroendocrine markers such as neuron-specific enolase (NSE), chromogranin, and synaptophysin.

There is evidence that the histologic grade of esthesioneuroblastoma influences biologic behavior, particularly as it relates to disease progression, local recurrence, and metastasis.[96] A study from the M.D. Anderson Cancer Center divided olfactory neuroblastomas into two groups: (1) neuroblastomas proper and (2) neuroendocrine carcinomas.[97] Neuroblastomas were subdivided into those manifesting olfactory differentiation and those without olfactory differentiation. Neuroblastomas without olfactory differentiation show a minimal tendency toward rosette formation; neuroendocrine carcinomas show no evidence of rosettes or pseudorosettes. Based on this histologic classification, it appears that well-differentiated tumors have a slower disease progression and fewer tendencies for local recurrence. Hyams from the Armed Forces Institute of Pathology (AFIP) introduced another histopathologic classification based largely on the level of cellular differentiation.[98] Four grades of differentiation were described based on growth, architecture, mitotic activity, necrosis, nuclear pleomorphism, rosette formation, and fibrillary stroma. Features designating higher grades in the Hyams systems have been found to correlate with a rapid clinical progression and reduced survival. Whatever system is used, it seems that high-grade tumors have the worst prognosis and probably should be more aggressively treated with combined modality therapy.

The prognosis of patients with esthesioneuroblastoma is also significantly related to the extent of disease. Several clinical staging systems have evolved over the years to help clinicians in planning treatment and predicting prognosis of patients with esthesioneuroblastoma. At least three staging classifications have been proposed. In 1976, Kadish

TABLE 9-2 TNM Staging of Esthesioneuroblastoma

Primary Tumor (T)

T1 Tumor involving the nasal cavity and/or paranasal sinuses (excluding sphenoid), sparing the most superior ethmoidal cells

T2 Tumor involving the nasal cavity and/or paranasal sinuses (including the sphenoid), with extension to or erosion of the cribriform plate

T3 Tumor extending into the orbit or protruding into the anterior cranial fossa, without dural invasion

T4 Tumor involving the brain

Regional Lymph Nodes (N)

N0 No cervical lymph node metastasis

N1 Any form of cervical lymph node metastasis

Distant Metastasis (M)

M0 No metastasis

M1 Distant metastasis

From Dulguerov P, Calcaterra T: Esthesioneuroblastoma: The UCLA experience 1970–1990. Laryngoscope 102:843–849, 1992.

introduced the first and most commonly used system.[99] It consists of three groups: tumors in group A are confined to the nasal cavity, tumors in group B involve the paranasal sinuses, and tumors in group C extend beyond the limits of the sinonasal cavity (e.g., intracranial or orbital). More recently, Foote and colleagues modified the Kadish system by adding a stage D, which included metastasis to the cervical lymph nodes or distant sites.[100] The third classification system described by Dulguerov and Calcaterra is based on the TNM system (Table 9–2).[101] This staging system, which relies on high-resolution imaging before therapy, proved to be more reliable than the Kadish system in assessing prognosis. This classification recognizes the early involvement of the cribriform plate, but it allows for tumors that arise below the cribriform plate and that can be treated in a more conservative fashion to be staged separately. Also, a stage is included at which a tumor is intracranial but remains extradural, and is therefore likely to have a better prognosis than a tumor that has invaded the brain.

Adequate surgical resection is the treatment of choice for olfactory neuroblastoma. Several surgical approaches have been described. Whatever approach is used, the goal of surgery must be complete surgical resection with tumor-free margins. This offers the best chance for both locoregional control and survival. Because the tumor originates from the olfactory epithelium, most tumors arise close to or within the nasal roof (Fig. 9–13). The cribriform plate will usually need to be resected en bloc with the tumor for adequate surgical margins to be achieved.[96] The most commonly used approach for adequate resection of tumors in these locations is a combined anterior craniofacial resection. Recent progress in surgery of the anterior cranial base has improved the survival of patients with esthesioneuroblastoma, through improved local control.[1]

Other surgical approaches, such as the transnasal route, whether through an external approach (e.g., a lateral rhinotomy) or an endoscopic approach, have been used successfully by some surgeons for well-selected cases. A recent report from the University Medical School of Graz, Austria, described the use of endoscopic resection followed by gamma-knife stereotactic radiosurgery in selected patients

with esthesioneuroblastoma.[102] The selection criteria included tumors without deep infiltration into the orbit or into the pterygopalatine fossa and without any involvement of the posterior wall of the frontal sinus. Excellent outcomes were reported in this small cohort of patients; because of the minimally invasive character of this treatment, it was recommended as an alternative to craniofacial resection and postoperative radiation in patients with localized disease. However, for more advanced lesions, anterior craniofacial resection allows better exposure and more adequate resection of the disease. In the UCLA experience, patients who were treated with craniofacial resection had a significantly higher rate of locoregional control than did patients who had a lateral rhinotomy, medial maxillectomy, and ethmoidectomy.[101]

Adjuvant postoperative radiation therapy is commonly used in most patients with esthesioneuroblastoma. Biller and colleagues questioned the need for routine combined therapy.[103] In their series of 20 patients with extracranial disease, combined craniofacial resection without radiotherapy was used. There was one local recurrence. However, several other studies have shown that the combination of surgery and radiation therapy appears to provide the most favorable long-term outcome for patients with esthesioneuroblastoma.[100, 101] Patients with limited disease (e.g., Kadish stage A or T1 lesions) that has been completely resected with adequate surgical margins, however, may not need additional treatment. In the University of Virginia experience, surgery combined with postoperative radiation therapy resulted in a 5-year survival rate for stage A tumors close to 100%, diminishing to 75% in stage B tumors.[104] A relatively high incidence of distant metastases (10%–20%) and local recurrence was found in stage C tumors. This has prompted the emergence of protocols incorporating the use of systemic chemotherapy.

Chemotherapy historically has been used for unresectable tumors, recurrence, or metastatic disease. Anecdotal reports suggest response rates that are high enough to warrant inclusion of chemotherapy in a multimodal strategy.[96] Inclusion of chemotherapy in such cases has been used for patients with advanced-stage tumors and a high histopathologic grade. In such cases, the inclusion of a multimodal approach has provided improved locoregional control and survival. Recently, workers at the Mayo Clinic reported their experience with adjuvant chemotherapy in 10 patients with stage C disease.[105] Tumor regression was more likely in patients with high-grade tumors. Despite sensitivity to platinum-based chemotherapy, patients with high-grade tumors, however, had a much more aggressive treatment program than did those with lower-grade tumors. The authors concluded that Hyams' grading of esthesioneuroblastoma tumors seems to be important in predicting response to chemotherapy. This series suggests that cisplatin-based chemotherapy is active in advanced, high-grade esthesioneuroblastoma and is a reasonable choice in the systemic treatment of these patients.[105]

Sarcomas

RHABDOMYOSARCOMA

Rhabdomyosarcoma involves the head and neck region in about 35% to 45% of cases. The sinonasal tract is involved

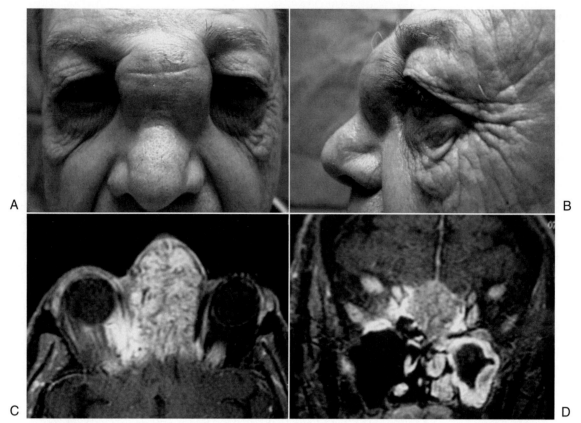

FIGURE 9–13 A 71-year-old patient who presented with progressive nasal obstruction and an enlarging mass at the upper nasal region. Biopsy was consistent with esthesioneuroblastoma. *A* and *B*, Clinical photographs showing the mass centered around the nasion, and causing widening of the interpalpebral distance (telecanthus). The mass shows involvement of the overlying skin and destruction of the underlying nasal bone. *C* and *D*, T1-weighted MRI with gadolinium in the axial *(C)* and coronal *(D)* projections, demonstrating the lesion to arise from the region of the cribriform plate and extend intracranially. The patient underwent a craniofacial resection and postoperative radiation therapy.

in about 10% of cases affecting the head and neck.[17] Sinonasal rhabdomyosarcoma involving nonorbital parameningeal sites demonstrates a more aggressive biologic behavior than do those arising in other sites.[43] Histologically, rhabdomyosarcoma is classified into embryonal, alveolar, and pleomorphic types. The embryonal and alveolar types are more common in the pediatric population, whereas the pleomorphic variety is more common among adults.[17, 106]

In 1987, the Intergroup Rhabdomyosarcoma Study reported remarkable improvement in survival—from 51% to 81%—with the use of intensive chemotherapy and radiation therapy in patients with nonorbital parameningeal rhabdomyosarcoma.[107] These results, however, were derived from the pediatric population, and similar results in adults had not yet been confirmed. A recent study from the M.D. Anderson Cancer Center reported the outcome of 37 pediatric and adult patients with sinonasal rhabdomyosarcoma.[106] Overall 5-year survival was 44%. For patients treated with a combination of chemotherapy and radiotherapy with or without surgery, 5-year survival was 60%, compared with 19% for patients treated with other forms of therapy. Factors associated with poorer survival were adult onset of disease, alveolar histology, and treatment with systemic chemotherapy for less than 1 year.

Patients receiving chemotherapy for longer than 1 year had a 5-year survival of 82%, compared with 71% for those with less than 1 year of treatment. Improved survival was associated with a lower incidence of distant metastasis.[106]

These data indicate that a combination of chemotherapy and radiotherapy may provide the best means of obtaining locoregional control for rhabdomyosarcoma arising in the nose and paranasal sinuses. Because the risk of regional disease is high, comprehensive radiotherapy to the neck in addition to the primary site should be considered. Surgical resection should be reserved for patients with residual disease after chemotherapy and radiotherapy. Administration of chemotherapy for longer than 1 year is associated with improved survival because of a decreased incidence of distant metastasis.[106]

CHONDROSARCOMA, CHORDOMA, AND OSTEOGENIC SARCOMA

Primary chondrosarcomas of the facial bones are typically of low grade and most often occur in the maxillary sinus or mandible. Mandibular tumors most frequently involve the body of the mandible, and maxillary tumors most commonly originate from the alveolar ridge and involve the maxillary sinus. Treatment is usually surgical resection, with postoperative radiation therapy provided for high-grade tumors. Secondary sarcomas of the facial skeleton may be radiation-induced or may arise in association with Maffucci's syndrome or Ollier's disease.[108, 109]

Chordomas are locally aggressive tumors that originate from embryonic remnants of the notochord. They are closely related to and are sometimes indistinguishable from low-grade chondrosarcomas. Chordomas most commonly arise from the clivus and frequently involve the nasopharynx, the paranasal sinuses, especially the sphenoid sinus, and the nasal cavity (Fig. 9–14). Primary chordomas

of the paranasal sinuses are extremely rare.[110] Surgical resection is the primary treatment, and unless the tumor is completely resected, recurrence is common. Postoperative radiation is recommended for advanced, recurrent, or incompletely resected tumors.[111] Proton irradiation has shown promising results in the treatment of these tumors.

Osteogenic sarcoma arising from the facial skeleton constitutes about 10% of all osteosarcomas. Histopathologic types include chondroblastic, osteoblastic, fibroblastic, and malignant fibrous histiocytoma–like. Despite the invasive

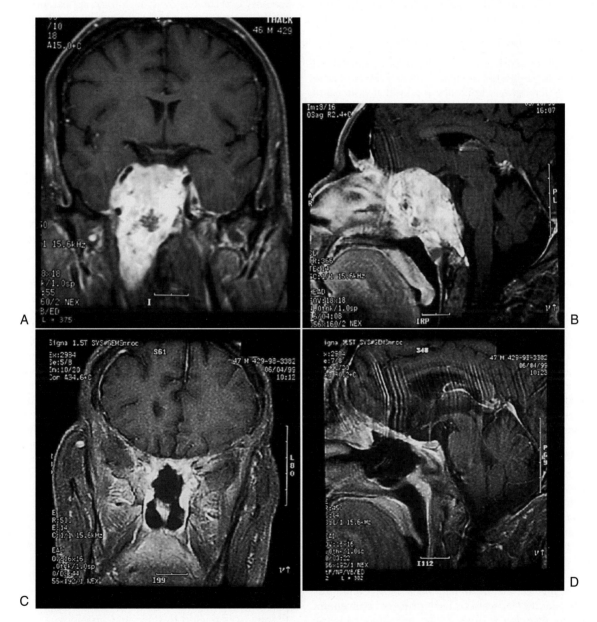

FIGURE 9–14 A 46-year-old patient presented with headache and diplopia. Nasal endoscopy revealed a mass filling the posterior nasal cavity and nasopharynx. Biopsy revealed chordoma. T1-weighted MRI with gadolinium in the coronal (A) and sagittal (B) planes, showing an intensely enhancing mass centered, arising from the clivus, and involving the sphenoid sinus, nasopharynx, and posterior nasal cavity. The tumor invades the skull base and extends intracranially to involve both cavernous carotid arteries. C and D, The patient underwent tumor resection through a combined craniofacial approach, followed by adjuvant radiation therapy. At 1 year postoperatively, the coronal and sagittal MRIs show no evidence of recurrent tumor. At 3 years follow-up, the patient has no evidence of disease.

and high-grade nature of some of these tumors, the long-term prognosis for patients with tumors in these locations is better than for those with tumors arising in the long bones. The most successful treatment appears to be wide surgical resection with postoperative radiation therapy. The role of chemotherapy in treatment of patients with osteosarcoma of the facial bones is less clear than its role in those with osteosarcoma of the long bones.[112] In a multi-institutional analysis of patients with sarcoma of the facial bones, neutron beam irradiation resulted in significant improvement in locoregional control.[113] For sarcomas arising in the maxillary sinus, it is more difficult to achieve a total gross resection than it is for those involving the mandible.

DESMOID FIBROMATOSIS AND FIBROSARCOMA

Desmoid fibromatosis comprises a group of nonmetastasizing, well-differentiated, nonencapsulated fibrous tissue proliferations that have a tendency for local invasion and recurrence. Biologically, they fall into an intermediate category between benign fibrous lesions and fibrosarcoma. The occurrence of this lesion in the head and neck is rare. A recent study reviewed the files of the Armed Forces Institute of Pathology and reported 25 cases of fibromatosis involving the sinonasal and nasopharyngeal areas that occurred between 1885 and 1985.[114] The maxillary sinus was the site most frequently involved (22 patients), followed by the nasal cavity (5 patients), the ethmoid sinus (4 patients), the orbit (4 patients), the sphenoid and frontal sinuses (2 patients each), and the nasopharynx (1 patient). The recurrence rate after treatment was 20%, and some patients had multiple recurrences. None of the patients died of the disease.

Fibrosarcoma encompasses a spectrum of low- and high-grade tumors. Histologic grading is difficult, and misdiagnosis is common. For the low-grade variety, wide local excision is the treatment of choice. Recurrences are treated with either reexcision or radiation therapy. High-grade tumors are more locally aggressive, metastasize more frequently, and are less radioresponsive. Wide surgical resection is the treatment of choice. Postoperative radiation is indicated for positive margins.[115]

ANGIOSARCOMA

Angiosarcomas are very rare but highly malignant soft tissue tumors derived from the vascular endothelium. Tumor cells form anastomosing vascular spaces and exhibit immunoreactivity for CD31.[116] This tumor is most commonly found in the skin, where it exhibits horizontal spread with indistinct margins. Angiosarcoma is known to cause early and widespread metastases, leading to a very poor prognosis.[117]

Angiosarcoma of the head and neck most commonly involves the skin of the scalp or face; primary involvement of the sinonasal region is exceedingly rare. Surgery is the primary method of treatment. Because the tumor may spread within the underlying dermis for a considerable distance, total surgical excision using frozen section control before reconstruction may offer the best chance for control of disease. The reported 2-year survival rate was 50%, and the 5-year survival rate was 22%.[118] Regional metastases were seen in 18% of patients.

Sinonasal angiosarcomas tend to develop at a younger age and are associated with a lower incidence of metastasis than is the cutaneous variety.[119] Surgical resection with adjunctive radiation therapy is the treatment of choice.[117]

HEMANGIOPERICYTOMA

These tumors are of vascular origin and arise from the capillary pericytes of Zimmermann. There is lack of uniformity in both the histologic appearance and biologic behavior of hemangiopericytomas. Benign and malignant varieties have been described. The biologic behavior of the tumor cannot be predicted by its histologic appearance. However, all these tumors should be regarded as at least low-grade malignancies.[17] Electron microscopy and immunohistochemical techniques are sometimes needed for diagnosis and to distinguish hemangiopericytomas from other mesenchymal tumors.[120] Primary treatment consists of wide surgical excision. Radiation therapy reduces the size of the tumor but rarely results in cure.[121, 122]

Lymphomas

Extranodal non-Hodgkin's lymphoma (NHL) of the head and neck is relatively uncommon. Most reported studies of NHL of the head and neck have included a relatively small number of patients, have used different modalities of therapy, and have not included all head and neck sites. Also, over the past 3 decades, a variety of systems, including the Rappaport, Luke-Collins, and Working Formulation classifications, have been used to classify extranodal NHLs. These factors make comparisons between different studies difficult and limit uniform characterization of the biologic behavior of NHL in the head and neck.

To address these limitations, a recent study from the Cleveland Clinic reviewed 98 patients with NHL of the head and neck and uniformly classified them according to the most current system—the Working Formulation—regardless of the time of diagnosis.[123] The sinonasal tract was the most commonly involved site (25%). Approximately 50% of patients had associated nodal disease, and only 20% had systemic or B symptoms. Three fourths of patients had stage I or II disease, and approximately two thirds had intermediate-grade lymphoma. Radiation therapy was the primary modality of therapy for localized disease (stages I and II), especially for low-grade lymphomas. Combination chemotherapy with or without radiation was used for more advanced disease and for intermediate- and high-grade lymphomas. Two thirds of patients had a remission after initial therapy. Two thirds of these patients had no further relapse. Three fourths of patients with relapse after initial remission died of their disease. The overall and disease-free survival rates for all patients were 60% and 50%, respectively. Outcome of therapy was related to stage and histologic grade. Patients with lymphomas of high histopathologic grade and those with recurrent and disseminated disease had the poorest prognosis.[123]

The Revised European American Lymphoma (REAL) classification is the most recently developed system for classifying NHL. A recent study investigated the clinical characteristics and the prognosis of 53 patients with sinonasal lymphomas according to REAL classification.[124] Using the Ann Arbor staging system, 30 patients were determined to have stage IE, 13 to have stage IIE, 4 to have stage IIIE, and 6 to have stage IVE lymphomas. B-symptoms were present in 40% of patients. Primary sites were the nasal cavity (68%), maxillary sinus (20%), ethmoid sinus (10%), and frontal sinus (2%). All lymphomas showed a diffuse growth pattern. Based on the type of tumor cells, patients were classified into five groups according to the REAL classification: diffuse large B-cell lymphoma (22%), peripheral T-cell lymphoma (15%), angiocentric lymphoma (36%), and other lymphomas and unclassified types (27%). Cumulative 5-year survival rates were 28% for all of the types, 55% for diffuse large B-cell lymphoma, 33% for peripheral T-cell lymphoma, and 20% for angiocentric lymphoma. Results suggest that conventional combined treatment (CHOP chemotherapy [cyclophosphamide, doxorubicin, vincristine, and prednisolone] + radiotherapy) is ineffective for NHL of the sinonasal tract, especially so for NHL with positive T-cell markers, angiocentric lymphoma, NHL with disease stage greater than IIE, and NHL with B-symptoms.[124]

"Lethal midline granuloma" is a clinical term that was used to describe progressive, destructive lesions affecting the midline of the face. This term is a misnomer because these lesions are actually sinonasal lymphomas. Most of these tumors exhibit a polymorphous pattern of proliferation; thus they were called *polymorphic reticulosis*. Recently, they have been categorized as sinonasal natural killer (NK)/T-cell lymphomas and defined as angiocentric lymphomas in the REAL classification.[125] They are more prevalent in Asia than in Europe or North America and are associated with EBV infection. Sinonasal NK/T-cell lymphomas in the United States most often occur in ethnic groups from areas of reported high frequency (e.g., Asia, Central and South America), although they are less common in endemic populations and are otherwise similar phenotypically. These tumors are typically located in the nasal cavity and have an aggressive, angioinvasive growth pattern that often results in necrosis and bony erosion.[126]

Treatment of destructive T/NK lymphomas of the midface involves a combination of local radiation therapy and chemotherapy with an anthracycline-based regimen.[127, 128] Of 13 patients treated at M.D. Anderson Cancer Center, 11 were initially treated with doxorubicin-based chemotherapy with or without radiotherapy. Eight patients (62%) responded to therapy—six (46%) with complete response and two (16%) with partial response. Five patients (38%) were alive—four with no evidence of disease at 1, 2, 3, and 9 years after treatment—and one patient was alive with disease. Six patients had disease progression to extranodal sites, including testis, central nervous system, lung, bone marrow, liver, peripheral blood, and skin. The authors concluded that these patients' response to doxorubicin-containing regimens was inferior to that of patients with other non-Hodgkin's lymphomas and similar prognostic factors. Because the disease is associated with EBV in 90% to 100% of cases and because the prognosis is poor, innovative therapies should be tried, including immunotherapy that targets the expression of EBV by the tumor with or without myeloablative procedures.[125]

Extracranial Meningiomas

Extracranial meningiomas of the sinonasal tract are rare. These tumors are frequently misclassified, resulting in inappropriate clinical management. Thirty cases of sinonasal tract meningiomas diagnosed between 1970 and 1992 were reported from the files of the Otorhinolaryngic Registry of the AFIP.[129] Men and women were equally affected. Age range was from 13 to 88 years (mean, 47.6 years). Patients presented clinically with a mass, epistaxis, sinusitis, pain, visual changes, or nasal obstruction, depending on the anatomic site of involvement. Symptoms were present for an average of 31 months. The tumors affected the nasal cavity (n = 14), nasopharynx (n = 3), frontal sinus (n = 2), sphenoid sinus (n = 2), or a combination of sites (n = 9). Radiographic studies demonstrated a central nervous system connection in only six cases. Bony erosion of the sinuses and extension to the surrounding soft tissues, the orbit, and occasionally the base of the skull were common. Histologically, the tumors demonstrated features similar to those of intracranial meningiomas, including whorled growth pattern and psammoma bodies. A majority were of the meningothelial type, although there were three atypical meningiomas. Immunohistochemical studies confirmed the diagnosis of meningioma with positive reactions for epithelial membrane antigen (EMA) and vimentin. The differential diagnosis includes paraganglioma, carcinoma, melanoma, psammomatoid ossifying fibroma, and angiofibroma. Surgical excision was used in all patients. Three patients died with recurrent disease (mean, 1.2 years), one was alive with recurrent disease (25.6 years), and the remaining 24 patients were alive or had died of unrelated causes (mean, 13.9 years) at the time of last follow-up. The authors concluded that the overall prognosis is good, without a difference in outcome between benign and atypical meningiomas.[129]

Metastasis to the Sinonasal Tract

Renal cell carcinoma is the most common source of distant metastasis to the sinonasal tract, followed by adenocarcinoma of the lungs, breast, and gastrointestinal tract.[15] Metastasis of prostatic and hepatocellular carcinoma to the paranasal sinuses is rare but has been reported.[130, 131] Metastasis to the sinonasal region may be the first clinical evidence of the primary tumor, or it might appear after treatment of the primary neoplasm. Although the maxillary antrum is the most frequent site of metastasis, any area of the sinonasal tract may be involved.[130, 131] The clinical picture of metastatic lesions is similar to that of primary sinonasal malignancy. Treatment is palliative and is indicated for the relief of pain, bleeding, or orbital complications. Excellent local symptom control may be achieved with the use of radiation therapy for sinonasal metastasis from renal cell carcinoma.[132]

Cancer of the Orbit

A majority of malignant tumors involving the orbit represent direct extension of tumors of the sinonasal tract. Cancers arising primarily within the orbit are less common and may be classified broadly into pediatric and adult groups.

Further subclassification may be assigned according to site of origin, histologic type, or both.

The most common intraocular tumor seen in children is *retinoblastoma,* which usually presents by the third year of life.[133] Common signs include strabismus and a white pupil (leukocoria). The diagnosis of retinoblastoma carries significant genetic implications, and family members of patients should receive genetic counseling. Treatment modalities include enucleation, radiation, and chemotherapy.[134] In a recent study of 1506 children with retinoblastoma (816 of whom had bilateral tumors), children surviving retinoblastoma had an increased incidence of radiation-induced second tumor, most often sarcoma of the facial skeleton and soft tissue.[135] However, no increased risk was observed for tumors outside of the field of radiation. This study also demonstrated that the risk for tumors in the field of radiation is heavily dependent on the age at which radiation is given; it may be acceptably small in patients receiving radiation after the age of 12 months.[135]

Other common tumors in the orbit in children include rhabdomyosarcoma, neuroblastoma, lymphoma, and leukemia.[136] Rhabdomyosarcoma (Fig. 9–15) is the most common primary orbital cancer of childhood. The average age of presentation is 7 years. Embryonal rhabdomyosarcoma is the most common type, alveolar rhabdomyosarcoma is the most aggressive, and pleomorphic rhabdomyosarcoma is associated with the best outcome. The botryoid type of rhabdomyosarcoma does not present primarily in the orbit.[137] Treatment is primarily a combination of radiation and chemotherapy.[138] Surgical resection is reserved for residual disease.

Neuroblastoma is the most common metastatic cancer to the orbit in children. Treatment is directed at the primary tumor. Granulocytic sarcoma as a primary orbital neoplasm may precede or follow systemic leukemia.[139] Primarily found in children with myelogenic leukemia, this tumor rarely occurs in adults.[140] Intraocular leukemic infiltrates have been found in more than 30% of leukemic patients at autopsy.[141] In addition to systemic management of leukemia, radiation therapy may be considered for local tumor control.

In adults, approximately 65% of orbital tumors are malignant.[142] Malignant tumors of the lacrimal gland are most commonly lymphomas or tumors of salivary gland origin. Overall, lymphoma is the most common tumor arising in the orbit in adults. The main differential diagnosis is lymphoid hyperplasia and orbital pseudotumor.[142, 143] Malignant salivary gland tumors of the lacrimal gland include adenoid cystic carcinoma, malignant mixed cell tumor, and mucoepidermoid carcinoma (Fig. 9–16).[144, 145]

Neoplasms of the lacrimal sac include squamous cell carcinoma, adenocarcinoma, transitional cell carcinoma, salivary gland carcinoma, and poorly differentiated carcinoma.[146]

Cancers of the skin of the eyelid include basal cell carcinoma, squamous cell carcinoma, sebaceous cell carcinoma, and malignant melanoma, any of which may invade the orbit. Sebaceous cell carcinoma is particularly treacherous because it may masquerade as a simple chalazion, leading to significant delay in diagnosis.

Tumors arising from the conjunctiva that may also invade the orbit include malignant melanoma, squamous carcinoma, and lymphoma. Choroidal melanoma is the most common of all *intraocular* malignancies and is biologically distinct from conjunctival or cutaneous melanoma.

Primary *intraorbital* malignancies in adults are rare. Malignant neurogenic tumors of the orbit are uncommon, but those of peripheral nerve sheath origin predominate. They most commonly represent malignant degeneration in patients with multiple benign neurofibromatosis. Other sarcomas that infrequently arise within the orbit include osteosarcoma, chondrosarcoma, malignant fibrous histiocytoma, hemangiopericytoma, and liposarcoma.[147] Multiple myeloma may present in the orbit as a solitary plasmacytoma, or the orbit may be involved as part of disseminated disease.[148] Hematogenous metastasis to the orbit most commonly originates from a primary in the lung or prostate in men. In women, carcinoma of the breast is the most common source of metastasis to the orbit.

SPREAD OF CANCER

Local Spread

The most common route of local spread of cancer of the sinonasal tract is through direct extension. Because most sinonasal cancers are relatively asymptomatic when small, it is often the manifestation of local spread that prompts patients to seek medical attention. In the maxillary sinus, direct extension may occur anteriorly into the soft tissues of the cheek; superiorly into the orbit with resultant proptosis and diplopia (see Fig. 9–10); inferiorly into the oral cavity; or posteriorly into the pterygomaxillary space, where it may spread along the branches of the maxillary division of the

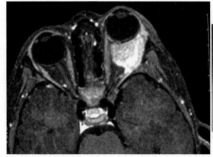
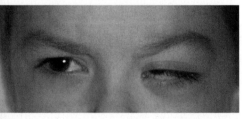

FIGURE 9–15 A 6-year-old boy presented with left lid ptosis and ophthalmoplegia. MRI revealed a left orbital tumor, which on biopsy revealed embryonal rhabdomyosarcoma. Treatment consisted of radiation and chemotherapy.

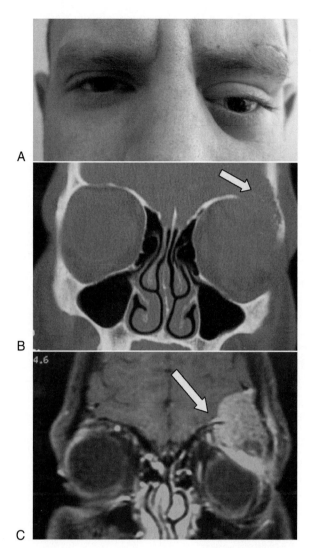

FIGURE 9–16 A 25-year-old patient who presented with a swelling of the left lacrimal gland and diplopia. *A*, Clinical examination revealed downward and medial displacement of the globe. The scar over the lateral brow resulted from a recent biopsy, which revealed adenoid cystic carcinoma. *B*, Coronal CT scan revealed bony destruction of the superior lateral orbital wall *(arrow)*. *C*, Coronal T1 MRI revealed the tumor to invade the superior orbit and extend intracranially. Tumor resection was done through a combined craniotomy and lateral orbitotomy. The tumor involved the dura but not the brain, and it invaded the periorbita but not the orbital fat or muscles. The eye was preserved, and the patient received postoperative adjuvant radiation therapy.

trigeminal nerve (V2). Cancer of the frontal sinus is quite rare, but the most significant direct extension occurs posteriorly to the frontal lobes. Cancer of the ethmoid sinus often presents with medial extension to the orbit, superior extension to the cribriform plate, and posterior extension into the sphenoid sinus and nasopharynx (see Fig. 9–13).[149] Cancers involving the sphenoid sinus may quickly become problematic because of proximity to the optic nerves, the cavernous sinus, and the pituitary fossa (see Fig. 9–5).[16]

In addition to direct local extension, cancer of the paranasal sinuses can spread to nearby structures via the many fissures and foramina located in this region. Cancer of the maxillary sinus frequently erodes posteriorly into the pterygopalatine fossa (PPF) (see Fig. 9–6). Once in the PPF, the tumor may extend laterally through the pterygomaxillary fissure into the infratemporal fossa; superiorly into the orbit via the inferior orbital fissure or into the middle cranial fossa through the foramen rotundum; posteriorly into the vidian canal with extension to the petrous portion of the temporal bone; or inferiorly into the oral cavity by way of the palatine canal or the sphenopalatine foramen (see Figs. 9–4 and 9–6).

From the frontal sinus, cancer may extend into the nasal cavity through the nasofrontal duct. Cancer of the ethmoid sinuses may also extend into the nasal cavity through the middle meatus and the sphenoethmoid recess, posteriorly into the nasopharynx and along the eustachian tube, or inferiorly along the nasolacrimal duct (see Fig. 9–2).

Lymphatic Spread

The lymphatic drainage of the posterior nasal cavities and paranasal sinuses goes primarily to the retropharyngeal and lateral pharyngeal nodes at the base of the skull, and then to the upper jugular lymph nodes. Cancers of the anterior nasal cavity and those that erode through the maxilla into the soft tissues of the face spread to the submandibular and upper jugular lymph nodes.

Regional metastases from paranasal sinus cancer are relatively uncommon and have been characterized to a greater extent for maxillary sinus cancer than for other paranasal sites.[45] Regional disease is evident on initial presentation in approximately 10% of patients; an additional 15% of patients will develop lymph node metastasis at some point after treatment. In patients with squamous cell carcinoma (SCC) of the maxillary sinus, the risk of having lymph node metastasis on presentation correlates with extension of the primary tumor to the nasopharynx or oral cavity. The risk of developing regional metastasis after treatment correlates with local tumor recurrence. The role of elective neck dissection or radiation has yet to be defined in patients with cancer of the maxillary sinus. Aggressive treatment to achieve maximum local control of the primary may be more important than elective neck treatment in prevention of nodal metastasis. Development of regional metastasis, however, is clearly a very poor prognostic indicator. In one study, the overall 5-year survival rate for node-positive patients was only 17%, and for node-negative patients 31%.[45]

Distant Spread

Although distant metastasis from cancer of the paranasal sinus does occur, failure to control the disease secondary to local recurrence is far more common. For squamous cell carcinoma of the maxillary sinus, the rate of distant metastasis is approximately 10%; it rarely occurs in the absence of local recurrence.[150] Cancer of the ethmoid sinus has a similar rate of distant metastasis, with adenocarcinoma having a slightly higher rate than squamous cell cancer

(15%–20% vs. 10%). In general, the most common sites for metastasis are the lung and bone.[150]

STAGING

In 1933, Ohngren proposed a method of classification for cancer of the antrum.[151] He divided the antrum into anteroinferior and superoposterior sections by an imaginary line drawn from the angle of the mandible to the medial canthus of the eye. Patients with cancer located above Ohngren's line (suprastructure) had a significantly worse prognosis than those with cancer located below it (infrastructure). The proximity of cancer of the suprastructure to major vascular, neural, and intracranial structures makes resection with negative margins very difficult, which explains the tendency for local recurrence and a worse prognosis.

Ohngren's original classification has proved to be very useful and represents the basis on which subsequent classifications, including the most current, have evolved. Despite its utility, this system was neither easily reproducible nor particularly precise. In 1963, Sisson and coworkers proposed a modification of Ohngren's system in an attempt to more accurately classify cancers of the maxillary antrum.[152] In this system, tumors were classified roughly as in Ohngren's system, but involvement of critical contiguous structures was included in the staging format. Since then, several staging systems have been proposed, including those of Lederman in 1970,[153] Rubin in 1972,[154] Harrison in 1978,[155] and Ellingwood and Million in 1979.[156] This evolution in the clinical staging of cancer of the paranasal sinuses reflects the difficulty and imprecision inherent in classifying these tumors. For example, according to several of these systems, it is difficult to distinguish T1 from T2 tumors, or T3 from T4 tumors. Also, most of these systems apply only to tumors of the maxillary sinus.

Currently, the most widely used system for classifying cancers of the paranasal sinuses is the American Joint Committee on Cancer (AJCC) staging system; the most recent version published in 2002.[157] This system is based on the tumor, node, metastasis (TNM) staging method, and it distinguishes in its (T) stage tumors arising from the maxillary sinus from those arising from the ethmoid sinuses (Table 9–3). Assessment of the primary tumor (T) is based on inspection and palpation (including examination of the orbits, nasal and oral cavities, and nasopharynx) and on neurologic evaluation of the cranial nerves. According to this classification, cross-sectional imaging with magnetic resonance imaging (MRI) or computed tomography (CT) is mandatory for accurate pretreatment staging of malignant tumors of the sinuses. If available, MRI more accurately depicts tumor involvement of the cranial base and intracranial structures and differentiation of fluid from solid tumor (vide infra). Lymph node metastasis (N) is also evaluated by palpation and imaging. Examinations for distant metastases (M) include appropriate radiographs, blood chemistries, blood count, and other routine studies as indicated. The updated 1997 AJCC staging system proved to be superior to previous staging systems in predicting local control, metastasis, and survival of patients with sinus cancer.[158] The 2002 guidelines further clarify the 1997 staging guidelines.

TABLE 9-3 Definition of TNM for Cancer of the Paranasal Sinuses

Primary Tumor (T)

TX   Primary tumor cannot be assessed
T0   No evidence of primary tumor
Tis Carcinoma in situ

Maxillary Sinus

T1   Tumor limited to maxillary sinus mucosa with no erosion or destruction of bone
T2   Tumor causing bone erosion or destruction, including extension into the hard palate and/or the middle nasal meatus, except extension to posterior wall of maxillary sinus and pterygoid plates
T3   Tumor invades any of the following: bone of the posterior wall of maxillary sinus, subcutaneous tissues, skin of cheek, floor or medial wall of orbit, pterygoid fossa, ethmoid sinuses
T4a Tumor invades anterior orbital contents, skin of cheek, pterygoid plates, infratemporal fossa, cribriform plate sphenoid or frontal sinuses
T4b Tumor invades any of the following: orbital apex, dura, brain, middle cranial fossa, cranial nerves other than maxillary division of trigeminal nerve (V_2), nasopharyx, or clivus

Nasal Cavity and Ethmoid Sinus

T1   Tumor restricted to any one subsite, with or without bony invasion
T2   Tumor invading two subsites in a single region or extending to involve an adjacent region within the nasothmoidal complex, with or without bony invasion
T3   Tumor extends to invade the medial wall or floor of the orbit, maxillary sinus, palate, or cribriform plate
T4a Tumor invades any of the following: anterior orbital contents, skin of nose or cheek, minimal extension to anterior cranial fossa, pterygoid plates, sphenoid or frontal sinuses
T4b Tumor invades any of the following: orbital apex, dura, brain, middle cranial fossa, cranial nerves other than V_2, nasopharynx, or clivus

Regional Lymph Nodes (N)

NX   Regional lymph nodes cannot be assessed
N0   No regional lymph node metastasis
N1   Metastasis in a single ipsilateral lymph node, 3 cm or less in greatest dimension
N2   Metastasis in a single ipsilateral lymph node, more than 3 cm but not more than 6 cm in greatest dimension, or in multiple ipsilateral lymph nodes, none more than 6 cm in greatest dimension, or in bilateral or contralateral lymph nodes, none more than 6 cm in greatest dimension
N2a Metastasis in a single ipsilateral lymph node, more than 3 cm but not more than 6 cm in greatest dimension
N2b Metastasis in multiple ipsilateral lymph nodes, none more than 6 cm in greatest dimension
N2c Metastasis in bilateral or contralateral lymph nodes, none more than 6 cm in greatest dimension
N3   Metastasis in a lymph node, more than 6 cm in greatest dimension

Distant Metastasis (M)

MX   Distant metastasis cannot be assessed
M0   No distant metastasis
M1   Distant metastasis

Stage Grouping			
Stage 0	Tis	N0	M0
Stage I	T1	N0	M0
Stage II	T2	N0	M0
Stage III	T3	N0	M0
	T1	N1	M0
	T2	N1	M0
	T3	N1	M0
Stage IVA	T4a	N0	M0
	T4a	N1	M0
	T1	N2	M0
	T2	N2	M0
	T3	N2	M0
	T4a	N2	M0
Stage IVB	T4b	Any N	M0
	Any T	N3	M0
Stage IVC	Any T	Any N	M1

Used with the permission of the American Joint Committee on Cancer (AJCC), Chicago, Illinois. The original source for this material is the *AJCC Cancer Staging Manual, Sixth Edition* (2002) published by Springer-Verlag New York, www.springer-ny.com.

■ PATIENT EVALUATION

Clinical evaluation of patients with cancer of the nasal cavity, paranasal sinuses, and orbit should help to achieve three objectives: (1) establishment of the diagnosis, (2) determination of the extent of disease, and (3) development of a plan for treatment. These objectives are usually achieved through a detailed history, comprehensive clinical examination of the head and neck, imaging, and biopsy.

History and Clinical Examination

The signs and symptoms of *early* sinonasal tumors are very subtle and nonspecific. Early lesions are often completely asymptomatic, or they mimic more common benign conditions such as chronic sinusitis, allergy, or nasal polyposis. Because early detection of sinonasal tumors is probably the most important factor in improving prognosis, a high degree of suspicion is necessary for the diagnosis of smaller lesions. Common symptoms include nasal obstruction, "sinus pressure" or pain, nasal discharge that may be bloody, anosmia, and epistaxis. Failure of these symptoms to respond to adequate medical therapy or the presence of unilateral signs and symptoms should alert the physician to the possibility of malignancy; further investigation by high-resolution imaging is warranted. Comprehensive examination of the nasal cavity should be done after topical decongestion and anesthesia using rigid or flexible endoscopy. The presence of intranasal masses, ulcers, or areas of contact bleeding may indicate a malignant tumor. Although unilateral "polyps" may be inflammatory, they are more commonly neoplastic (Fig. 9–17). Tumors may also present as submucosal masses without changes in the mucosa, other than displacement. Any suspicious lesions should be biopsied, preferably after high-resolution imaging has been obtained so that severe bleeding and/or CSF leak can be avoided (as discussed later).

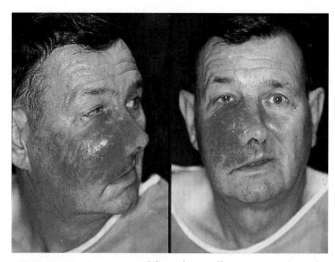

FIGURE 9–18 Carcinoma of the right maxillary sinus involving the overlying skin of the face. Note swelling and discoloration of the right cheek. Note also elevation of the right eye.

Extension of sinonasal tumors to adjacent structures renders the diagnosis obvious but is a late manifestation of the disease. Soft tissue swelling of the face may indicate tumor extension through the anterior bony confines of the nose and sinuses (Fig. 9–18). Inferior extension toward the oral cavity may present with an ulcer or a submucosal mass in the palate or the alveolar ridge (Fig. 9–19). Middle ear effusion may indicate tumor involvement of the nasopharynx, eustachian tube, pterygoid plates, or tensor veli palatini muscle. Extension to the skull base may lead to involvement of the cranial nerves, causing anosmia, blurred vision, diplopia, or hypoesthesia along the branches of the trigeminal nerves (see Fig. 9–12). Associated neck masses usually represent metastatic disease in the cervical lymph nodes.

Orbital involvement is common in patients with cancer arising from the ethmoid, sphenoid, and suprastructure of the maxillary sinuses (see Fig. 9–10).[16, 159] Less commonly,

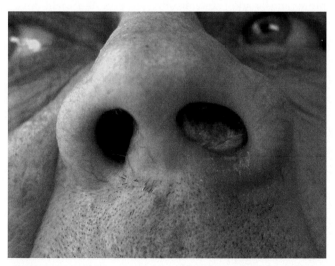

FIGURE 9–17 This patient presented with a unilateral nasal mass. His referring physician had previously treated him for a nasal "polyp." Biopsy revealed moderately differentiated squamous cell carcinoma.

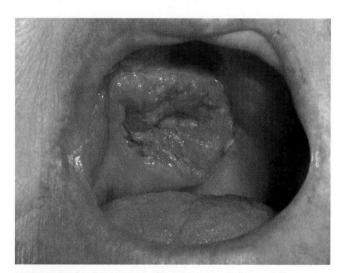

FIGURE 9–19 Squamous cell carcinoma of the maxillary sinus with invasion of the palate and ulceration into the oral cavity.

the orbit is involved with a primary tumor of the eye or its adnexa (see Figs. 9–15 and 9–16). Signs and symptoms of tumors in the orbit are usually due to mass effect or neuromuscular dysfunction. The patient may complain of proptosis, irregular shape of the eyelid, or blepharoptosis. Epiphora usually indicates involvement of the nasolacrimal duct. Double vision may result from compression or infiltration of ocular nerves or muscles. Visual loss secondary to optic nerve involvement is usually a late sign, although more subtle signs of optic nerve dysfunction, including afferent pupillary defect, loss of color vision, and visual field defect, are more frequently encountered. Finally, orbital involvement may be asymptomatic and is discovered only on CT or MRI evaluation of patients with sinonasal complaints.

Evaluation of patients with suspected primary or secondary malignancy in the orbit should include a detailed neuro-opthalmologic examination. This usually involves detailed assessment of visual acuity, visual fields, and ocular motility. Other ophthalmologic evaluation includes careful pupillary examination for afferent pupillary defect or anisocoria and external examination to include Hertel's exophthalmometry and marginal reflex distance as an indicator of eyelid position. Slit lamp examination of the conjunctivae, cornea, anterior chamber, and lens is appropriate. Finally, detailed examination of the fundus may reveal compressive effect, intraocular malignancy, or an unrelated reason for visual loss. Formal testing of color vision and automated visual fields is commonly appropriate.

Imaging

Imaging of the nasal cavity, paranasal sinuses, and orbit is indicated whenever there is clinical suspicion of a neoplastic process. Imaging is also indicated for obtaining pretreatment information regarding the location, size, extent, and invasiveness of the primary tumor, as well as the presence of regional and distant metastasis. Such information is crucial for decision making regarding therapeutic options and for proper preoperative planning of the optimal surgical approach. Imaging also plays an important role in post-treatment follow-up, indicating areas of residual or recurrent disease and defining suspicious areas for biopsy.[160]

Several imaging modalities are available for evaluation of sinonasal tumors. A combination of CT and MRI has now been established as the optimum radiologic assessment of sinonasal malignancy.[160] CT and MRI are of particular value in assessing the cranial base, orbit, and pterygopalatine and infratemporal fossae. CT is better in evaluating bone destruction, whereas MRI is better in delineating soft tissue detail; commonly, these studies are complementary (see Fig. 9–16).[161] Both spiral CT and 3-D MRI offer excellent opportunities for the clinician to obtain consecutive volume data sets and to visualize these data via 2-D or 3-D post-processing. 3-D reconstruction of the skull base region adds a different perspective to the data set than what is usually presented in the axial or coronal plane. It demonstrates simultaneously in a single illustration the spatial relationship of bone, tumor, vessels, and ventricles.[162] 3-D images can also assist the clinician in planning the surgical approach; data can be transferred directly into networked mobile computer systems for use in computer-assisted surgery.[163, 164]

However, in view of the current milieu of cost containment and in order to avoid redundancy in imaging studies requested, all advantages, limitations, and indications of these studies should be considered.

Computed Tomography

When a sinonasal tumor is suspected, CT scan in both the axial and coronal planes is the initial study of choice. Unilateral opacification of the sinus is not infrequently associated with a neoplastic process that may be malignant. In a recent prospective study, 43% of patients with unilateral opacification of the paranasal sinuses had a disease process other than chronic sinusitis, most commonly a neoplasm.[165] The incidence of significant disease other than chronic sinusitis rises strikingly as patient age increases. For instance, diseases other than chronic sinusitis were found in 14% of patients in the under-age-16 group, in 27% of patients in the 16-to-60 group, and in 86% of patients in the over-age-60 group.[165]

The main advantage of CT scans lies in their delineation of the architecture of bones, with the use of "bone windows."[163] The addition of contrast enhancement improves tumor definition from adjacent soft tissue, especially intracranially. Bone destruction and soft tissue invasion suggest an aggressive lesion, usually a malignant neoplasm (Fig. 9–20).[166] Coronal images best delineate involvement of the orbital floor and invasion of the skull base, particularly of the cribriform plate (Fig. 9–21). Axial images are particularly helpful in demonstrating tumor extension through the posterior wall of the maxillary sinus into the pterygopalatine fossa and the infratemporal fossae (see Fig. 9–20). Widening or sclerosis of the foramina of the infraorbital, vidian, mandibular, or maxillary nerves may indicate perineural spread (see Fig. 9–12A).

Magnetic Resonance Imaging

MRI is unsurpassed in delineating soft tissue detail, both intracranially and extracranially (see Figs. 9–15 and 9–16). The obliteration of fat planes in the pterygopalatine fossa, infratemporal fossa, and nasopharynx usually indicates tumor transgression along these boundaries and is best visualized by MRI.[167] Involvement of critical structures such as the brain and carotid artery is best delineated by MRI (see Figs. 9–13 and 9–14). Dural thickening or enhancement is usually an indication of tumor involvement and is best demonstrated with high-quality MRI (see Fig. 9–10). Similarly, enhancement or thickening of cranial nerves indicates perineural spread, which is better detected on MRI than on CT (see Fig. 9–12).[69] Perhaps one of the most significant advantages of MRI is its ability to distinguish tumor from retained secretions secondary to obstruction of sinus drainage (Fig. 9–22).

MRI is also particularly helpful in monitoring patients during the postoperative follow-up period, although this role may be supplanted in the near future by positron emission tomography (PET) scans because of their ability to distinguish between tumor recurrence and post-treatment fibrosis. Postoperative surveillance using MRI is best achieved with three planar T1-weighted images, with and

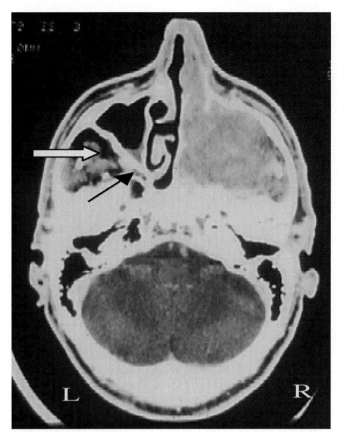

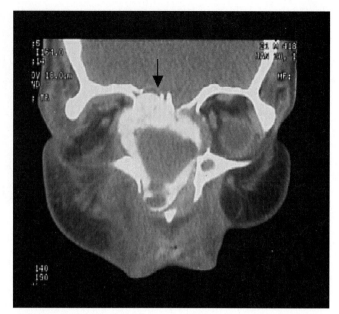

FIGURE 9–21 Coronal CT of a patient with sinonasal osteosarcoma (osteoblastic variety), demonstrating involvement of both medial orbital walls as well as the skull base, including the fovea ethmoidalis and the cribriform plate *(arrow)*.

FIGURE 9–20 Axial CT scan showing, on the left, the anatomy of the normal lateral nasal wall, delineating the inferior and middle turbinates. Both medial and posterior walls of the maxillary sinus are intact. The normal tissue densities of the pterygopalatine fossa *(black arrow)* and the infratemporal fossa *(white arrow)* are seen. In contrast, the right side shows a lesion in the maxillary sinus with evidence of bony destruction of both the medial maxillary wall and the lateral nasal wall. The lesion also invades the posterior maxillary wall and extends to and obliterates the pterygopalatine fossa and the infratemporal fossa. Both bony destruction and soft tissue invasion are characteristic of malignant tumors in this region.

without gadolinium, and with axial T2-weighted sequences (see Fig. 9–14). The subtraction of the T1 before and after gadolinium T1 sequences can be of particular value in delineating recurrence.[160] The accuracy of MRI in predicting recurrent tumor with this subtraction technique approaches 95%.[168] Additional advantages of MRI include avoidance of image degradation caused by dental filling artifact, imaging in the sagittal plane, and nonexposure to ionizing radiation. Sagittal images are particularly helpful in evaluating extension along the cribriform plate, planum sphenoidale, and clivus (see Fig. 9–14). These advantages have to be weighed against the increased expense and time that most MRI studies require.

Angiography

Angiography is not indicated in the routine assessment of patients with neoplasms of the nose, paranasal sinuses, and orbit. In certain selected cases, however, angiography may be necessary. These cases include vascular neoplasms of the sinonasal region, in which angiography not only delineates the tumor extent and the blood supply but also permits the use of selective embolization of the vascular supply to the tumor. This reduces intraoperative blood loss, facilitating surgical resection. Angiography is also indicated in sinonasal malignancy when the lesion is near the internal carotid artery. Angiography in these cases helps in evaluating the extent of carotid artery involvement. The adequacy of collateral cerebral blood supply through the contralateral carotid system is best assessed using balloon occlusion testing coupled with xenon-enhanced CT scans. This approach is very helpful in predicting the feasibility of carotid artery resection and the need for vascular reconstruction.

Biopsy

The definitive diagnosis of a neoplasm of the nasal cavity, paranasal sinuses, or orbit relies on removal of representative tissue from the tumor and its submission for histopathologic examination. This not only confirms the diagnosis but also, by indicating the type of neoplasm, guides the treating physician(s) in choosing the best therapeutic option(s).

Biopsy of Tumors of the Nasal Cavity

A vast majority of sinonasal neoplasms are accessible for biopsy through a strictly endonasal approach. A wide variety of rigid nasal endoscopes offer superb visualization of intranasal lesions with a high degree of optical resolution and bright illumination. The application of topical anesthetics and decongestants improves visualization and allows

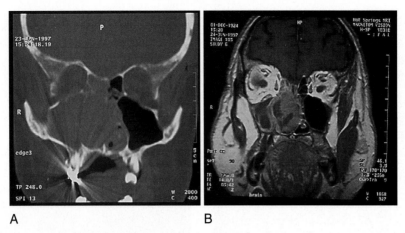

A   B

FIGURE 9–22   *A,* Coronal CT scan of a patient with sinonasal melanoma demonstrating opacification of the right nasal cavity as well as of the maxillary and ethmoid sinuses. There appears to be destruction of the lateral nasal wall and the nasal septum. The lesion is abutting the orbital floor and the cribriform plate, but it is unclear whether these structures are involved. *B,* Coronal T1-weighted MRI with gadolinium of the same patient revealing that the lesion is limited to the nasal cavity and ethmoid sinuses and that the changes in the maxillary sinuses are due to retained secretions secondary to obstruction of the ostium, rather than to soft tissue involvement. It also demonstrates that the lesion does not invade the orbit or the cranial base. The presence of low signal areas within the lesion gives it a heterogeneous appearance, which is characteristic of sinonasal melanoma.

thorough examination of the nasal cavity. The site of origin of the lesion and its relation to the nasal walls (i.e., septum, floor, roof, and lateral nasal wall) should be noted. An adequate specimen should be obtained (crushing of tissue should be avoided) and submitted for histopathologic examination. If the diagnosis of lymphoma is suspected, fresh tissue should be sent in saline, rather than fixed in formalin.

Usually mild bleeding occurs from the biopsy site and is easily controlled with cauterization or the application of light pressure for several minutes. Oxidized regenerated cellulose (Surgicel) may also be applied to the biopsy site, and in most cases, these simple measures will control bleeding. Occasionally, anterior nasal packing is needed to stop the bleeding. Most endonasal biopsies can be performed in the outpatient office with minimal discomfort to the patient. In certain cases, the diagnosis of a highly vascular neoplasm, such as angiofibroma, may be suspected on clinical grounds. Under these circumstances, it is prudent to postpone performing the biopsy until imaging and angiography (possibly with embolization) are performed. Preoperative biopsy can then be performed in the operating room under controlled conditions to confirm the diagnosis before surgical resection. If a nasal mass is suspected to have an intracranial communication (i.e., encephalocele, meningocele, nasal glioma), this should be confirmed with imaging; a biopsy is contraindicated to avoid the attendant risks of cerebrospinal fluid (CSF) leaks and subsequent meningitis.

Biopsy of Tumors of the Paranasal Sinuses

In the unusual case in which a paranasal sinus neoplasm is confined to the sinus cavity and does not present itself intranasally, a biopsy should be obtained by direct access to the involved sinus. Tumors of the maxillary sinus can still be

accessed through an endoscopic approach by creation of a wide antrostomy in the region of the natural ostium. Otherwise, the maxillary sinus is accessible through a sublabial incision in the canine fossa via an anterior antrostomy. The ethmoid sinus can be approached endonasally through an endoscopic ethmoidectomy. Alternatively, an external ethmoidectomy approach provides direct access via a Lynch incision.

The sphenoid sinus is easily approached endoscopically in the vast majority of cases. C-arm fluoroscopy or more recently computer-assisted 3-D intraoperative imaging is sometimes used in patients with difficult access or unusual anatomy. Isolated tumors of the frontal sinus are rare. A trephination through the floor of the sinus is used for biopsy of lesions within its cavity.

Biopsy of Orbital Lesions

In most cases of primary intraorbital tumor, the approach used to obtain a biopsy is dictated by the location of the tumor. Lesions in the superior orbit may be addressed by a coronal flap or through a brow incision (modified Kronlein or Stallard-Wright incision).[169] Lateral orbital lesions may require removal of the orbital rim. The transconjunctival approach, with detachment of the lateral canthal tendon, provides access to the orbital floor. The medial orbit may be entered through a modified Lynch or transcaruncular incision. Lesions within the muscle cone may be addressed by elevation of conjunctiva and Tenon's capsule from the globe and detachment of the necessary rectus muscle. Lacrimal gland lesions are best approached through the upper eyelid crease. Care must be taken with this approach not to disturb the palpebral lobe of the lacrimal gland so that interference with lacrimal secretory function can be prevented.

⬤ TREATMENT

Surgical Treatment

Indications

Surgical resection, alone or more commonly combined with adjunctive therapy, remains the mainstay of treatment of cancers of the sinonasal tract. This approach seems to provide the best chances for cure or control of disease.[19, 38, 170] Surgery is indicated whenever there is adequate evidence that the tumor can be completely resected with acceptable morbidity. The development of new combined craniofacial approaches has extended the indications of surgery to include some patients with skull base and even limited intracranial extension.[171–173] The advent of new reconstructive techniques, including microvascular free flaps, pericranial flaps, and prosthetic rehabilitation, has reduced morbidity and improved rehabilitation following extensive resection of advanced sinonasal cancer.

Surgery may be contraindicated in the presence of distant metastasis, extensive intracranial involvement, bilateral cavernous sinus extension, or disease involving both orbits,. However, in selected cases, surgery may still offer the most effective palliation even in the presence of extensive disease.

Preoperative Preparation

A thorough preoperative assessment should determine the candidacy of a patient for surgical management of his or her neoplasm. This involves careful "mapping" of the tumor extent, as well as evaluation of the general medical condition and functional status of the patient. This is usually accomplished by a detailed history and physical examination, as well as comprehensive examination of the head and neck region, including endoscopy of the sinonasal region. Cranial nerve examination and ophthalmologic evaluation should be done to evaluate cranial base and orbital extension, respectively. High-resolution imaging should be obtained using CT or MRI, or both, to accurately assess the tumor extent. In certain cases, angiography will be needed to determine the extent of carotid arterial involvement. The balloon occlusion test should be performed if carotid artery resection or reconstruction is contemplated. Preoperative embolization may be indicated in certain vascular tumors.

Neurosurgical consultation is needed if a combined craniofacial approach is anticipated. If free vascularized flaps will be used for reconstruction, expertise with microvascular surgery is needed, and appropriate consultation should be obtained. Evaluation by a maxillofacial prosthodontist is required in most patients so that preoperative dental impressions can be obtained and surgical obturators or splints can be designed for maintenance of proper dental occlusion and oral rehabilitation. Similar expertise is essential if prosthetic orbital, nasal, or facial rehabilitation is required. Consultations with medical and radiation oncology colleagues should be done so that incorporation of chemotherapy or radiation in the treatment plan can be considered. Radiation and/or chemotherapy may be used preoperatively as induction (neoadjuvant) therapy or postoperatively as adjuvant therapy. This is particularly important in patients with advanced-stage disease (e.g., dural or orbital involvement) or high-grade lesions (e.g., SNUC). In selected cases, chemotherapy and/or radiation may be a reasonable alternative to surgery. Such decisions are best discussed in the format of a multidisciplinary tumor board. If surgery is chosen as a treatment modality, the plan for the surgical approach, the extent of resection, and reconstructive options should then be formulated. This plan should be communicated clearly among the various members of the surgical team, particularly the otolaryngologists–head and neck surgeons, neurosurgeons, and plastic and reconstructive surgeons.

Careful assessment of the patient's general medical condition should be carried out before surgery is undertaken. Preoperative chest radiography, blood counts, liver and renal function tests, blood glucose level, electrolytes, coagulation studies, and an electrocardiogram (ECG) should be performed routinely. Appropriate consultation from medical colleagues should be obtained so that the patient's medical status before surgery can be optimized and so that help in management can be obtained postoperatively. The patient's nutritional status should be evaluated, and if indicated, enteral or parenteral feeding may be considered. High-resolution imaging for metastatic workup is not routinely performed unless indicated by history, clinical examination, chest radiograph results, or blood test abnormalities.

Finally, the surgical team should discuss with the patient and family the nature of the disease, the evaluation, and the indications, risks, possible complications, sequelae, and alternatives of therapy. The expected postoperative course, including length of stay in the hospital, feeding, rehabilitation, and need for adjunctive therapy, should be described. This ongoing communication should be maintained in a clear, honest, and sympathetic fashion throughout the course of patient care.

Surgical Approach Versus Extent of Resection

When addressing the subject of surgical treatment of sinonasal cancer, a distinction has to be made between the terminology used to describe the surgical approach on the one hand, and the extent of resection on the other hand. A surgical approach describes the various incisions, soft tissue dissection, and skeletal osteotomies required to expose the tumor and adjacent structures so that a complete and safe resection can be performed. On the other hand, extent of tumor resection describes the various structures that need to be surgically extirpated so that total tumor removal with tumor-free margins can be achieved. Obviously, the surgical approach and the extent of resection are closely related and vary according to the extent of tumor, its aggressiveness, and related critical structures. Without this distinction in terminology, however, considerable confusion exists in the nomenclature of surgical procedures used in the treatment of patients with sinonasal tumors.

SURGICAL APPROACHES

Endonasal. There is no doubt that the development of rigid nasal endoscopy with its superb illumination and optical resolution has allowed more precise visualization of intranasal abnormalities. The advantages of this technology in the *evaluation and biopsy* of neoplasms of the sinonasal tract were discussed in earlier sections (see the section on biopsy). The role of endoscopic *treatment* of nasal neoplasms, however, remains undefined. The use of this modality in the treatment of limited inverted papilloma of the nasal cavity has already been discussed (see section on inverted papilloma). Several recent studies have described the use of endonasal resection of malignant tumors of the sinonasal tract; it has been reported, in well-selected patients, that disease control and survival rates are comparable to those associated with more extensive open approaches.[174–177]

The largest series was from two Belgian institutions and included 66 patients who underwent endoscopic resection of malignant sinonasal tumors. This study reported local recurrence in 20%, distant metastasis in 8%, and simultaneous local recurrence and distant metastases in 9% of patients.[174] The 2-year and 5-year survival rates of the whole group were 73% and 52%, respectively. Patients with adenocarcinoma had a better prognosis than those with other histologic types, with 2-year and 5-year survival rates of 90% and 64%, respectively. The authors indicated that endoscopic resection was adequate, provided clear margins and en bloc removal in most cases, and was associated with minimal morbidity.[174] They concluded that in selected cases the endonasal approach is a reliable alternative to external approaches. The use of endonasal approaches has also been reported as an adjunct to external approaches in resection of tumors involving the cranial base.[175, 176]

Advantages of using an endonasal approach include the lack of external skin incisions and relatively lower morbidity compared with the open approaches. The keys to adequate oncologic results with the use of the endonasal approach include good selection of patients and the surgeon's vast surgical experience with this approach.[177] The endonasal approach should probably be limited to tumors without evidence of extensive involvement of the paranasal sinuses, orbit, or cranial base; it should be practiced in centers where there is extensive experience with this technique.[175]

Lateral Rhinotomy. This is the standard incision for exposure of sinonasal tumors through a transfacial approach. It can be used alone, or various extensions of the basic incision may be added for further exposure, depending on the extent of tumor.[178] This approach allows adequate exposure of the nasal cavity, lateral nasal wall, nasal septum, nasal roof, maxillary sinus, pterygopalatine fossa, pterygoid plates, ethmoid sinuses, medial and inferior orbital walls, sphenoid sinus, nasopharynx, clivus, and medial aspect of the infratemporal fossa. It is ideally suited for exposure of tumors of the nasal cavity and paranasal sinuses.

The skin incision begins beneath the medial aspect of the eyebrow and continues along a line halfway between the medial canthus and the midline on the nasal dorsum. The incision is carried down over the nasal bone and extends inferiorly to join the medial aspect of the alar crease. The incision then follows the alar crease to the philtrum (Fig. 9–23). Placing the incision in the alar crease helps to hide the scar. The nasal cavity is entered by incising the nasal mucosa at the level of the rim of the pyriform aperture.

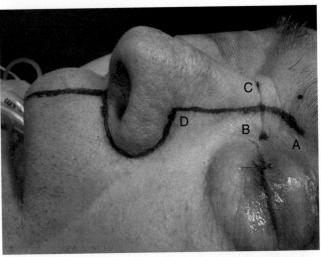

FIGURE 9–23 The lateral rhinotomy incision. The incision is outlined using three surface points. The first point (A) is marked at the inferior hairline of the medial eyebrow about 1 cm lateral to its medial end. The second point is marked halfway between the medial canthus (B) and the midline (C). The last point (D) is the medial end of the alar crease where the crease blends with the skin of the nasal tip. The incision starts by connecting the first two points with a gentle curve at the medial canthal area, corresponding to the concavity of this region. The second and the third points are then connected with a straight line. The incision follows the alar crease, turns toward the midline, makes a right angle inferiorly at the columellar base, and continues as a lip-splitting incision at the midline. Alternatively, the lip-splitting incision may be done along the philtrum.

Elevation of the soft tissues of the cheek is done in a subperiosteal plane over the maxilla and around the inferior orbital nerve. The attachment of the medial canthal tendon to the nasal bone is released. The periorbita is elevated over the medial orbital wall, exposing the lacrimal crest, the lamina papyracea, and the frontoethmoid suture. This suture serves as a landmark for the position of the floor of the anterior cranial fossa; when followed posteriorly, it leads to the anterior and posterior ethmoid foramina. The anterior and posterior ethmoid arteries are cauterized with the bipolar electrocautery, clipped or ligated, and transected. The optic nerve is located 4 to 5 mm posterior to the posterior ethmoid artery. The orbital floor should be dissected as far lateral as the inferior orbital fissure. The lacrimal sac is identified in its fossa between the anterior and posterior lacrimal crests. If a medial maxillectomy is performed, the lacrimal sac is elevated from the fossa and the lacrimal duct is transected; the sac is marsupialized into the nasal cavity so that adequate drainage of the lacrimal system is provided and stenosis is prevented.

The lateral rhinotomy approach allows adequate exposure for a medial maxillectomy and a complete sphenoethmoidectomy. This approach can be extended by adding lip-splitting, sublabial, and palatal incisions to accommodate a total maxillectomy.[178] Meticulous closure of the lateral rhinotomy incision usually results in excellent wound healing and aesthetic appearance (Fig. 9–24).

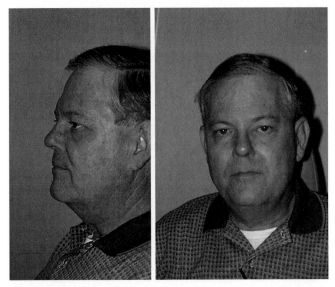

Figure 9–24 Postoperative photograph showing excellent healing and good aesthetic outcome of the lateral rhinotomy incision.

Transoral or Transpalatal Approach. The transoral approach is ideally suited for exposure of the palate, alveolar ridge, and inferior maxilla. The approach uses a combination of the sublabial gingivobuccal sulcus incision and a palatal incision. It is most commonly applied for inferior (infrastructure) maxillectomy. It can also be used for tumors limited to the upper alveolar ridge and hard palate.

The transpalatal approach is usually performed by elevating a posteriorly based palatal flap and removing the posterior aspect of the hard palate to expose the posterior choanae and nasopharynx. It allows adequate exposure for excision of limited tumors of the posterior nasal cavity and nasopharynx, such as juvenile nasopharyngeal angiofibroma.

Midfacial Degloving. The midfacial degloving approach is increasing in popularity in the management of extensive benign lesions of the sinonasal region and skull base, for treatment of selected malignancy in this area, and to afford access to the nasopharynx and infratemporal fossa.[179, 180] The main advantage of the degloving approach is that an external facial incision is avoided. Another advantage is that simultaneous exposure to the inferior and medial maxilla is provided bilaterally. This is particularly helpful when tumors with bilateral involvement of the nasal cavity and maxillary sinus are approached. A major disadvantage, however, is the limited superior, and occasionally posterior, exposure. Another disadvantage is that it is more technically difficult than a lateral rhinotomy and requires constant retraction of the soft tissue envelope for continued adequate exposure.

The midfacial degloving approach requires a basic level of proficiency and understanding of closed rhinoplasty incisions.[180] It involves a complete transfixion incision of the membranous septum (Fig. 9–25A). This is joined endonasally with a bilateral intercartilaginous incision (Fig. 9–25B), with soft tissue elevation over the nasal dorsum as far superior as the nasal root. The nasal skeleton is therefore "degloved" of overlying soft tissues as far lateral as the pyriform aperture. A gingivobuccal incision extends

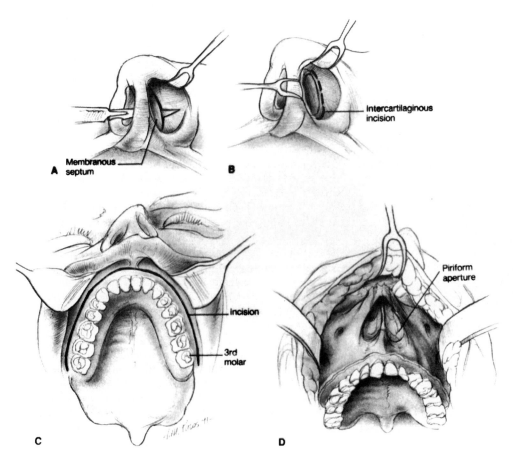

Figure 9–25 Midfacial degloving. (From Myers EN, Carrau RL: Neoplasms of the nose and paranasal sinuses. In Bailey BJ: Head and Neck Surgery–Otolaryngology, vol 2. Philadelphia, JB Lippincott, 1993, p. 1098).

bilaterally across the midline to both maxillary tuberosities laterally (Fig. 9–25C). Subperiosteal dissection is continued cephalad over the face of both maxillas. The dissection joins the nasal degloving with the use of sharp dissection over the pyriform aperture attachments (Fig. 9–25D).

Weber-Fergusson Approach. The incision consists of lateral rhinotomy, lip-splitting, gingivobuccal, palatal, and subciliary (or transconjunctival) incisions. The subciliary incision is thought to allow more lateral exposure of the maxilla and orbit. The lip-splitting incision, which may be done along the philtrum or in the midline, connects the lateral rhinotomy with the sublabial incision, thus allowing more lateral elevation of the facial flap. Transection of the infraorbital nerve allows even more lateral and posterior elevation of the soft tissues, to expose the entire maxillary bone as far lateral as its zygomatic extension and posteriorly to the pterygomaxillary fissure and over the pterygoid plates.

The sublabial incision is made through the gingivobuccal mucosa, starting from the lip-splitting incision and extending as far laterally as the region of the first molar and over the lateral surface of the maxillary tuberosity. In patients undergoing total maxillectomy, a midline or paramedian palatal incision is performed over the hard palate, extending from an interincisor space anteriorly to the junction of the soft and hard palate posteriorly. The incision then continues laterally between the hard and the soft palates to curve posterolaterally around the maxillary tuberosity, meeting the gingivobuccal incision (Fig. 9–26).

Combined Craniofacial Approach. This approach is used whenever a combined anterior craniofacial resection is indicated. In addition to facial incisions (e.g., lateral rhinotomy or facial degloving), a bicoronal incision is made. This incision is started at the level of the zygoma in a

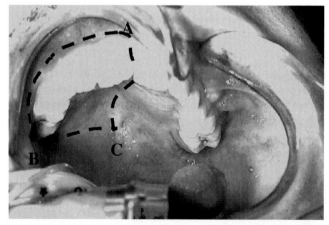

Figure 9–26 Intraoral incisions for a total maxillectomy. The gingivobuccal sulcus incision extends from A to B. Behind the last molar and around the maxillary tuberosity, the incision turns medially between the hard and soft palates (from B to C).The median or paramedian palatal incision extends from C to A. If there is adequate space between the central incisors, the osteotomy may be performed using a microreciprocating saw in the interincisor space. Otherwise, the ipsilateral central incisor should be extracted and the osteotomy placed in the tooth socket in order to avoid loss of bony support to the remaining contralateral incisor.

preauricular crease anterior to the tragus (Fig. 9–27A). Starting the incision as far posterior as the coronal plane preserves the anterior branches of the superficial temporal artery (STA), enhancing the viability of the scalp flap. The incision is extended in the coronal plane, staying behind the hairline along its entire course to the contralateral zygoma (Fig. 9–27B).

Some surgeons prefer to elevate the galea and pericranium with the scalp flap (rather than leaving it on the calvarium), to maintain its vascularity and prevent its drying and desiccation during surgery. After tumor resection has been completed, the vascularized galea–pericranial flap can be elevated off the scalp flap for reconstruction of the cranial base. Alternatively, the scalp flap is elevated in a plane superficial to the pericranium, both anteriorly toward the orbital rims and posteriorly toward the vertex. A pericranial incision is made as far posteriorly as is necessary to provide adequate length for the pericranial flap, which is dissected free from the bone and is reflected anteriorly along the superior temporal line bilaterally. The advantage of the latter technique is that the length of the pericranial flap is not dependent on placement of the scalp incision. Whatever technique is used, careful dissection and preservation of the supraorbital neurovascular pedicles is necessary in providing a well-vascularized pericranial flap for reconstruction of the cranial base defect (Fig. 9–27C).

The supraorbital nerves and vessels are located along the medial third of the superior orbital rim. Elevation of the supraorbital rim periosteum begins laterally and proceeds medially, until the margin of the supraorbital groove is carefully exposed with a fine elevator. The nerve and vessels may exit the skull through either a notch or a true foramen. If a notch is present, the nerve can be dissected free without difficulty. If a foramen rather than a notch is found, the floor of the foramen is removed with a fine osteotome. This liberates the pedicle; further elevation of the superior periorbita is then achieved.

Lateral to the superior temporal lines, an incision is made through the superficial layer of the temporalis fascia 1 to 1.5 cm posterior to the superior orbital rim; it extends posteriorly parallel to the course of the zygomatic arch (Fig. 9–27D). Dissection proceeds at the plane of the deep layer of the temporalis fascia to preserve the frontal branch of the facial nerve, which is superficial to the fascia. The muscle is then dissected off the lateral orbital wall and rim in a subperiosteal fashion and is reflected with the skin flap. The temporalis muscle is then cut at its attachment along the superior temporal line and is reflected inferiorly to expose the frontozygomatic suture line. We prefer to leave a cuff of fascia adherent to the bone so the muscle can be reattached at the conclusion of the procedure.

A frontal craniotomy is then done to expose the floor of the anterior cranial fossa, including the crista galli, cribriform plate, fovea ethmoidalis, orbital roof, and planum sphenoidale. Alternatively, a subfrontal approach may be used by adding osteotomies that allow incorporation of the superior orbit and/or nasal bone to the craniotomy.[181, 182] These skeletal elements may be removed in several subunits or as a single bone flap. Subfrontal approaches have the advantage of minimizing brain retraction by providing wider and more direct exposure of the floor of the anterior cranial

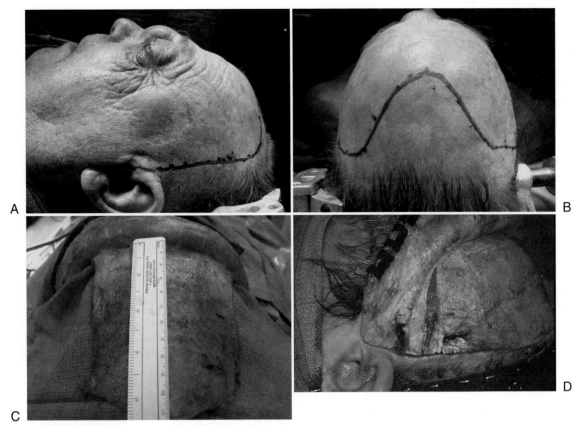

Figure 9–27 Anterior craniofacial approach. *A* and *B*, Bicoronal incision in the patient with esthesioneuroblastoma (Fig. 9–13). *C*, The pericranial flap. Adequate length and good vascular supply of the flap are prerequisites for effective reconstruction of the skull base defect. *D*, Incision of the superficial layer of the deep temporalis fascia. Further dissection is done deep to this plane to preserve the frontal branch of the facial nerve.

fossa. This is especially helpful in more posteriorly located lesions, such as those involving the planum sphenoidale, clivus, orbital apex, and optic chiasm.

EXTENT OF RESECTION

Medial Maxillectomy. This includes removal of the lateral nasal wall, as well as the medial maxillary segment bounded laterally by the infraorbital nerve. In addition, a complete sphenoethmoidectomy is usually performed. The most common indication for medial maxillectomy is the treatment of tumors of the nasal cavity, lateral nasal wall, and medial maxillary sinus (see Fig. 9–22). The incision most commonly used for exposure is the lateral rhinotomy (see Fig. 9–23). Alternatively, a midfacial degloving can be used, which is preferable if bilateral medial maxillectomy is needed (see Fig. 9–25).

After soft tissue exposure has been completed as discussed in the previous section, osteotomies are done as shown in Figure 9–28, and the anterior wall of the maxillary sinus above the level of the dental roots and medial to the infraorbital nerve is removed. Lateral to the infraorbital foramen, the antrostomy may be enlarged to expose the zygomatic recess of the antrum.

Resection of the lateral nasal wall begins with an inferior osteotomy along the nasal floor below the attachment of the

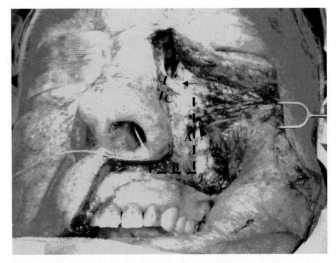

Figure 9–28 Medial maxillectomy. Osteotomies are done (A) vertically medial to the infraorbital foramen (*arrowhead*), (B) horizontally above the level of dental roots and into the pyriform aperture, and (C) obliquely along the nasomaxillary suture line. If the lateral nasal wall is to be resected, the lacrimal sac (*arrow*) is transected and marsupialized into the nasal cavity.

inferior turbinate, starting at the pyriform aperture and moving posteriorly to the posterior maxillary wall. With the orbit retracted laterally and protected with a malleable brain retractor, the lamina papyracea is identified and, if necessary, resected. A complete sphenoethmoidectomy is done, staying below the level of the frontoethmoid suture to avoid injury to the floor of the anterior cranial fossa. The superior attachment of the middle turbinate is then transected along the roof of the nose. Posteriorly, the lateral nasal wall cuts are connected with right-angled scissors behind the turbinates. The specimen is thus delivered and examined for margins with frozen section control. If the tumor involves the nasal septum, it should be included in the resection specimen by the addition of appropriate septal cuts to allow for tumor-free margins.

Closure is begun by reattachment of the medial canthal tendon to the nasal bone in its anatomic position. Meticulous multilayered closure of the lateral rhinotomy is performed (see Fig. 9–24). Adequate nonadherent nasal packing may be left for 1 to 2 days.

Inferior Maxillectomy. This procedure involves resection of the inferior maxillary sinus below the plane of the infraorbital nerve. It is most commonly used for neoplasms of the alveolar process of the maxilla with minimal extension to the maxillary antrum. Similarly, lesions of the hard palate sparing the antrum can be treated by an inferior maxillectomy.

A combination of sublabial and palatal incisions is usually used for exposure, and osteotomies are done around the lesion, ensuring an adequate margin of resection (Fig. 9–29). Alternatively, a midfacial degloving can be used for lesions crossing the midline and involving the inferior maxilla bilaterally. Reconstruction of the inferior maxillary or palatal defect is most simply and effectively achieved using a prosthetic obturator. This can be incorporated in a full or partial denture. Obviously, preoperative consultation with a maxillofacial prosthodontist for dental impressions and obturator design should be obtained.

Total Maxillectomy. Total maxillectomy is indicated for treatment of malignant tumors of the maxillary antrum. For years, the Weber-Fergusson incision was considered by many to be the standard approach for a total maxillectomy. However, we have recently reported the advantages of using the extended lateral rhinotomy instead of the classic Weber-Fergusson incision in patients undergoing total maxillectomy.[178] First, avoiding a subciliary incision eliminates any disruption to the lower lid skin-muscle-tarsus complex. This minimizes lower eyelid complications, particularly ectropion and prolonged eyelid edema. Additionally, its postoperative cosmetic appearance is superior to that of the Weber-Fergusson incision (see Fig. 9–24). Another advantage of the extended lateral rhinotomy incision is that it avoids a trifurcation or an acute angle at the medial canthal region. This reduces the frequency of skin breakdown and cheek flap tip necrosis at the medial canthal area. This is especially important for previously irradiated patients, who are more prone to develop medial canthal dehiscence. Similarly, because the vascularity of the thin lower eyelid skin is not affected by the lateral rhinotomy incision, patients who undergo orbital floor reconstruction with implants such as titanium mesh or porous

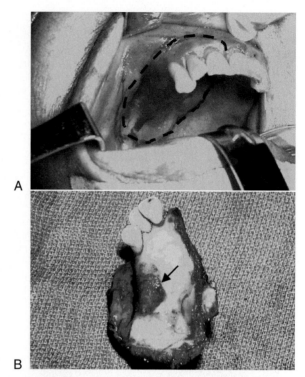

FIGURE 9–29 Inferior maxillectomy. Osteotomies are done around the lesion as shown in *A*. If there is adequate space between the central incisors, the osteotomy may be performed using a microreciprocating saw in the interincisor space. Otherwise, the ipsilateral central incisor should be extracted and the osteotomy placed in the tooth socket in order to avoid loss of bony support to the remaining contralateral incisor. *B*, Inferior maxillectomy specimen showing adequate surgical margins around an upper alveolar ridge carcinoma (*arrow*).

polyethylene (Medpore) have less chance to develop implant exposure.

The extended lateral rhinotomy incision has several functional and cosmetic advantages and provides an adequate approach for a safe oncologic resection. Extension of the lateral rhinotomy incision beneath the medial eyebrow shifts the fulcrum of rotation of the soft tissue flap superiorly and laterally, which enhances lateral exposure. In fact, the lateral extent of exposure obtained by the extended lateral rhinotomy is not different from that obtained with a classic Weber-Fergusson incision (Fig. 9–30).[178]

Whichever incision is used, elevation of the facial flap is usually done in the subperiosteal plane. However, if the tumor has invaded the anterior wall of the maxillary antrum, a supraperiosteal plane is used. Occasionally, if it is involved with tumor, the skin overlying the maxilla is included with the specimen. With the globe protected with a temporary tarsorrhaphy stitch, the periorbita is dissected along the medial, inferior, and lateral orbital walls.

Lateral osteotomies are performed along the frontal and temporal processes of the zygoma (see Fig. 9–30). Osteotomies are done along the frontal process of the maxilla and along the medial orbital wall just inferior to the frontoethmoid suture, extending posteriorly to the level of

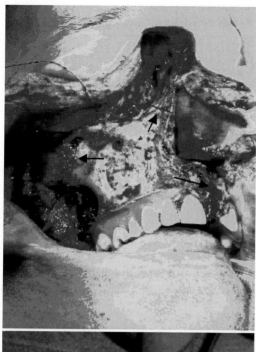

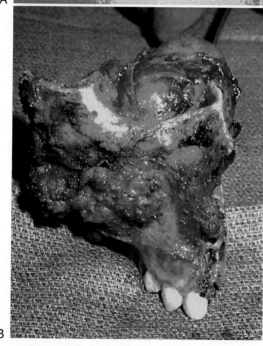

Figure 9–30 Total maxillectomy. *A*, The exposure offered through an extended lateral rhinotomy shown in this figure is not less than that offered by the Weber-Fergusson incision. The advantage of the former is avoiding a subciliary incision and its potential for lower eyelid ectropion and edema. Osteotomies have been performed *(arrows)*. *B*, En-bloc resection specimen. Note tumor involvement of the orbital floor, which had to be resected. Because the tumor did not transgress the periorbita, the eye was preserved.

the posterior ethmoid foramen. The medial and lateral osteotomies are then connected superiorly across the orbital floor along the inferior orbital fissure. Inferiorly, a midline sagittal osteotomy is made across the hard palate. The

ipsilateral central incisor should be preserved, if possible, to enhance prosthesis retention. Finally, after the internal maxillary artery has been identified at its entrance through the pterygomaxillary fissure and has been ligated and transected, a posterior osteotomy is done to disarticulate the maxilla from the pterygoid plates. The maxilla is delivered by anteroinferior traction, while remaining soft tissue attachments are cut with a curved heavy scissors (see Fig. 9–30). Bleeding is usually encountered at this point and is controlled by temporary packing of the cavity, followed by electrocoagulation of bleeding mucosal surfaces or ligature of bleeding points. The pterygoid plexus of veins may be a source of persistent bleeding and can be managed by hemostatic figure-of-8 sutures and Surgicel packing. Bleeding is usually minimized if the internal maxillary artery is ligated before the posterior osteotomy has been done along the pterygomaxillary fissure.

Any remnants of bone and mucosa of the ethmoid air cells are thoroughly removed, and a wide sphenoidotomy is performed. The pterygoid plates are then removed with a burr or bone rongeurs. The pterygoid musculature is then sewn over the bony remnants of the pterygoid plates. The surgical defect is lined with a split-thickness skin graft covering the periorbita, pterygoid musculature, and deep aspect of the cheek flap (Fig. 9–31). This minimizes the formation of granulation tissue in the surgical cavity, prepares the surgical defect to receive an obturator, and reduces soft tissue contracture of the overlying cheek. A bolster formed of iodoform (Xeroform) gauze is used to pack the cavity, aiding in hemostasis and skin graft immobilization. A preformed surgical prosthesis is then wired or screwed to the remaining contralateral maxilla. Alternatively, it can be wired to the remaining dentition. The obturator helps in stabilizing the bolster, as well as in promoting early postoperative speech and swallowing rehabilitation.

As an alternative to a prosthetic obturator, the palatal and maxillary defects may be reconstructed with the use of microvascular free flaps.[183] Reconstruction of the orbital floor may be necessary to provide adequate support of the eye, especially if the periorbita has been resected. The indications and pros and cons of the various reconstructive options are discussed later under Reconstruction and Rehabilitation. The medial canthal ligament is reattached to the nasal bone in its anatomic position to prevent telecanthus. Closure of the facial incisions is done in a meticulous multilayered fashion. The temporary tarsorrhaphy stitch is removed at the end of surgery.

Anterior Craniofacial Resection. Combined extracranial and intracranial (craniofacial) approaches allow en bloc extirpation of paranasal malignancies that abut or penetrate the skull base. When these were combined with appropriate adjuvant therapy, cure rates for such tumors rose from below 20% in the 1950s to 60% to 85% by 2000.[184–187] En bloc resection of the anterior cranial base, therefore, is commonly indicated for patients with sinonasal tumors involving the cribriform plate or fovea ethmoidalis. This is done, by definition, for most cases of esthesioneuroblastoma, as well as carcinoma of the ethmoid or maxillary sinus approaching or involving the anterior cranial base (see Fig. 9–13).[188–191] In a review of 86 consecutive patients

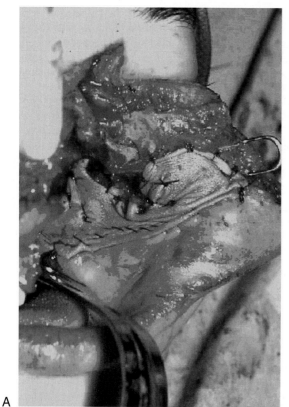

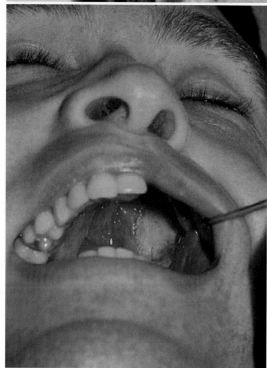

FIGURE 9–31 *A*, A split-thickness skin graft (STSG) is used to line the surgical cavity and the deep aspect of the cheek flap. Once healed, the STSG minimizes granulation tissue formation in the surgical cavity, prepares the surgical defect to receive an obturator, and reduces soft tissue contracture of the overlying cheek (*B*).

TABLE 9–4 Resection of Malignant Tumors of the Anterior Skull Base: Surgical Principles

- Adequate oncologic resection
- Minimal brain retraction
- Protection of critical neurovascular structures
- Meticulous reconstruction of the anterior cranial base
- Optimal aesthetic outcome

with advanced (T3/T4) sinonasal cancer treated at the University of Arkansas between 1988 and 1998, craniofacial resection was performed in one third of patients.[18]

Tumors transgress the cribriform plate either by direct bony invasion or by perineural spread along the filaments of the olfactory nerves. The dura of the anterior cranial fossa forms a barrier that, to a certain extent, delays brain invasion. Dural resection in patients with intracranial but extradural disease or patients with limited dural involvement often provides an adequate oncologic margin. However, malignant tumors that transgress the dural barrier and involve the underlying brain parenchyma are usually associated with poor prognosis.[171–173, 192]

Surgical exposure is achieved using a combination of a transfacial approach and a bicoronal incision, as described in the section on approaches (see Fig. 9–27). Whatever approach is used, certain surgical principles should be followed so that the best possible outcome is achieved (Table 9–4). If the extent of resection involves only the ipsilateral ethmoid sinus with the overlying cribriform plate, then a lateral rhinotomy incision is used (see Fig. 9–23). If the entire ethmoid labyrinth needs to be removed bilaterally, then a contralateral Lynch incision is needed to dissect the medial orbital wall by elevating the contralateral periorbita. If the resection also involves the maxillary sinus, orbital exenteration, or infratemporal fossa dissection, then the facial incision should be modified to a Weber-Fergusson, or preferably, extended lateral rhinotomy, as was discussed in the previous section (see Surgical Approaches). The need for wide exposure in these cases cannot be overemphasized.

The craniotomy may be done through an osteoplastic flap with removal of the posterior wall of the frontal sinus, if the frontal sinus is large. This avoids burr holes in the forehead area. If, however, the frontal sinus is small, an anterior bifrontal craniotomy can be done. The lower horizontal osteotomy should be kept as inferior as possible (within 1 cm of the supraorbital rims) to minimize the need for posterior retraction of the frontal lobes. Alternatively, a subfrontal approach that incorporates the superior orbit and nasal bone with the craniotomy can be performed (Fig. 9–32). These skeletal elements can be removed in several subunits or as a single bone flap. The advantage of subfrontal approaches is that they allow wider exposure of the anterior skull base while minimizing brain retraction. This is especially helpful in more posteriorly located lesions such as those involving the planum sphenoidale, clivus, orbital apex, cavernous sinus, and optic chiasm.[181, 182]

Brain "relaxation" is achieved by withdrawing 25 to 50 mL of CSF from the lumbar subarachnoid drain, achieving hypocapnia through controlled hyperventilation, using mannitol diuresis, or administering steroids. Brain relaxation

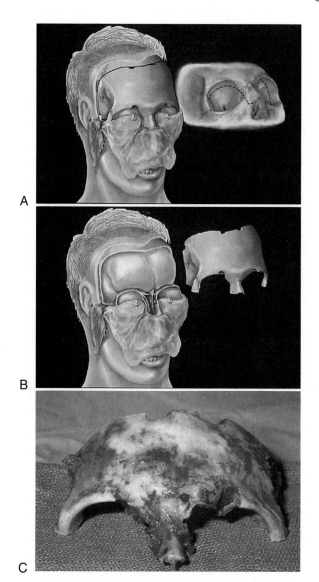

A

B

C

FIGURE 9–32 Subfrontal approach. Osteotomies are made to incorporate the superior orbital and nasal skeleton with the frontal craniotomy (*A*). These subunits can be removed separately or as a single bone flap (*B* and *C*). Subfrontal approaches have the advantage of minimizing brain retraction by providing wider and more direct exposure of the floor of the anterior cranial fossa.

also lessens the need for brain retraction, which minimizes postoperative brain edema. Next, the neurosurgeon elevates the frontal lobes from the anterior cranial fossa floor by severing the olfactory nerves, exposing the cribriform plate. This breaks the dural barrier and always results in some CSF leakage, which must be subsequently repaired by either direct dural suture or a dural patch using temporalis fascia or pericranium. Dural elevation is continued to expose the fovea ethmoidalis and orbital roofs. Posteriorly, the planum sphenoidale and the base of the anterior clinoid process may be exposed as dictated by the extent of the tumor.

With simultaneous exposure provided superiorly through the intracranial approach and inferiorly through the

extracranial approach, osteotomies of the cranial floor around the tumor can be safely completed. Malleable retractors are used to protect the brain and the orbit as osteotomies are made. The placement of osteotomies and the extent of resection are dictated by the extent of tumor involvement and are tailored in each case. Typically, however, osteotomies are made from the planum sphenoidale, along the roof of the ethmoid, and forward to the front of the cribriform plate. Frozen section control of the margins should be done to ensure adequacy of the resection. Watertight reconstruction of the skull base defect should be done to prevent CSF leak and meningitis. This is usually achieved with the use of a vascularized pericranial flap (see Fig. 9–27C).[193, 194] Occasionally, if the cranial base defect is too large or if there is exposure of carotid artery, the temporalis muscle flap or a microvascular free flap may be needed to obliterate dead space and provide adequate coverage of major neurovascular structures.[195, 196]

MANAGEMENT OF THE ORBIT

Surgical exenteration of the orbit carries with it significant emotional burden for patients and their families. Sometimes, this issue alone deters some patients from pursuing treatment altogether, or from choosing nonsurgical modalities of therapy regardless of the chances for cure. Over the past 4 decades, the indications for orbital exenteration have been more clearly defined. In the 1960s, orbital exenteration was almost routinely performed for patients with cancer of the sinonasal tract abutting or invading the bony orbital walls. Most surgeons now believe that the orbit can be safely preserved if cancer does not transgress the periorbita.[197-200]

A recent study from the University of Pittsburgh investigated whether surgery sparing the orbit influenced the rate of local recurrence or survival in patients with SCC of the sinonasal tract.[197] Fifty-eight patients with bone and/or soft tissue invasion of the orbit were included in the study. Patients presenting with invasion of the bony orbit *without* soft tissue invasion were treated with surgical resection, sparing the orbital contents. Patients presenting with invasion of the orbital bones *and* soft tissues were treated with en bloc resection, including orbital exenteration. At 3 years' follow-up, 52% of the patients whose orbit was exenterated were alive and without evidence of disease, compared with 59% of the patients whose orbit was spared. This difference was not statistically significant. Similarly, the rate of local recurrence was not significantly different between both groups. A meta-analysis of the literature revealed similar results.[197] In another recent study, histopathologic sections demonstrated that the periorbita, even when invaded, is an effective barrier against further cancer penetration into the periocular fat.[198] The study also demonstrated the presence of a thin, distinct fascial layer, which surrounds the periocular fat and separates it from the periorbita. These data suggest that sparing of the soft tissues of the orbit when cancer has not transgressed the periorbita does not compromise cure or local control of the disease.

Orbital exenteration is usually indicated when there is gross invasion of the periocular fat, extraocular muscles, or optic nerve.[197-200] Although orbital exenteration can provide good local control of the disease, gross invasion of the orbital contents is an indication of aggressive tumor behavior and is associated with poor prognosis.[172, 201] There is some evidence to indicate that the use of preoperative neoadjuvant therapy in such cases may improve the chances of orbital preservation and control of the disease (see Fig. 9–10).[199, 202]

Despite better definition of the indications for orbital exenteration, the decision as to whether the orbit should be preserved or sacrificed is sometimes difficult to make before surgery has been undertaken. Proptosis or diplopia may be due to displacement rather than to invasion of the intra-orbital contents. Decreased visual acuity or visual fields or the presence of an afferent pupillary defect usually indicates gross invasion of the orbit. In the absence of any ocular signs or symptoms, however, evaluation of the extent of orbital involvement relies mainly on imaging. The accuracy of imaging in detecting invasion of the periorbita is not completely reliable. In a recent study, neither clinical examination nor imaging could predict orbital invasion with absolute accuracy.[198] In many instances, the definitive and most accurate assessment of the extent of orbital invasion and whether the eye can be preserved has to be made intraoperatively.

Another important and frequently overlooked consideration is the functional outcome of the preserved eye. The detrimental effects of postoperative radiation on visual function have to be taken into account when the eventual functional outcome of the preserved eye is predicted. In a study from the M.D. Anderson Cancer Center, a very high rate of ocular complications was reported in patients treated with postoperative radiation therapy.[203] Ocular function in the ipsilateral eye was lost in as many as 79% of patients. The incidence of complications varied with the different techniques of shielding the globe. Patients shielded with only a small lens block had a higher complication rate than did those whose eye was completely shielded.

Another important factor influencing postoperative ocular function is extent of resection and method of reconstruction of the orbital floor. In a report of 28 patients with SCC of the maxillary sinus who underwent maxillectomy with preservation of orbital contents at the M.D. Anderson Cancer Center, 18 patients had part of or the entire orbital floor resected. Adjuvant postoperative radiation therapy was used in 9 of the 18 patients who underwent resection of the orbital floor. Although ocular function was slightly better in patients who did not receive adjuvant radiation therapy, only 3 of the 18 patients (17%) retained significant function in the ipsilateral eye. Ocular problems included ectropion, lymphedema of the eyelid, keratopathy, cataracts, diplopia on upward gaze, and optic atrophy. A significant number of patients patched the eye at all times. Three patients had no light perception in the ipsilateral eye, and two patients underwent enucleation for a painful eye. Based on these data, the authors concluded that strong consideration should be given to orbital exenteration at the time of surgery when the orbital floor has been resected, especially if postoperative radiation fields will include the globe.[204] It is important to note, however, that none of the patients who were treated with resection of the orbital floor underwent reconstruction of the floor of the orbit with bone. We believe that when a significant portion of the bony orbital floor is resected, especially if it includes the periorbita, a split-thickness skin graft does not provide adequate support for the globe. Without skeletal reconstruction of the orbital floor with bone, enophthalmos, ectropion, and diplopia are predictable sequelae. These complications may significantly compromise the functional outcome of the preserved eye, which may have been responsible for the exceedingly high rate of nonfunctional vision in this group of patients reported by the M.D. Anderson Cancer Center.[204]

We believe that every effort should be made to preserve the eye as long as preservation does not compromise the adequacy of oncologic resection. When a significant portion of the floor of the orbit is resected, we recommend reconstruction of the floor with bone to provide adequate support of the globe. Precise radiation dosimetry and proper shielding of the eye should be planned to minimize ocular complications secondary to radiation injury. The use of 3-D conformal radiation therapy (3-D CRT) or intensity-modulated radiation therapy (IMRT) is particularly helpful in delivering effective radiation doses to the tumor bed while sparing ocular contents.[205] With the use of these strategies, we were able to achieve a high rate (80%) of preservation of the orbital contents with good functional outcome in patients with advanced cancer of the sinonasal tract.[18]

If a decision has been made to exenterate the orbit, supraciliary and subciliary incisions are made around the upper and lower eyelids, respectively. This allows for preservation of the eyelids, which can be used to line the orbit. If the eyelids are involved with cancer, they must be included in the resection (Fig. 9–33). The periorbita is incised over the superior and lateral orbital rims. Dissection continues along the roof of the orbit and lateral walls until the superior orbital fissure and the optic foramen are exposed. Lidocaine is injected around these structures to block any autonomically induced cardiac arrhythmias. To prevent troublesome bleeding, the neurovascular structures in the superior orbital fissure are slowly and carefully isolated, ligated or clipped, and transected. The optic nerve and the ophthalmic artery are then managed in a similar fashion. The extraocular muscles are transected at their origin in the orbital apex. The medial and inferior orbit may be left attached to the specimen if en bloc resection of the eye in patients with sinonasal cancer is indicated. Osteotomies are done as previously described for total maxillectomy, except that the orbital bony cuts are connected at the orbital apex, rather than at the inferior orbital fissure. A split-thickness skin graft or the preserved eyelid skin is used to line the cavity. This skin-lined cavity tolerates a prosthetic eye very well.

RECONSTRUCTION AND REHABILITATION

The goals of reconstruction of surgical defects created from surgical ablation of sinonasal tumors must include the following:

1. Oronasal separation
2. Cranionasal separation
3. Eye and cheek support
4. Dental restoration
5. Restoration of facial defects

These goals must be tailored to the needs of individual patients. Options include prosthetic rehabilitation, surgical reconstruction, or a combination of both.

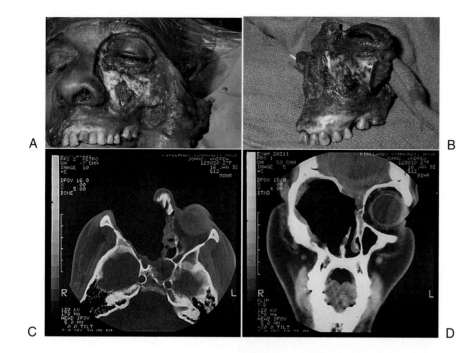

FIGURE 9–33 Orbital exenteration. *A,* The lateral rhinotomy is extended around the lids and included in the resection. *B,* En-bloc resection of the maxilla and the eye, which was extensively involved with carcinoma. *C* and *D,* Axial and coronal CT scans showing no evidence of recurrent cancer at 3 years of follow-up.

Oronasal Separation. Separation between the oral and nasal cavities is essential for effective speech and deglutition. Palatal defects resulting from a maxillectomy are simply and effectively sealed with the use of a prosthetic obturator. Preoperatively, the oromaxillofacial prosthodontist takes dental impressions and designs a *surgical* obturator, which is used at the end of surgery to seal the palatal defect (Fig. 9–34A).[206] The surgical obturator can be slightly modified intraoperatively to custom-fit the defect. The advantages of this immediate reconstruction are early postoperative restoration of normal speech and oral feeding. This minimizes the early postoperative morbidity of surgery and obviates the need for enteral feeding. The obturator is retained by an attachment to the remaining dentition with clasp wires. Its retention is enhanced by preserving, if possible, the ipsilateral incisor(s).[207] In edentulous patients, the surgical obturator can be temporarily fixed to the remaining hard palate with lag screws (see Fig. 9–34A). Preoperatively, clear communication between the head and neck surgeon and the maxillofacial prosthodontist concerning the anticipated maxillary defect is required for optimal results. An additional advantage of the surgical obturator is its ability to support the surgical packing used to immobilize the skin graft lining the cheek flap (see Fig. 9–34A). This epithelial lining, when completely healed, minimizes granulation tissue formation, provides a smooth mucosal lining, reduces scar contracture of the cheek, provides a scar band to support the obturator, and facilitates good hygiene of the cavity (see Fig. 9–31B).

At the end of the first postoperative week, and after removal of the surgical packing, the surgical obturator is replaced with an *interim* obturator (Fig. 9–34B and C). This is used for several weeks after the patient has been discharged from the hospital and after completion of adjuvant therapy, allowing the surgical cavity to heal completely. Patients are instructed to remove the obturator periodically and clean the cavity with saline irrigation. At follow-up visits, the obturator is removed and is cleaned of any crusts or debris. Finally, a *permanent* obturator is designed to custom-fit the cavity after it has matured to its final shape and dimensions. The acrylic dome incorporated into its design provides some cheek support (Fig. 9–34D). In addition to being a simple and effective method of reconstruction of palatal defects, permanent obturators can also provide full dental restoration (Fig. 9–34E). At follow-up visits, removal of the obturator allows for easy inspection of the cavity for any evidence of recurrent disease. Surgical reconstruction of palatal defects with tissue flaps eliminates the need for regular hygiene of the surgical cavity.[208, 209] Flap reconstruction, however, requires more extensive surgery, adds donor site morbidity, does not allow rapid dental restoration, and conceals the surgical cavity from inspection for recurrent tumor. These disadvantages make prosthetic obturators the method of choice for reconstruction of surgical defects of the palate. The use of tissue flaps is usually reserved for patients who need additional reconstruction in the maxillary skeleton, orbital floor, or cranial base.[210]

Cranionasal Separation. Whenever the cranial and nasal cavities are joined by a surgical defect, as is the case with anterior craniofacial resection, watertight cranionasal separation is mandatory to reduce the risk of CSF leak, meningitis, and pneumocephalus. All dural tears should be closed meticulously. Larger defects of the dura should be repaired with temporalis fascia, pericranium, or fascia lata grafts. Although bony reconstruction of the anterior skull base using vascularized and nonvascularized bone grafts[211] and bone cement[212] has been described, reconstruction of the bone defect is not routinely necessary in most patients. The vascularized galea–pericranial flap is currently the most frequently used flap for reconstructing defects of the floor of the anterior cranial fossa (see Fig. 9–27C).[193, 194] Certain technical considerations should be kept in mind when the

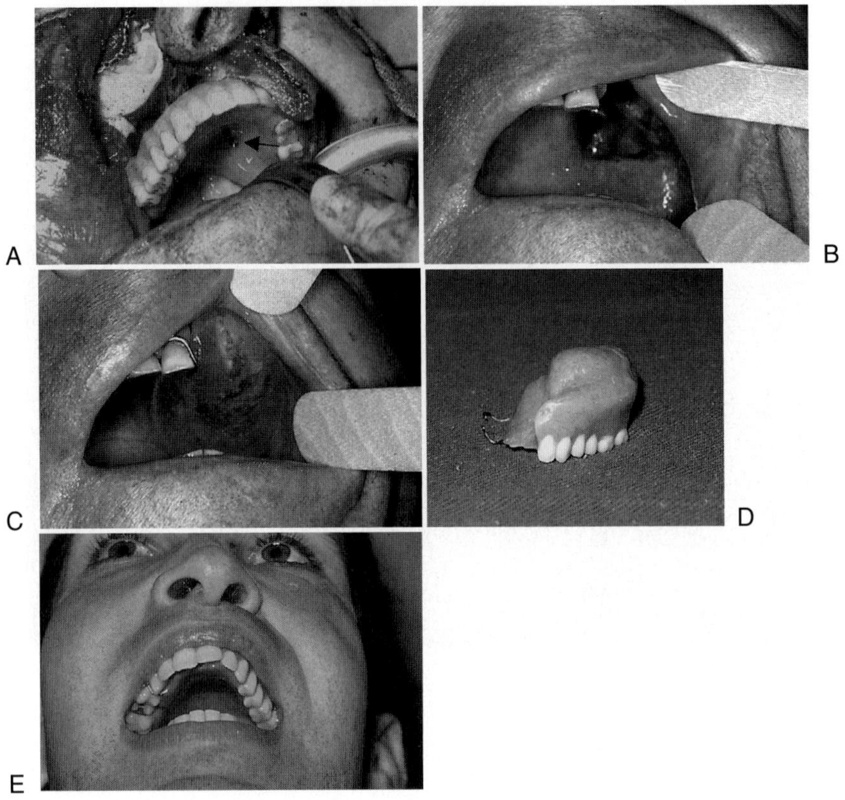

FIGURE 9–34 Prosthetic rehabilitation of postmaxillectomy palatal defect. *A,* A surgical obturator fixed to the palate with a lag screw *(arrow)* provides immediate rehabilitation and supports the surgical packing. *B* and *C,* Interim obturator is used for several weeks until the cavity is completely healed. *D* and *E,* The permanent obturator has an acrylic dome to provide some cheek support. It also provides adequate dental restoration.

bicoronal incision is planned, to ensure adequate flap length and viability (see under Combined Craniofacial Approach). Flap handling and suturing should be meticulously done so that a watertight seal is achieved. Fibrin glue and tissue adhesives do not compensate for an imperfect closure. Lumbar subarachnoid drainage for several days postoperatively helps to reduce CSF pressure and the possibility of a leak. However, aggressive lumbar drainage should be avoided because it may encourage the development of pneumocephalus.

Occasionally, more bulk is needed to reconstruct the surgical cavity and reduce dead space, such as with extensive defects of the cranial base. Regional flaps, such as the temporalis muscle, are usually adequate for this purpose. If muscle bulk is inadequate or if its blood supply has been sacrificed, a microvascular free flap is used.[195, 196] Vascularized tissue may also be needed to protect the carotid artery if it has been exposed to the surgical defect. This is done to prevent desiccation of the arterial wall and carotid artery blowout. This is particularly important if the patient has previously received radiation therapy or will receive postoperative adjuvant radiation.

Eye and Cheek Support. The maxilla has three bony buttresses—the nasomaxillary, zygomaticomaxillary, and pterygomaxillary. In addition to a palatal defect, total maxillectomy results in resection of all three buttresses and loss of adequate skeletal support to the soft tissues of the cheek. Loss of the zygomaticomaxillary buttress results in inferior displacement of the orbit and flattening of the malar eminence. Loss of the nasomaxillary buttress results in superior and posterior deviation of the alar base of the nose. Loss of the pterygomaxillary buttress results in superior and posterior

deviation of the upper lip.[213] Resection of the inferior orbital rim and floor results in loss of skeletal support to the eyelid and globe. Lack of adequate orbital support results in unacceptable aesthetic and functional outcomes of the preserved eye resulting from enophthalmos, ectropion, hypoglobus, and diplopia. The combined effects of loss of support of the eye and cheek result in the "typical" postmaxillectomy deformity (Fig. 9–35A). Although a split-thickness skin graft and a palatal obturator are commonly used in reconstruction after maxillectomy, these methods of reconstruction do not provide adequate support for the cheek and eye.

Skeletal reconstruction of the maxillary and orbital defects may be done using bone grafts, most commonly autogenous calvarial grafts. Demineralized and banked bone grafts, which are available in a variety of shapes and sizes, may also be used. Alternatively, alloplastic implants may be used for reconstruction of the maxillary buttresses, orbital rim, or orbital floor.[214] Titanium mesh, bone cement, and porous polyethylene have all been successfully used in orbital and maxillary bony reconstruction (Fig. 9–35B through E).[212, 215, 216]

Whatever method is used for bone reconstruction, adequate coverage with well-vascularized soft tissue is essential to prevent resorption of bone grafts and infection or extrusion of alloplastic implants. The pedicled temporalis muscle flap, temporoparietal fascial flap, or septal mucosal flap is most commonly used for this purpose.[195, 214, 217] Alternatively, microvascular free flaps may be used to provide soft tissue coverage of bone grafts or implants, or composite vascularized bone flaps may be used for full reconstruction of both soft tissue and bone defects.[213, 218]

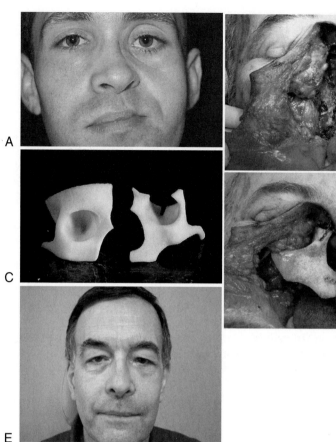

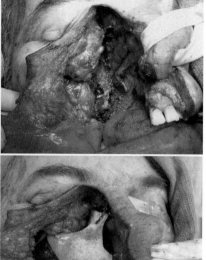

FIGURE 9–35 Orbital reconstruction. *A,* "Typical" postmaxillectomy deformity due to lack of support of the orbit and cheek. There is downward displacement of the orbit and medial canthus. Note the presence of enophthalmos, as evidenced by a prominent upper eyelid sulcus. There is flattening of the cheek and deviation of the nasal tip. The patient had significant diplopia. These deformities can be avoided with adequate bony reconstruction. *B,* Post total maxillectomy defect showing loss of orbital floor and periorbita. *C,* Porous polyethylene orbital implants (full and lower two-thirds). *D,* Primary reconstruction of the defect. The implant was covered with a temporoparietal fascial flap internally and with the cheek skin flap externally. *E,* Postoperative appearance showing good position of the eye, cheek, and nose.

Primary reconstruction of defects of the maxilla and orbit at the time of maxillectomy is easier and results in better aesthetic and functional outcomes than are provided with delayed reconstruction. Although secondary reconstruction after globe-sparing maxillectomy is feasible, it is often difficult, and the results are limited by excessive scarring and soft tissue contracture, especially in patients who have undergone adjuvant radiation therapy. These patients may benefit more from free-tissue transfer reconstruction.[214]

Dental Restoration. Prosthetic rehabilitation using partial or full upper dentures is the easiest method of dental restoration in patients who have undergone maxillectomy (see Fig. 9–34). Remaining contralateral teeth facilitate retention of partial dentures. In edentulous patients, dental fixatives can be used, but denture retention is more difficult. A soft palate "band" at the posterior edge of the defect may provide enough of a ledge to enable retention of the prosthesis. Retention of the prosthesis in edentulous patients who have undergone an extended resection including the soft palate may be extremely difficult. In such cases, the use of osteointegrated implants facilitates prosthetic dental restoration.

Another important aspect of the rehabilitation of patients who have undergone maxillectomy is the prevention of trismus. Patients who have undergone resection of the pterygoid plates or muscles of mastication are particularly prone to develop trismus. This may be severe enough to interfere with inserting and wearing a denture-bearing obturator. Early postoperative jaw opening exercises using "stacked" wooden tongue blades or commercially available devices (e.g., Therabite) are extremely important in preventing or minimizing postoperative trismus (Fig. 9–36).

Restoration of Facial Defects. Smaller defects of the face are optimally reconstructed with the use of local flaps. Local skin flaps provide the best thickness and color match for facial defects. Reconstruction of more extensive facial defects may require regional or microvascular free flaps, but less optimal aesthetic outcomes are achieved owing to color or thickness mismatch between the donor and defect sites (Fig. 9–37). Facial defects resulting from orbital exenteration or total rhinectomy are best managed with prosthetic restoration (Fig. 9–38).

CERVICAL METASTASIS

The incidence of palpable cervical metastasis on initial presentation of patients with cancer of the nasal cavity or paranasal sinuses ranges from 3% to 16%, with most series reporting an average incidence of around 10%. The development of nodal metastasis during the course of the disease is higher, ranging from 10% to 45%.[44, 45, 219] Although the most frequently reported sites of lymphatic metastasis are levels I and II,[44] a significant part of the lymphatic drainage

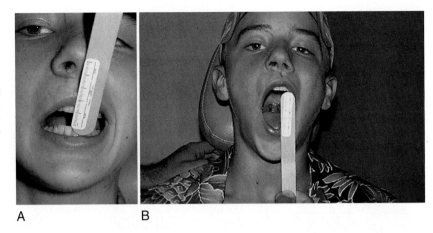

FIGURE 9–36 This 15-year-old boy underwent resection of a nasopharyngeal angiofibroma, which involved the pterygoid plates. Postoperatively, he had significant trismus, (*A*) which resolved with mouth-opening exercises (*B*).

of the paranasal sinuses and the nasal cavity is directed to the retropharyngeal lymph nodes, which are inaccessible for palpation and are frequently overlooked. It is possible, therefore, that the true incidence of lymphatic spread of sinonasal malignancy is underestimated. The retropharyngeal lymph nodes are best evaluated with high-resolution imaging (CT or MRI).

The overall risk of nodal involvement either at diagnosis or on follow-up may depend on the histology and the stage and extent of the primary tumor. In a recent report of 97 patients with carcinoma of the maxillary sinus treated at Stanford University, the risk of nodal metastasis was 28% for SCC, 25% for adenocarcinoma, 12% for undifferentiated carcinoma, and 10% for adenoid cystic carcinoma. All patients with nodal involvement had T3–T4 tumors.[44] Tumor extension into the oral cavity and nasopharynx is associated with increased risk of nodal metastasis.[45]

Lymphatic metastasis to the cervical lymph nodes carries with it a poor prognosis in patients with cancer of the sinonasal tract. Patients with nodal relapse have a significantly higher risk of distant metastasis. In one study, the 5-year actuarial risk of distant relapse was 30% for patients

with neck control versus 80% for patients with neck failure.[44] A trend for decreased survival was also noted with nodal relapse. The 5-year actuarial survival was 37% for patients with control of the neck and 0% for patients with relapse in the neck.

In patients with no clinical evidence of neck metastasis (N0) from sinonasal cancer, elective radiation of the neck (ENI) effectively reduces relapse in the neck.[219] In patients with cancer of the maxillary sinus, the 5-year actuarial risk of nodal relapse was 20% for patients without ENI and 0% for those with ENI.[44] For patients with clinical evidence of nodal metastasis on presentation, combined modality treatment with neck dissection and postoperative adjuvant radiation with or without chemotherapy offers the best chance for control of the disease.[45]

The prognostic significance of cervical metastasis at the time of initial presentation is controversial. Some authors have reported that the presence of nodal metastasis on initial diagnosis was associated with a dismal prognosis.[78, 79] Others have found no such correlation between nodal disease at presentation and survival.[58] The relatively low incidence of cervical metastasis from sinonasal malignancy

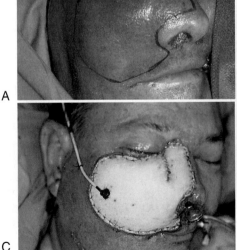

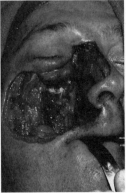

FIGURE 9–37 *A*, Maxillary sinus cancer involving the overlying cheek skin. *B*, Maxillectomy and facial defect. *C*, Reconstruction with a rectus abdominis free flap. Note the color and thickness mismatch.

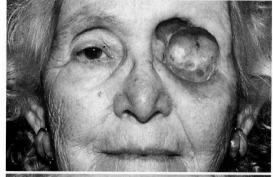

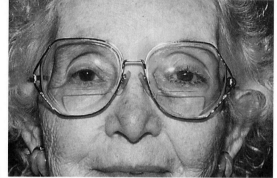

FIGURE 9-38 *A,* Orbital exenteration defect. *B,* Prosthetic restoration.

TABLE 9-5 Morbidity and Mortality of Anterior Craniofacial Resection

Study	Number of Patients	Morbidity	Mortality
Catalano et al 1994[221]	73	63%	2.7%
Shah et al 1997[171]	115	35%	3.5%
Dias et al 1999[220]	104	48.6%	7.6%
Solero et al 2000[190]	168	30%	4.7%

does not warrant the routine use of elective neck dissection. Additionally, the primary echelon for lymphatic spread from tumors of the paranasal sinuses—the retropharyngeal nodes—is not included in standard neck dissections. If these lymph nodes are deemed metastatic based on imaging criteria, they should be incorporated in radiation therapy fields used as a single or adjuvant modality of treatment. Palpable cervical lymphadenopathy is not a contraindication to radical treatment of the primary tumor, and its presence should be addressed with a therapeutic neck dissection.

COMPLICATIONS

The rate of complications following maxillectomy is relatively low. Intraoperative bleeding can occasionally be troublesome. Measures to reduce excessive bleeding include preoperative embolization for vascular tumors and early intraoperative identification and control of the internal maxillary artery. Postoperative bleeding is best prevented by meticulous intraoperative hemostasis and adequate surgical packing during the early postoperative period. Treatment usually requires identification and electrocautery or ligation of the source of bleeding. Wound complications are relatively uncommon. The risk of wound infection is reduced by the use of perioperative antibiotics and by meticulous postoperative care of the surgical cavity. Partial or total loss of the split-thickness skin graft lining the cavity is usually due to technical errors in the harvest, inset, or immobilization of the graft. The loss of epithelial lining complicates postoperative care of the surgical cavity owing to excessive granulation tissue formation and crusting. Treatment is conservative and requires frequent cleaning of the cavity, cauterization of granulation tissue, and meticulous removal

of crusts. Postoperative trismus is common and is prevented by early mouth opening exercises.

The risk of complications is higher with craniofacial resection. Despite its widespread application, the reported incidence of significant morbidity and even mortality associated with anterior craniofacial resection is relatively high (Table 9–5). The rate of major complications correlates with the type of surgical approach,[182] the extent of resection,[220] and the experience of the surgical team.[221] Complications can be divided into those related to the intracranial or to the extracranial approach (Table 9–6). Cerebrospinal fluid leak, pneumocephalus, and transient alteration in mental status were the most common intracranial complications.[190, 220] Transient mental status changes were attributed to contusion or edema of the brain or hematoma. These complications are less likely to occur when brain retraction is minimized, which is one of the main advantages of subfrontal approaches.[182] Invasion of the dura and the type of reconstruction of the anterior skull base were the most important factors related to cerebrospinal fluid leak and meningitis.[220] Overall, infectious complications were the most devastating, and bacterial contamination leading to septic complications was the principal cause of morbidity, accounting for more than half of the major complications.[220, 221] CSF leak is best prevented by meticulous watertight repair of dural tears and effective cranionasal separation. Most mild CSF leaks respond to conservative treatment, which includes bed rest, elevation of the head of the bed, avoidance of straining, and the use of gentle lumbar drainage. Persistent leaks usually require surgical exploration and closure of the dural defect. Endoscopic nasal approaches are rapidly gaining popularity as the primary treatment of postoperative CSF leaks because of their high success rate (approaching 95%) and low morbidity.[222]

Tension pneumocephalus occurs if air leaks from the sinonasal tract and is trapped within the cranial cavity. This

TABLE 9-6 Complications of Anterior Craniofacial Resection

Intracranial Approach	Extracranial Approach
Brain contusion/hematoma	Epiphora
CSF leak	Telecanthus
Pneumocephalus	Ectropion
Meningitis/Abscess	Enophthalmos
Cranial nerve deficits	Dystopia
Cerebrovascular accidents	Palatal fistula
Frontal sinus mucocele	Malocclusion
Osteomyelitis of the frontal bone	Facial deformity

CSF, cerebrospinal fluid.

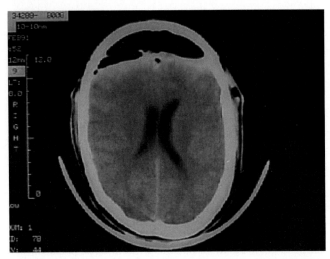

FIGURE 9–39 Tension pneumocephalus after anterior craniofacial resection.

can lead very quickly to serious brain compression and deterioration of neurologic status (Fig. 9–39). The risk of pneumocephalus following craniofacial procedures is significant and may be increased by the use of lumbar drainage of CSF intraoperatively. In one series, the use of lumbar CSF drainage during the operation correlated most strongly with the development of pneumocephalus.[223] Tension pneumocephalus is potentially devastating and usually presents with rapid neurologic deterioration. It requires prompt recognition and treatment to minimize permanent neurologic deficits. Diagnosis is confirmed by urgent imaging. Emergency treatment consists of release of intracranial air using a large-bore needle introduced through one of the preexisting burr holes over the entrapped air. Definitive treatment may necessitate reexploration, identification, and sealing of the site(s) of cranionasal defect(s).

Ocular complications are frequent after resection of cancer of the sinonasal tract. In one series of 58 patients, ocular complications occurred in more than 40% of patients and consisted of epiphora in 21 patients, diplopia in 8, vision loss in 6, and pain and enophthalmos in 2.[224] Twelve patients required revision surgery consisting of dacryocystorhinostomy in 8, repair of ectropion in 3, drainage of orbital mucocele in 1, and corneal transplant in 1. Ocular complications, particularly loss of vision, are more common among patients treated with postoperative radiation therapy. During surgery, delicate handling of the orbital contents, adequate corneal protection, accurate reconstruction of the bony orbit, and meticulous repair of the medial canthal ligament and lacrimal system can minimize ocular complications, and functional vision can be preserved in most patients.

Radiation Therapy

Radiation therapy is frequently incorporated in the overall management of patients with cancer of the nasal cavity and paranasal sinuses. Radiation therapy may be given with curative intent,[225] or as an adjuvant therapy before[79, 226] or after[38, 46] surgery. Radiation therapy may also be combined with chemotherapy either as definitive treatment or as an adjunct to planned surgical resection.[42, 227] Radiation therapy may also be used in the palliation of recurrent or unresectable tumors. Regardless of the treatment strategy, there is almost universal agreement that patients with advanced-stage tumors are best treated with multimodal therapy, including surgery, radiation, and in some cases, chemotherapy.[38, 42, 46, 79, 226–230]

A recent report from the University of Toronto, Ontario, Cancer Institute and Princess Margaret Hospital described the outcomes of 29 patients with carcinoma of the ethmoid sinus treated with curative intent using primary radiation therapy with salvage surgery for persistent or progressive disease.[225] Tumors included SCC, adenocarcinoma, and undifferentiated carcinoma. Two thirds of patients had T4 tumors. The most common radiation dose regimens were 60 Gy in 30 daily fractions over 6 weeks, and 50 Gy in 20 daily fractions over 4 weeks. With a median follow-up of 4 years, the 5-year local progression-free survival was 40%. Local progression was the major cause of treatment failure and was documented in 15 of 29 patients treated (52%). A total of 18 of 29 patients died during the period of review. Of these, 12 deaths were due to ethmoid cancer.[225] In another report from the same institution, patients treated with salvage surgery for recurrent sinonasal cancer who had failed primary radiation had poor 5-year survival (22%).[231] These data indicate that the use of primary radiation as the only method of treatment for advanced sinonasal cancer results in poor local control of the disease, with more than 50% of patients eventually dying from cancer.

There is strong evidence that the use of combined surgery and adjuvant radiation therapy results in better tumor control and survival than does radiation alone in patients with cancer of the maxillary[229] and ethmoid sinuses.[232] In a report of 73 patients with advanced carcinoma of the paranasal sinuses, the 5-year local control was 65% with combined surgery and radiation, in comparison with 47% with radiotherapy alone. Combined treatment resulted in significantly better 5-year overall and disease-free survival than did radiation therapy alone (60% vs. 9%, $P = 0.001$; and 53% vs. 6%, $P < 0.0001$, respectively).[228] Other studies have demonstrated that combined surgery and adjuvant radiation is the treatment modality of choice, particularly for advanced tumors, whereas surgery alone may be sufficient for small, well-localized, or low-grade tumors.[38, 229, 230]

Delivery of effective doses of radiation (60–70 Gy) for treatment of advanced sinonasal cancer using conventional radiotherapy is associated with serious morbidity, including blindness and brain necrosis.[46, 228] The use of 3-dimensional conformal radiotherapy (3D-CRT) and intensity-modulated radiotherapy (IMRT) increases treatment accuracy by delivering tumoricidal doses to the tumor bed while reducing radiation doses to nearby critical structures, such as the optic nerves and the brain.[233–235] In a recent study, 3D-CRT and IMRT significantly reduced radiation doses to the brain and ipsilateral parotid gland compared with conventional treatment of maxillary sinus cancer. IMRT reduced doses to both optic nerves while delivering radiation with improved homogeneity and coverage of the tumor bed.[205] Recent refinements in IMRT include the application of new tools such as the Segment Outline and Weight Adapting Tool (SOWAT)[236] and the Anatomy-Based Segmentation Tool (ABST).[237]

Brachytherapy using 3-dimensional CT planning has also been used effectively, either alone or in combination with external beam radiation therapy, in the treatment of sinonasal cancer.[238] This approach allows reliable and precise placement of brachytherapy after the use of load probes, avoiding the inaccuracy of traditional methods of brachytherapy placement. However, some radiation oncologists are reluctant to employ brachytherapy because of the complexity of the treatment and postoperative management, as well as concerns about radiation safety. Recently, the American Brachytherapy Society (ABS) developed guidelines for high-dose-rate (HDR) brachytherapy of the head and neck, which eliminates unwanted radiation exposure and thereby permits unrestricted delivery of clinical care to patients.[239] The ABS made specific recommendations for patients with previously untreated and recurrent cancer of the head and neck regarding patient selection, implant techniques, target volume definition, and HDR treatment parameters (such as time, dose, and fractionation schedules). Suggestions were provided for treatment with HDR alone and in combination with external beam radiation therapy.

Fast-neutron radiation therapy has shown promising results in the palliative treatment of patients with unresectable, inoperable, residual, or recurrent adenoid cystic carcinoma of the sinonasal tract and skull base. The results and outcome of this treatment were previously discussed under Adenoid Cystic Carcinoma.

Chemotherapy

In an effort to improve local control and survival rates, chemotherapy is being increasingly incorporated in the management of patients with cancer of the sinonasal tract and cranial base. Chemotherapy has been included in the treatment of SCC, SNUC, neuroendocrine carcinoma, esthesioneuroblastoma, and salivary gland carcinoma of the paranasal sinuses.[105, 240] Chemotherapy may be given as induction (neoadjuvant), adjuvant, maintenance, or palliative treatment. It may be combined with radiation in a sequential or concurrent fashion. Routes of administration include systemic (intravenous or oral), regional (intra-arterial), and local (topical).

The incorporation of chemotherapy with radiation in a multimodality treatment approach seems to further enhance local control and perhaps disease-specific survival in patients with advanced or high-grade cancer of the sinonasal tract. A recent report described the outcome of 59 of 74 patients with advanced cancer of the maxillary sinus who underwent multimodality therapy consisting of preoperative radiation therapy with concomitant intramaxillary arterial infusion of 5-fluorouracil, followed by total or partial maxillectomy. The patients who underwent multimodality therapy showed significantly better 5-year overall survival, disease-free survival, and local control rates than did those who underwent radiotherapy alone (68.5% vs. 9.1%, 73.2% vs. 18.2%, 84.0% vs. 18.2%, respectively).

Multivariate analysis revealed that T classification and treatment modality are independent predictors for disease-free survival.[42]

Excellent long-term local control, overall survival, and disease-free survival were also achieved in patients with locoregionally advanced paranasal sinus cancer treated with induction chemotherapy, followed by surgery and postoperative concomitant chemoradiotherapy.[227] Induction chemotherapy consisted of three cycles of cisplatin and 5-fluorouracil. Induction chemotherapy achieved a clinical response in 87% of patients, and a complete histologic response was documented at the time of surgery in half of these patients. The 10-year overall survival, disease-free survival, and local control rates were 56%, 73%, and 79%, respectively.[227] These results are encouraging and may be superior to those achieved with surgery and radiation therapy. Further investigation of incorporation of chemotherapy with radiation and surgery in a multimodal approach is warranted.

Recently, the use of long-term maintenance oral chemotherapy has been shown to result in more durable local disease control and improved survival after definitive treatment of patients with advanced cancer of the maxillary sinus. Chemotherapy consisted of uracil and tegaful (UFT), the active metabolites of 5-fluorouracil, given orally at a dose of 300 or 400 mg/day for longer than 1 year.[241, 242]

Several reports from Japan have described the use of regional or local chemotherapy in addition to radiation in reducing the extent of surgical resection of maxillary sinus cancer; these demonstrated equal (and sometimes better) cure rates than with conventional treatment consisting of radical surgery followed by radiation therapy. For example, a recent report described the outcome of 75 patients with cancer of the maxillary sinus treated with surgery through a sublabial incision and tumor debridement, radiotherapy, and regional chemotherapy.[47] All 23 patients with orbital involvement retained the orbital contents, and a majority demonstrated adequate ocular function. The authors concluded that combined therapy with conservative surgery, radiotherapy, and regional chemotherapy appears to be an effective method for local control and preservation of ocular function.[47]

The addition of neoadjuvant chemotherapy to radiation in the palliative management of patients with inoperable maxillary sinus cancer was recently investigated. Despite a higher response rate to neoadjuvant chemotherapy, there was no significant difference in 5-year actuarial survival or disease-free survival between the two treatment groups.[243]

◾ OUTCOME AND PROGNOSIS

Although the literature is replete with reports describing the outcome and prognosis of patients with sinonasal cancer, several confounding factors make meaningful interpretation of the results extremely difficult. Such factors include diversity of histologic diagnoses, site of origin, extent of tumor invasion, previous therapy, extent of surgical resection, status of surgical margins, adjuvant therapy, and length of follow-up. Despite these limitations, several recent reports have demonstrated that aggressive multimodality therapy offers good local control of disease and acceptable survival rates, ranging from 60% to 75%.[18, 42, 171, 172, 185, 189, 227, 230, 232] A systematic review of published articles on patients with malignancies of the nasal and paranasal sinuses during the past 40 years demonstrated a progressive improvement in results for patients with squamous cell and adenocarcinoma, primary cancer of the maxillary and ethmoid sinus, and the use of most treatment modalities.[1] The main pattern of treatment failure is still local recurrence, and efforts to further improve survival should be directed toward improvement of local control.[229, 230, 232]

Several factors influence the prognosis and outcome of patients with cancer of the nasal cavity, paranasal sinuses, and orbit. These include tumor stage, site of origin, histology, extent of resection, surgical margins, adjuvant therapy, and the patient's performance status. In a recent report describing the outcome of 220 patients with sinonasal cancer, the 5-year actuarial survival rate for the whole group was 63%, and the local control rate was 57%.[1] Major factors influencing prognosis included T stage, histology, site of origin, and treatment modality. The influence of these factors on 5-year survival rates is shown in Table 9–7.

In a recent review of 86 consecutive patients with advanced cancer of the sinonasal tract treated at the University of Arkansas between 1988 and 1998 with a minimum follow-up of 2 years, disease-specific survival for all patients was 65%.[18] The stage of disease and the status of surgical margins had the most significant impact on survival. Regardless of the extent of surgery (partial maxillectomy, total maxillectomy, or craniofacial resection) or the use of adjuvant therapy, 5-year survival of patients with tumor-free surgical margins was 66%, compared with 28% in patients

TABLE 9-7 Factors Influencing Survival in Patients With Cancer of the Nasal Cavity and Paranasal Sinuses

Factor	5-Yr Actuarial Survival Rate
Histology	
Glandular carcinoma	79%
Adenocarcinoma	78%
Squamous cell carcinoma	60%
Undifferentiated carcinoma	40%
T Classification	
T1	91%
T2	64%
T3	72%
T4	49%
Site of Origin	
Nasal cavity	77%
Maxillary sinus	62%
Ethmoid sinus	48%
Treatment Modality	
Surgery only	79%
Radiation only	57%
Combined surgery and radiation	66%

From Dulguerov P, Jacobsen MS, Allal AS, et al: Nasal and paranasal sinus carcinoma: Are we making progress? A series of 220 patients and a systematic review. Cancer 92:3012–3029, 2001.

TABLE 9-8 Disease-Specific Survival of Patients Treated With Anterior Craniofacial Resection of Malignant Sinonasal Tumors Involving the Anterior Cranial Base

Study	Number of Patients	5-Year	10-Year
Shah et al 1997[171]	115	58%	48%
Lund et al 1998[172]	167	44%	32%
Bridger et al 2000[185]	73	69%	69%

with positive surgical margins. Similarly, the 5-year survival for patients with early-stage (T1–T2) disease was 80%, compared with 46% for advanced-stage (T3–T4) disease, regardless of histology, site of origin, and extent of resection. These data illustrate that earlier detection of sinonasal cancer is by far the best strategy for improving the outcomes of patients with cancer of the nasal cavity and paranasal sinuses.

Although patients with sinonasal cancer that extended to or invaded the cranial base were generally thought to have poor prognosis, recent improvements in cranial base surgery have changed the outcome of these patients. Several recent reports have demonstrated that combined craniofacial approaches for resection of malignant tumors of the anterior cranial base offer good local control of disease and acceptable survival rates, which are not significantly different from those of patients with sinonasal cancer in general (Table 9–8).

Tumor grade and histology, however, have a significant impact on disease control and survival in patients treated with craniofacial resection of anterior skull base malignancy. Sekhar and others have found that 64% of patients with low-grade malignancies and 44% of patients with high-grade lesions were alive with no evidence of disease at an average follow-up of 26 months after craniofacial resection.[181] Eibling and others performed a meta-analysis of the outcome of anterior cranial base resection and reported longer than 2-year survival in 64% of patients with SCC, compared with only 45% for those with undifferentiated carcinoma.[244] The lowest survival rate was observed in patients with mucosal melanoma, and the highest was seen in those with esthesioneuroblastoma.[171, 192]

In another study of patients who underwent anterior craniofacial resection, a statistically significant difference was noted between the 5-year disease-free survival for patients having esthesioneuroblastoma and those with tumors other than esthesioneuroblastoma (90% vs. 59%, $P = 0.028$), and aggressive salvage therapy appeared to be a more successful option in the patients with esthesioneuroblastoma.[245] Invasion of the dura, brain involvement, and positive resection margins, however, were significantly correlated with poorer prognosis, regardless of histology.[173, 192, 232]

Survival of patients undergoing craniofacial resection also depends on their functional status and the presence or absence of comorbidity. For example, in a study of 73 patients treated with craniofacial resection, Bridger and colleagues found that the 5-year *cancer-specific* survival was 69%, which was unchanged at 10 years.[185] By contrast, the *overall* survival at 5 and 10 years was 61% and 48%, respectively. This highlights the fact that a significant number of patients die of comorbidities not related to cancer.

SUMMARY

Progress in the prognosis of patients with nasal and paranasal carcinoma has been made during the past 40 years. This is probably due to advances in both the evaluation and treatment of these patients. Office endoscopy and high-resolution imaging allow better assessment of the extent of disease and hence better treatment planning. Advances in cranial base surgery and microvascular reconstruction have allowed more adequate resection of advanced sinonasal cancer, even if it involves the cranial base. Improvements in the delivery of radiation therapy using 3D-CRT and IMRT have allowed more targeted and homogenous dosimetry to the tumor with sparing of nearby critical structures. The integration of more effective chemotherapeutic agents in the overall management of patients with sinonasal cancer has improved local control of the disease.

Despite these improvements, cancer of the paranasal sinuses remains a difficult and challenging problem. A vast majority of patients still present with advanced-stage disease, and the paucity and nonspecific nature of their signs and symptoms from smaller tumors hamper early diagnosis of the disease. The propensity for early spread to surrounding critical structures, such as the cranial base, orbit, and brain, increases the complexity and morbidity of treatment while reducing its efficacy. These factors continue to impede further improvement of treatment outcome, and a significant number of patients still die from the disease. Therefore, the most effective strategy for further improving the treatment outcome of patients with cancer of the nasal cavity and paranasal sinuses is earlier detection of disease.

REFERENCES

1. Dulguerov P, Jacobsen MS, Allal AS, et al: Nasal and paranasal sinus carcinoma: Are we making progress? A series of 220 patients and a systematic review. Cancer 92:3012–3029, 2001.
2. Anderhuber W, Walch C, Fock C: [Configuration of ethmoid roof in children 0–14 years of age.] [German.] Laryngorhinootologie 80:509–511, 2001.
3. Lateral nasal wall and sinus surgical anatomy: Contemporary understanding. In Gluckman JL (ed): Renewal of Certification Study Guide in Otolaryngology—Head and Neck Surgery. Nose and Paranasal Sinuses. Alexandria, Va, American Academy of Otolaryngology—Head and Neck Surgery, 1998, pp 171–181.
4. Sunderman FW Jr: Nasal toxicity, carcinogenicity, and olfactory uptake of metals. Ann Clin Lab Sci 31:3–24, 2001.
5. Hernberg S, Westerholm P, Schultz-Larsen K, et al: Nasal and sinonasal cancer. Connection with occupational exposures in Denmark, Finland and Sweden. Scand J Work Environ Health 9:315–326, 1983.
6. Selden AI, Westberg HB, Axelson O: Cancer morbidity in workers at aluminum foundries and secondary aluminum smelters. Am J Ind Med 32:467–477, 1997.
7. Mannetje A, Kogevinas M, Luce D, et al: Sinonasal cancer, occupation, and tobacco smoking in European women and men. Am J Ind Med 36:101–107, 1999.
8. Gordon I, Boffetta P, Demers PA: A case study comparing a meta-analysis and a pooled analysis of studies of sinonasal cancer among wood workers. Epidemiology 9:518–524, 1998.
9. Stoll D, Bebear JP, Truilhe Y, et al: [Ethmoid adenocarcinomas: Retrospective study of 76 patients.] [French.] Rev Laryngol Otol Rhinol 122:21–29, 2002.
10. Demers PA, Kogevinas M, Boffetta P, et al: Wood dust and sino-nasal cancer: Pooled reanalysis of twelve case-control studies. Am J Ind Med 28:151–166, 1995.
11. Ward EM, Burnett CA, Ruder A, et al: Industries and cancer. Cancer Causes Control 8:356–370, 1997.
12. Luce D, Gerin M, Morcet JF, et al: Sinonasal cancer and occupational exposure to textile dust. Am J Ind Med 32:205–210, 1997.
13. Calderon-Garciduenas L, Delgado R, Calderon-Garciduenas A, et al: Malignant neoplasms of the nasal cavity and paranasal sinuses: A series of 256 patients in Mexico City and Monterrey. Is air pollution the missing link? Otolaryngol Head Neck Surg 122:499–508, 2000.
14. Benninger MS: The impact of cigarette smoking and environmental tobacco smoke on nasal and sinus disease: A review of the literature. Am J Rhinol 13:435–438, 1999.
15. Manuel J: Double exposure. Environmental tobacco smoke. Environ Health Perspect 107:A196–A201, 1999.
16. DeMonte F, Ginsberg LE, Clayman GL: Primary malignant tumors of the sphenoidal sinus. Neurosurgery 46:1084–1091, 2000.
17. Barnes L: Surgical Pathology of the Head and Neck, 2nd ed. New York, Marcel Dekker, 2001.
18. Hanna E, Vural E, Teo C, et al: Sinonasal tumors: The Arkansas experience. Skull Base Surg 8:15, 1998.
19. Waldron JN, O'Sullivan B, Gullane P, et al: Carcinoma of the maxillary antrum: A retrospective analysis of 110 cases. Radiother Oncol 57:167–173, 2000.
20. Osguthorpe JD, Richardson M: Frontal sinus malignancies. Otolaryngol Clin North Am 34:269–281, 2001.
21. Kraft M, Simmen D, Casas R, et al: Significance of human papillomavirus in sinonasal papillomas. J Laryngol Otol 115:709–714, 2001.
22. Buchwald C, Lindeberg H, Pedersen BL, et al: Human papilloma virus and p53 expression in carcinomas associated with sinonasal papillomas: A Danish epidemiological study 1980–1998. Laryngoscope 111: 1104–1110, 2001.
23. Batsakis JG, Suarez P: Schneiderian papillomas and carcinomas: A review. Adv Anat Pathol 8:53–64, 2001.
24. Seshul MJ, Eby TL, Crowe DR, et al: Nasal inverted papilloma with involvement of middle ear and mastoid. Arch Otolaryngol Head Neck Surg 121:1045–1048, 1995.
25. Shohet JA, Duncavage JA: Management of the frontal sinus with inverted papilloma. Otolaryngol Head Neck Surg 114:649–652, 1996.
26. Vural E, Suen JY, Hanna E: Intracranial extension of inverted papilloma: An unusual and potentially fatal complication. Head Neck 21:703–706, 1999.
27. Yiotakis I, Psarommatis I, Manolopoulos L, et al: Isolated inverted papilloma of the sphenoid sinus. J Laryngol Otol 115:227–230, 2001.
28. Elner VM, Burnstine MA, Goodman ML, et al: Inverted papillomas that invade the orbit. Arch Ophthalmol 113:1178–1183, 1995.
29. Lawson W, Ho BT, Shaari CM, et al: Inverted papilloma: A report of 112 cases. Laryngoscope 105:282–288, 1995.
30. Myers EN, Fernau JL, Johnson JT, et al: Management of inverted papilloma. Laryngoscope 100:481–490, 1990.
31. Sanderson RJ, Knegt P: Management of inverted papilloma via Denker's approach. Clin Otolaryngol Allied Sci 24:69–71, 1999.
32. Sukenik MA, Casiano R: Endoscopic medial maxillectomy for inverted papillomas of the paranasal sinuses: Value of the intraoperative endoscopic examination. Laryngoscope 110:39–42, 2000.
33. Lund VJ: Optimum management of inverted papilloma. J Laryngol Otol 114:194–197, 2000.
34. Bertrand B, Eloy P, Jorissen M, et al: Surgery of inverted papillomas under endoscopic control. Acta Otorhinolaryngol Belg 54:139–150, 2000.
35. Han JK, Smith TL, Loehrl T, et al: An evolution in the management of sinonasal inverting papilloma. Laryngoscope 111:1395–1400, 2001.
36. Dictor M, Johnson A: Association of inverted sinonasal papilloma with non-sinonasal head-and-neck carcinoma. Int J Cancer 85:811–814, 2000.
37. Krouse JH: Development of a staging system for inverted papilloma. Laryngoscope 110:965–968, 2000.

38. Tufano RP, Mokadam NA, Montone KT, et al: Malignant tumors of the nose and paranasal sinuses: Hospital of the University of Pennsylvania experience 1990–1997. Am J Rhinol 13:117–123, 1999.

39. Kida A, Endo S, Iida H, et al: Clinical assessment of squamous cell carcinoma of the nasal cavity proper. Auris Nasus Larynx 22:172–177, 1995.

40. Wieneke JA, Thompson LD, Wenig BM: Basaloid squamous cell carcinoma of the sinonasal tract. Cancer 85:841–854, 1999.

41. Ram B, Saleh HA, Baird AR, et al: Verrucous carcinoma of the maxillary antrum. [See comments.] J Laryngol Otol 112:399–402, 1998.

42. Hayashi T, Nonaka S, Bandoh N, et al: Treatment outcome of maxillary sinus squamous cell carcinoma. Cancer 92:1495–1503, 2001.

43. Tiwari R, Hardillo JA, Mehta D, et al: Squamous cell carcinoma of maxillary sinus. Head Neck 22:164–169, 2000.

44. Le QT, Fu KK, Kaplan MJ, et al: Lymph node metastasis in maxillary sinus cancer. Int J Radiat Oncol Biol Phys 46:541–549, 2000.

45. Kim GE, Chung EJ, Lim JJ, et al: Clinical significance of neck node metastasis in squamous cell carcinoma of the maxillary antrum. Am J Otolaryngol 20:383–390, 1999.

46. Ogawa K, Toita T, Kakinohana Y, et al: Postoperative radiotherapy for squamous cell carcinoma of the maxillary sinus: Analysis of local control and late complications. Oncol Rep 8:315–319, 2001.

47. Nishino H, Miyata M, Morita M, et al: Combined therapy with conservative surgery, radiotherapy, and regional chemotherapy for maxillary sinus carcinoma. Cancer 89:1925–1932, 2000.

48. Itami J, Uno T, Aruga M, et al: Squamous cell carcinoma of the maxillary sinus treated with radiation therapy and conservative surgery. Cancer 82:104–107, 1998.

49. Kawashima M, Ogino T, Hayashi R, et al: Influence of postsurgical residual tumor volume on local control in radiotherapy for maxillary sinus cancer. Jpn J Clin Oncol 31:195–202, 2001.

50. Levine PA, Frierson HF Jr, Stewart FM, et al: Sinonasal undifferentiated carcinoma: A distinctive and highly aggressive neoplasm. Laryngoscope 97:905–908, 1987.

51. Gorelick J, Ross D, Marentette L, et al: Sinonasal undifferentiated carcinoma: Case series and review of the literature. Neurosurgery 47:750–754, 2000.

52. Sharara N, Muller S, Olson J, et al: Sinonasal undifferentiated carcinoma with orbital invasion: Report of three cases. Ophthal Plast Reconstr Surg 17:288–292, 2001.

53. Cerilli LA, Holst VA, Brandwein MS, et al: Sinonasal undifferentiated carcinoma: Immunohistochemical profile and lack of EBV association. Am J Surg Pathol 25:156–163, 2001.

54. Houston GD, Gillies E: Sinonasal undifferentiated carcinoma: A distinctive clinicopathologic entity. Adv Anat Pathol 6:317–323, 1999.

55. Shinokuma A, Hirakawa N, Tamiya S, et al: Evaluation of Epstein-Barr virus infection in sinonasal small round cell tumors. J Cancer Res Clin Oncol 126:12–18, 2000.

56. Deutsch BD, Levine PA, Stewart FM, et al: Sinonasal undifferentiated carcinoma: A ray of hope. Otolaryngol Head Neck Surg 108:697–700, 1993.

57. Spiro JD, Soo KC, Spiro RH: Nonsquamous cell malignant neoplasms of the nasal cavities and paranasal sinuses. Head Neck 17:114–118, 1995.

58. Khan AJ, DiGiovanna MP, Ross DA, et al: Adenoid cystic carcinoma: A retrospective clinical review. Int J Cancer 96:149–158, 2001.

59. Chummun S, McLean NR, Kelly CG, et al: Adenoid cystic carcinoma of the head and neck. Br J Plast Surg 54:476–480, 2001.

60. Toyoshima K, Kimura S, Cheng J, et al: High-molecular-weight fibronectin synthesized by adenoid cystic carcinoma cells of salivary gland origin. Jpn J Cancer Res 90:308–319, 1999.

61. Kimura S, Cheng J, Toyoshima K, et al: Basement membrane heparan sulfate proteoglycan (perlecan) synthesized by ACC3, adenoid cystic carcinoma cells of human salivary gland origin. J Biochem 125:406–413, 1999.

62. Kimura S, Cheng J, Ida H, et al: Perlecan (heparan sulfate proteoglycan) gene expression reflected in the characteristic histological architecture of salivary adenoid cystic carcinoma. Virchows Arch 437:122–128, 2000.

63. Irie T, Cheng J, Kimura S, et al: Intracellular transport of basement membrane-type heparan sulphate proteoglycan in adenoid cystic carcinoma cells of salivary gland origin: An immunoelectron microscopic study. Virchows Arch 433:41–48, 1998.

64. Fordice J, Kershaw C, El-Naggar A, et al: Adenoid cystic carcinoma of the head and neck: Predictors of morbidity and mortality. Arch Otolaryngol Head Neck Surg 125:149–152, 1999.

65. Renehan AG, Gleave EN, Slevin NJ, et al: Clinico-pathological and treatment-related factors influencing survival in parotid cancer. Br J Cancer 80:1296–1300, 1999.

66. Therkildsen MH, Reibel J, Schiodt T: Observer variability in histological malignancy grading of adenoid cystic carcinomas. APMIS 105:559–565, 1997.

67. Kim GE, Park HC, Keum KC, et al: Adenoid cystic carcinoma of the maxillary antrum. Am J Otolaryngol 20:77–84, 1999.

68. Hutcheson JA, Vural E, Korourian S, et al: Neural cell adhesion molecule expression in adenoid cystic carcinoma of the head and neck. Laryngoscope 110:946–948, 2000.

69. Hanna E, Janecka IP: Perineural spread in head and neck and skull base cancer. Crit Rev Neurosurg 4:109–115, 1994.

70. Vural E, Hutcheson J, Korourian S, et al: Correlation of neural cell adhesion molecules with perineural spread of squamous cell carcinoma of the head and neck. Otolaryngology Head Neck Surg 122:717–720, 2000.

71. Iannetti G, Belli E, Marini Balestra F, et al: [Lymph node metastasis of adenoid cystic carcinoma.] Minerva Stomatol 50:85–89, 2001.

72. Jones AS, Hamilton JW, Rowley H, et al: Adenoid cystic carcinoma of the head and neck. Clin Otolaryngol Allied Sci 22:434–443, 1997.

73. Lopes MA, Santos GC, Kowalski LP: Multivariate survival analysis of 128 cases of oral cavity minor salivary gland carcinomas. Head Neck 20:699–706, 1998.

74. Le QT, Birdwell S, Terris DJ, et al: Postoperative irradiation of minor salivary gland malignancies of the head and neck. Radiother Oncol 52:165–171, 1999.

75. Anderson JN Jr, Beenken SW, Crowe R, et al: Prognostic factors in minor salivary gland cancer. Head Neck 17:480–486, 1995.

76. Spiro RH: Distant metastasis in adenoid cystic carcinoma of salivary origin. Am J Surg 174:495–498, 1997.

77. Naficy S, Disher MJ, Esclamado RM: Adenoid cystic carcinoma of the paranasal sinuses. Am J Rhinol 13:311–314, 1999.

78. Pitman KT, Prokopakis EP, Aydogan B, et al: The role of skull base surgery for the treatment of adenoid cystic carcinoma of the sinonasal tract. Head Neck 21:402–407, 1999.

79. Konno A, Ishikawa K, Numata T, et al: Analysis of factors affecting long-term treatment results of adenoid cystic carcinoma of the nose and paranasal sinuses. Acta Otolaryngol Suppl 537:67–74, 1998.

80. Prott FJ, Micke O, Haverkamp U, et al: Results of fast neutron therapy of adenoid cystic carcinoma of the salivary glands. Anticancer Res 20:3743–3749, 2000.

81. Huber PE, Debus J, Latz D, et al: Radiotherapy for advanced adenoid cystic carcinoma: Neutrons, photons or mixed beam? Radiother Oncol 59:161–167, 2001.

82. Buchholz TA, Laramore GE, Griffin BR, et al: The role of fast neutron radiation therapy in the management of advanced salivary gland malignant neoplasms. Cancer 69:2779–2788, 1992.

83. Hocwald E, Korkmaz H, Yoo GH, et al: Prognostic factors in major salivary gland cancer. Laryngoscope 111:1434–1439, 2001.

84. Airoldi M, Pedani F, Succo G, et al: Phase II randomized trial comparing vinorelbine versus vinorelbine plus cisplatin in patients with recurrent salivary gland malignancies. Cancer 91:541–547, 2001.

85. Airoldi M, Brando V, Giordano C, et al: Chemotherapy for recurrent salivary gland malignancies: Experience of the ENT Department of Turin University. J Otorhinolaryngol 56:105–111, 1994.

86. Airoldi M, Fornari G, Pedani F, et al: Paclitaxel and carboplatin for recurrent salivary gland malignancies. Anticancer Res 20:3781–3783, 2000.

87. Conley J, Casler J: Data and statistics. In Casler Ca (ed): Adenoid Cystic Cancer of the Head and Neck. New York, Thieme Medical Publishers, 1991, pp 21–25.

88. Prokopakis EP, Snyderman CH, Hanna EY, et al: Risk factors for local recurrence of adenoid cystic carcinoma: The role of postoperative radiation therapy. Am J Otolaryngol 20:281–286, 1999.

89. Westerveld GJ, van Diest PJ, van Nieuwkerk EB: Neuroendocrine carcinoma of the sphenoid sinus: A case report. Rhinology 39:52–54, 2001.

90. Gallo O, Franchi A, Fini-Storchi I, et al: Prognostic significance of c-erbB-2 oncoprotein expression in intestinal-type adenocarcinoma of the sinonasal tract. Head Neck 20:224–231, 1998.

91. Perez P, Dominguez O, Gonzalez S, et al: ras Gene mutations in ethmoid sinus adenocarcinoma: Prognostic implications. Cancer 86:255–264, 1999.

92. Knegt PP, Ah-See KW, vd Velden LA, et al: Adenocarcinoma of the ethmoidal sinus complex: Surgical debulking and topical fluorouracil may be the optimal treatment. Arch Otolaryngol Head Neck Surg 127:141–146, 2001.

93. Batsakis JG, Suarez P, El-Naggar AK: Mucosal melanomas of the head and neck. Ann Otol Rhinol Laryngol 107:626–630, 1998.

94. Regauer S, Anderhuber W, Richtig E, et al: Primary mucosal melanomas of the nasal cavity and paranasal sinuses. A clinicopathological analysis of 14 cases. APMIS 106:403–410, 1998.

95. Lund VJ, Howard DJ, Harding L, et al: Management options and survival in malignant melanoma of the sinonasal mucosa. Laryngoscope 109:208–211, 1999.

96. Girod D, Hanna E, Marentette L: Esthesioneuroblastoma. Head Neck 23:500–505, 2001.

97. Silva EG, Butler J, Mackay B, et al: Neuroblastomas and neuroendocrine carcinomas of the nasal cavity. Cancer 50:2388–2405, 1982.

98. Hyams VJ: Olfactory neuroblastoma (case 6). In Batsakis JG, Hyams VJ, Morales AR (eds): Special Tumors of the Head and Neck. Chicago, American Society of Clinical Pathologists Press, 1992, pp 24–29.

99. Kadish S, Goodman M, Wang CC: Olfactory neuroblastoma. A clinical analysis of 17 cases. Cancer 37:1571–1576, 1976.

100. Foote RL, Morita A, Ebersold MJ, et al: Esthesioneuroblastoma: The role of radiation therapy. Int J Radiat Oncol Biol Phys 27:835–842, 1993.

101. Dulguerov P, Calcaterra T: Esthesioneuroblastoma: The UCLA experience 1970–1990. Laryngoscope 102:843–849, 1992.

102. Walch C, Stammberger H, Unger F, et al: [A new therapy concept in esthesioneuroblastoma.] [German.] Laryngorhinootologie 79:743–748, 2000.

103. Biller HF, Lawson W, Sachdev VP, et al: Esthesioneuroblastoma: Surgical treatment without radiation. Laryngoscope 100:1199–1201, 1990.

104. Levine PA, McLean WC, Cantrell RW: Esthesioneuroblastoma: The University of Virginia experience 1960–1985. Laryngoscope 96:742–746, 1986.

105. McElroy EA Jr, Buckner JC, Lewis JE: Chemotherapy for advanced esthesioneuroblastoma: The Mayo Clinic experience. Neurosurgery 42:1023–1027, 1998.

106. Callender TA, Weber RS, Janjan N, et al: Rhabdomyosarcoma of the nose and paranasal sinuses in adults and children. Otolaryngol Head Neck Surg 112:252–257, 1995.

107. Raney RB, Tefft M, Newton WA, et al: Improved prognosis with intensive treatment of children with cranial soft tissue sarcomas arising in nonorbital parameningeal sites. A report from the Intergroup Rhabdomyosarcoma Study. Cancer 59:147–155, 1987.

108. Gadwal SR, Fanburg-Smith JC, Gannon FH, et al: Primary chondrosarcoma of the head and neck in pediatric patients: A clinicopathologic study of 14 cases with a review of the literature. Cancer 88:2181–2188, 2000.

109. Galera-Ruiz H, Sanchez-Calzado JA, Rios-Martin JJ, et al: Sinonasal radiation-associated osteosarcoma after combined therapy for rhabdomyosarcoma of the nose. Auris Nasus Larynx 28:261–264, 2001.

110. Loughran S, Badia L, Lund V: Primary chordoma of the ethmoid sinus. J Laryngol Otol 114:627–629, 2000.

111. Fischbein NJ, Kaplan MJ, Holliday RA, et al: Recurrence of clival chordoma along the surgical pathway. AJNR Am J Neuroradiol 21:578–583, 2000.

112. Mardinger O, Givol N, Talmi YP, et al: Osteosarcoma of the jaw. The Chaim Sheba Medical Center experience. Oral Surg Oral Med Oral Pathol Oral Radiol Endod 91:445–451, 2001.

113. Laramore GE, Griffith JT, Boespflug M, et al: Fast neutron radiotherapy for sarcomas of soft tissue, bone, and cartilage. Am J Clin Oncol 12:320–326, 1989.

114. Gnepp DR, Henley J, Weiss S, et al: Desmoid fibromatosis of the sinonasal tract and nasopharynx. A clinicopathologic study of 25 cases. Cancer 78:2572–2579, 1996.

115. Olekszyk J, Siliunas V, Mauer T, et al: Fibrosarcoma of the nose and the paranasal sinuses. J Am Osteopath Assoc 89:901–904, 1989.

116. Wong KF, So CC, Wong N, et al: Sinonasal angiosarcoma with marrow involvement at presentation mimicking malignant lymphoma: Cytogenetic analysis using multiple techniques. Cancer Genet Cytogenet 129:64–68, 2001.

117. Haferkamp C, Pressler H, Koitschev A: [Angiosarcoma of the frontal sinus. Case report and review of the literature.] [German.] HNO 48:684–688, 2000.

118. Panje WR, Moran WJ, Bostwick DG, et al: Angiosarcoma of the head and neck: Review of 11 cases. Laryngoscope 96:1381–1384, 1986.

119. Bankaci M, Myers EN, Barnes L, et al: Angiosarcoma of the maxillary sinus: Literature review and case report. Head Neck Surg 1:274–280, 1979.

120. Herve S, Abd Alsamad I, Beautru R, et al: Management of sinonasal hemangiopericytomas. Rhinology 37:153–158, 1999.

121. Abdel-Fattah HM, Adams GL, Wick MR: Hemangiopericytoma of the maxillary sinus and skull base. Head Neck 12:77–83, 1990.

122. Gotte K, Hormann K, Schmoll J, et al: Congenital nasal hemangiopericytoma: Intrauterine, intraoperative, and histologic findings. Ann Otol Rhinol Laryngol 108:589–593, 1999.

123. Hanna E, Wanamaker J, Adelstein D, et al: Extranodal lymphomas of the head and neck. A 20-year experience. Arch Otolaryngol Head Neck Surg 123:1318–1323, 1997.

124. Hatta C, Ogasawara H, Okita J, et al: Non-Hodgkin's malignant lymphoma of the sinonasal tract—treatment outcome for 53 patients according to REAL classification. Auris Nasus Larynx 28:55–60, 2001.

125. Rodriguez J, Romaguera JE, Manning J, et al: Nasal-type T/NK lymphomas: A clinicopathologic study of 13 cases. Leuk Lymphoma 39:139–144, 2000.

126. Gaal K, Sun NC, Hernandez AM, et al: Sinonasal NK/T-cell lymphomas in the United States. Am J Surg Pathol 24:1511–1517, 2000.

127. Hongyo T, Li T, Syaifudin M, et al: Specific c-kit mutations in sinonasal natural killer/T-cell lymphoma in China and Japan. Cancer Res 60:2345–2347, 2000.

128. Vidal RW, Devaney K, Ferlito A, et al: Sinonasal malignant lymphomas: A distinct clinicopathological category. Ann Otol Rhinol Laryngol 108:411–419, 1999.

129. Thompson LD, Gyure KA: Extracranial sinonasal tract meningiomas: A clinicopathologic study of 30 cases with a review of the literature. Am J Surg Pathol 24:640–650, 2000.

130. Kleinjung T, Held P: [Metastasis in the frontal skull base from hepatocellular carcinoma.] [German.] HNO 49:126–129, 2001.

131. Jimenez OV, Lazarich VA, Davila MA, et al: [Frontal ethmoid metastases of prostatic carcinoma. Report of one case and review of the literature.] [Spanish.] Acta Otorrinolaringol Esp 52:151–154, 2001.

132. Simo R, Sykes AJ, Hargreaves SP, et al: Metastatic renal cell carcinoma to the nose and paranasal sinuses. Head Neck 22:722–727, 2000.

133. Wilson ME, Buckley EG, Kivlin JD, et al: Pediatric Ophthalmology and Strabismus, Section 6. San Francisco, Calif, The Foundation of the American Academy of Ophthalmology, 2001, p 325.

134. Padula GD, McCormick B, Abramson DH, et al: Brain necrosis after enucleation, external beam cobalt radiotherapy, and systemic chemotherapy for retinoblastoma. Arch Ophthalmol 120:98–99, 2002.

135. Abramson DH, Frank CM: Second nonocular tumors in survivors of bilateral retinoblastoma: A possible age effect on radiation-related risk. Ophthalmology 105:573–579; discussion 579–580, 1998.

136. Kodsi SR, Shetlar DJ, Campbell RJ, et al: A review of 340 orbital tumors in children during a 60-year period. Am J Ophthalmol 117:177–182, 1994.

137. Kersten RC, Bartley GB, Nerad JA, et al: Orbit, Eyelids, and Lacrimal System. San Francisco, Calif, The Foundation of the American Academy of Ophthalmology, 2001.

138. Crist WM, Anerson JR, Meza JL, et al: Intergroup rhabdomyosarcoma study-IV: Results for patients with nonmetastatic disease. J Clin Oncol 19:3091–3102, 2002.

139. Stockl FA, Dolmetsch AM, Saornil MA, et al: Orbital granulocytic sarcoma. Br J Ophthalmol 81:1084–1088, 1997.

140. Brock WD, Brown HH, Westfall CT: Extramedullary myeloid cell tumor in an elderly man. Arch Ophthalmol 119:1861–1864, 2001.

141. Leonardy NJ, Rupani M, Dent G, et al: Analysis of 135 autopsy eyes for ocular involvement in leukemia. Am J Ophthalmol 109:436–444, 1990.

142. Demirci H, Shields CL, Shields JA, et al: Orbital tumors in the older adult population. Ophthalmology 109:243–248, 2002.

143. Margo CE, Mulla ZD: Malignant tumors of the orbit. Analysis of the Florida Cancer Registry. Ophthalmology 105:185–190, 1998.

144. Shields JA, Shields CL, Eagle RC Jr, et al: Adenoid cystic carcinoma of the lacrimal gland simulating a dermoid cyst in a 9-year-old boy. Arch Ophthalmol 116:1673–1676, 1998.

145. Dithmar S, Wojno TH, Washington C, et al: Mucoepidermoid carcinoma of an accessory lacrimal gland with orbital invasion. Ophthal Plast Reconstr Surg 16:162–166, 2000.

146. Stefanyszyn MA, Hidayat AA, Pe'er JJ, et al: Lacrimal sac tumors. Ophthal Plast Reconstr Surg 10:169–184, 1994.

147. Rootman J: Diseases of the Orbit. Philadelphia, JB Lippincott, 1998.

148. Ezra E, Mannor G, Wright JE, et al: Inadequately irradiated solitary extramedullary plasmacytoma of the orbit requiring exenteration. Am J Ophthalmol 120:803–805, 1995.

149. Devos A, Lemmerling M, Vanrietvelde F, et al: Leptomeningeal metastases from ethmoid sinus adenocarcinoma: Clinico-radiological correlation. JBR-BTR Org Soc Roy Belg Radiol 82:285–287, 1999.

150. Lund VJ: Distant metastases from sinonasal cancer. J Otorhinolaryngol 63:212–213, 2001.

151. Ohngren LG: Malignant tumors of the maxillo-ethmoidal region. Acta Otolaryngol 19:476, 1933.

152. Sisson GA, Johnson NE, Amir CS: Cancer of the maxillary sinus: Clinical classification and management. Ann Otol Rhinol Laryngol 72:1050–1059, 1963.

153. Lederman M: Tumours of the upper jaw: Natural history and treatment. J Laryngol Otol 84:369–401, 1970.

154. Rubin P: Cancer of the head and neck: Nose, paranasal sinuses. J Am Med Assoc 219:336–338, 1972.

155. Harrison DF: Critical look at the classification of maxillary sinus carcinomata. Ann Otol Rhinol Laryngol 87:3–9, 1978.

156. Ellingwood KE, Million RR: Cancer of the nasal cavity and ethmoid/sphenoid sinuses. Cancer 43:1517–1526, 1979.

157. Paranasal sinuses. In Fleming ID, Cooper JS, Earl Henson D, et al (eds): Amercian Joint Committee on Cancer (AJCC): Manual for Staging Cancer, 5th ed. Philadelphia, Lippincott-Raven, 1997, pp 47–52.

158. Le QT, Fu KK, Kaplan M, et al: Treatment of maxillary sinus carcinoma: A comparison of the 1997 and 1977 American Joint Committee on cancer staging systems. Cancer 86:1700–1711, 1999.

159. Srinivasan S, Fern AI, Wilson K: Orbital apex syndrome as a presenting sign of maxillary sinus carcinoma. Eye 15:343–345, 2001.

160. Lloyd G, Lund VJ, Howard D, et al: Optimum imaging for sinonasal malignancy. J Laryngol Otol 114:557–562, 2000.

161. Curtin HD, Rabinov JD: Extension to the orbit from paraorbital disease. The sinuses. Radiol Clin North Am 36:1201–1213, 1998.

162. Elolf E, Tatagiba M, Samii M: Three-dimensional computed tomographic reconstruction: Planning tool for surgery of skull base pathologies. Comput Aid Surg 3:89–94, 1998.

163. Sievers KW, Greess H, Baum U, et al: Paranasal sinuses and nasopharynx CT and MRI. Eur J Radiol 33:185–202, 2000.

164. Damilakis J, Prassopoulos P, Mazonakis M, et al: Tailored low dose three-dimensional CT of paranasal sinuses. Clin Imaging 22:235–239, 1998.

165. Lehnerdt G, Weber J, Dost P: [Unilateral opacification of the paranasal sinuses in CT or MRI: An indication of an uncommon histological finding.] [German.] Laryngorhinootologie 80:141–145, 2001.

166. Kubal WS: Sinonasal imaging: Malignant disease. Semin Ultrasound CT MR 20:402–425, 1999.

167. Chan LL, Chong J, Gillenwater AM, et al: The pterygopalatine fossa: Postoperative MR imaging appearance. AJNR Am J Neuroradiol 21:1315–1319, 2000.

168. Lund VJ, Lloyd GA, Howard DJ, et al: Enhanced magnetic resonance imaging and subtraction techniques in postoperative evaluation of craniofacial resection for sinonasal malignancy. Laryngoscope 106:553–558, 1996.

169. Harris GJ, Logani SC: Eyelid crease incision for lateral orbitotomy. Ophthal Plast Reconstr Surg 15:9–16; discussion 16–18, 1999.

170. Yucel T, Cinar C, Aydin Y, et al: Malignant tumors requiring maxillectomy. J Craniofac Surg 11:418–429, 2000.

171. Shah JP, Kraus DH, Bilsky MH, et al: Craniofacial resection for malignant tumors involving the anterior skull base. Arch Otolaryngol Head Neck Surg 123:1312–1317, 1997.

172. Lund VJ, Howard DJ, Wei WI, et al: Craniofacial resection for tumors of the nasal cavity and paranasal sinuses—a 17-year experience. Head Neck 20:97–105, 1998.

173. Rutter MJ, Furneaux CE, Morton RP: Craniofacial resection of anterior skull base tumours: Factors contributing to success. ANZ J Surg 68:350–353, 1998.

174. Goffart Y, Jorissen M, Daele J, et al: Minimally invasive endoscopic management of malignant sinonasal tumours. Acta Otorhinolaryngol Belg 54:221–232, 2000.

175. Stammberger H, Anderhuber W, Walch C, et al: Possibilities and limitations of endoscopic management of nasal and paranasal sinus malignancies. Acta Otorhinolaryngol Belg 53:199–205, 1999.

176. Thaler ER, Kotapka M, Lanza DC, et al: Endoscopically assisted anterior cranial skull base resection of sinonasal tumors. Am J Rhinol 13:303–310, 1999.

177. Rice DH: Endonasal approaches for sinonasal and nasopharyngeal tumors. Otolaryngol Clin North Am 34:1087–1093, 2001.

178. Vural E, Hanna E: Extended lateral rhinotomy incision for total maxillectomy. Otolaryngol Head Neck Surg 123:512–513, 2000.

179. Howard DJ, Lund VJ: The role of midfacial degloving in modern rhinological practice. J Laryngol Otol 113:885–887, 1999.

180. Browne JD: The midfacial degloving procedure for nasal, sinus, and nasopharyngeal tumors. Otolaryngol Clin North Am 34:1095–1104, 2001.

181. Sekhar LN, Nanda A, Sen CN, et al: The extended frontal approach to tumors of the anterior, middle, and posterior skull base. J Neurosurg 76:198–206, 1992.

182. Raveh J, Laedrach K, Speiser M, et al: The subcranial approach for fronto-orbital and anteroposterior skull-base tumors. Arch Otolaryngol Head Neck Surg 119:385–393, 1993.

183. Butler CE: Skin grafts used in combination with free flaps for intraoral oncological reconstruction. Ann Plast Surg 47:293–298, 2001.

184. Osguthorpe JD, Patel S: Craniofacial approaches to tumors of the anterior skull base. Otolaryngol Clin North Am 34:1123–1142, 2001.

185. Bridger GP, Kwok B, Baldwin M, et al: Craniofacial resection for paranasal sinus cancers. Head Neck 22:772–780, 2000.

186. Hao SP, Chang CN, Hsu YS, et al: Craniofacial resection for tumors of the nasal cavity and paranasal sinuses. J Formos Med Assoc 99:914–919, 2000.

187. Fukuda K, Saeki N, Mine S, et al: Evaluation of outcome and QOL in patients with craniofacial resection for malignant tumors involving the anterior skull base. Neurol Res 22:545–550, 2000.

188. Girod D, Hanna E, Marentette L: Esthesioneuroblastoma. Head Neck 23:500–505, 2001.

189. Cantu G, Solero CL, Mariani L, et al: Anterior craniofacial resection for malignant ethmoid tumors—a series of 91 patients. Head Neck 21:185–191, 1999.

190. Solero CL, DiMeco F, Sampath P, et al: Combined anterior craniofacial resection for tumors involving the form plate: Early postoperative complications and technical considerations. Neurosurgery 47:1296–1304, 2000.

191. Salvan D, Julieron M, Marandas P, et al: Combined transfacial and neurosurgical approach to malignant tumours of the ethmoid sinus. J Laryngol Otol 112:446–450, 1998.

192. Bilsky MH, Kraus DH, Strong EW, et al: Extended anterior craniofacial resection for intracranial extension of malignant tumors. Am J Surg 174:565–568, 1997.

193. Snyderman CH, Janecka IP, Sekhar LN, et al: Anterior cranial base reconstruction: Role of galeal and pericranial flaps. Laryngoscope 100:607–614, 1990.

194. Cantu G, Solero CL, Pizzi N, et al: Skull base reconstruction after anterior craniofacial resection. J Craniomaxillofac Surg 27:228–234, 1999.

195. Atabey A, Vayvada H, Menderes A, et al: A combined reverse temporalis muscle flap and pericranial flap for reconstruction of an anterior cranial base defect: A case report. Ann Plast Surg 39:190–192, 1997.

196. Hochman M: Reconstruction of midfacial and anterior skull-base defects. Otolaryngol Clin North Am 28:1269–1277, 1995.

197. Carrau RL, Segas J, Nuss DW, et al: Squamous cell carcinoma of the sinonasal tract invading the orbit. Laryngoscope 109:230–235, 1999.

198. Tiwari R, van der Wal J, van der Waal I, et al: Studies of the anatomy and pathology of the orbit in carcinoma of the maxillary sinus and their impact on preservation of the eye in maxillectomy. Head Neck 20:193–196, 1998.

199. Perry C, Levine PA, Williamson BR, et al: Preservation of the eye in paranasal sinus cancer surgery. Arch Otolaryngol Head Neck Surg 114:632–634, 1988.

200. Larson DL, Christ JE, Jesse RH: Preservation of the orbital contents in cancer of the maxillary sinus. Arch Otolaryngol 108:370–372, 1982.

201. Mouriaux F, Martinot V, Pellerin P, et al: Survival after malignant tumors of the orbit and periorbit treated by exenteration. Acta Ophthalmol Scand 77:326–330, 1999.

202. Sisson GA, Toriumi DM, Atiyah RA: Paranasal sinus malignancy: A comprehensive update. Laryngoscope 99:143–150, 1989.

203. Jiang GL, Ang KK, Peters LJ, et al: Maxillary sinus carcinomas: Natural history and results of postoperative radiotherapy. Radiother Oncol 21:193–200, 1991.

204. Stern SJ, Goepfert H, Clayman G, et al: Orbital preservation in maxillectomy. Otolaryngol Head Neck Surg 109:111–115, 1993.

205. Adams EJ, Nutting CM, Convery DJ, et al: Potential role of intensity-modulated radiotherapy in the treatment of tumors of the maxillary sinus. Int J Radiat Oncol Biol Phys 51:579–588, 2001.

206. Dexter WS, Jacob RF: Prosthetic rehabilitation after maxillectomy and temporalis flap reconstruction: A clinical report. J Prosthet Dent 83:283–286, 2000.

207. Pigno MA, Funk JJ: Augmentation of obturator retention by extension into the nasal aperture: A clinical report. J Prosthet Dent 85:349–351, 2001.

208. Dumbrigue HB, Arcuri MR, Funk GF, et al: Impression technique for nonosseous free-tissue transfer reconstruction after cranioorbito-maxillary resection: A clinical report. J Prosthet Dent 76:4–7, 1996.

209. Freije JE, Campbell BH, Yousif NJ, et al: Reconstruction after infrastructure maxillectomy using dual free flaps. Laryngoscope 107:694–697, 1997.

210. Davison SP, Sherris DA, Meland NB: An algorithm for maxillectomy defect reconstruction. Laryngoscope 108:215–219, 1998.

211. Hasegawa M, Torii S, Fukuta K, et al: Reconstruction of the anterior cranial base with the galeal frontalis myofascial flap and the vascularized outer table calvarial bone graft. Neurosurgery 36:725–729, 1995.

212. Nakajima T, Yoshimura Y, Nakanishi Y, et al: Anterior cranial base reconstruction using a hydroxyapatite-tricalciumphosphate composite (Ceratite) as a bone substitute. J Craniomaxillofac Surg 23:64–67, 1995.

213. Yamamoto Y, Minakawa H, Kawashima K, et al: Role of buttress reconstruction in zygomaticomaxillary skeletal defects. Plast Reconstr Surg 101:943–950, 1998.

214. Pollice PA, Frodel JL Jr: Secondary reconstruction of upper midface and orbit after total maxillectomy. Arch Otolaryngol Head Neck Surg 124:802–808, 1998.

215. Kessler P, Hardt N: The use of micro-titanium mesh for maxillary sinus wall reconstruction. J Craniomaxillofac Surg 24:317–321, 1996.

216. Roux FX, Brasnu D, Menard M, et al: Madreporic coral for cranial base reconstruction. 8 years experience. Acta Neurochir 133:201–205, 1995.

217. Bozza F, Tauro F, Ruscito P, et al: The osteo-chondro-mucous flap of the nasal septum in orbital reconstruction. J Exp Clin Cancer Res 19:401–403, 2000.

218. Kyutoku S, Tsuji H, Inoue T, et al: Experience with the rectus abdominis myocutaneous flap with vascularized hard tissue for immediate orbitofacial reconstruction. Plast Reconstr Surg 103:395–402, 1999.

219. Jeremic B, Shibamoto Y, Milicic B, et al: Elective ipsilateral neck irradiation of patients with locally advanced maxillary sinus carcinoma. Cancer 88:2246–2251, 2000.

220. Dias FL, Sa GM, Kligerman J, et al: Complications of anterior craniofacial resection. Head Neck 21:12–20, 1999.

221. Catalano PJ, Hecht CS, Biller HF, et al: Craniofacial resection. An analysis of 73 cases. Arch Otolaryngol Head Neck Surg 120:1203–1208, 1994.

222. Schick B, Ibing R, Brors D, et al: Long-term study of endonasal duraplasty and review of the literature. Ann Otol Rhinol Laryngol 110:142–147, 2001.

223. Yates H, Hamill M, Borel CO, et al: Incidence and perioperative management of tension pneumocephalus following craniofacial resection. J Neurosurg Anesthesiol 6:15–20, 1994.

224. Andersen PE, Kraus DH, Arbit E, et al: Management of the orbit during anterior fossa craniofacial resection. Arch Otolaryngol Head Neck Surg 122:1305–1307, 1996.

225. Waldron JN, O'Sullivan B, Warde P, et al: Ethmoid sinus cancer: Twenty-nine cases managed with primary radiation therapy. Int J Radiat Oncol Biol Phys 41:361–369, 1998.

226. Konno A, Ishikawa K, Terada N, et al: Analysis of long-term results of our combination therapy for squamous cell cancer of the maxillary sinus. Acta Otolaryngol Suppl 537:57–66, 1998.

227. Lee MM, Vokes EE, Rosen A, et al: Multimodality therapy in advanced paranasal sinus carcinoma: Superior long-term results. Cancer J Sci Am 5:219–223, 1999.

228. Jansen EP, Keus RB, Hilgers FJ, et al: Does the combination of radiotherapy and debulking surgery favor survival in paranasal sinus carcinoma? Int J Radiat Oncol Biol Phys 48:27–35, 2000.

229. Paulino AC, Marks JE, Bricker P, et al: Results of treatment of patients with maxillary sinus carcinoma. Cancer 83:457–465, 1998.

230. Stavrianos SD, Camilleri IG, McLean NR, et al: Malignant tumours of the maxillary complex: An 18-year review. Br J Plast Surg 51:584–588, 1998.

231. Curran AJ, Gullane PJ, Waldron J, et al: Surgical salvage after failed radiation for paranasal sinus malignancy. Laryngoscope 108:1618–1622, 1998.

232. Jiang GL, Morrison WH, Garden AS, et al: Ethmoid sinus carcinomas: Natural history and treatment results. Radiother Oncol 49:21–27, 1998.

233. Claus F, De Gersem W, De Wagter C, et al: An implementation strategy for IMRT of ethmoid sinus cancer with bilateral sparing of the optic pathways. Int J Radiat Oncol Biol Phys 51:318–331, 2001.

234. Pommier P, Ginestet C, Sunyach M, et al: Conformal radiotherapy for paranasal sinus and nasal cavity tumors: Three-dimensional treatment planning and preliminary results in 40 patients. Int J Radiat Oncol Biol Phys 48:485–493, 2000.

235. Brizel DM, Light K, Zhou SM, et al: Conformal radiation therapy treatment planning reduces the dose to the optic structures for patients with tumors of the paranasal sinuses. [See comments.] Radiother Oncol 51:215–218, 1999.

236. De Gersem W, Claus F, De Wagter C, et al: Leaf position optimization for step-and-shoot IMRT. Int J Radiat Oncol Biol Phys 51:1371–1388, 2001.

237. De Gersem W, Claus F, De Wagter C, et al: An anatomy-based beam segmentation tool for intensity-modulated radiation therapy and its application to head-and-neck cancer. Int J Radiat Oncol Biol Phys 51:849–859, 2001.

238. Kremer B, Klimek L, Andreopoulos D, et al: A new method for the placement of brachytherapy probes in paranasal sinus and nasopharynx neoplasms. Int J Radiat Oncol Biol Phys 43:995–1000, 1999.

239. Nag S, Cano ER, Demanes DJ, et al: The American Brachytherapy Society recommendations for high-dose-rate brachytherapy for head-and-neck carcinoma. Int J Radiat Oncol Biol Phys 50:1190–1198, 2001.

240. Diaz EM Jr, Kies MS: Chemotherapy for skull base cancers. Otolaryngol Clin North Am 34:1079–1085, 2001.

241. Fujii M, Ohno Y, Tokumaru Y, et al: Adjuvant chemotherapy with oral tegaful and uracil for maxillary sinus carcinoma. Oncology 55:109–115, 1998.

242. Fujii M, Ohno Y, Tokumaru Y, et al: UFT plus carboplatin for head and neck cancer. Oncology (Huntington) 14:72–75, 2000.

243. Kim GE, Chang SK, Lee SW, et al: Neoadjuvant chemotherapy and radiation for inoperable carcinoma of the maxillary antrum: A matched-control study. Am J Clin Oncol 23:301–308, 2000.

244. Eibling DE, Janecka IP, Snyderman CH, et al: Meta-analysis of outcome in anterior skull base resection for squamous cell and undifferentiated carcinoma. Skull Base Surg 3:123–129, 1993.

245. Levine PA, Debo RF, Meredith SD, et al: Craniofacial resection at the University of Virginia (1976–1992): Survival analysis. Head Neck 16:574–577, 1994.

CHAPTER 10

Surgery of the Anterior and Lateral Skull Base

Ricardo L. Carrau
Carl H. Snyderman
Daniel W. Nuss

◐ INTRODUCTION

Until the 1960s, invasion of the cranial base by upper aerodigestive tract neoplasms was considered a contraindication for surgery and patients were deemed incurable. During the 1960s, several reports advocated the use of anterior cranial base resection; thus, sinonasal tumors invading the anterior skull base, but not invading the pterygopalatine fossa or the cranial cavity, were considered adequate indications for surgery. The survival rate of this patient population was approximately 50% at 24 months of follow-up.[1] However, the morbidity and mortality associated with these procedures were extremely high, with a large percentage of patients suffering major complications such as cerebrospinal fluid (CSF) leak, stroke, wound infection with loss of the craniofacial skeleton, or death.

During the 1970s and 1980s, advances in imaging (including computed tomography [CT] and magnetic resonance imaging [MRI]), advances in interventional radiology, and the development of craniofacial disassembly techniques and free-flap reconstructions facilitated the expansion of indications for skull base surgery. Patients with tumors invading the cranial cavity, pterygopalatine fossa, and infratemporal fossa were considered candidates for surgical extirpation. During this time period, the 3-year survival rate ranged from 55% to 60%, and the frequency and severity of complications decreased considerably.

In the 1990s, further refinements in surgical approaches, a better understanding of anatomy, and the development of novel technologies, such as intraoperative navigational devices and endoscopic techniques, decreased the cosmetic and functional morbidity associated with these procedures. The importance of the development of multidisciplinary teams could not be overstated. The organization of teams that include head and neck surgeons, neurosurgeons, head and neck radiologists, neuroradiologists, interventional radiologists, pathologists, and prosthodontic and rehabilitation experts has led to a better oncologic and functional outcome for patients who undergo cranial base surgery. Refinements in adjunctive therapy have also added to the improvements in results. Advances in radiotherapy, including proton therapy, neutron therapy, intensity-modulated radiation therapy (IMRT), and stereotactic radiosurgery, are important adjuncts for the curative therapy of patients with malignant tumors of the skull base and/or for the palliative treatment of inoperable patients; these advanced approaches have a reduced incidence of complications as compared with conventional radiation therapy.[1]

◐ ANATOMY

Anterior Cranial Base

The anterior cranial fossa comprises the frontal, ethmoid, and sphenoid bones.[2] Laterally the floor of the anterior cranial cavity corresponds to the roof of the orbits, and centrally it corresponds to the vault of the nasal cavity and the fovea ethmoidalis. The floor of the anterior cranial cavity is concave, with the medial or central area (i.e., cribriform plate) located at a lower level than the lateral area. A slant from anterior (higher) to posterior (lower) is also noted.

At the central region of the anterior skull base, the most prominent structure is the cribriform plate, which contains multiple foramina, through which the branches of the olfactory nerve pass into the nasal cavity. Branches of the anterior ethmoid artery penetrate the vertical lamina of the cribriform plate. This area marks the weakest point in the anterior skull base. Anterior to the cribriform plate and just posterior to the foramen cecum, a tooth-shaped prominence, the crista galli, is found. In small children, the foramen cecum, anterior to the crista galli, may contain a vein that connects to the superior sagittal sinus. The planum sphenoidale denotes the area posterior to the cribriform plate and marks the posterior boundary of the anterior cranial fossa. The average distance between the foramen cecum and the tuberculum sella ranges between 28 and 50 mm, with an average distance of 42.5 cm.[2]

The anterior skull base is affected most commonly by tumors arising in the paranasal sinuses, skin, or orbit.[3] The most common indication for an anterior craniofacial resection (ACR) is resection of tumors of the sinonasal tract (SNT) that invade the anterior skull base. Tumors of the SNT occur most commonly among white patients during the fifth to seventh decades; their incidence among men is twice that in women.[4–6] Overall, tumors of the SNT account for 8% of the malignancies of the upper aerodigestive tract (UAT).

Epithelial neoplasms are most common, and a majority of series demonstrate a preponderance of squamous cell carcinoma (SCC). This corresponds to the preponderance of SCC in the antrum, which is the most common site of origin of SNT tumors. In our experience, the histopathology of malignant neoplasms of the ethmoid sinuses is equally divided between SCCs and other malignancies such as sinonasal and salivary tumors, carcinomas, sarcomas, and melanomas. Similarly, cancer of the frontal sinuses, which are extremely rare, involve an equal number of SCCs and adenoid cystic carcinomas.

The prognosis of patients with lesions that require an ACR is highly dependent on the histologic diagnosis and the completeness of the resection. Patients with high-grade sarcomas and melanomas have a dismal prognosis owing to their propensity for early metastasis and high rate of local recurrence (i.e., <10% of patients are alive and without evidence of disease at 5 years). Patients with squamous cell carcinoma have an overall survival rate of 50% to 60% at 5 years.[3, 7, 8] Adenoid cystic carcinoma involving the base of the skull is somewhat unpredictable but behaves more aggressively than adenoid cystic carcinoma in other sites in the head and neck.[9]

Infratemporal Fossa/Middle Cranial Fossa

The infratemporal fossa (ITF) is a potential space bounded by the temporal bone and the greater wing of the sphenoid bone superiorly; by the superior constrictor muscle, the pharyngobasilar fascia, and the pterygoid plates medially; by the zygoma, mandible, parotid gland, and masseter muscle laterally; by the pterygoid muscles anteriorly; and by the articular tubercle of the temporal bone, glenoid fossa, and styloid process posteriorly. Thus, the ITF includes the parapharyngeal space containing the internal carotid artery, internal jugular vein, and cranial nerves IV to XII, and the masticator space containing the V3, the internal maxillary artery, the pterygoid venous plexus, and the pterygoid muscles.

Multiple foramina (i.e., carotid canal, jugular foramen, foramen spinosum, foramen ovale, foramen lacerum) connect the ITF with the middle cranial fossa. Medially, the ITF communicates with the pterygopalatine fossa via the pterygomaxillary fissure, which is continuous with the inferior orbital fissure and, thus, the orbit.

A tumor may originate from any of the structures within or surrounding the ITF. Although it occurs rarely, the ITF may also be invaded by metastatic tumors. Benign tumors tend to respect the boundaries of the ITF and expand in the direction of either the soft tissue planes or the preexisting pathways (e.g., foramen and fissure). Conversely, malignant tumors can infiltrate and destroy any of the structures within the ITF and adjacent spaces.

Evaluation of patients with ITF tumors requires the identification of the nature, origin, and extent of the tumor. Selection of surgical approach is influenced by these factors as well as by the biologic behavior of the tumor, the needs of the patient, comorbidities, patient demands, and the training and experience of the surgeon. A multidisciplinary team is critical for ensuring adequate diagnosis, staging, tumor extirpation, and administration of adjuvant therapies, and for the reconstruction and/or repair of cosmetic and functional deficits.

CLINICAL ASSESSMENT

Tumors arising in the SNT often cause symptoms of nasal obstruction, anosmia, facial pressure or pain, epistaxis, and nasal discharge. Because these are similar to the symptoms of chronic sinusitis, there is usually a delay in the diagnosis of sinonasal tumors. These patients frequently report a history of prolonged and repeated treatment for a presumptive "sinusitis." Even more challenging is that approximately 10% of patients with these tumors are asymptomatic, thus significantly delaying adequate diagnosis and treatment.[10, 11] Even advanced tumors of the SNT invading the anterior cranial fossa and/or the frontal lobe often produce very subtle neurologic deficits that go undetected.

A detailed physical examination of patients with symptoms related to the SNT should focus on the upper aerodigestive tract, the orbits, and the cranial nerves and should include nasal endoscopy. Orbital findings, such as limitation of extraocular muscle movements, chemosis, ocular displacement, or proptosis, should raise the level of suspicion for a neoplasm. Similarly, loose dentition—a mass effect in the cheek, nose, forehead, palate, or upper gingivobuccal sulcus commonly presents as ill-fitting dentures—also suggests the presence of an SNT neoplasm (Fig. 10–1). Sensory dysfunction of the first or second division of the trigeminal nerve suggests invasion of these nerves by a malignant neoplasm rather than inflammatory disease of the paranasal sinuses. Although tumors of the paranasal sinuses, even when they are advanced at initial presentation, are usually confined to the local site and rarely present with cervical lymphadenopathy, a detailed examination of the neck is mandatory.

Similarly, patients with ITF tumors can present with a variety of symptoms according to the structures affected. Mass effect, eustachian tube dysfunction, trismus, and cranial neuropathies are common signs of ITF lesions. A physical examination by itself is insufficient for full evaluation of the three-dimensional extent of tumors involving the skull base. Therefore, diagnostic imaging is a critical component of the clinical evaluation.

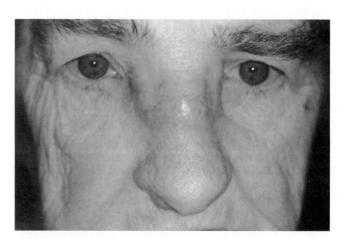

FIGURE 10–1 Patient with expansion of the glabella and nasal bridge due to an extensive carcinoma of the ethmoid sinus.

◻ IMAGING

Extent of Tumor

CT and MRI offer complementary information; therefore, both are recommended to delineate the extent of the tumor, especially in areas that are not amenable to endoscopic examination, such as the cranial cavity, brain, orbit and its contents, paranasal sinuses, and soft tissues of the face and pterygopalatine and infratemporal fossae.

CT scan is superior to MRI in defining bony boundaries (Fig. 10–2A). Intravenous contrast used during CT scanning demonstrates the degree of vascularity of the neoplasm and its relationship to adjacent neurovascular structures such as dura, brain, cranial nerves, internal carotid arteries, the internal jugular vein, and major venous sinuses.

MRI does not use ionizing radiation and better defines the soft tissue interfaces and perineural spread; it also differentiates tumor from retained secretions within the paranasal sinuses (Fig. 10–2B). MRI is usually reserved for imaging of patients who present with tumors that invade soft tissues, most importantly the orbit and brain, and/or for distinguishing tumor from retained secretions or inflammatory disease within the SNT.

Despite its superior soft tissue definition, MRI may not distinguish scar or reconstructive flaps from tumor. Distinguishing tumor from post-treatment fibrosis can be done with the use of a guided biopsy, positron emission tomography (PET) scanning, or sequential imaging to monitor changes or growth and thus establish the presence or absence of tumor.

Vascular Imaging

Vascular Anatomy

Angiography is rarely necessary in the evaluation of malignant tumors of the SNT. It is indicated in patients who present with vascular tumors and only when embolization is being considered. Angiography, however, is important in patients who present with sellar or parasellar lesions that approximate, enclose, or invade the internal carotid artery (ICA). Noninvasive methods such as MR angiography (MRA) or CT angiography (CTA) are adequate for delineating the vascular anatomy of the affected area (i.e., sphenoid sinus invasion).

MRA and CTA are noninvasive tests that demonstrate the arterial anatomy of the ITF and brain. Angiography is preferred over MRA and CTA when preoperative embolization of the tumor is indicated (e.g., juvenile angiofibromas, paragangliomas). Angiography can delineate the vascularity of the tumor and its relationship to the ICA and demonstrates the cerebral circulation and its collateral vasculature. Neither of these "anatomic" tests, however, predicts the adequacy of the intracranial collateral blood supply after sacrifice of the ICA.

Blood Supply

Adequacy of the collateral blood supply to the brain is better evaluated with the use of single-photon emission computed tomography (SPECT) with balloon occlusion, transcranial Doppler, or an angiography-balloon occlusion with xenon computed tomography (ABOX-CT) scan.[12] These tests predict the probability of ischemia when the ipsilateral ICA is sacrificed and, therefore, are indicated when the risk for injury or the need for sacrifice of the ICA is high. Technically and logistically, the ABOX-CT scan is more complex than other tests; however, it is our preferred method owing to its superior sensitivity and specificity.

During the ABOX-CT scan, a catheter with a nondetachable balloon is inserted into the ICA via the femoral artery. The balloon is inflated for 15 minutes, while the awake patient is monitored for changes in neurologic status

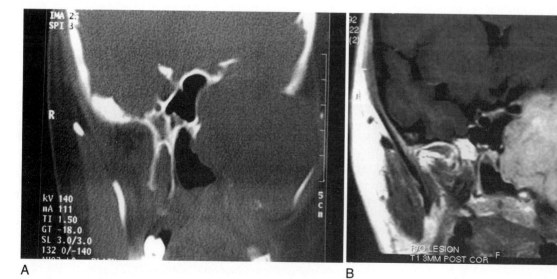

A   B

FIGURE 10–2 *A,* Coronal CT scan shows a large expanding lesion in the left infratemporal fossa. Note the remodeling of the lateral wall of the left sphenoid sinus and the destruction of the lateral skull base. *B,* Coronal MRI T1-weighted image demonstrates a mass in the middle cranial fossa and infratemporal fossa, displacing brain, internal carotid artery (intracranial), and muscles of the infratemporal fossa (extracranial). Note the precise definition of the soft tissue interfaces.

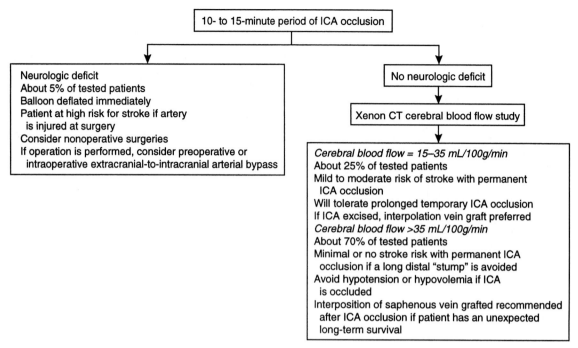

FIGURE 10–3 Algorithm for results of balloon occlusion test of the internal carotid artery (ICA).

(Fig. 10–3). Any neurologic deficit warrants aborting the test. Patients who develop any clinical deficit are classified in a high-risk category. If no neurologic deficits (clinical examination or neurophysiologic monitoring) develop, the balloon is deflated, and a mixture of 32% xenon/68% oxygen is administered via face mask for 4 minutes; the patient is then transferred to a CT suite. CT demonstrates the cerebral distribution of xenon, which reflects the blood flow and thus provides a quantitative assessment measured as cubic centimeters of blood flow per minute per 100 grams of brain tissue (mL/min/100 g). This process is then repeated after the ICA is occluded by reinflation of the balloon. Special software calculates the differential of the xenon diffusion in the brain before and after the balloon inflation. With this information, the baseline status of the brain can be established and the authors can identify those patients at risk for an ischemic injury if the ipsilateral ICA should be sacrificed.

Despite a completely negative test, patients can suffer a stroke because of embolic phenomena or because of the loss of collateral vessels in "watershed" areas that are not evaluated by balloon occlusion testing. In addition, it should be recognized that the ABOX-CT scan is performed under ideal and controlled circumstances and does not account for possible episodes of hypoxia, hypovolemia, hypotension, or electrolyte/acid-base disturbance, which may alter brain hemodynamics. Some advocate the use of controlled hypotension during balloon inflation to increase the sensitivity of the test. In any event, preservation of the ICA is the preferred option whenever possible.

◼ BIOPSY/STAGING

The transnasal approach is the preferred method of biopsying tumors of the paranasal sinuses. We prefer to defer the biopsy until the imaging evaluation has been completed, thus avoiding surgical artifacts caused by the biopsy or by nasal packing. A punch biopsy is typically performed in the office. However, vascular tumors or tumors that require multiple biopsies or extensive sampling (e.g., lymphomas, sarcomas, neuroendocrine tumors) are biopsied in a safer and more adequate manner in the operating room. In these patients, a frozen section analysis of the biopsy is advised to ascertain whether the sample is adequate.

Whenever possible, a histologic diagnosis should be established before the extirpative surgery of tumors involving the ITF. Most tumors are amenable to punch or open biopsy. Some tumors (e.g., angiofibromas, some neurilemmomas) can be diagnosed based on their clinical and imaging characteristics. Tumors in the deeper planes may be sampled by fine-needle aspiration biopsy (FNAB). In the rare instance that an adequate biopsy cannot be obtained, a frozen section analysis may be obtained via a skull base approach. If the histologic diagnosis can be established with a high degree of confidence, the tumor may be resected within the same surgery. However, a frozen section analysis is not without limitations. Thus, sacrifice of critical neurovascular structures (e.g., ICA, orbit, cranial nerves [CNs]) based solely on a frozen section analysis is not prudent. An extirpative procedure is deferred until the final histologic diagnosis has been obtained.

The staging evaluation is tailored to the histologic type, extent, and site of origin of the tumor. A CT scan of the neck is recommended to rule out regional lymph node metastasis. A metastatic evaluation, including a CT scan of the chest and abdomen, a bone scan, and a spine MRI, may be recommended for patients who present with tumors that metastasize hematogenously (i.e., sarcoma, melanoma, or adenoid cystic carcinoma). Patients with a sarcoma or other high-grade malignancies invading the dura are advised to undergo a lumbar puncture to obtain CSF for cytologic analysis. In addition, these patients should undergo an MRI of the brain and spine to rule out meningeal carcinomatosis or "drop metastasis."

■ PREOPERATIVE CONSIDERATIONS

Preoperative functional and neurologic deficits have a significant impact on the surgical planning, postoperative recovery, and functional rehabilitation of the patient. Preexistent lower cranial neuropathies (e.g., CNs IX to XII) are common in patients with tumors of the parapharyngeal space and/or tumors that extend to the jugular foramen. These patients present a wide spectrum of swallowing and speech problems, including hypernasal or slurred speech, nasal regurgitation, dysphagia, aspiration, and dysphonia (CNs X and XII).

Patients with lower cranial neuropathies who present with aspiration have life-threatening consequences. Findings on physical examination reflect the dysfunction of specific CNs and include decreased elevation of the ipsilateral palate (i.e., deviation of the uvula to the nonaffected side—CN X), decreased mobility/strength of the tongue (i.e., deviation to the involved side upon protrusion—CN XII), decreased supraglottic sensation, pooling of secretions in the hypopharynx, ipsilateral vocal cord paralysis (CN X), and atrophy and paralysis of the sternocleidomastoid and trapezius muscles (CN XI).

Lateral deviation of the jaw upon opening may be due to paralysis or invasion by tumor of the pterygoid muscles or to problems of the temporomandibular joint (TMJ). Trismus may be caused by the mechanical tethering caused by the bulk of the tumor, tethering of the muscles due to scarring or tumor invasion, ankylosis, destruction of the TMJ, or pain. The occurrence of trismus, along with factors related to its severity and cause, influence the perioperative management of the airway. Trismus produced by pain resolves with the induction of general anesthesia. Thus, if the extirpative surgery is expected to correct the trismus, the patient's airway can be maintained with an endotracheal tube that is removed at the end of the surgery. However, if the trismus is expected to persist even after removal of the tumor, the patient may require a tracheotomy, which can be performed under local anesthesia.

Limitations in extraocular movement may be the result of direct tumor invasion of the orbit and/or extraocular muscles, or to invasion or compression of CNs III, IV, and VI. We recommend a neuro-ophthalmologic evaluation to clarify these problems and to provide objective measures of the deficit. Similarly, patients with optic nerve problems or with tumor adjacent to the optic nerve, chiasm, or optic tract are also referred for neuro-ophthalmologic evaluation.

According to the vascularity of the tumor, its extent, and its association with neurovascular structures, the need for blood replacement should be anticipated. Preoperatively, the patient should be typed and crossmatched for 2 to 6 units of packed red blood cells (PRBCs) according to the extent and nature of the tumor and the surgery. Autologous blood banking is used when feasible, although it is frequently impractical. A cell saver/autotransfusion device may be used during the resection of benign vascular tumors.

Cranial base surgery is generally considered to be a clean-contaminated procedure for which perioperative prophylactic antibiotics are recommended. Wide-spectrum perioperative antibiotic prophylaxis with good penetration of the blood-brain barrier is administered before the surgery and is continued for 48 hours postoperatively.[17]

A variety of factors influence the choices of anesthetic agents and technique. Thus, a thorough preoperative discussion between the surgeon and the anesthesiologist is necessary regarding the extent of intracranial dissection, the potential for brain or vascular injury, the status of systemic hemodynamics, the need for monitoring of cortical and brain stem functions (e.g., brain stem–evoked response, somatosensory-evoked potential [SSEP], electroencephalogram [EEG]), and the need for CN monitoring (i.e., CNs VII, X–XII).

SSEP monitoring of the median nerve is indicated whenever surgical manipulation of the ICA or the temporal lobe is anticipated. Monitoring of the lower cranial nerves is not employed routinely, although it may be useful for identification of nerves when the tumor is nearby. Facial nerve monitoring, however, is used routinely for transparotid or transtemporal approaches.

Fixation of the endotracheal tube to the premolars or molars with a circumdental or circummandibular wire ligature (e.g., No. 26 stainless steel wire) provides a secure airway. Usually, the patient is extubated at the end of the surgery. A tracheotomy is performed when the patient has permanent trismus, when a free-flap reconstruction for prolonged mechanical ventilation is anticipated, or when tracheal-bronchial toilette is performed. Ultimately, the decision to perform a tracheotomy should take into consideration characteristics of the health care institution such as "after hours" coverage and level of intensive care provided, as well as the experience of the surgical team.

A lumbar spinal drain is indicated when intradural dissection is anticipated. Aggressive spinal drainage, however, may precipitate tension pneumocephalus and should be avoided. Other measures to diminish the intracranial pressure, such as hyperventilation, osmotic diuresis, or corticosteroids, are used as needed.

Other procedures to be considered include the insertion of a nasogastric tube for postoperative enteral feeding and a Foley catheter for monitoring of urinary output. Antiembolic sequential compression stockings are recommended to prevent deep venous thromboses.

The head should be positioned on a horseshoe-shaped head holder, or alternatively with three-pin fixation, if microsurgical work is anticipated. The use of "egg-crate" padding helps prevent ischemic ulcers of the scalp or back during a lengthy surgery. When the need for proximal control of the ICA is anticipated, the head should be positioned in slight extension to facilitate access to the neck. The cornea should be protected with the use of temporary tarsorrhaphy sutures. The scalp should be shaved, following the planned incision line (e.g., bicoronal), and the incision line should be infiltrated with a solution of lidocaine and epinephrine (1:100,000 to 1:400,000).

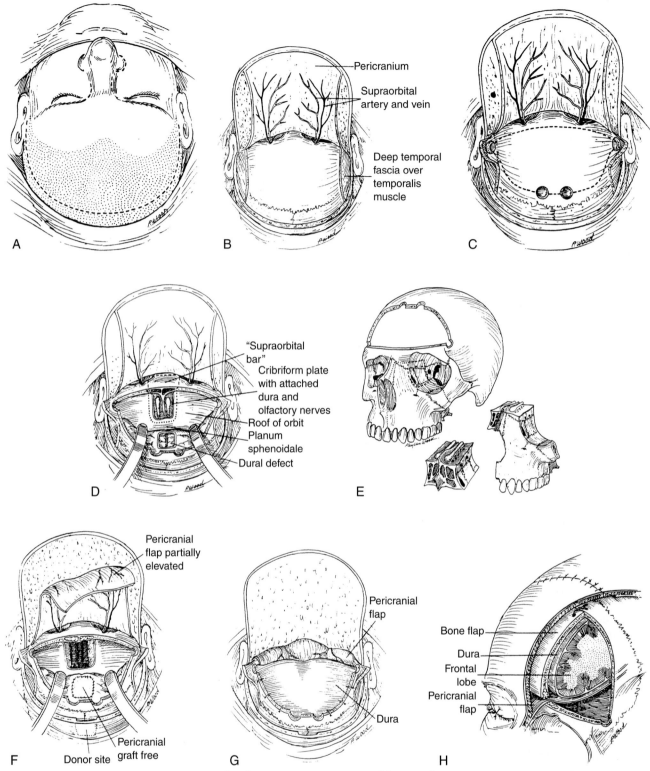

FIGURE 10–4 Anterior craniofacial resection. *A*, Incisions. High bicoronal incision preserves an optimal length of galea and pericranium for use as a reconstructive flap. Facial incisions usually include lateral rhinotomy and contralateral Lynch incisions as shown, but they may be modified to suit the clinical situation. *B*, Elevation of bicoronal scalp flap. Pericranium must be incised bilaterally at the superior temporal lines to separate it from the deep temporal fascia. Supraorbital vessels have been released from supraorbital foramina to allow exposure of the superior orbital rims. *C*, Bifrontal craniotomy. Temporalis muscles have been partially elevated so that burr holes may be placed below the temporal lines; superior burr holes are placed above level of frontal hairline. Such placement helps to minimize postoperative

Continued

SURGERY

Anterior Craniofacial Resection

Historical Perspective

In 1954, Smith[18] reported the first ACR in a patient presenting with a tumor of the frontal sinus. In 1963, Ketcham and associates[19] reported a critical analysis of their experience with ACR for carcinoma of the ethmoid sinuses, including indications, morbidity, and outcome. The oncologic principle for an anterior craniofacial resection remains, as described by Ketcham, an en bloc resection of the tumor that usually involves the anterior skull base between the medial orbital walls extending back to the planum sphenoidale, including the ethmoid sinuses and superior nasal septum.[19, 20] An ACR can be extended laterally to include parts of the orbit (anterolateral craniofacial resection). Subsequent modifications incorporated technical advances brought to craniofacial surgery by Tessier, such as the use of the subfrontal technique, which was subsequently adopted for craniofacial oncologic surgery by Derome.[7, 21-28] These modifications involve the removal of the supraorbital block to improve visualization of the tumor while decreasing the need for brain retraction, thus reducing its inherent morbidity.

A surgical approach is chosen on the basis of tumor extent, vascularity, and relationship to neurovascular structures, as well as surgeon or patient preference. After the extirpative surgery has been completed, the surgeon should restore the separation of the cranial cavity and the upper aerodigestive tract to provide an acceptable cosmetic and functional outcome.

Surgical Approach

The extirpative phase begins with exposure of the neoplasm. Wide exposure facilitates a complete resection, preserving normal tissue and protecting important neurovascular structures such as the brain, carotid artery, and cranial nerves. A subfrontal approach is the preferred technique for resection of the anterior cranial base because it avoids retraction of the frontal lobes and thus decreases the possibility of edema, contusion, or necrosis. It also facilitates reconstruction of the skull base and preserves the cosmesis of the craniofacial region, thereby meeting the previously mentioned surgical criteria.

An anterior subfrontal approach usually involves a combination of facial/oral incisions and/or scalp incisions and osteotomies to expose the intracranial and extracranial

components of the tumor (Fig. 10–4). A bicoronal incision exposes the upper face and cranium, and its resulting scar is hidden inside the hairline. A lateral rhinotomy, facial gingivobuccal degloving incisions, or endoscopically guided intranasal incisions are used to complement the cranial exposure. A medial maxillectomy may be completed with the use of any of these three approaches. We prefer the endoscopic technique because it leaves no facial scars. However, the choice is highly dependent on the surgeon's training and experience, as well as on the degree of tumor extension (i.e., intraorbital tumor) and the need for reconstruction after completion of the resection (i.e., orbital walls). Patients undergoing a total maxillectomy will require a lateral rhinotomy or a Weber-Fergusson incision or a gingivobuccal degloving incision. In patients presenting with neoplasms that invade the skin, incisions can be made directly over the margins of the tumor.

The bicoronal incision divides the scalp, following a true bicoronal plane that extends from the superior and anterior aspect of one auricle to the other (Fig. 10–5). If the surgical exposure should extend below the level of the glabella, the arc of rotation of the bicoronal scalp flap is improved by extending the incision inferiorly, following the preauricular crease. The incision is carried through the subcutaneous tissue, galea, and superficial temporal fascia laterally, and through the pericranium centrally (i.e., between the temporalis muscles). Hemostatic clamps or cautery can be used to control scalp bleeding. The scalp is then elevated in a subpericranial plane, transecting the pericranium at its junction with the deep temporal fascia around the superior border of the temporalis muscle (i.e., temporal line) (Fig. 10–6).

Once the supraorbital rims have been exposed, the supraorbital neurovascular bundle is dissected from the supraorbital notches to facilitate exposure of the superior orbits and glabella (Fig. 10–7). When a true supraorbital foramen is present, it may be opened inferiorly with the use of a small 3- to 6-mm osteotome. After this maneuver, the bicoronal approach should have exposed the superior cranium and frontal area, glabella, nasal bones, temporalis muscles, and temporal fossae, as well as the superior two thirds of the orbits.

A bifrontal craniotomy is then opened according to the extent of the lesion as a transfrontal sinus craniotomy, or as a craniotomy that follows the margins of the tumor (i.e., when the frontal bone has been invaded) (Fig. 10–8). The craniotomy can be extended laterally for tumors extending into the orbit or infratemporal fossa, or inferiorly to include the orbital rims as a monobloc bone graft. Alternatively,

cosmetic deformity. Paramedian positioning of superior burr holes aids in protection of the superior sagittal (venous) sinus while bone flap is being cut. *D,* Intracranial view of the anterior fossa floor just before tumor resection. Note that the olfactory nerves and adjacent dura will be included with the specimen as an oncologic margin. *E,* Outline of osteotomies for en bloc ethmoidectomy *(dashed lines)* and for extended resection when maxillectomy is also performed *(dotted lines)*; respective resection specimens are shown at right. *F,* View of defect in the anterior fossa floor after resection of the tumor. A pericranial flap is being developed to reconstruct the defect. The dural defect has been patched with a free graft of pericranium to achieve a watertight closure. *G,* The pericranial flap has been inserted beneath the frontal lobes. *H,* Cutaway view of the pericranial flap in the final position.

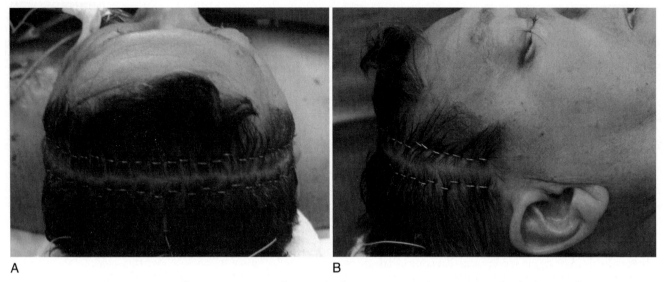

FIGURE 10–5 *A* and *B,* Intraoperative photographs demonstrating scalp preparation for the bicoronal incision. The hair is parted, not shaved, following the planned incision line. Staples keep hair out of the incision line.

the supraorbital block may be removed separately from the craniotomy. This latter technique facilitates inclusion of the posterior orbital roofs in the supraorbital bone graft.

A lateral rhinotomy exposes the medial maxilla, thus providing ample exposure for the resection of neoplasms that involve the ethmoid sinuses and lateral nasal wall. During the lateral rhinotomy, the medial attachment of the nasal ala, as well as its corresponding subcutaneous tissue and muscles, is preserved to support the nasal ala so that subsequent ala retraction and deformity can be prevented. This

preserves the support of the nasal ala. Furthermore, this perialar component of the lateral rhinotomy is not necessary for tumors that are located in the superior SNT, such as tumors of the ethmoid sinuses or nasal vault. A Weber-Fergusson incision or a transconjunctival, subciliary, and/or gingivobuccal incision facilitates the exposure for a total or radical maxillectomy (Fig. 10–9).

Gingivobuccal degloving incisions can be used in combination with the bicoronal incision to avoid facial incisions. In general, however, it is somewhat cumbersome to approach

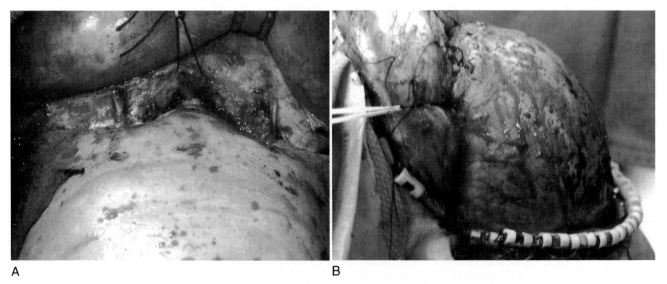

FIGURE 10–6 *A,* Intraoperative photograph demonstrating the surgeon's view of the frontal area, supraorbital rims, and cranium. *B,* Intraoperative photograph, lateral view of the bicoronal exposure. The scalp flap has been dissected anteriorly and inferiorly and is retracted using rubber bands.

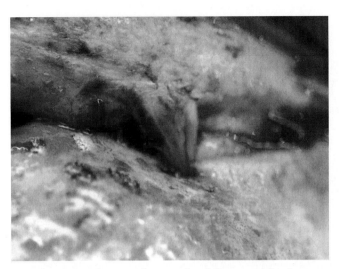

FIGURE 10–7 Close-up photograph of the supraorbital neurovascular bundle after mobilization from the supraorbital foramen.

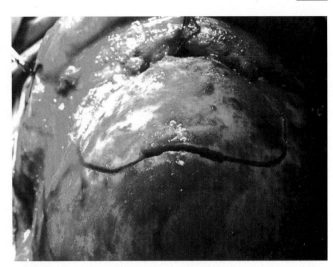

FIGURE 10–8 Intraoperative photograph: bifrontal craniotomy.

the ethmoid sinuses through a degloving approach because the cheek flaps are tethered by the infraorbital neurovascular bundles. In selected patients, intranasal incisions and osteotomies can be performed under endoscopic guidance, thereby avoiding any type of facial or intraoral incision.

Typically, a pericranial flap is used to restore the separation of the cranial cavity from the upper aerodigestive tract. The pericranium is elevated as a vascularized flap based on the supraorbital vessels to cover defects that include the cribriform plate, the fovea ethmoidalis, and the planum sphenoidale. We prefer to elevate the pericranial flap after the extirpative phase of the surgery has been completed. This avoids desiccation of the flap or accidental tearing or avulsion during resection of the tumor. Following the repair of any dural defect, the pericranial flap is rotated beneath the supraorbital and craniotomy bone grafts and the brain. All craniotomy and orbital bone grafts are stabilized with titanium alloy adaptation plates. Although titanium alloy plates are preferred over wires or sutures owing to their superior stability, cost and availability may dictate the use of the latter.

In patients who require resection of the orbital roof, a temporalis muscle flap may be used to reinforce the pericranial flap and protect the eye against the pulsations of the brain. A temporalis muscle flap may also be used to reinforce the pericranial flap in patients who require an orbital exenteration.

Free microvascular flaps are reserved for patients in whom the dura mater and/or brain and facial skin have been sacrificed or for patients who require extensive resection, including the infratemporal fossa, resulting in a large dead space. The most commonly used free microvascular flaps are the rectus abdominis muscle and radial forearm fasciocutaneous flaps.

In patients requiring the resection of craniofacial bones that may result in a cosmetic defect (e.g., frontal, nasal, facial), the defect may be reconstructed with autogenous bone grafts that can be harvested from the inner table of the craniotomy flap. If the bone defect is extensive or if cranial bone grafts are inadequate, the defect can be bridged with titanium mesh.

Approaches to the Intratemporal Fossa

Historical Perspective

Fairbanks-Barbosa[29] was the first to report an ITF approach for the resection of advanced tumors of the maxillary sinus. Transtemporal approaches described by Fisch,[30] preauricular approaches described by Sekhar and Schramm,[31] and transmaxillary approaches described by Terz,[32] Janecka,[33] Cocke,[34] and Catalano[35] validated the efficacy and clarified the indications of surgery for resection of tumors of the ITF fossa.

The presence of neurovascular structures within the ITF (e.g., ICA) or adjacent to it (e.g., CN VII) limits the exposure of any particular surgical approach to the ITF. Thus, surgical approaches are designed not only to remove the tumor but also to preserve and identify these neurovascular entities.

An ITF approach is a complex procedure involving significant time, effort, and cost; under most circumstances, the procedure itself constitutes only one part of a multimodality therapeutic plan.

An ITF approach may provide the access required for resection of the tumor, or it may be adjunctive to other approaches, such as transcranial-subtemporal, Le Fort I, transmaxillary, or anterior subfrontal approaches. Infrequently, an ITF approach is used to obtain an adequate biopsy and only when an FNAB, Tru-Cut biopsies, and other means have failed to obtain an adequate sample.

Indications for a preauricular approach include tumors originating in the ITF and intracranial tumors that originate at the anterior aspect of the temporal bone or greater wing of the sphenoid bone and that extend into the ITF. A preauricular approach may be combined with other approaches to expose tumors that arise from the SNT but extend posteriorly and/or laterally to involve the ITF. The preauricular approach, however, provides inadequate exposure for the

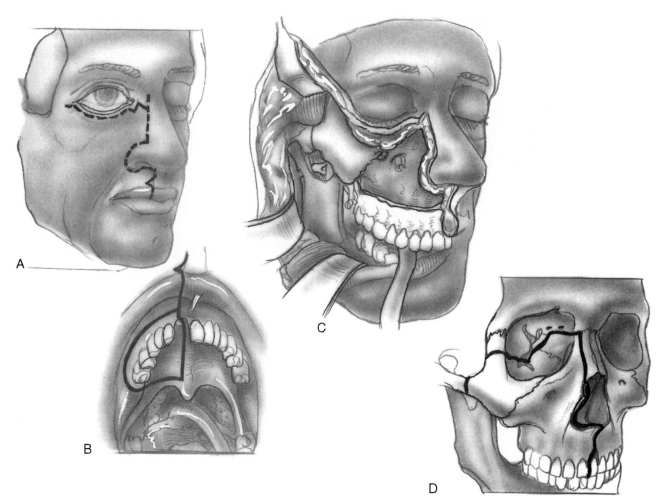

FIGURE 10-9 A total maxillectomy with preservation of the orbit can be performed using incisions identical to lateral rhinotomy incisions with a lip-splitting extension. Alternatively, a lateral rhinotomy incision may be combined with an ipsilateral degloving approach. *A,* If increased exposure is necessary, the facial incisions may be modified. The superior incision begins at the lateral canthus and extends medially, passing 3 to 4 mm below the ciliary line. The eye is protected by a temporary tarsorrhaphy stitch. A transconjunctival incision may be substituted for this incision. The subciliary limb is joined to a lateral rhinotomy incision. The orbicularis oculi muscle is incised with an inferiorly directed slant, exposing the orbital septum. The gingivobuccal incision is extended laterally to the ipsilateral maxillary tuberosity. *B,* The soft palate is incised at the junction with the hard palate, and its attachments are sharply transected. The mucoperiosteum of the hard palate is incised following a paramedian line ipsilateral to the lesion. The paramedian strip of mucosa will be later imbricated over the bony edge of the hard palate to facilitate the fitting of a prosthesis. *C,* The orbital contents are dissected from the medial inferior and lateral walls, exposing the lacrimal sac, the anterior and posterior ethmoid arteries, and the infraorbital fissure. *D,* The body and frontal process of the zygoma are divided with the saw. The maxilla is severed from the nasal bones with the saw, and the osteotomy is extended superiorly to the frontoethmoid suture. A superior osteotomy is carried out posteriorly to a point 3 to 4 mm posterior to the ethmoid artery. An osteotomy is performed to connect the lateral and medial wall osteotomies across the inferior orbital fissure. The hard palate is transected with a Gigli or a sagittal saw. The maxilla is detached from the skull by the tapping of a chisel placed into the ptergomaxillary fissure in a posterosuperior direction. The superior attachments of the turbinates are sharply severed as for a medial maxillectomy. The specimen is removed by anteroinferior traction. Remnants of ethmoid sinus mucosa are removed in a piecemeal fashion. The coronoid process of the mandible is removed to avoid displacement of the prosthesis when the mandible is opened.

Continued

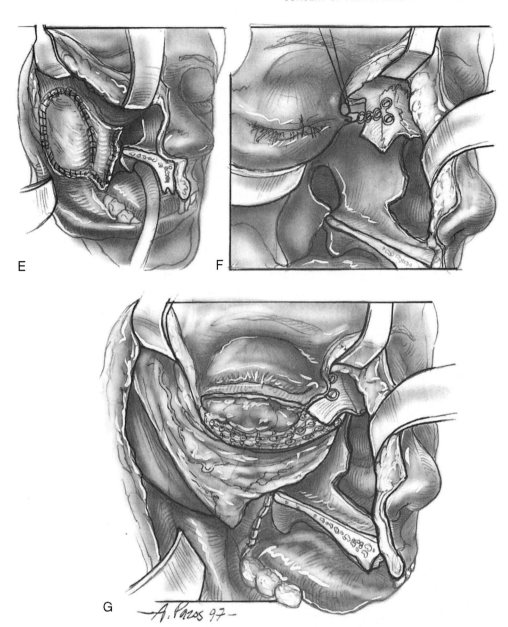

E

F

G   A. Pazos 97

FIGURE 10–9, Cont'd   *E,* The exposed facial and pterygoid muscles and the periorbita are lined with a split-thickness skin graft that is 0.35 to 0.45 mm thick. The obturator or denture is wired to the remaining dentition or is suspended from the zygomatic arch and pyriform aperture or is lag-screwed to the remaining hard palate. *F,* A medial canthopexy is done with the use of a Y-shaped titanium plate fastened to the nasal bones. A figure-of-8 nonabsorbable suture is used to medialize the medial canthal tendon. *G,* The floor and medial walls of the orbit are reconstructed with titanium mesh. This is then covered by a vertically split temporalis muscle flap. The anterior half is used for reconstruction, and the posterior half is transposed to the anterior temporal fossa to obliterate the defect. (From Carrau RL, Myers RN: Neoplasms of the nose and paranasal sinuses. In Bailey BJ [ed]: Head and Neck Surgery— Otolaryngology. Baltimore, Lippincott Williams & Wilkins, 2001, pp 1247–1265.)

resection of tumors that invade the temporal bone and does not provide adequate access to the infratemporal facial nerve or jugular bulb. The postauricular approach is designed to expose and resect those lesions that involve the temporal bone and that extend into the ITF.

A transfacial approach is best used to approach sinonasal tumors invading the ITF, the masticator space, or the pterygomaxillary fossa and for tumors of the nasopharynx that extend into the ITF. We reserve its use, however, for cancer of the antrum that extends into the ITF.

Poor candidates for an ITF approach and/or dissection include patients with lymphoreticular tumors, which are best treated with radiation and/or chemotherapy; patients who are poor surgical risks because of pulmonary, cardiac, renal, or other significant comorbidities; and patients with disseminated disease. The main limiting factor in choosing an ITF approach is the degree of extension of the tumor and its relationship to neurovascular structures.

Surgical Approaches

PREAURICULAR (SUBTEMPORAL) APPROACH TO THE INFRATEMPORAL FOSSA/MIDDLE CRANIAL FOSSA[31]

A hemicoronal or bicoronal incision is carried through the subcutaneous tissue, galea, and pericranium. Over the temporal area, the incision extends to the deep layer of the temporal fascia (Fig. 10–10). On the affected side, the incision is extended by following the preauricular crease down to the level of the tragus. Whenever possible, the anterior branches

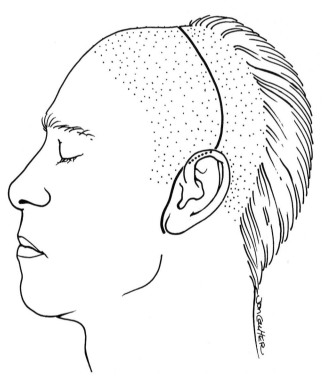

FIGURE 10–10 The coronal scalp incision may be extended in a preauricular skin crease to provide additional lateral exposure. (From Snyderman CH, Carrau RL: Anterior cranial base. In Myers EN [ed]: Operative Laryngology—Head and Neck Surgery. Philadelphia, WB Saunders, 1997, pp 808–834.)

of the superficial temporal artery are preserved to maximize blood supply to the scalp flap. Alternatively, the incision is carried throughout the subcutaneous tissue, and a temporoparietal facial flap is then dissected. For proximal control of the ICA, the incision is extended into the neck using a lazy-S pattern or using a separate horizontal incision that follows a neck crease. The scalp is evaluated from the cranium following a subpericranial plane, and the attachments of the pericranium to the deep layer of the temporal fascia are transected.

Superficial and deep layers of the deep temporal fascia attach to the lateral and medial surfaces of the zygomatic arch, respectively. To expose the zygoma, the superficial layer of the deep temporal fascia is incised, following an imaginary line from the superior orbital rim to the zygomatic temporal root. The superficial layer of the deep temporal fascia and the periosteum are elevated en bloc with the scalp flap to protect the frontal branches of the facial nerve and to expose the orbitozygomatic complex. This exposure allows for the dissection of the periorbita from the lateral orbital walls (i.e., from the trochlea to the inferior orbital fissure).

By means of electrocautery, the remaining fascial attachments of the temporalis muscle to the zygomatic arch and to the cranium are transected, and the muscle is elevated off the temporal fossa. If the temporalis muscle will be returned to its original position, a curved titanium plate is screwed to the temporal line. The fascia of the temporalis muscle may then be sutured to the plate. We obtain better and more reliable results with this technique than by leaving a fascial cuff or using drill holes through the bone to reattach the muscle.

Then, the masseteric fascia is dissected from the masseter muscle, thus elevating the overlying parotid gland, with a broad periosteal elevator. Although it is seldom necessary, the arc of rotation of the scalp flap may be increased by transecting the soft tissues anterior to the tympanic bone. A cuff of soft tissue around the main trunk of the facial nerve is preserved to prevent a traction injury.

When necessary, the internal, common, and external carotid arteries, along with the internal jugular vein (IJV) and CNs X to XII, are exposed, dissected, and controlled by the cervical incision. Orbitozygomatic osteotomies are performed (1) posteriorly, at the zygomatic root; (2) superiorly, at the zygomaticofrontal suture; and (3) medially, at the malar eminence at the level of the zygomaticofacial foramen. An assistant protects the soft tissues of the orbit using a malleable or orbital retractor, and the surgeon places the tip of the reciprocating saw at the lateral aspect of the inferior orbital fissure; then an osteotomy is completed through the lateral orbital wall, and the inferior orbital fissure is joined with the osteotomy performed at the frontozygomatic suture.

Accidental entry into the maxillary sinus is inconsequential unless intradural dissection creates the potential for a CSF leak. The antrostomy is closed by means of fascial and/or pericranium free grafts that are held in place by compression against the opening when the orbitozygomatic complex is plated in its original position.

All of these osteotomies may be modified to account for tumor involvement of any portion of the orbitozygomatic complex (OZC). In cases requiring both intracranial and extracranial exposure, the superior and lateral orbital osteotomies should be made after the craniotomy has been completed so that the superior and lateral orbital walls can be included in the orbitozygomatic graft. With the use of both intracranial and extracranial exposures, osteotomies can be made through the superior and lateral orbital walls to remove the orbitozygomatic bone segment.

As was previously described, one assistant protects and retracts the orbital soft tissues and another assistant protects the frontal lobe while the surgeon completes the osteotomies. The bone graft is kept in saline solution until the tumor is removed. A mandibular coronoidectomy, performed after the removal of the OZC, increases the arc of rotation of the temporalis muscle. Then, the temporalis muscle is dissected inferiorly until the infratemporal crest is fully visualized. A subperiosteal plane is then followed medially to dissect the soft tissues from the infratemporal skull base.

Dissection of the soft tissues from the infratemporal skull base usually is associated with troublesome bleeding arising from the pterygoid plexus. Bleeding may be controlled with the use of bipolar cautery (unipolar cautery stimulates V3, causing contraction of the mastication muscles and occasional cardiac arrhythmias) and/or cottonoids moistened in oxymetazoline 0.05% and/or Surgicel/Avitene packing. Removal of the skull base at the subtemporal area (subtemporal craniectomy) facilitates identification and dissection of neurovascular structures.

The lateral pterygoid plate is identified anteriorly. Anatomic relationships that are useful for the identification of infratemporal skull base structures include (in an anterior to posterior direction) (1) the posterior aspect of the lateral pterygoid plate, which is aligned with the foramen ovale, (2) the foramen spinosum, and (3) the spine of the sphenoid bone. These structures lie in a straight "line of sight" that is lateral to the canal of the ICA.

The pterygoid plates also provide a route of access to the inferolateral aspect of the sphenoid sinus, which may be entered between the second and third divisions of the trigeminal nerve. After these neurovascular structures have been identified and preserved, extirpation of the tumor can proceed. This approach provides excellent access to the infratemporal skull base, orbital apex, and lateral maxilla. Tumors that do not involve the temporal bone or petrous portion of the ICA are adequately exposed with this approach. Dissection of the petrous ICA requires removal of the glenoid fossa as part of the OZC graft.

A temporal craniotomy is used for exposure of the superior aspect of the glenoid fossa. The capsule of the TMJ should be dissected free from the fossa and should displace it inferiorly. Then, with the use of a reciprocating saw, osteotomies that incorporate the lateral two thirds of the fossa are made. It should be remembered that the ICA is located medial to the fossa. Preserving the lateral two thirds provides stability for the mandibular condyle following its reconstruction. The condyle, however, will be prone to anterior dislocation. Accidental injury to the cochlea is possible if the osteotomies are made too posteriorly. If additional exposure of the carotid canal and extratemporal ICA is necessary, the neck of the condyle can be transected at the level of the sigmoid notch to remove the contents of the condylar fossa; then its anterior and medial walls are drilled.

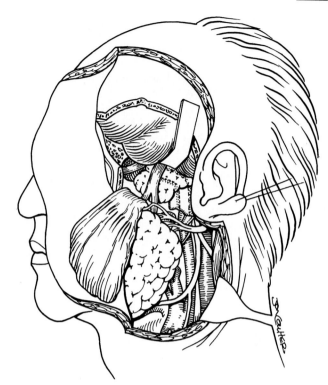

FIGURE 10–11 This illustration demonstrates a tumor medial to the mandibular division of the trigeminal nerve and near the petrous portion of the ICA. Additional exposure of the ICA and removal of the tumor often necessitate transection of the mandibular division of the trigeminal nerve. (Redrawn from Sekhar LN, Janecka IP: Surgery of Cranial Base Tumors. New York, Raven Press, 1993.)

Additionally, to attain dissection of the petrous segment of the ICA, the mandibular division of the trigeminal nerve should be dissected at the foramen ovale. Once the ICA has been mobilized from its horizontal canal, it can be transposed and/or retracted to facilitate resection of tumor or to gain access to the petrous apex (Fig. 10–11).

A variety of modifications to this approach are possible and can be used according to tumor extent and other clinical circumstances. A parotidectomy also may be performed to obtain negative margins or to enhance the exposure. Similarly, tumors that invade the mandible require a partial mandibulectomy.

Following removal of the tumor, it is necessary for the surgeon to close any communication with the upper aerodigestive tract. A temporoparietal fascial flap and/or temporalis muscle flap may be used to obliterate the dead space and to protect the ICA (Fig. 10–12). (The temporalis muscle can be divided vertically, and the anterior half of the muscle may be transposed to obliterate the defect, while the posterior half of the muscle is transposed anteriorly to fill the temporal fossa defect.) The orbital floor may be reconstructed with titanium mesh and then covered with a temporoparietal fascia flap or a temporalis muscle transposition flap. Similarly, defects of the lateral orbital wall can be reconstructed with titanium mesh. In selected patients, a pericranial or a temporoparietal flap may be used to provide protection of the infratemporal skull base. Extensive soft

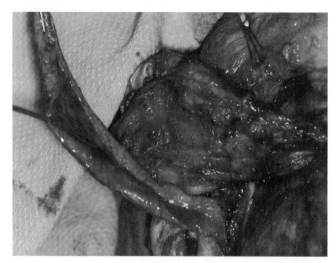

FIGURE 10–12 Intraoperative photograph: temporoparietal fascia flap and temporalis muscle, after dissection from the temporal fossa.

tissue defects are best reconstructed with microvascular free-tissue flaps. The bone grafts then are replaced and fixed in their original position by means of titanium alloy adaptation plates, wire, or braided nylon sutures.

Plating is preferred because it provides greater stability. If resection of the mandibular condyle is necessary to expose the petrous ICA, no attempt should be made to reconstruct the TMJ. Reconstruction of the TMJ after oncologic exenteration of the ITF does not significantly improve postoperative function and may actually lead to scarring, ankylosis, and trismus. Periosteal and muscular attachments to the craniofacial skeleton should be repaired to prevent retraction and/or sagging of the muscles and other soft tissues. The skin and mucosal incisions should be closed using a multilayered technique.

POSTAURICULAR (TRANSTEMPORAL) APPROACH[36]

A "question mark" or C-shaped incision in the temporal area is extended postauricularly into the mastoid region, curving down to follow a horizontal skin crease of the middle neck (Fig. 10–13). If the middle ear is sacrificed as part of the approach or the tumor resection and if the patient is at risk for a postoperative CSF leak, the external auditory canal (EAC) should be permanently closed to prevent CSF otorrhea. The EAC is divided at the bony-cartilaginous junction and is closed with the use of everting stitches. This closure is reinforced with a myoperiosteal U-shaped flap based on the posterior margin of the EAC. Alternatively, if the middle ear is spared, the canal may be preserved by placing the incisions in the conchal area.

The incision follows the margin of the conchal bowl and tragus, so that the scar is hidden. In the conchal area, the skin, cartilage, and perichondrium are incised to meet the retroauricular plane of dissection. An incision inside the EAC is difficult to suture in a watertight fashion and tends to stenose. These incisions, placed laterally, facilitate the anastomosis of the EAC to the pinna at the end of the extirpative procedure. A Penrose drain can be inserted through

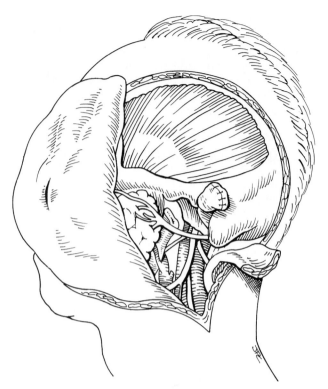

FIGURE 10–13 The facial flap is reflected anteriorly with exposure of the temporalis muscle, orbitozygomatic bone, masseteric fascia, mandible, parotid gland and facial nerve, and cervical vessels and nerves. The conchal tissues of the auricle are temporarily sewn together to maximize the operative exposure. (From Carrau RL, Snyderman CH: Surgical approaches to the infratemporal fossa. In Myers EN [ed]: Operative Otolaryngology—Head and Neck Surgery. Philadelphia, WB Saunders, 1997, pp 835–867.)

the conchal defect in the skin/auricle flap to facilitate its retraction. The cervicofacial flap is elevated following a subplatysmal plane in the cervical area and a suprasuperficial musculoaponeurotic system (supra-SMAS) plane over the parotid area. Elevation of the cervicofacial flap follows the deep layer of the deep temporal fascia over the cranium.

The main trunk of the facial nerve is identified, anterior to the EAC just distal to the stylomastoid foramen, as described for a parotidectomy. If circumferential mobilization of the main trunk is not necessary, a cuff of soft tissue is preserved around the main trunk to minimize the possibility of traction injury when the facial flap is retracted anteriorly. A "tail" (i.e., superficial) parotidectomy enhances access to the retromandibular area. A total parotidectomy is indicated when an epithelial malignancy of the parotid gland is to be removed. Skeletonization of the main trunk of the facial nerve and its branches facilitates their retraction and thus enhances access to the ITF (Fig. 10–14).

Resection of the main trunk of the facial nerve and its branches (i.e., radical parotidectomy) is indicated when the nerve has been invaded by the tumor. In these cases, direct attention is paid to the cervical exposure to obtain proximal control of the common, internal, and external carotid arteries, IJV, and CNs X to XII. The sternocleidomastoid and

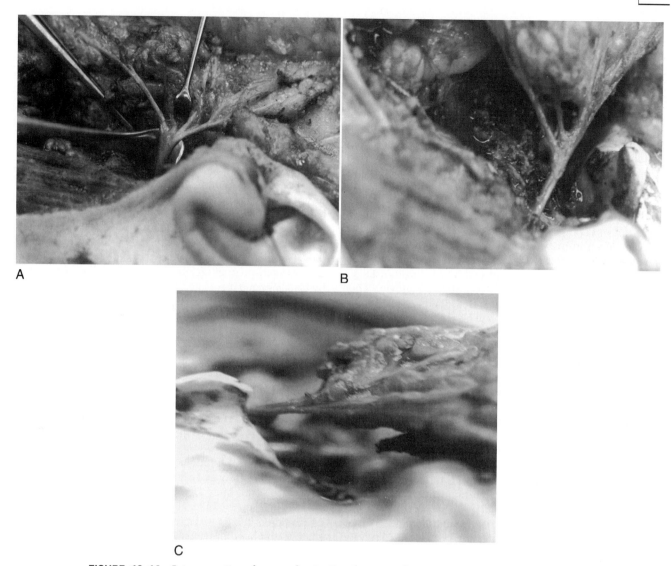

FIGURE 10-14 Intraoperative photograph. *A,* Facial nerve after total parotidectomy. *B,* Inferior ("worm's eye") view of facial nerve after radical parotidectomy, mandibular condylectomy, OZC osteotomies, and ITF exenteration. *C,* Superior ("bird's eye") view.

digastric muscles from the mastoid bone are transected. The stylohyoid and stylopharyngeus muscles are transected and the styloid process is removed. CN IX usually can be identified at this time because it crosses lateral to the ICA. Mastoidectomy and dissection of the vertical portion of the facial nerve allow transposition of the facial nerve, thus providing a wider access to the ITF.

In patients who require a radical parotidectomy, a mastoidectomy provides the means of obtaining proximal control of the margins of the resected facial neura and of inserting a nerve graft. Mastoidectomy also provides access to the jugular bulb and adjacent lower CNs. Orbitozygomatic osteotomies may be performed as described earlier in the chapter (preauricular approach). After the orbitozygomatic complex has been removed, the anterior, superior, medial, and posterior boundaries of the ITF are well exposed, and all major vessels are exposed.

An infratemporal skull base approach, including a temporal craniotomy, proceeds as described in the previous section. Extirpation of the tumor can now proceed, including the involved soft tissue and bone. Reconstruction of the defect follows the principles outlined in previous sections.

FISCH APPROACHES[30]

Fisch described several lateral ITF approaches that use subtemporal exposure and rerouting of the facial nerve.

The Fisch A approach is indicated for lesions within the temporal bone, such as glomus tumors. This approach involves the exenteration of the middle ear, a subtotal petrosectomy, and a permanent anterior transposition of the facial nerve. The lower CNs, ICA, and IJV are controlled in the neck early during the procedure. The external ear canal is closed as a blind pouch.

The Fisch B and C approaches are designed to approach more anteriorly located disease involving the petrous apex and clivus. The critical maneuvers in the type B ITF approach are the reflection of the zygomatic arch and temporalis muscle inferiorly and the removal of the bone of the skull base floor to provide access to the ITF. A key to this extradural exposure is the subtotal "petrosectomy." This step involves a canal wall–down mastoidectomy, including complete skeletonization of the labyrinth, facial nerve, sigmoid sinus, middle and posterior fossa dura, and jugular bulb, as well as exenteration of all hypotympanic air cells and skeletonization of the ICA.

The TMJ is disarticulated by incising the capsule and removing the articular disc. At this point, the bone of the glenoid fossa and the root of the zygoma are removed completely. Further skeletonization of the carotid artery is possible along the lateral and anterior canal of the ICA. Complete exposure of the carotid artery permits its mobilization out of the carotid canal, providing free access to the petrous apex and clivus. The eustachian tube must be sutured closed to prevent infection of the nasal cavity. The bone defect is filled with abdominal fat; temporalis muscle is used to cover the fat and is placed inferior to the skeletonized middle fossa dura and mandibular condyle. The orbitozygomatic graft is plated and the skin closed in a multilayered fashion.

The type C approach is an extension of the type B and is used for lesions of the anterior ITF, sella, and nasopharynx. Resection of the pterygoid plates distinguishes the type C from the type B approach. This resection permits exposure of the lateral wall of the nasopharynx, eustachian tube orifice, posterior maxillary sinus, and posterior nasopharyngeal wall past the midline. Following completion of the type B approach, the lateral surface of the pterygoid process is identified and soft tissues are elevated. In this fashion, the bases of both medial and lateral plates of the pterygoid processes can be drilled away, exposing the lateral wall of the nasopharynx. The exposure permits full visualization of the peritubal area, which can be resected en bloc. A "watertight" reconstruction of the resulting defect after type C ITF surgery is more difficult than in type B. Although mobilization of the entire temporalis muscle or a temporoparietal flap into the wound is a feasible technique, vascularized free flaps are often necessary to provide adequate closure.

The type D approach is a preauricular ITF approach that uses orbitozygomatic osteotomies and resection of the floor of the middle fossa to expose the medial middle cranial fossa without a lateral temporal craniotomy. During the type D approach, the middle ear and eustachian tube are not obliterated, and conductive hearing is not sacrificed. In addition, the intratemporal facial nerve is not rerouted, and the petrous ICA is not fully exposed. Subtype D1 addresses tumors of the anterior ITF, and subtype D2 is designed for lateral orbital wall lesions and high pterygopalatine fossa tumors. Although these preauricular approaches do not include a temporal craniotomy, the floor of the skull base can be drilled away to allow full access to the ITF.

ANTERIOR TRANSFACIAL APPROACH (FACIAL TRANSLOCATION)[24, 25, 33] (Fig. 10–15)

A Weber-Fergusson incision is made and is extended down to the periosteum of the maxilla, nasal bones, and orbital rim. The "traditional" translocation approach involves a horizontal incision over the superior edge of the zygomatic bone, extending into the lateral canthus to meet the Weber-Fergusson incision. The frontal branches of the facial nerve are dissected, entubulated with silicone tubing, and transected. These nerve branches are reconstructed using an entubulation technique. Subperiosteal dissection of the anterior maxilla exposes the infraorbital nerve, which then is transected and tagged. Next, an inferiorly based flap comprising the upper lip, cheek, lower eyelid, parotid gland, and facial nerve is reflected inferiorly. A frontotemporal scalp flap is elevated in a subpericranial plane and is reflected anteriorly to expose the supraorbital rims.

Alternatively, exposure can be achieved without the temporal incision by combining the preauricular approach with the anterior exposure provided by the Weber-Fergusson incision. Orbitozygomatic osteotomies are performed and joined with maxillary osteotomies to free the anterior face of the ipsilateral maxilla en bloc with the orbitozygomatic complex. Alternatively, the maxillary bone graft can be elevated as a vascularized graft attached to the cheek flap, as described by Catalano and associates.[35]

The temporalis and masseter muscles are dissected from the zygomatic bone with electrocautery. Osteotomies are completed, as required for the removal of the maxilla, and the bone graft is removed. A temporal-subtemporal craniotomy is performed, and the temporalis muscle is reflected inferiorly. After these steps have been completed, the anterior, medial, and lateral boundaries of the ITF are well exposed. The pterygoid plates can be removed to provide further access to the medial ITF or the nasopharynx. Their base can be removed to allow their resection en bloc with the maxilla.

A temporal-subtemporal craniotomy provides additional exposure superiorly and allows the dissection of intracranial structures. Following tumor resection, the temporalis muscle may be used to obliterate the surgical defect and provide separation of the cranial cavity from the upper aerodigestive tract, as has been previously described. Periosteal and muscular attachments are repaired and the incisions are closed with the use of a multilayer technique. The conjunctiva is repaired with running 6–0 fast-absorbing suture. The lacrimal canaliculi are stented with Crawford silicone tubing, which is tied to itself in the nasal cavity. The eye is closed with a temporary tarsorrhaphy for 10 to 14 days to prevent a lower-eyelid ectropion.

TRANSORBITAL APPROACH[36]

A transorbital approach may be used to complement the exposures obtained with one of the previous approaches, thus enhancing the exposure of the orbital apex and cavernous sinus. This approach should be reserved for patients with benign tumors of the orbital apex and cavernous sinus who have lost vision because of tumor growth. A transorbital approach may also be employed for low-grade malignant neoplasms with minimal involvement of the orbital soft apex or optic nerve to obtain complete tumor removal.

Extensive involvement of the orbital soft tissues requires an orbital exenteration. This approach consists of the transection of the orbital tissues posterior to the globe with preservation of the attachments of the orbital soft tissues (including the globe) to the scalp flap. The orbital apex is removed to provide direct anterior access to the cavernous sinus and the cavernous ICA. The advantages of this

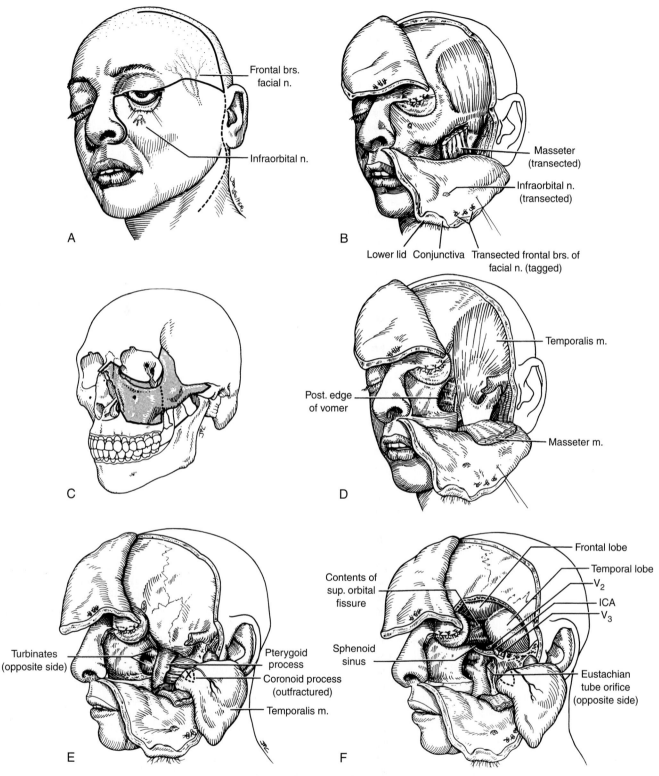

FIGURE 10–15 *A to F,* Surgical steps depicted in drawings of facial translocation procedure.

approach include improved cosmesis allowed by preservation of the globe, and excellent anterior and lateral exposure of the cavernous sinus and its associated structures.

One should address functional and cosmetic deficits created by the tumor or by the intervention in a single-stage surgery if it is safe for the patient. If temporary facial palsy is anticipated, corneal protection using lubricants and/or a temporary lateral tarsorrhaphy is usually adequate. Grafting of the facial nerve, however, involves a longer recovery period. Thus, insertion of a gold weight into the upper eyelid is advisable. Static fascial slings or muscle transpositions are indicated when immediate reconstruction of the facial nerve is not possible.

A temporalis muscle transposition flap is adequate to separate the cranial cavity from the upper aerodigestive tract and to obliterate the dead space. Microvascular free flaps, such as the rectus abdominis flap (for soft tissue defects), the latissimus dorsi flap (for myocutaneous or massive defects), or the iliac composite flap (for defects requiring bone reconstruction), are indicated when the temporalis muscle or its blood supply will be sacrificed as part of the oncologic resection; when the patient requires a complex resection involving composite tissue flaps with skin and/or bone; or when the extirpative surgery leads to a massive soft tissue defect and dead space. These needs usually are anticipated during the surgical planning, and the patient and consultants (e.g., microvascular surgeon) are informed accordingly.

■ IMMEDIATE POSTOPERATIVE MANAGEMENT

Postoperatively, the patient should be admitted to an intensive care unit for continuous cardiovascular and neurologic monitoring. Appropriate laboratory tests are carried out to rule out postoperative anemia and electrolyte imbalance. Patients who required multiple blood transfusions should be screened for transfusion-induced coagulation disorders. A mild narcotic analgesia should be provided. Sedation that could interfere with the neurologic evaluation should be avoided.

If the ICA was dissected, ligated, or grafted, close monitoring of the patient's hemodynamic status and fluid balance is essential. A CT scan of the brain (without contrast) should be ordered on the first or second postoperative day to screen for intracranial complications, such as cerebral contusion, edema or hemorrhage, fluid collections, or pneumocephalus. When grafting of the ICA is performed, an angiogram should be obtained in the early postoperative period to assess the patency of the graft and to detect formation of a pseudoaneurysm.

The scalp and other wound drains should be kept on bulb suction until the drainage is less than 30 mL/day. The drain should be removed and the wound closed by means of an encircling stitch, which is placed at the time of surgery. If the cranial cavity is entered, wall suction is contraindicated owing to the risk of direct negative pressure on the central nervous system.

In most cases, the spinal lumbar drain is needed only during the extirpative surgery and may be removed upon completion of the procedure. If a significant risk of postoperative CSF leak exists, the spinal drain should be kept at the level of the patient's shoulder, and 50 mL should be removed every 8 to 12 hours. The lumbar drain is removed 3 to 5 days after surgery, and the lumbar puncture site is closed with an encircling stitch of 2–0 nylon placed at the time of surgery.

Follow-up is dictated by the nature of the tumor, the need for postoperative radiotherapy and/or chemotherapy, and the adequacy of the resection. In general, patients with high-grade malignancies should be examined every 6 to 8 weeks, patients with low-grade malignancies every 2 to 3 months, and patients with benign tumors every 6 to 12 months. An MRI should be obtained 3 months after completion of treatment and should be repeated in 6 to 12 months.

■ REHABILITATION

A tracheotomy for tracheal toilette and a gastrostomy tube for nutrition and hydration are often necessary during the perioperative period. Alternatively, patients with a proximal vagal paralysis may benefit from a medialization laryngoplasty and an arytenoid adduction procedure. Laryngeal framework surgery may be performed concurrent with tumor removal or during the early postoperative period.[13, 14] Laryngeal framework surgery improves the glottic closure, thus decreasing the risk for aspiration and restoring an adequate cough and voice. These improvements often obviate the need for a tracheotomy for the sole purpose of tracheopulmonary toilette.

Laryngeal framework surgery, however, does not improve the sensory deficits produced by denervation of the afferent pathways. Thus, patients with lower cranial neuropathies remain at risk for aspiration, nutritional deficiencies, and dehydration even after the glottic insufficiency has been corrected. An experienced speech-language pathologist can assist with the monitoring of the patient, recommend diet modifications, and provide intensive swallowing therapy.[15, 16]

Velopharyngeal insufficiency may be corrected by the use of a palatal lift prosthesis. Alternatively, a pharyngeal flap or a palatopexy (palatal adhesion procedure) may be performed in patients who do not tolerate the prosthesis.

A tumor in the ITF may cause eustachian tube dysfunction, which leads to conductive hearing loss. Preexistent presbycusis also may compound the hearing loss. A myringotomy for middle ear effusion and/or amplification facilitates communication for the patient. Some tumors may destroy the temporal bone or posterior cranial fossa, which leads to sensorineural hearing loss.

Patients with neoplastic invasion of the facial nerve may have facial weakness or paralysis, facial spasms, and epiphora. A gold weight (implanted in the upper eyelid) or surgical tightening of the lower lid may be necessary to protect the cornea. Corneal anesthesia associated with lagophthalmos due to facial nerve palsy or other causes requires aggressive measures (e.g., tarsorrhaphy) to prevent corneal injury. Trigeminal sensory dysfunction commonly is underdiagnosed. Preoperative evaluation of corneal sensation and the protective mechanisms of the eyelids will help in the planning of corrective measures.

COMPLICATIONS

Wound

Elevation of the scalp flap superficial to the galea compromises the blood supply to the remaining scalp. Patients who have been irradiated preoperatively and who also undergo a galeal flap or galeopericranial flap are at risk for necrosis of the scalp flap. Prolonged use of hemostatic clamps (e.g., Raney clamps) also can result in necrosis of the scalp. Debridement and reconstruction with the use of posteriorly based scalp flaps often are required to close the secondary defect.

Postoperative infection is most commonly the result of an inadequate separation of the cranial or orbital bone grafts from the SNT, a large dead space, a noncompliant patient, or partial necrosis of the scalp flap. Late wound complications are usually the result of osteoradionecrosis. Correction of the primary problem (e.g., communication with the SNT, loss of flap), debridement (usually requiring the removal of the bone flaps), and prolonged antibiotics for osteomyelitis (45 days, guided by culture and sensitivities) are the treatments of choice (Fig. 10–16).

Necrosis of the scalp is rare and is most often the result of poorly designed incisions and the prolonged use of hemostatic clamps. The latter may result in areas of ischemia,

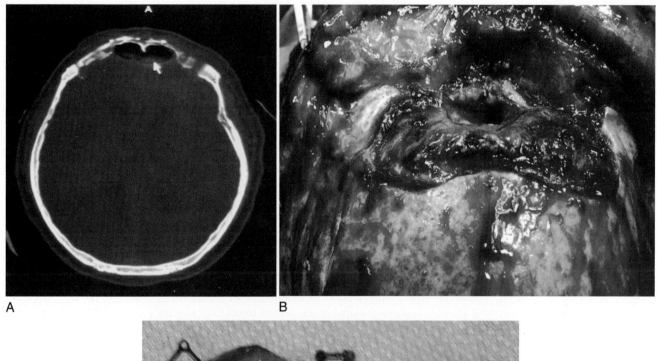

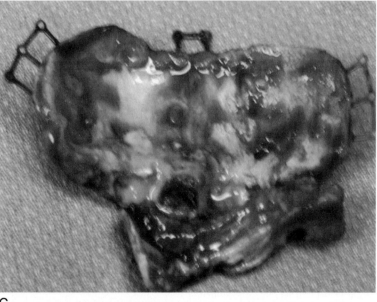

FIGURE 10–16 *A*, Coronal CT scan demonstrating epidural air and resorption of supraorbital bone graft in a patient with osteomyelitis after ACR. This patient lost the pericranial flap and hence the nasocranial separation. *B*, Intracranial view of the epidural cavity (bicoronal approach) after removal of the infected bone grafts. *C*, Note the abundance of granulation tissue.

particularly around the auricle, that can make the tissue susceptible to secondary infection.

Postoperative Sinonasal Bleeding

Postoperative bleeding from the SNT is usually self-limited or is easy to control with the use of topical vasoconstrictors and/or packing with hemostatic materials or self-expanding sponges. Significant postoperative nasal bleeding most commonly arises from a branch of the internal maxillary or anterior ethmoid arteries. If easily identifiable, the vessel may be clipped under endoscopic assistance. Angiography with embolization is reserved for patients in whom the bleeding site is not readily apparent—for example, patients who have undergone a reconstruction using a microvascular free flap. Postoperative bleeding from branches of the internal carotid artery (e.g., ethmoid, ophthalmic), however, is not usually amenable to embolization and may lead to an intracranial hematoma, requiring surgical exploration.

Trismus

Postoperative trismus is a common occurrence caused by postoperative pain and scarring of the pterygoid musculature and TMJ. Trismus improves dramatically if patients regularly perform stretching exercises for the jaw using devices such as the Therabite appliance.

Neurovascular Complications

Postoperative cerebral ischemia may result from surgical occlusion of the ICA, temporary vasospasm, and thromboembolic phenomena. Surgical dissection of the ICA can injure the vessel walls, resulting in immediate or delayed rupture and hemorrhage. In the event that a repair of the ICA is not possible, the ICA should be permanently occluded by ligation or by the placement of a detachable balloon or vascular coil. The occlusion should be performed as distal as possible (near the origin of the ophthalmic artery). The potential for thrombus formation decreases with a short column of stagnant blood above the level of occlusion.

Cranial Neuropathies

Deficits of the trigeminal nerve are the most common morbidity of surgery of the ITF. The loss of corneal sensation, especially in someone with facial nerve dysfunction, greatly increases the risk of corneal abrasion or exposure keratitis. Facial anesthesia may predispose the patient to self-inflicted injuries, including neurotrophic ulcers. The loss of motor function of the mandibular nerve causes asymmetry of the jaw opening and decreased force of mastication on the operated side, which may be further impaired by resection of the TMJ or mandibular ramus. Some report recovery of fifth nerve function after iatrogenic transection in a significant proportion of cases.

Temporary or permanent facial nerve dysfunction is common after transposition for ITF dissection and tumor removal. The facial nerve can suffer an ischemic injury caused by devascularization of its infratemporal segment or by traction to the extratemporal segments. A temporary paresis of the facial nerve with mobilization of the mastoid segment of the facial nerve should be expected. Frontal branches of the facial nerve are at risk for injury during elevation of the temporal scalp flap. Injury is usually the result of dissection in a plane that is superficial to the superficial layer of the deep temporal fascia, or it may be the result of compression during retraction of the flap.

Cerebrospinal Fluid Leak

A watertight dural closure may be difficult to achieve around nerves and vessels. Most CSF leaks can be managed nonsurgically by placement of a pressure dressing and a spinal drain to diminish the CSF pressure. Surgical exploration and repair of the dural defect may be necessary if the CSF leak does not resolve within a week.

We have encountered lateral skull base resection patients who developed profuse unilateral rhinorrhea postoperatively that was misinterpreted as a CSF leak. These cases were all associated with surgical dissection of the petrous ICA and probably were due to loss of the sympathetic fibers that travel along the ICA en route to the nasal mucosa. This situation produces vasomotor rhinitis that may be treated with the use of anticholinergic nasal sprays or botulinum toxin injections. Testing of the fluid for β_2-transferrin, however, is mandatory to rule out a CSF leak.

Tension Pneumocephalus

Intracranial air under pressure can act as a space-occupying lesion that compresses the brain parenchyma, causing lethargy, disorientation, slow mentation, or hemiparesis. A CT scan without contrast confirms the diagnosis. Initial treatment consists of aspiration of the air using a needle placed through a burr hole or osteotomy gap. In a rapidly deteriorating or unstable patient, this measure can be life saving. Recurrence of the tension pneumocephalus is rare and is usually associated with an inadequate cranionasal separation (e.g., loss of the pericranial flap), or it may be due to a noncompliant patient who blows the nose. Recurrent pneumocephalus may require bypassing the airway (i.e., tracheotomy or intubation) and/or surgical exploration to close any communication between the cranial cavity and the SNT.

A postoperative CSF leak is managed conservatively with bed rest, stool softeners, and a lumbar drain (50 mL every 6 to 8 hours). Persistence of the leak beyond 3 to 5 days, unabated by conservative measures, indicates the need for surgical repair. Surgical exploration, however, may be indicated as an initial therapy if loss of the reconstructive flap or dehiscence of the dural repair is suspected.

Meningitis/Abscess

Similar to pneumocephalus, CSF leak, and osteomyelitis, meningitis is the result of an inadequate separation of the cranial cavity from the SNT. However, it is important to recognize that meningitis can occur in the absence of a CSF leak and that its presentation may be atypical and caused by the use of perioperative prophylactic antibiotics. A CT scan followed by a lumbar puncture confirms the diagnosis.

Intravenous antibiotics with adequate CSF penetration are the treatment of choice. Any persistent communication between the cranial cavity and the upper aerodigestive tract should be closed as soon as the patient is stable enough to tolerate the surgery.

Management of intracranial/cerebral abscess is similar to treatment for meningitis. Abscess, however, usually requires drainage. Epidural abscesses usually require the removal of contaminated free bone grafts. This creates a deformity that should be corrected in a secondary surgical procedure.

Cerebral Edema/Contusion

Cerebral edema or contusion usually occurs as a result of excessive brain retraction. Systemic corticosteroids, stabilization of any hemodynamic problems, and correction of the electrolyte-fluid balance are essential for avoidance of further brain injury brought by the parenchymal swelling and subsequent increased intracranial pressure. Medical prophylaxis for seizures is recommended when there is a contusion of the brain parenchyma, or if brain has had to be removed as part of the oncologic surgery.

Orbital Complications

Epiphora

A dacryocystorhinostomy (DCR) diminishes the incidence of epiphora after resection of the medial maxilla. A DCR is performed by marsupializing the lacrimal sac after it has been transected from the lacrimal duct. Occasionally, stenoses of the DCR may require stenting of the lacrimal duct (e.g., Crawford tubes) or even a revision DCR. Another cause of epiphora is failure to restore the medial canthus, causing laxity and failure of the lacrimal pump mechanism. Similarly, a lax lower eyelid caused by paralysis of the facial nerve or failure to fix the lateral canthus may lead to lagophthalmos and epiphora. Tarsal strip surgery and canthopexy are indicated to resolve this problem.

Extraocular Muscle Limitation

Diplopia caused by dissection of the trochlea, postoperative edema, or removal of the orbital walls occurs in most patients in a self-limited fashion that typically lasts less than 4 weeks. Physicians should consider other causes for diplopia, however. Reconstructive grafts over the orbital walls may entrap the medial, lateral, or inferior rectus muscles, resulting in restriction of the range of motion and diplopia. Intraorbital dissection, such as that required when the periorbita is resected, or surgery of the cavernous sinus may injure the motor innervation of these muscles. A forced duction test helps to differentiate these two problems.

Enophthalmos

Enophthalmos is the result of expansion of the volume of the orbital cavity caused by resection of the orbital walls and is more pronounced when the periorbita is resected. It is best to prevent this complication by reconstructing the orbital walls with autogenous bone or titanium mesh (i.e., rigid reconstruction).

Blindness

Unexpected blindness after an anterior craniofacial resection is the result of injury to the optic nerve or interference with its blood supply caused by direct arterial injury, compression, or elevated intraorbital pressure. High-dose steroids and immediate orbital and/or optic nerve decompression are indicated for compression problems.

Endocrine/Electrolyte Abnormalities

Hyponatremia (serum sodium <130 mg/dL) may result from excessive fluid replacement or from the syndrome of inappropriate antidiuretic hormone (SIADH), which usually is caused by cerebral edema. SIADH is usually self-limited and may be treated by fluid restriction. However, administration of hypertonic (3%) saline solution is indicated when neurologic symptoms such as disorientation, irritability, changes in consciousness or mentation, and seizures are present.

Conversely, ischemia or traction injury to the hypothalamus may lead to diabetes insipidus (DI), which is caused by insufficient production of the antidiuretic hormone. DI is manifested by the inability to concentrate urine, resulting in voiding of large volumes that leads to hypernatremia and hypovolemia. Serum sodium greater than 145 mg/dL and a urine specific gravity greater than 1.020 mg/dL confirm the diagnosis. Aggressive fluid replacement and aqueous vasopressin (2.5 units every 4 hours) constitute the initial treatment.

Patients with diabetes mellitus should be monitored closely, especially if corticosteroids are being administered. Regular insulin, administered according to a sliding scale, commonly is required to control the glycemia.

Other electrolyte disorders, such as hypocalcemia, hypomagnesemia, and hypophosphatemia, may be encountered in patients who require extensive skull base surgery. These electrolytes should be replaced immediately using calcium gluconate 10% (10 mL at a rate of <1 mL/min), phosphate solution (10 to 15 mmol of sodium phosphate in 250 mL of 5% dextrose solution over 6 hours), and magnesium sulphate (2 to 4 g in 100 mL of normal saline solution over 30 minutes). Because of the prolonged nature of some cranial base surgeries, these electrolyte deficiencies may develop intraoperatively or during the immediate postoperative period. This is especially true in patients who require transfusion of more than 5 units of packed red blood cells.

REFERENCES

1. Janecka IP: Introduction. In Janecka IP, Tiedemann K (eds): Skull Base Surgery: Anatomy, Biology and Technology. New York, Raven Press, 1997, p 1.
2. Lang J: The anterior and middle cranial fossae including the cavernous sinus and orbit. In Sekhar LN, Janecka IP (eds): Surgery of Cranial Base Tumors. New York, Raven Press, 1993, p 99.
3. Snyderman CH, Sekhar LN, Sen CN: Malignant skull base tumors. Neurosurg Clin N Am 1:243–249, 1990.

4. Lewis JS, Castro EB: Cancer of the nasal cavity and paranasal sinuses. J Laryngol Otol 86:255–262, 1972.

5. Lund VJ, Harrison DF: Craniofacial resection for tumors of the nasal cavity and paranasal sinuses. Am J Surg 156(3 Pt 1):187–190, 1988.

6. Carrau RL, Myers EN: Neoplasms of the nose and paranasal sinuses. In Bailey BJ (ed): Head and Neck Surgery—Otolaryngology, vol 2. Philadelphia, Lippincott Williams and Wilkins, 1993, pp 1247–1265.

7. Schramm VL Jr, Myers EN, Maroon JC: Anterior skull base surgery for benign and malignant disease. Laryngoscope 89(7 Pt 1):1077–1091, 1979.

8. Shah JP, Sundaresan N, Galicich J, et al: Craniofacial resections for tumors involving the base of the skull. Am J Surg 154:352–358, 1987.

9. Pitman KT, Carrau RL: Endoscopic surgical anatomy of the paranasal sinuses. In Jho H-D (ed): Endoscopic Neurological Surgery. Switzerland, Karger Publishing (in press).

10. Frazell E, Lewis JS: Cancer of the nasal cavity and accessory sinuses: A report on the management of 416 patients. Cancer 16:1293, 1963.

11. Jackson RT, Fitz-Hugh GS, Constable WC: Malignant neoplasms of the nasal cavities and paranasal sinuses: (A retrospective study). Laryngoscope 87(5 Pt 1):726–736, 1977.

12. Snyderman CH, Carrau RL, deVries I: Carotid artery resection: Update on preoperative evaluation. In Instructional Courses, vol 6. St. Louis, CV Mosby, 1993, pp 341–344.

13. Pou AM, Carrau RL, Eibling DE: Laryngeal framework surgery for the management of aspiration in high vagal lesions. Am J Otolaryngol 19:1–7, 1998.

14. Netterville JL, Jackson CG, Civantos F: Thyroplasty in the functional rehabilitation of neurotologic skull base surgery patients. Am J Otol 14:460–464, 1993.

15. Murry R, Carrau RL: Clinical Manual for Swallowing Disorders. San Diego, California, Singular Publishing Co, 2001.

16. Carrau RL, Murry T (eds): Comprehensive Management of Swallowing Disorders. San Diego, California, Singular Publishing Co, 1998.

17. Carrau RL, Snyderman CH: Antibiotic prophylaxis in cranial base surgery. Infect Dis Dig 3:22–23, 1992.

18. Smith RR, Klopp CT, Williams JM: Surgical treatment of cancer of the frontal sinus and adjacent areas. Cancer 7:991–994, 1954.

19. Ketcham AS, Wilkins RH, Van Buren JM: A combined intracranial facial approach to the paranasal sinuses. Am J Surg 106:698–703, 1963.

20. Ketcham AS, Van Buren JM: Tumors of the paranasal sinuses: A therapeutic challenge. Am J Surg 150:406–413, 1985.

21. Tessier P, Guiot G, Derome P: Orbital hypertelorism. II. Definite treatment of orbital hypertelorism (OR.H.) by craniofacial or by extracranial osteotomies. Scand J Plast Reconstr Surg 7:39–58, 1973.

22. Panje WR, Dohrmann GJ 3d, Pitcock JK, et al: The transfacial approach for combined anterior craniofacial tumor ablation. Arch Otolaryngol Head Neck Surg 115:301–307, 1989.

23. Raveh J, Turk JB, Ladrach K, et al: Extended anterior subcranial approach for skull base tumors: Long-term results. J Neurosurg 82:1002–1010, 1995.

24. Nuss DW, Janecka IP, Sekhar LN: Craniofacial disassembly in the management of skull base tumors. Management of head and neck neoplasms. Otolaryngol Clin North Am 14:1465–1497, 1991.

25. Janecka IP: Surgery of Cranial Base Tumors. New York, Raven Press, 1992, pp 157–223.

26. Blacklock JB, Weber RS, Lee YY, et al: Transcranial resection of tumors of the paranasal sinuses and nasal cavity. J Neurosurg 71:10–15, 1989.

27. Cheeseman AD, Lund VJ, Howard DJ: Craniofacial resection for tumors of the nasal cavity and paranasal sinuses. Head Neck Surg 8:429–435, 1986.

28. Clifford P: Transcranial–facial approach for tumors of superior paranasal sinuses and orbit. J R Soc Med 73:413–419, 1980.

29. Fairbanks-Barbosa J: Surgery of extensive cancer of paranasal sinuses. Presentation of a new technique. Arch Otolaryngol 73:129–138, 1961.

30. Fisch U: The infratemporal fossa approach for the lateral skull base. In The Otolaryngologic Clinics of North America. Symposium of Skull Base Surgery. Philadelphia, WB Saunders, 1984, pp 513–552.

31. Sekhar LN, Schramm VL, Jones NF: Subtemporal-preauricular infratemporal fossa approach to large lateral and posterior cranial neoplasms. J Neurosurg 67:499, 1987.

32. Terz JJ, Young HF, Lawrence W Jr: Combined craniofacial resection for locally advanced carcinoma of the head and neck II. Carcinoma of the paranasal sinuses. Am J Surg 140:618–624, 1980.

33. Janecka IP, Sen CN, Sekhar LN: Facial translocation: A new approach to the cranial base. Otolaryngol Head Neck Surg 103:413–419, 1990.

34. Cocke EW Jr, Robertson JH, Robertson JT: The extended maxillotomy and subtotal maxillectomy for excision of skull base tumors. Arch Otolaryngol Head Neck Surg 116:92–104, 1990.

35. Catalano PJ, Biller HF: Extended osteoplastic maxillotomy. A versatile new procedure for wide access to the central skull base and infratemporal fossa [see comments]. Arch Otolaryngol Head Neck Surg 119:394–400, 1993.

36. Carrau RL. Snyderman CH: Surgical approaches to the infratemporal fossa (Chapter 84). In Myers EN (ed): Operative Otolaryngology–Head and Neck Surgery. Philadelphia, WB Saunders, 1997, pp 835–867.

CHAPTER 11

Cancer of the Nasopharynx

William Ignace Wei
Jonathan Shun Tong Sham

INTRODUCTION

Neoplasms of the nasopharynx encompass all malignant tumors arising from the epithelial lining, lymphoid tissue, and connective tissue, such as lymphomas and sarcomas. However, the most frequently encountered malignancies are those that arise from the epithelial lining, and these are referred to as nasopharyngeal carcinoma (NPC). These tumors exhibit varying degrees of differentiation.

The first clinical description of NPC appeared in the literature in 1837.[1] An article entitled "Primary Carcinoma of the Nasopharynx. A Table of Cases" that reported 14 patients suffering from NPC was published by Chevalier Jackson in 1901 in the United States.[1] A comprehensive report on 79 patients that emphasized their clinical features and the origin of the NPC was subsequently published.[2] In Asia, despite the marked geographic prevalence of NPC, especially in the Southeast China province of Guangdong, where NPC is designated as Guangdong tumor, there had been little published information on the disease until 1941. That year, Digby and colleagues[3] published a paper based on 114 patients with NPC whom they encountered in Hong Kong. The authors stated categorically the origin of the tumor and described, in detail, its clinical and pathologic features.

The management of NPC was mainly palliative in the early years, especially before the days of radiotherapy. Following the introduction of radium in 1924, radiotherapy was used for the treatment of NPC; however, the outcome was not favorable.[3] Curative treatment with long-term survival was possible only after the introduction of the linear accelerator in 1953.

EPIDEMIOLOGY AND ETIOLOGY

Nasopharyngeal carcinoma is an uncommon neoplasm in most parts of the world. The age-adjusted incidence for both sexes is less than 1 per 100,000 of the population per year in many countries.[4] This incidence varies from region to region and is highest in China,[5] Africa, and Alaska. Incidence also varies among different ethnic populations. For example, it is high among Greenland Eskimos[6, 7] and ethnic Southeastern Chinese, especially inhabitants of Guangdong province,[8, 9] where the reported incidence for men and women is 10 to 20 per 100,000 and 5 to 10 per 100,000, respectively.[4] A high frequency of NPC is also noted in Chinese immigrants to Southeast Asia[10] and California,[11] as well as to other parts of the world.[12] The incidence among Chinese born in North America, however, is lower than for those born in China.[13] These findings suggest that geographic, ethnic, and environmental influences are among the etiologic factors.

Consumption of salted fish has been suggested as a possible causative dietary factor because NPC is common among people whose diet contains a high proportion of salted fish.[14] A case-control study has shown that frequent consumption of salted fish before 10 years of age is associated with an increased risk of developing NPC.[15] This may be related to the presence of nitrosamine compounds in salted fish.[16]

Epstein-Barr virus (EBV) has a strong association with NPC and has also been associated with Burkitt's lymphoma.[17] This virus has been hypothesized to play an oncogenic role in NPC, in that the EBV genome and its associated antigens are consistently identified in biopsy specimens.[17,18] Patients with NPC also have higher serum EBV antibody titers, particularly of the IgA class, than do controls.[19,20] EBV, however, is unlikely to be the sole causative factor of NPC because it is widely present in all human populations. The high incidence of NPC among Southeastern Chinese and their descendants[12] suggests the presence of genetic factors, a suggestion that is further supported by the fact that NPC is four times more common in first-degree relatives of patients with the carcinoma than in controls.[21] Specific haplotypes (whole or part of the chromosome) of the human lymphocyte antigen (HLA) have been found to be associated with an increased risk of developing NPC.[22,23] The loci of these HLA have been localized to the short arm of chromosome 6. Studies based on affected sibling pairs have also shown the existence of a susceptibility gene that confers an increased risk for the development of NPC.[24] More recent studies of genetic alterations in NPC using comparative genomic hybridization have demonstrated alterations at multiple chromosomes. Defects include deletion of regions at 1p, 3p, 14q, 16p, and 16q, as well as amplification of 1q, 3q, 12p, and 12q.[25]

ANATOMY

The nasopharynx is the transitional area between the nasal cavity and the oropharynx. The average anteroposterior distance is 2 to 3 cm, and both the transverse and vertical diameters are 3 to 4 cm, with considerable individual variation.[26]

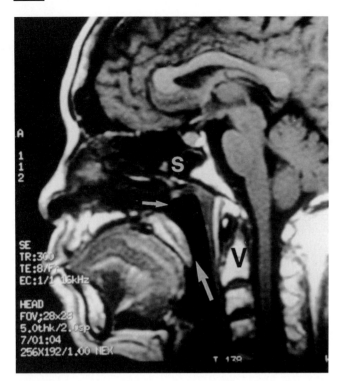

FIGURE 11–1 Magnetic resonance imaging. Sagittal section showing the boundaries of the nasopharynx. The posterior edge of the nasal septum *(horizontal arrow)* forms the anterior limit, and the sphenoid sinus (S) the superior limit. The superior cervical vertebra (V) and the soft palate *(vertical arrow)* form the posterior and inferior boundaries, respectively.

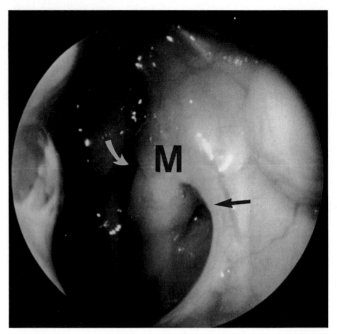

FIGURE 11–2 Endoscopic view of the right nasopharynx showing the eustachian tube orifice *(straight arrow)* and the medial crura (M). The space medial to the medial crura is the fossa of Rosenmüller *(curved arrow)*.

Anteriorly, the nasopharynx opens into the two choanae, which are separated from each other by the posterior edge of the nasal septum. The roof is formed by the undersurface of the body of the sphenoid, which slopes backward and downward to merge with the posterior wall formed by the arch of the atlas and the upper portion of the body of the axis. The floor opens into the oropharynx, and when upward movement of the soft palate closes this pharyngeal isthmus, the soft palate also becomes the floor (Fig. 11–1).

The lateral wall of the nasopharynx is formed by the orifices of the eustachian tube superiorly and the superior constrictor muscle inferiorly. The pharyngeal openings of the auditory tube are formed by an incomplete cartilaginous ring that is deficient inferolaterally. The cartilage on the medial side of the opening forms an elevation of mucosa called the *torus tubarius*. Medial to this elevation is the pharyngeal recess or fossa of Rosenmüller, which is a slitlike space of variable size and depth. The recess may be wide or narrow, and the recess may extend laterally—sometimes superior to the superior constrictor muscle. NPC is found most commonly in the fossa of Rosenmüller (Fig. 11–2). Early on, tumor in the fossa may infiltrate nearby structures rather than grow into the lumen of the nasopharynx. Because of the close proximity of the fossa to structures at the skull base, these may be affected early in the course of the disease, contributing to the presenting clinical features.

Near the choana, pseudostratified ciliated columnar cells are the main component of the epithelium of the nasopharynx. However, most of the lining of the epithelium in the posterior wall is made up of stratified squamous cells. There is a distinct basement membrane, and the lamina propria contains abundant lymphoid tissue. The muscular layer comprises the superior constrictor muscle, which is deficient in the superior aspect of the lateral wall where the auditory tube passes through it. Medial to the muscle is the pharyngobasilar fascia, which covers the posterior and lateral walls. This fascia is attached to the basiocciput superiorly and forms a median raphe in the posterior midline. Laterally, it is attached to the medial pterygoid plate, and inferiorly, it merges with the buccopharyngeal fascia. The fascial spaces around the nasopharynx contain important structures that influence the route of tumor spread:

1. The retropharyngeal space is located between the pharyngobasilar fascia and the prevertebral fascia and is a part of the retrostyloid portion of the paranasopharyngeal space. It is paramedian in location, lying lateral to the median raphe of the pharyngobasilar fascia. The retropharyngeal space contains the lymph node of Rouvière, which may be affected by lymphatic metastases (Fig. 11–3).

2. The parapharyngeal space is lateral to the pharynx and is divided by the styloid process and its attachments into the prestyloid and retrostyloid compartments. The former is lateral to the fossa of Rosenmüller and contains the maxillary artery and nerves. The retrostyloid compartment is located more posteromedially and contains the contents of the carotid sheath, the last four cranial nerves, the sympathetic trunk, and the upper deep cervical lymph nodes (see Fig. 11–3). Tumors can involve the prestyloid compartment by direct extension; once there, they can infiltrate the trigeminal nerve. The retrostyloid compartment can be affected by either

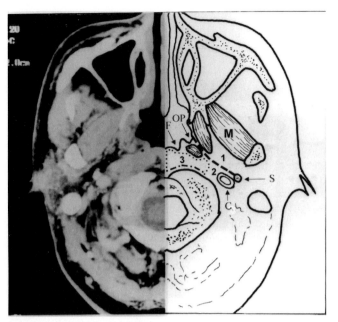

FIGURE 11–3 Cross-section of the nasopharynx showing the paranasopharyngeal spaces. C, carotid sheath; F, fossa of Rosenmüller; M, medial pterygoid muscle; OP, opening of the eustachian tube, S, styloid process. The *broken line* is the imaginary line joining the medial pterygoid plate to the styloid process. This separates the paranasopharyngeal space into the prestyloid space (1) and the poststyloid space (2). The *dotted line* is the pharyngobasilar fascia, which is also attached to the medial pterygoid plate and joins with the opposite side to form the median raphe. This fascia, together with the prevertebral fascia (*dash-dot line*), forms the retropharyngeal space (3).

direct invasion or lymphatic spread, leading to associated symptoms that may reflect the involvement of the respective cranial nerves.[9–12]

The arteries supplying the nasopharynx are the ascending pharyngeal, ascending palatine, and pharyngeal branches of the sphenopalatine artery, all of which are branches of the external carotid artery. The venous plexus beneath the mucous membrane communicates with the nearby pterygoid plexus. There is a well-developed submucosal plexus of lymph vessels that drains into the retropharyngeal lymph nodes. Efferents from this group of nodes, together with some lymphatics that drain into the nasopharynx directly, pass to the deep cervical lymph nodes.

☐ HISTOPATHOLOGY

NPC can be classified histologically according to the features seen under light microscopy and their response to treatment.[27–34] The most widely accepted classification has been established by the World Health Organization (WHO)[27] and includes three histologic types:

1. Keratinizing squamous cell carcinoma (WHO type 1). The characteristic feature of this type of carcinoma is squamous differentiation with the presence of intercellular bridges or keratinization over most of its extent (Fig. 11–4).

2. Nonkeratinizing squamous cell carcinoma (WHO type 2). This type of carcinoma shows evidence of a maturation sequence but does not exhibit definite squamous differentiation under light microscopy. The tumor cells have moderately well defined cell margins and show a stratified or pavement arrangement. There is no glandular formation or mucin secretion (Fig. 11–5).

3. Undifferentiated or poorly differentiated carcinoma, including lymphoepithelioma and anaplastic variants (WHO type 3). The tumor cells have indistinct cell margins with hyperchromatic nuclei, and some cells are spindle shaped. These cells either present as loose strands or form irregular masses lying within a lymphoid stroma (Fig. 11–6). When the density of the lymphocytic stroma increases to dominate the histologic picture, the term *lymphoepithelioma* is used.

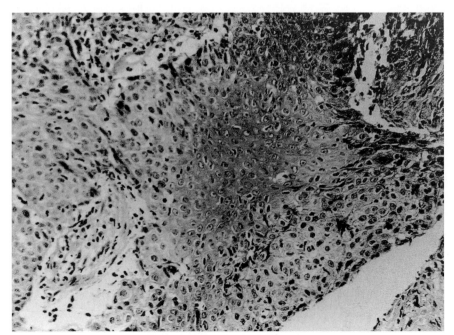

FIGURE 11–4 WHO classification type 1 carcinoma (hematoxylin-eosin, ×400).

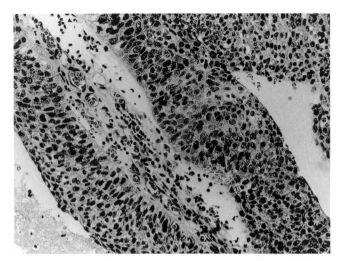

FIGURE 11–5 WHO classification type 2 carcinoma (hematoxylin-eosin, ×400).

This term, however, is inappropriate because the lymphocytic infiltration is not neoplastic, although there is also evidence to suggest that the lymphocytic infiltration plays a role in the pathogenesis of NPC.[28]

Over the years, modifications of the WHO classification have been proposed; subgroups with or without lymphocytic infiltration were added because these might be associated with prognosis.[29, 30] In 1991, the WHO revised its classification of NPC into two groups—squamous cell carcinoma and nonkeratinizing carcinoma. The latter group is further subdivided into differentiated and undifferentiated carcinoma.[31] The previous type 2 tumor is now a subgroup of the undifferentiated carcinoma. The revised classification takes into consideration that nonkeratinizing carcinoma, whether differentiated or undifferentiated, is associated with a better prognosis than is squamous cell carcinoma.[32] Nonkeratinizing

carcinoma is more sensitive to radiotherapy, which is the primary treatment modality,[33] and is also noted to be associated with characteristic anti-EBV serologic features.[34]

◨ CLINICAL FEATURES

Nasopharyngeal carcinoma affects relatively younger patients, compared with other malignancies of the head and neck region. In most reports, the male-to-female ratio is 3:1, with a median age of about 50 years.[11, 35] The symptoms of NPC are related to the location of the tumor, the degree of tumor infiltration into surrounding structures, and metastases.

Early symptoms are often trivial and are often ignored by the patient or misinterpreted by the physician. The most common mode of presentation of NPC is a painless unilateral metastatic cervical lymph node.[14, 36] Bilateral nodal involvement is not uncommon because the nasopharynx is a midline structure that has a rich bilateral lymphatic drainage. The lymph nodes around the digastric muscle and upper jugular groups are most frequently involved; these are often the largest nodes in the neck. These upper neck lymph nodes are nearly always affected before those of the middle and lower neck.[37] This orderly involvement of lymph nodes down the neck has been shown to be of prognostic significance.[38] Computed tomography (CT) is more sensitive than clinical examination in the evaluation of cervical lymph node involvement, and a significant proportion of patients are upstaged when CT examination is used as part of the evaluation.[39]

Nasal symptoms, in the form of unilateral nasal obstruction or blood-stained nasal discharge, are common when the tumor reaches a significant size and becomes ulcerated. Epistaxis is rarely severe and more frequently occurs as the presence of blood in the early-morning postnasal discharge.

Aural symptoms include hearing loss, tinnitus, and, less frequently, otalgia. Because the tumor originates from the fossa of Rosenmüller, close to the eustachian tube, it is not

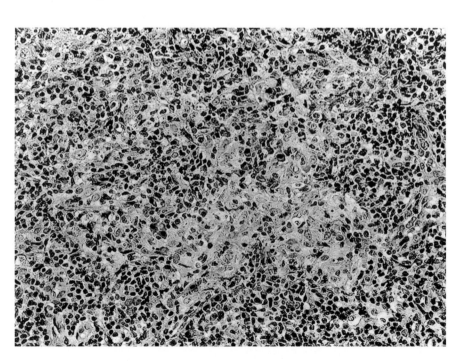

FIGURE 11–6 WHO classification type 3 carcinoma (hematoxylin-eosin, ×400).

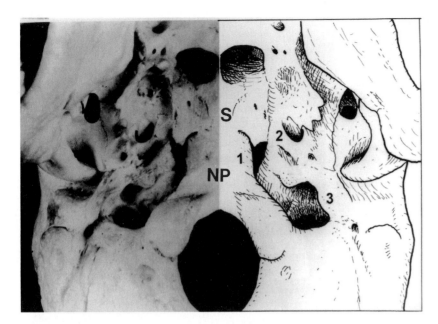

FIGURE 11–7 Base of skull showing the proximity of the nasopharynx to apertures where the cranial nerves pass through. NP, nasopharynx; S, posterior edge of the nasal septum; 1, foramen lacerum; 2, foramen ovale; 3, carotid canal.

surprising that the function of the auditory tube is often affected.[40] This leads to the development of fluid in the middle ear, which is responsible for the conductive hearing loss and, occasionally, tinnitus. Middle ear effusion is present in more than 40% of patients at diagnosis. For Chinese patients, the presentation of middle ear effusion after childhood should alert the attending clinician to the possible diagnosis of NPC.[41]

The incidence of cranial nerve involvement on presentation is about 20% and is related to direct tumor infiltration.[42] For some patients, this is the only presenting symptom.[43] Cranial nerves III, IV, and VI are involved when a tumor extends superiorly and affects the cavernous sinus. The trigeminal nerve is affected around the foramen ovale area, and cranial nerves IX to XII are affected at the parasopharyngeal space below the base of the skull, where the nerves lie near the tumor (Fig. 11–7). The incidence of single and multiple cranial nerve involvement is similar.

Other less frequent symptoms, such as trismus and headache, are related to extensive tumor infiltration of the pterygoid muscles and skull base, respectively. The incidence of distant metastasis on presentation in most patients is about 5%. Radiologically, the lesions may be lytic (66.0%), sclerotic (21.2%), or a mixture of lytic and sclerotic (12.8%).[44] Common sites of metastasis are the vertebrae and the femoral head. The main symptom associated with these metastases is severe bone pain. Less frequent sites of metastasis are the lungs and liver. Patients with metastases to these sites may develop pulmonary symptoms or altered hepatic function, respectively.

◼ DIAGNOSIS

Clinical Findings

Symptoms vary greatly in different patients with NPC, even when their disease is of similar stage. Some symptoms may be trivial; therefore, it is difficult to arrive at the diagnosis by history taking only. A full clinical examination of the head and neck region is essential, and particular effort should be exercised to detect cervical lymphadenopathy (Fig. 11–8), middle ear effusion, and cranial nerve involvement. Whenever NPC is suspected, a detailed examination of the nasopharynx is mandatory. The posterior nasal space in some patients can be adequately examined with a mirror. However, in other patients, this technique may be limited by anatomic variation of the nasopharynx and by the presence of excessive gag reflex.

Direct examination of the nasopharynx under topical anesthesia can be performed with the use of either the rigid or flexible endoscope. When a suspicious lesion is seen, a biopsy can be taken at the same time. Rigid 0-degree and 30-degree Hopkins rod endoscopes provide an excellent view of the nasopharynx on the side of the insertion (Figs. 11–9 and 11–10). The 70-degree endoscope can be used to view the opposite side of the nasopharynx when an anatomic variation,

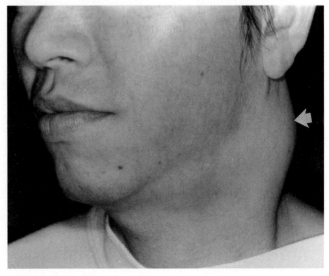

FIGURE 11–8 Clinical photograph of a patient with metastasis to a cervical lymph node *(arrow)*.

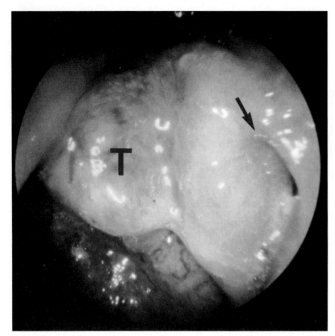

FIGURE 11–9 Endoscopic view (0° scope) of the left nasopharynx showing eustachian tube opening *(arrow)* and tumor (T).

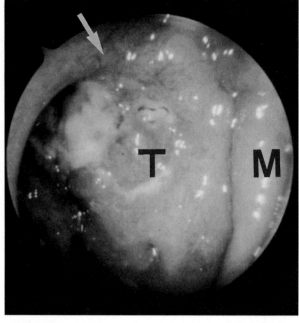

FIGURE 11–10 Endoscopic view (30° scope) of left nasopharynx showing medial crura of the eustachian tube (M) and tumor (T) in the posterior wall encroaching onto the septum *(arrow)*.

such as a deviated nasal septum, precludes introduction of the endoscope (Fig. 11–11). Alternatively, the 70-degree endoscope introduced through the mouth beyond the soft palate can provide a view of the entire nasopharynx (Fig. 11–12). These rigid endoscopes have no suction or biopsy channel. Therefore, a separate catheter has to be inserted alongside the endoscope to remove blood or mucus for an unobstructed view. A forceps also has to be inserted separately alongside the endoscope, or through the other nasal cavity, for biopsy.

A flexible endoscope with a suction and biopsy channel can be used to examine the nasopharynx more thoroughly than can be done with a rigid endoscope. However, the image obtained is inferior to that obtained with the rigid endoscope. The flexible endoscope can be inserted through one nasal cavity and then turned behind the nasal septum to examine the opposite nasopharynx. Thus, the entire nasopharynx can be adequately examined with only one passage of the endoscope. When there is difficulty in passing the

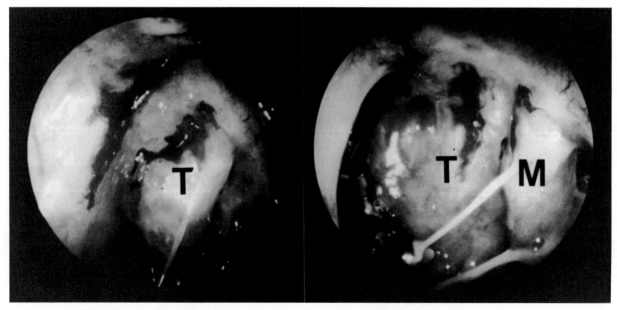

FIGURE 11–11 *Right*, Endoscopic view (0° scope) of the left nasopharynx, showing the medial crura of the eustachian tube (M) and tumor (T) in the posterior wall of the nasopharynx. *Left*, Endoscopic view (70° scope) inserted through the right nasal cavity, showing the same tumor (T) from the right side.

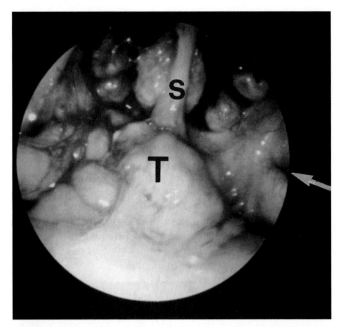

FIGURE 11–12 Nasopharyngeal carcinoma (T) seen with a 70° endoscope inserted behind the soft palate. The eustachian tube orifice (*arrow*) and the posterior edge of the nasal septum (S) can be identified.

endoscope through the nasal cavity owing to the presence of a large tumor or other anatomic variation, the flexible endoscope can be inserted through the mouth and manipulated to a position above the soft palate. Excessive mucus is removed by suction, and a biopsy is taken from the suspicious area as seen through the endoscope. Because only a small biopsy forceps can be inserted through the narrow channel of the endoscope, the tissue obtained may not be sufficient for diagnosis. However, the small size of the biopsy forceps means that it is useful for taking biopsies from the narrow confines of the pharyngeal recess. Therefore, the mucosa should be broken with the forceps before one of its jaws is inserted into the submucosa so that more tissue can be obtained for a more accurate biopsy.[45]

Serology

EBV is ubiquitous and affects the human population in many different ways. It may cause infections such as infectious mononucleosis and has also been found to be associated with Burkitt's lymphoma and NPC. The EBV is a double-stranded DNA virus that belongs to the herpes virus family. EBV-specific antigens in infected cells can be grouped into latent-phase antigens, early replicative antigens, and late antigens. Latent-phase antigens consist of the EBV-associated nuclear antigen (EBNA) and the latent membrane proteins (LMPs).[46] The early antigens include the early membrane antigen (EMA) and the early intracellular antigen (EA).[47] The late antigens are the viral capsid antigen (VCA) and the late membrane antigen (LMA).[48]

The immunologic response of a patient infected by EBV varies according to the associated disease that is manifested. Patients with NPC have a high level of immunoglobulin A (IgA) response to VCA and EA. This can be used as a diagnostic indicator.[49] The IgA anti-VCA is a more sensitive, but less specific, test than is the IgA anti-EA. Determination of levels of these antibodies has been used in the screening of NPC in endemic areas. Endoscopic examination and biopsy of the nasopharynx, aimed at early detection of NPC, have been carried out in patients with high IgA levels.[50]

A seroepidemiologic prospective study was carried out in Guangdong province in Southeast China to evaluate the efficacy of endoscopy versus biopsy in the diagnosis of subclinical NPC.[51] A total of 67,891 healthy persons between 30 and 59 years of age were tested for IgA levels against the VCA of the EBV. A total of 6102 (9%) subjects were found to have an elevated serum antibody titer. On clinical examination, 48 (0.8%) of the seropositive subjects had NPC, which was subsequently confirmed by histologic study. However, these patients had no symptoms related to the nasopharynx. Of the remaining 6054 seropositive patients, 130 were randomly recruited for endoscopic examination and biopsy of the nasopharynx. Complete clinical examination, including mirror examination of the postnasal space, was performed to exclude any obvious tumor in the nasopharynx. The patients then underwent fiberoptic endoscopic examination of the nasopharynx, and biopsies were performed under topical anesthesia. Biopsies of all patients were taken, using the technique described earlier,[45] from the same six sites—both pharyngeal recesses, both sides of the roof, and both sides of the posterior wall. Each biopsy specimen included both mucosa and submucosal tissue for histologic examination.

From these 130 subjects, a total of 780 biopsy specimens were obtained. The age of the subjects ranged from 30 to 61 years (median, 44 years). There were 71 men and 59 women. NPC was detected in 11 biopsy specimens obtained from seven patients. Of the 11 positive biopsy specimens, seven were from the pharyngeal recess (i.e., the fossa of Rosenmüller), three were from the roof, and one was from the posterior wall. In the biopsy specimens of four patients, carcinoma cells were present at one site in the nasopharynx; two patients had positive biopsies at two sites. In the remaining patients, three of the six biopsy sites in the nasopharynx revealed presence of tumor cells. Six of the seven patients with a positive biopsy had at least one positive specimen from the pharyngeal recess.

The endoscopic appearance of the nasopharyngeal mucosa of these 130 subjects revealed normal mucosal lining in 85.5%; among these, seven positive biopsy specimens were obtained. Other endoscopic findings, such as lymphoid hyperplasia, submucosal bulge, and erythematous mucosa, were noted in 14.5% of the biopsy specimens. Among these, four biopsy specimens showed the presence of tumor. Thus, the incidence of a positive biopsy is not related to the endoscopic appearance of the nasopharyngeal mucosa.[45]

From this prospective study, subclinical NPC was diagnosed in 5.4% of patients with elevated IgA titer against EBV. Based on this experience, we recommend that in high-risk regions, patients with elevated antibody levels should undergo an endoscopic examination of the nasopharynx. Regardless of whether the appearance of the mucosa is unremarkable, biopsy should be taken, especially from the pharyngeal recess. This will allow NPC to be detected early and, with prompt administration of treatment, the chance of eradicating the tumor is higher.

The level of IgA anti-EBV has also been shown to be related to the stage of the tumor, which is proportionate to the tumor burden.[52, 53] Although the level of IgA anti-VCA has been shown to decrease in NPC patients whose tumors have been eradicated,[53] its value in the monitoring of recurrences has yet to be established.[54] Recent studies have detected circulating cell-free EBV DNA in the plasma. Its quantity correlated with tumor recurrence; therefore, this may become a tumor marker for NPC.[55]

Cytology

Cytology may be helpful in the diagnosis of NPC in two ways. First, exfoliative cytology is employed for the detection of tumor cells from the primary lesion in the nasopharynx. In addition, fine-needle aspiration biopsy of cervical lymph nodes can lead to the diagnosis of metastasis to the neck.

The sensitivity of exfoliative cytology in the detection of NPC has been reported to range between 75% and 88%.[56, 57] This procedure involves scraping the mucosal surface of the nasopharynx with a swab, followed by cell collection, either transnasally or transorally. At present, because a biopsy of the nasopharynx can be easily obtained with the endoscope, exfoliative cytology is seldom used for diagnostic purposes. In view of the simplicity of exfoliative cytology, this technique is useful as a screening measure in NPC-endemic regions. Studies have shown that nasopharyngeal brushing along with polymerase chain reaction (PCR) may be a sensitive method of diagnosing NPC.[58]

Fine-needle aspiration of enlarged cervical lymph nodes has a high success rate in the diagnosis of metastatic NPC at the time of presentation.[59] However, the use of cytology in the diagnosis of recurrent cervical lymphadenopathy after radiotherapy is not as sensitive.[60] This is not surprising because it can be difficult to obtain a positive cytologic diagnosis after radiation when other head and neck malignancies are involved. The recent use of in situ hybridization for the determination of Epstein-Barr virus EBER1 RNA may improve the sensitivity and specificity of cytologic diagnosis of metastasis to the cervical lymph nodes.[61]

Radiology

CT is superior to conventional radiography for the imaging of NPC. CT is able to demonstrate soft tissue infiltration (a revelation that is not possible even with multidirectional tomography) (Fig. 11–13)[62] and is much more sensitive than conventional radiography in detecting erosion of the skull base.[63] The limitation of CT in the assessment of tumors in the nasopharynx lies in its poor tumor enhancement. Magnetic resonance imaging (MRI) is superior to CT in terms of multiplanar capabilities (Figs. 11–14, 11–15, and 11–16), better tissue specificity, and enhanced ability to delineate fascial planes and to distinguish tumor from inflammation within sinuses.[64] It is generally agreed that CT is more sensitive in demonstrating subtle bone erosion, which is not possible with MRI. However, in experienced hands, the reverse of this may be true.[65] Therefore, CT and MRI are more likely to be complementary, rather than competing, imaging techniques used to evaluate the deep tissue planes of the nasopharynx and the superior tip of the lateral pharyngeal recess.[66] This information cannot be obtained by endoscopic examination of the nasopharynx (Fig. 11–17).

The major contribution of cross-sectional imaging such as CT and MRI in NPC lies in determination of the extent of disease, including cervical nodal involvement after the diagnosis has been confirmed. CT and MRI are significantly

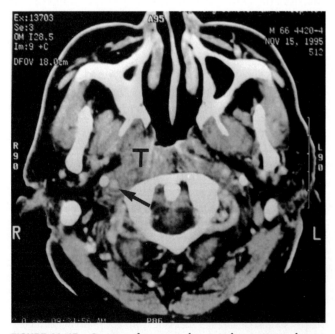

FIGURE 11–13 Computed tomography scan showing nasopharyngeal carcinoma (T) extending into the paranasopharyngeal space and encasing the internal carotid artery (*arrow*).

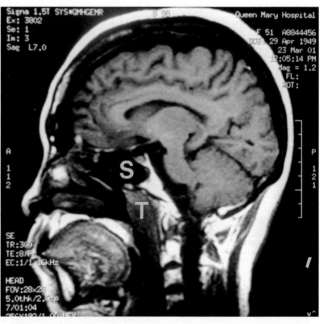

FIGURE 11–14 Magnetic resonance image; sagittal view shows tumor (T) below the sphenoid sinus (S).

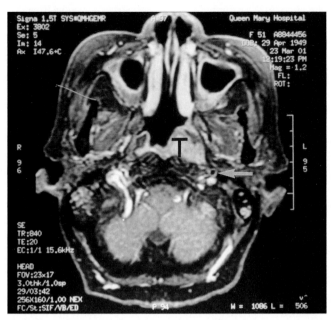

FIGURE 11–15 Magnetic resonance image; axial view shows tumor (T) extending into the paranasopharyngeal space close to the internal carotid artery (*arrow*).

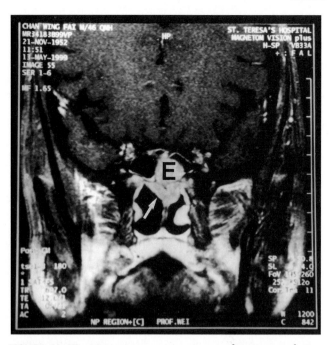

FIGURE 11–17 Magnetic resonance image; direct coronal view shows tumor (*arrow*) in the nasopharynx and its extension into the sphenoid sinus (E).

more accurate than clinical examination in the detection of tumor involvement in the following regions—the paranasopharyngeal space, oropharynx, nasal cavity, and choanae, and the ethmoid, maxillary, and sphenoid sinuses.[67–69] Accurate detection of tumor involvement is essential in the proper staging of NPC.[70] Identification of tumor extension into the paranasopharyngeal space, which is associated with the development of middle effusion, has been recognized as an independent adverse prognostic factor.[71] The two groups

of lymph nodes that are common sites of metastasis for NPC are the retropharyngeal nodes of Rouvière and the most cranially situated cervical nodes. These lymph nodes are readily identified by CT or MRI but are not accessible through clinical examination (Fig. 11–18).[72] Information gained through CT has resulted in a T-stage conversion in 23% of patients[66] and upstaging of N0 to N1 in 29.7% of patients.[72] Accurate identification of tumor extent by CT or MRI is also invaluable in the planning of radiotherapy.[72]

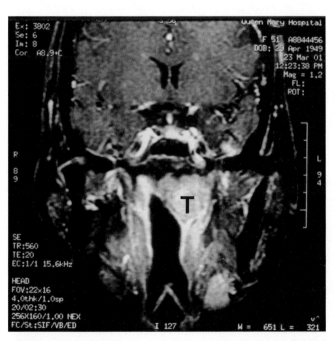

FIGURE 11–16 Magnetic resonance image; direct coronal view shows tumor (T).

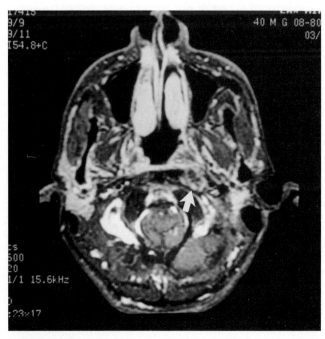

FIGURE 11–18 Magnetic resonance image shows enlarged left retropharyngeal lymph node (*arrow*).

▢ STAGING

As with other malignancies, a clinical staging system is essential in planning and evaluating the results of treatment for NPC. A simple classification for the staging of NPC was first described in 1952.[73] However, each stage described by this classification covered too wide a range of tumor involvement. Other frequently used clinical staging systems include the Union International Contre le Cancer (UICC),[74] the American Joint Committee on Cancer (AJCC),[75] and the Ho system.[76] Compared with other tumors of the head and neck, there is no widely accepted staging classification of NPC. The lack of a universally accepted staging system reflects, to some extent, the inadequacies of the various existing staging classifications.[77]

Previously, there was great disparity between the AJCC and Ho staging systems, but revision of the AJCC systemically in 1978 has made the two systems more similar. In more recent years, the experience of centers in endemic regions of Asia was incorporated into the UICC/AJCC stage classification system. These include grouping together tumors with upper and midneck nodal involvement; classifying tumors with paranasopharyngeal extension as advanced disease, similar to skull base erosion and/or cranial nerve involvement; and incorporating nodal level and laterality in the staging system.[78, 79] Therefore, in 1997, the AJCC stage classification was extensively revised,[80] with T1 and T2 tumors being grouped together as T1 tumor. Stage T2 tumor in the new staging system refers to disease that has extended to involve the nasal fossa, oropharynx, and/or paranasopharyngeal space. T3 refers to disease extension to the skull base and/or other paranasal sinus; T4 refers to tumor extension to the infratemporal fossa, orbit, or hypopharynx, or intracranially, or it denotes the presence of cranial neuropathy. For cervical lymph neck node metastasis, N1 refers to unilateral nodal metastasis, and N2 refers to bilateral nodal metastasis that has not reached the N3 designation, irrespective of the nodal size, number, and anatomic site. N3 in the new system refers to a nodal size larger than 6 cm (N3a) or extension to the supraclavicular fossa (N3b). The validity and superiority of the 1997 system, in terms of better prediction of survival across different stage groups, have been reported by a number of groups.[81–83]

A criticism common to the various N-staging systems is that the retropharyngeal nodes, which are the first-echelon nodes, are not taken into account by any staging system. These nodes, although difficult to examine clinically, can now be assessed by CT or MRI.[84, 85] There is, however, general agreement on M-staging, wherein M1 represents distant metastases, including any lymph node involvement below the level of the clavicle.

▢ MANAGEMENT

Radiotherapy

Because of the location of the nasopharynx and its relationship to many important structures, complete surgical excision is extremely challenging. In addition, NPC has a propensity to infiltrate surrounding tissues, making surgical clearance difficult. Fortunately, this tumor is radiosensitive;

therefore, the primary treatment modality for NPC is radiotherapy. For radiation treatment of NPC, the primary tumor and its direct extensions must be encompassed in the radiation field. The lymphatics in the upper neck are usually treated in the same target volume as the primary tumor.

Before radiotherapy begins, patients should be referred to the dentist for treatment of dental caries or tooth extractions and improvement of oral hygiene. Patients should also be instructed on the use of fluoride to prevent caries. This reduces the incidence of dental problems during and after radiotherapy.

The radiation dose given to the primary tumor is in the range of 66 to 70 Gy, with 60 Gy given to the neck. The delivery of this dose is usually in 1.8- to 2-Gy daily fractions, through two lateral opposing fields, with or without an anterior field (Fig. 11–19).[86, 87] The spinal cord is shielded from radiation when its tolerance is reached at 40 to 45 Gy. Because there is a high incidence of subclinical cervical node metastasis, even in the absence of palpable cervical lymph nodes, prophylactic radiation of the neck is performed and has been shown to improve survival.[88] The radiation dose delivered to the neck for this purpose is about 50 Gy.

The delivery of an adequate dose of radiation to the nasopharynx while sparing surrounding organs such as the brain stem, pituitary gland, temporal lobes, eyes, and ears has remained a challenge for radiation oncologists. Early reactions, such as swelling of the parotid glands, mucositis, altered taste sensation, and varying degrees of malaise, are not uncommon. These, however, nearly always subside with conservative management. After radiotherapy has been completed, skin reactions, submental edema, and facial puffiness may take a few months to subside.

Serious complications such as panhypopituitarism, encephalomyelitis, and temporal lobe necrosis are occasionally encountered and require appropriate treatment.[89, 90] Because of better understanding of the behavior of NPC, improvement in imaging techniques, and advances in radiotherapy

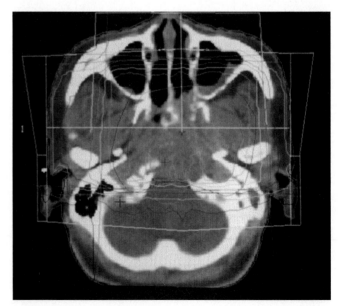

FIGURE 11–19 Radiation fields to the nasopharynx and neck for delivery of radical radiotherapy.

equipment, these complications can now be reduced or avoided. Minor problems such as increased dental caries and dry mouth related to radiation of the salivary glands are frequently encountered. Long-term complications related to radiotherapy are not infrequently encountered and include trismus due to fibrosis of the pterygoid muscles, osteoradionecrosis of the facial bones,[91] and neuritis that affects the last four cranial nerves. Long-term sequelae such as radiation sarcoma of the maxilla and soft tissues in the neck region are rare.[92] In recent years, the extent of tumor has been more accurately delineated by CT or MRI, which has allowed better planning of the delivery of radiation. Shielding of normal structures around the nasopharynx such as the pituitary and hypothalamus is now possible and has resulted in a reduced complication rate.[93]

Accurate delineation of the primary tumor with CT and MRI also allows three-dimensional conformal radiotherapy treatment. This achieves better tumor dose coverage while simultaneously reducing the dose to normal tissue. Studies on three-dimensional conformal radiotherapy have suggested improved treatment results.[94] The use of intensity-modulated radiotherapy (IMRT) improves target volume coverage and allows a greater dose to the gross tumor with significant sparing of the salivary glands and other critical normal structures and hence reduction in complications of treatment.[95, 96] Modification of the radiation therapy treatment schedule, for example, with the use of accelerated hyperfractionation, may also improve tumor control.[97]

Before the use of these precision radiotherapy modalities, the overall survival of patients with NPC was about 50%. The 5-year survival of patients diagnosed at the early stages ranges from 50% to 90%. For patients with more advanced disease, such as stage III or IV, the 5-year survival ranges from 17% to 80%.[83, 87, 94, 98, 99] Most recurrences occur within 2 to 3 years after cessation of treatment, and more than 90% of local and distant failures develop within 3 years.[100, 101]

Otologic Complications

The association of middle ear effusion with certain head and neck malignancies is well known.[102] Patients with NPC are particularly prone to middle ear effusion because the tumor, owing to its location, frequently causes eustachian tube dysfunction. This may result from mechanical or functional obstruction of the nasopharyngeal orifice of the auditory tube.[103] Middle ear effusion can also develop after radiotherapy because the radiation energy delivered to the nasopharynx probably contributes to eustachian tube dysfunction.[104] Myringotomy and insertion of a ventilation tube are the treatments of choice for middle ear effusion and should be performed before the start of radiotherapy. It has been shown that the rate of complications in the form of otalgia and persistent otorrhea is higher when the ventilation tube is inserted after radiotherapy.[105] For patients who develop middle ear effusion during or after radiation treatment, the insertion of a tube may not be beneficial. Although the ventilation tube will improve the patient's hearing immediately, approximately 29% of patients will subsequently develop perforation of the tympanic membrane and will later suffer from the hearing loss associated with tympanic membrane perforation. In addition, the risk

of these patients' developing intermittent otorrhea is 49%.[106] Careful judgment should be exercised before one resorts to insertion of a tube following radiotherapy. It may be more comfortable for the patient to have a dry ear—albeit with a mild hearing loss that could be managed with a hearing aid.

The cochlea and the brain stem auditory pathways are also located within the radiation field and may be affected by radiotherapy. Tinnitus is usually the presenting symptom, and evidence of inner ear damage can be reflected in abnormalities in auditory evoked response audiometry. Prolonged latency intervals are often present 1 year after completion of radiotherapy.[107] In a long-term prospective study of the effect of radiation on the inner ear, sensorineural hearing loss was noted in 14% of patients at 3 months following radiotherapy. Recovery in some patients was evident after 2 years, although 8% of patients developed progressive significant sensorineural hearing loss when seen at 4.5 years after completion of radiotherapy.[108] Administration of low-dose cisplatin before radiotherapy did not increase the rate of sensorineural hearing loss. Multivariate analysis has identified sex, age, and the development of postradiotherapy serous otitis media as significant prognostic factors for the development of persistent sensorineural hearing loss.[109]

Chemotherapy

Although patients with early NPC respond well to radiotherapy, those patients with more advanced disease are at high risk of local, regional, and distant failure when treated with radiation as a single modality. Because NPC is also chemosensitive, many attempts have been made to administer chemotherapy in addition to primary radiotherapy, with the goal of improving the treatment outcome. These attempts have included induction chemotherapy, concurrent chemoradiotherapy, adjuvant chemotherapy, or a combination of these. Results of many of these studies have been inconclusive because many trial participants had not been randomly assigned. A few randomized studies of induction chemotherapy have shown no significant improvement in survival in the arm that received chemotherapy.[110, 111] In addition, neither adjuvant chemotherapy[112] nor a combination of induction and adjuvant chemotherapy[113] has shown a difference in relapse-free survival or overall survival. With concurrent chemoradiotherapy and adjuvant chemotherapy, a prospective study of 147 patients reported a significant improvement in the 3-year progression-free survival (24% vs. 69%, $P < .001$) and in overall survival (47% vs. 78%, $P = .005$) compared with radiation alone. This North American study employed three courses of concurrent cisplatin with radiotherapy, followed by three courses of adjuvant chemotherapy using cisplatin and 5-fluorouracil.[114] The chemoradiation arm also demonstrated reductions in local, nodal, and distant relapse. This trial has been considered a breakthrough in the use of chemotherapy for NPC. However, there are concerns that treatment results of the radiation-alone arm were substantially worse than in many other reported studies. Moreover, many patients in the study had well-differentiated carcinoma, and there are still some doubts about the applicability of this treatment to endemic regions in which more than 95% of patients have undifferentiated carcinoma.

RECURRENT DISEASE

Diagnosis

Because both the primary NPC and its cervical metastases are radiosensitive, radiotherapy is the principal treatment for the disease. Radical doses of radiation are given to the nasopharynx and also to the neck because of the high incidence of cervical metastasis. Nevertheless, local failure in the form of persistent or recurrent tumor is not uncommon.[86] Regional recurrences range from 9.2% to 12%[115, 116] and may be associated with distant metastasis or tumor recurrence at the primary site.

For success to be attained in salvage treatment, early detection and treatment of persistent or recurrent local tumor are essential. When the target volume of the recurrence is small, eradication of the disease is still possible. Early treatment of persistent tumor also reduces the incidence of distant metastases. A prospective study was carried out to determine the efficacy of flexible endoscopic examination and biopsy in the detection of recurrent primary NPC, compared with the use of conventional mirror examination. The study also examined the regression time frame of NPC after radiotherapy.[117]

A total of 50 patients with NPC treated with a radical course of radiotherapy were studied. Examination and biopsy of the nasopharynx were performed starting from the second week after completion of radiation therapy. In 20 patients, examination was performed with a fiberoptic flexible endoscopy, and multiple biopsies were taken from suspicious areas in the nasopharynx. The size of each biopsy sample was usually 2 to 3 mm. In the other 30 patients, the examination was performed with a mirror, and the biopsy was taken with punch forceps inserted through the nasal fossae. The size of each biopsy specimen was approximately 4 to 5 mm. All patients had repeated examinations and biopsies performed every 2 weeks until their biopsy samples were negative on one or more occasions. The patients were then seen regularly every 6 weeks to 2 months for the first 2 years; the interval was extended to 3 months in the third year after treatment. All patients were followed for 21 to 31 months, with a median of 27 months.

The two groups of patients were comparable in terms of tumor stage and treatment techniques. Negative biopsy samples that were associated with abnormal macroscopic appearance occurred in both groups. These, however, were more frequently encountered in patients who were examined by the indirect nasopharyngeal mirror technique. Macroscopic abnormality was reported in 26 patients, three of whom (11.5%) also had a positive biopsy sample. Abnormal morphology was noted in 58 patients who were examined by fiberoptic endoscopy, and the biopsy samples of 24 patients (41.4%) revealed the presence of tumor. When the probability of positive biopsy obtained from the nasopharynx was plotted for the two groups of patients, conversion to negative biopsy was found to occur more quickly in the group assessed by mirror examination; the difference was significant ($P = .004$).[117] At 10 weeks after completion of radiotherapy, the overall probability of positive biopsy from the nasopharynx was approximately 10%; further analysis showed a 4% and 27% overall probability of positive biopsy for patients who underwent minor examination and fiberoptic endoscopy, respectively.

This study demonstrates that fiberoptic endoscopic examination and biopsy of the nasopharynx after radiotherapy are most effective in detecting persistent tumors early. It has also been shown that it takes about 10 weeks for the primary tumor to regress completely after radiotherapy. Therefore, it is appropriate for the nasopharynx to be examined at about 10 weeks after completion of radiotherapy for any persistent tumor to be detected. Treatment of residual tumor should be withheld unless the tumor persists beyond this period.[117]

Confirmation of tumor recurrence in the cervical lymph nodes is more difficult. Fine-needle aspiration is not helpful because the findings are frequently equivocal owing to the effects of radiotherapy. At this stage, even Tru-Cut biopsies may not be conclusive. CT may suggest recurrence of disease when it shows a hypodense center of the node and when the lesion size is seen to increase on follow-up. However, definitive diagnosis requires histologic confirmation.

[18]F fluorodeoxyglucose positron emission tomography ([18]FDG-PET) has been shown to be superior to CT in the detection of cervical lymph node metastases in nasopharyngeal carcinoma before radiotherapy, and it may be used to define tumor stage more accurately before treatment.[118] The efficacy of [18]FDG-PET in the detection of residual or recurrent tumor in the nasopharynx after radiotherapy has been documented,[119] with an accuracy of 97%; this is superior to CT.[120]

Treatment of Recurrent Tumor in the Nasopharynx

Recurrent tumor in the nasopharynx can be managed with a second course of radical external radiotherapy. The recommended radiation dose must exceed 60 Gy if the eradication of those tumor cells that survived the initial irradiation is to be achieved. In early reports, survival of up to 50% has been reported.[121] A large retrospective review of treatment results after local recurrence showed that successful local salvage was achieved in 32% of patients who received reradiation. The cumulative incidence of late post-reradiation sequelae was 24%, and treatment mortality was 1.8%.[122]

The response of surrounding tissues to further radiotherapy, however, limits the radiation dose that can be delivered. Even with a single dose of external radiation, neuroendocrine and soft tissue damage is not negligible.[89, 90] When the patient undergoes a second course of radiation, the incidence of complications can be expected to escalate. Certain neurologic complications, such as temporal lobe necrosis,[123] cranial nerve palsies, and brain stem damage, as well as other problems, such as trismus and deafness, can be incapacitating. However, the development of precision radiotherapy, including three-dimensional radiotherapy planning, intensity-modulated radiotherapy, and stereotactic radiotherapy, may mean that a second course of external radiotherapy can be given with sufficient efficacy and acceptable adverse effects. Nevertheless, long-term follow-up data are awaited regarding the benefits of their use in recurrent disease.[124]

Brachytherapy

Brachytherapy delivers a high dose of radiation to recurrent tumor. However, the amount of radiation delivered to adjacent tissues is less because a rapidly decreasing dosage is applied away from the radiation source. Brachytherapy has the added advantage of providing radiation at a continuous, slow dose rate, which may confer additional radiobiologic advantage over fractionated external beam radiation. Earlier experience with brachytherapy in the treatment of NPC was limited to intracavitary therapy.[125, 126] The radiation source of brachytherapy was placed in a tube or mold. Because of the irregular contour of the nasopharynx, it was sometimes difficult to apply the radiation source accurately to give the necessary tumoricidal dose. To circumvent this problem, interstitial implants have been used to manage small recurrent tumors in the nasopharynx.[127] For this form of application of brachytherapy to be effective, accurate insertion of the implant into the tumor is mandatory.

The most commonly employed radiation source implanted is the gold grain (^{198}Au). Although gold grains have been implanted transnasally with success,[128] they are more precisely inserted through the palate-splitting approach.[129] Radioactive gold grains are inserted according to a predefined geometric distribution so that a 1-cm-thick layer of tissue is treated with the implanted radiation source. Recurrent tumor in the nasopharynx is then exposed by splitting of the palate along the midline. In some instances, the posterior part of the hard palate is also removed so that an unobstructed view of the tumor can be gained. A specially designed introducer is loaded with gold grains and is placed through the mouth with the tip inserted into the tumor. The gold grains are then permanently implanted,

under direct vision, into the tumor. The number of gold grains implanted depends on the size and the location of the tumor (Figs. 11–20 and 11–21). After implantation of gold grains, the palatal wound is closed in layers. During the surgical procedure, lead shielding is required to protect all medical personnel in the operating room.

With this method of treatment, initial results showed that the probability of tumor control in the nasopharynx was 80% at 5 years for disease localized to the nasopharynx.[130] For this treatment to be effective, the recurrent tumor must be small and localized to the nasopharynx, with no invasion of bone. Long-term results of the treatment of 106 patients with gold grain implantation as the brachytherapy source showed that the 5-year local control rates for persistent disease and first recurrent disease were 87% and 63%, respectively. The 5-year disease-free survival rates for these two groups of patients were 68% and 60%, respectively.[131] Headache and palatal fistula occurred in about 28% and 19% of patients, respectively. The former can be managed conservatively and the palatal fistula can be closed surgically or, alternatively, the patient may elect to wear a palatal prosthesis. No other significant sequelae have been associated with this form of treatment, and this approach is recommended for management of small recurrent NPC localized in the nasopharynx.

Surgical Resection

When recurrent tumor in the nasopharynx has extended to the paranasopharyngeal space or has become too extensive

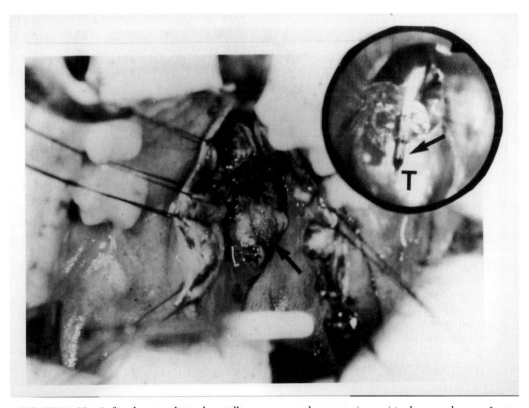

FIGURE 11–20   Soft palate is split in the midline to expose the tumor *(arrow)* in the nasopharynx. *Inset,* Flexible endoscope is inserted transnasally at the same time to monitor the accurate implantation of gold grains. The tip of the gold-grain introducer *(arrow)* is about to enter the tumor (T).

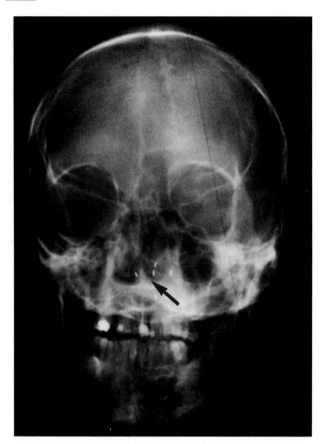

FIGURE 11–21 Plain radiograph of the skull following gold-grain (*arrow*) implantation.

to be treated by implantation of gold grains, or when the tumor has recurred after brachytherapy, the only chance of salvage without excessive risk of complications from a third course of radiotherapy is surgical resection.

The problems associated with surgical salvage of NPC lie in the fact that the nasopharynx is located in the center of the head, which makes it difficult to approach; it is also difficult to obtain adequate exposure of the region for a safe oncologic procedure. Recurrent tumors in the nasopharynx are located anterior to the brain stem and the upper cervical spine, which renders a posterior approach impractical. Intracranial approaches have been described for surgical resection of recurrent NPC. However, associated morbidities, such as cerebrospinal fluid (CSF) leak, meningitis, and encephalocele, are significant because the subarachnoid space is exposed to the pathogens of the nasal cavity.[132]

The various anterior approaches to the nasopharynx via the transantral or transnasal route do not provide adequate exposure for complete removal of tumor.[133] Even with downfracturing of the hard palate after transverse maxillary osteotomy,[134, 135] exposure of the lateral walls of the nasopharynx is not entirely satisfactory. The lateral approach to the nasopharynx has also been described. To reach the tumor, a radical mastoidectomy must be performed and exposure of the infratemporal fossa is necessary. Important anatomic structures, including the internal carotid artery, the fifth cranial nerve, and the floor of the middle cranial fossa, must be dissected and mobilized. Although tumors in

the nasopharynx and in the paranasopharyngeal space can be removed, the associated morbidity is not negligible.[136]

An approach from the inferior aspect to remove recurrent NPC employing the transpalatal, transmaxillary, and transcervical routes has been reported.[137, 138] However, the final exposure gained does not permit the dissection of paranasopharyngeal space under direct vision. This approach is applicable for tumors located in the central part of the nasopharynx; the resultant defect in the nasopharynx can be covered with a split-thickness skin graft. Morbidity associated with the operation is low provided that the internal carotid artery is protected.

We have described an anterolateral approach,[139] which provides adequate exposure of the nasopharynx and the paranasopharyngeal space using a "maxillary swing procedure." With the Weber-Fergusson incision, the soft tissue of the anterior wall of the maxilla is lifted just enough to allow osteotomy of the anterior wall of the maxilla. The mucoperiosteum over the hard palate is divided along the midline and the incision turned laterally to end behind the maxillary tuberosity. The soft palate is left intact. With the use of an oscillating saw, osteotomies over the anterior and posterior walls of the maxilla below the orbit are made together with the division of the hard palate along the midline. The maxillary tuberosity is also separated from the pterygoid plates

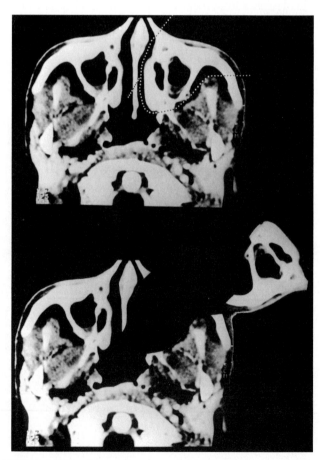

FIGURE 11–22 Schematic computed tomography scan. *Upper,* Planned osteotomy of the maxilla and the posterior part of the nasal septum (*dotted line*). *Lower,* The maxilla is swung laterally while remaining attached to the cheek flap.

by a curved osteotome. In this way, the entire maxilla is detached from the facial skeleton while retaining its blood supply from the anteriorly attached cheek flap (Fig. 11–22). When the entire osteocutaneous complex is swung laterally, wide exposure is obtained for the nasopharynx, the cartilaginous portion of the eustachian tube, and the paranasopharyngeal space tissue. The posterior part of the nasal septum, the rostrum, and the anterior wall of the sphenoid sinus can also be included in the resection. With the wide exposure, the internal carotid artery below the base of the skull can be dissected to effect a better tumor clearance. This approach allows for effective oncologic en bloc resection of a variety of tumors in the nasopharynx (Figs. 11–23 and 11–24).[140]

After tumor removal, the raw area created can be resurfaced with a graft using the mucosa from the inferior turbinate on the side of the swing. Well-vascularized flaps such as the temporalis flap or a microvascular free flap could also be used to cover the exposed critical microvascular structures, such as dura or carotid artery. The maxilla can then be returned and fixed onto the facial skeleton with miniplates. This wide exposure of the nasopharynx is necessary for tumor removal, with adequate margin, in the nasopharynx because pathologic study of nasopharyngectomy specimens has shown that tumors in the nasopharynx after radiation exhibit significant submucosal extension.[141] Results reported earlier on 45 patients who underwent nasopharyngectomy with this approach show a 5-year actuarial local tumor control rate of 52% and a 5-year actuarial disease-free survival of 43% (Fig. 11–25).[142]

Between February of 1989 and September of 1999, the maxillary swing nasopharyngectomy was employed in our hospital as the surgical salvage procedure for 71 patients with recurrent or persistent primary NPC after radiotherapy. Fifty-four patients had curative resection, and their follow-up period ranged from 6 to 125 months (median, 38 months). The 5-year actuarial local tumor control rate was 62%, and

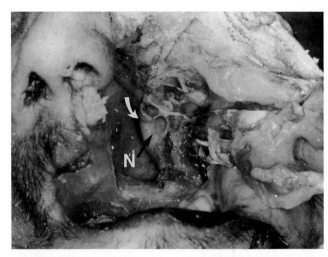

FIGURE 11–23 Postmortem dissection showing that when the maxilla is swung laterally, the nasopharynx (N), the fossa of Rosenmüller (*curved arrow*), and the opening of the eustachian tube (*straight arrow*) are exposed adequately.

the 5-year actuarial survival was 49%.[143] Approximately 25% of patients developed a palatal fistula, probably related to the previous radiotherapy and the surgical exposure. Surgical closure of these fistulas is possible when the fistula is small; for large palatal defects, the patient has to wear a palatal obturator for adequate swallowing and speech. More than 60% of patients developed some degree of trismus, which responded to conservative treatment. Overall, morbidity associated with this operation was not significant and was well tolerated (Fig. 11–26).

In summary, the difficulty in achieving local tumor control for patients who have recurrent NPC after radiotherapy is the inability to identify local recurrence early. If recurrences

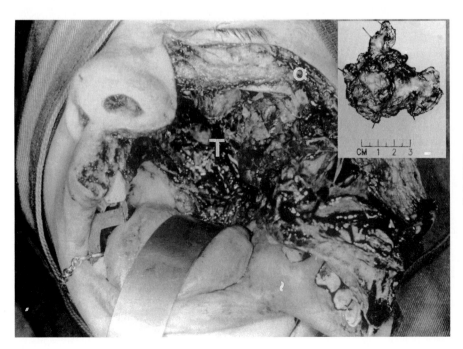

FIGURE 11–24 The right maxilla is swung laterally to expose the tumor (T) in the nasopharynx for resection. *Inset*, Resected specimen with tumor.

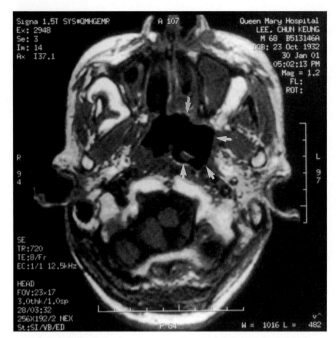

FIGURE 11–25 Postoperative magnetic resonance image shows soft tissue defect behind the left maxilla (*arrows*).

can be diagnosed when they are localized to the mucosa, interstitial brachytherapy offers a good chance that the tumor will be eradicated, with low morbidity. Larger tumors that are still localized to the nasopharynx and the paranasopharyngeal space are best managed with surgical resection.

Treatment of Recurrent Cervical Lymph Node Metastasis

Both sides of the neck are routinely included in the radiation field even if there are no palpable lymph nodes. Despite this, 9.2% to 12% of patients develop recurrence in the cervical lymph nodes.[115, 116] These patients frequently have distant metastases or recurrent tumors in the nasopharynx and generally have a poor prognosis. Isolated recurrent tumors confined to the neck are less common, ranging in incidence from 3% to 8%.[144, 145] When radiotherapy was combined with chemotherapy in the management of 1206 patients with NPC, the incidence of failure in the neck alone was reduced from 10% in 1978 to 5% in 1985.[146] In some of these patients, salvage therapy is possible.

When these cervical metastases were treated with further doses of external radiotherapy, the 5-year actuarial control rate of local disease for lymph nodes smaller than 4 cm in diameter was 51%. The overall 5-year survival rate was 19.7%.[147] In some institutes, excision of the lymph nodes followed by radiotherapy was the salvage treatment.[148] The number of patients reported was small, and the treatment plan was not uniform. Another therapeutic option was surgical salvage in the form of radical neck dissection. When this operation was carried out, the rate of control of disease in the neck was 66%, and the 5-year actuarial survival for this group of patients was 38%.[149]

The main criticism of the classical radical neck dissection as the treatment of choice for these patients is whether such an extensive operation is necessary to achieve control of the

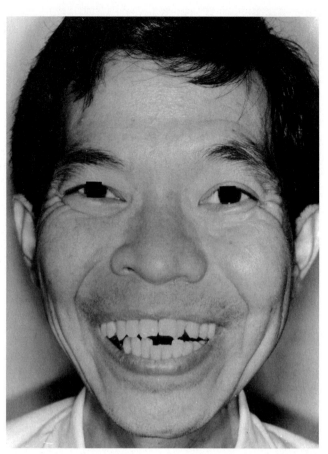

FIGURE 11–26 Postoperative view of a patient who underwent nasopharyngectomy employing the maxillary swing approach on the left side. The facial wound has healed and the teeth on the side of the swing are healthy.

neck disease. First, examination of the resected specimen following radical neck dissection sometimes revealed no tumor in any of the lymph nodes removed.[150] Second, in some patients, the cervical metastasis presented clinically as a solitary node, and it is thought that excision of the enlarged lymph node may be all that is necessary. Appropriate management of localized metastasis in the neck varies according to the pathologic behavior of the tumor. Assuming that tumor is present only in clinically positive lymph nodes, excision of these nodes would be adequate. As long as tumor does not extend beyond the capsule of the lymph nodes, selective neck dissection is adequate to clear the disease. Only when the tumor in the lymph nodes exhibits extracapsular spread should radical neck dissection be performed for salvage.

A prospective study was performed to evaluate the pathologic aspects of metastatic cervical lymph nodes in NPC after radiotherapy. The classical radical neck dissection was performed in 43 patients who developed localized disease in the neck after radiotherapy. After delivery, the entire radical neck dissection specimen was stretched out and pinned onto a foam board. The specimen was then immersed in 4% formaldehyde solution and, after complete fixation, the entire neck dissection specimen was cut into slices at 3-mm intervals (Fig. 11–27). The sequence of the tissue slices was recorded, and a histologic slide was made

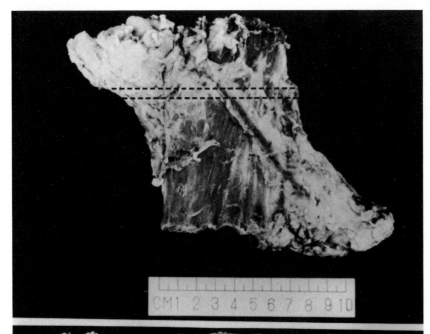

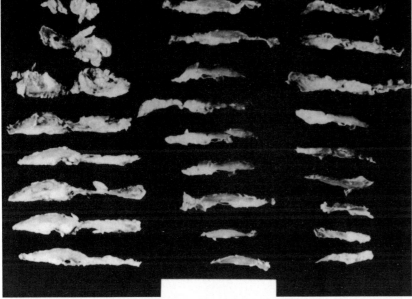

FIGURE 11–27 *Top,* Radical neck dissection specimen fixed in formaldehyde solution (formalin) and then cut into multiple parallel slices *(dotted line marks one slice). Bottom,* Consecutive slices obtained from one specimen, each 3 mm in thickness.

from each tissue block after processing. After microscopic examination of all the slides from one specimen, the total number of lymph nodes and the number of tumor-bearing lymph nodes in each patient can be determined. Consecutive histologic slides from this step-serial sectioning of the whole radical neck dissection specimen allowed spatial orientation of the tumor-bearing lymph nodes in relation to the surrounding structures to be reconstructed.

The number of histologic sections from each patient ranged from 18 to 36 (mean, 25). From 43 radical neck dissection specimens, a total of 1075 sections were obtained and a total of 2137 lymph nodes were identified. For each individual specimen, the number of nodes examined ranged from 17 to 110 (mean, 49.5). In three patients, the number of lymph nodes detected with the step-serial sectioning was 48, 58, and 76, respectively. However, no malignant cells

were identified in any of the nodes. Histologically, these lymph nodes showed only reactive hyperplasia with fibrosis.

For the remaining 40 patients who harbored tumor-bearing lymph nodes before operation, the number of nodes detected clinically ranged from 1 to 5 (mean, 1.5). The number of lymph nodes detected during surgery for this group of patients ranged from 1 to 8 (mean, 2.8). The number of lymph nodes that were histologically confirmed to harbor malignant cells ranged from 1 to 62 (mean, 7.4). Significantly more tumor-bearing lymph nodes were identified microscopically than were detected preoperatively and during surgery. Twenty-nine patients (73%) were found to have a greater number of tumor-bearing nodes in the neck dissection specimen than was clinically apparent (Fig. 11–28)[150]; the 294 tumor-bearing lymph nodes were subsequently found mostly in the superior aspect of the neck and in the posterior triangle. Step-serial

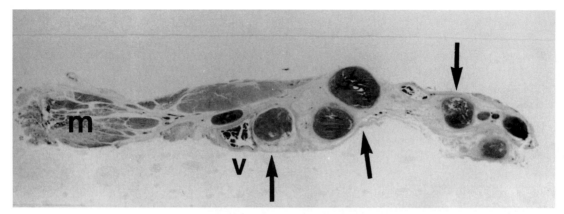

FIGURE 11–28 Histologic slide of neck dissection specimen showing more tumor-bearing lymph nodes *(arrows)* than were detected clinically. m, sternocleidomastoid muscle; v, internal jugular vein (hematoxylin-eosin, ×40).

sectioning examination showed that 38% (113/294) of the nodes were at level V, and 34% (99/294) were at level II. The respective figures for levels I, III, and IV were 5% (15/294), 16% (48/294), and 7% (19/294), respectively. Surgical clearance of lymph nodes of all levels in the neck is important, especially in the upper neck.

Microscopic examination of tumor-bearing lymph nodes showed that malignant cells destroy the intranodal structures and, in some nodes, the tumor breaches the capsule and infiltrates the surrounding tissue (Fig. 11–29). Of the 294 tumor-containing lymph nodes examined, 135 (45.9%) were discovered to have extracapsular spread. Of the 40 patients with lymph nodes that contained tumor, 28 patients (70%) harbored one or more lymph nodes that exhibited extracapsular spread. Another pathologic finding in 35% (14/40) of patients was the presence of isolated clusters of tumor within the stroma of the radical neck dissection specimen (Fig. 11–30).

These tumors could not be removed if selective or modified neck dissection was performed as the salvage procedure.

It was evident that metastasis in the cervical lymph nodes of NPC patients after radiotherapy is more extensive than was initially realized. A greater number of tumor-bearing lymph nodes were located in the neck than were clinically palpable. Radical neck dissection, which is associated with low morbidity and low mortality, is recommended for the treatment of cervical metastasis after radiotherapy in patients with NPC.

When the disease in the neck is extensive, such as when tumor-bearing nodes have infiltrated the overlying neck skin or have infiltrated the floor of the neck, then further brachytherapy following the radical neck dissection can be employed as the salvage procedure. The skin of the neck overlying the tumor is removed during the radical neck dissection, and hollow nylon tubes are placed precisely in the

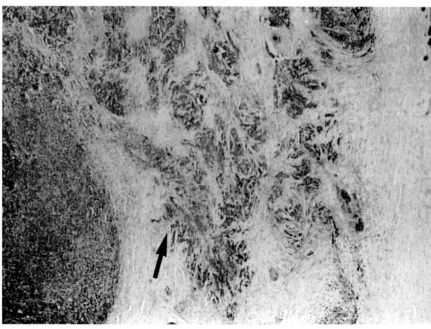

FIGURE 11–29 Histologic slide showing extracapsular spread of tumor *(arrow)* (hematoxylin-eosin, ×150).

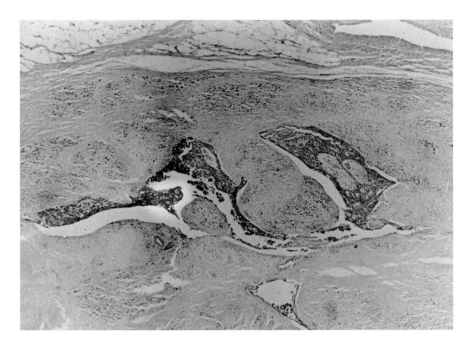

FIGURE 11–30 Histologic slide showing tumor cluster in tissue (hematoxylin-eosin, ×150).

operative site for afterloading of brachytherapy with iridium wire (Fig. 11–31). The cutaneous neck defect is then reconstructed with either a deltopectoral flap or a pectoralis major myocutaneous flap. The 5-year actuarial control of neck disease that was attained, with low morbidity, was around 60%.[151]

TREATMENT OF DISTANT METASTASES

Compared with other cancers of the head and neck region, NPC has a high propensity to develop distant metastases. The most common sites of distant spread are the liver, bones, and lungs. For a patient with a solitary metastasis to the lung, surgical removal may give worthwhile durable palliation.[152] NPC is sensitive to chemotherapy. With a combination of cisplatin, bleomycin, and 5-fluorouracil, a 75% response rate for recurrent and metastatic disease has been reported; 20% were complete responses.[153] Despite such good response, long-term survival for patients with distant metastases is, however, rare. A recent report suggests that long-term disease-free survival is possible in metastatic undifferentiated carcinoma of the nasopharynx when it is managed with a combination of chemotherapeutic agents.[154] In future trials to advance the treatment of metastatic diseases, more effective chemotherapeutic or biologically centered agents must be identified; alternatively, more effective administration regimens of existing agents may be developed.[155, 156]

REFERENCES

1. Jackson C: Primary carcinoma of the nasopharynx. A table of cases. JAMA 37:371–377, 1901.
2. New GB: Syndrome of malignant tumors of the nasopharynx, a report of seventy-nine cases. JAMA 79:10–14, 1922.
3. Digby KH, Fook WL, Che YT: Nasopharyngeal carcinoma. Br J Surg 28:517–537, 1941.
4. Muir C, Waterhouse J, Mack T, et al (eds): Cancer Incidence in Five Continents, vol 5, no. 88. Lyon, France, International Agency for Research on Cancer, 1987, pp 840–841.
5. Hirayama T: Descriptive and analytical epidemiology of nasopharyngeal cancer. In de-The G, Ito Y (eds): Nasopharyngeal Carcinoma: Etiology and Control, no. 20. Lyon, France, International Agency for Research on Cancer, 1978, pp 167–189.
6. Mallen RW, Shandro WG: Nasopharyngeal carcinoma in Eskimos. Can J Otolaryngol 3:175–179, 1974.
7. Nielsen NH, Mikkelsen F, Hansen JPH: Nasopharyngeal cancer in Greenland: The incidence in an arctic Eskimo population. Acta Pathol Microbiol Scand A 85:850–858, 1977.
8. Ho JHC: Nasopharyngeal carcinoma (NPC). Adv Cancer Res 15:57–92, 1972.
9. Ho HC: Epidemiology of nasopharyngeal carcinoma. J R Coll Surg Edinb 20:223–235, 1975.
10. Shanmugaratnam K: Cancer in Singapore—ethnic and dialect group variations in cancer incidence. Singapore Med J 14:69–81, 1973.

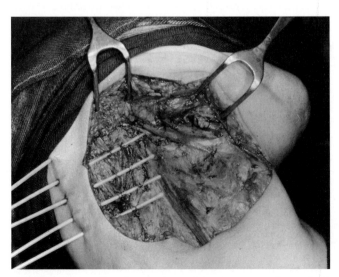

FIGURE 11–31 After the overlying skin was removed at radical neck dissection, hollow nylon tubes were placed over the tumor bed for afterloading brachytherapy.

11. Buell P: Nasopharynx cancer in Chinese of California. Br J Cancer 19:459–470, 1965.

12. Buell P: The effect of migration on the risk of nasopharyngeal cancer among Chinese. Cancer Res 34:1189–1191, 1974.

13. Dickson RI, Flores AD: Nasopharyngeal carcinoma: An evaluation of 134 patients treated between 1971–1980. Laryngoscope 95: 276–283, 1985.

14. Ho JHC: An epidemiologic and clinical study of nasopharyngeal carcinoma. Int J Radiat Oncol Biol Phys 4:183–197, 1978.

15. Yu MC, Ho JHC, Lai SH, et al: Cantonese-style salted fish as a cause of nasopharyngeal carcinoma: Report of a case-control study in Hong Kong. Cancer Res 46:956–961, 1986.

16. Fong YY, Chan WC: Bacterial production of demethylnitrosamine in salted fish. Nature 243:421–422, 1973.

17. Hausen HZ, Schulte-Holthausen H, Klein G, et al: EBV DNA in biopsies of Burkitt tumours and anaplastic carcinomas of the nasopharynx. Nature 228:1056–1058, 1970.

18. Huang DP, Ho HC, Henle W, et al: Presence of EBNA in nasopharyngeal carcinoma and control of patient tissues related to EBV serology. Int J Cancer 22:266–274, 1978.

19. Henle G, Henle W: Epstein-Barr virus-specific IgA serum antibodies as an outstanding feature of nasopharyngeal carcinoma. Int J Cancer 17:1–7, 1976.

20. Ho HC, Kwan HC, Ng MH, et al: Serum IgA antibodies to Epstein-Barr virus capsid antigen preceding symptoms of nasopharyngeal carcinoma. Lancet 1:436, 1978.

21. Yu MC, Garabrant DH, Huang TB, et al: Occupational and other non-dietary risk factors for nasopharyngeal carcinoma in Guangzhou, China. Int J Cancer 45:1033–1039, 1990.

22. Simons MJ, Wee GB, Chan SH, et al: Probable identification of an HLA second-locus antigen associated with a high risk of nasopharyngeal carcinoma. Lancet 1:142–143, 1975.

23. Zhu X, Chen R, Kong F, et al: Human leukocyte antigens-A, -B, -C and -DR and nasopharyngeal carcinoma in northern China. Ann Otol Rhinol Laryngol 99:286–287, 1990.

24. Lu SJ, Day NE, Degos L, et al: Linkage of a nasopharyngeal carcinoma susceptibility locus to the HLA region. Nature 346:470–471, 1990.

25. Fang Y, Guan X, Guo Y, et al: Analysis of genetic alterations in primary nasopharyngeal carcinoma by comparative genomic hybridization. Genes Chromosomes Cancer 30:254–260, 2001.

26. Adams WS: The transverse dimensions of the nasopharynx in child and adult with observations on its contractile functions. J Laryngol Otol 72:465–471, 1958.

27. Shanmugaratnam K: Histological typing of upper respiratory tract tumours. In Chr. Hedinger International Histological Classification of Tumours, no. 19. Geneva, World Health Organization, 1978, pp 32–33.

28. Zong YS, Lin H, Choy DTK, et al: Nasopharyngeal carcinoma and lymphoinfiltration. Oncology 48:290–296, 1991.

29. Hsu MM, Hsu HC, Lui LT: Local immune reaction in nasopharyngeal carcinoma, with special reference to its prognostic evaluation. Head Neck 11:505–510, 1989.

30. Reddy SP, Raslan WF, Gooneratne S, et al: Prognostic significance of keratinization in nasopharyngeal carcinoma. Am J Otolaryngol 16:103–108, 1995.

31. Shanmugaratnam K: Histological typing of tumors of the upper respiratory tract and ear. In Shanmugaratnam K, Sobin LH (eds): International Histological Classification of Tumors, 2nd ed. Geneva, World Health Organization, 1991, pp 32–33.

32. Nicholls JM: Nasopharyngeal carcinoma: Classification and histologic appearances. Adv Anat Pathol 4:71–84, 1997.

33. Shanmugaratnam K, Chan SH, de-The G, et al: Histopathology of nasopharyngeal carcinoma. Correlations with epidemiology, survival rates and other biological characteristics. Cancer 44:1029–1044, 1979.

34. Neel HB III, Pearson GR, Taylor WF: Antibodies to Epstein Barr virus in patients with nasopharyngeal carcinoma and in comparison groups. Ann Otol Rhinol Laryngol 93:477–482, 1984.

35. Sham JST, Wei WI, Tai PTH, et al: Multiple malignant neoplasms in patients with nasopharyngeal carcinoma. Oncology 47:471–474, 1990.

36. Huang SC: Nasopharyngeal cancer: A review of 1605 patients treated radically with cobalt 60. Int J Radiat Oncol Biol Phys 6:401–407, 1980.

37. Sham JST, Choy D, Wei WI: Nasopharyngeal carcinoma: Orderly neck node spread. Int J Radiat Oncol Biol Phys 19:929–933, 1990.

38. Sham JST, Choy D, Choi PHK: Nasopharyngeal carcinoma: The significance of neck node involvement in relation to the pattern of distant failure. Br J Radiol 63:108–113, 1990.

39. Sham JST, Cheung YK, Choy D, et al: Computed tomography evaluation of neck node metastases from nasopharyngeal carcinoma. Int J Radiat Oncol Biol Phys 25:787–792, 1993.

40. Su CY, Hsu SP, Lui CC: Computed tomography, magnetic resonance imaging, and electromyographic studies of tensor veli palatini muscles in patients with nasopharyngeal carcinoma. Laryngoscope 103: 673–678, 1993.

41. Sham JST, Wei WI, Lau SK, et al: Serous otitis media: An opportunity for early recognition of nasopharyngeal carcinoma. Arch Otolaryngol Head Neck Surg 118:794–797, 1992.

42. Neel HB III: A prospective evaluation of patients with nasopharyngeal carcinoma: An overview. J Otolaryngol 15:137–144, 1986.

43. Sham JST, Cheung YK, Choy D, et al: Cranial nerve involvement and base of skull erosion in nasopharyngeal carcinoma. Cancer 68: 422–426, 1991.

44. Sham JST, Cheung YK, Chan FL, Choy D: Nasopharyngeal carcinoma: Pattern of skeletal metastases. Br J Radiol 63:202–205, 1990.

45. Wei WI, Sham JST, Zong YS, et al: The efficacy of fiberoptic endoscopic examination and biopsy in the detection of early nasopharyngeal carcinoma. Cancer 67:3127–3130, 1991.

46. Reedman BM, Klein G: Cellular localization of an Epstein-Barr virus (EBV)-associated complement-fixing antigen in producer and non-producer lymphoblastoid cell lines. Int J Cancer 11:499–520, 1973.

47. Henle G, Henle W, Klein G: Demonstration of two distinct components in the early antigen complex of Epstein-Barr virus-infected cells. Int J Cancer 8:272–282, 1971.

48. Rowe M, Finke J, Szigeti R, et al: Characterization of the serological response in man to the latent membrane protein and the six nuclear antigens encoded by Epstein-Barr virus. J Gen Virol 69:1217–1228, 1988.

49. Ho JHC, Ng MH, Kwan HC, et al: Epstein-Barr-virus-specific IgA and IgG serum antibodies in nasopharyngeal carcinoma. Br J Cancer 34:655–660, 1976.

50. Zeng Y: Seroepidemiological studies on nasopharyngeal carcinoma in China. Adv Cancer Res 44:121–138, 1985.

51. Sham JST, Wei WI, Zong Y, et al: Detection of subclinical nasopharyngeal carcinoma by fibreoptic endoscopy and multiple biopsy. Lancet 335:371–374, 1990.

52. Henle W, Ho JHC, Henle G, et al: Antibodies to Epstein-Barr virus related antigens in nasopharyngeal carcinoma. Comparison of active cases and long-term survivors. J Natl Cancer Inst 51:361–369, 1973.

53. Henle W, Ho JHC, Henle G, et al: Nasopharyngeal carcinoma: Significance of changes in Epstein-Barr virus-related antibody patterns following therapy. Int J Cancer 20:663–672, 1977.

54. Lynn TC, Tu SM, Kawamura A: Long-term follow-up of IgG and IgA antibodies against viral capsid antigens of Epstein-Barr virus in nasopharyngeal carcinoma. J Laryngol Otol 99:567–572, 1985.

55. Lo YM, Chan LY, Chan AT, et al: Quantitative and temporal correlation between circulating cell-free Epstein-Barr virus DNA and tumor recurrence in nasopharyngeal carcinoma. Cancer Res 59: 5452–5455, 1999.

56. Lau SK, Hsu CS, Sham JST, et al: The cytological diagnosis of nasopharyngeal carcinoma using a silk swab stick. Cytopathology 2:239–246, 1991.

57. Dong HJ, Shen SJ, Huang SW, et al: The cytological diagnosis of nasopharyngeal carcinoma from exfoliated cells collected by suction method. An eight-year experience. J Laryngol Otol 97: 727–734, 1983.

58. Tune CE, Liavaag PG, Freeman JL, et al: Nasopharyngeal brush biopsies and detection of nasopharyngeal cancer in a high-risk population. J Natl Cancer Inst 91:796–800, 1999.

59. Chan MKM, McGuire LJ, Lee JCK: Fine needle aspiration cytodiagnosis of nasopharyngeal carcinoma in cervical lymph nodes. A study of 40 cases. Acta Cytol 33:344–350, 1989.

60. Cai WM, Zhang HX, Hu YH, et al: Influence of biopsy on the prognosis of nasopharyngeal carcinoma—a critical study of biopsy from the nasopharynx and cervical lymph node of 649 patients. Int J Radiat Oncol Biol Phys 9:1439–1444, 1983.

61. Dictor M, Siven M, Tennvall J, et al: Determination of nonendemic nasopharyngeal carcinoma by in situ hybridization for Epstein-Barr virus EBER1 RNA: Sensitivity and specificity in cervical node metastases. Laryngoscope 105:407–412, 1995.

62. Gonsalves CG, Briant TD, Harmand WM: Computed tomography of the paranasal sinuses, nasopharynx and soft tissues of the neck. Comput Tomogr 2:271–278, 1978.

63. Cheung YK, Sham JST, Cheung YL, et al: Skull base erosion in nasopharyngeal carcinoma: Comparison of plain radiographs and computed tomography. Oncology 51:422–446, 1994.

64. Chong VF, Fan YF, Khoo JB: Computed tomographic and magnetic resonance imaging findings in paranasal sinus involvement in nasopharyngeal carcinoma. Ann Acad Med Singapore 27: 800–804, 1998.

65. Chong VF, Fan YF: Skull base erosion in nasopharyngeal carcinoma: Detection by CT and MRI. Clin Radiol 51:625–631, 1996.

66. Mancuso AA, Bohman L, Hanafee W, et al: Computed tomography of the nasopharynx: Normal and variants of normal. Radiology 137: 113–121, 1980.

67. Yamashita S, Kondo M, Inuyama Y, et al: Improved survival of patients with nasopharyngeal squamous cell carcinoma. Int J Radiat Oncol Biol Phys 12:307–312, 1986.

68. Olmi P, Cellai E, Chiavacci A, et al: Computed tomography in nasopharyngeal carcinoma: Part I: T-stage conversion with CT-staging. Int J Radiat Oncol Biol Phys 19:1171–1175, 1990.

69. Sham JST, Cheung YK, Choy D, et al: Nasopharyngeal carcinoma: CT evaluation of pattern of tumor spread. Am J Neuroradiol 12: 265–270, 1991.

70. Chong VF, Mukherji SK, Ng SH, et al: Nasopharyngeal carcinoma: Review of how imaging affects staging. J Comput Assist Tomogr 23: 984–993, 1999.

71. Sham JST, Choy D: Prognostic value of paranasopharyngeal extension of nasopharyngeal carcinoma on local control and short-term survival. Head Neck 13:298–310, 1991.

72. Sham JST, Cheung YK, Choy D, et al: Computed tomography evaluation of neck node metastases from nasopharyngeal carcinoma. Int J Radiat Oncol Biol Phys 26:787–792, 1993.

73. Geist RM Jr, Portman UV: Primary malignant tumors of nasopharynx. AJR Am J Roentgenol 68:262–271, 1952.

74. International Union Against Cancer. In Hermanek P, Sobin LH (eds): TNM Classification of Malignant Tumors, 4th ed. Berlin, Springer-Verlag, 1987, pp 19–22.

75. American Joint Committee on Cancer: Manual for Staging of Cancer, 4th ed. Philadelphia, JB Lippincott, 1992, pp 34–35.

76. Ho JHC: Stage classification of nasopharyngeal carcinoma: A review. In de-The G, Ito Y (eds): Nasopharyngeal Carcinoma: Etiology and Control. Lyon, France, International Agency for Research on Cancer, 1978, pp 99–113.

77. Wei WI: A comparison of clinical staging systems in nasopharyngeal carcinoma. Clin Oncol 10:225–231, 1984.

78. Teo PM, Tsao SY, Ho JH, et al: A proposed modification of the Ho stage-classification for nasopharyngeal carcinoma. Radiother Oncol 21:11–23, 1991.

79. Lee AW, Foo W, Law CK, et al: N-staging of nasopharyngeal carcinoma: Discrepancy between UICC/AJCC and Ho systems. Union Internationale Contre le Cancer. American Joint Committee for Cancer. Clin Oncol 8:155–159, 1996.

80. American Joint Committee on Cancer. Manual for Staging of Cancer, 5th ed. Philadelphia, JB Lippincott, 1997.

81. Cooper JS, Cohen R, Stevens RE: A comparison of staging systems for nasopharyngeal carcinoma. Cancer 83:213–219, 1998.

82. Özyar E, Yildiz F, Akyol FH, et al: Comparison of AJCC 1988 and 1997 classifications for nasopharyngeal carcinoma. Int J Radiat Oncol Biol Phys 44:1079–1087, 1999.

83. Chua DT, Sham JST, Wei WI, et al: The predictive value of the 1997 American Joint Committee on cancer stage classification in determining failure patterns in nasopharyngeal carcinoma. Cancer 92: 2845–2855, 2001.

84. Chua DDT, Sham JST, Kwong DLW, et al: Retropharyngeal lymphadenopathy in patients with nasopharyngeal carcinoma: A computed tomography based study. Cancer 79:869–877, 1997.

85. King AD, Ahuja AT, Leung SF, et al: Neck node metastases from nasopharyngeal carcinoma: MR imaging of patterns of disease. Head Neck 22:275–281, 2000.

86. Mesic JB, Fletcher GH, Goepfert H: Megavoltage irradiation of epithelial tumors of the nasopharynx. Int J Radiat Oncol Biol Phys 7: 447–453, 1981.

87. Perez CA, Devineni VR, Marcial-Vega V, et al: Carcinoma of the nasopharynx: Factors affecting prognosis. Int J Radiat Oncol Biol Phys 23:271–280, 1992.

88. Lee AWM, Sham JST, Poon YF, et al: Treatment of stage I nasopharyngeal carcinoma: Analysis of the pattern of relapse and the results of withholding elective neck irradiation. Int J Radiat Oncol Biol Phys 17:1183–1190, 1989.

89. Lam KSL, Ho JHC, Lee AWM, et al: Symptomatic hypothalamic-pituitary dysfunction in nasopharyngeal carcinoma patients following radiation therapy: A retrospective study. Int J Radiat Oncol Biol Phys 13:1343–1350, 1987.

90. Woo E, Lam K, Yu YL, et al: Temporal lobe and hypothalamic-pituitary dysfunctions after radiotherapy for nasopharyngeal carcinoma: A distinct clinical syndrome. J Neurol Neurosurg Psychiatry 51: 1302–1307, 1988.

91. Peh WCG, Sham JST: Imaging of maxillary osteoradionecrosis. Australas Radiol 41:132–136, 1997.

92. Dickens P, Wei WI, Sham JST: Osteosarcoma of the maxilla in Hong Kong Chinese postirradiation for nasopharyngeal carcinoma. Cancer 66:1924–1926, 1990.

93. Sham JST, Choy D, Kwong PWK, et al: Radiotherapy for nasopharyngeal carcinoma: Shielding the pituitary may improve therapeutic ratio. Int J Radiat Oncol Biol Phys 29:699–704, 1994.

94. Leibel SA, Kutcher GJ, Harrison LB, et al: Improved dose distributions for 3D conformal boost treatments in carcinoma of the nasopharynx. Int J Radiat Oncol Biol Phys 20:823–833, 1991.

95. Lee N, Xia P. Quivey JM, et al: Intensity-modulated radiotherapy in the treatent of nasopharyngeal carcinoma: an update of the UCSF experience. Int J Radiat Oncol Biol Phys 53:12–22, 2002.

96. Hunt MA, Zelefsky MJ, Wolden S, et al: Treatment planning and delivery of intensity-modulated radiation therapy for primary nasopharynx cancer. Int J Radiat Oncol Biol Phys 49:623–632, 2001.

97. Wang CC: Accelerated hyperfractionation radiation therapy for carcinoma of the nasopharynx. Techniques and results. Cancer 63: 2461–2467, 1989.

98. Sham JST, Choy D: Prognostic factors of nasopharyngeal carcinoma: A review of 759 patients. Br J Radiol 63:51–58, 1990.

99. Schabinger PR, Reddy S, Hendrickson FR, et al: Carcinoma of the nasopharynx: Survival and patterns of recurrence. Int J Radiat Oncol Biol Phys 11:2081–2084, 1985.

100. Vikram B, Mishra UB, Strong EW, et al: Patterns of failure in carcinoma of the nasopharynx: I Failure at the primary site. Int J Radiat Oncol Biol Phys 11:1455–1459, 1985.

101. Vikram B, Mishra UB, Strong EW, et al: Patterns of failure in carcinoma of the nasopharynx: Failure at distant sites. Head Neck Surg 8:276–279, 1986.

102. Myers EN, Beery QC, Bluestone CD, et al: Effect of certain head and neck tumors and their management on the ventilatory function of the eustachian tube. Ann Otol Rhinol Laryngol 93(suppl 114):3–16, 1984.

103. Wei WI, Lund VJ, Howard DJ: Serous otitis media in malignancies of the nasopharynx and maxilla. J Laryngol Otol 102:129–132, 1988.

104. Brill AH, Martin MM, Fitz-Hugh GS, et al: Postoperative and postradiotherapeutic serous otitis media. Arch Otolaryngol 99: 406–408, 1974.

105. Wei WI, Engzell UCG, Lam KH, et al: The efficacy of myringotomy and ventilation tube insertion in middle-ear effusions in patients with nasopharyngeal carcinoma. Laryngoscope 97:1295–1298, 1987.

106. Ho WK, Wei WI, Yuen APW, et al: Otorrhea after grommet insertion for middle ear effusion in patients with nasopharyngeal carcinoma. Am J Otolaryngol 20:12–15, 1999.

107. Lau SK, Wei WI, Sham JST, et al: Early changes of auditory brain stem evoked response after radiotherapy for nasopharyngeal carcinoma—A prospective study. J Laryngol Otol 106:887–892, 1992.

108. Ho WK, Wei WI, Kwong DLW, et al: Long-term sensorineural hearing deficit following radiotherapy in patients suffering from nasopharyngeal carcinoma: A prospective study. Head Neck 21: 547–553, 1999.

109. Kwong DLW, Wei WI, Sham JST, et al: Sensorineural hearing loss in patients treated for nasopharyngeal carcinoma: A prospective study on the effect of radiation and cisplatin treatment. Int J Radiat Oncol Biol Phys 36:281–289, 1996.

110. International Nasopharynx Cancer Study Group: Preliminary results of a randomized trial comparing neoadjuvant chemotherapy (cisplatin, epirubicin, bleomycin) plus radiotherapy vs. radiotherapy alone in stage IV (> or = N2,M0) undifferentiated nasopharyngeal carcinoma: A positive effect on progression-free survival. International Nasopharynx Cancer Study Group. VUMCA I trial. Int J Radiat Oncol Biol Phys 35:463–469, 1996.

111. Chua DT, Sham JS, Choy D, et al: Patterns of failure after induction chemotherapy and radiotherapy for locoregionally advanced

nasopharyngeal carcinoma: The Queen Mary Hospital experience. Int J Radiat Oncol Biol Phys 49:1219–1228, 2001.

112. Rossi A, Molinari R, Boracchi P, et al: Adjuvant chemotherapy with vincristine, cyclophosphamide, and doxorubicin after radiotherapy in local-regional nasopharyngeal cancer: Results of a 4-year multicenter randomized study. J Clin Oncol 6:1401–1410, 1988.

113. Chan AT, Teo PM, Leung TW, et al: A prospective randomized study of chemotherapy adjunctive to definitive radiotherapy in advanced nasopharyngeal carcinoma. Int J Radiat Oncol Biol Phys 35: 569–577, 1995.

114. Al-Sarraf M, LeBlanc M, Giri PG, et al: Chemoradiotherapy versus radiotherapy in patients with advanced nasopharyngeal cancer: Phase III randomized Intergroup study 0099. J Clin Oncol 16: 1310–1317, 1998.

115. Hoppe RT, Goffinet DR, Bagshaw MA: Carcinoma of the nasopharynx: Eighteen years' experience with megavoltage radiation therapy. Cancer 37:2605–2612, 1976.

116. Chen WZ, Zhou DL, Luo KS: Long-term observation after radiotherapy for nasopharyngeal carcinoma (NPC). Int J Radiat Oncol Biol Phys 16:311–314, 1989.

117. Sham JST, Wei WI, Kwan WH, et al: Nasopharyngeal carcinoma. Pattern of tumor regression after radiotherapy. Cancer 65:216–220, 1990.

118. Kao CH, Hsieh JF, Tsai SC, et al: Comparison of 18-fluoro-2-deoxyglucose positron emission tomography and computed tomography in detection of cervical lymph node metastases of nasopharyngeal carcinoma. Ann Otol Rhinol Laryngol 109:1130–1134, 2000.

119. Peng N, Yen S, Liu W, et al: Evaluation of the effect of radiation therapy to nasopharyngeal carcinoma by positron emission tomography with 2-[F-18]fluoro-2-deoxy-D-glucose (PET-FDG). Clin Positron Imaging 3:51–56, 2000.

120. Kao CH, Tsai SC, Wang JJ, et al: Comparing 18-fluoro-2-deoxyglucose positron emission tomography with a combination of technetium 99m tetrofosmin single photon emission computed tomography and computed tomography to detect recurrent or persistent nasopharyngeal carcinomas after radiotherapy. Cancer 92:434–439, 2001.

121. Wang CC: Re-irradiation of recurrent nasopharyngeal carcinoma—treatment techniques and results. Int J Radiat Oncol Biol Phys 13: 953–956, 1987.

122. Lee AW, Law SC, Foo W, et al: Retrospective analysis of patients with nasopharyngeal carcinoma treated during 1976–1985: Survival after local recurrence. Int J Radiat Oncol Biol Phys 26:773–782, 1993.

123. Lee AWM, Ng SH, Ho JHC, et al: Clinical diagnosis of late temporal lobe necrosis following radiation therapy for nasopharyngeal carcinoma. Cancer 61:1535–1542, 1988.

124. Chua DTT, Sham JST, Hung KN, et al: Stereotactic radiosurgery as a salvage treatment for locally persistent and recurrent nasopharyngeal carcinoma. Head Neck 21:620–626, 1999.

125. Hilaris BS: Techniques of interstitial and intracavitary radiation. Cancer 22:745–751, 1968.

126. Wang CC, Busse J, Gitterman M: A simple afterloading applicator for intracavitary irradiation of carcinoma of the nasopharynx. Radiology 115:737–738, 1975.

127. Vikram B, Hilaris B: Transnasal permanent interstitial implantation for carcinoma of the nasopharynx. Int J Radiat Oncol Biol Phys 10: 153–155, 1984.

128. Harrison LB, Weissberg JB: A technique for interstitial nasopharyngeal brachytherapy. Int J Radiat Oncol Biol Phys 13:451–453, 1987.

129. Wei WI, Sham JST, Choy D, et al: Split-palate approach for gold grain implantation in nasopharyngeal carcinoma. Arch Otolaryngol Head Neck Surg 116:578–582, 1990.

130. Choy D, Sham JST, Wei WI, et al: Transpalatal insertion of radioactive gold grain for the treatment of persistent and recurrent nasopharyngeal carcinoma. Int J Radiat Oncol Biol Phys 25: 505–512, 1993.

131. Kwong DLW, Wei WI, Cheng ACK, et al: Long term results of radioactive gold grain implantation for the treatment of persistent and recurrent nasopharyngeal carcinoma. Cancer 91:1105–1113, 2001.

132. Van Buren JM, Ommaya AK, Ketcham AS: Ten years' experience with radical combined craniofacial resection of malignant tumors of the paranasal sinuses. J Neurosurg 28:341–350, 1968.

133. Wilson CP: Observations on the surgery of the nasopharynx. Ann Otol Rhinol Laryngol 66:5–40, 1957.

134. Belmont JR: The Le Fort I osteotomy approach for nasopharyngeal and nasal fossa tumors. Arch Otolaryngol Head Neck Surg 114:751–754, 1988.

135. Uttley D, Moore A, Archer DJ: Surgical management of midline skull-base tumors: A new approach. J Neurosurg 71:705–710, 1989.

136. Fisch U: The infratemporal fossa approach for nasopharyngeal tumors. Laryngoscope 93:36–44, 1983.

137. Fee WE Jr, Roberson JB Jr, Goffinet DR: Long-term survival after surgical resection for recurrent nasopharyngeal cancer after radiotherapy failure. Arch Otolaryngol Head Neck Surg 117: 1233–1236, 1991.

138. Morton RP, Liavaag PG, McLean M, et al: Transcervico-mandibulo-palatal approach for surgical salvage of recurrent nasopharyngeal cancer. Head Neck 18:352–358, 1996.

139. Wei WI, Lam KH, Sham JST: New approach to the nasopharynx, the maxillary swing approach. Head Neck 13:200–207, 1991.

140. Wei WI, Ho CM, Yuen PW, et al: Maxillary swing approach for resection of tumors in and around the nasopharynx. Arch Otolaryngol Head Neck Surg 121:638–642, 1995.

141. Wei WI Carcinoma of the nasopharynx. Adv Otolaryngol Head Neck Surg 12:119–132, 1998.

142. Wei WI: Salvage surgery for recurrent primary nasopharyngeal carcinoma. Crit Rev Oncol/Hematol 33:91–98, 2000.

143. Wei WI: Nasopharyngeal cancer: Current status of management. Arch Otolaryngol Head Neck Surg 127:766–769, 2001.

144. Bedwinek JM, Perez CA, Keys DJ: Analysis of failures after definitive irradiation for epidermoid carcinoma of the nasopharynx. Cancer 45:2725–2729, 1980.

145. Teo P, Ho JHC, Choy D, et al: Adjunctive chemotherapy to radical radiation therapy in the treatment of advanced nasopharyngeal carcinoma. Int J Radiat Oncol Biol Phys 13:679–685, 1987.

146. Huang SC, Lui LT, Lynn TC: Nasopharyngeal cancer: Study III. A review of 1206 patients treated with combined modalities. Int J Radiat Oncol Biol Phys 11:1789–1793, 1985.

147. Sham JST, Choy D: Nasopharyngeal carcinoma: Treatment of neck node recurrence by radiotherapy. Australas Radiol 35:370–373, 1991.

148. Tu GY, Hu YH, Xu GZ, et al: Salvage surgery for nasopharyngeal carcinoma. Arch Otolaryngol Head Neck Surg 114:328–329, 1988.

149. Wei WI, Lam KH, Ho CM, et al: Efficacy of radical neck dissection for the control of cervical metastasis after radiotherapy for nasopharyngeal carcinoma. Am J Surg 160:439–442, 1990.

150. Wei WI, Ho CM, Wong MP, et al: Pathological basis of surgery in the management of postradiotherapy cervical metastasis in nasopharyngeal carcinoma. Arch Otolaryngol Head Neck Surg 118:923–929, 1992.

151. Wei WI, Ho WK, Cheng AC, et al: Management of extensive cervical node metastasis in nasopharyngeal carcinoma after radiotherapy: A clinicopathological study. Arch Otolaryngol Head Neck Surg 127: 1457–1462, 2001.

152. Cheng LC, Sham JST, Chiu CSW, et al: Surgical resection of pulmonary metastases from nasopharyngeal carcinoma. Aust N Z J Surg 66:71–73, 1996.

153. Boussen H, Cvitkovic E, Wendling JL, et al: Chemotherapy of metastatic and/or recurrent undifferentiated nasopharyngeal carcinoma with cisplatin, bleomycin, and fluorouracil. J Clin Oncol 9:1675–1681, 1991.

154. Fandi A, Bachouchi M, Azli N, et al: Long-term disease-free survivors in metastatic undifferentiated carcinoma of nasopharyngeal type. J Clin Oncol 18:1324–1330, 2000.

155. Chua DT, Kwong DL, Sham JST, et al: A phase II study of ifosfamide, 5-fluorouracil and leucovorin in patients with recurrent nasopharyngeal carcinoma previously treated with platinum chemotherapy. Eur J Cancer 36:736–741, 2000.

156. Tan EH, Khoo KS, Wee J, et al: Phase II trial of a paclitaxel and carboplatin combination in Asian patients with metastatic nasopharyngeal carcinoma. Ann Oncol 10:235–237, 1999.

CHAPTER 12

Cancer of the Lip

Gregory J. Renner
Robert P. Zitsch III

◖ INTRODUCTION

The lip is a moderately common site for development of malignancy in the head and neck. Among cancers of the upper aerodigestive tract, cancer of the lip can be one of the most easily diagnosed and successfully treated. Even so, in as many as 15% of patients, the disease will prove to have an aggressive behavior manifested by recurrence, metastasis, and possible mortality.[1-4]

◖ ANATOMY OF THE LIP

The upper and lower lips are dominant features of the lower third of the face. The lips are formed embryologically by the union of five facial processes. Two lateral maxillary processes fuse with the centrally located frontomedian process to form the upper lip. Two mandibular processes fuse in the midline to form the lower lip. The lateral and superior borders of the upper lip are well defined by the melolabial (nasolabial) crease on each side and centrally by the base of the nose (Fig. 12–1). The peripheral border of the lower lip is also well defined by the mental crease.

The most characteristic feature of the lip is the vermilion (Fig. 12–2). It is a transitional mucosal surface that covers the free margin of the lip, bridging between the external skin and the internal buccal mucosa. The mucocutaneous junction forms the anterior vermilion border; the posterior point of contact of the lips, when they are held closed, marks the posterior vermilion border. The vermilion of the lip is the most anterior and proximal structure of the aerodigestive tract.

Another major feature of the lip is the orbicularis oris muscle, which derives from the second branchial arch. This muscle fills most of the body of the lip and completely encircles the mouth opening. It is a skeletal muscle and functions as a sphincter, which helps to regulate entrance into the mouth and to retain materials within the oral cavity. The orbicularis muscle of the lip is not a simple sphincter because in its periphery, it receives fibers from the many different surrounding facial muscles. These act together with the orbicularis to produce the various shapes and functions that are possible with the lips, such as smiling, frowning, kissing, blowing, whistling, articulating speech, and closing the lips.

Sensory innervation of the upper lip is supplied ipsilaterally by the second division of the trigeminal nerve, which enters the face as the infraorbital nerve. Sensory innervation of the lower lip is supplied on each side by the third division of the trigeminal nerve, which passes through the mandible as the inferior alveolar nerve and exits into the chin and lower lip as the mental nerve. The mental foramen is located in the outer cortex of the mandible, immediately below the second molar on each side.

The facial nerve supplies all motor innervation to the muscles of facial expression and to the orbicularis oris. The buccal branch of the facial nerve supplies the upper lip. Motor branches to the lower lip are supplied through the marginal mandibular branch.

Arterial supply to the lips is provided on each side principally by the facial artery, from which arise first the inferior and then the superior labial arteries. Both the inferior and the superior labial arteries pass medially through the lip in the submucosal plane, near the posterior vermilion line. Venous drainage of the lip is done by smaller vessels that drain principally in a lateral direction and into the facial vein on each side.

Lymphatic drainage from the lower lip originates as an interconnecting network of delicate vascular structures

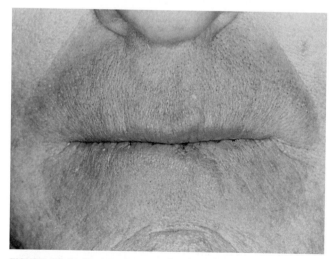

FIGURE 12–1 Patient 4 years after left V-lip excision; a distinct outline of the anatomic lip unit is demonstrated with melolabial and mental creases. Rhytid lines can be detected in a radiant pattern around the mouth opening.

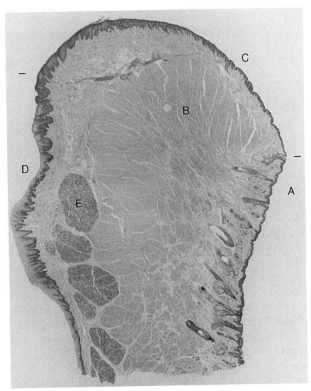

FIGURE 12–2 Histologic view of the lip in transection showing skin (A), orbicularis muscle (B), vermilion (C), mucosa (D), and minor salivary glands (E).

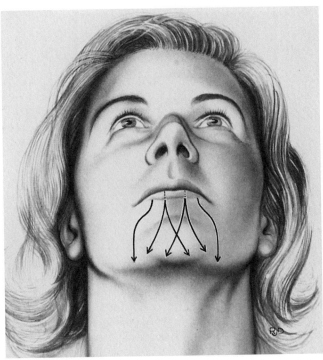

FIGURE 12–3 Patterns of lymphatic drainage from various portions of the lower lip. (From Zitsch RP III: Carcinoma of the lip. Otolaryngol Clin North Am 26:267–269, 1993.)

found in both the submucosal and the subcutaneous tissue planes. This lymphatic vascular plexus gives rise to approximately five lymphatic collecting trunks, which terminate in the regional lymph nodes.[5] Lymphatic trunks from the central third of the lower lip drain principally to the submental lymph nodes and occasionally also to the submandibular lymph nodes (Fig. 12–3). Lymphatic trunks from the lateral third of the lip on each side drain nearly always to the respective ipsilateral submandibular lymph nodes.[5]

Lymphatic drainage of the upper lip originates also as an interconnecting network of delicate vascular structures in the submucosal and subcutaneous planes. These connect into approximately five collecting trunks on each side, which then drain laterally from the midline and into the regional lymph nodes.[5] Most drainage from these trunks goes to the ipsilateral submandibular lymph nodes (Fig. 12–4). In some patients, limited lymphatic drainage to the preauricular or infra-auricular parotid lymph nodes may also occur. Lymphatic drainage from the upper lip may infrequently have connection even to the submental lymph nodes.[5] Lymphatic drainage of the upper lip, in contrast to that of the lower lip, does not cross over between left and right sides except in the very central part of the lip. This lack of crossover should naturally be expected, considering that embryonic fusion of the upper lip includes central insertion of the frontomedian process.

The submental, submandibular, and parotid lymph nodes make up the first echelon of lymphatic drainage from the lips. The submandibular and parotid lymph nodes next drain to the ipsilateral upper jugular cervical lymph nodes. Second-echelon drainage from the submental lymph nodes is most often directed to the submandibular nodes on each side, although it can also be directed to the upper jugular lymph nodes.

Oncologic Classification

For purposes of oncologic categorization, malignant tumors arising in different regions of the lip are placed into separate and distinct classifications. The American Joint Committee on Cancer (AJCC) defines the lip as "begins at the junction of the vermilion border with the skin and includes only the vermilion surface or that portion of the lip that comes into contact with the opposing lip."[6] The same definition is also supported by the Union International Contre le Cancer (UICC).[7] This definition recognizes the uniqueness of the vermilion epithelial surface and excludes cancers arising from the adjacent skin or the buccal mucosa.

Malignant tumors that arise in or principally involve the cutaneous portion of the lip are considered skin malignancies. They can also be categorized more specifically as "skin of the lip" malignancies. Malignancies arising from the buccal mucosa of the lip are considered by many to be oral cavity cancers. *The International Classification of Diseases for Oncology Manual*, which is published by the World Health Organization, considers malignant tumors involving the labial buccal mucosa as lip cancers, but in a special subcategory.[8] Reporting of lip malignancies for the Cancer Surveillance, Epidemiology, and End Results (SEER) Reporting Program of the National Institutes of

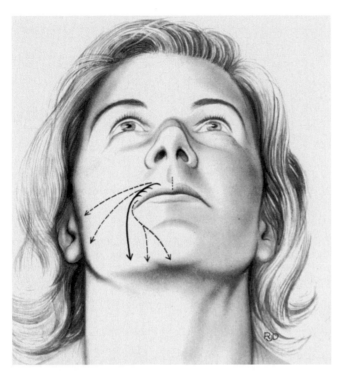

FIGURE 12–4 Patterns of lymphatic drainage from the upper lip. (From Zitsch RP III: Carcinoma of the lip. Otolaryngol Clin North Am 26:267–269, 1993.)

Health (NIH) includes tumors of the vermilion, as well as tumors of the mucosal surface of the lip, although some distinction is made with subcategorization.[9] In earlier years cancers of the skin of the lip were also included. Unfortunately, inconsistencies in what is reported as lip cancer have led to some confusion in the published data, particularly with regard to basal cell carcinoma.[10–13]

Cancer of the lip is commonly grouped with cancer of other oral cavity sites when reported. Traditional anatomic teaching considers the region between the posterior vermilion line and the central plane of the teeth and alveolar processes as the vestibular or buccal cavity. The region from the teeth and alveolar processes to the anterior limit of the soft palate and the palatoglossal arch is properly called the *cavum oris proprium*, or the oral cavity proper.[15] For oncologic purposes, the American Joint Committee on Cancer defines the oral cavity as extending "from the skin-vermilion junction of the lips to the junction of the hard and soft palate above and to the line of circumvallate papillae below."[6] In this context, cancer of the lip accounts for 25% to 30% of oral cavity malignancies.[16, 17] In actuality, malignancies arising from the vermilion of the lip could be considered as a unique group of tumors because they derive from a modified and externally exposed mucosal tissue that experiences a very different set of environmental challenges than do other sites of the oral cavity.

◼ ETIOLOGY OF CANCER OF THE LIP

An understanding of carcinogenesis and its relationship to the lip is not yet complete. A number of identified factors are felt to have some association with the development of lip cancer, although few at this time can be convincingly proved to be a distinct cause of cancer of the lip. The factor that so far has been most consistently associated with development of cancer of the lip is cumulative exposure to ultraviolet light, most of which comes from the sun.[18–23]

Much of the evidence that has implicated ultraviolet light exposure as etiologic in cancer of the lip is derived from associations that have been made in numerous case series studies and epidemiologic surveys. It has been consistently found that at least a third of patients who develop cancer of the lip have outdoor occupations, which presumably are associated with substantial exposure to ultraviolet light.[18, 22–29] Generalized changes attributable to chronic solar injury can be detected in the vermilion and skin of most patients who develop cancer of the lip. Typical findings include generalized atrophy of the vermilion, with substantial loss of elastic fibers and cellular changes such as hyperkeratosis and atypia. Advanced chronic actinic injury to the lip often produces fading of the sharp color contrast normally seen at the mucocutaneous line. Areas of the vermilion that have sustained particularly severe solar injury may display areas of chronic scaling or crusting that are referred to as *actinic cheilitis* and are analogous to actinic keratoses found in sun-damaged skin. Patients with cancer of the lip often have other sun-induced malignancies and premalignant changes in the surrounding vermilion and facial skin.[21, 28, 29]

Because the lips are located on the face, they sustain much greater exposure to ultraviolet light than do most other areas of the body. The lower lip is outwardly projected, with a downward angulation that favors direct exposure of the vermilion to overhead sunlight.[30] This is believed to be the principal reason why a much larger number of cancers (88% to 98%) arise in the vermilion of the lower lip.[1, 4, 22, 26, 31–33] Although the upper lip is also outwardly projected, its vermilion surface faces downward and is relatively more protected from direct sunlight.

Exposure to ultraviolet light has been shown to produce alterations in both local and systemic immune responses.[19, 34, 35] Such exposure has been shown to cause suppression in both contact hypersensitivity and delayed-type immunity. Exposure to ultraviolet light has been shown in animal studies to suppress rejection of transplanted tumors, even in body sites that were not directly exposed.[34]

Cancer of the lip is principally a disease of people with light skin complexion. It is much more common in whites than in those with darker skin color and is extremely rare among blacks.[1, 18, 25, 28, 29, 31] Explanation for this difference is thought to be that those of dark skin have significantly greater amounts of pigment within their vermilion, which can provide some protection from ultraviolet light, particularly in the wavelength range of 2900 to 3300 Å.[11, 13, 23] Some studies, however, do not show clear association of cancer of the lip with geographic or other variation in solar exposure, necessitating further study on this.[36, 37]

A variety of other factors have been reported to have some association with development of cancer of the lip. These include tobacco use, pipe smoking, thermal injury, mechanical irritants, trauma, use of alcohol, poor oral hygiene, chemical exposure, immunosuppression, influence of various infectious diseases, and prolonged exposure to harsh weather conditions (e.g., wind, cold, dryness).[36-39] Again, most of these can be considered only as associations, because well-designed and controlled studies that could possibly establish a firm causative relationship with cancer of the lip are lacking.

Exposure to tobacco products has clearly been shown, both in laboratory animal and in human clinical studies, to increase the risk for malignancy, particularly in the oral cavity.[33, 35] Association of tobacco with the development of cancer of the lip is less clear. This association has so far been based primarily on information obtained from various case series that have identified a large proportion of patients with cancer of the lip who have regularly used tobacco products.[25, 28, 40-42] Case-control studies by Dardanoni and by Blomquist have failed to support a distinct relationship of tobacco use with cancer of the vermilion of the lip.[43]

Use of a pipe in smoking, rather than the actual use of tobacco itself, has also been implicated as a possible causative agent in development of cancer of the lip. Support for this is found in studies by Broders and others in which pipe smoking was observed with greater frequency in patients with cancer of the lip (78%) than among the general population (38%).[40, 42, 44] Molnar reported that the incidence of cancer of the lip was higher among Irish, Swedish, and black women who smoked pipes.[22] Additionally, a case-control study by Spritzer demonstrated an increased risk of cancer of the lip among pipe smokers, which was not observed among those using tobacco in other forms.[45] It has been speculated that the carcinogenic effect may be due to some combination of chemical, mechanical, and thermal influences related to the use of a pipe in smoking.[12, 23]

An association of cancer of the lip with chronic alcohol use has also been suspected.[1, 18, 29] Molnar and coworkers reported that 47% of 2623 patients with cancer of the lip were habitual users of alcohol.[22] However, available data have not yet made the exact association clear. Poor oral and dental hygiene has also been implicated and is reported to be present in as many as 85% of patients with cancer of the lip.[18, 28, 46]

Patients who are immunosuppressed show a markedly increased risk for development of malignancies, particularly squamous cell carcinoma (SCC) of the exposed cutaneous surfaces. Patients who have had a renal transplant are pharmacologically immunosuppressed and have been found to be significantly more likely to develop cutaneous carcinoma, particularly SCC.[34, 47] The incidence of malignancy rises over time as patients continue to be immunosuppressed. Patients who are medically immunosuppressed for reasons other than organ transplant with the use of agents such as azathioprine or cyclophosphamide have also been shown to be more likely to develop cutaneous SCC.[34, 47] The increased incidence of cancer of the lip among renal allograft patients may be as great as 30-fold over a period of years.[48] Patients with immunocompromise are more likely to develop SCC of the lip at a relatively earlier age and also are more likely to develop multiple malignancies of the lip (Fig. 12–5).[49]

Chronic infection with human papilloma virus (HPV) has also been suspected of playing a role in oncogenesis of the lip and other tissues. A high incidence of HPV has been found in some subsets of patients with cutaneous SCC.[34]

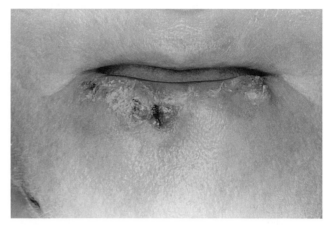

FIGURE 12–5 Rapid development of multiple squamous cell carcinomas of the lip is demonstrated in a 32-year-old woman with severe diabetes, who is also considered to be immunocompromised.

Barr identified the presence of HPV in 60% of cases of cutaneous SSC in patients with renal transplants.[50] In a matched control group of patients who did not develop SCC, the incidence of HPV was lower. A higher incidence of HPV was noted in patients with SCC of the oral cavity, cervix, penis, and digits.[26] It is possible, however, that oncogenic viruses such as HPV may simply become more active in patients who are immunocompromised.[50, 51]

Several authors in the past have considered syphilis to be a promoting factor in the pathogenesis of cancer of the lip.[28, 31, 46] Clear statistical proof showing that the incidence of lip cancer in seropositive patients is truly greater than in a similar population without positive serology, or that the rate of positive serology is significantly greater among lip cancer than among non–lip cancer patients, is lacking.[18, 20, 31, 33] In a similar manner, some have reported a higher frequency of infections with herpes simplex virus among patients with cancer of the lip, although this also remains to be proved with good scientific study.[12, 43, 50, 52]

● EPIDEMIOLOGY OF CANCER OF THE LIP

The incidence of cancer of the lip is quite varied throughout the world, presumably owing to factors such as race, environment, and personal habits.[12, 28, 53-55] In most parts of the world, cancer of the lip occurs very infrequently.[12] Relatively high rates have been identified in southern Australia (13 per 100,000 population) and among certain populations in northern Spain (11 per 100,000).[12] The highest rate found in a specific population has been identified in fishermen of Newfoundland, whose annual incidence is reported to be in excess of 50 cases per 100,000.[49] In some parts of the world, the incidence of reported cancer of the lip has increased; however, there is felt to be an overall trend of decreasing incidence in many parts of the world, with the most notable decline found in Great Britain.[12, 55-57]

Overall incidence of cancer of the lip in the United States has been reported to be 1.8 per 100,000 population; however, there is significant geographic variation.[11, 13, 54] The highest regional rate has been reported in Utah, where it has been documented at 12 per 100,000.[36] The American Cancer Society, using data collected from the National Cancer Institute's Surveillance, Epidemiology, and End Results (SEER) Reporting Program projected that 2590 new cases of carcinoma of the lip would occur in the United States in 1996.[56] Of these, 1900 were estimated to occur in men and 690 in women. It was also projected that 75 patients would die of cancer of the lip during that year, and one third of them would be women.[56]

Cancer involving the vermilion of the lip is predominantly a disease of men. The male-to-female ratio has varied somewhat among different case series but is consistently weighted to men, with a ratio that is roughly 20 to 50:1 (95% to 98%), based on reported series (a higher male ratio than is reflected in the American Cancer Society and SEER data).[1, 4, 20, 26, 31, 58–66] In a study done in Canada in 1964, MacKay and Seller[58] reported a male-to-female ratio of 79:1 for cancer of the lower lip, and 5:1 for cancer of the upper lip. These authors found an overall male-to-female ratio of 50:1 but noted that this was adjusted to 30:1 when only later years were reviewed separately.[58] A 1994 study at the University of Missouri by Zitsch and others, which reviewed a total of 1036 patients with cancer involving the vermilion of the lip, found that in 1001 patients with cancer of the lower lip, the male-to-female ratio was 36:1, and in 39 patients with cancer of the upper lip, the ratio was 5.5:1.[4]

Cancer of the vermilion is most commonly found in white men during their sixth decade of life.[16, 18] The usual age for patients with cancer of the lip is between 50 and 70 years, with more than 50% of cases occurring within this span.[22, 31, 59, 62, 67] The reported mean age at time of diagnosis has varied from 54 to 65 years of age.[1, 18, 23, 36, 51, 52, 63] Although it is uncommon, cancer of the lip has been found repeatedly in patients younger than 30 years of age; it has been found with less frequency in patients younger than 20 years of age; and it has been found very rarely even in some patients who are younger than 10 years of age.[4, 22, 31, 49, 50, 60–62, 67]

Cancer arising in the vermilion is much more frequent in the lower lip, occurring in between 88% and 98% of cases.[1, 4, 22, 26, 30–33] Malignancy arising in the upper lip vermilion constitutes only 2% to 7% of reported cases.[1, 26, 31, 68] Cancer arises in the commissure of the lip in no more than 1% of cases, a rate that is roughly proportionate to the actual surface area of exposed vermilion at the commissures.[4, 26, 31, 42, 58]

Patients who have developed either a cancer of the lip or a cancer of the skin have an increased chance of developing a second primary cancer in these sites.[26, 58] Based on a review of his own patient series, Baker[26, 58] determined that patients with cancer of the lip and significant occupational sun exposure have a 3.4 times greater chance of developing a later second primary cancer of the lip. Those with severe solar skin changes and a cancer of the lip have a 2.5 times greater chance of developing a second primary cancer of the lip, and they have a 5.5 times greater chance if they have an initial primary cancer of the lip and a concomitant second primary cancer of the skin.[29] The risk for second primary cancer of the lip is also significantly increased for patients who are immunocompromised.[47, 48]

Over the past several decades in many parts of the world, changes have been noted in the demographics of skin cancer, with suggestions of change in sites of occurrence and a trend of increasing overall incidence for all major histologic types.[56, 69–71] A study by Rowe and coworkers,[72] which reviewed his population of patients who had been referred for and treated with Mohs' micrographic surgery and then compared them with several other populations, revealed data that suggested an increased incidence of cutaneous basal cell carcinoma of the lip and a surprising predominance of this tumor in women. In their series of 4650 cases of basal cell carcinoma treated with Mohs' surgery, 3.7% involved the perioral region, a proportion consistent with other reports. Of the 136 cases involving the skin of the upper lip, a 3.5:1 female-to-male ratio was found, with an even higher ratio of 16:1 in young women (ages 30 to 39).[72] Basal cell carcinoma of the melolabial fold was found to be a little more common among men, and that of skin of the lower lip showed a higher incidence among women.

HISTOLOGY OF THE LIP

The lips are a composite soft tissue structure, of which the principal components are skin, muscle, and mucosa (see Fig. 12–2). They also contain nerves, vascular structures, glands, fat, and connective tissues. The lip is covered by three fairly distinct epithelial surfaces. The external cutaneous surface displays typical skin histology, with a keratinizing, stratified squamous epithelium and a rich complex of hair follicles, sweat, and sebaceous glands in the dermis.

The vermilion of the lip is a mucosal surface that is specially adapted for external exposure. It is made of nonkeratinizing, stratified squamous epithelium. The submucosal layer contains essentially no hair follicles or glandular structures, which allows the vermilion surface to remain smooth and dry.[73] The characteristic pink or red color that is seen in the vermilion of those with lighter skin tone is due to the presence of many elongated, vascular, connective tissue papillae that project into the epithelial layer.[73]

The labial buccal mucosa is also made of nonkeratinizing, stratified squamous epithelium with prominent underlying vascular papillae. In its submucosal layer are many serous, mucous, and mixed salivary glands, which serve to keep the epithelial surface moist.

HISTOPATHOLOGY OF CANCER OF THE LIP

Cancers of the lip encompass a variety of histopathologic types, each with a different clinical behavior. SCC stands out clearly as the most common type of carcinoma to involve the vermilion portion of the lip. Verrucous, spindle cell, and adenoid squamous are variant forms of SCC, all of which occur infrequently in the lip. Melanoma can arise in the vermilion, as well as in the cutaneous or mucosal portions of the lip. Basal cell carcinoma is the most frequent type of malignancy arising in the cutaneous portion of the lip; SCC is second. It is debated whether basal cell carcinoma can actually arise from the vermilion of the lip in regions separate from the mucocutaneous junction. Malignant salivary gland tumors can arise from the submucosal portion of the lip. Very rarely, malignancies can develop from other tissues of the lip, producing tumors such as malignant fibrous histiocytoma, leiomyosarcoma, fibrosarcoma, lymphoma, angiosarcoma, rhabdomyosarcoma, and Merkel cell carcinoma.[40, 74–78]

Squamous Cell Carcinoma

SCC accounts for the greatest majority of cancers of the lip, accounting for at least 95% and usually more in all reported case series.[1, 4, 20, 22, 25, 26] Because SCC makes up such a commanding proportion of cancer of the lip, nearly all that is described concerning behavior and treatment of lip cancer is a description of SCC of the lip.

SCC of the lip has an appearance that may vary from a small, superficial ulceration to a very prominent, exophytic growth (Fig. 12–6). It may be impossible to distinguish clinically between actinic cheilitis and early carcinoma, with both tending to display only superficial ulceration. This presents a strong indication for biopsy. Most actinic cheilitis occurs near the mucocutaneous border of the vermilion.

Leukoplakia and erythroplakia are morphologically defined lesions that may be found on the lip (Fig. 12–7).[79] The terms literally mean "white lesion" and "red lesion," respectively, and as such have no exact histopathologic correlation or relation to any specific clinical behavior. There is not even complete agreement as to which lesions qualify for these terms. Leukoplakic lesions commonly display histologic findings such as epithelial hyperplasia, parakeratosis, epithelial atrophy, and submucosal inflammation.[80] These sites are believed to have a greater tendency for malignant

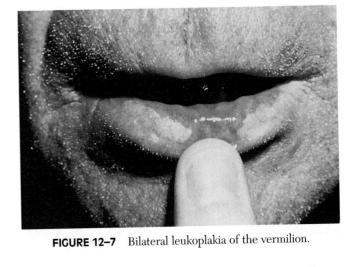

FIGURE 12–7 Bilateral leukoplakia of the vermilion.

transformation and, in some cases, they do actually represent SCC. Erythroplakic lesions have an even greater chance of representing invasive SCC.[80]

As lesions grow, three principal morphologic forms of SCC are recognized that have some tendency for variation in clinical behavior, at least in earlier stages. Tumors may be classified as exophytic, ulcerative, or verrucous.[18] Attempts have been made to assign considerable importance to distinguishing among these types; however, morphology alone, with some exception for verrucous carcinoma, does not significantly alter the need for adequate treatment.

SCCs demonstrating the exophytic form of growth typically begin as an area of thickened epithelium that slowly develops as a raised, papillary growth (Figs. 12–8 and 12–9). With continued growth, there is a tendency for the base of the tumor to become dislike in shape as the margins extend both laterally and deeper into the lip.[18] The papillary surface may become very irregular with many projections and clefts.[18] Lesions that display exophytic growth may actually become several centimeters in size and still have very

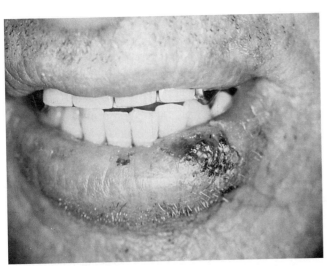

FIGURE 12–6 Vermilion with a region of broad, shallow ulceration that proved on biopsy to be squamous cell carcinoma.

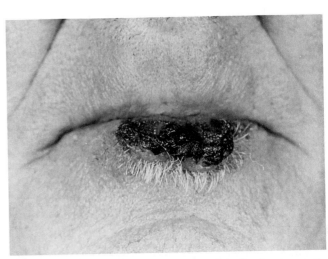

FIGURE 12–8 Squamous cell carcinoma of the lip that is remarkably exophytic in its growth. Although this lesion was quite thick, there was relatively little deep invasion.

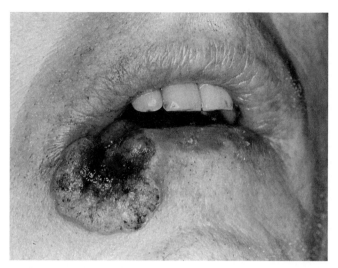

FIGURE 12–9 Squamous cell carcinoma of the lip that is also exophytic but is beginning to show central ulceration; it showed fairly deep invasion into the body of the lip.

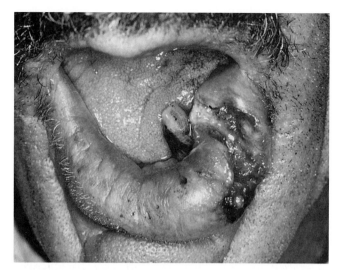

FIGURE 12–11 Another ulcerative squamous cell carcinoma with considerable deep invasion and surrounding inflammation.

limited invasion.[18, 31] They also tend to be of larger relative size before they metastasize. Eventually, these tumors achieve deeper levels of invasion, and metastasis becomes more likely.

SCCs of the lip displaying the ulcerative form of growth usually begin as an area of epithelial thickening that ulcerates as it progresses (Figs. 12–10 and 12–11). They may begin as an area of superficial ulceration that continues to enlarge. Further growth of the lesion tends to be more endophytic, displaying a relatively greater degree of invasion when compared with a tumor of comparable size with exophytic growth.[31, 40] Tumors of the ulcerative form are more likely to be of higher histologic grade than those of the exophytic or verrucous form.[18] They may be a little more likely than the other forms to metastasize while still in a stage of relatively low tumor volume.

Verrucous Carcinoma

Verrucous carcinoma is a special form of SCC that is unique in both its morphology and clinical behavior. Verrucous carcinoma typically appears as a distinct, raised,

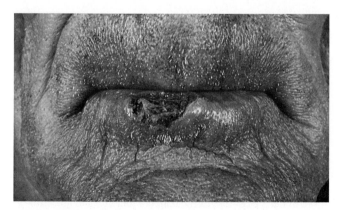

FIGURE 12–10 Squamous cell carcinoma of the lip that demonstrates an ulcerative morphology.

white or pink lesion with a warty or papillary surface.[80] Lesions usually have broad bases and are locally invasive. Most are slow growing, although some can display rapid growth.[81] It is also possible for a phase of relatively slow growth to be followed by one of rapid expansion.[81]

Histologic examination reveals a well-differentiated SCC with few malignant features other than invasion.[82] Lesions typically exhibit orderly maturation, with a thickened zone of nonproliferative, nonkeratinizing cells in their center.[81] Mitoses are uncommon, and there is a noted lack of S-phase cells, which are otherwise distributed throughout all nonkeratinized regions in other forms of SCC.[81] Near the surface, nearly all lesions display hyperkeratosis and often parakeratosis.[82] Rete pegs are typically swollen and voluminous.[82]

The margins of invasion with verrucous carcinoma are typically more "pushing" than they are with other forms of SCC.[80, 81] A special feature found commonly in verrucous carcinoma is integrity of the basement membrane throughout most or all of the tumor, even when there is considerable invasion into deeper tissues.[82] Verrucous carcinomas rarely metastasize, even when there is relatively deep invasion into muscle or bone.[82]

Verrucous carcinoma is predominantly a mucosal lesion, but it can arise rarely on a skin surface.[81] It may arise at any site along the upper aerodigestive tract, but it occurs most commonly in the oral cavity, particularly on the buccal wall, and next most commonly on the gingiva.[81–84] Verrucous carcinoma arising from the vermilion portion of the lip is much less common.[83, 84]

It is not unusual for verrucous carcinoma to arise within a field of previously existing leukoplakia.[18, 81] The relationship of verrucous carcinoma to other forms of hyperkeratosis or hyperplasia remains unclear.[81] There may even be some relationship to more invasive SCC. It has been suggested that some verrucous carcinomas could be part of a spectrum of disease. Hansen and coworkers[85] have attempted to describe a special "proliferative oral leukoplakia." It is their contention that some forms of leukoplakia have a strong tendency to progress to verrucous carcinoma, and they make the argument that this may represent a "continuum of hyperkeratotic disease, ranging from simple hyperkeratosis at one end to invasive SCC at the other."[85] Medina and colleagues,[84] in a review of 104 oral verrucous carcinomas that included tumors from the lip, identified in 20% of those studied foci of less well-differentiated, more traditional SCC with a more aggressively infiltrating margin. A few cases have been reported of a more aggressive SCC developing within a tumor that was initially identified as a verrucous carcinoma.[81, 83, 84] More needs to be done to clarify whether there is a true association. Because verrucous carcinoma is not commonly found on the lip, it is even less clear whether this concept has any real meaning in relation to verrucous carcinoma of the lip.

Any biopsy taken of a suspected verrucous carcinoma should include the full thickness of the lesion and a segment of adjacent, uninvolved mucosa.[81–83] It is possible otherwise for the diagnosis to be confused with other forms of hyperplasia and hyperkeratosis or some forms of SCC. Clinical correlation can sometimes be helpful to the pathologist in establishing the diagnosis of verrucous carcinoma.[81–83]

Spindle Cell Carcinoma

Spindle cell carcinoma is a variant form of SCC in which the epithelial cells appear spindled, resembling a sarcoma.[80] It has been reported to occur in the vermilion, as well as in other body sites.[80, 86, 87] In the oral cavity, it most commonly involves the lower lip, tongue, and gingiva.[87] Most present as a polypoid mass, and others present with ulceration.[80, 87] Microscopic diagnosis requires a biphasic histology with SCC and a malignant spindle cell stroma.[80, 87] All histologic grades of infiltrative SCC may be found in these tumors.[80] Spindle cell carcinomas of the oral cavity are in general highly aggressive, with an overall mortality rate reported at 42% to 61%.[80, 87] They have a strong tendency for deep infiltration and perineural invasion.[87] McClatchey and Zorbo[80] report that no histologic feature (including morphology or grade) has so far been clearly linked to prognosis in oral lesions.[87] Ellis and Corio[87] found that spindle cell carcinomas involving the lower lip had a somewhat better prognosis than did those of other sites in the oral cavity.[80]

Adenoid Squamous Cell Carcinoma

Adenoid SCC is an uncommon variant of SCC that has been reported by several authors to arise also within the vermilion and the skin of the lip, as well as in other cutaneous sites.[88, 89] These tumors appear to be strongly associated with chronic solar injury and are often preceded by actinic keratosis.[86–90] Lesions typically appear hyperkeratotic and nodular and are commonly also ulcerated.[90] Microscopic features reveal invasion of the corium by proliferating atypical epithelial cells, which form an adenoid-type pattern caused by acantholysis.[89] This pathology is distinguished from true adenosquamous carcinoma of the skin or mucosa, which derives from glandular structures, is mucin producing, and is more aggressive.[80, 86]

Weitzner reviewed 18 cases of adenoid SCC, all involving the vermilion, and found no metastases or deaths.[88] A review by Johnson of 155 patients with a total of 213 tumors, involving all body sites, found 3 patients with metastasis and 2 with direct extension, all of whom died of their disease.[90] A 14% incidence of fatal metastasis was reported by Wick, again including all skin sites.[91] Prognosis is felt to be worse in those lesions greater than 1.5 cm in diameter.[86, 91]

Basal Cell Carcinoma

A considerable amount of confusion and controversy pervades the medical literature as to the relative incidence and even the true existence of basal cell carcinoma that arises as a primary tumor of the vermilion portion of the lip. Basal cell carcinoma has sometimes been described as being the most frequent malignant tumor of the upper lip, which is true for tumors arising in the skin of the upper lip, but not for tumors of the upper lip vermilion. After a review of cases in 1941, Hayes Martin wrote: "In our opinion, the reported instances of basal cell carcinoma occurring in the lip should not be included . . . they obviously arise in the skin apart from the vermilion border and, therefore, should be classified with other facial skin cancers."[31] Proper classification becomes less certain when basal cell carcinoma arises near the mucocutaneous border and involves a portion of the vermilion.

Indeed nearly all basal cell carcinomas that are found to involve the vermilion have actually arisen from the cutaneous portion of the lip, originating at or near the mucocutaneous border (Fig. 12–12). Only a few cases of basal cell carcinoma have been reported, and these were believed to have actually originated within the vermilion of the lip, separate from the mucocutaneous junction.[62, 92, 93] A few case reports have also suggested that basal cell carcinoma has been found as a primary tumor arising from the gingiva of the mandible and the maxilla.[94] Some believe that those tumors that have been reported to arise from the gingiva may actually be forms of peripheral ameloblastoma.[80, 95] A variety of tumors, including several of salivary gland origin, can display features that may resemble basal cell carcinoma.[80]

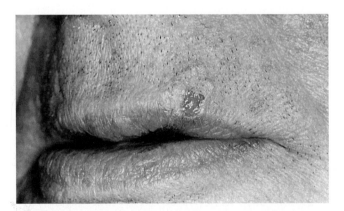

FIGURE 12–12 Basal cell carcinoma of the upper lip that has arisen in the area of the mucocutaneous junction and now involves the skin and, to a lesser extent, the vermilion. This should be classified as a skin cancer with secondary invasion of the vermilion.

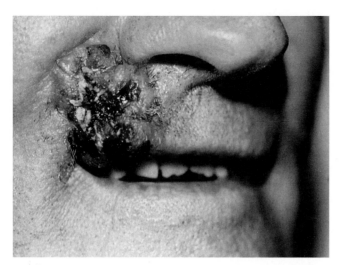

FIGURE 12–13 A remarkably advanced basal cell carcinoma that has now become a full-thickness lesion in the upper lip, involving skin, muscle, mucosa, and vermilion. This would be classified as a skin cancer with extensive invasion. (From Zitsch RP III: Carcinoma of the lip. Otolaryngol Clin North Am 26:267–269, 1993.)

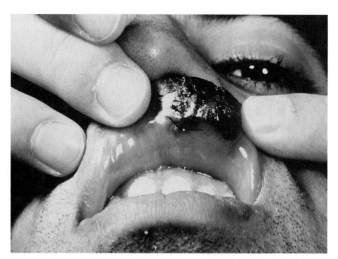

FIGURE 12–14 Young man with mucosal melanoma of the upper lip. Metastasis to the bowel was found 3 years after wide local excision.

Tumors reported as basal cell carcinoma of the lip represent no more than 1% of lip cancers (Fig. 12–13).[4, 24, 58] They occur with roughly equal frequency in the upper and lower lips; however, they are a little more common, and their relative proportion is greater among cancers of the upper lip.[4, 28, 96]

Melanoma

Melanocytes are normally present in the cutaneous, vermilion, and mucosal portions of the lip, allowing melanoma to arise in any of these sites. With the exception of acral lentigines, any of the other forms of cutaneous melanoma can arise in the skin of the lip. Melanoma arising within the vermilion of the lip is usually considered a mucosal melanoma because its appearance and behavior are similar. Mucosal melanoma is most frequently found in the palatal or gingival mucosa and is found with less frequency in the buccal mucosa and vermilion.[97, 98] In a review of several reported series of oral melanoma, Batsakis and coworkers[99] found that of 373 cases, 37 (10%) involved the lip and 25 (7%) involved the buccal mucosa.

Melanoma of both the vermilion and the buccal portions of the lip typically presents as a smooth, black or blue submucosal nodule that is covered by a thin, intact mucosa (Fig. 12–14). Before a mucosal melanoma is accepted as being a primary tumor, careful screening of other body sites is required to confirm that it does not actually represent a metastasis from a distant primary melanoma.

Salivary Gland Carcinoma

Numerous minor salivary glands are present immediately beneath the buccal mucosa of both the upper and lower lips; essentially, no salivary glands are present beneath the vermilion. Malignant tumors arising from the minor salivary glands have been found in the lip. Classic presentation for a tumor arising in the minor salivary glands of the lip is development of a firm submucosal nodule that enlarges slowly. Ulceration is not usually present unless a biopsy has been done.[98, 100] In general, these tumors arise beneath the labial buccal mucosa and, according to AJC and UICC rules, would not be properly classified as lip cancer, but instead as oral cancer.

In a review by Byers and colleagues[100] at the M.D. Anderson Cancer Center, 15 cases of minor salivary gland tumor were found in a series of 1308 lip malignancies, constituting approximately 1% of the series. In a later study of 50 minor salivary gland tumors reviewed at that same institution by Weber and coworkers,[101] a total of 19 patients were identified with tumors of the minor salivary glands of the lip and 31 patients with tumors in other portions of the buccal mucosa. A study of 2807 patients with salivary neoplasms done by Spiro[102] at the Memorial Sloan-Kettering Cancer Center identified 73 patients with tumors of the lips and cheeks, with no distinction made between these. Spiro reported a total of 63 salivary gland tumors of the lips and cheeks, only 13 of which were benign.[102] In 1982, Owens and Calcaterra[103] reported on 5 patients with salivary gland tumors of the lip and reviewed a total of 307 additional cases that had been reported in the English literature up to that time. In this more extensive series, 251 benign tumors (207 being pleomorphic adenoma) were documented, and only 58 were found to be malignant.[103]

In the studies of Byers[100] and Weber,[101] the most common type of salivary gland cancer found in the lip was the adenoid cystic carcinoma. There is disagreement regarding the reported incidence of adenocarcinoma; the later study by Weber and coworkers appears to have further subcategorized the previously reported adenocarcinomas. The next most common malignant tumor in both reports was mucoepidermoid carcinoma.[100, 101] Spiro reported relative numbers for adenoid cystic carcinoma, mucoepidermoid carcinoma, and adenocarcinoma of the lip and cheek at 12:23:20.[102] In the larger review by Owens and Calcaterra,[103] the relative frequencies for adenoid cystic carcinoma, mucoepidermoid carcinoma, and adenocarcinoma were 20:18:14.[103] It appears from these data that the relative frequencies for each of these three malignant salivary gland tumors in the lip are roughly equal. Other salivary gland malignancies that have been reported in the lip, but with less frequency, include clear cell carcinoma, terminal duct carcinoma, malignant papillary cystadenocarcinoma, carcinoma ex pleomorphic adenoma, and acinic cell carcinoma.[101, 103]

For reasons that are unclear, salivary gland tumors have been found more commonly in the upper lip than in the lower lip. Owens and Calcaterra determined that 85% of benign tumors and 61% of malignant salivary gland tumors occur in the upper lip.[103] They found that tumors occur in patients between ages 14 and 87, with a median of 46 years of age.[103] They also found no age distinction between those with benign and those with malignant tumors, as had been reported by some others.[103] No clear sex predominance was reported either, although a greater number of malignant tumors were identified in men (16:6).[103]

With respect to the lip, no extensive data exist concerning prognosis for each of the various minor salivary gland malignancies. In the study by Byers and colleagues, 8 of 15 patients were found to have evidence of invasion, and 5 were found to have positive cervical nodes, with an overall patient survival of only 20%; however, most of the patients in this series were referred for treatment of recurrent disease.[100] Tumors of at least several of these types, most notably mucoepidermoid carcinoma, can be identified as of high or low grade. Perineural invasion is also a moderately common feature, at least for adenoid cystic carcinoma; when present, it marks a poorer prognosis.

Owens and Calcaterra have advised that of minor salivary gland tumors in the lip, adenocarcinoma has the worst prognosis in that it is noted to develop recurrence and metastasis.[103] Adenoid cystic carcinomas have a somewhat better prognosis, although rates of recurrence are high.[103] Mucoepidermoid carcinomas are more commonly of low grade and show less tendency to recur or metastasize.[103]

◨ PROGNOSTIC FEATURES ASSOCIATED WITH SQUAMOUS CELL CARCINOMA

SCC of the lip is not typically aggressive early in its course. Most tumors grow slowly, usually favoring lateral growth and tending to remain localized to the vermilion and immediate submucosal tissues until later in the course.[13] Meaningful comparison of information from the many reported studies of SCC of the lip is somewhat difficult because of past differences in the treatments delivered, particularly with radiotherapy, and because of differences in the way data have been collected and reported.

A difference in outcome has been noted for SCCs that arise in the three major subsites of the lip (i.e., lower lip, upper lip, and commissures). Five-year disease-free survival rates reported for SCC of the lower lip have been reported in a range of 70% to more than 90%, and for cancer of the upper lip in a range of 40% to 60%.[2, 3, 18, 22, 24, 31] Cancers limited to the commissure are rare, and survival rates have been reported at 34% to 84%.[2, 16, 46] In the University of Missouri study, a 77% overall 5-year survival was found for 62 patients with SCC involving the upper lip or the commissure.[4] The oral commissure is quite small; consequently, a majority of cancers of the lip that are reported to be of the commissure actually also involve significant portions of the upper or lower lip or both.[4]

SCC of the lip is thought to be more aggressive when it arises in young patients. Boddie and coworkers[61] reported a higher incidence of cervical lymph node metastasis and higher disease-related mortality among patients who were younger than 40 years of age who had developed SCC of the lip. Young patients with cancer of the lip are more likely to be immunocompromised or to have other predisposing conditions such as xeroderma pigmentosum.[49, 104]

Tumor Size

Size of the primary cancer is one of the most significant factors that can be associated with prognosis and is one of the principal factors used in determination of clinical stage (T1–T4).[6, 7] For cancer with a greatest diameter less than 2 cm (T1), almost all reported 5-year survival rates exceeded 90%, whether treatment was with surgery or radiation.[1, 4, 16, 26, 58, 104] With progressively larger cancers, the rates of control diminish. Jorgensen and colleagues[26] reported persistent or recurrent disease in 7.4% of lip cancers that were larger than 2 cm in diameter or had deep infiltration. Older reports by Cross and coworkers[46] (1948) and Ward and Hendrick[33] (1950) indicate 5-year determinate survival rates for a T2 tumor to be in a range of approximately 40% to 60%. More current reports by Cruse and Radocha[2] (1987) and Heller and Shah[3] (1979) show survival rates for T2 tumors in a range of 71% to 83%.

Five-year determinate survival rates for tumors larger than 4 cm (T3) have been reported in a range of approximately 40% to 60%.[2, 33] Control rates for T4 tumors have been reported in a range of 40% to 50%.[1–3] In the University of Missouri study, those with tumors smaller than 3 cm had a 5-year determinate survival of 91%; for those with tumors larger than this, the rate was 64% ($P < .001$).[4] Unfortunately, there is so far no good way to clinically determine a three-dimensional or full-volume measurement of cancer of the lip; this would likely have more meaning than a one-dimensional measurement. Some tumors can be quite extensive but remain very superficial; others invade deeply. The earlier UICC staging system had considered degree of tumor invasion as well as horizontal tumor size in its primary tumor (T) classification (see under Staging).[105] Frierson and Cooper[66] have evaluated tumor thickness and found that metastasis occurred in 75% of patients whose cancer was greater than 6 mm in thickness; they concluded that this was a useful measurement from which to help determine prognosis.

Tumor Grading

Broders,[42] in 1920, first described a system for classification of SCCs of the lip based principally on the degree of cellular differentiation and to a lesser extent on the number of mitoses that were found. He wrote: "It is a well established fact that some cancers of the lip are fatal to patients and others are not."[42] He hypothesized that this fact could be explained by an observation of differing "degrees of cellular activity," noting that "the cells of some epitheliomas of the lip show a marked tendency to differentiate" while "in other squamous epitheliomas, there is no differentiation whatever."[42] He correlated mortality rate with histopathologic grade and found that the highest disease-specific mortality rates occurred with the least-differentiated cancers. Many other case series have corroborated this observation. They have also shown correlation of cancers that are more poorly differentiated with higher rates of both local recurrence and cervical lymph node metastasis.[1, 4, 21, 22, 58, 59, 64, 66, 106]

Broders assigned a grade of I, II, III, or IV to a given tumor, depending on its degree of cellular differentiation.[42] Those tumors with a very high degree of cellular differentiation, which as a group are noted to be more low grade in their appearance, are classified as grade I. Those found with progressively less differentiation or greater degrees of de-differentiation are assigned the higher grades. Very similar to Broders' classification, most pathologists currently classify SCCs of the lip as well differentiated, moderately differentiated, poorly differentiated, or undifferentiated. This system of descriptive grading is accepted for reporting by the American Joint Committee on Cancer.[6]

In his original series of 537 patients with SCC of the lip, Broders reported 16% as grade I, 62% as grade II, 21% as grade III, and 1% as grade IV.[42] Subsequent reports by others have shown some variation in these numbers but overall general agreement, with approximately 80% to 85% commonly found to be low-grade (I and II) and frankly anaplastic tumors that account for only approximately 2% of all tumors.[20, 31, 59, 107] Unfortunately, no uniform agreement has been reached among pathologists as to their interpretation or even exact criteria for interpretation of these distinctions in grade. Some pathologists have preferred other grading systems—some with division into only 2 or 3 separate grades.[23, 47, 58, 62, 64, 108, 109] With further advances in histopathology, it is hoped that this ambiguity will be eliminated.

More recent studies have been done to attempt to correlate various other features such as total DNA content (ploidy) with prognosis.[106, 110, 111] Several have noted poorer prognosis for SCCs with greater degree of aneuploidy, which generally are associated with lesser degrees of cellular differentiation. Most work concerning nuclear ploidy and SCC has been done with a mix of oral cavity sites; very little has been done with cancer of the lip specifically.[106, 110–114] Some of these data have been contradictory. Evaluation of DNA with the use of flow cytometry has not at this time become a widely accepted tool for the rating or grading of lip cancers.

Tumor Invasion

Patterns of invasion may be associated with outcome. Those with a more "pushing" pattern of invasion, as are seen most commonly with verrucous carcinoma, have a more favorable prognosis. Frierson and Cooper[66] have grouped SCCs of the lip into three pattern types, according to features of invasion. Pattern 1 cancers with pushing borders were generally found to be well-differentiated tumors that had no metastases. Pattern 2 cancers showed discrete islands and nests of malignant cell with multiple budlike protrusions and were typical of most invasive lip cancers. They found a 97% rate of metastases in those considered pattern 2. Pattern 3 cancers showed diffuse or disorganized features of growth, lacked well-defined borders, and often showed isolated strands or clusters of cells, or single, dissociated malignant cells. Pattern 3 was associated with a 77% incidence of metastasis and was found in 48% of the tumors that were at least 6 mm in thickness. Lund has used mode of invasion as one of the parameters to help determine his own histologic grading of 1 to 4 for lip cancers.[108]

Because the vermilion is thin, extension of cancer into at least the superficial portion of the orbicularis muscle is common. Superficial invasion into muscle has not proved to be of prognostic significance, but deep invasion into muscle is associated with poorer prognosis and may advance the clinical stage to T4.[47, 66] Attempts have been made to evaluate the inflammatory response seen in the submucosa of those with cancer of the lip, but as yet, no significant correlation with prognosis has been identified.[66] Angiolymphatic invasion has not been reported in most series, and the significance of its occurrence in lip cancers, although likely to be unfavorable, is not at this point completely clear.[66]

Perineural Invasion

SCC and other malignancies of the lip may invade the mandible by perineural spread along the mental nerve and less commonly by direct extension into bone (Figs. 12–15 and 12–16). Invasion of the maxilla can also occur via the infraorbital nerve. Some SCCs have a greater tendency to be neurotropic. A higher proportion of spindle cell carcinomas and some of the minor salivary gland tumors tend to be more neurotropic.[87, 101, 115] The presence of perineural or intraneural invasion has been clearly associated with poorer prognosis.[4, 66] Byers and colleagues[116] identified a 2% incidence of perineural invasion in a series of 1308 cases of SCC of the lower lip. Of the 20 patients with follow-up, 12 of whom had received prior radiotherapy for cancer of the lip, 80% developed cervical lymph node metastasis; the 5-year

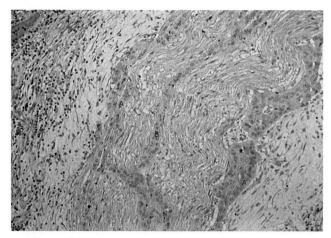

FIGURE 12–15 Hematoxylin-eosin histologic section revealing both perineural and intraneural invasion of squamous cell carcinoma.

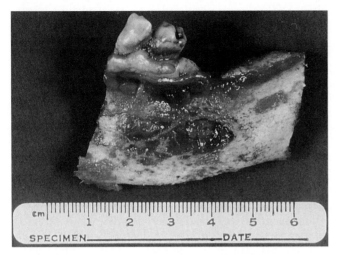

FIGURE 12–16 Segmental mandibular resection demonstrating considerable erosion of the mental foramen caused by transneural invasion by squamous cell carcinoma originating in the lower lip.

rate of survival was only 35%.[116] Frierson and Cooper found a 60% rate of cervical lymphatic metastasis associated with perineural invasion and noted a higher likelihood for metastasis when the degree of perineural invasion was greater.[66] In their report, Ballantyne and coworkers reveal an overall poor likelihood for the disease to be controlled when there is perineural involvement.[117] With tumor involvement of the mandible, Creely and Peterson have reported a 3-year survival rate of only 33%.[24] Tingling, numbness, or pain is a clinical sign of perineural involvement that cannot be relied upon as an early indicator. Several cases have been reported of SCC originating in the lip, with spread along the full length of the inferior alveolar nerve, through the foramen ovale, and into the cranial cavity.[117, 118] Some of these have occurred despite the clinical presence of primary tumors that were not particularly large.[118, 119] With perineural spread of tumor along the inferior alveolar nerve, other branches of the trigeminal nerve can become involved; in rare cases, this can be demonstrated by the loss of sensation in other facial regions, or by denervation atrophy of the ipsilateral muscles of mastication.[117, 120]

Lymphatic Metastasis

The presence of regional lymphatic metastases and failure of the clinician to manage them successfully are two of the primary factors associated with poor outcome in cancer of the lip. Determination of the presence of regional lymph node metastasis is an important component of clinical staging because it has a major impact on the rate of 5-year disease-free survival. Lymphatic metastasis of SCC to regional lymph nodes is less frequent from primary tumors of the lip than it is from primary tumors of other sites in the upper aerodigestive tract. When it does occur, however, the negative prognostic impact is similar. In general, patients who have regional lymphatic metastasis are reported to have 5-year determinate cure rates in a range of 30% to 70%.[1, 20, 26, 121, 122] Stoddart reported control of neck disease in 47% of those patients with cervical lymph node metastasis found at the time of initial lip cancer diagnosis;

control of the neck was attained in 50% of patients with lymph node metastasis found some time after the original treatment for cancer of the lip.[109]

An understanding of the patterns of lymphatic drainage from the lip is necessary for comprehensive tumor assessment and effective treatment planning. Metastasis of SCC and most other malignant tumors of the lip are almost always initially to the adjacent or regional lymph nodes, which reflects the known patterns of lymphatic drainage from the perioral region.

Based on limited reported data, metastasis to the submandibular nodes is found in approximately 70% to 90% of patients who have metastatic disease from cancer of the lower lip; in approximately 75% of such patients, these are the only nodes involved.[26, 42, 107, 123] The submental nodes are involved in approximately 25% to 45% of patients with nodal disease and are more likely to be involved when the cancer involves the central portion of the lower lip.[26, 42, 107, 123] Cervical metastases are likely to involve both submandibular and submental nodes in approximately 30% of patients.[26, 123] Metastases from the upper lip and commissures are most often reported to occur in the submandibular lymph nodes and in the lower parotid lymph nodes.[31] However, Zitsch and associates[124] found no contralateral or parotid metastasis among their reported cases with metastatic upper lip cancer.

Lymph node metastasis to the upper jugular chain nodes is found in approximately 15% to 25% of all patients who have lymph node metastases.[26, 42] Involvement of these nodes occurs most often in conjunction with ipsilateral submandibular lymph node metastasis.[26, 123] Lower jugular chain lymph node metastases are very uncommon, except in advanced-stage disease.[125] Bilateral lymph node metastases are observed in approximately 10% to 25% of patients with metastases, whereas contralateral metastases are found in only 5% to 10% of patients.[22, 26, 32, 107, 126]

The large review of cervical lymph node metastasis from SCC of the lip by Zitsch and colleagues[124] showed metastatic rates to ipsilateral, contralateral, and bilateral lymph nodes of 84%, 10%, and 6%, respectively, for cancers arising from the lateral third of the lip. Bilateral metastases occurred in 23% of cases of metastases from cancers of the central third of the lip.

Metastasis of SCC to regional lymph nodes may be found at the time of original cancer diagnosis or may be found at some later time interval after the original cancer has been managed. The finding of clinically positive lymph nodes at the time of initial diagnosis occurs in approximately 2% to 15% of patients, although a few have reported it to be higher.[1–4, 13, 20, 26, 31, 33, 121, 123–125, 127–129] Clinically positive lymph nodes are found later in the course in approximately 3% to 13% of patients with lip cancer.[1–4, 13, 20, 26, 29, 33, 46, 58, 62, 121, 123, 125, 127, 129] Most patients with positive lymphadenopathy are identified within the first year following treatment for cancer of the lip; nearly all are found within 2 years.[18, 26, 46, 128] With SCC, metastases are occasionally found as late as 5 years following initial treatment, and rarely beyond that time.[104] Therefore, most follow-up for patients with cancer of the lip should continue for at least 5 years. With local recurrence of cancer of the lip, the reported rates for metastasis to regional lymph nodes range from 15% to 26%.[1, 26, 124]

The finding of clinically enlarged or otherwise suspicious lymph nodes does not always correlate with the presence of actual tumor metastasis.[2, 22, 33, 125, 127] Heller and Shah[3] found that 7 of 17 patients who were identified with clinically positive cervical lymphadenopathy and who underwent lymphatic dissection did not have confirmed histologic evidence of metastatic disease. Zitsch and Renner reported a series in which 158 patients underwent some form of lymphatic dissection, but in only 95 patients was histologic evidence of metastatic tumor confirmed.[4] Rates for false-positive cervical lymphadenopathy, based on clinical examination alone, have been reported by other authors to be 17% to 25%.[2, 125, 129] Patients whose tumors are larger and more ulcerative or who have poor oral hygiene have a greater chance for nonmalignant, inflammatory lymphadenopathy. Ability to clinically assess cervical lymphatic disease has now been improved with the use of diagnostic imaging (e.g., ultrasound, computed tomography, magnetic resonance imaging) and fine-needle aspiration biopsy. On the other hand, Wilkinson and Hause[130] have reported that without serial- or step-sectioning, there can be a greater than 30% false-negative pathologic interpretation of lymph nodes studied for the presence of tumor.[130]

Several factors that correlate with increased risk for lymphatic metastasis from cancer of the lip have been identified. One is the actual site of the cancer on the lip. Metastasis has often been described as being more likely with SCC of the upper lip.[18] Several authors have reported this to occur in as many as 50% of patients.[13, 31] When reviewed in several larger series, however, the incidence does not seem to vary appreciably from that of the lower lip.[1, 2, 4, 22, 31, 58, 109] The possibility of lymphatic metastasis has also been described as greater with primary cancers of the oral commissure. Of 23 cases reported by Zitsch and colleagues in which the commissure was identified as being involved, 16 had involvement also of either the upper (3) or the lower (13) lip as well, and metastasis was more frequent in these than it was in the 7 patients who had tumors limited to the commissure.[4] Overall statistical information related to cancer of the commissure is not yet clear, but it appears that SCC of the lip that originates in or involves the commissure may have a somewhat greater risk for metastasis, with reported frequencies ranging from 15% to 50%.[2, 4, 58, 128]

As has already been discussed, the size of the primary tumor bears some correlation with increased chances for lymphatic metastasis. Martin and colleagues[31] found metastasis in approximately 3% of their patients with lip tumors smaller than 1 cm; they found that it increased proportionately with tumors of larger size. Cross and coworkers found no cervical metastasis in patients with primary cancer of the lip smaller than 0.5 cm, but they found it to occur in 15% of those 0.5 to 2 cm in size, in 24% of those 2 to 4 cm, and in 33% of those larger than 4 cm.[46] Luce reports that the rate of nodal metastasis is 4% with primary tumors less than 2 cm, 35% with tumors 2 to 4 cm, and 63% with tumors greater than 4 cm.[14] Most patients with lymph node metastasis have primary tumors that are larger than 2 cm.[2, 4, 41, 62, 126, 128] The concurrent or delayed finding of lymphatic metastasis is reported to occur in 16% to 35% of patients in whom the primary tumor size is larger than 2 cm, with a comparative rate of 4% to 7% for those with tumors smaller than 2 cm.[4, 14, 23, 64]

SCCs of the lip of higher histologic grade have a proportionately greater chance for metastasis to regional lymph nodes.[46] Taylor and Nathanson and others[1, 22, 131, 132] reported a 6% incidence of lymph node metastasis in lip cancers of low grade, 30% in those of medium grade, and 52% in those of high grade. The identified rate of metastasis that can be determined in Broders' patients is 0.0% for grade I, 11% for grade II, 56% for grade III, and 50% for the few patients with grade IV.[42] Frierson and Cooper[66] found cervical metastasis in 4% of grade II lip cancers, 34% of grade III, and 92% of those considered grade IV. Of interest, Cross and coworkers found 7 cases in which the metastatic lip tumor was of higher pathologic grade than was the primary lip carcinoma.[46]

Other features of primary lip cancer that are associated with a higher rate of regional lymphatic metastasis include more aggressive patterns of invasion, greater tumor thickness, presence of neural invasion, and, with less importance, ulcerative morphology.[66]

Factors that could help predict the presence of relatively infrequent occult lymph node metastasis have been evaluated in one retrospective study.[124] The authors concluded that the high risk for occult regional metastasis could be predicted by a primary tumor size greater than 3 cm, by high histologic grade, or by locally recurrent tumor.

Staging

For purposes of treatment planning and tumor reporting, a clinical stage should be determined for every cancer of the lip and its metastases. Similar rules for staging of lip cancer with a TNM system, which considers the primary cancer of the lip (T), regional lymph node status (N), and presence of distant metastasis (M), have been separately adopted by both the American Joint Committee on Cancer (AJCC, formerly the American Joint Committee for Cancer Reporting and End Results Reporting) and the International Union Against Cancer (UICC, Union International Contre le Cancer) (Table 12–1).[6, 7] The current rules for staging cancer of the lip are similar to those applied to cancer of the oral cavity.

Separate pathologic staging may also be done, following surgical treatment and based on histologic examination of a fully resected tissue specimen. When multiple primary cancers of the lip are present, each should be staged independently. A new and separate staging is also advised for cancer that is recurrent. In addition to TNM classification and stage grouping, information considered useful in reporting cancer of the lip at this time includes exact tumor site, morphologic characteristics of the cancer, rating of histologic differentiation, and factors such as degree of infiltration or evidence of bone erosion.[6]

When reviewing information on cancer of the lip, it is necessary for clinicians to determine exactly what rules for staging were used because prior to 1988, there were differences in those advocated by the AJCC and the UICC (see Table 12–1). In 1967, when the American Joint Committee for Cancer Staging and End Results Reporting first introduced its staging for cancer of the oral cavity, cancer of the vermilion was not included.[133] Some authors, however, used these rules also for staging of cancer of the lip.[24] In 1968,

TABLE 12-1 Rules for Staging of Lip Cancer (American Joint Committee on Cancer [AJCC], Union International Contre le Cancer [UICC])

	TIS	T1	T2	T3	T4
AJCC (1967)[132] oral cancers (excludes lip)	In situ	<2 cm	2 cm–4 cm	>4 cm	—
UICC (1968)[106, 124]	In situ	<2 cm, strictly superficial or exophytic	<2 cm, minimal infiltration in depth	>2 cm *or* deep infiltration irrespective of size	Tumor involving bone
AJCC (1976)[133] task force on lip	In situ	<1 cm	1 cm–3 cm	>3 cm	Deep invasion of bone and muscle
AJCC (1976)[133] task force on head/neck sites	In situ	<2 cm	2 cm–4 cm	>4 cm	>4 cm with deep invasion
UICC/AJCC [6, 7, 134, 135] (1977-78 to present [2003])	In situ	<2 cm	2 cm–4 cm	>4 cm	>4 cm with deep invasion (1977/78) Invades adjacent structures (1992) (no size limit, does not include simple invasion of muscle)

Measurements are made of greatest tumor diameter.

the UICC adopted rules for staging of cancer of the lip that differed from those presently used.[123, 127] Consideration was given to degree of invasion, as well as tumor diameter, in all primary tumor categories (T1–T4).[123, 127] In 1976, the AJCC had independent task forces for head and neck sites and for the lip, each adopting rules for staging of cancer of the lip that differed concerning measurement of the primary tumor (T), with both sets of rules being initially published.[105, 134] Uniform agreement on rules for primary tumor staging were adopted by the AJCC and the UICC in 1977, and they continue to be used. Rules for staging of regional lymph node metastasis have gone through considerable evolution over the past three decades. The UICC and AJCC reached similar agreement on nodal (N) staging in 1992.[6, 7, 105, 127, 134, 140]

Previous confusion concerning rules for staging of cancer of the lip poses some difficulties when reviews or comparisons are made with older reported data. In the large Danish series reported by Jorgensen and colleagues[26] in 1973, which used 1968 UICC rules, those lip cancers reported as T2 would be larger T1 tumors by current rules, and those reported as T3 would now be considered as T2 tumors.[123, 127] Excellent studies by Hendricks and coworkers[59] (1977) and by Baker and Krause[1] (1980) demonstrate the confusion created by publishing of conflicting systems by two separate AJCC task forces in 1976; both studies consequently applied T classifications to primary lip tumors of smaller size. Several other staging systems have also been used by various authors in the past.[22, 62, 127]

◘ MANAGEMENT OF CANCER OF THE LIP

A lesion of the lip that is nonhealing or in any other way suspicious for malignancy should be biopsied so that a proper diagnosis can be firmly established. Once histopathologic verification of a cancer diagnosis has been made, a plan for treatment must be formulated. This must include curative management for the primary cancer and for any regional metastasis that may be present. If distant metastasis has already occurred, treatment will essentially be palliative.

A more aggressive treatment may be considered for those patients whose tumors are identified as having more aggressive features.

A variety of therapeutic methods have been employed over the past century in the management of cancer of the lip. Treatments have principally included topical application of destructive agents, electrical or thermal tissue destruction, radiotherapy, and surgical excision. In the treatment of smaller lesions, most of these methods can be very effective. Choice of treatment is most apt to be based on the preferences of both the physician and the patient, the likelihood that lip function and/or cosmesis can be preserved or restored, the relative ease of treatment delivery, and considerations of time and cost.

Surgery and radiotherapy are presently the principal modalities employed in treatment of cancer of the lip. The reported rates of control with both modalities have been remarkably similar, although rates becomes less similar when radiotherapy is used in the treatment of advanced tumors.[1, 18]

Radiation Therapy

Treatment with radiation therapy can be very effective in the management of cancer of the lip. Most studies have shown that treatment with radiation therapy can produce results that are nearly equal to those achieved with surgical treatment of most cancers of the lip, particularly those of small size and without metastasis.[1, 18, 26, 64, 141, 142] Techniques of radiotherapy have gone through considerable evolution over the past century.[143] Radiation therapy is currently delivered in several ways for treatment of lip cancer.

Brachytherapy is a method of radiation therapy that employs the use of interstitial placement of radioactive implants. These are placed directly into the cancer and are carefully positioned to give a planned therapeutic dose to all parts of the cancer. In the past, treatment was most often done with placement of radium needles, which are a high-energy source of photons that can also pose a radiation hazard to both the patient and those who must handle or come near the material.[32, 33, 144] Current practice favors the use of lower-energy radioisotopes such as iridium-192, which are placed in a manner called *afterloading*.[144, 145] First, hollow, nonradioactive needles or tubes that can be filled with a nonradioactive dummy are placed and checked radiographically for proper placement. The radioactive source is placed later under a more controlled setting. Placement of multiple needles may be required; proper positioning is critical to ensure that an effective treatment dose is well distributed. Several applications may be required. Because of the complexities associated with brachytherapy, treatment with external beam is now more commonly preferred.[18, 32, 109]

Radiation therapy can be delivered to the lip from an external source in several ways. The type of beam used can vary, as can the configuration or pattern of the treatment field.[146] *Contact therapy,* a method that uses low-energy x-rays applied directly against the lip, has been used in the past and is still an acceptable means of treatment for smaller lesions.[32, 149] Higher-energy treatment is now generally preferred, particularly for tumors larger than 1.5 cm.[18] Currently, the types of beam most often used are orthovoltage x-rays (100–250 kV) or electrons (which have higher energy).[141, 147]

Treatment dosages typically vary from approximately 5000 cGy for a small cancer of the lip to as much as 7000 cGy for a cancer that is larger and more infiltrative.[18, 33, 109, 145, 148] Treatment is fractionated into schemes of 4 to 6 weeks for most tumors.[141] Treatment with smaller daily fractions that are spread over a longer course generally results in fewer adverse long-term tissue changes, such as atrophy, fibrosis, and telangiectasia.[18, 141, 147]

Osteoradionecrosis can develop when high-dose external beam therapy is given to the entire lip and the underlying portion of the mandible.[141, 145] Protective lead shields may be placed behind the lip during treatment to protect the mandible and other structures of the oral cavity.[141] Divided treatment, using an external beam to deliver the initial and the majority of treatment, followed by use of interstitial implants to deliver additional treatment to the main body of the cancer, may be used and may offer the best overall bone preservation and local tumor control, and possibly the best cosmesis with radiotherapy.[141, 145]

For the past several decades, most cancers of the lip have been treated with surgery; consequently, information on the results of treatment using current methods of radiation therapy is more limited, particularly regarding the treatment of more advanced cancer. Numerous authors have reported that determinate survival at 5 years is greater than 90% for cancers smaller than 2 cm and has been approximately 80% to 90% for primary cancer of the lip larger than this.[1, 18, 26, 60, 62, 64, 141, 145, 149, 150] Gladstone and Kerr[60] reported a successful 3-year determinate control of 92% for cancers of the lip smaller than 2 cm, and 76% for those larger than 2 cm. Jorgensen reported a nearly 25% failure to completely eradicate the primary tumor with radiation therapy for lesions larger than 2 cm or with deep infiltration.[26] In 1964, MacKay and Seller[58] reported that in 2415 patients with cancer of the lip with no clinically detected cervical lymphadenopathy who were treated with radiotherapy alone, an 85% overall 5-year rate of control was noted, with an additional 8% 5-year rate of control with subsequent treatment. In patients with advanced cancer of the lip (T3–T4) and clinically positive nodes who were treated only with radiotherapy, Petrovich and coworkers reported a 5-year actuarial survival of 40%.[151]

A principal advantage of radiation therapy as a choice for treatment of cancer of the lip is that it is much less invasive. Radiation therapy could be considered more often in treatment of cancer of the lip that is relatively superficial but involves an area encompassing more than one third of the lip, for cancers that involve the commissure and significant portions of either lip, for some cancers that are recurrent, and for treatment in patients who either refuse or otherwise cannot undergo surgery.[145]

A significant disadvantage of the use of radiation therapy for management of cancer of the lip is the prolonged time interval necessary for completion of treatment. Also, there is no histologic specimen from which to study the features of or to histologically determine the appropriateness of treatment field margins. A patient who has received radiotherapy requires greater protection from further environmental injury.[141]

The role of radiation therapy in the treatment of verrucous carcinoma has been debated; a higher incidence of local failure has been noted with this tumor. A few cases of anaplastic transformation found with recurrence of oral verrucous carcinoma following radiotherapy have been sufficiently documented, although this has also been documented in several patients who had not previously received radiotherapy.[81, 83] Medina and coworkers[84] have found that at least among oral lesions, there was a definite tendency for recurrences to be less differentiated and nonverrucous, regardless of the initial treatment modality. Reviews by these authors and by McDonald and colleagues[83] have led to the conclusion that radiotherapy should still be considered a generally effective alternative treatment for verrucous carcinoma. With regard to spindle cell carcinoma, data on oral tumors by Ellis and Corio[87] and on laryngeal tumors by Hyams[152] indicate that radiotherapy is not a generally effective treatment modality. It is also not generally favored as primary treatment for malignant salivary gland tumors of the lip.[103]

Surgery

Surgery is the most commonly chosen form of treatment for cancer of the lip. It offers the advantages of rapid treatment and generally complete excision of the tumor. In treatment of larger cancers, the chance for cure is best with wide surgical excision. Surgical excision results in a tissue specimen from which the full scope of favorable or unfavorable histopathologic features can be assessed. Rehabilitation of the patient is generally rapid with immediate reconstruction of the lip. The adjacent uninvolved tissues of the lip do not incur the chronic effects of ionizing radiation. Functional and cosmetic results can be very good to excellent in most cases with surgery.

The major disadvantage of surgery in treatment of cancer of the lip is that it is an invasive procedure, with potentially greater risk for morbidity. It results in a greater loss of nonmalignant tissue than does the use of radiation therapy. In some cases, the ultimate cosmetic or functional results may not be as good as would be possible with the use of radiation therapy.[141]

Any surgical procedure chosen for the management of cancer of the lip must focus on complete, en bloc removal of the tumor with additional normal tissue at all margins of the resection. Anything less than this is oncologically insufficient and would likely result in treatment failure. Preservation or restoration of lip function and cosmesis are important secondary considerations.

Most surgical resections for primary cancer of the vermilion require some form of full-thickness excision of the involved portion of the lip. The most frequently selected configurations of excision are V-shaped, W-shaped, or rectangular. The converging lines of a V or a W excision must not be allowed to come too close to the lateral margins of the tumor. Cosmetically, it is ideal if the unit of lip resection can be confined to within the borders of the anatomic lip unit (e.g., mental crease, melolabial crease, base of nose). With resection of larger cancers, the more vertically directed margins of a W or rectangular design can allow a more comfortable unit of resection.

What constitutes an adequate margin of normal tissue when a cancer of the lip is excised is determined somewhat arbitrarily. Detailed studies comparing the adequacy of various margin sizes during excision of cancer of the lip have not really been done. Most head and neck surgeons who confront this issue have advised that clinical margins of resection for SCC of the lip should be a minimum of 5 to 10 mm.[2, 11, 13, 14, 16, 17, 23, 31] Brodland and Zitelli,[153] using Mohs' micrographic surgery, have attempted to identify comfortable margins of resection for SCC of the skin with a tumor clearance standard of 95% or more. Margins of 4 mm were required to achieve a greater than 95% overall clearance in the 141 tumors studied. It was found that 6-mm margins were required, however, to clear 95% of the tumors that were 2 cm or larger and for tumors of histologic grades 2 to 4.[153] Davidson and coworkers,[154] in review of a series of 111 cases of head and neck mucosal SCCs resected with a modified form of Mohs' surgery, found that 70% of the tumors revealed subclinical peripheral extension of at least 1 cm beyond the clinical margin; in 50%, the margin was found to be at least 1.5 cm, and in 17%, it was found to be as much as 2 cm.

Mohs' Micrographic Excision

An alternative method of surgical excision of cancer of the lip that has gained favor in recent years is Mohs' micrographic resection. This is a method of soft tissue tumor excision that has evolved through several stages of development since it was initially described by Dr. Frederick Mohs in the 1930s.[155–157] It is a method of tumor excision that allows maximal study of tissues at the margins of resection. It was initially performed as a "fixed tissue" technique that required initial in situ chemical fixation of the lip tissue with a zinc chloride paste. The method of Mohs' surgery has now evolved to a "fresh tissue" technique, no longer requiring in situ fixation.[155–157] Microscopically controlled study is done with sampling that is horizontally shaved from all margins of the resected specimen. A system designed to maintain geographic orientation of the specimen makes use of colored stains and division of the specimen into a grid-type pattern of smaller pieces that are carefully mapped as they are individually studied.

Mohs' micrographic resection has become an accepted method of surgical excision for cutaneous malignancies.[156–158] It has become the favored method of resection for cutaneous basal cell carcinomas and SCCs that recur following previous surgery or radiation. It is also favored in the treatment of cutaneous malignancies that display aggressive patterns of growth (such as sclerosing basal cell carcinoma), are located in areas prone to deep invasion or high rates of local recurrence (such as the upper lip, near the nasal base), or are located in cosmetically sensitive areas where minimal resection is desired.[157] The usefulness of Mohs' micrographic resection is predicated on continuity of the tumor as it grows.[157] With much greater caution, it can also be useful in excision of tumors that are multicentric or that have reasonably limited degrees of discontinuity.

The first application of Mohs' micrographic resection in treatment of SCC involving the vermilion portion of the lip was done in 1936 by Dr. Mohs.[155] In 1985, Mohs and Snow reported on his series of 1448 patients with SCC of the lip who had been treated with his technique, noting a 94% overall rate of cure.[155] Mehregan and Roenigk[159] reported that they found no recurrences in a study of 41 patients who had been followed from 13 to 42 months. Cancers of the lip in this second group were all well differentiated, T1 or T2 in stage, and less than 2.5 mm in thickness.[159] In the series reported by Mohs and Snow,[155] 83% of lip tumors were smaller than 2 cm, and in this group, there was a 96.6% 5-year survival rate. For those with tumors larger than 2 cm, the survival rate was found to be 59.6%.[142] Also in this series, tumors assigned a Broders' grade of I or II had a 5-year survival rate of 96.3%, and those with a Broders' grade of III or IV had a 5-year survival rate of only 66.7%. Among 65 patients reported as treatment failures, 20 had positive lymph nodes at the time of resection and 37 displayed positive lymph nodes after treatment.[155] In 1992, Rowe and colleagues[47] performed a literature review and determined that treatment of SCC of the lip with non-Mohs' modalities had a combined long-term recurrence rate that varied from 7.6% with follow-up less than 5 years to 10.5% with longer follow-up; the recurrence rate with Mohs' micrographic surgery was 2.3%.

A disadvantage of the Mohs' micrographic approach is that the total operative time can sometimes become prolonged when several stages are required. Mohs' surgery may also prove to be more expensive than other traditional forms of surgical excision in the treatment of smaller lesions. Although Mohs' surgery is by design more tissue-sparing, in the treatment of larger lesions, it may still prove to be necessary to extend the volume of resection to the peripheral margins of the lip so that restoration may be done with the use of full anatomic or aesthetic subunits.

Presently, for the treatment of high-risk lip cancers, a multidisciplinary approach is favored.[157] Mohs' micrographic resection is currently considered a useful method of surgical treatment for at least smaller malignant tumors involving the vermilion of the lip.[47, 157, 159] Its role in the treatment of larger and high-risk lip cancers is less clear, yet its use is favored by some. More data on Mohs' surgery for treatment of cancer of the lip, particularly those that are larger or of high risk, must be evaluated. Mohs' surgery is frequently preferred for resection of both basal cell carcinoma and SCC involving the skin of the lip in the nasal base region.

Treatment of the Neck

Cervical lymphadenectomy is appropriate treatment when metastasis is present in cervical lymph nodes. In general, when metastatic disease is present in neck nodes, a comprehensive or complete neck dissection is favored. When metastasis is present in the parotid nodes, a parotidectomy, normally with preservation of the facial nerve, should be done in conjunction with a neck dissection. With discretion, it may be acceptable to perform a neck dissection that preserves structures such as the internal jugular vein, spinal accessory nerve, or sternocleidomastoid muscle, but the task of complete lymphatic dissection must be accomplished without compromise. Again, it is important for clinicians to understand that not all detectable lymphadenopathy is found to be metastatic disease, and confirmation with some form of node biopsy may be indicated.

There is considerable controversy regarding the best management of the clinically negative neck. Approximately 80% of patients with cancer of the lip will not develop cervical metastasis in the course of their disease; therefore, they require no treatment to the neck. Elective neck dissection has been advocated by some, particularly when the primary cancer of the lip is large or has more aggressive features.[2, 12, 13, 17, 22, 25, 41, 59, 65, 129, 160] Thus far, there have been limited data supportive of elective neck dissection in the treatment of cancer of the lip, and most authors have not supported the routine practice of elective neck dissection related to carcinoma of the lip.[10, 13, 17, 23, 31, 59, 106, 110, 122, 126, 160–162] Past studies by several authors provide evidence to suggest that the cure rate for therapeutic neck dissection compares favorably with that for elective dissection with confirmed occult metastasis.[17, 58, 67, 122, 126] However, based on their findings, Zitsch and colleagues recommended that patients with poorly differentiated lip carcinoma or locally recurrent carcinoma should be considered for elective neck treatment.[124] Elective treatment of the neck may be favored for patients at higher risk for regional metastasis if good follow-up evaluations cannot be ensured.

Supraomohyoid dissection may be considered a means of assessing metastatic disease in the neck in some patients.[41, 46, 65, 126, 129] If metastatic disease is clearly identified, complete cervical lymphatic dissection is then normally preferred. Supraomohyoid dissection involves complete removal of nodes from levels I, II, and III of the neck.[122] It is a much more complete node-sampling process than is accomplished with a suprahyoid (level I) dissection. In the past, suprahyoid dissection (unilateral or bilateral) had been favored by many authors.[2, 3, 11, 13, 16, 33, 129] Metastatic disease can sometimes be found in the upper cervical nodes when it is not present in the submandibular nodes, making suprahyoid dissection a much less adequate sampling.[3, 127, 163, 164] Bilateral supraomohyoid dissection should be considered when high-risk tumors involve the central portion of the lower lip. The functional and cosmetic consequences of supraomohyoid dissection can be kept to a minimum. If bilateral metastases are found, full bilateral neck dissection is indicated, normally with an attempt to preserve the internal jugular vein on at least one side. With cancer of the upper lip, an ipsilateral dissection of the superficial or lateral lobe of the parotid gland may also be indicated.

Radiotherapy could also be used for elective treatment of the neck in selected high-risk patients.[116] Radiotherapy to the neck is more commonly used as adjuvant treatment following neck dissection with high-risk features, such as in the identification of multiple nodes or nodes with extracapsular invasion. Very little has so far been reported about results with the use of adjuvant radiotherapy following neck dissection related to cancers of the lip. Older data by Ward and Hendrick[33] and by Cross and coworkers[46] indicate a 3-year survival rate of 58%, and a 5-year rate of approximately 51%.

Lymphatic mapping and sentinel lymphadenectomy is a novel approach that has been used to address the controversy over the use of elective lymphadenectomy for cutaneous melanoma and for cancer of the breast. This is a surgical staging procedure that, in theory, can predict which patients need treatment of the regional lymphatics by confirmation of metastasis in the radiolocalized, excised sentinel lymph node. This approach has been tested with promising results in some small pilot studies for oral and pharyngeal SCCs.[165–168] None of these studies, however, included cancers of the lip. Yet, from a technical standpoint, the lip readily lends itself to the identification of lymph node metastasis with this technique. Patients with large or poorly differentiated lip cancers are the ones for whom this technique would have the best potential for a beneficial impact on management.[124]

Cervical lymph node metastasis has a significant impact on prognosis. With cervical metastasis, the expected 5-year survival rate has been reported variously from 29% to 68%.[1, 18, 20, 26, 32, 121–123, 127] Stoddart[109] has reported control of neck disease in 47% of patients identified with cervical metastasis at the time of initial diagnosis of lip cancer; control of neck disease was achieved in 50% of those presenting with cervical metastasis some time after the original lip cancer treatment. Most authors have reported 5-year survival rates for those treated with positive cervical metastatic disease to be in the range of 40% to 50%.[1, 2, 20, 26, 67, 105, 118, 125] Results are poorer in those with more advanced neck disease.

Treatment of Advanced Tumors

Lip cancers that are deeply invasive, especially those that involve the mandible or mental nerve or that have metastasized to regional lymph nodes, must be considered serious disease that requires aggressive treatment (Fig. 12–17).[116] Surgical resection is usually considered necessary for curative treatment. Adjuvant treatment with radiation therapy should be considered for the treatment of locally advanced lip cancers (T4 and many T3). Radiation therapy should be given serious consideration when tumors are recurrent, when there have been positive surgical margins, when there is perineural spread of the lip cancer, or when tumors are poorly differentiated.[16, 125] Adjuvant radiation therapy may also be used for the treatment of nonepidermoid lip cancers that are of high grade, are known to generally have aggressive biologic behavior, and are known to be radiosensitive.

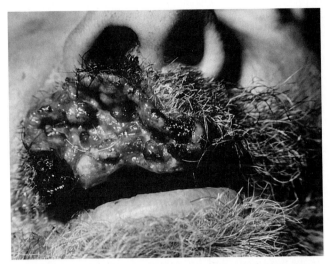

FIGURE 12–17 Patient with advanced squamous cell carcinoma of the upper lip. Treatment involved surgical excision with local flap repair and radiotherapy. No further disease was reported after more than 5 years.

Radiographic evaluation of the mandible is better done with computed tomography (CT scan) than with Panorex or other plain film study, but with all of these, considerable bone erosion must occur before involvement with tumor can be clearly identified.[120, 169] Bone scans can show evidence that suggests malignant involvement of the mandible at an earlier stage, but they cannot identify neural involvement or clearly distinguish cancerous invasion from inflammatory changes. Magnetic resonance imaging (MRI), with the use of contrast-enhancing agents such as gadolinium-diethylenetriamine pentaacetic acid, can be a better way of showing evidence of neural involvement, but it cannot yet clearly define the microscopic peripheral extent of disease.[121, 170] Newer forms of scanning, such as positron emission tomography, may be found useful.

Surgical resection in this setting should be performed with wide margins.[16] Biopsy of the mental (and much less commonly the infraorbital) nerve may be necessary. If tumor is found at the foramen, segmental bone resection is indicated with study of the revised distal nerve stump to help determine if further resection and/or other treatments are needed.[117, 170]

When tumors directly encroach onto the alveolar process or the outer cortex of the mandible, composite resection should include at least a marginal mandibulectomy. For malignant tumors that actually invade the mandible, a generous segmental resection is indicated (see Fig. 12–16). When invasion of the mandible has occurred, the prognosis is extremely poor. Adjuvant radiotherapy is usually provided. The 5-year survival rate is only approximately 30%.[24, 116, 123] In malignant tumors arising from the minor salivary glands of the lip that have shown tendency to perineural and mandibular invasion, rates of cure are generally no better.[100, 101]

Recurrence

Recurrent disease is most likely to present in the primary field of the lip or as regional lymphatic metastasis or as both. Recurrence at distant sites is extremely rare for cancer of the lip that is locally and regionally controlled. Local recurrence of cancer of the lip following initial treatment with surgery or radiation ranges from approximately 5% to 25% overall and is the most common form of treatment failure for this disease.[1, 3, 24, 25, 33, 46, 47, 58–60, 63, 64] As might be expected, the rate of local recurrence tends to increase proportionally with the size of the original lip cancer.[2, 18, 24, 26] Baker and Krause[1] noted local recurrence in approximately 10% of lesions smaller than 3 cm, in 21% of those larger, and in 91% of those with deep invasion.[1] In addition, the specific lip subsite of involvement has been associated with varied chances for local recurrence of lip cancer—the highest incidence has been noted with cancer of the commissure, and the lowest with cancer of the lower lip.[2, 46, 128]

Recurrence in the lip is best managed with aggressive surgical resection, incorporating the use of intraoperative margin assessment to ensure as completely as possible total clearance of the tumor. Strong consideration should be given to elective neck dissection because up to one fourth of these patients are likely to present with subsequent cervical lymph node metastases.[1] Surgical management of local recurrences of lip cancer can be successful in a range of approximately 60% to 85% of the time, as long as there has not been bone involvement.[2, 24, 116, 171] The salvage rate is considerably lower if the local recurrence is associated with cervical lymph node metastases. With a limited sampling, Baker and Krause[1] have shown that rates of recurrence in the neck following cervical node treatment vary proportionately with the initial clinical neck stage, ranging from 40% for N1 disease to nearly 100% for N3 disease in their series.

Alternative Forms of Management

In addition to radiotherapy and surgery, there are a number of other possible modalities that are not standard but in selected cases could be considered for treatment of cancers of the lip. Topical application of a wide variety of caustic agents such as arsenic paste and nitric acid has historically been used for attempted treatment of cancers of the lip, as well as other surface sites, but with limited success.[172–175] Such topical therapy is difficult to control, and its tumoricidal activity is least effective at the deep margins of the tumor, where cancer invasion is of greatest concern.

Cryotherapy

In unusual circumstances, cryotherapy could be considered in the treatment of smaller lip cancers, although no clear data have yet been reported on its use. When tumor cells are exposed to temperatures lower than −40°C, they are effectively destroyed.[143] The most commonly used cryogenic agent is liquid nitrogen (−195.6°C) because it is readily available and can be effective in achieving adequate therapeutic tissue temperatures.[143] Application of cryogen to the tumor results in a growing "iceball." A greater degree of tissue destruction occurs with a rapid freeze. Repeated freezing also results in greater destruction. Thermocouples could be placed into the deep margins of the tumor to further ensure adequacy of treatment in the base portions of the lesion.

Cryotherapy is most commonly used in the treatment of various benign skin lesions and, less commonly, for treatment of smaller skin malignancies. Skin cancers smaller than 1.5 cm have been successfully treated with cryotherapy, with recurrence rates reported to be lower than 5%.[143] A fairly significant edema may be present for at least several days following cryotherapy, and an eschar is formed that tends to weep. Healing typically takes several weeks and often results in a scar that is atrophic and hypopigmented. The lip is not an ideal structure for treatment with cryotherapy because of the discomfort associated with healing and the potential for development of a poor-quality scar.

Electrotherapy

Electrotherapy has been used in the past and could still be used in the treatment of lip cancer.[47, 170, 176] It is most commonly used for destructive treatment of various benign skin lesions and less commonly for small skin cancers. Electrotherapy makes use of thermal injury to destroy tissue lesions. Four modalities available for electrical tumor destruction are electrocautery, electrocoagulation, electrofulguration, and electrodesiccation.[143] Most treatment has been done with electrodesiccation.[47, 143, 170] Physical curettage may also be used to facilitate removal of eschar, allowing improved access to deeper portions of the tumor and removal of malignant tissue. Reported cure rates are as high as 95% for cutaneous carcinomas that are smaller than 1.5 cm.[47, 143] Electrotherapy creates an eschar that tends to weep. Healing is principally completed in several weeks. Dissatisfaction with scarring and poor ability to satisfactorily control completeness of treatment make this method of treatment less ideal for cancers involving the vermilion of the lip.

Chemotherapy

Chemotherapy may be considered in treatment of cancer of the lip, but no method has as yet emerged that can offer satisfactory or consistent curative results. Attempts have been made to treat smaller cancers of the skin with repeated topical application of 5-fluorouracil. Satisfactory response has reportedly been found only in the treatment of superficial basal cell carcinoma and SCC in situ (Bowen's disease), with reported 5-year cure rates of approximately 80%.[143] Topical 5-fluorouracil is available for treatment in concentrations of 5% to 20% in a hydrophilic base. Treatment for cancer requires numerous repeated daily applications, preferably kept under some form of occlusion and continued for a period of as long as 1 to 3 months. Such treatment for cancer of the vermilion of the lip is particularly difficult. Topical chemotherapy at this time offers very little for treatment of cancer of the vermilion portion of the lip.

α-Interferon has been under investigational use for the treatment of primary cutaneous malignancies. It has both antiproliferative and immunomodulatory effects that are felt to be useful in the treatment of malignancies.[143] Pilot studies have reportedly produced some encouraging responses in the treatment of nodular and superficial types of basal cell carcinoma.[143] Adverse reactions to treatment have included local pain, erythema, flulike symptoms (e.g., fever, chills, myalgias, fatigue, headache), leukocytopenia, and thrombocytopenia.[143] This form of treatment could be considered for use in some malignancies of the skin of the lip, but no data have so far been reported showing its use in the treatment of malignant tumors of the lip vermilion.

Systemically administered chemotherapy has also been used in the treatment of lip cancer. A variety of chemotherapeutic agents have been used, most often in a multiagent combination.[148, 177] Currently, chemotherapy is used as either an adjuvant treatment for advanced disease or, more commonly, palliative treatment of disease that is otherwise deemed incurable.

Photodynamic Therapy

Photodynamic therapy employs a photosensitizing agent that preferentially localizes within tumors and becomes activated upon exposure to some form of light, resulting in tumor necrosis. A variety of photosensitizing agents have so far been tried. Light activation is usually done with some form of laser, often transferred through a fiberoptic system. It may be administered as surface illumination or with interstitial implantation in the treatment of larger lesions. Photodynamic therapy has been used, at least experimentally, in the treatment of a wide variety of malignant tumors of many body sites, such as the lung, esophagus, and bladder. It has been used by investigators in treatment of cancers of the skin, with mixed results.[178, 179] In the attempted treatment of melanoma, responses have reportedly been noted to be more dramatic in those tumors that are lighter in pigmentation.[178]

Photodynamic therapy has been used in the treatment of cancer of the vermilion of the lip, but so far very little has been reported on this. In a phase II trial Kubler and associates[180] treated 25 patients with primary SSL of the lip, using Foscan-mediated photodynamic therapy and reported a 96% (24/25) complete response rate at 12 weeks, all supported by biopsy. With a mean follow-up of 424 days for this series, there was one patient who was found with a single site of cervical nodal metastasis 7 months after therapy. At present it appears that photodynamic therapy may have a useful place in treatment of cancers of the lip; however, more investigation needs to be done. Photodynamic therapy can be considered for palliative treatment in some patients.

◼ LIP RECONSTRUCTION

Reconstruction of the lip is necessary after excision of the cancer. This requires an understanding of the anatomy and physiology of the lip. Reconstruction should be planned to provide optimal preservation and restoration of anatomic and cosmetic subunits of the lip. Aesthetically, it is best if all incisions can be placed along the peripheral borders of the lip unit (mental and melolabial creases) or parallel with the lines of relaxed skin tension of the lips (see Fig. 12–1). For adequate function of the lip, it is best if continuity of the orbicularis muscle sphincter can be restored in some fashion, particularly in the lower lip.

In reconstruction of the lip, the first consideration should be methods that use tissues from within the anatomic lip unit. In general, there is no better substitute for lip tissue than lip tissue. Because it has no skeletal parts, the lip displays a remarkable tolerance for stretching, which is very useful in reconstruction. A wide variety of techniques can be used in reconstruction of the lips. Examples of some of the more favored methods are provided here.

Reconstruction of simple cutaneous defects can usually be done in routine fashion with fusiform closure, of which the long axis should be directed in parallel with the relaxed skin tension lines. Cosmetically, it is desirable if the unit of tissue resection can be designed to avoid crossing the mental or melolabial crease when possible. M-plasty may be used on one or the other end, but it makes orientation of closure lines somewhat more complicated. Skin grafts may be placed on the lip but are likely to be cosmetically inferior to what can be achieved with local flap repair. Full-thickness skin grafts are normally preferred.

For cutaneous reconstruction for defects of the upper lip, we favor flap transfer of skin and subcutaneous tissue from below and lateral to the oral commissure, where tissue redundancy is usually greatest[181-183] (Fig. 12–18A–D). The outline for this flap is designed as an inferolateral continuation of the melolabial cease. So that appropriate flap width is maintained, it may be necessary for the outline to encroach a short distance laterally into the cheek in those whose crease passes close to the commissure. Transfer of the flap involves both rotation and advancement as the tissue is brought up and around the commissure. It becomes progressively more difficult to reconstruct defects that are

more medial in the lip because distortion of the commissure becomes an increasing problem as the flap is transferred. Second-stage revision of the commissure could be performed, but it is not commonly needed; many times, the commissure tends to self-correct with time because it is greatly influenced by the muscle activity of the lip. Closure of the upper lip defect can be made easier with simultaneous use of a more conservative, laterally directed rotation advancement of tissue from the medial portion of the lip, with great care taken to minimize distortion of the philtrum or the base of the nose. If the defect extends into the cheek, closure may also be facilitated by simultaneous direct medial advancement of tissue from the melolabial fold.[181-183]

Defects of the vermilion are most often restored by forward advancement of the buccal mucosa (Fig. 12–19). Dissection for this flap is done in the submucosal plane. Neural and vascular connections can be preserved and stretched forward with the advancing flap, optimizing sensory function for the restored vermilion.[11, 13, 16-18, 181-186] Alternative reconstructions for the vermilion include transfer of mucosa with the use of pedicled flaps from the opposing lip or from the tongue, requiring second-stage pedicle release.[181, 184, 186, 187]

In full-thickness lip repair, V-shaped closure can be done for defects of up to one third of the lip. Meticulous approximation of all tissue layers should be done to optimize the cosmetic result, with special care to approximate precisely

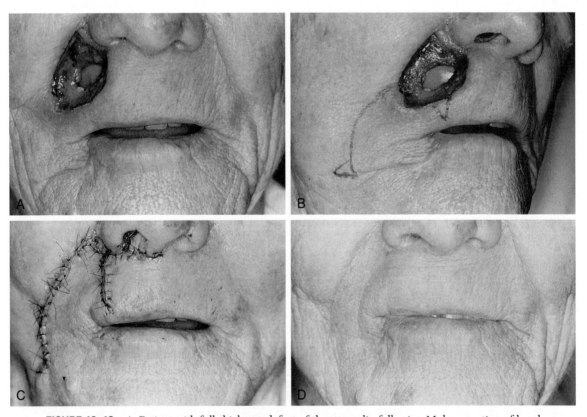

FIGURE 12–18 *A,* Patient with full-thickness defect of the upper lip following Mohs resection of basal cell carcinoma of the upper lip. *B,* Outline is made for a labial rotation/advancement flap from the lateral portion of the lip. *C,* Flap has been transferred. A smaller rotation/advancement flap from the central portion of the lip has also been used, with care to avoid distortion to the base of the nose. Note that the right oral commissure has been turned up. *D,* The surgical result at 4 weeks. The lip unit shows good overall symmetry, and the oral commissure has corrected itself.

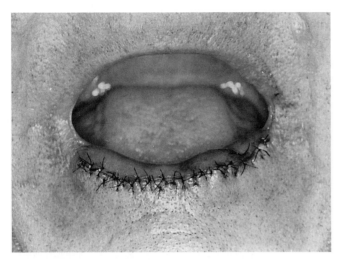

FIGURE 12–19 Resurfacing of the vermilion is demonstrated with anterior advancement of the buccal mucosa.

the anterior vermilion line.[11, 13, 16, 18, 181, 186–188] V-shaped closure should be oriented so that the line of closure is parallel with the relaxed skin tension lines for that portion of the lip, which means that it should be more obliquely oriented in more lateral portions of the lip.

Closure following W-shaped excision is similar. The principal line of closure should also be oriented in parallel with the lines of relaxed skin tension. In general, it is best if the two points of the W can be placed at the mental or melolabial crease.[13, 183, 186] If the resection has extended beyond the creases, the apex of the central triangle should be brought back to the crease line, so that there is a single line of scar in the lip, and so that the diverging distal scar lines remain outside the lip unit in a way that can be better masked.[181, 188]

Reconstruction of rectangular full-thickness defects of the lip requires some form of flap repair. Defects of as much as 50% of the lower lip can often be satisfactorily reconstructed with simultaneous, bilateral advancement of the remaining lip segments, with a releasing incision made along the mental crease (Fig. 12–20A and B).[11, 16, 181–184, 186, 183, 189] The same concept can be used in reconstruction of the upper lip, but it requires the removal of small crescent-shaped units of tissue from the cheek, taken immediately lateral to the nasal ala on each side, which then allows a more natural tissue advancement beneath the nose (Fig. 12–21).[181, 184, 188] This form of reconstruction is obviously best suited to restoration of defects of the more central portion of the lip.

A significant advancement in the reconstruction of larger defects of the lip was described by Karapandzic in 1974 (Fig. 12–22A–D).[190] This actually further refined a method of reconstruction initially described by von Bruns in 1857, which involves simultaneous bilateral, full-thickness, circumoral flaps.[15, 181, 184] Releasing incisions are placed around the peripheral margins of the anatomic lip unit and should be masked within the mental and melolabial creases as much as possible.[17, 181–183, 186, 189] Karapandzic's unique contribution to this reconstruction was to describe the isolation and preservation as much as possible of neural and vascular structures that are encountered in the plane of dissection, so that motor and sensory functions are preserved.[11, 181, 188–192] In the dissection, the muscles of facial expression are carefully separated from the orbicularis muscle and then are later reattached at anatomically correct relative positions after the orbicularis has been adjusted for restoration of the sphincter. Transfer of the flaps involves a unique combination of advancement and rotation around the mouth opening.

The Karapandzic reconstruction has now become one of the principal methods of major lip reconstruction. It can be used to comfortably restore defects of up to 60% to 70% of either lip.[14, 16–18, 141, 181–183, 186, 190–192] The relatively long outlining incision requires particularly meticulous closure so that the circumoral line of scar does not detract from the appearance. There is some tendency for blunting of the oral commissures, although this is not usually a major problem. The only real limit to this method of reconstruction is the degree to which the mouth opening will be narrowed, particularly in those who wear dentures.[184, 186] It is possible

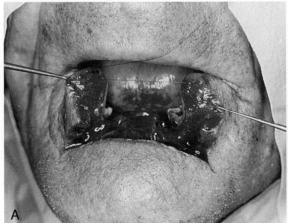
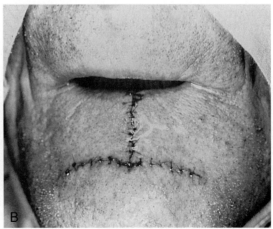

FIGURE 12–20 *A*, Patient with large rectangular defect of the central lower lip. Releasing incisions have been made bilaterally along the mental crease. A suture tag marks the anterior vermilion line on both sides. *B*, Lip is repaired with bilateral advancement of the flaps. (From Zitsch RP III: Carcinoma of the lip. Otolaryngol Clin North Am 26:267–269, 1993.)

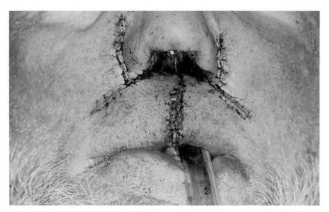

FIGURE 12-21 Patient after resection of carcinoma of the central upper lip and nasal base. Crescent-shaped excisions of skin were taken on each side of the nose to allow easier advancement of opposing flaps beneath the nose.

to enlarge the mouth opening over time with use of an expanding appliance or manual stretching techniques.[193]

Reconstruction of large, full-thickness lip defects can in many cases also be accomplished with some form of cross-lip flap (Fig. 12-23A and B).[11, 13, 16-18, 24, 181-184, 186, 188, 189] This concept of reconstruction has evolved since its first intro-

duction by Sabatinni in 1836.[184] More popularized descriptions of these flaps with separate variations were later reported by Estlander in 1872 and Abbe in 1898.[184, 194, 195] These have traditionally been taken as triangular or V-shaped flaps that are kept viable with a small pedicle that contains the labial artery. Cross-lip flaps may be transferred around the commissure as a single-stage procedure, or across the mouth opening as a two-stage procedure, with release of the pedicle at 2 to 3 weeks. Transfer of the flaps around the commissure typically results in blunting of the angle, which may be improved later with a commissureplasty.[13, 181, 188] Attempts have been made to transfer these as a free composite graft with some success; however, viability has not proved to be dependable.[196]

Cross-lip flaps may be designed with a rectangular approach, or with a W shape when desired.[18, 181-183, 186, 188, 197] They may be combined with other forms of reconstruction, and multiple cross-lip flaps may be used simultaneously. The biggest drawback to the use of cross-lip flaps is the total denervation that occurs as they are transferred. Some degree of motor and sensory function redevelops within these flaps over the course of several months to a year.[181, 198, 199] Because these flaps are almost totally surrounded by scar, there is a strong tendency for them to appear thickened and for the scar to appear sunken (Fig. 12-24). A cross-lip flap may

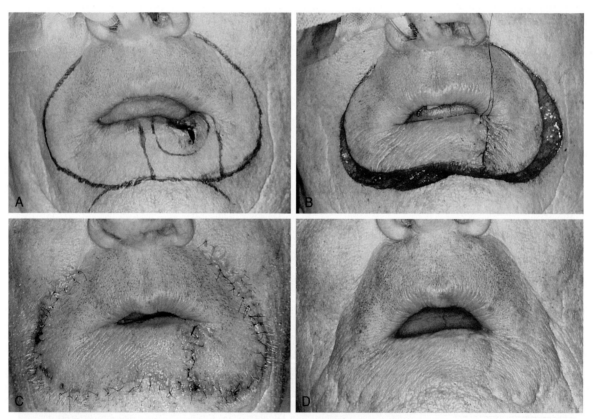

FIGURE 12-22 *A,* Plan for excision of a large cancer of the lower lip to be followed by Karapandzic-type flap repair. The mental and melolabial creases are used as much as possible, but the outline must be taken into the cheek, slightly lateral to the oral commissure on each side, to maintain roughly uniform flap width. *B,* After the Karapandzic flaps have been brought together, the entire lip unit can be adjusted to the best overall position before the lateral flap margins are closed. *C,* Same patient at 1 week after surgery. Exacting technique is required in tissue closure so that the perioral scar creates minimal deformity. *D,* Patient at approximately 9 months, with reasonably little deformity and excellent lip function.

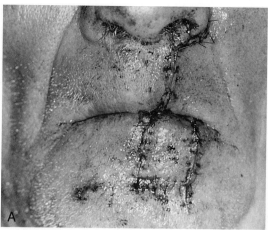 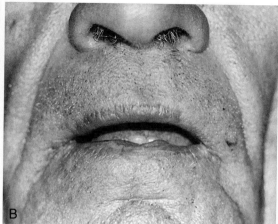

FIGURE 12–23 *A*, Patient immediately after transfer of a rectangular cross-lip flap. *B*, Same patient 6 months after completed transfer of the cross-lip flap. (From Zitsch RP III: Carcinoma of the lip. Otolaryngol Clin North Am 26:267–269, 1993.)

be used in combination with other forms of lip advancement.[16, 18, 188] Multiple (bilateral) cross-lip flaps may also be used for repair of some larger lip defects.[32, 200]

In the mid-19th century, Bernard and von Burow separately described a method for reconstruction of major full-thickness defects of the lip.[184] It involves direct medial advancement of tissue from the cheeks, which is facilitated by removal of strategically placed triangles of skin that allow for a more even redistribution of the facial tissues (Fig. 12–25*A–C*).[11, 16–18, 24, 32, 161, 181, 184, 186, 188, 189] This concept of reconstruction is often referred to as "Bernard cheiloplasty," and von Burow's eponymous credit comes with the term "Burow's triangle." The procedure was originally done with full-thickness incisions but was later modified to minimize disruption of the facial musculature. Other surgeons, most notably Freeman and Webster, have described modifications that attempt to produce more favorable lines of scar and better muscle function.[181, 182, 188, 201–204] This type of reconstruction can be used to restore even total loss of

the lip and can be adapted to reconstruction of either the upper or the lower lip.[184] Overall functional and cosmetic results with this general method of reconstruction are occasionally good, but typically they are only fair because satisfactory restoration of the orbicularis sphincter is often difficult to achieve.[181]

The cheeks and, less commonly, the chin are the most natural sites from which to obtain additional tissue for reconstruction of the lip. A large variety of techniques have been described that can transfer tissue from these areas into the lip. The most commonly chosen method involves transposition of skin and subcutaneous tissue from the melolabial fold, using a pedicle that is either superiorly or inferiorly based.[11, 13, 14, 18, 181, 184, 205–207] The melolabial (nasolabial) flap is designed so that the donor site, as it is closed, is well hidden within the melolabial crease. Use of a superiorly based pedicle tends to cause greater cosmetic detraction because it disrupts the medial portion of the melolabial crease—a situation that can be improved later by placing an incision across the pedicle in a fashion that restores the full line of the crease.[181, 206]

Melolabial transposition may be used for cutaneous resurfacing of the lip and in some situations for full-thickness lip deficits. It is not capable of truly restoring orbicularis muscle but rather relies on a certain degree of tightness. It is therefore less ideal in full-thickness reconstruction of the lower lip. Surfacing for the underside of these flaps may be done either with a second flap, including the skin or oral mucosa, or with application of a graft of skin or mucosa.[184] A skin graft can be buried beneath the cheek flap in a "delayed" fashion for 2 to 3 weeks, allowing the combined tissues to be later transferred as a composite.[181]

Massive full-thickness defects of the lip may require reconstruction with some form of distant flap or with a microvascular free flap.[16, 184, 188] In general, all of these reconstructions are capable of providing tissue for wound closure and replacement of the lip, but with the possible exception of some uniquely arranged microvascular flaps,

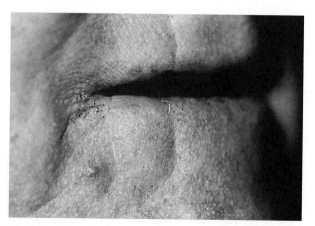

FIGURE 12–24 Persistent thickened appearance of a cross-lip flap after several years. Slight depression of the scar lines is noted in this patient.

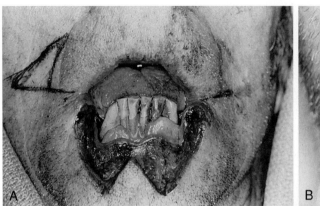
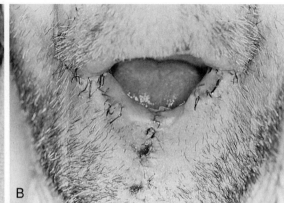
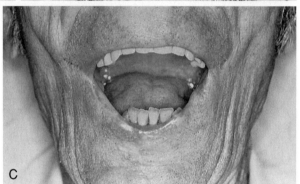

FIGURE 12–25 *A,* Patient who has lost essentially all of the lower lip after resection for recurrent cancer. Outline has been made for a modified Bernard-type repair. *B,* Result at 1 week. Lateral portions of the vermilion were reconstructed with buccal mucosa. *C,* Patient seen at 1 month, demonstrating good ability to open the mouth and place the upper denture. The central lower lip in this patient is extremely thin and has poor tone. He can close his mouth well, but some problems with oral continence are noted.

they have not so far been able to completely restore a fully functional lip.

REFERENCES

1. Baker SR, Krause CJ: Carcinoma of the lip. Laryngoscope 90:19–27, 1980.
2. Cruse CW, Radocha RF: Squamous cell carcinoma of the lip. Plast Reconstr Surg 80:787–791, 1987.
3. Heller KS, Shah JP: Carcinoma of the lip. Am J Surg 138:600–603, 1979.
4. Zitsch RP III, Park CW, Renner GJ, et al: Outcome analysis for lip carcinoma. Otolaryngol Head Neck Surg 113:589–596, 1995.
5. Feind CR: The head and neck. In Haagensen CD, Feind CR, Herter FP, et al: The Lymphatics in Cancer. Philadelphia, WB Saunders, 1972.
6. Greene FL, Page DL, Fleming ID, et al.: AJCC Cancer Staging Manual, 6th ed. New York, Springer-Verlag, 2002.
7. Sobine LH, Wittekind Ch: TNM Classification of Malignant Tumors, 5th ed. New York, Wiley-Liss, 1997.
8. Fritz A, Percy C, Jack A: International Classification of Diseases for Oncology, 3rd ed. Geneva, World Health Organization, 2000.
9. SEER Summary Staging Manual 2001 Codes and Coding Instructions. http://seer.cancer.gov/tools/ssm/.
10. Shambaugh EM, Weiss MA, Axtell LM: Summary Staging Guide for the Cancer Surveillance, Epidemiology and End Results Reporting (SEER) Program. US Department of Health and Human Services Publication No. (NIH)82–2313, 1983.
11. Bailey BJ: Management of carcinoma of the lip. Laryngoscope 87:250–260, 1977.
12. Blot WJ: Oral and pharyngeal cancers. In Doll R, Fraumeni JF, Muir CS (eds): Cancer Surveys: Trends in Cancer Incidence and Mortality, vol 19/20. New York, Cold Spring Harbor Laboratory Press, 1994.
13. Lore JM, Kaufman S, Graban JC, et al: Surgical management and epidemiology of lip cancer. Otolaryngol Clin North Am 12:81–95, 1979.
14. Luce EA: Carcinoma of the lower lip. Surg Clin North Am 66:3–11, 1986.
15. Goss CM: Gray's anatomy, 28th ed. Philadelphia, Lea & Febiger, 1966.
16. Esclamado RM, Krause GJ: Lip cancer. In Bailey BJ (ed): Head & Neck Surgery--Otolaryngology, vol 2. Philadelphia, JB Lippincott, 1993.
17. Holt GR: Surgical therapy of oral cavity tumors: Lip tumors. In Thawley SE, Panje WR (eds): Comprehensive Management of Head and Neck Tumors. Philadelphia, WB Saunders, 1987.
18. Baker SR: Cancer of the lip. In Myers EN, Suen JY (eds): Cancer of the Head and Neck, 2nd ed. New York, Churchill Livingstone, 1989.
19. Buzzell RA: Effects of solar radiation on the skin. Otolaryngol Clin 26:1–11, 1993.
20. Figi FA: Epithelioma of the lower lip. Surg Gynecol Obstet 59:810–819, 1934.
21. Dardanoni L, Lorenzo G, Rosario P, et al: A case-control study on lip cancer risk factors in Ragusa (Sicily). Int J Cancer 34:335–337, 1984.
22. Molnar L, Ronay P, Tapolesanji L: Carcinoma of the lip. Oncology 29:101–121, 1974.
23. Wurman LH, Adams GL, Meyerhoff WL: Carcinoma of the lip. Am J Surg 130:470–474, 1975.
24. Creely JJ, Peterson HD: Carcinoma of the lip. South Med J 67:779–784, 1974.
25. Bernier JL, Clark ML: Squamous cell carcinoma of the lip. A critical statistical and morphological analysis of 835 cases. Mil Surg 109:379–397, 1951.
26. Jorgensen K, Elbrond O, Andersen AP: Carcinoma of the lip. A series of 869 cases. Acta Radiol Ther Phys Biol 12:177–190, 1973.
27. Brownson RC, Reif JS, Chang JC, et al: Cancer risks among Missouri farmers. Cancer 64:2381–2386, 1989.
28. Keller AC: Cellular types, survival, race, nativity, occupations, habits, and associated diseases in the pathogenesis of lip cancer. Am J Epidemiol 91:486–499, 1969.
29. Baker SR: Risk factors in multiple carcinomas of the lip. Otolaryngol Head Neck Surg 88:248–251, 1980.
30. Ju DMC: On the etiology of cancer of the lower lip. Plast Reconstr Surg 52:151–154, 1973.
31. Martin HM, MacComb WS, Blady JV: Cancer of the lip. Part I. Ann Surg 114:226–242, 1941.
32. Martin HM, MacComb WS, Blady JV: Cancer of the lip. Part II. Ann Surg 114:341–368, 1941.

33. Ward CE, Hendrick JW: Results of treatment of carcinoma of the lip. Surgery 27:321–342, 1950.
34. Haydon RC: Cutaneous squamous carcinoma and related lesions. Otolaryngol Clin 26:57–71, 1993.
35. Granstein R: Photoimmunology. Semin Dermatol 9:16–24, 1990.
36. Douglass CW, Gammon MD: Reassessing the epidemiology of lip cancer. Oral Surg 57:631–642, 1984.
37. Lindquist C: Risk factors of lip cancer: A critical evaluation based on epidemiologic comparisons. Am J Public Health 69:256–260, 1979.
38. Sankaranarayanan R, Duffy SW, Padmakumary G, et al: Risk factors for cancer of the buccal and labial mucosa in Kerala, southern India. J Epidemiol Community Health 44:286–292, 1990.
39. Kaugars GE, Riley WT, Brandt RB, et al: The prevalence of oral lesions in smokeless tobacco users and an evaluation of risk factors. Cancer 70:2579–2585, 1992.
40. Brewer GE: Carcinoma of the lip and cheek. Surg Gynecol Obstet 36:169–184, 1923.
41. Kennedy RH: Epithelioma of the lip. With particular reference to lymph node metastases. Ann Surg 99:81–93, 1934.
42. Broders AL: Squamous cell epithelioma of the lip: A study of 537 cases. JAMA 74:656–664, 1920.
43. Blomquist G, Hirsch JM, Alberius P: Association between development of lower lip cancer and tobacco habits. J Oral Maxillofac Surg 49:1044–1047, 1991.
44. Ebenius B: Carcinoma of the lip. Acta Radiol (Stockh) Suppl 48, 1943.
45. Spritzer WO, Hill GB, Chambers LW, et al: The occupation of fishing as a risk factor in cancer of the lip. N Engl J Med 293:419–424, 1975.
46. Cross JE, Guralnick E, Daland EM: Carcinoma of the lip: A review of 563 case records of carcinoma of the lip at the Pondville Hospital. Surg Gynecol Obstet 87:153–162, 1948.
47. Rowe DE, Carroll RJ, Day CL: Prognostic factors for local recurrence, metastasis, and survival rates in squamous cell carcinoma of the skin, ear, and lip. J Am Acad Dermatol 26:976–990, 1992.
48. Penn I: Cancer in the immunosuppressed organ recipient. Transplant Proc 23:1771–1772, 1991.
49. Berger HM, Goldman R, Gonick HC, et al: Epidermoid carcinoma of the lip after renal transplantation: Report of two cases. Arch Intern Med 128:609–612, 1971.
50. Barr BB, Benton EC, McLaren K, et al: Human papilloma virus infection and skin cancer in renal allograft recipients. Lancet 1:124–128, 1989.
51. Bradford CR, Hoffman HT, Wolf GT, et al: Squamous carcinoma of the head and neck in organ transplant recipients: Possible role of oncogenic viruses. Laryngoscope 100:190–194, 1990.
52. Lindquist C: Risk factors in lip cancer: A questionnaire survey. Am J Epidemiol 109:521–530, 1979.
53. Grover R, Douglas RG, Shaw JHF: Carcinoma of the lip in Aukland, New Zealand, 1969–1987. Head Neck 11:264–268, 1989.
54. Szpak CA, Stone MJ, Frenkel EP: Some observations concerning the demographic and geographic incidence of carcinoma of the lip and buccal cavity. Cancer 40:343–348, 1977.
55. Levi F, La Vecchia C, Te VC, et al: Trends in lip cancer incidence in Vand, Switzerland. Br J Cancer 68:1012–1013, 1993.
56. American Cancer Society: Cancer Facts & Figures–1996. Atlanta, Publications of American Cancer Society, 1996.
57. American Cancer Society: Cancer Facts & Figures–1991. Atlanta, Publications of American Cancer Society, 1991.
58. MacKay EN, Seller AH: A statistical review of carcinoma of the lip. Can Med Assoc J 90:670–672, 1964.
59. Hendricks JL, Mendelson BC, Woods JE: Invasive carcinoma of the lower lip. Surg Clin North Am 57:837–844, 1977.
60. Gladstone WS, Kerr HD: Epidermoid carcinoma of the lower lip: Results of radiation therapy of the local lesion. Am J Roentgenol Radium Ther Nucl Med 79:101–113, 1958.
61. Boddie AW, Fischer EP, Byers RM: Squamous cell carcinoma of the lower lip in patients under 40 years of age. South Med J 70:711–712, 1977.
62. Burkell CC: Cancer of the lip. Can Med Assoc J 62:28–33, 1950.
63. Longenecker CG, Ryan RF: Cancer of the lip in a large charity hospital. South Med J 58:1459–1460, 1965.
64. Ashley FL, McConnell DV, Machida R, et al: Carcinoma of the lip: A comparison of five year results after irradiation and surgical therapy. Am J Surg 110:549–551, 1965.
65. Maroon SZ, Kennedy RH: Carcinoma of the lower lip: A ten year survey. Ann Surg 130:896–901, 1949.
66. Frierson HF, Cooper PH: Prognostic factors in squamous cell carcinoma of the lower lip. Hum Pathol 17:346–354, 1986.
67. Eckert CT, Petry JL: Carcinoma of the lip. Surg Clin 24:1064–1076, 1944.
68. Lindquist C, Teppo L: Is upper lip cancer "true" lip cancer? J Cancer Res Clin Oncol 97:187–191, 1980.
69. Rice DH, Spiro RH: Current concepts in head and neck cancer. Atlanta, Publications of American Cancer Society, 1989.
70. Glass AG, Hoover RN: The emerging epidemic of melanoma and squamous cell skin cancer. JAMA 262:2097–2100, 1989.
71. Czarnecki D, Mechan C, O'Brien T, et al: The changing face of skin cancer in Australia. Int J Dermatol 30:715–717, 1991.
72. Rowe D, Gallagher RP, Warshawski L, et al: Females vastly outnumber males in basal cell carcinoma of the upper lip. Am J Dermatol Surg Oncol 20:754–756, 1994.
73. Ham AW: Histology, 6th ed. Philadelphia, JB Lippincott, 1969.
74. Bailey BM: A rare malignant connective tumor arising in the upper lip. Br J Oral Surg 21:129–135, 1983.
75. Banuls J, Botella R, Sevila A, et al: Leiomyosarcoma of the upper lip. Int J Dermatol 33:48–49, 1994.
76. Miller RL: Non-Hodgkin's lymphoma of the lip: A case report. J Oral Maxillofac Surg 51:420–422, 1993.
77. Piatelli A, Tamborrino F, Tamborrino G: Angiosarcoma of the oral cavity: A clinical case report and review of the literature. Minerva Stomatol 39:951–957, 1990.
78. Piatelli A: Pleomorphic rhabdomyosarcoma of the upper lip in an adult patient. Acta Stomatol Belg 88:57–64, 1991.
79. Carey TE, Wennerberg J: Cellular and molecular biology of the cancer cell. In Yao-Shi F, Wenig BM, Abemeyer E, Wenig BL: Head and Neck Pathology with Clinical Correlations. New York, Churchill Livingstone, 2001.
80. McClatchey KD, Zarbo RJ: The jaws and oral cavity. In Sternberg SS, Antonioli DA, et al (eds): Diagnostic Surgical Pathology, 2nd ed. New York, Raven Press, 1994.
81. Batsakis JG, Hybels R, Crissman JD, et al: The pathology of head and neck tumors: Verrucous carcinoma. Head Neck Surg 5:29–38, 1982.
82. Harrison EG: Tumors and tumor-like conditions of the lips and cheeks. In Dockerty MB et al (eds): Tumors of the Oral Cavity and Pharynx. Washington, DC, Armed Forces Institute of Pathology, 1968.
83. MacDonald JS, Crissman JD, Gluckman JL: Verrucous carcinoma of the oral cavity. Head Neck Surg 5:22–28, 1982.
84. Medina JE, Dichtel W, Luna MA: Verrucous-squamous carcinomas of the oral cavity: A clinicopathologic study of 104 cases. Arch Otolaryngol 110:437–440, 1984.
85. Hansen LS, Olson JA, Silverman S: Proliferative verrucous leukoplakia. Oral Surg 60:285–298, 1985.
86. Rosai J: Ackerman's Surgical Pathology, 7th ed. St. Louis, CV Mosby, 1989.
87. Ellis GL, Corio RL: Spindle cell carcinoma of the oral cavity: A clinicopathologic assessment of fifty-nine cases. Oral Surg 50:523–534, 1980.
88. Weitzner S: Adenoid squamous-cell carcinoma of vermilion mucosa of lower lip. Oral Surg 37:589–593, 1974.
89. Lever WF, Schaumburg-Lever G: Histopathology of the Skin, 7th ed. Philadelphia, JB Lippincott, 1990.
90. Johnson WC, Helwig EB: Adenoid squamous cell carcinoma (adeno-acanthoma): A clinicopathologic study of 155 patients. Cancer 19:1639–1650, 1966.
91. Wick MR, Pettinato G, Nappi O: Adenoid (acantholytic) squamous carcinoma of the skin (abstract). J Cutan Pathol 15:351, 1988.
92. Weitzner S, Hentel W: Multicentric basal-cell carcinoma of vermilion mucosa and skin of lower lip: Report of a case. Oral Surg Oral Med Oral Pathol 26:269–272, 1968.
93. Keen, RR, Elzay RP: Basal cell carcinoma from mucosal surface of lower lip: Report of a case. J Oral Surg Anesth Hosp D Serv 22:453–455, 1964.
94. Williamson JJ, Cohney BC, Henderson BM: Basal cell carcinoma of the mandibular gingiva. Arch Dermatol 95:76–80, 1967.
95. Nguyen AV, Whitaker DC, Frodel J: Differentiation of basal cell carcinoma. Otolaryngol Clin 26:37–56, 1993.
96. Welton DG, Elliot JA, Kimmelstiel P: Epithelioma: Clinical and histologic data on 1,025 lesions. Arch Dermatol 60:277–293, 1949.
97. Strong EW, Spiro RH: Cancer of the oral cavity. In Myers EN, Suen JY (eds): Cancer of the Head and Neck, 2nd ed. New York, Churchill Livingstone, 1989.

98. Alvi A, Myers EN, Johnson JT: Cancer of the oral cavity. In Myers EN, Suen JY: Cancer of the Head and Neck, 3rd ed. Philadelphia, WB Saunders, 1996.

99. Batsakis JG, Regezi JA, Soloman AR, et al: The pathology of head and neck tumors: Mucosal melanomas, part 13. Head Neck Surg 4:404–418, 1982.

100. Byers RM, Boddie A, Luna MA: Malignant salivary gland neoplasms of the lip. Am J Surg 134:528–530, 1977.

101. Weber RS, Palmar JM, Adel E, et al: Minor salivary gland tumors of lip and buccal mucosa. Laryngoscope 99:6–9, 1989.

102. Spiro RH: Salivary neoplasms: Overview of a 35-year experience with 2,807 patients. Head Neck Surg 8:177–184, 1986.

103. Owens OT, Calcaterra TC: Salivary gland tumors of the lip. Arch Otolaryngol 108:45–47, 1982.

104. Shpitzer T, Stern Y, Segal K, et al: Carcinoma of the lip: Observations on its frequency in females. J Laryngol Otol 105:640–642, 1991.

105. Norante JD, Rubin P: Head and neck tumors. In Rubin P, Bakemeier RF (eds): Clinical Oncology for Medical Students and Physicians, 5th ed. Atlanta, Publications of American Cancer Society, 1978, p 169.

106. Beltrami CA, Desinan L, Rubini C: Prognostic factors in squamous cell carcinoma of the oral cavity. Pathol Res Pract 188:510–516, 1992.

107. Perras C: Carcinoma of the lip. Am J Surg 104:746–752, 1962.

108. Lund C, Sogaard H, Elbrond O, et al: Epidermoid carcinoma of the lip: Histologic grading in the clinical evaluation. Acta Radiol Ther Phys Biol 14:465–474, 1975.

109. Stoddart TG: Conference on cancer of the lip: Based on a series of 3166 cases. Can Med Assoc J 90:666–670, 1964.

110. Wang XL, Chen RM, Wang ZS, et al: Flow cytometric DNA-ploidy as a prognostic indicator in oral squamous cell carcinoma. Chin Med J-Peking 103:572–575, 1990.

111. Hemmer J, Kreidler J: Flow cytometric DNA ploidy analysis of squamous cell carcinoma of the oral cavity: Comparison with clinical staging and histologic grading. Cancer 66:317–320, 1990.

112. Suzuki K, Chen RB, Nomura T, et al: Flow cytometric analysis of primary and metastatic squamous cell carcinomas of the oral and maxillofacial region. J Oral Maxillofac Surg 52:855–861, 1994.

113. Balsara BR, Borges AM, Pradhan SA, et al: Flow cytometric DNA analysis of squamous cell carcinomas of the oral cavity: Correlation with clinical and histopathological features. Eur J Cancer 30:98–101, 1994.

114. Chen RB, Suzuki K, Nomura T, et al: Flow cytometric analysis of squamous cell carcinomas of the oral cavity in relation to lymph node metastasis. J Oral Maxillofac Surg 51:397–401, 1993.

115. Goepfert H, Dichtel WJ, Medina JE, et al: Perineural invasion in squamous cell skin carcinoma of the head and neck. Am J Surg 148:542–547, 1984.

116. Byers RM, O'Brien J, Waxler J: The therapeutic and prognostic implications of nerve invasion in cancer of the lower lip. Int J Radiat Oncol Biol Phys 4:215–217, 1978.

117. Ballantyne AJ, McCarten AB, Ibanez ML: The extension of cancer of the head and neck through peripheral nerves. Am J Surg 106:651–667, 1963.

118. Schmidseder R, Dick H: Spread of epidermoid carcinoma of the lip along the inferior alveolar nerve. Oral Surg 43:517–520, 1977.

119. Anderson C, Krutchkoff D, Ludwig M: Carcinoma of the lower lip with perineural extension to the middle cranial fossa. Oral Surg Oral Med Oral Pathol 69:614–618, 1990.

120. Kolin ES, Castro D, Jabour BA, et al: Imaging case of the month: Perineural extension of squamous cell carcinoma. Ann Otol Rhinol Laryngol 100:1032–1034, 1991.

121. Backus LH, DeFelice CA: Five year end results in epidermoid carcinoma of the lip with indications for neck dissections. Plast Reconstr Surg 17:58–63, 1956.

122. Medina JE, Byers RM: Supraomohyoid neck dissection: Rationale, indications and surgical technique. Head Neck Surg 11:111–122, 1989.

123. Sack JG, Ford CN: Metastatic squamous cell carcinoma of the lip. Arch Otolaryngol 104:282–285, 1978.

124. Zitsch RP, Lee BW, Smith RB: Cervical lymph node metastasis and squamous cell carcinoma of the lip. Head Neck 21:447–453, 1999.

125. Modlin J: Neck dissections in cancer of the lower lip. Surgery 28:404–412, 1950.

126. Marshall KA, Edgerton MT: Indications for neck dissection in carcinoma of the lip. Am J Surg 133:216–217, 1977.

127. Mahoney LJ: Resections of cervical lymph nodes in cancer of the lip: Result in 123 patients. Can J Surg 12:40–43, 1969.

128. Teichgraeber JF, Larson DL: Some oncologic considerations in the treatment of lip cancer. Otolaryngol Head Neck Surg 98:589–592, 1988.

129. Durkovsky J, Krajci M, Michalikova B: To the problem of the lip cancer metastases. Neoplasma 19:653–659, 1972.

130. Wilkinson EJ, Hause L: Probability in lymph node sectioning. Cancer 33:1269–1274, 1974.

131. Taylor, GW, Nathanson IT: Evaluation of neck dissection in carcinoma of the lip. Surg Gynecol Obstet 69:484–492, 1939.

132. Taylor GW, Nathanson IT: Lymph node metastases. New York, Oxford University Press, 1942.

133. Smith RR, Bullock WK, Friedman M, et al (eds): Clinical Staging System for Carcinoma of the Oral Cavity. Chicago, American Joint Committee, 1967.

134. American Joint Committee for Cancer Staging and End-Results Reporting: Classification and Staging of Cancer by Site: A Preliminary Handbook. Chicago, American Joint Committee, 1976.

135. Beahrs OH, Carr DT, Rubin P (eds): Manual for Staging of Cancer, 2nd ed. Chicago, American Joint Committee, 1978.

136. Harmer MH (ed): TNM Classification of Malignant Tumors, 2nd ed. Geneva, Union International Contre Le Cancer, 1978.

137. Hermanek P, Sobin L: TMN: Classification of Malignant Tumors, 4th ed. New York, Springer-Verlag, 1987.

138. Spiessl B, Beahrs OH, Hermanek P, et al: TNM Atlas: Illustrated Guide to the TNM/pTNM Classification of Malignant Tumors, 3rd ed. New York, Springer-Verlag, 1989.

139. Beahrs OH, Myers MH (eds): Manual for Staging of Cancer, 2nd ed. Philadelphia, JB Lippincott, 1983.

140. Beahrs OH, Henson D, Hutter RVP, et al (eds): Manual for Staging of Cancer, 3rd ed. Philadelphia, JB Lippincott, 1988.

141. Million RR, Cassisi NJ: Management of Head and Neck Cancer: A Multidisciplinary Approach, 2nd ed. Philadelphia, JB Lippincott, 1994.

142. Lampe I: The place of radiation therapy in the treatment of carcinoma of the lower lip. Plast Reconstr Surg 24:34–44, 1959.

143. Limmer BL, Clark D: Nonsurgical management of primary skin malignancies. Otolaryngol Clin North Am 26:167–184, 1993.

144. Bhadrasain V: General principles of radiation therapy for head and neck cancer. In Myers EN, Suen JY (eds): Cancer of the Head and Neck, 2nd ed. New York, Churchill Livingstone, 1989.

145. Wang CC: Radiation Therapy for Head and Neck Neoplasms: Indications, Technique, and Results, 2nd ed. Chicago, Yearbook Medical Publishers, 1990.

146. Almond PR: Physics of radiation therapy of head and neck tumors. In Thawley SE, Panje WR (eds): Comprehensive Management of Head and Neck Tumors. Philadelphia, WB Saunders, 1987.

147. Westgate SJ: Radiation therapy for skin tumors. Otolaryngol Clin North Am 26:295–309, 1993.

148. Zagars GK, Novante JD, Smith JL, et al: Tumors of the head and neck. In Rubin P (ed): Clinical Oncology, 7th ed. Philadelphia, WB Saunders, 1993.

149. Lampe I: The place of radiation therapy in the treatment of carcinoma of the lower lip. Plast Reconstr Surg 24:34–44, 1959.

150. Schreiner BF, Christy CJ: Results of irradiation treatment of cancer of the lip: Analysis of 636 cases from 1926–1936. Am J Roentgenol Radiol Ther 39:293–297, 1942.

151. Petrovich Z, Kuisk H, Tobochnik N, et al: Carcinoma of the lip. Arch Otolaryngol 105:187–191, 1979.

152. Hyams VJ: Spindle cell carcinoma of the larynx. Can J Otolaryngol 4:307–313, 1975.

153. Brodland DG, Zitelli JA: Surgical margins for excision of primary cutaneous squamous cell carcinoma. J Am Acad Dermatol 27:241–248, 1992.

154. Davidson TM, Haghighi P, Astarita R, et al: Mohs for head and neck mucosal carcinoma: Report on III patients. Laryngoscope 98:1078–1083, 1988.

155. Mohs FE, Snow SN: Microscopically controlled surgical treatment for squamous cell carcinoma of the lower lip. Surg Gynecol Obstet 160:37–41, 1985.

156. Stone JL: Mohs micrographic surgery: A synopsis. Hawaii Med J 52:134–139, 1993.
157. Clark D: Cutaneous micrographic surgery. Otolaryngol Clin 26:185–202, 1993.
158. Miller PK, Roenigk RK, Brodland DG, et al: Cutaneous micrographic surgery: Mohs procedure. Mayo Clin Proc 67:971–980, 1992.
159. Mehregan DA, Roenigk RK: Management of superficial squamous cell carcinoma of the lip with Mohs micrographic surgery. Cancer 66:463–468, 1990.
160. Zitsch RP: Carcinoma of the lip. Otolaryngol Clin 26:265–277, 1993.
161. Lee ES: Cancer of the lip. Proc R Soc Med 63:685–690, 1970.
162. Lyall D, Robson W, Grier N: Experiences with squamous carcinoma of the lip with special reference to the role of neck dissection. Ann Surg 152:1067–1070, 1960.
163. McGregor GI, Davis NL, Hay JH: Impact of cervical lymph node metastases from squamous cell cancer of the lip. Am J Surg 163:469–471, 1992.
164. Baker SR: Current management of cancer of the lip. Oncology 4:107–120, 1990.
165. Zitsch RP III, Todd DW, Renner GJ, et al: Intraoperative radio-lymphoscintigraphy for detection of occult nodal metastasis in patients with head and neck squamous cell carcinoma. Otolaryngol Head Neck Surg 122:662–666, 2000.
166. Stoeckli SJ, Steinert H, Pfaltz M, et al: Sentinel lymph node evaluation in squamous cell carcinoma of the head and neck. Otolaryngol Head Neck Surg 125:221–226, 2001.
167. Shoaib T, Suotar DS, Prosser JE, et al: A suggested method for sentinel node biopsy in squamous cell carcinoma of the head and neck. Head Neck 21:728–733, 1999.
168. Alex JC, Sasaki CT, Krag DN, et al: Sentinel lymph radiolocalization in head and neck squamous cell carcinoma. Laryngoscope 110:198–203, 2000.
169. Curtin HD, Tabor EK: Radiologic evaluation. In Myers EN, Suen JY (eds): Cancer of the Head and Neck, 2nd ed. New York, Churchill Livingstone, 1989.
170. Brown RG, Poole MD, Calamel PM, et al: Advanced and recurrent squamous carcinoma of the lower lip. Am J Surg 132:492–497, 1976.
171. Dickie WR, Colville J, Graham WJH: Recurrent carcinoma of the lip. Oral Surg Oral Med Oral Path 24:449–454, 1967.
172. Bryant T: Cancer of the lips. In Bryant T (ed): A Manual for the Practice of Surgery. Philadelphia, Lea's Son & Co, 1885.
173. Taylor JM, Freeman FE: Mouth, lips, jaws, diseases. In Sajons CE, Sajons LT (eds): Sajons's Analytic Cyclopedia of Practical Medicine, 7th ed, vol 6. Philadelphia, FA Davis, 1914.
174. Stille A, Maisch JM, Caspari C, et al: The National Dispensatory, 5th ed. Philadelphia, Lea Brothers & Co, 1894.
175. Potter SOM: Materia Medica, Pharmacy and Therapeutics, 9th ed. Philadelphia, Blakiston's Son & Co, 1902.
176. Prinz H, Greenbaum SS: Diseases of the Month and Their Treatment. Philadelphia, Lea & Febiger, 1939.
177. Grau JJ, Palombo H, Estape J, et al: Carboplatin plus Ftorafur as a palliative treatment in locally advanced cancer of the oral cavity and lip. Am J Clin Oncol 17:134–136, 1994.
178. Gluckman JL, Portugal LG: Photodynamic therapy for cutaneous malignancies of the head and neck. Otolaryngol Clin 26:311–318, 1993.
179. Gross DJ, Waner M, Schosser RH, et al: Squamous cell carcinoma of the lower lip involving a large cutaneous surface: Photodynamic therapy as an alternative therapy. Arch Dermatol 126:1148–1150, 1990.
180. Kubler AC, de Carpentier J, et al.: Treatment of squamous carcinoma of the lips using Foscan-mediated photodynamic therapy. Intl J Oral Maxillof Surg 30:504-509, 2001.
181. Renner G: Reconstruction of the lip. In Baker SR, Swanson NA (eds): Local Flaps in Facial Reconstruction. St. Louis, Mosby, 1995.
182. Renner G: Carcinoma of the lip. In Gates GA (ed): Current Therapy in Otolaryngology Head and Neck Surgery, vol 4. Philadelphia, BC Decker, 1990.
183. Renner G, Zitsch RP: Reconstruction of the lip. Otolaryngol Clin 23:975–990, 1990.
184. Mazzola RF, Lupo G: Evolving concepts in lip reconstruction. Clin Plast Surg 11:583–617, 1984.
185. Spira M, Hardy B: Vermilionectomy: Review of cases with variations in technique. Plast Reconstr Surg 33:39–46, 1964.
186. Calhoun KH, Stiernberg CM (ed): Surgery of the Lip (American Academy of Facial Plastic and Reconstructive Surgery). New York, Thieme Medical Publishers, 1992.
187. McGregor IA: The tongue flap in lip surgery. Br J Plast Surg 19:253–263, 1966.
188. Zide BM: Deformities of the lips and cheeks. In McCarthy JG (ed): Plastic Surgery, vol 3. Philadelphia, WB Saunders, 1990.
189. Smith PG, Muntz HR, Thawley SE: Local myocutaneous advancement flaps: Alternatives to cross-lip and distant flaps in the reconstruction of ablative lip defects. Arch Otolaryngol 108:714–718, 1982.
190. Karapandzic M: Reconstruction of lip defects by local arterial flap. Br J Plast Surg 27:93–97, 1974.
191. Jabaley ME, Clement RL, Orcutt TW: Myocutaneous flaps in lip reconstruction: Applications of the Karapandzic principle. Plast Reconstr Surg 59:680–688, 1977.
192. Clairmont AA: Versatile Karapandzic lip reconstruction. Arch Otolaryngol 103:631–633, 1977.
193. Panje WR: Lip reconstruction. Otolaryngol Clin 15:169–178, 1982.
194. Estlander JA: Einc methode aus der cinen lippe substanzverluste der anderen zu ersetzen (Archiv fur Klinishe Chirurgie 14:622, 1872). Translated by Sundell B: The classic reprint. Plast Reconstr Surg 42:361–366, 1968.
195. Abbe RA: A new plastic operation for the relief of deformity due to double harelip. Med Record 53:477–478, 1898.
196. Flanagin WS: Free composite grafts from lower to upper lip. Plast Reconstr Surg 17:376–380, 1956.
197. Templer J, Renner G, Davis WE, et al: A modification of the Abbe-Estlander flap for defects of the lower lip. Laryngoscope 91:153–156, 1981.
198. Takahashi S, Kato K: Functional return of tissue transplanted by Abbe-Estlander operation: Sensory and motor function. Bull Tokyo Dent Coll 7:183–201, 1966.
199. DePalma AT, Leavitt LA, Hardy SB: Electromyography in full thickness flaps rotated between upper and lower lips. Plast Reconstr Surg 21:448–452, 1958.
200. Murray JF: Total reconstruction of a lower lip with bilateral Estlander flaps: Case report. Plast Reconstr Surg 49:658–660, 1972.
201. Freeman BS: Myoplastic modification of the Bernard cheiloplasty. Plast Reconstr Surg 21:453–460, 1958.
202. Webster JP: Crescentic peri-alar cheek excision for upper lip flap advancement with a short history of upper lip repair. Plast Reconstr Surg 16:434–464, 1955.
203. Webster RE, Coffey RJ, Kellcher RE: Total and partial reconstruction of the lower lip with innervated muscle-bearing flaps. Plast Reconstr Surg 25:360–371, 1960.
204. Meyer R, Failat ASA: New concepts in lower lip reconstruction. Head Neck Surg 4:240–245, 1982.
205. Langdon JD, Ord RA: The surgical management of lip cancer. J Craniomaxillofac Surg 15:281–287, 1987.
206. Paletta FX: Early and late repair of facial defects following treatment of malignancy. Plast Reconstr Surg 13:95–108, 1954.
207. Schewe EJ: A technique for reconstruction of the lower lip following extensive excision for cancer. Ann Surg 146:285–290, 1957.

CHAPTER 13

Cancer of the Oral Cavity

Eugene N. Myers
Alfred A. Simental, Jr.

INTRODUCTION

Cancer of the oral cavity accounts for 2% to 6% of all cancers diagnosed annually in the United States and accounts for 30% of all cancers of the head and neck. Each year, 4000 to 8000 deaths are attributed to cancer of the oral cavity.[1] In the United States in 1997, 20,900 new cases of cancer of the oral cavity and 5600 deaths were reported among males, as well as 9850 new cases and 2840 deaths among females. Males are two to three times more likely to be affected than females, largely owing to their higher intake of alcohol and tobacco and their greater exposure to sunlight (predisposing to cancer of the lip). That trend is changing as the number of women using tobacco increases.[2] In India, females have a higher incidence of oral cavity cancer than do men, which is attributed to the use of betel nuts.

Worldwide, the incidence of cancer of the oral cavity varies greatly. In western Europe and Australia, the incidence closely approximates that in the United States, accounting for less than 5% of all cancers. France, India, Brazil, and central and eastern Europe have the highest rates of cancer of the oral cavity in the world. In France, this is the third most common form of cancer in males and the second most common cause of death from cancer.[3] India has the highest rate of cancer of the oral cavity of any country in Asia.[4] The differing social customs are likely responsible for these regional variations in disease incidence. The high rates of oral cancer in France and eastern Europe have historically been linked to heavy consumption of alcohol and tobacco in these countries. In parts of Asia, the habit of chewing betel nut leaves rolled with lime and tobacco, a mixture known as pan, results in prolonged contact of the carcinogens with the buccal mucosa and is thought to be the principal cause of oral cancer in India. The practice of reverse smoking, whereby the lighted end of the cigarette is held in the mouth, also contributes to the higher incidence of cancer of the palate in these countries. Even within the United States, there is a fivefold variation in mortality rates from cancer of the oral cavity between different states as a result of ethnic differences, socioeconomic status, and the more prevalent use of smokeless tobacco in the South.[3]

ANATOMY

The oral cavity encompasses the areas from the vermilion border of the lips to an imaginary plane drawn between the junction of the hard and soft palates and the circumvallate papillae inferiorly. It comprises seven anatomic subsites, including the lips, buccal mucosa, upper and lower alveolar ridges, floor of the mouth (FOM), anterior two thirds of the tongue, retromolar trigone, and hard palate (Fig. 13–1). Lymphatic drainage of the mucosal surfaces of the head and neck occurs by way of relatively constant and predictable routes (Fig. 13–2).[5] Lindberg demonstrated that the superior deep jugular nodes are those most frequently involved in patients with cancer of the oral cavity.[6]

The relative predictability of lymphatic drainage from the oral cavity has led to the popularization of the supraomohyoid neck dissection, in which the lymph nodes in levels I to III, which are most frequently involved with metastatic carcinoma, are selectively removed in those patients with

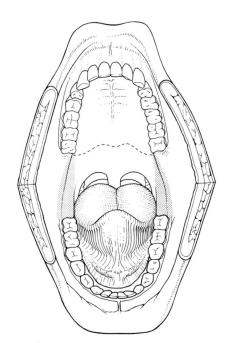

FIGURE 13–1 The oral cavity extends from the vermilion border of the lips to the posterior margin of the hard palate and the line of the circumvallate papillae of the tongue. The *stippled area* corresponds to the retromolar gingiva. The soft palate and base (pharyngeal portion) of the tongue are oropharyngeal sites.

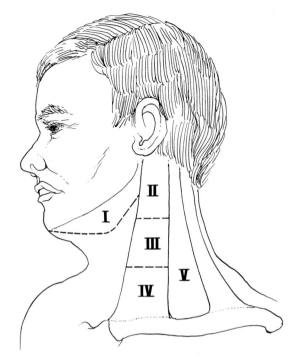

FIGURE 13–2 Levels of cervical lymph nodes. Level I includes the submental and submandibular nodes; levels II, III, and IV (the upper, middle and lower thirds, respectively) the internal jugular nodes; and level V, the nodes of the posterior triangle.

cancer of the oral cavity who have a clinically negative neck (N0).[7] In recent studies, the observation that cancer of the lateral aspect of the oral tongue may metastasize to level IV nodes without involving levels I, II, and III suggests the existence of separate lymphatic channels draining from the oral tongue directly to level IV nodes. Byers and associates found that almost 16% of patients with squamous cell carcinoma (SCC) of the oral cavity had solitary metastasis in level III or IV without involvement of the nodes in levels I or II.[8] These cases of "skip metastases" suggest that level IV lymph nodes should be included in elective neck dissections for these cancers of the oral tongue.[8]

Lips

The lips begin at the junction of the vermilion border with the skin and form the anterior border of the oral vestibule. The oral cavity portion of the lip includes the vermilion surface, or that portion of the lip that comes in contact with the opposing lip. The lymphatics of the medial portions of the lower lip drain primarily into the submental lymph nodes, and the lateral portions drain primarily into the lymph nodes of the submandibular triangle. The lymphatic drainage of the lip emanates from a capillary network beneath the vermilion border; numerous anastomoses exist between lymphatic channels near the midline and account for the bilateral metastasis of cancer that is close to or crosses the midline. Unlike the lower lip, there is sparse crossing of the mucosal lymphatics in the midline upper lip. The upper lip primarily drains into the preauricular, periparotid, submental, and submandibular lymph nodes (level I). These nodes in turn drain into the superior and middle deep jugular nodes (level II/III).

Buccal Mucosa

The buccal mucosa includes the mucosal surfaces of the cheek and lips extending from the line of contact of the opposing lip to the pterygomandibular raphe posteriorly. It extends to the line of attachment of the mucosa of the upper and lower alveolar ridge superiorly and inferiorly. The buccinator muscle forms the lateral wall of the oral vestibule. Cancer extending through the buccinator muscle can involve the buccal fat pad and the subcutaneous tissue and skin over the cheek. Lymphatics from the buccal mucosa drain to the periparotid, submental, and submandibular nodes (level I).

Alveolar Ridge

The alveolar ridges include the alveolar processes of the mandible and maxilla and the overlying mucosal covering. The mucosal covering of the lower alveolar ridge extends from the buccal sulcus to the mucosa of the FOM. The lower alveolar ridge extends to the ascending ramus of the mandible posteriorly. The mucosal coverage of the superior alveolar ridge extends from the buccal sulcus to the hard palate. The superior alveolar ridge extends to the superior end of the pterygopalatine arch posteriorly. Because of the relatively thin layer of mucosa covering the alveolar processes, cancer arising in the superior alveolar ridge can readily invade into the maxillary antrum or floor of nose. Lymphatics of the buccal aspect of the superior and inferior alveolar ridges drain to the submental and submandibular nodes (level I). The lingual aspects of the upper and lower alveolar ridges pass directly to the superior deep jugular and retropharyngeal nodes. Lymphatics of the lingual surface of the inferior alveolar ridge may also drain into the nodes in the submandibular triangle.

Floor of the Mouth

The FOM is a crescent-shaped space extending from the lower alveolar ridge to the ventral surface of the tongue. It overlies the mylohyoid and hyoglossus muscles. Its posterior limit is the anterior tonsillar pillar. The mucosa of the FOM also overlies the mylohyoid and hyoglossus muscles. It is divided anteriorly by the lingual frenulum into right and left sides. Sublingual caruncles are found on each side of the frenulum anteriorly, and the superior portions of the sublingual glands are located posterolaterally.

A muscular sling formed by a pair of mylohyoid muscles extending from the mandible laterally to the hyoid bone medially supports the anterior FOM. Medially, the hyoglossus, styloglossus, and genioglossus muscles are found between the mylohyoid muscle and the mucosa of the FOM. The hyoglossus muscle supports the posterior FOM. The sublingual gland, the lingual nerve, and the hypoglossal nerve are lateral to the hyoglossus muscle, whereas the lingual artery lies medial to this muscle.

Injection studies have demonstrated separate superficial and deep collecting lymphatic systems in the FOM.[9] The superficial system crosses randomly in the midline and drains into both the ipsilateral and contralateral submandibular nodes (level I). The deep system penetrates the mandibular periosteum and drains into the ipsilateral submandibular and superior jugular nodes. The most anterior deep lymphatic system can also cross the midline to drain to the contralateral nodes. Lymphatics from the posterior portion of the FOM drain directly into the jugulodigastric and jugulocarotid nodes. Cancer of the FOM can secondarily involve the ventral tongue or can extend along the lingual nerve, submandibular duct, or into the lingual cortex of the mandible.

Tongue

The mobile two thirds of the tongue anterior to the circumvallate papillae is considered part of the oral cavity; the base of tongue, which is that part posterior to the circumvallate papillae, is considered part of the oropharynx. The oral tongue includes four anatomic areas: the tip, lateral borders, and dorsal and ventral surfaces. Six paired muscles form the mobile tongue—three extrinsic and three intrinsic. Extrinsic muscles include the genioglossus, hyoglossus, and styloglossus muscles. Intrinsic muscles include the lingual, vertical, and transverse muscles. Extrinsic muscles primarily move the body of the tongue; intrinsic muscles alter the shape of the tongue during speech and swallowing.

Lymphatic drainage from the tongue is extensive and is divided into anterior, lateral, central, and posterior groups that drain to the deep jugular nodes between the digastric and omohyoid muscles. The lymphatics are arranged so that the more anterior lymphatic channels drain to the lower first-echelon cervical lymph nodes: The anterior tongue drains into submental nodes that ultimately drain to lower jugulo-omohyoid nodes, and the posterior group drains into the upper jugulodigastric nodes. The central group drains along the lingual artery into the upper jugular nodes. The rich lymphatics of the tongue also provide extensive communication across the midline; cancer of the tongue may occasionally metastasize bilaterally.

Retromolar Trigone

The retromolar trigone (RMT) is a triangular area overlying the ascending ramus of the mandible. The base of the triangle is formed by the last molar tooth, and its apex terminates at the maxillary tuberosity. The base of the triangle is contiguous with the gingivobuccal sulcus laterally and the gingivolingual sulcus medially. The lateral side of the triangle is continuous with the buccal mucosa, and the medial side continues into the anterior tonsillar pillars. The retromolar trigone mucosa is tightly adherent to the underlying mandible; it is not unusual for bony invasion to occur, even in early-stage tumors. The lymphatic drainage of the RMT passes primarily to the superior deep jugular nodes, although some channels can also drain into the periparotid and retropharyngeal nodes.

Hard Palate

The hard palate comprises the primary palate formed by the fusion of the palatine processes of the maxillae, and a secondary palate formed by the fusion of the horizontal laminae of palatine bones. The hard palate extends from the inner surface of the superior alveolar ridge to the posterior edge of the palatine bone. Although the dense mucoperiosteum of the hard palate is relatively resistant to tumor invasion, several pathways allow tumor to spread beyond the hard palate. The primary palate and the secondary palate are fused at the incisive fossa, which can act as a pathway into the nasal cavity. Similarly, the greater palatine foramina allow the spread of tumor posteriorly into the pterygopalatine fossa and skull base. The lymphatic drainage basins of the hard palate include the submandibular (level I) and superior deep jugular (level II) lymph nodes.

ETIOLOGY

Tobacco

Large epidemiologic studies continue to confirm the correlation between the use of tobacco and cancer of the head and neck. More than 300 carcinogens have been identified in tobacco smoke.[10] Of these, the aromatic hydrocarbons benzpyrene and tobacco-specific nitrosamines (TSNs) act locally on keratinocyte stem cells. Once absorbed, these compounds produce DNA adducts that interfere with DNA replication.[10] A review of studies worldwide conducted between 1994 and 2001 indicates a strong causal relationship between smoking and the incidence of cancer of the oral cavity.[11–14] Smoking was an independent risk factor in 80% to 90% of patients with cancer of the oral cavity,[11–14] and the relative risk of developing cancer of the oral cavity is six to eight times greater among smokers than among nonsmokers.[15–17] Kurumatani and colleagues reported a twofold increase in deaths due to cancer of the oral cavity in Japan from 1950 to 1994, which directly correlates with an increase in annual consumption of cigarettes over the same time period.[12]

Exposure to tobacco is thought to result in morphologic changes within the mucosa of the oral cavity that culminate in malignant transformation. These changes are reversible with the elimination of tobacco use. Tobacco cessation is associated with a rapid and marked decline in risk of cancer of the oral cavity.[11, 13, 16, 18] Cessation of smoking resulted in a 30% reduction of risk of cancer in those quitting for 1 to 9 years, and a 50% reduction for those who quit for longer than 9 years.[11] In patients who quit smoking for longer than 20 years, the relative risk of developing cancer of the oral cavity declines to 1.5 times that of nonsmokers.[18]

All forms of tobacco use are associated with cancer of the oral cavity. Cancer of the lip has been associated with pipe smoking, wherein the permeability of the pipe stem and its temperature are cofactors in carcinogenesis.[19] In one study in northern Italy, pipe smoking was associated with a higher risk than cigarettes for the development of oral and esophageal cancers.[19] The resurgence of smokeless tobacco and snuff as "safe" alternatives to smoking has been associated with an increase in cancer of the buccal mucosa.[20] The quid of snuff is usually held between the mucosa of the cheek or lower lip and the jaw, resulting in prolonged close contact with the carcinogens. Studies have shown that exposure to snuff can result in hyperkeratosis, dysplasia, and

SCC.[21] A case-control study in North Carolina found that the risk of cancer of the oral cavity increased four times among users of smokeless tobacco.[20] In addition to the risk of cancer, the use of snuff has been associated with abnormal salivary flow, gingival recession, and nicotine dependence and addiction.[21]

In India and other parts of southeast Asia, a similar habit uses a mixture of dried and cured tobacco leaf, betel nut, and slaked lime (pan) as a stimulant. The slaked lime lowers pH and accelerates the release of alkaloids from the tobacco and the nut. Worldwide, approximately 220 million people practice this habit. In one study, the incidence of cancer of the oral cavity was found to be 123-fold higher in patients who smoked and chewed betel quid than in those who did not.[22] Even without tobacco, the swallowing of betel nut juice or unripened betel fruit in the quid seemed to enhance the risk for cancer of the oral cavity.[22]

In recent years, the increasing popularity of cigar smoking has raised new concerns. In North America, the prevalence rate of the regular use of cigars increased by 133% between 1989 and 1993,[23] and adult cigar use in California increased twofold from 1990 to 1996.[24] Most new cigar smokers reported no previous use of cigarettes.[24] Contrary to popular belief, cigars are not a safe alternative to cigarettes; cigar smokers are four to twenty times more likely to develop cancer of the oral cavity than are nonsmokers,[25] and smoking two cigars a day has been found to be equivalent to smoking a pack of cigarettes daily, in terms of relative risk of developing cancer of the oral cavity.[26] Cigar smoking is also increasing among women. Studies have shown that adolescent girls are being targeted by advertisers with images of cigar-smoking women promoting lifestyles and nontobacco products, much as cigarette ads in the 1960s and 1970s promoted sexual equality and women's liberation.[27] The increase in tobacco use among women is even more alarming in light of studies that seem to indicate sex differences in smoking risk for cancer of the oral cavity: For all levels of tobacco consumption, women appear to be twice as likely as matched groups of men to develop cancer of the oral cavity.[28]

Marijuana

Conclusive links between the use of marijuana and cancer of the oral cavity have yet to be established.[29] Recreational use of marijuana is often combined with alcohol and tobacco, making independent analysis difficult. However, given that the same carcinogens found in tobacco smoke are also found in marijuana, a theoretical risk does exist.

Alcohol

The relationship of alcohol use, particularly hard liquor, to carcinogenesis has long been recognized. Approximately 75% to 80% of all patients who develop cancer of the oral cavity consume alcohol,[30] and the disease is six times more common among drinkers than nondrinkers. The role of alcohol consumption in the etiology of cancer of the oral cavity appears to exist independent of cigarette smoking. Even after adjustments were made for tobacco use, alcohol use in England closely matched the trends in cancer of the oral cavity mortality over the past century.[31] In individuals with extreme alcohol consumption (more than 55 drinks/week), the risk is actually greater than for tobacco alone.[32] Indirectly, alcoholism may result in impaired metabolism resulting from liver dysfunction and nutritional deficiencies that may promote carcinogenesis.

Alcohol and tobacco have a synergistic rather than a cumulative effect on the risk of carcinogenesis. The risk for a smoker who also drinks is 15 times that for one who does not drink.[33] Pooling in saliva of carcinogens from both tobacco and alcohol gives rise to cancers in dependent areas of the mouth, including the FOM, at much higher rates than those associated with either risk factor alone. Eighty percent of patients in Scotland with cancer of the FOM had both a strong smoking history and a higher than average consumption of alcohol.[34]

Ultraviolet Radiation

Outdoor workers have an increased risk for cancer of the lower lip from exposure to ultraviolet radiation. In countries closer to the equator, such as rural Greece, in which there are long daily periods of sunshine, cancer of the lip represents 60% of all cancers of the oral cavity.[35] Prolonged exposure to sunlight has been shown to cause hyperkeratosis and atrophy of fat and glandular elements within skin. The lips are especially vulnerable to ultraviolet radiation because they lack a pigmented layer for protection and are constantly exposed to sunlight. Studies have shown that early life exposures, especially those associated with sunburn, contribute to the formation of cancer of the lip. In southern California, the risk of a woman's developing cancer of the lip is strongly related to her lifetime exposure to solar radiation.[36] Whites in New Zealand have a four times relative risk of developing lip cancer compared with whites in England; migrants to both countries have an intermediate risk.[37] Blacks have some pigment in their lips, which may explain the fact that cancer of the lip is a rare occurrence in this population.

Human Viruses

Patients with recurrent herpes stomatitis develop cancer of the oral cavity even in the absence of other risk factors. Herpes simplex virus (HSV) has been shown to act as a cocarcinogen with tobacco and ultraviolet radiation in certain animal models,[38, 39] suggesting that prolonged HSV exposure may sensitize the mucosa to the carcinogens in tobacco. With the advent of improved polymerase chain reaction (PCR) assays, human papillomavirus (HPV) has been detected in cancer of the cervix and cancer of the oral cavity. HPV-6 and -16 are the most common types associated with cancer of the oral cavity. HPV-16 is twice as likely to be present in precancerous oral mucosa and five times as likely to be present in cancer of the oral cavity than in normal mucosa[40]; men with HPV-6 infection are three times as likely to develop oral cancer as noninfected men.[41] Although high-risk HPV types are known to immortalize human oral epithelial cell cultures,[42] additional exposure to tobacco-related chemicals is required for induction of a malignant transformation.[43] Although studies have detected high-risk

HPV in almost 50% of cancers of the oral cavity, it is still unclear whether infection with high-risk HPV is sufficient to induce the development of cancer of the oral cavity, or whether the detection of HPV in at-risk individuals is predictive of carcinogenesis.

Diet and Nutrition

Certain dietary deficiencies such as iron and vitamins A, C, and E have been associated with oral cancers. Chronic iron deficiency anemia as seen in Plummer-Vinson syndrome or Paterson-Brown Kelly syndrome is associated with dysphagia, glossitis, and atrophy of oral and pharyngeal mucosa. The high incidence of cancer of the oral cavity and pharynx in this group may be due to changes in the mucosa associated with iron deficiency.[44] Several large studies have demonstrated the protective benefits of a diet high in carotenoids, vitamin C, and the fiber found in green vegetables and fruit.[45–47] It has been estimated that the addition of a serving of fruit or vegetables per day is associated with a 50% reduction in the risk of oral cancer.[45] In addition, a high intake of dark yellow, cruciferous, and green leafy vegetables reduced the risk of second primary cancers by 40% to 60% among patients with oral and pharyngeal cancers.[48] Conversely, riboflavin deficiencies related to alcoholism are associated with dysplasia of the oral mucosa and may explain the association between alcoholism and oral cancer.

Dental Factors

Poor oral and dental hygiene is often associated with cancer of the oral cavity. Compared with the control population, patients with cancer of the oral cavity have a higher incidence of advanced dental caries, plaque, and gingival inflammation, and they make fewer visits to the dentist.[49] Although poor oral hygiene is correlated with alcohol and tobacco abuse, some dental factors appear to be independent factors in oral carcinogenesis. The enzymatic conversion of ethanol by oral microflora can lead to an accumulation of acetaldehyde, a known carcinogen in the oral cavity.[50] Poor oral hygiene has been correlated with higher levels of oral microflora and a twofold increase in salivary acetaldehyde production.[50] Oral sores from ill-fitting dentures were associated with a twofold increase in cancer of the tongue, although lifelong denture usage itself was not a risk factor.[51] Although the presence of broken teeth was not an independent risk factor for cancer of the oral cavity,[51] it is reasonable to hypothesize that any persistent irritation to the oral mucosa can lead to dysplastic changes in the epithelium.

GENETIC CHANGES IN ORAL CARCINOGENESIS

As described by Fearon and Vogelstein,[52] the concept of multistep carcinogenesis in colon cancer as it progresses from precancerous polyps to invasive carcinoma has been applied to the clinical, pathologic, and molecular events that occur during the formation of cancer of the oral cavity.[53, 54]

The recent characterization of some of these early molecular changes in the progression of cancer of the oral cavity has improved our understanding of this complex process and may ultimately lead to novel diagnostic and therapeutic interventions. A more detailed coverage of this topic can be found in Chapter 2, "Pathogenesis and Progression of Squamous Cell Carcinoma of the Head and Neck." Some important molecular alterations in oral carcinogenesis include those discussed in the following paragraphs.

EGFR/TGF-α. Epidermal growth factor receptor (EGFR) is a transmembrane tyrosine kinase receptor that can bind to ligands such as EGF and transforming growth factor alpha (TGF-α) and is related to the erbB family of oncogenes.[55] Studies have demonstrated that increased production of EGFR and TGF-α is an early event in head and neck carcinogenesis[56]; tumor levels of EGFR and TGF-α are significant predictors of disease-free and cause-specific survival.[57] Recently, Ford and Grandis suggested that EGFR is upregulated in head and neck SCC, and that blocking EGFR at the level of the receptor or its pathways may offer therapeutic benefit.[58] In addition, Myers and coworkers reported in vitro arrest of oral cancer cells in athymic nude mice with EGFR blockade.[59] This clearly may represent the most recent breakthrough in molecular therapy for squamous cell carcinoma of the head and neck (SCCHN).

TP53 **Gene.** Approximately half of all cancers of the head and neck studied contain a mutation of the *TP53* gene.[58] Cancers of the head and neck have either a high level of abnormal *TP53* expression and/or mutation of the *TP53* gene.[60] The loss of *TP53* function can result in an accumulation of cells with defective DNA, increasing the likelihood of genetic abnormalities and a transformation from preinvasive to invasive lesions.[61] The insertion of wild-type *TP53* into defective head and neck cancer cell lines via an adenovirus-mediated vector can induce apoptosis, which leads to an inhibition of tumor growth in vivo and in vitro.[62]

TP16 **and Cyclin D1.** Both *TP16* and cyclin D1 are involved in regulation of the cell cycle. Many early cancers of the head and neck demonstrate the loss of chromosomal region 9p21, which causes the inactivation of *TP16*.[63] Similarly, amplification of cyclin D1, which constitutively activates cell-cycle progression, is seen in 33% to 68% of cancers in the head and neck; elevated levels of cyclin D1 are associated with more invasive disease.[64–66] Elevated levels of cyclin D1 and a lack of *TP16* expression are correlated with reduced disease-free and overall survival rates in patients with cancer of the tongue.[67]

BAX/BCL2. The apoptotic mechanism of the cell is regulated by a balance of the proapoptotic *BAX* and the antiapoptotic *BCL2* subfamily of molecules.[68–71] Activation of *BAX* and other proapoptotic molecules increases the permeability of the mitochondrial outer membrane, causing a release of cytochrome *c* into the cell.[70] Several studies have demonstrated a differential expression of *BCL2* and *BAX* in oral cavity cancer.[72–74] In general, overexpression of *BCL2* was seen in more poorly differentiated cancer and in dysplastic epithelium adjacent to invasive cancer; *BAX* expression levels were reduced in the same areas.[73, 74] Patients with high *BCL2/BAX* ratios had significantly poorer prognosis than did those with lower ratios.[72]

▣ SECOND PRIMARY CANCERS

A second primary cancer is differentiated from recurrent tumor by temporal or geographic separation. In general, a temporal span of 5 years, a geographically distinct site, or a distance of at least 2 cm from the original primary should suffice as evidence of a second primary. The concept of "field cancerization," first proposed by Slaughter and associates in 1953,[75] has frequently been cited to explain the occurrence of multiple cancers in the head and neck region and recurrence following complete resection of the original cancer. Slaughter and colleagues reviewed specimens from patients with oral and oropharyngeal SCC and found an 11% incidence of multiple cancers.[75] They also noted that even epithelium found some distance from the main cancer contained foci of dysplasia.

These histologic changes seen by Slaughter support the multistep progression of carcinogenesis in the head and neck. In this model, inciting environmental events alter the histologic makeup of the primary cancer and the surrounding mucosa, giving rise to a larger area of "condemned mucosa" that is at increased risk for tumor formation. When this concept is applied to the molecular level, early genetic changes evident in the altered expression levels of molecules critical in the regulation of growth and apoptosis are seen to occur throughout the entire upper aerodigestive tract (UADT), even in histologically normal-appearing mucosa. These areas of biologically condemned mucosa are then at risk of becoming future foci of additional primary cancers in the oral cavity.

The risk for developing a second primary cancer varies from 10% to 40%, depending on the site of the initial cancer. In a meta-analysis,[76] patients with cancer of the oral cavity had the highest rate of second primaries (14%). Most of these second cancers were in the UADT, including the head and neck, lung, and esophagus. In general, at least 50% of all second primary cancers appear within 2 years after initial therapy. The risk for developing a second primary cancer is approximately 5% to 6% per year after treatment of the initial cancer.[77] Second primary cancers have an adverse effect on prognosis, frequently negating any benefit from successful control of the initial cancer. Second primary cancers are the chief cause of treatment failure and death in patients who present with early-stage disease.[78]

▣ PATHOLOGY

Several premalignant and malignant lesions can be found in the oral cavity. More than 90% of all oral cavity carcinomas are SCCs. Other malignancies include tumors of the minor salivary glands, Kaposi's sarcoma, melanoma, and lymphoma. A number of benign lesions can be confused with squamous cell carinoma of the oral cavity (SCCOC) and should be considered in the differential diagnosis, including pyogenic granuloma, keratoacanthoma, necrotizing sialometaplasia, follicular lymphoid hyperplasia, granular cell tumor, and tuberculous ulcers.

Premalignant Lesions

Leukoplakia

Oral leukoplakia is defined as a white keratotic plaque or patch that cannot be rubbed off and cannot be given another diagnostic name.[79] Leukoplakia is unrelated to the presence or absence of dysplasia but is considered a premalignant condition arising from chronic irritation of the oral mucosa. Although it is primarily a clinical description, oral leukoplakia has several key pathologic features, including hyperkeratosis (thickening of the stratum corneum), parakeratosis (increased number of nucleated cells near the surface), and acanthosis (elongation of rete pegs into the submucosa), that are all considered benign findings. Homogeneous oral leukoplakia is a uniformly white, flat lesion that is prevalent in the buccal mucosa and usually has a low potential for malignancy. In contrast, high-risk oral leukoplakia shows abnormal orientation of cells, nuclear hyperchromatism, increased numbers of mitotic figures, and altered nuclear-cytoplasmic ratio. Clinically, these lesions may present a verrucous or speckled pattern, central erosion or ulcer, red patches (erythroplakia), or a peripheral nodule (Fig. 13–3). Follow-up studies indicate that 4% to 18% of these lesions eventually transform into invasive cancer; therefore, they should be treated aggressively.[80]

Smoking, alcohol consumption, chronic cheek biting, ill-fitting dentures, sharp teeth, syphilitic glossitis, candidal infection, and vitamin A and B deficiencies have all been cited as risk factors for the development of oral leukoplakia.[81] Several recent studies have shown a significant correlation between heavy smoking (>20 cigarettes/day), heavy use of snuff, and the prevalence of oral leukoplakia.[82, 83] The role of ill-fitting dentures or poor dentition has not been established as a significant factor in malignant transformation. Moreover, although it is often seen in association with oral leukoplakia, the mutagenicity and carcinogenicity of *Candida albicans* has not been shown.[84]

The natural behavior of oral leukoplakia is unpredictable, and there is little standardization of treatment. Leukoplakia has been shown to regress spontaneously without any specific therapy; conversely, lesions that have been excised have been reported to recur in up to 35% of cases. A baseline biopsy is reasonable for the purposes of establishing a

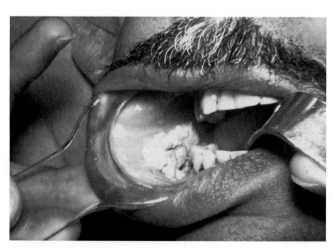

FIGURE 13–3 Verrucous hyperplasia of the buccal mucosa.

diagnosis and ensuring that malignant transformation has not occurred. Leukoplakia with clinically or histologically aggressive features, that is, moderate to severe dysplasia, should be excised. Larger areas of leukoplakia may require extensive excision of the mucosa and grafting. Cryotherapy ablation and carbon dioxide laser ablation have also been employed in the treatment of more extensive areas of leukoplakia. Low-dose β-carotene treatments have produced sustained remissions for up to a year.[85] Regardless of treatment, careful long-term follow-up is essential to ensure that invasive carcinoma does not arise in previously treated areas.

Lichen Planus

Lichen planus is implicated as a premalignant lesion with lymphyocytic infiltrate in the epithelial layers. The cause is unknown. The condition is clinically manifested as lacy white lines on the buccal mucosa with a violaceous background. Occasionally, pain and burning can be associated with this entity. Topical steroids, topical cyclosporine, and retinoids have been used in the treatment of this disease. The prevention of malignant degeneration is an attractive concept known as chemoprevention (see Chapter 32, Chemoprevention).

Erythroplakia

Erythroplakia is defined as a red mucosal plaque most commonly found on the soft palate and tonsillar pillars that does not arise from an obvious mechanical or inflammatory cause and cannot be ascribed to another clinical or pathologic condition. Erythroplakia is associated with a higher risk of malignant transformation than is leukoplakia. The rate of carcinogenesis in erythroplakic lesions has been estimated to be seven times that in homogeneous oral leukoplakia (9.1% vs. 1.3%).[84] Erythroplakia can also be seen in conjunction with leukoplakia in 1% to 3% of cases.[86] These "mixed lesions" have a fivefold increase in malignant transformation over homogeneous oral leukoplakia.[87] Other lesions of the oral cavity can have a reddened appearance and should be considered in the differential diagnosis. These include Kaposi's sarcoma, hemangiopericytoma, and leukemia. Because of their increased malignant potential, all oral erythroplakic lesions should be biopsied for histologic analysis.

Dysplasia

Unlike *leukoplakia* and *erythroplakia*, both of which are clinical terms, *dysplasia* is a histologic term that describes degrees of cellular aberration and abnormal maturation. These changes include an increased nuclear-cytoplasmic ratio, increased rate of mitotic figures, cellular pleomorphism, and an abnormal progression of cells from the basal layer to the more superficial layers. Dysplasia is graded as mild, moderate, or severe, depending on the extent of epithelial involvement: Mild dysplasia describes changes limited to the lower or basal layer of the epithelium; moderate dysplasia involves up to two thirds of the epithelium; and severe dysplasia involves from two thirds to almost the complete thickness of the epithelium. Full-thickness dysplasia is often referred to as *carcinoma in situ* and is characterized by an intact basement membrane. Histologically, the presence of dysplasia suggests a premalignant condition. Although one thinks of the progression of disease from mild dysplasia to carcinoma in situ to invasive carcinoma, full-thickness dysplasia is not a prerequisite for the development of invasive SCC. SCC can arise in any epithelial layer without overlying dysplastic epithelial changes. The reported risk of malignant transformation in oral dysplasia varies from 10% to 14%,[84] but the subjective nature of grading degrees of dysplasia and the lack of orderly progression from mild dysplasia to invasive carcinoma make difficult the assessment of malignant risk in these patients.

Malignant Lesions

Squamous Cell Carcinoma

SCC of the oral cavity exhibits ulcerative, infiltrative, and exophytic growth patterns. Ulcerative forms usually present as round or oval ulcerations with heaped-up edges that bleed easily. This is the most common form of SCC in the oral cavity; it has a tendency for deeper infiltration and higher histologic grade than are seen with infiltrative or exophytic types. Infiltrative growth is common in the tongue and presents as a firm mass or plaque with deep extension into the underlying submucosa. The overlying mucosa is not elevated initially. As the tumor grows, ulcerative or exophytic lesions may appear on the mucosa. The exophytic type is less common and carries a better prognosis.[88] Exophytic lesions have a more superficial growth pattern and gradually become more infiltrative as the tumor progresses. These tumors have a tendency to heap up and may become quite bulky with little invasion of surrounding tissues. This is the most common type arising on the lip; it has a tendency to metastasize later than the other types. The infiltrative type is aggressive, often exhibiting invasion of muscle and mandible. Occasionally, this type of cancer can exhibit perineural invasion.

HISTOLOGIC GRADING

Broders established a histologic grading of SCC based on microscopic evaluation of the tumor.[89] In this system, the percentage of cellular differentiation based on the degree of nuclear pleomorphism, frequency of mitoses, and extent of keratinization is used to classify tumors into four groups from well-differentiated (grade I) tumors with few mitoses and little pleomorphism, to poorly differentiated (grade IV) tumors with high degrees of mitosis and pleomorphism. Broders theorized that the more poorly differentiated carcinoma would have a worse prognosis. It is still widely used today; however, the prognostic value of the Broders grading system is unclear owing to the variability in pathologic interpretation.[90] Other authors have attempted to increase the prognostic value of histologic grading by including other factors such as pattern of invasion, stage of invasion, and presence of angiolymphatic invasion, or by assessing tumor thickness, DNA content, or various other cellular and serum markers.[90, 91]

Verrucous Carcinoma

Verrucous carcinoma refers to an exophytic squamous mucosal or cutaneous tumor that is heaped above the epithelial surface with a papillary micronodular appearance.[92] It is a variant of SCC and presents with a sharply circumscribed deep margin, often described as a "pushing border." Verrucous carcinoma represents less than 5% of all cancers of the oral cavity.[93] Clinically, these lesions can extend deeply into the underlying connective tissue and cause extensive local destruction because of their large size. The histologic appearance is that of a hyperplastic epithelium that pushes toward an intact basement membrane with little or no mitotic activity that classifies them as well-differentiated carcinomas.[94] The hybrid form of verrucous carcinoma contains foci of SCC and can behave aggressively, with the SCC portion having a higher tendency to recur locally and to have the ability to metastasize (Fig. 13–4).[95] Cigarettes, smokeless tobacco, betel nut chewing, and poor dental hygiene have all been implicated in the development of verrucous carcinoma.[96–98]

In a recent review of 2350 cases of verrucous carcinoma of the head and neck in the National Cancer Data Base, the most frequent site of involvement was the oral cavity (55.9%) with gingival and buccal mucosae as the most common subsites.[92] The highest incidence of verrucous carcinoma of the oral cavity was associated with female sex (78%) and advanced age (75% of patients older than 75 years of age). Treatment consisted of surgical excision in the majority of cases (69.7%), with primary radiation therapy (10%) or combination therapy (10%) used infrequently.[92] The infrequent use of radiation therapy in the treatment of verrucous carcinoma may reflect the belief that it is more radioresistant than conventional SCC[99] or that it may dedifferentiate into a more anaplastic carcinoma.[95] Although some studies have reported a 7% anaplastic transformation rate after radiation therapy,[99] recent studies have not reported a significant risk of progression with radiation.[100, 101] In fact, the consensus of many studies now suggests that the development of dedifferentiated carcinoma within verrucous carcinoma after radiation therapy probably reflects an initial sampling error at the time of diagnosis, which failed to identify foci of SCC within a hybrid verrucous carcinoma.[100, 101]

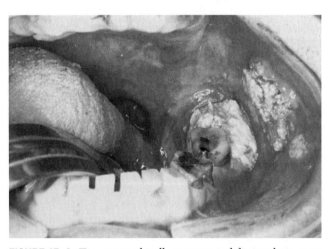

FIGURE 13–4 Two geographically separate and distinct lesions are shown. The lesion on the buccal mucosa is a verrucous carcinoma, with foci of less differentiated SCC present within the lesion. The lesion on the retromolar trigone is invasive SCC.

The 5-year absolute survival rate for verrucous carcinoma has been found to be 61.1% with an adjusted survival rate of 77.9%.[92] Five-year relative survival among localized cases is better for surgery alone (88.9%) than for radiation alone, leading many authors to strongly favor surgical excision in the initial treatment of verrucous carcinoma. Locally confined cancer represented 92.4% of cases in this series; the remaining cases of metastatic disease may have been mistakenly staged clinically based on the pathologic finding that most of the enlarged lymph nodes draining verrucous carcinoma are hyperplastic rather than neoplastic.[92] Because of their indolent biologic behavior, pure verrucous carcinomas rarely metastasize, and elective neck dissection is indicated only in those cases of documented hybrid tumors or when hybrid tumor is strongly suspected.

Basaloid Squamous Cell Carcinoma

Basaloid SCC is an aggressive variant of SCC that is characterized by basaloid cells arranged in nests or cords with pseudoglandular spaces and a high mitotic rate. Clinically, it is described as an ulcerative lesion that cannot be distinguished from other SCCs. Features such as perineural invasion and a duplicated basal lamina make this a distinct entity from acinic cell carcinoma or adenosquamous carcinoma of the minor salivary glands.[102] Basaloid SCC is generally thought to have a higher recurrence rate and a worse prognosis than other SCCs. Patients with basaloid SCC tend to present with more advanced disease and develop distant metastasis more frequently.[103] Histologically, the degree of basaloid differentiation of this cancer can be correlated with its aggressiveness.[102]

Nonepidermoid Malignancies

Nonepidermoid cancers make up less than 10% of all cancers arising in the oral cavity. Most are of minor salivary gland origin, but melanoma, Kaposi's sarcoma, and lymphoma may also occur. Unlike tumors of major salivary glands, approximately 80% of minor salivary gland tumors are malignant.

Adenoid Cystic Carcinoma

Adenoid cystic carcinoma (ACC) accounts for less than 1% of all cancers of the head and neck; however, it is the malignancy most commonly arising from the minor salivary glands, and it represents 30% to 40% of minor salivary gland cancers of the oral cavity.[104, 105] Weber and coworkers found a 42% incidence of ACC in a review of tumors arising from minor salivary glands in the oral cavity.[104] A majority of these tumors occur in the hard palate; they account for 46% of all salivary gland malignancies of the palate.[106] The inferior alveolar nerve is commonly involved by tumor, resulting in numbness in its distribution. ACC is a biologically aggressive cancer characterized by slow growth, local infiltration, and perineural invasion in 5% to 73% of patients.[107, 108] Perineural invasion is common in cancers with local extension and positive margins and has been associated with the development of distant metastasis in patients with ACC. ACC most commonly presents as an asymptomatic mass on the hard palate

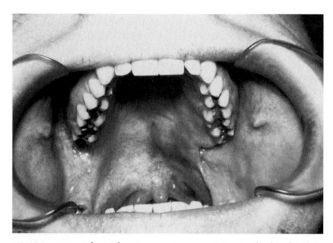

FIGURE 13–5 Adenoid cystic carcinoma arising in the hard palate.

(Fig. 13–5). Regional metastases of this tumor type are less common than distant metastases. In fact, only 14% of patients with cancers of minor salivary gland origin have initial evidence of cervical metastasis on presentation[106]; distant metastasis may occur in up to 50% of patients, with metastasis to the lungs, brain, or bone by the time of death.[108]

Surgery is the treatment of choice for ACC arising from the intraoral minor salivary glands. Combined therapy of surgery followed by radiotherapy results in better local control than is achieved with surgery or radiation therapy alone,[104, 109–111] although surgery alone may be adequate for small T1 cancers. Intraoperative frozen section biopsy of involved or nearby nerves and tissue margins is often employed. If the cancer is near the lingual nerve, the submandibular ganglion may be biopsied for evaluation of invasion by the cancer. If the inferior alveolar nerve is involved, it should be removed from its canal and followed in a retrograde fashion until negative margins are obtained. Neck dissection is reserved for patients with palpable metastasis.

Nearly 15% of these cancers recur more than 5 years after diagnosis; therefore, long-term follow-up is needed. It is not uncommon to see recurrences after as long as 15 to 20 years. The 5-, 10-, and 15-year survival rates are 45%, 33%, and 21%, respectively.[106] These survival rates are significantly better for ACC occurring in the oral cavity than for other sites in the head and neck. Only 22% of patients with oral ACC had recurrence, compared with 56% of patients with involvement of other sites.[112] Treatment failure is usually local; however, when metastasis does occur, it is likely to be associated with a fatal outcome.[113] The well-differentiated histologic pattern seems to predict far less aggressive cancer. However, patients with ACC can live for long periods with even extensive pulmonary metastases. Currently, no systemic therapy has been shown to be effective in treating this cancer. Primary radiation alone has shown good results in some cases, irrespective of tumor stage.[110] In unresectable or recurrent tumors, better locoregional control was achieved with neutron radiotherapy than with photon irradiation in a randomized Radiation Therapy Oncology Group (RTOG) clinical trial.[114] Because most patients with ACC unfortunately will not survive their disease, every effort should be made to treat the primary cancer aggressively to prevent local recurrence.

Kaposi's Sarcoma

Before the advent of acquired immunodeficiency syndrome (AIDS), Kaposi's sarcoma was primarily endemic to elderly men of Mediterranean descent whose disease remained confined to the lower extremities. Kaposi's sarcoma (KS) now is the most common malignancy associated with AIDS. Instead of the indolent course found in the most endemic forms, AIDS-associated KS is a progressive disease that can widely metastasize and involve multiple organ systems. Approximately 50% of patients with AIDS-related KS have oral cavity involvement, and oral KS may be the first manifestation of AIDS (see Chapter 25, Cancer of the Head and Neck in HIV-Infected Patients).

Lesions often involve the perioral skin, hard palate, gingiva, or tongue. Oral lesions range from asymptomatic plaques to ulcerative lesions that bleed or make speaking and eating difficult. Histologically, KS appears as a vascular proliferation with prominent endothelial cells and extravasated erythrocytes. No histologic distinction can be made between endemic and AIDS-related forms of KS. Asymptomatic lesions are usually followed clinically and do not require therapy until symptoms develop. Symptomatic lesions have been treated by primary excision, cryotherapy, laser ablation, and injection of chemotherapeutic agents. Intralesional injection of vinblastine has been used with some success.[115] Systemic chemotherapy has been used in cases of widespread KS.

AIDS-related KS is thought to have a viral etiology (Kaposi's sarcoma herpesvirus/human herpesvirus-8) resulting in malignant degeneration. The use of antiretroviral agents and decreasing human immunodeficiency virus-1 (HIV-1) viral load are associated with a decreased incidence of AIDS-related sarcoma and regression of existing cases.[116]

Lymphoma

Most primary lymphomas of the head and neck arise in Waldeyer's ring. Cervical adenopathy can be found in up to 80% of patients with non-Hodgkin's lymphoma (NHL); 10% have extranodal disease.[117] Of these, only 2% involve the oral cavity.[117] In primary extranodal NHL of the oral cavity, the palate and gingiva are most commonly involved.[118] Secondary extension of NHL from the base of the tongue into the tongue or from the submandibular glands into the FOM may occur. Lymphoma of the oral cavity can present as a painless swelling, although sore throat, dysphagia, pain, and paresthesia are late symptoms. Involvement of cervical lymph nodes may not be evident initially. Fever, night sweats, weight loss, and painless enlargement of lymph nodes may occur in patients with advanced disease.

Lymphoma of the oral cavity is surgically excised for diagnostic purposes only. Further staging of lymphoma includes a complete blood count, liver function tests, chest and abdominal computed tomography (CT), and bone marrow biopsy. Clinical staging, however, plays a less important role in treatment decisions and in determination of prognosis than does histologic classification. The differential diagnosis includes malignant melanoma, anaplastic carcinoma, Wegener's granulomatosis, and benign lymphoepithelial lesion. Early-stage disease (stages I and II) can be treated with radiotherapy with or without chemotherapy. Advanced disease (stages III and IV) is treated with combination radiotherapy and chemotherapy. In Barker's series of 37 lymphomas of the oral cavity, the 5-year survival rate was approximately 50%.[119] More detailed information in reference to lymphoma of the oral cavity can be found in Chapter 26, Lymphomas Presenting in the Head and Neck: Current Issues in Diagnosis and Management.

Melanoma

Melanoma of the oral cavity is extremely rare and represents only 0.2% to 8% of all melanomas.[120] This incidence is somewhat higher in Japan, approximately 11%.[121] The palate, gingiva, buccal mucosa, and lip are the most common subsites of involvement (Fig. 13–6).[122, 123] Early malignant melanoma of the oral cavity is asymptomatic, but as the disease progresses, it can produce ulceration, swelling, loose teeth, and pain. Most (95%) melanomas of the oral cavity are pigmented,[120] and the differential diagnosis should include other pigmented lesions such as amalgam deposits, hemangioma, KS, and benign melanosis. Preexisting benign melanosis is present in approximately one third of patients, and malignant transformation to melanoma has been reported.[124] Therefore, newly found pigmented lesions of the oral cavity should be biopsied. There is no evidence that incisional biopsy causes dissemination of the melanoma. Histologically, mucosal melanoma is indistinguishable from its cutaneous counterpart. Special staining and monoclonal antibody techniques have shown that the S-100 protein and the HMB-45 protein are useful diagnostic indicators of melanoma.[120]

It is important that primary melanoma of the oral cavity be distinguished from metastatic melanoma of the oral cavity. Patton and associates found that 15 of 24 cases of

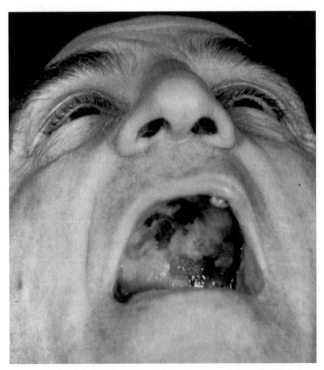

FIGURE 13–6 Malignant melanoma of the palate.

malignant melanoma were metastatic to the oral cavity.[125] A mean of 4.2 years elapsed between the discovery and treatment of the primary melanoma and the diagnosis of metastasis to the oral cavity. Preoperative metastatic evaluation should include chest radiographs, liver function tests, and CT scanning of the head and neck. The prognosis for melanoma of the oral cavity, as for all mucosal sites in the head and neck, is worse than for cutaneous melanoma. This poor prognosis has been attributed to late diagnosis and systemic dissemination due to the rich blood and lymphatic supply of the oral cavity. In one study, 31% of patients with localized melanoma survived for 5 years, and only 5.2% of patients with nodal metastasis survived for 5 years.[126] In most patients, treatment failure occurs locally and is often associated with distant metastasis. Regional recurrence is uncommon, but once metastasis has occurred, the average survival time is 6 months.[120] Most patients die within 1 to 2 years after onset of the disease. Long-term follow-up of patients with oral melanoma is needed because recurrence has been reported as late as 10 years or longer after initial therapy. The principles and rationale for treatment of melanomas of the head and neck are detailed in Chapter 8, Melanoma of the Head and Neck.

◘ REGIONAL METASTASIS

The single most reliable prognostic factor in patients with SCC of the oral cavity is the presence of cervical metastasis. In patients with cervical metastasis, 5-year survival is reduced by approximately 50%.[127] The prognosis is even worse for those with multiple levels of nodal involvement or extracapsular spread.

The risk of cervical node metastasis depends on multiple factors, including the primary site and stage of disease. In patients with SCCOC, cervical metastasis is noted in approximately 30% of patients on initial evaluation. The metastatic rates for SCC of the lips are closer to 10%. However, tumors of the oral commissure have as high as a 20% metastatic rate at time of presentation.[128] In the FOM, the rate of occult metastatic nodal disease is between 25% and 50%, and contralateral metastases are not uncommon from lesions close to the midline.[129] Nodal disease is seen in 30% of patients with carcinoma of the alveolar ridge with an occult metastatic rate of 15%.[130] Cancer of the buccal mucosa can be locally aggressive, with an occult metastatic rate of 10%, increasing to 20% for larger primary tumors.[131] Similar rates for occult metastasis occur for carcinoma of the RMT, but because more patients tend to present with advanced disease, the rates of regional metastasis are somewhat higher.[132] In contrast, owing to the rich lymphatics of the oral tongue, as many as 66% of patients with cancer of the oral tongue can present with occult metastasis.[133] Cervical metastasis from cancer of the oral tongue occurs more frequently than from any other site in the oral cavity. It has been reported that 20% to 50% of patients will eventually develop cervical node metastasis, including those with early-stage primary cancer.[134]

In addition to clinical nodal status, other features of regional metastasis may be related to prognosis in SCC of the oral cavity. The impact of extracapsular spread (ECS) of tumor on patient survival has been reported by other authors.[127, 135, 136] If the tumor is limited to the node, 5-year survival rates range from 50% to 70%; however, if ECS is present, 5-year survival is reduced to 25% to 30%.[127, 135] ECS may indicate an underlying depressed immunologic surveillance and an overall failure to contain tumor spread. In general, the incidence of ECS seems to be related to nodal size, with lymph nodes larger than 3 cm exhibiting ECS in approximately 75% of cases.[135] Other nodal features that carry a poor prognosis include multiple nodal involvement, large nodal size, and fixation of nodes.[137] According to some authors, involvement of inferior cervical nodes (levels IV and V) suggests greater systemic involvement,[137] although the recognition of some oral SCCs with "skip metastases" involving isolated level III or IV nodes may bring this concept into question.[8] The immunomorphology of the lymph nodes may also have prognostic significance. A node with a lymphocyte-predominant pattern suggestive of an active immune response is associated with a 70% to 80% 5-year survival rate versus a 0% to 20% 5-year survival rate for a lymphocyte-depleted pattern.[137]

DISTANT METASTASIS

SCC of the oral cavity tends to remain localized above the clavicle until advanced stages. Distant metastasis eventually occurs in 15% to 20% of patients who die of their disease. Survival is extremely poor after distant metastasis is discovered and may affect surgical treatment planning in these patients. The incidence of distant metastases is primarily affected by tumor location, initial stage, and presence or absence of regional control above and below the clavicles.[138] Distant metastasis rarely occurs in the absence of nodal disease. The presence of ECS and the involvement of more than two lymph nodes increase the incidence of distant metastasis. One notable exception is ACC, which has a tendency for distant metastasis even at early stages. Because of its long indolent course, long-term survival is possible even in the presence of pulmonary metastasis.

The most common sites of distant metastasis include the lung (66%), bone (22%), and liver (9.5%).[139] Disease stage correlates well with the rate of distant metastasis (stage I [1%], stage II [14%], stage III [15%], and stage IV [20%]). Histopathologic evidence of lymphatic or vascular invasion and ECS was also associated with increased rates of distant metastasis.[140] More than 90% of patients die of their disease within 2 years of diagnosis of distant metastasis.[140] Regional dermal metastasis usually results from aberrant lymphatic spread rather than from hematogenous seeding of skin, and this finding also portends an extremely poor prognosis.[141] It is usually seen in the setting of recurrent cancer or advanced disease.

Tumor surveillance should incorporate the risk of distant metastases. In patients (stages I to III) with a low risk of distant metastasis (3%), yearly tests should include a chest radiograph and liver enzymes when indicated.[139] In patients who have advanced-stage cancer or those with locoregional failure, the risk of distant metastasis is approximately 10%, and positron emission tomography (PET) or CT scans of the lungs are recommended.[139] More

extensive procedures, including bone marrow biopsies and bronchoscopies, are not generally recommended as routine screening methods.

DIAGNOSIS AND EVALUATION

Evaluation of a patient with cancer of the oral cavity should include a thorough history and physical examination, dental assessment, radiographic evaluation, tissue biopsy, and intraoperative visualization where indicated. Usually, the most common symptom is a painful lesion in the mouth. Other symptoms may include a persistent or bleeding ulcer, loose teeth, ill-fitting dentures, pain in the mandible, trismus, or hypoesthesia due to perineural involvement. As the tumor extends into the posterior oral cavity and oropharynx, dysphagia, drooling, voice change, and even respiratory distress can occur. Otalgia indicates involvement of the ninth and tenth cranial nerves. As the disease progresses, weight loss, malnutrition, and dehydration due to dysphagia can exacerbate existing comorbidities and must be taken into consideration in the treatment plan.

Physical examination begins with a thorough visual inspection of the oral cavity. Size, location, and appearance of the primary lesion are noted. Mobility of the tongue, elevation of the soft palate, and trismus, indicating pterygoid muscle involvement, are also noted. Bimanual palpation is used to evaluate the depth of invasion of the musculature of the tongue and FOM, as well as any invasion of the bone. Palpation of the neck is critical in assessing for nodal disease and for accurate staging of the tumor. Indirect or fiberoptic laryngoscopy can provide visualization of the extent of posterior oral cavity and oropharyngeal involvement.

Several imaging techniques can be helpful in visualization of the primary tumor and any nodal disease. A chest radiograph should be done routinely to assess for metastatic disease and second primary cancers. CT is the modality most often used in cancers of the oral cavity to assess the extent of soft tissue and bony involvement. The extent of invasion into deep tongue musculature, FOM, and adjacent structures can be assessed by CT scan. In addition, invasion of the mandible, palate, and pterygomaxillary fossa can be readily seen with this technique.

If CT scanning is not available, a dental panoramic radiograph or panorex can be effective in demonstrating mandibular invasion. Magnetic resonance imaging (MRI) can be used in conjunction with or in place of CT. In certain cases, invasion of the base of the tongue can be more accurately evaluated on MRI than on CT, and perineural invasion along the inferior alveolar nerve or the greater palatine nerve can best be visualized on postcontrast MRI.[142] MRI is also superior in cases where dental amalgams can result in CT artifacts.

Ultrasound (US) has recently been used to screen for nodal disease that is not otherwise palpable clinically; it provides the advantage of not exposing the patient to additional radiation. When the technique is combined with fine-needle aspiration (FNA), the specificity of US-guided cytology can approach 90%.[143] Newer techniques such as PET are being used to identify nodal metastases and recurrent disease.[144, 145] The overall sensitivity and specificity of PET have been reported to be equal to or even superior to those of CT and MRI, especially in cases of previous radiotherapy or chemotherapy.[146] The role of PET scanning in head and neck cancers continues to evolve as more experience is acquired with this modality.

Whenever possible, a biopsy specimen should be obtained at the time of initial evaluation. Many lesions of the oral cavity are amenable to biopsy under local anesthesia. A submucosal mass or suspicious lymph node can be diagnosed by FNA rather than by open biopsy. In cases where the lesion cannot be adequately palpated on physical examination, a CT- or US-guided FNA can be used to increase the likelihood of diagnosis. Intraoperative evaluation may be necessary in some patients who cannot be adequately examined owing to pain, trismus, or extensive disease. A thorough examination, including complete visualization and palpation of the oral cavity and neck, is performed with the patient under general anesthesia. In most cases, direct laryngoscopy and esophagoscopy are also indicated for evaluation of the extent of disease, as well as the presence of second primary cancers. The placement of a surgical airway and/or feeding tube should be anticipated and, if indicated, should be performed while the patient is under this anesthesia.

◼ CLINICAL STAGING

The clinical staging of oral cavity cancer follows the tumor, node, metastasis (TNM) staging system from the American Joint Committee for Cancer (AJCC) Staging and End-Results Reporting guidelines (Table 13–1).[147] This is a clinical staging system that is defined by the anatomic extent of the tumor based on physical examination, diagnostic tests, and imaging studies. In the oral cavity, TNM staging is limited to SCCs. *T* refers to the size of the primary tumor, *N* to the status and size of the cervical lymph nodes, and *M* to the presence or absence of distant metastasis. This staging system is based on the assumption that small cancers with no cervical metastasis have a better prognosis than large tumors with metastasis. It suggests a logical progression of cancer from the primary tumor (T) to the neck (N), and then to distant metastasis (M). TNM staging is further divided into four stages (I, II, III, and IV). Stage I and II tumors are confined to the primary site. Stage III tumors may represent large primary tumors or those with ipsilateral cervical metastasis. Stage IV tumors are massive primary tumors, or they may have extensive regional or distant metastases.

Although the AJCC staging system is useful for standardizing the description and reporting of oral cavity cancers, it does not take into account other important host factors known to affect survival and outcome, such as the patient's performance status, comorbidities, nutritional status, and immune status.[148, 149] Pathologic features such as the presence of perineural invasion and ECS are also not taken into account. Perineural invasion and ECS are both known to affect prognosis: Approximately 50% reduction in survival is seen in patients with nodes with ECS compared with survival in patients whose nodes do not reveal ECS.[150, 151] Lymph nodes larger than 3 cm exhibit ECS in approximately 75% of cases,[150] but this is not reflected in the current staging system.

Other important prognostic factors such as fixation of nodes and level of nodal disease are also not included in the

TABLE 13-1 Definition of TNM for Cancer of the Oral Cavity

Primary Tumor (T)

TX	Primary tumor cannot be assessed
T0	No evidence of primary tumor
Tis	Carcinoma in situ
T1	Tumor 2 cm or less in greatest dimension
T2	Tumor more than 2 cm but not more than 4 cm in greatest dimension
T3	Tumor more than 4 cm in greatest dimension
T4 (lip)	Tumor invades through cortical bone, inferior alveolar nerve, floor of mouth, or skin of face, i.e., chin or nose
T4a	(oral cavity) Tumor invades adjacent structures (e.g., through cortical bone, into deep [extrinsic] muscle of tongue [genioglossus, hyoglossus, palatoglossus, and styloglossus], maxillary sinus, skin of face)
T4b	Tumor invades masticator space, pterygoid plates, or skull base and/or encases internal carotid artery

Note: Superificial erosion alone of bone/tooth socket by gingival primary is not sufficient to classify a tumor as T4.

Regional Lymph Nodes (N)

NX	Regional lymph nodes cannot be assessed
N0	No regional lymph node metastasis
N1	Metastasis in a single ipsilateral lymph node, 3 cm or less in greatest dimension
N2	Metastasis in a single ipsilateral lymph node, more than 3 cm but not more than 6 cm in greatest dimension; or in multiple ipsilateral lymph nodes, none more than 6 cm in greatest dimension; or in bilateral or contralateral lymph nodes, none more than 6 cm in greatest dimension
N2a	Metastasis in single ipsilateral lymph nodes, none more than 3 cm but not more than 6 cm in greatest dimension
N2b	Metastasis in multiple ipsilateral lymph nodes, none than 6 cm in greatest dimension
N2c	Metastasis in bilateral or contralateral ipsilateral lymph nodes, 6 cm in greatest dimension
N3	Metastasis in a lymph node, more than 6 cm in greatest dimension

Distant Metastasis (M)

MX	Distant metastasis cannot be assessed
M0	No distant metastasis
M1	Distant metastasis

STAGE GROUPING

Stage 0	Tis	N0	M0
Stage I	T1	N0	M0
Stage II	T2	N0	M0
Stage III	T3	N0	M0
	T1	N1	M0
	T2	N1	M0
	T3	N1	M0
Stage IVA	T4a	N0	M0
	T4a	N1	M0
	T1	N2	M0
	T2	N2	M0
	T3	N2	M0
	T4a	N2	M0
Stage IVB	Any T	N3	M0
	T4b	Any N	M0
Stage IVC	Any T	Any N	M1

Used with the permission of the American Joint Committee on Cancer (AJCC), Chicago, Illinois. The original source for this material is the *AJCC Cancer Staging Manual, Sixth Edition* (2002) published by Springer-Verlag New York, www.springer-ny.com.

staging system. In addition, staging relies heavily on clinical examination of the neck, which is known to be inaccurate in some cases. The incidence of a false-negative physical examination (i.e., with occult disease) varies in the literature from 16% to 60%.[152] CT scanning appears to be helpful in the diagnosis of cervical metastatic disease. Van den Brekel and colleagues compared the accuracy of palpation, US, US-guided fine-needle cytology, CT, and MRI in the diagnosis of cervical metastasis.[143] The highest rate of accuracy occurred with US-guided fine-needle cytology (93%), followed by MRI (82%), CT (78%), US (75%), and palpation (69%).

Although the current clinical staging system is not perfect, it does allow the clinician to design treatment strategies, compare results, and assess the prognosis of patients with cancer.[147] Future staging systems will, no doubt, incorporate new insights into the changes that occur even at the molecular level of head and neck cancer.

TREATMENT

A number of treatment options are available for the management of oral cavity cancer. These include surgery, radiation, chemotherapy, or a combination of these treatments. The choice of therapy depends on multiple factors, including the site and stage of disease; the patient's physical, social, and personal status; and the physician's experience and skill. In all but the earliest-stage tumors, a combination of treatment modalities is usually used.

Surgery and radiation are equally effective in treating early (T1–T2) oral cavity cancers. In the choice between surgery and radiation, some general considerations should be taken into account. With surgery, patients with small tumors of the oral cavity amenable to local resection require less treatment time than is required by a full course of radiotherapy, allowing a faster rehabilitation and holding this other modality in reserve for the treatment of a second primary tumor of the UADT. Most early-stage oral cavity lesions do not require extensive reconstructive techniques. The degree of functional disability associated with surgery is directly related to the extent of tongue or mandible involvement, and rehabilitation becomes more difficult with extensive soft tissue or bony involvement. Radiotherapy can be used when there is a significant risk associated with general anesthesia, or when a patient refuses surgery. Functional disability (speech and deglutition) is usually less pronounced with radiotherapy than with surgery, although this may not be necessarily true with small tumors.

Radiotherapy

Radiotherapy should be used when survival and morbidity rates are better or equal to those for surgical therapy. In general, SCCs that are vascularized and well oxygenated tend to be the most radiosensitive. Deep invasion of muscle or bone tends to decrease response to radiotherapy; large cervical metastatic nodes are best managed by a combination of surgery and radiation rather than by radiation alone. Radiotherapy is most commonly given as external beam radiation. It is usually given as a 5- to 7-week course to a total dose of 65 to 75 Gy. A lower dose of radiation can be given if previous surgery has been performed.

The consequences of radiotherapy include xerostomia, mucositis, and temporary or permanent dysgeusia. Osteoradionecrosis (ORN) is a significant complication of radiation therapy that is related to carious teeth in the radiation field. ORN results from decreased production of saliva and damage to the microvasculature of the mandible and maxilla. This problem is best managed by prevention with prophylactic dental care. Some patients may even require full dental extraction before radiotherapy. In addition, the extended treatment time can be a significant burden for some patients.

Modifications to conventional radiotherapy have been made to maximize locoregional control while minimizing complications. Hyperfractionation, or the giving of smaller dose fractions twice daily, has been shown to improve locoregional control in some studies,[153] although it is unclear if rates of late complications are increased with hyperfractionation versus conventional radiotherapy. Other modifications include three-dimensional conformal radiotherapy that uses computer-assisted treatment planning to limit the radiation dose given to surrounding normal tissues. Intensity-modulated radiation therapy (IMRT) employs computer technology and sleeves to block individual fields and calculate dose based on adverse effects to normal tissue. This allows the maximum radiation to be delivered to the primary tumor while minimizing damage to critical structures such as the salivary glands, brain, orbit, brachial plexus, or spinal cord.

Interstitial radiation (brachytherapy) is often used in conjunction with external beam radiation therapy or with surgery for cancer of the oral cavity. With this combination method, larger doses of radiation can be given to localized areas of tissue. This produces a greater radiobiologic effective dose at the primary while sparing the patient approximately 2500 rads of external beam radiation therapy, thus decreasing the chances for adverse effects such as xerostomia, fibrosis, and trismus. Local control with brachytherapy has been reported to be between 10% and 80% depending on the series and the extent of follow-up.[154] A disadvantage associated with this technique is that it requires general anesthesia for placement of the catheters. An elective tracheotomy should be used as a precautionary measure to ensure airway maintenance should intraoral swelling or bleeding occur. Concentrating the radiation dose may increase the risk of hemorrhage, mucositis, and osteoradionecrosis in the treatment area.

Regardless of the dose and type of radiation chosen, this treatment plan must consider that a second course of external beam irradiation cannot be given should a patient develop a recurrence, and that salvage surgery after radiation failure is associated with low survival and high morbidity.

Chemotherapy

The use of chemotherapy as a single-modality agent for the treatment of SCCOC has produced dismal results. However, chemotherapy has gained recognition in the treatment of head and neck cancer through its use as an adjuvant agent.[155–157] Adjuvant chemotherapy has been reported to improve the rate of organ preservation, with no change in overall survival.[158–161] Many studies report the fact that chemotherapy does not increase overall survival in head and neck cancer patients,[162, 163] although a statistically significant improvement is seen in disease-free survival with the use of adjuvant chemotherapy.[155, 162]

Johnson and coworkers have reported a significant benefit in regional control and survival with the use of post-operative chemotherapy and radiation in patients with ECS.[164] In patients with neck dissection specimens demonstrating ECS, the addition of chemotherapy to standard radiation improved disease-free survival from 34% to 53%. Of the 131 patients in the surgery followed by the chemoradiation arm, 22% developed distant metastases. This suggests that the beneficial action of chemotherapy is related to radiosensitization. Although this study is encouraging, this was a nonrandomized trial, and randomized studies in France and those performed by the RTOG (95-01) have yielded conflicting results regarding the risks and benefits of adjuvant chemoradiotherapy versus radiotherapy alone.

Chemotherapy is often employed in the palliative setting in patients with recurrent, unresectable, or distant disease.

Induction Chemotherapy

Chemotherapy has been given before surgery, radiation, or even chemoradiation in an effort to improve rates of locoregional control and distant metastasis in head and neck cancers. However, studies have not demonstrated any benefit in survival with the use of induction chemotherapy.[158, 165] The Department of Veterans Affairs Laryngeal Study Group evaluated induction chemotherapy as a strategy for preserving the larynx in patients with advanced resectable glottic and supraglottic cancer.[158] No difference in 3-year survival rates was seen in patients treated with chemotherapy versus the surgically treated group. A decreased distant metastatic rate but an increased local failure rate among chemotherapy patients was noted in this study. Meta-analysis of adjuvant chemotherapy in head and neck cancer indicates that the impact of chemotherapy on overall survival, although small, is greater with concurrent chemotherapy than with induction chemotherapy (12% vs. 4%).[166]

Adjuvant Chemotherapy

In a study of patients with resectable cancer of the head and neck, Jacobs and Makuch showed a statistically significant improvement in disease-free survival with the use of chemotherapy, although the overall or absolute survival was unchanged.[162] Another study on the use of adjuvant chemotherapy in head and neck cancer found that among 3977 patients available for analysis, no significant change in survival was demonstrated in patients treated in chemotherapy programs versus standard therapy programs.[163] Although overall survival may not be improved, the use of adjuvant chemotherapy seems to decrease the incidence of distant metastasis.[167]

Concurrent Chemotherapy

It seems apparent that chemotherapy is most beneficial in the concurrent application of radiation, rather than in the inductive setting. Kohno and associates reported the results of 40 patients with unresectable head and neck SCC treated with concurrent chemoradiation.[168] A total of 50% of patients had a complete response with a median survival of 34 months, compared with 4-month survival in nonresponders.

This finding was supported by the work of Adelstein and colleagues, who reported on a phase III intergroup trial with unresectable SCC of the head and neck.[169] The addition of concurrent cisplatin to conventional radiation significantly improved survival over radiation alone (37% vs. 23% 3-year survival). In another report, both relapse-free survival (60% vs. 40%) and 3-year locoregional control (70% vs. 45%) were improved with concurrent chemoradiation versus conventional radiotherapy.[170] Locoregional control rates of 90% have been reported with concurrent hyperfractionated chemoradiation, although these regimens were toxic, with 12% to 50% of patients developing severe mucositis, neutropenia, and thrombocytopenia.[171] Concurrent chemoradiation protocols have improved locoregional control and reduced the development of distant disease, although many patients still die of distant disease.

Combined Therapy

In advanced disease (stages III and IV), a combination of surgery and radiation is often employed, although debate continues over the timing of the radiation. Advocates of preoperative radiotherapy point out that before surgery, tumors are well oxygenated and more radiosensitive, resulting in less likelihood of tumor seeding at the time of surgery and fewer viable tumor cells within surrounding lymphatics and vasculature that can metastasize. However, wound-healing problems such as fibrosis, infection, or fistula occur more frequently with total radiation doses exceeding 40 Gy and when surgery is performed more than 6 weeks after the completion of radiotherapy. Although uncommon, flap necrosis and carotid artery rupture can also occur. With preoperative radiotherapy, fibrosis and inflammation can make the assessment of tumor margins more difficult at the time of resection.

Postoperative radiotherapy has the theoretical advantages of a smaller microscopic tumor burden; intraoperative mapping that allows for better targeting of the radiotherapy; and better assessment of tumor margins. Wound healing is well under way before radiotherapy is begun, allowing for a safer administration of a larger total dose of radiation. A disadvantage with this protocol is that wound breakdown or other surgical complications can delay or prevent the delivery of radiation. Theoretically, any tumor remaining after resection is less vascular and less radiosensitive than before surgery and will require a higher total dose of radiation.

In studies, both preoperative and postoperative radiotherapy have been shown to improve locoregional control. In one RTOG study, Kramer and coworkers performed a randomized clinical trial in which patients received either preoperative or postoperative radiation.[172] The postoperative radiation group had better locoregional control, but no significant difference was noted in overall survival. Conventional combined therapy for oral cavity cancer currently involves the use of postoperative radiation to avoid potential wound-healing complications and to deliver a higher total dose of radiation than is possible with planned preoperative radiotherapy. Many surgeons also prefer to have the ability to obtain clear surgical margins without concern for the histologic changes brought on by preoperative radiotherapy that obscures the diagnosis.

Surgery

Many cancers of the oral cavity are amenable to surgical excision. These lesions are usually small (<2 cm) and are located anteriorly, allowing them to be resected perorally. The surgical defect may be closed primarily, skin grafted, or allowed to heal by second intention with minimal functional impairment. In addition, a specimen obtained for pathologic examination can give significant prognostic information, as well as objective assessment of the adequacy of the resection. Surgical resection is also preferred in patients who are at increased risk for developing radiation-induced complications and for those with second primary cancers of the UADT due to their excessive consumption of tobacco and alcohol. In these patients, adequate surgical resection can avoid the potential adverse effects of radiotherapy while preserving radiation for future treatment protocols.

The disadvantages of surgery are the potential risk associated with anesthesia; the resultant functional disability, which is directly related to the extent of resection; and the cost. In general, the larger the cancer, the greater the number of potential problems with deglutition and speech. It is important to involve speech and swallowing therapists before treatment for preoperative counseling and early after surgery for initiating the rehabilitation of these patients.

Mandible

Oral cavity cancers can involve the mandible in three major ways: (1) encroachment or abutting of bone; (2) direct invasion of bone; and (3) prevention of surgical access. Surgical management of oral cavity cancer must take into account the degree of involvement of the mandible.

Bone Involvement

A high incidence of microscopic invasion of the periosteum or cortical layer of the mandible is seen with tumors that encroach on the mandible even in the absence of radiographic findings. Conventional radiographs, including dental panorex views, are helpful in determining bony invasion. However, it is estimated that 30% of patients with encroachment on bone and normal radiographs have microscopic invasion of the mandible. If the cancer is immobile from the mandible or directly abuts it, invasion should be suspected. Technetium-99m bone scans are more sensitive than conventional radiographs but lack the specificity to differentiate between tumor, infection, and inflammation. Currently, CT is the preferred adjunctive diagnostic test for the assessment of mandibular invasion. Highly precise multiplanar reformatting CT (Dentascan) can provide specific spatial information about cortical destruction and associated structures such as the inferior alveolar canal and nerve, as well as the alveolar ridge.[173]

In cases of microscopic invasion of bone or bony encroachment that does not allow an adequate surgical margin, marginal resection of the inner or outer cortex of the mandible may provide an adequate margin around the tumor while still preserving the continuity of the mandible (Fig. 13–7). Marginal mandibulectomy should be considered for tumors that are clinically mobile from the mandible or that have normal mucosa between tumor and mandible. This is based on the observation that the mandibular periosteum may be a barrier to tumor involvement, and when clinically normal tissue exists between the primary cancer and the mandible, neither the mandible nor its periosteum demonstrates microscopic involvement. The oncologic efficacy of marginal mandibulectomy has been borne out by subsequent authors. In several studies, locoregional control rates with marginal mandibulectomy were equal or superior to those achieved with segmental resection.[174, 175]

Direct Invasion

Direct cortical invasion of the mandible, whether detected clinically, radiographically, or intraoperatively, requires an en bloc segmental mandibulectomy (see Fig. 13–7). Intraoperative techniques of frozen section analysis of the remaining bone are not currently feasible. Touch preparations or frozen section examinations of marrow scrapings may be useful when positive. The inferior alveolar nerve should be examined by frozen section to rule out any perineural invasion or invasion of the marrow space. The degree of functional impairment associated with segmental

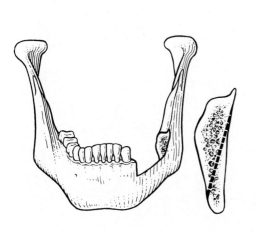

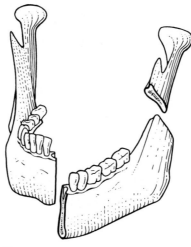

FIGURE 13–7 Mandible resection may be either marginal or rim (A) or segmental (B). Marginal mandibulectomy is appropriate when the tumor approaches (or minimally erodes) but does not invade bone. In selected patients, surgery can be performed via the peroral approach. When bone is invaded, segmental mandibulectomy is required, usually necessitating an external approach for adequate exposure.

A   B

mandibulectomy varies with the location of the bone defect. Even small anterior arch defects can produce considerable speech and swallowing disability, as well as cosmetic deformity, and require primary reconstruction in most cases. By contrast, lateral mandibular defects are well tolerated by most patients. The entire body and ascending ramus of the mandible may be removed without resultant significant swallowing disability. With lateral mandibular defects, a reconstruction plate is often used as a spacer to maintain proper dental alignment, but no further soft tissue reconstruction is needed in most cases. In our experience, lateral mandibular defects can be reconstructed with a split-thickness skin graft with excellent cosmetic and functional results.[176]

Surgical Access

A mandibular osteotomy or "mandibular swing" approach may be required to improve exposure and facilitate access to some oral cavity cancers. This approach requires a midline lip-splitting incision with exposure of the mandibular symphysis (Fig. 13–8). Mandibular osteotomy is performed in the midline or paramedian position, depending on the

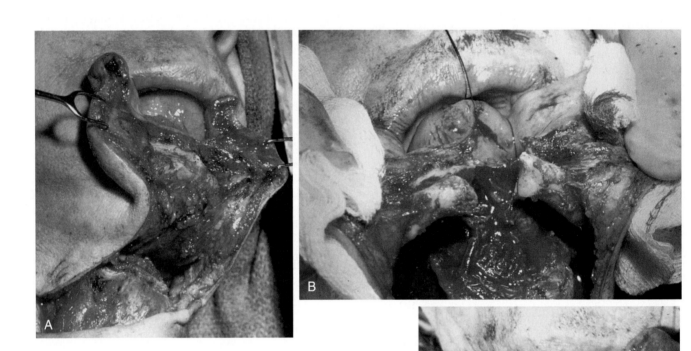

FIGURE 13–8 *A*, Midline lip-splitting incision in preparation for mandibular osteotomy. *B*, Mandibular osteotomy is carried out and the mandibular fragments are spread for wide exposure of the oral cavity. *C*, Wire and plating are used to stabilize the mandibular fragments following osteotomy.

location of the tumor. The mylohyoid muscle must be divided to allow the mandible to "swing." The mandible is stabilized by means of reconstruction plates. Potential disadvantages to this approach include scarring or paresthesia of the lip-splitting incision, malunion of the mandible, and loss of teeth due to injury of the tooth root during the osteotomy.

A visor flap approach is another mandible-sparing approach wherein the skin and soft tissues are incised and dissected free of the intact mandible and are elevated superiorly (Fig. 13–9). This technique provides access to the anterior and lateral oral cavity. Disadvantages associated with this approach include poor exposure to the posterior oral cavity, resection of the mental nerves, and potential compromise of the blood supply to the mandible.

Cervical Metastasis

Since radical neck dissection (RND) was first described by Crile[177] in 1906 for excision of head and neck cancer and was later popularized by Hayes Martin,[178–180] it has survived for generations as the gold standard for comprehensive oncologic clearance of cervical metastasis from cancer of the UADT. This operation includes removal of cervical nodes in levels I to V and the nonlymphatic structures of the neck (sternocleidomastoid muscle, internal jugular vein, spinal accessory nerve). Following this operation, patients experience chronic shoulder pain, numbness, fibrosis, immobility, and cosmetic deformity. In patients with advanced neck

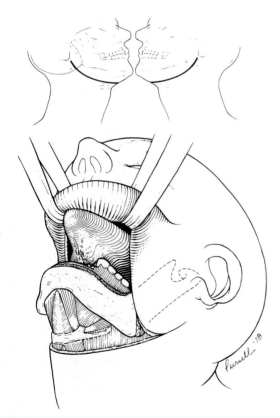

FIGURE 13–9 Visor flap approach to the anterior oral cavity requires extensive dissection in both sides of the neck for adequate exposure but avoids a midline lip-splitting incision.

metastasis (N2, N3), it is accepted that RND is the most appropriate operation to ensure clearance of malignant disease, which is often adherent to the spinal accessory nerve or the internal jugular vein. Nonetheless, many surgeons realized that the morbidity placed upon patients with minimal cervical disease by this procedure (i.e., N0 or N1) was excessive[181]; therefore, many surgeons adopted the modified radical neck dissection (MRND), which spared some or all of the nonlymphatic structures of the neck while providing comprehensive clearance of cervical nodal basins.[182–185] The functional results of MRND were found to be superior to those of traditional RND, especially with preservation of cranial nerve (CN) XI[186]; oncologic outcomes remained virtually unchanged. The MRND remains the current cornerstone of modern oncologic clearance of clinically positive cervical nodal disease. The cosmetic morbidity resulting from MRND, although better than that from RND, is still believed to be excessive in patients with clinically negative neck (N0) disease.

Over the past decade, the greatest advance in the surgical management of the neck has been increasing use of selective neck dissection (SND) (i.e., supraomohyoid neck dissection) for the surgical management of the N0 neck in patients with carcinoma of the oral cavity. The occult metastatic rate in patients with cancer of the oral cavity is reported to be approximately 31%.[7, 187, 188] Many surgeons began reporting their observations of certain lymph node groups with increasing frequency of metastatic disease.[6, 183, 189–191] Metastasis to cervical lymph nodes from cancer of the oral cavity occurs most often in levels I to III, with level IV involved to a lesser extent in cancer of the lateral aspect of the oral tongue and level V involvement of approximately 1%. This has resulted in surgeons' not only sparing the nonlymphatic structures of the neck but also leaving levels IV and V undisturbed because of the rarity of pathologic involvement.[192] Many studies have shown that SND is a reliable staging tool,[7, 193] has a low incidence of cervical recurrence,[194, 195] and results in less morbidity[186, 196, 197] and hospitalization time than either the MRND or the RND.[198] Kowalski reported a 29% ipsilateral regional recurrence in patients with oral carcinoma after observation versus 4% in those treated with SND.[199]

Approximately 30% to 35% of patients with N0 clinical cervical staging (cN0) are found to indeed have positive histologic evidence of malignancy in the cervical nodes (pN+). Patients treated with SND and found to be pN0 or pN+ with small single lymph nodes and no evidence of ECS are often successfully managed by observation alone. In many of these patients with early pN+ disease the disease never recurs in the neck and is in fact controlled by SND alone. Patients found to have adverse prognostic factors such as ECS,[127, 200, 201] N2 neck metastasis, and more than two positive lymph nodes should be treated with postoperative radiation therapy.[194, 202] The realization that SND was inadvertently being used with good results on patients with cN0 but pN+ neck disease, often with N2 disease, led to interest in systematically applying SND to patients with clinically early metastatic disease (N1). It was originally believed that if an intraoperative frozen section analysis confirmed the presence of metastatic disease, a comprehensive neck dissection (ND) should be performed.[203]

Early reports of SND cited regional failure rates of 15% to 29% at 2 years in patients with pathologically involved nodes treated with supraomohyoid neck dissection (SOHND), despite the addition of postoperative radiation therapy.[175] Chu and Strawitz reported recurrence rates higher after SOHND than after comprehensive ND.[204] Frequently, these recurrences were within the lymph node groups adjacent to the levels of dissection encompassed by the selective ND. Recent experience has revealed that the addition of postoperative radiation therapy to the N+ neck after SND results in improved regional control.[205] In addition, Anderson and associates reported a regional control rate of 94% with the use of SND in patients with clinically evident early neck disease.[206] Recent reports suggest that postoperative physical therapy decreases pain and shoulder disability after ND.[207]

A major concern for clinicians advocating SND rather than MRND involves the interpretation and application of SND by clinicians. Certainly, most oncologically oriented surgeons perform comprehensive clearance of lymph nodes in high-risk areas, and others simply perform "node plucking" from these areas. This practice of node plucking is to be discouraged for several reasons. First, if all the lymph nodes from high-risk regions are not removed, then the potential for false-negative results is increased secondary to sampling error. The ability of even highly trained cancer surgeons to reliably identify lymph nodes involved with cancer is less than satisfactory.[208–210] A second denouncement of node plucking is that surgical management of cervical recurrence in a previously operated field is difficult for the salvage surgeon and puts the patient at higher risk for neurovascular injury.

Lymphoscintigraphy and Sentinel Lymph Node Metastasis

The latest frontier in the surgical management of the N0 neck in oral cavity carcinoma involves the use of lymphoscintigraphy and the technique of sentinel lymph node biopsy (SLNB). The technique of SLNB has gained widespread acceptance in the field of surgical oncology for the management of cutaneous melanoma and breast cancer.[211, 212] Recently, Pitman and colleagues reported the use of lymphoscintigraphy and SLNB in 33 patients with SCC of the oral cavity who underwent immediate SND after SLNB.[213] In patients with N0 disease, the sentinel lymph node was accurately identified 95% of the time. On average, 2.9 sentinel lymph nodes were identified in 2.2 levels of the neck, including bilateral drainage in 20%. However, the sentinel lymph node was positive in only two of the three N0 patients with histologically confirmed neck metastasis, for a sensitivity of 66%. These authors currently use lymphoscintigraphy to determine the sites and levels of lymph nodes to be dissected, but we certainly are not advocating SLNB alone. Other authors have also reported encouraging preliminary data, with sensitivity ranging from 60% to 100%.[214–218] Future investigations must determine if there is decreased morbidity from the use of SLNB with little to no increase in regional failure to control neck disease. In addition, the proper application of additional surgery versus adjuvant therapy in the pN+ SLNB patient needs further investigation.

Advantages and Disadvantages of Surgery as Treatment

Surgical treatment of the N0 neck has its opponents, who favor observation or radiation therapy. Proponents of observation suggest that (1) morbidity is unnecessarily inflicted on 60% to 70% of N0 oral cavity patients who turn out to have a pN0 neck, (2) regional failures can be surgically salvaged, (3) neck dissection increases costs and length of hospital stay, and (4) survival advantage has not been proved with elective treatment of the N0 neck. It is estimated that 12% to 18% of patients undergoing SND still have residual tightness, numbness, and discomfort on long-term follow-up.[219]

Several reasons support the use of surgical treatment of the N0 neck: (1) This approach provides access for excision of cancer of the oral cavity that may require a cheek flap or a mandibulotomy approach; (2) the identification of microscopic metastasis guides the use of adjuvant or additional therapy; and (3) salvage surgery for neck recurrence is less than optimal.[220] Disadvantages of the observation approach are that it may not be feasible in a patient with a neck that is large, muscular, and difficult to examine, and it should not be used in patients who are unreliable for follow-up or in advanced cancers with a high rate of neck metastasis. Evidence suggests that although survival is unchanged with elective ND, patients who have regional recurrence have it at a higher stage and are thus potentially unsalvageable.[221, 222]

Proponents of radiation cite its decreased morbidity compared with that of neck dissection and the fact that many patients with advanced primary cancer need radiation treatments in addition to surgical treatment. Thus patients with high-stage primary cancer and an N0 neck can avoid the morbidity of surgery and still have the cervical lymphatics electively radiated along with the primary bed. In addition, primary radiation may be the best option in patients with systemic illness precluding general anesthesia. Primary radiation does have the disadvantages of no pathologic specimen, increased treatment time, and the potential for serious adverse effects in 13% of patients.[223] There is also the issue of second primary cancers. Comprehensive treatment of the initial primary often uses radiation therapy, which usually precludes its reapplication. This often mandates the management of second primaries with surgical modalities alone, although one often wishes that the opportunity for additional radiation therapy were available in the management of these often advanced cancers.

The issue of keeping the primary in continuity with the ND (en bloc) or discontinuous in the treatment of oral cavity cancer remains unclear. Discontinuity ND is an attractive option because it results in fewer postoperative wound and swallowing problems. Discontinuous ND is technically easier and allows for the use of skin grafting rather than flap reconstruction. The lymphatic drainage of the anterior oral cavity passes through the mylohyoid muscle[224] and the intervening tissues of the floor of the oral cavity before entering the neck. Failure to remove all lymphatic channels should theoretically result in missed in-transit tumors and thus a higher rate of recurrent disease.[225] It is likely that en bloc resection of the neck and primary site depends more on the primary cancer itself. With larger primary cancers of the

FOM and tongue, en bloc resection of the neck and primary provides for maximal clearance of the deep and lateral margins.

Leemans and coworkers compared in-continuity versus discontinuous ND in patients with T2 oral cavity SCC and found a regional relapse rate of 5.3% for the in-continuity group versus 19.1% for the discontinuity group, as well as decreased survival (63% vs. 80%).[226] Although Spiro and Strong found no adverse effects from discontinuity ND in patients treated for cancer of the tongue,[227] less advanced cases were more common in the discontinuity group than in the incontinuity group. Kaya and associates reported a 15% local recurrence rate in 58 patients treated with in-continuity glossectomy/neck dissection, 12% if margins were clear.[210] All nine patients with recurrence died of disease despite repeat radical surgery, radiation, and chemotherapy. In patients with positive margins, the recurrence rate was 50% despite irradiation.

Patients developing recurrent cancer in the neck after initial treatment have a poor outcome. Postsurgical and postradiation fibrosis, edema, and scarring make follow-up examination of the neck challenging. These patients tend to have recurrence with diffusely infiltrating disease that often involves dermal lymphatics. Tumor recurs around previously preserved structures such as the carotid artery and the cranial nerves; thus, salvage operations result in greater morbidity. Kowalski reported that 82 (16%) of 513 patients with oral cancer experienced recurrence in the neck.[199] Of these, only 44% were deemed to be salvageable, with a salvage rate of 6.6%.

◼ CANCER OF THE TONGUE

U.S. Surveillance, Epidemiology, and End Results (SEER) data from 1975 to 1998 report the incidence of cancer of the oral tongue to be higher than that of lip cancer, each accounting for roughly 20% of all oral cavity and pharyngeal cancers.[228] The SEER data also suggest a 5% to 10% increase among the white population; a 5% to 14% reduction has been seen in the black population.[228] An increase among patients 40 years of age and younger has also been reported.[229] Tobacco and excessive alcohol use are significant risk factors for the development of this cancer.

SCC of the tongue is often asymptomatic. The intrinsic tongue musculature provides little restriction to tumor growth; thus, cancers may enlarge considerably before producing symptoms. Local infiltration of the FOM, tongue base, and tonsillar pillars is common. Frequently, tongue cancer presents as a painless mass or ulcer that fails to heal after a minor trauma. With advancing disease, local pain, ipsilateral referred otalgia, and jaw pain are experienced by the patient.

Most cancers of the oral tongue occur on the lateral border of the tongue at the junction between the middle and posterior thirds (Fig. 13–10).[230] Approximately 30% of patients present with ipsilateral cervical node metastasis. When the cancer is in the midline, bilateral neck metastasis can occur. The primary basin for cervical lymphatic metastasis includes levels I to III, especially the superior deep jugular nodes (level II). It is rare for occult metastatic deposits to be found in level IV or V.[192] Cancer of the oral tongue is usually well differentiated and creates symptoms early, in contrast to cancer of the base of tongue, which is usually less differentiated and presents at a higher stage.[231] Patients should undergo endoscopy and biopsy of the cancer to assess the extent of the lesion and to rule out any second primary cancers. Radiologic studies such as CT or MRI complement the physical examination for prediction of depth of invasion, mandibular involvement, and the presence of cervical metastasis (Fig. 13–11).[232–234]

Treatment

Primary Cancer

Cancer of the tongue can be treated with either surgery or radiation with satisfactory results. Optimal management should address the primary cancer and any metastatic disease. Fortunately, most cancers of the oral tongue present at stages amenable to partial glossectomy. Surgical removal allows for evaluation of margins, perineural or lymphovascular invasion, and tumor depth, as well as accurate tumor staging. This allows for the application of multimodality therapy in advanced cases or in those with adverse prognostic indicators. Surgical resection for oral tongue cancer should be aggressive with planned margins of at least 1 cm. Initially positive margins, despite eventual clearance on final pathology, are predictive of poor outcome.[235] Unlike cutaneous or mucosal margins, the musculature of the tongue is unforgiving, with margins that are difficult to identify and orient after the tumor has been removed. It is possible that eventual clear margins in the tongue may indicate the surgeon's inability to locate the residual focus of carcinoma because of the elasticity of the tongue's muscle fibers and their tendency to retract after they are transected. Thus, any patient with initial or permanently positive margins should be strongly considered for postoperative radiation, regardless of tumor size.[235]

Many authors have reported on the efficacy of surgery for SCC of the oral tongue. Spiro and Strong reported a series of 185 patients with T1–T3N0 cancer of the oral tongue treated with partial glossectomy.[236] The local control rate was 79%, and the 5-year determinate survival rate was 62%. O'Brien and colleagues reported 97 stage I and II patients with tongue cancers followed for 2 to 20 years.[237] Local control was achieved in 91% of patients, resulting in a cancer mortality rate of 16%. However, cervical lymph node metastasis must be considered in the outcome of this disease. It appears that ECS is predictive of treatment failure in patients with SCC of the tongue.[201]

For patients with advanced cancer (stages III and IV), combined treatment with surgery and postoperative radiation provides the greatest chance for cure. In addition to partial glossectomy, these cancers may require labiomandibulotomy for optimal exposure to facilitate complete resection. The paramedian mandibulotomy gives excellent functional results because the attachments of the digastric muscles can be spared. Unfortunately, mylohyoid muscle transection is required to allow the mandible to swing, providing maximal access. When the cancer abuts or invades the mandible, marginal or segmental mandibulectomy may be necessary to ensure

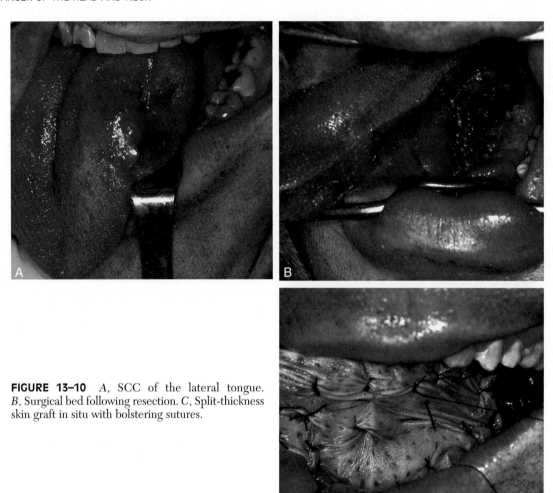

FIGURE 13–10 *A*, SCC of the lateral tongue. *B*, Surgical bed following resection. *C*, Split-thickness skin graft in situ with bolstering sutures.

adequate margins, especially if the mandible is clinically or radiographically involved.

Reconstruction of the tongue can be achieved with primary closure and local, regional, or distant flaps. For small defects, primary closure or a split-thickness skin graft can provide good speech and swallowing function (see Fig. 13–10). Healing by second intention may also work well for small defects, especially in the anterior tongue and FOM. This is usually used in patients treated with CO_2 laser excision. Large cancers requiring more extensive surgery, such as total glossectomy, require reconstruction with the use of regional or distant flaps to provide bulk and soft tissue (Fig. 13–12).

Radiation may be curative in early cancer (T1 and some T2) and may preserve maximal normal anatomy and function. Radiation can be provided in the form of external beam irradiation or interstitial irradiation (brachytherapy), or in combination. In exchange for the disadvantages of elective temporary tracheotomy for edema of the tongue and discomfort secondary to catheter placement, brachytherapy allows delivery of a large radiation boost to the primary tumor bed. This translates to improved local control with less toxic effect to the surrounding tissues than is achieved with traditional photons. In fact, brachytherapy can deliver as much as 100 Gy locally to the oral tongue; conventional irradiation techniques usually provide 65 to 70 Gy over a course of 5 to 6 weeks.

Benk and coworkers reported better local control rates in stage II SCC of the oral tongue treated exclusively with brachytherapy than in a group treated with external beam irradiation followed by an interstitial boost.[238] Piedbois and associates reported on 233 patients with stage I and II cancers of the oral cavity treated with brachytherapy (iridium-192 implants) with or without elective ND.[239] The local control rate was 87% at a minimum of 3 years' follow-up. Long-term sequelae may include xerostomia, loss of taste, exposed mandible, or osteoradionecrosis of the tissue.

Local control rates for T1 and T2 cancers of the oral tongue are between 60% and 80%. The 5-year disease-free survival ranges from 50% to 70%, but results as low as 30% for T2 cancer have also been reported.[237] These data suggest the importance of early treatment of cancer of the oral tongue. O'Brien and associates suggest that adjuvant treatment may not be needed in patients treated for early cancer of the tongue.[237] Careful follow-up examination is necessary

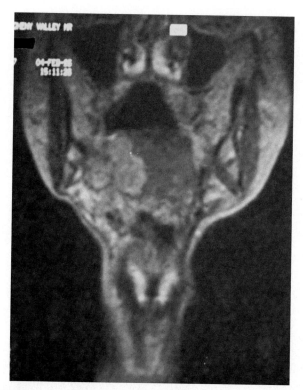

FIGURE 13–11 MRI demonstrates deeply infiltrative SCC of the tongue.

because these patients are at high risk for the development of metastasis to the neck, as well as second primary cancers.

Patients with locally advanced cancer usually require radical surgery, resulting in severe alterations in speech and swallowing. A 1991 study reported on the use of concomitant chemotherapy (cisplatin-5-fluorouracil) and radiation therapy for oncologic treatment of advanced cancers of the head and neck (tongue, hypopharynx, and larynx) with preservation of function.[240] Twelve of 29 patients had cancer of the tongue. Twenty-five of 29 patients (86%) had preservation of speech and swallowing function at a median follow-up of 5 years. Median survival was 45 months, with 14 (48%) of the patients currently disease-free. The authors concluded that concomitant chemotherapy and radiation therapy produce comparable control rates with those attained by surgery and radiation therapy for advanced cancers of the head and neck. Further controlled studies are needed to substantiate this conclusion.

Cancer of the Neck

The incidence of occult cervical metastasis in SCC of the oral tongue correlates with the size, grade, and depth of the primary tumor (T-stage). The particular site of cancer of the oral tongue is not considered an accurate predictor of cervical metastasis.[241] Cervical metastasis does not always correlate with T-stage. Even patients with T1 cancers have a significant risk of occult metastatic disease. Approximately 28% to 29% of T1 tumors, 43% to 47% of T2 tumors, and 56% to 77% of T3 tumors have pathologically positive cervical adenopathy when SNDs are performed.[236, 242]

Elective or therapeutic treatment of the cervical lymphatics is recommended for virtually all patients with cancer of the oral tongue. This is predicated on the notion that earlier treatment of cancer should result in improved outcome. It is also clear that the natural progression of disease over time involves increasing stage, and that increasing stage is associated with poorer outcome. However, only a trend toward improved survival has been seen, and the overall survival benefit of elective neck treatment may be small.[241, 243–246] In addition, many patients who are simply observed eventually are discovered to have cervical metastasis that is unresectable.[134, 244, 247] Thus, we favor elective ND rather than a wait-and-see policy. Selective ND of levels I to III, possibly level IV, at the time of primary tumor extirpation is recommended for N0 and selected N1 and N2 disease. It is recommended that patients with bulky metastatic deposits undergo standard radical dissection or MRND.

Regional failure continues to be a major factor in the treatment outcome of patients with tongue cancer. Many patients who develop metastasis to the neck during the follow-up period have unresectable disease, underscoring the importance of addressing the neck for treatment simultaneous with treatment of the primary. Cancer of the oral tongue is associated with a high incidence of clinically apparent and occult metastasis. In fact, up to 50% of patients have pathologically proven lymph node metastasis. The cervical lymphatics should be treated with the same modality used to treat the primary cancer, especially if the transcervical approach is necessary for resection of the cancer of the tongue.

Although several studies have shown that increasing grade of histologic differentiation correlates with cervical metastasis,[241, 248] the subjective interpretation of tumor grade may limit accurate prediction of cervical metastasis. Primary tumor thickness has also been shown to influence the risk of cervical node metastasis. Spiro and colleagues showed that patients with cancer of the tongue and FOM less than 2 mm in thickness had a treatment failure rate of 1.9% compared with 45.6% for patients whose primary cancer was greater than 2 mm in thickness.[249] Nearly 40% of patients with cancer greater than 2 mm in thickness had cervical lymph node metastasis. Thus, elective treatment of the neck based on the thickness of the cancer may provide an oncologically sound basis for decision making. However, accurate determination of histologic depth of invasion is often not available at the time of therapy planning, thus limiting its utility.

Cunningham and coworkers found a higher recurrence rate in patients who underwent therapeutic ND compared with those who received elective ND (42% vs. 11%, respectively).[134] The salvage rate among patients who developed cervical metastasis after initial therapy is poor. Johnson and associates reported a salvage rate of 35% in 40 patients (14/40) with T1N0 SCC of the oral tongue who developed cervical metastasis after initial therapy.[247] Similarly poor salvage rates have been reported by Whitehurst and Droubois (35%)[243] and Spiro and Strong (35% to 39%).[236] Survival after elective ND seems to be better than if the ND is performed after cervical metastasis becomes evident. Spiro and Strong reported a higher (70%) cervical metastatic rate in patients undergoing therapeutic ND as opposed

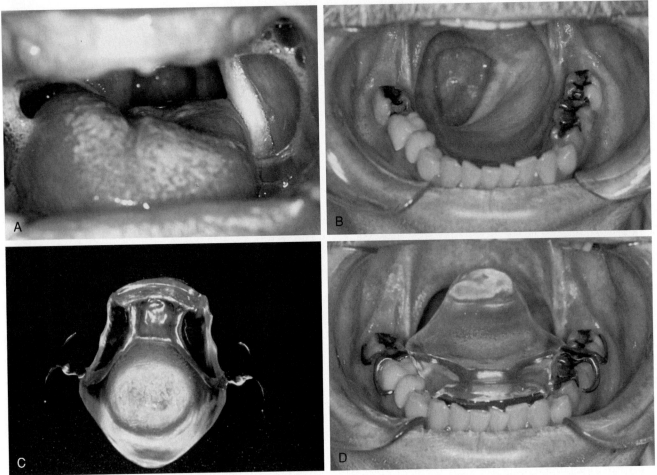

FIGURE 13–12 *A*, Almost complete destruction of the tongue by SCC. *B*, Reconstruction of the oral cavity with a pectoralis major myocutaneous flap following total glossectomy and neck dissections. *C*, Prosthesis designed to aid in speech and swallowing following total glossectomy. *D*, Prosthesis in place in the oral cavity.

to the elective ND group (50%).[236] Conversely, Jesse and colleagues were able to salvage 44 (70%) of 63 patients with delayed neck metastasis.[250] The authors estimated that only between 2.0% and 5.5% of patients would have benefited from elective treatment of the neck.

Alternatively, elective radiation therapy is an option for the treatment of the clinically N0 neck, especially in patients electing to undergo primary radiation treatment of their primary tumor. Mendenhall and coworkers demonstrated that elective neck radiation therapy significantly decreased the rate of neck recurrence.[251] Radiation can be given to bilateral necks with very little increase in morbidity and has been shown to decrease contralateral metastasis from 34% to 5% when compared with treatment in patients with unilateral neck dissection alone.[252] Higher failure rates of 14% to 16.6% with elective neck irradiation have been reported in patients with tongue cancer.[253] Radiation therapy may be preferable in patients in poor health, but it has the associated adverse effects of mucositis, taste change, xerostomia, and risk of osteoradionecrosis or radiation-induced tumors. Surgery seems to provide better overall cure rates and allows histologic examination of the neck specimen. Patients with smaller cancers should be considered for elective neck

treatment, especially if primary tumor characteristics such as poor differentiation, extension onto the FOM, and increased tumor thickness (>2 mm) are present.

Results of Treatment

The most common cause of death in patients with cancer of the oral tongue is locoregional failure. The 3-year survival rate for patients with cancer smaller than 4 cm is 70% to 80%. Patients with larger cancers have a 3-year survival rate of only 40% to 50%. Approximately 30% of patients develop second primaries. Lymph node metastasis decreases the survival rate to 15% to 30%.[230] The most common site for distant metastasis is the lung.[254]

Previous reports suggest that cancer of the oral tongue in patients younger than 40 years of age, for reasons that are unclear, is a more aggressive disease than that in older patients and may therefore warrant more aggressive treatment.[255] Investigators reported six patients with clear margins, although two patients had advanced-stage disease, resulting in a 33% survival rate. The report is limited by sample size; however, a literature review by these authors revealed that 57% of patients developed locoregional failure, and 47% of patients died of their cancer. Byers also reported decreased survival in patients younger than age 30 when compared with older patients (45% vs. 65% 2-year survival, respectively).[256] Recent studies reveal no significant difference in survival among younger patients in stage-matched analysis.[257–260] In fact, Myers and associates[229] and other authors[261–262] have reported a survival benefit in younger patients, which may be related to less comorbidity and hence an enhanced ability to tolerate treatment regimens.

CANCER OF THE LIP

U.S. SEER data from 1975 to 1998 report cancer of the lip as the second most common type of cancer of the oral cavity, accounting for 13.5% of all cancers of the oral cavity and pharynx.[228] During the same period, SEER data suggested that there had been a 37% to 45% reduction in incidence among black and white males, respectively. The National Cancer Institute estimated that the incidence of lip cancer for 1991 was 3600 cases, with a 6:1 male-to-female ratio.[263] SCC is the most common cancer of the lip. Cancers arising from the lower lip account for the majority of these cancers (88% to 98%), carcinomas in the commissure area account for less than 1% of all reported cases of cancer of the lip, and cancers of the upper lip account for 2% to 7% of cases.[263] The predilection for the lower lip has been attributed to solar exposure. More than one third of patients with cancer of the lip have outdoor occupations,[263] which suggests that sunlight may be an etiologic factor. Cancer of the lip occurs most commonly in fair-complexioned white men in their sixth decade of life.[264] Pigmented skin provides relative protection from ultraviolet (UV) damage, which may account for the rarity of cancer of the lip in the black population.

Carcinoma of the lip usually presents as a nonhealing erythematous lesion on the lower lip. Perioral chapping and crusting may also be seen in the early phase of progression. As the tumor progresses, ulceration and bleeding occur more frequently. Fortunately, cancer of the lip tends to be a localized disease in the majority of patients. Approximately 80% to 90% of these cancers present as T1 or T2 tumors. Superficial and lateral growth occurs initially rather than frank invasion of the musculature of the lip. However, cancer of the lip can invade not only the muscle but also the underlying bone of the maxilla or mandible. Loose dentition and numbness of the chin, lower lip, or cheek and lateral nose suggest perineural involvement, indicating advanced disease and warranting aggressive intervention. Most cancers of the lip are well differentiated and of the exophytic type. SCCs of the upper lip and oral commissure are more aggressive and less differentiated and present with earlier cervical metastasis.

Cervical metastasis is most often seen in advanced cancer of the lip. Cervical metastasis occurs in less than 10% of patients with cancer of the lower lip and in up to 20% of those with cancer of the upper lip and commissure.[265] Primary lymphatic drainage basins for cancer of the lip are found in level I, notably the submental, submandibular, and perivascular facial nodes. Carcinoma of the commissure and upper lip can also metastasize to the periparotid and preauricular nodes.

Bilateral metastasis may develop if the cancer is near to or crosses the midline of the lip. Crossover between the lymphatics of the right and left sides of the upper lip rarely occurs,[263] possibly because of embryonic fusion planes.

Treatment

Primary Cancer

Early cancer of the lip can be adequately treated with either surgery or radiation therapy. Local control rates exceed 90%. Surgery has the advantages of brevity, decreased cost, good cosmetic results, and a specimen available for pathologic analysis. However, cancer located at the commissure may be better treated with radiation therapy because the cosmetic and functional results are excellent. Advanced cancer of the lip (T3 or T4) should be treated with combined therapy (surgery and radiation therapy to achieve optimal local control).

Patients with carcinoma in situ or severe dysplasia can be managed with vermilionectomy (lip shave), with or without a small margin of muscle. Reconstruction with mucosal advancement is simple and highly successful and maintains the normal lip mucosa. Early cancer of the lip is usually excised with the patient under local anesthesia with a wedge excision in a V or W shape. This allows for adequate margins with the least sacrifice of normal tissue and markedly aids in reconstruction. For improved cosmesis, the point of the V or W should be kept at or above the submental crease. The wound should be closed in three or four layers, including the orbicularis oris muscle, mucosa, subcutaneous tissue, and skin. In general, a minimum of 1 cm of normal tissue should be resected.[263] Resection of 30% of the lip length can be repaired primarily; larger resections are best repaired with advancement or rotation flaps.

Large defects can be reconstructed through transfer of composite tissue on a pedicle from the uninvolved lip (Abbé-Estlander flap). The pedicle is divided within 2 weeks after flap transfer. Another favored method of reconstruction of large lip defects is the Karapandzic flap.[266] This is a bilateral, opposing, full-thickness myocutaneous advancement flap that maintains its neurovascular pedicle, ensuring the viability and sensory and motor functions of the flap. Unfortunately, microstomia often results from excision of cancer occupying more than 60% to 70% of the lip. Finally, large defects that leave less than one third of the lip intact require reconstruction with tissue outside the functional anatomic lip unit. This can be done with bilateral advancement flaps, nasolabial flaps, regional flaps, or free vascularized flaps.

Rarely, larger cancers involving skin, mandible, or mental nerve require composite resection, a marginal or segmental mandibulectomy, and postoperative radiation. Cutaneous and mucosal margins should be analyzed by means of frozen section analysis before the defect is repaired. In fact, if the margins are in question or if frozen section is not available, the wound may be left open and repaired a few days later when the margins have been finalized.

Radiation is highly effective in eradicating early cancer of the lip. Cerezo and associates reported 61 patients with T1 and T2 (99% of patients) cancer of the lip treated with radiation as a single modality.[267] With a median follow-up of

5.4 years, the overall survival rate was 81%. Local failure developed in four patients after radiation, three of whom were salvaged by surgery. Orrechia and colleagues reported 47 patients with early lower lip cancer (stage T1 or T2) treated with brachytherapy at doses ranging between 6000 and 8000 cGy.[268] Local control was achieved in 44 (93.6%) patients. The 5- and 10-year actuarial disease-free survival rates were 92% and 85%, respectively. However, there was a 10.6% incidence of mucosal necrosis. The cosmetic results of radiation are often poorer than those following surgery, and young patients are exposed to long-term effects of radiation.

Cancer of the Neck

Patients with early cancer of the lip do not benefit from elective treatment of the cervical lymph nodes because the rate of occult metastasis is low. The risk of cervical metastasis increases with poorly differentiated cancer, perineural invasion, deep invasion of lip muscle, recurrent cancer, and cancer that extends onto the buccal mucosa or involves the mandible. For cancer 2 to 4 cm in size, the reported delayed cervical metastatic rate has been between 35% and 40%.[263] Locally recurrent cancer of the lip has a 25% probability of occult cervical metastasis.[269] Therefore, elective ND of levels I to III (SOHND) is recommended in recurrent cancer, tumors larger than 4 cm, those with perineural involvement, or those with bone involvement. A superficial parotidectomy should be included for patients with advanced cancer of the upper lip and commissure. Clinically apparent lymph nodes require either radiation therapy or ND for N1 nodes, and combined therapy (ND and radiation therapy) for N2 and N3 nodes or nodes with ECS.[270]

Results of Treatment

Poor prognostic factors include a large cancer (>2 cm), poorly differentiated cancer, recurrent cancer, cancer of the upper lip and commissure, perineural invasion, muscular invasion, mandible invasion, and presence of cervical lymph node metastasis. The cure rates for T1 and T2 cancer without regional metastasis are greater than 90% with surgery or radiation therapy. The 5-year determinate survival is approximately 80%.[269] Cure rates for cancer of the lip have been reported to range between 83% and 96%, suggesting a better prognosis than other cancers of the oral cavity. Cancer involving the oral commissure is more aggressive, with 5-year cure rates ranging between 34% and 50%. Cancers larger than 2 cm have cure rates of less than 80%. Cancers that invade deeply to involve the mandible have a cure rate of less than 50%.[263] The primary cause of failure is local recurrence and not regional metastasis.[263, 271] Local recurrence correlates with the size of the original cancer and is seen in 5% to 15% of patients.[263]

The presence of cervical lymph node metastasis unquestionably affects survival. The average 5-year survival for patients with such metastasis is approximately 50% with a range of 29% to 68%. Recurrence rates in the neck after treatment of the regional metastasis are 40% for N1 cases and up to 100% for N3 cases[269] (see also Chapter 12, Cancer of the Lip).

■ CANCER OF THE BUCCAL MUCOSA

SCC of the buccal mucosa accounts for approximately 10% of all cancers of the oral cavity reported in the United States[272] and 41% of all cancers of the oral cavity in India. Although it is rare, recent data suggest a rise in incidence among American women over the past decade.[273] Risk factors such as tobacco and heavy alcohol use predispose patients to the development of cancer of the buccal mucosa. In addition, ill-fitting dentures, lichen planus, the use of smokeless tobacco,[274, 275] and betel nut chewing are associated with cancer of the buccal mucosa.[20, 272, 276–278]

Cancer of the buccal mucosa arises more commonly from preexisting leukoplakia than do other oral cavity cancers.[279] These cancers may commonly appear as an exophytic or verrucous mass (see Fig. 13–4), or they may simply present as a nonhealing ulcer, leukoplakia, trismus, cervical adenopathy, pain, or facial paralysis. The buccal region allows the cancer easy access laterally into the buccal fat and the underlying musculature, and enables spread to the mandible or maxilla (Fig. 13–13). Signs such as facial paralysis, induration or frank infiltration of the skin, and trismus indicate advanced disease. Approximately 65% of patients with cancer of the buccal mucosa have extensive disease beyond the mucosa.[278] Many series over the past 50 years have reported that nearly half of patients with buccal cancer present with stage III or IV disease.[278–283]

Treatment

Primary Cancer

Currently, the predominant treatment for carcinoma of the buccal mucosa is surgical excision with or without postoperative radiation. Small tumors located anteriorly are suitable for transoral excision and should include full-thickness mucosa down to the buccinator muscle. Buccal space involvement, even in T1 and T2 tumors, creates difficulty in adequate tumor clearance short of radical through-and-through resection of the skin of the cheek. The buccinator muscle is not a satisfactory barrier for preventing the spread of buccal cancer but should be removed as a deep margin. Tumors penetrating the buccinator muscle should be treated with postoperative radiation.

Larger tumors (T3 or T4) or those extending to the mandible or maxilla may require a lip-splitting approach, with or without mandibulectomy or maxillectomy, for obtaining adequate oncologic margins. Results of surgical treatment in buccal cancers requiring marginal mandibulectomy have been reported as an overall local control rate of 79%.[284] Identification of cortical mandibular invasion necessitates segmental resection of the mandible.

Early (T1 and T2) cancer can also be effectively treated with primary radiation. In fact, radiation may be preferred in cancer with indistinct margins or with surrounding areas of leukoplakia, in patients wishing to avoid cosmetic deformity, and in patients unfit for general anesthesia. Radiation therapy treats the entire buccal region at full-thickness depth and thus unrecognized disease in the buccal fat. However, radiation therapy does cause adverse effects such as dry mouth, dental caries, osteoradionecrosis, and trismus.

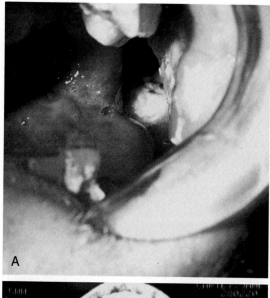

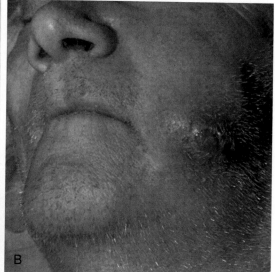

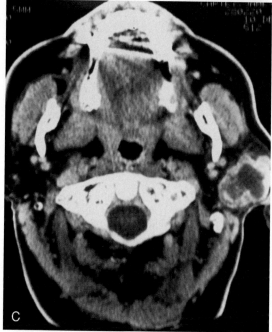

FIGURE 13–13 Infiltration of cancer of the buccal mucosa through the deep musculature *(A)* and the overlying skin of the cheek *(B)*. *C*, CT scan demonstrates the infiltrating cancer.

The major downside of primary radiation is that salvage after radiation failure is dismal.[283]

When possible, surgery combined with postoperative radiation is used in the management of advanced cancer (T3 and T4). This approach is especially favored in the treatment of patients with evidence of bone involvement because successful radiation is limited in this setting. Patients may present with such advanced disease that they are not surgical candidates. In fact, Pradhan and Rajpal deemed up to 50% of T4 cancers of the buccal mucosa as inoperable based on extensive fungation with edema, satellite nodules, pterygoid muscle involvement, severe trismus, and fixed metastatic nodes.[284] Trismus may represent masseteric inflammation or pterygoid fibrosis rather than absolute evidence of pterygoid invasion. Lesions that do not extend onto the RMT or maxillary alveolus are unlikely to have pterygoid muscle involvement.

A skin graft is most commonly used in the reconstruction of the defect following excision of T1 and T2 cancers. Often, a speech appliance may be required to improve speech or swallowing associated with oronasal fistula (Fig. 13–14). Small limited mucosal defects can heal by second intention, thus preventing the morbidity of skin grafting and the nuisance of bolster placement. However, trismus secondary to scar contracture related to this type of healing should not be overlooked. Larger tumors often require regional flap or free-tissue transfer for optimal reconstruction.

Cancer of the Neck

Approximately 50% of patients may present with clinical cervical adenopathy.[131] Therapeutic neck dissection should be performed in all patients with clinically positive disease. The primary lymphatic basin appears to comprise nodes in

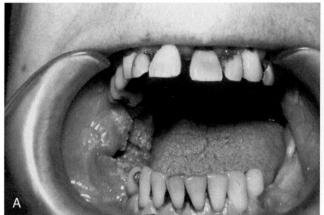
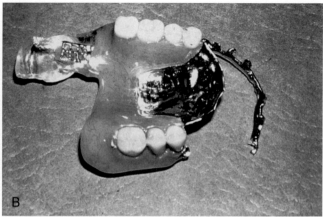
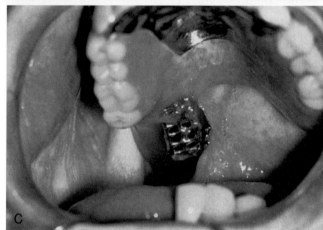

FIGURE 13–14 *A*, Extensive cancer of the buccal mucosa with infiltration into the underlying musculature. *B*, Speech appliance used to provide oronasal separation following resection of cancer of the buccal mucosa, including the palate. *C*, Dental appliance in place.

the submandibular space, as well as the superior deep jugular nodes. However, the periparotid and superior deep jugular nodes may constitute the primary lymphatic basin for more posteriorly located cancers of the buccal mucosa. Modified ND is performed for extensive or bulky nodal disease; SND of levels I to III is used for limited N1 disease confined to the upper neck.

The occult metastatic rate for carcinoma of the buccal mucosa is relatively low (10%).[131] Early cancers (T1 and T2) theoretically do not require elective ND.[131, 285] In a histopathologic study of 57 surgical specimens of T3 and T4 cancers of the buccal mucosa, occult metastases in patients to levels I and II were reported as 11.7% and 9.0%, respectively.[286] Nair and coworkers reported that 7.2% of patients with cancer of the buccal mucosa and a clinically N0 neck have occult metastasis.[287] SND in the setting of N0 disease should be performed in all patients because one cannot accurately select out those patients who do or do not require SND.

Results of Treatment

Improved outcomes for patients with buccal carcinoma have been reported with a change in primary treatment from radiation to surgical therapy.[273, 288] Overall 5-year cure rates following surgical therapy have been reported to be as low as 24%, with stage I and II being reported as 77% and 65%, respectively.[131] Surgical therapy has been reported as equal

to or better than radiation therapy for early-stage tumors[289] but superior to radiation for higher-stage disease.[279] In addition, patients with advanced buccal cancer have significantly improved 2-year disease-free intervals with surgery and postoperative radiation (33%) compared with patients with primary radiation (5%).[289] Vikram and Farr suggested improved control in patients with stage III and IV cancer with postoperative radiation (50 to 60 Gy/5 to 6 weeks).[290]

Some patients are treated with radiation initially in anticipation of avoiding morbidity and perceived disfigurement. Wang[285] and Pourquier and associates[291] reported primary treatment with radiation therapy and found overall 3- and 5-year cure rates of 40% and 26%, respectively, with especially poor results in patients with advanced disease. Nair and colleagues treated 234 patients with carcinoma of the buccal mucosa with primary radiation and reported disease-free intervals of 85%, 63%, 41%, and 15% for stages I to IV, respectively.[287] Overall 5-year survival rates with the use of all modalities are 52% to 60%.[281, 283, 292]

Local recurrence is a major problem in the treatment of cancer of the buccal mucosa. Reported local recurrence rates range from 37% to 45% depending on the stage of disease.[282, 293] Maccomb and Fletcher reported a lower incidence of 17%, probably because most of their patients had early-stage cancer.[294] However, Sieczka and coworkers reported a 40% local failure rate after surgery alone in T1–T2 buccal cancers despite pathologically clear margins.[282] Similarly, Strome and associates have reported local failure in 9 of 11 patients managed with surgical excision alone for T1–T2 disease despite clear margins.[281] It is possible that combined therapy would benefit all patients with buccal carcinoma. Fang and colleagues reported 64% locoregional control in 57 stage II to IV patients treated with surgery and postoperative radiation for buccal cancer.[295] Nair and coworkers reported that of 234 evaluable patients with cancer of the buccal mucosa treated with radiation therapy, local failure was seen in 27%, 43%, and 62% of patients with stages II through IV cancer, respectively.[287] Regional nodal failure was seen in 14%, 36%, and 42% of patients with stages II through IV cancer, respectively. Regional recurrence often occurs in combination with local recurrence (approximately 70%).[285, 293] Regional failure alone accounted for only 8% of patients in one study.[293] Results of salvage surgery are poor, with only 0% to 20% cure rates.[283, 293]

In a retrospective study of 162 cases of stage T4 carcinoma of the buccal mucosa, Pradhan and Rajpal showed that neck metastasis and positive margins predict locoregional recurrence.[284] However, the absence of these factors did not ensure locoregional control. Adverse local outcome is likely related to the sparsity of anatomic barriers in the buccal region. Once tumor enters the buccal fat, its biologic behavior is no longer predicted by T-stage. On multivariate analysis in two separate studies, poor prognosis was associated with involvement of the skin of the cheek[295] and tumor thickness.[296] Urist and associates in a study of 89 patients with SCC of the buccal mucosa demonstrated on multivariate analysis that only tumor thickness was an independent variable ($P < .0001$).[296] Patients with cancer less than 6 mm thick demonstrated better survival than did patients with cancer greater than 6 mm thick, regardless of stage.

Distant metastasis with buccal cancer is infrequent, occurring in 2% to 10% of patients.[273, 279, 281, 295] Although response rates to chemotherapy have been reported as 70% to 88% in patients with buccal carcinoma, overall survival rates remain poor.[297, 298] Schuller and colleagues suggested chemotherapy as part of adjuvant treatment for advanced buccal cancer.[298]

▢ CANCER OF THE FLOOR OF THE MOUTH

Over the past century, the percentage of women constituting the population of those with cancer of the FOM has risen from 6% to nearly 33%.[228, 299] This has been attributed to the increased use of tobacco and alcohol in this population, as has also been reported in cancer of the buccal mucosa in women.[273] The dependent location of the FOM allows prolonged contact with carcinogens such as alcohol or smokeless tobacco. In addition, a slow increase in tumor stage has been noted during the same period.[300] However, U.S. SEER data suggest an overall 30% reduction in the incidence of cancer of the FOM among whites and blacks over the past decade.[228]

Cancer of the FOM is often asymptomatic in the early stages of disease. These tumors may arise in regions of erythroplakia or leukoplakia. As the tumor enlarges, bleeding, ulceration, pain, and submandibular duct obstruction become more common. Deep infiltration of the FOM and tongue is suggested by weakness of the hypoglossal nerve, restricted tongue mobility, and numbness of the lingual nerve or mental nerves. Restricted motion of the tongue manifests itself as a change in quality of speech and difficulty with articulation. With lateral growth of the cancer, the ventral tongue or mandibular alveolus, including the RMT and tonsillar pillars, becomes involved. Despite the fact that the cancer abuts the mandible, the periosteum can be an effective barrier to tumor invasion.[301]

Patients with cancer of the FOM present with stage I/II disease as frequently as they present with stage III/IV disease.[299, 300, 302, 303] The incidence of clinically apparent cervical metastasis at presentation is approximately 30% to 40%, often with multiple levels of nodal involvement.[299, 300, 302–304] Patients with cancer of the FOM have a 17% to 62% incidence of occult cervical disease[299,302] and a 4% incidence of synchronous primary neoplasms.[300] Hicks and colleagues reported the occult cervical disease rate to be 21% for T1 tumors and 62% for T2 tumors.[302]

Treatment

Primary Cancer

Early cancer of the FOM can be effectively treated with either surgery or radiation. The transoral approach provides visualization of the oral cavity sufficient for the surgeon to obtain adequate tissue margins. Cancers of the FOM are often underestimated, with 30% to 37% of patients having positive margins on permanent section analysis.[300, 302] Planned margins of at least 1 cm, including the deep margin, should be delineated; this often involves sacrifice of one or both submandibular ducts.[305] The submandibular duct can be reimplanted posteriorly or can be ligated because the submandibular gland will likely be included in level I dissection. The sublingual glands are taken to form the deep margin of resection. Tumor involving the orifice of the duct may result in resection of the duct and submandibular and sublingual gland on the affected side because tumor can spread along the duct. Steinhart and Kleinsasser reviewed 48 specimens and observed that cancer of the FOM may invade through the sublingual gland and the intrinsic muscles of the tongue.[306] In cases requiring exposure only, midline mandibulotomy provides excellent exposure for resection of the primary and for reconstruction with minimal long-term morbidity.

Although many of these defects heal satisfactorily by secondary intention, the application of a split-thickness skin graft speeds healing, decreases bleeding, and results in less contraction of the healed surface and less interference with articulation. In previously irradiated patients or those with significant exposure of the mandible, vascularized tissue reconstruction is recommended. For localized FOM lesions, the split-thickness skin graft is simple and results in excellent functional outcome (Fig. 13–15).

For tumors of advanced stage, resection of part of the tongue or mandible is often required. In the anterior FOM, marginal or segmental mandibulectomy may be required to obtain an adequate margin of resection, especially with cancer abutting or adherent to the mandibular periosteum

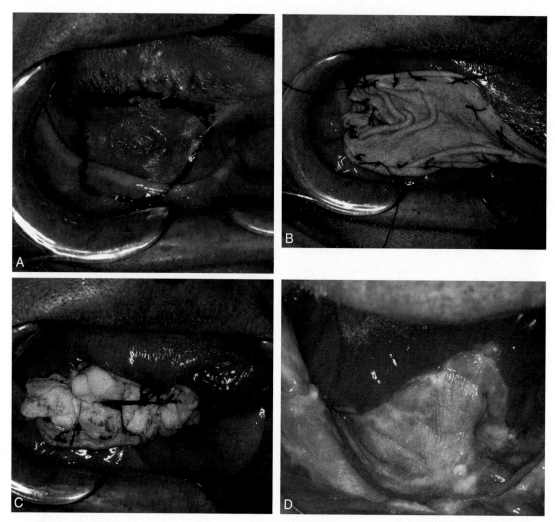

FIGURE 13–15 *A*, Floor-of-the-mouth cancer with intended resection, *B*, Split-thickness skin graft in situ. *C*, Iodoform bolster affixing skin graft in place, *D*, Final result of skin grafting with recontouring of natural sulcus.

(Fig. 13–16). Marginal mandibulectomy is defined as excision of the alveolar process. Segmental mandibulectomy has been shown to be oncologically safe in large series[232, 307, 308] and results in shorter operating times, likely providing superior functional results, especially when a portion of the mylohyoid or digastric muscle remains attached to the mandible. Werning and coworkers reported 86% 2-year local control in 222 patients receiving marginal mandibulectomy.[232] Shaha reported 2-year local control rates of 100%, 85%, and 60% for stages I through III, respectively, in a series of 65 patients with cancer of the FOM in which 44 underwent marginal mandibulectomy.[307] Beecroft and associates reported a 5-year determinate survival rate of 84% in 34 patients treated with marginal mandibulectomy.[308] For patients with clinical or radiologic evidence of mandibular invasion, segmental mandibulectomy is necessary.

Cole[309] and Rodgers[310] and colleagues reported 162 and 194 patients, respectively, with cancer of the FOM. Single-modality treatment was usually adequate for stages I and II, but locoregional control for stages III and IV was improved with the addition of postoperative irradiation. Postoperative irradiation is recommended for close or positive margins, nodal disease, ECS, and T3 or T4 disease.[309–312] Postoperative irradiation has been found to result in good local control in patients with cancer of the FOM, but patients are at risk for distant metastasis in up to 30% of cases.[311]

Primary radiation can result in control rates comparable with those of surgery for early FOM cancer. This may be given in the form of external beam or brachytherapy. Aygun and coworkers reported 166 patients with cancer of the FOM treated with primary brachytherapy with or without external beam irradiation.[313] Local control rates were 83%, 85%, 42%, and 21% for stages I through IV, respectively. The 5-year determinate survival rates were 79% and 77% for stages I and II, respectively, but dropped significantly to 26% and 14% for stages III and IV cancer, respectively. Brachytherapy is associated with a 17% to 40% severe complication rate, which includes necrosis of soft tissue and bone.[303, 313] Mazeron and associates reported on a series of 117 patients with T1 or T2 SCC of the FOM treated with iridium-192 implantation brachytherapy.[314] Primary local

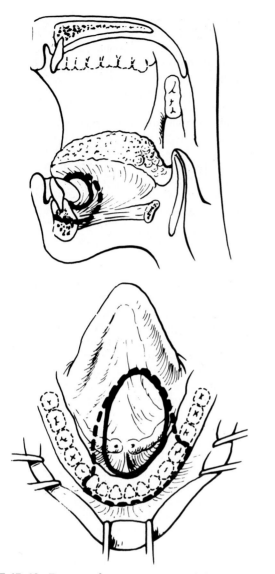

FIGURE 13–16 Diagram showing resection of the soft tissues of the floor of the mouth, including marginal mandibulectomy.

control was achieved in 93.5% of T1 patients, 74.5% of T2 patients, and 65% of patients with T2 N1–N3 disease. Control rates were lower than 58% in patients with lesions larger than 3 cm or with gingival extension. Salvage after radiation failure is poor.[302]

Cancer of the Neck

The primary tumor and metastases should be simultaneously addressed with the same treatment modality. Approximately 30% to 42% of patients with carcinoma of the FOM have clinically positive nodes at presentation.[300, 302, 304] The most common nodal basins of FOM cancer account for levels I and II.[6] Traditionally, any N+ disease is managed by surgery or radiation. The MRND has become the gold standard for oncologic clearance of the N+ neck. However, for early N+ disease, SND of levels I to III may be sufficient, especially with the use of planned postoperative radiation. The main advantage of this technique is improved

functional results, as were described earlier in this chapter. For lymph node metastasis larger than 2 cm or multiple in nature, MRND is most frequently advocated.

The incidence of occult metastasis ranges from 10% to 30%.[129] Elective treatment of the neck appears warranted in patients with T3 or T4 cancer.[305, 315] Recommendations for management of the N0 neck in patients with T1–T2 cancer vary from observation to elective ND to radiation therapy. Review of the literature reveals that the incidence of cervical node metastasis after initial treatment of cancer of the FOM ranges from 15% to 38%. Nason and associates state that they perform elective ND in patients with early cancers that are deeply infiltrative, in most patients with large cancers, and when patients are not amenable to close follow-up.[305]

The use of elective ND results in improved locoregional control, which likely translates to improved overall cure rates because salvage is relatively poor.[129, 227] Spiro and Strong documented increased survival in those patients undergoing elective ND and suggested a beneficial effect for removal of occult metastasis.[227] In contrast, studies by Jesse[250] and Schramm and colleagues[316] have provided data to suggest that surgical salvage rates of neck metastasis are acceptable and that the occult metastatic rate is low enough that routine elective ND is not warranted. However, in a recent retrospective analysis of a series of 129 patients with cancer of the FOM and N0 necks treated with surgery, McGuirt and colleagues observed that 23% of patients had occult metastatic disease. Recurrence in the neck developed in 36% of 103 patients who did not undergo ND.[129] Fifty-nine percent of those patients with failure of treatment in the neck were salvaged. The authors recommend elective ND in patients with cancer of the FOM.

Therapeutic neck dissection in the form of MRND or SND is recommended for N+ disease. Additionally, elective ND of at least levels I to III, bilateral if necessary, is recommended for all patients undergoing surgical treatment for their primary tumor.

Results of Treatment

Overall 5-year survival rates for cancer of the FOM range from 31% to 76%, including 64% to 95% for stage I, 61% to 86% for stage II, 28% to 82% for stage III, and 6% to 52% for stage IV cancer.[300, 302, 305, 310] Locoregional recurrence remains a major source of treatment failure in patients with cancer of the FOM. Positive margins are clearly associated with high risk of locoregional recurrence and decreased survival.[300, 302, 317] Hicks and coworkers reported that in patients treated with surgery alone, positive margins decreased the local control rate from 87% to 62%.[302] Shons and associates reported 68% and 48% locoregional control rates in stage III and IV cancer of the FOM, despite excision of the primary cancer with 2-cm margins and 89% of patients having mandible resection.[315] Ninety-one percent of patients had radical ND, and 15% received adjuvant radiation therapy. The overall incidence of regional recurrence is 13% to 18%.[300, 302] The incidence of distant metastasis ranges from 10% to 30%.[300] The efficacy of chemotherapy in the treatment of locoregional and distant metastases is not clear.

CANCER OF THE RETROMOLAR TRIGONE

The RMT is referred to as the gingiva covering the ascending portion of the mandible, immediately posterior to the last molar. Primary cancer of the RMT is rare. These tumors often present at advanced stages because they are usually ulcerative and camouflaged by molars. These cancers quickly spread to invade the mandible, which is covered by mucosa and periosteum. Pathologically proven invasion of the mandible of cancers arising in the RMT ranges from 12% to 50%[318, 319] and may be detected on CT with 61% sensitivity and a specificity of 91%. The soft tissue of the soft palate, tonsillar pillar, tongue, FOM, and pterygoid musculature often become involved with advancing disease. Pterygoid involvement is usually heralded by trismus. Pain and burning from a nonhealing ulcer are common retrospective symptoms reported by patients. Ear complaints can occur and range from referred otalgia to hearing loss from nasopharyngeal extension and eustachian tube involvement. The inferior alveolar nerve may become involved by direct mandibular invasion; alternatively, such invasion may spread along the ramus of the mandible to the lingula and is suggested by ipsilateral numbness of the lower teeth and lip.

Although RMT cancer is in an oral cavity location, its behavior is often aggressive, and it may behave similarly to oropharyngeal cancer. The common nodal basins for metastasis include the superior deep jugular nodes (level II), followed by level III. Because the RMT is an extension of the lower alveolar ridge, it is not surprising that the incidences of cervical metastasis are similar in these sites (39% with RMT and 30% with alveolar ridge).[318] The occult metastatic rate is 10% to 20%.[320] Pathologically, invasion of the mandible by cancer arising in the RMT varies from 12% to 50%.[318, 319]

Treatment

Primary Cancer

T1 and T2 cancer can be treated effectively with either radiation or surgery. Surgery is preferred as the initial treatment in cancers that are deeply infiltrative and in those causing trismus. Often, surgery involves at least a marginal mandibulectomy to obtain clear margins. Exposure of the RMT is limited with a strictly transoral approach; thus, adequate access to the RMT may require either a lip-splitting incision and cheek flap or a visor flap. When mandibulotomy is required, thought should be given to the position of the initial osteotomy. If a midline or paramedian mandibulotomy is performed and the tumor requires segmental resection of bone, the entire hemimandible may be lost. Yet, if segmental resection of bone is not performed, but lateral mandibulotomy is performed, medial exposure is more limited than with either a median or paramedian mandibulotomy with swing.

Because speech and swallowing dysfunction can result from surgery, some use radiation therapy as initial treatment for these cancers. In our experience, this treatment is more successful with small exophytic rather than ulcerative or infiltrative tumors in this area.

Stage III and IV cancers are managed with a combination of surgery and radiation therapy. In addition to segmental mandibulectomy, resection of tongue, floor of mouth, soft palate, and oropharynx is often necessary. Defects can rarely be closed primarily, and most often these lateral defects are repaired with a skin graft or a myocutaneous flap. Flaps with too much bulk, such as pectoralis myocutaneous or rectus abdominis, may actually impede swallowing and phonation. The radial forearm flap is ideal because it provides thin, pliable skin and a high degree of reliability with minimal donor site morbidity. Because lateral mandibular defects usually do not cause long-term speech and swallowing dysfunction, bony mandibular reconstruction is not necessary, except in younger patients in whom cosmesis may be a factor. Oral prostheses may be used to provide oronasal separation when soft palate defects occur.

Huang and colleagues reported 65 patients with RMT cancer treated with various regimens of radiation.[321] Patients treated with radiation alone experienced a local recurrence rate of 44% compared with rates of 10% to 23% in those receiving combined surgery and radiation. They reported severe complications of trismus and bone or soft tissue necrosis in roughly 11% of patients receiving radiation alone or postoperative radiation. It is interesting to note that no radiation-related complications were reported in patients receiving preoperative radiation, likely because unradiated soft tissue reconstruction was provided after radiation.

Cancer of the Neck

Patients treated with a transcervical surgical approach for the primary tumor with N0 neck should also undergo at least elective ND. Patients with palpable metastatic neck cancer are best managed with therapeutic ND and postoperative irradiation. In addition, it is recommended that patients with stage II or higher RMT cancer should undergo elective treatment of the neck with either surgery or irradiation. Overall survival is reportedly adversely affected by increasing N-stage.[321]

Results of Treatment

Byers and coworkers retrospectively reviewed 110 patients with SCC originating in the RMT treated with surgery or radiation or both.[318] Initial local control with mandibular conservation surgery alone was 92% (11/12 patients). Local control rates were 87.5% (42/48 patients) for segmental mandibulectomy and 80% (12/15) in patients with cortical bone invasion. Regional control in surgically treated patients was 84%. Absolute 5-year survival overall was 26%, which reflected the poor salvage of second primaries and a high incidence of intercurrent disease.

Kowalski and associates reviewed 114 cases of patients with cancer of the RMT treated with composite resection with or without radiation therapy.[322] Sixty-six patients underwent postoperative radiation therapy. Forty-one patients had a total of 50 cancer recurrences: 31 local, 9 in the dissected neck, 3 in the contralateral neck, and 7 distant metastases. The 5-year actuarial survival rates were 80% (T1), 57.8% (T2), 46.5% (T3), and 65.2% (T4). The 5-year overall survival rate was 55.3%. Owing to the high rate of local recurrence, the authors recommended that patients with advanced cancer (stage III or IV) should have adjunctive irradiation. Huang and colleagues reported improved outcomes with the use of combined-modality treatment for RMT.[321]

CANCER OF THE ALVEOLAR RIDGE

SCC of the alveolar ridge accounts for approximately 10% of all malignancies occurring in the oral cavity. These cancers usually arise on the inferior alveolar ridge and in the region of the posterior dental arch. Cancer of the alveolar ridge occurs most often in edentulous areas and at the free margin of the gingiva. Most cancers extend beyond the alveolus to involve adjacent soft tissue structures such as the buccal mucosa and FOM. This cancer usually occurs in men, with a 4:1 ratio over women, and predominates in the sixth and seventh decades of life.[323] Smoking, alcohol use, and ill-fitting dentures have been associated with these cancers.[130] Approximately 35% to 50% of patients have mandibular invasion demonstrated radiographically or histologically.[130, 324] Clinical evidence of metastasis is present or becomes apparent over the course of the disease in 30% of cases,[130] with an occult metastatic rate of 15%. Metastasis is usually to the superior deep jugular nodes.

Patients usually complain of loosening of the teeth or ill-fitting dentures associated with a nonhealing lesion. Pain, difficulty in mastication, and bleeding are common. Numbness of the lower teeth suggests mandibular invasion involving the inferior alveolar nerve. Cancer originating on the maxillary alveolar ridge can invade into the maxillary sinus.

Treatment

Primary Cancer

Early-stage cancers of the alveolar ridge may be managed effectively with surgery alone. Cancer involving the maxillary alveolar ridge can be excised via a transoral approach, and the soft tissue skin grafted. Larger cancers require a partial maxillectomy (Fig. 13–17). Although radiation has the ability to cure early cancers of the alveolar ridge, its use often leaves exposed intraoral bone, which is at increased risk for osteoradionecrosis. In addition, the efficacy of radiation in eradicating tumor that has invaded cortical bone is limited; this is best treated with surgery followed by radiation.

Careful assessment of the mandible and of the presence of perineural invasion is needed before treatment is provided for cancer of the inferior alveolar ridge. The mandibular periosteum provides a barrier to invasion of the mandible, but radiation therapy may remove this barrier,

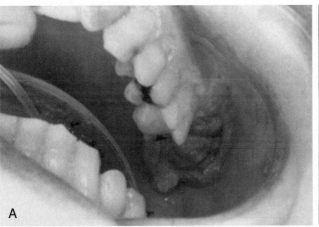
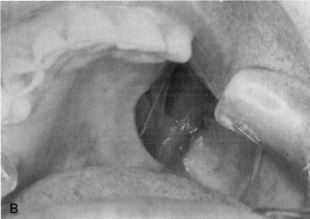
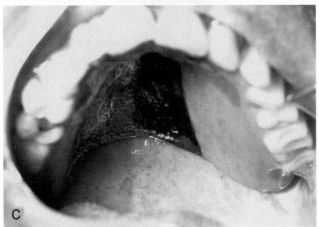

FIGURE 13–17 *A*, SCC of the alveolar ridge treated by transoral partial maxillectomy. *B*, Maxillary defect and skin graft resurfacing of the soft tissues. *C*, Partially removable prosthesis, which provides oronasal separation.

making the extent of cancer invasion less predictable. In the nonirradiated mandible, invasion occurs either through open tooth sockets or through small defects in the edentulous mandibular ridge more often than through the lingual or buccal cortical plates. If the cancer is large, however, the cortex can be invaded.[325] Radiographic evidence should be interpreted with caution because of the possibility of false-negative and false-positive data. Recent experience suggests that clinical evaluation is as accurate as radiologic studies in the assessment of bone invasion.[326] Early cancers can be effectively managed with marginal mandibulectomy and primary closure. Tight closures may tether the tongue and FOM, thus obliterating the natural sulcus. This results in poorer functional results, and a skin graft may be used to reconstruct the sulcus. Cancers demonstrating invasion of the cortical bone require segmental mandibulectomy. Small cancers of the superior alveolar ridge can be excised transorally. More advanced cancers of the superior alveolus may require a lateral rhinotomy or a midface degloving incision for exposure. In patients with loose dentition or recent extraction during the initial management of the tumor,

invasion of the mandible is likely, and segmental mandibulectomy should be performed.

Lateral defects of the mandible cause few functional deficits, and reconstruction should be individualized. However, anterior and hemimandibular resections require reconstruction so that speech, swallowing, and cosmetic dysfunction can be avoided (Fig. 13–18). Preferred reconstruction is provided with a fibula free flap, although various other free-tissue transfer flaps or myocutaneous pedicled flaps can be used in combination with reconstruction plates or trays. This latter approach, however, has been associated with a high rate of plate exposure and/or fracture.[327]

Cancer of the Neck

Therapeutic ND is indicated in all patients with clinically palpable cervical nodes. Stage I cancer likely does not benefit from elective ND. Byers and associates found a 29% incidence of nodal metastasis, and elective ND was not suggested, in patients with T1 carcinoma of the alveolar ridge.[130] However, elective ND should be employed in

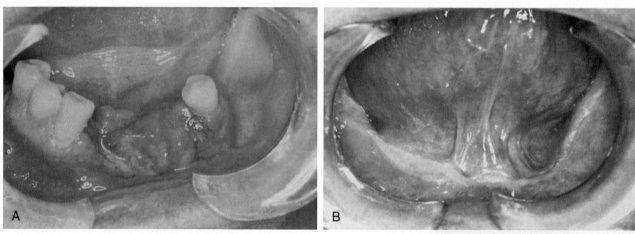

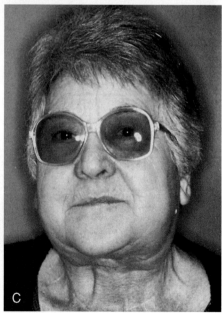

FIGURE 13–18 *A,* SCC destroying the alveolar ridge and invading the mandible anteriorly. *B,* Patient underwent bilateral selective dissections and anterior mandibulectomy reconstruction with a fibular osteocutaneous free flap; nicely healed oral cavity is seen. *C,* Normal projection of mandible following this type of reconstruction.

patients with T2–T4 cancer, in any patient requiring a transcervical approach for resection of a primary, and in any patient in whom radiation therapy has failed.

Results of Treatment

Overall 5-year survival rates for patients with carcinoma of the alveolar ridge range from 50% to 65%. No significant difference in survival has been demonstrated between upper and lower ridge malignancies. Soo and associates found that advanced stage, previous dental extraction, bone invasion, and positive surgical margins were predictive of a lower survival rate in patients with cancer of the alveolar ridge.[326] Byers and associates, in a review of a series of 67 patients with SCC of the lower alveolar ridge treated with surgery or radiation therapy or both, reported an overall survival rate of 67%.[130] The 2-year disease-free survival rates were 79% for T1, 69% for T2, 62% for T3, and 42% for T4 cancers. The local control rate was 98% with a local or regional failure rate of 5%. The authors recommended adjuvant radiation therapy when extensive nodal metastasis, perineural spread, or inadequate margins of resection were present. They stated, however, that surgery alone can provide satisfactory local control rates for T3 and T4 lesions. Surgery alone seems to be superior to radiation alone. Cady and Catlin, in a review of a series of 606 patients with SCC of the alveolar ridge treated over a 20-year period, reported an increased absolute survival rate ranging from 27% in patients treated primarily with radiation therapy to 50% in patients treated primarily with surgery.[328]

The presence of cervical metastases, however, definitely decreases survival in these patients. Backstrom and coworkers reviewed 125 patients with SCC of the alveolar ridge and observed that the 5-year determinate survival rate decreased from 41% in patients without neck metastasis to only 7% in patients with cervical metastasis.[329] Distant metastasis is rare in tumors of the alveolar ridge and is reported at a rate of approximately 3% to 4%.[130, 330]

CANCER OF THE HARD PALATE

SCC of the hard palate is rare, constituting only 0.5% of all oral cancers in the United States. In India, however, it represents approximately 40% of all oral cancers.[331] Minor salivary gland tumors occur in the hard palate with similar frequency as SCCs. Petruzzelli and Myers, in a study of 51 patients with cancer of the hard palate and alveolar ridge, reported that only 27 patients had SCC.[332] Most cancers of the hard palate are well differentiated and of the ulcerative type.

Patients with cancer of the hard palate usually present with a painless mass in the roof of the mouth or the alveolar ridge. Pain, bleeding, and ill-fitting dentures are less common presenting symptoms. The cancer is rarely localized to the hard palate and is often surrounded by areas of leukoplakia. The periosteum of the palate acts as a barrier to invasion of the bone, which occurs late in the disease (Fig. 13–19). Tumors may spread superiorly over the anterior maxilla, creating numbness, cheek swelling, or nasal obstruction. Lateral spread of tumor along the palate may result in invasion of the pterygomasseteric sling, causing trismus. Nonmalignant tumors of salivary gland origin, necrotizing sialometaplasia, granular cell tumor, and pseudoepitheliomatous hyperplasia should be included in the differential diagnosis.

The clinical metastatic rate is approximately 10% to 25% among patients with hard palate carcinoma who have clinical evidence of cervical metastasis.[333, 334] Metastasis to levels I and II lymph nodes is most common, although retropharyngeal nodes or prevascular facial nodes may also be involved.

Treatment

Primary Cancer

Patients with early cancer of the hard palate can be effectively treated with surgery or radiation therapy. However,

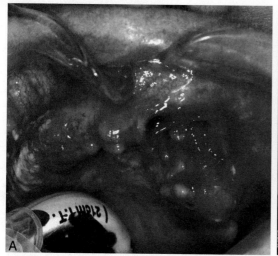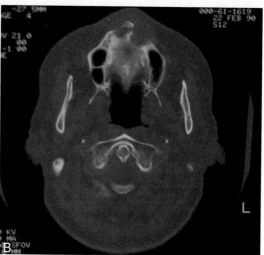

FIGURE 13–19 *A,* Advanced cancer of the hard palate. *B,* CT scan with evidence of maxillary invasion.

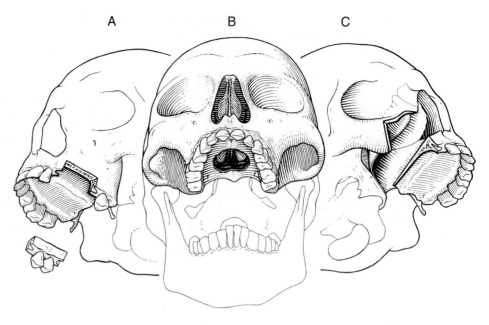

FIGURE 13–20 Maxillary alveolectomy (*A*) or partial palatectomy (*B*) for limited upper alveolar or hard palate cancer may be possible with the peroral approach. *C*, More extensive partial maxillectomy usually requires an upper cheek flap approach.

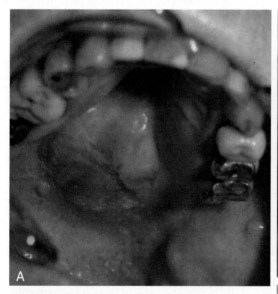

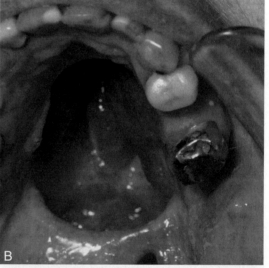

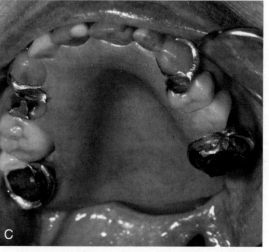

FIGURE 13–21 *A*, Submucosal tumor of the hard palate. *B*, Palatal defect following surgical resection with large oronasal fistula. *C*, Dental obturator in situ obliterating oronasal fistula, which improves speech and swallowing.

radiation often leaves exposed bone, which leaves the patient at risk for osteoradionecrosis. A majority of tumors can be excised via the transoral approach, which can be easily augmented by a lateral rhinotomy or a midfacial degloving incision. Surgery for small and superficial cancers consists of wide local excision, which granulates well. A split-thickness skin graft must be applied to the cheek flap for prevention of skin contracture. Most frequently, the safest approach is to remove the underlying bone, thus exposing the maxillary sinus to the oral cavity. This improves oncologic clearance and allows for improved surveillance of the sinus.

More advanced tumors require partial or total maxillectomy via the transoral approach, possibly augmented by a lateral rhinotomy incision or midfacial degloving (Fig. 13–20). All mucosa must be removed from the remaining maxillary sinus cavity and orbital floor to facilitate fit of the prosthesis. The cheek flap is lined by skin graft. Use of regional flaps or free-tissue transfer often creates unnecessary bulk and results in difficult dental rehabilitation. The use of a dental prosthesis is simple and again allows for improved surveillance of the surgical bed without the use of imaging. Smaller defects heal satisfactorily by second intention. Partial palatal defects are satisfactorily reconstructed with a dental obturator (Fig. 13–21). Total palatal defects can be reconstructed with regional flaps such as temporalis muscle flap or with free-tissue transfer (Fig. 13–22). Dental and cosmetic rehabilitation are often less than optimal in these patients.

Cancer of the Neck

Few published data exist regarding treatment of the neck in cancer of the hard palate. The traditional belief is that the incidence of occult metastasis is low and elective ND does not improve control or survival in these patients.[332] For the last 4 to 5 years, elective ND has been our routine practice in patients with T1–T4 SCC of the hard palate. Initial unpublished analyses of hard palate and maxillary alveolar ridge cancer suggest that occult metastasis among 34 patients occurred at a rate of 25%. Patients with clinically evident disease should be managed with a therapeutic ND.

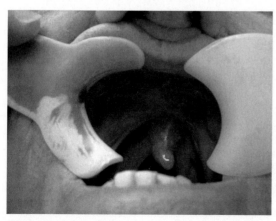

FIGURE 13–22 Total palatal defect reconstructed with temporalis flap and skin graft provides excellent soft tissue coverage, although dental rehabilitation is limited.

Results of Treatment

Evans and Shah reported on 392 patients with cancer of the palate, including 62 with untreated SCC of the hard palate.[335] All patients were treated with surgery; those with stages I and II received single-modality treatment, and stage III and IV patients were treated with single or combined therapy (radiation therapy). Fifty-three percent of these patients developed local recurrence, 30% developed regional recurrence, 10% developed local and regional recurrence, 7% developed locoregional and distant recurrence, and no patients developed solitary distant metastasis. Patients with lesions larger than 3 cm had marked reduction in 5-year cure rates (54% vs. 16%).

Chung and associates reported 32 patients with SCC of the hard palate treated primarily with radiation therapy.[333] Approximately 30% of patients experienced local recurrence, and one patient developed regional recurrence. The 5-year absolute and determinate survival rates were 44% and 75%, respectively, in patients without nodal metastasis, and 25% and 33%, respectively, in patients with nodal metastasis. No patients developed distant metastasis.

REFERENCES

1. American Cancer Society: Cancer facts and figures. Atlanta, American Cancer Society, 1996.
2. Costantinides MS, Rothstein SG, Persky MS: Squamous cell carcinoma in older patients without risk factors. Otolaryngol Head Neck Surg 106:275–277, 1992.
3. Johnson N: Tobacco use and oral cancer: A global perspective. J Dent Educ 65:328–339, 2001.
4. Malaowalla AM, Silverman S, Mani NJ, et al: Oral cancer in 57,518 industrial workers of Gujarat, India. Cancer 37:1882–1886, 1976.
5. Rouviere H: Anatomy of the Human Lymphatic System. Ann Arbor, Edward Brothers, 1938.
6. Lindberg R: Distribution of cervical lymph node metastasis from squamous cell carcinoma of the upper respiratory and digestive tracts. Cancer 29:1446–1449, 1972.
7. Spiro JD, Spiro RH, Shah JP, et al: Critical assessment of supraomohyoid neck dissection. Am J Surg 156:286–289, 1988.
8. Byers RM, Weber RS, Andrews T, et al: Frequency and therapeutic implications of "skip metastases" in the neck from squamous cell carcinoma of the oral tongue. Head Neck 19:445–446, 1997.
9. Ossoff RH, Bytell DE, Hast MH, et al: Lymphatics of the floor of mouth and periosteum: Anatomic studies with possible clinical correlations. Otolaryngol Head Neck Surg 88:652–660, 1980.
10. International Agency for Research on Cancer: Tobacco Smoking. IARC Monogr Eval Carcinog Risk Chem Hum 38. Lyon, IARC, 1986.
11. Macfarlane GJ, Zheng T, Marshall JR, et al: Alcohol, tobacco, diet and the risk of oral cancer: A pooled analysis of three case-control studies. Eur J Cancer B Oral Oncol 31B:181–187, 1995.
12. Kurumatani N, Kirita T, Zheng Y, et al: Time trends in the mortality rates for tobacco- and alcohol-related cancers within the oral cavity and pharynx in Japan, 1950–94. J Epidemiol 9:46–52, 1999.
13. EU-Working Group on Tobacco and Oral Health: Tobacco and oral diseases—report of EU Working Group, 1999. J Ir Dent Assoc 46:12–19, 22, 2000.
14. Boyle P, Macfarlane GJ, Scully C: Oral cancer: Necessity for prevention strategies. Lancet 342:1129–1133, 1993.
15. Buudgaard T, Wildt J, Frydenberg M, et al: Case-control study of squamous cell cancer of the oral cavity in Denmark. Cancer Causes Control 6:57–67, 1995.
16. Jaber MA, Porter SR, Gilthorpe MS, et al: Risk factors for oral epithelial dysplasia—the role of smoking and alcohol. Oral Oncol 35:151–156, 1999.
17. Moreno-Lopez LA, Esparaza-Gomez GC, Gonzalez-Navarro A, et al: Risk of oral cancer associated with tobacco smoking, alcohol consumption and oral hygiene: A case control study in Madrid, Spain. Oral Oncol 36:170–174, 2000.

18. Schlecht NF, Franco EL, Pintos J, et al: Effect of smoking cessation and tobacco type on the risk of cancers of the upper aerodigestive tract in Brazil. Epidemiology 10:412–418, 1999.

19. Franceschi S, Talamani R, Barra S, et al: Smoking and drinking in relation to cancers of the oral cavity, pharynx, larynx, and oesophagus in Northern Italy. Cancer Res 50:6502–6507, 1990.

20. Winn DM, Blot WJ, Shy CM, et al: Snuff dipping and oral cancer among women in the southern United States. N Engl J Med 305:745–749, 1986.

21. National Institutes of Health Consensus Development Conference Statement: Health implications of smokeless tobacco use. CA Cancer J Clin 36:310, 1986.

22. Ko YC, Huang YL, Lee CH, et al: Betel quid chewing, cigarette smoking and alcohol consumption related to oral cancer in Taiwan. J Oral Pathol Med 24:450–453, 1995.

23. Hyland A, Cummings KM, Shopland DR, et al: Prevalence of cigar use in 22 North American communities: 1989 and 1993. Am J Public Health 88:1086–1089, 1998.

24. Gilpin EA, Pierce JP: Patterns of cigar use in California in 1999. Am J Prev Med 21:325–328, 2001.

25. Shapiro JA, Jacobs EJ, Thun MJ: Cigar smoking in men and risk of death from tobacco-related cancers. J Natl Cancer Inst 92:333–337, 2000.

26. Garrote LF, Herrero R, Reyes RM, et al: Risk factors for cancer of the oral cavity and oropharynx in Cuba. Br J Cancer 85:46–54, 2001.

27. Feit MN: Exposure of adolescent girls to cigar images in women's magazines, 1992–1998. Am J Public Health 91:286–288, 2001.

28. Muscat JE, Richie JP, Thompson S, et al: Gender differences in smoking and risk for oral cancer. Canc Res 56:5192–5197, 1996.

29. Firth NA: Marijuana use and oral cancer: A review. Oral Oncol 6:398–401, 1997.

30. Rothman KJ, Keller AZ: The effect of joint exposure to alcohol and tobacco on the risk of cancer of the mouth and pharynx. J Chron Dis 25:711–716, 1972.

31. Hindle I, Downer MC, Moles DR, et al: Is alcohol responsible for more intra-oral cancer? Oral Oncol 36:328–333, 2000.

32. Brugere J, Guenel P, Leclerc A, et al: Differential effects of tobacco and alcohol in cancer of the larynx, pharynx and mouth. Cancer 57:391–395, 1986.

33. Cancer statistics. CA Cancer J Clin 35:19, 1985.

34. Llewelyn J, Mitchell R: Smoking, alcohol and oral cancer in south east Scotland: A 10-year experience. Br J Oral Maxillofac Surg 32:146–152, 1994.

35. Antoniades DZ, Styanidis K, Papanayatou P, et al: Squamous cell carcinoma of the lips in northern Greek population: Evaluation of prognostic factors on five year survival rate. Eur J Cancer Oral Oncol 31B:333–339, 1995.

36. Pogoda JM, Preston-Martin S: Solar radiation, lip protection and lip cancer risk in Los Angeles county women. Cancer Causes Control 7:458–463, 1996.

37. Swerdlow AJ, Cooke KR, Skegg DC, et al: Cancer incidence in England and Wales and New Zealand and in migrants between the two countries. Br J Cancer 75:236–243, 1995.

38. Larsson PA, Johansson SL, Vahlne A, et al: Snuff tumorigenesis: Effects of long term snuff administration after initiation with 4-nitro-quinolone N-oxide and herpes simplex virus type 1. J Oral Pathol Med 18:187–192, 1989.

39. Burns JC, Murray BK: Conversion of herpetic lesions to malignancy by ultraviolet exposure and promoter application. J Gen Virol 55:305–313, 1981.

40. Miller CS, Johnstone BM: Human papillomavirus as a risk factor for oral squamous cell carcinoma: A meta-analysis, 1982–1997. Oral Surg Oral Med Oral Pathol Oral Radiol 91:622–635, 2001.

41. Maden C, Beckmann AM, Thomas DB, et al: Human papillomaviruses, herpes simplex viruses, and the risk of oral cancer in men. Am J Epidemiol 135:1093–1102, 1992.

42. Park NH, Min BM, Li SL, et al: Immortalisation of normal human oral keratinocytes with type 16 human papillomavirus. Carcinogenesis 12:1627–1631, 1991.

43. Shin KH, Tannyhill RJ, Liu X, et al: Oncogenic transformation of HPV-immortalized human oral keratinocytes is associated with genetic instability of cells. Oncogene 12:1089–1096, 1996.

44. Larsson LG, Sandstrom A, Westling P: Relationship of Plummer-Vinson disease to cancer of the upper alimentary tract in Sweden. Cancer Res 35:3308–3316, 1975.

45. Levi F, Pasche C, La Vecchia C, et al: Food groups and risk of oral and pharyngeal cancer. Int J Cancer 77:705–709, 1998.

46. Negri E, Franceschi S, Boscetti C, et al: Selected micronutrients and oral and pharyngeal cancer. Int J Cancer 86:122–127, 2000.

47. Zheng T, Boyle P, Willett WC, et al: A case-control study of oral cancer in Beijing, People's Republic of China. Associations with nutrient intakes, foods and food groups. Eur J Cancer Oral Oncol 29B:45–55, 1993.

48. Day GL, Shore RE, Blot WJ, et al: Dietary factors and second primary cancers: A follow-up of oral and pharyngeal cancer patients. Nutr Cancer 21:223–232, 1994.

49. Maier H, Zoller J, Herrmann A, et al: Dental status and oral hygiene in patients with head and neck cancer. Otolaryngol Head Neck Surg 108:655–661, 1993.

50. Homann N, Tillonen J, Rintamaki H, et al: Poor dental status increases acetaldehyde production from ethanol in saliva: A possible link to increased oral cancer risk among heavy drinkers. Oral Oncol 37:153–158, 2001.

51. Velly AM, Franco EL, Schlecht N, et al: Relationship between dental factors and risk of upper aerodigestive tract cancer. Oral Oncol 34:284–291, 1998.

52. Fearon ER, Vogelstein B: A genetic model for colorectal tumorigenesis. Cell 6:759–767, 1990.

53. Califano J, van der Riet P, Westra W, et al: Genetic progression model for head and neck cancer: Implications for field cancerization. Cancer Res 56:2488–2492, 1996.

54. Slaughter DP, Southwick HW, Smejkal W.: "Field cancerization" in oral stratified squamous epithelium: Clinical implications of multicentric origin. Cancer 6:963–968, 1953.

55. Downward J, Yarden Y, Mayes E, et al: Close similarity of epidermal growth factor receptor gene and v-erb-B oncogene protein sequences. Nature 307:521–527, 1984.

56. Grandis JR, Tweardy DJ: Elevated levels of transforming growth factor alpha and epidermal growth factor receptor messenger RNA are early markers of carcinogenesis in head and neck cancer. Cancer Res 53:3579–3584, 1993.

57. Grandis JR, Melhem MF, Gooding WE, et al: Levels of TGF-alpha and EGFR protein in head and neck squamous cell carcinoma and patient survival. J Natl Cancer Inst 90:824–832, 1998.

58. Ford AC, Grandis JR: Targeting epidermal growth factor receptor in head and neck cancer. Head Neck 25:67–73, 2003.

59. Myers JN, Holsinger C, Bekele N, et al: Targeted molecular therapy for oral cancer with epidermal growth factor receptor blockade. Arch Otolaryngol Head Neck Surg 128:875–879, 2002.

60. Yao L, Iwai M, Furuta I: Correlations of bcl-2 and p53 expression with the clinico-pathological features in tongue squamous cell carcinomas. Oral Oncol 35:56–62, 1999.

61. Forastiere A, Koch W, Trotti A, et al: Head and neck cancer. New Engl J Med 345:1890–1900, 2001.

62. Liu TJ, El-Naggar AK, McDonnell TJ, et al: Apoptosis induction mediated by wild-type p53 adenoviral gene transfer in squamous cell carcinoma of the head and neck. Cancer Res 55:3117–3122, 1995.

63. Van der Riet P, Nawroz H, Hruban RH, et al: Frequent loss of chromosome 9p21-22 early in head and neck cancer progression. Cancer Res 54:1156–1158, 1994.

64. El-Naggar AK, Lai S, Clayman GL, et al: Expression of p16, Rb, and cyclin D1 gene products in oral and laryngeal squamous carcinoma: Biological and clinical implications. Hum Pathol 30:1013–1018, 1999.

65. Callender T, El-Naggar AK, Lee MS, et al: PRAD-1 (CCND1)/cyclin D1 oncogene amplification in primary head and neck squamous cell carcinoma. Cancer 74:152–158, 1994.

66. Jares P, Fernandez PL, Campo E, et al: PRAD-1/cyclin D1 gene amplification correlates with messenger RNA overexpression and tumor progression in human laryngeal carcinomas. Cancer Res 54:4813–4817, 1994.

67. Bova RJ, Quinn DI, Nankervis JS, et al: Cyclin D1 and p16INK4A expression predict survival in carcinoma of the anterior tongue. Clin Cancer Res 5:2810–2819, 1999.

68. Gallaher BW, Hille R, Raile K, et al: Apoptosis: Live or die—hard work either way! Horm Metab Res 33:511–519, 2001.

69. Antonsson B: Bax and other pro-apoptotic Bcl-2 family "killer proteins" and their victim, the mitochondrion. Cell Tissue Res 306:347–361, 2001.

70. Viera HL, Kroemer G: Pathophysiology of mitochondrial cell death control. Cell Mol Life Sci 56:971–976, 1999.

71. Xie X, Clausen OP, DeAngelis P, et al: The prognostic value of spontaneous apoptosis, Bax, Bcl-2, and p53 in oral squamous cell carcinoma of the tongue. Cancer 86:913–920, 1999.

72. Jordan RC, Catzavelos GC, Barrett AW, et al: Differential expression of bcl-2 and bax in squamous cell carcinomas of the oral cavity. Eur J Cancer B Oral Oncol 32B:394–400, 1996.

73. Chen Y, Kayano T, Takagi M: Dysregulation expression of bcl-2 and bax in oral carcinomas: Evidence of post-transcriptional control. J Oral Pathol Med 29:63–69, 2000.

74. Noutomi T, Chiba H, Itoh M, et al: Bcl-x(L) confers multi-drug resistance in several squamous cell carcinoma cell lines. Oral Oncol 38:41–48, 2002.

75. Slaughter DP, Southwick HW, Smejkal W. "Field cancerization" in oral stratified squamous epithelium: Clinical implications of multicentric origin. Cancer 6:963–968, 1953.

76. Haughey BH, Gates GA, Arfken CL, et al: Meta-analysis of second malignant in head and neck cancer: The case for an endoscopic screening protocol. Ann Otol Rhinol Laryngol 101:105–112, 1992.

77. Vikram B, Strong EW, Shah JP, et al: Second malignant neoplasms in patients successfully treated with multimodality treatment with advanced head and neck cancer. Head Neck 6:734–740, 1984.

78. Lippman SM, Hong WK: Second primary tumors in head and neck squamous cell carcinoma: The overshadowing threat for patients with early stage disease. Int J Radiat Oncol Biol Phys 17:691–694, 1989.

79. World Health Organization Collaborating Center for Oral Precancerous Lesions: Definition of leukoplakia and related lesions: An aid to studies on oral precancer. Oral Surg 46:518–539, 1978.

80. Kannan S, Balaram P, Pillai MR, et al: Ultrastructural variations and assessment of malignant transformation risk in oral leukoplakia. Pathol Res Pract 189:1169–1180, 1993.

81. Cawson RA, Odell EW: Essentials of Oral Pathology and Oral Medicine, 6th ed. New York, Churchill Livingstone, 1998.

82. Downer MC, Evans AW, Hughes Hallett CM, et al: Evaluation of screening for oral cancer and precancer in a company headquarters. Commun Dent Oral Epidemiol 23:84–88, 1995.

83. Winn DE: Relationship Between Tobacco Use and Oral and Dental Disease in the U.S. Tobacco and Oral Disease—Strategies for Dental Professional Interventions. Iowa City, Iowa, 2000.

84. Silverman S, Gorsky M, Lozada F: Oral leukoplakia and malignant transformation—a follow up study of 257 patients. Cancer 53:563–568, 1984.

85. Lippman SM, Batsakis JG, Toth BB, et al: Comparison of low-dose isotretinoin with beta carotene to prevent oral carcinogenesis. N Engl J Med 328:15–20, 1993.

86. Roed-Peterson B: Cancer development in oral leukoplakia: Follow up of 331 patients [abstract]. J Dent Res 50:711, 1971.

87. Kramer IRH, El-Lablan D, Lee KW: The clinical features and risk of malignant transformation in sublingual keratosis. Br Dent J 144:171–180, 1978.

88. Kokal WA, Gardine RL, Sheibani K: Tumor DNA content as a prognostic indicator in squamous cell carcinoma of the head and neck region. Am J Surg 156:276–280, 1988.

89. Broders AC: Squamous cell epithelioma of the lip. JAMA 74:656–664, 1920.

90. Anneroth G, Batsakis J, Luna M: Review of the literature and a recommended system of malignancy grading in oral squamous cell carcinomas. Scand J Dent Res 95:229–249, 1987.

91. Bryne M: Prognostic value of various molecular and cellular features in oral squamous cell carcinomas: A review. J Oral Pathol Med 20:413–420, 1990.

92. Koch BB, Trask DK, Hoffman HT, et al: National survey of head and neck verrucous carcinoma: Patterns of presentation, care and outcome. Cancer 92:110–120, 2001.

93. Kraus FT, Perez-Mesa C: Verrucous carcinoma: Clinical and pathological study of 105 cases involving oral cavity, larynx, and genitalia. Cancer 19:26–38, 1966.

94. Spiro RH: Verrucous carcinoma, then and now. Am J Surg 176:393–397, 1998.

95. Medina JE, Dichtel W, Luna MA: Verrucous squamous carcinomas of the oral cavity: A clinicopathological study of 104 cases. Arch Otolaryngol Head Neck Surg 110:437–444, 1984.

96. McGuirt WF: Snuff dipper's carcinoma. Arch Otolaryngol Head Neck Surg 109:757–760, 1983.

97. Wray A, McGuirt WF: Smokeless tobacco usage associated with oral carcinoma: Incidence, treatment, outcome. Arch Otolaryngol Head Neck Surg 119:929–933, 1993.

98. Shafer WG: Verrucous squamous carcinoma of the palate. Int Dent J 22:451, 1972.

99. Ferlito A, Rinaldo A, Mannara GM: Is primary radiotherapy an appropriate option for the treatment of verrucous carcinoma of the head and neck? J Laryngol Otol 112:132–139, 1998.

100. McCaffrey TV, Witte M, Ferguson MT: Verrucous carcinoma of the larynx. Ann Otol Rhinol Laryngol 107:391–395, 1998.

101. Tharp ME, Shidnia H: Radiotherapy in the treatment of verrucous carcinoma of the head and neck. Laryngoscope 104:391–396, 1998.

102. Coppola D, Catalano E, Tang C, et al: Basaloid squamous cell carcinoma of floor of mouth. Cancer 72:2299–2305, 1993.

103. Winzenburg SM, Niehans GA, George E, et al: Basaloid squamous cell carcinoma: A clinical comparison of two histologic types with poorly differentiated squamous cell carcinoma. Otolaryngol Head Neck Surg 119:471–475, 1998.

104. Weber RS, Palmer JM, El-Nagger A, et al: Minor salivary gland tumors of the lip and buccal mucosa. Laryngoscope 99:6–9, 1989.

105. Beckhardt RN, Weber RS, Zane R, et al: Minor salivary gland tumors of the palate: Clinical and pathologic correlates of outcome. Laryngoscope 105:1155–1160, 1995.

106. Spiro RH, Koss LG, Hajdu SI, et al: Tumors of the minor salivary gland origin: A clinicopathologic study of 492 cases. Cancer 31:117–129, 1973.

107. van der Waal JE, Snow GB, Karim A, et al: Intraoral adenoid cystic carcinoma: The role of postoperative radiotherapy in local control. Head Neck 11:497–499, 1989.

108. van der Waal JE, Snow GB, Van der Waal I: Intraoral adenoid cystic carcinoma—the presence of perineural spread in relation to site, size, local extension, and metastatic spread in 22 cases. Cancer 66:2031–2033, 1990.

109. Garden AS, Weber RS, Morrison WH, et al: The influence of positive margins and nerve invasion in adenoid cystic carcinoma of the head and neck treated with surgery and radiation. Int J Radiat Oncol Biol Phys 32:619–626, 1995.

110. Parsons JT, Mendenhall WM, Stringer SP, et al: Management of minor salivary gland carcinomas. Int J Radiat Oncol Biol Phys 35:443–454, 1996.

111. Prokopakis EP, Snyderman CH, Hanna EY, et al: Risk factors for local recurrence of adenoid cystic carcinoma: The role of postoperative radiation therapy. Am J Otolarygol 20:281–286, 1999.

112. Khan AJ, DiGiovanna MP, Ross DA, et al: Adenoid cystic carcinoma: A retrospective review. Int J Cancer 96:149–158, 2001.

113. Fuk KK, Leibel SA, Levine ML, et al: Cancer of the major and minor salivary glands: Analysis of treatment results and sites and causes of failure. Cancer 40:2882–2890, 1977.

114. Laramore GE, Krall JM, Griffin TW, et al: Neutron vs. photon irradiation for unresectable salivary gland tumors: Final report of an RTOG-MRC randomized clinical trial. Int J Radiat Oncol Biol Phys 27:235–240, 1993.

115. Nichols CM, Flaitz CM, Hicks MJ: Treating Kaposi's lesions in the HIV infected patient. J Am Dent Assoc 124:78–84, 1993.

116. Dezube BJ: Management of AIDS-related Kaposi's sarcoma: Advances in target discovery and treatment. Expert Rev Anticancer Ther 2:193–200, 2002.

117. Freeman C, Berg JW, Cutler SJ: Occurrence and prognosis of extranodal lymphomas. Cancer 29:252–260, 1984.

118. Takahashi N, Tsuda N, Tezuka F, et al: Primary extranodal non-Hodgkin's lymphoma of the oral region. J Oral Pathol Med 18:84–91, 1989.

119. Barker RG: Unifocal lymphomas of the oral cavity. J Oral Maxillofac Surg 22:426–430, 1984.

120. Smyth AG, Ward-Booth RP, Avery BS, et al: Malignant melanoma of the oral cavity—an increasing diagnosis? Br J Oral Maxillofac Surg 31:230–235, 1993.

121. Tanaka N, Amagasa T, Iwaki H, et al: Oral malignant melanoma in Japan. Oral Surg Oral Med Oral Pathol 78:81–90, 1994.

122. Rapini RP, Golitz LE, Greer RO, et al: Primary malignant melanoma of the oral cavity: A review of 177 cases. Cancer 55:1543–1547, 1985.

123. Shah JP, Huvos AG, Strong EW: Mucosal melanomas of the head and neck. Am J Surg 134:531, 1977.

124. Taylor CO, Lewis JS: Histologically documented transformation of benign oral melanosis into malignant melanoma. J Oral Maxillofac Surg 48:732–737, 1990.

125. Patton LL, Brahim JS, Baker AR: Metastatic melanoma of the oral cavity—a retrospective study. Oral Surg Oral Med Oral Pathol 78:51–56, 1994.

126. Liversedge RL: Oral malignant melanoma. Br J Oral Surg 13:40–46, 1975.

127. Johnson JT, Barnes L, Myers EN, et al: The extracapsular spread of tumors in cervical node metastasis. Arch Otolaryngol 107:725–729, 1981.

128. Mackay EN, Sellers AH: A statistical review of carcinoma of the lip. Can Med Assoc J 90:670–675, 1964.

129. McGuirt WF, Johnson JT, Myers EN, et al: Floor of mouth carcinoma: The management of the clinically negative neck. Arch Otolaryngol Head Neck Surg 121:278–282, 1995.

130. Byers RM, Newman R, Russell N, et al: Results of treatment of squamous carcinoma of the lower gum. Cancer 47:2236–2238, 1981.

131. Bloom ND, Spiro RH: Carcinoma of the cheek mucosa: A retrospective analysis. Am J Surg 140:556–560, 1980.

132. Baker SR: Malignant neoplasms of the oral cavity. In Cummings CW, Frederickson JM, Harker LA, et al (eds): Otolaryngology: Head and Neck Surgery, 2nd ed. St. Louis, Mosby–Year Book, 1993, pp 1248–1305.

133. Ho CM, Lam KH, Wei WI, et al: Occult lymph node metastasis in small oral tongue cancers. Head Neck 14:359–363, 1992.

134. Cunningham MJ, Johnson JT, Myers EN, et al: Cervical lymph node metastasis after local excision of early squamous cell carcinoma of the oral cavity. Am J Surg 152:361–366, 1986.

135. Johnson JT, Myers EN, Bedetti C, et al: Cervical lymph node metastasis. Arch Otolaryngol 11:534–537, 1985.

136. Snow GB, Annyes AA, Van Sloote EA, et al: Prognostic factors of neck node metastasis. Clin Otolaryngol 7:185–192, 1982.

137. Shah JP, Medina JE, Shaha AR, et al: Cervical lymph node metastasis. Curr Probl Surg 30:273–344, 1993.

138. Betka J: Distant metastasis from lip and oral cavity cancer. ORL J Otorhinolaryngol Relat Spec 63:217–221, 2001.

139. Ferlito A, Shaha AR, Silver C, et al: Incidence and sites of distant metastases from head and neck cancer. ORL J Otorhinolaryngol Relat Spec 63:202–207, 2001.

140. Holsinger FC, Myers JN, Roberts DB, et al: Clinicopathologic predictors of distant metastases from head and neck squamous cell carcinoma. Abstracts from the 5th International Conference on Head and Neck Cancer, 2000, San Francisco, Calif. Abstract 200.

141. Kmucha ST, Troxel JM: Dermal metastases in epidermoid carcinoma of the head and neck. Arch Otolaryngol Head Neck Surg 119:326–330, 1993.

142. Caldemeyer KS, Matthews VP, Righi PD, et al: Imaging features and clinical significance of perineural spread or extension of head and neck tumors. Radiographics 18:97–110, 1998.

143. van den Brekel MW, Castelijns JA, Stel HV, et al: Modern imaging techniques and ultrasound-guided aspiration cytology for the assessment of neck node metastases: A prospective comparative study. Eur Arch Otorhinolaryngol 250:11–17, 1993.

144. Farber LA, Benard F, Machtay M, et al: Detection of recurrent head and neck squamous cell carcinomas after radiation therapy with 2-18F-fluoro-2-deoxy-D-glucose positron emission tomography. Laryngoscope 109:970–975, 1999.

145. Anzai Y, Carroll WR, Quint DJ, et al: Recurrence of head and neck cancer after surgery or irradiation: Prospective comparison of 2-deoxy-2-[F-18] fluoro-D-glucose PET and MR imaging diagnoses. Radiology 200:135–141, 1996.

146. Berlangieri SU, Brizel DM, Scher RL, et al: Pilot study of positron emission tomography in patients with advanced head and neck cancer receiving radiotherapy and chemotherapy. Head Neck 16:340–346, 1994.

147. AJCC: American Joint Committee for Cancer Staging and End-Results Reporting. Chicago, American Joint Committee on Cancer, 1998.

148. Piccirillo JF: Purposes, problems, and proposals for progress in cancer staging. Arch Otolaryngol Head Neck Surg 121:145–149, 1995.

149. Pugliano FA, Piccirillo JF, Zequeira MR, et al: Clinical-severity staging system for oral cavity cancer: Five-year survival rates. Otolaryngol Head Neck Surg 120:38–45, 1999.

150. Johnson JT, Myers EN, Bedetti C, et al: Cervical lymph node metastasis. Arch Otolaryngol 11:534–537, 1985.

151. Snow GB, Annyes AA, Van Sloote EA, et al: Prognostic factors of neck node metastasis. Clin Otolaryngol 7:185–192, 1982.

152. Friedman M, Mafee MF, Pacella BL, et al: Rationale for elective neck dissection in 1990. Laryngoscope 100:54–59, 1990.

153. Hariot JC, LeFur R, N'Guyent T, et al: Hyperfractionation versus conventional fractionation in oropharyngeal carcinoma: Final analysis of a randomized trial of the EORTC cooperative group of radiotherapy. Radiother Oncol 25:231–241, 1992.

154. Langlois D, Hoffstetter S, Malissard L, et al: Salvage irradiation of oropharynx and mobile tongue with 192-iridium brachytherapy in Centre Alexis Vautrin. Int J Radiat Oncol Biol Phys 14:849–853, 1988.

155. Tishler RB, Norris CM, Colevas AD, et al: A phase I/II trial of concurrent docetaxel and radiation after induction chemotherapy in patients with poor prognosis squamous cell carcinoma of the head and neck. Cancer 95:1472–1481, 2002.

156. Ampil FL, Mills GM, Caldito G, et al: Induction chemotherapy followed by concomitant chemoradiation-induced regression of advanced cervical lymphadenopathy in head and neck cancer as a predictor of outcome. Otolaryngol Head Neck Surg 126:602–606, 2002.

157. Johnson JT, Myers EN, Schramm VL Jr, et al: Adjuvant chemotherapy for high-risk squamous-cell carcinoma of the head and neck. J Clin Oncol 5:456–458, 1987.

158. Department of Veterans Affairs Laryngeal Study Group: Induction chemotherapy plus radiation compared with surgery plus radiation in patients with advanced laryngeal cancer. N Engl J Med 324:1685–1690, 1991.

159. Poole ME, Sailer SL, Rosenman JG, et al: Chemoradiation for locally advanced squamous cell carcinoma of the head and neck for organ preservation and palliation. Arch Otolaryngol Head Neck Surg 127:1446–1450, 2001.

160. Licitra L, Grandi C, Guzzo M, et al: Primary chemotherapy in resectable oral cavity squamous cell cancer: A randomized controlled trial. J Clin Oncol 21:327–333, 2003.

161. Vokes EE, Stenson K, Rosen FR, et al: Weekly carboplatin and paclitaxel followed by concomitant paclitaxel, fluorouracil, and hydroxyurea chemoradiotherapy: Curative and organ-preserving therapy for advanced head and neck cancer. J Clin Oncol 21:320–326, 2003.

162. Jacobs C, Makuch R: Efficacy of adjuvant chemotherapy for patients with resectable head and neck cancer: A subset analysis of the Head and Neck Contracts Program. J Clin Oncol 8:838–847, 1990.

163. Stell PM: Adjuvant chemotherapy in head and neck cancer. Semin Radiat Oncol 2:195–205, 1992.

164. Johnson JT, Wagner RL, Myers EN: A long-term assessment of adjuvant chemotherapy on outcome of patients with extracapsular spread of cervical metastases from squamous carcinoma of the head and neck. Cancer 77:181–185, 1996.

165. Schuller DE, Metch B, Stein DW, et al: Preoperative chemotherapy in advanced resectable head and neck cancer: Final report of the Southwest Oncology Group. Laryngoscope 98:1205–1211, 1988.

166. Munro AJ: An overview of randomized controlled trials of adjuvant chemotherapy in head and neck cancer. Br J Cancer 71:83–91, 1995.

167. Laramore GE, Scott CB, al-Sarraf M, et al: Adjuvant chemotherapy for resectable squamous cell carcinoma of the head and neck: Report on Intergroup Study 0034. Int J Radiat Oncol Biol Phys 23:705–713, 1992.

168. Kohno N, Kitahara S, Tamura E, et al: Concurrent chemoradiotherapy with low-dose cisplatin plus 5-fluorouracil for the treatment of patients with unresectable head and neck cancer. Oncology 63:226–231, 2002.

169. Adelstein DJ, Li Y, Adams GL, et al: An intergroup phase III comparison of standard radiation therapy and two schedules of concurrent chemoradiotherapy in patients with unresectable squamous cell head and neck cancer. J Clin Oncol 21:92–98, 2003.

170. Brizel DM, Albers ME, Fisher SR, et al: Hyperfractionated irradiation with or without concurrent chemotherapy for locally advanced head and neck cancer. N Engl J Med 338:1798–1804, 1998.

171. Vokes EE, Kies MS, Haraf DJ, et al: Concomitant chemoradiotherapy as primary therapy for locoregionally advanced head and neck cancer. J Clin Oncol 18:1652–1661, 2000.

172. Kramer S, Gelber RD, Snow GB, et al: Combined radiation therapy and surgery in the management of advanced head and neck cancer: Final report of study 73-03 of the Radiation Therapy Oncology Group. Head Neck Surg 10:19–30, 1987.

173. King JM, Caldarelli DD, Petasnick JP: Dentascan (TM): A new diagnostic method for evaluating mandibular and maxillary pathology. Laryngoscope 102:379–387, 1992.

174. Flynn MB, Moore C: Marginal resection of the mandible in the management of squamous cancer of the floor of mouth. Am J Surg 128:490–493, 1987.

175. Bartellbort SW, Bahn SL, Ariyan S: Rim mandibulectomy for cancer of the oral cavity. Am J Surg 154:423–428, 1987.

176. Zieske LA, Johnson JT, Myers EN, et al: Composite resection reconstruction: Split thickness skin graft—a preferred option. Otolaryngol Head Neck Surg 98:170–173, 1988.

177. Crile G: Excision of cancer of the head and neck: With special reference to the plan of dissection based on 132 operations. JAMA 47:1780–1785, 1906.

178. Martin H, Del Valle B, Ehrlich HE, et al: Neck dissection. Cancer 4:441–449, 1951.

179. Martin H: The case for prophylactic neck dissection. Cancer 4:92–97, 1951.

180. Martin H: Radical neck dissection. Clin Symp 13:103–120, 1961.

181. Myers EN, Gastman BR: Neck dissection: An operation in evolution. Arch Otolaryngol Head Neck Surg 129:14–25, 2003.

182. Bocca E, Pignataro O, Oldini C, et al: Functional neck dissection: An evaluation of review of 843 cases. Laryngoscope 94:942–945, 1984.

183. Byers RM, Wolf PF, Ballantyne AJ: Rationale for elective modified neck dissection. Head Neck Surg 10:160–167, 1988.

184. Byers RM: Modified neck dissection: A study of 967 cases from 1970–1980. Am J Surg 150:414–421, 1985.

185. Anderson PE, Shah JP, Cambronero E, et al: The role of comprehensive neck dissection with preservation of the spinal accessory nerve in the clinically positive neck. Am J Surg 168:499–502, 1994.

186. Terrell JE, Welsh DE, Bradford CR, et al: Pain, quality of life, and spinal accessory nerve status after neck dissection. Laryngoscope 110:620–626, 2000.

187. Bradfield JS, Scruggs RP: Carcinoma of the mobile tongue: Incidence of cervical metastasis in early lesions related to method of primary treatment. Laryngoscope 93:1332–1336, 1983.

188. Teichgraeber JF, Clairmont AA: Incidence of occult metastasis for cancer of the oral tongue and floor of mouth: Treatment rationale. Head Neck Surg 7:15–21, 1984.

189. Shah JP, Candela FC, Poddar AK: The patterns of cervical lymph node metastasis from squamous carcinoma of the oral cavity. Cancer 66:109–113, 1990.

190. Shah JP, Cendon RA, Farr HW, et al: Carcinoma of the oral cavity: Factors affecting treatment failure at the primary site and neck. Am J Surg 132:504–507, 1976.

191. Davidson BJ, Kulkarny V, Delacure MD, et al: Posterior triangle metastases of squamous cell carcinoma of the upper aerodigestive tract. Am J Surg 166:395–398, 1993.

192. Khafif A, Lopez-Garza JR, Medina JE: Is dissection of level IV necessary in patients with T1-T3 N0 tongue cancer? Laryngoscope 111:1088–1090, 2001.

193. Pitman KT, Johnson JT, Myers EN: Effectiveness of selective neck dissection for management of the clinically negative neck. Arch Otolaryngol Head Neck Surg 123:917–922, 1997.

194. Hosal AS, Carrau RL, Johnson JT, et al: Selective neck dissection in the management of the clinically node-negative neck. Laryngoscope 100:2037–2040, 2000.

195. Shah JP, Anderson PE: The impact of patterns of nodal metastasis on modifications of neck dissection. Ann Surg Oncol 1:521–532, 1994.

196. Chepeha DB, Taylor RJ, Chepeha JC, et al: Functional assessment using Constant's Shoulder Scale after modified radical and selective neck dissection. Head Neck 24:432–436, 2002.

197. Cheng PT, Hao SP, Lin YH, et al: Objective comparison of shoulder dysfunction after three dissection techniques. Ann Otol Rhinol Laryngol 109(8 pt 1):761–766, 2000.

198. Urquhart AC, Berg RL: Neck dissections: Predicting postoperative drainage. Laryngoscope 112(7 pt 1):1294–1298, 2002.

199. Kowalski LP: Results of salvage treatment of the neck in patients with oral cancer. Arch Otolaryngngol Head Neck Surg 128:58–62, 2002.

200. Ferlito A, Rinaldo A, Devaney KO, et al: Prognostic significance of microscopic and macroscopic extracapsular spread from metastatic tumor in the cervical lymph nodes. Oral Oncol 38:747–751, 2002.

201. Myers JN, Greenberg JS, Mo V, et al: Extracapsular spread. A significant predictor of treatment failure in patients with squamous cell carcinoma of the tongue. Cancer 92:3030–3036, 2001.

202. Kolli VR, Datta RV, Orner JB, et al: The role of supraomohyoid neck dissection in patients with positive nodes. Arch Otolaryngol Head Neck Surg 126:413–416, 2000.

203. Kowalski LP, Magrin J, Waksman G, et al: Supraomohyoid neck dissection in the treatment of head and neck tumors. Arch Otolaryngol Head Neck Surg 119:958–963, 1993.

204. Chu W, Strawitz JG: Results in suprahyoid, modified radical, and standard radical neck dissections for metastatic squamous cell carcinoma: Recurrence and survival. Am J Surg 136:512–515, 1978.

205. Byers RM, Clayman GL, McGill D, et al: Selective neck dissections for squamous carcinoma of the upper aerodigestive tract: Patterns of regional failure. Head Neck 21:499–505, 1999.

206. Anderson PE, Warren F, Spiro J, et al: Results of selective neck dissection in management of the node-positive neck. Arch Otolaryngol Head Neck Surg 128:1180–1184, 2002.

207. Salerno G, Cavaliere M, Foglia A, et al: The 11th nerve syndrome in functional neck dissection. Laryngoscope 112(7 pt 1):1299–1307, 2002.

208. Rassekh CH, Johnson JT, Myers EN: Accuracy of intraoperative staging of the N0 neck in squamous cell carcinoma. Laryngoscope 105(12 pt 1):1334–1336, 1995.

209. Wein RO, Winkle MR, Norante JD, et al: Evaluation of selective lymph node sampling in the node negative neck. Laryngoscope 112:1006–1009, 2002.

210. Kaya S, Yilmaz T, Gursel B, et al: The value of elective neck dissection in treatment of cancer of the tongue. Am J Otolaryngol 22:59–64, 2001.

211. Krag DN, Weaver DL, Alex JC, et al: Surgical resection and radiolocalization of the sentinel node in breast cancer using a gamma probe. Surg Oncol 2:335–340, 1993.

212. O'Brien CJ, Uren RF, Thompson JF, et al: Prediction of potential metastatic sites in cutaneous head and neck melanoma using lymphoscintigraphy. Am J Surg 170:461–466, 1995.

213. Pitman KT, Johnson JT, Brown ML, et al: Sentinel lymph node biopsy in head and neck squamous cell carcinoma. Laryngoscope 112:2101–2113, 2002.

214. Civantos FJ, Gomez C, Duque C, et al: Sentinel node biopsy in oral cavity cancer: Correlation with PET scan and immunohistochemistry. Head Neck 25:1–9, 2002.

215. Shoaib T, Soutar DS, MacDonald DG, et al: The accuracy of head and neck carcinoma sentinel lymph node biopsy in the clinically N0 neck. Cancer 91:2077–2083, 2001.

216. Zitsch RP 3rd, Todd DW, Renner GJ, et al: Intraoperative radiolymphoscintigraphy for detection of occult nodal metastasis in patients with head and neck squamous cell carcinoma. Otolaryngol Head Neck Surg 122:662–666, 2000.

217. Alex JC, Sakaki CT, Krag DN, et al: Sentinel lymph node localization in squamous cell carcinoma. Laryngoscope 110(2 pt 1):198–203, 2000.

218. Koch WM, Choti MA, Civelek AC, et al: Gamma probe-directed biopsy of the sentinel node in oral squamous cell carcinoma. Arch Otolaryngol Head Neck Surg 124:455–459, 1998.

219. Shah S, Har-El G, Rosenfeld RM: Short-term and long-term quality of life after neck dissection. Head Neck 23:954–961, 2001.

220. Vikram B, Strong EW, Shah JP, et al: Failure in the neck following multimodality treatment in advanced head and neck cancer. Head Neck Surg 6:724–729, 1984.

221. Anderson PE, Cambronero E, Shaha AR, et al: The extent of neck disease after regional failure during observation of the N0 neck. Am J Surg 172:689–691, 1996.

222. Kowalski LP, Bagietto R, Lara JR, et al: Prognostic significance of the distribution of neck node metastasis from oral carcinoma. Head Neck 22:207–214, 2000.

223. Wendt CD, Peters LJ, Delclos L, et al: Primary radiotherapy in the treatment of stage I and II oral tongue cancers: Importance of the proportion of therapy delivered with interstitial therapy. Int J Radiat Oncol Biol Phys 18:1287–1292, 1990.

224. Abe M, Murakami G, Noguchi M, et al: Afferent and efferent lymph-collecting vessels of the submandibular nodes with special reference to the lymphatic route passing through the mylohyoid muscle. Head Neck 25:59–66, 2003.

225. Dutton JM, Graham SM, Hoffman HT: Metastatic cancer to the floor of mouth: The lingual lymph nodes. Head Neck 24:401–405, 2002.

226. Leemans CR, Tiwari R, Nauta JJ, et al: Discontinuous versus in-continuity neck dissection in carcinoma of the oral cavity. Arch Otolaryngol Head Neck Surg 117:1003–1006, 1991.

227. Spiro RH, Strong EW: Discontinuous partial glossectomy and radical neck dissection in selected patients with epidermoid carcinoma of the mobile tongue. Am J Surg 126:544–546, 1973.

228. Canto MT, Devesa SS: Oral cavity and pharynx cancer incidence rates in the United States, 1975–1998. Oral Oncol 38:610–617, 2002.

229. Myers JN, Elkins T, Roberts D, et al: Squamous cell carcinoma of the tongue in young adults: Increasing incidence and factors that predict treatment outcomes. Otolaryngol Head Neck Surg 122:44–51, 2000.

230. Krupala JL, Gianoli R: Carcinoma of the oral tongue. J La State Med Soc 145:421–426, 1993.

231. Nason RW, Anderson BJ, Gujrathi DS, et al: A retrospective comparison of treatment outcome in the posterior and anterior tongue. Am J Surg 172:665–667, 1996.

232. Werning JW, Byers RM, Novas MA, et al: Preoperative assessment for and outcomes of mandibular conservation surgery. Head Neck 23:1024–1030, 2001.

233. Tsue TT, McCulloch TM, Girod DA, et al: Predictors of carcinomatous invasion of the mandible. Head Neck 16:116–126, 1994.

234. Piollet H, Lufkin R, Steckel RJ, et al: Magnetic resonance imaging to distinguish tumor persistence from delayed fibrosis in carcinoma of the tongue and floor of mouth. Ann Otol Rhinol Laryngol 99:753–755, 1990.

235. Scholl P, Byers RM, Batsakis JG, et al: Microscopic cut-through of cancer in the surgical treatment of squamous carcinoma of the tongue. Am J Surg 152:354–360, 1986.

236. Spiro RH, Strong EH: Epidermoid carcinoma of the mobile tongue treated by partial glossectomy alone. Am J Surg 122:707–710, 1971.

237. O'Brien CJ, Lahr CJ, Soong SJ, et al: Surgical treatment of early stage carcinoma of the oral tongue—would adjuvant treatment be beneficial? Head Neck Surg 8:401–408, 1986.

238. Benk V, Mazeron JJ, Grimard L, et al: Comparison of curietherapy versus external irradiation combined with curietherapy in stage II squamous cell carcinomas of the mobile tongue. Radiother Oncol 18:339–344, 1990.

239. Piedbois P, Mazeron JJ, Haddad E, et al: Stage I–II squamous cell carcinoma of the oral cavity treated by iridium-192: Is elective neck dissection indicated? Radiother Oncol 21:100–106, 1991.

240. Hirsch SM, Caldarelli DD, Hutchinson JC, et al: Concomitant chemotherapy and split course radiation for cure and preservation of speech and swallowing in head and neck cancer. Laryngoscope 101:583–586, 1991.

241. Mendelson BC, Woods JE, Beahrs OH, et al: Neck dissection in the treatment of carcinoma of the anterior two thirds of the tongue. Surg Gynecol Obstet 143:75–80, 1976.

242. Fujitani T, Ogasawara H, Hattori H, et al: Seventeen years experience in the treatment of carcinoma of the mobile tongue. Auris Nasus Larynx 13:43–52, 1986.

243. Whitehurst JO, Droubois CA: Surgical treatment of squamous cell carcinoma of the oral tongue. Arch Otolaryngol 103:212–215, 1977.

244. Silver CE, Moisa II: Elective treatment of the neck in cancer of the oral tongue. Semin Surg Oncol 7:14–19, 1991.

245. Perzik SL, Jorgensen EJ, Carter RP, et al: End results in carcinoma of the oral cavity. Arch Surg 76:677–681, 1958.

246. Van den Brouk C, Sancho-Garnier H, Chassogne D, et al: Elective versus therapeutic radical neck dissection in epidermoid carcinoma of the oral cavity—results of a randomized clinical trial. Cancer 41:386–390, 1980.

247. Johnson JT, Liepzig B, Cummings CW: Management of T1 carcinoma of the anterior aspect of the tongue. Arch Otolaryngol 106:249–251, 1980.

248. Shear M, Hawkins DM, Farr HW: The prediction of lymph node metastasis from oral squamous carcinoma. Cancer 37:1901–1907, 1976.

249. Spiro RH, Huvos AG, Wong GY, et al: Predictive value of tumor thickness in squamous cell carcinoma confined to the tongue and floor of the mouth. Am J Surg 152:345–350, 1986.

250. Jesse RH, Barkley HT, Lindberg RD, et al: Cancer of the oral cavity: Is elective neck dissection beneficial? Am J Surg 120:505–508, 1970.

251. Mendenhall WM, Million RR, Cassisi NJ: Elective neck irradiation in squamous cell carcinoma of the head and neck. Head Neck Surg 3:15–20, 1980.

252. Northrop M, Fletcher GH, Jesse RH, et al: Evolution of neck disease in patients with primary squamous cell carcinoma of the oral tongue, floor of mouth, and palatine arch, and clinically positive neck nodes either fixed or bilateral. Cancer 29:23–30, 1972.

253. Meoz RT, Fletcher GH, Lindberg R: Anatomical coverage in elective irradiation of the neck for squamous cell carcinoma of the oral tongue. Int J Radiat Oncol Biol Phys 8:1881–1885, 1982.

254. Takagi M, Kayano T, Yamamato H, et al: Causes of oral tongue cancer treatment failures. Cancer 69:1081–1087, 1992.

255. Sarkaria JN, Harari PM: Oral tongue cancer in young adults less than 40 years of age: Rationale for aggressive therapy. Head Neck 16:107–111, 1994.

256. Byers R: Squamous cell carcinoma of the oral tongue in patients less than 30 years of age. Am J Surg 130:475–478, 1975.

257. Pitman KT, Johnson JT, Wagner RL, et al: Cancer of the tongue in patients less than 40. Head Neck 22:297–302, 2000.

258. Friedlander PL, Schantz SP, Shaha AR, et al: Squamous cell carcinoma of the tongue in young patients: A matched pair analysis. Head Neck 20:363–368, 1998.

259. Atula S, Grenman R, Laippala P, et al: Cancer of the tongue in patients younger than 40 years: A distinct entity. Arch Otolaryngol Head Neck Surg 122:1313–1319, 1996.

260. Siegelman-Danieli N, Hanlon A, Ridge J, et al: Oral tongue cancer in patients less than 45 years old: Institutional experience and comparison with older patients. J Clin Oncol 16:745–753, 1998.

261. Verschuur HP, Irish JC, O'Sullivan B, et al: A matched control study of treatment outcome in young patients with squamous cell carcinoma of the head and neck. Laryngoscope 109:249–258, 1999.

262. Davidson BJ, Root WA, Trock BJ: Age and survival from squamous cell carcinoma of the oral tongue. Head Neck 23:273–279, 2001.

263. Zitsch RP: Carcinoma of the lip. Otolaryngol Clin North Am 26:265–277, 1993.

264. Baker SR: Risk factors in multiple carcinomas of the lip. Can Med Assoc J 90:670–675, 1964.

265. Jorgensen K, Elbrond O, Anderson AP: Carcinoma of the lip: A series of 869 cases. Acta Radiol 12:177–180, 1973.

266. Karapandzic M: Reconstruction of lip defects by local arterial flaps. Br J Plast Surg 27:93–97, 1974.

267. Cerezo L, Liu FF, Tsang R, et al: Squamous cell carcinoma of the lip: Analysis of the Princess Margaret Hospital experience. Radiother Oncol 28:142–147, 1993.

268. Orecchia R, Rampino M, Gribaudo S, et al: Interstitial brachytherapy for carcinomas of the lower lip. Results of treatment. Tumor 77:336–338, 1991.

269. Baker SR, Krause CJ: Carcinoma of the lip. Laryngoscope 90:19–25, 1980.

270. Duplechain G, Amedee RG: Carcinoma of the lip. J La State Med Soc 144:441–442, 1992.

271. Krabel MR, Koranda FC, Panje WR, et al: Squamous cell carcinoma of the upper lip. J Dermatol Surg Oncol 8:487–490, 1982.

272. Holmstrup P, Thorn JJ, Rindum J, et al: Malignant development of oral lichen planus affected oral mucosa. J Oral Pathol 17:219–225, 1988.

273. Ildstad ST, Bigelow ME, Remensnyder JP: Clinical behavior and results of current therapeutic modalities for squamous cell carcinoma of the buccal mucosa. Surg Gynecol Obstet 160:254–258, 1985.

274. Guggenheimer J, Weissfeld JL, Kroboth FJ: Who has the opportunity to screen for oral cancer? Cancer Causes Control 4:63–66, 1993.

275. Borges AM, Shrikhande SS, Ganesh S: Surgical pathology of squamous carcinoma of the oral cavity: Its impact on management. Semin Surg Oncol 5:310–317, 1989.

276. Jusawalla DJ, Despandi VA: Evaluation of cancer risk in tobacco chewers and smokers. An epidemiologic assessment. Cancer 28:244–252, 1971.

277. Tobacco Habits Other Than Smoking, Betel Quid and Areca Nut Chewing, and Some Related Nitrosamines, Monograph 37. Lyon, International Agency for Research on Cancer, 1985.

278. Martin HE, Pfluger OH: Cancer of the cheek (buccal mucosa): A study of 99 cases with results of treatment at end of 5 years. Arch Surg 30:731–736, 1935.

279. Vegers JWM, Snow GB, Van der Waal I: Squamous cell carcinoma of the buccal mucosa. Arch Otolaryngol 105:192–195, 1979.

280. Conley J, Sadoyama JA: Squamous cell cancer of the buccal mucosa: A review of 90 cases. Arch Otolaryngol 97:330–333, 1973.

281. Strome SE, To W, Strawderman M, et al: Squamous cell carcinoma of the buccal mucosa. Otolaryngol Head Neck Surg 120:375–379, 1999.

282. Sieczka E, Datta R, Singh A, et al: Cancer of the buccal mucosa: Are margins and T-stage accurate predictors of local control? Am J Otolaryngol 22:395–399, 2001.

283. Chhetri DK, Rawnsley JD, Calcaterra TC: Carcinoma of the buccal mucosa. Otolaryngol Head Neck Surg 123:566–571, 2000.

284. Pradhan SA, Rajpal RM: Marginal mandibulectomy in the management of squamous cancer of the oral cavity. Indian J Cancer 24:167–171, 1987.

285. Wang CC: Radiation therapy for head and neck neoplasms. Boston, Wright, 1983, pp 112–121.

286. Dhawan IK, Verma K, Khazanchi RK, et al: Carcinoma of the buccal mucosa: Incidence of regional lymph node involvement. Indian J Cancer 30:176–180, 1993.

287. Nair NK, Sankaranarayanan R, Padmanabhan TK: Evaluation of the role of radiotherapy in the management of carcinoma of the buccal mucosa. Cancer 61:1326–1331, 1988.

288. O'Brien PH, Catlin D: Cancer of the cheek (mucosa). Cancer 18:1326–1331, 1965.

289. Chaudary AJ, Pande SC, Sharma V, et al: Radiotherapy of carcinoma of the buccal mucosa. Semin Surg Oncol 5:322–326, 1989.

290. Vikram B, Farr HW: Adjuvant radiation therapy in locally advanced head and neck cancer. CA Cancer J Clin 33:134–138, 1983.

291. Pourquier H, Dubois JB, Querrier B, et al: Epitheliomas du trigone retromolare et de la face infere des joues. Etude de 53 cas (1959–1972). Ann Otolaryngol 94:95–106, 1977.

292. Ash CL: Oral cancer. A twenty-five year study. AJR Am J Roentgenol 87:417–430, 1962.

293. Pop LAM, Eijkenboom WMH, deBoer MF, et al: Evaluation of treatment results of squamous cell carcinoma of the buccal mucosa. Int J Radiat Oncol Biol Phys 16:483–487, 1989.

294. Maccomb WS, Fletcher OH: Cancer of the Head and Neck. Baltimore, Williams & Wilkins, 1967, pp 133–140.

295. Fang F, Leung SW, Huang C, et al: Combined-modality therapy for squamous carcinoma of the buccal mucosa: Treatment results and prognostic factors. Head Neck 19:506–512, 1997.

296. Urist MM, O'Brien CJ, Soong S, et al: Squamous cell carcinoma of the buccal mucosa: Analysis of prognostic factors. Am J Surg 154:411–414, 1987.

297. Bahadur S, Chatterjee TK: Chemotherapy in buccal mucosa cancer. J Surg Oncol 32:245–247, 1986.

298. Schuller DE, King GW, Smith RE, et al: Combination therapy protocol for stage III or IV carcinoma of the oral cavity, oropharynx, and hypopharynx. Laryngoscope 90:1265–1270, 1980.

299. Shaha A, Spiro R, Shah J, et al: Squamous carcinoma of the floor of the mouth. Am J Surg 148:455–459, 1984.

300. Sessions DG, Spector GJ, Lenox J, et al: Analysis of treatment results for floor-of-mouth cancer. Laryngoscope 110:1764–1772, 2000.

301. Komisar A, Barrow HN: Mandible preservation in cancer of the floor of the mouth—anatomical and oncological considerations. Arch Otolaryngol Head Neck Surg 120:1197–1200, 1994.

302. Hicks WL, Loree TR, Garcia RI, et al: Squamous cell carcinoma of the floor of mouth: A 20-year review. Head Neck 19:400–405, 1997.

303. Guillamondegui OM, Oliver B, Hayden R: Cancer of the anterior floor of mouth: Selective choice of treatment and analysis of failures. Am J Surg 140:560–562, 1980.

304. Hudson DA, Stannard CE, Binnewald B, et al: The role of suprahyoid block dissection in carcinoma of the floor of the mouth. J Surg Oncol 55:20–23, 1994.

305. Nason RW, Sako K, Beecroft WA, et al: Surgical management of squamous cell carcinoma of the floor of the mouth. Am J Surg 158:292–296, 1989.

306. Steinhart H, Kleinsasser O: Growth and spread of squamous cell carcinoma of the floor of mouth. Eur Arch Otorhinolaryngol 250:358–361, 1993.

307. Shaha A: Marginal mandibulectomy for carcinoma of the floor of the mouth. J Surg Oncol 49:116–119, 1992.

308. Beecroft WA, Sako K, Razack MS: Mandible preservation in the treatment of cancer of the floor of the mouth. J Surg Oncol 19:171–175, 1982.

309. Cole DA, Patel PM, Matar JR, et al: Floor of mouth cancer. Arch Otolaryngol Head Neck Surg 120:260–263, 1994.

310. Rodgers LW, Stringer SP, Mendenhall WM, et al: Management of squamous cell carcinoma of the floor of mouth. Head Neck 15:16–19, 1993.

311. Zelefsky MJ, Harrsion LB, Fass DE, et al: Postoperative radiotherapy for oral cavity cancers: Impact of anatomic subsite on treatment outcome. Head Neck 12:470–475, 1990.

312. Klotch DW, Muro-Cacho C, Gal TJ: Factors affecting survival for floor-of-mouth carcinoma. Otolaryngol Head Neck Surg 122:495–498, 2000.

313. Aygun C, Salazar OM, Sewchand W, et al: Carcinoma of the floor of the mouth: A 20 year experience. Int J Radiat Oncol Biol Phys 10:619–626, 1984.

314. Mazeron JJ, Grimaid L, Raynal M, et al: Iridium-192 curietherapy for T1 and T2 epidermoid carcinomas of the floor of the mouth. Int J Radiat Oncol Biol Phys 18:1299–1306, 1990.

315. Shons A, Magallanes F, McQuarrie D: The results of aggressive regional operation in the treatment of cancer of the floor of the mouth. Surgery 96:29–34, 1984.

316. Schramm VL, Myers EN, Sigler BA: Surgical management of early epidermoid carcinoma of the anterior floor of mouth. Laryngoscope 90:207–216, 1980.

317. Fu K, Lichter A, Galante M: Carcinoma of the floor of the mouth: An analysis of treatment results and the sites and causes of failures. Int J Radiat Oncol Biol Phys 1:829–837, 1976.

318. Byers RM, Anderson B, Schwarz EA, et al: Treatment of squamous carcinoma of the retromolar trigone. Am J Clin Oncol 7:647–652, 1984.

319. Lane AP, Buckmire RA, Mukherji SK, et al: Use of computed tomography in the assessment of mandibular invasion in carcinoma of the retromolar trigone. Otolaryngol Head Neck Surg 122:673–677, 2000.

320. Shumrick DA, Quenelle DJ: Malignant disease of the tonsillar region, retromolar trigone and buccal mucosa. Otolaryngol Clin North Am 12:115–120, 1979.

321. Huang CJ, Chao KS, Tsai J, et al: Cancer of the retromolar trigone: Long-term radiation therapy outcome. Head Neck 23:758–763, 2001.

322. Kowalski LP, Hasimoto I, Magrin J: End results of 114 extended "commando" operations. Am J Surg 166:374–379, 1993.

323. Batsakis JG: Tumors of the Head and Neck, 2nd ed. Baltimore, Williams & Wilkins, 1979.

324. Swearingen AG, McGrew JP, Palumbo VD: Roentgenograph-pathologic correlation of carcinoma involving the mandible. AJR Am J Roentgenol 96:15–20, 1966.

325. McGregor AD, MacDonald DG: Routes of entry of squamous cell carcinoma to the mandible. Head Neck Surg 10:294–297, 1988.

326. Soo KC, Spiro RH, King W, et al: Squamous carcinoma of the gingiva: An update. Am J Surg 156:281–289, 1988.

327. Blackwell KE, Lacombe V: The bridging lateral mandibular reconstruction plate revisited. Arch Otolaryngol Head Neck Surg 125:988–993, 1999.

328. Cady R, Catlin D: Epidermoid carcinoma of the gum—a 20 year survey. Cancer 23:551–569, 1969.

329. Backstrom A, Jakobsson PA, Nathanson A, et al: Prognosis of squamous cell carcinoma of the gums with cytologically verified cervical lymph node metastasis. J Laryngol Otol 89:391–396, 1975.

330. Love R, Stewart IF, Coy P: Upper alveolar carcinoma—a 30 year survey. J Otolaryngol 6:393–398, 1977.

331. Ramulu C, Reddy CM: Carcinoma of the hard palate and its relationship to reverse smoking. Int Surg 57:636–640, 1972.

332. Petruzzelli GJ, Myers EN: Malignant neoplasms of the hard palate and upper alveolar ridge. Oncology 8:43–48, 1994.

333. Chung CK, Johns ME, Cantrell RW, et al: Radiotherapy in the management of primary malignancies of the hard palate. Laryngoscope 90:576–584, 1980.

334. Patzer ER, Schweitzer RJ, Frazell EL: Epidermoid carcinoma of the palate. Am J Surg 119:294–298, 1970.

335. Evans HL, Shah JP: Epidermoid carcinoma of the palate. Am J Surg 142:451–458, 1981.

CHAPTER 14

Cancer of the Oropharynx

Merrill S. Kies

K. Kian Ang

Gary L. Clayman

◨ INTRODUCTION

Approximately 5000 new cases of oropharyngeal malignancy are diagnosed each year in the United States.[1] These cancers have a strong association with chronic alcohol and tobacco use. Squamous cell carcinoma is the predominant histologic type; minor salivary gland cancer, melanoma, lymphoma (including Hodgkin's disease), and sarcoma are seen much less frequently. Lymphoepithelioma and small cell carcinoma are also uncommon, but their recognition is important because the differences in their natural history have important implications for therapy.

Cancers of the oropharynx pose diagnostic and therapeutic challenges that necessitate an individualized, multidisciplinary approach to management. Head and neck surgeons, radiation and medical oncologists, speech pathologists, and dental oncologists must work in concert with the common goal of curing these cancers and functionally rehabilitating these patients. Because these tumors have a tendency to be deeply invasive and may present initially with an advanced-stage primary and/or with ipsilateral or bilateral lymph node metastasis, locoregional control is a primary therapeutic goal. Despite evolving expertise in locoregional therapy, however, overall survival rates have changed little over 30 years and remain unsatisfactory. Furthermore, distant metastases and second primary malignancies remain appreciable problems for patients whose primary cancer was treated successfully. Finally, mortality rates in patients with these cancers are escalated because of intercurrent cardiovascular disease and other chronic effects resulting from alcohol and tobacco abuse. Therapeutic measures must therefore recognize these major comorbidities.

◨ ANATOMY

The oropharynx includes the soft palate, tonsils, base of tongue, and pharyngeal walls bounded superiorly by the nasopharynx and inferiorly by the pharyngoepiglottic fold (Fig. 14–1). The soft palate, including the uvula, partially separates the oral cavity from the nasopharynx, forming the roof of the oropharynx and the floor of the nasopharynx. It attaches anteriorly to the hard palate and laterally joins the tonsillar pillars. The palatine (or faucial) tonsils, located on the lateral walls of the oropharynx, are oval-shaped lymphoid structures embedded in a fibrous capsule. The tonsillar fossae, which encase the palatine tonsils, are bounded by anterior and posterior pillars. These comprise the palatoglossus and palatopharyngeus muscles, respectively, and converge superiorly to form the soft palate. The inferior portion of the fossa is known as the glossopalatine sulcus.

The base of the tongue extends from the circumvallate papillae to the vallecula at the base of the epiglottis, encompassing the glossoepiglottic and pharyngoepiglottic folds. Laterally, this structure extends to the glossopalatine sulcus. The pharyngeal wall starts at the inferior aspect of the nasopharynx in the region of the soft palate and extends to the level of the epiglottis inferiorly, including the posterior and lateral surfaces of the oropharynx. The pharyngeal constrictor muscles form the scaffolding of the pharyngeal wall. This structure relates to the second and third cervical vertebrae and contains squamous epithelium and pharyngobasilar fascia. Posterior to these structures are the retropharyngeal space, longus capitus and colli muscles, and prevertebral fascia. The lateral pharyngeal wall becomes the pharyngoepiglottic fold, which then further descends to become the lateral aspect of the pyriform sinus. Innervation is provided by cranial nerves IX and X.

The most important functions of the oropharynx are speech and swallowing. The soft palate provides oronasal separation by closing off the nasopharynx from the oropharynx during swallowing to prevent nasopharyngeal regurgitation. The tongue base plays a critical role in propelling the food bolus into the hypopharynx. The soft palate and base of tongue also have important functions in phonation.

Lymphatic drainage of the oropharynx and neck is also important to consider in patients with oropharyngeal cancers (Fig. 14–2) because the lymphatic drainage of this area is rich.[2] The lymph node areas are mapped as shown in Figure 14–3. Primary drainage of the oropharynx is to the superior internal jugular lymphatics in level II. The lymphatics of the posterior soft palate, tonsillar area, base of tongue, and oropharyngeal walls also drain to the retropharyngeal and parapharyngeal lymph nodes. Drainage may be bilateral, as is most often seen with tumor infiltration of midline structures. Risk of nodal involvement relates to the differentiation, grade, and size of the primary tumor. Lymphatic spread most often progresses in an orderly fashion from upper echelon nodes of level II to middle and inferior lymph nodes of levels III and IV, respectively. Nodal levels I and V represent secondary stations; isolated

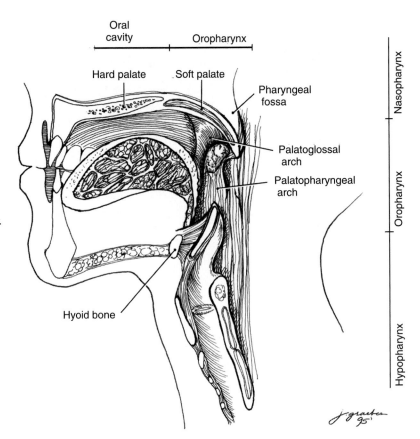

FIGURE 14–1 Oropharynx: surface anatomy.

involvement of these levels by oropharyngeal primary tumor is rare.

ETIOLOGY, PATHOLOGY, AND MOLECULAR BIOLOGY

Squamous cell carcinoma accounts for more than 90% of cancers of the oropharynx.[3] In the United States, cancer of the tonsil is the most common, followed by cancers of the base of tongue, oropharyngeal wall, and soft palate. These cancers tend to be moderately or poorly differentiated and are often locally advanced at the time of diagnosis. Although uncommon, malignant melanoma, minor salivary gland cancer, lymphoma, small cell carcinoma, and sarcoma are other primary malignancies of the oropharynx. Management for these less common malignancies must be considered on an individual basis and after consultation with appropriate

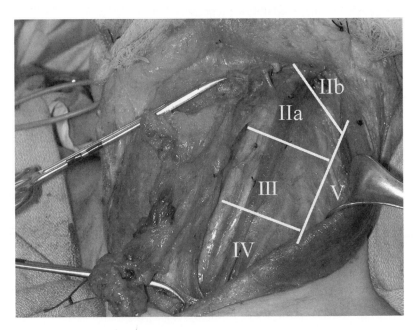

FIGURE 14–2 Patient undergoing elective dissection of levels II through IV. The anterior component of level V is included in this dissection, as is the submuscular recess of level IIb. Anatomically preserved structures—sternocleidomastoid muscle, internal and external carotid arteries, internal jugular vein, cranial nerve IX, and cervical rootlets—are shown.

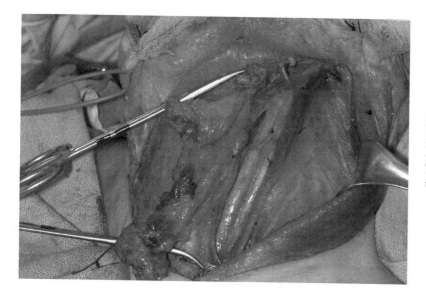

FIGURE 14-3 Demonstration of the lymphatic basins that should be resected in elective dissection for oropharyngeal cancers. The retropharyngeal and parapharyngeal nodes are generally not resected because radiotherapy to the primary site addresses these echelons.

specialty medical services. Our discussion here focuses on squamous cell cancers. Chapter 3 provides a more detailed review of pathology that may affect the oropharynx.

Etiology—Risk Factors

Understanding of the causes of oropharyngeal cancer is incomplete, but certain identifiable environmental risk factors are associated with these diseases. Moreover, the presence of concomitant mucosal dysplasia in tissues adjacent to primary malignancies and the high incidence of second primary cancers are indicative of a generalized mucosal "field defect" that can be attributed to longstanding exposure to carcinogens.[4] Most clearly, tobacco use and excessive alcohol consumption are major determinants of upper aerodigestive tract cancers, probably accounting for 80% of oropharyngeal malignancies.[5–9] Tobacco and alcohol are independent carcinogens, and combined use results in a synergistic effect on cancer incidence.[5, 6, 8] Although cigarette smoking is most strongly correlated with oropharyngeal cancer, cigar and pipe smoking, tobacco chewing, and smoking marijuana are also clearly identified risk factors for cancer of the head and neck.[10]

Epidemiologic evidence implicates dietary deficiencies, including carotenes, vitamin A, and alpha-tocopherol, in the development of cancer of the oropharynx.[11, 12] The use of mouthwash and poor oral hygiene are more controversial factors. Recent evidence suggests that human papilloma virus (HPV) may have a role in the development of a minority of oropharyngeal squamous cell cancers, with subtypes 16 and 18 most frequently reported.[13] The prognosis of HPV-related oropharyngeal cancer may be better than that of oropharyngeal cancers not related to HPV.[14] Host-specific factors presumably also influence the likelihood of cancer development. Considering that only a fraction of individuals exposed to tobacco and alcohol actually develop clinical cancer, there may be heritable differences in susceptibility in almost every phase of carcinogenesis. Emerging data reveal interindividual heterogeneity in the ability to metabolize carcinogens, in DNA repair capacity, and in genomic instability; these factors, along with alterations in the expression of oncogenes and/or tumor suppressor genes, may contribute to risk for individual patients. Sturgis and Wei nicely reviewed this important concept of "genetic susceptibility."[15]

Tumor and Molecular Biology

Our understanding of the initiation and progression of carcinogenesis continues to evolve with advances in molecular biology and biotechnology. Mutations in the tumor suppressor gene *TP53* (formerly known as *p53*) occur in 50% of head and neck cancers.[16, 17] Boyle and associates reported that 20% of premalignant head and neck lesions, including carcinoma in situ and moderate to severe dysplasia, have also been found to contain *TP53* mutations.[18] Mutations of *TP53* are more common among smokers than in nonsmokers,[19] and time to recurrence has been found to be shorter for tumors that overexpress TP53 protein. A model of progressive molecular abnormalities has been identified that may reflect critical genetic changes in the evolution of invasive cancer from premalignant lesions.[20, 21] The oncogene cyclin D1 is amplified in approximately one third of head and neck squamous cell carcinomas.[22, 23] Ongoing studies are addressing other alterations, including the tumor suppressor gene *RB* and oncogenes such as *mutated RAS, MYC,* and *BCL2,* as potential predictors of phenotypic behavior and of responsiveness to therapy.[24, 25] Molecular abnormalities also represent potential "targets" for novel therapeutic approaches.

Recent advances have led to the identification of areas of frequent chromosomal loss in cancer of the head and neck. Called loss of heterozygosity (LOH), these losses most frequently are found in two loci—3p14 and 9p21.[25] Further understanding of the progression to malignancy and identification of putative tumor suppressor genes in these malignancies may emerge from these studies. Multistep carcinogenesis and field carcinogenesis are important considerations relative to oropharyngeal cancers because the carcinogens that initiate tumorigenesis also affect nontransformed surrounding tissues. Supporting the field hypothesis are chromosome labeling and LOH studies showing that LOH at 9p and abnormalities in chromosome 11 are present in histologically normal mucosa adjacent to malignant tumors.[25]

Tumor growth rate, invasiveness, and metastatic pattern depend on the interactions of a complex set of biologic factors. Growth and invasiveness appear to be affected by interaction of microenvironmental components such as degradative enzymes (including collagenases), matrix metalloproteinases, plasminogen activators and cathepsins, and angiogenic factors, as well as by growth factors, cytokines, and concentrations of related receptors. The metastatic process also may be affected by cell surface properties and motility factors. In addition, perineural tumor cell infiltration, presence or absence of natural fascial barriers, tumor-associated and tumor-infiltrating lymphocytes, and other factors combine to create a biologic environment that profoundly influences the metastatic process, response to therapy, and ultimate outcome.

◼ CLINICAL PRESENTATION AND STAGING

Oropharyngeal cancers tend to be relatively asymptomatic in early stages, which may extend over months to a year or longer, and many of these tumors are initially identified after a patient presents for evaluation of a painless neck mass. Once the cancer reaches a significant size, initial complaints may be of a nonspecific soreness or fullness in the region of the primary tumor. Masses in the tonsil and soft palate are often detected by the patient, dentist, or a general physician, but lesions of the base of tongue and pharyngeal wall are not easily visible. With advanced disease at the primary site, patients may complain of a foul odor of their breath, worsening sore throat, otalgia, dysphagia, and/or trismus. Tethering appears with deeply infiltrating cancer of the tongue. Patients with persistent sore throat for longer than 2 weeks or a mass in the neck must undergo a comprehensive head and neck examination for the evaluation of potential sites of primary disease.

Cancer of the soft palate tends to occur on the inferior surface and may spread in a centrifugal fashion to adjacent structures. Primary lymphatic drainage is to level II nodes. Cancer of the tonsil most often presents with involvement of the anterior tonsillar pillar. These cancers are frequently exophytic and tend to spread anterolaterally to the retromolar and buccal regions. Extension to the base of the tongue is also common. Posterior and deep extension may involve the pterygoid musculature, with consequent pain and trismus. Primary lymphatic drainage of such extensions is also to level II.

Cancers of the base of the tongue may be highly invasive and insidious, and they frequently are asymptomatic until an advanced stage because nerve fibers are scant in this region. Because lymphatics are plentiful and bilateral, patients may present with cervical lymphadenopathy. Expertise in the examination of the head and neck is required for tumors to be detected. With a large cancer, patients may complain of difficulty swallowing, dysphagia, or alteration of speech. Pain is also common. The cancer may extend anteriorly to involve the mobile tongue or laterally to the tonsillar region. Lymph node metastases with involvement of levels II, III, and IV are common. Referred pain in the ear is also a common symptom.

Cancer of the lateral and posterior pharyngeal walls also is usually diagnosed at an advanced stage. The presenting complaint may be of pain or cervical adenopathy. Primary cancer may extend superiorly to the nasopharynx or inferiorly to the hypopharynx. Because cancers of the pharynx are often advanced, extending past the midline, bilateral cervical adenopathy may be present at diagnosis.

The evaluation of the head and neck should include a complete history and physical examination, direct visualization of the oral cavity and oropharynx, indirect mirror examination of the oropharynx and hypopharynx, and fiberoptic endoscopic examination when necessary. The staging evaluation also should routinely include a complete blood count, a routine chemistry panel, and appropriate imaging studies. Computed tomographic (CT) scan or magnetic resonance imaging (MRI) studies are also useful in defining the anatomic extent of the primary tumor and metastatic spread. Chest CT and bone scanning are obtained as indicated. The role of positron emission tomographic (PET) scanning is currently being studied.

Physical evaluation includes assessment of the site and extent of the primary cancer and the presence/location of pathologic lymphadenopathy. Primary lesions and enlarged lymph nodes should be palpated and measured. Impairment of tongue mobility is an important sign of deep muscular invasion into the root of the tongue. Trismus reflects the presence of disease infiltrating the pterygoid muscles and should be documented by a measurement of the distance between the upper and lower gums. Assessment of cranial nerves V and VII is also important.

The 2000 American Joint Commission on Cancer (AJCC) staging system for oropharyngeal carcinoma is shown in Table 14–1. All available information obtained before treatment, including findings on CT and/or MRI scans, is used to define disease stage. T-stage is based largely on tumor size. However, for a tumor to be classified as T4, invasion of deep muscular structures should be demonstrated, such as pterygoid involvement that results in substantial trismus or bone involvement. Similarly, significant deviation or impaired mobility of the tongue would indicate extension of the tumor into the deep muscles.

◼ CYSTIC METASTASIS TO THE NECK OF UNKNOWN PRIMARY

Patients with oropharyngeal cancer frequently present with a neck mass from an "unknown primary" tumor. Such neck masses must be considered as originating from a primary cancer in the oropharynx until proven otherwise. Thorough investigation of the oropharyngeal sites, specifically the lateral pharyngeal wall and tonsil, the glossopharyngeal sulcus, and the base of the tongue, must be undertaken with consideration of cystic metastasis to the neck from an unknown primary tumor. Sometimes these circumstances may be complicated even further by a presentation such as squamous cell carcinoma as a "branchial cleft cyst." This pathology should be reviewed thoughtfully. In patients in whom a primary cannot be identified, tonsillectomy and biopsy of the base of the tongue should be considered; in fact, contemporary molecular characterization may also be considered, including

TABLE 14-1 Definition of TNM for Cancer of the Oropharynx

Primary Tumor

TX	Primary tumor cannot be assessed
T0	No evidence of primary tumor
Tis	Carcinoma in Situ

Nasopharynx

T1	Tumor confined to the nasopharynx
T2	Tumor extends to soft tissues
	T2a Tumor extends to the oropharynx and/or nasal cavity without parapharyngeal extension°
	T2b Any tumor with parapharyngeal extension°
T3	Tumor involves bony structures and/or paranasal sinuses
T4	Tumor with intracranial extension and/or involvement of cranial nerves, infratemporal fossa, hypopharynx, orbit, or masticator space

°Note: Parapharyngeal extension denotes posterolateral infiltration of tumor beyond the pharyngobasilar fascia.

Oropharynx

T1	Tumor 2 cm or less in greatest dimension
T2	Tumor more than 2 cm but not more than 4 cm in greatest dimension
T3	Tumor more than 4 cm in greatest dimension
T4a	Tumor invades the larynx, deep/extrinsic muscle of tongue, medial pterygoid, hard palate, or mandible
T4b	Tumor invades lateral pterygoid muscle, pterygoid plates, lateral nasopharynx, or skull base or encases carotid artery

Hypopharynx

T1	Tumor limited to one subsite of hypopharynx and 2 cm or less in greatest dimension
T2	Tumor invades more than one subsite of hypopharynx or an adjacent site, or measures mor than 2 cm but not more than 4 cm in greatest diameter without fixation of hemilarynx
T3	Tumor more than 4 cm in greatest dimension or with fixation of hemilarynx
T4a	Tumor invades thyroid/cricoid cartilage, hyoid bone, thyroid gland, esophagus, or central compartment soft tissue°
T4b	Tumor invades prevertebral fascia, encases carotid artery, or involves mediastinal structures

°Note: Central compartment soft tissue includes prelaryngeal strap muscles and subcutaneous fat.

Regional Lymph Nodes (N)

Nasopharynx

The distribution and the prognostic impact of regional lymph node spread from nasopharynx cancer, particularly of the undifferentiated type, are different from those of other head and neck mucosal cancers and justify the use of a different N classification scheme.

NX	Regional lymph nodes cannot be assessed
N0	No regional lymph node metastasis
N1	Unilateral metastasis in lymph node(s), 6 cm or less in greatest dimension, above the supraclavicular fossa°
N2	Bilateral metastasis in lymph node(s), 6 cm or less in greatest dimension, above the supraclavicular fossa°
N3	Metastasis in a lymph node(s)°>6 cm and/or to supraclavicular fossa
	N3a Greater than 6 cm in dimension
	N3b Extension to the supraclavicular fossa°°

°Note: Midline nodes are considered ipsilateral nodes.
*°°Supraclavicular zone or fossa is relevant to the staging of nasopharyngeal carcinoma and is the triangular region originally described by Ho. It is defined by three points: (1) the superior margin of the sternal end of the clavicle, (2) the superior margin of the lateral end of the clavicle, (3) the point where the neck meets the shoulder. Note that this would include caudal portions of Levels IV and V. All cases with lymph nodes (whole or part) in the fossa are considered N3b.

Oropharynx and Hypopharynx

NX	Regional lymph nodes cannot be assessed
N0	No regional lymph node metastasis
N1	Metastasis in a single ipsilateral lymph node, 3 cm or less in greatest dimension
N2	Metastasis in a single ipsilateral lymph node, more than 3 cm but not more than 6 cm in greatest dimension, or in multiple ipsilateral lymph nodes, none more than 6 cm in greatest dimension, or in bilateral or contralateral lymph nodes, none more than 6 cm in greatest dimension
N2a	Metastasis in a single ipsilateral lymph node more than 3 cm but not more than 6 cm in greatest dimension
N2b	Metastasis in multiple ipsilateral lymph nodes, none more than 6 cm in greatest dimension
N2c	Metastasis in bilateral or contralateral lymph nodes, none more than 6 cm in greatest dimension
N3	Metastasis in a lymph node more than 6 cm in greatest dimension

Distant Metastasis (M)

MX	Distant metastasis cannot be assessed
M0	No distant metastasis
M1	Distant metastasis

STAGE GROUPING: NASOPHARYNX

Stage 0	Tis	N0	M0
Stage I	T1	N0	M0
Stage IIA	T2a	N0	M0
Stage IIB	T1	N1	M0
	T2	N1	M0
	T2a	N1	M0
	T2b	N0	M0
	T2b	N1	M0
Stage III	T1	N2	M0
	T2a	N2	M0
	T2b	N2	M0
	T3	N0	M0
	T3	N1	M0
	T3	N2	M0
Stage IVA	T4	N0	M0
	T4	N1	M0
	T4	N2	M0
Stage IVB	Any T	N3	M0
Stage IVC	Any T	Any N	M1

STAGE GROUPING: OROPHARYNX, HYPOPHARYNX

Stage 0	Tis	N0	M0
Stage I	T1	N0	M0
Stage II	T2	N0	M0
Stage III	T3	N0	M0
	T1	N1	M0
	T2	N1	M0
	T3	N1	M0
Stage IVA	T4a	N0	M0
	T4a	N1	M0
	T1	N2	M0
	T2	N2	M0
	T3	N2	M0
	T4a	N2	M0
Stage IVB	T4b	Any N	M0
	Any T	N3	M0
Stage IVC	Any T	Any N	M1

microsatellite analysis and HPV analysis. In the rare circumstance of a patient with cystic metastasis to the neck in whom a primary cannot be located despite exhaustive workup, the primary should be presumed to be of oropharyngeal origin and the disease managed in this light.

◖ THERAPY

Surgery and radiation therapy, either alone or in combination, had been the mainstays of treatment for squamous cell carcinoma of the oropharynx for many years. Although our therapeutic approaches for squamous cell carcinoma of the oropharynx have evolved to feature radiotherapy and radiation-sensitizing approaches in patients with intermediate or advanced disease, some centers continue to use surgery as a primary therapeutic approach in these patients. Owing to the complexity and duration of care required by the patient with cancer of the oropharynx, an interdisciplinary team, including head and neck surgeons, reconstructive surgeons, radiation therapists, medical oncologists, dental oncologists, and speech-language pathologists, offers the patient the best opportunity for comprehensive treatment and long-term care. Clearly, the optimal therapeutic approach for each patient depends on multiple factors, including the patient's desires, biologic potential of the neoplasm, stage of disease, and comorbid medical conditions; more defined predictors of tumor biology do not yet exist to help in selection of therapy.

Surgical Management

Although a variety of surgical techniques have been employed and described for excision of primary cancer in the oropharynx, patients with squamous cell carcinoma of the oropharynx, even early stage T1 and T2 lesions that can be completely excised, are also at significant risk for metastasis to the regional lymph nodes. Despite the feasibility of selective neck dissection of levels II, III, and IV for oropharyngeal cancer, these dissections fail to address the additional lymphatic basins at risk, including the retropharyngeal and parapharyngeal lymphatics. Moreover, with more extensive cancers or those that approach the midline, the risk for bilateral involvement is significant, increasing both the difficulty of the procedure and the risk of operative complications.

Recognition of the problems inherent in the surgical approach led to the plan now in use at the University of Texas M.D. Anderson Cancer Center, which applies radiotherapy in the management of primary and regional squamous cell carcinoma of the oropharynx. Whether lymphoscintigraphy and/or lymphatic mapping could have an impact on the revitalization of surgery in oropharyngeal squamous cell carcinomas is a subject of conjecture.[26]

Extension of the primary cancer into the poststyloid compartment or prevertebral fascia, or involvement of the carotid artery, is clearly indicative of an aggressive process and thus warrants thoughtful consideration of the goals of resection. Our previous analysis of patients with deeply invasive squamous cell cancer of the oropharynx suggested that patients with trismus or decreased tongue protrusion had better outcomes with radiotherapy.[27] Patients with T3 and T4 cancer of the base of the tongue, who may require laryngectomy with long-term dependence on tracheotomy and gastric tube feedings, fared similarly. Successful resection of cancers of the oropharynx requires adequate exposure and three-dimensional comprehensive resection with free margins. A thorough understanding of the propensity of these cancers for submucosal extension as well as perineural invasion needs to be considered by the oncologic surgeon contemplating such a resection.

The cancer should be resected with at least a 1-cm margin of normal-appearing tissue, with comprehensive frozen section analysis of all margins, including the deep margins of resection. Although microscopically positive margins should be re-resected, circumvention of carcinoma in situ or severely dysplastic tissues by such an approach may not be possible. Molecular pathologic studies clearly suggest that the genetic profile of malignancy may be found quite distant from the epicenter of these tumors.[28]

Cancer of the oropharynx can generally be resected through one of several different surgical techniques—transoral, transpharyngeal, and transmandibular approaches. Selection of the optimal approach must take into account the size and extent of the cancer, consideration of concomitant neck dissection, and involvement of osseous structures, as well as the expertise and clinical experience of the surgeon.

Transoral Approaches

Transoral approaches to the oropharynx involve resection of the neoplasm through the open mouth without an external incision. The success of this approach is dependent on the size and location of the cancer as well as on the actual surgical technique used. Adequate assistance and retraction are mandatory to facilitate this process. Self-retaining retractors may facilitate the approach. Intact dentition may, in fact, impair the surgeon's ability to adequately visualize or resect specific areas. Trismus would be a relative contraindication. Resection is relatively quick and frequently offers rapid recovery to the patient. However, careful consideration of deep and undissected structures, as well as of the technical difficulty of three-dimensional comprehensive excision, needs to be given when transoral excision of a cancer of the oropharynx is contemplated.

TRANSORAL AND LASER EXCISION OF TONGUE BASE AND PHARYNGEAL CANCERS

Transoral microscopic laser surgical approaches to the oropharynx can be performed successfully by surgeons who are experienced with using these approaches. The learning curve can be quite steep, and the less experienced laser surgeon should attempt the transoral excision only for very favorable lesions. The surgeon using this approach should be familiar with the special instrumentation such as laser coagulation and with control techniques, microvessel clip ligature, and microscopic dissection of the lingual and ascending pharyngeal arteries via the transoral endoscopic approach. Transition to an open approach must be available to surgeons with limited expertise in this technique.

Skilled microlaryngeal surgeons have extensively supported transoral microlaser-assisted surgical techniques through the use of extended approaches that require specialized retractors and microdissection techniques.[29] Only the most skilled microlaser surgeons should consider these approaches.

The more experienced surgeon can consider extended transoral approaches. Comprehensive excision of tissues affected by oropharyngeal cancer, including the lingual cortex of the mandible, maxilla (partial maxillectomy), soft palate, and even nasopharynx, can be performed in selected patients. Thoughtful consideration of three-dimensional anatomy and of lymphatic basins at potential risk owing to the histologic type of cancer is necessary.

Transcervical Approach

LINGUAL MANDIBULAR RELEASE

The lingual mandibular release is a transcervical approach that may be considered for cancer of the oropharynx, although as a general recommendation, we do not advocate this approach. The technique involves making a complete incision through the floor of the mouth from anterior tonsillar pillar to anterior tonsillar pillar. It offers little benefit over other approaches, except in cancers that involve midline structures when mandibulotomy is best avoided.

Transpharyngeal Approaches

SUPRAHYOID (TRANSHYOID) PHARYNGOTOMY

The suprahyoid approach is generally most appropriate for small neoplasms of the base of tongue and pharyngeal walls. (For such small neoplasms, transoral approaches in and of themselves may offer equal visualization and less morbidity than the transpharyngeal approaches.) The procedure is performed transcervically by making an incision above the hyoid bone and entering the vallecula. When performed in conjunction with neck dissections, an apron flap is recommended together with a tracheotomy. This approach is most appropriate for lesions in the midline or in the posterior pharyngeal wall. In addition, the pharyngotomy can be extended laterally and inferiorly to provide even wider exposure. These defects can usually be closed primarily.

LATERAL PHARYNGOTOMY AND "DROP-THROUGH" APPROACHES

The lateral pharyngotomy can be performed for access to the pharyngeal wall and the base of the tongue. If more extensive resection of the base of the tongue is necessary, a "delivery" approach should be considered. A release of the floor of mouth and oral cavity should be performed on the homolateral side and extended past the midline. The periosteum should be elevated along the medial aspect of the mandible and the floor of mouth released to the genial tubercle. Extension past the midline and delivery of oral cavity and tongue base into the neck can then be performed easily. In these circumstances, resection of the lingual and hypoglossal nerves is frequently necessary for homolateral tongue-based lesions. The surgeon must be thoughtful and resourceful in utilization of these approaches. Sometimes, combination approaches using transoral and cervical delivery techniques allow adequate three-dimensional excision of the primary tumor with functional sparing of critical organs. The disadvantages of this approach include limited superior visualization and likely risk to the hypoglossal nerve. The superior laryngeal nerves should be anatomically visualized and preserved.

Transmandibular Approaches

Most transmandibular approaches require a lip-splitting incision. Depending on the prominence of the mental crease, generally a curvilinear incision around the mentum is recommended to optimize cosmetic outcome. A step along the vermilion border facilitates aesthetic vermilion restitution and prevents unfavorable contraction. Other surgeons prefer a midline lip-splitting incision.

MIDLINE LABIAL MANDIBULAR GLOSSOTOMY

The midline labial mandibular glossotomy, frequently described as the "Trotter" approach, is rarely used in oropharyngeal cancers. It is indicated primarily for small midline tongue-based and posterior pharyngeal wall lesions that are not amenable to transoral approaches. Bleeding and deficits are minimal because the hypoglossal nerves and lingual arteries are not transected, except along their cross-innervating components. This approach does not provide access to the parapharyngeal space or lateral oropharyngeal sites and is described in the management of oropharyngeal cancers primarily for historical purposes.

MANDIBULAR SWING APPROACH

The mandibular swing approach provides wide exposure of the entire oropharynx and allows comprehensive three-dimensional excision of the cancer and draining lymphatics while sparing the mandible. Multiple modifications and descriptions have been exhaustively documented for this approach.[30] Stepwise osteotomy should be performed anterior to the mental foramen so that the sensory innervation of the lip is spared. The stepped osteotomy is performed following predrilling of the mandibular fixation plate. This ensures adequate restitution of the maxillomandibular relationship as well as maintenance of the subtleties of occlusion. The floor of mouth is released along with the lateralized mandibular segment. Although the lingual nerve can be spared, maintenance of the nerve prevents extreme lateralization of the mandibular segment. If resection of the cancer will require resection of the lingual nerve, this should be performed promptly to facilitate utilization of this approach.

Only experienced surgeons should perform the mandibular swing. If the surgeon does not adequately investigate the patient preoperatively, and if previously unsuspected mandibular involvement is noted during the procedure, a large mandibular segment may be lost. This problem generally can be avoided by thoughtful preoperative evaluation.

The other significant disadvantage of the mandibular swing is the trauma to the temporomandibular joint and the muscles of mastication. Lateralization of the temporomandibular joint in combination with postoperative radiation therapy generally induces significant trismus and long-term functional disturbance of the joint. When surgery alone can be performed, the long-term functional aspects of the temporomandibular joint tend to be more favorable.

MANDIBULECTOMY

Composite resection of the mandible and pharynx may be required for the management of some advanced cancers of the oropharynx. For cancer that obviously invades bone, concomitant neck dissection with mandibulectomy and pharyngectomy should be considered. The anterior

TABLE 14-2 Therapeutic Outcomes of Soft Palate Cancer by Treatment Modality and T-Stage

	Number of Patients (number with disease control)					
	Stage					Total
	Tx	T1	T2	T3	T4	
Primary treatment						
Surgery	2 (2)	9 (9)	12 (11)	4 (4)	1 (0)	28 (26)
Radiation	4 (3)	24 (21)	79 (60)	30 (23)	13 (4)	150 (111)
Surgery + radiation	—	1 (1)	1 (0)	5 (3)	3 (2)	10 (6)
Total	6 (5)	34 (31)	92 (71)	39 (30)	17 (6)	188 (143)

Modified from Weber RS, Peters LG, Wolf P, et al: Squamous cell carcinoma of the soft palate, uvula, and anterior faucial pillar. Otolaryngol Head Neck Surg 99:16–23, 1988.

osteotomy is performed so that adequate margins of resection are ensured and generally should be placed at least 2 cm anterior to areas that have gross or radiographic suggestion of bony involvement. The proximal mandibular osteotomy must be performed at a similar distance from the disease process. When trismus and/or involvement of the ascending ramus of the mandible is noted, surgical resection should include disarticulation of the temporomandibular joint. Failure to adequately excise the ptyergoid musculature, which may be infiltrated with these cancers, can cause trismus and may leave bulky unresected disease within the surgical site. This should be avoided whenever surgery is considered as a definitive modality.

The mandibulotomy should be considered as a gold standard for three-dimensional excision of cancer of the oropharynx. Once the osteotomies have been made, three-dimensional excision of the primary cancer can proceed safely. The carotid sheath should be the deep margin of the excision. The primary disadvantages of mandibulectomy are the resultant functional and cosmetic deficits, although the latter have certainly been relieved by the appreciation of osteocutaneous free-tissue transfer (see Chapter 28).

Chemoradiation

Early and Intermediate Stages

Single-modality therapy with radiation or surgery can achieve similar locoregional control rates for early (T1N0-1) and intermediate (T2N0-1 and exophytic T3N0) cancers. Table 14–2 illustrates this point for cancer of the soft palate with some bias for the selection of more superficial tumors for surgical therapy.[31] However, radiotherapy generally yields better functional outcomes; moreover, a sizable percentage of patients undergoing surgical resection end up receiving adjuvant radiation because of the presence of adverse pathologic features (e.g., positive nodes, extracapsular spread, or perineural invasion). Therefore, many oncologists recommend radiotherapy as the treatment of choice.

The policy at M.D. Anderson is to treat patients with early-stage cancers with conventionally fractionated radiotherapy to a cumulative dose of 66 Gy over 6.5 weeks. On the basis of results of clinical trials on altered fractionation (see Chapter 31, General Principles of Radiation Therapy for Cancer of the Head and Neck), patients with intermediate-stage cancers are treated preferentially with the concomitant

boost regimen to a cumulative dose of 72 Gy over 6 weeks, which incorporates twice-a-day irradiation during the last 2.5 weeks of radiotherapy. Table 14–3 shows the local control rates achieved by this regimen in the treatment of patients in various stages of oropharyngeal cancer. Notably, only selected patients with T4 disease were treated with primary radiotherapy.

Clinical investigations for early- and intermediate-stage cancer of the oropharynx now focus on testing the role of high-precision conformal radiation technology in enhancing the quality of life by reducing annoying sequelae such as xerostomia, fibrosis, and trismus.

Advanced Disease

Fifty percent of patients with squamous cell carcinoma of the oropharynx present with T3 or T4 disease, and only a small percentage of these patients have demonstrable distant metastases.[32] Traditional therapy for advanced disease has consisted of surgical resection with postoperative radiation. Although this approach is often effective in locoregional control of disease, it can have devastating effects on personal appearance and critical functions such as speech and swallowing. Patients whose disease is considered to be unresectable owing to site (e.g., T4 base of tongue) or massive size have been treated historically with radiation alone. Unfortunately, treatment goals in this setting are usually palliative. Notably, criteria for tumor resectability vary considerably from center to center.

For patients with stage III or IV disease who are treated with surgical resection and postoperative radiation, long-term survival rates are generally low, ranging from 30% to

TABLE 14-3 Outcomes Associated With Radiation Boost Technique in Patients With Oropharyngeal Cancer

T-Stage	Number of Patients	5-Year Actuarial Control
T1	13	92%
T2	84	94%
T3	91	73%
T4	8	50%

Primary control of 200 patients treated between 1984 and 1994 at M.D. Anderson Cancer Center.

40%.[32, 33] Despite the diversity of these patients, recurrence patterns are more often locoregional than systemic,[34, 35] although systemic recurrence remains an important issue. Recent molecular studies demonstrated persistent *TP53* mutations specific for the primary tumor at resection sites, even in those with negative surgical margins after routine histologic assessment.[36] As a consequence, radiotherapy is a logical postoperative approach for treatment of a wide field. Despite postoperative radiation, one third of patients still develop locoregional recurrence. Postoperative findings of close surgical margins, perineural tumor infiltration, and lymph node metastases, especially with extracapsular spread, are prognostic features indicative of high risk of recurrence. This has led to trials of combined-modality therapy—that is, chemoradiotherapy—in an attempt to enhance locoregional control.

At M.D. Anderson, radiotherapy is the core of treatment for most patients with squamous cell carcinoma of the oropharynx. T3 and T4 cancers are the subjects of current clinical investigations. Induction chemotherapy with cisplatin and infusional 5-fluorouracil (5-FU) in previous studies,[37, 38] and more recently with paclitaxel, ifosfamide, and cisplatin,[39] has been used in sequence in a phase II trial with radiation as the definitive local treatment. Chemotherapy is active, inducing disease remission in 80% to 90% of previously untreated patients. However, randomized trials have failed to demonstrate a clear impact of inductive chemotherapy on local tumor control or overall survival.[32, 33, 37, 38] This approach does allow for preservation of the larynx in selected patients with stage III or IV laryngeal cancer.[37, 38] The induction treatment format also provides a useful instrument for evaluation of a novel drug or regimen.

Simultaneous or alternating administration of chemotherapy and radiation is a conceptually attractive application of the principle of "spatial cooperation."[40] Chemotherapy provides the potential for better regional and distant tumor control if systemically effective doses of active agents can be given. Moreover, concurrent administration of chemotherapy and radiation may markedly enhance the cytotoxicity of radiation, resulting in better local antitumor effect. Preclinical models have demonstrated mechanisms of interaction between chemotherapy and radiation, including cell-cycle synchronization, treatment of hypoxic cell populations, increased activity for tumor cells in S-phase, and inhibition of tumor cell repopulation between radiation treatment fractions. Locoregional control may be improved by these combinations, in part because most chemotherapy agents have independent activity. Of course, there is also the potential for increased local and systemic toxicity.

Concurrent Chemotherapy and Radiation

Concurrent administration of chemotherapy and radiation in oropharyngeal carcinoma has been under intense study for some years.[41] Chemoradiotherapy combinations clearly enhance tumor control and improve survival rates over radiation treatment alone. They also have substantially increased acute toxic effects, especially dermatitis and mucositis; with longer follow-up, evidence for increased late toxicity has begun to emerge.

Randomized studies have been performed to investigate the efficacy of concurrent chemotherapy and radiation (Table 14–4). As a generalization, patients admitted to these studies had variable head and neck primary T-sites, although oropharyngeal primaries tended to predominate. Brizel and colleagues compared a hyperfractionated radiotherapy regimen of total dose 75 Gy with the same radiation schedule to 70 Gy, and concurrent cisplatin 5-FU.[42] The concurrent combination treatment was followed by two cycles of adjuvant chemotherapy and yielded a statistically significant improvement in local disease control and a strong trend toward improved overall survival rate. In this trial, neck dissection was recommended in patients with N2-3 disease.

We recently reviewed our experience in examining the indications for neck dissection in this patient population. Our data suggest that neck dissections are required only when there is radiographic evidence of residual disease 6 to 8 weeks following the completion of definitive

TABLE 14–4 Selected Randomized Trials of Concomitant Chemotherapy and Radiation

Investigators	Patients	Experimental Arm	Outcome
Brizel[42]	"Advanced" multisite (n = 122)	RT 1.25 Gy bid to 70 Gy with cisplatin 12 mg/m²/d × 5 d and 5-FU 600 mg/m²/d × 5 d given during wk 1 and 6. Two adjuvant cycles cisplatin/5-FU followed.	LRC improved 70% vs. 44% (P = .01) and 3-yr survival rate 55% vs. 34% (P = .07)
Wendt[44]	Unresectable multisite (n = 298)	Split course, accelerated RT 70.2 Gy with cisplatin 60 mg/m², 5-FU 350 mg/m² IV, then 350 mg/m²/d and leucovorin infusions × 4 days given wk 1, 4, and 7.	LRC was 36% vs. 17% @ 3 yr (P < .004) OS rate was 48% vs. 24% (P < .004)
Calais[45]	Stage III/IV oropharynx (n = 226)	RT qd to 70 Gy carboplatin 70 mg/m²/d and 5-FU 600 mg/m²/d CI × 4 d, starting on d 1, 22, 43.	LRC improved 66% vs. 47%; OS rate was 51% vs. 31% (P = 0.02) @ 3 yr.
Jeremic[46]	Stage III/IV, multisite (n = 130)	Hfx to 77 Gy—cisplatin 6 mg qd.	Improved LRC 50% vs. 36% (P = .04); distant control 86% vs. 57% (P = .001); and OS rate 46% vs. 25% @ 5 yr

RT, radiotherapy; LRC, locoregional control; OS, overall survival; Hfx, hyperfractionated radiotherapy; bid, twice daily; qd, every day.

chemoradiation.[43] Wendt and coworkers reported a statistically significant 3-year survival advantage after concurrent use of cisplatin, 5-FU, and leucovorin given in a split-course, accelerated radiation format compared with the same radiation schedule given as a single therapeutic modality.[44] Calais and associates compared a more standard once-daily fractionation radiation schedule with a regimen combining the same radiotherapy schedule and concurrent carboplatin and 5-FU, demonstrating a statistically significant advantage in locoregional tumor control and overall survival rate at 3 years.[45] This report is particularly germane because the study group consisted only of patients with oropharyngeal cancer. Finally, Jeremic and colleagues compared the value of adding daily cisplatin to a hyperfractionated radiation therapy program with the same radiation schedule given alone in patients with locally advanced squamous cell cancer of the head and neck.[46] In this recent report, locoregional and distant disease control and overall survival rate were improved at the 5-year mark.

The clearest benefit in all four studies was an improvement in locoregional control that translated into a survival advantage. The combination regimens resulted in greater acute toxicity, especially mucositis and hematologic effects, but there was no obvious escalation of long-term sequelae. However, this potential problem area has not been fully studied. In aggregate, the overall 3-year survival rate exceeded 50% in these experimental programs, underscoring the potential therapeutic efficacy of concomitant chemotherapy and radiation in advanced cancer of the head and neck.

As was noted in the previous paragraph, concurrent chemotherapy, particularly with multiple drugs, leads to a marked increase in acute toxicity. "In-field" mucositis and dermatitis can be severe, are associated with much discomfort, and may lead to increased risk of infection, poor nutritional intake, and interruption of radiotherapy or dose reductions of chemotherapy. This may compromise tumor control and ultimate survival. There also is the potential for an increase in serious long-term toxic effects because survival is prolonged after these intensive treatment programs.[47] For optimal results, concurrent treatments should be administered in centers where oncology professionals have sufficient training and expertise, and experienced supportive care teams are available.

Despite some initial anxiety, innovative treatment programs in which radiotherapy is administered in split-course or cycling schedules have emerged. These trials have shown high complete remission rates and feasibility and have offered the promise of improved survival with organ preservation. Phase II trials from the Chicago group investigated the potential utility of a cisplatin-based induction regimen with concurrent chemotherapy consisting of infusional 5-FU, hydroxyurea, and radiation (FHX) in patients with stage IV disease.[48] The FHX regimen was given on days 1 to 5 every 14 days, in effect an alternate-week schedule. Organ preservation principles were maintained, with only a minority of patients undergoing limited surgery. Locoregional tumor control was achieved in 75% of patients and distant control in 90%. The 5-year survival rate exceeded 60%, with only a minority of patients undergoing limited surgery. This experience led to subsequent studies in which cisplatin or paclitaxel was added to the FHX regimen.[49, 50] With this third systemically active agent, the radiotherapy fractionation

schedule was intensified to twice-daily administration and the induction component was deleted. Locoregional control improved to 90%, providing increased evidence that the protraction or cycling of radiotherapy in the presence of concomitant chemotherapy is not detrimental and that locoregional control without surgery is feasible in patients with advanced-stage disease. An ancillary observation has been that the functional status for patients so treated is acceptable. Organ preservation does not necessarily correlate with preserved function, but a 2-year analysis indicated that 75% of surviving patients had acceptable speech and swallowing performance. Long-term follow-up data are awaited, and controlled trials are needed to assess the ultimate value of such regimens.

Not all patients with stage III or IV disease should receive chemoradiation. Multiple factors, including precise T and N staging, general medical condition, and expertise within the institution, must be considered before a specific treatment plan is designed. At M.D. Anderson, we often rely on radiotherapy for patients with T1-2N2-3 cancers of the oropharynx because definitive treatment is highly effective in sterilizing the T-site. Residual neck disease should be treated with salvage neck dissection. Complete radiographic response in the neck does not require planned postradiotherapeutic neck dissection.[43]

A multidisciplinary care group is necessary to optimize the outcomes of patients with cancer of the oropharynx. Rehabilitative therapy focusing on speech and swallowing functions, attention to dentition, and nutritional support, often with some form of gastric feeding tube, should be routine considerations. Longitudinal assessment of quality of life measures and functional parameters should be included in head and neck cancer trials. Social and psychological consultations are needed for many patients. Supportive measures (e.g., granulocyte/macrophage colony-stimulating factors to promote mucosal healing) and radioprotectants (e.g., amifostine) to enhance tolerance of therapy by normal tissues require further study. Advances in radiobiology and physics have led to sophisticated conformal and intensity-modulated treatment-planning techniques and hyperfractioned or concomitant boost dosing schedules. Integration of these approaches into combined treatment programs is anticipated, with or without sensitizing chemotherapy.

Salvage Surgery

Salvage surgery following failure of radiation therapy alone, radiation therapy in combination with chemotherapy, or radiation therapy in combination with biologic therapy has recently become an issue of importance in cancer of the oropharynx as the use of radiation-based approaches has become commonplace in the primary definitive management of these cancers. The oncologic surgeon must be cautious in consideration of surgical approaches in patients with persistent or recurrent disease in these sites. In today's clinical environment, failure to respond to radiation therapy must be considered a biologic indicator and a potential predictor of poor outcome. The grave consequence of primary oropharyngeal disease that persists following radiotherapy alone or concomitant chemotherapy and radiotherapy is known.[34] Surgical salvage may not benefit the patient by prolonging survival or improving quality of life, but it may provide palliation for patients with severe pain or draining wounds or necrotic bone.

Salvage Surgery for Residual Neck Disease

Evaluation of the results of a cooperative study and subsequent analyses of residual disease at laryngeal sites has provided evidence suggesting that surgical salvage of neck disease of N2a or higher stage should be performed following definitive radiation therapy to the neck. At M.D. Anderson Cancer Center, our multidisciplinary programmatic experience in oropharyngeal cancer did not appear to be consistent with these observations. We therefore sought to determine the role of salvage surgery in patients treated with definitive radiation and chemotherapy for cancers at these specific sites in the oropharynx.

In our report of radiation-based treatment for cancer of the oropharynx with advanced neck disease (stage N2a or greater), not all patients required salvage neck surgery.[31] Nevertheless, there was a clear subgroup that required neck dissection following radiation-based treatment. In patients with radiographic evidence of persistent disease (by CT scan, MRI, or ultrasound), neck dissection should be performed 6 to 10 weeks following completion of definitive radiation therapy. Dissections may require lymphadenectomy of levels I through V or a more extended approach that may require coverage of the great vessels and resurfacing of the neck in more advanced cases. In our experience, patients with radiographic evidence of residual disease who received planned postradiation/postsurgical treatment of the neck all obtained regional control. This occurred independent of the pretreatment stage of neck disease, which ranged from N2a to N3. Unfortunately, patients with incomplete radiographic response in the neck exhibited significantly compromised survival.

Surgical Salvage of Primary Tumor Site Following Definitive Radiation-Based Therapy

Centers in which radiation-based approaches to the treatment of cancer of the oropharynx have been commonplace for decades, including ours, have extensive experience with surgical salvage of the primary cancer site. Although surgery in these circumstances is sometimes considered the "last hope" for patients, the true aims of surgery must be considered carefully by the surgeon as well as by the patient and family members. In patients with an advanced primary cancer following definitive radiation therapy, surgical salvage for persistent or recurrent disease is fraught with failure—failure to obtain locoregional control and ultimately to cure the disease or provide palliation for the patient. In our experience with combination chemotherapy and radiation therapy, surgical salvage for persistent disease in the primary site was not observed.[34]

Although all oncologic head and neck surgeons have their unique fortunate patients who have successfully undergone salvage following radiation therapy to a primary tumor site in the oropharynx, the true success rate of primary site salvage is probably less than 15%.[26] Even small primary cancer that recurs or persists may require extensive resection and reconstruction despite the perceived limited localization of the disease. Patients with extensive locally persistent or recurrent disease should not undergo surgical resection in a "palliative" sense because, in our opinion, surgery plays no role in true palliation in this disease. Palliation in the sense of airway support and enteral supplementation is, nevertheless, frequently appropriate.

◼ RECONSTRUCTION

Reconstruction of the oropharyngeal cancer defect has been revolutionized over the past several decades. The "ladder" of reconstruction philosophy, ranging from healing by second intention to free-tissue transfer, must be available in the care of these patients. The objective of reconstruction must be to restore the integrity of the oropharynx in its essential functions of deglutition, respiration, and speech production, as well as in cosmesis. An intimate understanding of the impact of the defect, the maxillofacial prosthetic potential, and the functional and cosmetic roles of the ablated tissue must be considered in successful reconstruction. The advent of sensate flaps, mandibular reconstruction, and maxillofacial prosthetics all must be considered in conjunction with the multidisciplinary rehabilitation of the patient with oropharyngeal cancer.

◼ CONCLUSIONS

Advances in the treatment of patients with oropharyngeal carcinoma have been made through refinement of radiation therapy fractionation and technology and the combination of cytotoxic agents with radiation. Combined modality treatment with concurrent chemotherapy and radiation appears to have had a significant impact on locoregional disease control and overall survival rate in selected patients with advanced cancer of the oropharynx. However, a true standard program has not yet been identified. This approach to therapy is best offered in institutions with experienced multidisciplinary treatment teams, including not only surgical, radiation, and medical oncologists but also specialized head and neck nurses, oncologic dentists, and speech-language therapists. The toxic effects associated with intensive concurrent chemotherapy and radiation are formidable; therefore, performance of long-term outcome studies is imperative to assess general medical performance levels, quality of life, and disease control.

Support of clinical trials is important. Integration of more sophisticated radiation techniques and increased emphasis on rehabilitation strategies are anticipated. Therapeutic trials in the future can be expected to introduce novel biologic and chemotherapeutic drugs with the potential for increased efficacy and less toxicity. Investigator and patient participation in these activities is strongly encouraged so that this clinical science can be advanced.

REFERENCES

1. Greenlee RT, Hill-Harmon MB, Murray T, et al: Cancer statistics, 2001. CA Cancer J Clin 51:15–36, 2001.
2. Rouviere H: Anatomy of the human lymphatic system. Ann Harbor, Edwards Brothers, 1938.
3. Wenig BM: General principles of head and neck pathology (Chapter 15). In Head and Neck Cancer: A Multidisciplinary Approach. Philadelphia, Lippincott-Raven, 1999, pp 253–333.

4. Slaughter DP, Southwick HW, Smejkal W: "Field cancerization" in oral stratified squamous epithelium: Clinical implications of multicentric origin. Cancer 6:963, 1953.

5. Blot WJ, McLaughlin JK, Winn DM, et al: Smoking and drinking in relation to oral and pharyngeal cancer. Cancer Res 48:3282, 1988.

6. Graham S, Dayal H, Rohrer T, et al: Dentition, diet, tobacco, and alcohol in the epidemiology of oral cancer. J Natl Cancer Inst 59:1611, 1977.

7. Wynder EL, Stellman SD: Comparative epidemiology of tobacco related cancers. Cancer Res 37:4608, 1977.

8. Schottenfeld D, Gantt RD, Wynder EL: The role of alcohol and tobacco in multiple primary cancers of the upper digestive system, larynx and lung: A prospective study. Prev Med 3:277, 1974.

9. Moore C: Cigarette smoking and cancer of the mouth, pharynx and larynx. JAMA 218:553, 1971.

10. Spitz MR, Trizna Z: Molecular epidemiology and genetic predisposition for head and neck cancer (Chapter 2). In Head and Neck Cancer a Multidisciplinary Approach. Philadelphia, Lippincott-Raven, 1999, pp 11–22.

11. Higginson J, Terracini B, Agthe C: Nutrition and cancer: Ingestion of foodborne carcins. In Schottenfeld D (ed): Cancer Epidemiology and Prevention: Current Concepts. Springfield, Illinois, Charles C Thomas, 1974, p 177.

12. Sporn MB, Clamon GH, Dunlop NM, et al: Activity of vitamin A analogues in cell cultures of mouse epidermis and organ cultures of hamster trachea. Nature 253:47, 1975.

13. Gillison ML, Shah KV: Human papillomavirus–associated head and neck squamous cell carcinoma: Mounting evidence for an etiologic role for human papillomavirus in a subset of head and neck cancers. Curr Opin Oncol 13:183–188, 2001.

14. Gillison M, Koch W, Capone R, et al: Evidence for a causal association between human papillomavirus and a subset of head and neck cancers. J Natl Cancer Inst 92:709–720, 2000.

15. Sturgis EM, Wei Q: Genetic susceptibility—molecular epidemiology of head and neck cancer. Curr Opin Oncol (in press).

16. Hollstein M, Sidransky D, Vogelstein B, et al: p53 mutation in human cancers. Science 253:49–53, 1991.

17. Somers K, Merrick MA, Lopez ME, et al: Frequent p53 mutations in head and neck cancer. Cancer Res 52:5997–6000, 1992.

18. Boyle JO, Hakim J, Koch W, et al: The incidence of p53 mutations increases with progression of head and neck cancer. Cancer Res 53:4477–4480, 1993.

19. Brennan JA, Boyle JO, Koch WM, et al: Association between cigarette smoking and mutation of the p53 gene in squamous-cell carcinoma of the head and neck. N Engl J Med 332:712–717, 1995.

20. Califano J, van de Riet P, Westra W, et al: Genetic progression model for head and neck cancer: Implications for field cancerization. Cancer Res 56:2488–2492, 1996.

21. van der Riet P, Nawroz H, Hruban RH, et al: Frequent loss of chromosome 9p21–22 early in head and neck cancer progression. Cancer Res 54:1156–1158, 1994.

22. Berenson JR, Yang J, Michel RA: Frequent amplification of the bcl-1 locus in head and neck squamous cell carcinomas. Oncogene 4:1111–1116, 1989.

23. Callendar T, El-Naggar AK, Lee MS, et al: PRAD-1 (CCND1)/cyclin D1 oncogene amplification in primary head and neck squamous cell carcinoma. Cancer 74:152–158, 1994.

24. Hartwell LH, Kastan MB: Cell cycle control and cancer. Science 266:1821–1828, 1994.

25. Mao L, El-Naggar AK: Molecular changes in the multistage pathogenesis of head and neck cancer (Chapter 13). In Srivastava S, Henson DE, Gazdar AF (eds): Molecular Pathology of Early Cancer. Washington, DC, IOS Press, 1999.

26. Taylor RJ, Wahl RL, Sharma PK, et al: Sentinel node localization in oral cavity and oropharynx squamous cell cancer. Arch Otolaryngol Head Neck Surg 127:970–974, 2001.

27. Remmler D, Medina JE, Byers RM, et al: Treatment of choice for squamous carcinoma of the tonsillary fossa. Head Neck Surg 7:206–211, 1985.

28. Koch WM, Brennan JA, Zahurak M, et al: p53 mutation and locoregional treatment failure in head and neck squamous cell carcinoma. J Natl Cancer Inst 88:1580–1586, 1996.

29. Steiner W, Ambrosch P, Hess CF, et al: Organ preservation by transoral laser microsurgery in piriform sinus carcinoma. Otolaryngol Head Neck Surg 124:58–67, 2001.

30. Clayman GL, Adams GL: Modifications of the mandibular swing for preservation of occlusion and function. Head Neck 13:102–106, 1991.

31. Weber RS, Peters LG, Wolf P, et al: Squamous cell carcinoma of the soft palate, uvula, and anterior faucial pillar. Otolaryngol Head Neck Surg 99:16–23, 1988.

32. Forastiere A, Koch W, Trotti A, et al: Head and neck cancer. N Engl J Med 345:1890–1900, 2001.

33. Hong WK, Lippman SM, Wolf GT: Recent advances in head and neck cancer—larynx preservation and cancer chemoprevention: The Seventeenth Annual Richard Rosenthal Foundation Award Lecture. Cancer Res 53:5113–5120, 1993.

34. Tupchong L, Scott CB, Blitzer PH, et al: Randomized study of preoperative versus postoperative radiation therapy in advanced head and neck carcinoma: Long-term follow-up of RTOG study 73–03. Int J Radiat Oncol Biol Phys 20:21–28, 1991.

35. Hong WK, Bromer RH, Amato DA, et al: Patterns of relapse in locally advanced head and neck cancer patients who achieved complete remission after combined modality therapy. Cancer 56:1242–1245, 1985.

36. Brennan JA, Mao L, Hruban RH, et al: Molecular assessment of histopathological staging in squamous-cell carcinoma of the head and neck. N Engl J Med 332:429–435, 1995.

37. The Department of Veterans Affairs Laryngeal Cancer Study Group: Induction chemotherapy plus radiation in patients with advanced laryngeal cancer. N Engl J Med 324:1685–1690, 1991.

38. Lefebvre JL, Chevalier D, Luboinski B, et al: Larynx preservation in pyriform sinus cancer: Preliminary results of a European Organization for Research and Treatment of Cancer phase III trial. EORTC Head and Neck Cancer Cooperative Group. J Natl Cancer Inst 88:890–899, 1996.

39. Shin DM, Glisson BS, Khuri FR, et al: Phase II study of induction chemotherapy with paclitaxel, ifosfamide and carboplatin (TIC) for patients with locally advanced squamous cell carcinoma of the head and neck. Cancer (in press).

40. Vokes EE: Interactions of chemotherapy and radiation. Semin Oncol 20:70–79, 1993.

41. Kies MS, Bennett CL, Vokes EE: Locally advanced head and neck cancer. Curr Treatment Options Oncol 2:7–13, 2001.

42. Brizel DM, Albers ME, Fisher SR, et al: Hyperfractionated irradiation with or without concurrent chemotherapy for locally advanced head and neck cancer. N Engl J Med 338:1798–1804, 1998.

43. Clayman GL, Johnson CH, Morrison W, et al: The role of neck dissection after chemoradiotherapy for oropharyngeal cancer with advanced nodal disease. Arch Otolaryngol Head Neck Surg 127:135–139, 2001.

44. Wendt TG, Grabenbauer GG, Rodel CM, et al: Simultaneous radiochemotherapy versus radiotherapy alone in advanced head and neck cancer: A randomized multicenter study. J Clin Oncol 16:1318–1324, 1998.

45. Calais G, Alfonsi M, Bardet E, et al: Randomized trial of radiation therapy versus concomitant chemotherapy and radiation therapy for advanced-stage oropharynx carcinoma. J Natl Inst 91:2081–2086, 1999.

46. Jeremic B, Shibamoto Y, Milicic B, et al: Hyperfractionated radiation therapy with or without concurrent low-dose daily cisplatin in locally advanced squamous cell carcinoma of the head and neck: A prospective randomized trial. J Clin Oncol 18:1458–1464, 2000.

47. Eisbruch A, Lyden T, Bradford CR, et al: Objective assessment of swallowing dysfunction and aspiration after radiation concurrent with chemotherapy for head and neck cancer. Int J Radiat Oncol Biol Phys 53:23–28, 2002.

48. Kies MS, Haraf DJ, Athanasiadis I, et al: Induction chemotherapy followed by concurrent chemoradiation for advanced head and neck cancer: Improved disease control and survival. J Clin Oncol 16:2715–2721, 1998.

49. Vokes E, Kies M, Haraf D, et al: Concomitant chemoradiotherapy as primary therapy for locoregionally advanced head and neck cancer. J Clin Oncol 18:1652–1661, 2000.

50. Kies MS, Haraf DJ, Rosen F, et al: Concomitant infusional paclitaxel and fluorouracil, oral hydroxyurea, and hyperfractionated radiation for locally advanced squamous head and neck cancer. J Clin Oncol 19:1961–1969, 2001.

CHAPTER 15

Cancer of the Larynx

Ashutosh Kacker

Suzanne Wolden

David G. Pfister

Dennis H. Kraus

▣ INTRODUCTION

The incidence of laryngeal cancer has stabilized at approximately 10,000 cases reported in the United States per year. Thus, except for oral cavity cancer, it is the most frequent cancer arising in the upper aerodigestive tract. A significant evolution has occurred in the management of these neoplasms. Previously, treatment was surgically directed. Because of an increased knowledge base regarding causes, imaging, cancer biology, and treatment effect, a number of options now exist. The integration of chemotherapy and radiation therapy has expanded organ preservation options. The patient's perspective, with emphasis on retention of speech, swallowing, and quality of life, has affected the decision-making process for these neoplasms. Patient preference, local expertise, and the availability of a spectrum of treatment options ultimately have a large impact on therapy choices.

▣ EPIDEMIOLOGY

Cancer caused an estimated 553,400 deaths in the United States in 2001, that is, a death rate of about 174 per 100,000 population. Approximately 4000 of these deaths, or nearly 1% of all cancer-related deaths, were due to laryngeal cancer. In 2001, an estimated 10,000 new cases of laryngeal cancer were diagnosed nationwide. The estimated 5-year survival for cancer of the larynx as a whole, including all stages, is 65%, making it one of the more curable cancers of the upper aerodigestive tract (Tables 15–1 and 15–2).[1, 2] However this number has not changed significantly over the past 20 years.

A distinct male predominance is noted for cancer of the larynx, but recent data show that the ratio of affected males to females is decreasing as the result of an increasing incidence among women. In the 15-year periods from 1959 through 1973 and 1974 through 1988, the male-to-female ratio for cancer of the larynx in the United States decreased from 5.6:1 to 4.5:1; the absolute incidence increased over the same period from 6 to 10 cases per 100,000.[3]

The male-to-female ratio is greater for glottic (9.2:1 among whites and 11.8:1 among blacks) than for supraglottic carcinoma (3–5:1 for both races),[4] and women are more likely to develop supraglottic cancer than glottic.[5] Cancer of the larynx is a disease of the elderly, with the peak incidence in the sixth and seventh decades.[6] Less than 1% of cases occur in patients younger than 30 years of age, although it has been reported in children with no risk factors.[7–11]

No racial predominance in the United States has been demonstrated. Some evidence exists that blacks have a higher incidence at a younger age and a poorer outcome than whites, but this has not been uniformly established.[12, 13] The distribution of carcinoma among the supraglottis, glottis, and subglottis is reported by Austen to be 40:59:1.[6]

▣ RISK FACTORS

As with most tumors, multiple factors contribute to the development of cancer of the larynx. Foremost among them is tobacco use. Second is the synergistic effect produced when tobacco is combined with heavy alcohol intake. A case-control study on the Texas Gulf Coast revealed a dose-dependent effect for cigarette smoking. The risk of developing cancer of the larynx was 4.4 times greater for those who smoked up to a half pack per day and 10.4 times greater for those who smoked more than two packs per day. Risks were also shown to decline markedly following cessation of smoking, with risk returning to nearly that of nonsmokers by 15 years after cessation.[14]

Possible effects of secondhand smoking have not yet been carefully investigated for cancer of the larynx. The relationship of alcohol consumption to the relative risk is not clear; most studies show that it has a synergistic effect when combined with smoking, but others deny that alcohol alone is an independent risk factor.[14–17] Still others contend that alcohol is an independent risk factor only for cancers of the supraglottic larynx.[14, 18]

Certain occupations and exposures also pose a higher risk for subsequent cancer of the larynx. After provision of controls for smoking, alcohol consumption, and age, a significantly increased risk has been identified for painters, metal-working and plastic-working machine operators, construction workers, and those exposed to diesel and gasoline fumes, as well as for those exposed to therapeutic doses of radiation.[19–21] A specific increased risk has also been identified for those exposed chronically to wood dust. Asbestos is also a risk factor, but it is not nearly as strong for laryngeal cancer as it is for lung cancer.[22–24]

TABLE 15-1 Estimated New Cancer Cases and Deaths by Sex for All Sites (United States, 2001)

Site	Estimated New Cases			Estimated Deaths		
	Both Sexes	Males	Females	Both Sexes	Males	Females
All	1,268,000	643,000	625,000	553,400	286,100	267,300
Tongue	7,100	4,800	2,300	1,700	1,100	600
Mouth	10,500	6,000	4,500	2,300	1,300	1,000
Pharynx	8,400	6,300	2,100	2,100	1,500	600
Other oral cavity	4,100	3,100	1,000	1,700	1,200	500
Larynx	10,000	8,000	2,000	4,000	3,100	900

Data from American Cancer Society: Cancer Facts & Figures 2001. Atlanta, American Cancer Society, 2001.

Dietary factors have also been postulated to have significant influence. A protective effect of fruits and dark-green vegetables has been demonstrated in case-control studies, possibly due to their high concentrations of carotenoids. Salt-preserved meats and high dietary fats have been implicated in increased risks for cancer of the larynx.[25, 26] Gastroesophageal reflux disease has recently been identified in several studies as a significant risk factor for cancer of the larynx.[27–31] One study has provided evidence for a specific increase in cancers of the anterior two thirds of the glottis with reflux disease.[32]

Several other factors identified by laboratory investigation await clinical correlation. Notable are infection with human papilloma virus (HPV) (specifically, strains 16, 18, and 33)[33–36] and a genetically determined susceptibility to mutagens.[37–41]

Patient age and previous lifestyle factors such as tobacco and alcohol use contribute to a high rate of medical comorbidity and second primary cancers among these patients, thus complicating management and increasing mortality. Clearly, the development of cancer of the larynx is the result of a complex interaction between host and environmental factors that we are only beginning to understand.

ANATOMY AND EMBRYOLOGY

The larynx can be divided embryologically, clinically, and anatomically into a supraglottis, glottis, and subglottis (Figs. 15–1 and 15–2). The specific anatomic features of the larynx, such as the shapes and sizes of the cartilages and the origins and insertions of the intrinsic musculature, can be found in many anatomy texts. The purpose of this section is to describe laryngeal anatomy as it relates to the origin and spread of cancer to promote better understanding

TABLE 15-2 Five-Year Relative Survival Rates of Laryngeal Cancer by Stage at Diagnosis, 1989–1996

All Stages	Local	Regional	Distant
65%	81%	52%	41%

Data from Surveillance, Epidemiology, and End Results Program, 1973–1997. Bethesda, MD, Division of Cancer Control and Population Sciences, National Cancer Institute, 2000.

of why cancers of each subsite behave so differently and how different schemes of treatment have developed.

Supraglottis

The supraglottis subunit includes the lingual and laryngeal surfaces of the epiglottis, the aryepiglottic folds, the arytenoid cartilages, the false vocal folds, and the ventricle. During embryologic development, these structures are derived from the buccopharyngeal anlagen of branchial arches three and four. The glottic and subglottic subunit develop from the tracheobronchial anlagen of the fifth and sixth branchial arches. The embryonic fusion plane between the supraglottic subunit and the glottic and subglottic subunits is represented by a horizontal line drawn through the ventricle. This horizontal plane provides the anatomic and oncologic basis of supraglottic laryngectomy.

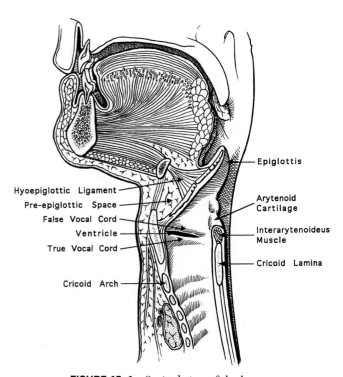

FIGURE 15–1 Sagittal view of the larynx.

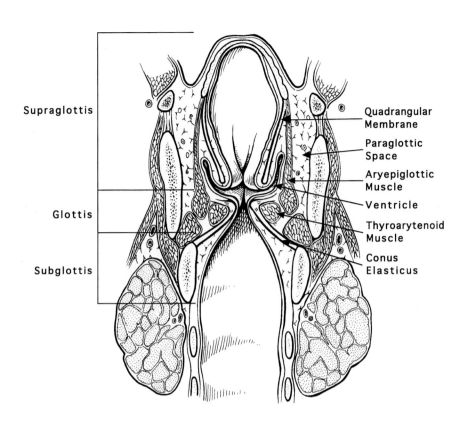

FIGURE 15–2 Coronal view of the larynx.

The supraglottic larynx comprises the suprahyoid epiglottis (both lingual and laryngeal surfaces), the infrahyoid epiglottis, the pre-epiglottic space, the laryngeal aspects of the aryepiglottic folds, the two arytenoids, and the ventricular bands (false cords). The vallecula is part of the oropharynx. The inferior boundary of the supraglottis, as defined by the American Joint Committee on Cancer (AJCC), is a horizontal plane passing through the apex of the ventricle of the larynx. This clinical definition is to be used for staging and in reporting results of cancer treatment. The anatomic division is located at the arcuate line, which marks the change from respiratory to squamous epithelium and is reliably located at the apex of the ventricle. Thus the roof of the ventricle is included in the supraglottis, and the floor belongs to the glottis.[42]

The "marginal zone" of the supraglottis is recognized because of the aggressive clinical behaviors of cancers arising in this area. It is composed of the suprahyoid epiglottis and the aryepiglottic folds. Because of their lack of embryologic separation from the adjacent hypopharynx, cancers in this zone behave similarly to the more aggressive cancers of the hypopharynx, and they carry a worse prognosis.

Histologically, the supraglottis is lined by ciliated columnar epithelium, as is the majority of the upper respiratory tract. Exceptions are the free edges of the epiglottis and the aryepiglottic folds, which are lined by stratified squamous mucosa. Mucous glands are abundant and are of greatest density in the saccule and the periarytenoid areas. Some authors relate the lymphatic spread of supraglottic cancer to the rich vascularity and lymphatics associated with these glands.[43]

Glottis

The glottic larynx includes the true vocal cords and the anterior and posterior commissures. The lower border is the horizontal plane passing 1 cm below the apex of the ventricle. Histologically, the vocal cords are covered by stratified squamous epithelium around the edges and pseudostratified ciliated epithelium at the superior and inferior aspects, where the glottis merges with the supraglottis and the subglottis, respectively. The lamina propria has (1) a superficial layer composed of loose fibrous tissues that make the Reinke's space, and (2) intermediate and deep layers of elastic and collagenous fibers that form the vocal ligament. Blood vessels and lymphatics are almost absent in Reinke's space, creating a resistance to the spread of early cancer of the glottis. No mucous glands are found on the free edge of the vocal cord, and only sparse glands are noted on the superior aspect. The conus elasticus extends upward from the superior border of the cricoid cartilage to merge with the inferior surface of the vocal ligament; it resists the extralaryngeal spread of glottic and subglottic cancer.[44]

Subglottis

The subglottic larynx has no subsites and is the area of the larynx inferior to the glottis down to the inferior rim of the cricoid cartilage. It is a rare site of origin of cancer of the larynx but is commonly involved by subglottic extension of glottic cancer. Tumors here have a higher incidence of extralaryngeal spread owing to the proximity of the cricothyroid membrane and the rich postcricoid lymphatics.

■ DIAGNOSIS

History, Physical Examination, and Laboratory Tests

The patient history should assess for risk factors such as the use of tobacco and alcohol, the occurrence and extent of weight loss, and all other medical conditions.

Common presenting symptoms include hoarseness, pain, sore throat, otalgia, odynophagia, dysphagia, and trismus. The proportion of early-stage lesions is greater among glottic tumors, and patients with a supraglottic tumor present more often with advanced-stage disease characterized by neck node metastases. Hoarseness is the most common symptom and is more prevalent among patients with a glottic tumor. The symptom patterns of supraglottic carcinoma are less well defined.

A complete examination of the head and neck, including examination of all areas of the oral cavity and pharynx, and indirect laryngoscopy must be performed. Indirect laryngoscopy is supplemented by fiberoptic examination and stroboscopy of the larynx and pharynx. Palpation of the floor of the mouth, tongue, base of the tongue, and/or tonsil is necessary for evaluation of the "base" or depth of the tumor and its proximity to the mandible, and for exclusion of a second primary. Examination should include an assessment of the status of the mandible and the dentition, as well as an evaluation of the status of the airway. Careful palpation of the neck bilaterally is important, as is documentation of the location (group or level I to VI), size, mobility, and relationship of the node(s) to adjacent structures. Staging of the primary and of the cervical lymph nodes must be documented.

Diagnosis of a neoplasm of the larynx usually requires direct laryngoscopy with the patient under general anesthesia. Direct laryngoscopy not only helps the clinician in making a diagnosis; it is also an important tool in proper mapping of the tumor for further management planning. The use of laryngeal telescopes allows adequate and thorough evaluation of the extent of glottic and supraglottic

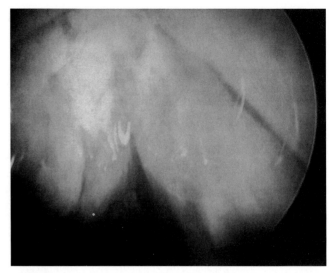

FIGURE 15–4 A 120-degree endoscope examining the same patient with 8 mm of subglottic extension.

neoplasms (Figs. 15–3 through 15–14). Many examiners advocate a bronchoscopy and esophagoscopy during the same anesthesia to help in mapping selected, more extensive tumors and in evaluating for concurrent cancers, although this practice has not been proved effective in this regard. Fine-needle aspiration biopsy of suspected metastatic disease can be performed in selected cases.

Laboratory tests are usually directed by the findings on history and physical examination. A pulmonary function test may be performed if partial laryngectomy is being considered. A chest radiograph and baseline liver function testing are performed to assess metastatic disease, a secondary primary, or other factors that may complicate treatment. Consultations with other services, including radiation therapy, medical oncology, dentistry, speech pathology, psychiatry, and general medical services, are obtained as indicated.

Radiographic Examination

Clinical/endoscopic examination alone often fails to reveal tumor invasion of the laryngeal cartilages and of the

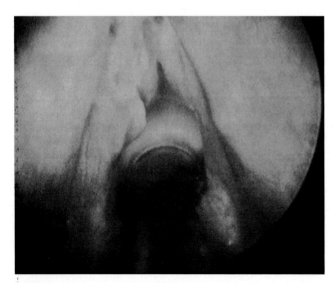

FIGURE 15–3 T1 glottic carcinoma visualized at the time of operative endoscopy with the 0-degree endoscope.

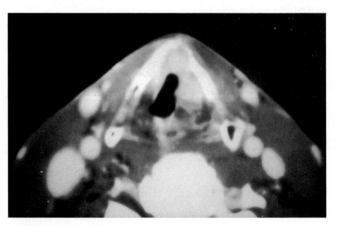

FIGURE 15–5 CT scan of the larynx reveals early destruction of the thyroid cartilage in the anterior commissure.

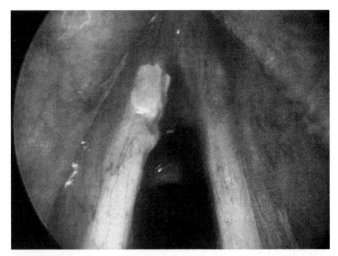

FIGURE 15–6 A 0-degree laryngeal telescope is used to visualize a T1 glottic cancer.

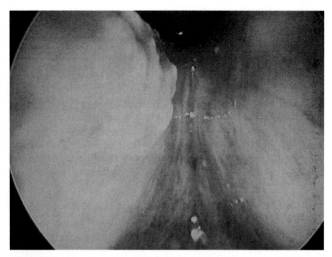

FIGURE 15–8 A 120-degree view confirming no evidence of significant subglottic extension.

extralaryngeal soft tissues, resulting in a low staging accuracy (57.5%). Many pT4 (according to the Union International Contre le Cancer [UICC] Tumor-Node-Metastasis [TNM] Staging System) tumors remain clinically unrecognized (Fig. 15–15). The combination of clinical/endoscopic evaluation and an additional radiologic examination, by either computed tomography (CT) or magnetic resonance imaging (MRI), results in significantly improved staging accuracy (CT scan improves imaging in 80% of patients, and MRI in 87.5%). MRI is significantly more sensitive but is less specific than CT in detecting cartilage invasion. Therefore, MRI tends to overestimate cartilage invasion and lead to overtreatment, whereas CT tends to underestimate cartilage invasion and may result in inadequate therapy.[45] A study by Stadler and colleagues revealed functional CT (spiral CT scans) to be more accurate than nonfunctional CT in the T-staging of laryngeal and hypopharyngeal carcinomas.[46] In a study from Toronto, the T classification was altered in 20.2% of those patients who underwent CT, with most being "upstaged."[47] The role of positron emission tomography (PET) scanning is

more controversial; the use of PET is currently limited to classifying equivocal findings on cross-sectional imaging and facilitating early detection of recurrent or persistent head and neck cancer after radiotherapy and/or chemotherapy has been administered.

In a study by Hollenbeak and colleagues, the PET scan was used for the purpose of evaluating patients with an N0 neck with squamous cell carinoma (SCC) of the upper aerodigestive tract. The incremental cost-effectiveness ratio for the PET strategy was $8718 per year of life saved, or $2505 per quality-adjusted life-year. This supports that a diagnostic and treatment strategy that proceeds from classification of N0 to a PET scan is cost-effective.[48]

Kresnik studied the usefulness of ^{18}F fluorodeoxyglucose ([18]FDG)-PET in the diagnosis and staging of primary and recurrent malignant head and neck tumors in comparison with conventional imaging methods (including ultrasonography,

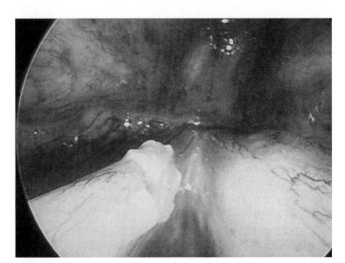

FIGURE 15–7 A 70-degree laryngeal telescope with limited infracord extension and no true subglottic involvement.

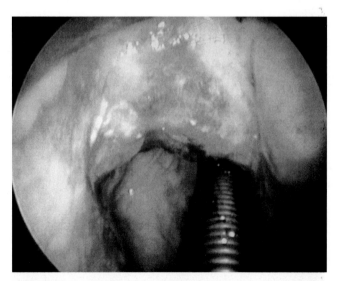

FIGURE 15–9 A 0-degree laryngeal telescope is used to visualize the laryngeal surface of the epiglottic primary. The relationship of the inferior aspect of the tumor to the anterior commissure is difficult to discern.

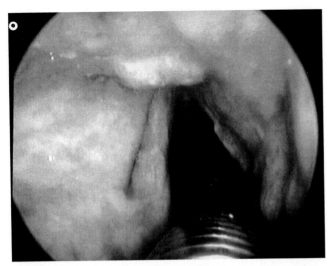

FIGURE 15–10 With a 70-degree laryngeal telescope, it remains difficult to discern the inferior aspect of the tumor in relationship to the anterior commissure.

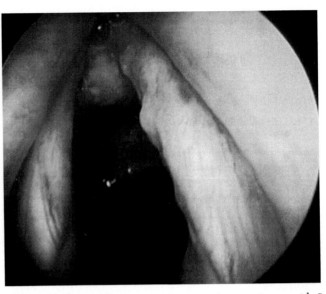

FIGURE 15–12 A 0-degree anterior commissure primary with 8 mm of subglottic extension.

radiography, CT, and MRI), physical examination, panendoscopy, and biopsy in clinical routine evaluation.[49] The study concluded that compared with conventional diagnostic methods, [18]FDG-PET provides additional and clinically relevant information in the detection of primary and metastatic carcinomas, as well as in the early detection of recurrent or persistent head and neck cancer after radiotherapy and/or chemotherapy has been administered. [18]FDG-PET should therefore be performed early in the clinical routine, usually before CT or MRI is provided.[49]

In a study by Stokkel and colleagues, the sensitivity for the detection of lymph node metastases per neck side was 96%, 85%, and 64% for [18]FDG-PET, CT, and ultrasound/fine-needle aspiration biopsy, respectively.[50] The specificity was 90%, 86%, and 100% for [18]FDG-PET, CT, and ultrasound/fine-needle aspiration biopsy, respectively.

In terms of the classification, [18]FDG-PET showed the best correlation with the histologic data. Finally, in nine patients (17%), a second primary tumor was detected by [18]FDG-PET and confirmed by histologic evaluation. The authors concluded that because of the high prevalence of second primary tumors detected by [18]FDG-PET and the decreased error rate in the assessment of lymph node involvement compared with CT and ultrasound, [18]FDG-PET should be routinely performed in patients with primary head and neck cancer.[50]

In another study by Kau and colleagues, the diagnostic accuracy of PET for detecting "neck sides" with malignant involvement was superior to that of morphologic procedures, with a sensitivity and specificity of 87% and 94%, respectively, compared with CT values of 65% and 47% and MRI values of 88% and 41%, respectively.[51] The authors advised that a short PET protocol suitable for routine

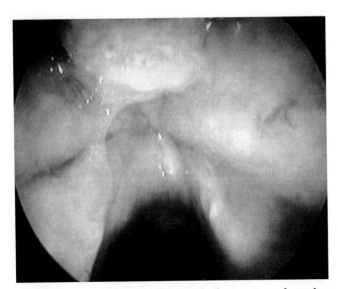

FIGURE 15–11 A 120-degree laryngeal telescope is used visualize a 5-mm border of normal mucosa between the inferior extent of the epiglottic primary and the anterior commissure.

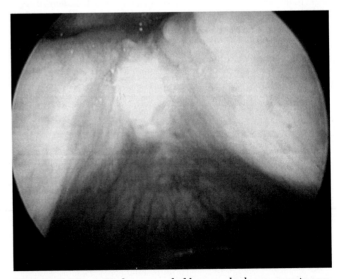

FIGURE 15–13 A 70-degree angled laryngeal telescope again confirms 8 mm of subglottic extension.

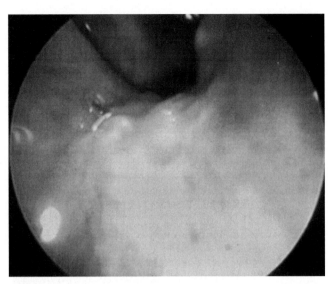

FIGURE 15–14 A 120-degree laryngeal telescope confirms considerable subglottic involvement.

clinical use is superior to morphologic procedures (CT and MRI) for the detection of lymph node involvement in head and neck SCCs.[51]

Although the PET scan is still in its infancy, data suggest that it should play an increasing role in the management of head and neck cancer patients.

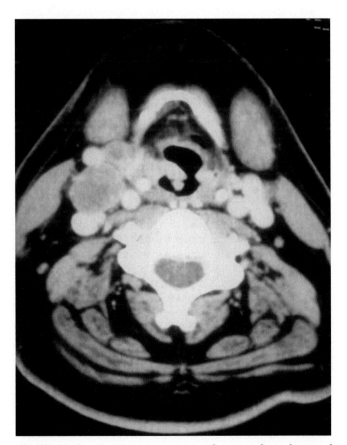

FIGURE 15–15 Contiguous extension of a supraglottic laryngeal primary with involvement of the soft tissues of the neck.

STAGING

Primary Site

The specifics of the primary staging system for the supraglottic, glottic, and subglottic larynx are listed later in the discussion of the TNM staging system.

Regional Lymph Nodes

The incidence and distribution of cervical nodal metastases from cancer of the larynx vary with the site of origin and the "T" classification of the primary tumor. The true vocal cords are nearly devoid of lymphatics, and tumors of that site alone rarely spread to regional nodes. In contrast, the supraglottis has a rich and bilaterally interconnected lymphatic network, and primary supraglottic cancers are commonly accompanied by regional nodal spread. Glottic tumors may spread directly to adjacent soft tissues and to prelaryngeal, pretracheal, paralaryngeal, and paratracheal nodes, as well as to upper, middle, and lower jugular nodes. Supraglottic tumors commonly spread to upper and middle jugular nodes and considerably less commonly to submental or submandibular nodes, but only occasionally do they spread to retropharyngeal nodes. Subglottic primary tumors, which are rare, spread first to adjacent soft tissues and prelaryngeal, pretracheal, paralaryngeal, and paratracheal nodes, then to middle and lower jugular nodes.

In clinical evaluation, the physical size of the nodal mass should be measured. It is recognized that most masses larger than 3 cm in diameter are not single nodes but confluent nodes or tumors in soft tissues of the neck. Clinically positive nodes are classified into three categories: N1, N2, and N3. N2a represents patients with a single ipsilateral lymph node larger than 3 cm but not larger than 6 cm in greatest dimension; N2b represents multiple ipsilateral lymph nodes, none larger than 6 cm in greatest dimension; N2c represents bilateral or contralateral lymph nodes, none larger than 6 cm in greatest dimension. Midline nodes are considered ipsilateral nodes.

In addition to the components used to describe the N category, regional lymph nodes should be described according to the level of the neck involved. Pathologic examination is necessary for documentation of such disease extent. Imaging studies showing amorphous spiculated margins of involved nodes or involvement of internodal fat, resulting in loss of normal oval to round nodal shape, strongly suggest extracapsular (extranodal) tumor spread. No imaging study can yet identify microscopic foci in regional nodes, nor can the distinction be made between small reactive nodes and small malignant nodes without central radiographic inhomogeneity.

Metastatic Sites

Distant spread is common among patients who have bulky adenopathy. When distant metastases occur, spread to the lungs is most common; skeletal or hepatic metastases occur less often. Patients with extracapsular spread have a high rate of metastasis to distant sites. Mediastinal lymph node metastases are considered distant metastases.

RULES FOR CLASSIFICATION

Clinical Staging

The larynx is assessed primarily by inspection, with the use of indirect mirror and direct endoscopic examinations. The tumor must be confirmed histologically, and any other data obtained by biopsy may be included. Cross-sectional imaging in laryngeal carcinoma is particularly recommended when the extent of the primary tumor is in question based on clinical examination; it is best accomplished with a high-resolution/fine-cut CT scan through the larynx. Radiologic nodal staging should be done simultaneously to supplement clinical examination. Endoscopic examination with the patient under general anesthesia is generally performed after completion of other diagnostic studies that accurately assess, document, and biopsy the tumor.

Pathologic Staging

All information used in clinical staging and in histologic study of the surgically resected specimen is also used for pathologic staging (Table 15–3). The surgeon's evaluation of gross unresected residual tumor must also be included. The pathologic description of any lymphadenectomy specimen should describe the size, number, and level of involved lymph nodes, as well as whether extracapsular spread is present.

A number of investigators have used grade of tumor as a prognostic factor. There is bias in the literature about high-grade tumors' having a poor prognosis, but this is controversial as there are no data to support this conception.

DEFINITION OF TNM[42]

Primary Tumor (T)

TX Primary tumor cannot be assessed
T0 No evidence of primary tumor
Tis Carcinoma in situ

Supraglottis

T1 Tumor limited to one subsite of supraglottis with normal vocal cord mobility
T2 Tumor invades mucosa of more than one subsite of supraglottis or glottis or region outside the supraglottis (e.g., mucosa of the base of tongue, vallecula, medial wall pyriform sinus) without fixation of the larynx
T3 Tumor limited to the larynx with vocal cord fixation and/or invades any of the following: postcricoid area, pre-epiglottic tissues
T4 Tumor invades through the thyroid cartilage and/or extends into soft tissues of the neck, thyroid, and/or esophagus

Glottis

T1 Tumor limited to the vocal cord(s) (may involve anterior or posterior commissure) with normal mobility
T1a Tumor limited to one vocal cord
T1b Tumor involves both vocal cords
T2 Tumor extends to supraglottis and/or subglottis and/or occurs with impaired vocal cord mobility
T3 Tumor limited to the larynx with vocal cord fixation
T4 Tumor invades through the thyroid cartilage and/or to other tissues beyond the larynx (e.g., trachea, soft tissues of neck, including the thyroid and pharynx)

Subglottis

T1 Tumor limited to the subglottis
T2 Tumor extended to vocal cord(s) with normal or impaired mobility
T3 Tumor limited to the larynx with vocal cord fixation
T4 Tumor invades through the cricoid or thyroid cartilage and/or to other tissues beyond the larynx (e.g., trachea, soft tissues of neck, including the thyroid and pharynx)

Regional Lymph Nodes (N)

NX Regional lymph nodes cannot be assessed
N0 No regional lymph node metastasis
N1 Metastasis in a single ipsilateral lymph node, 3 cm or smaller in greatest dimension
N2 Metastasis in a single ipsilateral lymph node, larger than 3 cm but not larger than 6 cm in greatest dimension; or in multiple ipsilateral lymph nodes, none larger than 6 cm in greatest dimension; or in bilateral or contralateral lymph nodes, none larger than 6 cm in greatest dimension
N2a Metastasis in a single ipsilateral lymph node larger than 3 cm but not larger than 6 cm in greatest dimension
N2b Metastasis in multiple ipsilateral lymph nodes, none larger than 6 cm in greatest dimension
N2c Metastasis in bilateral or contralateral lymph nodes, none larger than 6 cm in greatest dimension
N3 Metastasis in a lymph node larger than 6 cm in greatest dimension

Distant Metastasis (M)

MX Distant metastasis cannot be assessed
M0 No distant metastasis
M1 Distant metastasis

TABLE 15-3 Stage Grouping

Stage	T	N	M
0	Tis	N0	M0
I	T1	N0	M0
II	T2	N0	M0
III	T3	N0	M0
	T1	N1	M0
	T2	N1	M0
	T3	N1	M0
IVA	T4	N0	M0
	T4	N1	M0
	Any T	N2	M0
IVB	Any T	N3	M0
IVC	Any T	Any N	M1

Histopathologic Grade (G)

GX Grade cannot be assessed
G1 Well differentiated
G2 Moderately differentiated
G3 Poorly differentiated

NATURAL COURSE OF DISEASE

Nodal Metastases

Most nodal metastases are concentrated within level II, level III, and level IV; level I and level V are rarely involved.

Occult cervical lymph node metastases are often associated with cancer of the supraglottic larynx. The overall incidence of occult lymph node metastases in all stages of supraglottic carcinoma is approximately 27%. Based on the preoperative staging of the tumor, 14% of cases had occult metastases involving lymph nodes in T1 tumors, 21% in T2 tumors, 35% in T3 tumors, and 75% in T4 tumors. The incidence of occult metastases was higher for the less differentiated tumors and for the ones with a higher T value; the effects of both factors are combined, thereby increasing the rate of occult metastases.[52]

In a study from Washington University of 2550 patients with laryngeal cancer, the overall incidence of delayed regional metastases was 12.4% (317/2550 patients); distant metastases, 8.5% (217/2550); and second primary tumors, 8.9% (228/2550), with a 5-year disease-specific survival of 41%, 6.4%, and 35%, respectively. Delayed regional metastases and distant metastases were related to advanced primary disease (T4 stage), lymph node metastases (node positive [N+]), the tumor arising in the hypopharynx as the primary site, and locoregional tumor recurrence (*P* = .028). Advanced regional metastases at initial diagnosis (N2 and N3 disease) increased the incidence of delayed and distant metastases threefold (*P*=.017). Incidences of delayed regional metastases by anatomic location of the primary tumor were as follows: glottic, 4.4%; supraglottic, 16%; subglottic, 11.5%; aryepiglottic fold, 21.9%; pyriform sinus, 31.1%; and posterior hypopharyngeal wall, 18.5%. Delayed regional metastases to the ipsilateral treated neck had a significantly worse survival prognosis than did delayed metastases to the contralateral nontreated neck.[53]

Distant Metastases

Distant metastases are associated with a poor prognosis and seem to be on the rise with the improved locoregional control of laryngeal cancer. Prognostic factors must be delineated so that patients at highest risk for distant metastases can be identified. Among patients with cancers of the head and neck region, approximately 8% eventually develop distant metastases.[54]

The lung is the most common site of distant metastases in laryngeal SCC. Staging has been helpful in predicting distant metastases in that most cases occur during stages III and IV (85%). A supraglottic primary is the most common subsite at which patients with laryngeal cancer develop distant metastases.

In the Washington University study, the incidences of distant metastases were as follows: glottic, 4%; supraglottic, 3.7%; subglottic, 14%; aryepiglottic fold, 16%; pyriform fossa, 17.2%; and posterior hypopharyngeal wall, 17.6%. Seventeen patients with cancer of the hypopharynx (2%) presented with M1 disease.[47]

The overall 5-year disease-specific survival after patients developed distant metastases was 6.4%. Distant metastases were related to advanced local disease (T3 + T4), lymph node metastases at presentation (N+), tumor location (hypopharynx), and locoregional tumor recurrence (*P* = .028). A meta-analysis of variables that predispose to a higher incidence of distant metastases identified tumor location (hypopharynx > larynx), advanced primary disease (T3 + T4), regional disease (N+), locoregional recurrence, and advanced regional metastasis (N2 + N3).[55]

Second Primary Cancers

In a study of 514 cases of laryngeal cancer, the presence of second primary neoplasms was established in 42 (8.17%); 8 were synchronous and 34 were metachronous to the initial larynx primary. Respiratory and upper gastrointestinal sites were affected primarily, incidence was highest among septuagenarians, and staging of the index primary was found to be irrelevant to the incidence rates of second primaries. The modality of original treatment of the index primary did not statistically influence incidence rates.

In a retrospective study of 410 patients from France, the incidence of second primary tumors was 23.9% (98/410). Lung cancer was the most common second primary, and 68.4% (67/98) of patients who developed a second primary died of disease. The 10-year actuarial survival estimates were 24% for a lung second primary; 43.7% for a nonlung, non–upper aerodigestive tract second primary; and 63.4% for an upper aerodigestive tract second primary.[56]

In another retrospective review of 240 patients from Oregon with T1–T2 SCC of the larynx, 72% had glottic primaries, 27% had supraglottic tumors, and 1% had subglottic disease. With a median follow-up of 68 months, 68 patients (28%) have developed 72 other cancers. Ten of 68 presented with synchronous primaries (15%).[57]

PATHOLOGY

Keratosis

Keratosis of the larynx involves most commonly the true vocal cords and the interarytenoid area. It often occurs in smokers, singers, and professional voice users. It is grossly characterized as white, thickened plaques. Microscopically, keratotic lesions are characterized by increased thickness of a normally present keratin layer of the epithelium. Keratosis is more accurately defined as the presence of (1) a keratin layer in a normally nonkeratinized epithelium and (2) acanthosis.[58]

Dysplasia

Dysplasia refers to a microscopic change present in some cases of keratosis that is characterized by cellular atypia, loss of maturity, and loss of stratification. Three grades of dysplasia are defined by the World Health Organization (WHO) classification.[59]

1. Mild, in which changes are limited to the lower third of the epithelial thickness
2. Moderate, in which changes are limited to the lower two thirds of the epithelial thickness
3. Severe, in which changes involve more than the lower two thirds of the epithelial thickness, but the cells are less crowded as in classic carcinoma in situ (CIS) and usually reveal greater differentiation

Carcinoma In Situ

CIS may be present as the only lesion, or it may occur at the periphery of an invasive carcinoma. The standard criterion for diagnosis is the presence of atypical changes throughout the epithelium without evidence of surface maturation or invasion through the basement membrane.

Papillary CIS is a form of CIS characterized by papillary fronds with cytologic features of the classic CIS. An unknown number of untreated cases of CIS progress to invasive carcinoma. CIS of the larynx can be treated by means of biopsy, local excision, laryngofissure, stripping, or radiation.[60]

Invasive Squamous Cell Carcinoma

Microscopically, more than 90% of laryngeal carcinomas are SCCs. They are graded into well-, moderately-, and poorly differentiated lesions based on the degree of differentiation, cellular pleomorphism, and mitotic activity.[61]

Postirradiation persistence of SCC is often difficult to diagnose because postirradiation atypia is difficult to differentiate from tumor recurrence. Immunoreactivity for keratin is universally present, and cells also express epidermal growth factor receptors.[62, 63]

Prognostic indicators that have been reported in the literature for invasive SCC include the following:

1. Clinical stage and site
2. Microscopic grade
3. Field size
4. DNA ploidy
5. Lymph nodes
6. Host reaction
7. Keratin expression (controversial)
8. Perineural spread

Variants of Squamous Cell Carcinoma

1. Papillary SCC is characterized by an exophytic pattern of growth and is distinguished from verrucous carcinoma on the basis of cellular atypia.
2. Sarcomatoid carcinoma is composed of a small SCC with a pleomorphic sarcoma–like component.[64]
3. Basaloid SCC is characterized by a predominance of basaloid features in the epithelium.

Verrucous Carcinoma

Clinically, verrucous carcinoma is a slow-growing, locally aggressive tumor with an exophytic, fungating, warty, gray-white appearance and well-defined margins. Because it produces few early symptoms, patients often present with a bulky cancer. Histologically, this cancer is composed of elongated papillary fronds of well-differentiated squamous epithelium with extensive keratinization. Cytologic abnormalities are absent. The margins of the tumor show "pushing" rather than infiltrative growth that is usually accompanied by an exuberant host response of inflammatory cells. Regional lymph nodes are commonly enlarged and raise suspicion for occult malignancy within the lesion, but this cancer does not metastasize, and enlarged lymph nodes are invariably a part of the host inflammatory response. Diagnosis requires close cooperation between the surgeon and the pathologist and often multiple biopsies because the cancer exhibits growth characteristics of invasive carcinoma but histologically lacks the conventional features of SCC. The combination of the gross appearance of the cancer and the suggestive histologic findings is usually sufficient for the clinician to make the diagnosis.[65]

In the past, ambiguity existed in the classification of verrucous carcinoma tumors, especially those that were predominantly verrucous carcinoma with small foci of higher-grade SCC. It is noteworthy that among the verrucous carcinoma cases assigned a grade in the National Cancer Data Base (NCDB) for the years 1985 to 1990, 18.6% were grade II or higher. Newer clinicopathologic characteristics support the division of papillary SCC from other exophytic SCCs, including verrucous carcinoma. The characteristics of papillary SCC, including minimal to absent keratin production, solitary or clustered papillary lesions, and cytomorphology-like CIS, help in differentiating verrucous carcinoma from papillary SCC.[66]

Verrucous carcinoma constitutes from 1% to 3% of all laryngeal carcinomas. The larynx is the second most common site of origin in the head and neck, with the oral cavity being the most common site. Within the larynx, a majority of these cancers arise from the glottis, and the remainder almost all begin in the supraglottis.[67]

The typical patient is a man in his fifties or sixties who has been hoarse for at least a year before presentation. Rarely, hemorrhage or airway obstruction is the presenting symptom.[68] Smoking is a known risk factor, as with SCC. Overall prognosis is excellent with proper treatment, even among patients with locally advanced cancer. Several studies have linked HPV infection with the pathogenesis of verrucous carcinoma, especially infection with types 16 and 18.[69, 70] Fliss and coworkers found 13 of 29 patients (45%) with verrucous carcinoma of the larynx to have HPV detectable in their cancer by the polymerase chain reaction, all of which cases of HPV were either type 16 or 18.[71] Other researchers studying verrucous carcinoma in other sites of the body, however, have not found this association to be reliable.[72, 73] Anderson and coworkers, studying verrucous cancer of the oral cavity, found an association between simultaneous HPV infection and transfection with an activated RAS gene with oral lesions, supporting a multi-hit hypothesis for the development of this tumor.[74]

Treatment has consisted of radiation and surgery used as single agents. In 1993, Hagen and colleagues reviewed the literature on reported cases of verrucous carcinoma of the larynx.[75] Among 37 patients treated with primary radiation therapy, 18 (49%) were cured by radiation, all stages included. Of the 19 treatment failures, 12 cancers were surgically salvaged and 4 (11%) developed anaplastic transformation; all 4 patients subsequently died from disease. Of 12 radiation failures with T1 or T2 lesions, 7 patients required total laryngectomy for salvage. The same study also reviewed the reported cases of surgical treatment, ranging from vocal cord stripping to total laryngectomy. Of 144 patients, 133 (92%) were initially cured and 5 (3.5%) ultimately died from cancer.

Lundgren and coworkers reviewed their series of 44 patients with laryngeal verrucous carcinoma.[76] Of 28 who received radiotherapy, 12 were cured, 13 experienced treatment failure but were surgically salvaged, and 3 declined further treatment. One patient underwent malignant transformation of the tumor and was the only mortality from disease. Of 16 who received primary surgery, all were without evidence of disease or died from intercurrent disease at last follow-up. The authors concluded that surgery should be the primary modality of treatment unless it would require a total laryngectomy, in which case a trial of radiation therapy should be considered.

The debate concerning anaplastic transformation of verrucous carcinoma following radiation therapy remains unsettled. The early literature reports incidences of anaplastic transformation as high as 30% among those patients treated with radiation.[77] Opponents of this opinion believe that nonrepresentative biopsies that geographically miss the area of less differentiated carcinoma, as well as misclassification of well-differentiated SCC, account for the reported high incidence of supposed malignant transformation.[65] In 1998, Ferlito and colleagues reviewed 148 previously published reports of verrucous carcinoma and concluded that verrucous carcinoma was more resistant to radiation than was conventional SCC. In this review, the investigators reported a 6.7% rate of anaplastic transformation after irradiation.[78]

A recent review based on data from the NCDB included 2350 cases of verrucous carcinoma of the head and neck diagnosed between 1985 and 1996. Tumors originated most frequently in the oral cavity (55.9%) and larynx (35.2%). The most prevalent treatment was surgery alone (69.7%), followed by surgery combined with irradiation (11.0%), and irradiation alone (10.3%). Most laryngeal tumors were treated with surgery (60.3% for early and 55.6% for advanced disease), but compared with oral cavity cases, a higher proportion received radiation alone or surgery combined with radiation.[66]

Nonsquamous Tumors

Nonsquamous cancers account for less than 5% of all laryngeal malignancies. Among these, salivary or mucous gland tumors, cartilaginous tumors, sarcomas, and neuroendocrine tumors have been the most common.

Adenocarcinoma

Laryngeal adenocarcinoma is one of the three commonly reported carcinomas arising from the glandular tissues of the larynx. The other two types, adenoid cystic and mucoepidermoid carcinoma, are discussed separately. These cancers follow the distribution of the laryngeal mucous glands and are primarily supraglottic and subglottic in origin. Adenocarcinomas are most often supraglottic. Male predominance has also been reported. Clinically, the cancers appear as submucosal, nonulcerated masses. Symptoms are the same as for carcinomas of the larynx.

Most adenocarcinomas of the larynx present with advanced disease, and cervical metastases are common during the course of the disease. Distant metastases to the liver and lung account for the dismal 5-year survival of 12% to 17%.[79] Because of this aggressive behavior, most authors have recommended radical surgery, which invariably consists of total laryngectomy and radical neck dissection, except in the unusual early case. Postoperative radiotherapy is usually given, although the numbers of cases are too small to know if this confers a survival benefit. Patients die from both locoregional failure and distant metastases.

Adenoid Cystic Carcinoma

Just over 100 cases of adenoid cystic carcinoma of the larynx have been reported to date, and these represent an estimated 0.6% of all laryngeal malignancies. The most common site of origin is the subglottis, but supraglottic primaries have also been reported. Like adenoid cystic carcinoma elsewhere in the head and neck, these cancers produce only vague symptoms of pain and fullness for long periods while they spread in a perineural and infiltrative growth pattern. Patients usually present with involvement of the laryngeal framework, trachea, thyroid gland, and esophagus, especially when the primary originates from the subglottis.[80]

Extensive microscopic perineural invasion makes clear surgical margins difficult to obtain. Metastasis to the lung is common for this cancer, and patients may present with pulmonary lesions. These metastases, however, tend to be asymptomatic and indolent, allowing extended survival despite their presence. In the series of Cohen and associates,[81] patients survived an average of 3 years after the appearance of pulmonary metastasis, and 5- and 15-year survivals have been reported. Thus, most authors recommend surgery for the local and regional control of cancer, even in the presence of distant metastases. Total laryngectomy is required for subglottic cancers. Conservation surgery for supraglottic primaries and tracheal resection for lesions below the subglottis are often possible, with completion laryngectomy reserved for local recurrence.[81]

Neck dissection is indicated only for palpable or radiographically suspected metastasis. Because adenoid cystic carcinoma is characterized as radiosensitive, most authors recommend that it be used for palliation or postoperatively, as is often indicated in patients with positive or close margins. Resection of pulmonary metastases is controversial.[82]

Mucoepidermoid Carcinoma

Mucoepidermoid carcinoma of the larynx is an uncommon tumor, with a predominance in older males.[83] The supraglottis is the primary site. As with mucoepidermoid carcinoma elsewhere, low, intermediate, and high grades of malignancy have been identified, with worse prognosis among patients with high-grade lesions. Low-grade cancer rarely spreads beyond the confines of the larynx, and conservation surgery without neck dissection is often curative.[84] Radiation has not been shown to be effective when used as a single modality.

The management of high-grade mucoepidermoid carcinoma is similar to that of SCC, and the extent of surgery is dictated by the extent of the cancer. Elective neck dissection is recommended even for smaller cancers because of the risk of occult neck disease. Radiation therapy is usually administered postoperatively.[85]

The management of intermediate-grade cancer is controversial, and many authors tend to follow a more aggressive approach than that used for low-grade tumors. Surgery is the mainstay of therapy, and the use of postoperative radiation therapy varies according to the surgical margins and other factors, such as the patient's age and the presence or absence of regional metastases.[86, 87]

Cartilaginous Tumors

Cartilaginous tumors of the larynx are uncommon. A literature review disclosed approximately 250 cases since 1816; the cricoid cartilage is the most common site of occurrence.[88]

Chondrosarcoma

Chondrosarcoma is the most common sarcoma of the larynx. Its incidence is difficult to know because the low-grade form of this tumor is often confused with a benign chondroma. It predominantly affects men (3:1 male-to-female ratio) between the ages of 50 and 70 years. Chondrosarcomas arise from the hyaline cartilages of the larynx.[89]

ORIGIN

The most common of these sites are the cricoid (especially the posterior lamina) (70%), the thyroid (20%), and the body of the arytenoid cartilage (10%). Some authors believe that tumors arising from the elastic cartilages of the larynx, which form the epiglottis and the vocal process of the arytenoid, are really just focal areas of metaplastic cartilage,[90] whereas others believe that these are true low-grade chondrosarcomas.[91]

PRESENTATION

Symptoms are similar to those of laryngeal carcinomas. Chondrosarcoma arising from the cricoid cartilage tends to grow into the airway and cause progressive obstruction, whereas chondrosarcoma arising from the thyroid cartilage typically protrudes laterally and presents as a firm mass in the neck. Endoscopically, the tumor appears as a firm, submucosal mass that is difficult to biopsy because it is so dense. Radiographically, these lesions are typically hypodense, well-circumscribed masses containing mottled calcifications with smooth walls centered within the cartilage.[92]

Macroscopically, the tumor develops within the cartilage of origin and only rarely extends beyond the external perichondrium into the surrounding tissues. Microscopically, the tumors are divided into low, medium, and high grade (myxoid), and histologic grade correlates directly with prognosis.[93]

Regional and distant metastasis occurs in 8% to 14% overall. The lung is the most common site of metastasis, followed by the cervical lymph nodes. Nakayama and colleagues reported a "dedifferentiated" chondrosarcoma, which contains additional mesenchymal components such as fibrosarcoma or osteosarcoma.[94]

This subtype accounts for 6% to 10% of all chondrosarcomas and has an extremely poor prognosis, with a mean survival of only 6 months.

MANAGEMENT

The management of chondrosarcoma varies with the grade and extent of the tumor. The primary modality is surgery because both radiation and chemotherapy are thought to be ineffective. For low-grade and some medium-grade tumors, local control is the goal, and most authors recommend partial laryngectomy with voice preservation and reoperation if the tumor recurs. Challenges arise with cricoid tumors, and a variety of techniques have been described to reconstruct the larynx following partial resection with reconstruction of the cricoid, using hyoid bone, rib, and strap muscle. High-grade chondrosarcomas usually require total laryngectomy, but neck dissection is generally reserved for clinical or radiographic evidence of metastasis.[91]

Five-year survival rates are not useful data for chondrosarcomas of the larynx, especially with low-grade tumors, because recurrences and subsequent mortality may occur well beyond this time point.[89]

Neuroendocrine Tumors

Neuroendocrine neoplasms of the larynx have been divided into those of epithelial and neural origin. Those of neural origin consist of paragangliomas; the epithelial origin group can be divided into typical and atypical carcinoids and small cell neuroendocrine carcinomas, the latter consisting of the oat cell type, the intermediate cell type, and the combined cell type. There are now more than 500 cases of neuroendocrine neoplasms of the larynx in the literature.[95]

Differences in nomenclature have made difficult the systematic study of neuroendocrine tumors of the larynx. In 1991, Moisa reviewed the world literature to date and compiled all reported cases into three groups: 68 paragangliomas (neural origin), 42 large cell neuroendocrine carcinomas (Kulchitsky cell origin), and 74 small cell neuroendocrine carcinomas (also of Kulchitsky cell origin).[96]

In 1992, Batsakis and coworkers reported on an additional 200 cases and included in this classification the atypical carcinoid, a tumor also of Kulchitsky cell origin, which histologically and biologically lies between the large cell neuroendocrine tumor (also called typical carcinoid) and the small cell neuroendocrine tumor (also called oat cell). Each of these subtypes is discussed separately.[97]

Paraganglioma

Paraganglioma of the larynx arises from the paired, bilateral paraganglia within the larynx. The superior paraganglia are located in subepithelial tissue on each side of the midline just above the anterior ends of the false vocal cords, associated with the internal branch of the superior laryngeal nerve. This is the most common site of origin of paraganglioma of the larynx, specifically from the aryepiglottic fold and false cord region. The inferior paraganglia are located more variably from the inferior border of the thyroid cartilage to the cricotracheal junction, producing the less common subglottic tumors.[98]

Although the tumor cells contain neurosecretory granules and stain positively for serotonin metabolites, clinically functional paragangliomas have not been reported. They arise in adults, with a 1:3 male-to-female ratio.[95, 97] The typical endoscopic appearance is a reddish or bluish submucosal mass of the supraglottis. Bleeding is often profuse with biopsy.

Recent studies of paragangliomas of the larynx by Ferlito and colleagues,[98] Sanders and colleagues,[99] and Barnes[100] have independently refuted the traditional belief that these tumors act more aggressively and metastasize more commonly than do other paragangliomas of the head and neck. The authors state that many paragangliomas have been confused with atypical carcinoids, which behave in a more aggressive fashion. Local recurrence after excision of true paraganglioma is reported in 17% of cases, and in only 1 of 34 cases has it been reported to metastasize.

The vascular nature of neuroendocrine tumors prevents preoperative pathologic diagnosis. Radiologic features demonstrating a vascular mass with a dominant feeder vessel by the superior or inferior thyroid artery may help in the clinical diagnosis of paraganglioma of the larynx.[99]

The preferred treatment is surgery, and many successful voice-sparing procedures have been described. Preoperative embolization is not routinely recommended because of the ease associated with ligating the superior laryngeal artery. Elective neck dissection is not recommended given the rarity of cervical metastases. No proven role of radiotherapy or chemotherapy has been reported. In the review by Ferlito and coworkers of 62 cases in which the diagnosis of paraganglioma was confirmed retrospectively, the only patient who developed metastatic disease was a female who had a metastasis to the lumbar spine 16 years after initial diagnosis.[98]

Large Cell Tumor

Also known as a carcinoid, large cell neuroendocrine tumors of the larynx are extremely rare. In a critical review of the literature up to 1991, Batsakis and colleagues found only 13 cases of true carcinoid of the larynx.[97]

Only one of the patients was female. None had regional metastases at the time of diagnosis, four developed distant metastases during the course of their disease, and only one died from this disease. Most tumors arose from the arytenoid and the aryepiglottic fold. The treatment is surgical excision with adequate margins of clinically normal tissue to include perineural spread.[95]

Neck dissection is indicated only for obvious metastasis. Neither radiation nor chemotherapy has been shown to be effective,[101] although the development of new chemotherapeutic agents may provide future direction.

ATYPICAL CARCINOID

In stark contrast to the typical carcinoid, atypical carcinoids are clinically far more aggressive. Woodruff and Senie,

in their review of 127 reported cases, found cervical metastases in 43%, skin and subcutaneous metastases in 22%, and distant metastases in 44%. Survival was 48% at 5 years and 30% at 10 years. Surgery was the primary therapy, and radiation therapy did not appear to affect survival.[102]

Clinically, atypical carcinoids usually occur during the sixth and seventh decades in a 3:1 male-to-female ratio. A vast majority (96%) arise from the supraglottic larynx. Elevated calcitonin levels are so common that it is now regarded as a specific marker for atypical carcinoid of the larynx.[98] In a review by Ferlito and Friedmann[103] of distant metastases in 29 cases, 5 patients underwent total laryngectomy, and local control was achieved in all cases.

In the 22 patients undergoing partial laryngectomy, 9 tumors recurred locally; 7 of the patients underwent salvage surgery, suggesting that conservation laryngeal surgery is appropriate in properly selected cases. In the same study, 5 of 6 patients who developed cervical metastasis eventually died of their disease. It is recommended that ipsilateral selective neck dissection be performed for N0 disease and radical neck dissection for patients with N+ necks.[104] The integration of chemotherapy and/or radiation again is a potential future direction.

Small Cell Tumor

Small cell cancer, also known as oat cell carcinoma, is the most lethal neoplasm of the larynx. The most common presentation is a man in his fifties or sixties who is a heavy smoker. Fifty percent present with cervical metastasis, and 75% overall will die distant metastasis to the liver and bone. The 5-year survival rate is a dismal 5%.[105]

Patients must be presumed to have disseminated disease on presentation, and a full metastatic evaluation must be performed first. Although some authors still favor radical surgery, most believe that systemic chemotherapy with radiation to the larynx and neck appears to offer the least disabling and most efficacious form of therapy.[106]

◼ GENERAL GUIDELINES FOR TREATMENT OF CANCER OF THE LARYNX

Early cancer of the larynx (stage I or II) is usually treated with single-modality therapy involving surgery or radiotherapy. Although controversy exists regarding the relative merits of either treatment modality, the rates of cancer control are similar, and patients should be made aware of the options available. Surgical options include endoscopic laser partial laryngectomy/laser cordectomy, open partial laryngectomy, and total laryngectomy.

In contrast, advanced cancer of the larynx requires multimodality therapy employing different combinations of surgery, radiation therapy, and chemotherapy. Modalities may be combined to treat the primary site and the draining lymphatic basin. The combination of surgery with postoperative radiation therapy is used if there are positive margins, cartilage invasion, or bulky disease in the primary site; if multiple regional lymph nodes are involved; or if evidence of extracapsular spread is found in the cervical nodes.

Radiotherapy with or without chemotherapy is used as the primary modality to treat both the primary site and the lymphatic basin with planned postirradiation neck dissection for N2–N3 disease; controversy exists regarding whether to perform neck dissection for N1 disease when there has been complete regression of lymphadenopathy. Some authors have demonstrated that positive nodes are found in some cases when neck dissections have been carried out in patients undergoing salvage laryngectomy with elective neck dissection.[107]

Locoregionally advanced laryngeal cancer has been historically treated with either surgery and adjuvant radiotherapy, or radiotherapy alone with surgery for salvage. Recently, chemoradiotherapy with surgery for salvage has been demonstrated to yield disease control comparable to that achieved with primary surgical management, but with better larynx preservation rates than result from radiation alone.

SURGICAL TREATMENT

A spectrum of treatment plans, including surgical procedures, is available for management of laryngeal cancer. The approach of chemotherapy and irradiation, or irradiation alone, followed by total laryngectomy for failure is often employed by present-day clinicians; however, the options of conventional (open) conservation surgery (CCS), transoral endoscopic laser surgery (TLS), and supracricoid partial laryngectomy (SCPL) provide a wide choice of treatments that may help in attaining the goal of cure with preservation of laryngeal function and integrity of the airway.

Although CCS has been supplanted for many early-stage lesions by TLS and for more advanced stages by SCPL, centers throughout the world have reported favorable results with CCS, which is often modified to include resection of more extensive tumors than was previously possible. During the past decades, a number of extended CCS procedures have been developed for management of glottic cancer involving both vocal cords and the anterior commissure, for cancer in the paraglottic space with vocal cord fixation, and for supraglottic tumors involving the glottis or hypopharynx.

TLS has proved to be an effective, minimally invasive, and functionally satisfactory procedure for management of selected T1 and T2 glottic cancers, as well as for T1–T3 supraglottic cancers. The procedure may be effectively employed in combination with neck dissection and postoperative radiotherapy when necessary, particularly for moderately advanced supraglottic carcinomas. Controversy exists surrounding the role of endoscopic laser surgery as a curative modality of treatment, with endoscopic surgery favored more in Europe than in North America.

SCPL has proved effective in the management of glottic and supraglottic cancers of all stages, even with involvement of the paraglottic space and the thyroid cartilage, provided at least one arytenoid unit can be preserved with clear margins. Invasion of the cricoid cartilage is the most significant limitation of this procedure.

All three surgical approaches have been employed for radiation failure, but with increased failure and complication rates compared with the results of treatment of nonirradiated patients. Thus, a decision to treat laryngeal cancer initially with radiation may preclude a satisfactory result from salvage partial laryngectomy. The treatment of laryngeal cancer should be individualized with various treatment modalities and surgical procedures according to the size and extent of the tumor, the age and physical condition of the patient, and the skill and experience of the treating physicians.

In 1866, Patrick Watson of Edinburgh performed the first laryngectomy. The patient was a 36-year-old man whose larynx was being destroyed by syphilis. He survived the operation but died several weeks later from pneumonia; after his death, the procedure was condemned. In 1873, Billroth of Vienna performed what is considered to be the first successful laryngectomy. Since then, laryngeal surgery for cancer has seen significant advances that have made the surgery both safe and reliable.[108]

Glottic Carcinoma

Endoscopic Resection

The European Laryngological Society has proposed a classification of different laryngeal endoscopic cordectomies in order to ensure better definitions of postoperative results; the word *cordectomy* is used even for partial resections because it is the term most often used in the surgical literature. The classification includes eight types of cordectomies: (1) subepithelial cordectomy (type I), which is resection of the epithelium; (2) subligamental cordectomy (type II), which is resection of the epithelium, Reinke's space, and the vocal ligament; (3) transmuscular cordectomy (type III), which proceeds through the vocalis muscle; (4) total cordectomy (type IV); (5) extended cordectomy that encompasses the contralateral vocal fold and the anterior commissure (type Va); (6) extended cordectomy that includes the arytenoid (type Vb); (7) extended cordectomy that encompasses the subglottis (type Vc); and (8) extended cordectomy that includes the ventricle (type Vd). These operations are classified according to the surgical approach used and the degree of resection. Each surgical procedure ensures that a specimen is available for histopathologic examination.[109]

Vertical Partial Laryngectomies

The central concept in all types of vertical partial laryngectomy is vertical transection of the thyroid cartilage and the paraglottic space. The extent of resection depends on the extent of the lesion.

LARYNGOFISSURE AND CORDECTOMY

This procedure is reserved for T1 glottic lesions involving the mid true vocal cord and results in cure rates of greater than 90% in selected patients. An endoscopy is performed before the laryngofissure is undertaken, and the tumor is mapped for the suitability of laryngofissure and cordectomy, following which a tracheotomy is performed. A horizontal incision involving a major skinfold in the neck is used; this is separate from the tracheotomy incision. Superior and inferior flaps are raised and the larynx is exposed in the midline by separation of the strap muscles. A midline thyrotomy is then performed and the larynx opened via a cricothyrotomy;

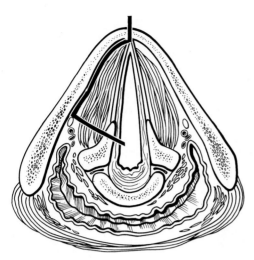

FIGURE 15–16 Cordectomy, axial view.

the anterior commissure is released. The lesion is then visualized and removed (Fig. 15–16). The specimen is sent for examination by frozen section. The anterior commissure is reconstructed by anchoring the anterior end of the uninvolved cord to the thyroid lamina. The perichondrium and the strap muscles are closed, and the incision is closed over suction with drains. The increased use of endoscopic cordectomy has resulted in the decreased use of the open procedure.

VERTICAL HEMILARYNGECTOMY (VH)

This procedure is reserved for T1 and T2 lesions of the true vocal cords; success rates of greater than 90% have been reported. The results of VH for selected T3 and T4 lesions have also provided acceptable outcomes. An endoscopy is performed before the VH is completed, and the cancer is mapped for the suitability of the procedure, following which a tracheotomy is performed. A horizontal incision that is separate from the tracheotomy incision is used. Superior and inferior flaps are raised. The strap muscles are retracted. The external perichondrium overlying

the thyroid cartilage to be removed is incised; the perichondrium and musculature are elevated as a single flap, and the larynx is skeletonized. At this point, midline thyrotomy, cricothyroidotomy, and incision across the petiole are performed to provide visualization of the lesion. The lesion and the thyroid cartilage are then resected (Fig. 15–17). The muscle and perichondrial flap are then used for creating a neoglottis. The wound is closed over a suction drain.

EXTENDED VERTICAL HEMILARYNGECTOMY

1. Frontolateral vertical hemilaryngectomy—Used for lesions involving the anterior commissure and the anterior contralateral cord (Fig. 15–18)
2. Posterolateral vertical hemilaryngectomy—Used for lesions involving the ipsilateral arytenoid cartilage

The systematic use of frozen section control of margins cannot be overemphasized in this type of precision surgery. If frozen sections are not used and the permanent sections indicate that the margins are positive, the rate of recurrence is intolerably high. Three options are then available:

1. Reoperation with more extended partial surgery
2. Radiation therapy. This is unlikely to control the cancer and has a high probability of resulting in a nonfunctioning larynx
3. Total laryngectomy

Supraglottic Carcinoma

Studies performed by Pressman in 1956 to map laryngeal barriers lent support to the oncologic safety of supraglottic laryngectomy by demonstrating that dyes injected submucosally into the supraglottis did not spread inferior to the ventricle.[110, 111] Pressman also studied the lymphatic drainage of the subunits and showed that the lateral structures of the aryepiglottic folds and false cords were found to demonstrate ipsilateral lymphatic drainage, and that the midline epiglottis drainage pattern was bilateral. The superficial lymphatic channels in the supraglottis had bilateral

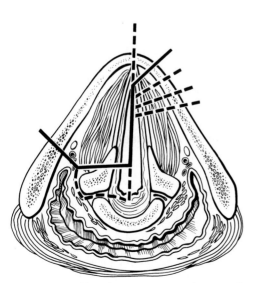

FIGURE 15–17 Vertical hemilaryngectomy, axial view, with multiple variations.

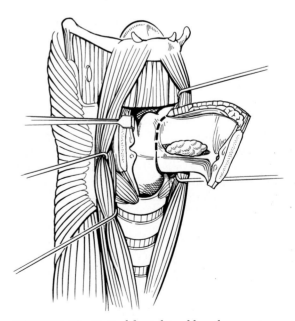

FIGURE 15–18 Vertical frontolateral hemilaryngectomy.

drainage, and the deep lymphatic channels were side specific. The lymphatic vessels traverse the thyrohyoid membrane, alongside the superior thyroid artery and vein, and empty into the jugulodigastric (level II) and midjugular (level III) lymph nodes.[110, 111]

Fibroelastic membranes within the laryngeal framework serve as functional barriers and prevent the spread of tumor from one subunit to another. These barriers include the thyrohyoid membrane, the hyoepiglottic ligament, the thyroepiglottic ligament, the conus elasticus, and the quadrangular membrane; all serve to divide the larynx into two three-dimensional compartments—the pre-epiglottic space and the paraglottic space. Cancer initially invading the pre-epiglottic space can directly extend into the paraglottic space; in this situation, the use of supraglottic laryngectomy is precluded (Figs. 15–19 through 15–21). Involvement of these spaces by supraglottic cancer has a direct effect on the potentially conservative surgical management of supraglottic cancer.

Endoscopic Resection

The concept of endoscopic management of supraglottic lesions began in 1939 when Jackson described the use of a laryngoscope and punch biopsy forceps to resect cancer of the suprahyoid epiglottis.[112] Endoscopic management fell into disrepute owing to the poor results and morbidity associated with it. The advent of the operating microscope,

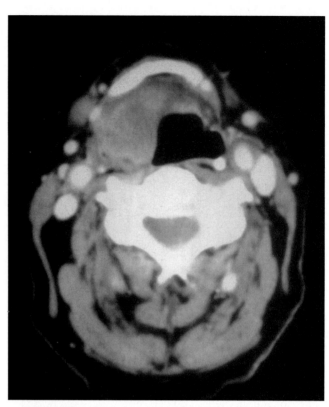

FIGURE 15–20 Inferior section of patient shown in Figure 15–19, showing direct extension to the right paraglottic space.

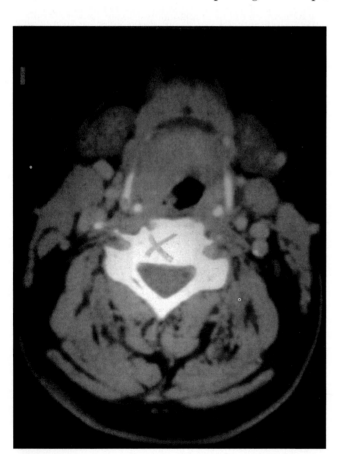

FIGURE 15–19 Cross-sectional CT reveals tumor involvement of the pre-epiglottic space.

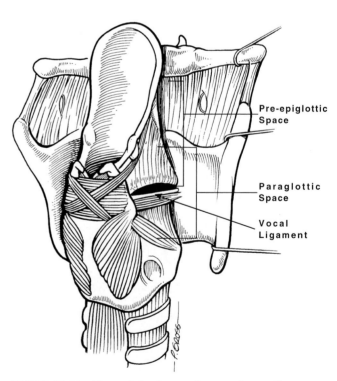

Pre-epiglottic Space

Paraglottic Space

Vocal Ligament

FIGURE 15–21 View of the larynx showing the confluent pre-epiglottic and paraglottic spaces.

suspension microlaryngology, and the carbon dioxide (CO_2) laser over the past decade has led to the renewed popularity of endoscopic management of laryngeal cancers, both in Europe and the United States.

The potential advantages of endoscopic management over open surgery include elimination of the need for tracheotomy, shorter operating times, and earlier rehabilitation of swallowing function. Disadvantages include the need for specialized equipment, prolonged healing time in that the defect is allowed to heal by second intention, and poor exposure that often leads to inadequate removal of the lesion. The CO_2 laser combined with an operating microscope is the most frequently used instrumentation. The quality of voice following laser surgery for supraglottic cancer should be unchanged. Studies from Europe have shown that the results of endoscopic laser surgery are comparable to those of radiation therapy, with the latter type of treatment being more convenient for patients and less expensive for society.

The use of endoscopic laser resection with intent to cure is dependent on the size, location, and extent of tumor. T1 and T2 lesions located on the suprahyoid epiglottis, aryepiglottic fold, and vestibular fold with minimal pre-epiglottic and no paraglottic involvement may be treated with endoscopic resection. Cancers arising on the infrahyoid epiglottis and false cord are less amenable to endoscopic resection owing to their tangential relationship to the distal lumen of the laryngoscope. The most important factor in endoscopic laser surgery is adequate exposure. The use of the Weerda Bivalved Laryngopharyngoscope (Karl Storz Endoscopy America, Charlton, Massachusetts) more than triples the operative field and allows optimal exposure. The superior blade is placed into the vallecula, and the lower blade pushes the endotracheal tube against the posterior pharyngeal wall. The laryngoscope is repositioned as needed to maintain optimal exposure throughout the procedure.

The CO_2 laser is the laser of choice for endolaryngeal surgery. Advantages of the CO_2 laser include its superficial effect, which helps to minimize damage to surrounding normal tissue, and its ability to be used as a cutting tool in the focused mode and as a coagulation tool in the defocused mode.

Small cancers on the suprahyoid epiglottis or the aryepiglottic fold may be resected en bloc with the laser, but a majority of supraglottic cancers are excised piecemeal. The epiglottis is split sagittally in the midline with resection of the suprahyoid division first, followed by the infrahyoid component. The pre-epiglottic fat is then encountered and removed until the thyroid cartilage is identified.

Resection is then continued inferiorly to include the aryepiglottic folds and false cords as needed. Frozen sections are taken from the specimens, and additional resection is performed for positive margins. The defect is allowed to granulate and heal by second intention.

Potential complications of endoscopic excision include intraoperative or postoperative hemorrhage and infection of the exposed laryngeal cartilage.[112] Radiation may be used approximately 2 to 4 weeks following resection of the primary. The patient is readmitted for neck dissections. At that time, further resection can be carried out if permanent sections reveal positive margins.

Supraglottic Laryngectomy

Supraglottic laryngectomy is indicated in patients in whom the cancer arises from the epiglottis, aryepiglottic folds, and false vocal cords. This procedure minimizes morbidity and maintains the three primary functions of the larynx—airway protection, respiration, and phonation (Figs. 15–22 through 15–25). Supraglottic laryngectomy (in a two-stage procedure) was first introduced by Alonzo in 1947 as an alternative to prevailing primary treatment for supraglottic tumors, which included total laryngectomy and radical neck dissection. Modifications made by Ogura in 1958 and later by Som in 1959 converted supraglottic laryngectomy to a one-stage procedure.[112]

INDICATIONS

The most important factor influencing the success of supraglottic laryngectomy is appropriate patient selection based on both host (patient) and tumor factors. Every patient undergoing supraglottic laryngectomy will experience temporary aspiration postoperatively, thus making the patient's cardiopulmonary reserve an important factor in patient selection. Patients must have a reasonably good cough mechanism or they will aspirate, will not be able to swallow properly, and will develop recurrent aspiration pneumonia.

Tumor factors are equally important in the selection process; established contraindications are based on anatomic considerations, including involvement by cancer of the thyroid cartilage or the anterior commissure, vocal cord fixation due to involvement of the paraglottic space, and involvement of the pyriform apex or postcricoid mucosa. Such patients are at an unacceptable risk because of the potential for recurrent cancer, as well as the potential for postoperative aspiration and dysphagia. In patients with involvement of the base of the tongue, primary closure can be difficult, resulting in increased dysphagia and aspiration.

PROCEDURE

Suspension microlaryngoscopy is performed before the definitive procedure, and the extent of cancer is mapped to

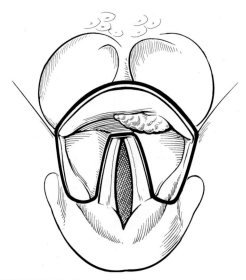

FIGURE 15–22 Supraglottic laryngectomy, axial view.

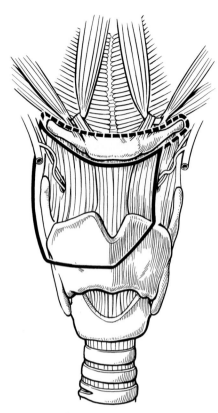

FIGURE 15–23 Supraglottic laryngectomy, frontal view of a right-sided malignant lesion.

reconfirm the suitability of the cancer for a supraglottic laryngectomy. A superiorly based apron skin incision is designed, and flaps are elevated to above the hyoid superiorly; the inferior and posterior limits of skin flap elevation

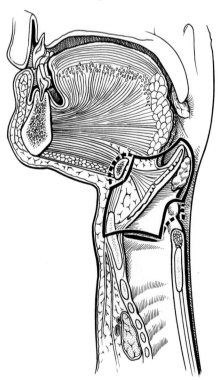

FIGURE 15–24 Supraglottic laryngectomy, sagittal view.

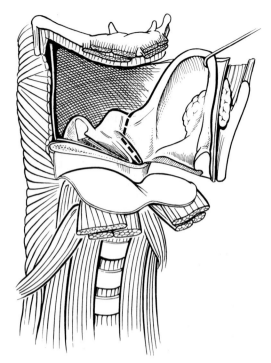

FIGURE 15–25 Supraglottic laryngectomy specimen.

are dictated by the type of neck dissection to be performed. Neck dissections are carried out before the supraglottic laryngectomy is performed. A tracheotomy is then completed to provide maximum visualization of the cancer at the time of resection.

The suprahyoid muscles are released from the hyoid bone; the infrahyoid muscles are divided 1 cm below the hyoid and are reflected inferiorly. The greater cornu is skeletonized bilaterally with preservation of the hypoglossal nerves and the lingual arteries. The outer thyroid perichondrium is incised along its superior aspect and elevated inferiorly but is left attached to the cartilage. After the thyroid cartilage has been skeletonized, transverse incisions are made at the junction of the upper third and the lower two thirds of the thyroid cartilage. This incision, which coincides with the superior surface of the true vocal cords, extends through the cartilage; the inner perichondrium should be left intact at this time. The incisions are extended posteriorly to include the superior cornu of the thyroid cartilage. Care is taken to preserve the contralateral superior laryngeal nerve, if possible. Entry into the pharynx is dictated by tumor location but may occur through the vallecula or the contralateral pyriform sinus. Mucosal incisions begin anterior to the arytenoid on the side of least involvement. The mucosal incision is made perpendicularly across the aryepiglottic fold inferiorly to the level of the ventricle. The mucosal incision is then continued horizontally through the ventricle under direct vision. This incision proceeds anteriorly to the midline, thereby opening the larynx like a book and allowing resection of the more involved side with maximal visualization.

During the process of making mucosal incisions, it is important that the surgeon attempt to leave the mucosa over the arytenoids intact. If this is not possible, all exposed cartilage should be covered by the mucosa from the adjacent pyriform sinus. After it has been ascertained that the margins of resection are clear on frozen section, the wound is then closed by reapproximating the thyroid perichondrium to the tongue base. If the perichondrium is insufficient, drill holes are made through the thyroid cartilage for suture placement. It is important that the bites through the tongue base include the deep musculoaponeurotic layer to increase the strength of the closure, incorporating the preserved hypoglossal nerves bilaterally. Tying of the sutures is delayed until the patient has been taken out of extension. This effectively reduces tension on the closure, which is then reinforced by approximating the suprahyoid and infrahyoid musculature. Drains are inserted and the skin closed in layers.

Modifications of this procedure advocated by some authors include suspending the remaining thyroid cartilage to the mandible and inferiorly releasing the larynx by dividing the infrahyoid strap muscles. These additions have not demonstrated significantly improved postoperative rehabilitation. The simultaneous performance of a cricopharyngeal myotomy is controversial. Some clinicians believe that it improves postoperative swallow, but others state that it increases the risk of postoperative aspiration by increasing the propensity for laryngopharyngeal reflux.

Supracricoid Partial Laryngectomy

Supracricoid partial laryngectomy (SCL) is a variation of the horizontal partial laryngectomy (supraglottic laryngectomy) technique; it is extended to provide an oncologically sound removal of certain laryngeal cancers in an attempt to preserve voice and avoid a permanent tracheotomy. Supracricoid laryngectomy was first introduced in Vienna in 1959 by Majer and Reider. Tucker, Labayle, and Bistmuth and Piquet refined the procedure in the 1970s, and it has been recently popularized by Weinstein in the United States and Laccourreye in Europe.[113]

SCL can be divided into two main categories—supracricoid partial laryngectomy with cricohyoidopexy (SCL-CHP) and the supracricoid partial laryngectomy with cricohyoidoepiglottopexy (SCL-CHEP)—depending on the extent of lesion, the extent of resection, and the degree of subsequent reconstruction. SCL-CHP is typically used in supraglottic lesions, and SCL-CHEP is used in glottic cancers.

In SPL-CHP, the entire supraglottis, the false and true vocal cords, and the thyroid cartilage, including the paraglottic and pre-epiglottic spaces, are removed (Figs. 15–26 and 15–27). The procedure can be extended to resect one involved arytenoid cartilage. The cricoid cartilage, hyoid bone, and at least one arytenoid are saved. Phonatory and swallowing functions are maintained by the movement of the spared arytenoid against the tongue base. Respiratory function is dependent on preservation of the cricoid cartilage.

In SCL-CHEP, the false and true vocal cords and the thyroid cartilage, including the paraglottic, are removed. Reconstruction is performed by suturing the hyoid bone and the remnants of the epiglottis to the cricoid cartilage. SCL-CHEP is the most common extended partial laryngectomy performed in the United States and Europe.

INDICATIONS

SCL can be used as a primary treatment modality or as a salvage option after failure of organ preservation therapy (radiation therapy or radiation therapy with chemotherapy). SCL-CHP has a high rate of failure (aspiration and tracheotomy dependence) after radiation therapy with chemotherapy. SCL is used for supraglottic cancers that

1. Involve the glottis and the anterior commissure
2. Invade the ventricle
3. Invade the thyroid cartilage
4. Are associated with impaired vocal cord mobility
5. Have paraglottic invasion
6. Have moderate pre-epiglottic space involvement
7. Are transglottic

Patient selection for SCL is similar to that in patients undergoing supraglottic laryngectomy.

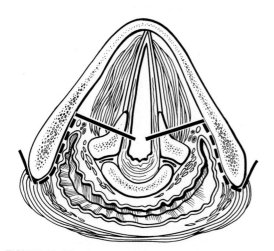

FIGURE 15–26 Supracricoid laryngectomy, axial view.

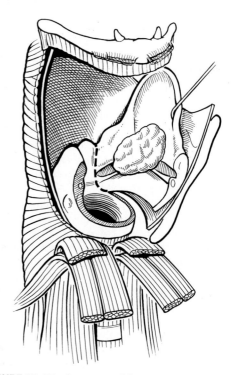

FIGURE 15–27 Supracricoid laryngectomy specimen.

PROCEDURE

The procedure of SCL begins with a direct microlaryngoscopy to evaluate resectability of the tumor with an SCL. All patients undergoing any type of open partial laryngectomy are approved for a total laryngectomy if it is required for complete resection of the tumor. A standard apron incision is used; the skin flaps are elevated superiorly to 1 cm above the hyoid and inferiorly to the clavicles. Appropriate neck dissections are then carried out.

A tracheotomy is performed through the same incision. The sternohyoid and thyrohyoid muscles are transected along the superior border to the thyroid cartilage. The medial laryngeal vessels are then ligated, and the sternothyroid muscles are transected along the inferior border of the thyroid cartilage. Next, the inferior constrictor muscles and the external thyroid perichondrium are transected along the posterior border of the thyroid cartilage. Care is taken to preserve the internal branch of the superior laryngeal nerve by incising the constrictor muscles right on the thyroid cartilage. The pyriform sinuses are dissected off the thyroid cartilage as in a total laryngectomy. The cricothyroid joints are disarticulated, with care taken to stay right on the joint, thereby avoiding damage to the recurrent laryngeal nerve. The isthmus of the thyroid gland is transected, and blunt dissection along the anterior tracheal is performed to help mobilize the trachea to avoid tension on the final anastomosis. The periosteum of the hyoid bone is incised, and a sharp elevator is used to dissect the pre-epiglottic space from the posterior surface of the hyoid bone. The larynx is entered through the vallecula superiorly and inferiorly through the cricothyroid membrane immediately above the cricoid. The larynx is grasped with an Allis clamp, and the endolaryngeal incisions are made.

The endolaryngeal incision is begun on the side of least tumor involvement. A vertical incision is made anterior to the arytenoid from the aryepiglottic fold to the cricoid with scissors. The pyriform sinus is spared. The entire paraglottic space is anterior to the incision, and care must be taken to adequately resect the entire paraglottic space because disease left at this site contributes to local failure. This incision and the cricothyroid incision are connected by transection of the cricothyroid muscle along the superior border of the cricoid. The thyroid cartilage is grasped and fractured along the midline so that it opens like a book. Excision of the tumor-bearing side is completed under direct visualization by the cricothyroid incision on that side and a vertical prearytenoid incision, or if need be, by resection of a portion or all of the arytenoid on that side.

Following receipt of the frozen section diagnosis, closure of the mucosa of only the upper part of the arytenoids is performed with sutures. The hyoid bone and cricoid cartilage are then secured with three to five submucosal sutures of 0 polypropylene. The midline suture is placed first with care taken to include a portion of tongue base with this suture. The lateral sutures are placed 1 cm from the midline. The sutures are tagged with clamps. Care must be taken to ensure that the cricoid and hyoid anterior borders are well aligned. The sternohyoid muscles are reconstituted and the incision is closed in two layers. Cricopharyngeal myotomy should be avoided in these patients because it predisposes them to gastroesophageal reflux disease, which can lead to aspiration. The wound is then closed in layers over suction drains, and a tracheotomy tube is inserted.

Total Laryngectomy

INDICATIONS

Despite the advances made in organ preservation treatment protocols, total laryngectomy (TL) is a viable option in certain patients, including those with locally advanced cancer of the larynx with cartilage destruction; recurrent or persistent disease after conservative treatment (surgery, radiation therapy, or chemoradiotherapy); and advanced malignant tumors of certain histologic types such as spindle cell carcinoma, adenocarcinoma, and others that respond poorly to radiation therapy and/or chemotherapy. It is also appropriate for those with benign processes such as chronic severe aspiration or radionecrosis of the larynx refractory to more conservative management.

Criteria for patient selection for TL include the ability of the patient to undergo general anesthesia and to care for the stoma, as well as the psychological capability for adjusting to a laryngectomy.

PROCEDURE

The patient is placed under general anesthesia via either tracheotomy or endotracheal intubation (unobstructed larynx). He or she is then positioned on the operating table with proper extension of the neck for adequate exposure. At this time, the skin incision and the stoma incisions are marked. An apron flap is used for exposure of the larynx, and the neck dissections are carried out, if necessary. The skin flaps are elevated and anchored. The investing fascia overlying the sternocleidomastoid muscle is raised on both sides. The omohyoid muscle is transected to obtain exposure to the visceral compartment of the neck. The strap muscles are then divided near their sternal attachments, and the thyroid gland is exposed.

The thyroid lobe and the tracheoesophageal lymphatics on the side of the tumor are resected in continuity with the larynx. The contralateral lobe and contralateral parathyroids are preserved on their vascular pedicle. The hyoid bone is skeletonized by detaching the mylohyoid, the geniohyoid, the hyoglossus, and the diagastric sling. The infrahyoid muscles are left intact. The posterior border of the thyroid lamina is rotated anteriorly, and constrictor muscles are released on the unaffected side. The pharynx is entered either superiorly or laterally on the unaffected side. Mucosal incisions are made to release the lateral pharynx from the larynx. The incision from the vallecula to the pyriform sinus is made, and the postcricoid mucosa is exposed. At this time, a beveled incision of the trachea is performed and the larynx is removed with the ipsilateral thyroid cartilage. Hemostasis is achieved and the wound irrigated.

Following confirmation of clear margins by frozen section technique, pharyngeal closure is carried out. Tension-free closure is achieved by means of either horizontal or T-shaped closure of the pharynx. The pharyngeal wall is closed in a single layer with an interrupted inversion stitch. This repair is done after a nasogastric feeding tube is inserted and a primary tracheoesophageal puncture (if indicated) is carried out.

TABLE 15-4 Results of Surgery for Advanced Cancer of the Larynx

Reference	Year	Selection Criteria	Procedure	Absolute Survival	Disease Specificity
Pradhan[114]	2002	T3/T4 primary or salvage	Near-total laryngectomy		70.1% (3-year)
Shenoy[115]	2002	T3/T4	Near-total laryngectomy		74% (3-year)
Schwaab[116]	2001	Majority T2/T3	CHP		88% (5-year)
Lassaletta[117]	2001	T3	Total laryngectomy	58.1% (5-year)	66.8% (5-year)
Lima[118]	2001	T2	CHEP		79% (3-year)
Lima[118]	2001	T3	CHEP	75% (3-year)	
Bron[119]	2001	T2/T3/T4	CHEP/CHP	68% (5-year)	
Watters[120]	2000	T1–T4 salvage	Vertical or horizontal partial laryngectomy		97%
Laccourreye[121]	1998	T1–T4	CHEP/CHP	68% (5-year)	93.9%% (5-year)
Chevalier[122]	1997	T2 (primary)	CHEP	81.3% (5-year)	96% (5-year)
Chevalier[122]	1997	T3 (primary)	CHEP	85.5% (5-year)	94.1% (5-year)
Laccourreye[123]	1996	Salvage	CHEP/CHP		83% (3-year)

CHP, partial laryngectomy with cricohyoidopexy; CHEP, partial laryngectomy with cricohyoidoepiglottopexy.

A tracheostoma is created after the pharynx is closed. The beveled end of the trachea is sutured to the skin, with interrupted horizontal mattress sutures, in a tension-free fashion. The wound is irrigated and closed in layers over a suction drain. A laryngectomy tube is essential after the endotracheal tube has been removed.

Surgical Outcomes

We have presented a number of series dealing with the primary surgical management of patients with intermediate to advanced SCC of the larynx treated with a variety of surgical procedures (Table 15–4).[114–123] We think that these results represent the best outcomes that can be anticipated when surgical management is used for cancer of the larynx. One must remember that a number of selection criteria are in place when these patients are managed, and these selection criteria may differ from group to group. These results are provided for the purposes of comparison with subsequent data that will be presented on the use of radiation therapy alone or chemoradiation as part of an organ preservation protocol for intermediate to advanced SCC of the larynx. The management of advanced SCC of the larynx at Memorial Sloan-Kettering Cancer Center has evolved to the predominant use of primary chemoradiation with surgery for salvage. Although many capable surgeons are able to perform these elegant procedures, patient factors, patient preference, and treating physician bias have led to the use of cheomoradiation with surgery for salvage in our institution, as well as in many other institutions throughout the world.

COMPLICATIONS OF LARYNGECTOMY

Early Complications

- Hematoma formation
- Pharyngocutaneous fistula
- Infection
- Wound breakdown

Early complications of laryngectomy include infection, stomal crusting, and fistula formation. Perioperative antibiotics have significantly decreased the incidence of infection. Crusts around the stoma are removed at least once a day to prevent airway obstruction.

Fistula formation occurs in 15% to 40% of cases, depending on whether regional flaps are used for pharyngeal closure and whether the tissues have been previously irradiated.[124] The fistula itself is conservatively managed with drainage, irrigation, and packing; most heal spontaneously. Preoperative radiation, short interval between radiation therapy and operation, and cobalt/roentgen radiation instead of photons predispose to this complication (Figs. 15–28 through 15–30). The fistulas in this group of patients appeared earlier; they were significantly larger in patients who had undergone previous irradiation than in patients who had not received preoperative irradiation.[125]

Free-tissue transfer reconstruction of the hypopharynx is the preferred method of reconstruction following combined chemotherapy and radiation therapy protocols. Surgical complications such as pharyngocutaneous fistulas are significantly reduced, and hospital stays are minimized.[126]

The most feared complication of a salivary fistula is carotid artery blowout from contact or exposure of the artery, with salivary drainage due to necrosis of the skin flaps. The high morbidity and mortality associated with urgent carotid ligation have led many to advocate routine carotid artery coverage in all cases in which laryngectomy is performed after radiation therapy is provided. The sternocleidomastoid muscle often provides adequate coverage. If the muscle has been removed during a concomitant radical neck dissection, dermal grafts, the levator scapulae muscle, and regional flaps have all been described to either provide coverage for the artery or direct fistula flow away from the artery. Surgical salvage procedures performed after induction chemotherapy and definitive radiation therapy are associated with a high rate of major wound complications.[127]

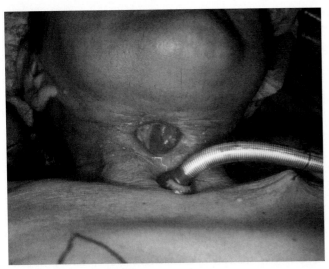

FIGURE 15–28 Pharyngocutaneous fistula after surgical salvage for radiation failure with inability to heal spontaneously.

Late Complications

- Stomal stenosis
- Pharyngeal stenosis

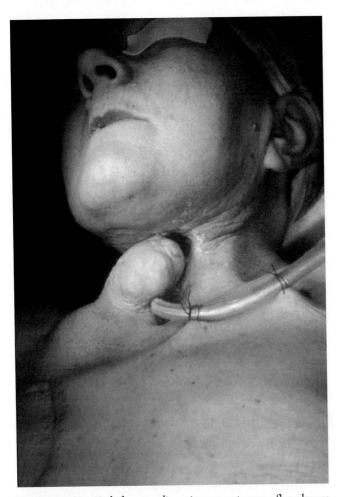

FIGURE 15–29 Failed pectoralis major myocutaneous flap closure of fistula, with persistent pharyngocutaneous fistula track.

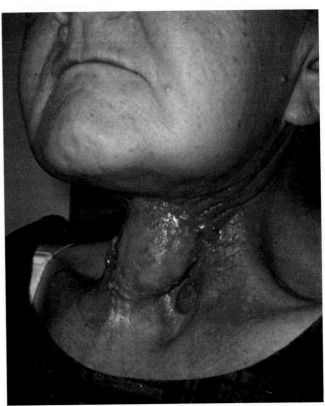

FIGURE 15–30 Revision of pectoralis major myocutaneous flap with closure of the fistula site and resumption of oral intake.

- Delayed pharyngocutaneous fistula
- Hypothyroidism

Late complications following laryngectomy include stomal stenosis and hypopharyngeal stricture with dysphagia. Stenosis of the tracheostoma is a frequent complication following total laryngectomy that results in reduced air flow. Many authors have attempted to identify factors associated with stomal stenosis; a number of procedures have been recommended for the surgical correction of such stenosis.[128, 129]

Dysphagia that gradually develops during the postoperative period is often a sign of pharyngeal stenosis; however, one must first rule out recurrent cancer. Barium esophagram is helpful in revealing the site of narrowing, but operative endoscopy with biopsy under general anesthesia is required to determine if the stricture is recurrent cancer or benign scarring. (Recurrent cancer is discussed under Stomal Recurrence.) Benign strictures can usually be managed with serial dilations, but occasionally, patients require excision of the stenotic pharynx with pharyngoesophageal reconstruction and regional or free-tissue transfer.[130]

◘ VOICE REHABILITATION AFTER TOTAL LARYNGECTOMY

A major challenge faced by the head and neck surgeon and the speech pathologist in treating a patient who has had a total laryngectomy is the restoration of speech. The first artificial larynx was devised by Gussenbauer in 1874. Artificial instruments were introduced by Western Electric, and the esophageal voice became better understood as a means of voice rehabilitation. Voice restoration using the fistula technique was reintroduced by Asai in 1965. In 1979, Singer and Blom introduced the tracheoesophageal puncture (TEP) and silicone prosthesis for generating tracheo-esophageal voice.[131]

The patient who is undergoing a total laryngectomy is offered three options: the artificial larynx or electrolarynx, esophageal voice, tracheoesophageal voice.

Electrolarynx

The artificial larynx is available as an external device that is placed against the neck, or as an oral type. Both types are electrically driven and produce a mechanical sound. This sound is articulated by the tongue, lips, and teeth as under-standable speech. Advantages of the electrolarynx include the short learning time required for its use, its ability to be used during the immediate postoperative period, and its rel-ative availability and low cost. Disadvantages include its mechanical sound and dependence on batteries, as well as the need for maintenance of the intraoral tubes.

Esophageal Voice

A speech pathologist or another laryngectomee usually teaches the patient insufflation behavior in acquiring esoph-ageal speech. This entails trapping air in the mouth or pharynx and propelling it into the esophagus. This produces a belchlike sound that can be articulated by the tongue, lips, and teeth. The patient learns how to rapidly insufflate and eject air through the esophagus to produce understandable speech.

Tracheoesophageal Voice

In the opinion of one author (D.K.), tracheoesophageal speech is the preferred modality for rehabilitation of a laryn-gectomy patient. It is based on the concept of shunting of tracheal air to the pharynx through a fistulous tract during exhalation to produce sound through vibration of the mucosa of the upper esophageal segment. Speech is pro-duced by articulation of this sound at the level of the oral cavity.[132]

Technique of Tracheoesophageal Puncture

TEP can be performed at the time of laryngectomy (pri-mary TEP) or later as an independent procedure (secondary TEP). The timing of TEP is another area of debate and appears to be the surgeon's preference. Primary TEP offers the advantages of avoiding a secondary procedure and pro-viding early voice rehabilitation; the transesophageal fistula can be used temporarily as a feeding esophagostome. Primary TEP is performed after the stoma has been constructed and before the pharynx has been closed.[133]

It is the practice of one author (D.K.) to perform primary TEP only in patients who have received no previous therapy or radiation, and to perform secondary TEP in patients undergoing salvage laryngectomy for chemo-radiotherapy failure or in those requiring flap closure (Figs. 15–31 through 15–40).

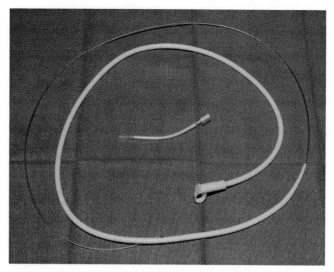

FIGURE 15–31 Blom-Singer TEP placement set for tracheo-esophageal puncture. (Inhealth Technologies, Carpinteria, Calif.)

COMPLICATIONS

The most common problem following TEP is failure of voice restoration. Studies have shown that failure rates range from 3% to 15%. Some of the common causes of failure of voice restoration following TEP include inadequate patient motivation and learning capabilities. In addition, patients with poor vision, arthritis, or neurologic disabilities have been found to be poor candidates for the procedure. In many instances, patients may be fitted with a hands-free, self-retaining unit that precludes the need for digital manip-ulation of the stoma (Fig. 15–41). These conditions should be considered during the preoperative evaluation of the patient by a speech pathologist.

Another cause of failure is pharyngoesophageal spasm, which appears to be caused by reflex contraction of crico-pharyngeal constrictor muscles when the midesophagus is distended with air. It is believed to be a cause of TEP speech

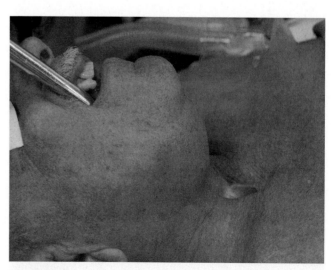

FIGURE 15–32 Placement of short Jesberg esophagoscope with illumination of the posterior wall of the stoma and the anterior wall of the cervical esophagus.

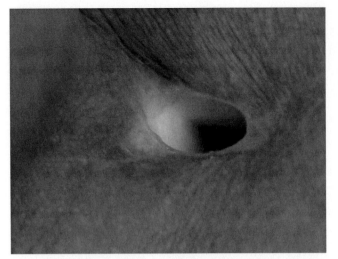

FIGURE 15–33 Transillumination of stoma (closeup).

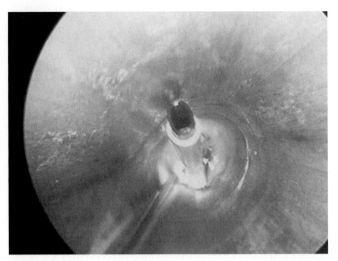

FIGURE 15–35 Intraluminal appearance of introducer needle within the distal aspect of the esophagoscope.

failure in 10% to 12% of patients. Therapeutic options for pharyngoesophageal spasm include cricopharyngeal and constrictor myotomies, pharyngeal neurectomies, and injection of the pharyngeal muscle with botulinum toxin.

Other complications resulting from TEP include bleeding from around the tract (usually granulation tissue), air in the stomach, salivary leakage around or through the prosthesis, and aphonia during radiation therapy. More serious and potentially life-endangering, although fortunately rare, complications include mediastinitis, cervical cellulitis, cervical spine fracture, and aspiration of the prosthesis.[134]

RADIATION THERAPY FOR CANCER OF THE LARYNX

Radiation therapy plays an important role in the treatment of cancer of the larynx. Radiation may be used alone as definitive therapy, or it may be combined with surgery and/or chemotherapy, depending on patient and disease factors.

Indications

Early Glottic Lesions

Radiation therapy alone is a standard treatment option for stage T1–T2 glottic cancer. The rates of local control following radiation with and without surgical salvage from three large series are presented in Table 15–5. Rates of local control with laryngeal preservation at 5 years compare favorably with surgical series, and severe late complication rates are lower than 1%.[135] Nearly all nonbulky T1–T2 tumors are suitable for radiation alone. Impaired vocal cord mobility has been reported as an adverse factor in some series, but this is not evident in others.[136] The cost of radiation therapy for early glottic carcinoma is estimated to be half the cost of open surgery,[137] although the comparison of cost assessment and the use of changes as opposed to true

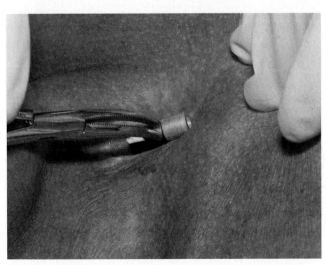

FIGURE 15–34 Placement of introducer needle.

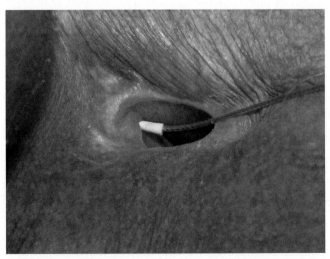

FIGURE 15–36 Removal of inner cannula with threading of leader cable.

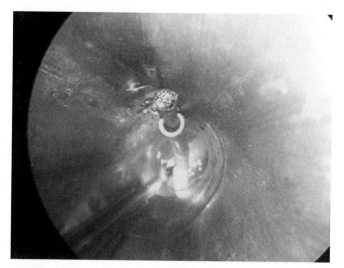

FIGURE 15–37 Intraluminal appearance of leader cable through the introducer needle as visualized through the distal end of the esophagoscope.

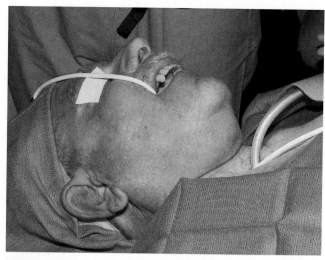

FIGURE 15–39 Silicone catheter with division of the distal leader cable.

costs make this literature difficult to interpret. In a study by Myers and colleagues, which compared the use of direct microlaryngoscopy and excision of glottic carcinoma with external beam radiation therapy, the estimated cost of radiation therapy was four to five times as high as the cost of the microscopic procedure.[138]

Advanced Glottic Lesions

Radiation as a primary modality has also been studied for advanced-stage, T3–T4 glottic cancer. Results from series of selected patients from the University of Florida and Massachusetts General Hospital, along with those from a relatively unselected population (Princess Margaret Hospital), are displayed in Table 15–5. In the Florida experience, the ultimate voice preservation rate with primary radiation therapy and surgical salvage is 66%.[139] CT scan

findings associated with increased local failure include arytenoid or paraglottic space involvement, multiple involved sites, and tumor volume greater than 3.5 mL.[140] Harwood and colleagues showed that local control was 67% for T4 lesions based on cartilage invasion when only 19% of the pyriform sinus was involved.[141] No randomized trials of total laryngectomy versus radiation alone for advanced cancer of the larynx have been undertaken, but overall survival appears to be slightly lower in the primary radiation group in retrospective reports.[142] Thus, the role of this therapeutic option remains controversial. Radiation therapy alone may be considered for patients who have T3 lesions with favorable features, such as unilateral tumor, exophytic growth pattern, absence of nodal involvement, and an adequate airway. For more advanced cases, radiation therapy alone may be considered for patients who cannot tolerate or who refuse surgery and chemotherapy.

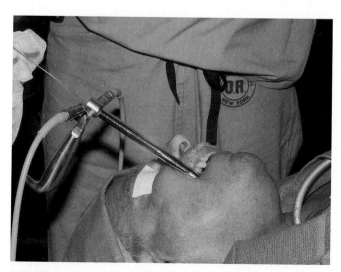

FIGURE 15–38 Leader cable threaded via the esophagoscope through the oral cavity.

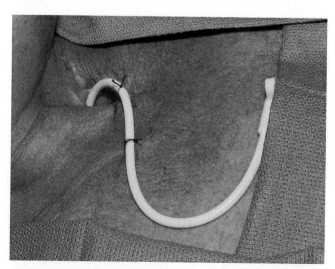

FIGURE 15–40 Silicone catheter in place after passage under direct vision into the distal esophagus. Patient underwent placement of self-retaining transesophageal puncture device 3 days later as an outpatient.

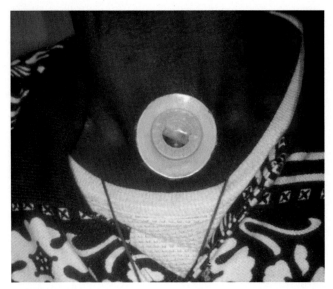

FIGURE 15–41 Self-retaining tracheostoma housing unit that allows for hands-free speech in a patient with a tracheoesophageal puncture.

Cancer of the Supraglottic Larynx

Radiation alone is an alternative to surgery for stage T1 to early T3 supraglottic cancers.[143] Ultimate local control with voice preservation has been reported to be 100% for T1, 87% for T2, 69% for T3, and 57% for T4 tumors in the University of Florida experience.[144] The complication rate in this series was 3% for T1–T3 cancers and 29% for T4 tumors. CT scan tumor volume of less than 6 mL is associated with improved local control.[145] As in glottic cancer, radiation alone should be considered for unfavorable stage T3 and T4 tumors only when the patient is unable to undergo surgery or chemoradiotherapy.[146]

Techniques

Planning

Before beginning a course of radiation therapy, patients must undergo a planning session, called *simulation*. The patient is positioned supine with the head hyperextended.

TABLE 15–5 Local Control for Squamous Cell Carcinoma of the Glottic Larynx Following Primary Radiation Therapy (RT) and With Surgical Salvage (SS)

Reference	T1 RT	T1 SS	T2 RT	T2 SS	T3 RT	T3 SS	T4 RT	T4 SS
University of Florida (Mendenhall[139, 142])	95	98	82 (a) 76 (b)	95 (a) 90 (b)	62	81	—	—
Massachusetts General Hospital (Wang[152])	93	98	75	89	57	79	67	—
Princess Margaret Hospital (Harwood[136, 141])	—	—	69	—	51	77	56	—

An immobilization device such as an aquaplast mask may be used to ensure reproducible positioning throughout treatment. The traditional technique for 2-dimensional (2D) simulation uses fluoroscopy and plain radiographs of the intended treatment field. Wires should be placed around palpable lymph nodes to indicate their location on the films. Movement of the larynx with respiration and swallowing is noted, and an adequate margin should be used to allow for such movement during treatment. Right and left lateral fields are used to treat the larynx and upper neck. These fields are matched, below the cricoid, to an anterior field when treatment of the lower neck is indicated. An axial contour of the neck at the level of the larynx is taken so that appropriate wedges or tissue compensators can be used to decrease dose inhomogeneity (hot and cold spots) within the larynx (Fig. 15–42). CT scan–based simulation is becoming increasingly popular, although the use of conformal radiation therapy for larynx cancer is not widely practiced.

Patients with cancer of the larynx should be treated with relatively low energy beams such as Co-60 or 4- to 6-MV photons. Bolus material may be required with 6-MV beams for superficial sparing. This is especially important for patients with cancer involving the anterior commissure, in whom a lower control rate with 6-MV beams has been reported.[147] Electron beams, usually of 6 to 9 MeV, are used to treat the posterior neck after a spinal cord block has been placed; they may also be used to boost superficial lymph nodes.

Treatment Volumes

Because of the remarkably low risk of lymph node metastasis with stage T1–T2 vocal cord lesions (2% to 7%), the regional lymph nodes are not included in the treatment field. A pair of small, approximately 5 × 5-cm lateral fields may be used to encompass the glottic larynx. Field borders typically extend from the hyoid bone superiorly to the cricoid bone inferiorly. The anterior beam edge flashes the skin, and the posterior edge is near the anterior edge of the vertebral bodies. These borders should be individualized according to the extent of cancer.

Treatment of all other cancers of the larynx, including stage III to IV glottic as well as all supraglottic and subglottic tumors, requires inclusion of the cervical lymph nodes in the radiation fields, whether or not nodal involvement exists. The larynx and upper neck nodes are treated in the lateral fields that typically extend from the skull base to below the cricoid, and the supraclavicular nodes are treated in a matching anterior field. A small spinal cord block must be placed throughout treatment at the bottom of the lateral fields to prevent overlapping beams on the cord. A full spinal cord block is later placed in the lateral beams at approximately 40 Gy (Fig. 15–43). The remainder of the prescribed dose may then be given to the posterior neck with matching electron fields.

A "boost" field is used in every case to deliver a larger dose to areas at highest risk such as the primary site or involved nodes. The boost to the larynx may be accomplished by using smaller lateral fields that include the entire larynx. More creative techniques may be necessary for boosting postoperative patients or those with extensive

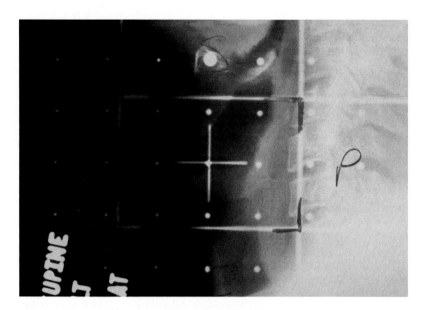

FIGURE 15–42 Radiation field for stage I or II glottic cancer. Treatment is given through opposed lateral fields with the use of appropriate wedges. Cervical lymph nodes are not included.

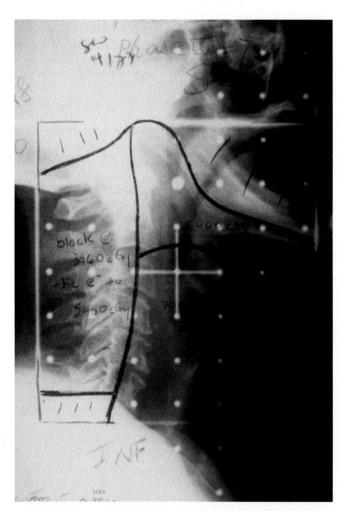

FIGURE 15–43 Radiation fields for stage III or IV laryngeal cancer. The upper neck is treated with opposed lateral fields matched to an inferior field for treatment of the lower neck. A shrinking field technique is used to block the spinal cord and boost the tumor at appropriate dose levels.

nodal disease. In patients with a tracheotomy, the stoma is almost always treated because this area is at high risk for recurrence if a patient has stage T3–T4 disease, extensive subglottic involvement of a glottic carcinoma, or primary cancer of the subglottis. Stomal recurrences are very difficult to salvage; therefore, radiation is used in an effort to prevent this problem.

Dose and Fractionation

The current standard of care for stage I and II laryngeal cancer involves standard fractions of 2 Gy daily. Single institutions have published favorable results with the use of alternative fractionation schemes, but these have never been studied in a randomized trial for early-stage disease.[148] The total dose prescribed for gross disease may vary slightly from institution to institution but is approximately 66 to 70 Gy. For early-stage supraglottic cancer, electively treated lymph node regions should receive approximately 50 Gy, and a dissected neck or tumor bed should receive a dose of approximately 60 Gy to counteract postsurgical hypoxia. Radiation therapy should begin within 6 weeks of surgery, provided that wound healing is adequate. A delay in the initiation of radiation and breaks during treatment are known to adversely impact local control. Overall treatment time is an important prognostic factor.[135]

A recent phase III Radiation Therapy Oncology Group (RTOG) study (9003) proved that accelerated fractionation is superior to standard fractionation for stage III to IV laryngeal cancer when radiation alone is used as definitive therapy.[149] This four-arm trial showed that intensification of radiation with either hyperfractionation (1.2 Gy twice daily to 81.6 Gy) or accelerated fractionation with concomitant boost (1.8 Gy per day and 1.5 Gy per day as a second daily fraction for the last 12 treatments to 72 Gy) significantly improved 2-year locoregional control (54.4% and 54.5%, respectively) compared with standard fractionation (46%) and accelerated fractionation with split (47.5%; $P < .05$). As a result, these regimens have now been adopted as the gold standard for definitive treatment with radiation alone. It remains to be seen whether intensified radiation schedules will be feasible on a widespread basis when concurrent chemotherapy is added, and whether there are incremental benefits with the combination of the two approaches. Single-institution data are promising[150, 151] but results of a phase II RTOG study are pending.[152]

▣ CHEMOTHERAPY/RADIATION FOR CANCER OF THE LARYNX

A number of drugs have demonstrated activity against SCC of the larynx. Many of the supporting data, however, are derived from studies that are not site-specific. Among the most commonly used agents are cisplatin, carboplatin, 5-fluorouracil, methotrexate, paclitaxel, docetaxel, and ifosfamide.[153] Anticipated response rates vary depending on the amount of previous treatment and whether combination or single-agent chemotherapy is applied. For example, major response rates in the 60% to 90% range can be anticipated with cisplatin-based combination chemotherapy in patients with previously untreated, locoregionally advanced disease, but this number drops to 30% to 40% in patients with recurrent disease. Toxicity is less with single-agent chemotherapy,[154] but response rates are also lower, being approximately one half of that expected with a combination of drugs. Besides having their own activity, these drugs may also be used as radiation sensitizers.[155]

Historically, chemotherapy had been used mostly with palliative intent. Most major responses to chemotherapy are not durable and generally last weeks to months in the absence of other therapy. Consistent with this observation is that when patients with recurrent or distant metastatic disease are treated with chemotherapy as their principal anticancer therapy, median survivals are consistently less than 1 year.[154–158] As a result, clinical trials evaluating new agents deserve particular consideration in this group of patients with a poor prognosis.

Although chemotherapy has not been viewed as a curative modality by itself, the impressive responses commonly seen in previously untreated patients have supported initiatives to improve tumor control rates by incorporating chemotherapy in different ways with surgery and/or radiation. This approach has evolved over the past 30 years and has varied with the resectability of the cancer and the goals of treatment.[153–159] In patients in whom resection for cure was possible, chemotherapy was integrated initially with surgery and radiation in a sequential manner, as either induction/neoadjuvant or maintenance/adjuvant chemotherapy, or both. The principal goal of these studies was improvement in survival. Subsequently, organ preservation, and most relevant here, larynx preservation without compromise in survival (thus reserving surgery for patients with recurrent cancer) became important endpoints. Among patients with unresectable disease or in whom nonsurgical management was preferred, radiation as a single modality had been the historical treatment option. With the goal of improving the results of treatment, the addition of chemotherapy to radiation in either a sequential or concomitant fashion was investigated. Insights gained from studies in patients with unresectable tumors have subsequently led to investigation of the role of chemoradiotherapy in laryngeal preservation in patients with locally advanced but resectable cancer.

With the exception of larynx preservation trials, most of the literature in phase III/randomized studies used to assess the potential role of chemotherapy combined with traditional locoregional management in patients with larynx cancer is derived from non–site-specific studies. Also, the risk of type II error is a frequent concern, given the prognostic heterogeneity of entered patients and the competing causes of mortality related to medical comorbidity and second primary cancers.[160, 161] Despite these limitations, important lessons that guide current management and future research directions have been derived from these clinical trials.

▣ IMPROVEMENT IN SURVIVAL AS AN ENDPOINT

Sequential chemotherapy combined with planned surgery and radiation in resectable patients has yielded disappointing results, and its use outside of a clinical trial is not supported by the available data.[162–164] Individual studies demonstrate that the pattern of failure may be affected by the incorporation of chemotherapy with a decrease in distant metastases, but there has been no significant improvement in overall survival. A recent meta-analysis quantitated the absolute improvement in overall survival associated with induction chemotherapy at 5 years to be 2% ($P = .10$); it is only 1% for adjuvant chemotherapy ($P = .74$).[165] Poor compliance may compromise the results obtained with adjuvant chemotherapy in that patient tolerance after locoregional treatment is often suboptimal.[162]

Results integrating chemotherapy with radiation have yielded much more encouraging results, particularly with the concomitant incorporation of chemotherapy.[166, 167] On meta-analysis, the estimated absolute improvement in overall survival with the concomitant use of chemotherapy with radiation was quantitated at 8% ($P < .0001$), although there was significant heterogeneity among the combined trials.[164] Selected studies have compared the same drugs given either sequentially or concomitantly with radiation.[168–171] Overall, these trials favor the concomitant arms with regard to a variety of intermediate endpoints, although improvement in overall survival has been more elusive. A meta-analysis of these studies yields a hazard ratio of 0.91 ($P = .23$) favoring a concomitant approach.[165] For patients with unresectable cancer who are chemotherapy candidates, concomitant chemotherapy and radiation deserves consideration and is appropriately viewed as a standard treatment option.

Given these results, concurrent chemotherapy/radiation has been increasingly investigated in patients with resectable cancer, both as an organ preservation strategy, discussed later, and as an adjuvant. In the latter context, two recent randomized trials are of particular interest. Both the Radiation Therapy Oncology Group trial (RTOG 9501) and the European Organization for Research and Treatment Cancer (EORTC) trial 22931 compared concurrent cisplatin 100 mg/m² on days 1, 22, and 43 with radiation (60 to 66 Gy, depending on the study) versus the same radiation dosing alone in patients with poor-risk, resected SCC of the head and neck.[172, 173] The proportions of patients with cancer of the larynx entered into each study were similar (21% to 23%). The RTOG study demonstrated a significant improvement with chemotherapy and radiation in disease-free survival (54% vs. 43% at two years, P = .05), but not in locoregional control or overall survival. The EORTC study, on the other hand, demonstrated significant improvements in all three of these endpoints in favor of the combined-modality arm. The studies used different stratification and criteria for poor-risk cases, which led to some differences in the study populations and may explain in part the observed differences in results. Further follow-up and analysis should provide additional insights.

Larynx Preservation

Initial studies that looked to improve upon anticipated organ preservation results obtained with radiation alone used chemotherapy in a neoadjuvant manner. This strategy was built on the results of previous studies demonstrating that the use of initial chemotherapy did not significantly increase the morbidity associated with subsequent surgery and/or radiation, as well as on an apparent correlation between response to chemotherapy and the likelihood of complete response with subsequent radiation.[174] A number of single-arm studies proved the feasibility of an approach whereby induction chemotherapy and radiation were applied, with surgery to the primary site reserved for nonresponse to induction chemotherapy or disease persistence.[175, 176] Historical comparisons suggested that survival outcomes were not compromised. These pilot data provided the basis for a series of randomized trials that warrant more detailed discussion.

The Veterans Administration (VA) larynx preservation study[177] randomly assigned 332 patient with T2–T4 SCC to either induction cisplatin and 5-fluorouracil for three cycles followed by radiation, with surgery reserved for less than a partial response at the primary site, persistent cancer, or salvage at relapse, or to total laryngectomy followed by radiation. On long-term follow-up, no significant difference in overall survival was noted between the groups, and approximately two thirds of surviving patients randomly assigned to treatment with chemotherapy and radiation avoided total laryngectomy. Delayed surgery because of lack of response to induction chemotherapy did not adversely affect survival outcomes. Follow-up of a subgroup of 46 surviving patients indicated that quality of life scores were better and depression was less common among those treated with larynx preservation intent, although it was curious that communication scores were similar between the two groups.[178]

The Group d'Etude des Tumeurs de la Tete et du Cou (GETTEC) performed a much smaller randomized study (n = 68) to evaluate similar treatment arms.[179] The patients who entered into this study differed from those in the VA study in that eligibility required that patients have T3 disease. A review of baseline characteristics indicates that the GETTEC study had more patients with glottic/transglottic versus supraglottic primaries. Furthermore, the criteria to proceed to definitive radiation were more stringent in that greater than 80% response to induction was required. Unlike the VA study, the GETTEC investigators reported that local, regional, and distant failures and survival endpoints were all superior with primary surgical management.

A third study, done under the auspices of the EORTC,[180] compared treatment strategies similar to those used in the VA and GETTEC studies; enrollment primarily included patients with advanced pyriform sinus cancer, but 22% of enrollees had cancer of the aryepiglottic fold. This study also used different response criteria from the other two in terms of what allowed the patient to proceed to definitive radiation—a complete response at the primary, including restoration of vocal cord mobility, was required. As was the case with the VA study, no significant difference in survival was noted between the treatment groups; a significant proportion of surviving patients treated with chemotherapy and radiation avoided total laryngectomy and were without tracheotomy or feeding tube afterward; and lack of response to chemotherapy and related delayed surgery did not adversely affect survival outcomes.

A meta-analysis of these three studies found a 6% absolute decrement in survival in the chemotherapy and radiation group (P = .10); this was associated with a 58% larynx preservation rate.[165] To what extent some of the described differences in study population and design among the three studies account for the variation in results, particularly in the GETTEC study, requires further study. Certainly, these data fail to indicate any survival advantage with the chemotherapy and radiation approach outlined. Because patients destined to fail chemotherapy and radiation are arguably best served by primary surgical management, strategies to optimize patient selection are receiving increased attention.[181, 182]

These larynx preservation trials used sequential chemotherapy and radiation, yet as was noted earlier, non–site-specific randomized data suggest that the concurrent integration of these modalities may be superior. In a study including a spectrum of primary sites, Adelstein and colleagues[183] reported a superior organ preservation rate with concurrent cisplatin, 5-fluorouracil, and radiation compared with radiation alone, although when the contribution of surgical salvage was incorporated, overall survival was equivalent on the two arms. An important intergroup randomized study, RTOG 91-11, evaluated different approaches to modality integration with eligibility limited to patients with T2-favorable T4 larynx cancer.[184] The three treatment arms included (1) induction chemotherapy with standard dose cisplatin (100 mg/m^2) and infusional 5-fluorouracil (1000 mg/m^2/day, days 1 to 5) for three cycles followed by definitive radiation (70 Gy); (2) radiation alone to 70 Gy; and (3) concurrent cisplatin (100 mg/m^2) on days 1, 22, and 43 with radiation to 70 Gy. The fraction size was 2 Gy once daily on all arms, as was the option of salvage surgery. No difference in overall survival was noted among the arms, but laryngectomy-free survival favored the concurrent arm (58% vs. 52% vs. 66%, respectively), as did time to laryngectomy. Accordingly, a concurrent chemotherapy and radiation strategy has displaced the other two as the preferred organ preservation option, as long as patients are chemotherapy candidates and can tolerate the expected added toxicity associated with the integration of chemotherapy.

A number of initiatives are under investigation with the intention of improving the efficacy of combined-modality therapy incorporating chemotherapy in both resectable and unresectable settings. These include but are not limited to the use of intra-arterial chemotherapy with radiation,[185] integrating chemotherapy with altered fractionation[151] radiation based on the apparent therapeutic superiority of selected altered fractionation schedules to standard once-daily fractionation,[149] primary chemotherapy leading to a modification in surgical management,[186] and a potential growing role for targeted therapy.[187, 188] Further investigation is necessary if the role of such approaches outside the clinical trial setting is to be determined.

Few data in the literature address the function of the preserved larynx after chemotherapy as part of an organ preservation approach. Most patients who are rendered disease-free do retain good function with intact speech, swallowing, and quality of life. However, some patients either retain their tracheotomy tube or require replacement of a tracheotomy tube owing to airway insufficiency at the level of the glottis secondary to scarring and stenosis. Moreover, many patients remain gastrostomy tube dependent as a consequence of fibrosis and scarring of the constrictor muscles, as well as glottic insufficiency (Figs. 15–44 and 15–45). Many of these events are a consequence of both local tumor destruction and secondary scarring and fibrosis from the effects of chemotherapy and radiation (Figs. 15–46 through 15–52). Future studies must focus on ways to predict which patients will obtain satisfactory outcomes from organ preservation and the implementation of strategies to prevent these quality of life–impairing sequelae of treatment.[181]

Early Glottic Cancer: Surgery Versus Radiation

Both surgery and radiation therapy are recognized treatments for T1–T2 SCC of the larynx (Table 15–6).[189–206] Many studies have analyzed and compared the oncologic outcomes of patients treated in a single institution by either endoscopic surgery or partial laryngectomy versus radiation therapy. These studies have shown similar 5-year

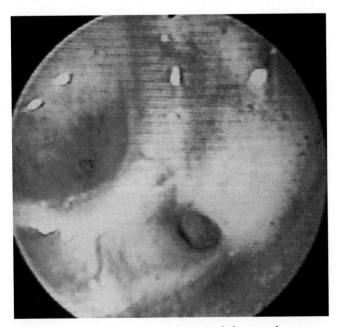

FIGURE 15–44 Endoscopic visualization of pharyngeal stricture.

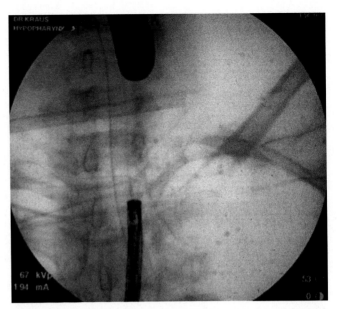

FIGURE 15–45 A 5-cm pharyngeal stricture confirmed by both antegrade and retrograde esophagoscopies with an intervening stricture that prevented cannulation or dilation.

cause-specific survival rates. Anterior commissure infiltration has been reported to represent a negative predictive factor of local control for radiation therapy, although with modern radiation therapy techniques, it should not significantly affect treatment outcome.

Radiation therapy had a local control rate of 79%, which increased to 90% with salvage surgery, and a high larynx preservation rate (83%). Partial laryngectomy (PL) offered a better initial local control rate of 84%, which increased to 88% with salvage surgery, and functional results were also good (80%).[194, 200] The treatment approach for laryngeal cancer is often a compromise between oncologic efficiency and preservation of function. Radiation therapy and surgery yield similar local control and survival rates.

T1 to T2 Glottic Cancer: Comparison of Surgery Versus Radiation Therapy Voice Outcome

Voice quality remains the issue often used to support preference for radiation therapy in the treatment of early glottic cancer. In a study by Verdonck-De Leeuw and colleagues, voice characteristics of patients were analyzed following radiation therapy for early glottic cancer through a multidimensional analysis protocol, including vocal function and voice quality measures.[207] Voice analyses were performed for 60 patients treated with radiation therapy (66 Gy/33 fractions, 60 Gy/30 fractions, or 60 Gy/25 fractions) for early T1 glottic cancer and 20 matched control speakers. Data revealed that the voice characteristics of patients were decreased before radiation therapy, improved after treatment, and became comparable to the voice characteristics of control speakers in at least 55% of patients. Following radiation therapy, deviant voice quality was attributed to increased age and stripping of the vocal cord for initial diagnosis.[207]

Delsupehe and colleagues compared perceptual voice in 2 groups—one treated with radiation therapy for malignant

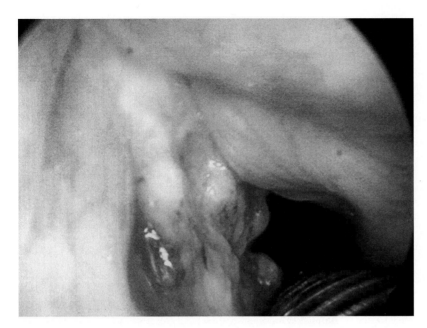

FIGURE 15–46 Transglottic carcinoma with involvement of the anterior commissure and subglottic extension.

disease and the other with narrow margin laser cordectomy for either malignant or extensive benign lesions.[208] Sequential patients, 12 treated with radiation therapy and 30 with CO_2 laser excision, were included. Data demonstrated that voice deteriorated temporarily after surgery as compared with the radiated group; however, at 6 and 24 months, no significant differences were seen. These authors recommended preferential use of narrow margin laser cordectomy for specific early glottic tumors for oncologic reasons, but also on the basis of voice results, cost, and efficiency considerations.[208]

Hirano and colleagues compared vocal function following laser surgery in 17 patients with glottic T1a carcinoma and vocal function following radiation therapy in 14 patients.[209] The results of this study demonstrated the following: (1) A slight degree of hoarseness was found more frequently following laser surgery than following radiation therapy. The quality of hoarseness was rough and breathy in most cases. (2) In stroboscopic examination, incomplete

glottal closure and diminution or lack of vibration of the operated vocal fold were frequently observed following laser surgery. (3) No marked difference was seen in maximum phonation time, mean air flow rate, fundamental frequency, range of phonation, intensity range of phonation, and intensity-to-flow ratio between the laser and radiation therapy groups. On the basis of these results, the authors concluded that there is little difference in vocal function as far as conversational voice is concerned between postlaser and post–radiation therapy patients.[209]

Schuller and colleagues studied perception of lifestyle change among laryngeal cancer patients.[210] Seventy-five patients (total laryngectomy 35, supraglottic laryngectomy 15, hemilaryngectomy 12, radiation therapy 8, laser cordectomy 5) and close relatives responded to a questionnaire and interview eliciting perception of the following: (1) post-treatment voice quality; (2) vocational and social adverse effects of treatment; and (3) degree of vocal or communicative change

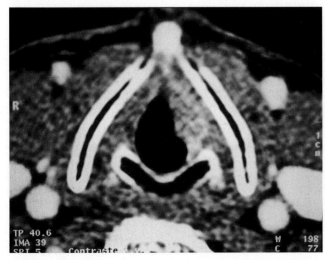

FIGURE 15–47 CT scan reveals involvement of the transglottic larynx.

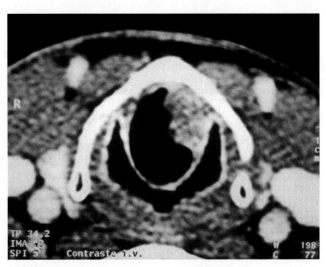

FIGURE 15–48 Subglottic extension with tumor extending to the level of the superior border of the cricoid cartilage.

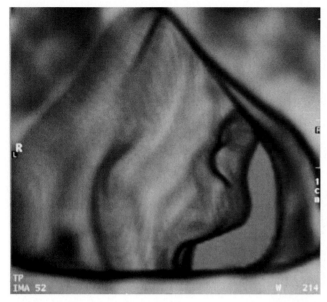

FIGURE 15–49 Three-dimensional renderings of the CT scan confirm transglottic carcinoma with 1 cm of subglottic extension.

associated with vocational or social change. Overall, 43% of patients reported vocational change, 37% reported social change, and 88% expressed satisfaction with their voices after cessation of treatment.[210]

As is evident from the data discussed earlier, no clear significant difference in objective voice quality is seen between surgery in appropriately selected patients and radiation therapy for early glottic cancers based on available voice assessment methodology data.

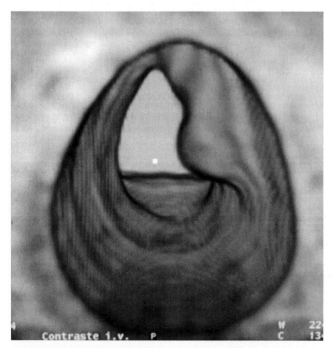

FIGURE 15–50 Three-dimensional renderings of the CT scan confirm transglottic carcinoma with 1 cm of subglottic extension.

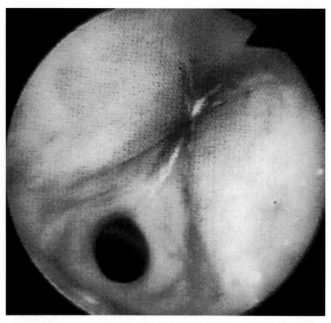

FIGURE 15–51 Anterior and posterior commissure stenosis after successful chemotherapy/radiation. Patient retains mobile arytenoids and the ability to approximate the vocal cords. Although the patient acknowledges a hoarse voice, he has intact speech and swallowing and no ventilatory embarrassment.

Early Supraglottic Cancer: Surgery Versus Radiation

Controversy exists as to whether partial laryngectomy or radiation therapy is the treatment modality of choice in the early stages of SCC of the supraglottic larynx. Radiation therapy had a local control rate of 79%, which increased to 90%

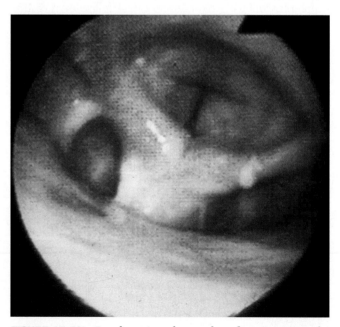

FIGURE 15–52 On phonation, the vocal cords approximate the midline.

with salvage surgery, and a high larynx preservation rate (83%).[211] PL offered a better initial local control rate of 84%, which increased to 88% with salvage surgery, and functional results were also reported as good (80%). No statistically significant differences were found between radiation therapy and PL. Radiation therapy was less costly and produced moderate morbidity and sequelae; also, local recurrence was easier to salvage. However, it is a once-only application technique. PL showed higher immediate postoperative morbidity and involved higher costs but had fewer sequelae, offered the best initial local control, and was reported to have been used on multiple occasions. No clear oncologic arguments are available to define whether PL or radiation therapy is the treatment of choice for early supraglottic carcinoma. Both are effective therapies. Secondary factors such as suitability for treatment, morbidity, cost, and applicability should be individually evaluated when the type of treatment is chosen. If the laser endoscopic approach decreases morbidity and costs and has comparable oncologic outcomes in comparison with radiation therapy, it could provide a compelling option.

Cancer of the Subglottis

The rarity of primary subglottic cancer, along with the varied definitions of the anatomic confines of this region, has limited our understanding of the patterns of tumor spread within the subglottis. A pattern of disease progression has been identified, defined by the cartilaginous laryngeal framework with the fibroelastic barriers susceptible to tumor invasion. Although cartilaginous laryngeal structures are preserved until late in the disease course, the ability of tumors to invade the fibroelastic membranes provides them with an insidious means of escape. Specifically, tumor progression occurs primarily within the paraglottic space and extralaryngeal compartments; the potential for mucosal spread is limited. The lack of mucosal disease in patients whose cartilaginous laryngeal structures are intact may present a facade of normality in patients with advanced disease and perhaps delays the early diagnosis of subglottic malignancies by physical and radiologic examination. In a study by Stell and Tobin, 32% of patients with subglottic carcinoma required an emergent tracheotomy.[212]

The combination of primary radiation therapy and surgery has been used to treat cancer of the subglottic larynx with varying results. A retrospective study of 39 patients with primary subglottic cancer seen between 1955 and 1988 was conducted at Washington University. Overall 5-year survival was 57.7%, and disease-free survival was 46.2%. Patients treated with radiation therapy alone, surgery alone, or both had disease-free 5-year survival rates of 22.2%, 41.7%, and 100%, respectively.[213] Shaha and Shah reviewed a series of 16 patients at Memorial Sloan-Kettering Cancer Center treated with partial laryngectomy for early disease and total laryngectomy with or without neck dissection for advanced disease; they recommended laryngectomy with thyroidectomy and paratracheal neck dissection (as the incidence of paratracheal nodal metastasis is estimated at 50%) as optimal treatment of subglottic carcinoma with postoperative radiation therapy for most of the advanced lesions.[214]

A retrospective study performed at the Princess Margaret Hospital Center to evaluate outcomes after radical radiation therapy and surgical salvage and to assess the risk of late toxicity for patients with primary subglottic SCC revealed that local control was achieved with radiation

TABLE 15-6 Comparison of Surgery Versus Radiation Therapy for Early Glottic Carcinoma

Study	Year	Patients (n)	Stage	Dose (Gy)	Surgery	2-Year Survival	5-Year Disease-Free Survival
Garcia-Serra[189]	2002	30	Tin	60			100%
Fein[190]	1993	19	Tin	56		100%	
Smitt[191]	1994	29	Tin	62			100%
Rothfield[192]	1991	20	Tin		Vertical partial laryngectomy		90%
Kersh[193]	1990	95	T1	60		100%	
Terhaard[194]	1991	194	T1	66		97%	
Small[195]	1992	103	T1	64			97%
Rudholtz[196]	1993	91	T1	64			92%
Barthel[197]	2001		T1	64			87.5%
Haugen[198]	2002	92	T1	62.4			85%
Ton-Van[199]	1991	206	T1		Cordectomy	87%	84%
Johnson[200]	1993	54	T1		Hemilaryngectomy	98%	
Daniilidis[201]	1990	94	T1		Cordectomy		93%
Steiner[202]	1993	96	T1		CO_2 laser		87%
Myers[138]	1994	50	T1		CO_2 laser	100%	
Thomas[203]	1994	159	T1		Laryngofissure	91%	84%
Smith[204]	2002	54	T1		Surgery	100%	
Howell-Burke[205]	1990	114	T2	56–78			92%
Kersh[193]	1990	53	T2	60		86%	
Pellitteri[206]	1991	48	T2	64–70			79%
Barthel[197]	2001		T2	64			75%
Haugen[198]	2002	45	T2	62.4			88%
Johnson[200]	1993	31	T2		Hemilaryngectomy	84%	
Steiner[202]	1993	34	T2		CO_2 laser	78%	

therapy alone in 24 (56%) of the 43 patients: 7 of 11 with T1, 8 of 12 with T2, 4 of 8 with T3, and 5 of 12 with T4.[215] The 5-year actuarial local relapse-free rate was 52%. Subsequent local control was achieved in 11 of the 13 patients with failed radiation therapy and attempted surgical salvage, for an ultimate local control rate of 81.4% (35 of 43).

The 5-year overall and cause-specific actuarial survival rates were 50.3% and 66.9%, respectively. No patients developed late radiation morbidity. Based on these data, the authors support the use of primary radiation therapy in the treatment of patients with primary SCC of the subglottis as an appropriate treatment approach that provides an option for laryngeal conservation.[215]

TUMORS OF THE LARYNX IN THE PEDIATRIC AGE GROUP

Malignant tumors of the larynx in children are rare, with the embryonal variant of rhabdomyosarcoma being the most common followed by SCC. Several risk factors have been mentioned, such as radiation therapy for juvenile laryngeal papillomatosis, intrauterine exposure to ionizing radiation, and chemical carcinogens. History of smoking or tobacco use is usually absent in this group. The management of malignant tumors of the larynx is more difficult in children than adults for several reasons, including the following: (1) the aggressive nature of a tumor, which is often diagnosed late in children; (2) the delicacy of pediatric anatomic structures; (3) long-term post-treatment complications; and (4) psychological factors peculiar to children. Choice of therapy depends on the clinical stage, the histologic type, and the potential radiochemosensitivity of the tumor.[7–10]

QUALITY OF LIFE OUTCOME

Quality of life outcome is very important in the formulation of treatment protocols. In a study from Europe, the quality of life assessment included five treatment groups: cordectomy, PL, irradiation as primary therapy, laryngectomy, and combined laryngectomy and radiation therapy. Evaluation of the functional scales of the European Organization for Research and Treatment of Cancer Quality of Life Questionnaire (EORTC QLQ-C 30) revealed a higher quality of life of patients with a maintained larynx compared with laryngectomized patients. On the symptom scales, patients after laryngectomy and/or radiation therapy suffered more from fatigue, pain, and appetite loss. Laryngectomees stated enhanced financial difficulties. Evaluation of the ENT-specific EORTC module showed that patients after laryngectomy reported increased symptoms. Typical symptoms after radiation therapy included dry mouth, sticky saliva, and coughing.[216]

SALVAGE SURGERY AFTER CHEMOTHERAPY/RADIATION THERAPY

After treatment of locally advanced cancer of the larynx with induction chemotherapy and radiation therapy, some patients suffer a local or regional failure that requires salvage surgery. A retrospective study was performed involving a cohort of 110 patients diagnosed between 1989 and 1996 with locally advanced cancer of the larynx (T3–T4) treated with induction chemotherapy and radiation therapy.[217] Forty-two patients presented a local and/or a regional recurrence of the tumor: 26 patients in the larynx, 8 in the neck, and 8 in both the larynx and the neck. Salvage surgery was carried out in 28 patients (67%) and consisted of total laryngectomy with neck dissection (24 cases), endoscopic resection of tumor (1 case), and radical neck dissection (3 cases). Five-year adjusted survival for the 42 patients with recurrence was 38%. Five-year survival for the 28 patients treated with salvage surgery was 57%. Five patients had postoperative complications: 4 had a pharyngocutaneous fistula and 1 had a wound infection. The authors concluded that after a local and/or a regional recurrence, 67% of patients with advanced laryngeal carcinoma treated with induction chemotherapy and radiation therapy were candidates for salvage surgery.[217]

In a recent series from Denmark, 1005 consecutive patients treated during the period between 1965 and 1998 were reviewed.[218] Salvage surgery was performed if patients had residual tumor or developed recurrence. Disease-specific survival and crude survival after 5 years, among 643 patients with glottic carcinomas treated with curative radiation therapy, were 88.6% and 65.3%, respectively. Among T1 glottic carcinomas, the locoregional control rate was 88% (i.e., 88% of patients were cured after radiation therapy alone), and the rate of disease-specific survival was 99% after 5 years (i.e., salvage surgery added approximately 11% to the survival of T1 glottic patients). Only 4% (12/312) of T1 glottic patients underwent laryngectomy. Locoregional control among T2 glottic cases was 67%, and the disease-specific survival was 88%, but 18% (41/233) of patients lost their larynx. The corresponding results among T3 glottic cases were 30% and 59%, respectively (i.e., organ preservation was close to 50%). Among patients with supraglottic carcinomas, the two estimates were 44% and 63%, respectively.[218]

STOMAL RECURRENCE

Stomal recurrence refers to carcinoma's arising from the margins of the tracheal or pharyngeal resection, or from the soft tissues or lymph nodes of the peristomal area, after a total laryngectomy. This disappointing result has a dismal prognosis, even with the most aggressive therapy, and many investigations have been undertaken to understand its pathogenesis for the purpose of preventing its occurrence.

Classification

The classification system of Sisson and colleagues[219] describes in the following ways the location of the recurrent tumor for the purposes of staging and prognosis:

Type I   Tumor involves the superior half of the stoma without esophageal involvement

Type II   Tumor involves the superior half of the stoma with esophageal involvement

Type III   Tumor involves the inferior half of the stoma and extends into the mediastinum

Type IV   Tumor extends out laterally underneath the clavicles

Incidence

In their comprehensive review of references encompassing 4281 laryngectomies, Esteban and coworkers calculated the overall incidence of stomal recurrence to be 6%. Of the many risk factors identified, subglottic extension of tumor is the one factor unanimously agreed upon as a significant risk.[220]

Muntz and Sessions reported that 19% of their patients with carcinoma of the glottis with subglottic extension had recurrence of cancer, most of which was local and varied with the amount of subglottic extension as follows: 10% for 5 to 14 mm, 29% for 15 to 19 mm, and 42% for greater than 20 mm.[221] Yuen and coworkers reported a 29% locoregional failure rate with subglottic extension greater than 1 cm compared with 19% for those with extension less than 1 cm.[222] Rubin and coworkers studied line-independent variables with multivariate analysis and found that cancer involving the subglottis and the size of the primary cancer (stage T4) were the only significant predictors of stomal recurrence.[223]

A controversial issue is whether emergent tracheotomy performed before definitive treatment of the larynx increases the incidence of stomal recurrence. Earlier reports in the literature estimate stomal recurrence to occur about 10% more frequently when preceded by emergent tracheotomy, citing cancer seeding into the trachea and peristomal soft tissues as the causes.[224–226] Some even advocate "emergency laryngectomy," performed in the same setting as the tracheotomy for the obstructing cancer, to help prevent stomal recurrence. However, recent studies have failed to show previous tracheotomy to be an independent risk factor. Rubin and coworkers, in a study of 444 laryngectomy patients, found no difference in stomal recurrence rate among the subglottic cancers that required emergent tracheotomy.[223] They proposed that the size and location of cancer of the subglottis made it more prone to both stomal recurrence and the need for urgent tracheotomy, and that the tracheotomy itself was not an independent risk factor. Other risk factors identified include metastasis to cervical lymph nodes, paratracheal lymph nodes, and the thyroid gland.[227–229]

Prevention

Efforts to prevent stomal recurrence focus on two interventions. First is the use of postoperative radiation to the stoma. Weber and colleagues studied 141 patients who underwent total laryngectomy, hemi- or total thyroidectomy, and paratracheal lymph node dissection for carcinoma of the larynx, hypopharynx, or cervical esophagus.[227] Stomal recurrence developed in 6 of 76 patients who did not receive radiation to the stoma and in 0 of 65 who did.[227]

The second intervention used to decrease stomal recurrence is the addition of paratracheal lymph node dissection in all cases of cancer of the larynx with subglottic extension.[229] A recent study from Japan, which evaluated stomal recurrence after total laryngectomy, revealed that primary site, preoperative tracheotomy, and paratracheal lymph node metastasis are significant risk factors for stomal recurrence.[230]

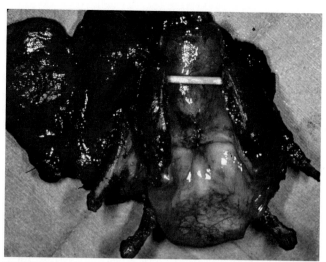

FIGURE 15–53 Salvage laryngectomy, ipsilateral tracheoesophageal groove dissection, and lateral neck dissection for patient who initially presented with a T1 glottic cancer. Patient had failed radiation therapy and presented with an ipsilateral vocal cord paralysis. All surgical margins were negative, and there was no evidence of metastatic disease in the dissected lymph nodes.

Hosal and coworkers reported a decline in stomal recurrence among 488 laryngectomy patients, from 11.5% in cases before 1968 to 2.7% in subsequent cases with the routine addition of pretracheal and paratracheal lymph node dissection in both primary and secondary subglottic cancer.[231] Rockley and coworkers compared a group of patients with T3N0M0 glottic cancer receiving emergent tracheotomy and subsequent laryngectomy with a matched group of patients with T3N0M0 cancer of the glottis treated with laryngectomy alone. The former group demonstrated an increase not only in mortality and stomal recurrence but also in regional metastases, suggesting that subclinical paratracheal and low cervical lymph node involvement was a possible factor in treatment failure, more so than the tracheotomy itself.[232] Rubin and colleagues pointed out that

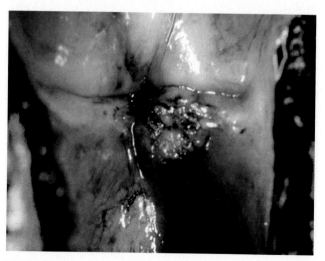

FIGURE 15–54 Close-up of Figure 15–53 shows 1.5 cm of subglottic extension of the primary lesion at the time of laryngectomy.

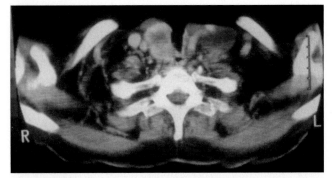

FIGURE 15–55 CT scan shows contralateral parastomal recurrence with no obvious involvement of the carotid artery system.

patients with primary cancer confined to the glottis and supraglottis have also had recurrences at the stoma, indicating that factors other than subglottic extension alone, such as subclinical paratracheal node metastases, also contribute to this event.[223]

Management

The management of stomal recurrence is primarily surgical. Currently, mediastinal dissection is recommended for type I and type II stomal recurrence, with postoperative radiation if this modality has not already been used. Patients with type III and type IV disease can be offered surgery if they are medically fit and are willing to accept higher morbidity and mortality rates. Radiation therapy has been

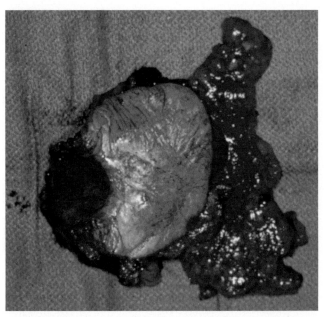

FIGURE 15–57 Parastomal resection specimen consisting of a portion of the trachea, the parastomal skin, the contralateral thyroid lobe, and the contralateral neck contents.

reported to provide palliation but is ineffective when used as a single agent. Furthermore, many patients have already had full-course radiation to control their primary cancer and are not able to receive further therapeutic doses. Combinations of radiation and chemotherapy when feasible have been used with encouraging early results.

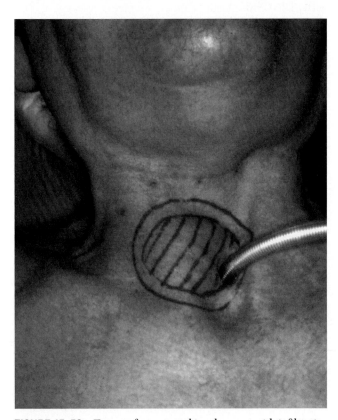

FIGURE 15–56 Extent of parastomal involvement with infiltration of the overlying skin.

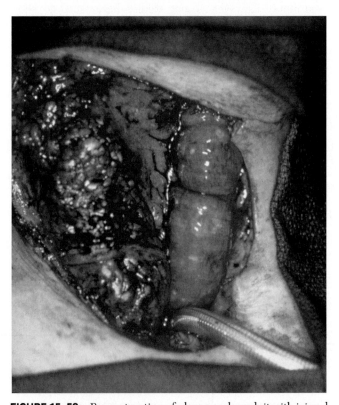

FIGURE 15–58 Reconstruction of pharyngeal conduit with jejunal free-flap reconstruction.

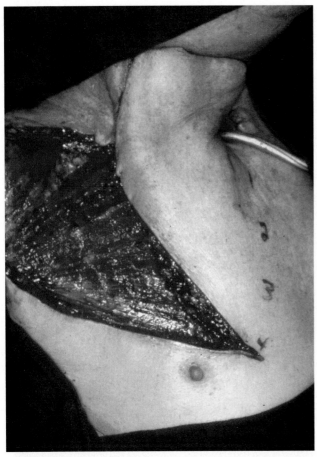

FIGURE 15–59 Elevation of deltopectoral flap for the purpose of reconstructing the cervical skin defect.

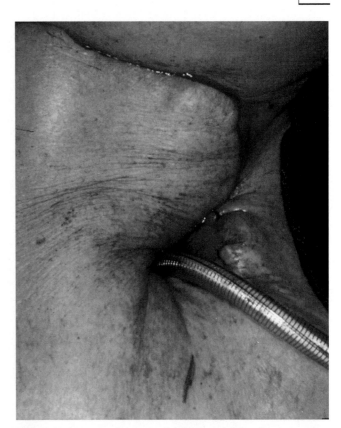

FIGURE 15–60 Deployment of deltopectoral flap for reconstruction of the cervical skin defect in the peristomal region with reconstruction of the stoma.

Surgery includes resection of the tracheostoma and the surrounding skin, mediastinal dissection with removal of the manubrium (with or without removal of the heads of the clavicles), and resection of involved pharyngoesophageal segments with reconstruction and obliteration of dead space using various flaps (Figs. 15–53 through 15–60).[233] Perioperative mortality approaches 15%, and death most often results from mediastinitis and rupture of the great vessels. Gluckman and coworkers reported the results of 41 mediastinal dissections for stomal recurrence of all types. Overall survival was a dismal 16% with a 24% determinate survival rate. Survival among types I and II lesions was 45%, but among types III and IV, it was only 9%. Acceptable palliation of pain and airway obstruction was achieved in the nonsurvivors.[234]

◘ PET SCANNING FOR POST-TREATMENT EVALUATION IN PATIENTS WITH CANCER OF THE LARYNX

[18]FDG is a radiolabeled glucose analogue that is taken up by cells through the glucose transporter and is subsequently phosphorylated by hexokinase. [18]FDG distribution within the body is a measure of glucose metabolism and may be assessed by PET. Because cancer cells generally exhibit increased glucose metabolism, PET imaging with [18]FDG may be used for the detection and localization of a wide variety of malignancies.[235]

Several small retrospective reports have suggested that [18]FDG-PET may be fairly accurate in detecting recurrent head and neck SCC. These studies have reported sensitivities ranging from 84% to 100%, and specificities ranging from 61% to 93%.[235–240]

In a review of 36 patients, Greven and colleagues also noted that the timing of the PET scan following radiation therapy may affect its accuracy.[240] PET scans performed at 4 months following the completion of radiation therapy demonstrated fewer false-positive findings than those performed at 1 month.[240] Two prospective studies have also supported the use of PET in the routine surveillance for recurrent head and neck SCC.[240, 241] Lowe and colleagues evaluated 44 patients with stage III or IV head and neck cancer following therapy with PET, physical examination, and correlative imaging.[241] Only PET detected all of the recurrences (16) in the first year following therapy. Terhaard and colleagues examined 75 patients with PET scan following radiation therapy for laryngeal or pharyngeal cancers and noted a sensitivity of 92% and a specificity of 63% on the initial PET scan.[242]

Wong retrospectively reviewed 143 patients who underwent 181 PET scans to detect recurrent head and neck cancers.[243] In this review, the overall sensitivity of PET

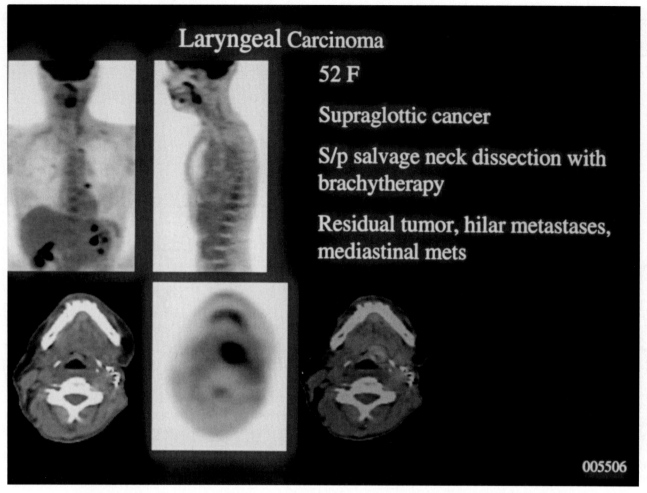

FIGURE 15–61 This 52-year-old white female initially presented with metastatic supraglottic cancer that was treated with chemotherapy and radiation, followed by salvage neck dissection with brachytherapy. The patient now presents with residual tumor in her supraglottic larynx. PET CT scan was performed to determine the local extent of invasion and to exclude metastatic disease. A PET fusion study confirms residual tumor at the primary site, with hilar metastasis and mediastinal metastatic lymph nodes.

was 96%, with a specificity of 72%. False-positive findings were most likely to occur at local sites of disease. PET was both highly sensitive and specific at both regional and distant sites. Furthermore, PET and standardized uptake value were found to be strong predictors of clinical outcome. An increase in standardized uptake value by 1 unit increased the relative risk of relapse by 11%, and the relative risk of death by 14%. A positive PET interpretation increased the relative risk of relapse fourfold and increased that of death sevenfold. These findings suggest that PET has an important diagnostic and prognostic value in the detection of recurrent head and neck cancers (Figs. 15–61 and 15–62).

■ TREATMENT OF THE NECK

Surgical Treatment of the Neck in Cancer of the Larynx

Controversy abounds regarding current concepts in the management of the clinically negative and clinically positive neck in cancer of the larynx. Occult disease in the neck not detected by physical and radiographic examination may be difficult to identify on routine histologic examination. Immunohistochemistry or molecular analysis may detect metastatic involvement not apparent by light microscopy. The surgeon should be aware of the relatively high incidence of micrometastasis in patients with cancer of the larynx, particularly for supraglottic primaries, so that optimal treatment approaches are established. Elective treatment of the neck is recommended for supraglottic cancers staged T2 or higher, and for glottic or subglottic tumors staged T3 or higher. The neck may be treated electively by either surgery or radiation, with radiation employed for cases in which that modality is employed for the primary cancer.

Elective neck dissection provides important information for prognostic purposes and therapeutic decisions by establishing the presence, number, location, and nature of occult lymph node metastases. Selective lateral neck dissection (levels II, III, and IV), unilateral or bilateral, is the procedure of choice for elective treatment. Paratracheal nodes (level VI) should be dissected in cases of advanced glottic

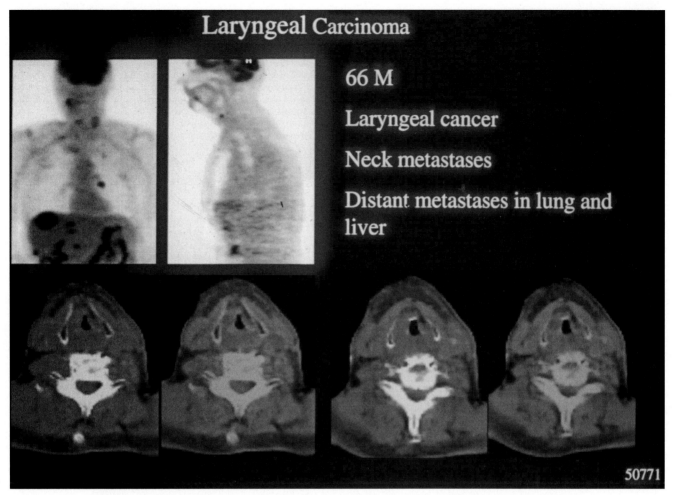

FIGURE 15–62 This 66-year-old male presents with laryngeal cancer treated with chemotherapy and radiation therapy with residual neck mass upon completion of treatment. Patient underwent PET CT fusion for assessment of locoregional extent of disease. Residual disease is found both in the larynx and in the contralateral neck. Patient also has distant metastasis to his lung and liver.

and subglottic cancer. Complete radical or functional neck dissections are often excessive in extent in that levels I and V are rarely involved. Sentinel lymph node biopsy procedures have not been shown to be effective for laryngeal primary cancers at this time. The clinically involved neck is usually treated by complete radical or functional neck dissection of levels I through V.

Selective neck dissection has been employed successfully in selected cases, particularly for N1 or occasionally N2 nodal involvement. Selective neck dissection can be extended to include structures at risk. More advanced disease has been treated in this manner, often in association with adjuvant chemotherapy and/or irradiation. Although the benefit of adjuvant treatment is difficult to assess, it appears most useful in cases with extranodal spread of disease—a factor associated with the worst prognosis.

Either modified type III radical neck dissection (MRND) or lateral neck dissection (LND) is considered valid treatment for patients with laryngeal carcinoma with clinically negative neck findings (N0) who are undergoing surgical management of the primary. A prospective study was performed to compare complications, neck recurrences,

and survival results of elective MRND and LND on the management of laryngeal cancer patients. A total of 132 patients were included in the trial. All patients had previously untreated T2–T4 N0M0 supraglottic or transglottic SCC. Seventy-one patients underwent MRND (13 bilateral) and 61 underwent LND (18 bilateral). The rate of occult metastasis detected on histologic examination was 26%, and most positive nodes occurred at levels II and III.[244]

Treatment of the Neck in Supraglottic Cancer

Controversy exists regarding the role of neck dissection as well as the extent of neck dissection after definitive radiation therapy in patients with supraglottic carcinoma specifically for N0 and N1 disease. Regional response has been related to the size of lymph nodes at presentation. Most patients with nodal size of 3 cm or less had a complete response, whereas patients with nodal size greater than 3 cm had a partial response. For patients with complete response in whom post–radiation therapy neck dissection was withheld, regional control rates were 75% and 86% for N1 and N2, respectively. In multivariate analysis, significant favorable factors predictive for regional control were female sex, accelerated hyperfractionation, and complete response; factors predictive for overall survival were Karnofsky Performance Scale score and regional response. Isolated regional relapse is not common among patients with supraglottic carcinoma when a complete response is achieved at 4 to 6 weeks after definitive radiation therapy is provided and post–radiation therapy neck dissection is not performed.[245]

Salvage Surgery of the Neck After Organ Preservation Protocols

As more and more patients are undergoing organ preservation protocols for laryngeal cancer, new issues have arisen with respect to the surgical management of the neck.

In a study from Memorial Sloan-Kettering Cancer Center, between 1983 and 1989, 80 patients were entered into larynx preservation protocols involving one to three cycles of cisplatin-based induction chemotherapy followed by radiation therapy with or without neck dissection.[246] Overall, there were 54 patients with clinically positive necks to treatment, of whom 44% (24/54) had a complete response and 20% (11/54) had a partial response to chemotherapy in the neck. In 22 of these 35 patients with clinically positive necks who achieved either a complete or a partial (75%) neck response to chemotherapy, radiation therapy (median 66 Gy) was used as the only subsequent treatment of the neck. At a median follow-up of 25 months (range, 7 to 83 months), neck control for this subset was 91% (20/22). Neck failure occurred in 20% (1/5) of patients with a partial response to chemotherapy treated without neck dissection and 6% (1/17) of node-positive patients with a complete response. Patients treated with radiation to the neck as the sole therapy experienced a 9% (2/22) rate of failure in the neck. No difference in survival rates was noted between groups. These results suggest that patients with clinically palpable cervical nodal metastases who have a complete response to chemotherapy and receive high-dose radiation therapy have excellent control of the neck and may not need neck dissection.[246]

The development of a recurrence in the neck after treatment of head and neck SCC is associated with a poor prognosis.[247] It has been shown that surgical salvage after radiation is more successful than surgical salvage after a surgical failure; this provides a rationale for attempting surgical salvage after failure of an organ preservation approach.[248, 249] A recent multicenter study involving 77 patients who underwent salvage surgery for isolated cervical recurrence after therapy showed an improved disease-free survival.[250] Complication rates among patients who have undergone previous organ preservation therapy are higher than among untreated patients, which should be kept in mind when surgical salvage is planned.[251]

REFERENCES

1. American Cancer Society: Cancer Facts & Figures 2001. Atlanta, American Cancer Society, 2001.
2. Surveillance, Epidemiology, and End Results Program, 1973–1997. Bethesda, MD, Division of Cancer Control and Population Sciences, National Cancer Institute, 2000.
3. DeRienzo DP, Greenberg SD, Fraire AE: Carcinoma of the larynx. Changing incidence in women. Arch Otolaryngol Head Neck Surg 117:681, 1991.
4. Yang PC, Thomas DB, Daling JR, et al: Differences in the sex ratio of laryngeal cancer incidence rates by anatomic subsite. J Clin Epidemiol 43:729, 1990.
5. Stephenson WT, Barnes DE, Holmes FF, et al: Gender influences subsite of origin of laryngeal carcinoma. Arch Otolaryngol 117:774, 1991.
6. Austen DF: Larynx. In Schottenfeld D, Fraumani JF (eds): Cancer Epidemiology and Prevention. Philadelphia, WB Saunders, 1982.
7. Simon M, Kahn T, Schneider A, et al: Laryngeal carcinoma in a 12-year-old child. Association with human papillomavirus 18 and 33. Arch Otolaryngol Head Neck Surg 120:277, 1994.
8. Ohlms LA, McGill T, Healy GB: Malignant laryngeal tumors in children: A 15-year experience with four patients. Ann Otol Rhinol Laryngol 103:686, 1994.
9. Bindlish V, Papsin BC, Gilbert RW: Pediatric laryngeal cancer: Case report and review of literature. J Otolaryngol 30:55, 2001.
10. Prasad KC, Abraham P, Peter R: Malignancy of the larynx in a child. Ear Nose Throat J 80:508, 2001.
11. Barnes C, Sexton M, Sizeland A, et al: Laryngo-pharyngeal carcinoma in childhood. Int J Pediatr Otorhinolaryngol 61:83, 2001.
12. Wasfie T, Newman R: Laryngeal carcinoma in black patients. Cancer 61:167, 1988.
13. Roach M III, Alexander M, Coleman JL: The prognostic significance of race and survival from laryngeal carcinoma. J Natl Med Assoc 84:668, 1992.
14. Falk RT, Pickle LW, Brown LM, et al: Effect of smoking and alcohol consumption on laryngeal cancer risk in coastal Texas. Cancer Res 49:4024, 1989.
15. Spitz MR, Fueger JJ, Goepfert H, et al: Squamous cell carcinoma of the upper aerodigestive tract. A case comparison analysis. Cancer 61:203, 1988.
16. Hedberg K, Vaughan TL, White E, et al: Alcoholism and cancer of the larynx: A case-control study in western Washington. Cancer Causes Control 5:3, 1994.
17. Zheng W, Blot WJ, Shu XO, et al: Diet and other risk factors for laryngeal cancer in Shanghai, China. Am J Epidemiol 136:178, 1992.
18. Brugers J, Guenel P, Leclerc A, et al: Differential effects of tobacco and alcohol in cancer of the larynx, pharynx, and mouth. Cancer 57:391, 1986.
19. Wortley P, Vaughan TL, Davis S, et al: A case-control study of occupational risk factors for laryngeal cancer. Br J Ind Med 49:837, 1992.
20. Brown LM, Mason TJ, Pickle LW, et al: Occupational risk factors for laryngeal cancer on the Texas Gulf Coast. Cancer Res 48:1960, 1988.
21. Amendola BE, Amendola MA, McClatchey KD: Radiation induced carcinoma of the larynx. Surg Gynecol Obstet 161:30, 1985.
22. Muscat JE, Wynder EL: Tobacco, alcohol, asbestos, and occupational risk factors for laryngeal cancer. Cancer 69:2244, 1992.
23. Smith AH, Handley MA, Wood R: Epidemiological evidence indicates asbestos causes laryngeal cancer. J Occup Med 32:499, 1990.
24. Chan CK, Gee JB: Asbestos exposure and laryngeal cancer: An analysis of the epidemiologic evidence. J Occup Med 30:23, 1988.
25. Freudenheim JL, Graham S, Byers TE, et al: Diet, smoking, and alcohol in cancer of the larynx: A case-control study. Nutr Cancer 17:33,1992.
26. Mackerras D, Buffler PA, Randall DE, et al: Carotene intake and the risk of laryngeal cancer in coastal Texas. Am J Epidemiol 128:980, 1988.
27. Olson NR: Laryngopharyngeal manifestations of gastroesophageal reflux disease. Otolaryngol Clin North Am 24:1201, 1991.
28. Koufman JA: The otolaryngologic manifestations of gastroesophageal reflux disease (GERD): A clinical investigation of 225 patients using ambulatory 24-hour pH monitoring and an experimental investigation of the role of acid and pepsin in the development of laryngeal injury. Laryngoscope 101:1, 1991.
29. Ward PH, Hanson DG: Reflux as an epidemiologic factor in carcinoma of the laryngopharynx. Laryngoscope 99:666, 1989.
30. El-Serag HB, Hepworth EJ, Lee P, et al: Gastroesophageal reflux disease is a risk factor for laryngeal and pharyngeal cancer. Am J Gastroenterol 96:2013, 2001.
31. Harrill WC, Stasney CR, Donovan DT: Laryngopharyngeal reflux: A possible risk factor in laryngeal and hypopharyngeal carcinoma. Otolaryngol Head Neck Surg 120:598, 1999.

32. Morrison MD: Is chronic gastroesophageal reflux a causative factor in glottic carcinoma? Otolaryngol Head Neck Surg 99:370, 1988.

33. Brandwein MS, Nuovo GJ, Biller H: Analysis of prevalence of human papillomavirus in laryngeal carcinomas. Study of 40 cases using PCR and consensus primers. Ann Otol Rhinol Laryngol 102:309, 1993.

34. Dayman GL, Stewart MG, Weber RS, et al: Human papillomavirus in laryngeal and hypopharyngeal carcinomas. Arch Otolaryngol Head Neck Surg 120:743, 1994.

35. Almadori G, Cadoni G, Cattani P, et al: Human papillomavirus infection and epidermal growth factor receptor expression in primary laryngeal squamous cell carcinoma. Clin Cancer Res 7:3988, 2001.

36. Kaya H, Kotiloglu E, Inanli S, et al: Prevalence of human papillomavirus (HPV) DNA in larynx and lung carcinomas. Pathologica 93:531, 2001.

37. Spitz MR, Fueger JJ, Halabi S, et al: Mutagen sensitivity in upper aerodigestive tract cancer: A case-control analysis. Cancer Epidemiol Biomarkers Prev 2:329, 1993.

38. Bondy ML, Spitz MR, Halabi S, et al: Association between family history of cancer and mutagen sensitivity in upper aerodigestive tract cancer patients. Cancer Epidemiol Biomarkers Prev 2:103, 1993.

39. Spitz MR. Fueger JJ, Beddingfield NA, et al: Chromosome sensitivity to bleomycin-induced mutagenesis, an independent risk factor for upper aerodigestive tract cancers. Cancer Res 49:4626, 1989.

40. Lynch HT, Kriegler M, Christiansen TA, et al: Laryngeal carcinoma in a Lynch syndrome II kindred. Cancer 62:1007, 1988.

41. Gallo O, Santoro R, Lenzi S, et al: Increased mutagen-induced chromosome damage in patients with transformed laryngeal precancerosis. Int J Cancer 68:700, 1996.

42. American Joint Committee on Cancer: Manual for Staging of Cancer, 5th ed. Philadelphia, Lippincott-Raven, 1997.

43. Nassar VH, Bridger GP: Topography of the laryngeal mucous glands. Arch Otolaryngol 94:490, 1971.

44. Kirchner JA: Vocal Fold Histopathology. San Diego, College Hill Press, 1986.

45. Zbaren P, Becker M, Lang H: Staging of laryngeal cancer: Endoscopy, computed tomography and magnetic resonance versus histopathology. Eur Arch Otorhinolaryngol 254(suppl 1):117, 1997.

46. Stadler A, Kontrus M, Kornfehl J, et al: Tumor staging of laryngeal and hypopharyngeal carcinomas with functional spiral CT: Comparison with nonfunctional CT, histopathology, and microlaryngoscopy. J Comput Assist Tomogr 26:279, 2002.

47. Barbera L, Groome PA, Mackillop WJ, et al: The role of computed tomography in the T classification of laryngeal carcinoma. Cancer 91:394, 2001.

48. Hollenbeak CS, Lowe VJ, Stack BC Jr: The cost-effectiveness of fluorodeoxyglucose 18-F positron emission tomography in the N0 neck. Cancer 92:2341, 2001.

49. Kresnik E, Mikosch P, Gallowitsch HJ, et al: Evaluation of head and neck cancer with 18F-FDG PET: A comparison with conventional methods. Eur J Nucl Med 28:816, 2001.

50. Stokkel MP, ten Broek FW, Hordijk GJ, et al: Preoperative evaluation of patients with primary head and neck cancer using dual-head 18fluorodeoxyglucose positron emission tomography. Ann Surg 231:229, 2000.

51. Kau RJ, Alexiou C, Laubenbacher C, et al: Lymph node detection of head and neck squamous cell carcinomas by positron emission tomography with fluorodeoxyglucose F 18 in a routine clinical setting. Arch Otolaryngol Head Neck Surg 125:1322, 1999.

52. Esposito ED, Motta S, Cassiano B, et al: Occult lymph node metastases in supraglottic cancers of the larynx. Otolaryngol Head Neck Surg 124:253, 2001.

53. Spector JG, Sessions DG, Haughey BH, et al: Delayed regional metastases, distant metastases, and second primary malignancies in squamous cell carcinomas of the larynx and hypopharynx. Laryngoscope 111:1079, 2001.

54. Taneja C, Allen H, Koness RJ, et al: Changing patterns of failure of head and neck cancer. Arch Otolaryngol Head Neck 128:324, 2002.

55. Spector GJ: Distant metastases from laryngeal and hypopharyngeal cancer. ORL J Otorhinolaryngol Relat Spec 63:224, 2001.

56. Laccourreye O, Veivers FD, Hans S, et al: Metachronous second primary cancers after successful partial laryngectomy for invasive squamous cell carcinoma of the true vocal cord. Ann Otol Rhinol Laryngol 111:204, 2002.

57. Holland JM, Arsanjani A, Liem BJ, et al: Second malignancies in early stage laryngeal carcinoma patients treated with radiotherapy. J Laryngol Otol 116:190, 2002.

58. Goodman ML: Keratosis (leukoplakia) of the larynx. Otolaryngol Clin North Am 17:179, 1984.

59. Shanmugaratnam K: Histological Typing of the Tumors of the Upper Respiratory Tract and Ear. Berlin, Springer-Verlag, 1991.

60. Crissman JD, Gnepp DR, Goodman ML, et al: Preinvasive lesions of the upper aerodigestive tract: Histologic definitions and clinical implications (a symposium). Pathol Annu 22:311, 1987.

61. Chung CK, Stryker JA, Abt AB, et al: Histologic grading in the clinical evaluation of laryngeal carcinoma. Arch Otolaryngol 106:623, 1980.

62. Mallofre C, Cardesa A, Campo E, et al: Expression of cytokeratins in squamous cell carcinomas of the larynx: Immunohistochemical analysis and correlation with prognostic factors. Pathol Res Pract 189:275, 1993.

63. Scambia G, Panici PB, Battaglia F, et al: Receptors for epidermal growth factor and steroid hormones in primary laryngeal tumors. Cancer 67:1347, 1991.

64. Randall G, Alonso WA, Ogura JH: Spindle cell carcinoma (pseudosarcoma) of the larynx. Arch Otolaryngol 101:63, 1975.

65. Batsakis JG (ed): Tumors of the Head and Neck. Baltimore, Williams & Wilkins, 1979.

66. Koch BB, Trask DK, Hoffman HT, et al: National survey of head and neck verrucous carcinoma: Patterns of presentation, care, and outcome. Cancer 92:110, 2001.

67. Batsakis JG, Hybek R, Crissman JD, et al: The pathology of head and neck tumor: Verrucous carcinoma. Head Neck Surg 5:29, 1982.

68. Ferlito A, Recher G: Ackerman's tumor (verrucous carcinoma) of the larynx. A clinicopathologic study of 77 cases. Cancer 46:1617, 1980.

69. Abramson A, Brandsma J, Steinberg B, et al: Verrucous carcinoma of the larynx: Possible human papillomavirus etiology. Arch Otolaryngol 111:709, 1985.

70. Sllamniku B, Bauer W, Painter C, et al: Clinical and histopathological considerations for the diagnosis and treatment of verrucous carcinoma of the larynx. Arch Otorhinolaryngol 246:126, 1989.

71. Fliss DM, Noble-Topham SE, McLachlin M, et al: Laryngeal verrucous carcinoma: A clinicopathologic study and detection of human papilloma virus using polymerase chain reaction. Laryngoscope 104:146, 1994.

72. Bradford CR, Zacks SE, Androphy EJ, et al: Human papillomavirus DNA sequences in cell lines derived from head and neck squamous cell carcinomas. Otolaryngol Head Neck Surg 104:303, 1991.

73. Chan KW, Lam KY, Lau P, et al: Prevalence of human papillomavirus types 16 and 18 in penile carcinoma: A study of 41 cases using PCR. J Clin Pathol 47:823, 1994.

74. Anderson JA, Irish JC, McLachlin CM, et al: H-ras oncogene mutation and human papillomavirus infection in oral carcinomas. Arch Otolaryngol Head Neck Surg 120:755, 1994.

75. Hagen P, Lyons GD, Haindel C: Verrucous carcinoma of the larynx: Role of human papillomavirus, radiation, and surgery. Laryngoscope 103:253, 1993.

76. Lundgren J, Van Nostrand A, Harwood A, et al: Verrucous carcinoma (Ackerman's tumor) of the larynx: Diagnostic and therapeutic considerations. Head Neck Surg 9:19, 1986.

77. Demian S, Bushkin F, Echevarria R: Perineural invasion and anaplastic transformation of verrucous carcinoma. Cancer 32:395, 1973.

78. Ferlito A, Rinaldo A, Mannara GM: Is primary radiotherapy an appropriate option for the treatment of verrucous carcinoma of the head and neck? J Laryngol Otol 112:1329, 1998.

79. Haberman PJ, Haberman RS: Laryngeal adenocarcinoma. Not otherwise specified, treated with carbon dioxide laser excision and postoperative radiotherapy. Ann Otol Rhinol Laryngol 101:920, 1992.

80. Serafini I, Lucioni M, Bittesini L, et al: Treatment of laryngeal adenoid cystic carcinoma. Acta Otorhinolaryngol Ital 11:13, 1991.

81. Cohen J, Guillamondegui OM, Batsakis JG, et al: Cancer of the minor salivary glands of the larynx. Am J Surg 150:513, 1985.

82. Ferlito A, Bames L, Myers EN: Neck dissection for laryngeal adenoid cystic carcinoma: Is it indicated? Ann Otol Rhinol Laryngol 99:277, 1990.

83. Snow RT, Fox AR: Mucoepidermoid carcinoma of the larynx. J Am Osteopath Assoc 91:182, 1991.

84. Damiani JM, Damiani KK, Hauck K, et al: Mucoepidermoid-adeno-squamous carcinoma of the larynx and hypopharynx: A report of 21 cases and a review of the literature. Otolaryngol Head Neck Surg 89:235,1981.

85. Moisa II, Mahadevia P, Silver CE: Unusual tumors of the larynx. In Silver CE (ed): Laryngeal Cancer. New York, Thieme, 1991.

86. Mahlstedt K, Ussmuller J, Donath K: Malignant sialogenic tumours of the larynx. J Laryngol Otol 116:119, 2002.

87. Jones AS, Beasley NJ, Houghton DJ, et al: Tumours of the minor salivary glands. Clin Otolaryngol 23:27, 1998.

88. Thome R, Thome DC, de la Cortina RA: Long-term follow-up of cartilaginous tumors of the larynx. Otolaryngol Head Neck Surg 124:634, 2001.

89. Bogdan CJ, Maniglia AJ, Eliachar I, et al: Chondrosarcoma of the larynx: Challenges in diagnosis and management. Head Neck 16:127, 1994.

90. Fechner RE: Chondrometaplasia of the larynx. Arch Otolaryngol 110:554, 1984.

91. Nicolai P, Sasaki CT, Ferlito A, et al: Laryngeal chondrosarcoma: Incidence, pathology, biological behavior, and treatment. Ann Otol Rhinol Laryngol 99:515, 1990.

92. Wang SJ, Borges A, Lufkin RB, et al: Chondroid tumors of the larynx: Computed tomography findings. Am J Otolaryngol 20:379, 1999.

93. Moran CA, Suster S, Carter D: Laryngeal chondrosarcomas. Arch Pathol Lab Med 117:914, 1993.

94. Nakayama M, Brandenburg JH, Hafez GR: Dedifferentiated chondrosarcoma of the larynx with regional and distant metastases. Ann Otol Rhinol Laryngol 102:785, 1993.

95. Ferlito A, Barnes L, Rinaldo A, et al: A review of neuroendocrine neoplasms of the larynx: Update on diagnosis and treatment. J Laryngol Otol 112:827, 1998.

96. Moisa II: Neuroendocrine tumors of the larynx. Head Neck 13:498, 1991.

97. Batsakis JG, El-Naggar AK, Luna MA: Neuroendocrine tumors of larynx. Ann Otol Rhinol Laryngol 101:710, 1992.

98. Ferlito A, Barnes L, Wenig BM: Identification, classification, treatment, and prognosis of laryngeal paraganglioma. Ann Otol Rhinol Laryngol 103:525, 1994.

99. Sanders KW, Abreo F, Rivera E, et al: A diagnostic and therapeutic approach to paragangliomas of the larynx. Arch Otolaryngol Head Neck Surg 127:565, 2001.

100. Barnes L: Paraganglioma of the larynx. A critical review of the literature. ORL J Otorhinolaryngol Relat Spec 53:220, 1991.

101. El-Naggar AK, Batsakis JG: Carcinoid tumor of the larynx. A critical review of the literature. ORL J Otorhinolaryngol Relat Spec 53:188, 1991.

102. Woodruff JM, Senie RT: Atypical carcinoid tumor of the larynx. A critical review of the literature. ORL J Otorhinolaryngol Relat Spec 53:194, 1991.

103. Ferlito A, Friedman I: Review of neuroendocrine carcinomas of the larynx. Ann Otol Rhinol Laryngol 98:780, 1989.

104. Laccourreye O, Brasnu D, Camot F, et al: Carcinoid (neuroendocrine) tumor of the arytenoid. Arch Otolaryngol Head Neck Surg 117:1395, 1991.

105. Gnepp DR: Small cell neuroendocrine carcinoma of the larynx. A critical review of the literature. ORL J Otorhinolaryngol Relat Spec 53:210, 1991.

106. Baugh RF, Wolf GT, Krause CJ, et al: Small cell carcinoma of the larynx: Results of therapy. Laryngoscope 96:1283, 1986.

107. Wax MK, Touma J: Management of the N0 neck during salvage laryngectomy. Laryngoscope 109:4, 1999.

108. Shedd SP: Historical Landmarks in Head and Neck Cancer Surgery. Pittsburgh, PA, American Head and Neck Society, 1999.

109. Remacle M, Eckel HE, Antonelli A, et al: Endoscopic cordectomy. A proposal for a classification by the Working Committee, European Laryngological Society. Eur Arch Otorhinolaryngol 257:227, 2000.

110. Pressman JJ: Submucosal compartmentation of the larynx. Ann Otol Rhinol Laryngol 65:766, 1956.

111. Pressman JJ: Further studies upon the submucosal compartments and lymphatics of the larynx by the injection of dyes and radioisotopes. Ann Otol Rhinol Laryngol 65:963, 1956.

112. Zeitels SM: Surgical management of early supraglottic cancer. Otolaryngol Clin North Am 30:59, 1997.

113. Weinstein GS, Laccourreye O: Supracricoid laryngectomy with cricohyoidoepiglottopexy. Otolaryngol Head Neck Surg 111:684, 1994.

114. Pradhan SA, D'Cruz AK, Pai PS, et al: Near-total laryngectomy in advanced laryngeal and pyriform cancers. Laryngoscope 112:375, 2002.

115. Shenoy AM, Sridharan S, Srihariprasad AV, et al: Near-total laryngectomy in advanced cancers of the larynx and pyriform sinus: A comparative study of morbidity and functional and oncological outcomes. Ann Otol Rhinol Laryngol 111:50, 2002.

116. Schwaab G, Kolb F, Julieron M, et al: Subtotal laryngectomy with cricohyoidopexy as first treatment procedure for supraglottic carcinoma: Institut Gustave-Roussy experience (146 cases, 1974–1997). Eur Arch Otorhinolaryngol 258:246, 2001.

117. Lassaletta L, Garcia-Pallares M, Morera E, et al: T3 glottic cancer: Oncologic results and prognostic factors. Otolaryngol Head Neck Surg 124:556, 2001.

118. Lima RA, Freitas EQ, Kligerman J, et al: Supracricoid laryngectomy with CHEP: Functional results and outcome. Otolaryngol Head Neck Surg 124:258, 2001.

119. Bron LP, Soldati D, Zouhair A, et al: Treatment of early stage squamous-cell carcinoma of the glottic larynx: Endoscopic surgery or cricohyoidoepiglottopexy versus radiotherapy. Head Neck 23:823, 2001.

120. Watters GW, Patel SG, Rhys-Evans PH: Partial laryngectomy for recurrent laryngeal carcinoma. Clin Otolaryngol 25:146, 2000.

121. Laccourreye O, Brasnu D, Perie S, et al: Supracricoid partial laryngectomies in the elderly: Mortality, complications, and functional outcome. Laryngoscope 108:237, 1998.

122. Chevalier D, Laccourreye O, Brasnu D, et al: Cricohyoidoepiglottopexy for glottic carcinoma with fixation or impaired motion of the true vocal cord: 5-year oncologic results with 112 patients. Ann Otol Rhinol Laryngol 106:364, 1997.

123. Laccourreye O, Weinstein G, Naudo P, et al: Supracricoid partial laryngectomy after failed laryngeal radiation therapy. Laryngoscope 106:495, 1996.

124. Kraus DH, Pfister DG, Harrison LB, et al: Salvage laryngectomy for unsuccessful larynx preservation therapy. Ann Otol Rhinol Laryngol 104:936, 1995.

125. Virtaniemi JA, Kumpulainen EJ, Hirvikoski PP, et al: The incidence and etiology of postlaryngectomy pharyngocutaneous fistulae. Head Neck 23:29, 2001.

126. Teknos TN, Myers LL, Bradford CR, et al: Free tissue reconstruction of the hypopharynx after organ preservation therapy: Analysis of wound complications. Laryngoscope 111:1192, 2001.

127. Sassler AM, Esclamado RM, Wolf GT: Surgery after organ preservation therapy. Analysis of wound complications. Arch Otolaryngol Head Neck Surg 121:162, 1995.

128. Giacomarra V, Russolo M, Tirelli G, et al: Surgical treatment of tracheostomal stenosis. Laryngoscope 111:1281, 2001.

129. Wax MK, Touma BJ, Ramadan HH: Management of tracheostomal stenosis. Laryngoscope 109:1397, 1999.

130. Davis RK, Vincent ME, Shapshay SM, et al: The anatomy and complications of "T" versus vertical closure of the hypopharynx after laryngectomy. Laryngoscope 92:16, 1982.

131. Singer MI, Blom ED: An endoscopic technique for restoration of voice after laryngectomy. Ann Otol Rhinol Laryngol 89:529, 1980.

132. McAuliffe MJ, Ward EC, Bassett L, et al: Functional speech outcomes after laryngectomy and pharyngolaryngectomy. Arch Otolaryngol Head Neck Surg 126:705, 2000.

133. Kao WW, Mohr RM, Kimmel CA, et al: The outcome and techniques of primary and secondary tracheoesophageal puncture. Arch Otolaryngol Head Neck Surg 120:301, 1994.

134. Izdebski K, Reed CG, Ross JC, et al: Problems with tracheoesophageal fistula voice restoration in totally laryngectomized patients. A review of 95 cases. Arch Otolaryngol Head Neck Surg 120:840, 1994.

135. Mendenhall WM, Amdur RJ, Morris CG, et al: T1–2N0 squamous cell carcinoma of the glottic larynx treated with radiation therapy. J Clin Oncol 19:4029, 2001.

136. Harwood AR, Beale FA, Cummings BJ, et al: T2 glottic cancer: An analysis of dose-time-volume factors. Int J Radiat Oncol Biol Phys 7:1501, 1981.

137. Mittal B, Rao DV, Marks JE, et al: Role of radiation in the management of early vocal cord carcinoma. Int J Radiat Oncol Biol Phys 9:997, 1983.

138. Myers EN, Wagner RL, Johnson JT: Microlaryngoscopic surgery for T1 glottic lesions: A cost-effective option. Ann Otol Rhinol Laryngol 103:28, 1994.

139. Mendenhall WM, Parsons JT, Stringer SP, et al: Stage T3 squamous cell carcinoma of the glottic larynx: A comparison of laryngectomy and irradiation. Int J Radiat Oncol Biol Phys 23:725, 1992.

140. Lee WR, Mancuso AA, Saleh EM, et al: Can pretreatment computed tomography findings predict local control in T3 squamous cell carcinoma of the glottic larynx treated with radiotherapy alone? Int J Radiat Oncol Biol Phys 25:683, 1993.

141. Harwood AR, Beale FA, Cummings BJ, et al: T4N0M0 glottic cancer: An analysis of dose-time volume factors. Int J Radiat Oncol Biol Phys 7:1507, 1981.

142. Mendenhall WM, Million RR, Sharkey DE, et al: Stage T3 squamous cell carcinoma of the glottic larynx treated with surgery and/or radiation therapy. Int J Radiat Oncol Biol Phys 10:357, 1984.

143. Mendenhall WM, Parsons JT, Mancuso AA, et al: Radiotherapy for squamous cell carcinoma of the supraglottic larynx: An alternative to surgery. Head Neck 18:24, 1996.

144. Mendenhall WM, Parsons JT, Stringer SP, et al: Carcinoma of the supraglottic larynx: A basis for comparing the results of radiotherapy and surgery. Head Neck 12:204, 1990.

145. Freeman DE, Mancuso AA, Parsons JT, et al: Irradiation alone for supraglottic larynx carcinoma: Can CT findings predict treatment results? Int J Radiat Oncol Biol Phys 19:485, 1990.

146. Weems DH, Mendenhall WM, Parsons JT, et al: Squamous cell carcinoma of the supraglottic larynx treated with surgery and/or radiation therapy. Int J Radiat Oncol Biol Phys 13:1483, 1987.

147. Akin Y, Tokita N, Ogino T, et al: Radiotherapy of T1 glottic cancer with 6MeV x-rays. Int J Radiat Oncol Biol Phys 20:1215, 1991.

148. Parsons JT, Mendenhall WM, Stringer SP, et al: Twice-a-day radiotherapy for squamous cell carcinoma of the head and neck: The University of Florida Experience. Head Neck 15:87, 1993.

149. Fu KK, Pajak TF, Trotti A, et al: A Radiation Therapy Oncology Group (RTOG) phase III randomized study to compare hyperfractionation and two variants of accelerated fractionation to standard fractionation radiotherapy for head and neck squamous cell carcinomas: Preliminary results of RTOG 9003. Int J Radiat Oncol Biol Phys 45:145, 1999.

150. Harrison LB, Raben A, Pfister DG, et al: A prospective phase II trial of concomitant chemotherapy and radiotherapy with delayed accelerated fractionation in unresectable tumors of the head and neck. Head Neck 20:497, 1998.

151. Brizel DM, Albers ME, Fisher SR, et al: Hyperfractionated irradiation with or without concurrent chemotherapy for locally advanced head and neck cancer. N Engl J Med 338:1798, 1998.

152. Wang CC: Carcinoma of the larynx. In Wang CC (ed): Radiation Therapy for Head and Neck Neoplasms, 3rd ed. New York, Wiley-Liss, 1997, pp 221–255.

153. Maluf FL, Sherman E, Pfister DG: Chemotherapy and chemoprevention in head and neck cancer. In Shah JP (ed): Cancer of the Head and Neck. Hamilton, ON, BC Decker, 2001, p 444.

154. Browman GP, Cronin L: Standard chemotherapy in squamous cell head and neck cancer: What we have learned from randomized trials. Semin Oncol 21:311, 1994.

155. Vokes EE, Weichselbaum RR: Concomitant chemoradiotherapy: Rationale and clinical experience in patients with solid tumors. J Clin Oncol 8:911, 1990.

156. Jacobs C, Lyman G, Velez-Garcia E, et al: A phase III randomized study comparing cisplatin and fluorouracil as single agents and in combination for advanced squamous cell carcinoma of the head and neck. J Clin Oncol 10:257, 1992.

157. Forastiere AA, Metch B, Schuller DE, et al: Randomized comparison of cisplatin plus fluorouracil and carboplatin plus fluorouracil versus methotrexate in advanced squamous cell carcinoma of the head and neck: A southwest oncology group study. J Clin Oncol 10:1245, 1992.

158. Clavel M, Vermorken JB, Cognetti F, et al: A randomized comparison of cisplatin, methotrexate, bleomycin and vincristine (CABO) versus cisplatin and 5-fluorouracil (CF) versus cisplatin in recurrent or metastatic squamous cell carcinoma of the head and neck. Ann Oncol 5:521, 1994.

159. Pfister DG, Shaha AR, Harrison LB: The role of chemotherapy in the curative treatment of head and neck cancer. Surg Oncol Clin N Am 6:749, 1997.

160. Piccirillo JF: Inclusion of comorbidity in a staging system for head and neck cancer. Oncology 9:831, 1995.

161. Shaha AR, Hoover EL, Marti JR, et al: Synchronicity, multicentricity, and metachronicity of the head and neck cancer. Head Neck 10:225, 1988.

162. Adjuvant chemotherapy for advanced head and neck squamous carcinoma. Final report of the Head and Neck Contracts Program. Cancer 60:301, 1987.

163. Laramore GE, Scott CB, Al-Sarraf M, et al: Adjuvant chemotherapy for resectable squamous cell carcinomas of the head and neck: Report on intergroup study 0034. Int J Radiat Oncol Biol Phys 23:705, 1992.

164. Paccagnella A, Orlando A, Marchiori C, et al: Phase III trial of initial chemotherapy in stage III and IV head and neck cancers: A study by the Gruppo di Studio sui Tumori della Testa e del Collo. J Natl Cancer Inst 86:265, 1994.

165. Pignon JP, Bourhis J, Domenge C, et al, on behalf of the MACH-NC Collaborative Group: Chemotherapy added to locoregional treatment for head and neck squamous-cell carcinoma: Three meta-analyses of updated individual data. Lancet 355:949, 2000.

166. Merlano M, Vitale V, Rosso R, et al: Treatment of advanced squamous-cell carcinoma of the head and neck with alternating chemotherapy and radiotherapy. N Engl J Med 327:1115, 1992.

167. Adelstein DJ, Adams GL, Li Y, et al: A phase III comparison of standard radiation therapy (RT) versus RT plus concurrent cisplatin (DDP) versus split-course RT plus concurrent DDP and 5-fluorouracil (5FU) in patients with unresectable squamous cell head and neck cancer (SCHNC): An intergroup study. Proc Am Soc Clin Oncol 19:411a, 2000.

168. South-East Co-operative Oncology Group: A randomized trial of combined multidrug chemotherapy and radiotherapy in advanced squamous cell carcinoma of the head and neck. An interim report from the SECOG participants. Eur J Surg Oncol 12:289, 1986.

169. Adelstein DJ, Sharan VM, Earle AS, et al: Simultaneous versus sequential combined technique therapy for squamous cell head and neck cancer. Cancer 65:1685, 1990.

170. Merlano M, Rosso R, Sertoli MR, et al: Randomized comparison of two chemotherapy, radiotherapy schemes for stage III and IV unresectable squamous cell carcinoma of the head and neck. Laryngoscope 100:531, 1990.

171. Taylor SG IV, Murthy AK, Vannetzel JM, et al: Randomized comparison of neoadjuvant cisplatin and fluorouracil infusion followed by radiation versus concomitant treatment in advanced head and neck cancer. J Clin Oncol 12:385, 1994.

172. Bernier J, Domenge C, Eschwege F, et al: Chemo-radiotherapy, as compared to radiotherapy alone, significantly increases disease-free and overall survival in head and neck cancer in patients after surgery: Results of EORTC phase III trial 22931. Int J Radiat Oncol Biol Phys 51:3, 2001. Abstract, Plenary #1.

173. Cooper JS, Pajak TF, Forastiere AA, et al: Postoperative concurrent radiochemotherapy in high risk SCCA of the head and neck: Initial report of RTOG 9501/intergroup phase III trial. Proc Am Soc Clin Oncol 21:226a, 2002.

174. Pfister DG, Harrison LB, Strong EW: Current status of larynx preservation with multimodality therapy. Oncology 6:33, 1994.

175. Pfister DG, Strong E, Harrison L, et al: Larynx preservation with combined chemotherapy and radiation therapy in advanced but resectable head and neck cancer. J Clin Oncol 9:850, 1991.

176. Karp DD, Vaghan CW, Carter R, et al: Larynx preservation using induction chemotherapy plus radiation therapy as an alternative to laryngectomy in advanced head and neck cancer. A long-term follow-up report. Am J Clin Oncol 14:273, 1991.

177. The Department of Veterans Affairs Laryngeal Cancer Study Group: Induction chemotherapy plus radiation compared with surgery plus radiation in patients with advanced laryngeal cancer. N Engl J Med 324:1685, 1991.

178. Terrell JE, Fischer SG, Wolf GT, for the Veterans Affairs Laryngeal Cancer Study Group: Long-term quality of life after treatment of laryngeal cancer. Arch Otolaryngol Head Neck Surg 124:964, 1998.

179. Richard JM, Sancho-Garnier H, Pessey JJ, et al: Randomized trial of induction chemotherapy in larynx cancer. Oral Oncol 34:224, 1998.

180. Lefebvre J-L, Chevalier D, Luboinsk B, et al: Larynx preservation in pyriform sinus cancer: Preliminary results of a European Organization for Research and Treatment of Cancer phase III trial. J Natl Cancer Inst 88:890, 1996.

181. Sherman EJ, Pfister DG, Venkatraman E, et al: TALK score: A prognostic model used to predict successful larynx preservation. Proc Am Soc Clin Oncol 18:392a, 1999.

182. Osman I, Sherman E, Singh B, et al: Inactivation of p53 pathway in squamous cell carcinoma of the head and neck: Impact on treatment outcome in patients treated with larynx preservation intent. J Clin Oncol (in press).

183. Adelstein DJ, Saxton JP, Lavertu P, et al: A phase III randomized trial comparing concurrent chemotherapy and radiation therapy with radiation therapy alone in resectable stage III and IV squamous cell head and neck cancer: Preliminary results. Head Neck 19:567, 1997.

184. Forastiere AA, Berkey B, Maor M, et al: Phase III trial to preserve the larynx: Induction chemotherapy and radiotherapy versus concomitant chemoradiotherapy versus radiotherapy alone, intergroup trial R91-11. Proc Am Soc Clin Oncol 20:2a, 2001.

185. Samant S, Kumar P, Wan J, et al: Concomitant radiation therapy and targeted cisplatin chemotherapy for the treatment of advanced pyriform sinus carcinoma: Disease control and preservation of organ function. Head Neck 21:595, 1999.

186. Laccourreye O, Brasnu D, Biacabe B, et al: Neoadjuvant chemotherapy and supracricoid partial laryngectomy with cricohyoidopexy for advanced endolaryngeal carcinoma classified as T3–T4: 5-year oncologic results. Head Neck 20:595, 1998.

187. Huang SM, Bock JM, Harari PM: Epidermal growth factor receptor blockade with C225 modulates proliferation, apoptosis, and radiosensitivity in squamous cell carcinomas of the head and neck. Cancer Res 59:1935, 1999.

188. Fan Z, Baselga J, Masui H, et al: Antitumor effect of anti-epidermal growth factor receptor monoclonal antibodies plus cisdiaminedichloroplatinum on well established A431 cell xenografts. Cancer Res 53:4637, 1993.

189. Garcia-Serra A, Hinerman RW, Amdur RJ, et al: Radiotherapy for carcinoma in situ of the true vocal cords. Head Neck 24:390, 2002.

190. Fein DA, Mendenhall WM, Parsons JT, et al: Carcinoma in situ of the glottic larynx: The role of radiotherapy. Int J Radiat Oncol Biol Phys 27:379, 1993.

191. Smitt MC, Goffinet DR: Radiotherapy for carcinoma in situ of the glottic larynx. Int J Radiat Oncol Biol Phys 28:251, 1994.

192. Rothfield RE, Myers EN, Johnson JT: Carcinoma in situ and microinvasive squamous cell carcinoma of the vocal cords. Ann Otol Rhinol Laryngol 100:793, 1991.

193. Kersh CR, Kelly MD, Hahn SS, et al: Early glottic carcinoma: Patterns and predictors of relapse after definitive radiotherapy. South Med J 83:374, 1990.

194. Terhaard CH, Snippe K, Ravasz LA, et al: Radiotherapy in T1 laryngeal cancer: Prognostic factors for locoregional control and survival, uni-multivariate analysis. Int J Radiat Oncol Biol Phys 21:1179, 1991.

195. Small W Jr, Mittal BB, Brand WN, et al: Results of radiation therapy in early glottic carcinoma: Multivariate analysis of prognostic and radiation therapy variables. Radiology 182:789, 1992.

196. Rudholtz MS, Benammar A, Mohiuddin M: Prognostic factors for local control and survival in T1 squamous cell carcinoma of the glottis. Int J Radiat Oncol Biol Phys 26:767, 1993.

197. Barthel SW, Esclamado RM: Primary radiation therapy for early glottic cancer. Otolaryngol Head Neck Surg 124:35, 2001.

198. Haugen H, Johansson KA, Merke C: Hyperfractionated-accelerated or conventionally fractionated radiotherapy for early glottic cancer. Int J Radiat Oncol Biol Phys 52:109, 2002.

199. Ton-Van J, Lefebvre JL, Stern JC, et al: Comparison of surgery and radiotherapy in T1 and T2 glottic carcinomas. Am J Surg 162:337, 1991.

200. Johnson JT, Myers EN, Hao SP, et al: Outcome of open surgical therapy for glottic carcinoma. Ann Otol Rhinol Laryngol 102:752, 1993.

201. Daniilidis J, Nikolaou A, Symeonidis V: Our experience in surgical treatment of T1 carcinoma of the vocal cord. J Laryngol Otol 104:222, 1990.

202. Steiner W: Results of curative laser microsurgery of laryngeal carcinomas. Am J Otolaryngol 14:116, 1993.

203. Thomas JV, Olsen KD, Neel HB 3rd, et al: Early glottic carcinoma treated with open laryngeal procedures. Arch Otolaryngol Head Neck Surg 120:264, 1994.

204. Smith JC, Johnson JT, Myers EN: Management and outcome of early glottic carcinoma. Otolaryngol Head Neck Surg 126:356, 2002.

205. Howell-Burke D, Peters LJ, Goepfert H, et al: T2 glottic cancer. Recurrence, salvage, and survival after definitive radiotherapy. Arch Otolaryngol Head Neck Surg 116:830, 1990.

206. Pellitteri PK, Kennedy TL, Vrabec DP, et al: Radiotherapy. The mainstay in the treatment of early glottic carcinoma. Arch Otolaryngol Head Neck Surg 117:297, 1991.

207. Verdonck-De Leeuw IM, Hilgers FJ, Keus RB, et al: Multidimensional assessment of voice characteristics after radiotherapy for early glottic cancer. Laryngoscope 109:241, 1999.

208. Delsupehe KG, Zink I, Lejaegere M, et al: Voice quality after narrow-margin laser cordectomy compared with laryngeal irradiation. Otolaryngol Head Neck Surg 121:528, 1999.

209. Hirano M, Hirade Y, Kawasaki H: Vocal function following carbon dioxide laser surgery for glottic carcinoma. Ann Otol Rhinol Laryngol 94:232, 1985.

210. Schuller DE, Trudeau M, Bistline J, et al: Evaluation of voice by patients and close relatives following different laryngeal cancer treatments. J Surg Oncol 44:10, 1990.

211. Orus C, Leon X, Vega M, et al: Initial treatment of the early stages (I, II) of supraglottic squamous cell carcinoma: Partial laryngectomy versus radiotherapy. Eur Arch Otorhinolaryngol 257:512, 2000.

212. Stell PM, Tobin KE: The behavior of cancer affecting the subglottic space. Can J Otolaryngol 4:612, 1975.

213. Dahm JD, Sessions DG, Paniello RC, et al: Primary subglottic cancer. Laryngoscope 108:741, 1998.

214. Shaha AR, Shah JP: Carcinoma of the subglottic larynx. Am J Surg 144:456, 1982.

215. Paisley S, Warde PR, O'Sullivan B, et al: Results of radiotherapy for primary subglottic squamous cell carcinoma. Int J Radiat Oncol Biol Phys 52:1245, 2002.

216. Muller R, Paneff J, Kollner V, et al: Quality of life of patients with laryngeal carcinoma: A post-treatment study. Eur Arch Otorhinolaryngol 258:276, 2001.

217. Leon X, Quer M, Orus C, et al: Results of salvage surgery for local or regional recurrence after larynx preservation with induction chemotherapy and radiotherapy. Head Neck 23:733, 2001.

218. Jorgensen K, Godballe C, Hansen O, et al: Cancer of the larynx—treatment results after primary radiotherapy with salvage surgery in a series of 1005 patients. Acta Oncol 41:69, 2002.

219. Sisson GA, Bytell DE, Becker SP: Mediastinal dissection—1976: Indications and newer techniques. Laryngoscope 87:751, 1977.

220. Esteban F, Moreno JA, Delgado-Rodriguez M, et al: Risk factors involved in stomal recurrence following laryngectomy. J Laryngol Otol 107:527, 1993.

221. Muntz H, Sessions D: Surgery of laryngopharyngeal and subglottic cancer. In Bailey B, Biller H (eds): Surgery of the Larynx. Philadelphia, WB Saunders, 1985, pp 293–315.

222. Yuen A, Medina JE, Goepfert H, et al: Management of stage T3 and T4 glottic carcinomas. Am J Surg 148:467, 1984.

223. Rubin J, Johnson JT, Myers EN: Stomal recurrence after laryngectomy: Interrelated, risk factor study. Otolaryngol Head Neck Surg 103:805, 1990.

224. Weisman RA, Colman M, Ward PH: Stomal recurrence following laryngectomy: A critical evaluation. Ann Otol Rhinol Laryngol 88:855, 1979.

225. Davis RK, Shapshay SM: Peristomal recurrence: Pathophysiology, prevention, treatment. Otolaryngol Clin North Am 13:499, 1980.

226. Bignardi L, Gavioli C, Staffieri A: Tracheostomal recurrences after laryngectomy. Arch Otorhinolaryngol 238:107, 1983.

227. Weber RS, Marvel J, Smith P, et al: Paratracheal lymph node dissection for carcinoma of the larynx, hypopharynx, and cervical esophagus. Otolaryngol Head Neck Surg 108:11, 1993.

228. Gilbert RW, Cullen RJ, van Nostrand AW, et al: Prognostic significance of thyroid gland involvement in laryngeal carcinoma. Arch Otolaryngol Head Neck Surg 112:856, 1986.

229. Brennan JA, Meyers AD, Jafek BW: The intraoperative management of the thyroid gland during laryngectomy. Laryngoscope 101:929, 1991.

230. Imauchi Y, Ito K, Takasago E, et al: Stomal recurrence after total laryngectomy for squamous cell carcinoma of the larynx. Otolaryngol Head Neck Surg 126:63, 2002.

231. Hosal IN, Onerci M, Turan E: Peristomal recurrence. Am J Otolaryngol 14:206, 1993.

232. Rockley TJ, Powell J, Robin PE, et al: Post-laryngectomy stomal recurrence: Tumour implantation or paratracheal lymphatic metastasis? Clin Otolaryngol 16:43, 1991.

233. Krespi YP, Wurster CF, Sisson GA: Immediate reconstruction after total laryngopharyngoesophagectomy and mediastinal dissection. Laryngoscope 95:156, 1985.

234. Gluckman JL, Hamaker RC, Schuller DE, et al: Surgical salvage for stomal recurrence: A multi-institutional experience. Laryngoscope 97:1025, 1987.

235. Phelps ME: Positron emission tomography provides molecular imaging of biological processes. Proc Natl Acad Sci U S A 97:9226, 2000.

236. Lonneaux M, Lawson G, Ide C, et al: Positron emission tomography with fluorodeoxyglucose for suspected head and neck tumor recurrence in the symptomatic patient. Laryngoscope 110:1493, 2000.

237. Stokkel MP, Terhaard CH, Hordijk GJ, et al: The detection of local recurrent head and neck cancer with fluorine-18 fluorodeoxyglucose dual-head positron emission tomography. Eur J Nucl Med 26:767, 1999.

238. Lapela M, Eigtved A, Jyrkkio S, et al: Experience in qualitative and quantitative FDG PET in follow-up of patients with suspected recurrence from head and neck cancer. Eur J Cancer 36:858, 2000.

239. Farber LA, Benard F, Machtay M, et al: Detection of recurrent head and neck squamous cell carcinomas after radiation therapy with 2-^{18}F-fluoro-2-deoxy-D-glucose positron emission tomography. Laryngoscope 109:970, 1999.

240. Greven KM, Williams DW, McGuirt WF, et al: Serial positron emission tomography scans following radiation therapy of patients with head and neck cancer. Head Neck 23:942, 2001.

241. Lowe VJ, Boyd JH, Dunphy FR, et al: Surveillance for recurrent head and neck cancer using positron emission tomography. J Clin Oncol 18:651, 2000.

242. Terhaard CH, Bongers V, van Rijk PP, et al: F-18-Fluorodeoxy glucose positron-emission tomography scanning in detection of local recurrence after radiotherapy for laryngeal/pharyngeal cancer. Head Neck 23:933, 2001.

243. Wong RJ, Lin DT, Schöder H, et al: Diagnostic and prognostic value of 18-fluorodeoxyglucose positron emission tomography for recurrent head and neck squamous cell carcinoma. J Clin Oncol 20:4199, 2002.

244. Brazilian Head and Neck Cancer Study Group: End results of a prospective trial on elective lateral neck dissection vs type III modified radical neck dissection in the management of supraglottic and transglottic carcinomas. Head Neck 21:694, 1999.

245. Chan AW, Ancukiewicz M, Carballo N, et al: The role of postradiotherapy neck dissection in supraglottic carcinoma. Int J Radiat Oncol Biol Phys 50:367, 2001.

246. Armstrong J, Pfister D, Strong E, et al: The management of the clinically positive neck as part of a larynx preservation approach. Int J Radiat Oncol Biol Phys 26:759, 1993.

247. Grandi C, Mingardo M, Guzzo M, et al: Salvage surgery of cervical recurrences after neck dissection or radiotherapy. Head Neck 15:292, 1993.

248. Kokal WA, Neifeld JP, Eisert DR, et al: Management of locoregional recurrent oropharyngeal carcinoma. Am J Surg 146:436, 1983.

249. Deutsch M, Leen R, Parsons JA: Radiotherapy for postoperative recurrent squamous cell carcinoma in head and neck. Arch Otolaryngol 98:316, 1973.

250. Krol BJ, Righi PD, Paydarfar JA, et al: Factors related to outcome of salvage therapy for isolated cervical recurrence of squamous cell carcinoma in the previously treated neck: A multi-institutional study. Otolaryngol Head Neck Surg 123:368, 2000.

251. Panje WR, Namon AJ, Vokes E, et al: Surgical management of the head and neck cancer patient following concomitant multimodality therapy. Laryngoscope 105:97, 1995.

CHAPTER 16

Cancer of the Hypopharynx and Cervical Esophagus

Jean-Louis Lefebvre
Dominique Chevalier
Bernard Coche-Dequeant

◼ INTRODUCTION

Cancer of the hypopharynx and cervical esophagus presents a major therapeutic challenge to head and neck specialists. Therapy for these tumors requires a multidisciplinary approach that must involve surgeons (i.e., head and neck surgeon, reconstructive and plastic surgeon, thoracic surgeon), radiation oncologists, and medical oncologists, as well as radiologists and speech pathologists. This multidisciplinary approach enables tailoring of the treatment for each patient with two primary goals—cure and functional rehabilitation.

These cancers often occur in debilitated patients with serious comorbidities. They are usually of advanced primary stage with a high tendency for submucosal spread and enlarged ipsilateral or bilateral cervical lymph node deposits. These features combine to make locoregional control of these cancers difficult. Although the ability to achieve locoregional control and/or preservation of organ function has improved, survival rates remain essentially unchanged. This is attributed to the rising incidence of distant metastases and intercurrent diseases, as well as to second primary malignancies.

◼ ANATOMY

Hypopharynx

The hypopharynx, or laryngopharynx, is interposed between the oropharynx and the esophagus. It extends from the level of the hyoid bone down to the upper esophageal sphincter (which corresponds approximately to the sixth cervical vertebra) and lies posterior to the larynx and partially surrounds it on each side. The hypopharynx includes the posterior pharyngeal wall, the pyriform sinuses, and the postcricoid area (Fig. 16–1). The cervical esophagus extends from the lower edge of the cricoid cartilage to the thoracic inlet.

The lumen of the hypopharynx is cone shaped. The superior margin of the pyriform sinus begins at the level of the pharyngoepiglottic fold, and each pyriform sinus is made up of an anterior dihedral angle between a lateral wall and a medial wall that narrows inferiorly to the apex. The hypopharyngeal lumen becomes narrow in the postcricoid and cervical esophageal areas. The anterior portion of the hypopharynx opens directly into the larynx, from which it is separated by the epilarynx.

The wall of the hypopharynx is composed of four layers— (1) an inner mucosal lining of stratified squamous epithelium over a loose stroma; (2) a fibrous layer of pharyngeal aponeurosis; (3) a muscular layer formed by the inferior constrictor muscle and, in the upper part, by the distal portion of the middle constrictor (the most distal fibers of the inferior constrictor condense into the cricopharyngeus muscle; just proximal to this muscle on the posterior wall is an area of relative weakness known as Killian's triangle); and (4) an outer layer of fascia that derives from buccopharyngeal fascia.

The pyriform sinuses are divided into a superior or membranous part, and an inferior or cartilaginous part. The superior aspect of the pyriform sinus is bounded by the thyrohyoid membrane, through which passes the internal branch of the superior laryngeal nerve. Sensory axons of this nerve synapse superiorly in the jugular ganglion along with sensory nerves of the external auditory canal (Arnold's nerve), which accounts for the referred otalgia frequently seen with tumors of the pyriform sinus. The lower portion of the pyriform sinus is bounded by the ala of the thyroid cartilage.

The postcricoid area corresponds to the posterior surface of the arytenoid cartilages and the posterior aspect of the cricoid ring. It terminates inferiorly at the pharyngoesophageal junction and is intimately related to the apex of each pyriform sinus laterally.

The hypopharyngeal portion of the posterior wall of the pharynx extends from the level of the hyoid bone to the pharyngoesophageal junction and is in continuity laterally with the lateral wall of each pyriform sinus. It is related posteriorly to the retropharyngeal space.

The terminal branches of the recurrent laryngeal nerve pass through the fibers of the cricopharyngeus muscle and the posterior cricoarytenoid muscles of the larynx. Motor and sensory innervation of the hypopharynx occurs via the pharyngeal plexus, which is formed by branches of cranial nerves IX and X. The arterial supply arises from branches of the superior thyroid arteries along with collateral vessels from the lingual and ascending pharyngeal arteries.

The junction between the postcricoid area and the cervical esophagus is the narrowest portion of the upper alimentary tract; it acts like a sphincter and is controlled by the

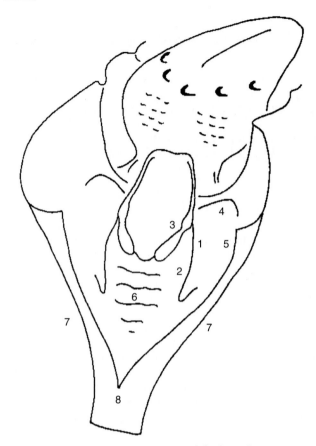

FIGURE 16–1 Posterior view of the hypopharynx.

cricopharyngeus muscle. The cervical esophagus is lined by nonkeratinizing squamous epithelium over a loose stroma and a muscular layer consisting of an inner circular and an outer longitudinal layer covered by a fascial sheath. Between the cricopharyngeus and the upper portion of the esophageal musculature is Lanier's triangle. The outermost layer of the cervical esophagus is continuous with the buccopharyngeal fascia. This layer separates the esophagus posteriorly from the retroesophageal space, which is continuous with the retropharyngeal space above and with the posterior mediastinum below. Anteriorly, the cervical esophagus is in direct relation to the trachea, although it deviates slightly to the left of this organ. In the tracheoesophageal groove on both sides are the recurrent laryngeal nerves and the paratracheal lymph nodes. The lateral aspect of the thyroid gland and, more laterally, the carotid sheaths and their contents are related to the cervical esophagus. This anatomic proximity allows direct extension of tumors of the esophagus to the thyroid gland.

Branches of the recurrent laryngeal nerves provide the nerve supply, and branches of the inferior thyroid arteries and ascending vessels from the thoracic esophagus provide the vascular supply.

Lymphatics

The hypopharynx and the cervical esophagus are richly supplied with lymphatics. Major lymphatic drainage channels terminate in the lymph nodes along the jugular vein (levels II, III, and IV) and appear to a lesser extent in the nodes along the spinal accessory nerve (level V) and even less frequently in the submandibular area (level I). Significant lymphatic drainage from the posterior pharyngeal wall travels to the retropharyngeal lymph nodes. Lymphatics from the inferior portion of the pyriform sinuses, the postcricoid area, and the cervical esophagus often drain to the nodes along the recurrent nerves to the paratracheal lymph nodes (level VI).

◼ EPIDEMIOLOGY

Descriptive Epidemiology

The incidence of hypopharyngeal cancer is much higher in men than in women, although the incidence in women is rising as more women are smoking. The annual incidence is evaluated at 1 per 100,000 persons and corresponds to 8% to 10% of head and neck malignancies. France and India are known for their high incidence of hypopharyngeal cancer, with an annual incidence ranging between 8 and 15 per 100,000 men.[1] These cancers usually occur during the second half of life, with a peak incidence in the fifth and sixth decades (on the average at around 55 years for men and 60 years for women). They occur mainly among men (around 95%), but in Anglo-Saxon countries, there is a higher incidence of postcricoid cancers (up to 30%) among women. Increased incidence of cancer of the hypopharynx is closely associated with lower socioeconomic classes and lower levels of education.

Analytic Epidemiology

The etiology of hypopharyngeal cancer is definitively linked to the excessive use of both tobacco and alcohol, which are in general the prime etiologic factors for squamous cell carcinoma (SCC) of the upper aerodigestive tract. In a prospective epidemiologic study of 339 consecutive patients with newly diagnosed cancer of the hypopharynx at Centre Oscar Lambret, the average daily consumption of tobacco was 0.84 ounce (range, 0.11 to 2.12) for a total consumption of 699 pounds (range, 29 to 2200) before diagnosis. The average alcohol consumption was as high as 4.87 ounces (range, 1.41 to 19.04) of ethanol for a cumulative consumption of 3646 pounds (range, 121 to 13,391) before diagnosis. Dietary deficiencies may also contribute to the establishment of cancer, but the exact role of such deficiencies is not well understood.

The possibility of a genetic predisposition to the development of cancer of the hypopharynx and cervical esophagus continues to be investigated. Genotypic and phenotypic deficiencies in the metabolism of tobacco-related and other carcinogens, as well as abnormalities in DNA repair mechanisms, may also be involved in the predisposition to pharyngeal cancers.

The Plummer-Vinson or Paterson-Brown Kelly syndrome represents a combination of dysphagia, hypopharyngeal web, weight loss, and iron deficiency anemia, usually occurring in nonsmoking women between the ages of 30 and 50 years. Patients with this syndrome are at a higher risk of developing cancer of the hypopharynx, particularly in the postcricoid region.

PATHOLOGY AND CLASSIFICATION

Macroscopic Pathology

In the United States, the most common site of origin of cancer of the hypopharynx is the pyriform sinus (66% to 75%), followed by the posterior pharyngeal wall (20% to 25%) and the postcricoid region. In Europe, the proportion of cancer of the pyriform sinus is even higher, except in northern Europe, where cancer in the postcricoid area may be as frequent as 30% of cases. Most of the tumors are ulcerated and infiltrative, and local infection is a common feature. Macroscopic margins are often poorly defined, in particular on the posterior wall (so-called *carpet carcinoma*).

Histopathologic Description

By far (in at least 90% of cases), the most frequent histologic type of cancer in the hypopharynx and cervical esophagus is SCC. Cancer arising from submucosal minor salivary glands is occasionally encountered, and malignant mesenchymal or neuroendocrine tumors and lymphomas are rare. Submucosal spread around the macroscopic margins of the tumor is a frequent feature either in direct continuity with the cancer or at some distance (skip metastases).

Routes of Spread

Cancer of the medial wall of the pyriform sinus may spread superficially toward the lateral epilarynx (aryepiglottic fold, arytenoids). It may infiltrate deeply to the pharyngolaryngeal wall, including the cricoarytenoid joint. Involvement of the paraglottic and pre-epiglottic spaces explains the frequency of early vocal cord fixation. Involvement of the recurrent laryngeal nerve beneath the mucosa of the pyriform sinus may also fix the hemilarynx. Tumors of the lateral wall spread rapidly to the ala of the thyroid cartilage and thereafter to the ipsilateral thyroid lobe.

Cancer of the postcricoid area frequently invades the posterior cricoarytenoid muscles and the cricoid and arytenoid cartilages. The apex of the pyriform sinus terminates in the postcricoid area and is often invaded early. Advanced tumors may totally encircle the hypopharyngeal lumen.

Cancer of the posterior pharyngeal wall usually manifests as ulcerating infiltrating lesions that spread both superficially and submucosally to the entire posterior pharyngeal wall from the nasopharynx to the cervical esophagus. These lesions may spread posteriorly to the prevertebral muscles and the retropharyngeal space, but vertebral bone extension is rare. Carcinomas of the pharyngeal wall spread laterally to both pyriform sinuses.

In our experience at Centre Oscar Lambret, review of a series of 652 consecutive patients with newly diagnosed cancer of the hypopharynx revealed cancer of the pyriform sinuses in 83% of patients, cancer of the postcricoid area in 9%, and cancer of the posterior wall in the remaining 8%. Cancer of the pyriform sinus extended to the larynx in 76% of cases, to the postcricoid and cervical esophagus in 20%, to the oropharynx in 14%, and to the soft tissues of the neck in 10%. Cancer of the postcricoid area extended to the pyriform sinuses in 89% of cases, to the larynx in 62%, to the cervical esophagus in 52%, and to the soft

tissues of the neck in 5%. Finally, cancer of the posterior wall extended to the pyriform sinuses in 77% of cases, to the pharyngoesophageal junction in 36%, and to the oropharynx in 21%.

In up to 80% of patients, metastatic lymph nodes are found either on physical examination or by imaging at first presentation. In the previously mentioned series, 78% of the patients had clinically (via palpation and imaging) metastatic lymph nodes at presentation. In the ipsilateral neck, level I was involved in 3% of patients, level II in 49%, level III in 38%, level IV in 14%, and level V in 4%. In the contralateral neck, level I was involved in none of patients, level II in 6%, level III in 3%, level IV in 3%, and level V in 1%. Direct metastases to level IV without involvement of levels I to III (skip metastases) were found in 9% of patients.

Distant metastases are a common feature during the evolution of carcinoma of the hypopharynx. Figures as high as 50% have been reported in the literature when autopsies were performed. As for most upper aerodigestive tract tumors, patients with locally advanced diseases and/or lymph node metastases had the highest risk for distant metastases (mainly in the lung, followed by the liver, bone, and brain).

A majority of patients with cancer of the hypopharynx present with advanced stages of the disease. In our series, 4% of patients presented with stage I, 3% with stage II, 40% with stage III, and 53% with stage IV. In addition, 54% of patients had documented serious comorbidities at presentation (consisting of cirrhosis of the liver in 11% of patients).

Classification

Primary cancers of the hypopharynx are classified as follows[2]:

Tis   Carcinoma in situ
T1   Tumor limited to one subsite of hypopharynx
T2   Tumor invades more than one subsite of hypopharynx or an adjacent site, without fixation of hemilarynx
T3   Tumor invades more than one subsite of hypopharynx or an adjacent site, with fixation of hemilarynx
T4   Tumor invades adjacent structures, for example, cartilage or soft tissues of neck

For cancer of the cervical esophagus, the recommended staging is identical to that for the intrathoracic esophagus:

Tis   Carcinoma in situ
T1   Tumor invades lamina propria or submucosa
T2   Tumor invades muscularis propria
T3   Tumor invades adventitia
T4   Tumor invades adjacent structures

The nodal classification for the hypopharynx is the same as that for other sites in the head and neck. For the cervical esophagus, the nodal classification differs as follows:

N0   No regional lymph node metastasis
N1   Regional lymph node metastasis

PATIENT EVALUATION

Presenting Symptoms

Patients with cancer of the hypopharynx commonly present with a history of sore throat, dysphagia, referred otalgia, hoarseness, and/or a neck mass. Dysphagia is a common symptom. Initially vague throat pain, usually unilateral, is indicative of an early cancer, when associated with intermittent difficulties while swallowing saliva. Patients often complain of feeling a foreign body in the throat. Progressive dysphagia, initially for solids foods and later for liquids, is frequently seen in patients with hypopharyngeal cancer. Severe dysphagia and odynophagia are symptoms of advanced-staged cancer that invades the inferior aspects of the hypopharynx or the cervical esophagus. Hoarseness is often associated with cancer of the hypopharynx that invades the larynx or the recurrent laryngeal nerve in the postcricoid region or cervical esophagus. Dyspnea is uncommon in the early stages but may occur later because of infiltration of the larynx or bilateral involvement of the recurrent laryngeal nerves. Weight loss is common in patients with hypopharyngeal cancer and is even more common among patients with cervical esophageal lesions. Weight loss resulting from obstruction of the pharynx or the upper esophagus adds to the patient's underlying malnutrition resulting from inadequate diet and excessive alcohol intake. A nutritional assessment must be documented. Such information is necessary at the time of therapeutic decision making.

Cervical lymphadenopathy is frequent at the time of diagnosis and is most often seen in the subdigastric and midjugular nodal levels. Careful examination must be performed in every patient who presents with enlarged lymph nodes, persistent sore throat, otalgia, and dysphagia, particularly when known risk factors (alcohol abuse and/or tobacco consumption) are recorded in the patient's history.

Clinical Findings

The oral cavity and the oropharynx are examined so that possible second primary cancer can be detected and the patient's dental status assessed. A panoramic and dynamic visual examination is mandatory. Indirect pharyngolaryngoscopy remains the basic diagnostic procedure. Examination is performed with a laryngeal mirror, followed when necessary by examination with a rigid endoscope or a flexible fiberoptic scope. The fiberoptic laryngoscope gives a less precise view of the mucosa, but its use is necessary in patients with an uncontrollable gag reflex. On the other hand, videoscopic examination with the rigid endoscope is a procedure of better quality; it also allows for photography and videography of the tumor. Patients must be examined during both respiration and phonation. This indirect pharyngolaryngoscopy provides global information on the site and size of the tumor and the mobility of the vocal cords. Although tumors of the posterior wall or the upper pyriform sinus are usually easily visualized by this indirect mirror examination, tumors of the apex of the pyriform sinus or of the postcricoid region and cervical esophagus may escape detection. Attention must be paid to indirect signs such as edema, erythema, and pooling of secretions, which may reveal an underlying abnormality and indicate that further investigation should be initiated.

Vocal cord mobility and laryngeal function should be carefully assessed. Laryngeal invasion with limited mobility, which suggests more advanced disease, is significant and must be considered at the time of therapeutic decision.

Bilateral immobility is encountered in cases of bilateral invasion of the recurrent laryngeal nerves and is more often seen in cancer of the cervical esophagus.

Palpation of the neck is necessary to detect adenopathy. All cervical areas, including the supraclavicular areas, are carefully examined bilaterally. The size, site, and mobility of all nodes should be documented. Examination of the neck may also reveal signs of direct extension of the cancer into the tissues of the neck, but this condition may be difficult to differentiate from adjacent lymph node metastasis. Pain generated by the movement of the thyroid cartilage is highly suggestive of an extension to the neck. Nodal involvement may be the presenting symptom of an early primary cancer. In such cases, careful clinical examination is necessary to visualize the primary cancer.

Direct Pharyngolaryngoscopy

Direct endoscopic examination of the pharynx, larynx, and esophagus is performed with the patient under general anesthesia. It is conducted with rigid endoscopes and with rigid telescopes for enhanced quality of the mucosal assessment, particularly in the case of a small cancer. It is an indispensable diagnostic tool that has several goals:

- It allows multiple biopsies for histologic examination.
- It provides an accurate evaluation of superficial tumor spread.
- Systematic examination of the entire upper aerodigestive tract and the esophagus allows for detection of synchronous cancers.
- Palpation of the neck with the patient under general anesthesia reveals more detailed information on the possible continuity between a mass in the neck and the primary cancer.

Diagnostic Imaging

Imaging techniques are becoming more precise and are now routinely used in conjunction with clinical and endoscopic assessments for complete evaluation of patients with hypopharyngeal and/or upper esophageal carcinomas.

Computed tomography (CT) is at the moment the most useful imaging modality used in the initial evaluation of patients with cancer of the hypopharynx. Helical CT is simple and fast and allows multiplanar reconstruction.[3] The goals of CT are to accurately assess the location and size of the primary cancer and to evaluate extension to the neck, either directly or by lymphatic metastasis. CT examination must be performed from the nasopharynx to the upper mediastinum, first without and thereafter with intravenous contrast enhancement. CT is preferably performed before the endoscopy and the biopsies to avoid inflammation, which may result in an overestimation of the cancer infiltration. Helical CT also allows dynamic maneuvers such as the Valsalva maneuver, which by opening the pyriform sinuses provides excellent analysis of the hypopharynx and the epilarynx (Fig. 16–2). It also provides useful information regarding laryngeal mobility and possible extension to laryngeal structures including the bottom of the ventricle and the postcricoid area.

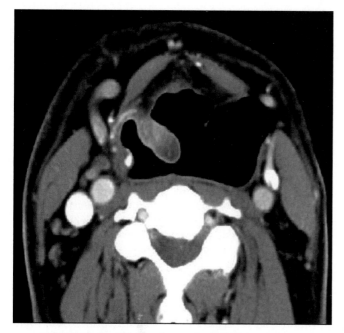

FIGURE 16–2 CT scan during the Valsalva maneuver.

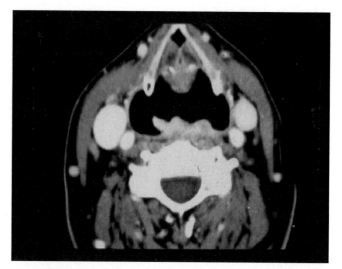

FIGURE 16–4 CT scan for cancer of the posterior wall.

It is important that the clinician carefully assess superior extension of cancer of the hypopharynx to the oropharynx and the nasopharynx. Inferior extension into the esophagus may be more difficult to evaluate. Mucosal contrast enhancement is usually a sign of local extension. A cancer of the pyriform sinus may extend into the paraglottic space or even into the pre-epiglottic space in the case of a large cancer. This pre-epiglottic extension is easily detected after image reconstruction in the sagittal plane. Laterally, cancer of the pyriform sinus may extend to the thyroid cartilage, which acts as a temporary barrier against extension to the neck. CT usually demonstrates cartilage destruction when it is massive; however, it often fails to detect limited invasion of cartilage, which may be indicated only by cartilage sclerosis.[4] The postcricoid area and the posterior wall of

the hypopharynx are also better assessed during the Valsalva maneuver (Figs. 16–3 and 16–4).

CT is also helpful in the evaluation of patients with carcinoma of the cervical esophagus (Fig. 16–5). An anteroposterior diameter of the esophagus greater than 24 mm must be considered abnormal. The average thickness of the wall is 4.8 mm laterally and 3.8 mm posteriorly.[5] Two criteria with the best sensitivity are any thickening of the wall and effacement of the fat plane, with a reported sensitivity of 93%; another criterion is circumferential mass that surrounds the esophagus by greater than 180 or 270 degrees, with a reported sensitivity of 100%.[6] CT also evaluates extraesophageal extension and/or extension to the posterior wall of the trachea.

In addition to clarification with respect to local tumor extent, CT also provides information about tumor extension of cancer into the neck (Fig. 16–6). Metastatic lymph nodes are frequently encountered with carcinoma of the

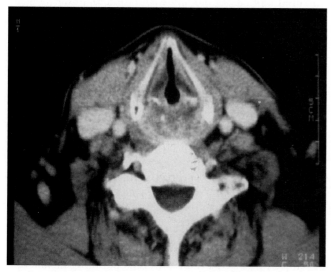

FIGURE 16–3 CT scan for cancer of the posterior wall.

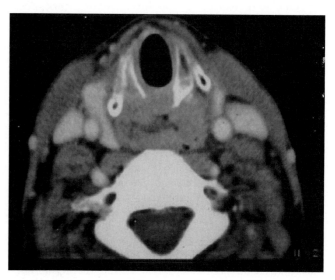

FIGURE 16–5 CT scan for cancer of the cervical esophagus.

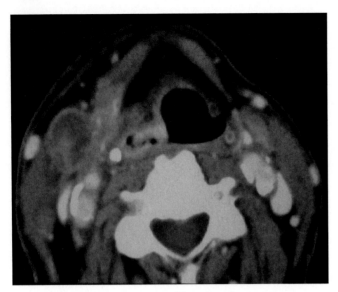

FIGURE 16–6 CT scan and lymph node metastases.

hypopharynx. The probability of metastatic involvement of a lymph node is associated with the following criteria seen on imaging: Size greater than 10 mm (12 mm in the subdigastric area), central necrosis with heterogeneity and peripheral enhancement, and circular shape (see Fig. 16–4).[7] In the evaluation of carcinoma of the cervical esophagus, CT scan yields important information regarding superior mediastinal and retropharyngeal lymph nodes when clinical examination is not feasible.

Magnetic resonance imaging (MRI) is performed with an anterior neck coil; the protocol usually consists of axial T2-weighted fast spin-echo and T1-weighted spin-echo images. Then, after intravenous administration of gadolinium, axial, sagittal, and coronal T1-weighted spin-echo images are obtained.[8] MRI is more sensitive than CT in detecting minimal neoplastic invasion to the cartilage, but CT is more specific.[4] MRI has superior resolution for demonstrating soft tissue details. Nevertheless, owing to its susceptibility to motion-induced artifact, MRI is not routinely performed in the staging of cancer of the hypopharynx and cervical esophagus.

Older methods of imaging such as soft tissue films of the neck, contrast laryngograms, and laryngeal tomograms have been largely supplanted by current imaging techniques (CT and MRI). The barium swallow esophagram, however, remains a useful tool, when esophagoscopy is not feasible, for determining the extent of mucosal disease and the presence of a second primary cancer in the esophagus. Mucosal irregularity, aspiration of barium, and impaired filling of esophageal segments are suspicious signs of tumor involvement. However, esophagrams are inefficient in demonstrating the thickness of the cancer and the presence of upper mediastinal node extension.

Ultrasonography is helpful in assessment of the cervical lymph nodes. It is a simple, noninvasive, rapid, high-sensitivity technique for the detection of subclinical lymph node metastasis, but its reliability is operator dependent. It is a useful method for follow-up and can be combined with fine-needle aspiration to confirm histologic invasion.

▣ THERAPEUTIC OPTIONS

Surgery

Partial Pharyngectomy via External Approaches (Fig. 16–7)

Several partial pharyngectomy procedures are available for the extirpation of hypopharyngeal cancers with preservation of the pharynx and pharyngeal function. Many of these require a temporary tracheotomy and a nasogastric tube. Because occult cervical metastasis is frequent, neck dissection should be performed simultaneously regardless of clinical nodal status. Only a few patients are amenable to partial pharyngectomy, and although these procedures are associated with good local control of disease, patients have a poor overall prognosis caused by the high incidence of second primary tumors, comorbidities, and metastasis.

PARTIAL LATERAL PHARYNGECTOMY (TROTTER)

By means of a lateral approach, the posterior two thirds of the thyroid cartilage and the greater cornu of the hyoid bone are resected. Then the lateral wall of the pyriform sinus is resected, as are the deep fascia and the thyrohyoid muscle. Primary closure is usually possible, but reconstruction with a local muscular flap is sometimes necessary. This procedure is indicated for limited cancer to the lateral wall of the pyriform sinus.

PARTIAL PHARYNGOLARYNGECTOMY (ANDRE, PINEL, LACCOURREYE)

With a lateral approach, the ispsilateral thyroid ala and half of the hyoid bone are resected. Then the entire pyriform sinus and the ispsilateral hemilarynx above the cricoid cartilage are removed with the tumor. The true and false vocal cords are resected with half of the epiglottis and the pre-epiglottic space. The defect is covered by apposition of the edges, after mobilization of the prevertebral muscle insertions, which are sutured to the posterior border of the infrahyoid muscles. This procedure is indicated for cancer limited to the medial wall of the pyriform sinus without impaired mobility of the larynx and located above the level of the superior border of the cricoid cartilage. The postoperative course is often marked by slow recovery of swallowing ability and the risk of aspiration and bronchopulmonary infections. In a series of 34 patients with cancer of the pyriform sinus staged as T2, Laccourreye confirmed the reliability of this technique with 5-year actuarial local and 5-year actuarial regional control rates of, respectively, 96.6% and 93.7%.[9]

SUPRAGLOTTIC HEMIPHARYNGOLARYNGECTOMY

This varies from the previous procedure only in that both true vocal cords are conserved. Only half of the thyroid cartilage is resected. Closure is achieved by apposition of the mucosal edges or use of a subhyoid muscle flap. This procedure is indicated for limited cancer of the superior part of the pyriform sinus, particularly in cases of macroscopic ulceration. In a series of 45 patients[10] who underwent this procedure in association with postoperative radiotherapy, a high local control rate (97.8%) was reported.

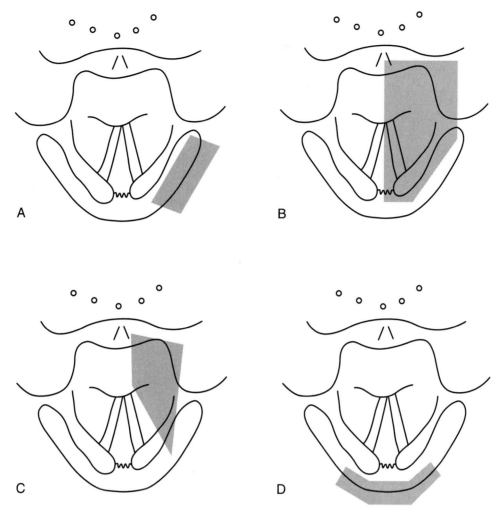

FIGURE 16–7 Partial pharyngectomy via external approaches. *A*, Partial lateral pharyngectomy, *B*, Partial pharyngolaryngectomy. *C*, Supraglottic hemipharyngolaryngectomy. *D*, Posterior partial pharyngectomy.

POSTERIOR PARTIAL PHARYNGECTOMY

The pharynx is opened anteriorly through a transhyoid approach. The posterior wall of the hypopharynx is exposed and the tumor is resected down to the prevertebral fascia. Reconstruction is performed with a flap or a skin graft, or the wound may be left to heal by second intention. This procedure is indicated for the rare cancer that is limited to the upper posterior wall of the pharynx.

ENDOSCOPIC SURGERY

Endoscopic excision using a CO_2 laser is advocated by several authors, particularly in Germany.[11] This technique requires optimal exposure of the larynx and hypopharynx to achieve resection of the tumor with satisfactory margins. Specific laryngopharyngoscopes and multiple changes of the position of the endoscope are often necessary. The CO_2 laser coupled to an operating microscope is the most useful type of laser for these procedures. The lesions are resected with a margin of at least 5 mm for small cancers and 10 mm for larger ones. During the resection, bleeding of large vessels is controlled by electrocautery. Steiner has published a series on 129 patients.[11] Neck dissection was performed in

85.3% of the cases, most often 10 days after resection of the cancer. The vast majority of patients in this series underwent postoperative radiotherapy. Functional results were better with this technique, with a median duration of nasogastric feeding of less than 7 days, and no tracheotomy was necessary. The 5-year recurrence-free survival rate was 95% for stages I/II and 69% for stages III/IV. This technique is not widely used because it is technically difficult to perform and requires special expertise in endoscopic laser surgery.

Radical Surgery

TOTAL LARYNGECTOMY WITH PARTIAL PHARYNGECTOMY

Despite an increasing trend toward organ preservation, this operation is still commonly performed for advanced SCC of the pyriform sinus. En bloc neck dissections are systematically performed. This procedure combines a total laryngectomy and a partial hypopharyngectomy with surgical margins of at least 10 mm. The extent of the pharyngeal resection varies, but in many cases, a primary pharyngoesophageal closure is allowed. A permanent tracheostoma is created. Voice rehabilitation requires, if it is not contraindicated, a tracheoesophageal puncture with insertion of a voice prosthesis. When surgery is performed after radiation failure, a muscular flap may be used to protect the mucosal suture line and the carotid artery.

NEAR-TOTAL LARYNGECTOMY

This surgical technique is usually indicated for the treatment of SCC of the larynx,[12] but it may be indicated in selected patients with SCC of the pyriform sinus. These indications are T2 or T3 cancers that involve the apex of the pyriform sinus with fixation of the ipsilateral hemilarynx. The surgical procedure involves removal of a large part of the larynx and the entire pyriform sinus with the cancer. The vocal shunt is performed with the contralateral hemilarynx. Pearson[12] conducted a review of 75 patients with pyriform SCC whom he had treated with this technique. Voice was produced with the tracheolaryngeal shunt and was used by 85% of patients. Local recurrences occurred in only 3 of these 75 patients, which confirms that this operation did not alter the local control rate. This technique requires that the patient have a permanent tracheotomy.

CIRCUMFERENTIAL TOTAL LARYNGOPHARYNGECTOMY

This procedure is used for more advanced cancer that is massively invading the postcricoid area and/or the posterior pharyngeal wall, thus requiring complete resection of the hypopharyngeal mucosa. The resection includes the hypopharynx and the larynx between the hyoid bone and the second tracheal ring. Many options are available to reconstruct this defect. A tubed pectoralis major myocutaneous flap sutured to the prevertebral musculature is the simplest option, but it is not often used because postoperative strictures and fistulas are common. The radial forearm free flap offers the combined advantages of a rapid harvest, a long and large-caliber vascular pedicle, and a high flap viability rate. The length is compatible with the large pharyngolaryngeal resection. The radial forearm free flap has had one of the highest success rates of any microvascular free flap, generally higher than 95% in most series.[13] The jejunum is another free flap commonly used for reconstruction of the pharynx and cervical esophagus. The segment is harvested through a midline laparotomy, and a long pedicle should be obtained. The required length of the jejunum is the measured length of the defect, which is approximately 8 cm. Mortality and morbidity rates are currently low.[14] The success rates of microvascular free-tissue transfers are high, ranging between 90% and 97%.[14, 15]

TOTAL ESOPHAGOPHARYNGOLARYNGECTOMY

Surgical resection includes circumferential pharyngolaryngectomy and a total esophagectomy. This procedure is indicated for lesions involving and infiltrating the cervical esophagus (either hypopharyngeal SCC invading the cervical esophagus or cervical esophageal SCC invading the inferior part of the hypopharynx). Such extensive cancer carries a very poor prognosis. The goals of this surgery are to remove the larynx, the hypopharynx, and the esophagus, and to restore the digestive tract with the lowest morbidity and mortality, the shortest hospital stay, and the earliest oral feeding recovery possible.

Reconstruction of the upper digestive tract is achieved either by a gastric pullup or gastric tube, or by a colon transposition into the posterior mediastinum.[16] Gastric pullup, a reliable method of reconstruction, has been used since the 1960s.[17, 18] Gastric pullup, along with esophagectomy, is one of the classic methods of reconstruction. This technique has many advantages. It is a one-stage method of reconstruction that involves only one anastomosis. It allows dissection of the paratracheal lymph nodes. The stomach has a very good blood supply that promotes rapid healing. However, regurgitation of the gastric contents and the development of dumping syndrome are not uncommon, and the combined abdominal, thoracic, and cervical dissection carries an increased morbidity. Despite these complications, Triboulet[19] demonstrated in a recent study the reliability of this reconstruction with acceptable morbidity and mortality. The significant adverse factors affecting survival were cervical localization, postoperative complications, T3–T4 tumors, and incomplete resection.

Colon interposition is another option of reconstruction. The considerable length of the colon transplant and the absence of peptic digestion of the colonic-gastric anastomosis and of stricture formation are notable advantages, but this reconstruction has a tendency to become inert; therefore, three anastomoses are required, which leads to a greater risk of wound infection.

Nevertheless, despite a large resection in combination with postoperative radiotherapy, oncologic results are poor regardless of the technique of reconstruction that is used. Triboulet,[19] in an analysis of 209 cases, found a local recurrence rate of 59.3% occurring at 19 months on average.

Neck Dissection

Partial and radical surgical excision of the primary cancer is always combined with radical or modified homolateral neck dissection, even in cases of clinically negative necks, because histologically proven occult metastasis to cervical lymph nodes in as many as 38% of cases has been reported.[20] Contralateral dissection is necessary each time the lesion reaches the midline.

The type of neck dissection required is dictated by the nodal status, as defined both clinically and on imaging.

- In cases of N0 necks, a selective neck dissection may be performed, consisting of at least a lateral neck dissection in which the nodes in levels II to IV are removed. In cases of cancer of the hypopharynx involving the oropharynx, level Ib should also be resected.
- In cases of N1 necks, a posterolateral neck dissection in which levels II to V are removed must be performed because in these cases, the risk of level V involvement may be higher than 10%. Again, in cases of hypopharyngeal tumor involving the oropharynx, level Ib should be resected as well.
- In cases of N2a or N2b, a near-comprehensive neck dissection in which levels Ib to V are removed must be performed. The radicality or lack of it with these neck dissections depends on the size of the biggest node and its possible close contact with the internal jugular vein.

- In cases of N2c necks, each neck must be considered individually.
- In case of N3 necks, a classical radical neck dissection is indicated.
- Whatever the N status, level VI must be dissected each time the pharyngoesophageal junction is reached or involved.

Risk of metastases to the retropharyngeal lymph nodes has been reported to be as high as 9%.[21] This level is systematically resected in case of circumferential pharyngo-laryngectomy or in cases of total laryngectomy with partial pharyngectomy extended to the posterior wall. Finally, the mediastinorecurrent chains are also resected in circumferential total pharyngolaryngectomy, particularly for the treatment of cervical esophagus carcinomas.

Radiation Therapy

As for other cancers of the head and neck, radiation therapy may be used in various settings. Definitive radiation therapy has been proposed mainly for early cancer of the hypopharynx, with oncologic results comparable to those obtained with partial surgery.[22] Reported local control rates[23, 24] for advanced cancer were less satisfactory than those obtained with combined surgery and radiation.[25] It must be stressed that definitive radiotherapy series often mixed potentially operable diseases and nonoperable diseases, either because of the locoregional extension or because of the poor performance status of the patients (and often as a result of both concerns).

In the absence of a randomized trial comparing both approaches in comparable groups of patients, no definitive conclusion can be made. However, it seems that patients with advanced cancer are not good candidates for conventional radiation therapy. Local control is poorly achieved; also, salvage surgery after full-dose radiation carries a high morbidity and results in low success rates.

Combined surgery and radiation therapy may consist of either preoperative or postoperative radiation. Results gained with preoperative radiation are controversial in terms of local control, but the indisputably higher morbidity of surgery following radiation (even in cases of low-dose preoperative radiation, i.e., delivering 40 to 50 Gy) has led most multidisciplinary teams to recommend surgery with postoperative radiation therapy. In addition, the surgical specimen provides precise data, particularly on the nodal status, which provides radiation therapists with information that allows better treatment planning.

As with other patients receiving radiation therapy to the head and neck, pretreatment dental care is mandatory, including extraction of carious teeth and fluoride gel prophylaxis. Patients with nutritional deficits benefit from intensive nutritional therapy. Treatment of comorbidities and optimization of performance status are mandatory. Treatment planning requires a CT scan performed in the treatment position, use of a simulator, and immobilization with thermoplastic masks. Either Cobalt 60 or photon X of 4- to 6-MV linear accelerators may be used.[26]

The target volume includes the primary cancer bed as well as lymph node metastases. Two major concerns make the radiated volume larger than that defined by the clinical examination. Submucosal extension around the macroscopic limits of the tumor is very common and is not well defined with imaging. In addition, a vast majority of patients present with metastatic lymph nodes, and the frequency of occult metastases in N0 neck patients is as high as 40%.[27] Finally, except for level I (submandibular lymph nodes), all other nodal levels are at risk, including levels II to V and level VI (prelaryngeal/paratracheal nodes) and the retropharyngeal nodes. As a result, the radiated volume encompasses the pharynx, from the oropharynx to the pharyngoesophageal junction and both necks. This usually encompasses the spinal cord, the larynx, and the thyroid gland. To avoid radiation to these structures, the spinal cord is shielded after a dose of 40 Gy has been reached (and posterior electron beams are used to cover the posterior node areas). In the same way, the anterior skin of the neck, as well as the anterior part of the glottis, may be spared whenever local extension makes it possible.

Whether radiation is given as primary or adjuvant therapy, patients are treated in a supine position with three fields—two opposed lateral beams for the upper neck, and one anterior and inferior field for the lower neck. In cases of definitive radiation, a dose of 55 to 60 Gy is given to the overall volume, with a boost of 10 to 15 Gy to the primary tumor and grossly involved nodal areas. The flat aspect of the dose-response curve after 70 Gy does not justify higher doses, even for advanced disease. For postoperative irradiation, a total dose of 50 to 60 Gy is given, with a boost of 10 to 15 Gy to the primary tumor surgical bed in cases of positive margins, and to areas of extranodal extension in the neck. Patients are usually treated with a conventional radiation schedule—one 2-Gy fraction per day, 5 days a week.

Altered fractionation schedules (i.e., bifractionated or accelerated or concomitant boost techniques) have been explored in the treatment of cancer of the head and neck.[28–30] Only rarely have these published series focused on hypopharyngeal cancers alone.[31] Both hyperfractionated radiation and the concomitant boost technique appeared to improve local control, but both acute and late toxicities were higher.[28] The acute toxicity is manageable provided that appropriate supportive care is implemented. Late toxicity is less controllable and may make surgery in radiated fields difficult or nonfeasible.

Chemotherapy is another option for improving results achieved by radiation therapy. Organ preservation is discussed in the chemotherapy section. Concurrent chemoradiotherapy seems to be promising, either for definitive or for postoperative radiation. Different schedules may be used. Chemotherapy may be delivered at low daily doses as a radiosensitizer. This schedule is rarely used in the treatment of cancer of the head and neck. Chemotherapy is usually administered at classic dosages before, during, or after radiotherapy. Adjuvant chemotherapy has failed to improve survival and disease control.[32] Induction chemotherapy, after a period of enthusiasm, did not improve patients' outcome.[32]

The most promising schedule is concurrent chemoradiotherapy, either as the definitive treatment or as a postoperative therapy.[32, 33] Although concurrent chemoradiotherapy may enhance locoregional control of cancer of the hypopharynx, this treatment regimen is associated with increased morbidity, which may not be tolerated by some patients. Whenever resectable, cancer-extensive soft tissue infiltration or obvious destruction of the cartilage(s) remains better controlled by surgery and postoperative radiation.

Finally, new radiotherapeutic modalities, such as intensity-modulated radiation therapy (IMRT) or fractionated stereotactic radiation therapy,[34] may be used for the reradiation of recurrences occurring in previously radiated fields.

Chemotherapy

For a long time, owing to its poor activity in the treatment of cancer of the head and neck, chemotherapy was used primarily for palliative purposes. A new era in the management of cancer of the head and neck was initiated in the early 1980s with the introduction of platinum-based chemotherapeutic regimens. Actually, clinical studies using cisplatin as a single agent or more often in combination with other drugs have demonstrated partial response rates of 40% to 50%, and complete response rates of 26% to 50%, for an overall response rate ranging between 78% and 94%.[35, 36] These impressive response rates in previously untreated patients generated intensive clinical research to evaluate the role of chemotherapy in therapeutic protocols with curative intent. In the early 1990s, it appeared obvious that this approach had not provided any improvement in survival benefit for most patients. This was clearly demonstrated by the major meta-analysis carried out at the Institut Gustave Roussy (Meta-analysis of Chemotherapy in Head and Neck Cancer [MACH-NC]),[32] which included more than 10,000 patients enrolled in randomized trials comparing conventional treatment with the same treatment combined with chemotherapy (adjuvant or induction or concomitant chemotherapy). The conclusion of this meta-analysis was that adjuvant chemotherapy, as well as induction chemotherapy (4%), produced a nonsignificant increase in survival (1%). On the contrary, concomitant chemoradiotherapy resulted in a significant increase in survival of 8%, but this group had a mixture of definitive and postoperative radiation trials. However, additional trials of concurrent chemoradiation as the first line of treatment that were published after this meta-analysis confirmed the trend toward an improved outcome. As a result, concurrent chemoradiation remains an important challenge currently under evaluation for advanced cancer. As far as cancer of the hypopharynx is concerned, it must be underscored that (1) this site is rarely studied separately, (2) in cases of mixed sites, hypopharynx represents just a few cases, (3) little is known about the selection of patients with cancer of the hypopharynx (detailed locoregional extension, performance status), and (4) no information is provided about the possibilities of surgical salvage.

The potential goals of induction chemotherapy were to increase disease-free survival time, possibly to render unresectable tumors resectable, and to preserve function. When it appeared that the first two goals had not been reached, clinical research focused on only the last one. The hypothesis that chemosensitive tumors should also be radiosensitive was confirmed in a number of cases, which suggested the ability of induction chemotherapy to predict radiosensitivity. This led some teams to use a scheme of induction chemotherapy as a selective test for two groups of patients—good responders as candidates for subsequent radiation therapy, and poor responders still as candidates for subsequent surgery. The larynx has been the primary site investigated most often for this new approach in noncontrolled trials using historical comparisons with surgical series.

Only two randomized trials had focused on cancer of the hypopharynx. The first trial was conducted by the European Organization for Research and Treatment of Cancer (EORTC)[37] on cancer of the hypopharynx eligible for total laryngectomy with partial pharyngectomy. Two hundred two patients were enrolled in this study, which compared the standard treatment (surgery and postoperative radiation) with two or three cycles of chemotherapy, followed in clinically complete responders at the primary site by irradiation or, for other patients, by the conventional treatment. There was a notable difference in median survival favoring the experimental arm (44 months) when compared with the surgery arm (25 months). This difference in median survival was explained only by the fact that distant metastases appeared later after chemotherapy, leading to a better survival at 3 years, which was not shown at 5 years. However, at 3 and 5 years, half the survivors in the chemotherapy arm had retained their larynx.

The second trial[38] compared patient outcome with resectable cancer of the hypopharynx amenable only to total laryngectomy/pharyngectomy with the outcome of patients randomly assigned to receive induction chemotherapy. Chemotherapy was followed in one arm by surgery and postoperative radiation therapy, and in the other arm by radiation with surgery reserved for salvage. With a median follow-up of 92 months in the 92 randomly assigned patients, a better 5-year survival (37%) and a better local control (63%) in the surgery arm when compared with the radiotherapy arm (19% 5-year survival and 39% local control) were observed. Comparison of this trial with the EORTC trial suggests that sensitivity of the cancer to chemotherapy must be taken into account before subsequent radiation therapy is chosen instead of surgery.

In addition, many published series[39-45] had assessed in a nonrandomized fashion the reliability of induction chemotherapy–based protocols. They usually reported small series of cases mixing laryngeal, hypopharyngeal, and oropharyngeal tumors, or tumors amenable to partial surgery and to radical surgery. In addition, the concept of organ preservation and/or preservation of function was unclear. Finally, larynx preservation rates were presented under different forms—for the overall population at a precise follow-up time or for survivors at that time, or according to a median follow-up. All in all, larynx preservation could be achieved in one third to one half of patients, according to the patient selection.

However, the discussion about larynx preservation regardless of the primary site but particularly with regard to the hypopharynx is not closed. As has already been mentioned, promising data have been compiled with concurrent chemoradiation. The questions are these: (1) How many patients in daily community practice are able to undergo such toxic treatments? (2) What is the highest disease stage amenable to larynx-preserving strategies? (Are clinically defined T4 or large necrotic lymph nodes acceptable?) (3) What are the most appropriate tools for detecting as early as possible residual diseases to be treated by salvage surgery? (4) What would be the postoperative morbidity of this salvage surgery? These concerns are of the utmost importance if the cancer is initially operable. Radical surgery has indisputably a negative impact on quality of life but is able to control the disease above the clavicle in the vast majority of cases. Nothing, even the loss of the larynx, would be worse than dying of a locoregionally uncontrolled disease. Finally, it must be emphasized that cancer originating on or involving the cervical esophagus is never included in larynx preservation approaches.

In the case of unresectable recurrent or metastatic cancer for which reradiation cannot be delivered, chemotherapy remains the sole option, other than supportive and palliative care. In such situations, whatever the regimen, the median duration of survival is about 6 months. Chemotherapy in this case should be discussed according to the patient's wishes and performance status. New drugs or new administration modalities are often assessed in these clinical situations, again in the framework of clinical research. Attention must be paid to proposal of a tracheotomy and/or a gastrostomy (either percutaneous endoscopic gastrostomy [PEG] or percutaneous radiologic gastrostomy [PRG]).

Decision Making

Appropriate therapy for cancer of the hypopharynx and cervical esophagus depends on several factors, including extent of disease, laryngeal involvement, presence and extent of lymph node metastasis, patient's performance status, and foreseeable compliance. Decision making is particularly difficult and requires expertise in the management of patients with cancer of the hypopharynx who present with advanced disease and serious comorbidities. Treatment selection must be tailored to each patient by a multidisciplinary team, including a head and neck surgeon, a radiation oncologist, and a medical oncologist.

OUTCOME

The overall prognosis of patients with cancer of the hypopharynx and the cervical esophagus remains poor because a majority of patients are diagnosed at an advanced stage and have a poor performance status. Most of them are not amenable to therapy with curative intent. When they are treated with palliative intent, the median survival is very short and does not exceed 1 year.

Generally, patients with advanced cancer treated with curative intent have a 5-year survival of approximately 35%. The most frequent causes of death are distant metastases and intercurrent diseases. The 5-year survival for patients with early cancer does not exceed 50%, and most of these patients die of second primary cancers and, to a lesser extent, distant metastases.

At the moment, no data clearly show a real improvement in survival; improved locoregional disease control has not translated into improved survival owing to the multiple causes of death. However, even if ultimately the outcome will remain poor, all efforts must be pursued to improve disease control above the clavicles and to enhance patient quality of life.

Emerging data show that combined chemoradiotherapy could reach this goal, at least for moderately advanced cancer. For patients with advanced cancer that is still operable, organ-preserving strategies should be discussed whenever possible, except in cases of extension to the neck. In such cases, more extensive radical surgery and postoperative radiation therapy remain the best way to manage these patients.

CONCLUSION

Despite notable advances in biologic knowledge, modern imaging, new surgical procedures, and new chemoradiotherapeutic concepts, the prognosis of patients with cancer of the hypopharynx and cervical esophagus remains unchanged in terms of overall survival. For patients amenable to treatments with curative intent, less than one of two are still alive at 5 years, although locoregional control might be as high as 80%. For patients with more advanced cancer treated with palliative intent, both survival and quality of life are very poor. The anatomic complexity of these primary sites, which overlap the neck and the upper mediastinum; the very high tendency for cervical and distant metastases; and the poor performance status and late presentation of most of these patients are factors that lead to a poor outcome. To date, prevention and early diagnosis, both of which have remained unattainable goals, offer more realistic approaches to solving the problems of cancer at these sites.

REFERENCES

1. Parkin DM, Muir CS, Whelan SL, et al: Cancer Incidence in Five Continents, vol VI. Lyon, IARC Scientific Publications, 1992.
2. Bearhrs OH, Henson DE, Hutter RVP, et al: Manual for Staging of Cancer, 4th ed. Philadelphia, Lippincott, 1992.
3. Robert Y, Rocourt N, Chevalier D, et al: Helical CT of the larynx: A comparative study with conventional CT scan. Clin Radiol 51:882, 1996.
4. Castelijns JA, Gerritsen GJ, Kaiser MC, et al: Invasion of laryngeal cartilage by cancer: Comparison of CT and MRI imaging. Radiology 167:199, 1988.
5. Schmalfuss IM, Mancuso AA, Tart RP: Postcricoid region and cervical esophagus: Normal appearance at CT and MR imaging. Radiology 214:237, 2000.
6. Roychowdury S, Loevner LA, Yousem DM, et al: MR imaging for predicting neoplastic invasion of the cervical esophagus. Am J Neuroradiol 21:1681, 2000.
7. Steinkamp HJ, Hosten N, Richter C, et al: Enlarged cervical lymph nodes at helical CT. Radiology 191:795, 1994.
8. Zbären P, Becker M, Läng H: Pretherapeutic staging of hypopharyngeal carcinoma. Arch Otolaryngol Head Neck Surg 123:903, 1997.
9. Laccourreye O, Merite-Drancy A, Brasnu D, et al: Hemilaryngopharyngectomy in selected pyriform sinus carcinoma staged as T2. Laryngoscope 103:1373, 1993.
10. Chevalier D, Watelet JB, Darras JA, et al: Supraglottic hemilaryngectomy plus radiation for the treatment of early lateral margin and pyriform sinus carcinoma. Head Neck 19:1, 1997.
11. Steiner W, Ambrosch P, Hess CF, et al: Organ preservation by transoral laser microsurgery in piriform sinus carcinoma. Otolaryngol Head Neck Surg 124:58, 2001.

12. Pearson BW, DeSanto LW, Olsen KD, et al: Results of near-total laryngectomy. Ann Otol Rhinol Laryngol 107:820, 1998.

13. Anthony JP, Singer MI, Deschler DG, et al: Long term functional results after pharyngoesophageal reconstruction with the radial forearm free flap. Am J Surg 168:441, 1994.

14. Theile DR, Robinson DW, Theile DE, et al: Free jejunal interposition reconstruction after pharyngolaryngectomy: 201 consecutive cases. Head Neck 17:83, 1995.

15. Chevalier D, Triboulet JP, Patenotre P, et al: Free jejunal graft reconstruction after total pharyngolaryngeal resection for hypopharyngeal cancer. Clin Otolaryngol 22:41, 1997.

16. Surkin MI, Lawson W, Biller HF: Analysis of the methods of pharyngoesophageal reconstruction. Head Neck 6:953, 1984.

17. Ong GB, Lee TC: Pharyngo-gastric anastomosis after oesopharyngectomy for carcinoma of the hypopharynx and cervical oesophagus. Br J Surg 48:193, 1960.

18. LeQuesne LP, Ranger D: Pharyngolaryngectomy with immediate pharyngogastric anastomosis. Br J Surg 53:105, 1966.

19. Triboulet JP, Mariette C, Chevalier D, et al: Surgical management of carcinoma of the hypopharynx and cervical esophagus: Analysis of 209 cases. Arch Surg 136:1164, 2001.

20. Pillsbury HC, Clark M: A rationale for therapy of the N0 neck. Laryngoscope 107:1294, 1997.

21. McLaughlin MP, Mendenhall WM, Mancuso AA, et al: Retropharyngeal adenopathy as a predictor of outcome in squamous cell carcinoma of the head and neck. Head Neck 17:190, 1995.

22. Spector GJ, Sessions DG, Emami B, et al: Squamous cell carcinoma of the pyriform sinus: A non-randomized comparison of therapeutic modalities and long-term results. Laryngoscope 105:397, 1995.

23. Bataini P: Results of radical radiotherapeutic treatment of carcinoma of the pyriform sinus: Experience of the Institut Curie. Int J Radiat Oncol Biol Phys 8:1277, 1982.

24. Dubois JB, Guerrier B, Di Ruggiero JM, et al: Cancer of the piriform sinus: Treatment by radiation therapy alone and with surgery. Radiology 160:377, 1993.

25. Kraus DH, Zelefski MJ, Brock HAJ, et al: Combined surgery and radiation therapy for squamous cell carcinoma of the hypopharynx. Otolaryngol Head Neck Surg 116:637, 1997.

26. Aref A, Berkey BA, Schwade JG, et al: The influence of beam energy on the outcome of postoperative radiotherapy in head and neck patients: Secondary analysis of RTOG 85-03. Int J Radiat Oncol Biol Phys 47:389, 2000.

27. Pillsbury HC, Clark M: A rationale for therapy of the N0 neck. Laryngoscope 107:1294, 1997.

28. Fu KK, Pajak TF, Trotti A, et al: A radiation therapy oncology group (RTOG) phase III randomized study to compare hyperfractionation and two variants of accelerated fractionation to standard fractionation radiotherapy for head and neck squamous cell carcinomas: First report of RTOG 9003. Int J Radiat Oncol Biol Phys 48:7, 2000.

29. Garden AS, Morisson WH, Kian Ang K, et al: Hyperfractionated radiation in the treatment of squamous cell carcinomas of the head and neck: A comparison of two fractionation schedules. Int J Radiat Oncol Biol Phys 31:493, 1995.

30. Jackson SM, Weir LM, Hay JH, et al: A randomized trial of accelerated versus conventional radiotherapy in head and neck cancer. Radiother Oncol 43:34, 1997.

31. Allal AS, Dulguerov P, Bieri S: Assessment of quality of life in patients treated with accelerated radiotherapy for laryngeal and hypopharyngeal carcinomas. Head Neck 22:288, 2000.

32. Pignon JP, Bourhis J, Domenge C, et al, on behalf of the MACH-NC Collaborative Group: Chemotherapy added to locoregional treatment for head and neck squamous-cell carcinoma: Three meta-analyses of updated individual data. Lancet 355:949, 2000.

33. Bernier J, van Glabbeke M, Domenge C, et al: Results of EORTC phase III trial 22 931 comparing postoperatively, radiotherapy (RT) to concurrent chemo-radiotherapy (RT-CT) with high dose cisplatin in locally advanced head and neck (H&N) carcinoma (SCC). In Proceedings of the 11th. European Conference on Clinical Oncology (ECCO 11), October 2001, Lisbon, Portugal.

34. Ahn YC, Lee KC, Kim DY, et al: Fractionated stereotactic radiation therapy for extracranial head and neck tumors. Int J Radiat Oncol Biol Phys 48:501, 2000.

35. Jacobs JR, Weaver A, Ahmed K, et al: Proto-chemo-therapy in advanced head and neck cancer. Head Neck 10:93, 1987.

36. Hill BT, Price LA, McRae K: Importance of primary site in assessing chemotherapy response and 7-year survival data in advanced squamous-cell carcinomas of the head and neck treated with initial combination chemotherapy with cisplatin. J Clin Oncol 4:1340, 1986.

37. Lefebvre JL, Chevalier D, Luboinski B, et al: Larynx preservation in pyriform sinus cancer: Preliminary results of a European Organization for Research and Treatment of Cancer phase III study. J Natl Cancer Inst 13:890, 1996.

38. Beauvillain C, Mahe M, Bourdin S, et al: Final results of a randomized trial comparing chemotherapy plus radiotherapy with chemotherapy plus surgery plus radiotherapy in locally advanced resectable carcinomas. Laryngoscope 107:648, 1997.

39. Karp DD, Vaughan CW, Carter R, et al: Larynx preservation using induction chemotherapy plus radiation therapy as an alternative to laryngectomy in advanced head and neck cancer. A long-term follow-up report. J Clin Oncol 14:273, 1991.

40. Pfister DG, Strong E, Harrison L, et al: Larynx preservation with combined chemotherapy and radiation therapy in advanced but resectable head and neck cancer. J Clin Oncol 9:850, 1991.

41. Price LA, Hill BT: Larynx preservation after initial chemotherapy plus radiotherapy as opposed to surgical intervention with or without radiotherapy in previously untreated advanced head and neck cancer: Final analysis. Proc Am Soc Clin Oncol 11:785, 992.

42. Demard F, Chauvel P, Schneider M, et al: Induction chemotherapy for larynx preservation in laryngeal and hypopharyngeal cancers. In Johnson JT, Didolkar MS (eds): Head and Neck Cancer, vol III. Amsterdam, Elsevier, 1993, pp 3–10.

43. Shirinian MH, Weber RS, Lippman SM, et al: Laryngeal preservation by induction chemotherapy plus radiotherapy in locally advanced head and neck cancer: The MD Anderson Cancer Center experience. Head Neck 16:39, 1994.

44. Kraus DH, Pfister DG, Harrison LB, et al: Larynx preservation with combined chemotherapy and radiation therapy in advanced hypopharynx cancer. Otolaryngol Head Neck Surg 111:31, 1994.

45. Zelepski MJ, Kraus DH, Pfister DG, et al: Combined chemotherapy and radiotherapy versus surgery and postoperative radiotherapy for advanced hypopharyngeal cancer. Otolaryngol Club J 4:23, 1997.

CHAPTER 17

Tumors of the Cervical Trachea

Zane T. Hammoud

Hermes C. Grillo

Douglas J. Mathisen

INTRODUCTION

Primary tumors in the trachea are relatively uncommon, with an estimated 2.7 new cases per million per year. A recent survey from the United Kingdom disclosed only 321 patients with primary tracheal tumors over a 10-year period.[1] The rarity of these tumors explains the relatively small experience that has been accumulated even in major referral centers. Owing to their rare occurrence, the diagnosis of a tumor of the trachea requires a high index of suspicion. Patients with a tumor of the trachea often have a range of symptoms, including dyspnea on exertion and inspiratory wheezing, with a normal chest radiograph; these patients may be diagnosed and treated as having adult-onset asthma long before further investigations determine the presence of an obstructing tumor of the trachea. Therefore, maintaining a high index of suspicion for a tumor in the trachea allows for earlier detection and the best chance for cure in these patients.

Techniques that allow resection and reconstruction of the trachea at any level have been developed.[2–8] However, only a few institutions have had sufficient experience to make meaningful conclusions about these techniques in the management of tumors of the trachea and to provide long-term follow-up information. At the Massachusetts General Hospital, more than 250 patients with a primary tumor of the trachea have been treated over the past 35 years. The data presented here represent a detailed analysis of our experience with 198 tumors of the trachea treated over a 27-year period (1963–1990).[9] This relatively small number, constituting the largest experience in a single center in the world, combined with the variable biologic behavior of some of these tumors, makes it difficult to derive definitive conclusions regarding the treatment of these tumors. Therefore, the management of each case must be individualized.

The surgical approach to tumors involving the cervical trachea differs from the approach used for tumors of the distal trachea or carina. Although this chapter is directed toward the special problems of the cervical trachea, generalizations must be made from the total experience with tracheal tumors. It is a fallacy in most cases to consider the treatment of tumors of the cervical trachea apart from the general problem of management of tumors of the trachea as a whole.

SURGICAL ANATOMY OF THE TRACHEA

The trachea begins at the lower border of the cricoid cartilage. It terminates where the lateral walls of the right and left main bronchi flare out from the lower trachea. The carinal spur is useful as a definite landmark for the termination of the trachea because it is clearly seen both bronchoscopically and radiologically. The average adult human trachea measures 11 cm in length, with slight variation in proportion to the height of the individual.[10] There are approximately two tracheal cartilaginous rings per centimeter of trachea. Except for some cases of congenital stenosis with circumferential rings of the trachea, the cricoid is the only completely circular cartilage in the upper airway.[11]

The potential for presentation of the trachea in the neck is of critical importance, both for surgical access to the trachea and for ease of reconstruction following resection. In young people, hyperextension of the neck frequently delivers in excess of 50% of the trachea into the neck.[12, 13] Conversely, in an aged, kyphotic individual, even the most vigorous hyperextension may fail to deliver any of the trachea into the neck. The anatomic position of the trachea changes from an essentially subcutaneous position at the level of the cricoid to a prevertebral position at the level of the carina; thus, the course of the trachea is normally caudad and dorsal.

The blood supply of the trachea is of critical importance in resection and reconstruction of the trachea. The upper trachea is supplied primarily by branches of the inferior thyroid artery.[14] The lower trachea is supplied by branches of the bronchial artery, with contributions from the subclavian, supreme intercostal, internal thoracic, and innominate arteries.[15] The vessels supply branches anteriorly to the trachea and posteriorly to the esophagus; these arrive at the trachea through lateral pedicles of tissue. The longitudinal anastomoses between these vessels are fine, and transverse intercartilaginous arteries branch ultimately into a submucosal capillary network. Excessive division of the lateral tissues by circumferential dissection of the trachea risks disruption of this network and may lead to serious complications, for example, nonhealing anastomosis.

The trachea is also intimately related to several critical structures. These include the recurrent laryngeal nerves, the esophagus, and the thyroid gland. Detailed knowledge of these anatomic relationships is mandatory before any attempt can be made at resection and reconstruction.

CLASSIFICATION OF TUMORS

Primary neoplasms of the trachea can be grouped into three main categories—malignant (squamous carcinoma), intermediate malignant (adenoid cystic), and miscellaneous. In our series, adenoid cystic carcinoma (cylindroma) was the most common primary tumor of the trachea, closely followed by squamous cell carcinoma (Table 17–1).[9] In other series, squamous cell carcinoma has predominated.[1] Many other tumors are encountered much less frequently and are of varying malignant potential (Table 17–2). Many of these

TABLE 17-1   Primary Tracheal Tumors

	Squamous	Adenoid Cystic	Other	Total
Number of cases	70	80	48	198
Percent of total	36	40	24	
Surgical treatment	50	65	43	158
Excised	44	60	43	147
Explored	6	5	0	11
Resection				
With reconstruction	41	50	41	132
Trachea	32	22	28	82
Carina	9	28	13	50
Laryngotracheal	1	4	2	7
Staged	2	6	0	8

Data from Grillo HC, Mathisen DJ: Primary tracheal tumors: Treatment and results. Ann Thorac Surg 49:69, 1990.

TABLE 17-2   Primary Tracheal Tumors Other than Squamous Cell and Adenoid Cystic

Type	Number of Patients
Benign	
Squamous papilloma	4
Pleomorphic adenoma	2
Granular cell tumor	2
Fibrous histiocytoma	1
Leiomyoma	2
Chondroma	2
Chondroblastoma	1
Schwannoma	1
Paraganglioma	2
Hemangioendothelioma	1
Vascular malformation	2
Intermediate	
Carcinoid	10
Mucoepidermoid	4
Plexiform neurofibroma	1
Pseudosarcoma	1
Malignant	
Adenocarcinoma	1
Adenosquamous carcinoma	1
Small cell carcinoma	1
Apical carcinoid	1
Melanoma	1
Chondrosarcoma	1
Spindle cell sarcoma	2
Rhabdomyosarcoma	1

Data from Grillo HC, Mathisen DJ: Primary tracheal tumors: Treatment and results. Ann Thorac Surg 49:69, 1990.

represent one-of-a-kind tumors. Some tumors, such as tumors of the larynx and thyroid, may secondarily involve the trachea by direct extension; rarely, tumors may also metastasize to the submucosa of the trachea.

The peak incidence of squamous cell carcinoma of the trachea is between 50 and 60 years of age, whereas adenoid cystic carcinoma has a fairly even distribution from the third to the seventh decades of life. Preceding or subsequent primary neoplasms in the aerodigestive tract are quite common with squamous cell carcinoma of the trachea. In our series, 16 of 40 patients who had resection of a tracheal squamous cell carcinoma had a previous history, a concurrent finding, or a later occurrence of squamous cell carcinoma elsewhere in the aerodigestive tract.[9] Primary tracheal tumors, regardless of histology, are distributed throughout the entire length of the trachea without a predilection for one location over another.

PRESENTATION

Primary squamous cell carcinoma of the trachea may present as an exophytic lesion that is circumscribed, or as a spreading lesion that involves a considerable length of the trachea. It may also present as an ulcerative lesion. The tumor may grow into the mediastinum and may be noted radiographically as a bulky extratracheal mass. Metastases to paratracheal and subcarinal lymph nodes as well as direct invasion of mediastinal structures may also occur. This tumor occurs predominantly in males, and all patients in our series were cigarette smokers.

Adenoid cystic carcinoma may present as an exophytic lesion, frequently with poorly defined margins. A bulky extratracheal mass may be demonstrated. At exploration, the tumor mass is often found to have compressed and displaced adjacent structures within the mediastinum rather than to have invaded those structures directly. In the cervical trachea, however, the thyroid gland may be directly invaded. The esophagus may also be invaded. Although adjacent lymph nodes may be involved by metastatic tumor, this occurs with less frequency than in squamous cell carcinoma. This tumor is histologically characterized by submucosal extension and perineural invasion over long distances of trachea. The submucosal extent is often not visible to the naked eye, even after transection of the trachea. Frozen section control during surgery is critical, and the extent of the tumor may present the surgeon with a problem not predictable preoperatively. There appears to be a wide variation in the metastatic potential of adenoid cystic carcinoma. Distant metastases occur with more aggressive tumors. These may not become apparent until many years following treatment of the primary tumor. Unlike squamous cell carcinoma, there appears to be no sex predilection, and smoking was an incidental finding.

The group of miscellaneous tumors includes a wide variety of tumors of varying malignant potential. Owing to the relatively low numbers of individual types of tumor, it is difficult to predict the biologic behavior of these tumors. Our institution applies an aggressive surgical approach to many such tumors because there is anecdotal evidence in the literature that some of these tumors continue to grow and cause obstruction of the trachea.

Tumors may also involve the trachea secondarily. Carcinoma of the lung may present with direct proximal extension of a main bronchial lesion, or it may invade the trachea through involvement of paratracheal lymph nodes. Carcinoma of the esophagus may invade the trachea at any point from the cricoid to the carina; fistulization from spontaneous necrosis or following irradiation may occur. A variety of carcinomas of the thyroid may also involve the trachea; these patients may even present with hemoptysis. Often, invasion of the trachea is seen after incomplete surgical removal of the primary tumor, with the surgeon aware of having "shaved" a tumor off the trachea.

▣ EVALUATION OF PATIENTS

Symptoms of a tumor in the trachea, even in the presence of a high degree of airway obstruction, may be insidious. Most commonly, patients with a tumor in the trachea present with dyspnea, hemoptysis, cough, wheezing, dysphagia, change in voice or hoarseness, stridor, and pneumonia.[16] In one series, productive cough and shortness of breath were the most common symptoms.[17] A history of slowly progressive dyspnea on exertion is often present. Many patients with a malignant neoplasm present with hemoptysis. This often leads to appropriate bronchoscopic diagnosis. An irritative cough, which may or may not be productive, and which may in time be associated with hemoptysis, is sometimes also seen. Involvement of one of the recurrent nerves leads to hoarseness; this may be insidious in onset. Stridor may be detected later in the course of the disease. Some patients, particularly those with tumors in the distal trachea, may present with unilateral or, at times, bilateral pneumonitis; this will often respond to antibiotics, only to recur later. All too often, especially with slowly growing tumors such as adenoid cystic carcinoma, the patient who has developed slowly progressive shortness of breath and wheezing will have an apparently normal chest radiograph. This leads to the diagnosis of adult-onset asthma, with some patients treated with steroids for a prolonged period of time before the slowly growing tumor is recognized.

In general, the more aggressive tumors are diagnosed earlier owing to their propensity to present with prominent symptoms, for example, hemoptysis. In one study, the mean duration of symptoms before diagnosis in patients with squamous cell carcinoma of the trachea was 4 months, whereas the mean duration of symptoms before diagnosis in adenoid cystic carcinoma of the trachea was 18 months. It is important to note that all patients with a tumor of the trachea who are being considered for resection and reconstruction should be weaned from steroids and should not be required to use postoperative mechanical ventilation so that the risk of subsequent tracheal separation or stenosis can be reduced. Also, previous irradiation carries an excessive risk for primary healing and must be carefully considered.

▣ DIAGNOSTIC STUDIES

The primary diagnostic modalities for delineating tracheal abnormalities are radiologic studies and bronchoscopy.

These studies define the presence and extent of tumor in almost every case. The following studies are often helpful:

1. Chest radiograph (posteroanterior, lateral, and oblique) centered high enough to obtain good views of the trachea
2. Anteroposterior overpenetrated view, including the larynx and trachea down to the carina
3. Lateral view of the neck in extension with swallowing to elevate the upper trachea
4. Fluoroscopy of the larynx and trachea with necessary spot films and opacification of the esophagus with barium
5. If necessary, additional anteroposterior, lateral, and oblique linear tomography of the trachea
6. Computed tomography (CT), helpful for defining extratracheal involvement and for detecting the presence of lymph node involvement

All too often, the plain chest radiograph is considered normal. However, on closer inspection, an abnormality of the tracheal air column is seen. The overpenetrated anteroposterior view is often most helpful in providing a general picture of the extent of tumor and its involvement in the trachea. The lateral view, with the neck in extension, is useful in delineating abnormalities of the upper trachea. Fluoroscopy may provide information on involvement of the recurrent laryngeal nerves, variability in the airway, and involvement of the esophagus. Laminography may provide additional information about invasion of the walls of the trachea and larynx and the extent of mediastinal and carinal involvement.

Additional radiographic studies may be obtained. If there is any question of involvement of the superior vena cava, innominate arteries, or pulmonary arteries, angiography may prove helpful. Barium esophagram may demonstrate esophageal involvement by extrinsic compression and/or invasion. Magnetic resonance imaging offers the advantage of sagittal and coronal views of the trachea; however, it is costly and offers little advantage over CT. Recently, the use of spiral or helical CT has been advocated.[18, 19] This CT technique offers the advantage of multiplanar and 3-dimensional reconstruction with resolution that is equal to that of conventional CT. This may be helpful in individual cases.

Functional studies are of limited usefulness. They may, at times, call attention to an obstructing lesion when clinical signs and symptoms are subtle. Functional studies may also give information about the status of the lung parenchyma; this, however, is rarely useful because the presence of an obstructing airway lesion requires treatment regardless of the state of the lung parenchyma.

All patients suspected of having or known to have a tumor of the trachea require endoscopy at some point during their evaluation. Great caution must be taken with the use of flexible bronchoscopy in these patients. Instrumentation of a nearly obstructed trachea may lead to bleeding, edema, or increased secretions that may precipitate sudden airway compromise. No effort should be made to employ instrumentation or to pass beyond a tumor if there is a high degree of obstruction unless preparations have been made to proceed directly with surgical correction of the lesion. It is preferable to simply identify the presence of the tumor and to defer any further evaluation and biopsy until appropriate arrangements have been made to manage the airway in the event of problems.

In general, the rigid bronchoscope is preferred when tumors of the trachea are studied. The need to establish an airway by removal of bits of tumor or to obtain more adequate biopsy for diagnosis by frozen section justifies the use of the rigid bronchoscope (with appropriate magnifying telescopes) rather than the flexible bronchoscope. If necessary, the flexible bronchoscope may be passed through the rigid instrument for the evaluation of disease distal to the carina. Careful measurements must be taken to determine the extent of tracheal involvement as well as to determine the amount of trachea remaining available for reconstruction. It is best to record the distance from the incisors to the carina, to the inferior aspect of the tumor, to the superior aspect of tumor, and to the vocal cords.

AIRWAY MANAGEMENT

Adequate control of the airway is of critical importance in the management of all tumors of the trachea. Tumors of the trachea may present with airway obstruction, and endotracheal intubation may prove impossible. Control of the airway is best accomplished in the operating room, where an assortment of rigid bronchoscopes, dilators, biopsy forceps, and instruments for emergency tracheotomy are readily available.[20, 21] Sedation with a short-acting intravenous agent such as propofol is often helpful. Anesthesia is best accomplished by inhalational induction with a volatile anesthetic.[22] This requires patience on the part of the anesthesiologist as well as the surgeon because induction deep enough to allow rigid bronchoscopy may take as long as 20 minutes. Paralytic agents are to be avoided because these may lead to a potentially lethal combination of airway obstruction and apnea.

Initial evaluation should be done with a rigid bronchoscope carefully inserted through the vocal cords, stopping just proximal to the level of obstruction. Rigid telescopes may then be inserted through the bronchoscope to assess the degree of obstruction. A rigid bronchoscope can be passed beyond most tumors, even those causing near-complete airway obstruction. Once the status of the distal airway has been assessed, partial removal of the tumor with biopsy forceps can be done in order to determine its consistency and vascularity. If a tumor appears to be very vascular, it may be wiser to forgo biopsy, proceed with the necessary surgical exposure, and obtain a histologic diagnosis later when the field is under direct control. For the vast majority of tumors, the tip of the rigid bronchoscope can be used to "core out" most of the tumor; the tumor may then be grasped with the biopsy forceps and removed. If bleeding is noted in the airway, the bronchoscope can be passed into the distal airway, thus ensuring adequate ventilation as well as serving to tamponade the bleeding. On occasion, one may have to use gauze soaked in epinephrine to control bleeding. Rarely, cautery (with insulated electrodes) may have to be used. The use of the laser has become increasingly popular in the management of tracheal obstruction, as well as in coagulation of bleeding sites. In our experience, however, the use of the laser has proved time-consuming, costly, and

rarely advantageous compared with the mechanical technique delineated earlier.

A variety of nonresectional techniques have been described in the management of tracheal tumors.[23, 24] Recently, the use of argon plasma coagulation through a flexible bronchoscope has been reported.[25] Endotracheal removal of malignant tumors, either mechanically or by other means, is only a temporary measure. However, the use of such techniques in emergent situations may allow for further evaluation of the patient in a relatively elective setting; it also may allow surgery to be performed in an elective manner. Many patients with low-grade tumors are receiving steroids at the time of presentation, having been treated for refractory "asthma." When an airway has been established, the steroids may be tapered and discontinued, thus obviating the threat of impaired wound healing at the time of surgery. Multiple core-outs of the tumor may be necessary during the interval of steroid tapering. Similar airway control maneuvers may be used at the time of surgery, even if the patient has presented with a stable airway, because these may allow adequate assessment of the distal airway, as well as the placement of a large enough endotracheal tube to prevent CO_2 accumulation during surgery.

ANESTHESIA

Anesthesia for tracheal reconstruction, especially if there is a high degree of airway obstruction, is best administered by inhalation of a volatile anesthetic.[22] An experienced anesthesiology team working in close cooperation with the surgical team is essential. As noted before, slow induction may be necessary and paralytic agents are to be avoided. The surgeon should be in the operating room with an array of rigid bronchoscopes, including pediatric sizes, as induction commences. The residual airway through which the patient is breathing may be as small as 2 to 3 mm in diameter. In most cases, tumors of the trachea are not circumferential, unlike the circumferential stenoses seen in some inflammatory lesions. After bronchoscopy, a small endotracheal tube can often be inserted past a highly obstructing tumor. In some cases, the tube may be left above the tumor; in others, it may be necessary to remove bits of tumor with a biopsy forceps so that a lumen large enough to accommodate an endotracheal tube may be created.

Epidural anesthesia significantly decreases thoracotomy pain. When maintenance of the airway is a concern, a breathe-down with an inhalation agent is employed, and paralytic agents are given once the airway is secured. Anesthesia is maintained with intravenous anesthesia given in short-acting agents such as remifentanil and propofol. This allows immediate extubation at the completion of the procedure. Endotracheal intubation is accomplished with an extra-long armored endotracheal tube. The flexibility of such a tube allows bronchoscopic placement into one of the mainstem bronchi. After transection of the airway, the orotracheal tube is pulled back into the trachea, and intermittent ventilation is performed with sterile cross-field equipment. Intraoperative deoxygenation can be alleviated by periodic partial inflation of a single lung. The orotracheal tube is again advanced once the anastomosis is complete.

On occasion, the technique of high-frequency jet ventilation is employed. Cardiopulmonary bypass is not helpful and introduces unnecessary risks.

The patient should be extubated and should breathe spontaneously at the conclusion of the procedure. It is undesirable to have even a low-pressure cuff lying in contact with the anastomosis.

◨ SELECTION OF TREATMENT

Treatment of Localized Tumors

There is no question that the best treatment for a benign tumor of the trachea is complete surgical extirpation with primary end-to-end reconstruction.[9, 26–28] This is almost always feasible for benign lesions, even if they are relatively extensive. Complete removal by circumferential segmental resection must be emphasized. There is little, if any, role for lateral resection.

The same rationale applies to low-grade malignant tumors. Segmental resection and reconstruction performed in a single stage seems to offer the best chance for cure or extended palliation. Few true cures have been achieved by radiation alone. However, there is some evidence that radiation may play a role in the neoadjuvant or adjuvant setting.

Tracheal resection and reconstruction has limited application for tumors that involve the trachea secondarily. When the primary tumor is localized and is a low-grade malignancy (e.g., papillary thyroid carcinoma), tracheal resection may lead to either cure or long-term palliation. We have treated 52 patients with thyroid cancer invading the trachea.[29] Our results indicate that resection and primary reconstruction of the trachea invaded by thyroid carcinoma should be done in the absence of extensive metastases when technically feasible. It offers prolonged palliation, avoidance of suffocation caused by bleeding or obstruction, and an opportunity for cure.

Treatment of Extensive Contained Disease

This applies principally to adenoid cystic carcinoma. Involvement of the majority of the trachea by longitudinal extension of this tumor creates a special problem. Modern techniques of resection and primary reconstruction with the patient's own tissues do not usually allow for removal of more than approximately one half of the trachea. When primary reconstruction is not feasible, palliative measures should be used. These include T tubes, tracheal stents, tracheotomy, laser therapy, and radiation. Each case must be individualized.

Treatment of Advanced Invasive Disease

In our 27-year experience, a group of 70 patients with primary squamous cell carcinoma of the trachea were seen. In 44 of these patients, surgical extirpation was attempted; the remaining 26 carcinomas were deemed unresectable. The decision against surgery was usually made on the basis of tumor involvement of a long segment of trachea or carina (>50%), extension into the mediastinum (determined radiographically), or extension into the mainstem bronchi. The patients in our series with unresectable disease were treated by irradiation. In some of these patients, the tumor was cored out through the rigid bronchoscope so that an adequate airway could be provided.

Treatment of an unresectable tumor is particularly relevant in those tumors located in the lower trachea because a simple tracheotomy will not resolve obstruction even if a long tube is used. If massive tumor is present in the upper trachea, one may insert a tracheotomy tube into normal trachea below the level of the tumor; at times, it may be necessary to core out the tumor so that the tube passes into normal trachea. Radiation can then be given with the tube in place. Earlier in our experience, some patients underwent mediastinal tracheotomy distal to an obstructing tumor. However, in view of the final expectations, we deemed such a procedure unjustified because, as in carcinoma of the lung, distant metastases may occur to any of the usual sites and these patients ultimately die of local extension of disease.

Eighty patients with adenoid cystic carcinoma were treated during the same 27-year period. Of these, 60 underwent attempted surgical extirpation; only 12 were treated primarily by irradiation. In 6 patients, exploration revealed such extensive disease as to preclude resection.

Both squamous cell carcinoma and adenoid cystic carcinoma are generally responsive to irradiation. Recurrence occurs earlier after irradiation in squamous cell tumors than in adenoid cystic carcinoma. Whereas prolonged palliation may be obtained from full-dose irradiation in adenoid cystic carcinoma, when squamous cell carcinoma extensively involves the mediastinum, little palliation can be expected. When carcinoma of the lung or of the esophagus involves the trachea extensively, little can be done therapeutically. Most of the other types of primary tumors of the trachea, whether benign or of low-grade malignancy, produce symptoms of airway obstruction relatively early in the disease and are therefore often amenable to therapy.

◨ SURGICAL TECHNIQUES

The initial operation is usually the best opportunity for the clinician to resect a tumor of the trachea. The surgeon should have a full understanding of the techniques of management of the entire upper airway. Knowledge of the larynx, various release maneuvers, ways to obtain a tension-free anastomosis, and methods for obtaining access to all parts of the trachea is necessary. The surgeon must know the blood supply of the trachea, the course of the recurrent laryngeal nerves, and the acceptable types of reconstruction. Each case must be carefully studied and each operation carefully planned before such a reconstruction is undertaken.

Positioning/Incision

The patient must be positioned to allow full access to the operative field. A cervical collar incision is used for relatively limited tumors located in the upper half of the trachea. This incision may be extended through the upper portion of the sternum if access to the mediastinal trachea is

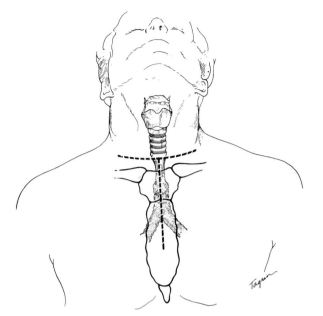

FIGURE 17–1 Reconstruction of the upper trachea. Collar incision and extension for upper sternotomy. Essentially, all benign strictures as well as upper tracheal neoplasms may be most easily reconstructed through this approach.

mandated (Fig. 17–1). Exposure to the larynx may be attained either beneath the upper flap of the collar incision or through a separate, small incision above the hyoid. If the tumor appears to be extensive, as is sometimes the case with adenoid cystic carcinoma, the patient should be positioned in a manner that allows extension of the incision into the right fourth interspace to the posterior axillary line. For this reason, the right arm is draped and kept within the field so that it can be moved back and forth as necessary.

The preferred approach to tumors of the lower trachea and carina is through a high right posterolateral thoracotomy. The right arm is draped into the operative field. The entire neck is also prepped into the field for access to the hyoid region, the larynx, and the trachea if cervical mobilization and laryngeal release maneuvers become necessary. In rare instances, individual incisions are made. If subtotal removal of the trachea or a laryngotracheiectomy is necessary, a long, somewhat lower collar incision is used. Vertical incisions are to be avoided so that the possibility of mediastinal tracheotomy is preserved. Although this is rarely needed, it must be planned for in advance.

Resection

During the dissection of the tumor, every effort is made to remove as much surrounding tissue as possible at the level of the tumor. The trachea is approached above and below the lesion, and these areas are cleared first. If the primary tumor is a thyroid cancer, it may be necessary to remove the strap muscles en bloc; this may also be accompanied by a partial neck dissection. With other primary tumors of the cervical trachea, resection of one or both lobes of the thyroid on the side of the tumor may be required to avoid the possibility of exposing tumor that may have invaded the

tracheal wall at that point. Each case must be considered individually.

The surgical approach for benign tumors of the trachea varies somewhat more than that for malignant tumors. For benign tumors, dissection remains close to the trachea, and recurrent laryngeal nerves encased in scar may not be visualized; this is a safe technique as long as dissection is maintained on the surface of the trachea. When malignant tumors are dissected, the recurrent laryngeal nerves are identified at a distance away from the tumor and are followed toward the area of the tumor. It may be necessary to sacrifice a recurrent laryngeal nerve on the side of the tumor owing to its involvement with tumor, even if no functional paralysis is observed. Special care must be observed in the right transthoracic approach to avoid injury to the left recurrent nerve as the aortic arch is approached. Adjacent lymph nodes should be included in any dissection for a malignant tumor. However, such a dissection should be limited because it may endanger the blood supply to the trachea. A compromise must be made between leaving behind paratracheal tissue that may contain positive lymph nodes and avoiding devascularization of the trachea. Circumferential dissection of the trachea over a great distance should be avoided because this may endanger the blood supply and can lead to problems with healing and/or stenosis. It is best not to circumferentially free more than 1 to 2 cm of trachea from the point at which the trachea is to be transected.

Once the trachea has been identified, the entire pretracheal plane is freed bluntly to the carina and often down the proximal anterior surfaces of the mainstem bronchi. Care is taken to spare the lateral pedicles because these contain the blood supply to the trachea. Isolation of the portion of the trachea containing the tumor is begun on the side of the trachea away from the tumor, and an effort is made to include appropriate lymph nodes. Once the inferiormost extent of tumor is identified, midlateral traction sutures of 2–0 Vicryl (polyglactin 910) are placed through the full thickness of the tracheal wall, approximately 1 to 2 cm distal to the anticipated line of transection. Preparations are then made for transection. Sterile connecting tubing is passed to the anesthesiologist, and a sterile cuffed endotracheal tube (flexible armored Tovell tube) is brought into the operative field. The trachea is then opened in a transverse manner immediately distal to the inferior aspect of the tumor, and the lumen is carefully inspected. If it seems that the division will occur at an appropriate level, the transection is completed; if the level is inappropriate, a more distal level is chosen under direct vision.

After transection of the distal trachea, the airway is intubated across the field with the flexible endotracheal tube. At this point, the orotracheal tube may be withdrawn to a level proximal to the anticipated proximal extent of tumor; it is wise to suture a catheter to the tip of the tube so that if it is withdrawn above the vocal cords, it may be reintroduced with ease at the end of the case. An assistant usually exerts traction on the previously placed sutures, thus keeping the cuffed flexible tube at an appropriate position in the trachea and hence keeping blood and secretions out of the distal airway. A small portion of tracheal tissue distal to the line of transection is removed and sent for frozen section analysis so that the adequacy of the distal margin can be determined.

The transected end of trachea is now grasped with forceps and is placed on gentle traction to facilitate proximal dissection. The esophagus is usually left intact. However, it may be necessary to include a full-thickness segment of the anterolateral wall of the esophagus; at other times, only the muscularis may be excised. Any defect in the esophagus is repaired primarily in two layers with fine interrupted sutures and is reinforced with autologous tissue such as a strap muscle. Preoperative studies can usually predict when a segment of esophagus must be excised, so that appropriate preparations can be made for gastric pullthrough or for colon interposition.

With the dissection carried proximally, the proximal extent of tumor is identified from within the tracheal lumen and a point of transection is chosen. At times, it may be necessary to bevel obliquely a portion of the inferior aspect of the larynx, such as half or more of the cricoid cartilage, to obtain an adequate proximal margin. Once the proximal point of transection is determined, traction sutures are placed in the proximal trachea in a manner similar to those placed distally; if the transection point is relatively high, the sutures may be placed in the larynx. The trachea is then transected, and a specimen is submitted for frozen section analysis of the proximal margin.

Reconstruction

After removal of the specimen and after establishment of clear margins of resection both proximally and distally, reconstruction can begin (Fig. 17–2). The anesthesiologist is asked to temporarily flex the neck as the surgeon and assistant simultaneously draw together the traction sutures on each side of the trachea. Gentle traction on the sutures should approximate the two ends of the trachea. At times, however,

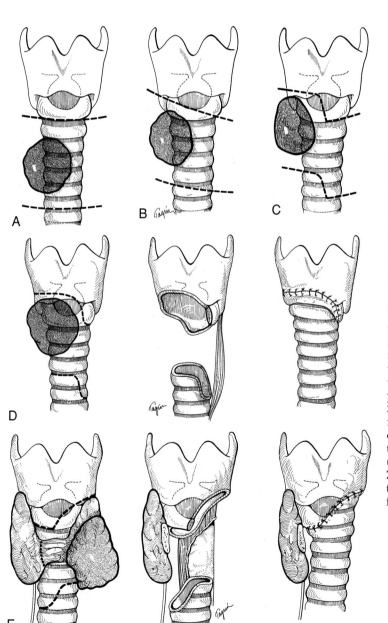

FIGURE 17–2 Types of resection. *A,* Sleeve resection of the trachea. In some cases, the proximal transection was at the lower border of the cricoid cartilage. *B,* Beveled resection of the cricoid to provide a margin on the side where the lower border of that cartilage was involved by tumor. The recurrent laryngeal nerve may or may not be involved in such a resection. *C,* Bayonet line of resection where tumor extended above the level of the upper border of the cricoid cartilage anterolaterally or laterally. The upper margin of transection through the lateral thyroid cartilage lay beneath the vocal cord in every instance. The line of distal tracheal resection was shaped to mortise into the laryngeal defect. It was extended over only two cartilages to maintain suitable stability. In these patients, the recurrent laryngeal nerve was usually paralyzed prior to resection or necessarily sacrificed on one side because of tumor involvement. *D* and *E,* Examples of the complex type of resection shown in *C. D,* Resection of mixed papillary and follicular carcinoma following recurrence 2 years after total thyroidectomy. *E,* Mixed papillary and follicular carcinoma (not previously treated) managed by complex resection as diagrammed, including removal of the anterolateral muscular wall of the esophagus. (Reprinted from Ann Thorac Surg, v. 42: Grillo HC, Zannini P: Resectional management of airway invasion by thyroid carcinoma. Pp 287–298, 1986, with permission from "The Society of Thoracic Surgeons.")

excessive tension is noted during this maneuver. Although there is no absolute rule as to how much trachea may be safely resected and reconstructed, intraoperative assessment of tension is essential in determining the extent of resection and the need for possible release maneuvers. Excessive tension on the anastomosis markedly increases the likelihood of separation or stenosis, both potentially disastrous complications. If further relaxation is deemed necessary to avoid excessive tension, a variety of release maneuvers may be used. The suprahyoid laryngeal release (Montgomery release) is particularly effective, especially after resection of the proximal trachea.[30] This maneuver usually obtains an additional 1 to 2.5 cm of tracheal length proximally, but it is of little use in resection of the distal trachea or carina. Other maneuvers may be performed, but they require entry into the thoracic cavity. These include mobilization of the inferior pulmonary ligament,[11] intrapericardial release of the right hilum, and, rarely, bronchial transplantation.

Once it has been demonstrated that tracheal approximation can be obtained without excessive tension, the neck is again extended and the anastomosis completed. The anastomosis is performed with coated 4–0 Vicryl suture. The use of such absorbable suture material has reduced to zero the incidence of suture line granulomas, a problem that was encountered early in our experience with the use of nonabsorbable suture. All sutures are placed individually in a circumferential manner, beginning posteriorly and working anteriorly, first on one side and then on the other. The sutures are placed approximately 4 mm apart and approximately 3 mm from the cut edge of trachea. Anterolaterally, the sutures are placed through cartilage. No effort is made to pass sutures submucosally. All sutures are sequentially and carefully clipped to the drapes so that they will not become entangled and/or the order confused.

Once all sutures have been placed, the endotracheal tube is removed from across the operative field, and the orotracheal tube is once again advanced and placed into the distal airway under direct vision. The neck is then securely supported in flexion by the anesthesiologist. The lateral traction sutures are pulled together and tied, approximating but not intussuscepting the tracheal ends. The anastomotic sutures are tied sequentially from front to back on each side, with each suture being cut after it is tied. Saline is then instilled over the anastomosis, and airtightness is tested by deflating the cuff of the endotracheal tube and applying high airway pressures. If the anastomosis is high and if the thyroid isthmus is intact, the isthmus may be sutured over the anastomosis. Although it is not necessary to interpose a pedicled strap muscle between the innominate artery and the anastomosis, some surgeons may wish to do so to add a measure of security that this may afford.

Suction drains are placed in the substernal and/or paratracheal areas and the incision is closed in layers, with wiring of the sternum if it has been divided. A heavy suture is placed from the crease below the chin to the presternal skin. This serves as a guardian suture in the postoperative phase, reminding the patient not to suddenly hyperextend the neck. The suture is usually removed on postoperative day 7, after a satisfactory anastomosis has been documented bronchoscopically. Except in rare circumstances, every effort is made to extubate the patient at the conclusion of the operation.

If the tumor involves the carina, various techniques are used. Unless the tumor is small, it is rarely possible to reconstruct the airway by forming a neocarina from the right and left mainstem bronchi. Such a reconstruction anchors the carina low in the mediastinum, and if more trachea has been excised, approximation is not possible. More commonly, either the right or left mainstem bronchus is sutured to the trachea, and a lateral anastomosis of the other mainstem bronchus to the lower portion of the tracheal wall above the initial anastomosis is performed.

The principles and technique of anastomosis in carinal reconstruction are as described previously for tracheal resection and reconstruction. Management of the airway is somewhat more challenging and therefore requires even closer cooperation with the anesthesiologist. In some instances, jet ventilation has proved useful in complex reconstructions. All intrathoracic anastomoses are covered with a second layer of either pedicled pleura or pericardial fat pad. It is important to interpose tissue between the airway suture line and adjacent pulmonary vessels. If previous irradiation has been given, then the omentum is used.

◨ POSTOPERATIVE CARE

Throughout the performance of tracheal resection and reconstruction, care is taken to avoid the entry of blood and secretions into the tracheobronchial tree. This helps to prevent postoperative pneumonitis and shunting, the end result of which may be a requirement for mechanical ventilation, which is an extremely hazardous procedure for a patient with a recently completed tracheal reconstruction. During the operation, the assistant must be vigilant in the clearance of blood and secretions by careful suctioning and must not allow them entry into the airway (even in the presence of an inflated cuff). Postoperatively, the patient is instructed to maintain airway clearance with gentle coughing and other chest physical therapy maneuvers. If these techniques are inadequate, gentle tracheal suctioning is performed. If all of these maneuvers prove unsuccessful, then the flexible bronchoscope is used to clear secretions. In our experience, most of the difficulty in maintaining airway clearance is encountered in patients who have undergone complex carinal reimplantations.

As has been noted previously, cervical fixation with sutures is maintained for approximately 1 week after surgery. After removal of the suture(s), the patient is instructed not to extend the neck for another week. After this second week, there is no need for any further restriction. Occasionally, when the trachea has been markedly shortened, the patient may have to swallow with the neck in a slightly flexed position.

◨ REVIEW OF TREATMENT RESULTS IN ONE SERIES

Of the 198 tumors of the trachea in the series at Massachusetts General Hospital, 147 were treated by resection and reconstruction of trachea or carina, laryntotracheal resection with or without cervicomediastinal exenteration, or staged reconstruction with excision of the tumor, in the hope of restoring airway continuity with cervical cutaneous tubes. Eleven patients underwent exploration only, with or without placement of a tracheotomy or a T tube. Patients who underwent coring out of the tumor and placement of a tracheotomy or a T tube as the only treatment are not listed as having been surgically treated. This report focuses on the 132 patients who underwent resection and primary reconstruction. Seven patients underwent laryngectomy and resection of the trachea because of extensive involvement of the larynx. Eight patients underwent staged reconstruction. These procedures were performed when the extent of possible resection was being explored. Because of the great number of complications, the high mortality, and the small number of patients who could be followed to completion, staged reconstruction was abandoned. Most patients whose tumor was unresectable were referred for irradiation.

An approximately equal number of patients with squamous cell carcinoma, adenoid cystic carcinoma, and other types of cancer were eligible for primary resection and reconstruction (41, 50, and 41 patients, respectively). The number of patients subjected to resection of the trachea, as opposed to carinal resection, varied markedly within each of these categories. Overall, only 37% of patients who had primary reconstruction underwent resection of the carina; however, more than 50% of patients with adenoid cystic carcinoma were so treated. Only 9 of the 41 patients with squamous cell carcinoma had resection of the carina, reflecting the differing distribution of these tumors.

◨ SURGICAL APPROACH

Operations were planned flexibly so that the approach would be adequate if more trachea was involved with tumor than was anticipated. Tumors of the upper trachea were explored through a cervical collar incision, with the option of extending the incision through the superior portion of the sternum if necessary. For tumors in the midtrachea, the operative field was such that the surgeon kept open the option of a full sternotomy and use of a transpericardial approach or a "trapdoor" incision through the right fourth interspace. For tumors of the lower trachea, a right thoracotomy was used. Early in our experience, the trapdoor incision was used because this allows access to the entire trachea. Although a median sternotomy with a transpericardial approach was used, this offered less adequate exposure for extensive tumors.

Carinal resection was approached most often through a right posterolateral thoracotomy. In selected cases, carinal resection was approached through a left thoracotomy or through bilateral thoracotomies (if a left pneumonectomy was anticipated). Figure 17–3 shows the modes of reconstruction.

Technical Features

In 10 patients (1 squamous, 3 adenoid cystic, 6 other), a laryngoplasty, or partial resection of the larynx, was necessary for adequate margins to be obtained. Each of these cases was individualized. The trachea was tailored appropriately to mortise into the irregular defect created in the larynx. The recurrent laryngeal nerve was preserved. We have described this type of resection for the management of secondary invasion of the airway by thyroid carcinoma.

In some cases, adjunctive procedures were used to decrease tension on the anastomosis. Laryngeal release was performed in 7 patients who underwent tracheal resection and in 5 patients who underwent carinal resection. We have since concluded that laryngeal release does not translate into additional tracheal relaxation in patients undergoing carinal resection only. However, laryngeal release may be helpful in patients undergoing resection of the midtrachea and the carina. Hilar release, which involves making a U-shaped incision in the pericardium below the inferior pulmonary vein or complete circumcision of the pericardium at the hilum, was performed in 12 of 32 patients undergoing transthoracic resection of the trachea and in 23 of 50 patients undergoing carinal resection. In addition, 4 patients with adenoid cystic carcinoma who had carinal resection underwent both laryngeal and hilar release.

Ten patients had varying degrees of thyroid resection performed concomitantly. Resection of the esophagus, either full-thickness or muscularis only, was performed in 9 patients (7 tracheal resections and 2 carinal resections). A recurrent laryngeal nerve was deliberately sacrificed in 4 tracheal resections and in 1 carinal resection. Omentum was used as tissue reinforcement of the anastomosis in 4 patients; all had received previous irradiation. In 2 patients with adenoid cystic carcinoma who presented with tracheoesophageal fistula, colon interposition was used for reconstruction.

Operative Results

Complications

Stenosis of the anastomotic site developed in two patients who underwent resection of the trachea. One case of stenosis occurred in a patient after a transient air leak; the other occurred in a patient who was operated on while receiving high-dose steroids.[31] Both patients later underwent a successful re-resection. Stenosis of the anastomosis also developed in four patients after carinal resection. Two of these patients had undergone carinal pneumonectomy; re-resection of the anastomosis, one through a cervical collar incision, was successful in both cases. The two remaining patients required upper lobectomy of the reimplanted right lung with reattachment of the bronchus intermedius or of the lower lobe; both were successful. Three air leaks were managed nonoperatively with success. Four patients developed granulomas of the suture line; all occurred in the era before the use of absorbable suture and all were managed by bronchoscopy. One patient, after laryngoplasty, had an elevation of the posterior mucosal flap; this healed in place after brief intubation. One esophageal fistula occurred in a patient in whom extensive full-thickness resection of the esophageal wall was performed. Another small fistula occurred and healed spontaneously. Vocal cord paralysis, reversible with time in most cases, occurred in eight patients undergoing tracheal or carinal resection for adenoid cystic carcinoma. Six patients experienced aspiration on deglutition, principally after undergoing laryngeal release; most

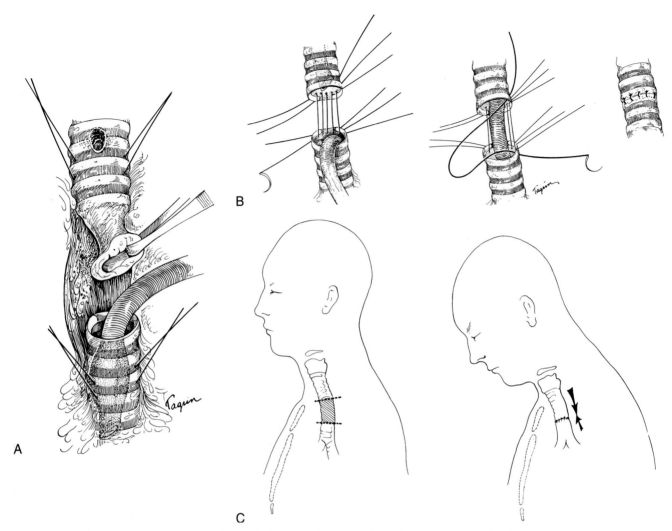

FIGURE 17–3 *A*, Circumferential dissection has been carried out only immediately beneath the lowermost level of the pathologic lesion. Traction sutures are in place and the patient has been intubated distal to the lesion. The lesion is now being retracted upward to facilitate dissection from the underlying esophagus. *B*, Details of the anastomotic technique. The sutures are first placed posteriorly and are then worked in an anterior fashion. There has been a tendency to place all of the sutures prior to advancing the tube from above into the distal trachea. All of the knots are on the outside. The diagrammatic representation must be recognized not to indicate complete circumferential dissection of the lengths of trachea shown. *C*, This diagram indicates that the maximum amount of approximation is obtained by cervical flexion rather than by upward traction on the carina in the anterior approach. (*A* from Myers EN, Suen JY: Cancer of the Head and Neck, ed 3. Philadadelphia, WB Saunders, 1996; *B* from Grillo HC: Surgery of the trachea. Curr Probl Surg July 1970, pp 3–59; *C* from Grillo HC: Congenital lesions, neoplasms, and injuries of the trachea. In Sabiston DC Jr, Spencer FC [eds]: Gibbon's Surgery of the Chest, 3rd ed. Philadelphia, WB Saunders, 1976.)

resolved in time, although some patients required a temporary gastrostomy. One patient, who underwent transthoracic tracheal resection, experienced a small empyema, which required drainage. Guillain-Barré syndrome developed in one patient. Acute pulmonary edema developed in two patients who had undergone right carinal pneumonectomy. Pneumonia developed in three patients. Hypoxia was noted in a patient who had undergone carinal resection with reattachment of the right main bronchus and exclusion of the left lung; the pulmonary artery had not been ligated. This patient later underwent left pneumonectomy for removal of the nonfunctioning but shunting lung.

Deaths

A total of 7 (5%) deaths occurred among the 132 patients who underwent primary resection and reconstruction. One death occurred in the 82 patients undergoing tracheal resection, and 6 deaths occurred in patients undergoing carinal resection. The highest mortality was noted among patients who underwent carinal resection for adenoid cystic carcinoma; this is probably the result of excessive anastomotic tension after the extended resection that is at times required in this infiltrating disease.[6] The death after resection of the trachea occurred in a patient who experienced an anastomotic leak followed by pneumonia. Among the deaths after carinal resection, 2 patients experienced respiratory failure after an anastomotic leak, respiratory failure from pulmonary edema developed in 1 patient, and in 1 patient, massive hemorrhage occurred on the ninth postoperative day, presumably from a pulmonary artery.

There were no deaths among the 7 patients with laryngotracheal tumor (with or without cervicomediastinal exenteration). Mortality (5 of 8) was unacceptably high in those patients undergoing staged reconstruction, and this procedure has been abandoned. Three deaths occurred among the 9 patients who underwent exploration only; 2 died of respiratory failure, and 1 died of a presumed tracheoinnominate fistula. Two additional deaths were attributed to technical failure of the operation, although both occurred many months after surgery, and the patients had been treated elsewhere. One of these patients had undergone a carinal resection, and the other had undergone a staged reconstruction. Stenosis developed in both patients, and one may have experienced continued aspiration secondary to laryngeal malfunction; further surgical management would have been advisable in both patients.

Oncologic Results

Of the 147 patients who underwent resection of tumor, either with or without primary reconstruction, 135 survived surgery. As of last follow-up, 70% were alive without tumor. Of those patients with a diagnosis of squamous cell carcinoma, 49% were alive; of those with adenoid cystic carcinoma, 75% were alive; and of those with other tumors, 83% survived. Table 17–3 shows the number of patients in each category who died of tumor or of other causes as well as the number who are alive with known carcinoma. It must be noted that interpretation of these figures is rather difficult because the cases are scattered over many years. The fact that more patients have been referred for treatment in the past 10 years reflects favorably on the number of patients living without known disease (i.e., assumed cured). These figures are encouraging.

If we consider 20 patients who had squamous cell carcinoma and are living without known disease, ten were operated on longer than 3 years ago; four were disease free at the time of death from other disease or had been followed for 5, 7, 8, and 15 years without evidence of disease (Table 17–4). This likely represents 14 patients in whom cure had been achieved. An additional 10 patients were free of disease but have been followed for only 3 years. Although this interval seems short, it is clinically significant for squamous cell carcinoma of the trachea because this disease tends to recur early, in a time frame similar to that of squamous cell carcinoma of the lung.

Adenoid cystic carcinoma has a proclivity for a long clinical course, at times recurring many years after initial resection; this makes it difficult for clinicians to interpret results of resection for this disease (see Table 17–4). The first patient in this series treated for adenoid cystic carcinoma underwent carinal resection; recurrence was discovered at the suture line 17 years later. Because resection margins and lymph nodes had been negative at the time of surgery, no irradiation was given. Bronchoscopic follow-up had been terminated after 10 years.

Sixteen patients with adenoid cystic carcinoma were alive without evidence of disease 5 years after resection. Twenty-three additional patients who underwent resection were free of disease at less than 5-year follow-up. The long-term outlook for adenoid cystic carcinoma is somewhat difficult to determine. Five patients were free of disease at 10-year follow-up. Of these five patients, four later died of metastatic disease or of recurrent disease. Three patients died of metastatic disease or of recurrent disease between 3 and

TABLE 17-3 Results of Surgical Treatment of Primary Tracheal Tumors

Variable	Squamous Cell	Adenoid Cystic	Other	Total
Number of tumors resected	44	60	43	147
Operative deaths (resection)	3	8	1	12
Resection, with reconstruction				
Trachea	1	0	0	1
Carina	1	4	1	6
Laryngotracheal	0	0	0	0
Staged procedures	1 of 2	4 of 6	0	0
Exploration only	2 of 6	1 of 3	0	3
Survival (resected tumors)				
Dead				
Of tumor	13	7	3	23
Of other cause	6	5	1	12
Alive				
With tumor	0	1	0	1
Without tumor	20	39	35	94
Lost to follow-up	2	0	3	5

Data from Grillo HC, Mathisen DJ: Primary tracheal tumors: Treatment and results. Ann Thorac Surg 49:69, 1990.

TABLE 17-4 Survival After Resection of Tracheal Carcinoma

Variable	Tumor Type*	
	Squamous Cell	Adenoid Cystic
Operative deaths	3	8
Alive without carcinoma (yr)		
>10	3 (9)	5 (11)
5–10	4 (10)	11 (12)
3–5	3 (6)	10 (11)
0–3	10 (11)	13 (13)
Died of carcinoma (yr)		
>10	0	4
5–10	0	1
3–5	5	2
0–3	8	0
Died without carcinoma; lost to follow-up (yr)		
>10	1	0
5–10	3	0
3–5	1	1
0–3	3	4
Alive with carcinoma	0	1

*Original number of operative survivors, excluding those who died later of the other causes, is shown in parentheses.

Data from Grillo HC, Mathisen DJ: Primary tracheal tumors: Treatment and results. Ann Thorac Surg 49:69, 1990.

10 years after resection, and an additional 21 patients were free of disease during a similar period of follow-up. These figures emphasize the fact that patients with adenoid cystic carcinoma may remain free of disease for a prolonged period, yet they still are threatened by late recurrence.

In the heterogeneous group of tumors, outcome tends to be quite good, because many of these tumors were either benign or of low-grade malignancy. Of the 11 carcinoids in the group, 1 was highly atypical and had metastasized to regional lymph nodes. All mucoepidermoid tumors behaved in a benign manner. One adenocarcinoma occurred in the membranous wall of the carina at the base of a cyst; the affected child was free of disease at later than 3.5 years follow-up. One patient had an adenosquamous carcinoma that required simultaneous laryngeal resection; this patient died of metastatic disease 4.7 years after resection. A single patient with small cell carcinoma limited to the trachea underwent adjuvant chemoradiation; he was free of disease after 3.7 years' follow-up. A single patient with melanoma who had no evidence of primary disease elsewhere was free of disease after a brief follow-up period. The patient with pseudosarcoma remained free of disease at 19 years' follow-up. Several patients with similar disease in the era before tracheal resection died of strangulation from local growth of tumor. The patient with chondrosarcoma died 5 years after resection. The patient with rhabdomyosarcoma died of osteogenic sarcoma, which likely was due to the radiation treatments the patient had received in early childhood for a cervical rhabdomyosarcoma. One early death occurred in the patient with a spindle cell sarcoma of the carina.

Five patients were referred after operations for tumor at another institution. Three of these patients had undergone incomplete resection of a carcinoid tumor that had recurred between 10 and 14 years after resection. An 8-year-old girl had undergone incomplete resection of a carinal malignant fibrous histiocytoma. She underwent re-resection and was free of disease at 3 years' follow-up. Another patient had had a pneumonectomy performed for a fibrous tumor and had residual disease at the carina. He remains free of disease at nearly 2 years after carinal resection. Two patients were lost to follow-up. One of these had a low-grade spindle cell sarcoma and was free of disease at 10 years' follow-up; the other had a solitary squamous papilloma and was free of disease at 7 years' follow-up. One patient had a granular cell tumor high in the trachea involving the larynx. He was later found to have a granular cell tumor in the bronchus intermedius; this was removed by sleeve resection.

◼ IMPORTANCE OF TUMOR AT RESECTION MARGINS AND IN LYMPH NODES

The finding of tumor at the resection margins, even microscopically by frozen section, is of particular importance in airway reconstruction. Because the airway must be reconstructed, it may be impossible to resect any additional airway without creating excessive tension on the anastomosis. Furthermore, extensive lymph node dissection is to be

TABLE 17–5 Effect on Survival of Tumor at Margins and in Lymph Nodes at Resection*

Variable	Died with Cancer	Alive, No Cancer
Squamous cell (no.)	13	22
Nodes positive	6	2
Margins positive		
Invasive	4	1
In situ	0	6
Nodes, margins negative	3	12
Adenoid cystic (no.)	7	38
Nodes, margins positive	3	16
Nodes, margins negative	4	22

*Almost all patients received postoperative radiotherapy.
Data from Grillo HC, Mathisen DJ: Primary tracheal tumors: Treatment and results. Ann Thorac Surg 49:69, 1990.

avoided because it may disrupt the blood supply of the trachea and ultimately lead to necrosis at the anastomosis, followed by irreparable stenosis. Therefore, only immediately adjacent lymph nodes are taken with the specimen. Table 17–5 shows the distribution of involved lymph nodes and margins for squamous cell carcinoma and for adenoid cystic carcinoma in two groups of patients—those who died of cancer and those who were alive and cancer free. The clinical significance of these findings appears to differ among the two types of tumors.

In squamous cell carcinoma, positive lymph nodes were found more commonly in patients who later died with cancer than in those who ultimately survived cancer free. A total of 6 of 13 patients who died with this tumor had positive lymph nodes; only 2 of 20 patients who remained disease free had positive lymph nodes. Furthermore, the finding of invasive carcinoma at the resection margin is of more serious consequence than that found with in situ carcinoma; 4 of 5 patients with invasive carcinoma died of their disease, but all 6 patients with in situ carcinoma were disease free at last follow-up. Almost all of these patients received radiotherapy, with doses ranging from 4500 to 6500 cGy. It was impossible to control for irradiation dose or portal differences in these patients because their therapy was administered at several centers.

In adenoid cystic carcinoma, positive lymph nodes and/or margins proved of little significance with regard to outcome. Owing to the proclivity of this tumor to extend for long distances, the finding of malignant cells at a distance from the gross tumor is all too common. A compromise between total resection and safety must be made in many cases. All patients with adenoid cystic carcinoma now receive postoperative irradiation. Suture line recurrences have been rare, but late recurrences have occurred in lung, bone, liver, and brain. In contrast, primary irradiation of these tumors is characterized by nearly uniform local recurrence within 3 to 5 years, in spite of a good early response.

Sixteen of 40 patients (40%) who underwent resection for squamous cell carcinoma of the trachea had a previous history, a concomitant finding, or a later occurrence of squamous cell carcinoma elsewhere in the respiratory tract. One patient was found to have a concomitant squamous cell carcinoma of the tongue. One patient had a squamous cell carcinoma of the larynx treated before tracheal resection, and another patient had a similar cancer after tracheal resection. A second tracheal squamous cell carcinoma developed in another patient at a site remote from the previously resected tumor. Seven patients had undergone surgical resection of a squamous cell carcinoma of the lung, and 5 later developed such a cancer. This group of 12 patients included 2 patients who had carcinoma of opposite lungs after extended intervals, 3 patients who died of recurrent tracheal carcinoma, 1 who died of recurrence of a previously treated lung carcinoma, 1 who died of lung carcinoma that developed subsequent to tracheal resection, and 1 patient who died of a second primary lung carcinoma in whom a tracheal resection had been performed after treatment of the initial lung carcinoma. Four patients who underwent lung resection for carcinoma either before or after tracheal resection were disease-free at 2.5 to 15 years follow-up after tracheal resection.

ROLE OF IRRADIATION

Because of the limited margins that are often obtainable in resection of the trachea, even when margins and lymph nodes are histologically negative, it may be prudent to give postoperative irradiation in the treatment of squamous cell carcinoma and adenoid cystic carcinoma. Both tumors are radiosensitive, particularly adenoid cystic carcinoma. Irradiation alone as primary therapy has been used in the treatment of tumors of the trachea.[32] We compared patients who underwent resection, with and without postoperative irradiation, with those who received radiotherapy alone. A few of the patients who had irradiation alone also underwent exploration. The principal parameter for assigning patients to the radiotherapy alone category was extent of tumor. This extent, however, was frequently longitudinal extent only and did not necessarily indicate a large mass. Table 17–6 shows the number of patients who died of disease, as well as the number who are alive and free of disease for longer than 1 year for each type of tracheal carcinoma and for each treatment method (resection plus radiation vs. radiation alone). These patients were seen over many years, a fact that may diminish the accuracy of the comparison.

Of those 29 patients with squamous cell carcinoma who underwent resection followed by radiotherapy, 11 eventually died of their disease and 18 remained alive for longer than 1 year without evidence of disease. In contrast, 16

TABLE 17-7 Palliative Value of Operation and Radiation for Tracheal Squamous Cell Carcinoma

Time to Death (mo)	Radiation Only	Resection (+radiation)
<12	5	1
12–24	3	2
24–36	1	4
36–48	0	4
>48	1	0

Data from Grillo HC, Mathisen DJ: Primary tracheal tumors: Treatment and results. Ann Thorac Surg 49:69, 1990.

patients who received radiotherapy as primary treatment died of their disease, and only 1 remained alive without evidence of disease (7 years after treatment).

Patients with adenoid cystic carcinoma were divided into those who died of carcinoma and those who were alive without known disease. Analysis in this group of patients was more difficult because this type of tumor may have long periods of apparent control after resection or irradiation, only to recur later. Of 45 patients treated with resection, usually followed by irradiation, 7 died of carcinoma and 38 were alive without known disease. In the irradiation-alone group, 9 died of carcinoma and 3 were alive without known disease.

In an effort to determine whether resection (with radiotherapy), with its attendant risks, is of any palliative benefit versus radiotherapy alone, we compared the survival of patients with squamous cell carcinoma who received one or the other form of treatment but who nonetheless died of their disease. Table 17–7 shows the number of surviving patients in 12-month periods. Our data show that the results of irradiation alone for squamous cell carcinoma of the trachea are similar to those obtained in lung cancer—that is, most tumors will recur within 2 years. In contrast, patients who undergo resection followed by radiotherapy survive disease-free for longer than 2 years. Because the course of adenoid cystic carcinoma is so prolonged, we examined similar treatment groups with the same endpoint of death from squamous or adenoid cystic carcinoma but compared median and average survival in months (Table 17–8). Our results, given the limits of this nonrandomized comparison, indicate that resection plus radiotherapy triples the survival time in squamous cell carcinoma and at least triples the survival time in adenoid cystic carcinoma.

TABLE 17-6 Treatment of Tracheal Tumor: Resection Versus Radiation

Tumor Type	Dead of Carcinoma	Alive Without Carcinoma (>1 yr)
Squamous cell		
Resection (+/− irradiation)	11	18
Radiation (+/− exploration)	16	1
Adenoid cystic		
Resection (+/− irradiation)	7	38
Radiation (+/− exploration)	9	3

Data from Grillo HC, Mathisen DJ: Primary tracheal tumors: Treatment and results. Ann Thorac Surg 49:69, 1990.

TABLE 17-8 Duration of Survival (in Months) After Irradiation or Resection

Tumor Type	Median Survival	Average Survival
Squamous cell		
Irradiation only	10	11
Resection (+/− irradiation)	34	31
Adenoid cystic		
Irradiation only	28	39
Resection (+/− irradiation)	118	107

Data from Grillo HC, Mathisen DJ: Primary tracheal tumors: Treatment and results. Ann Thorac Surg 49:69, 1990.

The analysis of our 26-year experience with surgical management of primary tumors of the trachea appears to confirm and extend conclusions based on previously reported experiences. Eschapasse collected 152 primary tracheal tumors from multiple teams in France and the Soviet Union.[26] In 1974, he reported on 121 patients surgically treated, with 75 reconstructed after cylindrical resection and anastomosis (47 cases) or carinal resection (28 cases). Thirteen deaths occurred among the 121 patients. Five of 19 patients who had adenoid cystic tumors were alive and free of disease for 3 to 9 years, and 11 of 27 patients who had squamous cell carcinoma were alive and free of disease for 7 months to 16 years. Pearson and colleagues reported surgical treatment of 44 patients between 1963 and 1983.[28] Twenty-nine patients underwent reconstruction, including 16 sleeve resections and 13 carinal resections, with 2 deaths. Nine patients with adenoid cystic carcinoma were alive without disease at 1 to 20 years after surgery; 3 patients died 6 to 18 years after surgery; and 2 remained alive with disease. Four of 6 patients with squamous cell carcinoma who underwent resection were alive at 6 to 56 months.

In 1987, Perelman and Koroleva also reported a 20-year experience (1963–1983) with 116 open operations in 135 patients[33]; of these, 75 were treated by sleeve resection (41) or by carinal resection (34). Eleven deaths were reported. Overall survival for squamous cell carcinoma was 27% at 3 years and 13% at 5 and 10 years; for adenoid cystic carcinoma, survival was 71% at 3 years, 66% at 5 years, and 56% at 10 years and at 15 years.

In 1996, Maziak and associates updated the 32-year experience (1963–1995) of the Toronto group, focusing on adenoid cystic carcinoma.[34] Of their 38 patients, 32 were treated with resection and reconstruction. Three deaths occurred within 30 days of operation. Of the 14 patients who had complete resections, the mean survival was 9.8 years. Of the 15 patients with incomplete resections, the mean survival was 7.5 years. In 6 patients who were treated with irradiation only, mean survival was 6.2 years.

Regnard and colleagues reported the results of 208 patients with tracheal tumors collected from 26 centers in France.[35] This series included 94 patients with squamous cell carcinoma, 4 with adenocarcinoma, 65 with adenoid cystic carcinoma, and 45 with miscellaneous tumors. Operative mortality was 10.5%. Overall survival for adenoid cystic carcinoma was 73% at 5 years and 57% at 10 years. In the remaining cancers of the trachea, the corresponding survival was 47% and 36%. Among those patients with cancers of the trachea, the 5-year survival for complete and for incomplete resection was 55% and 25%, respectively. Postoperative radiotherapy was used in 59% of patients who had tracheal cancers and in 43% of patients who had adenoid cystic carcinomas. The authors believed that the benefit of postoperative radiotherapy was inconclusive except in those patients who had undergone an incomplete resection.

Rafaely and Wessberg reported 22 tracheal resections for tumor.[36] One operative death was reported. Of the 12 survivors with adenoid cystic carcinoma, 2 patients, neither of whom received postoperative radiotherapy, died of metastatic disease, and 9 patients who received postoperative radiotherapy were living free of disease. Among the 5 patients with squamous cell carcinoma, 1 died of another cause,

1 had a local recurrence and was alive at 3.3 years and receiving radiotherapy, and 3 were without evidence of disease at 5 to 11 years.

Schneider reported a series of 14 tumors of the trachea treated with resection and reconstruction, both with and without irradiation.[37] There were 2 postoperative deaths, one of which was due to mediastinitis from an anastomotic leak. Of the remaining 12 patients, 9 were alive and recurrence-free after long-term follow-up (3 adenoid cystic carcinoma, 2 mucoepidermoid carcinoma, 1 squamous cell carcinoma, 1 carcinoid, and 2 benign).

Based on our experience, as well as that of others, several recommendations appear justified in the treatment of tumors of the trachea. Benign primary tumors and tumors of intermediate aggressiveness are best treated by surgical resection and reconstruction. Primary squamous cell carcinoma and adenoid cystic carcinoma are also best treated by resection and reconstruction if this can be safely accomplished; in these patients, resection should be followed in most cases by mediastinal irradiation. Malignant primary tumors of other types should also be treated by resection and reconstruction, again if this can be safely accomplished; most of these patients should also receive postoperative radiotherapy.

Surgical morbidity and mortality in tracheal resection can undoubtedly be improved. Tracheal resection and reconstruction, particularly if extensive or if it involves the carina, is probably best accomplished at centers with considerable experience and expertise in this type of surgery.

REFERENCES

1. Gelder CM, Hetzel MR: Primary tracheal tumors: A national survey. Thorax 48:688, 1993.
2. Grillo HC: Surgery of the trachea. In Keen G (ed): Operative Surgery and Management, 2nd ed. Bristol, Wright, 1987, pp 776–784.
3. Grillo HC: The trachea. In Ravitch MM, Steichen FM (eds): Atlas of General Thoracic Surgery. Philadelphia, WB Saunders, 1988, pp 293–331.
4. Pearson FG: Resection of the trachea for stricture. In Jackson JW (ed): Rob and Smith's Operative Surgery, 3rd ed. London, Butterworths, 1978, pp 373–380.
5. Grillo HC: Primary reconstruction of airway after resection of subglottic and upper tracheal stenosis. Ann Thorac Surg 33:39, 1982.
6. Grillo HC: Carinal reconstruction. Ann Thorac Surg 34:356, 1982.
7. Mitchell JD, Mathisen DJ, Wright CD, et al: Clinical experience with carinal resection. J Thorac Cardiovasc Surg 117:39, 1999.
8. Kutlu CA, Goldstraw P: Tracheobronchial sleeve resection with the use of a continuous anastomosis: Results of one hundred consecutive cases. J Thorac Cardiovasc Surg 117:1112, 1999.
9. Grillo HC, Mathisen DJ: Primary tracheal tumors: Treatment and results. Ann Thorac Surg 49:69, 1990.
10. Grillo HC, Dignan EF, Miura T: Extensive resection and reconstruction of mediastinal trachea without prosthesis or graft: An anatomical study in man. J Thorac Cardiovasc Surg 48:741, 1964.
11. Grillo HC: Terminal or mural tracheostomy in the anterior mediastinum. J Thorac Cardiovasc Surg 51:422, 1966.
12. Grillo HC: Congenital lesions, neoplasms and injuries of the trachea. In Sabiston DC Jr, Spencer FC (eds): Gibbon's Surgery of the Chest, 3rd ed. Philadelphia, WB Saunders, 1976, p 256.
13. Harris RS: The effect of extension of the head and neck upon the infrahyoid respiratory passage and the supraclavicular portion of the human trachea. Thorax 14:176, 1959.
14. Miura T, Grillo HC: The contribution of the inferior thyroid artery to the blood supply of the human trachea. Surg Gynecol Obstet 123:99, 1966.
15. Salassa JR, Pearson BW, Payne WS: Gross and microscopical blood supply of the trachea. Ann Thorac Surg 24:100, 1977.

16. Weber AL, Grillo HC: Tracheal tumor: Radiological, clinical and pathologic evaluation. Adv Otorhinolaryngol 24:170, 1978.
17. Licht PB, Friis S, Pettersson G: Tracheal cancer in Denmark: A nationwide study. Eur J Cardiothorac Surg 19:339, 2001.
18. Whyte RI, Quint LE, Kazerooni EA, et al: Helical computed tomography for the evaluation of tracheal stenosis. Ann Thorac Surg 60:27, 1995.
19. LoCicero J III, Costello P, Campos CT, et al: Spiral CT with multiplanar and three dimensional reconstructions accurately predicts tracheobronchial pathology. Ann Thorac Surg 62:818, 1996.
20. Mathisen DJ, Grillo HC: Endoscopic relief of malignant airway obstruction. Ann Thorac Surg 48:469, 1989.
21. Daddi G, Puma F, Avenia N, et al: Resection with curative intent after endoscopic treatment of airway obstruction. Ann Thorac Surg 65:203, 1998.
22. Behringer EC, Wilson RS: Tracheal resection and reconstruction. In Cohen E (ed): The Practice of Thoracic Anesthesia. Philadelphia, JB Lippincott, 1995, pp 531–561.
23. Brutinet WM, Cortese DA, McDougall JC, et al: A two year experience with the neodymium-YAG laser in endobronchial obstruction. Chest 91:159, 1987.
24. Marasso A, Gallo E, Massaglia GM, et al: Cryosurgery in bronchoscopic treatment of tracheobronchial stenosis: Indications, limits, personal experience. Chest 103:472, 1993.
25. Okada S, Yamauchi H, Ishimori S, et al: Endoscopic surgery with a flexible bronchoscope and argon plasma coagulation for tracheobronchial tumors. J Thorac Cardiovasc Surg 121:180, 2001.
26. Eschapasse H: Les tumeurs tracheales primitives. Traitment chirurgical. Rev Fr Mal Respir 2:425, 1974.
27. Grillo HC: Tracheal tumors: Surgical management. Ann Thorac Surg 26:112, 1978.
28. Pearson FG, Todd TR, Cooper JD: Experience with primary neoplasms of the trachea and carina. J Thorac Cardiovasc Surg 88:511, 1984.
29. Grillo HC, Zannini P: Resectional management of airway invasion by thyroid carcinoma. Ann Thorac Surg 42:287, 1986.
30. Montgomery WW: Suprahyoid release for tracheal anastomosis. Arch Otolaryngol 99:255, 1974.
31. Grillo HC, Zannini P, Michelassi F: Complications of tracheal reconstruction: Incidence, treatment, and prevention. J Thorac Cardiovasc Surg 91:322, 1986.
32. Makarewicz R, Mross M: Radiation therapy alone in the treatment of tumors of the trachea. Lung Cancer 20:169, 1998.
33. Perelman MI, Koroleva NS: Primary tumors of the trachea. In Grill HC, Eschapasse H (eds): International Trends in General Thoracic Surgery, vol 2. Philadelphia, WB Saunders, 1987, pp 91–106.
34. Maziak DE, Todd TR, Keshavjee SH, et al: Adenoid cystic carcinoma of the airway: Thirty-two year experience. J Thorac Cardiovasc Surg 112:1522, 1996.
35. Regnard JF, Fourquier P, Levasseur P: Results and prognostic factors in resections of primary tracheal tumors: A multicenter restrospective study. The French Society of Cardiovascular Surgery. J Thorac Cardiovasc Surg 111:808, 1996.
36. Rafaely Y, Weissberg D: Surgical management of tracheal tumors. Ann Thorac Surg 64:1429, 1997.
37. Schneider P, Schirren J, Muley T, et al: Primary tracheal tumors: Experience with 14 resected patients. Eur J Cardiothorac Surg 20: 12, 2001.

CHAPTER 18

Cancer of the Neck

Javier Gavilán

Jesús J. Herranz-Gonzalez

Eric J. Lentsch

■ INTRODUCTION

Tumors of the neck encompass a heterogeneous group of neoplasms ranging from benign neoplasms, to primary malignancies such as lymphoma and sarcomas, to the most common clinical situation—metastatic disease from a primary site usually located within the head and neck. In adults, the most common entity is squamous cell carcinoma of the head and neck (SCCHN). In patients with SCCHN, approximately 50% have regional lymphatic involvement—either clinical or occult—at the time of diagnosis.[1] Because lymph node metastasis is a frequent occurrence, and because the presence of cervical lymphadenopathy is the single most significant prognostic variable in determining survival of patients with SCCHN, diagnosis and treatment of this problem are among the most important roles of the head and neck oncologist. In this chapter, we discuss the approach to evaluation of the patient with a mass in the neck, and we describe the treatment of primary malignancies and metastatic disease in the neck from a variety of primary sites.

■ ANATOMY

The cervical lymphatic system is a rich network of lymphatic channels that drain into numerous lymph nodes scattered throughout the face, scalp, and neck. About one third of all lymph nodes in the body are located in the neck.[2] They act as filters within the lymphatic circulatory system and constitute important sites of antibody production and antigen-antibody interaction.

The anatomy of the cervical lymphatics is complex and varied among individuals (Fig. 18–1). It consists of two different networks—the superficial and the deep cervical nodes. The superficial cervical lymph nodes, which drain the skin of the head and neck region, are located along the external and anterior jugular veins. They include the facial, external jugular, anterior jugular, occipital, mastoid, and parotid lymph nodes. The deep cervical lymph nodes drain the mucous membrane of the upper aerodigestive tract, as well as organs such as the thyroid. This network includes the following nodes: deep jugular chain, spinal accessory, transverse cervical, retropharyngeal, and deep anterior chain.

Fascial Compartments

The fascial layers of the neck create compartments that contain the lymphatic tissue of the neck (Fig. 18–2). This concept of fascial compartmentalization is the rationale for use of the various modifications of the classic radical neck dissection—including the modified radical neck dissection, selective neck dissections, and the so-called functional neck dissection. The neck has two different fascial layers—the superficial and the deep cervical fascia. The superficial cervical fascia corresponds to the subcutaneous tissue. The deep cervical fascia can be divided into a superficial and a deep or prevertebral layer.

Superficial Layer of Deep Cervical Fascia. The superficial layer of deep cervical fascia, also known as the investing fascia, completely envelops the neck with the exception of the skin, platysma muscle, and superficial fascia. This layer splits to enclose the trapezius, the portion of the omohyoid muscle that crosses the posterior triangle of the neck, and the sternocleidomastoid muscle. In a similar way it envelops the strap muscles before ending in the mandible. The superficial veins of the neck lie on this superficial layer of the deep cervical fascia.

Middle Layer of Deep Cervical Fascia. The middle layer of deep cervical fascia, also known as the visceral fascia, forms the pretracheal fascia, which overlies the trachea and the midline pharyngeal structures, including the pharynx, larynx, and esophagus. In addition, this layer envelops the thyroid and parathyroid glands.

Deep Layer of Deep Cervical Fascia. The deep layer of deep cervical fascia, also known as the prevertebral fascia, covers the muscles that enter into the neck immediately deep to the trapezius muscle (splenius and levator scapulae). This fascial layer splits into a deep prevertebral layer and a more superficial alar layer, creating a potential space between the layers. Laterally, the spinal accessory nerve crosses the posterior triangle within this layer, along with some lymph nodes. At the lower end, both fascial layers further separate, with the deep layer covering the scalene muscles; the superficial layer, however, remains attached to the trapezius muscle and clavicle. The phrenic nerve runs inferiorly on the anterior aspect of the scalene group, covered by the deep fascial layer.

Carotid Sheath. The carotid sheath comprises all three layers of the deep cervical fascia. It runs from the base of the skull to the root of the neck and has independent compartments for the internal jugular vein, the carotid artery, the vagus nerve, and the ansa cervicalis. The cervical portion of the sympathetic trunk runs posterior to the carotid sheath.

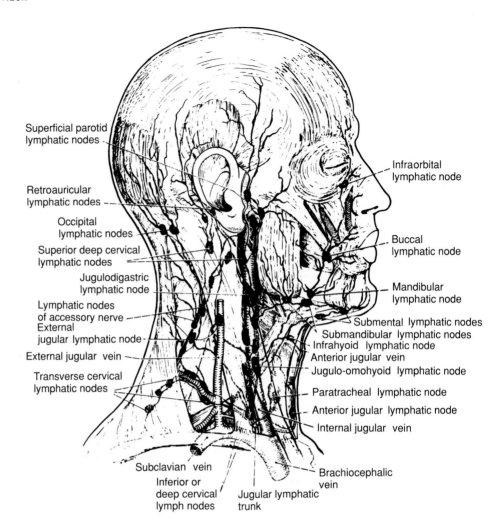

FIGURE 18–1 The lymphatic structures of the neck.

Labels on figure:
Superficial parotid lymphatic nodes
Retroauricular lymphatic nodes
Occipital lymphatic nodes
Superior deep cervical lymphatic nodes
Jugulodigastric lymphatic node
Lymphatic nodes of accessory nerve
External jugular lymphatic node
External jugular vein
Transverse cervical lymphatic nodes
Subclavian vein
Inferior or deep cervical lymph nodes
Jugular lymphatic trunk
Infraorbital lymphatic node
Buccal lymphatic node
Mandibular lymphatic node
Submental lymphatic nodes
Submandibular lymphatic nodes
Infrahyoid lymphatic node
Anterior jugular vein
Jugulo-omohyoid lymphatic node
Paratracheal lymphatic node
Anterior jugular lymphatic node
Internal jugular vein
Brachiocephalic vein

Nodal Groups

For the purpose of standardizing clinical observations and surgical reports, the Union International Contre le Cancer (UICC), the American Joint Committee on Cancer (AJCC), and the American Academy of Otolaryngology–Head and Neck Surgery (AAO-HNS) adopted the classification of cervical lymph nodes into specific groups, based on anatomic location.[3, 4] This classification was suggested by Suen and Goepfert in 1987,[5] based on the classification used in the Memorial Sloan-Kettering Cancer Center.[6] This regional lymph node classification is intended to provide a uniform, standardized nomenclature that can facilitate the reporting and analysis of treatment results (Figs. 18–3 and 18–4). Each lymph node group, or level, has specific anatomic, clinical, and radiologic boundaries, which are described in the following paragraphs.

Level I. This level consists of the submental (IA) and the right and left submandibular (IB) groups. The boundaries of this level are as follows:

- *Anatomic*—Lymph nodes within the triangular boundaries of the anterior belly of the digastric muscles and the hyoid bone (Ia), the lymph node between the anterior and posterior bellies of the digastric muscle and the body of the mandible, and nodes along the facial vessels lateral to the mandible (Ib)

- *Clinical*—Same
- *Radiologic*—This includes all the nodes above the level of the hyoid bone, superficial to the mylohyoid muscles, and anterior to a transverse line drawn through the posterior edge of the submandibular gland

Level II. Level II includes the superior jugular nodes. This consists of two subdivisions—those nodes anterior to the spinal accessory nerve (IIa) and those posterior to the spinal accessory nerve (IIb). The boundaries of this level are as follows:

- *Anatomic*—Lymph nodes anterior to and behind the great vessels extending from the skull base to the carotid bifurcation and between the sternohyoid muscle anteriorly and the posterior border of the sternocleidomastoid muscle posteriorly

- *Clinical*—Lymph nodes along the superior aspect of the jugular vein, extending from the skull base to the hyoid bone and between the sternohyoid muscle anterior and the posterior border of the sternocleidomastoid muscle posteriorly

- *Radiologic*—Lymph nodes along the superior aspect of the jugular vein, extending from the skull base to the inferior aspect of the hyoid bone and between the back of the submandibular gland anteriorly and the posterior border of the sternocleidomastoid muscle posteriorly

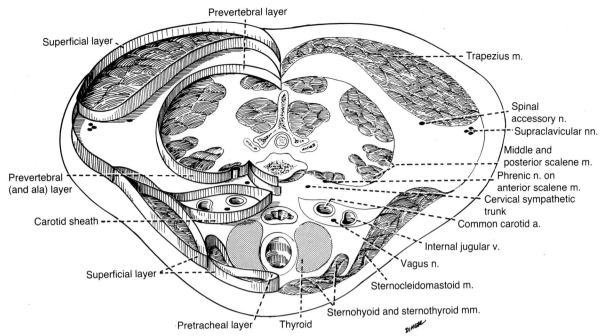

FIGURE 18–2   Compartments of the deep cervical fascia.

Level III. Level III includes the midjugular nodes. The boundaries of this level are as follows:
- *Anatomic*—Lymph nodes along the middle third of the jugular vein, extending from the carotid bifurcation to the omohyoid muscle and between the sternohyoid muscle anterior and the posterior border of the sternocleidomastoid muscle posteriorly

- *Clinical*—Lymph nodes along the middle third of the jugular vein and sternocleidomastoid muscle, between the sternohyoid muscle anterior and the posterior border of the sternocleidomastoid muscle posteriorly
- *Radiologic*—Lymph nodes along the middle third of the jugular vein, extending from the bottom of the hyoid bone to the bottom of the cricoid arch, and between the sternohyoid muscle anterior and the posterior border of the sternocleidomastoid muscle posteriorly

Level IV. Level IV includes the inferior jugular nodes. The boundaries of this level are as follows:
- *Anatomic*—Lymph nodes along the inferior aspect of the jugular vein, extending from the omohyoid muscle to the clavicle, and between the sternohyoid muscle anterior and the posterior border of the sternocleidomastoid muscle posteriorly
- *Clinical*—Lymph nodes along the inferior aspect of the jugular vein, extending from about the cricothyroid notch to the clavicle, and between the sternohyoid muscle anterior and the posterior border of the sternocleidomastoid muscle posteriorly
- *Radiologic*—Lymph nodes along the inferior aspect of the jugular vein, extending from the inferior aspect of the cricoid arch to the clavicle, and lying anterior to a line connecting the posterior border of the sternocleidomastoid muscle and the posterolateral border of the anterior scalene muscle

Level V. Level V includes the posterior triangle nodes. It consists of two subdivisions—those nodes superior to the level of the cricoid cartilage (Va) and those inferior to the level of the cricoid cartilage (Vb). The boundaries of this level are as follows:
- *Anatomic*—Lymph nodes bounded anteriorly by the sternocleidomastoid muscle, posteriorly by the trapezius muscle, and inferiorly by the clavicle

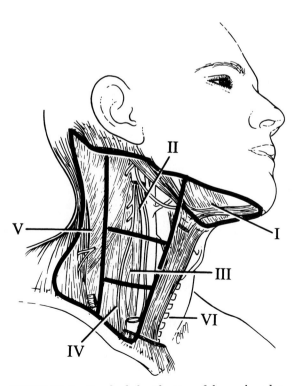

FIGURE 18–3   Standard classification of the neck nodes.

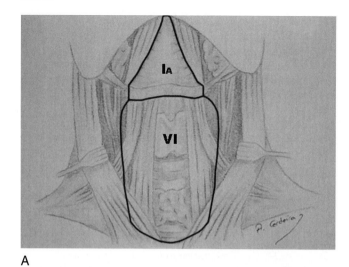

A

B

FIGURE 18–4 Subdivisions of levels I, II, and V. (From Robbins KT, Denys D: The American Head and Neck Society's revised classification for neck dissection. Proceedings of the 5th International Conference on Head and Neck Cancer, July 29–Aug. 2, 2000, San Francisco, pp 365–371.)

- *Clinical*—Same
- *Radiologic*—Lymph nodes bounded posteriorly by the trapezius muscle, inferiorly by the clavicle, and anteriorly by the posterior border of the sternocleidomastoid above the inferior border of the cricoid arch, and to a line connecting the posterior border of the sternocleidomastoid muscle and the posterolateral border of the anterior scalene muscle below the cricoid arch

TABLE 18-1 Relationship Between Location of Primary Tumor and Nodal Groups at High Risk for Metastasis

Levels	Location of Primary Tumor
Level I	
Submental nodes	Floor of the mouth, anterior oral tongue, anterior mandibular alveolar ridge, lower lip
Submandibular nodes	Oral cavity, anterior nasal cavity, soft tissues and structures of the midface, submandibular gland, maxillary sinus
Level II	Oral cavity, nasal cavity, nasopharynx, oropharynx, hypopharynx, larynx, parotid gland
Level III	Oral cavity, nasopharynx, oropharynx, hypopharynx, larynx
Level IV	Hypopharynx, larynx, cervical esophagus
Level V	Nasopharynx, oropharynx
Level VI	Thyroid gland, larynx (glottic and subglottic), apex of the pyriform sinus, cervical esophagus

Level VI. Level VI includes the central compartment nodes. The boundaries of this level are as follows:

- *Anatomic*—Lymph nodes bounded by the carotid arteries laterally, the hyoid superiorly, and the suprasternal notch inferiorly
- *Clinical*—Paratracheal lymph nodes, often difficult to palpate
- *Radiologic*—Lymph nodes bounded by the carotid arteries laterally, the hyoid superiorly, and the top of the manubrium inferiorly

Retropharyngeal Nodes (Nodes of Rouvière). These nodes are often forgotten because they are not apparent on clinical examination. The boundaries of this area are as follows:

- *Anatomic*—Lymph nodes posterior to the nasopharynx and oropharynx and medial to the carotid sheath
- *Clinical*—Rarely clinically apparent; when large, may cause retro-ocular pain and prevertebral muscle spasm
- *Radiologic*—Seldom clinically apparent; these nodes require special imaging studies

The rationale for grouping lymph nodes by levels is that under normal conditions, the lymph flow follows a predictable course. Based on this observation, the treatment of the neck in cancer of the head and neck can be tailored to the high-risk areas of metastasis.[1, 7] These high-risk areas of metastasis according to the primary location are shown in Table 18–1. However, it must be remembered that the predictability of normal lymph flow may be modified by factors related to the tumor itself, the anatomic characteristics of the patient, and the influence of external factors such as previous treatments. Thus, treatment of the neck should be carefully planned according to the surgical procedure and the personal experience of the surgeon.

■ EVALUATION OF THE MASS IN THE NECK

The diagnostic approach to a mass in the neck depends on a variety of factors, including the age of the patient, the time

TABLE 18-2 Differential Diagnosis of the Mass in the Neck

Inflammatory
    Lymphadenopathy
        Bacterial
        Viral
        Granulomatous
    Abscess
Congenital
    Thyroglossal duct cyst
    Branchial cleft cyst
    Dermoid cyst
    Laryngocele
    Thymic cyst
Neoplastic
    Benign
        Paraganglioma
        Schwannoma
        Hemangioma/lymphangioma
        Lipoma
    Malignant
        Primary tumor
            Lymphoma
            Salivary gland tumor
            Thyroid carcinoma
            Sarcoma
        Metastatic carcinoma
            From a head and neck primary (SCCHN, thyroid, salivary gland, cutaneous, unknown primary)
            From an infraclavicular primary (lung carcinoma, gastric carcinoma, renal cell carcinoma)

SCCHN, squamous cell carcinoma of the head and neck.

of evolution of the lesion, the topographic location of the mass, and the associated symptoms. The differential diagnosis includes a wide variety of entities, usually divided into inflammatory, congenital, and neoplastic conditions (Table 18–2). A majority of masses in the neck in patients younger than 40 years of age are benign; they are usually inflammatory in origin or derived from embryologic remnants. Malignant masses in children are usually determined to be a lymphoma or a sarcoma and are often located in the posterior triangle. In patients older than age 40, a majority of masses in the neck are malignant. By means of a thorough history and physical examination, and with the judicious use of laboratory studies and imaging, an accurate diagnosis can be made in the vast majority of cases.

The combination of history and physical examination may suggest the nature of the mass (i.e., inflammatory, congenital, or neoplastic) and may also suggest further studies that may be needed to confirm the diagnosis. Laboratory tests may on occasion be useful in the diagnosis of a mass in the neck, such as when a granulomatous lymphadenitis is suspected (e.g., typical or atypical tuberculosis, actinomycosis, sarcoidosis, or cat-scratch fever). However, complete evaluation of a mass in the neck requires some form of imaging and a histopathologic evaluation.

History

History of Present Illness

The time and course of illness, including specifics about the size and growth rate of the mass or masses, may give important information about the causes and/or aggressiveness of the tumor. A longstanding mass that has not significantly changed suggests, but does not guarantee, a benign process. An acute and painful enlargement usually is indicative of an inflammatory disorder. Associated symptoms such as malaise, weight loss, hemoptysis, dysphagia, odynophagia, hoarseness, otalgia, or an ulceration that does not heal should be regarded as suspicious for cancer of the upper aerodigestive tract metastatic to the lymph nodes in the neck. Information about personal habits, sexual exposures, recent dental work, exposure to radiation, previous surgery, or recent travel to a foreign country may serve as a valuable key to a correct diagnosis.

Certain symptoms are important when a mass in the neck is evaluated. Pain usually indicates pressure on or invasion of neighboring nerves. Otalgia, as the manifestation of referred pain, may be the first indication of primary cancer in the upper aerodigestive tract. Dysphagia may be associated with growth of a primary cancer that is deforming or invading the alimentary tract. Sore throat is often a presenting symptom in cancers of the oral cavity, oropharynx, hypopharynx, and larynx. Shortness of breath often indicates growth of cancer that is deforming or invading the airway. Dysphonia suggests involvement of structures in the oral cavity or larynx. Nonhealing sores are not an infrequent symptom in patients with skin or oral cavity carcinoma. Nasal symptoms such as unilateral nasal obstruction, discharge, or epistaxis suggest the presence of a mass. Hearing loss, especially unilateral hearing loss due to middle ear effusion, may suggest obstruction of the eustachian tube from a tumor in the nasopharynx. Weight loss, especially when otherwise unexplained, often accompanies malignancy. Hemoptysis or blood-tinged saliva may suggest a cancer of the oral cavity, pharynx, or larynx. Bone pain, jaundice, neurologic disorders, and hemoptysis are symptoms that may indicate systemic disease and the need for a metastatic evaluation.

Past Medical History

A complete review of all medical problems should be obtained in every case. Surgical history, especially any previous head or neck surgery, is very important. Also, history of previous cancers of the skin or lesions and any past history of radiation to the neck should be elicited.

Social History

The single most important risk factor for SCCHN is tobacco use.[8] It is important to document the date the smoking habit began and the number of packs smoked per day. Also, inquiry as to other forms of tobacco use—pipe or cigar smoking, chewing tobacco, or smokeless tobacco—must be made. Although it is difficult to prove, passive or "secondhand" smoke exposure may also be a risk factor for malignancy and should be asked about. Aside from tobacco use, alcohol history is also important. This is so, first, because alcohol represents a significant risk factor for SCCHN,[9] and second, because if dependence is severe, the risk of alcohol-related complications, such as delirium tremens, can be estimated and such complications possibly prevented following cancer surgery.

Family History

A family history of cancer may lead to important clues about genetic predisposition to cancer—such as in medullary cancer of the thyroid. In addition, it is important to inquire because other diseases diagnosed in family members (such as coronary artery disease, diabetes, and hypertension) may predispose to medical comorbidities.

Physical Examination

Physical examination of a patient with a mass in the neck should include a systematic and complete examination of the head and neck area. This includes inspection of the skin of the face and scalp as well as of all mucosal surfaces of the upper aerodigestive tract. Palpation of the neck, along with examination of the nose, nasopharynx, oral cavity, oropharynx, hypopharynx, and larynx, is a vital part of a thorough head and neck examination. Accurate description of the location, size, consistency, and mobility of the mass; color of or fixation of the overlying skin; evidence of pulsation; or presence of an audible bruit should be recorded. The use of mirror and fiberoptic examination of the head and neck can be invaluable. In patients with an "unknown" primary cancer, the precise site of the neck mass is important because it may be predictive of the site of the primary (see Table 18–1).

Imaging Studies

Imaging of masses in the neck plays a vital role in the diagnosis and treatment of these lesions. For suspected primary lesions of the neck, such as paragangliomas, the diagnosis is sometimes made by radiologic evaluation alone. In other cases, radiologic tests provide a useful tool for diagnosis, a helpful "road map" for future surgical intervention, or a necessary baseline examination for the evaluation of future treatment efficacy. In patients with cancer of the head and neck, imaging of the cervical lymphatics is almost always performed. Careful study has demonstrated that imaging of the cervical lymphatics alters the estimated clinical stage in 20% to 30% of patients.[10]

In the clinically N0 neck, imaging is used to evaluate subclinical disease and to verify the absence of contralateral disease. In the clinically N+ neck, imaging should be considered to assess resectability in advanced nodal disease, to assist in the detection of primary tumors not identified on physical examination, and to act as a baseline study for palpable tumors when nonsurgical therapy is contemplated. In addition, imaging should be used to assess carotid artery invasion and retropharyngeal and paratracheal node involvement.

There is some controversy in the literature concerning the optimal imaging modality for tumors of the head and neck. This choice should be based on various parameters, including the preference of the surgeon, clinical strengths of the available radiologists, technology available, and clinical variables related to the patient and the tumor itself. The most commonly used imaging modalities are ultrasound, computed tomography (CT), and magnetic resonance imaging (MRI). Newer modalities, including positron emission tomography (PET-CT scan) and lymphoscintigraphy, are emerging and currently have specific, though limited, roles in the evaluation of masses in the neck. Advantages and disadvantages of each are described below and are listed in Table 18–3.

Ultrasound is a fast, safe, and inexpensive study that helps in the differentiation of solid from cystic masses. It is especially useful in the diagnosis of thyroid nodules. In some centers, it is used with great accuracy in the screening and evaluation of cervical lymphatics[11]; however, it is highly operator-dependent, and radiologists inexperienced with the technique are often uncomfortable with its use, preferring CT or MRI instead. As described by several authors, ultrasound can be combined with fine-needle aspiration to increase the sensitivity and specificity of the test.[11, 12]

CT is probably the most commonly used imaging modality in the evaluation of the cervical lymphatics. It is often used in the evaluation of the neck in patients at risk for cervical node involvement but with no appreciable signs on physical examination. In this regard, CT has been shown to be a useful tool because it is more sensitive and specific than physical examination alone.[13] It also allows accurate assessment

TABLE 18-3 Imaging Modalities Used in the Evaluation of Masses in the Neck

Modality	Advantages	Disadvantages	Sensitivity	Specificity
Ultrasound	Noninvasive Inexpensive Often used for FNA	Operator-dependent Poor for deep nodes	50%–58%	75%–82%
CT	Noninvasive Relatively inexpensive Easy to perform Easy to interpret	Exposes patient to ionizing radiation Iodine in contrast media may conflict with thyroid workup	40%–68%	78%–92%
MRI	Noninvasive Multiplanar examination No radiation MRI angiography possible	Expensive Subject to motion artifact	55%–66%	82%–92%
PET	Noninvasive May have increased ability to detect recurrences	Expensive Poor resolution	67%–90%	94%–100%

FNA, fine-needle aspiration.

of involved structures in the patient with clinically evident lymphadenopathy and often plays an important role in treatment planning. Used with newer scanners, it is a fast procedure that is relatively easy to interpret and is therefore less likely than ultrasound to be subject to "operator dependence." Disadvantages include the fact that optimal examination requires the introduction of intravenous contrast (and its attendant risk of allergic response), as well as the fact that the patient must be exposed to low doses of ionizing radiation.

MRI remains less used than CT, mainly owing to its high cost and greater difficulty in interpretation. It has the advantage of being a multiplanar examination that does not require the patient to be exposed to ionizing radiation. The soft tissue detail afforded by MRI is significantly better than provided by CT or ultrasound. In addition, it is the best method for the evaluation of perineural invasion. However, it remains a relatively difficult examination for patients to tolerate owing to the claustrophobic confines of the machinery and the need for the patient to remain still for long periods. This can become significant because any motion artifact may render the examination uninterpretable.

The newest commonly used imaging modality is PET. PET differs from other imaging techniques in that it evaluates metabolic activity, rather than anatomic structures. PET relies on the fact that different tissues will take up metabolic tracers at different rates, depending on how metabolically active they are. PET, therefore, is a physiologic or functional study. Despite this advantage, however, several factors have limited its widespread use. First, the test is expensive, especially when compared with ultrasound or CT. Second, PET scanners are currently available only in large research centers. Lastly, it has a very low resolution when compared with CT or MRI and therefore is less useful in operative planning.[14] This limitation is starting to be overcome with the advent of combined-modality imaging, which combines the physiologic data of PET scanning with the anatomic detail of CT (see Chapter 5). Currently, PET appears most useful in the detection of occult primary tumors and in the evaluation of recurrent disease after treatment with radiation, chemotherapy, surgery, or combinations thereof.[15]

Other imaging studies are occasionally useful for the evaluation of the mass in the neck. Arteriography may be useful for diagnosing certain primary tumors in the neck such as the carotid body paraganglioma, in which the classic "lyre sign" (bowing of the internal and external carotid arteries around the tumor) is pathognomonic.[16] Arteriography may also be useful for assessing carotid artery involvement by tumor. Balloon occlusion arteriography and single photon emission computed tomography (SPECT) or xenon CT scanning may be helpful in assessment of the feasibility of carotid resection in selected cases for which this may be considered.[17] Lymphoscintigraphy is becoming more widespread in the evaluation of cutaneous malignancies, especially melanoma. It is most commonly used to identify sentinel nodes that may then be biopsied to assess the risk of regional spread of melanoma.[18] This technique has become the standard of care for truncal and extremity melanomas and is being evaluated in the treatment of the head and neck as well.[19]

Regardless of the type of imaging, several criteria have been developed to aid in determining if cervical nodes are pathologic. They include the following: (1) a node larger than 1.0 cm (or >1.5 cm in the jugulodigastric region), especially when round, (2) decreased central attenuation in a node, (3) a poorly defined mass in a lymph node–bearing region, and (4) the combination of ill-defined borders and loss of plane between mass and normal adjacent neck structures. If any of these criteria is present, the cervical nodes must be considered to harbor metastasis.[20]

Pathologic Assessment

The primary dilemma in evaluating patients with a mass in the neck is determining whether the lesion is benign or malignant. If analysis of the information obtained from the history, physical examination, laboratory tests, and imaging studies does not allow the physician to make a definitive diagnosis, fine-needle aspiration (FNA) is the next step in the diagnostic evaluation.[21, 22] Since it was first described in 1930 by Hayes Martin,[23] FNA has become the "gold standard" in establishing the diagnosis of the mass in the neck. For squamous cell carcinoma, FNA approaches a 99% sensitivity and specificity.[24] For a mass in the thyroid, its accuracy is in the range of 95%.[25] Controversy still exists concerning the diagnosis of salivary gland tumors.[26] The reported figures of the accuracy of FNA in this field have a direct relationship to the skills of the cytopathologist and the quality of the material obtained. For lesions that are difficult to access, ultrasound or CT guidance may be helpful.[27]

If no definitive diagnosis is obtained after repeated FNAs, the last step is an open biopsy. Open biopsy of a neck mass should be considered only as a last resort in any diagnostic protocol. Hayes Martin's 1944 admonition still rings true:

> Incisional biopsy for the removal of a portion or of the whole of a cervical tumor should never be made until other methods have been unsuccessful. One of the most reprehensible surgical practices is the immediate incision or excision of a cervical mass for diagnosis without any preliminary investigation for a possible primary growth. There can be no better example of ill-advised and needless surgery.[28]

Although some controversy exists concerning the real harm of open biopsy of neck masses, it is generally accepted that it should never be the first step in the diagnostic approach to a neck mass. Some authors have associated the practice of open cervical node biopsy with increased rates of local complications, local recurrences, and distant metastases.[29] However, others state that although it is important to refrain from proceeding with an open biopsy until after a complete head and neck evaluation has been done, violation of the neck does not imply a poorer prognosis as long as adequate treatment is subsequently given.[30, 31] From a practical standpoint, open biopsy may not usually provide any different information than a simple FNA, and it can sometimes compromise further treatment. The approach to the neck that has been previously violated may include more extensive surgery, such as the resection of structures that could otherwise have been preserved. This fact, in the era of nonradical, conservative neck dissections, may be a stronger argument against open cervical node biopsy than the traditional concept of increased distant metastasis.[32] Currently, open biopsy is used primarily in patients suspected of having lymphoma.

◼ PRIMARY TUMORS OF THE NECK

As was indicated in Table 18–2, the differential diagnosis of a mass in the neck includes primary as well as metastatic tumors. Primary tumors in the neck include lymphoma, salivary gland neoplasms, thyroid tumors, and soft tissue neoplasms.

Lymphoma

Lymphomas of the head and neck are the most common malignancies in the neck encountered in the pediatric population, representing about 10% of all childhood malignancies.[33] They are equally divided between Hodgkin's and non-Hodgkin's types. Hodgkin's lymphoma is more frequent in those between 5 and 30 years of age, with a higher incidence among males. Non-Hodgkin's lymphomas are more frequent during the older decades of life and have a similar incidence among males and females.[34]

About 75% of patients with Hodgkin's disease present with a mass in the neck, whereas only 30% to 40% of non-Hodgkin's patients present this way. Systemic symptoms are infrequent in cervical lymphoma. However, because non-Hodgkin's lymphoma may affect the head and neck region, especially the structures constituting Waldeyer's ring, a head and neck examination should be performed in all patients with lymphoma. The nodes in lymphoma are usually discrete, multiple, rubbery to the touch, and nontender. Although the treatment of lymphoma is nonsurgical, an open biopsy is required to confirm the diagnosis and to provide enough tissue for flow cytometric analysis so that the histologic type can be determined.

Neoplasms of the Salivary Glands

Neoplasms of the salivary glands account for 5% of all tumors of the head and neck.[35] The parotid gland is the most frequent location, followed by the submandibular gland and the minor salivary glands. Tumors of the parotid gland are usually located in the tail of the gland; approximately 80% are benign. This proportion changes when the primary tumor is located in the submandibular gland, where only 50% of the lesions are benign. A majority of masses in the minor salivary glands (~80%) are malignant. Although FNA provides accurate diagnosis of most tumors of the salivary glands, controversy exists regarding the use of FNA versus tumor removal via gland excision.[36, 37] Slow-growing tumors of the salivary glands may correspond to low-grade mucoepidermoid carcinoma, acinic cell carcinoma, or low-grade adenocarcinoma, giving the false impression of a benign lesion. Pain, facial palsy, a fixed firm mass, and cervical metastasis must be considered as characterizing a malignant tumor.

The most common benign parotid tumor is pleomorphic adenoma.[38] It is more common among women, with a peak incidence during the fifth decade of life. Pleomorphic adenoma usually presents as a painless, mobile, well-demarcated, slow-growing mass in the parotid gland. In rare instances, these tumors may undergo malignant degeneration.

Warthin's tumor is far more frequent among men, with a peak incidence during the fifth and sixth decades of life.[38] The lesions are often cystic, and FNA may reveal a characteristic thick, turbid fluid. The lesion can present as bilateral or multicentric lesions.

Mucoepidermoid carcinoma is the most common cancer of the parotid gland.[38] It is more frequent among females and can be associated with previous irradiation. The peak age of incidence ranges between the third and fifth decades of life. It usually presents as an asymptomatic mass, solid or cystic, with 30% to 40% of the patients having node metastasis at the time of diagnosis. Low-, intermediate-, and high-grade variants are described, with the latter group being much more aggressive and having a high incidence of metastasis.[39] High-grade mucoepidermoid cancer has the highest rate of metastasis to the neck of all cancers of the parotid gland.

Adenoid cystic carcinoma is also a prevalent salivary gland cancer; it is the most common malignancy of the submandibular gland and minor salivary glands.[38] Its propensity for perineural spread is well known and probably accounts for the difficulty often associated with gaining local control of the tumor. Regional metastases are rare; in fact, it is more common for a patient to die from distant metastases than from regional metastases.[40]

Tumors of the Thyroid

Thyroid nodules, benign or malignant, may present as a mass in the neck. The diagnostic approach should be directed toward confirming the presence of a malignant tumor. A malignant tumor should be suspected especially in young patients with history of previous irradiation who present with a rapidly growing mass with palpable cervical nodes. A firm fixed node along with dysphonia is also highly suggestive of malignancy.

A careful history and physical examination, along with FNA, remains the most appropriate therapeutic approach. In cases of benign lesions, surgery may be indicated for cosmetic reasons or pathologic confirmation, or to relieve symptoms related with compression of the trachea or esophagus by the mass. If a malignant tumor is suspected, the approach will vary according to the histology of the lesion (differentiated vs. undifferentiated), the extension of the disease, and the policy of the institution.

Soft Tissue Neoplasms

Soft tissue tumors are rare in the neck. They may be benign (lipoma, fibroma, neurilemmoma) or malignant (fibrosarcoma, liposarcoma, rhabdomyosarcoma). The diagnosis is based on histologic studies. Neurilemmomas or schwannomas are encapsulated, firm, slow-growing solitary tumors that arise from the Schwann cells covering the axons. They can present as a neck mass, usually in the parapharyngeal space. They have a slight preference for women, with a peak age between 30 and 50 years. The vagus nerve, sympathetic trunk, and sensory cervical roots are the nerves most frequently involved in the neck. Imaging studies, especially MRI, may be helpful in the diagnosis. The treatment of choice for tumors of neural origin is surgical removal, with a low incidence of recurrence.

Carotid body tumors are nonchromaffin paragangliomas arising in the chemoreceptors of the carotid body.[41] Their peak prevalence is between the fourth and fifth decades of life. The typical carotid body tumor presents as a firm, rubbery, pulsatile, painless, slow-growing mass located in the upper anterior triangle of the neck. On palpation, it can be displaced laterally but not superiorly or inferiorly. The diagnosis should be suspected by the clinical symptoms and can be confirmed with imaging studies. MRI, with and without contrast, can identify carotid body tumors as small as 8 mm. Angiography should be carried out in all patients to assess the blood supply of the tumor and to determine whether encroachment of the artery, which is associated with infiltration of the wall of the carotid artery, is noted. The pathognomonic sign of a carotid body tumor on angiography is a mass displacing the internal carotid artery laterally, and widening of the carotid bifurcation. Multicentric lesions are present in 10% of cases. The ideal treatment for carotid body tumors is surgical removal. The assessment of serum catecholamines and urinary vanillylmandelic acid should be included in the preoperative study to rule out associated pheochromocytoma as well as the possibility of hormonal activity (less than 10% of cases).

Malignant soft tissue tumors, usually sarcomas, present difficult treatment dilemmas. These tumors usually present as painless, rapidly enlarging, submucosal or subcutaneous masses. Most commonly the masses are asymptomatic, but reported symptoms vary widely depending on tumor size and location. Routine evaluation usually includes history and physical examination, regional imaging, and a metastatic screen. Representative tissue for biopsy is vital because the diagnosis can be difficult for the pathologist. Sarcomas of the head and neck are best treated with multimodality therapy.[42] If resection is possible, surgery with or without postoperative radiotherapy is the best approach. Standardized neck dissections must often be modified to encompass the tumor with a wide excision because sarcomas often spread across normal tissue barriers. Also, the head and neck surgeon should be aware that negative margins commonly are not possible; therefore, combinations of surgery, radiation, and chemotherapy are usually employed.

■ METASTASIS FROM SQUAMOUS CELL CARCINOMA

A vast majority of malignant masses in the neck in adults represent metastasis from a carcinoma of the head and neck, usually squamous cell carcinoma. The complex underlying mechanisms of tumor cell invasion and metastasis are just now beginning to be understood. The specifics of mechanisms of metastasis are addressed in Chapter 2. However, regardless of the mechanism, the presence of cancer in cervical lymph nodes is known to be the most important prognostic factor in patients with SCCHN.

Predictive Factors of Neck Metastasis

Because regional lymph node metastasis is so important in SCCHN, the ability to accurately predict regional spread is critically important to the subsequent management of the patient. For most of the past century, investigators have attempted to delineate factors that predict regional metastasis. To date, no single factor has been unequivocally related to a patient's risk for regional spread; however, several factors appear to have some association with increased risk: site, tumor stage, tumor thickness, tumor differentiation, perineural invasion, and perivascular invasion.

Primary sites in the nasopharynx, oropharynx, and hypopharynx are more likely than other subsites to be associated with regional spread of disease—either clinically apparent disease or occult disease.[1] More advanced tumor stage is associated with a higher percentage of cervical metastasis.[43] Tumor thickness has been studied, and thicker tumors, especially in the oral cavity and skin, are usually associated with a higher rate of regional metastasis.[44] Although this concept is not completely accepted, tumor differentiation may be a factor in metastasis—that is, some high-grade or poorly differentiated cancers have higher rates of cervical metastasis.[45] Perineural invasion is associated with increased risk for cervical metastasis, as well as for local recurrence.[46, 47] Likewise, perivascular invasion is highly associated with increased rates of cervical metastasis.[48, 49] Recently, workers in genetic analysis have attempted to identify patients at high risk for cervical metastasis; this is discussed further in Chapter 2.

Staging

Pretreatment staging constitutes the basis for an adequate selection of therapy in patients with SCCHN. The clinical evaluation should include staging of the primary cancer and a careful search for regional lymph node involvement and distant metastasis. Because of its importance in treatment planning, clinical staging should be as accurate as possible. The currently used staging systems—the AJCC system and the UICC system—are based on the TNM staging system. That is, assessment of the primary tumor (T), the regional lymphatics (N), and distant spread (M) is required for accurate overall staging. These staging systems aid in treatment selection, provide prognostic information, help in the evaluation of treatment response, and make it possible for results to be compared between different institutions. The UICC and the AJCC have recently unified their classification systems to achieve a consensus.[50, 51] This is shown in Tables 18–4 and 18–5.

TABLE 18–4 UICC and AJCC Definitions of the Nodal Categories for all Head and Neck Sites (Except Thyroid)

Regional Lymph Nodes (N)

NX   Regional lymph nodes cannot be assessed
N0   No regional lymph node metastasis
°N1   Metastasis in a single ipsilateral lymph node, 3 cm or less in greatest dimension
°N2   Metastasis in a single ipsilateral lymph node, more than 3 cm but not more than 6 cm in greatest dimension; or in multiple ipsilateral lymph nodes, none more than 6 cm in greatest dimensions; or in bilateral or contralateral lymph nodes, none more than 6 cm in greatest dimension
°N2a   Metastasis in single ipsilateral lymph node more than 3 cm but not more than 6 cm in greatest dimension
°N2b   Metastasis in multiple ipsilateral lymph nodes, none more than 6 cm in greatest dimension
°N2c   Metastasis in bilateral or contralateral lymph nodes, none more than 6 cm in greatest dimension
°N3   Metastasis in a lymph node more than 6 cm in greatest dimension

°*Note:* A designation of "U" or "L" may be used to indicate metastasis above the lower border of the cricoid (U) or below the lower border of the cricoid (L).

TABLE 18-5 UICC and AUCC Definitions of the Nodal Categories for Thyroid Carcinomas

Regional Lymph Nodes (N)
Regional lymph nodes are the central compartment, lateral cervical, and upper mediastinal lymph nodes.
NX   Regional lymph nodes cannot be assessed.
N0   No regional lymph node metastatis
N1   Regional lymph node metastatis
N1a Metastasis to Level VI (pretracheal, paratracheal, and prelaryngeal/
        Delphian lymph nodes)
N1b Metastasis to unilateral, bilateral, or contralateral cervical or
        superior mediastinal lymph nodes

Used with the permission of the American Joint Committee on Cancer (AJCC), Chicago, Illinois. The original source for this material is the *AJCC Cancer Staging Manual, Sixth Edition* (2002) published by Springer-Verlag New York, www.springer-ny.com.

Management of the Clinically Negative (N0) Neck

If clinical examination, imaging, and pathologic assessment fail to detect any evidence of regional disease, the head and neck surgeon is faced with one of the most controversial issues in the field—management of the clinically N0 neck. Several important concepts must be understood when one is considering treatment for the N0 neck. First and foremost, in terms of overall survival, there are few significant clinical data that support elective treatment of the neck. Most trials have demonstrated that observation of the N0 neck with subsequent treatment for those that become N+ confers an overall survival on patients equal to that with elective treatment. Despite this, most oncologic surgeons feel that elective treatment decreases locoregional recurrence rates, allows for easier treatment of the neck, may decrease the risk for distant metastasis, and may add a survival benefit.[52, 53] Surgical treatment of the neck has the additional benefit of allowing pathologic staging of the regional nodes, which may change treatment planning. Therefore, in most institutions, elective treatment of the neck is recommended when the risk of occult metastasis is 15% to 20% or higher.

Treatment Options for the N0 Neck

If the decision is made to treat the N0 neck, two therapeutic options are possible: elective neck dissection and elective neck irradiation. These options are theoretically equally effective in controlling subclinical disease, with control rates on the order of 90%. Therefore, generally the treatment selected for the primary tumor should be used to treat the neck. A third option, sentinel lymph node biopsy (SLNB), has more recently become a choice for staging (not treating) the N0 neck in patients with melanoma. Some centers have broadened the indications to include SCCHN; however, detailed evidence of its efficacy is currently lacking for SCCHN.

ELECTIVE NECK DISSECTION

Elective neck dissection is usually chosen when the primary tumor is treated with surgery. There is no therapeutic advantage to treatment of the neck with surgery over radiotherapy; however, neck dissection gives important prognostic information that could be used for treatment

planning, such as the need for adjuvant treatment. Also, elective surgery does not "burn the bridges" for future treatments because surgery can be repeated if recurrence or second primaries develop in the area.

It is important that all surgeons treating cancer of the head and neck have a basic understanding of neck dissections, their classifications, and the underlying rationale behind each of them. Because there was significant confusion surrounding the terminology used in describing neck dissections, the American Academy of Otolaryngology–Head and Neck Surgery provided a classification schema for defining the types, scope, indications, and rationale of the various neck dissections.[54] These definitions distinguish *comprehensive* neck dissections (wherein nodal groups I to V and sometimes VI are removed) from *selective* neck dissections (in which only some nodal groups are removed and others are spared).

Comprehensive Neck Dissection. The comprehensive neck dissection entails the removal of all nodal groups on one side of the neck and is subdivided into radical neck dissection, extended radical neck dissection, bilateral radical neck dissection, and modified radical neck dissection.

Radical neck dissection (Fig. 18–5) refers to the removal of all lymph node groups extending from the inferior border of the mandible superiorly to the clavicle inferiorly, and from the lateral border of the sternohyoid muscle, hyoid bone, and contralateral anterior belly of the digastric muscle medially, to the anterior border of the trapezius muscle laterally. Included are all lymph nodes from levels I to V with sacrifice of the internal jugular vein, sternocleidomastoid muscle, and spinal accessory nerve.

Occasionally, the procedure must be extended to include the removal of one or more additional lymph node groups, nonlymphatic structures, or both, that are not usually encompassed by radical neck dissection. This then is called an extended radical neck dissection.

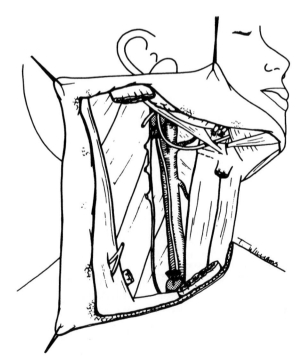

FIGURE 18–5   Schematic representation of radical neck dissection.

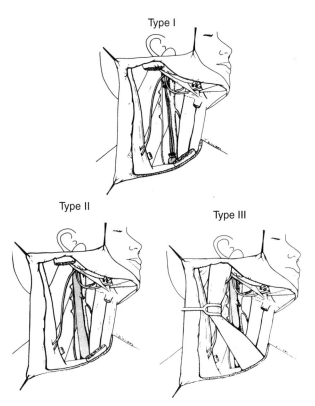

Type I

Type II

Type III

FIGURE 18–6 Schematic representation of modified radical neck dissections. Type I preserves only spinal accessory nerve. Type II preserves cranial nerve XI and the internal jugular vein. Type III preserves cranial nerve XI, internal jugular vein, and the sternocleidomastoid muscle.

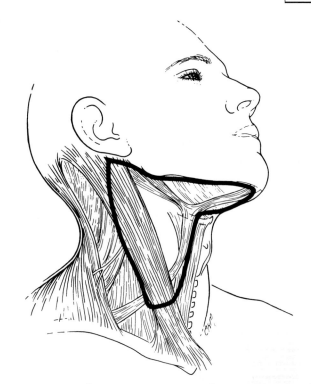

FIGURE 18–7 Schematic representation of supraomohyoid neck dissection.

Bilateral radical neck dissection may be necessary when bilateral N+ necks are encountered.

Modified radical neck dissection (Fig. 18–6) refers to an operation wherein all the lymph node groups that would be removed by the radical neck dissection are removed; however, one or more of the nonlymphatic structures (i.e., the spinal accessory nerve, the internal jugular vein, and the sternocleidomastoid muscle) are preserved.

Selective Neck Dissection. Selective neck dissection refers to any type of cervical lymphadenectomy in which one or more of the lymph node groups removed by the radical neck dissection are preserved. Various types of selective dissections have been described.

Supraomohyoid neck dissection (Fig. 18–7) refers to the removal of lymph nodes contained in levels I to III. The posterior limit of the dissection is marked by the cutaneous branches of the cervical plexus and by the posterior border of the sternocleidomastoid muscle. The inferior limit is the superior belly of the omohyoid muscle at which it crosses the internal jugular vein.

Occasionally, this dissection is extended to include level IV, in which case it is called an extended supraomohyoid neck dissection.

Posterolateral neck dissection (Fig. 18–8) refers to removal of the suboccipital lymph nodes, retroauricular lymph nodes, and lymph nodes in levels II to V—basically, all nodal groups except levels Ia and Ib.

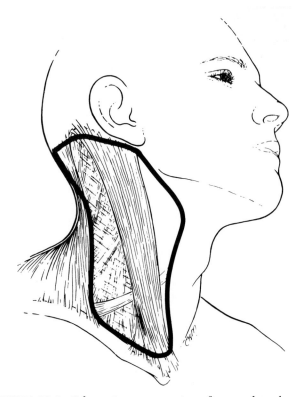

FIGURE 18–8 Schematic representation of posterolateral neck dissection.

Lateral neck dissection (Fig. 18–9) refers to the removal of lymph nodes in levels II to IV, along the internal jugular vein. It excludes nodes in levels Ia, Ib, and V.

Central compartment neck dissection (Fig. 18–10) refers to the removal of lymph nodes surrounding the midline visceral structures of the anterior neck—level VI. These lymph nodes include the pretracheal and paratracheal, precricoid (Delphian), and perithyroidal nodes. The superior limit of the dissection is the hyoid bone, the inferior limit is the suprasternal notch, and the lateral limits are the carotid arteries.

The phrase *functional neck dissection* (FND) is often used in the literature, especially in Europe. Practicing head and neck surgeons should be aware of the differences between the FND as described by its proponents, and the standard terminology used commonly in the United States. First introduced by Suárez in the 1960s[55] and popularized by Bocca[56] and Gavilán,[57] FND does not fit exactly within the AAO-HNS guidelines. A common misunderstanding among American head and neck surgeons is that FND is the same as a modified radical neck dissection. This is not precisely true because Suárez did not routinely remove levels I to V as part of his FND, instead tailoring the extent of the surgery to the patient's presentation and anatomy.[55] Gavilán and associates[58] suggested that the FND is not a modification of the radical neck dissection but rather is a different surgical procedure conceptually based on the fascial compartments of the neck.

ELECTIVE NECK IRRADIATION

As has been stated earlier, elective neck irradiation is generally performed when the primary tumor is treated by radiotherapy. As with neck dissections, radiation portals are determined by the site of the primary tumor and the predicted drainage patterns. For N0 necks, the recommended dose is 50 to 54 Gy in 25 to 30 fractions. This treatment was first proposed by Jesse and Fletcher,[59, 60] who showed that elective irradiation, consisting of 5000 cGy, would prevent metastasis from occurring in the N0 neck. Mantravadi and colleagues, in 1982, concluded that a radiation dose of 5000 cGy or more can eradicate 99% of subclinical carcinoma in lymph nodes.[61] This was based on comparison of the observed rate of conversion from N0 to N+ after elective irradiation of the neck, with a 20% to 40% incidence of occult disease in the neck. Arguments have been raised against the scientific data on which these affirmations are based because they are considered to be inferential data[62]; however, elective neck irradiation remains a well-accepted method of treating the N0 neck.

Some disadvantages are associated with elective neck irradiation. Because no specimen is available for histologic examination, no information regarding the pathologic stage of the neck is available either. Thus, an important prognostic factor is lost. If there is recurrence in the neck, salvage surgery is usually more difficult in an irradiated neck than in a previously untreated neck.[63] In addition, should a second primary tumor occur, irradiation would no longer be a therapeutic option. Likewise, if positive margins are found after salvage surgery is attempted, postoperative irradiation is usually not possible. Lastly, one should not underestimate the adverse effects of radiotherapy to the neck, which can include mucositis, xerostomia, chondronecrosis, and hypothyroidism.[64]

SENTINEL LYMPH NODE BIOPSY

The theoretical basis for SLNB, a newer option for staging of the neck, is that the first stop along the route of

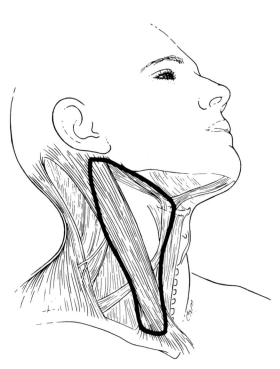

FIGURE 18–9 Schematic representation of lateral neck dissection.

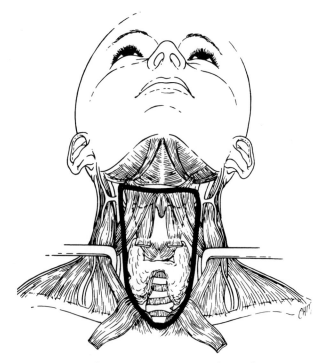

FIGURE 18–10 Schematic representation of central compartment neck dissection.

lymphatic drainage from a primary tumor is a limited set of regional lymph nodes. With the use of dyes, radiographic contrast agents, or radioactive tracers, these "sentinel" lymph nodes can be identified and removed. It is thought that close examination of these nodes can yield a better decision as to whether more extensive lymphadenectomy should be performed and/or systemic adjuvant therapy offered.

The main role of SLNB is in the treatment of melanoma. In fact, with regard to melanoma of the trunk and extremities, the status of the sentinel nodes is considered the strongest predictor of disease-free survival.[65] Despite its clear role in the management of melanoma of the trunk and extremities, the role of SLNB has not yet been fully defined in head and neck melanoma. The complexity of lymphatic drainage patterns and the frequent need to remove sentinel lymph nodes from the parotid gland, thus placing the facial nerve at risk, have made head and neck surgical oncologists slow to adopt this method. Currently, the data from studies of head and neck sites seem to indicate that sentinel nodes can be identified in about 95% of patients, and that the rates of false-negative results are low.[66, 67] Based on these data as well as its successful use in the trunk and extremities, SLNB is becoming more popular in the treatment of melanoma of the head and neck.

Several groups have attempted to extend the indications for SLNB to SCCHN, specifically the evaluation of early tumors of the oral cavity and oropharynx.[68, 69] Thus far these studies are promising, again indicating high success rates in identifying and biopsying the SLN and low false-negative rates.[70] However, the procedure needs much more study in SCCHN before it can be advocated for widespread use.

Treatment by Site of Primary

ORAL CAVITY

The rate of occult metastasis from cancer of the oral cavity ranges from 20% to 45%. Several studies have attempted to define predictive factors for metastasis from oral cavity sites. It appears that depth of invasion is a major criterion, with a depth of invasion greater than 2.0 mm being more likely to harbor occult metastases.[44, 71] Byers and coworkers showed that even patients with the most favorable status—depth of invasion less than 4 mm, clinically N0, and with a well-differentiated primary—still have a 14% chance of occult metastasis.[72] In most institutions, oral cavity cancers are treated surgically; therefore, the neck is treated surgically as well. In general, unless a patient has a small tumor with less than 2 mm of invasion, a supraomohyoid neck dissection (levels I to III) is performed. One caveat is that with a primary cancer of the tongue, it is necessary that level IV be included in the dissection because skip metastasis to this level may occur.[73] Rarely, if treatment of the cancer requires surgery that alters function, or if the patient is not a good surgical candidate, primary radiotherapy, with or without chemotherapy, is used. In these patients, elective neck irradiation is recommended.

OROPHARYNX

Oropharyngeal carcinomas have a rate of occult metastasis estimated to be between 30% and 35%.[1] In addition, the rate of bilateral metastasis is high (~20% in most series).

Therefore, in cancer of the oropharynx, elective treatment of the neck is warranted. The primary treatment for oropharyngeal cancer varies across different centers, with equal control and survival rates reported with the use of either surgery or irradiation. As is usually the case, the appropriate treatment of the neck is determined by the treatment of the primary. When surgery is the primary modality and the neck remains N0, supraomohyoid neck dissection (levels I to III) is recommended.[74] Bilateral dissections are usually performed, except for the most lateral primary lesions. Advanced cancer of the oropharynx may also be treated with a chemoradiation protocol. In this case, the radiotherapy component includes elective neck irradiation. In addition, some oropharyngeal sites, the soft palate in particular, are associated with a high rate of retropharyngeal adenopathy; these lymph nodes, in addition to the jugular chain and posterior triangle lymph nodes, need to be evaluated and treated.

HYPOPHARYNX

The hypopharynx has one of the highest rates of occult metastasis, ranging from 30% to 60%.[1] As with cancer of the oropharynx, the rate of bilateral metastasis is also high (up to 59%). In addition, retropharyngeal nodes are often involved (in up to 44% of patients). Owing to the high rate of regional metastasis, the neck should always be treated in patients with squamous cell carcinoma of the hypopharynx. In most centers, T1 and T2 hypopharyngeal cancers are treated with primary radiotherapy, which systematically includes elective irradiation of the neck. However, surgical treatment may also be considered, especially in advanced lesions, for which a lateral neck dissection (levels II to IV) is recommended.[75] Bilateral dissections are usually performed, except with the most lateral primary lesions. Advanced cancer of the hypopharynx may also be treated with a chemoradiation protocol. In this case, the radiotherapy component includes elective irradiation of the neck.

SUPRAGLOTTIC LARYNX

As with cancers of the oropharynx and hypopharynx, the rate of occult metastasis is high (estimated at 20% to 40%).[1] The rate of bilateral metastasis is also high. In addition, one third of patients with clinical nodal disease on one side have subclinical involvement on the contralateral side.[76] Therefore, elective treatment is routinely advised and should include both sides of the neck. As with other sites, supraglottic cancers are treated equally effectively by surgery or radiotherapy. When surgery is chosen, bilateral lateral neck dissections (levels II to IV) are recommended.[77, 78] This has been shown to decrease the regional failure rate from 20% to 9% with no increase in morbidity, as compared with patients whose necks were not dissected at the time of surgery.[79] When radiation is chosen, bilateral neck portals should be included.

GLOTTIC LARYNX

Unlike the supraglottic larynx, the glottic larynx has a comparatively low rate of occult metastasis (approximately 2% to 7%) for T1 and T2. These early cancers can be effectively treated with surgery or radiotherapy without the need for elective treatment of the neck. The rate of occult metastasis is higher in *recurrent* T1 and T2 tumors after radiotherapy (approximately 20%); thus, elective dissection of levels II to IV should be included in salvage therapy.[80] Most T3 and T4 cancers are treated surgically. Because the rate of occult metastasis is higher for these cancers (10% to 40%), elective lateral neck dissection (levels II to IV) is usually recommended.[81] Advanced cancer of the larynx may also be treated with a chemoradiation protocol, which includes elective irradiation of the neck in patients with a clinically negative neck.

SUBGLOTTIC LARYNX

This is a rare location for a primary cancer with few convincing data regarding treatment of the neck. The predominant routes of spread are to the paratracheal nodes and the recurrent laryngeal nerve nodes. It is generally accepted that a central compartment dissection, including an ipsilateral thyroidectomy, should be done at the time of treatment, followed by postoperative radiotherapy if any nodes are involved.[82, 83]

Management of the Clinically Positive (N+) Neck

Involvement of cervical nodes in patients with cancer of the head and neck is an ominous sign. Multiple studies have shown that survival is decreased by approximately 50% when cervical nodes are involved.[84, 85] Furthermore, when the involved node demonstrates extracapsular spread—as is the case in up to 23% of the smallest N1 nodes—overall survival is decreased by 50%.[86, 87] This is most likely a factor of the inherent ability of the cancer to spread to regional and eventually distant sites, thus making cure more difficult.

Based on this information, aggressive treatment is recommended in patients with involved cervical nodes. Several treatment options are available, including surgery, radiation, chemotherapy, and combined treatment. In general, the treatment modality selected for the primary cancer determines the treatment approach for neck metastasis. The generally accepted treatment approach for metastatic lymphadenopathy is surgery, usually with postoperative radiotherapy. However, it is important to realize that cancers in certain anatomic sites, such as the nasopharynx and oropharynx, respond well to irradiation; thus, cervical metastasis from these cancers may be treated by radiotherapy. Also, concomitant chemoradiotherapy under investigational protocols is an option for advanced cervical metastasis.

Surgery for Nodal Disease

The most common treatment for the N+ neck is surgery, usually with adjuvant radiotherapy. The type and extent of neck dissection performed are based on several factors, including site of primary cancer, treatment selected for the primary cancer, extent of cervical lymph node metastasis and structures invaded, history of prior treatment, and availability of adjuvant radiotherapy.

In general, treatment of the N1 neck rarely requires a radical neck dissection. A functional approach is often performed[88]; however, a selective neck dissection may also be effective treatment for patients with a single mobile node

located in the first echelon of lymphatic drainage.[89, 90] Usually, adjuvant radiation therapy is recommended if multiple nodes or levels are involved or if extracapsular spread is present.[91]

Patients with N2 disease have a varied treatment pattern. If the size, mobility, and anatomic site are suitable, a selective neck dissection with postoperative radiotherapy has been shown to be as efficacious as a modified radical neck dissection with postoperative radiotherapy.[92, 93] Often, however, the location of the cancer requires either a complete functional or a radical neck dissection with postoperative radiotherapy.

In the treatment of the N3 neck, modified radical neck dissection may be attempted, but radical neck dissection is often required, with the understanding that any cervical structures involved need to be resected as well. Patients with "fixed node(s)" are not candidates for neck dissection.

It should be mentioned that the number of metastatic nodes is not necessarily a contraindication for a functional approach, as long as all nodes are mobile and small. Similarly, those who advocate functional neck dissection indicate that because all the lymphatic tissue contained within the fascial system of the neck is removed with functional neck dissection, the indication for a functional approach to the neck is based on nodal size and mobility, not on the number of nodes.[94, 95] Modified radical neck dissection, or lesser dissections, may be considered for the least involved side of the neck in N2c disease. A vast majority of head and neck oncologists recommend adjuvant radiotherapy for patients with advanced nodal stages.[91]

Special Issues in Treatment of the N+ Neck

EXTRACAPSULAR SPREAD

It is generally accepted that the histologic identification of extracapsular spread (ECS) implies a higher risk for regional recurrence and distant metastasis.[86, 96] The definition of ECS requires the presence of invasive carcinoma on both sides of the capsule. ECS has been related to the size of the node, with an increasing incidence of ECS noted in larger nodes.[94, 97] The group from Amsterdam reported that 33% of nodes smaller than 2 cm had histologic ECS and that this was the most important single prognostic factor.[98] Histopathologic evidence in patients with ECS was associated with a statistically significant reduction in survival compared with patients without ECS. The disease-free interval between treatment and the development of recurrent disease was shorter for patients with ECS than for patients without ECS.

However, not all series arrive at the same conclusion. Mamelle and associates[99] and Pinsolle and colleagues[100] state that ECS per se was not a significant prognostic factor for recurrence in the neck, although most patients in this series underwent postoperative radiotherapy. Few data are available for determination of whether the degree of ECS, microscopic or macroscopic, is important; however, it appears that microscopic ECS has a 10 times lower risk of regional recurrence than does macroscopic ECS.[101] When the tumor was confined to the lymph node or when only a microscopic ECS was present, no significant difference was found in regional recurrence or in death rates.[102] Thus, when predicting the outcome for patients with nodal metastasis, it is important for clinicians to accurately establish the presence of ECS using objective data that indicate the degree of extension and the number of nodes affected.

MULTIPLE NODES

According to the TNM staging system, the presence of multiple metastatic nodes is considered a bad prognostic indicator. However, the real significance of multiple metastatic nodes has not been clearly established in the literature. Whereas in some series, the chances of survival are inversely related to the number of involved nodes,[103, 104] not all reported experiences have arrived at the same conclusion.[105]

LEVEL OF METASTASIS

The involvement of retropharyngeal nodes, inferior jugular nodes, or nodes in the posterior triangle indicates an important tumor burden that reduces the chances that the patient will survive the disease.[106, 107] Involvement of nodes at these levels is associated with a higher risk of metastasis at multiple levels.[108] Special interest should be given to the retropharyngeal region because the presence of metastasis at this level is related to a high risk of recurrence, even after radical operation followed by radiation therapy. Patients with retropharyngeal involvement may also have distant metastases simultaneously.[109]

RESECTABLE VERSUS UNRESECTABLE DISEASE

Resectability remains one of the most crucial surgical decisions that the head and neck surgeon must make. It should be emphasized that what is unresectable to one surgeon may be resectable to another; the surgeon must evaluate each case individually and use his or her best judgment in determining resectability. Major factors affecting the ability of the surgeon to resect cervical nodes include the level of invasion of (1) the skin, (2) the deep cervical fascia or vertebral body, (3) the carotid artery, (4) the brachial plexus, and (5) the base of the skull. Any of these features may render a node unresectable; however, it is also important to note that *unresectable* does not mean *untreatable.* Thus, other therapeutic modalities should be considered in those patients with borderline resectability.[110] In addition, *inoperable* does not necessarily mean *unresectable*—that is, patients may have comorbid factors that make them poor surgical candidates despite having resectable disease. Unfortunately for these patients, the same factors that make them poor surgical candidates often also make them poor candidates for nonsurgical treatments. Finally, *operable* does not necessarily mean *curable.* The head and neck surgeon must be aware of this and, after balancing the risks and benefits, must be prepared to offer these patients less aggressive, less morbid therapeutic options that are focused on palliation.

BILATERAL DISEASE

Bilateral nodal disease can also portend a poor prognosis.[111] However, it is nodal fixation, not simple bilaterality, that appears to be responsible for this poor prognosis[112]—that is, bilateral mobile nodes do not appear to have as significant an effect on survival as do unilateral or bilateral fixed nodes. Regardless of this, the standard treatment for bilateral nodal disease is bilateral neck dissection. However, the use of bilateral radical neck dissection, with simultaneous ligation of the internal jugular veins, can be associated with significant morbidity, including edema, increased intracranial pressure, syndrome of inappropriate antidiuretic hormone (SIADH) secretion, and stroke.[113] Therefore, many options for the treatment of bilateral disease have been developed. Simultaneous bilateral neck dissection, when performed, usually focuses on retaining at least one internal jugular vein. If this is not possible, staged bilateral neck dissections should be considered. Another option that is less commonly performed is reconstruction of the internal jugular vein.[114] If none of these is possible, it may be wise for the patient to forego surgical treatment in favor of radiation treatment and/or chemotherapy.

INVASION OF THE CAROTID ARTERY

Invasion of the carotid artery is associated with a very poor prognosis.[115] Much has been written to describe the options available for treatment of patients with involvement of the carotid artery; however, the head and neck surgeon must be prudent in weighing the risks and benefits of surgical treatment for patients with involvement of the carotid artery. Options for the treatment of carotid artery invasion include (1) no treatment, (2) tumor debulking (peeling the cancer off the carotid artery) with adjuvant therapy, (3) radiation therapy/chemoradiation, and (4) resection of the carotid artery with or without reconstruction. Although many surgeons consider invasion of the carotid artery to be a contraindication to curative surgical treatment of the neck, a meta-analysis of patients undergoing aggressive treatment of carotid artery invasion, including resection of the carotid artery, showed a 22% 2-year disease-free survival rate.[116] This indicates that with proper patient selection, experienced surgeons may consider aggressive treatment of patients in this poor prognostic group.

Radiotherapy for Nodal Disease

In the treatment of nodal disease, radiotherapy can be used alone, in combination with chemotherapy, or as an adjunct to surgery (preoperatively or postoperatively). It is rare that patients with cervical node involvement can be treated with primary radiotherapy; however, certain subsites such as the nasopharynx and oropharynx respond quite well to radiotherapy, and it may be considered as single-modality treatment for these patients. Nevertheless, a vast majority of patients with cervical node involvement require combined treatment, usually in the form of surgery and radiotherapy. By itself, functional and selective neck dissection is effective treatment for N0 and N1 disease if the node is less than 3 cm, does not adhere to any structures, and demonstrates no ECS.[90] Likewise, radical and modified radical neck dissections are effective forms of treatment for N1 disease without ECS; some would suggest that they are effective alone for N2 disease as well.[117] However, in patients with multiple nodes (more than two), nodes larger than 3 cm, and nodes with ECs, postoperative radiotherapy is usually recommended.[91] In general, higher doses are needed for eradication of gross nodal disease as opposed to subclinical deposits.

PRIMARY RADIOTHERAPY

If radiotherapy is used as primary treatment for control of cervical metastasis, several factors are important to consider. The first is *nodal size.* It is well known that control rates decrease as nodal size increases. For instance, nodes smaller than 3 cm have control rates of approximately 92%, whereas nodes 4 to 7 cm in size have control rates of approximately 80%, and nodes larger than 7 cm have control rates of approximately 60%.[118] Second, *nodal number* is important—that is, the more nodes that are involved, the lower the control rates.[119] *Nodal fixation* appears to be an independent factor, with fixed nodes faring worse than mobile nodes, mainly because of ECS.[117] The *duration of radiation* also appears to be important[116]—that is, given equivalent dosages, the shorter the duration of therapy, the better the control rates. This is best explained by the outgrowth of tumor clonogens that can repopulate the radiated field during treatment breaks.

The N1 neck is usually treated with a dosage of 66 to 70 Gy with conventional fractionation, or 72 Gy with a concomitant boost regimen.[120] With these regimens, regional control is achieved in 85% to 90% of patients. Treatment of the N2/N3 neck is rarely undertaken with radiotherapy alone (except with nasopharyngeal or selected oropharyngeal primaries). Again, doses of 70 Gy are given with conventional fractionation, or 72 Gy with a concomitant boost regimen.[118] Regional control is achieved in 70% to 80% of patients with N2 disease and in 40% to 50% of patients with N3 disease. Concomitant chemotherapy may improve response rates.

In patients treated with primary radiotherapy, residual nodal disease following treatment presents a diagnostic dilemma.[121] Some centers perform a planned neck dissection following radiotherapy, depending on factors related to the initial stage of the nodal disease.[122, 123] Others take a wait-and-see approach, with the understanding that a majority of these residual masses are "sterile."[124, 125] At the M.D. Anderson Cancer Center, patients are evaluated 4 to 6 weeks after treatment by means of physical examination and CT scanning. If no primary or nodal disease is noted on examination and imaging, the patient is observed. If the primary has resolved but residual nodal disease is evident on examination or imaging, a limited neck dissection is performed to remove all gross disease. More than 50% of these specimens are negative for cancer. If cancer is present at the primary site, salvage surgery that incorporates the appropriate neck dissection is considered. Using this algorithm, patients at highest risk for persistent disease are selected and treated early; however, a significant percentage of patients still receive unneeded surgery. Better methods of tumor assessment after radiotherapy are needed at this time.

ADJUVANT RADIOTHERAPY

When combined with surgery, preoperative versus postoperative radiotherapy is largely a matter of personal or institutional preference. RTOG trial 73-03 revealed a slight advantage in locoregional control with postoperative radiotherapy; however, there was no significant difference in overall survival.[126] When used preoperatively, radiotherapy dosage varies according to the size, location, and fixation of the node, as well as its response to treatment. In general, doses of 50 Gy are sufficient for mobile nodes smaller than 3 cm. However, 60 Gy or more may be required for larger nodes. Surgery is usually performed 6 weeks after the completion of radiotherapy. This "golden window" is important because it allows for resolution of the hyperemia associated with radiotherapy, yet it comes before the inevitable tissue fibrosis that obscures surgical planes. In addition, it allows minimal chance for tumor regrowth following radiotherapy. When used postoperatively, radiotherapy is usually given in dosages of 60 to 65 Gy. In this instance, all attempts should be made to begin radiotherapy 4 to 6 weeks after surgery; delays in treatment may decrease control and/or lead to the need for higher doses.[127]

◼ METASTASIS FROM AN UNKNOWN PRIMARY

In most patients with metastatic cervical lymph nodes, meticulous evaluation of the head and neck area identifies the primary site of cancer. However, in 2% to 8% of cases, no primary malignancy is ever identified.[128] This presents a difficult diagnostic and therapeutic dilemma.

Diagnostic Approach

As with all masses in the head and neck, evaluation includes a complete history and physical examination, which includes examination of the entire upper aerodigestive tract, thyroid gland, salivary glands, and skin. The most common sites for occult primary cancer are the tonsil, base of the tongue, nasopharynx, and pyriform sinus.[129] Quite often, the site of the nodal metastasis may give clues as to where the primary site is.[130] For instance, a node in the jugulodigastric area is suspicious for a primary site in the oropharynx, especially the base of the tongue or tonsil. Similarly, a node in the posterior triangle is a classic location for a cancer that arises in the nasopharynx. A node in the supraclavicular area should alert the clinician to a possible infraclavicular primary site (i.e., lung, breast, stomach, colon).

FNA biopsy should be performed to confirm the presence of metastatic cancer; it may also provide some information regarding the primary. As with other metastatic lesions in the neck, the predominant histologic type is squamous cell carcinoma; however, undifferentiated carcinoma, adenocarcinoma, melanoma, and thyroid cancer may also be found. The most common locations for squamous cell carcinoma are levels II, III, and V. Adenocarcinomas are frequently located in the supraclavicular fossa, with the origin being usually below the clavicles. Undifferentiated carcinomas and metastatic melanomas are distributed with equal frequency in the superior and inferior aspects of the neck.[131] The histologic characteristics obtained by special staining techniques (prostate-specific antigen, thyroglobulin, calcitonin) may help the clinician in determining the possible site of origin. If FNA demonstrates adenocarcinoma, then mammography, CT scan of the abdomen and pelvis, and GI imaging or endoscopic studies may be useful, depending on the location of the node, the patient's age, individual risk factors, and the results of pelvic/rectal examinations. If FNA shows poorly differentiated carcinoma, then cancer of the nasopharynx, base of the tongue, and tonsil should be suspected, and anti–Epstein-Barr virus antibodies may be useful for treatment planning and follow-up.[132] Cervical metastasis from undifferentiated tumors may need further differential diagnosis, including lymphoma, melanoma, metastatic oat cell tumor, and medullary carcinoma of the thyroid gland.[133]

In almost all cases, directed imaging (CT or MRI) is important in the evaluation; however, overuse of imaging (e.g., full body CT) should be discouraged. Imaging is useful for evaluating an occult primary, as well as for examining the neck for any evidence of further lymphadenopathy. The presence of cystic metastasis in the neck is strongly suggestive of a primary cancer in the tonsil.[134] Recently, PET scanning has been found to be helpful for use in evaluation of the unknown primary. Preliminary data are promising, showing that up to 37% of primary tumors may be revealed by PET.[135, 136] At this point, however, the use of this modality is limited by cost and availability.

Examination under anesthesia (EUA) is also important in the diagnostic evaluation. During EUA, it is important for the clinician to examine the nasopharynx, base of the tongue, tonsils, pyriform sinuses, and postcricoid regions because these are common sites of undiagnosed primaries. Biopsies of suspicious areas are recommended; however, random biopsies of these sites, when no visual or palpable abnormalities are present, have a very low pathologic yield and offer the potential for significant morbidity. Recently, tonsillectomy has been advocated at the time of EUA,[137, 138] the rationale being that between 10% and 18% of tonsillectomy specimens in this setting harbor an occult primary tumor. The authors of the study advocate bilateral tonsillectomy because 10% of the positive tonsils detected were from the contralateral tonsil.[139] Through this regimen of history, physical examination, FNA biopsy, guided imaging, and EUA with tonsillectomy, up to 50% of initially unknown tumors can be identified.[140, 141]

Management

If the primary site of cancer is not identified despite a thorough search, several treatment options are appropriate. These include surgery, radiotherapy, or a combination of both. Limited data exist regarding the benefits of systemic chemotherapy added to local therapy. Several areas of current controversy regarding the treatment of the unknown primary include (1) whether the treatment modality should be surgery, radiotherapy, or a combination, and (2) whether radiotherapy, when it is used, should be limited to the neck (or must it include areas of potential primaries?).

The treatment strategy employed by many centers includes a combination of surgery and postoperative radiotherapy. Data from the M.D. Anderson Cancer Center show that 2-year disease-specific survival was 82% with this protocol (which included elective irradiation to the entire upper aerodigestive tract).[142] Likewise, groups at the Mayo Clinic,[143] Memorial Sloan-Kettering Cancer Center,[144] and the University of Florida[145] have also recommended elective irradiation of the nasopharynx, oropharynx, supraglottis, and

hypopharynx because it significantly decreased the appearance of the occult primary (12% compared with 36%).

Other groups, however, have raised concerns about the use of elective radiation of the upper aerodigestive tract. Because radiation is associated with significant complications and will no longer be available if a second primary develops in the area, they recommend single-modality therapy when possible. Coster and coworkers,[146] in a review of the literature, concluded that there is no evidence to support elective mucosal radiation in an effort to lower the rate of primary tumor development. They recommend surgery alone for N1, leaving adjuvant radiotherapy for N2 or higher stages, evidence of extracapsular extension, and features suggesting primary nasopharyngeal tumor. Similarly, Wang and associates[147] recommend single-modality treatment, either surgery or radiotherapy, for N1 and N2a stages. No postoperative radiation is given to the neck or possible primary sites unless other risk factors are found (ECS, multiple levels affected, residual disease, or previous excisional biopsy). Glynne-Jones and colleagues[148] suggest that when radiotherapy is needed, a more conservative approach, without elective radiation of the naso-orohypopharynx, can give similar survival but will spare the morbidity of wide-field radiotherapy.

Settling this controversy is difficult. It is clear, however, that the choice of therapy depends on many factors, including histology, location of the mass, extension of the lesion, and the philosophy of the institution, as well as the preferences of the individuals involved in the treatment. Each patient must be considered individually, and surgeons should try not to be dogmatic.

Recommendations for some of the common clinical situations encountered include the following:

- For resectable disease smaller than 3 cm, the most commonly performed treatment is neck dissection, usually in the form of a functional neck dissection. If a single node is found with no ECS, no further treatment is required. If multiple nodes or ECS are noted, postoperative radiotherapy is recommended. However, in lieu of surgery, radiation may be used alone as definitive treatment with very good success.[144]
- For resectable disease larger than 3 cm, a neck dissection, either modified or radical, followed by postoperative radiotherapy, is usually recommended. Some centers have had success using a limited neck dissection (essentially removal of the positive node[s]) followed by postoperative radiotherapy.[139] Also, preoperative radiotherapy followed by neck dissection has been advocated.
- For unresectable disease, radiotherapy is usually recommended, often with chemotherapy.
- Lymphoepithelioma or poorly differentiated squamous cell carcinoma with a strong suspicion of nasopharyngeal origin (bilateral metastasis in the posterior cervical triangle, Chinese ethnic origin, age younger than 30 years, elevated Epstein-Barr virus titers) is usually treated with radiotherapy to the naso-oropharynx and both sides of the neck.[149]
- For adenocarcinoma located in the supraclavicular fossa, surgery is usually not recommended because this probably reflects systemic tumor dissemination from a primary tumor located below the clavicles, with a high chance of metastasis to other body sites.[150] Patients

with unilateral metastasis located above the cricoid cartilage have a significantly longer survival. If metastatic cancer is found only in the neck, surgery along with postoperative radiotherapy may be recommended.

◾ METASTASIS FROM NASOPHARYNGEAL CARCINOMA

According to Lindberg's classic study, nasopharyngeal carcinoma is associated with the highest incidence of cervical node involvement of any head and neck cancer subtype—approximately 87%.[1]

The patterns of lymphatic drainage from the nasopharynx are complex. Direct pathways exist to (1) the nodes of Rouvière in the lateral retropharyngeal space, (2) the jugulodigastric (level II) nodes, and (3) the upper posterior triangle group of nodes (level V). Because the location of the nasopharynx is midline, the incidence of bilateral cervical lymphadenopathy is also very high—up to 65%.[151] Although the most common site of metastatic spread of nasopharyngeal carcinoma is the retropharyngeal nodes (of Rouvière), because these are not palpable, the jugulodigastric or upper posterior cervical nodes are the most commonly encountered nodes clinically.[152] Therefore, CT and MRI are important in the evaluation of nasopharyngeal carcinoma because they remain the only way to assess retropharyngeal nodes.[153]

The mainstay of therapy is radiotherapy; therefore, cervical lymph node metastases are also usually treated with radiotherapy. Doses for N0 necks approximate 45 to 50 Gy, and N+ necks usually require between 60 and 75 Gy.[154] Control rates, even for large nodes, are excellent. One large series showed the following control rates: N0—100%, N1—90%, N2—88%, and N3—82%.[155] Concomitant chemoradiotherapy appears to show efficacy in advanced disease (stages III and IV) with significant improvement in disease-free survival and overall survival in the United States.[156] Surgery is usually reserved for regional failure, which occurs in approximately 10% of patients. Comprehensive neck dissection, either radical or functional, is the treatment of choice for persistent or recurrent cervical disease, if parapharyngeal nodes are controlled.[157]

◾ METASTASIS FROM CARCINOMA OF THE THYROID

As a group, thyroid carcinomas tend to have a high rate of regional spread, usually estimated at between 30% and 60%, depending on tumor type.[158] This is partially due to the highly vascular nature of the gland and its complex lymphatic drainage. Lymphatic drainage from the thyroid gland progresses in three major pathways. The basic echelons of lymphatic drainage are (1) into the perithyroid nodes, the pretracheal nodes, and the paratracheal nodes, commonly referred to as the central compartment nodes (medial to the internal jugular veins, caudal to the thyroid cartilage, and cephalic to the innominate vein; (2) to the level II, III, and IV jugular chain nodes; and (3) to the lower level V nodes via channels along the transverse cervical artery.

Papillary Carcinoma of the Thyroid

The incidence of cervical lymphatic metastasis is very high (56% at initial presentation; 5% develop subsequent metastasis).[159] Unlike SCCHN, a majority of studies have shown that the presence of cervical metastasis has *no substantiated effect* on prognosis in patients with differentiated thyroid cancer, except perhaps in patients older than 45 years of age.[160, 161]

Treatment of the N0 neck in patients with papillary carcinoma of the thyroid usually involves a central compartment dissection (including removal of superior mediastinal nodes) and examination of all nodes within the tracheo-esophageal groove and jugular chain. Suspicious nodes are biopsied, and if cancer is found, neck dissection should be performed. The type of dissection performed is usually functional and selective neck dissection, encompassing the major routes of lymphatic drainage described previously. Dissection of level I nodes is seldom required. Elective neck dissection in the absence of pathologically positive nodes is of dubious value.

Treatment of the N+ neck in patients with papillary carcinoma of the thyroid is usually provided in the form of a functional neck dissection. Postoperative radioactive iodine treatment is indicated in an effort to ablate any microscopic foci of tumor.[162] In addition, radiotherapy may be beneficial for a select group of patients with extensive disease and/or close or positive margins.[163]

Treatment of the neck in children and adolescents with papillary carcinoma of the thyroid can present a difficult dilemma. In this population, the rate of clinically apparent lymph node metastasis is 60%. Occult lymph nodes are found in 26% of clinically N0 patients. In addition, recurrence rates are highest in the neck, at 24%. For this reason, thorough, aggressive initial neck therapy is required (resist *"berry-picking"*). Most head and neck surgeons recommend total thyroidectomy with central compartment dissection and functional neck dissection, although selective neck dissection is a reasonable alternative with mobile nodes.[164, 165] Postoperative iodine-131 treatment is recommended in most patients, although the possibility of late adverse effects in females must be considered.

Follicular Carcinoma of the Thyroid

In patients with follicular carcinoma, the incidence of cervical lymphatic involvement is moderate (21% at initial presentation; 9% develop subsequent metastasis) compared with the rate in papillary carcinoma.[156] As with papillary carcinoma, cervical node status appears to have no effect on prognosis in these patients. Treatment of the neck is as described for papillary carcinoma. Treatment of children and adolescents is as described for papillary carcinoma.

Medullary Thyroid Carcinoma

In patients with medullary carcinoma, the incidence of cervical lymphatic involvement is very high—approximately 50%. Here, unlike with other forms of thyroid carcinoma, the presence of regional metastasis at the time of presentation decreases survival.[157]

The treatment of the N0 neck must be individualized. For patients with sporadic medullary thyroid carcinoma, in addition to total thyroidectomy, a meticulous central compartment dissection, including upper mediastinal nodes, and elective functional neck dissection on the side of primary disease are recommended. For familial medullary thyroid carcinoma (occurring in multiple family members; usually associated with mutation or alteration of the *RET* oncogene), the recommended treatment is as described previously, except that elective *bilateral* neck dissection is recommended.[162] This recommendation is based on the higher incidence of bilateral disease in this patient population. With the advent of molecular testing, a new group of patients requiring treatment is emerging—"*RET* oncogene carriers" (asymptomatic carriers of mutation or alteration of the *RET* oncogene). In these patients, a total thyroidectomy without node dissection is recommended.[166, 167]

Treatment of the N+ neck usually requires functional neck dissection, unless invasion of cervical structures requires radical neck dissection. In high-risk patients, postoperative external beam radiation treatment has been shown to decrease the locoregional recurrence rate, but it has little impact on survival.[168] Radioactive iodine treatments are rarely effective in the treatment of medullary thyroid carcinoma.[169]

Undifferentiated Carcinoma of the Thyroid

Undifferentiated carcinoma of the thyroid is not a surgical disease. This cancer usually presents with diffuse infiltration of many of the structures in the neck, including the larynx, trachea, and esophagus. Radiation combined with tracheotomy for airway protection is the preferred method of palliation. Most patients with undifferentiated carcinoma of the thyroid do not survive longer than 6 months.

▣ METASTASIS FROM CARCINOMA OF THE SALIVARY GLANDS

The rate of cervical node metastasis from carcinoma of the salivary glands is widely varied and is dependent on cell type. For instance, mucoepidermoid carcinoma has a rate of metastasis on the order of 45% to 70%.[170, 171] Conversely, adenoid cystic carcinoma has a regional metastasis rate of approximately 4% to 10%.[167, 172] Therefore, treatment must be individualized and based on the histology and the site of origin.

In general, there is agreement that the N+ neck should be treated surgically because radiotherapy is not very effective for gross disease. Usually, a functional neck dissection is appropriate. Postoperative radiotherapy is required.

Treatment of the N0 neck is more controversial. In general, elective treatment is not indicated for low-grade, small cancers. However, based on several retrospective studies, elective treatment is suggested for patients with high-grade cancer larger than 3 to 4 cm, facial paralysis, age older than 54 years, extraglandular extension, and perilymphatic invasion.[173, 174]

Treatment in this high-risk group is effectively provided by surgery or radiotherapy. Although some authors advocate surgery,[167] others feel that because the factors that would dictate the use of elective neck dissection are the same factors that would dictate postoperative radiation therapy to the primary site, elective neck dissection is rarely indicated.[172] Instead, they recommend removal of any easily accessible nodal groups at the time of primary tumor resection (e.g., removing level II nodes with the parotidectomy specimen, or level I and II nodes with submandibular gland excision), then the administration of postoperative radiotherapy to the neck and primary site in this group of high-risk patients.[175] Usually, a combination of photon and electron therapy is used. Fast-neutron radiotherapy has been studied with mixed results oncologically and findings of high morbidity.[176]

▣ METASTASIS FROM CUTANEOUS CANCER

Basal Cell Carcinoma

The most common cancer of the skin in North America, basal cell carcinoma, has an extremely low metastatic rate—less than 0.1%.[177] Factors associated with increased risk of metastasis include young age, multiple recurrences, large ulcerated primary lesions, and basalosquamous pathology.[178] Because of the extremely low rate of metastasis, there is no role for elective neck treatment. Neck dissection plus or minus parotidectomy is required for those rare tumors that present with metastatic spread.

Squamous Cell Carcinoma

Squamous cell carcinoma is the second most common skin cancer; similar to basal cell carcinoma, it has a very low rate of metastatic spread—2% to 5%.[179, 180] Several factors associated with increased risk for metastasis include recurrence, thickness greater than 6 mm, size larger than 2 cm, poorly differentiated tumors, an immunocompromised host, perineural invasion, tumor arising from a scar/burn, and a primary site on the ear, lip, or temple.[181, 182]

Because of the low incidence of metastasis, elective neck treatment for the N0 neck is not warranted. For those with palpable cervical lymphadenopathy, neck dissection is required. Generally, this takes the form of a modified radical neck dissection or selective neck dissection, depending on the site of the primary and the site and size of the involved node(s). Parotidectomy in continuity with neck dissection is suggested for those sites with a risk of spread to parotid and periparotid lymph nodes. Patients with metastasis to the parotid gland should have a parotidectomy and elective neck dissection. For primary tumors treated with definitive radiotherapy rather than surgery, the neck should be included in the treatment portals only if nodal disease is clinically evident.

Malignant Melanoma

Although it is highly curable in early stages, melanoma is difficult to cure in advanced stages, primarily owing to failure to control distant metastasis even when locoregional control has been achieved. Of utmost importance is the fact that the rates of metastasis, both regional and distant, are

TABLE 18-6 Rates of Regional and Distant Metastasis Based on Melanoma Thickness

Tumor Thickness	Regional Metastasis	Distant Metastasis
<0.75 mm	Rare	Rare
0.76–1.50 mm	25%	8%
1.51–4.00 mm	57%	15%
>4.00 mm	62%	72%

related to the thickness of the primary lesion (Table 18–6).[183] Similarly, the rate of occult nodal metastasis also correlates with thickness of the primary. Tumors smaller than 1.5 mm have an occult nodal metastatic rate of 8%; tumors larger than 1.5 mm have an occult nodal metastatic rate of 15%.[184] The presence of positive nodes is the single most important prognostic factor in patients with melanoma of the head and neck.[185]

Treatment of the N0 Neck

Most randomized prospective trials have demonstrated no efficacy in elective treatment of the neck in patients clinically staged at N0. Only one study—the Intergroup Melanoma Surgical Program[186]—has shown any benefit of elective treatment, and that was for a specific subgroup of patients younger than 60 years old with intermediate-thickness melanomas. Despite this, most surgical oncologists address the regional nodes when treating intermediate or thick lesions.

Elective Neck Dissection. The most commonly employed elective treatment of the neck is elective neck dissection. If elective neck dissection is undertaken, it should be based on a sound knowledge of the pathways of lymphatic spread. In general, tumors arising on the scalp and forehead anterior to a line drawn through the external auditory canal most commonly spread to the parotid/periparotid lymph nodes and upper jugular lymph nodes; therefore, parotidectomy and lateral neck dissection are recommended.[187] Tumors arising on the scalp and occiput posterior to a line drawn through the external auditory canal most commonly spread to the postauricular, suboccipital, and posterior triangle lymph nodes; therefore, a posterolateral neck dissection is recommended.[188] Tumors located anteriorly on the face and neck generally spread to the facial, submental, submandibular, and deep cervical nodes; therefore, a supraomohyoid neck dissection is recommended.[184]

Elective Neck Irradiation. Another option for treatment of the N0 neck is elective neck irradiation. Historically, melanoma was considered a radioresistant tumor. However, experience over the past 20 years has clearly shown that different dosimetry and fractionation schemes are required to treat cutaneous malignant melanoma (CMM) than are used to treat other tumors. With the advent of large-dose fractions, significant improvements in locoregional control have been noted with the use of adjuvant radiotherapy.[189] Data from the M.D. Anderson Cancer Center reveal that in the head and neck, 88% locoregional control is possible in patients with stage II disease when postoperative radiotherapy is used at a dose of 30 Gy given in five fractions.[190] Therefore, postoperative radiotherapy may be recommended for patients with stage II lesions in whom the regional lymphatics are not treated surgically.

Sentinel Lymph Node Biopsy. A newer option for evaluation of the neck is sentinel lymph node biopsy. The theoretical basis for sentinel lymph node biopsy has already been defined. Sentinel lymph node biopsy is a well-accepted procedure in the treatment of truncal and extremity melanoma; however, its role in the management of CMM of the head and neck is unclear at this time. The complexity of lymphatic drainage patterns and the frequent need to remove sentinel lymph nodes from the parotid gland, thus placing the facial nerve at risk, have made head and neck surgical oncologists slow to adopt this method. However, several centers have adopted sentinel lymph node biopsy for CMM of the head and neck and are reporting its efficacy. Thus far, it appears that sentinel lymph nodes can be identified reliably, and the false-negative rate (i.e., the rate of lymph node metastases in nonsentinel lymph nodes) is extremely low.[191, 192] At this time, sentinel lymph node biopsy for melanoma of the head and neck is promising, but more study is required before its widespread usage can be recommended.

Treatment of the N+ Neck

For patients with clinically positive nodes, a neck dissection is necessary. It is important to remember that in these patients, all intervening lymphatics between the primary and the node must be addressed. Thus, if a patient presents with a primary on the temple, anterior scalp, or face, along with a clinically positive node in level II, a parotidectomy must be performed along with the neck dissection. For primary sites on the chin or neck, a parotidectomy is not required. For posterior scalp lesions, the postauricular and suboccipital nodes must be addressed. The type of neck dissection must be tailored to the disease. All patients with regional metastasis should be considered for postoperative radiotherapy and systemic adjuvant treatment such as interferon α 2b.[193, 194]

CONCLUSIONS

The mass in the neck constitutes an important challenge for the head and neck surgeon. The varied histology and prognostic significance of cervical disease dictate a careful approach to the diagnosis and management of neck lesions. A thorough knowledge of the anatomy of the neck, especially the relations between the lymphatic system and the fascial planes within the neck, is crucial if an understanding of the clinical significance of tumors in the neck is to be acquired. A careful diagnostic approach requires the sequential use of the clinical tools currently available; the importance of a well-performed history and physical examination must be emphasized. Even in this era of modern technology, these remain the foundation for a correct diagnosis. Differentiating between benign and malignant, which may include primary and metastatic tumors, should be the first step in the diagnostic approach to the patient with a mass in the neck. Primary cancers are treated according to specific protocols for each tumor type. Metastatic tumors require careful thought as to the treatment modality that should be used for the primary lesion and knowledge of its effectiveness when used with clinically apparent or occult nodes. Use of all therapeutic modes available to the clinician, including surgery, radiotherapy, and chemotherapy, provides the best chance for cure of malignant lesions in the neck.

REFERENCES

1. Lindberg R: Distribution of cervical lymph node metastases from squamous cell carcinoma of the upper respiratory and digestive tracts. Cancer 29:1446–1449, 1972.
2. Lymphatics of the head and neck. In Hiatt JL, Gartner LP (eds): Textbook of Head and Neck Anatomy, 2nd ed. Baltimore, Williams & Wilkins, 1987.
3. Fleming ID, Cooper JS, Henson DE, et al (for the American Joint Committee on Cancer): AJCC Cancer Staging Manual. Philadelphia, Lippincott-Raven, 1997.
4. Robbins KT, Medina JE, Wolf GT: Standardizing neck dissection terminology. Arch Otolaryngol Head Neck Surg 117:601–605, 1991.
5. Suen JY, Goepfert H: Standardization of neck dissection nomenclature. Head Neck Surg 10:75–77, 1987.
6. Shah JP, Strong E, Spiro RH, et al: Surgical grand rounds. Neck dissection: Current status and future possibilities. Clin Bull 11:25–33, 1981.
7. Shah JP: Patterns of cervical lymph node metastasis from squamous carcinoma of the upper aerodigestive tract. Am J Surg 160:405–409, 1990.
8. Johnson N: Tobacco use and oral cancer: A global perspective. J Dent Educ 65:328–339, 2001.
9. Lewin F, Norell SE, Johansson H, et al: Smoking tobacco, oral snuff, and alcohol in the etiology of squamous cell carcinoma of the head and neck: A population-based case-referent study in Sweden. Cancer 82:1367–1375, 1998.
10. Stevens MH, Harnsberger HR, Mancuso AA, et al: Computed tomography of cervical lymph nodes. Staging and management of head and neck cancer. Arch Otolaryngol 111:735–739, 1985.
11. van den Brekel MW, Castelijns JA: Radiologic evaluation of neck metastases: The otolaryngologist's perspective. Semin Ultrasound CT MR 20:162–174, 1999.
12. van den Brekel MW, Castelijns JA, Stel HV, et al: Occult metastatic neck disease: Detection with US and US-guided fine-needle aspiration cytology. Radiology 180:457–461, 1991.
13. Merritt RM, Williams MF, James TH, et al: Detection of cervical metastases: A metanalysis comparing computed tomography and physical examination. Arch Otolaryngol Head Neck Surg 123:149–152, 1997.
14. Stokkel MP, tenBroek FW, van Rilk PP: The role of FDG PET in the clinical management of head and neck cancer. Oral Oncol 34: 466–471, 1998.
15. van den Brekel MW, Casteijns JA, Snow GB: Imaging of cervical lymphadenopathy. Neuroimaging Clin N Am 6:417–434, 1996.
16. Westerband A, Hunter GC, Cintora I, et al: Current trends in the detection and management of carotid body tumors. J Vasc Surg 28:84–92, 1998.
17. Eckard DA, Purdy PD, Bonte FJ: Temporary balloon occlusion of the carotid artery combined with brain blood flow imaging as a test to predict tolerance prior to permanent carotid sacrifice. AJNR Am J Neuroradiol 13:1565–1569, 1992.
18. O'Brien CJ, Uren RF, Thompson JF, et al: Prediction of potential metastatic sites in cutaneous head and neck melanoma using lymphoscintigraphy. Am J Surg 170:461–466, 1995.
19. Wagner JD, Park HM, Coleman JJ 3rd, et al: Cervical sentinel lymph node biopsy for melanomas of the head and neck and upper thorax. Arch Otolaryngol Head Neck Surg 126:313–321, 2000.
20. Curtin HD, Weissman JL: Radiologic evaluation of head and neck cancer. In Myers EN, Suen JY (eds): Cancer of the Head and Neck, 3rd ed. Philadelphia, WB Saunders, 1996, pp 50–78.
21. Frable MA, Frable WJ: Fine-needle aspiration biopsy revisited. Laryngoscope 92:1414–1418, 1982.
22. Rimm DL, Stastny JF, Rimm EB, et al: Comparison of the costs of fine-needle aspiration and open surgical biopsy as methods for obtaining a pathologic diagnosis. Cancer 81:51–56, 1997.
23. Martin HE, Ellis EB: Biopsy of needle puncture and aspiration. Ann Surg 92:169–181, 1930.
24. Feldman PS, Kaplan MJ, Johns ME, et al: Fine-needle aspiration in squamous cell carcinoma of the head and neck. Arch Otolaryngol 109:735–742, 1983.
25. Gharib H: Fine-needle aspiration biopsy of thyroid nodules: Advantages, limitations, and effect. Mayo Clin Proc 69:44–49, 1994.
26. Schindler S, Nayar R, Dutra J, et al: Diagnostic challenges in aspiration cytology of the salivary glands. Semin Diagn Pathol 18:124–146, 2001.
27. van den Brekel MWM, Stel HV, Castelijns JA, et al: Lymph node staging in patients with clinically negative neck examination by ultrasound and ultrasound-guided aspiration cytology. Am J Surg 162:362–366, 1991.
28. Martin H, Morfit HM: Cervical lymph nodes metastases as the first symptom of cancer. Surg Gynecol Obstet 78:133, 1944.
29. McGuirt WF, McCabe BF: Significance of node biopsy before definitive treatment of cervical metastatic carcinoma. Laryngoscope 88:594–597, 1978.
30. Robbins KT, Cole R, Marvel J, et al: The violated neck: Cervical node biopsy prior to definitive treatment. Otolaryngol Head Neck Surg 117:60–61, 1991.
31. Ellis ER, Mendenhall WM, Rao PV, et al: Incisional or excisional neck-node biopsy before definitive radiotherapy, alone or followed by neck dissection. Head Neck 13:177–183, 1991.
32. Collins SL: Controversies in management of cancer of the neck. In Thawley SE, et al (eds): Comprehensive Management of Head and Neck Tumors, 2nd ed. Philadelphia, WB Saunders, 1999, pp 1479–1563.
33. Bonilla JA, Healy GB: Management of malignant head and neck tumors in children. Pediatr Clin North Am 36:1443–1450, 1989.
34. Dailey SH, Sataloff RT: Lymphoma: An update on evolving trends in staging and management. Ear Nose Throat J 80:164–170, 2001.
35. Eveson JW, Cawson RA: Salivary gland tumors. A review of 2410 cases with particular reference to histological types, site, ages and sex. J Pathol 146:51–58, 1985.
36. Stewart CJ, MacKenzie K, McGarry GW, et al: Fine-needle aspiration cytology of salivary gland: A review of 341 cases. Diagn Cytopathol 22:139–146, 2000.
37. Cajulis RS, Gokaslan ST, Yu GH, et al: Fine needle aspiration biopsy of the salivary glands. A five-year experience with emphasis on diagnostic pitfalls. Acta Cytol 41:1412–1420, 1997.
38. Spiro RH: Salivary neoplasms: Overview of a 35-year experience with 2,807 patients. Head Neck Surg 8:177–184, 1986.
39. Batsakis JG, Luna MA: Histopathologic grading of salivary gland neoplasms: I. Mucoepidermoid carcinomas. Ann Otol Rhinol Laryngol 99(10 Pt 1):835–838, 1990.
40. Matsuba HM, Spector GJ, Thawley SE, et al: Adenoid cystic salivary gland carcinoma. A histopathologic review of treatment failure patterns. Cancer 57:519–524, 1986.
41. van der Mey AG, Jansen JC, van Baalen JM: Management of carotid body tumors. Otolaryngol Clin North Am 34:907–924, 2001.
42. Wanebo HJ, Koness RJ, MacFarlane JK, et al: Head and neck sarcoma: Report of the Head and Neck Sarcoma Registry. Society of Head and Neck Surgeons Committee on Research. J Sci Spec Head Neck 14:1–7, 1992.
43. Byers RM, El-Naggar AK, Lee YY, et al: Can we detect or predict the presence of occult nodal metastases in patients with squamous carcinoma of the oral tongue? Head Neck 20:138–144, 1998.
44. Spiro RH, Huvos AG, Wong GY, et al: Predictive value of tumor thickness in squamous carcinoma confined to the tongue and floor of the mouth. Am J Surg 152:345–350, 1986.
45. Rubio Bueno P, Naval Gias L, Garcia Delgado R, et al: Tumor DNA content as a prognostic indicator in squamous cell carcinoma of the oral cavity and tongue base. J Sci Spec Head Neck 20:232–239, 1998.
46. Goepfert H, Dichtel WJ, Medina JE, et al: Perineural invasion in squamous cell skin carcinoma of the head and neck. Am J Surg 148:542–547, 1984.
47. Fagan JJ, Collins B, Barnes L, et al: Perineural invasion in squamous cell carcinoma of the head and neck. Arch Otolaryngol Head Neck Surg 124:637–640, 1998.

48. Ozdek A, Sarac S, Akyol MU, et al: Histopathological predictors of occult lymph node metastases in supraglottic squamous cell carcinomas. Eur Arch Otorhinolaryngol 257:389–392, 2000.

49. Woolgar JA, Scott J: Prediction of cervical lymph node metastasis in squamous cell carcinoma of the tongue/floor of mouth. J Sci Spec Head Neck 17:463–472, 1995.

50. Fleming ID, Cooper JS, Henson DE, et al (for the American Joint Committee on Cancer): AJCC Cancer Staging Manual. Philadelphia, Lippincott-Raven, 1997.

51. Hermanek P, Hutter RVP, Sobin LH, et al: In Hermanek P, et al (eds): TNM Atlas: Illustrated Guide to the TNM/pTNM Classification of Malignant Tumours, 4th ed. New York, Springer, 1997.

52. Breau RL, Suen JY: Management of the N(0) neck. Otolaryngol Clin North Am 31:657–669, 1998.

53. Pillsbury HC, Clark M: A rationale for therapy of the N0 neck. Laryngoscope 107:1294–1315, 1997.

54. Robbins KT: Neck Dissection Classification and TNM Staging of Head and Neck Cancer. American Academy of Otolaryngology-Head and Neck Surgery Foundation, Inc, 1991.

55. Suárez O: El problema de las metástasis linfáticas y alejadas del cáncer de laringe e hipofaringe. Rev Otorrinolaringol (Santiago de Chile) 23:83–99, 1963.

56. Bocca E, Pignataro O, Oldini C, et al: Functional neck dissection: An evaluation and review of 843 cases. Laryngoscope 94:942–945, 1984.

57. Gavilán C, Gavilán J: Five-year results of functional neck dissection for cancer of the larynx. Arch Otolaryngol Head Neck Surg 115:1193–1196, 1989.

58. Gavilán J, Herranz J, DeSanto LW, Gavilán C: Functional and Selective Neck Dissection. New York, Thieme, 2002.

59. Fletcher GH: Elective irradiation of subclinical disease in cancers of the head and neck. Cancer 29:1450–1454, 1972.

60. Jesse RH, Fletcher GH: Treatment of the neck in patients with squamous cell carcinoma of the head and neck. Cancer 39(2 Suppl):868–872, 1977.

61. Mantravadi R, Katz A, Haas R, et al: Radiation therapy for subclinical carcinoma in cervical lymph nodes. Arch Otolaryngol 108:108–111, 1982.

62. DeSanto LW: Oncologic issues relating to neck dissection. In Pillsbury HC, Goldsmith MM (eds): Operative Challenges in Otolaryngology—Head and Neck Surgery. Chicago, Year Book Medical Publishers, 1990, pp 410–421.

63. Weiss MH, Harrison LB, Isaacs RS: Use of decision analysis in planning a management strategy for the stage N0 neck. Arch Otolaryngol Head Neck Surg 120:699–702, 1994.

64. Parsons JT: The effect of radiation on normal tissues of the head and neck. In Million RR, Cassisi NJ (eds): Management of Head and Neck Cancer. Philadelphia, JB Lippincott, 1989, pp 173–207.

65. Gershenwald JE, Thompson W, Mansfield PF, et al: Multi-institutional melanoma lymphatic mapping experience: The prognostic value of sentinel lymph node status in 612 stage I or II melanoma patients. J Clin Oncol 17:976–983, 1999.

66. Wells KE, Rapaport DP, Cruse CW, et al: Sentinel lymph node biopsy in melanoma of the head and neck. Plast Reconstr Surg 100:591–594, 1997.

67. Alex JC, Krag DN, Harlow SP, et al: Localization of regional lymph nodes in melanomas of the head and neck. Arch Otolaryngol Head Neck Surg 124:135–140, 1998.

68. Taylor RJ, Wahl RL, Sharma PK, et al: Sentinel node localization in oral cavity and oropharynx squamous cell cancer. Arch Otolaryngol Head Neck Surg 127:970–974, 2001.

69. Alex JC, Sasaki CT, Krag DN, et al: Sentinel lymph node radiolocalization in head and neck squamous cell carcinoma Laryngoscope 110(2 Pt 1):198–203, 2000.

70. Stoeckli SJ, Steinert H, Pfaltz M, et al: Sentinel lymph node evaluation in squamous cell carcinoma of the head and neck. Otolaryngol Head Neck Surg 125:221–226, 2001.

71. Mohit-Tabatabai MA, Sobel HJ, Rush BF, et al: Relation of thickness of floor of mouth stage I and II cancers to regional metastasis. Am J Surg 152:351–353, 1986.

72. Byers RM, El-Naggar AK, Lee YY, et al: Can we detect or predict the presence of occult nodal metastases in patients with squamous carcinoma of the oral tongue? Head Neck 20:138–144, 1998.

73. Byers RM, Weber RS, Andrews T, et al: Frequency and therapeutic implications of "skip metastases" in the neck from squamous carcinoma of the oral tongue. Head Neck 19:14–19, 1997.

74. Spiro JD, Spiro RH, Shah JP, et al: Critical assessment of supraomohyoid neck dissection. Am J Surg 156:286–289, 1988.

75. Candela FC, Kothari K, Shah JP: Patterns of cervical node metastases from squamous carcinoma of the oropharynx and hypopharynx. J Sci Spec Head Neck 12:197–203, 1990.

76. Gallo O, Fini-Storchi I, Napolitano L: Treatment of the contralateral negative neck in supraglottic cancer patients with unilateral node metastases (N1–3). J Sci Spec Head Neck 22:386–392, 2000.

77. Myers EN, Alvi A: Management of carcinoma of the supraglottic larynx: Evolution, current concepts, and future trends. Laryngoscope 106(5 Pt 1):559–567, 1996.

78. Anonymous: End results of a prospective trial on elective lateral neck dissection vs type III modified radical neck dissection in the management of supraglottic and transglottic carcinomas. Brazilian Head and Neck Cancer Study Group. J Sci Spec Head Neck 21:694–702, 1999.

79. Weber PC, Johnson JT, Myers EN: The impact of bilateral neck dissection on pattern of recurrence and survival in supraglottic carcinoma. Arch Otolaryngol Head Neck Surg 120:703–706, 1994.

80. Wax MK, Touma BJ: Management of the N0 neck during salvage laryngectomy. Laryngoscope 109:4–7, 1999.

81. Kligerman J, Olivatto LO, Lima RA, et al: Elective neck dissection in the treatment of T3/T4 N0 squamous cell carcinoma of the larynx. Am J Surg 170:436–439, 1995.

82. Ferlito A, Rinaldo A: The pathology and management of subglottic cancer. Eur Arch Otorhinolaryngol 257:168–173, 2000.

83. Hanna EY: Subglottic cancer. Am J Otolaryngol 15:322–328, 1994.

84. Schuller DE, McGuirt WF, McCabe BF, et al: The prognostic significance of metastatic cervical lymph nodes. Laryngoscope 90:557–570, 1980.

85. Johnson JT: Cervical lymph node metastases. Arch Otolaryngol 111:534–537, 1995.

86. Johnson JT, Barnes EL, Myers EN, et al: The extracapsular spread of tumors in cervical lymph node metastasis. Arch Otolaryngol 107:725–729, 1981.

87. Johnson JT, Myers EN, Bedetti CD, et al: Cervical lymph node metastasis: Incidence and implications of extracapsular carcinoma. Arch Otolaryngol 111:534–537, 1985.

88. Byers RM, Wolf PF, Ballantyne AJ: Rationale for elective modified neck dissection. Head Neck Surg 10:160–167, 1988.

89. Byers RM, Clayman GL, McGill D, et al: Selective neck dissections for squamous carcinoma of the upper aerodigestive tract: Patterns of regional failure. Head Neck 21:499–505, 1999.

90. Traynor SJ, Cohen JI, Gray J, et al: Selective neck dissection and the management of the node-positive neck. Am J Surg 172:654–657, 1996.

91. Amdur RJ, Parsons JT, Mendenhall WM, et al: Postoperative irradiation for squamous cell carcinoma of the head and neck: An analysis of treatment results and complications. Int J Radiat Oncol Biol Phys 16:25–36, 1989.

92. Chepeha DB, Hoff PT, Taylor RJ, et al: Selective neck dissection for the treatment of neck metastasis from squamous cell carcinoma of the head and neck. Laryngoscope 112:434–438, 2002.

93. Kolli VR, Datta RV, Orner JB, et al: The role of supraomohyoid neck dissection in patients with positive nodes. Arch Otolaryngol Head Neck Surg. 126:413–416, 2000.

94. Suárez C, Llorente JL, Nunez F, et al: Neck dissection with or without postoperative radiotherapy in supraglottic carcinomas. Otolaryngol Head Neck Surg 109:3–9, 1993.

95. Gavilán C, Gavilán J: Five-year results of functional neck dissection for cancer of the larynx. Arch Otolaryngol Head Neck Surg 115:1193–1196, 1989.

96. Snow GB, Annyas AA, van Slooten EA, et al: Prognostic factors of neck node metastasis. Clin Otolaryngol 7:185–192, 1982.

97. Cachin Y, Sancho-Garnier H, Micheau C, et al: Nodal metastasis from carcinomas of the oropharynx. Otolaryngol Clin North Am 12:145–154, 1979.

98. Snow GB, Balm AJM, Arendse JW, et al: Prognostic factors in neck node metastasis. In Larson DL, Ballantyne AJ, Guillamondequi OM (eds): Cancer in the Neck: Evaluation and Treatment. New York, Macmillan, 1986, pp 53–63.

99. Mamelle G, Pampurik J, Luboinski B, et al: Lymph node prognostic factors in head and neck squamous cell. Am J Surg 168:494–498, 1994.

100. Pinsolle J, Pinsolle V, Majoufre C, et al: Prognostic value of histologic findings in neck dissections for squamous cell carcinoma. Arch Otolaryngol Head Neck Surg 123:145–148, 1997.

101. Carter RL, Bliss JM, Soo KC, et al: Radical neck dissections for squamous carcinomas: Pathological findings and their clinical implications with particular reference to transcapsular spread. Int J Radiat Oncol Biol Phys 13:825–832, 1987.

102. Brasilino de Carvalho M: Quantitative analysis of the extent of extracapsular invasion and its prognostic significance: A prospective study of 170 cases of carcinoma of the larynx and hypopharynx. Head Neck 20:16–21, 1998.

103. Kalnins IK, Leonard AG, Sako K, et al: Correlation between prognosis and degree of lymph node involvement in carcinoma of the oral cavity. Am J Surg 134:450–454, 1977.

104. Ono I, Ebihara S, Saito H, et al: Correlation between prognosis and degree of lymph node involvement in carcinoma of the head and neck. Auris Nasus Larynx 12(suppl 2):85–89, 1985.

105. Gavilán J, Prim MP, De Diego JI, et al: Postoperative radiotherapy in patients with positive nodes after functional neck dissection. Ann Otol Rhinol Laryngol 109:884–888, 2000.

106. Kraus EM, Panje WR: Factors influencing survival in head and neck patients with giant cervical lymph node metastasis. Otolaryngol Head Neck Surg 90:296–304, 1982.

107. Schuller DE, McGuirt WF, McCabe BF, et al: The prognostic significance of metastatic cervical lymph node. Laryngoscope 90:557–570, 1980.

108. Shah JP: Patterns of cervical lymph node metastasis from squamous carcinoma of the upper aerodigestive tract. Am J Surg 160:405–409, 1990.

109. Collins SL: Controversies in management of cancer of the neck. In Thawley SE, et al (eds): Comprehensive Management of Head and Neck Tumors, 2nd ed. Philadelphia, WB Saunders, 1999, pp 1479–1563.

110. Catimel G: Head and neck cancer: Guidelines for chemotherapy. Drugs 51:73–88, 1996.

111. Ahn C, Sindelar WF: Bilateral radical neck dissection: Report of results in 55 patients. J Surg Oncol Suppl 40:252–255, 1989.

112. Jones AS, Stell PM: Is laterality important in neck node metastases in head and neck cancer? Clin Otolaryngol Allied Sci 16:261–265, 1991.

113. Razack MS, Baffi R, Sako K: Bilateral radical neck dissection. Cancer 47:197–199, 1981.

114. al-Ghamdi SA, Beecroft WA, Downs AR: Internal jugular vein reconstruction using a superficial femoral vein graft. Can J Surg 34:621–624, 1991.

115. Nayak UK, Donald PJ, Stevens D: Internal carotid artery resection for invasion of malignant tumors. Arch Otolaryngol Head Neck Surg 121:1029–1033, 1995.

116. Snyderman CH, D'Amico F: Outcome of carotid artery resection for neoplastic disease: A meta-analysis. Am J Otolaryngol 13:373–380, 1992.

117. Suárez C, Llorente JL, Nunez F, et al: Neck dissection with or without postoperative radiotherapy in supraglottic carcinomas. Otolaryngol Head Neck Surg 109:3–9, 1993.

118. Mendenhall WM, Million RR, Bova FJ: Analysis of time-dose factors in clinically positive neck nodes treated with irradiation alone in squamous cell carcinoma of the head and neck Int J Radiat Oncol Biol Phys 10:639–643, 1984.

119. Bataini JP, Bernier J, Asselain B, et al: Primary radiotherapy of squamous cell carcinoma of the oropharynx and pharyngolarynx: Tentative multivariate modelling system to predict the radiocurability of neck nodes. Int J Radiat Oncol Biol Phys 14:635–642, 1988.

120. Ang KK, Peters LJ, Weber RS: Concomitant boost radiotherapy schedules in the treatment of carcinoma of the oropharynx and nasopharynx. Int J Radiat Oncol Biol Phys 19:1339–1345, 1990.

121. Corry J, Smith JG, Peters LJ: The concept of a planned neck dissection is obsolete. Cancer J 7:472–474, 2001.

122. Lee HJ, Zelefsky MJ, Kraus DH, et al: Long-term regional control after radiation therapy and neck dissection for base of tongue carcinoma. Int J Radiat Oncol Biol Phys 38:995–1000, 1997.

123. Kaylie DM, Stevens KR Jr, Kang MY, et al: External beam radiation followed by planned neck dissection and brachytherapy for base of tongue squamous cell carcinoma. Laryngoscope 110(10 Pt 1):1633–1636, 2000.

124. Narayan K, Crane CH, Kleid S, et al: Planned neck dissection as an adjunct to the management of patients with advanced neck disease treated with definitive radiotherapy: For some or for all? J Sci Spec Head Neck 21:606–613, 1999.

125. Peters LJ, Weber RS, Morrison WH, et al: Neck surgery in patients with primary oropharyngeal cancer treated by radiotherapy. J Sci Spec Head Neck 18:552–559, 1996.

126. Tupchong L, Scott CB, Blitzer PH, et al: Randomized study of preoperative versus postoperative radiation therapy in advanced head and neck carcinoma: Long-term follow-up of RTOG study 73-03. Int J Radiat Oncol Biol Phys 20:21–28, 1991.

127. Peters LJ, Goepfert H, Ang KK, et al: Evaluation of the dose for postoperative radiation therapy of head and neck cancer: First report of a prospective randomized trial. Int J Radiat Oncol Biol Phys 26:3–11, 1993.

128. Fu KK: Neck node metastases from unknown primary. Controversies in management. Front Radiat Ther Oncol 28:66–78, 1994.

129. Johnson JT, Newman RK: The anatomic location of neck metastasis from occult squamous cell carcinoma. Otolaryngol Head Neck Surg 89:54–58, 1981.

130. Molinari R, Cantu G, Chiesa F, et al: A statistical approach to detection of the primary cancer based on the site of neck lymph node metastases. Tumori 63:267–282, 1977.

131. Spiro RH, DeRose G, Strong EW: Cervical node metastasis of occult origin. Am J Surg 146:441–446, 1983.

132. Lee WY, Hsiao JR, Jin YT, et al: Epstein-Barr virus detection in neck metastases by in-situ hybridization in fine-needle aspiration cytologic studies: An aid for differentiating the primary site. Head Neck 22:336–340, 2000.

133. Hainsworth JD, Wright EP, Johnson DH, et al: Poorly differentiated carcinoma of unknown primary site: Clinical usefulness of immunoperoxidase staining. J Clin Oncol 9:1931–1938, 1991.

134. Gourin CG, Johnson JT: Incidence of unsuspected metastases in lateral cervical cysts. Laryngoscope 110:1637–1641, 2000.

135. Safa AA, Tran LM, Rege S, et al: The role of positron emission tomography in occult primary head and neck cancers. Cancer J Sci Am 5:214–218, 1999.

136. Jungehulsing M, Scheidhauer K, Damm M, et al: 2[F]-fluoro-2-deoxy-D-glucose positron emission tomography is a sensitive tool for the detection of occult primary cancer (carcinoma of unknown primary syndrome) with head and neck lymph node manifestation. Otolaryngol Head Neck Surg 123:294–301, 2000.

137. Lapeyre M, Malissard L, Peiffert D, et al: Cervical lymph node metastasis from an unknown primary: Is a tonsillectomy necessary? Int J Radiat Oncol Biol Phys 39:291–296, 1997.

138. Randall DA, Johnstone PA, Foss RD, et al: Tonsillectomy in diagnosis of the unknown primary tumor of the head and neck. Otolaryngol Head Neck Surg 122:52–55, 2000.

139. Koch WM, Bhatti N, Williams MF, et al: Oncologic rationale for bilateral tonsillectomy in head and neck squamous cell carcinoma of unknown primary source. Otolaryngol Head Neck Surg 124:331–333, 2001.

140. Lee DJ, Rostock RA, Harris A, et al: Clinical evaluation of patients with metastatic squamous carcinoma of the neck with occult primary tumor. South Med J 79:979–983, 1986.

141. Mendenhall WM, Mancuso AA, Parsons JT, et al: Diagnostic evaluation of squamous cell carcinoma metastatic to cervical lymph nodes from an unknown head and neck primary site. Head Neck 20:739–744, 1998.

142. Colletier PJ, Garden AS, Morrison WH, et al: Postoperative radiation for squamous cell carcinoma metastatic to cervical lymph nodes from an unknown primary site: Outcomes and patterns of failure. J Sci Spec Head Neck 20:674–681, 1998.

143. Coster JR, Foote RL, Olsen KD, et al: Cervical nodal metastasis of squamous cell carcinoma of unknown origin: Indications for withholding radiation therapy. Int J Radiat Oncol Biol Phys 23:743–749, 1992.

144. Davidson BJ, Spiro RH, Patel S, et al: Cervical metastases of occult origin: The impact of combined modality therapy. Am J Surg 168:395–399, 1994.

145. Harper CS, Mendenhall WM, Parsons JT, et al: Cancer in neck nodes with unknown primary site: Role of mucosal radiotherapy. Head Neck 12:463–469, 1990.

146. Coster JR, Foote RL, Olsen KD, et al: Cervical nodal metastasis of squamous cell carcinoma of unknown origin: Indications for withholding radiation therapy. Int J Radiat Oncol Biol Phys 23:743–749, 1992.

147. Wang RC, Goepfert H, Barber AE, et al: Unknown primary squamous cell carcinoma metastatic to the neck. Arch Otolaryngol Head Neck Surg 116:1388–1393, 1990.

148. Glynne-Jones RG, Anand AK, Young TE, et al: Metastatic carcinoma in the cervical lymph nodes from an occult primary: A conservative approach to the role of radiotherapy. Int J Radiat Oncol Biol Phys 18:289–294, 1990.

149. Marcial-Vega VA, Cardenes H, Perez CA, et al: Cervical metastases from unknown primaries: Radiotherapeutic management and appearance of subsequent primaries. Int J Radiat Oncol Biol Phys 19:919–928, 1990.

150. Lee NK, Byers RM, Abbruzzese JL, et al: Metastatic adenocarcinoma to the neck from an unknown primary source. Am J Surg 162:306–309, 1991.

151. Morales P, Bosch A, Salaverry S, et al: Cancer of nasopharynx in young patients. J Surg Oncol Suppl 27:181–185, 1984.

152. Ballantyne AJ: Significance of retropharyngeal nodes in cancer of the head and neck. Am J Surg 108:500–504, 1964.

153. Som PM: Detection of metastasis in cervical lymph nodes: CT and MR criteria and differential diagnosis. AJR Am J Roentgenol 158:961–969, 1992.

154. Fu KK: Treatment of tumors of the nasopharynx: Radiation therapy. In Thawley SE, et al (eds): Comprehensive Management of Head and Neck Tumors, 2nd ed. Philadelphia, WB Saunders, 1999, pp 1479–1563.

155. Mesic JB, Fletcher GH, Goepfert H: Megavoltage irradiation of epithelial tumors of the nasopharynx. Int J Radiat Oncol Biol Phys 7:447–453, 1981.

156. Cooper JS, Lee H, Torrey M, et al: Improved outcome secondary to concurrent chemoradiotherapy for advanced carcinoma of the nasopharynx: Preliminary corroboration of the intergroup experience. Int J Radiat Oncol Biol Phys 47:861–866, 2000.

157. Wei WI, Lam KH, Ho CM, et al: Efficacy of radical neck dissection for the control of cervical metastasis after radiotherapy for nasopharyngeal carcinoma. Am J Surg 160:439–442, 1990.

158. Bumsted RM: Thyroid disease: A guide for the head and neck surgeon. Ann Otol Rhinol Laryngol Suppl 89:1–16, 1980.

159. Shaha AR, Shah JP, Loree TR: Patterns of nodal and distant metastasis based on histologic varieties in differentiated carcinoma of the thyroid. Am J Surg 172:692–694, 1996.

160. Grebe SK, Hay ID: Thyroid cancer nodal metastases: Biologic significance and therapeutic considerations. Surg Oncol Clin N Am 5:43–63, 1996.

161. Hughes CJ, Shaha AR, Shah JP, et al: Impact of lymph node metastasis in differentiated carcinoma of the thyroid: A matched-pair analysis. Head Neck 18:127–132, 1996.

162. Mazzaferri EL, Jhiang SM: Long-term impact of initial surgical and medical therapy on papillary and follicular thyroid cancer. Am J Med 97:418–428, 1994.

163. Mazzarotto R, Cesaro MG, Lora O, et al: The role of external beam radiotherapy in the management of differentiated thyroid cancer. Biomed Pharmacother 54:345–349, 2000.

164. Hallwirth U, Flores J, Kaserer K, et al: Differentiated thyroid cancer in children and adolescents: The importance of adequate surgery and review of literature. Eur J Pediatr Surg 9:359–363, 1999.

165. Gagel RF, Goepfert H, Callender DL: Changing concepts in the pathogenesis and management of thyroid carcinoma. CA Cancer J Clin 46:261–283, 1996.

166. Lallier M, St-Vil D, Giroux M, et al: Prophylactic thyroidectomy for medullary thyroid carcinoma in gene carriers of MEN2 syndrome. J Pediatr Surg 33:846–848, 1998.

167. Brandi ML, Gagel RF, Angeli A, et al: Guidelines for diagnosis and therapy of MEN type 1 and type 2. J Clin Endocrinol Metab 86:5658–5671, 2001.

168. Brierley J, Tsang R, Simpson WJ, et al: Medullary thyroid cancer: Analyses of survival and prognostic factors and the role of radiation therapy in local control. Thyroid 6:305–310, 1996.

169. Simpson WJ: Radioiodine and radiotherapy in the management of thyroid cancers. Otolaryngol Clin North Am 23:509–521, 1990.

170. Mcguirt WF: Management of occult metastatic disease from salivary gland neoplasms. Arch Otolaryngol Head Neck Surg 115:322–325, 1989.

171. Evans HL: Mucoepidermoid carcinoma of salivary glands: A study of 69 cases with special attention to histologic grading. Am J Clin Pathol 81:696–701, 1984.

172. Conley J, Dingman DL: Adenoid cystic carcinoma in the head and neck (cylindroma). Arch Otolaryngol 100:81–90, 1974.

173. Armstrong JG, Harrison LB, Thaler HT: The indications for elective treatment of the neck in cancer of the major salivary glands. Cancer 69:615–619, 1992.

174. Frankenthaler RA, Byers RM, Luna MA, et al: Predicting occult lymph node metastasis in parotid cancer. Arch Otolaryngol Head Neck Surg 119:517–520, 1993.

175. Frankenthaler RA, Luna MA, Lee SS, et al: Prognostic variables in parotid gland cancer. Arch Otolaryngol Head Neck Surg 117:1251–1256, 1991.

176. Krull A, Schwarz R, Brackrock S, et al: Neutron therapy in malignant salivary gland tumors: Results at European centers. Recent Results Cancer Res 150:88–99, 1998.

177. von Domarus H, Stevens PJ: Metastatic basal cell carcinoma. Report of five cases and review of 170 cases in the literature. J Am Acad Dermatol 10:1043–1060, 1984.

178. Randle HW: Basal cell carcinoma. Identification and treatment of the high-risk patient. Dermatol Surg 22:255–261, 1996.

179. Moller R, Reymann F, Hou-Jensen K: Metastases in dermatological patients with squamous cell carcinoma. Arch Dermatol 115:703–705, 1979.

180. Epstein E, Epstein NN, Bragg K, et al: Metastases from squamous cell carcinomas of the skin. Arch Dermatol 97:245–251, 1968.

181. Barksdale SK, O'Connor N, Barnhill R: Prognostic factors for cutaneous squamous cell and basal cell carcinoma. Determinants of risk of recurrence, metastasis, and development of subsequent skin cancers. Surg Oncol Clin N Am 6:625–638, 1997.

182. Rowe DE, Carroll RJ, Day CL Jr: Prognostic factors for local recurrence, metastasis, and survival rates in squamous cell carcinoma of the skin, ear, and lip. Implications for treatment modality selection. J Am Acad Dermatol 26:976–990, 1992.

183. Medina JE, Canfield V: Malignant melanoma of the head and neck. In Myers EN, Suen JY (eds): Cancer of the Head and Neck, 3rd ed. Philadelphia, WB Saunders, 1996, 160–183.

184. Weissmann A, Roses DF, Harris MN, et al: Prediction of lymph node metastases from the histologic features of primary cutaneous malignant melanomas. Am J Dermatopathol 6(suppl):35–41, 1984.

185. Fitzpatrick PJ, Brown TC, Reid J: Malignant melanoma of the head and neck: A clinicopathological study. Can J Surg 15:90–101, 1972.

186. Balch CM, Soong SJ, Bartolucci AA, et al: Efficacy of an elective regional lymph node dissection of 1 to 4 mm thick melanomas for patients 60 years of age and younger. Ann Surg 224:255–263, 1996.

187. Byers RM: Treatment of the neck in melanoma. Otolaryngol Clin North Am 31:833–839, 1998.

188. Goepfert H, Jesse RH, Ballantyne AJ: Posterolateral neck dissection. Arch Otolaryngol 106:618–620, 1980.

189. Ang KK, Byers RM, Peters LJ, et al: Regional radiotherapy as adjuvant treatment for head and neck melanoma. Preliminary results. Arch Otolaryngol Head Neck Surg 116:169–172, 1990.

190. Ang KK, Peters LH, Weber RS, et al: Postoperative radiotherapy for cutaneous melanoma of the head and neck region. Int J Radiat Oncol Biol Phys 30:795–798, 1994.

191. Wagner JD, Park HM, Coleman JJ 3rd, et al: Cervical sentinel lymph node biopsy for melanomas of the head and neck and upper thorax. Arch Otolaryngol Head Neck Surg 126:313–321, 2000.

192. Wells KE, Rapaport DP, Cruse CW, et al: Sentinel lymph node biopsy in melanoma of the head and neck. Plast Reconstr Surg 100:591–594, 1997.

193. Kirkwood JM, Strawderman MH, Ernstoff MS, et al: Interferon-alfa-2b adjuvant therapy of high risk resected cutaneous melanoma: The Eastern Cooperative Oncology Group Trial EST 1684. J Clin Oncol 14:7–17, 1996.

194. Kirkwood JM, Ibrahim JG, Sondak VK, et al: High- and low-dose interferon alfa-2b in high-risk melanoma: First analysis of intergroup trial E1690/S9111/C9190. J Clin Oncol 18:2444–2458, 2000.

Cancer of the Thyroid

Donald L. Bodenner
Randall L. Breau
James Y. Suen

INTRODUCTION

The uncommon nature and overall excellent prognosis of thyroid cancer have been both a blessing and a curse. Because of the low incidence and mortality, the large numbers of patients required to participate in prospective randomized clinical trials for optimal treatment strategies to be identified are not available. Consequently, these studies have not been performed and likely never will be. As a result, many widely accepted management practices are based on retrospective studies or case series, and the conclusions reached remain controversial. Nevertheless, a significant minority of patients with thyroid cancer will do poorly, with widespread disease refractory to all attempts at treatment. These circumstances place the treating physician in the uncomfortable position of deciding between often-conflicting management recommendations. In this chapter, we present many of these issues in light of the currently available evidence. In some situations, data are insufficient to warrant adopting one approach over another. In others, a consensus has developed regarding the optimal diagnostic or treatment approach.

SURGICAL ANATOMY OF THE THYROID GLAND

The head and neck surgeon must have a thorough knowledge of the surgical anatomy of the thyroid gland and its surrounding structures. The thyroid gland itself is composed of two lateral lobes, with a connecting bridge of tissue called the *isthmus*. Often, a finger-like projection of thyroid tissue, referred to as the *pyramidal lobe*, extends superiorly from this region. The posterior suspensory ligament (Berry's ligament) extends from the cricoid cartilage and the first tracheal ring to the posteromedial aspect of each thyroid lobe. It is frequently adherent in this area and is associated with arterial and venous plexuses or occasionally a branch of the inferior thyroid artery. The recurrent laryngeal nerve, with rare exceptions, courses deep to the ligament as it proceeds toward the larynx. In addition, thyroid tissue can often extend deep to the ligament and lateral to the recurrent laryngeal nerve, increasing the risk of damage to the nerve. Thyroid tissue in this area may be embedded in the ligament or otherwise difficult to remove, making a true total thyroidectomy difficult. This may account for the frequently found uptake of ^{131}I following a total thyroidectomy.[1]

Meticulous dissection and knowledge of vascular anatomy are necessary if a dry surgical field is to be maintained during surgical treatment of the thyroid gland. The superior thyroid artery arises as the first branch of the external carotid artery and enters the upper pole of the thyroid gland, usually in the anterior aspect. This artery may also send branches to the superior parathyroid gland before its entrance into the thyroid. The artery is important not only from a vascular standpoint but also because of its close relation to the superior laryngeal nerve. This relationship is highly variable, but most often the nerve courses superiorly and medially to the artery. The nerve also may be intertwined with branches of the artery; in this case, extensive caution is required when this area is dissected.

The inferior thyroid artery is a branch of the thyrocervical trunk and the second of the major arterial arteries supplying the thyroid gland. It is important for supplying both the thyroid and the parathyroid glands, and also because of its close association with the recurrent laryngeal nerve. The inferior thyroid artery passes deep to the carotid sheath and ascends anteriorly to a level above the inferior pole of the thyroid gland. Before entering at the midpoint in the gland, it frequently divides into several branches. Because of its close association with the recurrent laryngeal nerve and the importance of preserving the blood supply to the parathyroid glands, the inferior thyroid artery branches are ligated medially, close to their entrance into the thyroid lobe. Ligation of these branches is typically performed after exposure of the recurrent nerve by someone with knowledge of the location of the parathyroid glands.

Occasionally, a branch from the aorta or innominate artery will ascend in front of the trachea and supply the inferior portion of the thyroid gland. This artery, referred to as a thyroid ima artery, is more commonly found on the right side. Its origin is extremely variable, as is its size; it may be present in up to 10% of patients undergoing thyroidectomy.[1]

The recurrent laryngeal nerve is especially vulnerable to injury at several specific sites during thyroidectomy. The right recurrent laryngeal nerve leaves the vagus nerve at the base of the neck, loops around the subclavian artery, and then extends into the thyroid bed some 2 cm lateral to the trachea. Normally, the right nerve extends in a superiomedial direction to enter the larynx between the arch of the cricoid cartilage and the inferior cornu of the thyroid cartilage. The left recurrent laryngeal nerve leaves the vagus nerve at the level of the aortic arch, passing inferior and posterior to the arch, before extending into the tracheo-esophageal groove toward the larynx. The recurrent laryngeal nerve often branches before entering the larynx, with these branches in close association with the branches of the inferior thyroid artery. In most instances, the recurrent laryngeal nerve does not branch below the inferior thyroid artery. Therefore, identification of the nerve should be performed below this level. Rarely, and most often on the right side of the neck, a nonrecurrent nerve may extend off the vagus in the neck and enter the larynx directly. In this circumstance, there is usually an associated retroesophageal subclavian artery. Because this anomaly generally occurs on the right side, nonrecurrent laryngeal nerves are usually found on the right, except in cases of transposition of the great vessels.

The locations of the parathyroid glands vary somewhat but are predictable in most cases. Because of their embryologic migration, the parathyroid glands may be located anywhere from the level of the hyoid bone down into the mediastinum. The superior glands are the most consistent and are usually located on the undersurface of the thyroid gland, approximately 1 cm above the intersection of the recurrent laryngeal nerve and the inferior thyroid artery. These glands tend to lie posterior and medial to the recurrent laryngeal nerve and frequently within the fascia covering the thyroid gland between it and the thyroid capsule. Frequently a superior gland is found deep to the thyroid capsule, but only rarely are the superior parathyroids found entirely within the thyroid gland.[1] Of superior parathyroid glands, 12% may be located beneath the capsule of the thyroid; about 2% lie at the upper limits of the thyroid lobe; and only 0.8% are above this level. In up to 1% of cases, the superior parathyroid gland may be found in the retropharyngeal or retroesophageal space, and very occasionally (0.2%), superior parathyroids are located within the parenchyma of the gland itself.[2, 3]

The inferior parathyroid glands are much more variable in their anatomic location. They are usually located anterior and lateral to the recurrent laryngeal nerve. Of inferior parathyroid glands, 61% are located inferior, lateral, or posterior to the lower pole of the thyroid gland. They also may be located just inferior to the thyroid gland in close association with the cervical thymus (26%). They rarely extend their migration into the anterior mediastinum (0.5%). In less than 5% of cases, the inferior parathyroid glands are located above the intersection of the recurrent laryngeal nerve and the inferior thyroid artery.[2, 3]

◼ WELL-DIFFERENTIATED THYROID CANCER

Both papillary and follicular thyroid carcinoma originate from thyroid tissue and are often referred to together as well-differentiated thyroid cancer (WDTC). They share similar diagnostic and treatment algorithms and have an overall excellent prognosis when diagnosed early and treated appropriately.

Epidemiology

Thyroid nodules are extremely common. Imaging studies detect nodules in almost 50% of patients during middle age, and the prevalence increases linearly over time.[4] Clinically apparent thyroid cancer represents less than 1% of all cancers. The incidence of thyroid cancer varies widely around the world, ranging from 0.5 to 10 cases per 100,000 people.[5] Thyroid cancer is rare in children and adolescents, with a median age at diagnosis of 45 to 50 years. Thyroid carcinomas smaller than 1 cm are found incidentally at autopsy in up to 30% of adults.[6]

Between 75% and 85% of WDTCs are of the papillary type, with follicular cancer constituting the remainder.[7] Areas of the world in which the population has an adequate iodine intake have a slightly higher ratio of papillary to follicular carcinoma than do countries where iodine intake is low.[8] Approximately 3% of papillary carcinomas are familial.[9, 10]

Staging

Several staging methods have been devised for WDTC that identify disease characteristics helpful in managing care and in predicting outcomes. All of these systems incorporate size of the initial tumor, extension beyond the capsule of the thyroid gland, presence or absence of lymph node metastasis, distant metastasis, and age of the patient. The familiar tumor-node-metastasis (TNM) staging system is most widely applied (Table 19–1). Tumor size refers to the largest malignant lesion originating from the thyroid gland. Lymph nodes include regional lymphadenopathy in the neck and upper mediastinum. Metastatic lesions are those outside of the neck and upper mediastinum. Unlike with most cancers, the age of the patient at the time of diagnosis with thyroid cancer has a marked influence on outcome (Fig. 19–1). The TNM staging system reflects this by heavily weighting younger age toward a lower stage. Patients younger than

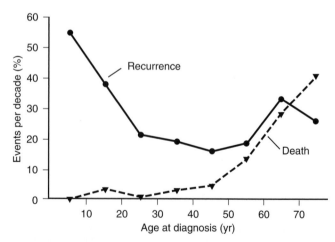

FIGURE 19–1 Tumor recurrence and cancer deaths according to patient age at the time of diagnosis. A total of 1355 patients were followed for a median of 15.7 years, with 79% papillary tumors and 21% follicular tumors. (Modified with permission by Excerpta Medica Inc. from Mazzaferri EL, Jhiang SM: Long-term impact of initial surgical and medical therapy on papillary and follicular thyroid cancer. Am J Med 97:418–428, 1994.)

TABLE 19-1 Definition of TNM for Papillary and Follicular Carcinoma

Primary Tumor (T)

Note: All categories may be subdivided: (a) solitary tumor, (b) multifocal tumor (the largest determines the classification).

TX   Primary tumor cannot be assessed
T0   No evidence of primary tumor
T1   Tumor 2 cm or less in greatest dimension limited to the thyroid
T2   Tumor more than 2 cm but not more than 4 cm in greatest dimension limited to the thyroid
T3   Tumor more than 4 cm in greatest dimension limited to the thyroid or any tumor with minimal extrathyroid extension (e.g., extension to sternothyroid muscle or perithyroid soft tissue)
T4a Tumor of any size extending beyond the thyroid capsule to invade subcutaneous soft tissues, larynx, trachea, esophagus, or recurrent laryngeal nerve
T4b Tumor invades prevertebral fascia or encases carotid artery or mediastinal vessels

All anaplastic carcinomas are considered T4 tumors.

T4a Intrathyroidal anaplastic carcinoma–surgically resectable
T4b Extrathyroidal anaplastic carcinoma–surgically unresectable

Regional Lymph Nodes (N)

Regional lymph nodes are the central compartment, lateral cervical, and upper mediastinal lymph nodes.

NX   Regional lymph nodes cannot be assessed.
N0   No regional lymph node metastatis
N1   Regional lymph node metastatis
N1a Metastasis to Level VI (pretracheal, paratracheal, and prelaryngeal/Delphian lymph nodes)
N1b Metastasis to unilateral, bilateral, or contralateral cervical or superior mediastinal lymph nodes

Distant Metastasis (M)

MX   Distant metastasis cannot be assessed
M0   No distant metastasis
M1   Distant metastasis

STAGE GROUPING

Separate stage groupings are recommended for papillary or follicular, medullary, and anaplastic (undifferentiated) carcinoma.

Papillary or Follicular
Under 45 years

Stage I	Any T	Any N	M0
Stage II	Any T	Any N	M1

Papillary or Follicular
45 years and older

Stage I	T1	N0	M0
Stage II	T2	N0	M0
Stage III	T3	N0	M0
	T1	N1a	M0
	T2	N1a	M0
	T3	N1a	M0
Stage IVA	T4a	N0	M0
	T4a	N1a	M0
	T1	N1b	M0
	T2	N1b	M0
	T3	N1b	M0
	T4a	N1b	M0
Stage IVB	T4b	Any N	M0
Stage IVC	Any T	Any N	M1

Used with the permission of the American Joint Committee on Cancer (AJCC), Chicago, Illinois. The original source for this material is the *AJCC Cancer Staging Manual, Sixth Edition* (2002) published by Springer-Verlag New York, www.springer-ny.com.

45 years are designated stage I despite large tumors or regional lymph node involvement and are assigned to stage II even with distant metastasis.

The clinical utility of the TNM staging system for estimating the prognosis of WDTC was evaluated in 700 patients.[11] Recurrence rates increased steadily with higher stage, as did mortality, with 1.7%, 15.8%, 30%, and 60.9% of patients dying of their disease in stages I through IV, respectively. Similar results were obtained in a series in which patients had a median follow-up of 15 years.[4]

Other staging systems incorporate the same essential variables, with modifications, that may be useful in determining prognosis in certain situations. The Mayo Clinic MACIS system is based on a score equal to the sum of numeric values assigned to several variables. The presence of *m*etastasis adds +3; *a*ge at diagnosis contributes +3.1 when the patient is younger than 40 years old, or 0.08 × age if the patient is older than 40 years; +1 if the resection was in*c*omplete; +1 for extrathyroidal *i*nvasion; and 0.3 × the initial tumor *s*ize.[12] These scores are divided into four groups, with group I consisting of patients with a score less than 6, group II including those with scores from 6.0 to 6.99, group III comprising those with scores of 7.0 to 7.99, and group IV including patients with scores of 8 or above. The 20-year mortality rate from thyroid cancer was statistically distinct between the groups and increased by group number, mortality being 1%, 11%, 44%, and 76% in groups I through IV, respectively.

Another method of staging thyroid cancer was developed at Ohio State University by a retrospective analysis of a series of 1355 patients.[13] Stage I patients were defined as those with tumors smaller than 1.5 cm. Stage II disease included tumors with any of the following characteristics: size between 1.5 and 4.4 cm, more than three intrathyroidal foci, or cervical metastasis. Patients with stage III disease had local tumor invasion or a tumor at least 4.5 cm. Patients with distant metastasis were classified as stage IV. Recurrence and mortality increased with higher stage. However, outcome was strongly influenced by factors not included in the staging method. Cancer-associated death was less in patients younger than 40 years of age and according to the extent of initial surgery. Radioiodine therapy reduced recurrence and cancer-related mortality by at least one half.

Each of the available staging systems has advantages and disadvantages. All indicate that age of the patient, tumor size, regional lymph node involvement, and distant metastasis have a strong impact on recurrence and prognosis. No statistically significant difference was found in a comparison of widely used staging systems for WDTC.[14] Thus, to ensure conformity in reporting and data collection, the TNM system of classification has been suggested as a standard.[15] Nevertheless, the prognosis of the individual patient will be affected by other factors, such as extension of the tumor through the thyroid capsule, or the presence of an aggressive type of WDTC such as the tall cell variant of papillary thyroid cancer. More extensive treatment or follow-up may be necessary when these variables are identified.

Prognosis and Risk Stratification

The overall prognosis of thyroid cancer is generally excellent. Several staging classifications have been developed to help clinicians in estimating prognosis (see under Staging). Certain patient and tumor characteristics are associated with a higher recurrence rate and risk of mortality. Foremost is patient age. Younger patients have less than a 2% to 3% long-term mortality, whereas up to 20% of middle-aged patients die of their disease. Mortality and recurrence markedly increase for patients older than 45 to 50 years of age. In the elderly, the mortality rate is even higher, approaching 40% if thyroid cancer is diagnosed over the age of 70.[16]

Size is also a strong predictor of a poorer outcome. Overall, patients with lesions smaller than 1.5 cm have a 5% to 10% risk of recurrence and a mortality rate less than 3%. If the tumor is larger than 4 cm, the recurrence rate increases to as high as 40%, and the mortality to as high as 20% of patients.[16] Follicular thyroid cancer has been shown in some, but not all, studies to pose an independent risk for poor outcome. The discrepancy may be secondary to the fact that follicular thyroid cancer typically occurs in patients of an older age group.[13]

Pathogenesis

Intensive research into thyrocyte signaling pathways has provided several clues and insights into events leading to dedifferentiation and carcinogenesis of thyroid tissue. Early events in this process can generally be viewed as either mutational activation of a protein within a mitogenic pathway, or mutational deactivation of proteins that function as repressors of cascades that induce proliferation and dedifferentiation. Thyroid hormone induces proliferation and differentiation of the thyrocyte through the thyroid-stimulating hormone (TSH) receptor/adenyl cyclase/protein kinase A pathway. Activating mutations of TSH receptors or the stimulatory G-proteins (Gs) have been identified in some toxic adenomas[17, 18] and in hyperfunctioning nodules in a multinodular goiter,[19] but as expected with activation of adenyl cyclase, these tumors are rarely malignant. Their biologic behavior is indistinguishable from that of toxic adenomas without a TSH receptor mutation.[20]

The tyrosine kinase receptor/RAS/mitogen-activated protein kinase pathway[21] triggers proliferation but also promotes loss of differentiation. Activation of this pathway can occur through mutation of any of several elements within the signaling cascade. Mutations of two tyrosine kinase receptors—RET and TRK—have been implicated as primary events in the development of papillary carcinoma.[22–24] Genetic rearrangement of the genes encoding these receptors results in a gene product in which the tyrosine kinase domain becomes fused to another protein, leading to dysregulation of the enzymatic activity of the kinase. The constitutive activity of the mutant hybrid receptors leads to uncontrolled growth and oncogenesis. Validation of this concept was demonstrated by the induction of papillary carcinoma in transgenic mice that overexpress the RET gene.[25, 26] It is interesting to note that TSH promoted the growth of the transgene-induced papillary carcinoma, possibly explaining the increased incidence[27, 28] and virulence[29–31] of WDTC in Graves' disease as observed by some investigators.

Clinically, the level of rearranged RET gene expression within papillary thyroid cancer correlates with increased virulence in some studies.[32–34] RET gene rearrangements may be associated with radiation exposure and have been detected in papillary cancers in children from Chernobyl.[35–37] The measurement of RET rearrangement has also been used as an aid in the diagnosis of papillary thyroid carcinoma. Rearranged RET was measured by reverse transcription polymerase chain reaction (RT-PCR) and was detected in 17 of 33 fine-needle aspirations (FNAs) performed on lesions that proved at surgery to be papillary thyroid carcinoma.[38] The presence of rearranged RET correctly identified papillary thyroid cancer in 15 specimens that were otherwise believed to be indeterminate or inadequate by routine cytologic analysis of the FNA biopsy specimen. There were no false-positives. Through an improved assay system, 85% of papillary carcinomas and no benign thyroid tissue samples were recently found to be positive for RET rearrangements.[39]

The RET rearrangement found in papillary cancer is highly specific and should not be confused with the RET mutations characteristic of familial forms of medullary thyroid carcinoma (discussed later). For example, RET rearrangements were found in 19% of 177 papillary carcinomas but in none of 109 other thyroid neoplasms that included medullary thyroid carcinoma.[40]

Mutation of RAS, a downstream component of the tyrosine kinase receptor/RAS/mitogen-activated protein kinase pathway, has been implicated in a variety of thyroid cancers.[41] These mutations constitutively activate the signal cascade, stimulate cell growth and loss of differentiation, and promote genetic instability. RAS mutations have been found in anaplastic,[41] follicular,[42] and papillary[43] thyroid carcinomas. Unlike RET mutations, RAS mutations have been found in benign follicular adenomas,[41] suggesting that RAS mutations occur early in the pathogenesis of follicular cancers.[44]

Inactivating mutations of the p53 tumor suppressor gene are rare in differentiated thyroid carcinoma but are commonly found in anaplastic thyroid carcinoma, suggesting that impaired p53 function may contribute to the undifferentiated and highly aggressive phenotype of these tumors.[45–48] Reintroduction of wild-type p53 has been shown to increase the sensitivity of anaplastic thyroid carcinoma cell lines to doxorubicin hydrochloride (Adriamycin) therapy[49, 50] and to induce the reexpression of TSH and thyroglobulin proteins associated with the differentiated state.[51] p53 mutations have been identified in WDTCs that years later undergo anaplastic dedifferentiation, and there is some evidence that this dedifferentiation is associated with radioiodine therapy.[52, 53] Others, however, have demonstrated no evidence of p53 mutation until after dedifferentiation occurred.[54–56] Loss of expression of other tumor suppressor genes seen in many types of cancer, including the p16 gene, is less commonly found in follicular and papillary thyroid carcinomas.[57]

Pathology

On gross pathologic examination, papillary carcinomas are often nonencapsulated and have a granular cut surface. They also often display foci of calcification and minor cystic changes. Microscopically, papillary thyroid carcinoma is characterized by intranuclear inclusions and grooves that are formed by invaginations of cytoplasm into the nucleus. The cell nuclei often overlap and have a ground glass or clear appearance. Chronic inflammatory cells can be observed in and around the tumor. Fibrosis can occur in an irregular pattern, and areas of dense fibrosis can frequently be identified.[58] Cytologic smears contain pronounced cellularity and tight clusters of neoplastic cells in a papillary arrangement. Nuclear grooves are infrequent, whereas intranuclear inclusions are often observed.

Variants of Papillary Carcinoma. Several histologic variants of papillary carcinoma have been recorded. The follicular variant has a histologic pattern of neoplastic follicles that can constitute up to 70% of the cellular material. The follicles are small and contain little colloid. Smears obtained after FNA are markedly cellular with small follicles that contain relatively fewer intranuclear inclusions or psammoma bodies. Biologic behavior and outcome are similar to the classic pattern of papillary thyroid carcinoma. The sclerosing variant of papillary carcinoma presents with little epithelium, dense fibrotic tissue, patchy infiltration, and abundant psammoma bodies.[59] It typically occurs in younger individuals and has a propensity to spread to cervical lymph nodes; in some studies, it carries a worse prognosis.[60, 61] The tall cell variant is defined as neoplastic cells in which the height is twice the width. These tumors are often large and contain extensive papillary structures.[62] The tall cell variant is uncommon, representing less than 5% of all papillary carcinomas.[63] It has a poor prognosis with frequent metastasis and early recurrence.[62–64] The columnar cell variant of papillary carcinoma is very rare, with only 24 reported cases. It is similar to the tall cell variant except that the height of the cells is three times the width. Other major differences are that the nuclei are stratified and the cytoplasm is clear.[65, 66] This rare variant has an aggressive course and a poor prognosis in the majority of cases studied.[66, 67]

Follicular Thyroid Carcinomas. Follicular thyroid carcinomas lack the nuclear features seen in papillary carcinoma. Grossly, these cancers are often thickly encapsulated with cystic changes and focal necrosis.[37] Cells of follicular carcinoma are small and monotonous, with central nucleoli and round nuclei. Papillae and psammoma bodies are rare, and the cells are organized into follicles that contain sparse colloid. Fine-needle aspirates of these tumors yield follicular cells arranged in microfollicles, rosettes, or spindles with little colloid present. These findings also occur in benign follicular neoplasms, and it is currently impossible to differentiate between the two on a cytopathologic basis. Only identification of capsular or vascular invasion after careful examination of multiple sections postoperatively can differentiate between benign and malignant follicular tumors.[68, 69]

Hürthle Cell Carcinoma. Hürthle cell carcinoma is a variant of follicular carcinoma; it accounts for 3% to 5% of all thyroid carcinomas and is composed of large acidophilic or oncocytic cells.[70] These tumors typically do not take up radioactive iodine as well as follicular carcinoma does, and they generally have a slightly worse prognosis than follicular carcinoma.[71, 72] As with more typical follicular lesions, the diagnosis of Hürthle cell carcinoma can be made only after surgical resection and permanent section pathologic analysis of the entire gland have been performed.

Insular or Poorly Differentiated Carcinoma. Although included as a variant of follicular carcinoma by the World Health Organization (WHO), insular or poorly differentiated carcinoma lacks the typical morphology associated with papillary or follicular carcinoma.[73] Only rare follicular structures are seen with limited staining for thyroglobulin. Cells are arranged in trabeculae or islands of cells separated by connective tissue. This cancer is rare, with 228 cases reported before 1996.[74] Although insular thyroid carcinomas frequently take up radioactive iodine,[74, 75] they are aggressive and have a mortality rate much higher than other forms of WDTC. One of the first reports of 25 patients described a high incidence of local invasion, with 44% of patients dead

of disease by 8 years.[76] In one recent series of 28 cases, the mortality rate was 46%.[77]

Evaluation of a Thyroid Nodule

Thyroid nodules are exceedingly common.[4] They are found more often in women and increase in prevalence with advancing age.[78] However, thyroid cancer is relatively uncommon and is found in only approximately 5% of thyroid nodules.[4, 79, 80] Despite numerous studies and published recommendations,[4, 78, 81–83] the optimal approach to and management of a thyroid nodule remain controversial. For example, the members of the European Thyroid Association were recently questioned regarding their evaluation of a solitary 2 × 3-cm thyroid nodule in a 42-year-old woman. Although 99% performed FNA, additional tests would have included a nuclear imaging study (66%), a thyroid ultrasound (80%), and measurement of thyroid autoantibodies (47%).[84] Despite a benign diagnosis on FNA, 23% recommended surgical removal.

History and Physical Examination

The initial physical examination and history often provide important information. A family history of thyroid cancer is important in that the hereditary nature of WDTC is well established.[85, 86] Inquiring about a history of radiation exposure, particularly during childhood, is extremely important because thyroid nodules are associated with radiation exposure in a linear fashion, up to approximately 1800 cGy.[87] Furthermore, radiation treatment of cutaneous hemangioma,[88] adenotonsillar hypertrophy,[89] and acne[90] has been associated with an increased risk of thyroid cancer. Children and adolescents have a particularly increased risk of neoplastic changes from external beam radiation.[91] In patients who received such radiation treatments in childhood, the risk of developing thyroid nodules approaches 30%, and up to 40% of these nodules are malignant.[89, 92] A majority of these are papillary thyroid cancer with a prognosis similar to that associated with papillary thyroid carcinoma arising in a nonirradiated gland.[93, 94] The risk of thyroid cancer following irradiation appears to peak after 30 years of exposure but remains elevated even 40 years after the event.[95]

Considerable controversy has arisen regarding the management of patients with a history of radiation exposure to the neck. Irradiated thyroid glands often are multinodular, and thyroid cancer is often found incidentally at surgery in a lesion not originally suspected as cancerous.[96] This, coupled with an up to 40% risk of malignancy, has led some to remove all nodular thyroid glands with a history of childhood radiation. On the other hand, papillary cancers are predominantly encountered with little change in their virulence compared with the classic form of the disease. Therefore, others propose close follow-up with FNA of the dominant nodules, as is practiced in the management of multinodular goiter.[89, 97] However, surgery is preferred with multiple lesions greater than 1.5 cm owing to the inherent difficulty in performing multiple biopsies and the increased likelihood of malignancy.[98]

A history of rapidly growing nodules with the development of hoarseness and chronic pain markedly increases the likelihood of malignancy. The sudden onset of pain, however, suggests a benign process, usually hemorrhage into a benign cyst or subacute viral thyroiditis.[99] In particular, hoarseness from recurrent laryngeal nerve involvement and the presence of a thyroid mass are strongly suggestive of the presence of thyroid cancer. The age and sex of the patient are also important diagnostic variables. Up to 24% of nodules in patients younger than 20 years of age will be malignant,[100] and males have a two- to threefold higher risk of malignancy than females.[79, 101, 102] The presence of these clinical findings obviously does not indicate that immediate surgery is in order; however, if any subsequent equivocation is noted in the cytopathologic diagnosis, these findings may be helpful in the decision of whether to remove a suspicious nodule.

Clinical signs and symptoms of thyroid dysfunction should be noted. Hyperthyroidism, as evidenced by tremor, weight loss, heat intolerance, or palpitations, holds out the possibility that the nodule may be a benign toxic adenoma. If these clinical findings are supported by biochemical evidence of hyperthyroidism, a thyroid scan before FNA is indicated to confirm the diagnosis. Toxic adenomas are almost always benign,[103] although thyroid carcinoma and toxic adenoma have been reported in the same gland.[78, 104–106] Most investigators believe that FNA under these circumstances is unnecessary for diagnostic purposes; however, a negative biopsy result can often be reassuring to the patient.

Laboratory Evaluation

Laboratory testing on the initial visit should consist only of a TSH and free thyroxine (T_4). A TSH level that is lower than the detectable assay limits in the laboratory employed indicates hyperthyroidism, and toxic adenoma should be ruled out. Nodularity of the thyroid is not uncommon in Graves' disease, and occasionally, undiagnosed patients are referred for evaluation. FNA is unnecessary if a homogeneous uptake is observed on the thyroid scan. However, up to 19% of cold thyroid nodules in a patient with Graves' disease are malignant.[27, 28] The virulence of these carcinomas is controversial, with some[29–31] but not all[106–109] investigators having shown these cancers to be more aggressive with a higher mortality rate than cancers found in patients without Graves' disease. Consequently, some recommend surgery for all patients with Graves' disease and a cold nodule in the thyroid gland.[28] We recommend that cold nodules in patients with Graves' disease initially undergo FNA under ultrasound guidance. Anything but a satisfactory sample with benign cytology should prompt surgical removal of the diseased lobe.

A high TSH level indicates thyroid failure and is often found in nodular goiters associated with Hashimoto's thyroiditis, which is a chronic autoimmune-mediated destruction of the thyroid gland. The presence of Hashimoto's thyroiditis is associated with neither an increased nor a decreased risk of WDTC[110]; the measurement of serum markers of this process, antithyroglobulin and antimicrosomal (TPO) antibodies, is therefore unwarranted. The exception is a rapidly growing nodule in a patient with Hashimoto's thyroiditis, which must be evaluated as a possible lymphoma (see under Lymphoma of the Thyroid). Hypothyroid patients with Hashimoto's thyroiditis require levothyroxine supplementation, and because the condition is often progressive, TSH levels should be assessed at regular intervals and levothyroxine dosage adjusted accordingly. Routine measurement of thyroglobulin levels is not indicated in the evaluation of a thyroid nodule. Thyroglobulin levels significantly overlap in patients with and without cancer before thyroidectomy; levels are often elevated in a variety of benign processes.

Imaging Studies

For decades, a thyroid scan using ^{123}I or Tc99m-labeled pertechnetate was the initial step in the evaluation of a thyroid nodule. These isotopes are taken up by normally functioning thyroid tissue, but only rarely are they taken up by thyroid cancers. Thus a "cold nodule" carries an increased risk of malignancy and was either biopsied or resected without further evaluation. However, benign lesions such as colloid nodules, cysts, and nodules in thyroid glands affected by Hashimoto's thyroiditis also appear cold with imaging and constitute the great majority of all cold nodules. Therefore, a cold nodule on thyroid scan is benign in the majority of cases, and the thyroid scan adds little diagnostic information. The argument can be made that scans are useful in detecting a nodule with increased metabolic activity, considered "hot" on scan, because these nodules are malignant far less often than are cold nodules.[4, 82] Among Europeans and other relatively iodine-deficient populations, this may be reasonable when the prevalence of hot nodules approaches 10%. In the United States, however, the prevalence is very low—in some series, 3% or less.[111] Therefore, 100 scans would be required to prevent one to three unnecessary FNAs. The ease, relatively low cost, and minimal discomfort of FNA have made the initial use of thyroid scans cost-ineffective; they should be reserved for use only in identification of a toxic adenoma when a follicular lesion has been identified by FNA (see under Fine-Needle Aspiration Biopsy).

Thyroid ultrasound is often obtained before FNA is performed. Current generations of ultrasound instruments have enhanced many aspects of the evaluation of a thyroid nodule. Improved resolution allows the accurate characterization and follow-up of lesions, but it also identifies many small nodules that are of little clinical significance and do not require further evaluation. Attempts have been made to use several sonographic characteristics of thyroid nodules as predictors of malignancy. These include the intensity of the echo, the presence of calcifications or a hypoechoic "halo," and the degree of encapsulation.[112–114] Malignant lesions are more hypoechoic, but their overlap with benign lesions is considerable. Likewise, the appearance of a lucent halo around a lesion is not specific enough to be helpful.[113]

The calcification pattern within a nodule can be useful in some situations. Rim or eggshell calcification is usually associated with a chronic, benign lesion. Large, scattered calcifications are seen in both malignant and benign nodules, whereas small, punctate calcifications are often associated with papillary carcinoma of the thyroid. With patients in whom there is diagnostic uncertainty regarding FNA results, these characteristics may influence the decision for or against surgery. Usually, however, these sonographic criteria overlap substantially between benign and malignant lesions and should not be exclusively relied on.[115] It should be added, however, that some investigators have recently used a constellation of sonographic criteria and have reported a sensitivity and a specificity of ultrasound alone that approach those of FNA.[116]

Ultrasound has significantly improved the diagnostic yield of FNA.[117–119] The beveled edge of the biopsy needle strongly reflects ultrasound and is clearly visible. The needle tip can be placed to within millimeters of the desired location, either freehand or with the use of a needle guide. FNA of small nodules and posterior lesions can therefore be performed with confidence.[120] This improved accuracy allows for effective sampling of several dominant nodules in a multinodular gland and is exceedingly helpful in assessing changes in the size of benign nodules to within 2 mm. Ultrasound is also particularly useful for sampling the solid component of a cystic nodule.[121]

Computed tomography (CT) and magnetic resonance imaging (MRI) are occasionally used before FNA in the evaluation of a thyroid nodule. They are most commonly employed as a complement to ultrasound in delineating thyroid architecture and evaluating substernal extension of a goiter. The major disadvantage of CT compared with MRI is the administration of iodine-containing contrast agents that prohibit the use of radioactive iodine for at least 8 weeks. MRI has been reported to differentiate benign and malignant lesions with relative accuracy, but these studies need further validation.[122] In general, MRI and CT imaging add little to the initial diagnosis of a thyroid nodule and should be reserved for patients in whom anatomic detail will aid in refining the surgical approach.

Fine-Needle Aspiration Biopsy

FNA is now accepted as the first procedure to be performed in the evaluation of a thyroid nodule after physical examination and laboratory determination of thyroid function have been completed. In multiple series, the sensitivity and specificity are greater than 90%, with some investigators reporting values close to 100%.[121, 123–126] FNA of the thyroid has decreased the number of unnecessary surgical procedures by 30% to 50% and has reduced the cost of diagnosis substantially.[127–129] Several caveats are associated with these remarkable results.

FNA is highly operator dependent, and as expected, the studies reporting extremely good results were conducted in institutions that perform hundreds of FNAs every year. Nondiagnostic samples increase, and sensitivity and specificity drop off dramatically, when practitioners perform the procedure infrequently. It is highly recommended that an individual perform at least 30 FNAs per year to remain competent in the procedure. A cytopathologist experienced in interpreting FNAs is also crucial to successful diagnosis. Close communication between the cytopathologist and the surgeon is extremely important; in small institutions with limited experience, a second opinion may be helpful in difficult cases.

FNA is relatively painless and complications are rare.[130] Slight bruising may occur approximately 20% of the time, and infection is extremely uncommon. Because of the small needle bore, serious bleeding is rarely seen, even after inadvertent puncture of a major vessel.[130] A few minutes of pressure is usually all that is required to stop the bleeding. The risk of bleeding is increased in patients who take anticoagulants, but

it is unnecessary to discontinue therapy before FNA is performed. These patients may require pressure over the biopsy site for 5 to 10 minutes, and observation in the waiting room for 30 to 60 minutes is recommended. The only major complication of FNA is the occurrence of bleeding into the nodule with esophageal or tracheal compression. All patients should be instructed to immediately report rapid enlargement of the nodule, choking sensations, or difficulty in breathing.

A variety of techniques are used to perform FNA, yet no good evidence indicates that one method is superior to another. Extensive sterile procedure is unnecessary. Swabbing with alcohol is sufficient, but care should be taken to allow the alcohol to completely evaporate so that burning sensations from the biopsy can be prevented. The use of sterile gloves is common, but some investigators feel that this also is unnecessary; increased rates of infection have not been reported when sterile gloves are not used.

The patient is typically positioned supine with the neck extended, but others prefer the patient to be sitting. A 25- or 21-gauge needle is most commonly used, and larger-bore biopsies should be avoided (this technique increases the risk of bleeding and does not improve diagnostic yield[131, 132]). Both open-bore syringes without applied suction and biopsy by syringe guns with negative pressure are common. Many physicians believe that suction produces a bloody specimen that hinders interpretation, but there is little evidence to support this contention. Conversely, others believe suction is important for maximizing the cellularity of the sample. If suction is employed, it should be discontinued before the needle is withdrawn. A common compromise is to perform several biopsies without suction and to reserve negative pressure for the final stick. Almost all agree, however, that a needle with a clear hub should be used and that the needle should be withdrawn when the first flash of blood is seen, regardless of whether suction is used. The sample should be immediately applied to a microscope slide and smeared with a coverslip or a second slide. Half of the samples should be air-dried and the other half immediately fixed. Diff-Quik is a common stain for air-dried samples, and fixed samples are stained with Papanicolaou stain. We commonly collect residual material from the needle by flushing with fixative and then cytospinning the preparation. The cellular material often yields additional diagnostic information. Fluid aspirated during FNA can be sent to the laboratory to be spun down and examined.

The cytologic results of the examination of an FNA fall into four main categories: benign, insufficient, indeterminate or suspicious, and malignant. Typical benign lesions include Hashimoto's thyroiditis and colloid nodules. Lymphocytes, occasional giant cells, Hürthle cells, and variable amounts of colloid characterize Hashimoto's thyroiditis. Benign colloid nodules include copious amounts of colloid and groups of benign-appearing follicular cells.

The reported percentage of insufficient samples varies from less than 1% to 25%.[133, 134] This wide range reflects the skill of the physician performing the FNA and also the cytologic criteria used to assess sufficiency. However, even physicians with considerable experience may obtain insufficient samples in up to one of five FNAs performed.[133] No criteria have been universally adopted for judging the adequacy of the FNA specimen. Some institutions require a total of five clusters of follicular cells for the entire procedure,[135] whereas others require up to 10 groups on each of two different slides.[130] It is often worthwhile to discuss criteria for sufficiency with the cytopathologist and to periodically review the number of insufficient samples obtained by individuals performing FNA. Simple adjustments in technique or the use of additional passes may improve sample sufficiency and reduce the need for repeat FNAs. FNA under ultrasound guidance has been reported to significantly decrease the number of insufficient samples and adds relatively little to the cost of the procedure.[118, 119]

Both the definition and the management of nodules that yield an insufficient sample remain controversial.[4, 82, 119, 134, 136] Some maintain that an insufficient specimen from a thyroid nodule suggests a lower potential for malignancy and recommend medical management.[134, 137, 138] However, in several studies, nodules that yielded insufficient samples were malignant up to 9% of the time.[139, 140] We recommend aggressive follow-up for nodules with insufficient cytology. Repeat FNA, which should be the initial step, is successful in obtaining an adequate sample 50% of the time.[141] If the reaspiration is again insufficient, a third attempt under ultrasound guidance may yet yield a diagnosis. If the biopsy remains insufficient after three attempts, a surgical approach is recommended.

A malignant FNA result most commonly indicates papillary carcinoma and its variants. Papillary fronds are virtually pathognomonic for the diagnosis. Nuclear inclusions and grooves are highly suggestive, but these features can be seen occasionally in biopsies from Hashimoto's thyroiditis. Follicular cells grouped into microfollicular architecture with scant colloid mark an indeterminate FNA. Indeterminate FNAs result from both follicular cancer and benign follicular lesions such as follicular neoplasm or hyperplastic nodules. Unfortunately, no cytologic criteria can definitively classify these follicular aspirates as benign or malignant. The diagnosis of follicular cancer can be made only after the tumor has been resected and vascular or capsular invasion has been identified. Often, this is not apparent on frozen section and must await final pathology. Of special note, however, are toxic adenomas that also yield follicular pattern on cytology but can be identified by thyroid scan. Most but not all investigators believe these nodules are virtually always benign and do not require resection.

It is not uncommon for small toxic adenomas or those early in their development that appear hot on scan to fail to suppress the TSH level or to produce clinical thyrotoxicosis. Therefore, a thyroid scan is recommended for all patients with an indeterminate follicular FNA. These issues are summarized in an algorithm for the approach to a thyroid nodule (Fig. 19–2).

Other Considerations in the Evaluation of Thyroid Nodules

Several unresolved issues remain regarding the best approach to management of a patient with a thyroid nodule. First, is there a minimal size of a palpable nodule above which a biopsy is indicated? Second, what are the indications for FNA of an "occult nodule" identified by imaging of the neck performed for other purposes? Third, what is the

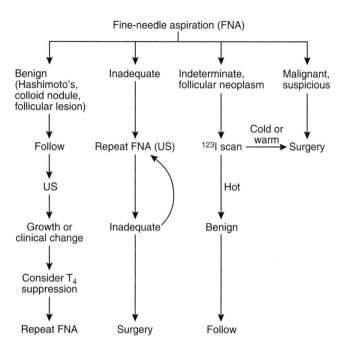

FIGURE 19–2 Algorithm for the evaluation of a thyroid nodule. (US, ultrasound.)

optimal approach for nodules within a multinodular gland? Fourth, what is the optimal diagnostic algorithm and treatment of thyroid cysts? Fifth, what is the appropriate follow-up for nodules judged benign by initial FNA?

Decision to Perform Biopsy. Most physicians biopsy all palpable nodules in a euthyroid patient, regardless of age. The decision to biopsy an occult nodule is more difficult. Nodules are extremely common, increasing almost linearly with age, so that by the age of 50 years, approximately 5% of patients have palpable thyroid nodule, and 30% to 50% have nodules apparent on ultrasound or other imaging modalities.[4] It is therefore impractical to biopsy every nodule identified by imaging performed for unrelated purposes. The size of a nodule is the selection criterion used most often for further evaluation by FNA. WDTC smaller than 1.5 cm has an overall excellent prognosis. Therefore, although recommendations vary, occult nodules larger than 1.5 cm should be biopsied with ultrasound guidance if necessary. Nodules smaller than 1.5 cm should be periodically followed by palpation or by ultrasound examination, initially at 6- to 9-month intervals for several years, and then yearly thereafter.[142] Although growth of a nodule does not correlate with malignancy in some studies,[143] we believe (1) that if no growth is noted on two sequential ultrasound examinations, then the interval can be further increased, and (2) that rapid growth of the nodule at any time warrants immediate FNA.

Approach to a Nodule Within a Multinodular Goiter. The management approach to a nodule within a multinodular goiter (MNG) has also evolved over time. Historically, the overall risk of malignancy was believed to be lower in an MNG than in a solitary nodule.[144, 145] This assumption has been challenged by several recent studies.[146–148] The most convincing of these is a study in which FNA was performed on more than 1500 nodules found in unselected sequential patients. The incidence of malignancy in solitary nodules

(4.7%) was not statistically different from that found in dominant nodules in an MNG (4.1%).[79] No agreement has been reached on the definition of a dominant nodule. Many physicians use the 1.5-cm cut-off proposed for occult nodules, whereas others use 2 cm, with the belief that an overwhelming number of nodules would be biopsied if these criteria were strictly applied to all MNGs (particularly if ultrasound is employed).

The follow-up of a solitary nodule or a dominant nodule in an MNG following a benign FNA is controversial. As was discussed earlier, the sensitivity and specificity of FNA are excellent in the experienced hands of a cytopathologist trained in FNA interpretation. Therefore, routine re-biopsy of a nodule after an FNA with benign cytology is rarely helpful.[149–152] Nonetheless, if the nodule continues to grow or if questions arise concerning the diagnostic accuracy of the FNA, a second biopsy is indicated.

Prevention of Future Growth of a Nodule or an MNG. Another controversial management issue is the prevention of future growth of a nodule or an MNG. Levothyroxine therapy in doses sufficient to reduce the TSH level to between .03 and 0.1 μIU/mL is commonly employed to shrink nodules, but the efficacy of this approach is extremely controversial. Little is known about the natural history of nodules, and few randomized studies have been performed to evaluate the efficacy of suppression therapy. Ultrasonography was used to follow patients with solitary nodules receiving suppressive L-thyroxine therapy, and the results were reported in three nonrandomized studies. Response rates varied widely from 34% to 56%.[153–155] Similar results were obtained in attempts to use suppression therapy to shrink nodules in an MNG[156] or to prevent new nodule occurrence.[157]

Much of this variability may stem from our general lack of knowledge concerning the natural history of thyroid nodules. In one study in which patients with a thyroid nodule were followed for an average of 15 years without therapy, 53% of nodules spontaneously decreased in size, with 11% of the total no longer seen by ultrasound. Only 13% of untreated nodules increased in size over the follow-up period.[158] The risks of suppression have not been well quantified in this setting; however, it is known that levothyroxine suppression of the TSH level below the detectable limits of standard assays results in a threefold increase in the incidence of atrial fibrillation[159] and a clinically significant reduction in the bone mineral density of postmenopausal women.[160]

With the uncertainties involved in estimating the future growth of a particular nodule and the limited efficacy of current therapy, several experienced clinicians advise against routine thyroid hormone suppression.[161, 162] An alternative conservative approach is to follow the size of the nodule or MNG by yearly ultrasound examinations and to institute suppressive therapy only if a gradual increase in size is seen. A relatively brief trial of thyroid hormone treatment for patients with mild obstructive symptoms such as dysphagia or dyspnea may be attempted, but improvement is uncommon. Patients with moderate to severe obstructive symptoms or rapid growth despite benign FNA results should proceed to surgery. Thyroid hormone suppression therapy is empirical, with the initial levothyroxine dose

between 75 and 125 μg per day, adjusted by 0.025 mg every 4 to 6 weeks until the desired TSH level is reached. If no response is observed within 4 to 6 months, therapy should be discontinued.

An alternative to thyroid hormone suppression of a benign MNG is treatment with radioactive iodide. Several recent studies show that administration of between 50 and 100 mCi reduces the size of an MNG by as much as 60%.[163, 164] Radiation thyroiditis is relatively common but manageable with acetaminophen or nonsteroidal anti-inflammatory drugs (NSAIDs). Dyspnea is extremely uncommon, even in substernal goiter,[165] and steroid therapy is rarely necessary.

Treatment of Thyroid Cysts. Thyroid cysts can pose difficult management decisions. Simple cysts are those that contain only fluid and are almost always benign. However, these are uncommon, representing as few as 1% of all cystic lesions.[78] A majority of cysts contain septations or other cellular material and are called *complex thyroid cysts.* The risk of malignancy in a complex cyst has approached 10% to 15% in several studies.[166, 167] Undoubtedly, there is a component of referral bias in these reports, but the risk of malignancy in all likelihood at least approaches that of a solitary nodule.

Diagnostic FNA of complex cysts is often difficult, and the cystic fluid obtained by aspiration is rarely helpful to the cytopathologist. A common approach is to aspirate the cyst dry, then biopsy the residual tissue. Several practical difficulties characterize this approach. When the FNA is performed by palpation, septated cysts are often difficult to drain completely. Moreover, after fluid has been removed with the first few passes, the residual tissue may be difficult to localize. Ultrasound-guided FNA is often helpful under these conditions. After drainage is complete, tissue in the wall of the cyst can be easily visualized and biopsied. Given that the risk of malignancy is similar to that associated with a solitary thyroid nodule, repeated FNAs are indicated if initial specimens are inadequate. Occasionally, repeated FNAs will be nondiagnostic, especially if the fluid recurs and the FNA is performed by palpation. In such cases, FNA under ultrasound guidance or surgical removal is appropriate. Injection of cysts with sclerosing agents is advocated by some,[168–170] but painful extravasation of sclerosing agents and occasional damage to the recurrent laryngeal nerve have limited widespread acceptance of this approach.[169]

Treatment of Well-Differentiated Thyroid Cancer

Medical Treatment for Thyroid Cancer

POSTOPERATIVE ^{131}I ABLATION

Ablation of residual thyroid tissue with ^{131}I following near-total thyroidectomy facilitates optimal follow-up. Subsequent radioiodine total body scan (TBS) will not be hindered by residual activity in the neck, and the absence of thyroglobulin production by normal thyroid tissue allows for sensitive detection of recurrence. ^{131}I ablation may also destroy occult metastatic lesions within the thyroid remnant or regional lymph nodes. There is considerable evidence that ^{131}I ablation significantly reduces the risk of recurrence and perhaps mortality (Fig. 19–3). In a retrospective study of 269 patients with papillary thyroid cancer, radioiodine

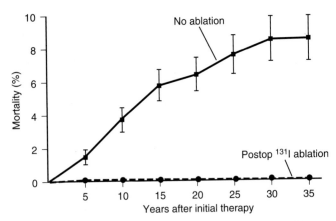

FIGURE 19–3 Effects of postoperative radioactive iodine ablation on mortality in well-differentiated thyroid cancer. Patients with stage II or stage III disease were treated either with (n = 350) or without (n = 802) [131]I after total or subtotal thyroidectomy. (Modified with permission by Excerpta Medica Inc. from Mazzaferri EL, Jhiang SM: Long-term impact of initial surgical and medical therapy on papillary and follicular thyroid cancer. Am J Med 97:418–428, 1994.)

ablation decreased recurrence in patients with lesions larger than 1 cm, and fewer patients with stage I or stage II tumors larger than 1 cm died of their disease.[171] A similar study of 138 patients revealed a 30% decrease in recurrence and no deaths in patients treated with postoperative ablation.[13] Subsets of patients who derived greatest benefit from ablation were identified in a study of 1004 patients with WDTC.[172] Patients with primary tumors larger than 1.5 cm had a threefold reduction in recurrence (P < .001), fewer distant metastases (P < .002), and reduced mortality (P < .001). These benefits were more pronounced in patients over the age of 45. These results strongly suggest that postoperative ablation is indicated in older patients and in younger patients with tumors larger than 1 to 1.5 cm at the time of resection. The need for ablation in younger patients with small lesions remains controversial, with the decision often colored by emotion. Despite statistics demonstrating extremely favorable prognosis in the event of a recurrence, many younger patients in our experience choose ablation. The ultimate decision is a difficult one for patient and physician, with the small risk afforded by the tumor balanced against the often equally small risk of potential harm from radioiodine therapy (see under Radioactive Iodine Therapy).

The dose of ^{131}I that is required for successful ablation is also controversial. A review of several studies was inconclusive in determining an advantage of single treatment with 100 and 200 mCi of ^{131}I postoperatively compared with repetitive treatment with doses between 25 mCi and 29 mCi.[173] Higher-dose radioiodine was successful in ablation of residual thyroid tissue in 87% of treated patients,[174] with no advantage observed at doses greater than 100 mCi of [131]I. The results of lower-dose remnant ablation are highly variable. In one study, radioiodine ablation with 29.9 mCi was successful in only 8% of treated patients.[175] However, ablation with 29.9 mCi of ^{131}I was successful in 77% to 95% of patients in whom the surgeon had left small (less than 2 g) remnants of thyroid tissue.[176–178] The advantage of ablation with 29.9 mCi

of ^{131}I or less is that hospitalization is not required and radiation exposure is minimized. However, recent regulatory changes have made outpatient administration of greater than 29.9 mCi feasible in most states. Because of the demonstrable prevention of thyroid cancer recurrence and the reduction in the number of repeated treatments needed to obtain complete ablation, most centers use between 70 and 150 mCi of ^{131}I as a routine ablative dose.

TBS should be routinely obtained after ^{131}I ablation. Several authors have demonstrated that postablation scanning is the most sensitive tool for localizing disease outside of the thyroid bed; disease not shown by diagnostic scanning with 2 to 5 mCi of ^{131}I is found in more than 50% of patients with elevated thyroglobulin (Tg) levels.[179–183]

ABLATION AFTER RECOMBINANT HUMAN TSH STIMULATION

The use of recombinant human TSH (rhTSH) for remnant ablation after thyroidectomy has also been studied (see later for details regarding rhTSH). Five men and five women had residual activity in the thyroid bed following an rhTSH-stimulated ^{131}I diagnostic TBS. Two patients also had cervical or lung uptake. A mean ablative dose of 110 mCi of ^{131}I was administered immediately after the TBS, and a second rhTSH-stimulated diagnostic TBS was performed an average of 9 months later. None of the patients, including those with disease outside of the thyroid bed at follow-up, had visible uptake. However, rhTSH-stimulated thyroglobulin levels were greater than 2 ng/mL in four patients at follow-up despite negative TBS. These patients were treated with high-dose ^{131}I; three of the four patients had metastatic lesions identified on post-treatment TBS.[184] Although it has not been approved for this use, this study of a limited number of patients demonstrates the possible use of rhTSH preparation for postoperative ablation.

RADIOACTIVE IODINE THERAPY

Therapy with radioiodine should always be distinguished from radioiodine ablation. Ablation refers to destruction of residual thyroid tissue after thyroidectomy, whereas therapy refers to treatment typically targeting persistent, recurrent, or metastatic disease.

Dosage. Several views have been put forth as to the optimal amount of ^{131}I to be employed in the treatment of recurrent or residual disease. Most widely used is a fixed-dose method, with the dosage increased incrementally according to the severity of disease.[185] Typically, 150 mCi of ^{131}I is administered for recurrent activity in the thyroid bed or lymph nodes in the neck, and 200 to 250 mCi of ^{131}I for distant metastasis.[186] Another approach is to administer a dosimetric amount of ^{131}I calculated from the expected dose that will be taken up by the tumor.[187–190] This method individualizes therapy according to the body clearance of ^{131}I and attempts to balance the risks of adverse effects with therapeutic efficacy. One of the initial validations of this technique can be seen in thyroid ablation after surgery, wherein approximately 84% of remnants were successfully ablated (47% of these patients were treated as outpatients).[176] With this method, 74% of patients with lymph node metastasis were successfully treated.[176] Patients with distant metastases may benefit most from the higher dose afforded by dosimetric calculations, but this has not been demonstrated. Dosimetry is recommended in patients with reduced clearance of ^{131}I. For example, patients on continuous peritoneal dialysis for end-stage renal disease who were administered 28 mCi of ^{131}I were shown to receive radiation exposure similar to a dose of 150 mCi in a patient with normal renal function.[191]

Disease Factors. The success of radioiodine treatment for metastatic thyroid cancer is highly dependent on the size and location of disease. Up to 40% of patients have lymph node involvement at the time of surgery.[13, 72] Although several studies indicate that lymph node involvement at the time of surgery did not affect life expectancy,[12, 192] a majority have found lymph node involvement to be associated with increased recurrence and mortality.[171, 16, 193–195] In one study, as many as 15% of patients with lymph node disease confined to the neck died of cancer-related causes, whereas none died in the absence of lymph node involvement.[196] A large study of outcomes in 2479 patients who had thyroid cancer showed a statistically and clinically significant increase in mortality with initial lymph node involvement.[194] Recurrence and death rates were reduced when these patients were treated with radioactive iodine.[13] In one study of 1599 patients, treatment with radioactive iodine was the single most powerful predictor of disease-free survival and recurrence.[72]

Extent of Metastasis. Radioiodine is least successful in patients with distant metastasis. Pulmonary metastasis is more common among younger patients, but mortality is lowest in this age group. The survival of patients under the age of 40 with pulmonary involvement treated with ^{131}I was 71% compared with 16% among patients older than 40, although radioactive iodine therapy significantly extended survival in both age groups.[197] Extent of metastasis at the time of discovery is highly associated with survival, suggesting that early detection is of paramount importance.[198] Bone metastasis is common in follicular thyroid cancer and is difficult to treat. Surgical debulking of bone metastasis appears to improve subsequent responses to radioactive iodine,[199] although only 17% of those with lesions that take up radioactive iodine have been cured.[200]

Stimulation by rhTSH. Stimulation by rhTSH shows promise as an alternative to thyroid hormone withdrawal in the treatment of thyroid cancer. Eleven patients with metastatic thyroid cancer who could not tolerate hypothyroidism or demonstrated no increase in TSH after withdrawal were treated with ^{131}I after rhTSH injection.[201] Although no direct comparison could be made with treatment after withdrawal, five patients showed a greater than 30% decrease in thyroglobulin levels, and three had stabilization or a decrease in tumor burden. A potential advantage of rhTSH administration may be that endogenous TSH-stimulated tumor growth and impingement of metastatic disease on vital structures such as the spinal cord are circumvented. However, a recent case report describes rapid growth of metastatic thyroid lesions after administration of rhTSH.[202]

Radioiodide Before Surgical Exploration. Recently, the preoperative administration of radioiodine has been used to help guide surgical exploration for small nodal or soft tissue recurrences.[203–205] ^{131}I was administered several days preoperatively. A TBS was obtained and a gamma probe was used intraoperatively to identify thyroid cancer tissue. This approach was successful in identifying recurrent or persistent disease within postoperative scar tissue, within the mediastinum, or behind vessels.[206] Lymph node involvement that persisted after two radioiodine treatments was localized with preoperative radioiodine and successfully resected in six of six patients approached with the intraoperative gamma probe.[205] However, these studies did not compare this technique with traditional surgical approaches, so the actual advantage is unknown. Nevertheless, this method may be useful in the resection of recurrent or residual disease when preoperative localization through standard imaging is inadequate. An additional advantage is that a postoperative TBS assesses completeness of the surgical dissection.

Risks Associated With Radioactive Iodine Therapy. The risks of radioactive iodine treatment are for the most part minor. The salivary glands concentrate iodide several times above plasma levels, and acute or chronic sialoadenitis may occur after ^{131}I treatment.[207] Symptoms usually occur within 1 week of treatment and consist of dry mouth, gland tenderness, and swelling. Salivary and parotid gland dysfunction were seen in 40% and 39%, respectively, in one study,[208] and in up to 72% of patients in another.[209] Chronic sialoadenitis, however, appears to be uncommon, occurring in 1 of 63 patients treated with an average ablative dose of 103 mCi.[210] Amifostine ameliorates sialoadenitis, but its effect on ^{131}I treatment efficacy has not been evaluated.[208]

The most important preventive therapy is to increase salivation, typically with the use of sour candies in the first few days following ^{131}I administration. Neck pain and tenderness following ^{131}I therapy for Graves' disease or multinodular goiter are relatively common, but they are rarely seen following near-total thyroidectomy. Nausea is the most common gastrointestinal adverse effect observed, occurring in up to 67% of patients treated with 150 mCi of ^{131}I.[211] ^{131}I therapy can induce a metallic taste, but this is almost always transient.[211] Pulmonary function can be affected by ^{131}I therapy, primarily when lung metastases are present. Radiation pneumonitis and fibrosis were noted in more than 10% of patients treated with high-dose ^{131}I.[188] This adverse effect can be minimized with the use of dosimetry to estimate which ^{131}I dose will decay to less than 80 mCi at 48 hours after administration. When this protocol was used, no instance of pneumonitis was noted in one large series,[212] and alveolar-capillary damage was rare when assessed by Tc99m-diethylenetriaminepentaacetic acid (DTPA) clearance.[213]

Decreased reproductive function and secondary malignancies are of concern to many patients. In men, dose-dependent decreases in sperm count have been observed.[214] Gonadotropin elevation, indicating testicular failure, was present in one third of patients treated with ^{131}I. Long-term fertility is not impaired in the majority of patients,[215] but permanent infertility after ^{131}I has been reported.[216] In women, transient ovarian failure lasting up to a year has been observed,[217] but no long-term infertility problems have been noted.[215, 218]

A slight association between very high cumulative doses of ^{131}I (800 to 1000 mCi) and an increased risk of developing leukemia or bladder cancer has been noted.[219, 220] However, no increased risk of leukemia has been observed with doses below this amount in some,[221] but not all, studies.[222] Weak associations between ^{131}I treatment and cancers of the intestine and bladder have also been described in some studies,[216] but not in others.[223]

In summary, at present, there appear to be few serious risks associated with radioactive iodine therapy. Transient infertility in both men and women is common, but permanent infertility is rare and seems to occur only in men. These risks and the opportunity to bank sperm before ^{131}I is given should be discussed with all men. [131]I treatment is associated with a slight increase in the risk for developing leukemia in some studies when the total dose is greater than 800 mCi. Pulmonary pneumonitis and fibrosis are uncommon when ^{131}I is used judiciously.

Surgical Management of Locally Invasive Thyroid Cancer

The proximity of the thyroid gland to the larynx, pharynx, cervical esophagus, and recurrent laryngeal nerve places these structures at high risk of involvement with thyroid cancers that extend beyond the gland. The choice of the proper surgical procedure is often difficult and depends on the extent of disease, the histopathologic tumor type, and other prognostic factors. Proper preoperative patient education and consent are imperative in the decision-making process.

The preoperative history and physical examination often points to potential involvement of surrounding structures in invasive thyroid carcinoma. CT and MRI scans also play a significant role in assessment and are reliable in documenting the extension of disease into the upper aerodigestive tract, as well as in revealing the extent of resection that will be required. MRI offers the additional advantage of not requiring iodinated contrast material, but both images are useful in preoperative planning.

In differentiated thyroid cancer, treatment involves conservative resection with an emphasis on maintaining function, if possible. Medullary thyroid carcinoma often requires a more extensive resection. Well-differentiated, locally invasive thyroid carcinomas can be resected with narrower margins than can squamous cell carcinoma of the upper aerodigestive tract.[224–227] Long-term survival can be attained in patients with invasive, well-differentiated thyroid carcinoma, even with microscopically positive margins.[224–227] Adjuvant therapy should be considered in all patients with invasive thyroid carcinoma, but especially in those with close or microscopically positive margins. This may include ^{131}I, external beam radiotherapy, or both.[228–230]

Fixation to the thyroid cartilage or trachea may require partial- or full-thickness removal of these structures. Every effort should be made to avoid leaving gross disease on these structures. The trachea can be partially resected when invasive thyroid carcinoma is removed. If the tracheal cartilage is removed with the underlying mucosa still intact, reconstruction can be performed by rotating adjacent soft tissues into the defect. Isolated full-thickness tracheal wall defects can be repaired with a mucosal-cartilage composite graft harvested from the nasal septum. With more extensive involvement, tracheal resection with end-to-end anastomosis can be performed.[231] Laryngeal conservation procedures are possible in most patients with well-differentiated thyroid cancer invading the laryngeal cartilage. Total laryngectomy is used on only the most severe cases of intralaryngeal extension.[232–234]

Invasion is often unilateral, and vertical hemilaryngectomy usually allows complete resection of the invasive tumor. Involvement of the subglottic region of cricoid cartilage makes reconstruction after resection more difficult. Reconstruction with myoperiosteal or myocutaneous flaps may be performed for laryngeal or tracheal defects.[235]

Local invasion of thyroid cancer into the wall of the pharynx or the esophageal wall is usually managed by conservative resection. The muscular wall and submucosa of the esophagus may be resected with little or no morbidity. Transluminal extension into the esophagus may require circumferential resection of a small part of the esophagus. Reconstruction of segmental resections of the esophagus in patients with thyroid cancer varies according to the length of the resected segment; in most cases, limited resections are reconstructed with end-to-end anastomosis. Less commonly, extensive resections are necessary and may require microvascular free-flap reconstruction or even gastric pullup.

Preservation of the recurrent laryngeal nerve should be attempted in all patients with invasive thyroid carcinoma; it is often possible, even in patients with circumferential tumor involvement. Gross tumor removal should be achieved with attempts to obtain a tumor-free margin. Microscopic residual disease along the course of the nerve necessitates the addition of postoperative adjuvant treatment.[1] Alternatively, a nerve involved with cancer can be excised and the voice rehabilitated with type I thyroplasty, immediate or delayed.

TOTAL VERSUS LESS THAN TOTAL THYROIDECTOMY

In all patients with follicular thyroid carcinoma and those patients with papillary thyroid carcinoma either larger than 1 to 1.5 cm or with lymph node metastasis, total or near-total thyroidectomy results in a decreased likelihood of recurrence and mortality.[13, 15, 171, 172, 236–239] This approach also allows for optimal follow-up. The remnant can be ablated with radioiodine, and residual disease or recurrence can be detected by an elevated thyroglobulin level or ^{131}I total body scan.

Whether total thyroidectomy is indicated in patients with occult (<1.0 cm) papillary carcinoma without lymph node metastasis or capsular involvement remains controversial. Although up to 32% of these patients with microcarcinoma will have lymph node involvement at the time of surgery,[240] the prognosis remains excellent, with a 30-year mortality rate lower than 3% independent of the extent of surgery or whether radioactive iodine ablation is performed postoperatively.[13, 172, 241] Despite earlier detection of recurrence in these low-risk patients who underwent total thyroidectomy, there is no evidence that mortality is lowered when compared with lobectomy and isthmectomy. In such cases, the uncommon but meaningful surgical complications of permanent hypoparathyroidism or recurrent laryngeal nerve involvement must be weighed against the small benefit. Patients should be advised of these considerations preoperatively and should be reminded that, unlike most cancers, lymph node recurrence in papillary thyroid carcinoma is treatable and does not typically herald a poor outcome. Occasionally, a patient will have lymph node involvement with extremely small primary lesions noted at the time of surgery. Such patients should undergo complete thyroidectomy and lymph node dissection.

THYROIDECTOMY

Thyroidectomy is usually performed with the patient under general anesthesia, although local anesthesia may be used on rare occasions.[242] After general endotracheal intubation has been achieved, a shoulder roll is placed under the patient, and the head is supported by a donut-shaped holder. The skin incision is centered in the midline and extends symmetrically in a natural skin crease approximately 1 to 2 fingerwidths above the clavicle. Laterally, the incision extends 1 to 2 cm posterior to the anterior edge of the sternocleidomastoid muscle. If a neck dissection is needed, the incision is extended more posteriorly and superiorly on one or both sides. The incision is carefully made through the platysma muscle, with care taken to avoid injury to the anterior jugular veins. The skin, subcutaneous tissue, and platysma muscle are elevated as a superior-based flap to the level of the hyoid bone. The inferior-based flap is elevated in a subplatysmal plane to the level of the clavicles. The strap muscles are divided in the midline, with the dissection carried between the posterior aspect of the strap muscles and the thyroid gland. The thyroid gland may also be approached laterally along the outer edge of the sternocleidomastoid muscle. This approach may prove beneficial in previously dissected glands.

After dissection of the midline, care is taken to separate both the sternohyoid and sternothyroid muscles from the underlying thyroid gland. Portions of the strap muscles may be resected if they are adherent to or infiltrated by tumor. The middle thyroid vein is then ligated, allowing increased exposure laterally. Blunt dissection is used to gently separate any remaining strap muscle fibers or loose areolar tissue from the thyroid lobe. Great care is taken to identify and gently separate the parathyroid glands from the thyroid gland. The carotid artery is then identified by means of continued blunt dissection. The superior pole vessels are individually isolated and ligated. This is aided by downward retraction of the thyroid lobe, with the use of great caution to avoid damage to the superior laryngeal nerves.[1, 243] Some surgeons prefer to identify the recurrent laryngeal nerve before addressing the superior pole vessels, believing that this is a safer technique.

The dissection of the thyroid gland is continued along the posterior aspect of the gland. The recurrent laryngeal nerve is identified in the tracheoesophageal groove inferior to the gland and is dissected superiorly. The nerve can also be located near the inferior thyroid artery. Caution must be maintained when this technique is used because of the high variability in the relationship between the inferior thyroid artery and the recurrent laryngeal nerve. Occasionally, a nonrecurrent inferior laryngeal nerve may be found coursing directly off the vagus nerve. This anomaly occurs infrequently but more often on the right side and is associated with an anomalous retroesophageal right subclavian artery. It occurs very rarely on the left side and only with situs inversus. Once the recurrent laryngeal nerve is identified, it is followed superiorly, with care taken to preserve all branches of the nerve. The branches of the inferior thyroid artery are individually ligated, with preservation of the vascular pedicle to the parathyroid glands and with care taken to avoid injuring the recurrent laryngeal nerve.

The lobe is completely mobilized by the division of the posterior suspensory (Berry's) ligament, with preservation of the recurrent laryngeal nerve as it enters the larynx. Dissection of the lateral lobe extends medially on the trachea, with dissection of a pyramidal lobe if present. The isthmus of the gland is divided and the lobe removed. A similar approach is performed on the opposite side to complete the total thyroidectomy procedure.

NECK DISSECTION

The decision to perform a neck dissection after a total thyroidectomy is dependent not only on the presence or absence of clinically metastatic disease but also on the histologic tumor type. Papillary and medullary thyroid carcinomas frequently metastasize to regional lymph nodes, whereas follicular carcinoma does so only rarely. Preoperative assessment by clinical examination and imaging studies with or without FNA is often useful in demonstrating metastatic disease and in determining whether a neck dissection is necessary. Even if preoperative workup demonstrates no evidence of metastatic disease, central compartment nodes (level VI) must be carefully evaluated after the diagnosis of thyroid cancer has been established. In the absence of palpable or otherwise demonstrable positive metastatic nodes, dissection beyond the central compartment is not required. If palpable nodes or otherwise demonstrable nodes are noted, then a modified neck dissection is performed. Elective neck dissection for differentiated thyroid carcinoma is of questionable value and has not conclusively proved to be more effective than observation and therapeutic dissection.[1]

A modified (selective) neck dissection of levels II to V with preservation of the internal jugular vein, the sternocleidomastoid muscle, and the spinal accessory nerves provides adequate removal of lymphatics at risk. Care must be taken to evaluate the area posterior to the carotid artery near the scalene muscles because this area is a common site of metastasis and represents the course of the inferior thyroid artery as it passes posterior to the carotid sheath.[244–246] Thyroid carcinoma rarely metastasize to the submandibular region, and removal of these nodes is not typically incorporated into a standard neck dissection for thyroid cancer.[1] Radical neck dissections are rarely required in the primary treatment of differentiated thyroid malignancy.

Complications of Thyroid Surgery

HEMORRHAGE

Significant hemorrhage is most likely to occur during the first few hours after a thyroidectomy, while the patient is still in the recovery room, but its onset may also be delayed. Significant postoperative hemorrhage is usually caused by an uncoupling of a ligature that was placed on an artery or vein during the procedure or is secondary to damage to a small vessel near the point in which the recurrent laryngeal nerve enters the larynx. Symptoms of a major hemorrhage may include stridor, hypoxia, or swelling in the anterior neck. Prolific drain output and soiling of the pressure dressing may also occur. This situation requires immediate attention, with removal of the sutures or surgical clips and evacuation of the hematoma. Once the immediate threat of airway compromise has been dealt with, the patient is taken back to the operating room for reintubation and control of the bleeding source.[231]

SEROMA

Wound seroma is periodically encountered in post-thyroidectomy patients, especially after resection of large tumors or goiters. Left undrained, this collection of fluid may cause a postoperative infection. Most seromas can be treated by repeated aspiration; only rarely is open drainage required.

PNEUMOTHORAX AND CHYLOUS FISTULAS

Pneumothorax and chylous fistulas have been reported after thyroidectomy, usually when extended thyroid resections or neck dissections have been performed. Management is similar to treatment of these complications during other procedures. A chest tube may be required in some patients, depending on the size of the pneumothorax and the patient's symptoms. Chylous fistula is often treated by closed suction drainage and pressure dressings. More extensive discussion of the treatment of chylous fistula is beyond the scope of this chapter.

INJURY TO THE RECURRENT LARYNGEAL NERVE

The frequency of trauma to the recurrent laryngeal nerve during the course of thyroid surgery has diminished during the past decade. Overall, the incidence of permanent injury to the recurrent laryngeal nerves is probably less than 1%.[247] The incidence of temporary unilateral vocal cord paresis or paralysis is between 2.5% and 5%.[248, 249] A higher incidence of recurrent nerve injury has been reported in thyroidectomy performed in combination with neck dissection, but this may reflect a more advanced stage of disease in these patients.[250]

Unilateral nerve injury resulting in vocal cord paralysis is the most common form of injury to the recurrent laryngeal nerve. The vocal cord is usually paralyzed in a median or paramedian position, with the patient experiencing a weak, breathy voice. If the ipsilateral superior laryngeal nerve has also been injured, the cord assumes a more lateral (intermediate) position and the voice is proportionately worse.[251] Unilateral vocal cord paralysis is only rarely associated with aspiration, and when this does occur, the superior laryngeal nerves have usually been concomitantly injured.

Recognition of intraoperative recurrent laryngeal nerve injury is important. If a nerve has been transected during thyroidectomy, microsurgical repair of the nerve is recommended to decrease the associated morbidity. Although the repair will not restore nerve function completely, it may aid in reducing the degree of vocal cord atrophy.[252, 253]

Management of unilateral vocal cord paralysis depends on the patient's level of morbidity. Patients with major problems of aspiration may require immediate intervention; those with limited symptoms may be observed for a variable length of time. This allows assessment for possible return of nerve function in those patients with neurapraxia and, more frequently, allows vocal cord compensation to occur. Over time, compensation may occur as the paralyzed cord moves medially, allowing better approximation by the opposite vocal cord. The patient may become relatively asymptomatic and require no further surgical intervention. A detailed description of the surgical management of unilateral vocal cord paralysis is beyond the scope of this chapter. Different forms of laryngoplasty with or without arytenoid adduction often provide excellent results.[254]

Bilateral vocal cord paralysis is much more problematic. Varying degrees of stridor may be noted in the postoperative period, often with a near-normal voice. This often requires immediate intervention, with control of the airway by either endotracheal intubation or tracheotomy. In some cases, bilateral recurrent laryngeal nerve paralysis may go unnoticed for years as patients assume a sedentary lifestyle and remain relatively asymptomatic. After airway control has been achieved, these patients may be monitored for 6 to 12 months so that return of nerve function can be assessed. Surgical procedures, such as cordotomy, arytenoidectomy, or nerve muscle pedicle renovation techniques, may be of benefit to some patients.[253–255]

SUPERIOR LARYNGEAL NERVE INJURY

Thyroidectomy is a common cause of superior laryngeal nerve injury, although the true incidence remains unknown. Patients with this type of injury experience a voice that is restricted in vocal range, rather than hoarse. Symptoms of superior laryngeal nerve injury include loss of control and variability of vocal pitch or a weak, breathy voice. Despite these symptoms, physical findings are often subtle. The affected vocal cord may be shorter or possibly at a different level when compared with the opposite vocal cord. Electromyography (EMG) may also be useful in revealing the diagnosis. Surgical intervention is usually not beneficial in these patients, although speech therapy may be helpful.[231]

METABOLIC COMPLICATIONS OF THYROIDECTOMY

Permanent hypocalcemia should be uncommon after an uncomplicated thyroidectomy but should be considered as a possibility in patients undergoing bilateral surgical procedures or in patients having a complete thyroid lobectomy. The incidence of permanent hypoparathyroidism is 1% to 10%, but it may be significantly higher when extensive dissection has to be performed during reoperation for a recurrent cancer in the thyroid bed.[1]

Hypoparathyroidism is the major cause of significant postoperative hypocalcemia, usually because of ischemic damage as well as actual resection of the parathyroid glands. Postoperative laboratory findings of hypoparathyroidism include hypocalcemia, hyperphosphatemia, metabolic alkalosis, hypocalciuria, and inappropriately low parathyroid (PTH) hormone levels. In patients with liver disease or malnutrition, magnesium deficiency causes impaired PTH secretion and end-organ resistance to the actions of PTH.

The patient's serum ionized calcium level should be measured every 12 hours for the first 2 days after thyroidectomy. Asymptomatic patients may be observed carefully without receiving therapy. Treatment for postoperative hypocalcemia should be tailored to the severity and expected duration of the calcium deficiency. In the setting of severe tetany, seizures, laryngospasm, or markedly prolonged electrocardiographic QT intervals, emergency therapy is indicated. Calcium gluconate, 10 mL of a 10% solution (or 0.2 mL/kg for children), should be infused intravenously over 10 minutes. Continued support should include 10% calcium gluconate, 1.5 mg/kg diluted in 500 mL of 5% dextrose empirically, with subsequent adjustments based on serial calcium levels. To avoid increased calcium binding to serum proteins and further reductions in ionized calcium, alkalosis should be carefully avoided.

Long-term vitamin D and calcium supplementation may be necessary in the treatment of prolonged hypocalcemia. Serum calcium levels should be maintained at no higher than 9.0 mg/dL so that significant hypercalciuria (which may result from lack of PTH-mediated calcium resorption) may be avoided. Vitamin D_2 (ergocalciferol), 50,000 to 100,000 IU (1.25–2.5 mg)/day, provides inexpensive long-term oral therapy for promoting enteric calcium absorption. Calcitriol (1,25-dihydroxyvitamin D_3), 0.5 to 2.0 µg/day, rapidly increases enteric calcium absorption and should be given on a short-term basis while the effects of ergocalciferol are awaited. Treatment may be tapered after several weeks so that the need for continued therapy can be assessed. Oral calcium salts, which provide 1 to 3 g/day of elemental calcium, are often necessary; calcium carbonate is usually the most cost-effective and has the highest percentage of elemental calcium content. Elderly patients and others who may be achlorhydric often do not absorb calcium carbonate and require therapy with an alternative salt, for example, calcium citrate. In patients who require liquid supplementation administered via feeding tubes, calcium glubionate is the drug of choice. Calcium acetate may be preferred for patients with concurrent renal insufficiency. When calciuria exceeds 300 to 400 mg/day, a thiazide diuretic may be added to promote calcium resorption and permit reduction of calcium and vitamin D doses. Patients with mild postoperative hypocalcemia may be treated with oral calcium supplementation alone.[1]

Chemotherapy and External Beam Radiation Therapy for Well-Differentiated Thyroid Cancer

Chemotherapy has a limited role in the treatment of thyroid cancer and is reserved for inoperable, advanced disease that does not concentrate [131]I. Doxorubicin hydrochloride was first used in a group of 30 patients diagnosed with all forms of thyroid cancer. Among the 10 patients with differentiated cancer, there were three partial responses; no change occurred in three patients; and four of the patients progressed.[256] A subsequent study examined 35 patients with inoperable disease that was radioiodine insensitive. Patients treated with doxorubicin alone or in combination with cisplatin demonstrated no statistical difference in response rate (17% and 26%, respectively).[257] Of note, five patients had a complete response in the combination group compared with none in the monotherapy group. However, a similar study with doxorubicin and cisplatin used in combination to treat 22 patients resulted in only two partial responses and overall severe toxicity.[258]

The primary indications for external beam radiation therapy (XRT) remain to be completely defined. Typically, this modality has been used to treat tumors that are locally invasive into the visceral compartments or deep muscles of the neck. Also, it has been used for tumors that recur after treatment with ^{131}I doses that exceed the cumulative maximal amount that one can safely give, and for lesions that do not accumulate ^{131}I or that progress despite treatment.

A majority of studies examining the role of XRT are retrospective. In one study, XRT was administered to 113 patients, with 74 receiving [131]I. Of patients with gross residual disease, 37% had complete regression. Of 25 patients with suspected and of 18 with definite microscopic disease,

8% and 29% had local recurrence, respectively.[259] In a large study of 1578 patients with WDTC thyroid cancer, XRT and ^{131}I demonstrated equivalent local control after surgery.[260] In a similar study of patients treated with XRT before administration of ^{131}I, no prolongation of survival was observed compared with ^{131}I alone.[261] In one small study, XRT was found to adversely affect outcome.[262] On the other hand, in a smaller retrospective study of patients who were treated with ^{131}I, 38 had also received XRT. These patients had a significantly smaller local recurrence rate than was seen in those receiving ^{131}I alone (3% vs. 21%), although survival was unchanged.[263] With more advanced disease at the time of surgery, radioiodine followed by XRT significantly improved local recurrence in patients older than 40 years of age with papillary thyroid cancer.[264] A combination of XRT and low-dose doxorubicin was prospectively studied in 22 patients with differentiated thyroid cancer.[265] Moderate tracheitis and pharyngoesophagitis that did not require cessation of treatment were encountered. Ninety-one percent had a complete response rate, with 50% survival at 5 years.

Follow-up of Well-Differentiated Thyroid Cancer

The follow-up of WDTC remains a controversial issue. The obvious goal is to use the most sensitive and specific method for detecting persistent or recurrent thyroid cancer. However, the low mortality and slow-growing characteristics of most WDTCs have made randomized trials virtually impossible to perform; consequently, current methods of follow-up are based on often-conflicting results from retrospective analyses of patient outcomes. The uncertainty in assessing the risks and benefits for an individual patient remains at the core of the controversy.

Thyroid-Stimulating Hormone Suppression Therapy

The trophic effects of TSH on WDTC are widely accepted and can occur after administration of rhTSH.[202, 267] The total number of recurrences and distant recurrences of WDTC has been shown to be significantly reduced by T_4 treatment alone after initial therapy.[13, 172] Yet the need for complete suppression of TSH to minimize adverse outcomes is controversial. Any derived benefit must be weighed against the increased risks for atrial fibrillation and osteoporosis when T_4 is administered in suppressive doses. Extremely elevated Tg levels have been shown to increase further in a single patient with WDTC when TSH levels rose from undetectable to levels still considered suppressed.[267]

In a study of 141 patients with WDTC who were free of disease, relapse occurred within a significantly shorter time in those with TSH levels greater than 1 mU/L compared with patients in whom the TSH level was consistently lower than 0.05 mU/L ($P < .01$).[268] Conversely, Tg levels were not shown to decrease significantly when the dosage of T_4 was increased to reduce TSH levels from an average of 0.26 mU/L to less than 0.1 mU/L.[269] Moreover, in a large study of 617 patients, TSH suppression did not reduce disease progression in low-risk patients, but in high-risk patients, a reduction was noted.[270] Taken together, these results suggest that a low-risk WDTC patient who has undergone thyroidectomy and ablative ^{131}I and then is treated with T_4 to maintain the TSH level just below the lower limit of normal will derive little benefit from further TSH suppression. Complete suppression of TSH should be considered in patients who are at high risk of recurrence or have demonstrable persistent disease.

Radioactive Iodine Total Body Scan

TSH stimulates the uptake and organification of iodine by thyroid tissue and the secretion of thyroglobulin. These characteristics are retained in most papillary and follicular thyroid cancers. An elevated TSH is therefore required for adequate amounts of ^{131}I to enter thyroid cancer cells and achieve therapeutic results. Until recently, levothyroxine withdrawal for 4 to 6 weeks has been the only means of increasing plasma TSH to adequate levels (>30 mU/L). Unfortunately, many patients respond very poorly to the hypothyroid state and develop loss of energy, impaired cognition, depression, muscle cramps, and other symptoms of hypothyroidism.[271] The mitogenic activity of TSH on thyroid follicular cells can also induce rapid growth of metastatic disease, which is of particular importance in patients with spinal cord compression or large lung metastasis.[272]

Treatment with triiodothyronine (T_3) at doses of 25 µg up to three times daily for 3 weeks after levothyroxine is stopped can minimize the symptoms of hypothyroidism. Discontinuation of T_3 for 2 or 3 weeks before ^{131}I TBS results in an adequate rise in TSH.[273] T_3 has a very short half-life and is rapidly cleared. However, the rapid rise in blood levels can precipitate cardiac arrhythmia or angina in patients with history of cardiac disease, requiring caution in the prescribing of T_3 to these patients. Despite the use of T_3 therapy in appropriate individuals, hypothyroidism is unavoidable for several weeks before the TBS and for the first week or two after replacement therapy with L-thyroxine is started. This interval can significantly disrupt the patient's life and limit the ability to function properly at work.

Recombinant Human TSH

Alternative methods by which to perform ^{131}I total body scanning without thyroid hormone withdrawal have been sought for several decades. The feasibility of raising TSH levels by direct injection was established with bovine TSH,[274] although systemic adverse effects[275] and the generation of neutralizing antibodies[276] with repeated doses prohibited widespread use. Recombinant human TSH (rhTSH) is now commercially available in injectable form with the approved algorithm for administration shown in Figure 19–4.

Initial clinical trials compared ^{131}I TBS after rhTSH administration and T_4 withdrawal sequentially in the same patient.[277] Two-day regimens of rhTSH injection resulted in TSH levels that exceeded those noted after T_4 withdrawal (220 mU/L vs. 77 mU/L). Scans were reviewed in a blinded fashion. rhTSH-stimulated scans were equivalent to withdrawal scans in 17 of 19 patients (87%). Iodine uptakes were lower in the rhTSH group, an occurrence that was later shown to be secondary to lower metabolism and excretion. Thyroglobulin levels were increased more than twofold in 58% of patients receiving rhTSH compared with 79% after withdrawal-induced hypothyroidism. It is important to note that no patients showed detectable levels of circulating antibodies against rhTSH. This phase I/II study demonstrated that rhTSH injection in preparation for TBS was nearly as efficacious as thyroid hormone withdrawal. However, approximately 10% of positive TBS identified by withdrawal were not identified by rhTSH preparation.

These promising results were extended in two phase III trials that were similar in design.[278, 279] Thyroid cancer patients received two or three consecutive intramuscular injections of 0.9 mg rhTSH while they were maintained on suppressive doses of thyroid hormone. Twenty-four hours after the final dose of rhTSH, 2 to 4 mCi of ^{131}I was administered, and TBS was performed 2 days later. Thyroglobulin was measured 48 and 72 hours after the last dose of rhTSH. Thyroid hormone was then stopped for 4 to 6 weeks until the TSH was sufficiently elevated, and a second ^{131}I TBS was performed together with thyroglobulin levels. Three reviewers interpreted whole body scans in a blinded fashion.

The first study of 152 patients showed rhTSH to be inferior to withdrawal TBS in 29% of positive scans.[278] One potential problem in the study design was the definition of discordance, given as any new area of uptake identified regardless of whether the difference changed tumor stage. A second problem was that the hypothyroid state decreased ^{131}I secretion, increasing counting efficiency relative to rhTSH. These issues were addressed in the second study wherein discordance was defined as a new area of uptake that altered the stage of disease, and a slower scanning speed was adopted with a minimal number of counts necessary to qualify as a successful scan. The second study of 226 patients demonstrated no statistically significant difference between rhTSH and withdrawal in the detection of disease (8% superiority of withdrawal). The detection of metastatic disease, defined as disease outside the thyroid bed on withdrawal-stimulated TBS or a thyroglobulin greater than 10 ng/mL, was also not statistically different between withdrawal and rhTSH-stimulated TBS (16% superiority of withdrawal). Of note, 20% of patients with thyroglobulin levels greater than 10 ng/mL had negative scans by either method.

The role of thyroglobulin in the follow-up of WDTC was examined in detail in the second study.[280] Fifteen percent of patients studied had antithyroglobulin antibodies and could not be evaluated. Basal and stimulated thyroglobulin levels were obtained in all patients who had undergone previous ablation of thyroid tissue. Thyroglobulin levels of 2 ng/mL and 5 ng/mL were used as cut-offs for the presence of

FIGURE 19–4 Method for the administration of recombinant human thyroid-stimulating hormone (rhTSH).

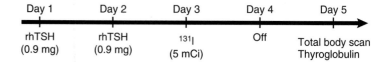

Day 1	Day 2	Day 3	Day 4	Day 5
rhTSH (0.9 mg)	rhTSH (0.9 mg)	131I (5 mCi)	Off	Total body scan Thyroglobulin

disease, based on evidence that any detectable serum Tg indicates the presence of thyroid tissue or thyroid cancer.[281] When the 2-ng/mL cut-off was used, only 22% of patients with uptake limited to the thyroid bed had elevated Tg while on suppression. Tg elevation above 2 ng/mL was similar after rhTSH or thyroid hormone withdrawal (52% vs. 56%). For metastatic disease, with the use of the same 2-ng/mL cut-off, 80% of patients had an elevated Tg while on suppression. rhTSH or thyroid hormone withdrawal detected elevated Tg in 100% of patients with metastases. It is important to note that 23% of total patients evaluated had elevated Tg levels and no uptake on TBS. Stimulated TBS and Tg levels were superior to each alone in the detection of disease. Again with the use of 2 ng/mL as a cut-off, rhTSH detected 93% of patients with thyroid bed uptake by withdrawal TBS and 100% who had metastatic disease. In all studies, the 5-ng/mL cut-off was marginally less sensitive than the 2-ng/mL cut-off.

Withdrawal and rhTSH-stimulated TBS detection of thyroid cancer were compared in a retrospective analysis of 289 patients.[282] The tumor characteristics and other demographics of the two groups were similar. The results convincingly showed that as in the earlier phase III study, rhTSH stimulation and thyroid hormone withdrawal followed by a combination of thyroglobulin levels greater than 2 ng/mL or ^{131}I TBS were equivalent in detecting residual or recurrent thyroid cancer outside of the thyroid bed. Similar results were obtained in 72 patients with WDTC and an undetectable Tg level after thyroidectomy and radioiodine ablation while suppressive doses of L-thyroxine were taken.[283] Measurement of thyroglobulin after rhTSH detected 100% of patients with local or distant metastasis identified by positive withdrawal TBS and elevated Tg. However, these studies were strictly designed to detect recurrent or residual cancer outside of the thyroid bed. Patients were excluded if they had uptake only within the thyroid bed (40% of patients who underwent withdrawal and 15% of patients receiving rhTSH). The clinical significance of thyroid bed uptake is unclear at present. The risk that this represents significant disease that will adversely affect outcome is almost certainly small, as is discussed later, except perhaps in high-risk patients.

In summary, TBS and thyroglobulin measurement after thyroid hormone withdrawal are marginally superior to those obtained after rhTSH in the detection of residual thyroid tissue following thyroidectomy. There appears to be no difference between withdrawal and rhTSH protocols in the identification of patients after thyroidectomy and radioiodine ablation who have disease outside of the thyroid bed. Patients with positive antithyroglobulin antibodies are not suitable for rhTSH scanning protocols. Moreover, the reproducibility and accuracy of thyroglobulin measurements differ markedly between laboratories; employing a laboratory that reliably measures thyroglobulin in the lower range is crucial.

Following Stimulated Thyroglobulin Levels Without a TBS

Recent evidence suggests that patients with very low or undetectable stimulated Tg levels after postoperative ^{131}I ablation may not require follow-up TBS. Pacini and associates retrospectively studied 315 patients with undetectable Tg levels while hypothyroid at the time of the first TBS following thyroid ablation.[284] Of these, 71.4% of patients had a negative TBS, and 28.6% had persistent uptake only in the thyroid bed. The patients were followed for between 9 and 19 years. In 89.2% of patients, the serum Tg level remained undetectable and the TBS was negative. Despite persistent activity in the thyroid bed, 9.2% of patients continued to have undetectable Tg levels. Only 0.6% of patients experienced recurrent disease in cervical lymph nodes, and in these patients, the recurrence was easily treated by surgery or ^{131}I therapy.

Cailleux and colleagues followed 210 patients in a similar manner.[179] All patients had Tg levels lower than 1 ng/mL while hypothyroid in preparation for the TBS. The first diagnostic TBS after thyroidectomy and ablation was positive in the thyroid bed in only 7.1% of these patients. Recurrent disease was detected in only 2 patients (0.9%) during follow-up, and again in both patients, the disease was easily treated.

Virtually identical results were obtained by measuring Tg after rhTSH stimulation. Mazzaferri and coworkers studied 107 patients clinically free of disease with low or undetectable Tg levels while receiving T_4 after thyroidectomy and ablation.[285] Fifty percent of patients were at high risk of recurrence (T3, T4, N1, or M1). All patients were administered rhTSH followed by ^{131}I TBS and measurement of Tg. Twenty patients had Tg levels greater than 2 ng/mL; persistent disease was identified in 10 of these patients through examination of the pathologic specimen, TBS activity outside of the thyroid bed, or positive CT scan of the chest. No persistent or recurrent cancer was found in any patient with rhTSH-stimulated Tg levels lower than 2 ng/mL. It is important to note that diagnostic TBS after rhTSH was falsely negative in 73% of patients with persistent disease.

These studies strongly suggest that TBS adds very little to the follow-up of patients with undetectable or low Tg measured after thyroid hormone withdrawal or the administration of rhTSH. These results also suggest that persistent activity in the thyroid bed is seldom clinically significant. It is notable that TBS failed to detect up to three fourths of patients with recurrent or residual cancer identified by stringent criteria. Therefore, measurement of Tg after thyroid hormone withdrawal or rhTSH stimulation is superior to TBS in differentiating between patients who will remain free of disease and those who will require further evaluation for recurrent or persistent thyroid cancer. The precise cut-off level of stimulated Tg to be used in this approach and whether such a level is identical after rhTSH or withdrawal stimulation are unclear. Nonetheless, from evidence available at present, stimulated Tg greater than 2 ng/mL by either thyroid hormone withdrawal or rhTSH injection will identify virtually all patients at risk for recurrent disease.

Basal Thyroglobulin Levels

The follow-up of WDTC routinely includes the periodic measurement of basal Tg levels obtained during T_4 therapy. Virtually everyone agrees that a basal Tg level greater than 5 ng/mL indicates clinically significant disease requiring prompt evaluation. Recent data suggest, however, that even a basal Tg level of 2.0 ng/mL obtained after surgery and ^{131}I ablation indicates the presence of persistent or recurrent cancer. Twenty percent of patients with metastatic disease had Tg levels equal to or less than 2 ng/mL in one study,[280] and 3 of 102 patients were found to have clinically identifiable persistent thyroid cancer with basal Tg levels between 0.5 and 1.0 ng/mL.[285] The crucial question is whether pushing the envelope of early detection results in enhanced survival. At present, the answer is unknown. However, as has been pointed out by Mazzeferri,[285] delayed initial diagnosis of WDTC,[286] delayed diagnosis of pulmonary metastasis,[287] and a large degree of tumor bulk[288] have all been shown to increase mortality. Thus, detection of disease at the earliest possible point during follow-up may indeed have an impact on prognosis.

Thyroglobulin-Positive/Total Body Scan–Negative Patients

A significant minority of patients with residual or recurrent WDTC will have elevated thyroglobulin levels but nondetectable disease on TBS following either endogenous TSH stimulation or injection with rhTSH. In a recent study comparing the two methods, 10 of 49 patients with metastatic disease had stimulated thyroglobulin levels greater than 10 ng/mL with negative TBS.[279] With the use of lower Tg cut-off levels, up to 75% of patients with recurrent or persistent disease had a negative diagnostic TBS but a Tg greater than 2 ng/mL after rhTSH stimulation.[285] Up to 80% of TBS-negative but Tg-positive patients will demonstrate uptake by the tumor after the administration of 100 mCi or more of [131]I.[213, 214, 289, 290] For example, Cailleux and associates found that three of nine patients with a negative diagnostic TBS with 2 to 5 mCi of ^{131}I and Tg levels greater than 10 ng/mL while hypothyroid showed uptake outside of the thyroid bed after administration of 100 mCi [131]I.[179] The explanation for this phenomenon is unclear but may involve disease foci too small to be detected by 2 to 5 mCi ^{131}I TBS, intake of dietary iodine that interferes with the TBS, stunning by diagnostic doses of ^{131}I, or dedifferentiation of the tumor with preservation of thyroglobulin synthesis but loss of iodine trapping.

Management of these patients is controversial, but several studies indicate a clinical response after the administration of 100 mCi or more of ^{131}I in these situations. Empirical high-dose ^{131}I was administered in 17 patients who had negative pretreatment TBS but elevated thyroglobulin levels. The post-treatment scan was positive in 16 of these patients. Thyroglobulin levels fell to less than 5 ng/mL in 8 patients, and post-treatment TBS converted to negative in 3 patients. However, 8 patients continued to have positive TBS after three treatments.[183] A similar approach was adopted in the treatment of thyroid cancer metastatic to the lung with low ^{131}I uptake. Despite uptake of less than 1% of the pretreatment scanning dose of ^{131}I, repeated doses of 100 mCi of ^{131}I led to negative post-treatment scans in 20 of 23 patients, with the disappearance of lung nodules in 7.[182]

Although the clinical response to this approach is not universal, an additional advantage is localization of metastases for possible surgical intervention. This has led some to recommend routine TBS after administration of 100 mCi of ^{131}I in all patients with thyroglobulin levels greater than 5 ng/mL

during thyroid hormone therapy, or greater than 10 ng/mL after TSH stimulation.[289]

Positron emission tomography (PET) with ^{18}F fluorodeoxyglucose ([18]FDG) has recently emerged as an alternative to the localization of metastatic WDTC that does not concentrate radioiodine. A distinct advantage to this approach is that it does not require thyroid hormone withdrawal. In one study, 6 of 12 thyroglobulin-positive ^{131}I scan–negative patients had their tumors identified, with thyroglobulin levels lower than 10 in the 6 PET scan–negative patients.[291] In a similar study of 37 patients, 71% of tumors were detected. Those tumors missed by PET scanning were small, stage I cervical lesions. The PET scan results changed management in almost 50% of the patients.[292] Another recent report found that PET scanning using [18]FDG detected 89% of known lesions and uncovered 11 new sites in 28 patients with metastatic WDTC.[293] In such patients, an effort to resect the tissues that do not take up ^{131}I is advisable. In ^{131}I scan–negative patients with known cervical disease, preoperative PET scan accurately identified 80% of the lymph nodes involved.[294] An intriguing recent study suggested that prognosis is poorer in metastatic WDTC that avidly takes up [18]FDG.[295]

Other alternative scanning methods have also been examined. [201]Tl demonstrated higher sensitivity and specificity than ^{131}I in the detection of recurrent or persistent disease. Of 14 ^{131}I scan–negative patients with known thyroid cancer, ^{201}Tl successfully detected lesions in 71%. These findings are not universal, however; in a similar study, ^{131}I was found to be superior.[296]

The use of Tc99m complexed to a variety of organic agents has also been evaluated for the follow-up of WDTC. Tc99m-hydroxy methylene diphosphate (HMDP) detected 14 of 14 bone metastases in patients with disease documented by ^{131}I scanning.[297] In a study of patients with local recurrence or lymph node involvement, Tc99m-sestamibi was superior to a ^{131}I scan, detecting 32 of 40 lesions, whereas ^{131}I identified 18 of 40.[297] Tc99m-sestamibi was equivalent to ^{131}I scanning when used to evaluate patients with lung, lymph node, and bone metastases,[298] and was in agreement with ^{131}I scans 96% of the time in 99 patients following thyroidectomy and radioiodine ablation.[299] Ng and colleagues found Tc99m-sestamibi to be less sensitive than ^{131}I in the imaging of thyroid remnants but superior in the identification of lymph node metastasis.[300]

Tc99m-tetrafosmin has shown promise as an imaging agent in the follow-up of WDTC. Seventeen of 23 radioiodine-negative metastases to bone and lungs were detected, and all radioiodine-sensitive lesions were identified.[301] In a recent study, Tc99m-tetrafosmin identified 89% of metastatic WDTC compared with 43% of lesions with [131]I. Tc99m-tetrafosmin identified 100% of lesions in the lung and mediastinum, and 85% of those in bone.[302]

Somatostatin receptor scintigraphy with octreotide has also shown advantages over radioiodine scanning. Octreotide successfully identified 12 of 16 thyroid cancers that were ^{131}I-negative and was 89% concordant with radioiodine-positive lesions.[303] Octreotide also successfully identified metastatic lesions in a patient with Hürthle cell carcinoma, in which radioiodine scanning is relatively ineffective.[304]

Another therapeutic approach in these patients is to redifferentiate the tumors and restore their iodine-trapping abilities. In one patient, retinoic acid administration increased ^{131}I uptake in distant metastasis, and FNA post therapy indicated a return of cells to a more differentiated state.[305] In two separate studies, a reinduction of iodine uptake was seen in up to 50% of patients after treatment with retinoic acid at a dose of 1.5 mg/kg body weight/day over 5 weeks.[306, 307] Eight of 20 patients treated with a similar regimen showed regression or stabilization of tumor size.[308] However, these findings are not universal. Only 2 of 12 patients with ^{131}I scan–negative WDTC became scan-positive after retinoic acid therapy in one study.[306]

The management of radioiodine scan–negative WDTC patients remains challenging for the physician and the patient. It is important to first determine with confidence that the situation exists. False-positive elevations in thyroglobulin must be ruled out by measuring circulating antithyroglobulin antibodies. Documentation of an adequately elevated TSH level and the absence of consumption of large amounts of iodine or injection of contrast material should be determined. An increasing number of alternative methods are becoming available for locating and following these tumors when standard imaging modalities fail. However, without evidence of progressive disease, the morbidity and costs of aggressive radioiodine therapy must be weighed against the present questionable benefits. Redifferentiation with retinoic acid is experimental, but in some circumstances, patients have few alternatives and the toxicity is low.

Summary of Follow-up of WDTC

The management of patients with WDTC has recently undergone dramatic change. Although no uniform recommendations are available that cover the long-term follow-up of all patients with WDTC, a reasonable algorithm given available data is outlined in Figure 19–5. The cut-off values for basal and stimulated Tg levels used are conservative, but it should be stressed that after successful ablation, any measurable Tg may indicate disease. However, the added benefit of aggressive treatment of patients with minimally elevated Tg levels has not been determined. The intensity of follow-up in the first few years after surgery should be modified according to the risk assessment of each patient. Low-intensity follow-up patients include those with Tg less than 1 ng/mL, a negative neck examination, and classic WDTC histology. These patients initially can be monitored every 9 to 12 months. High-intensity follow-up patients should be followed every 4 to 6 months and include those with Tg greater than 1 ng/mL during suppressive T_4 therapy, palpable lesions in the neck, or antibodies to Tg. High-risk patients with large tumors, capsular invasion, and aggressive histology, and those older than 45 years of age also fall into this category.

At each follow-up visit, all patients should undergo careful examination of the neck, determination of TSH and free T_4, and if Tg antibody–negative, a Tg measurement during T_4 therapy. Low-intensity patients should have Tg measured after rhTSH injection or thyroid hormone withdrawal. An elevated Tg level indicates the presence of disease and that an ultrasound of the neck should be performed. This will detect the majority of lymph node involvement, if present; the lymph node is the most common location of recurrent or persistent cancer in low-risk patients. High-intensity follow-up patients should proceed directly to neck ultrasound or CT. In either group, surgery after appropriate staging should be performed on any lesion found to be positive for cancer.

If imaging of the neck is negative, treatment doses of ^{131}I should be administered to low-intensity follow-up patients. High-intensity follow-up patients are approached according to the specifics of their presentation. Antibody-positive patients should undergo TBS after thyroid hormone withdrawal. Patients at high risk, with a Tg greater than 1 ng/mL, or those with suspicious findings on physical examination should have TBS after either rhTSH or T_4 withdrawal. A positive TBS or elevated Tg indicates significant disease, and treatment doses of ^{131}I should be administered.

A TBS 7 to 10 days after ^{131}I is imperative. Positive lesions not seen on pretreatment TBS may be detected. It is important to note that in patients with elevated Tg levels, a negative post-treatment scan signifies Tg-positive–TBS-negative disease, which requires additional imaging with PET or the alternative modalities discussed previously.

The proposed algorithm is applicable for the first few years after surgery. However, the optimal long-term follow-up after two or three stimulated Tg levels are obtained that are stable and less than 5 ng/mL is unknown. Six-month or yearly Tg measurement during levothyroxine suppressive therapy is a common practice. However, as has been discussed earlier, recent studies demonstrating the presence of significant disease despite low Tg levels during suppressive doses of thyroid hormone suggest that monitoring of stimulated Tg levels at 3-year intervals in the high-intensity group, and every 5 or 6 years in the low-intensity group, may be advisable for the detection of late recurrences.

HÜRTHLE CELL CARCINOMA

FNA may reveal a solitary nodule that consists almost entirely of Hürthle cells. Such Hürthle cell neoplasms are believed to be variants of follicular lesions, and if vascular or capsular invasion is detected, they are classified as Hürthle cell carcinomas. Hürthle cell carcinomas are uncommon, representing 3% to 5% of thyroid cancers.[309] As few as 9% of Hürthle cell carcinomas will concentrate radioiodine, but they typically retain the ability to synthesize thyroglobulin.[310–312] Although considered follicular variants, Hürthle cell carcinomas have been reported as more aggressive than follicular carcinomas, with frequent recurrences and higher mortality.[313, 314] Har-El and coworkers found 10- and 15-year cancer-related mortality rates of 36% and 75%, respectively.[312] This remains controversial, however, with other reports finding no significant difference in mortality between Hürthle cell carcinoma and WDTC.[315] Evans and associates at M.D. Anderson recently compared the outcomes of patients with Hürthle cell carcinoma with those with follicular carcinoma of equivalent initial tumor size and invasiveness and found no difference in mortality between the groups.[314]

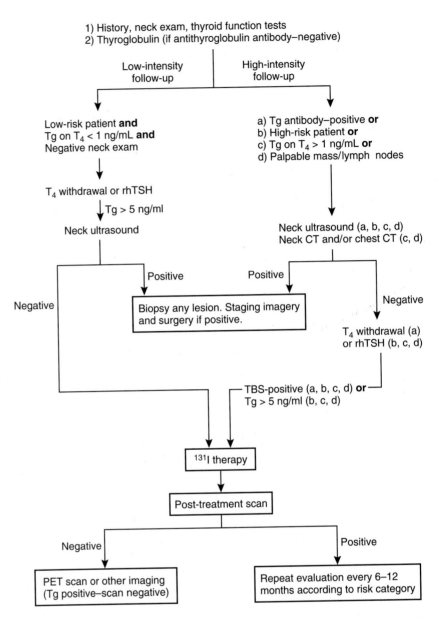

FIGURE 19–5 Algorithm for a follow-up visit for well-differentiated thyroid cancer (WDTC) patients with low-risk or high-risk disease, or positive antithyroglobulin antibodies. Conservative estimates were used for thyroglobulin (Tg) cut-off values used to initiate further evaluation. Recent evidence strongly suggests that total body scan (TBS) adds little information to Tg levels in management of thyroglobulin antibody–negative patients with WDTC. (CT, computed tomography; PET, positron emission tomography; rhTSH, recombinant human thyroid-stimulating hormone.)

Because of the frequent insensitivity to radioiodine and the often-aggressive nature of Hürthle cell carcinoma, close follow-up is recommended. Total thyroidectomy followed by radioiodine ablation should be performed. TSH-stimulated ^{131}I TBS and thyroglobulin measurement 9 to 12 months postoperatively will identify those patients with recurrent or persistent disease who can benefit from high-dose radioiodine treatment. Patients with negative ^{131}I TBS with elevated thyroglobulin should be imaged by CT or MRI for localization of disease. Although they have been less well studied than in other forms of WDTC, alternative imaging methods may also be helpful.[316] Follow-up of patients free of disease should include initial 6-month surveillance of serum thyroglobulin levels during L-thyroxine therapy and yearly monitoring after TSH stimulation for several years.

◾ MEDULLARY CARCINOMA OF THE THYROID

Classification

Medullary thyroid carcinoma (MTC) is an uncommon form of thyroid neoplasia that accounts for approximately 3% to 5% of all thyroid cancers. It typically is found in patients during their third to sixth decades of life. MTC arises from the parafollicular C-cells that are found predominantly in the upper two thirds of the thyroid gland.[317] These cells are of neural crest origin, belonging to the amine precursor uptake and decarboxylation (APUD) cell system. C-cells produce calcitonin and are not involved in thyroid hormone synthesis or secretion. Calcitonin is therefore a very useful plasma marker for MTC (see later).

Molecular Genetics

MTC is inherited through linkage with a mutation in the *RET* proto-oncogene in 20% to 30% of all occurrences. This was first established when it was demonstrated that the locus for inherited MTC resides on chromosome 10.[318] Several groups subsequently identified mutations within the RET protein that are responsible for the inherited forms of MTC.[319–321] This discovery has had a profound effect on the diagnostic evaluation and treatment of this disease.

The inherited form of MTC is associated with three autosomal dominant syndromes. Individuals affected with the most common syndrome, multiple endocrine neoplasia type 2A (MEN 2A), present with MTC 95% of the time, and with a lesser frequency, pheochromocytoma (50%) or hyperparathyroidism (15%). Hirschsprung's disease[322] and cutaneous lichen amyloidosis[323] are also associated with MEN 2A but are far less common. The second most common syndrome, multiple endocrine neoplasia type 2B (MEN 2B), also presents with MTC and pheochromocytoma. MEN 2B differs from MEN 2A in that there is an increased incidence of ganglioneuroma of the oral and gastrointestinal mucosa and a marfanoid body habitus without an increase in hyperparathyroidism. Familial MTC (FMTC) is the third and least common of the MTC-associated syndromes. FMTC presents only with MTC, without extrathyroidal manifestations.

All three syndromes are associated with mutations of the *RET* proto-oncogene. *RET* functions as a tyrosine kinase receptor for neurotrophic growth factor (GDNF), a member of the transforming growth factor-beta (TGF-β) subfamily of proteins that are important for the survival and proliferation of many neuronal cell types.[324, 325] GDNF ligands do not bind *RET* directly but act through the family of GFR (GDNF family receptor) coreceptors.[326] The GDNF/GFR complex binds to and activates RET.[326] In MEN 2A, the most common syndrome associated with MTC, more than 98% of affected family members will harbor a single mutation in the extracellular region of the receptor in codons 609, 611, 618, or 620 of exon 10, or in codon 634 of exon 11.[327, 328] Approximately 87% of MEN 2A mutations affect codon 634. Functionally, the mutations disrupt RET protein structure and allow uncontrolled dimerization between RET receptors, with resultant constitutive activation of the RET tyrosine kinase.

There is considerable overlap between mutations found in MEN 2A and FMTC. An exception is the mutation of codon 634 in exon 11, the most common mutation in MEN 2A, which is not found in FMTC. Eighty percent of FMTC families have one of the remaining four mutations described for MEN 2A.[328] FMTC-associated *RET* mutations have been described within exons 13,[329] 14,[330] and 15,[331] which code for intracellular *RET* domains. More than 90% of patients affected with MEN 2B have a single missense mutation of codon 918.[321, 332] Less commonly, mutation of codon 883 in exon 15 has been described.[333] These mutations alter the *RET* domain that recognizes substrate, allowing phosphorylation of substrates preferred by other tyrosine kinases such as c-*src* and c-*abl*.[334] A compilation of mutations found in both hereditary and sporadic MTC is shown in Figure 19–6.

Secretory Function

The primary product secreted by parafollicular C-cells is the hormone calcitonin. However, calcitonin is also secreted by neuroendocrine cells found in the pancreas, stomach, lungs, and adrenal medulla.[335] Neoplastic and non-neoplastic diseases stemming from these APUD-containing tissues, such as small cell lung cancer,[336] carcinoid tumor,[337] gastrinoma,[338] islet cell tumor of the pancreas,[339] renal failure,[340] and pulmonary inflammation,[323] can be associated with modest elevations in calcitonin, but substantial elevations are diagnostic of MTC. Calcitonin secretion is stimulated by the administration of calcium and pentagastrin. Before the identification of *RET* mutations associated with MTC and the feasibility of using this knowledge to genetically screen potentially affected family members, pentagastrin and calcium secretogogues were used for this purpose. Administration of 0.5 µg/kg of pentagastrin IV over 5 seconds and measurement of calcitonin at 0, 1.5, and 5 minutes after injection should not raise serum calcitonin levels above 100 pg/mL in patients without MTC. Likewise, calcitonin should be less than 100 pg/mL when measured at 0, 10, 20, and 30 minutes after the administration of 3 mg/kg of calcium IV over 10 minutes.[341]

MTC is of neuroendocrine origin and can secrete a variety of other polypeptide hormones, including gastrin-releasing peptide, substance P, adrenocorticotropic hormone (ACTH), somatostatin, and vasoactive intestinal peptide (VIP). Nonhormonal neuroendocrine substances also secreted by MTC include neural cell adhesion molecule (NCAM), chromogranin A, L-dopa decarboxylase, and neuron-specific enolase. Carcinoembryonic antigen (CEA) is secreted by MTC and has been used both as a tumor marker and for nuclear medicine imaging. The somatostatin receptor is also expressed in MTC; octreotide scanning is capable of detecting 60% to 80% of tumors.

Diagnosis

Both inherited and sporadic MTC will typically present as a thyroid nodule. The history and physical examination will reveal symptoms such as hoarseness, dysphagia, or painful lymph nodes in the 20% of patients who present with more advanced disease. A small percentage of patients with a large tumor burden will present with paraneoplastic manifestations. These may include hypercortisolism from ACTH production, VIP-induced secretory diarrhea, or flushing from calcitonin gene-related peptide.[342]

FNA is almost always the first procedure performed in keeping with the recommended diagnostic algorithm for any nodule. Characteristic histologic features of FNA specimens such as the nuclear grooves and inclusions found in papillary thyroid cancer are absent. Thus, it is not uncommon for MTC to be misdiagnosed as follicular, papillary, or even anaplastic carcinoma.[343, 344] Immunohistochemical analysis can detect calcitonin on FNA samples from MTC; however, because of cost considerations, this unfortunately is often not performed unless specifically requested. To minimize the risk of intraoperative emergencies from oversecretion by an undiagnosed pheochromocytoma in MEN patients, a family history should be obtained that specifically

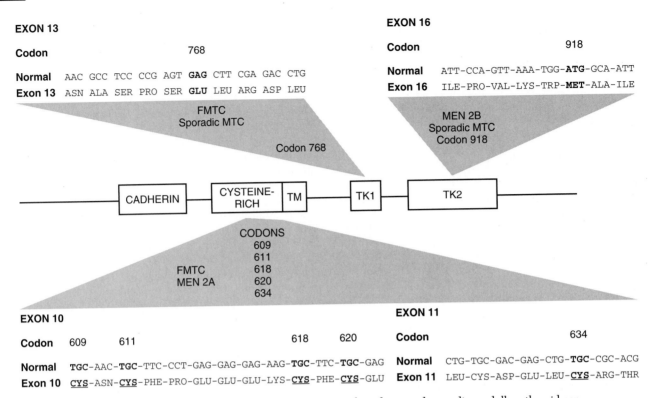

FIGURE 19–6 Mutations of the RET proto-oncogene in hereditary and sporadic medullary thyroid carcinoma (MTC). All hereditary MTC mutations are germline, whereas those associated with sporadic MTC occur only in the parafollicular cell. Mutations of codons 609, 611, 618, 620, 634, and 768 are associated with MEN 2A (multiple endocrine neoplasia type 2A) and FMTC (familial medullary thyroid carcinoma). Mutation of codon 918 is associated with multiple endocrine neoplasia type 2B (MEN 2B). Mutations of codons 768 and 918 have been found in sporadic MTC.

probes for a history compatible with hyperparathyroidism or pheochromocytoma, particularly in those patients with equivocal FNA findings.

Measurable serum calcitonin levels after thyroidectomy reliably indicate persistent or recurrent MTC. However, the use of calcitonin levels to diagnose MTC in patients with an intact thyroid is controversial. The low prevalence of MTC has been an argument against measuring calcitonin levels to screen patients with thyroid nodules or nodular goiter. However, a large prospective study of 1385 patients with thyroid nodules demonstrated that eight patients (0.57%) had calcitonin levels greater than 55 pg/mL with MTC confirmed at surgery.[344] In a similar study of 657 patients with nodular and non-nodular thyroid disease, four (0.84%) of the nodular and none of the non-nodular patients had elevated levels of calcitonin. All four of the surgical specimens immunostained positively for calcitonin after resection.[345]

Another large prospective study determined calcitonin levels in 1167 patients with nodules or goiter before thyroidectomy. MTC was histologically confirmed in 1.37% of patients. A calcitonin level greater than 35 pg/mL identified 75% of patients with MTC with no false-positives. The relative insensitivity of FNA in the diagnosis of MTC was emphasized by the fact that 50% of cases were missed or incorrectly diagnosed by cytologic analysis of the FNA specimen.[346] Several recent studies have substantiated these earlier findings. Among 1448 patients, an elevated calcitonin level identified 10 patients with MCT, 90% having

calcitonin levels greater than or equal to 30 pg/mL.[343] In another study, calcitonin levels greater than 100 pg/mL were detected in 4 of 773 patients, all of whom had MTC found at surgery. Although highly specific, false-negatives have been reported, with normal calcitonin levels measured despite large MTC tumors removed at surgery.[347]

In summary, FNA misdiagnoses MTC at least 50% of the time. In thousands of patients studied, an elevated calcitonin level correctly identifies MTC with a high sensitivity and no reported false-positives. Routine screening of patients with thyroid nodules by measurement of serum calcitonin levels remains controversial. However, as is discussed more fully in the following section, the long-term prognosis of patients with MTC is highly dependent on the extent of the initial surgery. Preoperative diagnosis is crucial for staging and in planning the surgical approach. Therefore, although the cost-effectiveness of calcitonin screening for MTC in nodular thyroid disorders has yet to be determined, routine calcitonin measurements in the evaluation of nodular thyroid disease should be considered and is strongly advocated by some investigators.[348]

Staging

The prognosis after the diagnosis of MTC depends on the extent of initial surgery, particularly when the disease is restricted to the neck. Moreover, metastasis is not uncommonly present when MTC presents as an asymptomatic solitary thyroid nodule. Preoperative staging should therefore include careful evaluation for the presence of metastasis to the neck, chest, mediastinum, liver, and bone. Typically, a combination of ultrasound, CT, or MRI is employed. Other methods that are complementary to traditional imaging include octreotide, dimercaptosuccinic acid (DMSA), and thallium scanning. Metastases to the liver are often difficult but important to detect. Such metastases discourage aggressive reoperation for recurrence, or repeat neck dissection for calcitonin elevations in the absence of other disease. Laparoscopic liver biopsy or hepatic vein sampling for calcitonin appears to be more sensitive than traditional imaging modalities; these approaches are advocated by some before extensive surgery is performed. Patients should preoperatively be evaluated for pheochromocytoma by urine testing for catecholamine excess, and for hyperparathyroidism by parathyroid hormone (PTH) and calcium analysis.

An important part of the staging process unique to MTC is the decision whether to test the patient for germline mutations of the *RET* gene. Traditionally, an elevated calcitonin level after pentagastrin or calcium stimulation was used to screen family members for syndromes associated with MTC. As has been noted earlier, more than 90% of inherited forms of MTC contain mutations detectable by DNA testing; consequently, germline mutation analysis has in most circumstances replaced routine calcitonin testing. These assays are now readily available, and all MTC patients with a family history of pheochromocytoma, hyperparathyroidism, or classic physical findings of MEN 2 should be tested. If positive, family members should be notified and the importance of *RET* testing discussed. It is often helpful to enlist the aid of genetic counselors in this process. However, for a variety of reasons, a negative family history does not preclude the presence of *RET* mutations. The mobile nature of the population and a de-emphasis on the nuclear family may result in an inability to recall a relative's specific medical history or cause of death. For example, even after a detailed family history that was negative for evidence of MEN in newly diagnosed MTC patients, 3% to 6% tested positive for a *RET* mutation.[349, 350] All patients with MTC should be presented with these issues and offered *RET* testing.

Although *RET* testing is very sensitive and accurate, several kindreds have been described that are *RET* negative but still have classic components of hereditary syndromes associated with MTC. Therefore, calcitonin measurement after pentagastrin or calcium stimulation testing of family members is indicated after a family history has been obtained that is suggestive of MEN in a seemingly sporadic case of MTC that tests *RET* negative.

The decision to perform prophylactic thyroidectomy in *RET*-positive family members remains somewhat controversial. MTC found in patients with MEN 2B is very aggressive and can occur before the age of 5. Thyroidectomy is recommended even without evidence of disease. MTC in patients with MEN 2A or FMTC can be indolent or can occur late in life. *RET*-positive patients in a kindred of FMTC were reported to die in their 70s without evidence of disease.[351] Regardless of these facts, the vast majority of *RET*-positive patients will develop MTC. In one study, 71 *RET*-positive MEN and FMTC patients younger than 20 years of age underwent thyroidectomy. All had MTC or C-cell hyperplasia, with 4 having lymph node metastasis.[352] In a similar, smaller study, 11 *RET*-positive MEN/FMTC patients all had either C-cell hyperplasia or MTC at the time of prophylactic thyroidectomy.[353] The overwhelming majority of *RET*-positive patients will develop MTC, and prophylactic thyroidectomy is strongly recommended.

Initial Surgical Management

Up to 40% of patients with MTC will present with palpable regional lymphadenopathy; microscopic lymph node involvement is even more frequent.[354] This early tendency to metastasize to local lymph nodes helps to explain the high rate of persistently elevated postoperative calcitonin levels that occurs in between 57%[355] and 80% of patients.[356] The standard surgical approach to MTC is total thyroidectomy and meticulous central neck dissection.[357] Ipsilateral modified neck dissection should be performed in patients with tumors larger than 2 cm and with cervical lymph node or central lymph node involvement. Parathyroid glands should be identified, and if vascular supply is compromised or threatened, these should be autotransplanted into the neck muscle. The exception is patients with MEN 2A. These patients have a propensity to develop hyperparathyroidism, and their parathyroid gland should be autotransplanted into the forearm.

Although the half-life of injected salmon calcitonin used in the treatment of osteoporosis is approximately 1 hour,[358] the clearance of endogenous calcitonin following resection of MTC can be highly variable. Fugazzola and associates found that normalization of calcitonin occurred quickly, within 15 days postoperatively in the majority of patients, although in one patient, 6 months was required.[359]

Follow-up and Prognosis

Persistent or recurrent medullary carcinoma is typically characterized by slow progression. Patients with no evidence of disease but elevated basal calcitonin levels have up to a 90% survival at 10 years.[360] Long-term survival was studied in 247 patients with MTC. Overall, 64% of patients were alive at 15 years. When hereditary forms of MTC were excluded, the 15-year survival was 54%. Age, tumor size, and stage were the only significant prognostic factors.[361] In a similar study of 899 patients, overall survival was 78% at 10 years, with 97% alive who had postoperative biochemical cures. Age and stage were the only significant predictors of survival by multivariate analysis.[355]

Given the slow progression of MTC, follow-up should be individualized for each patient according to age, stage, and other clinical parameters present at the time of initial resection. All patients require a periodic physical examination and history, with particular attention to symptoms of hoarseness, shortness of breath, dysphagia, bone pain, diarrhea, or abdominal pain. For patients with undetectable calcitonin levels after surgery, basal calcitonin levels and CEA should be initially measured at least at 6-month intervals. If levels are stable after 3 years, yearly calcitonin levels are sufficient. The frequency of imaging procedures for patients with detectable levels of calcitonin after surgery should be based on staging and the calcitonin level. Calcitonin levels roughly correlate with extent of disease, so CT or MRI of the neck is rarely helpful with levels lower than 200 pg/mL, and 6-month to yearly intervals are sufficient in the absence of clinical symptoms. Patients with obvious disease will need closer radiologic follow-up; this process should be tempered by the threshold adopted for reoperation. Complete cure or normalization of calcitonin levels is rare at this juncture. Tumor that threatens the major vessels in the neck or mediastinum or causes significant signs of obstruction should be resected. Resection of clinically "silent" lesions in the lung, neck, or liver is of doubtful utility.

One caveat to the previous approach is an attempted cure of patients with detectable calcitonin levels without extensive physical or radiographic evidence of disease. An initial report of reexploration and aggressive lymph node dissection in 11 patients with increased calcitonin levels following thyroidectomy resulted in normalization of calcitonin in three patients.[362] A similar study of 33 patients normalized the calcitonin in 33% and reduced the level by more than 40% in 39% of patients studied.[363] In a subsequent series, the same authors substantially increased the success rate by selecting patients without evidence of distant metastasis through measurement of stimulated calcitonin levels in hepatic vein catheterization samples.[364] A recent study found that aggressive initial surgery or reoperation for calcitonin positivity in the absence of obvious disease resulted in normalization in 29% of patients. Reoperation for bulky cervical lymphadenopathy was rarely curative.[365]

Other Forms of Treatment

Medullary carcinoma is only moderately radiosensitive, even less so than differentiated thyroid carcinoma. Several reports have shown improved local tumor control but no effect on survival.[366–368] The primary indication for external irradiation is palliation of brain metastasis, obstruction, or prevention of pathologic fracture in the case of bone metastasis.

Chemotherapy has a very limited role in the treatment of medullary carcinoma. Doxorubicin is the most effective agent, and there is no convincing evidence that the addition of other drugs increases efficacy. No cures have been reported, and response is typically defined as a decrease in calcitonin level for a few months. Doxorubicin at various doses alone produced responses in 11% to 60% of patients.[256, 257, 369] The response rate was similar when doxorubicin was combined with bleomycin (33%),[370] cisplatin (10%),[371] and streptozotocin (20%).[372] One promising regimen was a combination of doxorubicin, carboplatin, dacarbazine (DTIC), and vincristine; when this was given, 44% of patients responded with sustained decreases in calcitonin and CEA levels for 5 months. Octreotide provides symptomatic relief of diarrhea and reduction in calcitonin but no decrease in tumor mass.[373]

◻ ANAPLASTIC CANCER OF THE THYROID

Anaplastic or undifferentiated thyroid cancer is a lethal disease that commonly overcomes the patient within a few months of diagnosis. The patient usually presents with a rapidly growing mass in the anterior lower neck and has airway or swallowing difficulties. However, anaplastic thyroid cancer must be differentiated from lymphoma of the thyroid, which can have a similar presentation. Anaplastic thyroid carcinoma accounts for approximately 5% of primary malignant thyroid neoplasms.[374, 375] The frequency of this highly aggressive disease appears to be decreasing, which may be the result of the introduction of iodine supplementation in endemic goiter regions.[1] Compared with differentiated thyroid cancer, anaplastic carcinoma is mainly a disease of the elderly, with a peak incidence in the seventh decade of life.[374, 376] The cause of anaplastic carcinoma is uncertain but appears to be associated with existing thyroid disease. At least 20% of patients have a history of papillary or follicular carcinoma or preexisting goiter, and another 30% may have areas of well-differentiated carcinoma in the resected specimen. These findings support the theory that many anaplastic carcinomas arise as a result of dedifferentiation from more differentiated thyroid cancer,[377–380] although evidence of a triggering event or environmental risk factor is uncertain.

Pathology

Anaplastic thyroid carcinoma is usually an obviously infiltrating tumor that contains foci of necrosis and hemorrhage. Grossly, these tumors are gray/white in color and fibrous and may have areas that are calcified or ossified. Microscopic features characteristic of all anaplastic carcinomas are high mitotic activity, marked cellular pleomorphism, extensive necrosis, tumor emboli, and vascular invasions.[376] This malignancy is readily diagnosed by FNA biopsy, although immunohistochemical stains or electron microscopy may be necessary to distinguish this tumor from melanoma, lymphoma, MTC, and other poorly differentiated malignancies. Immunohistochemical staining of anaplastic thyroid carcinoma is often positive for thyroglobulin, indicating a thyroid epithelial cell origin, although negative staining does not exclude such an origin.[381, 382] Alternatively, tumors may stain for various epithelial sarcoma markers, such as epithelial membrane antigen, keratin, or 1-antichymotrypsin.[377, 383, 384]

Clinical Presentation

Clinical presentation in patients with anaplastic thyroid cancer includes a history of preexisting goiter of long duration that suddenly changes in clinical behavior, or possibly a history of a differentiated thyroid carcinoma. The most frequent presenting complaint is a rapidly growing mass, with tightness or pressure in the neck (Fig. 19–7). Other symptoms in decreasing order of frequency include dysphagia, hoarseness, dyspnea, neck pain, sore throat, and cough.[385, 386] An inflammatory component is often evident at presentation. Necrosis is a common event in these neoplasms, which may cause thyrotoxicosis secondary to thyroid tissue loss.[387]

On physical examination of the neck, the tumor is usually a large, irregular, firm mass that is fixed to surrounding or underlying structures, indicating extrathyroidal involvement. Metastatic cervical lymph nodes may be palpable.

are frequently used concomitantly to take advantage of the radiation-sensitizing properties of doxorubicin and the inhibiting effects of cisplatin on DNA repair mechanisms after radiation damage.

Although control of the primary tumor has improved with these varied approaches, mortality remains high. Despite this, a subset of patients are cured of this condition. The common underlying theme in these patients is localized disease, often with areas of dedifferentiated anaplastic carcinoma in an otherwise differentiated thyroid carcinoma specimen. Various combinations of surgery, radiation, and chemotherapy have been responsible for these cures, and we recommend that all patients with this diagnosis be given a chance to respond to a combination of radiation and chemotherapy.

☐ LYMPHOMA OF THE THYROID

Primary thyroidal lymphoma, once regarded as a rare disease, is now recognized to occur with greater frequency than anaplastic thyroid carcinoma, accounting for more than 5% of all thyroid malignancies.[1, 398–400] The incidence of thyroid lymphoma has increased in recent years, which may be a result of the rise in occurrence of Hashimoto's disease in many countries. Hashimoto's disease increases the patient's risk of thyroid lymphoma by approximately 70-fold.[401] Thus, histiocytic (large cell) lymphoma is almost always accompanied by clinical and histologic evidence of chronic lymphocytic thyroiditis.[399, 400]

Pathology

A vast majority of thyroid lymphomas are of the non-Hodgkin's B-cell type, with large cell lymphoma being more common than other histologic types. Hodgkin's disease extending from the cervical lymph nodes can also involve the thyroid secondarily. Grossly, the glands are enlarged and are replaced by gray/tan to gray/white firm tissue; extension into the adjacent tissues frequently is grossly visible.[402] Microscopically, lymphomas are recognized on the basis of the infiltrated growth pattern and the effacement of the thyroid tissue by monotonous or admixed small and large lymphoid cells.[403] Extension of lymphomatous infiltrates into the adjacent soft tissues and skeletal muscle is a common and helpful diagnostic finding. Evidence of lymphocytic thyroiditis can invariably be found in the preserved thyroid parenchyma, often making precise classification difficult. FNA can usually distinguish lymphoma from autoimmune thyroiditis, particularly if lymphocyte monoclonality can be established. Differentiation from anaplastic thyroid carcinoma may not be possible by FNA biopsy, and separation of these disorders may require open biopsy with tissue immunohistochemical staining.[404–406] The appropriate extent of the biopsy is controversial, but sufficient tissue should be obtained to allow the pathologist to type the lymphoma.

Clinical Presentation

Similar to anaplastic disease, symptoms of lymphoma are typically those of a rapidly expanding thyroid mass causing

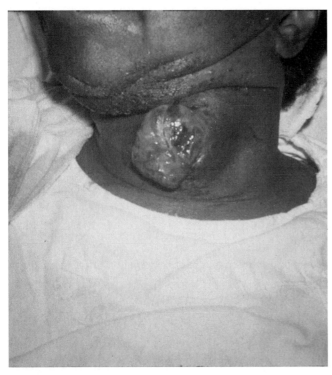

FIGURE 19–7 Patient with a rapidly growing thyroid mass with significant skin and extrathyroidal involvement. Biopsy demonstrated anaplastic carcinoma.

Tracheal invasion is found in up to 25% of patients, with 50% presenting with tumors larger than 5 cm in diameter.[1, 388] The larynx should be examined for vocal cord paralysis, which can be unilateral or bilateral. Patients presenting with dyspnea may have paralyzed vocal cords or tracheal obstruction by compression or direct invasion. Involvement of the esophagus may result in dysphagia. Distant metastasis occurs most often to the lung; however, spread has been documented to occur to multiple other organ sites, including the brain, esophagus, ribs, or small bowel.[388, 389]

Treatment

Single-modality treatment for anaplastic carcinoma is rarely effective in controlling this disease, and a multimodality regimen, although often ineffective also, has been found to be the most effective treatment. The sequence in which the different treatment modalities are applied varies with the stage of disease at presentation, and the initial goals of therapy should be to ensure airway protection and a route for nutritional support.[385] Surgery can play an important role, especially when complete surgical removal can be achieved; however, the extent of resection must be carefully weighed against its feasibility and the complications of treatment in these patients, who carry a dismal prognosis.

Doxorubicin has become established as a standard chemotherapy,[390–396] often in combination with cisplatin.[395, 397] There is no standard approach to the combined therapeutic efforts; some investigators prefer other chemotherapy agents and others prefer hyperfractionated radiation rather than standard dosing. Chemotherapy and radiation therapy

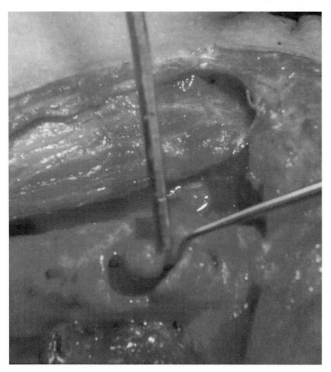

FIGURE 19–8 Patient with a diagnosis of thyroid lymphoma. Note intratracheal extension of tumor mass and subsequent removal.

compression of surrounding neck structures (Fig. 19–8). Occasionally, lymphoma presents as a solitary nodule rather than as a diffuse firm mass.[407] Most patients complain of swelling in the neck and tenderness, hoarseness, dysphagia, neck pressure, and/or vocal cord paralysis.[400] In addition to biopsy of the specimen for adequate typing of the lymphoma, staging should include a CT scan of the brain, head, neck, chest, abdomen, and pelvis; a bipedal angiogram; and a bone marrow biopsy. Some advocate a gastrointestinal tract contrast study to evaluate for mucosa associated lymphoid tissue (MALT) because thyroid lymphoma may have a common origin with these lymphomas that arise from MALT. Thyroid lymphoma is generally localized to the thyroid gland and is classified as stage IE (E = extranodal). If regional lymph nodes are involved, the disease is stage IIE.

Treatment

The treatment of thyroid lymphoma is controversial. After the sensitivity of lymphomas to radiation was demonstrated, this became the mainstay of therapy, either alone or in combination with chemotherapy. The success of combination chemotherapy in patients with advanced aggressive lymphomas has led to an increased use of chemotherapy in patients with clinically localized disease.[408] The most common chemotherapeutic regimens used are anthracycline-based (doxorubicin), such as cyclophosphamide, doxorubicin, vincristine, and prednisone (CHOP).

A study done at Yale University compared the incidences of local and distant relapse after radiation therapy, chemotherapy, or combined-modality treatment for stage I or II thyroid lymphoma; a patient series at that institution (N = 211) was used, as were series in the published literature. Distant and overall relapse rates were significantly lower in the group that received combined-modality treatment. Local relapse was less, but the difference was not statistically significant. In a small number of patients with disease confined to the neck, the results with radiation were similar to those with combined-modality treatment if the mediastinum was included in the treatment port. Overall, the relapse rates were 7.7% for combined-modality therapy versus 37.1% and 43% for radiation therapy alone and chemotherapy alone, respectively.[408–418]

Given the excellent results of either radiation or combined-modality therapy in patients with stage IE to IIE thyroid lymphoma (neck), and the low likelihood that the two treatments will be directly compared, the choice between the two treatments must be individualized. However, because chemotherapy offers the advantage of systemic treatment, combined-modality therapy is currently recommended in patients with good performance status and no contraindication to systemic chemotherapy.

REFERENCES

1. Callendar DL, Sherman SI, Gagel RF, et al: Cancer of the thyroid. In Myers EN, Suen JY (eds): Cancer of the Head and Neck, 3rd ed. Philadelphia, WB Saunders, 1996, pp 485–515.
2. Akerstrom G, Malmaeus J, Bergstrom R: Surgical anatomy of human parathyroid glands. Surgery 95:14, 1984.
3. Wang CA: The anatomic basis of parathyroid surgery. Ann Surg 183:271, 1976.
4. Mazzaferri EL: Management of a solitary thyroid nodule. N Engl J Med 328:553–559, 1993.
5. Parkin DM, Muir CS: Cancer Incidence in Five Continents. Comparability and Quality of Data. Lyon, IARC Scientific Publications, 1992, pp 45–173.
6. Bramley MD, Harrison BJ: Papillary microcarcinoma of the thyroid gland. Br J Surg 83:1674–1683, 1996.
7. Hay ID: Papillary thyroid carcinoma. Endocrinol Metab Clin North Am 19:545–576, 1990.
8. Franceschi S, Boyle P, Maisonneuve P, et al: The epidemiology of thyroid carcinoma. Crit Rev Oncog 4:25–52, 1993.
9. Musholt TJ, Musholt PB, Petrich T, et al: Familial papillary thyroid carcinoma: Genetics, criteria for diagnosis, clinical features, and surgical treatment. World J Surg 24:1409–1417, 2000.
10. Marchesi M, Biffoni M, Biancari F, et al: Familial papillary carcinoma of the thyroid: A report of nine first-degree relatives of four families. Eur J Surg Oncol 26:789–791, 2000.
11. Loh KC, Greenspan FS, Gee L, et al: Pathological tumor-node-metastasis (pTNM) staging for papillary and follicular thyroid carcinomas: A retrospective analysis of 700 patients. J Clin Endocrinol Metab 82:3553–3562, 1997.
12. Hay ID, Bergstralh EJ, Goellner JR, et al: Predicting outcome in papillary thyroid carcinoma: Development of a reliable prognostic scoring system in a cohort of 1779 patients surgically treated at one institution during 1940 through 1989. Surgery 114:1050–1057; discussion 1057–1058, 1993.
13. Mazzaferri EL, Jhiang SM: Long-term impact of initial surgical and medical therapy on papillary and follicular thyroid cancer. (See comments.) (Erratum appears in Am J Med 98:215, 1995.) Am J Med 97:418–428, 1994.
14. Brierley JD, Panzarella T, Tsang RJ, et al: A comparison of different staging systems: Predictability of patient outcome. Thyroid carcinoma as an example. Cancer 79:2414–2423, 1997.
15. DeGroot LJ, Kaplan EL, Straus FH, et al: Does the method of management of papillary thyroid carcinoma make a difference in outcome? World J Surg 18:123–130, 1994.
16. Salvesen H, Njolstad PR, Akslen LA, et al: Papillary thyroid carcinoma: A multivariate analysis of prognostic factors including an evaluation of the p-TNM staging system. Eur J Surg 158:583–589, 1992.

17. Russo D, Arturi F, Wicker R, et al: Genetic alterations in thyroid hyperfunctioning adenomas. J Clin Endocrinol Metab 80:1347–1351, 1995.

18. Nogueira CR, Kopp P, Arseven OK, et al: Thyrotropin receptor mutations in hyperfunctioning thyroid adenomas from Brazil. Thyroid 9:1063–1068, 1999.

19. Tonacchera M, Chiovato L, Pinchera A, et al: Hyperfunctioning thyroid nodules in toxic multinodular goiter share activating thyrotropin receptor mutations with solitary toxic adenoma. J Clin Endocrinol Metab 83:492–498, 1998.

20. Arturi F, Capula C, Chiefari E, et al: Thyroid hyperfunctioning adenomas with and without Gsp/TSH receptor mutations show similar clinical features. Exp Clin Endocrinol Diabetes 106:234–236, 1998.

21. Dent P, Grant S: Pharmacologic interruption of the mitogen-activated extracellular-regulated kinase/mitogen-activated protein kinase signal transduction pathway: Potential role in promoting cytotoxic drug action. Clin Cancer Res 7:775–783, 2001.

22. Bongarzone I, Pierotti MA, Monzini N, et al: High frequency of activation of tyrosine kinase oncogenes in human papillary thyroid carcinoma. Oncogene 4:1457–1462, 1989.

23. Grieco M, Santoro M, Berlingieri MT, et al: PTC is a novel rearranged form of the ret proto-oncogene and is frequently detected in vivo in human thyroid papillary carcinomas. Cell 60:557–563, 1990.

24. Jhiang SM, Caruso DR, Gilmore E, et al: Detection of the PTC/retTPC oncogene in human thyroid cancers. Oncogene 7:1331–1337, 1992.

25. Jhiang SM, Sagartz JE, Tong Q, et al: Targeted expression of the ret/PTC1 oncogene induces papillary thyroid carcinomas. Endocrinology 137:375–378, 1996.

26. Feunteun J, Michiels F, Rochefort P, et al: Targeted oncogenesis in the thyroid of transgenic mice. Horm Res 47:137–139, 1997.

27. Carnell NE, Valente WA: Thyroid nodules in Graves' disease: Classification, characterization, and response to treatment. Thyroid 8:647–652, 1998.

28. Kraimps JL, Bovia-Pineau MH, Mathonnet M, et al: Multicentre study of thyroid nodules in patients with Graves' disease. Br J Surg 87:1111–1113, 2000.

29. Pellegriti G, Belfiore A, Giuffrida D, et al: Outcome of differentiated thyroid cancer in Graves' patients. J Clin Endocrinol Metab 83:2805–2809, 1998.

30. McClellan DR, Francis GL: Thyroid cancer in children, pregnant women, and patients with Graves' disease. Endocrinol Metab Clin North Am 25:27–48, 1996.

31. Belfiore A, Garofalo MR, Giuffrida D, et al: Increased aggressiveness of thyroid cancer in patients with Graves' disease. J Clin Endocrinol Metab 70:830–835, 1990.

32. Kjellman P, Learoyd DL, Messina M, et al: Expression of the RET proto-oncogene in papillary thyroid carcinoma and its correlation with clinical outcome. Br J Surg 88:557–563, 2001.

33. Basolo F, Giannini R, Monaco C, et al: Potent mitogenicity of the RET/PTC3 oncogene correlates with its prevalence in tall-cell variant of papillary thyroid carcinoma. Am J Pathol 160:247–254, 2002.

34. Miki H, Kitaichi M, Masuda E, et al: ret/PTC expression may be associated with local invasion of thyroid papillary carcinoma. J Surg Oncol 71:76–81; discussion 81–82, 1999.

35. Ito T, Seyama T, Iwamoto KS, et al: Activated RET oncogene in thyroid cancers of children from areas contaminated by Chernobyl accident. Lancet 344:259, 1994.

36. Elisei R, Romei C, Vorontsova T, et al: RET/PTC rearrangements in thyroid nodules: studies in irradiated and not irradiated, malignant and benign thyroid lesions in children and adults. J Clin Endocrinol Metab 86:3211–3216, 2001.

37. Evans HL: Follicular neoplasms of the thyroid. A study of 44 cases followed for a minimum of 10 years, with emphasis on differential diagnosis. Cancer 54:535–540, 1984.

38. Cheung CC, Carydis B, Ezzat S, et al: Analysis of ret/PTC gene rearrangements refines the fine needle aspiration diagnosis of thyroid cancer. J Clin Endocrinol Metab 86:2187–2190, 2001.

39. Lahr G, Stich M, Schutze K, et al: Diagnosis of papillary thyroid carcinoma is facilitated by using an RT-PCR approach on laser-microdissected archival material to detect RET oncogene activation. Pathobiology 68:218–226, 2000.

40. Santoro M, Carlomagno F, Hay ID, et al: Ret oncogene activation in human thyroid neoplasms is restricted to the papillary cancer subtype. J Clin Invest 89:1517–1522, 1992.

41. Suarez HG, DuVillard JA, Caillou B, et al: Detection of activated ras oncogenes in human thyroid carcinomas. Oncogene 2:403–406, 1988.

42. Horie H, Yokogoshi Y, Tsuyuguchi M, et al: Point mutations of ras and Gs alpha subunit genes in thyroid tumors. Jpn J Cancer Res 86:737–742, 1995.

43. Hara H, Fulton N, Yashiro T, et al: N-ras mutation: An independent prognostic factor for aggressiveness of papillary thyroid carcinoma. Surgery 116:1010–1016, 1994.

44. Namba H, Rubin SA, Fagin JA: Point mutations of ras oncogenes are an early event in thyroid tumorigenesis. Mol Endocrinol 4:1474–1479, 1990.

45. Lo CY, Lam KY, Wan KY: Anaplastic carcinoma of the thyroid. Am J Surg 177:337–339, 1999.

46. Ito T, Seyama T, Mizuno T, et al: Unique association of p53 mutations with undifferentiated but not with differentiated carcinomas of the thyroid gland. Cancer Res 52:1369–1371, 1992.

47. Donghi R, Longoni A, Pilotti S, et al: Gene p53 mutations are restricted to poorly differentiated and undifferentiated carcinomas of the thyroid gland. J Clin Invest 91:1753–1760, 1993.

48. Fagin JA: Tumor suppressor genes in human thyroid neoplasms: p53 mutations are associated undifferentiated thyroid cancers. J Endocrinol Invest 18:140–142, 1995.

49. Blagosklonny MV, Giannakakou P, Wojtowicz M, et al: Effects of p53-expressing adenovirus on the chemosensitivity and differentiation of anaplastic thyroid cancer cells. J Clin Endocrinol Metab 83:2516–2522, 1998.

50. Nagayama Y, Yokoi H, Takeda K, et al: Adenovirus-mediated tumor suppressor p53 gene therapy for anaplastic thyroid carcinoma in vitro and in vivo. J Clin Endocrinol Metab 85:4081–4086, 2000.

51. Moretti F, Farsetti A, Soddu S, et al: p53 re-expression inhibits proliferation and restores differentiation of human thyroid anaplastic carcinoma cells. Oncogene 14:729–740, 1997.

52. Sera N, Ashizawa K, Ando T, et al: Anaplastic changes associated with p53 gene mutation in differentiated thyroid carcinoma after insufficient radioactive iodine (^{131}I) therapy. Thyroid 10:975–979, 2000.

53. Shingu K, Kobayashi S, Yokoyama S, et al: The likely transformation of papillary thyroid carcinoma into anaplastic carcinoma during postoperative radioactive iodine-131 therapy: Report of a case. Surg Today 30:910–913, 2000.

54. Matias-Guiu X, Cuatrecasas M, Musulen E, et al: p53 expression in anaplastic carcinomas arising from thyroid papillary carcinomas. J Clin Pathol 47:337–339, 1994.

55. Matias-Guiu X, Villanueva A, Cuatrecasas M, et al: p53 in a thyroid follicular carcinoma with foci of poorly differentiated and anaplastic carcinoma. Pathol Res Pract 192:1242–1249; discussion 1250–1251, 1996.

56. Nakamura T, Yana I, Kobayashi T, et al: p53 gene mutations associated with anaplastic transformation of human thyroid carcinomas. Jpn J Cancer Res 83:1293–1298, 1992.

57. Jones CJ, Shaw JJ, Wyllie FS, et al: High frequency deletion of the tumour suppressor gene P16INK4a (MTS1) in human thyroid cancer cell lines. Mol Cell Endocrinol 116:115–119, 1996.

58. Isarangkul W: Dense fibrosis. Another diagnostic criterion for papillary thyroid carcinoma. Arch Pathol Lab Med 117:645–646, 1993.

59. Carcangiu ML, Bianchi S: Diffuse sclerosing variant of papillary thyroid carcinoma. Clinicopathologic study of 15 cases. (See comments.) Am J Surg Pathol 13:1041–1049, 1989.

60. Fujimoto Y, Obara T, Ito Y, et al: Diffuse sclerosing variant of papillary carcinoma of the thyroid. Clinical importance, surgical treatment, and follow-up study. Cancer 66:2306–2312, 1990.

61. Albareda M, Puig-Domingo M, Wengrowicz S, et al: Clinical forms of presentation and evolution of diffuse sclerosing variant of papillary carcinoma and insular variant of follicular carcinoma of the thyroid. Thyroid 8:385–391, 1998.

62. Filie AC, Chiesa A, Bryant BR, et al: The tall cell variant of papillary carcinoma of the thyroid: Cytologic features and loss of heterozygosity of metastatic and/or recurrent neoplasms and primary neoplasms. Cancer 87:238–242, 1999.

63. Prendiville S, Burman KD, Ringel MD, et al: Tall cell variant: An aggressive form of papillary thyroid carcinoma. Otolaryngol Head Neck Surg 122:352–357, 2000.

64. Ostrowski ML, Merino MJ: Tall cell variant of papillary thyroid carcinoma: A reassessment and immunohistochemical study with comparison to the usual type of papillary carcinoma of the thyroid. Am J Surg Pathol 20:964–974, 1996.

65. Putti TC, Bhuiya TA: Mixed columnar cell and tall cell variant of papillary carcinoma of thyroid: A case report and review of the literature. Pathology 32:286–289, 2000.

66. Jayaram G: Cytology of columnar-cell variant of papillary thyroid carcinoma. Diagn Cytopathol 22:227–229, 2000.

67. Sobrinho-Simoes M, Nesland JM, Johannessen JV: Columnar-cell carcinoma. Another variant of poorly differentiated carcinoma of the thyroid. Am J Clin Pathol 89:264–267, 1988.

68. Kahn NF, Perzin KH: Follicular carcinoma of the thyroid: An evaluation of the histologic criteria used for diagnosis. Pathol Ann 18(Pt 1):221–253, 1983.

69. Lang W, Georgii A, Stauch G, et al: The differentiation of atypical adenomas and encapsulated follicular carcinomas in the thyroid gland. Virch Arch A Pathol Anat Histol 385:125–141, 1980.

70. Cooper DS, Schneyer CR: Follicular and Hurthle cell carcinoma of the thyroid. Endocrinol Metab Clin North Am 19:577–591, 1990.

71. McDonald MP, Sanders LE, Silverman ML, et al: Hurthle cell carcinoma of the thyroid gland: Prognostic factors and results of surgical treatment. Surgery 120:1000–1004; discussion 1004–1005, 1996.

72. Samaan NA, Schultz PN, Hickey RC, et al: The results of various modalities of treatment of well differentiated thyroid carcinomas: A retrospective review of 1599 patients. J Clin Endocrinol Metab 75:714–720, 1992.

73. Sakamoto A, Kasai N, Sugano H: Poorly differentiated carcinoma of the thyroid. A clinicopathologic entity for a high-risk group of papillary and follicular carcinomas. Cancer 52:1849–1855, 1983.

74. Burman KD, Ringel MD, Wartofsky L: Unusual types of thyroid neoplasms. Endocrinol Metab Clin North Am 25:49–68, 1996.

75. Papotti M, Botto Micca F, Favero A, et al: Poorly differentiated thyroid carcinomas with primordial cell component. A group of aggressive lesions sharing insular, trabecular, and solid patterns. Am J Surg Pathol 17:291–301, 1993.

76. Carcangiu ML, Zampi G, Rosai J: Poorly differentiated ("insular") thyroid carcinoma. A reinterpretation of Langhans' "wuchernde Struma." Am J Surg Pathol 8:655–668, 1984.

77. Sobrinho-Simoes M, Sambade C, Fonseca E, et al: Poorly differentiated carcinomas of the thyroid gland: A review of the clinicopathologic features of a series of 28 cases of a heterogeneous, clinically aggressive group of thyroid tumors. Int J Surg Pathol 10:123–131, 2002.

78. Mazzaferri EL, de los Santos ET, Rofagha-Keyhani S: Solitary thyroid nodule: Diagnosis and management. Med Clin North Am 72:1177–1211, 1988.

79. Belfiore A, LaRosa GL, LaPorta GA, et al: Cancer risk in patients with cold thyroid nodules: Relevance of iodine intake, sex, age, and multinodularity (see comments). Am J Med 93:363–369, 1992.

80. Rojeski MT, Gharib H: Nodular thyroid disease. Evaluation and management. N Engl J Med 313:428–436, 1985.

81. Sheppard MC, Franklyn JA: Management of the single thyroid nodule. Clin Endocrinol (Oxf) 37:398–401, 1992.

82. Ridgway EC: Clinical review 30: Clinician's evaluation of a solitary thyroid nodule. J Clin Endocrinol Metab 74:231–235, 1992.

83. Ridgway EC: Medical treatment of benign thyroid nodules: Have we defined a benefit? Ann Intern Med 128:403–405, 1998.

84. Bennedbaek FN, Perrild H, Hegedus L: Diagnosis and treatment of the solitary thyroid nodule. Results of a European survey. Clin Endocrinol 50:357–363, 1999.

85. Marchesi M, Biffoni M, Biancari F, et al: Familial papillary carcinoma of the thyroid: A report of nine first-degree relatives of four families. Eur J Surg Oncol 26:789–791, 2000.

86. Musholt TJ, Musholt PB, Petrich T, et al: Familial papillary thyroid carcinoma: Genetics, criteria for diagnosis, clinical features, and surgical treatment. World J Surg 24:1409–1417, 2000.

87. Ron E, Kleinerman RA, Boice JD Jr, et al: A population-based case-control study of thyroid cancer. J Natl Cancer Inst 79:1–12, 1987.

88. Lundell M: Thyroid cancer after radiotherapy for skin hemangioma in infancy. Radiat Res 140:334–339, 1994.

89. Schneider AB: Radiation-induced thyroid carcinoma. Clinical course and results of therapy in 296 patients. Ann Intern Med 105:405–412, 1986.

90. DeJong SA: Thyroid carcinoma and hyperparathyroidism after radiation therapy for adolescent acne vulgaris. Surgery 110:691–695, 1991.

91. Tucker MA: Therapeutic radiation at a young age is linked to secondary thyroid cancer. The Late Effects Study Group. Cancer Res 51:2885–2888, 1991.

92. DeGroot LJ, Reilly M, Pinnameneni K, et al: Retrospective and prospective study of radiation-induced thyroid disease. Am J Med 74:852–862, 1983.

93. Roudebush CP: Natural history of radiation-associated thyroid cancer. Arch Intern Med 138:1631–1634, 1978.

94. Samaan NA: A comparison of thyroid carcinoma in those who have and have not had head and neck irradiation in childhood. J Clin Endocrinol Metab 64:219–223, 1987.

95. Ron E: Thyroid cancer after exposure to external radiation: A pooled analysis of seven studies. Radiat Res 141:259–277, 1995.

96. Mortensen JD, Woolner LB, Bennett WA: Gross and microscopic findings in clinically normal thyroid glands. J Clin Endocrinol Metab 15:1270–1280, 1955.

97. DeGroot LJ: Clinical review 2: Diagnostic approach and management of patients exposed to irradiation to the thyroid. J Clin Endocrinol Metab 69:925–928, 1989.

98. Schneider AB: Radiation-induced tumors of the head and neck following childhood irradiation. Prospective studies. Medicine 64:1–15, 1985.

99. Singer PA: Thyroiditis. Acute, subacute, and chronic. Med Clin N Am 75:61–77, 1991.

100. Hung W, Hung W, Anderson KD, et al: Solitary thyroid nodules in 71 children and adolescents. J Pediatr Surg 27:1407–1409, 1992.

101. Wong TH, Ong CL, Tan WT, et al: The solitary thyroid nodule revisited. Ann Acad Med Singapore 22:593–597, 1993.

102. Messaris G, Kyriakou K, Vasilopoulos P, et al: The single thyroid nodule and carcinoma. Br J Surg 61:943–944, 1974.

103. Clark OH: Thyroid nodules and thyroid cancer: Surgical aspects. West J Med 133:1–8, 1980.

104. Pacini F, Elisei R, DiCoscio GC, et al: Thyroid carcinoma in thyrotoxic patients treated by surgery. J Endocrinol Invest 11:107–112, 1988.

105. Terzioglu T, Tezelman S, Onaran Y, et al: Concurrent hyperthyroidism and thyroid carcinoma. Br J Surg 80:1301–1302, 1993.

106. Ahuja S, Ernst H: Hyperthyroidism and thyroid carcinoma. Acta Endocrinol 124:146–151, 1991.

107. Hales IB, McElduff A, Crummer P, et al: Does Graves' disease or thyrotoxicosis affect the prognosis of thyroid cancer. J Clin Endocrinol Metab 75:886–889, 1992.

108. Behar R, Arganini M, Wu TC, et al: Graves' disease and thyroid cancer. Surgery 100:1121–1127, 1986.

109. Dobyns BM, Sheline GE, Workman JB, et al: Malignant and benign neoplasms of the thyroid in patients treated for hyperthyroidism: A report of the cooperative thyrotoxicosis therapy follow-up study. J Clin Endocrinol Metab 38:976–998, 1974.

110. Holm LE, Blomgren H, Lowhagen T: Cancer risks in patients with chronic lymphocytic thyroiditis. N Engl J Med 312:601–604, 1985.

111. DeGroot LJ, Larsen PR, Hennemann G: The Thyroid and Its Diseases. New York, Churchill Livingstone, 1996, p 494.

112. Aggarwal SK, Jayaram G, Kakar A, et al: Fine needle aspiration cytologic diagnosis of the solitary cold thyroid nodule. Comparison with ultrasonography, radionuclide perfusion study and xeroradiography. Acta Cytol 33:41–47, 1989.

113. Propper RA, Skolnick ML, Weinstein RJ, et al: The nonspecificity of the thyroid halo sign. J Clin Ultrasound 8:129–132, 1980.

114. Simeone JF, Daniels GH, Hall DA, et al: Sonography in the follow-up of 100 patients with thyroid carcinoma. AJR Am J Roentgenol 148:45–49, 1987.

115. Evans DM: Diagnostic discriminants of thyroid cancer. Am J Surg 153:569–570, 1987.

116. Katagiri M, Harada T, Kiyono T: Diagnosis of thyroid carcinoma by ultrasonic examination: Comparison with diagnosis by fine needle aspiration cytology. Thyroidology 6:21–26, 1994.

117. Braga M, Cavalcanti TC, Collaco LM, et al: Efficacy of ultrasound-guided fine-needle aspiration biopsy in the diagnosis of complex thyroid nodules. J Clin Endocrinol Metab 86:4089–4091, 2001.

118. Haber RS: Role of ultrasonography in the diagnosis and management of thyroid cancer. Endocrinol Pract 6:396–400, 2000.

119. Danese D, Sciacchitano S, Farsetti A, et al: Diagnostic accuracy of conventional versus sonography-guided fine-needle aspiration biopsy of thyroid nodules. Thyroid 8:15–21, 1998.

120. Hagag P, Strauss S, Weiss M: Role of ultrasound-guided fine-needle aspiration biopsy in evaluation of nonpalpable thyroid nodules. Thyroid 8:989–995, 1998.

121. Cochand-Priollet B, Guillausseau PJ, Chagnon S, et al: The diagnostic value of fine-needle aspiration biopsy under ultrasonography in nonfunctional thyroid nodules: A prospective study comparing cytologic and histologic findings (see comments). (Erratum appears in Am J Med 97:311, 1994.) Am J Med 97:152–157, 1994.

122. Blum M: Evaluation of thyroid function: Sonography, computed tomography and magnetic resonance imaging. In Becker KL (ed): Principles and Practice of Endocrinology and Metabolism. Philadelphia, Lippincott, 1990, pp 289–293.

123. Asp AA, Georgitis W, Waldron EJ, et al: Fine needle aspiration of the thyroid. Use in an average health care facility. Am J Med 83:489–493, 1987.

124. de los Santos ET, Keyhani-Rafagha S, Cunningham JJ, et al: Cystic thyroid nodules. The dilemma of malignant lesions. Arch Intern Med 150:1422–1427, 1990.

125. Hall TL, Layfield LJ, Philippe A, et al: Sources of diagnostic error in fine needle aspiration of the thyroid. Cancer 63:718–725, 1989.

126. Pepper GM, Zwickler D, Rosen Y: Fine-needle aspiration biopsy of the thyroid nodule. Results of a start-up project in a general teaching hospital setting. Arch Intern Med 149:594–596, 1989.

127. Al-Sayer HM, Krukowski ZH, Williams VM, et al: Fine needle aspiration cytology in isolated thyroid swellings: A prospective two year evaluation. Br Med J Clin Res Ed 290:1490–1492, 1985.

128. Caplan RH, Kisken WA, Strutt PJ, et al: Fine-needle aspiration biopsy of thyroid nodules. A cost-effective diagnostic plan (see comments). Postgrad Med 90:183–187, 1991.

129. Hamberger B, Gharib H, Melton LJ 3rd et al: Fine-needle aspiration biopsy of thyroid nodules. Impact on thyroid practice and cost of care. Am J Med 73:381–384, 1982.

130. Gharib H, Goellner JR, Johnson DA: Fine-needle aspiration cytology of the thyroid. A 12-year experience with 11,000 biopsies. Clin Lab Med 13:699–709, 1993.

131. Karstrup S, Balslev E, Juul N, et al: US-guided fine needle aspiration versus coarse needle biopsy of thyroid nodules. Eur J Ultrasound 13:1–5, 2001.

132. Nishiyama RH, Bigos ST, Goldfarb WB, et al: The efficacy of simultaneous fine-needle aspiration and large-needle biopsy of the thyroid gland. Surgery 100:1133–1137, 1986.

133. Gharib H, Goellner JR: Fine-needle aspiration biopsy of the thyroid: An appraisal (see comments). Ann Intern Med 118:282–289, 1993.

134. Burch HB, Burman KD, Reed HL, et al: Fine needle aspiration of thyroid nodules. Determinants of insufficiency rate and malignancy yield at thyroidectomy. Acta Cytol 40:1176–1183, 1996.

135. Damiani S, Dina R, Eusebi V: Cytologic grading of aggressive and nonaggressive variants of papillary thyroid carcinoma. Am J Clin Pathol 101:651–655, 1994.

136. Block MA, Dailey GE, Robb JA: Thyroid nodules indeterminate by needle biopsy. Am J Surg 146:72–78, 1983.

137. Schmidt T, Riggs MW, Speights VO Jr: Significance of nondiagnostic fine-needle aspiration of the thyroid. South Med J 90:1183–1186, 1997.

138. McHenry CR, Walfish PG, Rosen IB: Non-diagnostic fine needle aspiration biopsy: A dilemma in management of nodular thyroid disease. Am J Surg 59:415–419, 1993.

139. Chow LS, Gharib H, Goellner JR, et al: Nondiagnostic thyroid fine-needle aspiration cytology: Management dilemmas. Thyroid 11:1147–1151, 2001.

140. McHenry CR, Walfish PG, Rosen IB: Non-diagnostic fine needle aspiration biopsy: A dilemma in management of nodular thyroid disease. Am Surg 59:415–419, 1993.

141. Goellner JR, Gharib H, Grant CS, et al: Fine needle aspiration cytology of the thyroid, 1980 to 1986. Acta Cytol 31:587–590, 1987.

142. Burguera B, Gharib H: Thyroid incidentalomas. Prevalence, diagnosis, significance, and management. Endocrinol Metab Clin N Am 29:187–203, 2000.

143. Castillo L, Haddad A, Meyer JM, et al: (Predictive malignancy factors in thyroid nodular disease.) Ann Otolaryngol Chir Cervicofac 117:383–389, 2000.

144. Cerise EJ, Guansing AR, Oschner A: Carcinoma of the thyroid and nontoxic nodular goiter. Surgery 31:552–561, 1952.

145. Anglem TJ, Bradford ML: Nodular goiter and thyroid cancer. N Engl J Med 239:217–220, 1948.

146. Ma MK, Ong GB: Cystic thyroid nodules. Br J Surg 62:205–206, 1975.

147. Layfield LJ, Reichman A, Bottles K, et al: Clinical determinants for the management of thyroid nodules by fine-needle aspiration cytology. Arch Otolaryngol Head Neck Surg 118:717–721, 1992.

148. McCall A, Jarosz H, Lawrence AM, et al: The incidence of thyroid carcinoma in solitary cold nodules and in multinodular goiters. Surgery 100:1128–1132, 1986.

149. Merchant SH, Izquierdo R, Khurana KK: Is repeated fine-needle aspiration cytology useful in the management of patients with benign nodular thyroid disease? Thyroid 10:489–492, 2000.

150. Mittendorf EA, McHenry CR: Follow-up evaluation and clinical course of patients with benign nodular thyroid disease. Am Surg 65:653–657; discussion 657–658, 1999.

151. Erdogan MF, Kamal N, Aras D, et al: Value of re-aspirations in benign nodular thyroid disease. Thyroid 8:1087–1090, 1998.

152. Lucas A, Llatjos M, Salinas I, et al: Fine-needle aspiration cytology of benign nodular thyroid disease. Value of re-aspiration. Eur J Endocrinol 132:677–680, 1995.

153. Morita T, Tamai H, Ohshima A, et al: Changes in serum thyroid hormone, thyrotropin and thyroglobulin concentrations during thyroxine therapy in patients with solitary thyroid nodules. J Clin Endocrinol Metab 69:227–230, 1989.

154. Celani MF, Mariani M, Mariani G: On the usefulness of levothyroxine suppressive therapy in the medical treatment of benign solitary, solid or predominantly solid, thyroid nodules. Acta Endocrinol 123:603–608, 1990.

155. Kuo SW, Hu CA, Pei D, et al: Efficacy of thyroxine-suppressive therapy and its relation to serum thyroglobulin levels in solitary nontoxic thyroid nodules. J Formos Med Assoc 92:55–60, 1993.

156. Lima N, Knobel M, Cavaliere H, et al: Levothyroxine suppressive therapy is partially effective in treating patients with benign, solid thyroid nodules and multinodular goiters. Thyroid 7:691–697, 1997.

157. Papini E, Petrucci L, Guglielmi R, et al: Long-term changes in nodular goiter: A 5-year prospective randomized trial of levothyroxine suppressive therapy for benign cold thyroid nodules. J Clin Endocrinol Metab 83:780–783, 1998.

158. Kuma K, Matsuzuka F, Kobayashi A, et al: Outcome of long standing solitary thyroid nodules. World J Surg 16:583–587; discussion 587–588, 1992.

159. Sawin CT, Geller A, Wolf PA, et al: Low serum thyrotropin concentrations as a risk factor for atrial fibrillation in older persons (see comments). N Engl J Med 331:1249–1252, 1994.

160. Faber J, Galloe AM: Changes in bone mass during prolonged subclinical hyperthyroidism due to L-thyroxine treatment: A meta-analysis. Eur J Endocrinol 130:350–356, 1994.

161. Gharib HMD, Mazzaferri ELMD: Thyroxine suppressive therapy in patients with nodular thyroid disease. Ann Intern Med 128:386–394, 1998.

162. Hegedus L, Nygaard B, Hansen JM: Is routine thyroxine treatment to hinder postoperative recurrence of nontoxic goiter justified? J Clin Endocrinol Metab 84:756–760, 1999.

163. Huysmans D, Hermus A, Edelbroek M, et al: Radioiodine for nontoxic multinodular goiter. Thyroid 7:235–239, 1997.

164. Nygaard B, Hegedus L, Ulriksen P, et al: Radioiodine therapy for multinodular toxic goiter. Arch Intern Med 159:1364–1368, 1999.

165. Huysmans DA, Hermus AR, Corstens FH, et al: Large, compressive goiters treated with radioiodine. Ann Intern Med 121:757–762, 1994.

166. de los Santos ET, Keyhani-Rofagha S, Cunningham JJ, et al: Cystic thyroid nodules. The dilemma of malignant lesions (see comments). Arch Intern Med 150:1422–1427, 1990.

167. Rosen IB, Provias JP, Walfish PG: Pathologic nature of cystic thyroid nodules selected for surgery by needle aspiration biopsy. Surgery 100:606–613, 1986.

168. Cho YS, Lee HK, Ahn IM, et al: Sonographically guided ethanol sclerotherapy for benign thyroid cysts: Results in 22 patients. AJR Am J Roentgenol 174:213–216, 2000.

169. Zingrillo M, Torlontano M, Chiarella R, et al: Percutaneous ethanol injection may be a definitive treatment for symptomatic thyroid cystic nodules not treatable by surgery: Five-year follow-up study. Thyroid 9:763–767, 1999.

170. Monzani F, Lippi F, Goletti O, et al: Percutaneous aspiration and ethanol sclerotherapy for thyroid cysts. J Clin Endocrinol Metab 78:800–802, 1994.

171. DeGroot LJ, Kaplan EL, McCormick M, et al: Natural history, treatment, and course of papillary thyroid carcinoma. J Clin Endocrinol Metab 71:414–424, 1990.

172. Mazzaferri EL: Thyroid remnant 131I ablation for papillary and follicular thyroid carcinoma. Thyroid 7:265–271, 1997.

173. Roos DE, Smith JG: Randomized trials on radioactive iodine ablation of thyroid remnants for thyroid carcinoma—a critique. Int J Radiat Oncol Biol Phys 44:493–495, 1999.

174. Beierwaltes WH, Rabbani R, Dmuchowski C, et al: An analysis of "ablation of thyroid remnants" with I-131 in 511 patients from 1947–1984: Experience at University of Michigan. J Nucl Med 25:1287–1293, 1984.

175. Simpson WJ, Panzarella T, Carruthers JJ, et al: Papillary and follicular thyroid cancer: Impact of treatment in 1578 patients. Int J Radiat Oncol Biol Phys 14:1063–1075, 1988.

176. Maxon HR 3rd, Englaro EE, Thomas SR, et al: Radioiodine-131 therapy for well-differentiated thyroid cancer—a quantitative radiation dosimetric approach: Outcome and validation in 85 patients. J Nucl Med 33:1132–1136, 1992.

177. Comtois R, Theriault C, Del Vecchio P: Assessment of the efficacy of iodine-131 for thyroid ablation. J Nucl Med 34:1927–1930, 1993.

178. Leung SF, Law MW, Ho SK: Efficacy of low-dose iodine-131 ablation of post-operative thyroid remnants: A study of 69 cases. Br J Radiol 65:905–909, 1992.

179. Cailleux AF, Baudin E, Travagli JP, et al: Is diagnostic iodine-131 scanning useful after total thyroid ablation for differentiated thyroid cancer? J Clin Endocrinol Metab 85:175–178, 2000.

180. Sherman SI, Tielens ET, Sostre S, et al: Clinical utility of posttreatment radioiodine scans in the management of patients with thyroid carcinoma. J Clin Endocrinol Metab 78:629–634, 1994.

181. Tenenbaum F, Corone C, Schlumberger M, et al: Thyroglobulin measurement and postablative iodine-131 total body scan after total thyroidectomy for differentiated thyroid carcinoma in patients with no evidence of disease. Eur J Cancer 32A:1262, 1996.

182. Schlumberger M, Arcangioli O, Piekarski JD, et al: Detection and treatment of lung metastases of differentiated thyroid carcinoma in patients with normal chest X-rays. J Nucl Med 29:1790–1794, 1988.

183. Pineda JD, Lee T, Ain K, et al: Iodine-131 therapy for thyroid cancer patients with elevated thyroglobulin and negative diagnostic scan. J Clin Endocrinol Metab 80:1488–1492, 1995.

184. Robbins RJ, Tuttle RM, Sonenberg M, et al: Radioiodine ablation of thyroid remnants after preparation with recombinant human thyrotropin. Thyroid 11:865–869, 2001.

185. Beierwaltes WH: The treatment of thyroid carcinoma with radioactive iodine. Semin Nucl Med 8:79–94, 1978.

186. Beierwaltes WH, Nishiyama RH, Thompson NW, et al: Survival time and "cure" in papillary and follicular thyroid carcinoma with distant metastases: Statistics following University of Michigan therapy. J Nucl Med 23:561–568, 1982.

187. Maxon HR: Quantitative radioiodine therapy in the treatment of differentiated thyroid cancer. Q J Nucl Med 43:313–323, 1999.

188. Maxon HR, Thomas SR, Hertzberg VS, et al: Relation between effective radiation dose and outcome of radioiodine therapy for thyroid cancer. N Engl J Med 309:937–941, 1983.

189. Furhang EE, Larson SM, Buranapong P, et al: Thyroid cancer dosimetry using clearance fitting. J Nucl Med 40:131–136, 1999.

190. Reynolds JC: Percent 131I uptake and post-therapy 131I scans: Their role in the management of thyroid cancer. Thyroid 7:281–284, 1997.

191. Kaptein EM, Levenson H, Siegel ME, et al: Radioiodine dosimetry in patients with end-stage renal disease receiving continuous ambulatory peritoneal dialysis therapy. J Clin Endocrinol Metab 85:3058–3064, 2000.

192. Cady B, Rossi R: An expanded view of risk-group definition in differentiated thyroid carcinoma. Surgery 104:947–953, 1988.

193. Scheumann GF, Gimm O, Wegener G, et al: Prognostic significance and surgical management of locoregional lymph node metastases in papillary thyroid cancer. World J Surg 18:559–567; discussion 567–568, 1994.

194. Akslen LA, Haldorsen T, Thoresen SO, et al: Survival and causes of death in thyroid cancer: A population-based study of 2479 cases from Norway. Cancer Res 51:1234–1241, 1991.

195. Coburn MC, Wanebo HJ: Prognostic factors and management considerations in patients with cervical metastases of thyroid cancer. Am J Surg 164:671–676, 1992.

196. Sellers M, Beenken S, Blankenship A, et al: Prognostic significance of cervical lymph node metastases in differentiated thyroid cancer. Am J Surg 164:578–581, 1992.

197. Samaan NA, Schultz PN, Haynie TP, et al: Pulmonary metastasis of differentiated thyroid carcinoma: Treatment results in 101 patients. J Clin Endocrinol Metab 60:376–380, 1985.

198. Schlumberger M, Tubiana M, DeVathaire F, et al: Long-term results of treatment of 283 patients with lung and bone metastases from differentiated thyroid carcinoma. J Clin Endocrinol Metab 63:960–967, 1986.

199. Harness JK, Thompson NW, Sisson JC, et al: Proceedings: Differentiated thyroid carcinomas. Treatment of distant metastases. Arch Surg 108:410–419, 1974.

200. Proye CA, Dromer DH, Carnaille BM, et al: Is it still worthwhile to treat bone metastases from differentiated thyroid carcinoma with radioactive iodine? World J Surg 16:640–645; discussion 645–646, 1992.

201. Luster M, Lassmann M, Haenscheid H, et al: Use of recombinant human thyrotropin before radioiodine therapy in patients with advanced differentiated thyroid carcinoma. J Clin Endocrinol Metab 85:3640–3645, 2000.

202. Robbins RJ, Voelker E, Wang W, et al: Compassionate use of recombinant human thyrotropin to facilitate radioiodine therapy: Case report and review of literature. Endocr Pract 6:460–464, 2000.

203. Gallowitsch HJ: Gamma probe-guided resection of a lymph node metastasis with I-123 in papillary thyroid carcinoma. Clin Nucl Med 22:591–592, 1997.

204. Boz A: Gamma probe-guided resection and scanning with TC-99m MIBI of a local recurrence of follicular thyroid carcinoma. Clin Nucl Med 26:820–822, 2001.

205. Lippi F: Use of surgical gamma probe for the detection of lymph node metastases in differentiated thyroid cancer. Tumori 86:367–369, 2000.

206. Travagli JP: Combination of radioiodine (131I) and probe-guided surgery for persistent or recurrent thyroid carcinoma. J Clin Endocrinol Metab 83:2675–2680, 1998.

207. Lin WY, Shen YY, Wang SJ: Short-term hazards of low-dose radioiodine ablation therapy in postsurgical thyroid cancer patients. Clin Nucl Med 21:780–782, 1996.

208. Bohuslavizki KH, Klutmann S, Brenner W, et al: Radioprotection of salivary glands by amifostine in high-dose radioiodine treatment. Results of a double-blinded, placebo-controlled study in patients with differentiated thyroid cancer. Strahlenther Onkol 175(suppl 4):6–12, 1999.

209. Malpani BL, Samuel AM, Ray S: Quantification of salivary gland function in thyroid cancer patients treated with radioiodine. Int J Radiat Oncol Biol Phys 35:535–540, 1996.

210. DiRusso G, Kern KA: Comparative analysis of complications from I-131 radioablation for well-differentiated thyroid cancer. Surgery 116:1024–1030, 1994.

211. Van Nostrand D, Neutze J, Atkins F: Side effects of "rational dose" iodine-131 therapy for metastatic well-differentiated thyroid carcinoma. J Nucl Med 27:1519–1527, 1986.

212. Benua RS, Cicale NR, Sonenberg M: The relation of radioiodine dosimetry to results and complications in the treatment of metastatic thyroid cancer. Am J Radiol 87:171, 1962.

213. Samuel AM, Unnikrishnan TP, Baghel NS, et al: Effect of radioiodine therapy on pulmonary alveolar-capillary membrane integrity. J Nucl Med 36:783–787, 1995.

214. Handelsman DJ, Turtle JR: Testicular damage after radioactive iodine (I-131) therapy for thyroid cancer. Clin Endocrinol (Oxf) 18:465–472, 1983.

215. Sarkar SD, Beierwaltes WH, Gill SP, et al: Subsequent fertility and birth histories of children and adolescents treated with 131I for thyroid cancer. J Nucl Med 17:460–464, 1976.

216. Ahmed SR, Shalet SM: Gonadal damage due to radioactive iodine (I131) treatment for thyroid carcinoma. Postgrad Med J 61:361–362, 1985.

217. Raymond JP, Izembart M, Marliac V, et al: Temporary ovarian failure in thyroid cancer patients after thyroid remnant ablation with radioactive iodine. J Clin Endocrinol Metab 69:186–190, 1989.

218. Dottorini ME, Lomuscio G, Mazzucchelli L, et al: Assessment of female fertility and carcinogenesis after iodine-131 therapy for differentiated thyroid carcinoma. J Nucl Med 36:21–27, 1995.

219. Edmonds CJ, Smith T: The long-term hazards of the treatment of thyroid cancer with radioiodine. Br J Radiol 59:45–51, 1986.

220. Pochin EE: Radioiodine therapy of thyroid cancer. Semin Nucl Med 1:503–515, 1971.

221. Hall P, Holm LE, Lundell G, et al: Cancer risks in thyroid cancer patients. Br J Cancer 64:159–163, 1991.

222. Bitton R, Sachmechi I, Benegalrao Y, et al: Leukemia after a small dose of radioiodine for metastatic thyroid cancer. J Clin Endocrinol Metab 77:1423–1426, 1993.

223. Hall P, Holm LE, Lundell G, et al: Tumors after radiotherapy for thyroid cancer. A case-control study within a cohort of thyroid cancer patients. Acta Oncol 31:403–407, 1992.

224. Breaux E, Guillamondegui OM: Treatment of locally invasive carcinomas of the thyroid: How radical? Am J Surg 140:514, 1980.

225. Ballantyne AJ: Resections of the upper aerodigestive tract for locally invasive thyroid cancer. Am J Surg 168:636, 1994.

226. Friedman M, Shelton VK, Skolnick GM, et al: Laryngotracheal invasion by thyroid carcinoma. Ann Otol Rhinol Laryngol 91:363, 1982.

227. Lipton RV, McCaffrey TV, von Heerden JA: Surgical treatment of invasion of the upper aerodigestive tract by well differentiated thyroid carcinoma. Am J Surg 154:363, 1987.

228. Simpson WJ, Carruthers JS: The role of external radiation in the management of papillary and follicular thyroid cancer. Am J Surg 136:457, 1978.

229. Simpson WJ: Radioiodine and radiotherapy in the management of thyroid cancers. Otolaryngol Clin N Am 23:509, 1990.

230. Samaan NA, Schultz PN, Hickey RC, et al: The results of various modalities of treatment of well differentiated thyroid carcinoma: A retrospective review of 1599 patients. J Clin Endocrinol Metab 75:714, 1992.

231. Sessions RB, et al: Cancer of the thyroid gland. In Harrison LB, Sessions RB, Hong WK (eds): Head and Neck Cancer: A Multidisciplinary Approach. Philadelphia, Lippincott-Raven Publishers, 1999.

232. Ballantyne A: Resections of the upper aerodigestive tract for locally invasive thyroid cancer. Am J Surg 168:636, 1994.

233. Friedman M, Shelton V, Skolnick G: Laryngotracheal invasion by thyroid carcinoma. Ann Otol Rhinol Laryngol 91:363, 1982.

234. Lipton R, McCaffrey T, von Heerden J: Surgical treatment of invasion of the upper aerodigestive tract by well differentiated thyroid carcinoma. Am J Surg 154:363, 1987.

235. Friedman M, Toricimi DT, Owens R, et al: Experience with the sternocleidomastoid myoperiosteal flap for reconstruction of subglottic and tracheal defects: Modification of technique and report of long-term results. Laryngoscope 98:1003, 1988.

236. Demeure MJ, Clark OH: Surgery in the treatment of thyroid cancer. Endocrinol Metab Clin N Am 19:663–683, 1990.

237. Duren M, Yavuz N, Bukey Y, et al: Impact of initial surgical treatment on survival of patients with differentiated thyroid cancer: Experience of an endocrine surgery center in an iodine-deficient region. World J Surg 24:1290–1294, 2000.

238. McCaffrey TV, Bergstralh EJ, Hay ID: Locally invasive papillary thyroid carcinoma: 1940–1990. Head Neck 16:165–172, 1994.

239. Fujimoto Y, Obara T, Ito Y, et al: Aggressive surgical approach for locally invasive papillary carcinoma of the thyroid in patients over forty-five years of age. Surgery 100:1098–1107, 1986.

240. Hay ID, Grant CS, van Heerden JA, et al: Papillary thyroid microcarcinoma: A study of 535 cases observed in a 50-year period. Surgery 112:1139–1146; discussion 1146–1147, 1992.

241. Mazzaferri EL: Papillary thyroid carcinoma: Factors influencing prognosis and current therapy. Semin Oncol 14:315–332, 1987.

242. Hochman M, Fee WE Jr: Thyroidectomy under local anesthesia. Arch Otolaryngol Head Neck Surg 117:405, 1991.

243. Cernea CR, Ferraz AR, Nishio S, et al: Surgical anatomy of the external branch of the superior laryngeal nerve. Head Neck 14:380, 1992.

244. Samaan NAI, Schultz PN, Hickey RC: Medullary thyroid carcinoma: Prognosis of familial versus nonfamilial disease and the role of radiotherapy. Horm Metab Res Suppl 21:21, 1989.

245. Miller HH, Melvin KEW, Gibson JM, et al: Surgical approach to early familial medullary carcinoma of the thyroid gland. Am J Surg 123:438, 1972.

246. Tisell L, Hansson G, Jansson S, et al: Reoperation in the treatment of asymptomatic metastasizing medullary thyroid carcinoma. Surgery 99:60, 1986.

247. Flynn MB, Lyons KJ, Tartar JW, et al: Local complications after surgical resection for thyroid cancer. Am J Surg 168:404, 1994.

248. Pearson FG, Cooper JD, Nelems JM, et al: Primary tracheal anastomosis after resection of cricoid cartilage with preservation of recurrent laryngeal nerves. J Thorac Cardiovasc Surg 70:806, 1975.

249. Lore JM, Kim DJ, Elias S: Preservation of the laryngeal nerves during total thyroid lobectomy. Ann Otol Rhinol Laryngol 86:777, 1977.

250. Beahrs OM: Complications of surgery of the head and neck. Surg Clin N Am 57:823, 1977.

251. Dedo H: The paralyzed larynx: An electromyographic study in dogs and humans. Laryngoscope 80:1455, 1970.

252. Crumley RL, Izdensk K: Voice quality following laryngeal reinnervation by ansa hypoglossi transfer. Laryngoscope 96:611, 1986.

253. Tucker HM: Reinnervation of unilaterally paralyzed larynx. Ann Otol Rhinol Laryngol 86:789, 1977.

254. Netterville J, Aly A, Ossoff RH: Evaluation and treatment of complications of thyroid and parathyroid surgery. Otolaryngol Clin N Am 23:529, 1990.

255. Rice DH: Laryngeal reinnervation. Laryngoscope 92:1049, 1982.

256. Gottlieb JA, Hill CS: Chemotherapy of thyroid cancer with Adriamycin. Experience with 30 patients. N Engl J Med 290:193–197, 1974.

257. Shimaoka K, Schoenfeld DA, DeWys WD, et al: A randomized trial of doxorubicin versus doxorubicin plus cisplatin in patients with advanced thyroid carcinoma. Cancer 56:2155–2160, 1985.

258. Williams SD, Birch R, Einhorn LH: Phase II evaluation of doxorubicin plus cisplatin in advanced thyroid cancer: A Southeastern Cancer Study Group Trial. Cancer Treat Rep 70:405–407, 1986.

259. O'Connell ME, A'Hern RP, Harmer CL: Results of external beam radiotherapy in differentiated thyroid carcinoma: A retrospective study from the Royal Marsden Hospital. Eur J Cancer 30A:733–739, 1994.

260. Simpson WJ, Panzarella T, Carruthers JS, et al: Papillary and follicular thyroid cancer: Impact of treatment in 1578 patients. Int J Radiat Oncol Biol Phys 14:1063–1075, 1988.

261. Benker G, Olbricht T, Reinwein D, et al: Survival rates in patients with differentiated thyroid carcinoma. Influence of postoperative external radiotherapy. Cancer 65:1517–1520, 1990.

262. Mazzaferri EL, Young RL: Papillary thyroid carcinoma: A 10 year follow-up report of the impact of therapy in 576 patients. Am J Med 70:511–518, 1981.

263. Phlips P, Hanzen C, Andry G, et al: Postoperative irradiation for thyroid cancer. Eur J Surg Oncol 19:399–404, 1993.

264. Farahati J, Reiners C, Stuschke M, et al: Differentiated thyroid cancer. Impact of adjuvant external radiotherapy in patients with perithyroidal tumor infiltration (stage pT4). Cancer 77:172–180, 1996.

265. Kim JH, Leeper RD: Treatment of locally advanced thyroid carcinoma with combination doxorubicin and radiation therapy. Cancer 60:2372–2375, 1987.

266. Mazzaferri EL, Young RL: Papillary thyroid carcinoma: A 10 year follow-up report of the impact of therapy in 576 patients. Am J Med 70:511–518, 1981.

267. Spencer CA, LoPresti JS, Fatemi S, et al: Detection of residual and recurrent differentiated thyroid carcinoma by serum thyroglobulin measurement. Thyroid 9:435–441, 1999.

268. Pujol P, Daures JP, Nsakala N, et al: Degree of thyrotropin suppression as a prognostic determinant in differentiated thyroid cancer. J Clin Endocrinol Metab 81:4318–4323, 1996.

269. Kamel N, Gullu S, Dagci Ilgin S, et al: Degree of thyrotropin suppression in differentiated thyroid cancer without recurrence or metastases. Thyroid 9:1245–1248, 1999.

270. Cooper DS, Specker B, Ho M, et al: Thyrotropin suppression and disease progression in patients with differentiated thyroid cancer: Results from the National Thyroid Cancer Treatment Cooperative Registry. Thyroid 8:737–744, 1998.

271. Dow KH, Ferrell BR, Anello C: Quality-of-life changes in patients with thyroid cancer after withdrawal of thyroid hormone therapy. Thyroid 7:613–619, 1997.

272. Goldberg LD, Ditchek NT: Thyroid carcinoma with spinal cord compression. JAMA 245:953–954, 1981.

273. Singer PA, Cooper DS, Daniels GS, et al: Treatment guidelines for patients with thyroid nodules and well-differentiated thyroid cancer. American Thyroid Association. Arch Intern Med 156:2165–2172, 1996.

274. Hershman JM, Edwards CL: Serum thyrotropin (TSH) levels after thyroid ablation compared with TSH levels after exogenous bovine TSH: Implications for 131-I treatment of thyroid carcinoma. J Clin Endocrinol Metab 34:814–818, 1972.

275. Sherman WB, Werner SC: Generalized allergic reaction to bovine thyrotropin. JAMA 190:244–245, 1964.

276. Melmed S, Harada A, Hershman JM, et al: Neutralizing antibodies to bovine thyrotropin in immunized patients with thyroid cancer. J Clin Endocrinol Metab 51:358–363, 1980.

277. Meier CA, Braverman LE, Ebner SA, et al: Diagnostic use of recombinant human thyrotropin in patients with thyroid carcinoma (phase I/II study). J Clin Endocrinol Metab 78:188–196, 1994.

278. Ladenson PW, Braverman LE, Mazzaferri EL, et al: Comparison of administration of recombinant human thyrotropin with withdrawal of thyroid hormone for radioactive iodine scanning in patients with thyroid carcinoma. N Engl J Med 337:888–896, 1997.

279. Haugen BR, Pacini F, Reiners C, et al: A comparison of recombinant human thyrotropin and thyroid hormone withdrawal for the detection of thyroid remnant or cancer. J Clin Endocrinol Metab 84:3877–3885, 1999.

280. Haugen BR, Lin EC: Isotope imaging for metastatic thyroid cancer. Endocrinol Metab Clin N Am 30:469–492, 2001.

281. Spencer CA, Wang CC: Thyroglobulin measurement. Techniques, clinical benefits, and pitfalls. Endocrinol Metab Clin N Am 24:841–863, 1995.

282. Robbins RJ, Tuttle RM, Sharaf RN, et al: Preparation by recombinant human thyrotropin or thyroid hormone withdrawal is comparable for the detection of residual differentiated thyroid carcinoma. J Clin Endocrinol Metab 86:619–625, 2001.

283. Pacini F, Molinaro E, Lippi F, et al: Prediction of disease status by recombinant human TSH-stimulated serum Tg in the postsurgical follow-up of differentiated thyroid carcinoma. J Clin Endocrinol Metab 86:5686–5690, 2001.

284. Pacini F, Capezzone M, Elisei R, et al: Diagnostic 131-iodine whole-body scan may be avoided in thyroid cancer patients who have undetectable stimulated serum Tg levels after initial treatment. J Clin Endocrinol Metab 87:1499–1501, 2002.

285. Mazzaferri EL, Kloos RT: Is diagnostic iodine-131 scanning with recombinant human TSH useful in the follow-up of differentiated thyroid cancer after thyroid ablation? J Clin Endocrinol Metab 87:1490–1498, 2002.

286. Mazzaferri EL, Kloos RT: Clinical review 128: Current approaches to primary therapy for papillary and follicular thyroid cancer. J Clin Endocrinol Metab 86:1447–1463, 2001.

287. Kitamura Y, Shimizu K, Nagahama M, et al: Immediate causes of death in thyroid carcinoma: Clinicopathological analysis of 161 fatal cases. J Clin Endocrinol Metab 84:4043–4049, 1999.

288. Schlumberger M, Challeton C, DeVathaire F, et al: Radioactive iodine treatment and external radiotherapy for lung and bone metastases from thyroid carcinoma. J Nucl Med 37:598–605, 1996.

289. Schlumberger M, Mancusi F, Baudin E, et al: 131I therapy for elevated thyroglobulin levels. Thyroid 7:273–276, 1997.

290. Pacini F: Therapeutic doses of iodine-131 reveal undiagnosed metastases in thyroid cancer patients with detectable serum thyroglobulin levels. J Nucl Med 28:1888–1891, 1987.

291. Altenvoerde G, Lerch H, Kuwert T, et al: Positron emission tomography with F-18-deoxyglucose in patients with differentiated thyroid carcinoma, elevated thyroglobulin levels, and negative iodine scans. Langenbecks Arch Surg 383:160–163, 1998.

292. Wang W, Macapinlac H, Larson SM, et al: (18F)-2-fluoro-2-deoxy-d-glucose positron emission tomography localizes residual thyroid cancer in patients with negative diagnostic (131)I whole body scans and elevated serum thyroglobulin levels. J Clin Endocrinol Metab 84:2291–2302, 1999.

293. Helal BO, Merlet P, Taubert ME, et al: Clinical impact of (18)F-FDG PET in thyroid carcinoma patients with elevated thyroglobulin levels and negative (131)I scanning results after therapy. J Nucl Med 42:1464–1469, 2001.

294. Yeo JS, Chung JK, So Y, et al: F-18-fluorodeoxyglucose positron emission tomography as a presurgical evaluation modality for I-131 scan-negative thyroid carcinoma patients with local recurrence in cervical lymph nodes. Head Neck 23:94–103, 2001.

295. Wang W, Larson SM, Tuttle RM, et al: Resistance of (18F)-fluorodeoxyglucose-avid, metastatic thyroid cancer lesions to treatment with high-dose radioactive iodine. Thyroid 11:1169–1175, 2001.

296. Lorberboym M, Murthy S, Mechanick JI, et al: Thallium-201 and iodine-131 scintigraphy in differentiated thyroid carcinoma. J Nucl Med 37:1487–1491, 1996.

297. Alam MS, Takeuchi R, Kasagi K, et al: Value of combined technetium-99m hydroxy methylene diphosphonate and thallium-201 imaging in detecting bone metastases from thyroid carcinoma. Thyroid 7:705–712, 1997.

298. Miyamoto S, Kasagi K, Misaki T, et al: Evaluation of technetium-99m-MIBI scintigraphy in metastatic differentiated thyroid carcinoma. J Nucl Med 38:352–356, 1997.

299. Almeida-Filho P, Ravizzini GC, Almeida C, et al: Whole-body Tc-99m sestamibi scintigraphy in the follow-up of differentiated thyroid carcinoma. Clin Nucl Med 25:443–446, 2000.

300. Ng DC, Sundram FX, Sin AE: 99mTc-Sestamibi and 131I whole-body scintigraphy and initial serum thyroglobulin in the management of differentiated thyroid carcinoma. J Nucl Med 41:631–635, 2000.

301. Lind P, Gallowitsch HJ, Langsteger W, et al: Technetium-99m-tetrofosmin whole-body scintigraphy in the follow-up of differentiated thyroid carcinoma. J Nucl Med 38:348–352, 1997.

302. Gallowitsch HJ, Mikosch P, Kresnik E, et al: Thyroglobulin and low-dose iodine-131 and technetium-99m-tetrofosmin whole-body scintigraphy in differentiated thyroid carcinoma. J Nucl Med 39:870–875, 1998.

303. Baudin E, Schlumberger M, Lumbroso J, et al: Octreotide scintigraphy in patients with differentiated thyroid carcinoma: Contribution for patients with negative radioiodine scan. J Clin Endocrinol Metab 81:2541–2544, 1996.

304. Wilson CJ, Woodroof JM, Girod DA: First report of Hurthle cell carcinoma revealed by octreotide scanning. Ann Otol Rhinol Laryngol 107(10 Pt 1):847–850, 1998.

305. Koerber C, Schmutzler C, Rendl J, et al: Increased I-131 uptake in local recurrence and distant metastases after second treatment with retinoic acid. Clin Nucl Med 24:849–851, 1999.

306. Grunwald F, Menzel C, Bender H, et al: Redifferentiation therapy-induced radioiodine uptake in thyroid cancer. J Nucl Med 39:1903–1906, 1998.

307. Simon D, Kohrle J, Schmutzler C, et al: Redifferentiation therapy of differentiated thyroid carcinoma with retinoic acid: Basics and first clinical results. Exp Clin Endocrinol Diabetes 104(suppl 4):13–15, 1996.

308. Schmutzler C, Kohrle J: Retinoic acid redifferentiation therapy for thyroid cancer. Thyroid 10:393–406, 2000.

309. McDonald MP, Sanders LE, Silverman ML, et al: Hurthle cell carcinoma of the thyroid gland: Prognostic factors and results of surgical treatment. Surgery 120:1000–1004; discussion 1004–1005, 1996.

310. Grossman RF, Clark OH: Hurthle cell carcinoma. Cancer Control 4:13–17, 1997.

311. Cooper DS, Schneyer CR: Follicular and Hurthle cell carcinoma of the thyroid. Endocrinol Metab Clin North Am 19:577–591, 1990.

312. Har-El G, Hadar T, Segal K, et al: Hurthle cell carcinoma of the thyroid gland. A tumor of moderate malignancy. Cancer 57:1613–1617, 1986.

313. Samaan NA, Maheshwari YK, Nader S, et al: Impact of therapy for differentiated carcinoma of the thyroid: An analysis of 706 cases. J Clin Endocrinol Metab 56:1131–1138, 1983.

314. Evans HL, Vassilopoulou-Sellin R: Follicular and Hurthle cell carcinomas of the thyroid: A comparative study. Am J Surg Pathol 22:1512–1520, 1998.

315. Heppe H, Armin A, Calandra DB, et al: Hurthle cell tumors of the thyroid gland. Surgery 98:1162–1165, 1985.

316. Blount CL, Dworkin HJ: F-18 FDG uptake by recurrent Hurthle cell carcinoma of the thyroid using high-energy planar scintigraphy. Clin Nucl Med 21:831–833, 1996.

317. Guyetant S, Rousselet MC, Durigon M, et al: Sex-related C cell hyperplasia in the normal human thyroid: A quantitative autopsy study (see comments). J Clin Endocrinol Metab 82:42–47, 1997.

318. Mathew CG, Chin KS, Easton DF, et al: A linked genetic marker for multiple endocrine neoplasia type 2A on chromosome 10. Nature 328:527–528, 1987.

319. Mulligan LM, Kwok JB, Dealey CJ, et al: Germ-line mutations of the RET proto-oncogene in multiple endocrine neoplasia type 2A. Nature 363:458–460, 1993.

320. Donis-Keller H, Dou S, Chi D, et al: Mutations in the RET proto-oncogene are associated with MEN 2A and FMTC. Hum Mol Genet 2:851–856, 1993.

321. Hofstra RM, Landsvater RM, Ceccherini I, et al: A mutation in the RET proto-oncogene associated with multiple endocrine neoplasia type 2B and sporadic medullary thyroid carcinoma (see comments). Nature 367:375–376, 1994.

322. Smith DP, Eng C, Ponder BA: Mutations of the RET proto-oncogene in the multiple endocrine neoplasia type 2 syndromes and Hirschsprung disease. J Cell Sci Suppl 18:43–49, 1994.

323. Gagel RF, Levy ML, Donovan DT, et al: Multiple endocrine neoplasia type 2a associated with cutaneous lichen amyloidosis (see comments). Ann Intern Med 111:802–806, 1989.

324. Trupp M, Arenas E, Fainzilber M, et al: Functional receptor for GDNF encoded by the c-ret proto-oncogene (see comments). Nature 381:785–789, 1996.

325. Lin LF, Doherty DH, Lile JD, et al: GDNF: A glial cell line-derived neurotrophic factor for midbrain dopaminergic neurons (see comments). Science 260:1130–1132, 1993.

326. Baloh RH, Enomoto H, Johnson EM Jr, et al: The GDNF family ligands and receptors—implications for neural development. Curr Opin Neurobiol 10:103–110, 2000.

327. Eng C, Clayton D, Schuffenecker I, et al: The relationship between specific RET proto-oncogene mutations and disease phenotype in multiple endocrine neoplasia type 2. International RET mutation consortium analysis. JAMA 276:1575–1579, 1996.

328. Mulligan LM, Marsh DJ, Robinson BG, et al: Genotype-phenotype correlation in multiple endocrine neoplasia type 2: Report of the International RET Mutation Consortium. J Intern Med 238:343–346, 1995.

329. Bolino A, Schuffenecker I, Luo Y, et al: RET mutations in exons 13 and 14 of FMTC patients. Oncogene 10:2415–2419, 1995.

330. Fattoruso O, Quadro L, Libroia A, et al: A GTG to ATG novel point mutation at codon 804 in exon 14 of the RET proto-oncogene in two families affected by familial medullary thyroid carcinoma. Hum Mutat Suppl 1:S167–S171, 1998.

331. Hofstra RM, Fattoruso O, Quadro L, et al: A novel point mutation in the intracellular domain of the ret protooncogene in a family with medullary thyroid carcinoma. J Clin Endocrinol Metab 82:4176–4178, 1997.

332. Eng C, Smith DP, Mulligan LM, et al: Point mutation within the tyrosine kinase domain of the RET proto-oncogene in multiple endocrine neoplasia type 2B and related sporadic tumours. (Erratum appears in Hum Mol Genet 3:686, 1994.) Hum Mol Genet 3:237–241, 1994.

333. Gimm O, Marsh DJ, Andrew SD, et al: Germline dinucleotide mutation in codon 883 of the RET proto-oncogene in multiple endocrine neoplasia type 2B without codon 918 mutation. J Clin Endocrinol Metab 82:3902–3904, 1997.

334. Bocciardi R, Mograbi B, Pasini B, et al: The multiple endocrine neoplasia type 2B point mutation switches the specificity of the Ret tyrosine kinase towards cellular substrates that are susceptible to interact with Crk and Nck. Oncogene 15:2257–2265, 1997.

335. Becker KL, Snider RH, Moore CF, et al: Calcitonin in extrathyroidal tissues of man. Acta Endocrinol 92:746–751, 1979.

336. Becker KL, Nash D, Silva OL, et al: Increased serum and urinary calcitonin levels in patients with pulmonary disease. Chest 79:211–216, 1981.

337. Takayama T, Kameya T, Inagaki K, et al: MEN type 1 associated with mediastinal carcinoid producing parathyroid hormone, calcitonin and chorionic gonadotropin. Pathol Res Pract 189:1090–1096; discussion 1096–1100, 1993.

338. Cecchettin M, Albertini A, Bonora G, et al: Calcitonin, parathyroid hormone and insulin concentrations in sera from patients with gastrinoma. Adv Exp Med Biol 106:117–119, 1978.

339. Howard JM, Gohara AF, Cardwell RJ: Malignant islet cell tumor of the pancreas associated with high plasma calcitonin and somatostatin levels. Surgery 105(2 Pt 1):227–229, 1989.

340. Garancini S, Ballada L, Roncari G, et al: Calcitonin in chronic renal failure. Nephron 34:224–227, 1983.

341. Levine MA: Laboratory evaluation of calciotropic hormones and minerals. In Moore WT, Eastman RC (eds): Diagnostic Endocrinology. St. Louis, Missouri, Mosby, 1996, pp 411–438.

342. McEwan JR, Benjamin N, Larkin S, et al: Vasodilatation by calcitonin gene-related peptide and by substance P: A comparison of their effects on resistance and capacitance vessels of human forearms. Circulation 77:1072–1080, 1988.

343. Hahm JR, Lee MS, Min YK, et al: Routine measurement of serum calcitonin is useful for early detection of medullary thyroid carcinoma in patients with nodular thyroid diseases. Thyroid 11:73–80, 2001.

344. Pacini F, Fontanelli M, Fugazzola L, et al: Routine measurement of serum calcitonin in nodular thyroid diseases allows the preoperative diagnosis of unsuspected sporadic medullary thyroid carcinoma (see comments). J Clin Endocrinol Metab 78:826–829, 1994.

345. Rieu M, Lame MC, Richard A, et al: Prevalence of sporadic medullary thyroid carcinoma: The importance of routine measurement of serum calcitonin in the diagnostic evaluation of thyroid nodules. Clin Endocrinol (Oxf) 42:453–460, 1995.

346. Niccoli P, Wion-Barbot N, Caron P, et al: Interest of routine measurement of serum calcitonin: Study in a large series of thyroidectomized patients. The French Medullary Study Group (see comments). J Clin Endocrinol Metab 82:338–341, 1997.

347. Redding AH, Levine SN, Fowler MR: Normal preoperative calcitonin levels do not always exclude medullary thyroid carcinoma in patients with large palpable thyroid masses. Thyroid 10:919–922, 2000.

348. Horvit PK, Gagel RF: The goitrous patient with an elevated serum calcitonin—what to do? (letter; comment). J Clin Endocrinol Metab 82:335–337, 1997.

349. Marsh DJ, Andrew SD, Eng C, et al: Germline and somatic mutations in an oncogene: RET mutations in inherited medullary thyroid carcinoma. Cancer Res 56:1241–1243, 1996.

350. Gill JR, Reyes-Mugica M, Iyengar S, et al: Early presentation of metastatic medullary carcinoma in multiple endocrine neoplasia, type IIA: Implications for therapy. J Pediatr 129:459–464, 1996.

351. Hansen HS, Torring H, Godballe C, et al: Is thyroidectomy necessary in RET mutation carriers of the familial medullary thyroid carcinoma syndrome? Cancer 89:863–867, 2000.

352. Niccoli-Sire P, Murat A, Baudin E, et al: Early or prophylactic thyroidectomy in MEN 2/FMTC gene carriers: Results in 71 thyroidectomized patients. The French Calcitonin Tumours Study Group (GETC). Eur J Endocrinol 141:468–474, 1999.

353. Frank-Raue K, Hoppner W, Buhr H, et al: Results and follow-up in eleven MEN 2A gene carriers after prophylactic thyroidectomy. Exp Clin Endocrinol Diabetes 105(suppl 4):76–78, 1997.

354. Bergholm U, Adami HO, Bergstrom R, et al: Clinical characteristics in sporadic and familial medullary thyroid carcinoma. A nationwide study of 249 patients in Sweden from 1959 through 1981. Cancer 63:1196–1204, 1989.

355. Modigliani E, Cohen R, Campos JM, et al: Prognostic factors for survival and for biochemical cure in medullary thyroid carcinoma: Results in 899 patients. The GETC Study Group. Groupe d'etude des tumeurs a calcitonine. Clin Endocrinol 48:265–273, 1998.

356. Wells SA Jr, Dilley WG, Farndon JA, et al: Early diagnosis and treatment of medullary thyroid carcinoma. Arch Intern Med 145:1248–1252, 1985.

357. Tisell LE, Hansson G, Jansson S, et al: Reoperation in the treatment of asymptomatic metastasizing medullary thyroid carcinoma. Surgery 99:60–66, 1986.

358. Beveridge T, Niederer W, Nuesch E, et al: Pharmacokinetic study with synthetic salmon calcitonin (Sandoz). Z Gastroenterol Verh 10:12–15, 1976.

359. Fugazzola L, Pinchera A, Luchetti F, et al: Disappearance rate of serum calcitonin after total thyroidectomy for medullary thyroid carcinoma. Int J Biol Markers 9:21–24, 1994.

360. van Heerden JA, Grant CS, Gharib H, et al: Long-term course of patients with persistent hypercalcitoninemia after apparent curative primary surgery for medullary thyroid carcinoma. Ann Surg 212:395–400; discussion 400–401, 1990.

361. Bergholm U, Bergstrom R, Ekbom A: Long-term follow-up of patients with medullary carcinoma of the thyroid. Cancer 79:132–138, 1997.

362. Tisell LE, Hansson G, Jansson S, et al: Reoperation in the treatment of asymptomatic metastasizing medullary thyroid carcinoma. Surgery 99:60–66, 1986.

363. Moley JF, Wells SA, Dilley WG, et al: Reoperation for recurrent or persistent medullary thyroid cancer. Surgery 114:1090–1095; discussion 1095–1096, 1993.

364. Moley JF, Debenedetti MK, Dilley WG, et al: Surgical management of patients with persistent or recurrent medullary thyroid cancer. J Intern Med 243:521–526, 1998.

365. Fleming JB, Lee JE, Bouvet M, et al: Surgical strategy for the treatment of medullary thyroid carcinoma. Ann Surg 230:697–707, 1999.

366. Nguyen TD, Chassard JL, Lagarde P, et al: Results of postoperative radiation therapy in medullary carcinoma of the thyroid: A retrospective study by the French Federation of Cancer Institutes—the Radiotherapy Cooperative Group. Radiother Oncol 23:1–5, 1992.

367. Brierley J, Tsang R, Simpson WJ, et al: Medullary thyroid cancer: Analyses of survival and prognostic factors and the role of radiation therapy in local control. Thyroid 6:305–310, 1996.

368. Fersht N, Vini L, A'Hern R, et al: The role of radiotherapy in the management of elevated calcitonin after surgery for medullary thyroid cancer. Thyroid 11:1161–1168, 2001.

369. Droz JP, Rougier P, Goddefroy V, et al: Chimiotherapie des cancers medullaires de la thyroide. Essais phase II avec adriamycine et cis-platinum administres en monochimiotherapie. Bull Cancer 71:195–199, 1984.

370. De Besi P, Busnardo B, Toso S, et al: Combined chemotherapy with bleomycin, Adriamycin, and platinum in advanced thyroid cancer. J Endocrinol Invest 14:475–480, 1991.

371. Scherubl H, Raue F, Ziegler R: Combination chemotherapy of advanced medullary and differentiated thyroid cancer. Phase II study. J Cancer Res Clin Oncol 116:21–23, 1990.

372. Frame J, Kelsen D, Kemeny N, et al: A phase II trial of streptozotocin and Adriamycin in advanced APUD tumors. Am J Clin Oncol 11:490–495, 1988.

373. Mahler C, Verhelst J, de Longueville M, et al: Long-term treatment of metastatic medullary thyroid carcinoma with the somatostatin analogue octreotide. Clin Endocrinol 33:261–269, 1990.

374. Aldinger KA, Samaan NA, Ibanez ML, et al: Anaplastic carcinoma of the thyroid: A review of 84 cases of spindle and giant cell carcinoma of the thyroid. Cancer 41:2267, 1978.

375. Venkatesh YS, Ordonez NG, Schultz PN, et al: Anaplastic carcinoma of the thyroid. Cancer 66:321, 1990.

376. Austin JR, El-Naggar AK, Goepfert H: Thyroid cancers II medullary, anaplastic, lymphoma, sarcoma, squamous cell. Otolaryngol Clin N Am 29:611, 1996.

377. Venkatesh YSS, Ordonez NG, Schultz PN, et al: Anaplastic carcinoma of the thyroid: A clinicopathologic study of 121 cases. Cancer 66:321, 1990.

378. Carcangiu ML, Steeper T, Zampi G, et al: Anaplastic thyroid carcinoma: A study of 70 cases. Am J Clin Pathol 83:135, 1985.

379. Spires JR, Schwartz MR, Miller RH: Anaplastic thyroid carcinoma. Association with differentiated thyroid cancer. Arch Otolaryngol Head Neck Surg 114:40, 1988.

380. Demeter JG, DeJong SA, Lawrence AM, et al: Anaplastic thyroid carcinoma: Risk factors and outcome. Surgery 110:956, 1991.

381. Kobayashi S, Yamadori I, Ohmori M, et al: Anaplastic carcinoma of the thyroid with osteoclast-like giant cells: An ultrastructural and immunohistochemical study. Acta Pathol Jpn 37:807, 1987.

382. Ratnatnga N, Ramadasa S: Immunohistochemical staining for thyroglobulin in poorly differentiated carcinoma of the thyroid. Ceylon Med J 38:113, 1993.

383. Hurlimann J, Gardiol D, Scazziga B: Immunohistology of anaplastic thyroid carcinoma: A study of 43 cases. Histopathology 11:567, 1987.

384. LaVolsi VA, Brooks JJ, Arendash Durand B: Anaplastic thyroid tumors: Immunohistology. Am J Clin Pathol 87:434, 1987.

385. Moosa M, Mazzaferri EL: Management of thyroid neoplasms. In Cummings CW, Fredrickson JM, Harker LA, et al (eds): Otolaryngology—Head and Neck Surgery, 3rd ed. St. Louis, Missouri, Mosby, 1998, pp 2480–2518.

386. Aldinger KA, Samaan NA, Ibanez M, et al: Anaplastic carcinoma of the thyroid: A review of 84 cases of spindle and giant cell carcinoma of the thyroid. Cancer 41:2267, 1978.

387. Oppenheim A, Miller M, Anderson GH Jr, et al: Anaplastic thyroid cancer presenting with hyperthyroidism. Am J Med 75:702, 1983.

388. Shvero J, Gal R, Avidor I, et al: Anaplastic thyroid carcinoma: A clinical, histologic and immunohistochemical study. Cancer 62:319, 1988.

389. Phillips DL, Benner KG, Keeffe EB, et al: Isolated metastasis to small bowel from anaplastic thyroid carcinoma: With a review of extra-abdominal malignancies that spread to the bowel. J Clin Gastoenterol 9:563, 1987.

390. Prendiville S, Burman K, Ringeil M, et al: Prognostic implications of the tall cell variant of papillary thyroid carcinoma. Otolaryngol Head Neck Surg 122:352–357, 2000.

391. Crile G, Pontius K, Hawk W: Factors influencing the survival of patients with follicular carcinoma of the thyroid gland. Surg Gynecol Obstet 160:409, 1985.

392. Souhami L, Simpson W, Carruthers J: Malignant lymphoma of the thyroid gland. Int J Radiat Oncol Biol Phys 6:1143, 1980.

393. Burke J, Butler J, Fulleri L: Malignant lymphoma of the thyroid gland. Cancer 39:1587, 1977.

394. Hamburger J: Nontoxic Goiter. Springfield, Illinois, Charles C Thomas, 1973, p 108.

395. Holm L, Blomgren H, Lowhagen T: Cancer risks in patients with chronic lymphocytic thyroiditis. N Engl J Med 312:601, 1985.

396. Williams E: Malignant lymphoma thyroid. Clin Endocrinol Metab 10:379, 1981.

397. Watson R, Brennan M, van Heerden J: Invasive Hurthle cell carcinoma of the thyroid: Natural history and management. Mayo Clin Proc 59:850, 1984.

398. Anscombe AM, Wright DH: Primary malignant lymphoma of the thyroid: A tumor of mucosa-associated lymphoid tissue: Review of seventy six cases. Histopathology 9:81, 1985.

399. Hamburger JI, Miller JM, Kini SR: Lymphoma of the thyroid. Ann Intern Med 99:685, 1983.

400. Mazzaferri EL, Oertel YC: Primary malignant lymphoma and related lymphoproliferative disorders. In Mazzaferri EL, Samaan N (eds): Endocrine Tumors. Boston, Blackwell Scientific Publications, 1993.

401. Holm LE, Blomgren H, Lowenhagen T: Cancer risks in patients with chronic lymphocytic thyroiditis. N Engl J Med 312:601, 1985.

402. Compagno J: Diseases of the thyroid. In Barnes L (ed): Surgical Pathology of the Head and Neck, vol 2. New York, Marcel Dekker, 1985, pp 1435–1486.

403. Samaan NA, Ordonez NG: Uncommon types of thyroid cancer. Endocrinol Metab Clin N Am 19:637, 1990.

404. Burt AD, Kerr DJ, Brown IL, et al: Lymphoid and epithelial markers in small cell anaplastic thyroid tumours. J Clin Pathol 38:893, 1985.

405. Guarda LA, Baskin HJ: Inflammatory and lymphoid lesions of the thyroid gland: Cytopathology by fine-needle aspiration. Am J Clin Pathol 87:14, 1987.

406. Gatter KC, Alcock C, Heryet A, et al: The differential diagnosis of routinely processed anaplastic tumors using monoclonal antibodies. Am J Clin Pathol 82:33, 1984.

407. Andersson T, Biörklund A, Landberg T, et al: Combined therapy for undifferentiated giant and spindle cell carcinoma of the thyroid. Acta Otolaryngol 83:372, 1977.

408. Doria R, Jekel JF, Cooper DL: Thyroid lymphoma. The case for combined modality therapy. Cancer 73:200, 1994.

409. Tennval J, Cavallin-Stahl E, Akerman M: Primary localized non-Hodgkin's lymphoma of the thyroid: A retrospective clinico-pathological review. Eur J Surg Oncol 13:297, 1987.

410. Vigliotti A, Kong JS, Fuller LM, et al: Thyroid lymphomas stage IE and IIE: Comparative results for radiotherapy only, combination chemotherapy only, and multimodality treatment. Int J Radiat Oncol Biol Phys 12:1807, 1986.

411. Souhami L, Simpson J, Carruthers JS: Malignant lymphoma of the thyroid gland. Int J Radiat Oncol Biol Phys 6:1143, 1980.

412. Chak LY, Hoppe RT, Burke JS, et al: Non-Hodgkin's lymphoma presenting as thyroid enlargement. Cancer 48:2712, 1985.

413. Kapadia SB, Dekker A, Cheng VS, et al: Malignant lymphoma of the thyroid gland: A clinicopathologic study. Head Neck Surg 4:270, 1982.

414. Blair TJ, Evans RG, Buskirk SJ, et al: Radiotherapeutic management of primary thyroid lymphoma. Int J Radiat Oncol Biol Phys 11:365, 1985.

415. Tupchong L, Hughes F, Harmer CL: Primary lymphoma of the thyroid: Clinical features, prognostic factors, and results of treatment. Int J Radiat Oncol Biol Phys 12:1813, 1986.

416. Makepeace AR, Fermont DC, Bennet MH: Non-Hodgkin's lymphoma of the thyroid. Clin Radiol 38:277, 1987.

417. Skarsgard ED, Connors JM, Robins RE: A current analysis of primary lymphoma of the thyroid. Arch Surg 126:1199, 1991.

418. Leedman PJ, Sheridan WP, Downey WF, et al: Combination chemotherapy as single modality therapy for stage IE and IIE thyroid lymphoma. Med J Aust 152:40, 1990.

CHAPTER 20

Tumors of the Parathyroid Glands

Ashok R. Shaha

INTRODUCTION

A Swedish medical student, Ivar Sandstrom, described parathyroid glands in 1880.[1, 2] Interestingly, in 1849, Sir Richard Owen performed an autopsy on a rhinoceros and described the parathyroid glands as a "small yellow glandular body." However, Sandstrom suggested the name *glandulae parathyroideae*. Friedrich von Recklinghausen described characteristic bony disease, that is, fibrocystic disease caused by hyperparathyroidism. It was in 1926 at Massachusetts General Hospital that the first parathyroid surgical exploration was performed on a merchant marine captain, Charles Martell.[1, 2] He had undergone six explorations, and during his seventh exploration in 1932, an enlarged parathyroid gland was noted in the mediastinum. Unfortunately, he subsequently died from urinary complications. In 1934, Albright noted an association between renal stones and osteitis fibrosa cystica. Parathyroid hormone (PTH) was first isolated by Rasmussen and Craig in 1959, while Berson, Yallow, and colleagues reported radioimmunoassay for PTH.

Understanding of the anatomic development and physiologic function of the parathyroid glands is extremely important because these endocrine glands have very important biologic functions of regulating calcium and phosphorus metabolism. With the recent routine use of multichannel serum chemistry, parathyroid disorders in general, and hyperparathyroidism in particular, are often recognized before the onset of clinical symptoms or complications.

ANATOMY AND EMBRYOLOGY

The parathyroid glands develop during the sixth week of gestation. The superior parathyroid glands develop from the fourth branchial pouch, and the inferior parathyroid glands develop from the third pharyngeal pouch along with the thymus. The superior parathyroid gland develops in conjunction with the ultimobranchial body. Because of this relationship, the superior parathyroid gland remains near the superior pole of the thyroid lobe. Occasionally, the superior parathyroid gland may descend inferior to the inferior parathyroid gland. However, the gland may remain undescended near the hyoid bone or along with the pharyngeal musculature described as "parapharyngeous." The inferior parathyroid glands arise in conjunction with the thymus. The inferior parathyroid glands are more commonly found in ectopic sites. The most common ectopic location of the inferior parathyroid gland is within the thymic capsule or the superior mediastinum. Even though there are usually four parathyroid glands, approximately 10% of individuals may have between five and seven supernumerary parathyroid glands; rarely (in 2% to 3% of individuals), there may be fewer than four parathyroid glands.

An understanding of the embryologic development of the parathyroid glands is extremely important because the most common location of the superior parathyroid gland is in the posterior capsule of the superior pole of the thyroid behind the recurrent laryngeal nerve; the inferior parathyroid gland is generally in front of the recurrent laryngeal nerve near the lower pole of the thyroid gland. The average weight of the parathyroid gland is approximately 35 mg, and the diameter ranges between 1 and 5 mm.[2] These glands are generally tan-colored with variable shapes from oval to an irregular flat surface.

The parathyroid glands receive their blood supply mainly from the inferior thyroid artery. Invariably, there is a tiny branch of the inferior thyroid artery supplying the parathyroid before the inferior thyroid artery enters the thyroid gland. During total thyroidectomy, it is vital to preserve the blood supply to the parathyroid gland so that the function of the parathyroid glands is maintained. Occasionally, the superior parathyroid glands may receive their blood supply directly from the posterior branch of the superior thyroid artery.

Rarely, the parathyroid glands may receive their blood supply directly from the thyroid gland, and the glands may be located on the lateral or anterior surface of the thyroid gland. This anatomic variation is extremely important because the parathyroid glands may be injured during total thyroidectomy. In these rare situations, the parathyroid gland is best autotransplanted in the neck muscles after total thyroidectomy. Occasionally, the parathyroid glands may be in ectopic locations such as the superior mediastinum, the thymic capsule, behind the esophagus, inside the carotid sheath, or medial to the superior pole of the thyroid gland. Even more rarely, the parathyroid glands may be in more disparate locations, such as near the base of the skull, behind the angle of the mandible, or near the hyoid bone.

During surgical exploration, the parathyroid glands may be easily confused with fat, thyroid tissue, lymph node, or commonly, the thymic remnant. It is important for the surgeon to understand the normal size and weight of the parathyroid gland (35 to 50 mg) because the pathologically abnormal gland is much larger and heavier. In a majority of cases, the parathyroid gland is under the capsule of the thyroid or in the crypt of the thyroid gland; generally, it can be easily felt by careful evaluation of the thyroid surface. Rarely, the parathyroid gland may be truly intraglandular in the thyroid substance; this may lead to considerable confusion during primary surgical exploration.

◘ PARATHYROID DISORDERS

The management of patients with asymptomatic hyperparathyroidism is controversial because there are many asymptomatic patients with mild hypercalcemia who are diagnosed as having primary hyperparathyroidism.[3–7] To address this controversy, the National Institutes of Health (NIH) organized a consensus development conference in 1990 on the diagnosis and management of asymptomatic primary hyperparathyroidism.[8] In April of 2002, another consensus conference was held at the NIH, and new guidelines are expected to be published soon. Technologic developments, including the routine serum analysis of calcium and phosphorus, a relatively simple assay of PTH, and recent improvements in bone densitometry, have all had a major impact on the early diagnosis and management of parathyroid disorders.[9] In addition, there has been a paradigm shift in the surgical management of hyperparathyroidism, especially with the development of several new technologies, including sestamibi scan and "quick" PTH assay.

Types of Hyperparathyroidism

The most common disorder of the parathyroid gland is a hyperfunctioning parathyroid gland, which produces abnormally high quantities of PTH. Primary hyperparathyroidism is primarily related to hyperfunction of one or several parathyroid glands, with the hyperfunction most commonly resulting from parathyroid adenoma or hyperplasia. Secondary hyperparathyroidism is most commonly noted in patients with renal failure, in whom all four parathyroid glands are enlarged from compensatory hyperplasia, which results in an increase in the level of calcium in the blood. Rarely, the hyperplastic gland, owing to prolonged compensatory stimulation, may develop autonomous function referred to as tertiary hyperparathyroidism.

Primary Hyperparathyroidism

INCIDENCE

The average incidence of primary hyperparathyroidism is 1 in 700 individuals; it is most commonly noted in women over the age of 45.

ETIOLOGY

Even though the true cause of primary hyperparathyroidism remains unclear, an increased incidence of hyperparathyroidism has been noted in patients who have received low-dose irradiation, usually during childhood. Genetic studies have identified overexpression of the PRAD1 oncogene in parathyroid adenomas. Overexpression of PRAD1 leads to increased parathyroid cell division.

The most common cause of primary hyperparathyroidism is solitary adenoma, which is found in 85% of these patients. Histologic distinction between a parathyroid adenoma and hyperplasia can be difficult for the pathologist, but the presence of a true capsule with an identifiable normal parathyroid gland surrounding enlarged parathyroid tissue confirms the diagnosis of parathyroid adenoma.

CLINICAL PRESENTATION

Although patients with hyperparathyroidism may occasionally be reported to be asymptomatic, on detailed evaluation and questioning, patients usually present with some type of symptoms that generally improve remarkably after surgical intervention.[9]

The most frequent symptoms and signs of hyperparathyroidism include muscle weakness, gastrointestinal (GI) disturbance, nausea, constipation, and vague neuropsychiatric symptoms such as forgetfulness. The classic presentation of primary hyperparathyroidism heralded by complaints described best by the mnemonic, "bones, moans, fatigue, and psychic overtones" is rarely noted today because of early diagnosis of most patients with hyperparathyroidism. Renal complications such as nephrocalcinosis are another uncommon presentation of this disorder, and bone disorders such as osteitis fibrosa cystica are also rarely noted today. The GI manifestations of hyperparathyroidism are mainly related to peptic ulcer disease or pancreatitis. Patients with primary hyperparathyroidism may also develop psychiatric or neurologic disturbances.

Hyperparathyroidism may be one of the presenting signs of multiple endocrine neoplasia (MEN) type 1 or type 2. MEN type 1 includes Wermer's syndrome with pancreas, parathyroid, and pituitary adenomas. MEN type 2 includes Sipple's syndrome—medullary carcinoma of the thyroid, pheochromocytoma, and hyperparathyroidism.[2, 10]

Approximately 10% to 14% of patients who are hyperparathyroid may have multiple hyperplastic parathyroid glands. Multiglandular involvement is generally related to hyperplasia.

Approximately 3% to 4% of patients may present with multiple adenomas, which are a common cause of surgical failure.[11] Multiple adenomas are the most common cause of persistent or recurrent hyperparathyroidism after removal of a single enlarged parathyroid gland. This clinical situation has occurred more rarely since the advent of intraoperative PTH measurement and more precise preoperative localization studies.[11–15]

Parathyroid carcinoma is very uncommon, accounting for less than 1% of patients with primary hyperparathyroidism, and can be quite difficult to diagnose in the absence of nodal or distant metastasis or recurrent hyperparathyroidism.

LABORATORY FINDINGS

The most common laboratory finding in patients with hyperparathyroidism is persistent hypercalcemia. Primary

TABLE 20-1 Causes of Hypercalcemia

Metastatic cancer from lungs, kidneys, prostate, and breast
Primary hyperparathyroidism
Multiple myeloma
Paget's disease
Sarcoidosis
Thiazide diuretic therapy
Milk-alkali syndrome
Benign familial hypocalciuric hypercalcemia (BFHH)
Pseudohyperparathyroidism
Hyperproteinemia
Hypervitaminosis D
Immobilization
Acute Addison's disease
Chronic or acute leukemia

TABLE 20-2 Diagnostic Evaluation of Primary Hyperparathyroidism

Diagnostic triad
  High calcium
  Low phosphorus
  High PTH
Laboratory tests
  Blood
  Calcium
  Phosphorus
  Parathyroid hormone
  Chloride:phosphorus ratio
  Urinary cAMP
  Ionized calcium
  Tubular reabsorption of phosphorus
Bone analysis
  Photon beam bone densitometry
  Metacarpal bone thickness
  Quantitative bone histomorphometry
PTH—chemimmunoluminometric assay, N terminal, C terminal, intact
Localization studies—sestamibi scan

cAMP, cyclic adenosine monophosphate; PTH, parathyroid hormone.

hyperparathyroidism is the second most common cause of hypercalcemia after metastatic tumors (Table 20–1).

Secondary Hyperparathyroidism

Secondary hyperparathyroidism is mainly seen in patients with renal failure and those on chronic dialysis. Generally the diagnosis is made by mild hypercalcemia with high PTH levels. The main indication for surgery in secondary hyperparathyroidism is related to osteopenia (bony demineralization). One of the other indications for surgery in secondary hyperparathyroidism is severe pruritus. The surgical intervention generally includes either subtotal parathyroidectomy with removal of 3½ enlarged parathyroid glands or total parathyroidectomy along with autotransplantation of normal-sized parathyroid tissue in the forearm. The surgical procedure generally leads to considerable improvement in the symptom complex related to secondary hyperparathyroidism.

Tertiary Hyperparathyroidism

Tertiary hyperparathyroidism is occasionally seen in patients with chronic renal failure in whom a single gland autonomously grows into development of a parathyroid adenoma.

Laboratory Diagnosis of Hyperparathyroidism

Although the diagnostic triad of hyperparathyroidism consists of high calcium, low phosphorus, and high PTH, the best way of diagnosing hyperparathyroidism is through measurement of the serum level of PTH (Table 20–2). Other studies that may help to confirm the diagnosis include measurement of serum alkaline phosphatase, the calcium content of a 24-hour urinary collection, serum chloride/phosphorus ratio, urinary cyclic adenosine monophosphate (cAMP), and determination of bone densitometry. Some authors advocate the use of bone densitometry studies as a major indicator for surgical intervention in asymptomatic patients. Some patients may present with mild hypertension, which may be related to hyperparathyroidism.

The differential diagnosis of hyperparathyroidism includes metastatic carcinoma, milk-alkali syndrome, multiple myeloma, and sarcoidosis. Twenty-four-hour urine collection for urine calcium is important in patients undergoing reexploration so that familial benign hypocalciuric

hypercalcemia can be ruled out. Patients with parathyroid carcinoma invariably present with very high PTH and high calcium levels. A calcium level of more than 14 mg/dL should raise the clinician's level of suspicion for the diagnosis of parathyroid carcinoma.[2]

Localization Studies

Parathyroid localization studies may be divided into invasive and noninvasive studies.

Invasive studies generally include arteriography, selective venous catheterization, and digital subtraction angiography. Invasive studies are rarely performed today because newer noninvasive studies, especially the sestamibi scan, are so accurate and reliable, and because invasive methods are associated with risk for complications. Selective venous catheterization is extremely cumbersome, and very few centers can perform this technique reliably. However, angiography may be used occasionally in patients for whom open surgical intervention is contraindicated and in whom angiographic ablation of the enlarged parathyroid gland may be undertaken.

Among the variety of noninvasive studies, the most commonly performed tests include ultrasonography and sestamibi scanning. Imaging with computed tomographic (CT) scanning or magnetic resonance imaging (MRI) may be used occasionally; however, many false-positive and false-negative results are obtained with these tests. The CT scan is rarely used for parathyroid localization because of the considerable difficulty in distinguishing between thyroid and parathyroid abnormalities. The mediastinal glands are also difficult to evaluate on CT scan. However, MRI appears to be a good localization method, especially because the T2-weighted image generally highlights the enlarged parathyroid gland and may be helpful in localizing ectopic parathyroid glands, particularly undescended parathyroid or mediastinal glands.

The sestamibi scan appears to offer the best localization results and can identify an enlarged parathyroid gland in the mediastinum and in other ectopic locations. Several reports in the literature have revealed high accuracy and a positive predictive value for the sestamibi scan exceeding 80% to 90%.[11-18] It is also very helpful in locating ectopic parathyroid glands, either in the mediastinum or in undescended glands, that may be missed on ultrasound or CT scan.

The sestamibi scan can be performed by one of two different techniques. The first technique includes early and delayed images of the parathyroid gland. Approximately 20 to 25 μg of sestamibi is injected and a parathyroid scan is performed at intervals of 10 minutes, 30 minutes, and 2 hours, with a final scan performed after 4 to 6 hours. The sestamibi reveals a differential washout between the thyroid and parathyroid glands as the parathyroid retains the sestamibi, giving the delayed image of the parathyroid gland. This technique is used in most nuclear medicine departments. Oblique views are important for determining the exact location of the parathyroid gland. The addition of sestamibi single photon emission computed tomography (SPECT) imaging helps the clinician to localize the correct position of the enlarged parathyroid gland. The SPECT scan localizes the parathyroid in three dimensions and is also helpful to distinguish parathyroid from thyroid pathology. The sestamibi scan is extremely important for unilateral parathyroid exploration, gamma probe localization, and parathyroidectomy under local anesthesia.

The other technique of sestamibi scan is to use sestamibi along with radioactive iodine to subtract the thyroid image from the thyroid/parathyroid complex. However, this is generally not necessary unless the thyroid reveals clinically obvious abnormalities.

After sestamibi scanning, ultrasound is the preferred noninvasive method for intraoperative parathyroid localization. However, this test is limited by the experience of the ultrasonographer, and the presence of enlarged nodes or thyroid abnormalities can lead to difficulty in interpretation of the test. In addition, ultrasound may be difficult to interpret in patients with previous exploration because of scar tissue. Ultrasound-guided fine-needle aspiration can be performed to document the presence of an enlarged parathyroid gland with identifiable PTH in the washout of the aspirated material; cytology of the aspirated material can also be revealing. Recently, a few reports in the literature have used ultrasound-guided alcohol injection for parathyroid ablation.[19]

LOCALIZATION STUDIES IN PRIMARY EXPLORATION

The issue of parathyroid localization has been surrounded by considerable controversy, which has been exemplified

TABLE 20-3 Parathyroid Localization Studies

Noninvasive Studies	Invasive Studies
Esophagraphy	Arteriography
Ultrasound—US needle biopsy	Selective venous catheterization
Thallium-technetium scan	Digital subtraction angiography
CT scan	
MRI scan	
Sestamibi scan	
PET scan	
Monoclonal antibodies	

CT, computed tomography; MRI, magnetic resonance imaging; PET, positron emission tomography; US, ultrasound.

by the comments of Doppman, who stated that the only localization study indicated in patients with primary hyperparathyroidism is to localize an experienced parathyroid surgeon. Doppman and many endocrine surgeons had voiced strong opposition to the performance of any localization study before primary exploration was undertaken because surgical success was invariably higher than 95%. However, with improvements in technology over the past decade, interest has increased considerably in preoperative localization with imaging studies such as the sestamibi scan (Table 20-3). Localization studies are mandatory before reexploration so that the surgeon is aware of the exact location of the enlarged parathyroid gland.

Sestamibi, a radionuclide commonly used for cardiac evaluation, was first used for parathyroid scanning around 1989. Scanning with this radionuclide appears to be the most sensitive and specific parathyroid localization study; it also has a relatively low cost, which is critically important given that the cost of unsuccessful surgical exploration is quite high.[11-17] Because routine serum chemistry studies have led to the discovery of an increased number of patients with asymptomatic hyperparathyroidism, there is also considerable interest in sestamibi localization tests before neck exploration to ensure that surgical intervention is easy, accurate, and successful.

In addition to the sestamibi scan, which appears to be the most sensitive localization study, several other techniques, including intraoperative quick PTH assay, scan-directed unilateral parathyroid exploration, surgical exploration with gamma probe, and endoscopic parathyroidectomy, have been developed as major advances in parathyroid surgery (Table 20-4). These advances have led to a major shift over the past decade in the surgical management of hyperparathyroidism.

TABLE 20-4 Indications for Parathyroid Localization Prior to Primary Exploration

Patient Factors	Diagnostic Problems—Associated Malignancies	Technical Problems
Poor-risk patients in whom unilateral exploration is crucial	Mild asymptomatic hypercalcemia	Patients with previous neck or thyroid surgery
Poor-risk patients for whom surgery under local anesthesia is considered	Hypercalcemic crisis for urgent diagnosis	Obese individuals with a short neck Associated palpable thyroid abnormality
Difficult and uncooperative patient for better documentation		

LOCALIZATION STUDIES IN SECONDARY HYPERPARATHYROIDISM

Secondary hyperparathyroidism generally represents multiple gland hyperplasia, and the role of localization studies is quite limited. Ultrasound may be of greater value in documenting the enlarged parathyroid gland or the missing parathyroid gland after previous surgical exploration. Invariably, if the enlarged parathyroid gland is smaller than 300 to 500 mg, its localization with sestamibi scanning may be quite difficult.

LOCALIZATION STUDIES IN REEXPLORATION

If previous surgical exploration has failed to identify an enlarged parathyroid gland, future surgical procedures are generally complemented with one or more localization studies. The most common localization studies, again, under these circumstances are ultrasonography and sestamibi scanning. Rarely, an MRI may be of additional value. The most common sites for an undiscovered parathyroid gland are near the hyoid (parapharyngeal), behind the esophagus, in the carotid sheath, in the superior mediastinum, or rarely, in the posterior mediastinum. The undiscovered superior parathyroid gland may be inferior to the inferior parathyroid gland, and the undiscovered inferior parathyroid gland may be superior to the superior parathyroid gland. Accurate localization and confirmation of the parathyroid are extremely important before reexploration.[20, 21] Before surgical intervention, it is vital to confirm the diagnosis of primary hyperparathyroidism with 24-hour urinary calcium in order to rule out familial hypocalciuric hypercalcemia. The clinical utility of newer localization studies such as positron emission tomography (PET) scanning and the use of radiolabeled monoclonal antibodies need further evaluation before their clinical utility can be determined.

Surgical Treatment of Hyperparathyroidism

The surgical treatment of hyperparathyroidism consists of surgical exploration and removal of enlarged parathyroid glands. In the majority of cases, a single gland is enlarged; however, occasionally, multiple adenomas may be noted when bilateral surgical exploration is necessary.

The main treatment for primary hyperparathyroidism continues to be surgical exploration, except in poor-risk surgical patients. In the poor-risk patient, surgery may be performed using local anesthesia after previous accurate localization studies.

There continues to be controversy regarding bilateral or unilateral surgical exploration (Table 20–5). The dispute regarding unilateral versus bilateral exploration centers mainly on preoperative localization of the parathyroid adenoma. If an adenoma has not been clearly localized preoperatively and the patient has undergone unilateral exploration with removal of a slightly enlarged parathyroid gland, some surgeons believe that it is advisable to explore the other side to avoid missing an abnormal gland, which could lead to persistent hyperparathyroidism. Even with accurate localization of the unilaterally enlarged parathyroid gland, some surgeons still prefer bilateral exploration because 10% to 14% of patients may have multiglandular disease, and 3%

TABLE 20–5 Indications for Unilateral Versus Bilateral Parathyroid Exploration

Unilateral	Bilateral
Scan-directed exploration	Uniglandular versus multiglandular disease
Look for second normal gland on same side	Multiple adenomas
Less operating time	Examine the other side for abnormal glands
Reduced complications	Does not take too much extra time in the OR
	Easy to explore both sides in primary exploration

OR, operating room.

to 4% of patients may have multiple adenomas. These surgeons believe that not much extra time is needed in the operating room to check the other side and remove an enlarged gland if it is found. Biopsy of the other ipsilateral parathyroid gland is generally performed to compare the histology.

During surgery, the enlarged parathyroid gland can be identified by the size and color differences. Occasionally, a thyroid nodule or an enlarged lymph node may be confused with the parathyroid gland. Once the parathyroid gland has been removed, it is submitted for histopathologic evaluation to confirm that the tissue removed is the parathyroid gland. Frequently, the pathologist will not be able to clearly distinguish between the diagnoses of parathyroid adenoma and glandular hyperplasia. The specimen submitted for pathology should be weighed so that the exact weight of the enlarged parathyroid can be compared with that of the normal parathyroid gland. Because the parathyroid gland normally weighs 35 mg, glands weighing 35 to 300 mg are generally hyperplastic, and those parathyroid glands measuring more than 500 to 750 mg are more likely to be adenomas.

Uniglandular versus multiglandular disease needs to be determined. Although pathologists generally prefer to compare a normal parathyroid gland with the abnormal gland, biopsy of the normal parathyroid gland is not absolutely essential in every case. With primary hyperparathyroidism, biopsying normal parathyroid glands may lead to parathyroid dysfunction. In uniglandular pathology, the treatment of choice is to remove the abnormal parathyroid gland.

In multiglandular disease, two surgical options are available. The first includes subtotal parathyroidectomy whereby a normal-appearing parathyroid gland is left behind with its intact blood supply. There is a small risk that this parathyroid tissue will develop hyperplasia again, causing recurrent hyperparathyroidism. The other option includes total parathyroidectomy with autotransplantation of a small portion of the parathyroid gland in the arm. This approach is associated with a small risk that the implanted parathyroid gland will not function, which leads to permanent hypoparathyroidism. It is important to preserve the parathyroid gland with its blood supply. It is also essential to have the facilities for cryopreservation of the parathyroid tissue should the surgeon decide to perform total parathyroidectomy with autotransplantation, so that if the autotransplanted parathyroid tissue does not function, a previously preserved parathyroid gland can be re-autotransplanted in the forearm.

In the surgical procedure of parathyroid autotransplantation, generally the parathyroid is autotransplanted in the forearm rather than in the neck, so that blood can be drawn for the evaluation of parathyroid function from the forearm. In renal failure patients, total parathyroidectomy with autotransplantation is the preferred choice. However, there is a high incidence of autotransplanted parathyroid tissue's regrowing in the forearm, which can cause recurrent hyperparathyroidism. Because the parathyroid tissue is in the forearm, it can be easily removed with the patient under local anesthesia. It is important to confirm on frozen section that the tissue is parathyroid gland before the tissue in the forearm is autotransplanted to ensure this is not a lymph node, fat, or thyroid carcinoma.

Parathyroid Reexploration

The success of initial surgery exceeds 95%. There are several reasons for failed surgical exploration, including (1) multiglandular disease, (2) incorrect diagnosis, (3) undiscovered parathyroid gland in the mediastinum, or (4) parathyroid carcinoma.

It is extremely important in surgical reexploration to confirm the diagnosis of hyperparathyroidism by obtaining a 24-hour urinary calcium to rule out hypocalciuric hypercalcemia (Figs. 20–1 and 20–2).

Noninvasive localization studies are routinely performed to localize the enlarged parathyroid gland and to note any ectopic locations of the parathyroid gland. Usually the missing parathyroid gland is found in the neck, but occasionally it may be undescended or may be found in the mediastinum. Rarely, invasive studies such as angiography or selective venous PTH assay may be necessary. A majority of the superior mediastinal glands can be easily removed through a transcervical approach.[20, 21]

The sternal split is reserved for failed parathyroid reexploration or for documented enlarged parathyroid gland in the mediastinum. Approximately 1% of the parathyroid glands may be deep in the superior or posterior mediastinum and may require a sternal split. Rarely, the parathyroid gland may be deep in the mediastinum near the aortopulmonary window or inside the pericardium, requiring sternal split.

Minimal Access Parathyroid Surgery

With improved technology, there has been increasing interest in minimal access parathyroid surgery in an effort to minimize surgical exploration and reduce complications of parathyroid surgery, hopefully improving the quality of life of patients treated for this disorder. Several of these advances in minimal access parathyroid surgery are described in Table 20–6.

One of the major advances in parathyroid surgery is the applicability of quick chemimmunoluminescent PTH assay, which is completed in approximately 15 minutes and thus can be performed during parathyroid surgery. Irvin is credited for introducing this technology into clinical practice.[22, 23] Recently, Nichol's laboratory has made this test commercially available, and it has been approved by the U.S. Food and Drug Administration (FDA). Since the FDA's approval of the quick PTH assay, the approach described here has become a commonly practiced technique at many institutions. Availability of the quick PTH assay is particularly important during reexploration procedures.

To optimally use this assay, it is recommended that a preoperative sestamibi scan be obtained, along with a preoperative quick PTH assay. The localized gland is removed, and after the adenoma has been removed, a repeat PTH is performed 5 and 15 minutes after excision of an enlarged parathyroid gland. If the PTH level falls to less than 50% of the preoperative level, the surgical procedure is completed. This practice is associated with a 99% success rate. However, if the PTH level does not drop to the 50% level, bilateral exploration is indicated, and any other enlarged parathyroid gland is removed. After the other parathyroid gland or multiple enlarged parathyroid glands have been removed, a PTH assay should be performed to document a more than 50% drop.

Another major advance is radioguided parathyroid surgery, which has been reported extensively by Norman.[24, 25] This approach looks at parathyroid surgery physiologically rather than anatomically. Because a parathyroid adenoma would have high sestamibi activity (20% more than background activity), it can be used to identify an enlarged parathyroid gland with the help of a scan-directed gamma probe. In this technique, sestamibi is injected approximately 2 hours before surgery, and a parathyroid scan is performed. A gamma probe is inserted through a mini-incision of approximately 3 cm on the involved side, and the location of the enlarged parathyroid gland is noted by high radionuclide activity. Once the enlarged parathyroid gland has been removed, the background activity and the activity of the parathyroid gland are compared. If the radionuclide activity of the removed tissue is more than 20% of the background

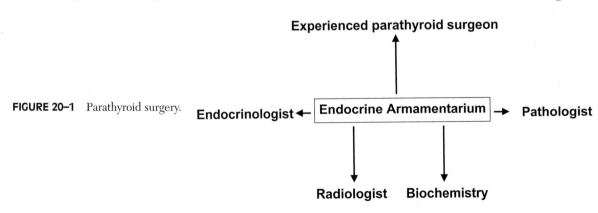

FIGURE 20–1 Parathyroid surgery.

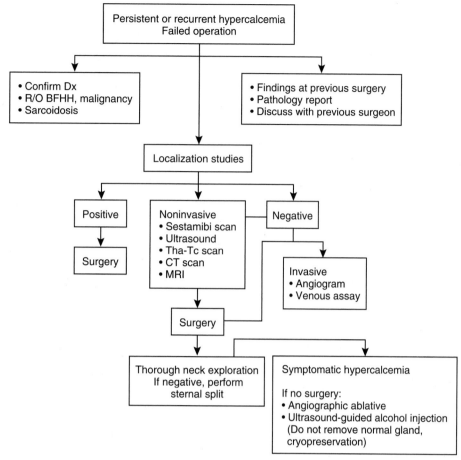

FIGURE 20–2 Parathyroid reexploration schema. BFHH, benign familial hypocalciuric hypercalcemia; Tha, thallium.

activity, indicating that it is parathyroid adenoma, the surgical procedure is terminated. Parathyroid hyperplasia generally gives activity of approximately 10%; fat and lymph nodes have minimal activity compared with the background activity.

However, very few reports in the literature have duplicated the results of Norman and associates.[24, 25] Our own experience revealed minimal applicability of gamma probe–directed parathyroid surgery because, in the majority of cases, preoperative sestamibi scan was sufficient to identify the parathyroid gland, and the gamma probe was not needed. When the parathyroid gland is not seen on the preoperative sestamibi scan, generally bilateral exploration is warranted.

TABLE 20–6 Types of Minimally Invasive Parathyroidectomy

Sestamibi-guided unilateral exploration
Scan-guided surgery with "quick" PTH
Outpatient parathyroidectomy
Parathyroidectomy under local anesthesia
Scan-directed parathyroidectomy with intraoperative gamma
  probe (physiologic approach to parathyroid surgery)
Endoscopic parathyroidectomy
  Cervical
  Mediastinal
Endoscopically assisted parathyroidectomy
  Sestamibi-assisted minimal incision approach

Under these circumstances, we have not found the gamma probe to be of great help.

In recent years, there has also been considerable interest in endoscopic parathyroidectomy. Although experience with this approach has been limited in the United States, considerable experience has been reported from France, Italy, and Japan. The first endoscopic parathyroidectomy was performed by Gagner at Cleveland Clinic in 1996. The initial technique involved the use of carbon dioxide for insufflation; however, this led to considerable subcutaneous emphysema and other problems related to carbon dioxide. The more recent technique involves a gasless procedure with the use of a special approach to lifting the cervical skin. The technique of endoscopic parathyroidectomy requires three or four mini-incisions, which may not be advantageous over the standard parathyroid mini-incision. There have been some reports in the Japanese literature regarding the infraclavicular incision or the transaxillary or submammary approach.[26] Miccoli and colleagues from Pisa, Italy, have described video-assisted parathyroid exploration.[27] They generally make a small incision, as in standard parathyroidectomy, and most of the dissection is performed with an endoscope. There has also been considerable interest in endoscopic parathyroidectomy for mediastinal enlarged parathyroid glands via the thoracoscopic approach; however, the role of endoscopic parathyroidectomy for enlarged cervical parathyroid glands needs expertise and further critical review.[28]

◼ PARATHYROID CARCINOMA

Parathyroid carcinoma is a rare clinical condition occurring in less than 1% of patients undergoing parathyroid surgery. There are only a few published series of small numbers of cases. Hundahl and coworkers recently published a large series in the United States of 286 patients from the National Cancer Data Base (NCDB).[29, 30] However, the information provided is mainly demographic and does not relate per se to the management of parathyroid cancer. Approximately 1000 cases are reported in the world literature, accounting for approximately 1% of parathyroid pathologies.[31–39] There appears to be equal sex distribution with a median age at diagnosis of approximately 55 years (14 to 88 years).

The clinical and histopathologic diagnoses may be quite complex, and the final diagnosis rests on the presence of local recurrence or nodal or distant metastasis.

Clinical Presentation

The major clinical finding in patients with parathyroid cancer is severe hypercalcemia and occasionally bony disease. The clinical features are mainly related to hyperparathyroidism; common presenting symptoms include fatigue, weight loss, psychiatric symptoms, muscular weakness, nephrolithiasis, and bone disease; certain abdominal symptoms such as abdominal pain, constipation, peptic ulcer disease, and pancreatitis may be associated. Obara and Fujimoto reported an incidence of 48% of patients with renal involvement and 39% with bone disease.[31] Occasionally, the parathyroid tumor may be clinically palpable, which may lead to a strong preoperative clinical suspicion of parathyroid carcinoma. Also, the serum calcium may be above 14 mg/dL, and the patient may present with hypercalcemic crisis. There appears to be a very low incidence of parathyroid carcinoma in patients with secondary hyperparathyroidism, especially in dialysis patients.

A preoperative diagnosis of parathyroid cancer is difficult unless there is a clinically palpable mass, metastatic disease to the lymph nodes, or distant metastasis (Table 20–7). This is a unique endocrine neoplasm in which occasionally the pathologist may find it difficult to confirm the diagnosis of malignancy on purely histologic criteria. Therefore, the clinical scenario is critically important in making the proper diagnosis. Frequent clinical correlates of malignant potential include the presence of lymph node metastasis, distant metastasis, or locally recurrent parathyroid tumor. Even though there is no definite etiologic factor, radiation is occasionally considered to be associated; however, radiation has also been associated with benign parathyroid adenoma.

The diagnosis of parathyroid carcinoma is based mainly on the intraoperative findings—invasion of the tumor into surrounding soft tissues such as the strap muscles, trachea, recurrent laryngeal nerve, esophagus, and thyroid gland. Histopathologic findings of mitosis or capsular and vascular invasion, rosette formation, presence of intraglandular fibrous bands, cellular pleomorphism, trabecular pattern, and atypia are also helpful to the clinician in making the proper diagnosis. The role of intraoperative frozen section analysis of the resected specimen continues to generate considerable controversy because the diagnosis of parathyroid carcinoma

TABLE 20–7 Diagnostic Criteria for Parathyroid Carcinoma

Preoperative	Intraoperative
• Ca > 14 mg/dL	• Hard mass
• Marked evaluation of PTH	• Invasion of surrounding structures
• Recurrent hypercalcemia	• Lymphadenopathy
• Bone changes	
• Recurrent urolithiasis	

Pathology	Confirmation
• Invasion into surrounding structures	• Positive lymph nodes
• Pseudorosette formation	• Vascular invasion
• Desmoplastic reaction	• Distant metastasis
• Mitosis	• Recurrent disease

is difficult on routine histopathology. Ancillary studies such as DNA ploidy may be helpful; however, they are not used on a routine basis. *TP53* gene mutation may be demonstrated in malignant parathyroid tumors.[40]

Treatment

The mainstay of the treatment of parathyroid cancer is surgical resection; data related to postoperative radiation therapy or adjuvant treatment are sparse. The initial surgical procedure should be adequate and radical enough to remove all gross tumor along with adjacent tissues such as the strap muscles, thyroid gland, and structures involved by the parathyroid. Ipsilateral thyroid lobectomy should be strongly considered along with resection of the strap muscles. If the recurrent laryngeal nerve is preoperatively involved or if the tumor appears to be surrounding the nerve, the nerve should be sacrificed. En bloc resection of the parathyroid with ipsilateral thyroid lobectomy is strongly recommended.

Because the diagnosis of carcinoma is often not known at the time of exploration, the finding of a parathyroid gland that is intimately adherent to or directly infiltrating into the thyroid should raise the level of suspicion for parathyroid cancer, and an ipsilateral thyroid lobectomy should be performed at the same time. It is extremely important at the time of surgery to avoid a capsular break or spillage of the tumor into the wound, which may lead to parathyrosis with multifocal recurrent tumor.

Even though there is no role for elective node dissection, paratracheal node clearance and central compartment clearance should be considered when there is clinical suspicion of parathyroid carcinoma. The jugular lymph nodes should be evaluated for suspicion of metastatic tumor. Although the role of neck dissection in this disease is controversial, modified or radical neck dissection is generally reserved for clinically palpable cervical lymph node metastasis or recurrent nodal disease.

After surgical intervention, the patient should be carefully followed for recurrence with serial serum calcium and PTH levels. Progressive hypercalcemia or hyperparathormonemia can indicate local recurrence, regional disease, or distant metastasis. Appropriate workup should be considered to rule out local recurrence or distant metastasis. Fraker reported a local and a regional recurrence of 36% and 14%, respectively, in his review of 163 patients.[28] The lung appears to be the most common site of distant metastasis (15%), and bone and liver are involved in 6% and 4% of patients, respectively. Resection of the recurrent parathyroid tumor appears to offer a survival advantage and offers symptomatic relief with normalization of the serum calcium level.

The role of postoperative radiation therapy remains undefined; however, it is generally considered in patients with high risk for local recurrence. Although there are some reports in the literature regarding chemotherapy with cyclophosphamide, fluorouracil, and dacarbazine, the therapeutic response appears to be limited. Hypercalcemia and its metabolic consequences and renal complications appear to be a major prognostic consideration. Rarely, the tumor may recur locally or in the paratracheal lymph nodes, leading to a frozen central compartment with involvement of the trachea and esophagus. Review of the NCDB data led to survival estimates of 85% and 49% at 5 and 10 years, respectively.[29] Sandelin reported a series of 95 patients with parathyroid carcinoma; prognostic factors considered are (1) age at the time of diagnosis; (2) extent of initial surgery; and (3) histopathologic review of definite invasive growth and or metastasis.[32] Local recurrence appears to be the most common site of treatment failure, and appropriate surgical consideration may be given if the recurrent tumor is resectable.

REFERENCES

1. Thompson NW: The history of hyperparathyroidism. Acta Chir Scand 156:5, 1990.
2. Wells SA, Leight GF, Ross A: Primary hyperparathyroidism. Curr Probl Surg 17:398–467, 1980.
3. Clark OH, Wilkes W, Siperstein AE, et al: Diagnosis and management of asymptomatic hyperparathyroidism: Safety, efficacy, and deficiencies in our knowledge. J Bone Miner Res 6:S135, 1991.
4. Scholz DA, Purnell DC: Asymptomatic primary hyperparathyroidism: 10-year prospective study. Mayo Clin Proc 56:473–478, 1981.
5. Wells SA: Surgical therapy of patients with primary hyperparathyroidism: Long-term benefits. J Bone Miner Res 6:S143, 1991.
6. Nussbaum SR: Pathophysiology and management of severe hypercalcemia. Endocrinol Metab Clin North Am 22:343, 1993.
7. Parisien M, Silverberg SJ, Shane E, et al: Bone disease in primary hyperparathyroidism. Endocrinol Metab Clin North Am 19:19, 1990.
8. Potts JT Jr, Ackerman IP, Barker CF, et al: Diagnosis and management of asymptomatic primary hyperparathyroidism: Consensus development conference statement. Ann Intern Med 114:593–597, 1991.
9. Clark OH. "Asymptomatic" primary hyperparathyroidism: Is parathyroidectomy indicated? Surgery 116:947, 1994.
10. van Heerden JA, Grant CS: Surgical treatment of primary hyperparathyroidism: An institutional perspective. World J Surg 15:688, 1991.
11. Shaha AR, Jaffe BM: Cervical exploration for primary hyperparathyroidism. J Surg Oncol 52:14, 1993.
12. Rodriguez JM, Tezelman S, Siperstein AE, et al: Localization procedures in patients with persistent or recurrent hyperparathyroidism. Arch Surg 129:870, 1994.
13. Shaha AR, La Rosa CA, Jaffe BM: Parathyroid localization prior to primary exploration. Am J Surg 166:289–294, 1993.
14. Duh QY, Uden P, Clark OH: Unilateral neck exploration for primary hyperparathyroidism—analysis of a controversy using a mathematical model. World J Surg 16:654–662, 1992.
15. Shaha AR, Sarkar S, Strashun A, et al: Sestamibi scan for preoperative localization in primary hyperparathyroidism. Head Neck 19:870–891, 1997.
16. Greene AK, Mowschenson P, Hodin RA: Is sestamibi-guided parathyroidectomy really cost-effective? Surgery 126:1036–1041, 1999.
17. Martin D, Rosen JB, Ichise M: Evaluation of single isotope technetium 99m-sestamibi in localization efficiency for hyperparathyroidism. Am J Surg 172:633–636, 1996.
18. Shaha AR, La Rosa CA, Jaffe BM: Parathyroid localization prior to primary exploration. Am J Surg 166:289–294, 1993.
19. Harman CR, Grant CS, Hay ID, et al: Indications, technique, and efficacy of alcohol injection of enlarged parathyroid glands in patients with primary hyperparathyroidism. Surgery 124:1011–1020, 1998.
20. Brennan MF, Norton JA: Reoperation for persistent and recurrent hyperparathyroidism. Ann Surg 201:40, 1985.
21. Brennan MF, Marx SJ, Doppman JL, et al: Results of reoperation for persistent and recurrent hyperparathyroidism. Ann Surg 194:671, 1981.
22. Irvin GL, Dembrow VD, Prudhomme DL: Operative monitoring of parathyroid gland hyperfunction. Am J Surg 162:299–302, 1991.
23. Irvin GL, Prudhomme DL, Periso GT, et al: A new approach to parathyroidectomy. Ann Surg 219:574–581, 1994.
24. Norman J, Denham D: Minimally invasive radioguided parathyroidectomy in the reoperative neck. Surgery 124:1088–1093, 1998.
25. Murphy C, Norman J: The 20% rule: A simple, instantaneous radioactivity measurement defines cure and allows elimination of frozen sections and hormone assays during parathyroidectomy. Surgery 126: 1023–1029, 1999.
26. Ikeda Y, Takmi H, Niimi M, et al: Endoscopic thyroidectomy and parathyroidectomy by the axillary approach. A preliminary report. Surg Endosc 16:92–95, 2002.
27. Miccoli P, Berti P, Conte M, et al: Minimally invasive video-assisted parathyroidectomy: Lessons learned from 137 cases. J Am Coll Surg 191:613–618, 2000.
28. Fraker DL: Update on the management of parathyroid tumors. Curr Opin Oncol 12:41–48, 2000.
29. Hundahl SA, Fleming ID, Fremgen AM, et al: Two hundred eighty-six cases of parathyroid carcinoma treated in the U.S. between 1985–1995: A National Cancer Data Base Report. The American College of Surgeons Commission on Cancer and the American Cancer Society. Cancer 86:538–544, 1999.
30. Shaha AR, Shah JP: Parathyroid carcinoma: A diagnostic and therapeutic challenge (editorial). Cancer 86:378–380, 1999.
31. Obara T, Fujimoto Y: Diagnosis and treatment of patients with parathyroid carcinoma: Update and review. World J Surg 15:738–744, 1991.
32. Sandelin K, Auer G, Bondeson L, et al: Prognostic factors in parathyroid cancer: A review of 95 cases. World J Surg 16:724–731, 1992.
33. Shantz A, Castleman B: Parathyroid carcinoma: A study of 70 cases. Cancer 31:600–605, 1973.
34. Koea JB, Shaw JHF: Parathyroid cancer: Biology and management. Surg Oncol 8:155–165, 1999.
35. Cordeiro AC, Montenegro FLM, Kulcsar MAV, et al: Parathyroid carcinoma. Am J Surg 175:52–55, 1998.
36. August DA, Flynn SD, Jones MA, et al: Parathyroid carcinoma: The relationship of nuclear DNA content to clinical outcome. Surgery 113:290–296, 1993.
37. Shortell CK, Andrus CH, Phillips CE Jr, et al: Carcinoma of the parathyroid gland: A 30-year experience. Surgery 110:704–708, 1991.
38. Cohn K, Silverman M, Corrado J, et al: Parathyroid carcinoma: The Lahey Clinic experience. Surgery 98:1095–1100, 1985.
39. Shaha AR, Ferlito A, Rinaldo A: Distant metastases from thyroid and parathyroid cancer. ORL J Otorhinolaryngol Relat Spec 63:243–249, 2001.
40. Cryns VL, Rubio MP, Thor AD, et al: p53 abnormalities in human parathyroid carcinoma. J Clin Endocrinol Metab 78: 1320–1324, 1994.

CHAPTER 21

Malignant Tumors of the Salivary Glands

Ehab Y. N. Hanna
James Y. Suen

◑ INTRODUCTION

For many years, our understanding of the biologic behavior of malignant tumors of the salivary glands was hampered by several factors. First, malignant neoplasms of the salivary glands constitute a large collection of highly heterogeneous tumors that exhibit a wide spectrum of biologic behavior, ranging from slow growth and indolence to highly aggressive behavior and rapid fatality. Second, the nomenclature used to classify these tumors has been, until recently, inconsistent. Third, malignant tumors of the salivary glands are relatively infrequent; hence, it is difficult for any single institution to compile a large enough experience to define optimal treatment strategies for these tumors.

Although at present some of these challenges still remain, several recent advances have allowed us to better understand the nature and behavior of cancer of the salivary glands. Some of these advances include the development of a standardized, clear, and rational classification system of salivary gland neoplasms. This classification system is based on a better understanding of the histogenesis and natural history of the various types of salivary gland tumors. Moreover, advances in molecular biology have allowed us to better characterize some of the genetic bases for the development of cancer of the salivary gland, as well as to define molecular markers associated with aggressive behavior. Such markers may be used in the future to further refine the classification of salivary gland tumors and to help with planning optimal treatment strategies, particularly adjuvant therapy. In addition to discussing these advances, this chapter discusses some of the current consensus (or controversy) regarding the diagnosis and treatment of patients with malignant tumors of the salivary glands.

◑ SURGICAL ANATOMY

The salivary glandular system is made of two types of glands. The *major* salivary glands are relatively large and anatomically distinct; they drain into the mouth via complex identifiable ductal systems. There are three pairs of major salivary glands—the parotid, submandibular, and sublingual glands (Fig. 21–1). In contrast, the *minor* salivary glands are much smaller and anatomically indistinct and lack an organized ductal excretory system. Numerous minor salivary glands are dispersed throughout the mucosal lining of the upper aerodigestive tract.

Parotid Gland

The parotid gland is the largest of the three major salivary glands and varies in weight from 14 to 28 g. It lies directly below and in front of the external ear. The main portion of the gland lies relatively flat over the ramus of the mandible and the masseter muscle (see Fig. 21–1). Above, it is broad and reaches nearly to the zygomatic arch; below, it tapers to form what is known as the "tail" of the parotid. This lower portion extends to a variable distance in the neck overlying the upper portion of the sternocleidomastoid muscle (SCM) and, more medially, the digastric muscle. The remainder of the gland is irregularly wedge shaped and extends deeply behind and medial to the mandible through the stylomandibular tunnel into the prestyloid compartment of the parapharyngeal space (Fig. 21–2). Because of the proximity of the gland to the lateral pharyngeal wall, tumors arising from or extending to the deep portion of the parotid gland may appear as a swelling in the oropharynx that pushes the tonsil or soft palate anteromedially. The mastoid and tympanic processes of the temporal bone form the posterior boundary of the parotid gland.

The parotid gland is enclosed within a capsule formed by the deep cervical fascia. Superficial to the fascial capsule, the gland is covered by the superficial musculoaponeurotic system (SMAS) in the face and by the platysma muscle in the neck. The parotid (Stensen) duct, which was discovered by and named after Dr. Niel Stensen in 1662,[1] crosses over the masseter and at the anterior border of this muscle turns inward nearly at a right angle, passes through the buccal fat pad of the cheek, and pierces the buccinator; it then runs for a short distance obliquely forward between the buccinator and the mucous membrane of the mouth, and it opens on the oral surface of the cheek by a small orifice, opposite the second upper molar. An accessory portion of the parotid gland, if present, is usually found adjacent to Stensen's duct in the buccal space.

Although the parotid gland is commonly described as consisting of two lobes, it is actually a unilobar gland. There

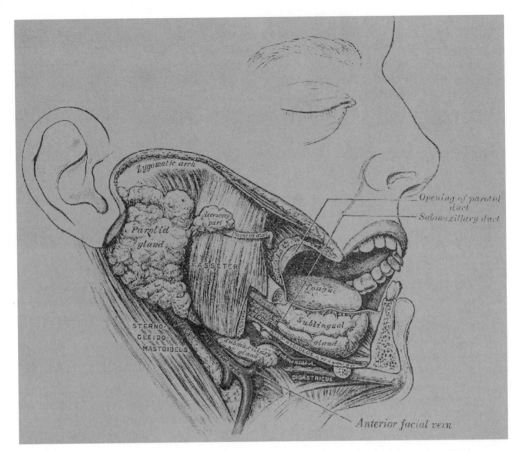

FIGURE 21–1 Dissection showing the anatomy of the major salivary glands. (From Gray H: Anatomy of the Human Body, 20th ed. Edited by WH Lewis. New York, Bartleby.com.)

is no true fascial separation between the superficial and deep portions of the gland. The facial nerve, which is the most critical structure within the parotid gland, divides the gland into two surgical zones. The main bulk (80%) of the parotid gland lies lateral to the facial nerve and is designated the *superficial lobe,* whereas a much smaller portion lies medial to the nerve and is designated the *deep lobe.* Accurate identification of the facial nerve is the most important step in any surgical procedure performed on the parotid gland. It is essential, therefore, for the clinician to know the surgical landmarks that facilitate the identification of the facial nerve, as well as the anatomic variations of the facial nerve.

The facial nerve exits the temporal bone through the stylomastoid foramen, which is located at the most medial aspect of the tympanomastoid fissure between the mastoid tip and the external auditory meatus. At this level, the stylomastoid artery travels just lateral to the main trunk of the extratemporal facial nerve.

The branches of the facial nerve supplying the posterior auricular muscle and the posterior belly of the digastric muscle usually arise from the main trunk, which is usually found 1 to 1.5 cm inferior and deep to the tragal "pointer." The main trunk divides in a variable pattern to provide motor innervation to the upper, middle, and lower portions of the face (Fig. 21–3). The point at which the main trunk separates into these two or three main divisions is designated the *pes anserinus.* The lower division contains the

branches to the platysma (cervical branch) and the marginal mandibular nerve, which supplies the muscles that depress the lower lip. The marginal mandibular nerve (ramus mandibularis) lies deep to the platysma muscle, and in its posterior-to-anterior course, it travels lateral to the retromandibular vein and the capsule of the submandibular gland. The midface division (i.e., zygomaticobuccal) supplies the buccal, zygomatic, and lower eyelid areas. The buccal branch is identified adjacent to the parotid salivary duct, which in turn may be identified at the anterior aspect of the masseter muscle (approximately 1 cm inferior and parallel to the zygomatic arch) before it pierces the buccinator muscle to enter the oral cavity. The surface anatomy of Stensen's duct corresponds to a line drawn from the tragal cartilage to the angle of the mouth. The upper face division (i.e., frontal branch) consists of one or more branches that supply the frontalis muscle and upper eyelid; it is located lateral to the superficial layer of the deep temporal fascia.

Other nerves related to the parotid gland include the greater auricular and auriculotemporal nerves. The greater auricular nerve is identified on the surface of the gland lateral to the parotid fascia and the SCM. It divides into anterior and posterior branches and provides sensation to the lower half of the auricle and adjacent skin. Preservation of the posterior branch is possible in selected patients undergoing parotidectomy, but whether this offers any advantage is uncertain.[2] The auriculotemporal nerve, a

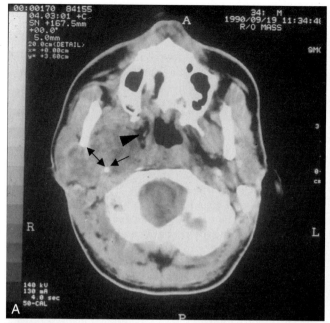

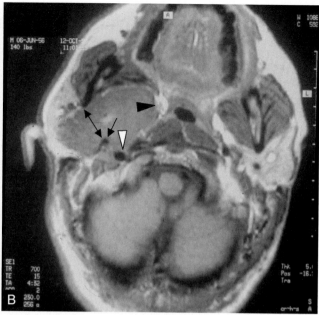

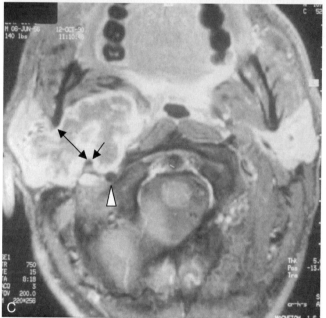

FIGURE 21–2 Large tumor of the partiod gland. Axial CT scan, *(A)* and T1-weighted MRI without *(B)* and with *(C)* gadolinium. The tumor, which involves both the superficial and the deep lobes of the parotid gland, lies anterior to the styloid process *(black arrow in A, B, and C)* in the prestyloid compartment of the parapharyngeal space. The fat of the parapharyngeal space is displaced medially *(black arrowhead in A and B),* and the internal cartoid artery (ICA) is displaced posteriorly *(white arrowhead in B and C).* The isthmus of tumor between the superficial and the deep components passes through the stylomandibular "tunnel" *(double arrow in A, B, and C)* and therefore is relatively narrow, giving the appearance of a dumbbell.

branch of the trigeminal nerve, courses superiorly on the posterior surface of the gland, along with the superficial temporal artery and vein. It is a sensory nerve to the temporal region, but it also carries parasympathetic fibers to the parotid gland from the otic ganglion. Cross-innervation between the sensory and parasympathetic nerve fibers may result in stimulation of the sweat glands of the temporal skin during mastication. This gustatory sweating is also known as Frey's syndrome. Prophylactic resection of the auriculotemporal nerve to prevent postparotidectomy Frey's syndrome has proved unsuccessful.[3]

The arterial supply to the parotid gland is provided from the superficial temporal and internal maxillary arteries; both are terminal branches of the external carotid artery, which traverses the deep portion of the gland. The main venous drainage flows from the superficial temporal vein and the internal maxillary vein to form the retromandibular vein (or posterior facial vein), which branches into anterior and posterior divisions. The anterior division joins the anterior facial vein to form the common facial vein, whereas the posterior division joins the posterior auricular vein to form the external jugular vein. Lymphatic drainage is directed into intraglandular and extraglandular lymph nodes. These nodes, which are located in the preauricular and infraauricular regions, receive primary lymphatic drainage from a large area of the scalp and face anterior to the coronal plane. Therefore, the differential diagnosis of any parotid mass should include metastasis from cutaneous malignancy of the face or scalp. Lymphatic drainage thereafter proceeds to the deep upper jugular lymph node chain.

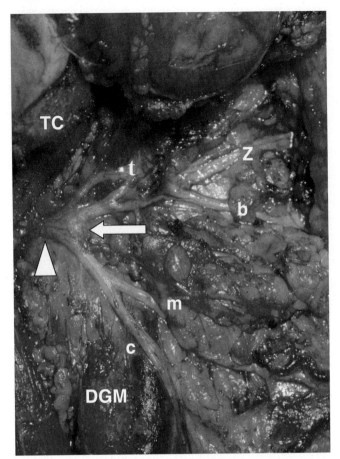

FIGURE 21–3 Intraoperative photograph demonstrating the anatomy of the extratemporal facial nerve. After exiting the temporal bone at the stylomastoid foramen, the main trunk of the facial nerve (*white arrowhead*) is located between the mastoid attachment of the posterior belly of the digastric muscle (DGM) and the tragal cartilage (TC). It usually lies 1.5 cm inferior and deep to the tragal "pointer," at the medial end of the tympanomastoid suture line (see Figs. 21–17D and 21–19). The main trunk divides in a variable pattern to provide motor innervation to the upper, middle, and lower portions of the face. The point at which the main trunk separates into these two or three main divisions is known as the pes anserinus (*white arrow*). In this patient, the lower division divides into the cervical branch (c), which supplies the platysma muscle, and the marginal mandibular branch (m), which supplies the muscles that depress the lower lip. The midface division (zygomaticobuccal) divides into the buccal (b) and zygomatic (z) branches. The upper face division, after receiveing a contribution from the middle division, yields the temporal branch (t), which provides several branches to the frontalis muscle and upper eyelid.

Submandibular Gland

The submandibular gland is mostly situated in the submandibular triangle, reaching forward to the anterior belly of the digastric and backward to the stylomandibular ligament, which intervenes between it and the parotid gland (see Fig. 21–1). Above, it extends medial to the body of the mandible; below, it usually overlaps the intermediate tendon of the digastric, the mylohyoid, and the hyoglossus muscles. The gland is covered by the skin, superficial fascia, platysma, and deep cervical fascia. The marginal mandibular

nerve lies superficially across the anterior facial vein as it crosses over the capsule of the gland. The facial artery is embedded in a groove in the posterior border of the gland.

The deep process of the submandibular gland extends from the main portion of the gland around the free posterior border of the mylohyoid muscle. This deep portion of the gland, which is insinuated between the mylohyoid and the hyoglossus, is related to the lingual nerve and the submandibular ganglion superiorly; it is related to the hypoglossal nerve and its accompanying vein inferiorly.

The submandibular duct (*Wharton's duct*) is about 5 cm long, and its wall is much thinner than that of the parotid duct. It begins by numerous branches from the deep surface of the gland and runs forward between the mylohyoid and the hyoglossus, and then between the sublingual gland and the genioglossus; it then opens by a narrow orifice on the summit of a small papilla, at the side of the frenulum linguae. On the hyoglossus, it lies between the lingual and hypoglossal nerves, but at the anterior border of the muscle, it is crossed laterally by the lingual nerve; the terminal branches of the lingual nerve ascend on its medial side.

The blood supply to the submandibular gland is provided by branches of the facial artery that enter the submandibular triangle just deep to the posterior belly of the digastric muscle. The artery then courses superiorly, becoming intimately associated with the medial aspect of the submandibular gland. As the artery approximates the mandible, it turns around its inferior edge to enter the face at the anterior border of the masseter muscle insertion. The parasympathetic innervation reaches the gland through the chorda tympani nerve via the lingual nerve, which carries the preganglionic fibers into the submandibular (submaxillary) ganglion. Postsynaptic fibers reach the gland via the ansa submandibularis, which connects the lingual nerve with the most superior aspect of the gland.

Sublingual Gland

The sublingual gland is the smallest of the three glands (see Fig. 21–1). It is situated beneath the mucous membrane at the side of the frenulum linguae, in contact with the sublingual depression of the medial surface of the mandible. It is narrow and flattened and weighs nearly 2 g. Above it is the mucous membrane; below it is the mylohyoid; behind it is the deep part of the submandibular gland; laterally from it is the mandible; and medial to it is the genioglossus, from which it is separated by the lingual nerve and the submandibular duct. Its excretory ducts are from 8 to 20 in number. Of the smaller sublingual ducts (*ducts of Rivinus*), some join the submandibular duct; others open separately into the mouth on the elevated crest of mucous membrane (lingual papilla, or *plica sublingualis*) (caused by the projection of the gland) on each side of the frenulum linguae. One or more join to form the larger sublingual duct (*duct of Bartholin*), which opens into the submandibular duct.

◼ EMBRYOLOGY AND HISTOLOGY

The major salivary glands originate from ectoderm and begin their development as solid ingrowths from the oral

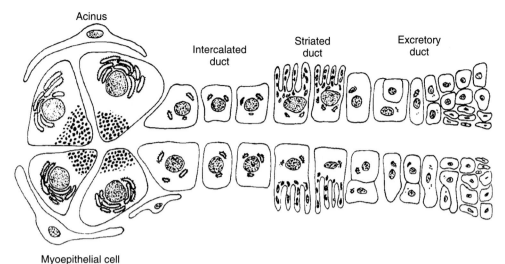

Acinus

Intercalated duct

Striated duct

Excretory duct

Myoepithelial cell

FIGURE 21–4 Basic structure of a salivary gland unit.

epithelium. These ingrowths continue to develop into tubules that later become the ductal system of the salivary glands.[4] In the major salivary glands, both serous and mucous cells are arranged into acini, which are drained by a series of ducts—an intercalated duct that drains into a striated duct, which empties into an excretory duct. Contractile myoepithelial cells surround the acini and intercalated ducts and help in draining saliva through the ductal system (Fig. 21–4). Serous acini predominate in the parotid gland, whereas mucinous acini are more abundant in the sublingual and the minor salivary glands scattered throughout the upper aerodigestive tract. The submandibular gland has both serous and mucous acini, although the latter are more numerous (Fig. 21–5).

◼ HISTOGENESIS OF SALIVARY GLAND TUMORS

The embryology and ultrastructure of the normal salivary gland provide the framework for our understanding of the histogenesis of the various types of salivary gland tumors. At least two theories of tumorigenesis have been proposed for salivary gland neoplasms.[5] In the *multicellular theory*, each type of neoplasm is thought to originate from a different cell type within the salivary gland unit. For example, Warthin's and oncocytic tumors are thought to arise from striated ductal cells, acinic cell tumors from acinar cells, squamous and mucoepidermoid carcinomas from excretory duct cells, and mixed tumors from intercalated duct and myoepithelial cells.[6] The experimental observation that all differentiated salivary cell types retain the ability to undergo mitosis and regenerate supports this theory and suggests that no limitations exist for a potential neoplastic cell of origin.[7, 8]

An alternative theory, the *bicellular reserve cell theory*, assumes that the origin of salivary neoplasms can be traced to the basal cells of either the excretory or the intercalated duct. Either of these two cells can act as a reserve cell with the potential for differentiation into a variety of epithelial cells.[9] Hence, despite the seeming heterogeneity of these tumors, all of them are predicted to arise from one of two pluripotential cell populations. In this model, *adenomatoid* tumors, including pleomorphic adenoma, oncocytic tumors, acinic cell carcinoma, and adenoid cystic carcinoma, are derived from the reserve cell of the intercalated duct, whereas *epidermoid* tumors, such as squamous cell carcinoma and mucoepidermoid carcinoma, are derived from the reserve cell of the excretory duct.[10] Recently, several studies have provided some molecular evidence to support the reserve cell theory of salivary gland tumorigenesis.[5, 11, 12]

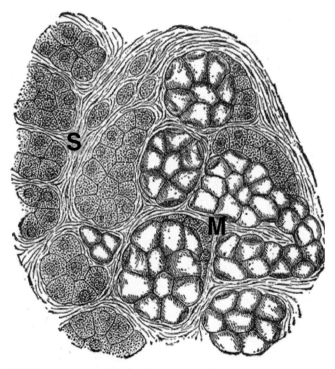

FIGURE 21–5 Histology of the submandibular gland, showing a mixture of mucous acini (M) and serous acini (S). (From Gray H: Anatomy of the Human Body, 20th ed. Edited by WH Lewis. New York, Bartleby.com.)

⬛ ETIOLOGY

The etiology of malignant tumors of the salivary gland, like most other types of cancer, remains unknown. However, there is growing evidence that some environmental factors such as radiation, viruses, diet, and certain occupational exposures may increase the risk for cancer of the salivary glands. Recently, the genetic abnormalities associated with the development of malignant tumors of the salivary glands have also been well characterized. The following section discusses both environmental and genetic risk factors associated with the development of salivary gland neoplasia.

Environmental Factors

Radiation

IONIZING RADIATION

There is increasing evidence to indicate that exposure to ionizing radiation may increase the risk for development of cancer of the salivary glands. In 1996, the Radiation Epidemiology Branch of the National Cancer Institute published a study on the risk among atomic bomb survivors of developing salivary gland tumors.[13] The study indicated that these patients had a higher radiation-related risk of developing both benign and malignant salivary gland tumors, when compared with the general population. Dose-response analyses found statistically significant increases in risk with increasing A-bomb dose for both cancer and benign tumors. The risk was higher for malignant tumors, especially mucoepidermoid carcinoma.

Radiation therapy to the head and neck, especially if it encompasses the salivary glands, may also be a risk factor in the development of salivary gland cancer.[14] The incidence of cancer of the salivary glands in patients with a previous history of radiation therapy to the head and neck was 4.5-fold that of matched controls.[15] The risk increased with increasing radiation doses. The mean latency period until tumor development was 11 years. These data suggest a possible role for radiation therapy in salivary gland carcinogenesis.

ULTRAVIOLET RADIATION

Exposure to ultraviolet radiation (UVR) may also be associated with an increased risk of salivary gland cancer. In investigation of this possible association, data from the Surveillance Epidemiology and End Results (SEER) program were analyzed to determine whether the incidence of salivary gland cancer exhibited the inverse correlation with geographic latitude that is characteristic of skin cancer incidence.[16] The SEER areas were grouped into three regions (north, central, and south), based on indices of UVR. The southern area had significantly higher rates of cancer of the salivary glands for white males and females than did with the northern area for all histologic subtypes combined. These data provide evidence of an association between skin and salivary neoplasms, with both exhibiting a pattern of incidence suggestive of susceptibility to UVR exposure.

Epstein-Barr Virus

There is some evidence to indicate that Epstein-Barr virus (EBV) may be implicated in the development of certain types of salivary gland neoplasms. Several studies have found a consistent association between EBV infection and lymphoepithelial carcinoma of the salivary glands.[17–21] The relatively high geographic concentration of lymphoepithelial carcinoma of the salivary glands among natives of Greenland,[21] southern China,[17, 18] and Japan[20] may be due to the high prevalence of EBV infections in these regions. The presence of the virus in a clonal form and the expression of its viral oncoprotein provide further evidence of the role of EBV in the oncogenesis of this tumor.[19, 22]

Other Factors

Occupational exposure to silica dust was linked to a 2.5-fold increased risk of cancer of the salivary gland.[23] The risk was also elevated among rubber workers exposed to nitrosamines.[24] Dietary analyses revealed a possible protective effect for a diet high in polyunsaturated fatty acids.[23, 25] As with breast cancer, women with history of early menarche and nulliparity had an increased risk of cancer of the salivary gland, which may be due to a hormonal effect.[26] Although tobacco use was not associated with a higher incidence of malignant salivary neoplasms, Warthin's tumor is strongly associated with cigarette smoking.[27] Despite concerns raised by cellular telephone users about the possible carcinogenic effects of radiofrequency signals from these phones, a recent nationwide study from Denmark showed that the risk of salivary gland cancer was not influenced by duration of cellular telephone use, time since first subscription, age at first subscription, or type of cellular telephone (analogue or digital).[28]

Genetic Factors

The genetic basis of cancer of the salivary glands continues to unfold. Data collected from comparative genomic hybridization indicate that different genetic alterations are present in the different types of salivary gland tumors and that these alterations involve several chromosomes.[29] Genetic alterations associated with the development of salivary neoplasms may include allelic loss and point mutation, structural rearrangement of chromosomal units (most commonly translocations), the absence of one chromosome (monosomy), or the presence of an extra chromosome (polysomy). Any of these factors may be present as the sole karyotypic abnormality as an early event in salivary gland carcinogenesis, or several genetic alterations may coexist, which is associated with tumor progression and more aggressive biologic behavior.[30, 31]

Allelic Loss

Tumors of salivary gland origin display allelic loss patterns different from those of many other tumor types, suggesting distinct genetic pathways in the initiation or progression of these tumors. The most significant allelic losses in adenoid cystic carcinoma are 1p, 2p, 6q, 17p, 19q, and 20p. Mucoepidermoid carcinoma has a 50% or greater loss at 2q, 5p, 12p, and 16q. Although losses at 9p, 3p, and 17p are common in squamous cell carcinoma of the head and neck, only carcinoma ex mixed tumors demonstrates loss at these loci.[32] Recently, investigators from the M.D. Anderson Cancer Center demonstrated that the most frequent alterations in acinic cell carcinoma involve chromosomes 4p, 5q, 6p, and 17p.[33] These regions showed the highest incidence of loss of heterozygosity (LOH), suggesting the presence of tumor suppressor genes associated with the oncogenesis of these tumors. LOH was significantly associated with tumor grade. More recently, the same group of investigators demonstrated that LOH at 12q loci may identify a subset of pleomorphic adenoma with potential progression to carcinoma; that acquisition of additional alterations at chromosome arm 17p loci might represent an event preceding malignant transformation and progression; and that 8q, 12q, and 17p regions may harbor tumor suppressor genes involved in the genesis of carcinoma ex pleomorphic adenoma.[31]

Point mutations of a variety of genes may also be involved in the initiation or promotion of cancer of the salivary glands. For example, the activation of the H-*RAS* oncogene is thought to be involved in the development and/or progression of mucoepidermoid carcinomas, and it is thought that a stepwise increase in the frequency of H-*RAS* mutations strongly correlates with tumor grade.[34] Overexpression of the c-kit protein, a tyrosine kinase receptor, has been implicated in the pathogenesis of several types of malignant tumors of the salivary glands.[35] Inactivation of tumor suppressor genes such as *TP16*[36] or *TP53*[37] may also be important in the development or progression of carcinoma of the salivary glands.

Monosomy and Polysomy

Trisomy 5 was described as the only karyotypic abnormality in a moderately differentiated primary mucoepidermoid carcinoma of minor salivary gland origin and may be an early event in the development of this tumor.[38] This finding was remarkably different from those of previous cytogenetic studies of mucoepidermoid carcinomas, which have shown heterogeneous and unrelated chromosomal aberrations. Other studies suggest that polysomy of both chromosomes 3 and 17 occurs during the development of salivary gland tumors, and its frequency is higher in adenoid cystic carcinoma as compared with pleomorphic adenoma. Monosomy of chromosome 17 could also be involved in the development of salivary gland tumors.[39]

Structural Rearrangement

The most common genetic structural rearrangement in salivary gland malignancy is translocation of genetic material involving chromosome 11. This finding was most commonly reported in mucoepidermoid carcinoma.[40] Cytogenetic analysis of mucoepidermoid carcinoma of the minor salivary glands demonstrated that chromosomal translocation (11,19)(q21; p13.1) is an early, and most likely a primary, event in the development of at least a subset of these neoplasms.[41] Similarly, a nonrandom pattern of translocations involving chromosomes 6q, 9p, and 17p was commonly found in adenoid cystic carcinoma.[42]

HISTOPATHOLOGIC CLASSIFICATION

Tumors of the salivary glands display a wide variety of histologic appearances and vary in behavior from totally benign to high-grade and usually fatal malignancies. Over the past 40 years, several classification schemes have been proposed, of which the most comprehensive and accurate are those of the Armed Forces Institute of Pathology (AFIP) and the World Health Organization (WHO).[43] The WHO classification is more concise, but both are readily applicable by practicing surgical pathologists and encompass most of the range of tumors likely to be encountered. The second edition of *The World Health Organization's Histological Classification of Salivary Gland Tumors* is more extensive and detailed than the previous edition, which was published more than 20 years ago. The revised edition is based on data regarding newly described tumor entities and the behavior and prognosis of previously classified tumors.[44]

Tumors of the salivary glands are broadly divided into benign neoplasms, tumorlike conditions, and malignant neoplasms (Table 21–1). Tumorlike conditions of the salivary glands may be confused with benign or malignant tumors. Malignant tumors of the salivary glands comprise carcinomas, malignant nonepithelial tumors, malignant lymphomas, and secondary tumors. New entities in the revised WHO classification include polymorphous low-grade adenocarcinoma, basal cell adenocarcinoma, salivary duct carcinoma, and malignant myoepithelioma. Carcinoma in pleomorphic adenoma can be distinguished as noninvasive and invasive carcinoma, and carcinosarcoma.[45] Malignant nonepithelial tumors are mostly malignant fibrous histiocytomas, malignant schwannomas, and rhabdomyosarcomas. A large majority of malignant lymphomas are non-Hodgkin's lymphomas with high differentiation. Many lymphomas are associated with Sjögren's syndrome. Secondary tumors are mostly metastases from primary squamous cell carcinomas or from melanomas of the skin of the head and neck. Hematogenous metastases are rare and originate mainly from lung, kidney, or breast.[44, 45]

INCIDENCE

Cancer of the salivary glands is relatively rare. According to the National Cancer Data Base (NCDB), cancer of the salivary glands accounts for between 0.3% and 0.9% of all cancers in the United States.[46, 47] A majority (70%) of salivary gland neoplasms arise in the parotid gland (Fig. 21–6). Whereas three fourths of parotid tumors are benign, a majority of tumors of the minor salivary glands are malignant (Fig. 21–7). In a review of the Memorial Sloan-Kettering experience with salivary neoplasms over a 35-year period, malignant neoplasms constituted 46% of all tumors, of which mucoepidermoid carcinoma and adenoid cystic carcinoma were the most common (Fig. 21–8).[48]

TABLE 21-1 The World Health Organization's Histologic Classification of Salivary Gland Tumors (1992)

1 Adenomas

  1.1 Pleomorphic adenoma
  1.2 Myoepithelioma (myoepithelial adenoma)
  1.3 Basal cell adenoma
  1.4 Warthin's tumor (adenolymphoma)
  1.5 Oncocytoma (oncocytic adenoma)
  1.6 Canalicular adenoma
  1.7 Sebaceous adenoma
  1.8 Ductal papilloma
      1.8.1 Inverted ductal papilloma
      1.8.2 Intraductal papilloma
      1.8.3 Sialadenoma papilliferum
  1.9 Cystadenoma
      1.9.1 Papillary cystadenoma
      1.9.2 Mucinous cystadenoma

2 Carcinomas

  2.1 Acinic cell carcinoma
  2.2 Mucoepidermoid carcinoma
  2.3 Adenoid cystic carcinoma
  2.4 Polymorphous low-grade adenocarcinoma (terminal duct adenocarcinoma
  2.5 Epithelial-myoepithelial carcinoma
  2.6 Basal cell adenocarcinoma
  2.7 Sebaceous carcinoma
  2.8 Papillary cystadenocarcinoma
  2.9 Mucinous adenocarcinoma
  2.10 Oncocytic carcinoma
  2.11 Salivary duct carcinoma
  2.12 Adenocarcinoma
  2.13 Malignant myoepithelioma (myoepithelial carcinoma)
  2.14 Carcinoma in pleomorphic adenoma (malignant mixed tumor)
  2.15 Squamous cell carcinoma
  2.16 Small cell carcinoma
  2.17 Undifferentiated carcinoma
  2.18 Other carcinomas

3 Nonepithelial tumors

4 Malignant lymphomas

5 Secondary tumors

6 Unclassified tumors

7 Tumorlike lesions

  7.1 Sialadenosis
  7.2 Oncocytosis
  7.3 Necrotizing sialometaplasia (salivary gland infarction)
  7.4 Benign lymphoepithelial lesion
  7.5 Salivary gland cysts
  7.6 Chronic sclerosing sialadenitis of submandibular gland (Kuttner's tumor)
  7.7 Cystic lymphoid hyperplasia in AIDS

From Seifert G, Sobin LH: The World Health Organization's Histological Classification of Salivary Gland Tumors. A commentary on the second edition. Cancer 70:379–385, 1992.

◘ PATIENT EVALUATION

Clinical Features

Parotid Gland. Both benign and malignant tumors of the parotid gland usually present as a painless swelling. However, certain clinical features associated with a parotid mass are usually indicative of malignancy, albeit advanced. These features include facial nerve paresis or paralysis, pain, fixation of the mass to the overlying skin or underlying

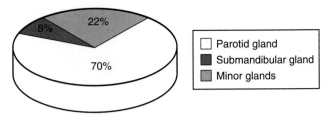

FIGURE 21-6 Site of origin of neoplasms of the salivary glands.

structures, and associated cervical adenopathy. It should be noted, however, that these findings usually indicate local or regional extension of advanced tumors. Therefore, the diagnosis of parotid malignancy should not await the development of these signs and symptoms but must be ruled out in patients presenting with any mass in the parotid gland. This usually requires histologic evaluation with a fine-needle biopsy (FNAB) and/or parotidectomy.

Patients presenting with a mass in the parotid gland should be asked about a history of cancer of the scalp or facial skin. Metastasis to the parotid gland from skin cancer, including melanoma, may be diagnosed by a careful examination of these areas for evidence of a skin cancer or a scar of previous excision. The oropharynx must also be examined carefully to rule out extension to the parapharyngeal space from a deep lobe parotid tumor. A mass in the deep lobe of the parotid gland, or a tumor arising from the minor salivary glands in the parapharyngeal space, may displace the soft palate or tonsil medially. This could be mistaken for tonsillar enlargement and could lead to an attempt at intraoral biopsy or excision. This may result in tumor seeding or mucosal scarring, making definitive resection through a transparotid/transcervical approach more difficult.

Submandibular Gland. Both benign and malignant tumors of the submandibular gland usually present as a painless, mobile mass in the submandibular triangle. Involvement of the overlying skin or fixation to the mandible usually indicates local extension of a malignant tumor. Ipsilateral weakness or numbness of the tongue indicates perineural spread of malignancy along the hypoglossal or lingual nerve, respectively. Enlargement of the submandibular or upper cervical lymph nodes may be due to reactive lymphadenopathy associated with submandibular sialadenitis, but it usually indicates regional metastasis of malignancy in the submandibular gland.

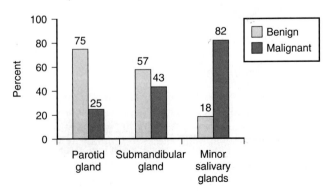

FIGURE 21-7 Distribution of benign and malignant salivary neoplasms according to site of origin.

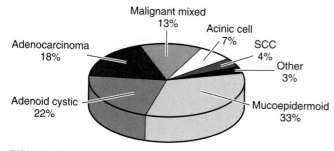

FIGURE 21–8 Incidence of malignant salivary neoplasms. SCC, Squamous cell carcinoma.

Minor Salivary Glands. The clinical presentation of malignant tumors of the minor salivary glands depends on the site of origin and does not differ from the presentation of other malignant tumors in these sites such as squamous cell carcinoma. The palate is the most common site of involvement, and adenoid cystic carcinoma is the most common histologic type encountered. Minor salivary gland tumors on the palate usually present either as a submucosal mass or as an ulcerative lesion (Fig. 21–9). The second most common site of involvement is the sinonasal tract; these patients usually present with nasal obstruction, epistaxis, or a nasal mass. Numbness or tingling in the distribution of the branches of the trigeminal nerve may indicate perineural spread, which occurs most frequently in patients with adenoid cystic carcinoma. Careful examination of the dermatomal distribution of the three divisions of the trigeminal nerve should be done, and any hypoesthesia or anesthesia should be considered evidence of perineural involvement.

Fine-Needle Aspiration Biopsy

The accuracy of FNAB in the diagnosis of tumors of salivary gland origin has been well established. The overall

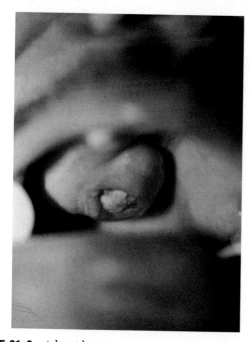

FIGURE 21–9 Adenoid cystic carcinoma of the hard palate presenting as an ulcerative mass.

sensitivity ranges from 85.5% to 99%, and the overall specificity ranges from 96.3% to 100%.[49-51] Diagnostic accuracy depends greatly on the experience of the cytopathologist[52] and on the overall volume of patients with salivary neoplasms evaluated in any given institution. The reported sensitivity and specificity were slightly lower in a community hospital setting than in a large academic center.[53] The most common source of diagnostic error of FNAB is inadequate sampling.[54] The use of ultrasound-guided FNAB may be of help when it is difficult to obtain a representative sample.[55]

In addition to being accurate, FNAB is safe, simple to perform, and relatively inexpensive. However, one essential question is worth asking: Is FNAB really necessary in the evaluation of salivary gland masses? Would it change the course of management based on clinical assessment? In an attempt to answer this question, Heller and colleagues performed a study to determine the impact of FNAB on patient management.[56] One hundred patients underwent FNAB of major salivary gland masses. The physician's initial clinical impression was compared with the FNAB diagnosis and the final diagnosis in each case. Overall, FNAB resulted in a change in the clinical approach to 35% of patients. Examples of such changes in the planned management included avoiding surgical resection for lymphomas and inflammatory masses, and adopting a more conservative approach with benign tumors in elderly and high-surgical-risk patients. FNAB also allows better preoperative counseling of patients regarding the nature of the tumor, the likely extent of resection, management of the facial nerve, and the likelihood of a neck dissection. Such information not only is important in treatment planning but also helps alleviate an already high level of anxiety in patients and their families. However, there are several caveats to the use of FNAB in the evaluation of parotid masses. Hemorrhage or inflammation at the biopsy site may obscure histologic patterns, thereby increasing the difficulty of making definitive diagnoses of smaller lesions. Also, these effects can make dissection of the facial nerve during definite resection technically more challenging.

Imaging

The routine use of imaging in small, well-defined masses of the superficial lobe of the parotid gland is probably not warranted because the results of imaging are not likely to change the treatment plan. However, tumors that present with clinical findings suggestive of malignancy, tumors arising from the deep lobe of the parotid gland or the parapharyngeal space, and tumors of the submandibular and minor salivary glands should be evaluated with high-resolution imaging. In such cases, imaging provides accurate delineation of the location and extent of tumor, its relation to major neurovascular structures, perineural spread, skull base invasion, and intracranial extension.

Computed Tomography and Magnetic Resonance Imaging

In evaluation of patients with tumors of the salivary glands, both computed tomography (CT) and magnetic resonance imaging (MRI) provide information that is superior to that provided by other imaging techniques or by physical examination.[57] The normal parotid gland has a high fat content and is easily visualized on both CT and MRI; therefore, both techniques can demonstrate whether a mass in that region is intraglandular or extraglandular. Only rarely does CT or MRI provide information regarding the specific histologic diagnosis. An example of such a rare scenario is lipoma of the parotid gland (Fig. 21–10). MRI is superior to CT in demonstrating the internal architecture of salivary gland tumors in a multiplanar fashion and in delineating the interface between tumor and normal salivary gland.[58] In contrast to benign tumors, which invariably have well-defined margins, malignant tumors may exhibit irregular margins (Fig. 21–11). Extension of the tumor beyond the fascial confines of the gland can be adequately seen on both CT and MRI and should raise the suspicion of malignancy.[59] Bone destruction of the mandible or skull base is best visualized

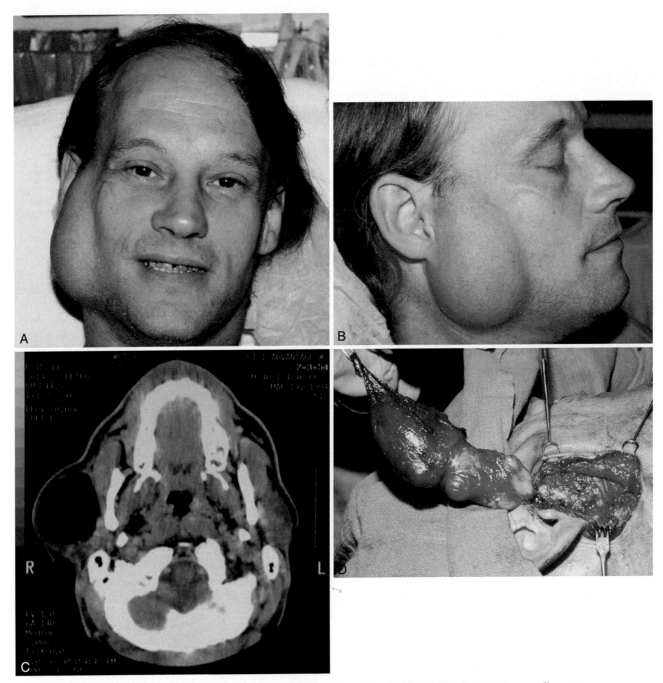

FIGURE 21–10 A 40-year-old man with a large, painless, slow-growing parotid mass. Fine-needle aspiration biopsy was indeterminate. *A,* Anterior view. *B,* Lateral view. *C,* An axial CT scan with IV contrast demonstrates a large, rounded, well-defined mass, with smooth borders in the parotid gland. The mass was nonenhancing and had the same density as the subcutaneous fat. These findings were pathognomonic of parotid lipoma. *D,* A superficial parotidectomy was performed, and the diagnosis was confirmed.

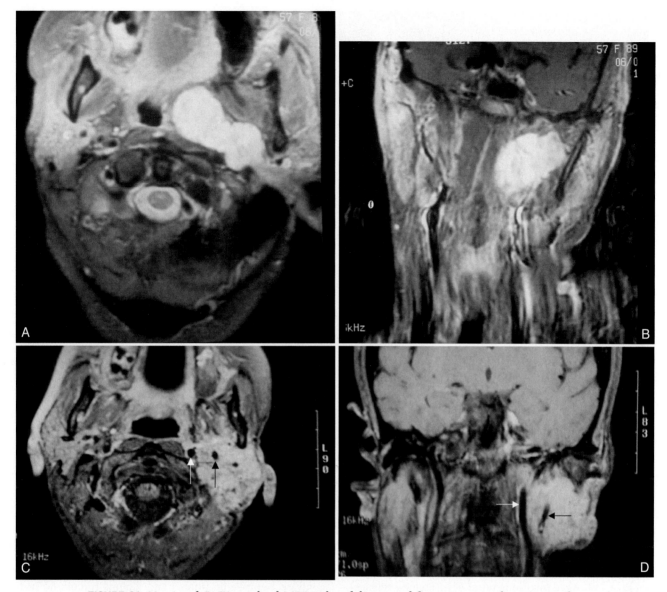

FIGURE 21–11 *A* and *B*, T1-weighted MRI with gadolinium and fat suppression of a patient with a dumbbell tumor (pleomorphic adenoma) of the parotid gland. Note the smooth and well-defined border of the tumor, which is easily delineated from the adjacent normal parotid tissue in both the axial *(A)* and coronal *(B)* images. *C* and *D*, In contrast, the T1-weighted MRI with gadolinium of a patient with mucoepidermoid carcinoma of the parotid shows the tumor to have an irregular border and to be indistinct from the normal parotid gland. Note complete encasement, rather than displacement of both the internal *(white arrow)* and external carotid arteries *(black arrow)*, in both the axial *(C)* and coronal *(D)* images.

on CT; bone marrow involvement is better demonstrated on MRI. Both studies can adequately evaluate the neck for metastatic adenopathy. CT is less expensive and more available than MRI. However, CT images are more susceptible to degradation by dental and motion artifact, although the latter has been greatly reduced with the introduction of high-speed spiral CT scanners.

High-resolution imaging is of paramount importance in detecting perineural involvement. Perineural spread is common in salivary gland malignancy, especially with adenoid cystic carcinoma. Perineural spread is a precursor of facial nerve and trigeminal ganglion infiltration, skull base invasion, and cavernous sinus involvement. These findings have

a profound negative impact on survival and may drastically change the therapeutic plan, including the surgical approach and adjuvant therapy.[60] Although perineural spread may present with sensory or motor deficits, it is often asymptomatic, hence the importance of high-resolution imaging.

MRI is superior to CT in early detection of perineural spread because of its better soft tissue delineation. The criteria of nerve nerve involvement seen with CT are bony changes in the foramina, fissures, or canals, through which nerves normally traverse the skull base. However, these changes, which include bone erosion, sclerotic margins, and widening of the normal diameter of these cranial base channels (Fig. 21–12A), are late indicators of perineural spread.

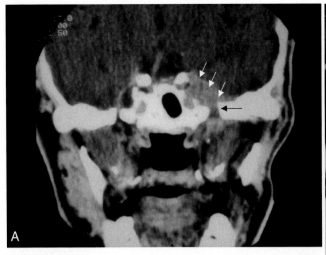

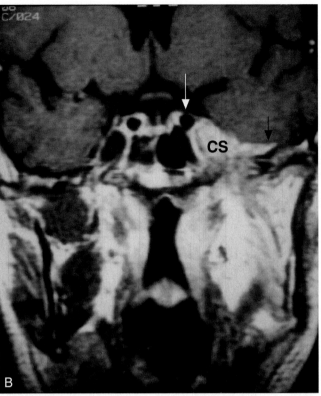

FIGURE 21–12 Imaging studies in a patient with perineural spread of adenoid cystic carcinoma along the third division of the trigeminal nerve (V3), involving the cavernous sinus and the dura of the middle cranial fossa. *A*, A coronal CT with IV contrast shows widening of the left foramen ovale *(black arrow)*, compared with the one on the right. There is also enhancement and thickening along the left Meckel's cave *(white arrows)*. *B*, A coronal T1-weighted MRI with gadolinium shows marked thickening and enchancement of V3, trigeminal ganglion, and lateral cavernous sinus (CS). The tumor abuts the cavernous carotid artery *(white arrow)*. There is enhancement of the dura along the floor of the middle cranial fossa *(black arrow)*. This "dural tail" is usually a sign of involvement of the dura with tumor.

The capability of MRI to detect the different signal intensities of tumor, fat, nerve, cerebrospinal fluid, meninges, and brain allows for better assessment of perineural spread. The criteria of nerve involvement on MRI include replacement of normal perineural fat with tumor, enhancement with gadolinium (regardless of size), and increased size of the nerve in question (regardless of enhancement) (Fig. 21–12*B*). According to these criteria, MRI is more sensitive and specific than CT in evaluating perineural spread.[60] MRI is also superior to CT in evaluating intracranial extension of tumor, especially in delineating the relationship of tumor to the cavernous carotid artery and the brain parenchyma (Fig. 21–13).

Although parapharyngeal space masses are well visualized by both techniques, they are better delineated with MRI than with CT (see Fig. 21–2). This is because of the different signal intensities of tumor, fat, and muscle on MRI. Most salivary tumors have low-to-intermediate T1 signal intensities and intermediate-to-high T2 signal intensities. The differential diagnosis of parapharyngeal masses includes deep lobe parotid tumors, minor salivary gland tumors, and neurogenic and vascular tumors. Deep lobe parotid tumors and minor salivary gland tumors of the parapharyngeal space lie in the prestyloid compartment, anterior to the carotid artery, and displace the parapharyngeal fat medially

(see Fig. 21–2). Deep lobe tumors are connected to the parotid gland at least in one imaging section, whereas minor salivary gland tumors are completely surrounded by fat. By contrast, neurogenic tumors and glomus tumors lie in the poststyloid compartment, posterior to the carotid artery, which is displaced anteriorly. Neurogenic tumors usually enhance intensely with gadolinium; glomus tumors have characteristic serpiginous flow voids (salt-and-pepper appearance) on MRI.

Ultrasonography

Ultrasonography is inexpensive, noninvasive, simple to perform, and virtually free of complications. It can be used to differentiate solid from cystic masses in the salivary glands. Its use is limited by its ability to visualize only relatively superficial masses. It has been supplanted by CT and MRI in the evaluation of salivary gland tumors. Ultrasound guidance may enhance the accuracy of FNAB in nonpalpable tumors and in masses with a highly heterogeneous architecture.[55]

Color Doppler Sonography

Color Doppler sonography has been recently used to evaluate the vascular anatomy of the salivary glands. It can

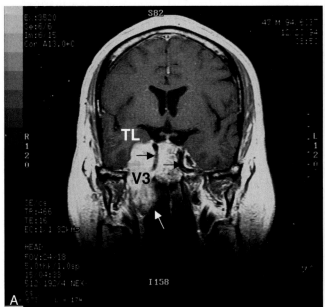
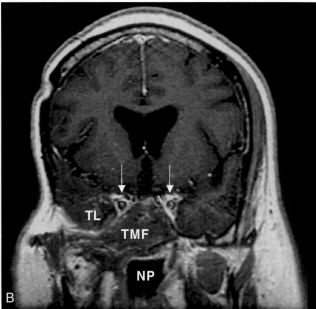

FIGURE 21–13 A 47-year-old patient who presented with headache and diplopia. On examination, he was found to have right abducent palsy and a polypoid mass in the right fossa of Rosenmüller. Biopsy showed adenoid cystic carcinoma. *A,* Coronal T1-weighted MRI with gadolinium showing the origin of the mass in the right nasopharynx (*white arrow*), with extension into the infratemporal and pterygopalatine fossae. There is destruction of the skull base and marked widening of the foramen ovale resulting from perineural spread along the third division of the trigeminal nerve (V3). More proximal perineural spread resulted in intracranial extension that elevated the temporal lobe (TL). There is evidence of involvement of the cavernous carotid artery bilaterally (*black arrows*). Surgical resection was done via a temporal-infratemporal fossa combined approach with gross total removal of tumor and temporalis muscle flap reconstruction. Postoperatively, the patient received 70 cGy of radiation. *B,* At 5-year follow-up, the coronal T1-weighted MRI shows no evidence of progressive local disease. Note the expansion of the temporal lobe (TL) to near-normal position. The temporalis muscle flap (TMF) provides well-vascularized coverage to the internal carotid arteries (*white arrows*) and adequate separation between the intracranial defect and the nasopharynx (NP).

distinguish between the physiologic changes that occur during salivary stimulation in normal subjects and the flow alterations that occur in diseased glands.[61] Specific patterns of peak systolic vascular shifts were described in various pathologic processes, including Sjögren's syndrome, pleomorphic adenoma, and malignant tumors.[61–63] Other vascular parameters such as the pulsatility and resistive indices have recently been described, and their predictive value in the diagnosis of malignant tumors of the salivary glands is surprisingly high.[62]

Positron Emission Tomography

Positron emission tomography (PET) scans have not gained wide application in the imaging of tumors of the salivary gland for several reasons. First, tumors of the salivary glands have a variable and inconsistent uptake of ^{18}F fluorodeoxyglucose (FDG), which is the radiotracer most commonly used with PET scans; therefore, [18]FDG-PET is unreliable both in tumor detection and in distinguishing benign from malignant salivary tumors.[64] Second, competing techniques such as CT, MRI, and even clinical examination already have a high degree of accuracy. Third, high-resolution studies such as CT and MRI provide the anatomic detail required for treatment planning that is unavailable from

[18]FDG-PET images. Finally, the high cost of [18]FDG-PET prohibits its widespread use.

Despite these limitations, because [18]FDG-PET offers a unique method of measuring metabolic activity in various tissues, it has proved superior to both CT and MRI in detecting recurrence and distinguishing tumor from post-treatment fibrosis.[65] Also, because [18]FDG-PET is able to measure tumor metabolism, it has the potential to evaluate various biologic parameters such as proliferation rates or tumor hypoxia. This information can then be used to optimize treatment strategies such as fractionation schemes for radiation therapy or the sequence of combined therapy. Clearly, considerable opportunity remains for further research on the use of [18]FDG-PET in patients with cancer of the head and neck.

◼ PATHOLOGY

Adenoid Cystic Carcinoma

Understanding the biologic behavior of adenoid cystic carcinoma (ACC) has been elusive for many decades, mainly owing to its highly variable natural history and relatively infrequent occurrence. It took almost 100 years for the capricious nature of ACC to be fully appreciated. In 1854, Lorain and Robin described an "unusual sinus tumor," which may have been the first description of ACC in the literature.[66] In 1856, Billroth coined the term *cylindroma* to describe the pathologic features of this rare salivary gland tumor,[67] but it was not until 1942 that the malignant nature of this disease was identified when Dockerty and Mayo described it as "adenocarcinoma, cylindroma type."[68] In 1953, Foote and Frazell coined the term *adenoid cystic carcinoma*, which best describes the histologic characteristics of this tumor.[69]

ACC accounts for approximately 10% of all nonsquamous carcinomas in the head and neck and for 15% of all neoplasms of the salivary glands.[70, 71] It is the second most common malignant tumor of salivary glands, after mucoepidermoid carcinoma. However, it is the most common malignant tumor in submandibular, sublingual, and minor salivary glands. It is slightly more common among females; approximately 90% of patients are between 30 and 70 years of age, with a peak incidence in the fifth and sixth decades of life. In a review of 242 patients with ACC, Spiro and associates found that more than two thirds of cases of ACC occurred in the minor salivary glands.[72] The most common site of origin is the oral cavity, (50%), followed by the sinonasal tract (18%).

ACC is described in three histologic subtypes based on tumor architecture—cribriform, tubular, and solid. The *cribriform* pattern, which is the most common subtype, has the classic "Swiss cheese" appearance in which the cells are arranged in nests separated by round or oval spaces (Fig. 21–14). It is suggested that this characteristic stromal architecture of ACC, represented by stromal pseudocysts, results from the ability of ACC cells to synthesize, secrete, and degrade basement membrane proteins such as fibronectin[73] and heparan sulfate proteoglycan.[74] The biosynthesis and secretion of these basement membrane proteins are regulated by the rate of cell growth, which may reflect the correlation between the histologic appearance and the biologic behavior of ACC.[75, 76] The *tubular* (or trabecular)

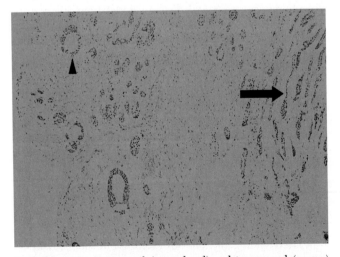

FIGURE 21–14 Perineural (*arrowhead*) and intraneural (*arrow*) spread of cribriform-type adenoid cystic carcinoma, which has the classic "Swiss cheese" appearance.

pattern has a more glandular architecture, and the *solid* (or basaloid) pattern shows sheets of cells with few or no luminal spaces. The tubular variety has the best prognosis, the solid variety has the worst, and the cribriform pattern has an intermediate prognosis.[77, 78] Most ACCs usually exhibit a mixed architecture of more than one pattern; their classification in such cases depends on the predominant histologic subtype.[79]

ACC has a peculiar tendency to spread along nerves. This neurotropic tendency has been reported to occur in 20% to 80% of patients.[80] Identification of perineural spread during histopathologic examination of ACC tumor specimens depends largely on the diligence of the pathologist, which explains, at least in part, the wide range of the reported incidence of perineural spread in ACC.[60]

The pathogenesis of perineural involvement is poorly understood; perineural involvement was initially thought to result from spread of tumor through perineural lymphatics. According to this theory, spread occurs by emboli along the perineural lymphatics; therefore, skip lesions can occur with no direct continuity with the main tumor mass. If this mechanism were true, the achievement of negative surgical margins via en bloc resection of ACC would be not only impossible to guarantee but also meaningless. However, this notion of perineural lymphatic emboli was dispelled by well-executed studies, which showed that neural spread occurs by direct invasion of malignant cells through the path of least resistance in the perineural and/or the endoneural spaces (see Fig. 21–14).[81, 82] This theory assumes microscopic continuity of perineural tumor with the primary tumor and provides the rationale for striving to achieve negative surgical margins of nerves involved by ACC. Recently, several studies have shown that neural cell adhesion molecules (NCAMs) may have a role in the pathogenesis of perineural spread of malignant tumors, including ACC and squamous cell carcinoma.[80, 83]

Perineural spread can occur in both an axial and a circumferential pattern along the involved nerve, and further spread can occur both in an antegrade and in a retrograde fashion. The most commonly involved nerves are the facial nerve and the mandibular (V3) and maxillary (V2) branches of the trigeminal nerve. Perineural spread of ACC along these nerves provides a pathway for invasion of the skull base.[60] Eventually, tumor cells may reach the trigeminal (gasserian) ganglion, the pterygopalatine ganglion, or the cavernous sinus (see Figs. 21–12 and 21–13). These neural pathways may act as "relay stations" and provide access for further perineural spread in a centripetal (toward the brain) or a centrifugal (peripheral) fashion. Achievement of negative surgical margins in such cases is difficult.[70, 84] This may be responsible for the poorer prognosis of patients with ACC who exhibit perineural involvement of major nerves.[71, 85–87] Perineural involvement is more frequent in advanced, recurrent, and high-grade tumors.

Lymphatic spread of ACC is uncommon. The incidence of lymph node metastasis from ACC, detected at presentation or developing later in the course of the disease, ranges from 10% to 30%.[88, 89] Metastasis to the regional lymphatics is more common among tumors originating from the parotid glands than from the minor salivary glands, and in those with solid rather than cribriform or tubular histopathologic pattern.[88] The development of lymph node metastasis was associated with poor outcomes despite aggressive therapy.[78, 89–92]

Although distant metastasis from ACC occurs most frequently in the first 5 years after diagnosis, the risk of developing systemic metastasis continues for up to 20 years or longer. Therefore, the true incidence of systemic metastasis in ACC is difficult to estimate; obviously, it depends on the length of follow-up of any particular group of reported patients. Recently, Spiro reviewed 196 patients with ACC who received definitive treatment at Memorial Sloan-Kettering Hospital between 1939 and 1986.[93] With a minimum follow-up of 10 years, the incidence of distant metastasis was 38% for all patients and 70% for those who died of disease. The incidence of distant metastasis correlated highly with the stage of disease (size of the primary tumor and status of the lymph nodes) on presentation. The lung was the most common site of distant metastasis (90%), either alone or in combination with other distant sites. Survival after the appearance of distant metastasis varied from 1 to 16 years (median, more than 3 years), being less than 3 years in 54% but more than 10 years in 10% of patients with distant metastasis. Approximately two thirds of patients with distant metastasis had associated local or regional recurrence. The high incidence of distant metastasis with locoregional failure confirms the importance of aggressive initial surgery combined with irradiation for high-stage tumors or involved surgical margins. Considering that lung metastases are usually multiple and that prolonged survival without treatment is not unusual, resection of pulmonary metastases may be hard to justify in patients with ACC. Similarly, chemotherapy for metastatic ACC is probably best withheld until symptoms appear.[93]

The reported prognosis of patients with ACC also depends on the length of follow-up. Unlike the survival curves of patients with squamous cell carcinoma of the upper aerodigestive tract, survival curves of patients with ACC do not show a plateau at 5 years, and survival continues to decline even after 20 years (see Fig. 21–22).[70] In a review of the outcomes of 406 patients with ACC, Conley and Casler reported that at 10 years, roughly one third of patients were free of disease, one third were dead of disease, and one third were alive with disease.[94] They commented, however, that undoubtedly if patient follow-up were longer, those who are free of disease would develop recurrences, and those who are alive with disease might end up dying from ACC. They projected that at 30 years of follow-up, 80% of patients would be dead of disease.

Several factors influence the survival and outcome of patients with ACC. These factors include stage of the disease, site of origin, histologic pattern, grade, surgical margins, the use of adjunctive radiation therapy, locoregional failure, and systemic metastasis.[70] These clinical factors as well as newly described biologic and molecular markers that affect the prognosis of patients with cancer of the salivary glands are detailed later in the chapter.

Mucoepidermoid Carcinoma

Overall, mucoepidermoid carcinoma (MEC) is the most common malignant tumor of the salivary glands.[95] It is the second most common malignancy (after ACC) of the submandibular and minor salivary glands. MEC constitutes approximately 35% of salivary gland malignancy, and 80% to 90% of MEC occurs in the parotid gland. As its name implies, mucoepidermoid carcinoma includes two major elements—mucin-producing cells and epithelial cells of the epidermoid variety. These two different cells may originate from an intermediate cell, which is also present in MEC. This dual cell type forms the basis of classifying MEC into a three-tiered histologic grading system: Grade I (low grade) are well differentiated, grade II (intermediate grade) are moderately differentiated, and grade III (high grade) are poorly differentiated tumors.[96] Grade I tumors show a predominance of mucus-secreting cells and well-differentiated epidermoid cells. Grade III tumors show few or no mucus-producing cells and poorly differentiated epidermoid cells. This variety can sometimes be mistaken for poorly differentiated squamous cell carcinoma. In such cases, meticulous search for any mucus-producing cells by a thorough microscopic examination, and in some cases, with the use of special stains for mucin, will usually provide the diagnosis of MEC.

The grading system of MEC not only classifies tumors according to histologic appearance but also correlates with prognosis. Patients with high-grade MEC tend to present with more advanced-stage disease and have a higher incidence of nodal involvement, positive surgical margins, locoregional recurrence, distant metastasis, and worse survival than do patients with low-grade MEC.[97] In a recent review of 80 patients with MEC, Brandwein and colleagues found that all patients with grade 1 MEC presented with stage I tumors, and none of these patients experienced tumor recurrence after treatment.[98] The local tumor recurrence rates at 75 months for grades II and III MEC were 30% and 70%, respectively. In another study, 5-year cumulative survival was 100% for grade I, 70.1% for grade II, and 47.2% for grade III.[99] These data illustrate the value of using the histologic grade of MEC as a guide for anticipating the clinical outcome of the disease.

One major limitation of the three-tiered grading system for MEC is the significant grading disparity even among experienced head and neck pathologists, especially with intermediate (grade II) tumors. The interobserver variation for pathologists was less when they used standardized criteria recommended by the AFIP than when they used their own criteria for grading MEC.[98] However, the AFIP-proposed criteria have a tendency to downgrade MEC. In 2001, Brandwein and colleagues proposed a modified grading schema, which includes other criteria such as vascular invasion and pattern of tumor infiltration.[98] It is hoped that this modified grading system will enhance predictability and provide much needed reproducibility in the classification of MEC.

Acinic Cell Carcinoma

Acinic cell carcinoma represents 3% of all salivary gland neoplasms and from 5% to 11% of malignant tumors of the salivary glands. The National Cancer Data Base (NCDB) identified 1353 patients with acinic cell carcinoma of the head and neck for the years 1985 to 1995.[47] Acinic cell carcinoma presents at a younger median age (52 years) than most other salivary gland cancers, affects women (58.8%) more commonly than men, and arises most commonly in the parotid gland (86.3%).

Grossly, acinic cell carcinoma appears fairly well circumscribed by a layer of surrounding dense fibrous tissue. Microscopic examination reveals nests of cells with basophilic cytoplasm and frequently an associated lymphoid infiltrate in the supporting stroma. Four histologic patterns are described—solid, microcystic, papillary-cystic, and follicular.[43–45] It is not uncommon for these patterns to coexist in the same tumor. Batsakis and coworkers demonstrated that varieties of acinic cell carcinoma occur within a histomorphologic spectrum defined by the lowest and highest grades.[100] Low-grade acinic cell carcinomas are broadly interpreted as those most closely resembling the architecture of a normal salivary lobule. High-grade acinic cell carcinomas are poorly differentiated and resemble the early phases of embryonic development of acini.

Unlike the situation with adenoid cystic or mucoepidermoid carcinoma, the correlation between histologic grade of acinic cell carcinoma and prognosis is not clear.[44, 101] It is generally believed that most patients with acinic cell carcinoma do well regardless of the histologic grade of the tumor. Wide acceptance of this concept has resulted in the practice of lumping all acinic cell carcinomas into the same favorable prognostic group as low-grade mucoepidermoid carcinoma and low-grade adenocarcinoma without further classification of acinic cell carcinoma according to grade. However, the recent study by Hoffman and colleagues of patients with acinic cell carcinoma registered in the NCDB clearly identified a correlation between histologic grade and prognosis. Patients with higher histologic grade had a significantly more advanced stage of disease and a higher incidence of metastatic disease at presentation.[47] Although the disease-specific 5-year survival was over 90%, patients with higher-grade tumors had worse survival. It is hoped that this report, which identifies a strong correlation between grade and aggressive behavior, will stimulate greater effort in establishing and recording grade for acinic cell carcinoma.

Malignant Mixed Tumor

As their name implies, malignant mixed tumors represent a malignancy with both epithelial and mesenchymal elements. They constitute 3% to 12% of salivary gland cancer, and about 75% of them arise in the parotid gland. When they arise from a preexisting pleomorphic adenoma, they are called *carcinoma ex pleomorphic adenoma*. The malignant components and metastasis of this variety are purely epithelial in origin. By contrast, *de novo malignant mixed tumor* is a true carcinosarcoma with malignant features of both the epithelial and mesenchymal elements, which are present in both the primary tumor and its metastases. The mesenchymal component shows mostly a chondrosarcomatous pattern. This rare true malignant mixed tumor is highly lethal, with a 5-year survival rate close to 0%.[44]

Carcinoma ex pleomorphic adenoma is more common than de novo malignant mixed tumor; the malignant transformation occurs in 3% to 4% of all benign mixed tumors. The risk of malignant transformation of a pleomorphic adenoma increases with the duration of disease. This risk is 1.5% within the first 5 years, but it increases to 9.5% after a pleomorphic adenoma has been present for longer than 15 years.[44, 45] Patients with malignant mixed tumors are 10 to 20 years older than those with benign mixed tumors. There is also an approximately 7% risk of associated carcinoma with recurrent pleomorphic adenoma. Findings suggesting malignant changes in a pleomorphic adenoma include microscopic foci of necrosis, hemorrhage, calcification, and/or excessive hyalinization. The presence and degree of local invasion and histologic differentiation allow the pathologist to distinguish between a noninvasive and an invasive variety of carcinoma in a pleomorphic adenoma. Noninvasive carcinoma consists of circumscribed malignant areas in a pleomorphic adenoma without infiltration of the surrounding tissue. Other terms used to describe this entity are *intracapsular carcinoma* and *carcinoma in situ*.[45] Complete surgical excision in these cases results in an excellent prognosis. The prognosis for invasive carcinoma depends on the degree of local infiltration. Lesions with less than 8 mm of invasion have a 5-year survival rate of 100%. By contrast, carcinomas that invade 8 mm or more have a 5-year survival rate of less than 50%.[44, 45]

The prognosis of patients with carcinoma ex pleomorphic adenoma is generally poor. In a recent study of 74 patients treated at the Mayo Clinic, overall survival was 39% at 3 years and 30% at 5 years. Of 66 patients with previously untreated tumors, 23% had local recurrence. Metastasis (either initial or delayed) occurred regionally in 56% and distantly in 44%. Important prognostic factors included tumor size, grade, and clinical and pathologic stage.[102, 103]

Epithelial-Myoepithelial Carcinoma

Epithelial-myoepithelial carcinomas (EMCs) account for approximately 1% of all salivary gland neoplasms.[104] Histopathologically, they are characterized by a dual cell population of epithelial (ductal) cells and myoepithelial cells.[105] These cells vary in their dominance and phenotypic expression. Like ACC, EMC may exhibit a solid, tubular, or cribriform pattern. Hyperplasia of the intercalated duct epithelium has been recently described in association with EMC and is thought to be a possible precursor lesion for EMC as well as other malignant tumors of the salivary glands.[106] EMC most commonly involves the parotid gland and mainly affects patients in their sixth to eighth decades. Although the overall mortality from EMC is low, its clinical course is characterized by a high incidence of local recurrence (50%) and not-infrequent distant metastasis (25%). The rate of recurrence and the development of metastasis may be related to the presence of DNA aneuploidy and a predominantly solid histologic pattern.[105]

Salivary Duct Carcinoma

Salivary duct carcinoma (SDC) is a high-grade aggressive malignancy that primarily affects the major salivary glands. Initially named after its resemblance to intraductal carcinoma of the breast, this entity derives its histogenesis from the excretory duct reserve cells, which are also the source of other biologically high-grade neoplasms. The microscopic features of SDC are remarkably similar to those of mammary ductal carcinoma, raising the question of whether these tumors also share common antigenic or hormonal features. However, investigators from the University of Pittsburgh recently demonstrated that the androgen receptor (AR), a marker frequently detected in prostatic carcinoma, is expressed in more than 90% of SDCs, whereas two common breast carcinoma markers—estrogen and progesterone receptors (ERs and PRs)—are expressed in only 1.3% and 6% of the tumors, respectively, by immunohistochemistry.[107–109] This hormonal profile suggests that SDC, in contrast to its histologic similarity to ductal carcinoma of the breast, is immunophenotypically more related to prostatic carcinoma. This immunophenotypic homology that exists between SDC and prostatic carcinoma also suggests that antiandrogen therapy as used in the treatment of prostatic carcinoma might be beneficial in patients with metastatic SDC.[108]

The clinical course of patients with SDC is characterized by a high incidence of local recurrence, regional lymph node metastasis, and systemic dissemination. More than two thirds of patients die within 4 years of initial diagnosis despite aggressive, combined surgical resection and radiotherapy.[107, 108] In a report of 26 cases of SDC of the major salivary glands treated at the Mayo Clinic from 1960 to 1989, 35% patients had local recurrence, 62% patients showed distant metastasis, and 77% of patients died of disease at a mean interval of 3 years after diagnosis.[110] Similarly, a study from M.D. Anderson Cancer Center reported regional metastases in 73%, systemic metastases in 43%, and local recurrences in 27% of patients with SDC of the major salivary glands.[111] A similarly poor prognosis was reported for patients with SDC of the minor salivary glands.[112] Because the prognosis of patients with SDC is generally poor, it is important for the pathologist to distinguish between this malignancy and more indolent neoplasms, such as polymorphous low-grade adenocarcinoma, previously known as *terminal duct carcinoma*.[113]

Polymorphous Low-Grade Adenocarcinoma

Polymorphous low-grade adenocarcinoma (PLGA), also known as terminal duct or lobular carcinoma, was first described in 1983.[114] Before that time, most of these neoplasms were diagnosed as pleomorphic adenomas, variants of monomorphic adenomas, malignant mixed tumor, adenoid cystic carcinomas, or adenocarcinoma not otherwise specified.[115] This may have been a result of its highly varied histologic pattern—hence the name *polymorphous*—including cords, tubules, papillae, glandular structures, and solid aggregates.[44, 45] Despite this varied histologic pattern, the tumor is characterized by cytologic uniformity, consisting mostly of myoepithelial or luminal ductal cells.

The overwhelming majority of PLGA originates in the oral cavity, mostly the palate (Fig. 21–15). Its clinical course is that of slow growth, and the tumor may be present for many years before diagnosis. Vincent and associates reviewed 204 cases reported in the literature (including 15 of their own).[115] In their report, PLGA was twice as common among females than among males. Forty-nine percent originated in the palatal mucosa. Lymph node metastasis

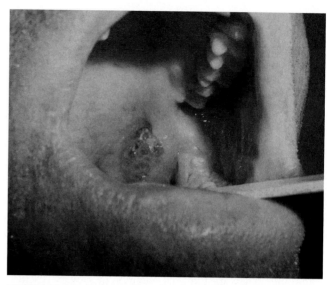

FIGURE 21–15 Polymorphous low-grade adenocarcinoma of the oral cavity.

occurred in 9% of patients, either at the time of presentation or during the course of their disease. The local recurrence rate was 17%, and most recurrences were at or beyond 5 years after the initial diagnosis. None of the 15 patients in their own series developed distant metastasis.[115]

More recently, a review of files from the AFIP revealed 164 patients with PLGA diagnosed between 1970 and 1994.[116] At an average of 115 months after presentation, approximately 97.5% of all patients either were alive or had died without evidence of recurrent disease after treatment with surgical excision only. These data illustrate that patients with PLGA have an excellent prognosis and that conservative but complete surgical excision is the treatment of choice for these slow-growing tumors. Adjuvant therapy does not appear to alter the prognosis.[116]

Hyalinizing Clear Cell Carcinoma

Milchgrub and colleagues coined the term hyalinizing clear cell carcinoma (HCCC) to distinguish this neoplasm from other clinicopathologic entities formerly described as *clear cell neoplasms*.[117] The majority of HCCC originates in minor salivary glands of the oral cavity.[118] Microscopically, these lesions are characterized by the formation of trabeculae, cords, islands, and/or nests of monomorphic clear cells that are glycogen rich and mucin negative; they are surrounded by hyalinized bands with foci of myxohyaline stroma. Cells with eosinophilic and granular cytoplasm were also noted. Both cell types show minimal nuclear pleomorphism and a very low mitotic index. Grossly, these neoplasms have infiltrative borders.[117] The clinical course of hyalinizing clear cell carcinoma is that of a low-grade malignancy. Less than 20% of cases show regional metastasis. Complete surgical excision is the treatment of choice.[117, 118]

Adenocarcinoma

The term *adenocarcinoma* implies an epithelial malignancy that originates from a glandular unit and, in its most differentiated form, maintains a glandular cytoarchitecture. Previously, a wide variety of heterogeneous tumors arising from salivary glandular subunits were collectively described as adenocarcinomas. With refinements in histopathologic examination, these tumors are now classified in more homogeneous subgroups that have specific histopathologic characteristics and share similar biologic behavior. Clinicopathologic entities such as *salivary duct carcinoma, terminal duct carcinoma,* and *epithelial-myoepithelial carcinoma* that were formerly classified as adenocarcinoma are examples of this refinement in classification.[119]

There remain, however, adenocarcinomas of salivary origin that cannot be accommodated in conventional classifications; these are collectively given the term *adenocarcinoma, not otherwise specified (NOS)*. The exact incidence of this subgroup of tumors is difficult to determine. As refinements in classification with clinicopathologic correlations proceed, the adenocarcinomas, NOS, of salivary tissue are reduced in number. They are the least common of salivary carcinomas and manifest a cytoarchitecture ranging from a well-differentiated, low-grade appearance to high-grade, invasive lesions.[119] However, they share some common salient features. They are more common in the major salivary glands and arise from the excretory or striated duct. They may exhibit a solid or a cystic pattern, which may be papillary or nonpapillary. Some tumors are mucin producing and others are not. Poor prognostic indicators include advanced stage, high histologic grade, infiltrative growth pattern, and tumor DNA content.[119]

Squamous Cell Carcinoma

Primary squamous cell carcinoma (SCC) of the parotid is rare. It should be distinguished from the more common metastatic SCC to the intraparotid lymph nodes from cutaneous malignancy of the face and scalp. It should also be distinguished from direct parotid involvement with cancer of the external ear or preauricular region (Fig. 21–16). Another differential diagnosis that should be ruled out is high-grade undifferentiated mucoepidermoid carcinoma, with little or no evidence of mucin-producing elements on light microscopy.[120] Under such circumstances, the use of electron microscopy and special stains for mucin may help establish the diagnosis. Recently, immunohistochemical testing for markers of glandular differentiation in salivary gland tumors has been described.[121, 122] Such markers may be useful in distinguishing undifferentiated mucoepidermoid carcinoma from squamous cell carcinoma of the salivary glands.

The exact incidence of primary SCC of the salivary glands is difficult to determine from published data. The reported incidence of SCC of the salivary glands varies from 0.5% to 9% in the parotid glands and from 2% to 11% in the submandibular glands. Batsakis and colleagues indicated that the true incidence of primary SCC of the salivary glands is only 0.3% to 1.5%.[123] Most patients present with advanced-stage disease, and nodal metastasis occurs in about half of patients.[124] This may explain, at least in part, the poor prognosis associated with primary SCC of the salivary glands. In a series of 50 patients reported by Shemen and coworkers, the incidence of locoregional failure was

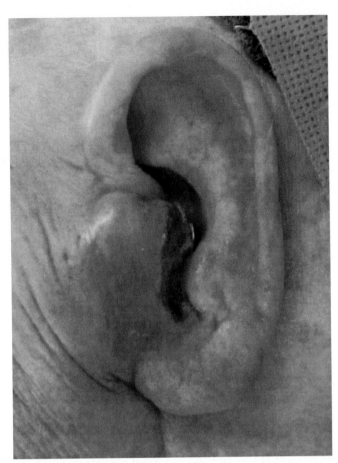

FIGURE 21–16 A patient with squamous cell carcinoma of the external ear invading the parotid gland.

51% for SCC of the parotid gland and 67% for SCC of the submandibular gland.[124]

Undifferentiated Carcinoma

The term *undifferentiated carcinoma* describes an epithelial malignancy that, because of lack of distinguishing histologic characteristics, could not be otherwise classified. The diagnosis of undifferentiated carcinoma will undoubtedly be used less as refinements in histopathologic diagnosis continue with the use of electron microscopy, special stains, and immunohistochemistry. A special subtype is the undifferentiated carcinoma with lymphoid stroma, which was previously described as a malignant lymphoepithelial lesion of the salivary gland.[44] This tumor has a relatively high incidence in Inuit and Chinese populations and is indistinguishable histologically from the lymphoepithelial-undifferentiated carcinoma of the nasopharynx. The cause of this tumor has been linked to Epstein-Barr virus.

Lymphoma

Lymphomas of the salivary glands may originate either from intraglandular lymph nodes (nodal) or from the lymphoid tissue dispersed within the salivary gland parenchyma (extranodal), which is considered a part of the mucosa-associated lymphoid tissue (MALT) system.[125] Lymphoma of the salivary gland can involve the salivary glands as the only manifestation of the disease (primary) or as a part of disseminated lymphoma.[126] Primary lymphomas of the salivary glands are usually associated with chronic immunosialadenitis (benign lymphoepithelial lesion or Sjögren's syndrome).[127] The risk of malignant lymphoma in patients with Sjögren's syndrome is 44-fold higher than that in the normal population.[128]

Approximately 5% of all extranodal lymphomas affect the salivary glands, and more than 90% of salivary gland lymphomas occur in the parotid.[44] This predilection for the parotid gland is undoubtedly due to the abundance of lymphoid aggregates within its salivary parenchyma. Most salivary gland lymphomas are of the non-Hodgkin's variety (85%). Salivary gland lymphomas associated with Sjögren's syndrome have a significantly worse prognosis than do those arising in normal glands, or in glands with benign lymphoepithelial lesions without the manifestations of Sjögren's syndrome.

Secondary (Metastatic) Tumors

Hematogenous metastases to the salivary glands from infraclavicular primaries are rare. These occur mainly from the lung, kidney, and breast. The parotid gland is the most common site of involvement.[129] An overwhelming majority of metastases to the salivary glands are due to lymphatic spread from cutaneous malignancy of the head and neck. This is due to the presence of intraparotid lymph nodes and reflects the lymphatic drainage pattern of the skin of the ear, face, and scalp. The area of skin that has the highest predilection of metastasis to the parotid gland is located anterior to the midcoronal plane and extends anteriorly to the oblique line corresponding to the course of the facial vessels. This underscores the importance of careful examination of the skin of the head and neck, particularly the ear, cheek, forehead, temple, and scalp, for evidence of cutaneous malignancy in any patient presenting with a parotid mass.

Metastatic tumors account for less than 10% of malignant parotid gland tumors; of these, 40% are squamous cell carcinomas, and 40% are melanomas. About two thirds of metastatic squamous cell carcinomas to the parotid occur within the first year after treatment of the primary skin cancer. The incidence of parotid metastasis from cutaneous melanoma of the head and neck correlates with the thickness of the primary tumor.[130]

◼ STAGING

In 2002, The American Joint Commission on Cancer updated the staging system for cancer of the major salivary glands.[131] The staging system follows the tumor, node, metastasis (TNM) system of staging tumors in other parts of the body. Primary tumor stage depends primarily on the size of the primary tumor, extraparenchymal extension, and involvement of the seventh cranial nerve or skull base (Table 21–2). Several recent studies compared the 1997 with the previous classification (published in 1987) and found that the updated classification better defines the prognosis for cancer of the parotid gland and should have a higher impact

TABLE 21-2 Definition of TNM for Major Salivary Gland Cancer

Primary Tumor (T)

TX   Primary tumor cannot be assessed
T0   No evidence of primary tumor
T1   Tumor 2 cm or less in greatest dimension without extraparenchymal extension°
T2   Tumor >2 cm but not >4 cm in greatest dimension without extraparenchymal extension°
T3   Tumor >4 cm and/or tumor having extraparenchymal extension°
T4a Tumor invades skin, mandible, ear canal, and/or facial nerve
T4b Tumor invades skull base and/or pterygoid plates and/or encases carotid artery

°*Note:* Extraparenchymal extension is clinical or macroscopic evidence of invasion of soft tissues. Microscopic evidence alone does not constitute extraparenchymal extension for classification purposes.

Regional Lymph Nodes (N)

NX   Regional lymph nodes cannot be assessed
N0   No regional lymph node metastasis
N1   Metastasis in a single ipsilateral lymph node, 3 cm or less in greatest dimension
N2   Metastasis in a single ipsilateral lymph node, >3 cm but not >6 cm in greatest dimension, or in multiple ipsilateral lymph nodes, none >6 cm in greatest dimension, or in bilateral or contralateral lymph nodes, none >6 cm in greatest dimension
N2a Metastasis in a single ipsilateral lymph node, >3 cm but not >6 cm in greatest dimension
N2b Metastasis in multiple ipsilateral lymph nodes, none >6 cm in greatest dimension
N2c Metastasis in bilateral or contralateral lymph nodes, none >6 cm in greatest dimension
N3   Metastasis in a lymph node >6 cm in greatest dimension

Distant Metastasis (M)

MX   Distant metastasis cannot be assessed
M0   No distant metastasis
M1   Distant metastasis

Stage Grouping			
Stage I	TI	N0	M0
Stage II	T2	N0	M0
Stage III	T3	N0	M0
	T1	N1	M0
	T2	N1	M0
	T3	N1	M0
Stage IVA	T4a	N0	M0
	T4a	N1	M0
	T1	N2	M0
	T2	N2	M0
	T3	N2	M0
	T4a	N2	M0
Stage IVB	T4b	Any N	M0
	Any T	N3	M0
Stage IVC	Any T	Any N	M1

Used with the permission of the American Joint Committee on Cancer (AJCC), Chicago, Illinois. The original source for this material is the *AJCC Cancer Staging Manual, Sixth Edition* (2002) published by Springer-Verlag New York, www.springer-ny.com.

on the clinical evaluation of patients with cancer of the major salivary glands.[132, 133] The 2002 guidelines further clarify the T3 and T4 stages. Minor salivary gland cancer is staged according to the staging system used to classify primary tumors in their particular sites of origin (e.g., oral cavity, oropharynx).

TREATMENT

Surgery

The principal treatment of cancer of the salivary glands is surgical resection, used either as a single modality or, in most cases, in conjunction with adjuvant radiation therapy. The goals of surgical treatment are complete excision of the tumor and avoidance of unnecessary morbidity. The surgical approach and the scope of resection vary according to the location and extent of tumor.

Treatment of Parotid Gland Tumors

Small (T1–T2) tumors of the superficial lobe of the parotid gland that are located lateral to the plane of the facial nerve may be adequately treated with a superficial parotidectomy. Larger tumors and tumors involving the deep lobe of the parotid gland usually require a total parotidectomy. The facial nerve is dissected and preserved, unless it has been directly infiltrated or encased by the tumor. Preoperative weakness or paralysis of the facial nerve usually indicates tumor involvement, and in these instances, the main trunk or the involved nerve branches may have to be sacrificed. The nerve and its involved branches should also be sacrificed if there is intraoperative evidence of gross invasion or microscopic infiltration of the nerve by tumor, even in the presence of normal preoperative facial nerve function. This is more likely to occur with larger and high-grade tumors and in tumors that extend from the superficial to the deep lobe, transgressing the plane of the facial nerve. Surgical margins on both the distal and the proximal nerve stumps should be checked because of the possibility of perineural spread for some distance from the area of the primary tumor. In certain cases, achieving negative surgical margins on the proximal stump of the facial nerve may require a mastoidectomy and facial nerve dissection along its course in the temporal bone. If the facial nerve is sacrificed, nerve repair may be done with the use of either direct neurorrhaphy of the cut edges or a cable graft, depending on the length of the resected segment. Tumors extending beyond the confines of the parotid gland may require resection of surrounding structures, including the skin, mandibular ramus, and masseter muscle; infratemporal fossa dissection; and/or subtotal petrosectomy.[134]

Treatment of Submandibular Gland Tumors

Surgical management of cancer of the submandibular salivary gland depends on the extent of the tumor. Small tumors confined to the gland itself are treated by resection of the submandibular gland. Tumors spreading beyond the confines of the gland to invade surrounding structures are treated with a wider en bloc excision. This may require removal of the contents of the submandibular triangle; resection of the floor of the mouth and the mylohyoid and digastric muscles; or marginal or segmental mandibulectomy, depending on the extent of the tumor.[135] Special attention should be given to the lingual, hypoglossal, mylohyoid, and marginal mandibular nerves because these may be involved through perineural spread of tumor. Thickening and nodularity of these nerves may indicate perineural involvement; in such cases, histologic

confirmation by frozen section may be useful in both establishing nerve invasion and obtaining negative surgical margins.

Treatment of Minor Salivary Gland Tumors

Surgical resection of cancer of the minor salivary gland depends on the site of origin and extent of disease. In the oral cavity, this may require only a wide local excision of localized low-grade tumors. Larger and/or high-grade tumors may require more radical excision, including marginal or segmental mandibulectomy and/or partial or total resection of the hard or soft palate.[136, 137] Salivary gland cancer involving the sinonasal tract is usually of high grade and presents at an advanced stage. Surgical resection may require partial or total maxillectomy, infratemporal fossa dissection, and/or anterior craniofacial resection. Palatal defects resulting from these resections are best managed by prosthetic rehabilitation. The branches of the second (V2) and third (V3) divisions of the trigeminal nerve are at high risk for perineural spread of minor salivary gland malignancy. These nerves may provide an avenue for early skull base invasion. Resection of the cranial base may be required in some cases to eradicate the tumor and obtain negative surgical margins.

Neck Dissection

In the presence of clinically evident metastasis in the cervical lymph nodes, a neck dissection is performed in conjunction with resection of the primary cancer. This usually involves a comprehensive cervical lymphadenectomy, either a modified radical or a radical neck dissection, according to the extent of disease. However, controversy still exists about the surgical management of the clinically negative neck (N0) in patients with cancer of the salivary glands.[138] Neither the indications for nor the type of elective neck dissection is well defined in the literature.

To better define the indications for elective neck treatment, Armstrong and colleagues studied the incidence of clinical and occult nodal disease in 474 patients with cancer of the salivary glands.[139] Clinically positive nodes were present in 14% of patients. Overall, clinically occult, pathologically positive nodes occurred in 12% (47 of 407) of patients who underwent an elective neck dissection. In view of the low frequency of occult metastases in the entire group, routine elective treatment of the neck was not recommended. However, the incidence of occult metastatic disease was significantly influenced by tumor size and histologic grade. Tumors 4 cm or larger had a 20% risk of occult metastases compared with a 4% risk for smaller tumors ($P < .00001$). High-grade tumors (regardless of histologic type) had a 49% risk of occult metastases, compared with a 7% risk for intermediate-grade or low-grade tumors ($P < .00001$). Similarly, Rodriguez-Cuevas and colleagues found an increased risk (50%) of occult node metastases in patients with high-grade carcinomas, although no cases were found in those with low-grade carcinomas ($P < .05$).[140]

More recently, in a total of 145 patients with cancer of the parotid gland with complete clinical and pathologic information, the following variables were significantly associated with risk of lymph node metastasis by univariate analysis: histologic type, T-stage, desmoplasia, facial palsy, perineural invasion, extraparotid tumor extension, and necrosis. By multivariate analysis, histologic type and T-stage had the highest correlation with lymph node metastasis.[86] These findings demonstrate that the incidence of occult regional disease in patients with advanced stage (T3–T4) or high-grade tumors (such as undifferentiated carcinoma, high-grade mucoepidermoid and adenoid cystic carcinoma, squamous cell carcinoma, adenocarcinoma, and salivary duct carcinoma) is relatively high and, therefore, an elective neck dissection should be considered in these patients.[141] A selective (supraomohyoid) neck dissection may be used as a staging procedure in such cases. Suspicious nodes should be sent for frozen section diagnosis, and if they are positive for metastatic carcinoma, a comprehensive neck dissection should be performed. Elective neck dissection seems not to be indicated for low-grade malignancy of the salivary glands.[139, 140]

Surgical Technique

PAROTIDECTOMY

The patient is placed in the supine position, with the head turned to the opposite side. The skin incision is placed in a preauricular crease that extends superiorly to the level of the root of the helix. The incision extends inferiorly around the lobule of ear over the mastoid tip. It then gently curves down along the sternocleidomastoid muscle, and then slightly forward in a natural skin crease in the upper neck (Fig. 21–17A). Skin flaps are elevated in the plane superficial to the parotid fascia in the preauricular region, and in the subplatysmal plane in the cervical portion of the incision (Fig. 21–17B).

The greater auricular nerve and the external jugular vein are identified over the sternocleidomastoid muscle and are divided to free the tail of the parotid gland (see Fig. 21–17B). In some cases the greater auricular nerve can be preserved, but whether this preservation has a significant impact on a patient's quality of life is debatable (see Chapter 37).[2, 142] The posterior belly of the digastric muscle is exposed proximal to its attachment to the mastoid bone. The fascia between the parotid gland and the cartilaginous external auditory canal is dissected, and the parotid gland is retracted anteriorly (Fig. 21–17C). This exposes the tragal pointer. The most common method of identifying the main trunk of the facial nerve is by following its course in the region located between the tragal pointer and the attachment of the posterior belly of the digastric muscle to the mastoid bone (Fig. 21–17D). Unless displaced by tumor, the nerve is usually located approximately 1 to 1.5 cm deep and inferior to the tragal pointer. Another reliable, and perhaps more constant, landmark for identification of the facial nerve is the tympanomastoid suture line, which could be followed medially to the main trunk of the nerve. The nerve is usually 6 to 8 mm deep to the tympanomastoid suture line.

In certain cases when the tumor is directly overlying the region of the main trunk of the facial nerve, one or more of the peripheral branches of the nerve are identified distally and traced proximally toward the main trunk.[143] The marginal mandibular branch can be identified below the lower border of the mandible because it crosses superficial to the facial vessels, in the plane immediately underneath the deep cervical fascia. Alternatively, the buccal branch can be identified underneath the parotidomasseteric fascia, coursing parallel to the parotid duct.

Once the facial nerve has been identified, the overlying parotid tissue is meticulously elevated from the nerve with a fine clamp, and the bridge of tissue between the blades of the clamp is carefully divided. If the main trunk of the nerve is identified first, the overlying parotid tissue is progressively dissected free of the nerve to the first branching of the nerve, usually into an upper and a lower division (see Fig. 21–17D). Subsequent branching of the nerve (pes anserinus) is sequentially dissected in a similar fashion until the entire superficial lobe of the parotid gland lying lateral to the facial nerve is delivered (Fig. 21–17E). This completes a *superficial* or *lateral parotidectomy*.

If a *total parotidectomy* is indicated, the procedure is extended by meticulous dissection of the main trunk and the branches of the facial nerve from the underlying parotid tissue in a gentle and atraumatic fashion. This allows the salivary tissue lying deep to the facial nerve to be delivered with preservation of the nerve and its function.

Complications

Facial Nerve Paresis or Paralysis. Facial nerve dysfunction may result from traction injury to the facial nerve during dissection. As long as the anatomic integrity of the nerve is preserved, this type of injury usually results in neurapraxia, so complete recovery is anticipated. The degree of weakness or paralysis may range from minimal partial weakness of one or more branches of the facial nerve to complete paralysis of all branches of the nerve. Recovery of facial nerve function may be prompt and complete within days, or it may be delayed for several months. In a study of 256 consecutive patients who underwent parotid surgery at the Cleveland Clinic over a period of 15 years, immediate postoperative facial nerve dysfunction was encountered frequently (46%), but permanent dysfunction was uncommon (4%).[144] The incidence of long-term dysfunction was higher in revision cases and when an extended (total or subtotal) parotidectomy was performed. To minimize facial nerve injury, the parotid surgeon should adhere to meticulous dissection and gentle handling of the facial nerve. Excessive traction on the nerve must be avoided, as should overzealous use of the nerve stimulator.

Transection of one or more of the branches of the facial nerve will result in paralysis of the corresponding muscles supplied by the injured nerve. The degree of paralysis may vary according to the presence and extent of cross-innervation of the involved muscle groups by the uninjured branches of the facial nerve. Complete transection of the main trunk of the facial nerve results in complete and permanent paralysis of all ipsilateral muscles of facial expression.

If the facial nerve has been sacrificed, nerve repair may be done with the use of either direct neurorrhaphy of the cut edges or a cable graft, depending on the length of the resected segment (Fig. 21–18). Immediate rehabilitation of the paralyzed face requires diligent eye care to prevent exposure keratitis. This involves liberal use of artificial tears, lubricating ointment, and protection with an appropriate

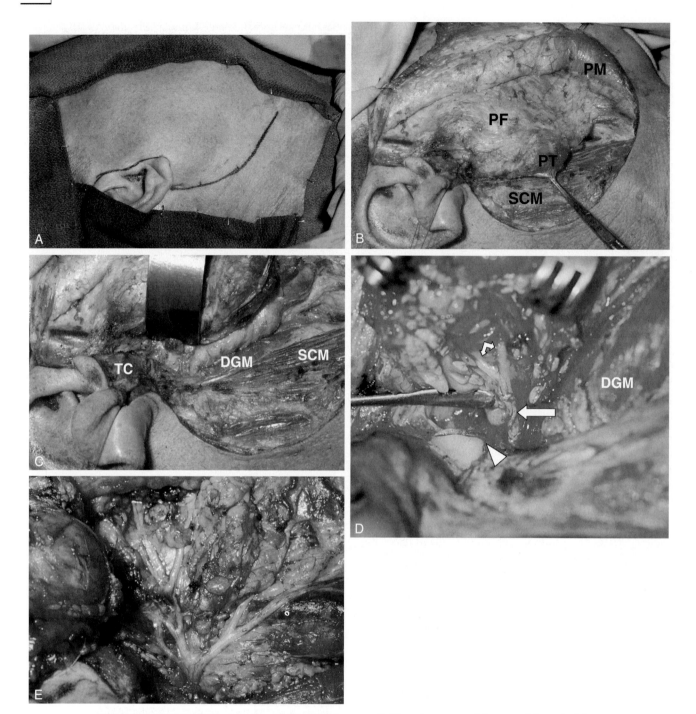

FIGURE 21–17 *A*, Skin incision for a right parotidectomy. *B*, Flap elevation and freeing of the tail of the parotid gland. PF, parotid fascia; PM, platysma muscle, PT, parotid tail; SCM, sternocleidomastoid muscle. *C*, Incision of the fascia between the parotid gland and the cartilaginous external auditory canal along with anterior retraction of the parotid gland. This exposes the tragal cartilage (TC) and the insertion of posterior belly of digastric muscle (DGM) to the mastoid bone. SCM, Sternocleidomastoid muscle. *D*, Identification of the main trunk of the facial nerve. The facial nerve is usually identified by dissecting the main trunk *(white arrow)* in the region located between the tragal pointer *(white arrowhead)* and the attachment of the posterior belly of the digastric muscle (DGM) to the mastoid bone. Unless displaced by tumor, the nerve is usually located approximately 1 to 1.5 cm deep and inferior to the tragal pointer. Dissection of the main trunk then proceeds distally until it branches *(double arrow)*; then all branches are sequentially and meticulously dissected. *E*, Complete dissection of all parotid tissue lateral to the facial nerve reveals the main trunk and the complex branching pattern of the facial nerve (pes anserinus).

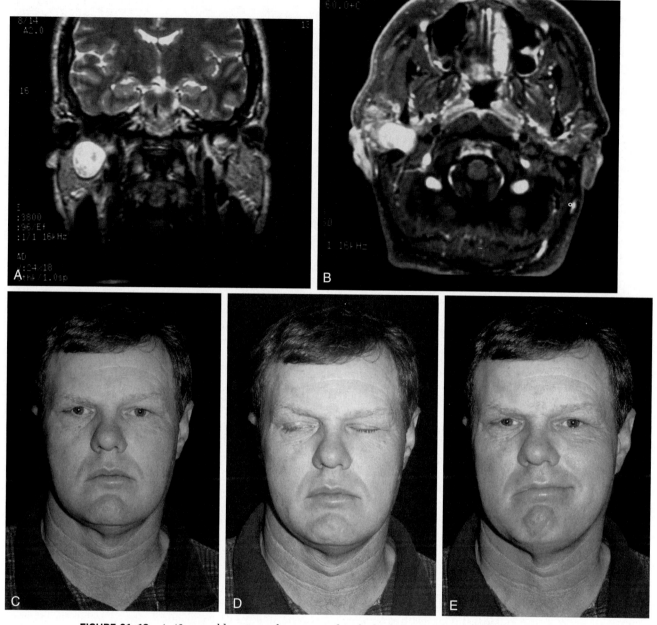

FIGURE 21–18 A 42-year-old patient who presented with slowly progressive right facial palsy and no palpable masses in the parotid gland. The T2-weighted coronal MRI (A) and the T1-weighted axial gadolinium-enhanced MRI (B) show a well-circumscribed rounded mass within the deep lobe of the parotid gland. Signal characteristics were consistent with a neurogenic tumor. The provisional diagnosis was that of a facial nerve schwannoma. Surgical exploration revealed the tumor to originate from and completely involve the main trunk of the facial nerve. The tumor extended across the stylomastoid foramen and along the vertical segment of the facial nerve within the mastoid process. The tumor, along with the involved segment of the nerve, was excised, and a cable graft from the greater auricular nerve was interposed between the cut edges of the facial nerve. Histopathologic examination of the tumor revealed neurofibroma Antoni type B. At 9 months postoperatively, the patient has good facial tone at rest (C), complete eye closure (D), and mild synkinesis when smiling (E). This result was classified as grade III House-Brackmann facial function.

eye dressing and eyewear. A gold weight implant should be used routinely in patients with complete facial paralysis. A temporary tarsorrhaphy may be needed for patients with lower eyelid ectropion. If the facial nerve has not been repaired or grafted, one or more of the various surgical procedures for static or dynamic rehabilitation of the paralyzed face may be indicated. The details of these procedures are described in Chapter 28.

Sensory Abnormalities Associated With Sacrifice of the Greater Auricular Nerve. The greater auricular nerve (GAN) is frequently divided during parotidectomy. This usually results in sensory deficits in the dermatomal distribution of the GAN, which includes the lower third of the pinna, including the earlobe, as well as the adjacent preauricular and postauricular skin. Some surgeons have suggested that preserving the posterior branches of the GAN reduces the area of postoperative anesthesia. Porter and Wood conducted a prospective study to compare the area of anesthesia and hypoesthesia in patients undergoing parotidectomy, with and without sacrifice of the GAN.[2] Mapping of the area of sensory loss at 2 weeks and 3, 6, 9, and 12 months showed that there was no difference between the two groups. The area of sensory loss decreased in an exponential fashion in both groups. The majority of the change occurred within 6 months. The authors concluded that preservation of the posterior branches of the GAN is unnecessary.

In a more recent study, Patel and colleagues evaluated the impact of sacrifice of the GAN during parotidectomy on patients' quality of life.[142] Although more than half of patients reported at least one abnormal sensory symptom, the number of symptoms decreased significantly over time. Even among patients experiencing symptoms, 77% reported only a little or no bother caused by the symptoms, and 90% reported no interference or almost none with their daily activities. The results suggest that although many patients experienced sensory deficits, their overall quality of life was not significantly affected by GAN sacrifice during parotidectomy.

Gustatory Sweating—"Frey's Syndrome." Patients with Frey's syndrome experience flushing and sweating of the ipsilateral facial skin during mastication (gustatory sweating). The symptoms may vary in severity from barely noticeable to severe and quite bothersome. The true incidence of postoperative Frey's syndrome is unknown, but it is estimated to be between 35% and 60%. The incidence would probably be higher if the syndrome could be searched for by directed symptom-specific questions.[145] The presumed pathophysiology of Frey's syndrome involves aberrant cross-reinnervation between the postganglionic secretomotor parasympathetic fibers to the parotid gland and the postganglionic sympathetic fibers supplying the sweat glands of the skin.

The diagnosis of Frey's syndrome depends largely on the patient's symptoms. An objective method of confirming the diagnosis is Minor's starch-iodine test. This involves painting the ipsilateral side of the face and neck with iodine solution, which is allowed to dry. Starch powder is then dusted over the painted area. The patient then chews on a sialagogue (e.g., lemon wedge) for several minutes. The appearance of dark blue spots along the face confirms gustatory sweating. This discoloration is the result of the reaction of the dissolved starch with iodine. In a recent German study, Minor's starch-iodine test revealed that 85% of patients who did not complain of Frey's syndrome after surgery actually had a subclinical manifestation of this complication.

If the symptoms are bothersome enough, treatment involves simply applying an antiperspirant over the involved skin. Glycopyrrolate (1%) roll-on lotion is also effective in controlling the symptoms. In cases not responding to these simple measures, surgical interruption of the secretory fibers may be attempted by a tympanic neurectomy. Recently, intracutaneous injection of botulinum toxin A has been described as an effective treatment in severe cases of Frey's syndrome.[145]

Salivary Fistula. This is an uncommon problem. It usually presents as a clear sialorrhea from the wound, or a fluid collection under the skin flaps. In the majority of cases, the problem is self-limiting. Management includes repeated aspiration, pressure dressing, wound care, and patience. Oral anticholinergics (e.g., glycopyrrolate) may be helpful in temporarily reducing salivary flow until healing is complete.

SUBMANDIBULAR GLAND EXCISION

A curvilinear incision is placed, preferably in a natural skin crease, 3 to 4 cm below the lower border of the mandible overlying the submandibular gland. The incision is carried down through the subcutaneous fat and the platysma muscle. Great care should be taken to avoid injury of the marginal mandibular nerve. This nerve lies immediately beneath the deep cervical fascia and can be identified crossing the anterior facial vein. The vein is doubly ligated and transected well below the nerve; upward retraction of the superior ligature displaces the nerve superiorly and protects it from injury during further dissection.

Superior dissection proceeds by double ligation and transection of the facial artery, which frees the superior attachment of the gland. The vessels to the mylohyoid muscle are divided anteriorly, and the gland is mobilized posteriorly, exposing the free edge of the mylohyoid muscle. The free (posterior) edge of the mylohyoid muscle is retracted anteriorly, and gentle posterior traction on the gland is maintained. This exposes the deep portion of the gland and its duct, the submandibular ganglion, and the lingual and hypoglossal nerves. These structures lie superficial to the hyoglossus muscle. The contribution of the lingual nerve to the submandibular ganglion is transected, and Warthin's duct is doubly ligated and divided. This delivers the deep portion of the gland. Care should be taken to avoid injury to the lingual and hypoglossal nerves. Finally, the facial artery is divided a second time, and the gland is removed.

EXCISION OF PARAPHARYNGEAL SALIVARY GLAND TUMORS

Salivary gland tumors located in the parapharyngeal space originate either from the parotid gland or from the extraparotid minor salivary glands scattered within the parapharyngeal space. Tumors arising from the parotid gland can originate entirely from the deep lobe of the gland or from its retromandibular portion and extend medially, passing posteroinferior to the stylomandibular ligament to expand the parapharyngeal space without a pre-tragal palpable component (see Fig. 21–18A and B). Alternatively, parotid tumors may involve both the superficial and the deep lobes with a connecting isthmus that passes through the narrow stylomandibular tunnel, giving the tumor a dumbbell appearance (see Fig. 21–2). The external component is usually palpable in the pre-tragal region, and the deep component, if it is large enough, may displace the palate/tonsil medially (see Figs. 21–11A and B and 21–12). Tumors originating from the minor salivary glands within the parapharyngeal space have no connection to the parotid gland. Whatever their site of origin, parapharyngeal salivary gland tumors are located in the prestyloid compartment of the parapharyngeal space (see Fig. 21–2).

Surgical excision of salivary gland tumors within the parapharyngeal space is best done via an external approach. The incision is that of a parotidectomy with a cervical extension. If the tumor involves the deep lobe of the parotid gland, a superficial parotidectomy is done first. If the tumor arises from the minor salivary glands of the parapharyngeal space, the inferior division of the facial nerve is identified and carefully preserved. Next, the sternocleidomastoid is retracted laterally, and the upper neck is dissected to expose the internal jugular vein, the external and internal carotid arteries, and the last four (IX, X, XI, and XII) cranial nerves. The posterior belly of the digastric muscle and the stylohyoid muscle are identified, are divided near their mastoid and styloid attachments, respectively, and are retracted medially. This allows further superior exposure of the internal carotid artery, the internal jugular vein, and adjacent nerves, as well as visualization of the stylomandibular ligament and the styloid process. The stylomandibular ligament is divided, which allows further anterior retraction of the mandible and provides a wide opening into the parapharyngeal space (Fig. 21–19). The styloid process may be resected for further exposure and to facilitate delivery of larger tumors. Through this exposure, the tumor can be easily visualized and safely excised.

In patients with malignant tumors located in the superior aspect of the parapharyngeal space approaching the eustachian tube and skull base, a *mandibulotomy* may be needed.[146] The enhanced exposure offered by the mandibulotomy allows the visualization necessary for resection of the tumor with adequate margins. Details of the mandibulotomy approach and of other approaches to the parapharyngeal space are discussed in Chapter 22.

Radiation Therapy

Adjuvant (Postoperative) Radiation Therapy

Several reports suggest that the use of adjuvant radiation therapy with surgery is superior to surgery alone in the treatment of high-grade and/or advanced cancers of the major and minor salivary glands.[71, 85] Theriault and Fitzpatrick reported the outcome of 271 patients with carcinoma of the parotid gland treated with surgery with and without postoperative adjuvant radiation therapy.[147] Tumor types among these patients included mucoepidermoid tumors with all degrees of differentiation (24%), adenocarcinomas (18%), malignant mixed tumors (15%), adenoid cystic carcinomas (14%), undifferentiated carcinomas (14%), acinic cell carcinomas (8%), and squamous cell carcinomas (7%). The prognostic characteristics were similar for the 67 (25%) patients treated by surgery alone and for the 169 (62%) patients treated with surgery and postoperative radiotherapy. Patients treated with combined therapy had a 10-year relapse-free rate of 62% compared with 22% for those treated by surgery alone (P = .0005).

Recently, Garden and associates reported the M.D. Anderson Cancer Center experience with adjuvant radiation therapy in the treatment of 160 patients with minor salivary gland cancers.[148] Microscopic positive margins were present in 40% of patients, and half of patients had pathologic evidence of perineural invasion. Radiation doses ranged from 50 to 75 Gy (median, 60 Gy). With a median follow-up of 110 months, 36% of patients experienced disease relapse. Local recurrence occurred in 12% of patients. Regional failures occurred in approximately 25% of patients with initially node-positive disease, but these were uncommon (less than 5%) in patients with node-negative disease, regardless of elective neck treatments. Distant metastases developed in 43 patients, mostly (79%) within 5 years of treatment. Actuarial overall survival rates at 5, 10, and 15 years were 81%, 65%, and 43%, respectively. The authors concluded that postoperative radiation therapy is effective in preventing local recurrence in most patients with minor salivary gland tumors after gross total excision. When local failure occurs, it tends to be a late event. For most patients, a postoperative dose of 60 Gy in 30 fractions to the operative bed is adequate; if there is named nerve invasion, the path of the nerve is treated electively to its ganglion.[148]

The addition of adjuvant radiation therapy should not be considered an adequate substitute for clear surgical margins; however, in some instances, it is not possible to obtain tumor-free margins of resection. In such cases, the use of postoperative radiation may enhance local control. The 5-year local disease control rate in patients with microscopic positive surgical margins who received postoperative radiation therapy is reported to be as high as 65%.[149] Meanwhile, patients with positive surgical margins have a higher incidence of distant metastasis, which is not influenced by the addition of postoperative adjuvant radiation therapy.[150] These findings underscore the importance of investigating other therapeutic modalities, such as chemotherapy, to reduce the occurrence of distant disease in such a high-risk patient population.

Wide-field radiation therapy to the parotid glands may result in significant complications, including severe xerostomia, sensorineural hearing loss, osteoradionecrosis of the temporal bone, and radiation injury to the temporal lobe. Recent advances in the delivery of radiation therapy, including three-dimensional conformal radiotherapy (3DCRT) and intensity-modulated radiotherapy (IMRT), have led to better tumor dosimetry and relative sparing of surrounding normal structures such as the oral cavity, cochlea, and brain.[151]

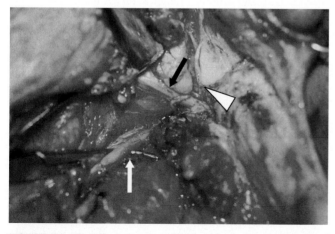

FIGURE 21–19 Intraoperative photograph during resection of a left parapharyngeal salivary gland tumor. The stylomandibular ligament (*white arrow*) is seen overlying the curved hemostat. The relationship of the main trunk of the facial nerve (*black arrow*) and the tragal "pointer" (*white arrowhead*) is also demonstrated.

In conclusion, postoperative radiation therapy is generally recommended for patients with poor prognostic indicators, including high-grade tumors, large primary lesions, perineural invasion, bone invasion, cervical lymph node metastasis, and positive margins. Although a clear-cut survival advantage has not been proved, the addition of postoperative radiation therapy improves locoregional control for patients with such adverse prognostic parameters.[152]

Radiation Therapy as a Single Modality

To compare the effectiveness of radiotherapy used alone or in combination with surgery in the treatment of minor salivary gland malignancy, Parsons and coworkers reported the results of treatment of 95 patients with minor salivary gland cancer.[136] Fifty-one patients were treated with radiotherapy alone, and 44 were treated with surgical resection plus radiotherapy. Although the tumor was locally controlled in 20 patients with previously untreated primary lesions after radiotherapy alone, freedom-from-relapse rates were significantly higher for patients who received combined treatment.

In another study, despite a high 5-year local disease control rate of 72% in patients with adenoid cystic carcinoma treated with radiation therapy alone, the disease-free survival rate at 10 years was only 20%.[153] These findings indicate that in resectable tumors, complete surgical excision followed by radiation therapy is the preferred treatment for high-grade and advanced tumors.

Radiation Therapy for Inoperable Tumors

Over the past decade, there has been substantial evidence that fast-neutron radiation therapy provides higher rates of locoregional control of unresectable cancer of the salivary glands than does photon or electron radiation therapy[154, 155] and perhaps should be considered the initial treatment of choice in some cases.[156] Buchholz and colleagues reported the outcome of 53 patients with locally advanced malignant neoplasms of the salivary glands treated with fast-neutron radiation therapy.[157] All patients received treatment for gross inoperable, residual unresectable, or recurrent disease.

With a median follow-up of 42 months and a minimum follow-up of 1 year, the overall locoregional tumor control rate was 77%. The 5-year actuarial overall locoregional control rate was 65%. With patients grouped according to previous treatment status, actuarial 5-year locoregional control rates were 92% for patients treated definitively (without a previous surgical procedure), 63% for those treated postoperatively for gross residual disease, and 51% for those treated for recurrent disease after a surgical procedure. This study suggested that neutron irradiation alone may be the therapy of choice in the treatment of some patients with unresectable advanced-stage salivary gland tumors, and that surgery should be limited to those patients in whom disease-free margins can be obtained. The potential morbidity of a "debulking" surgical procedure before neutron irradiation is not warranted by an improvement in locoregional control over that achievable with neutron therapy alone.[157] These impressive results are encouraging; however, the use of fast-neutron radiation therapy is hampered by the lack of its widespread availability. Currently, only a few facilities are equipped with the technology and expertise for delivery of fast-neutron radiation therapy.

Other investigators have described their experience with photon beam radiation therapy for the treatment of unresectable salivary gland cancer and have reported results comparable to those obtained by fast-neutron therapy. Wang and Goodman presented their experience with 24 patients with inoperable and/or unresectable cancer of the parotid (9 patients) or the minor salivary glands (15 patients), treated by photon irradiation.[158] The 5-year actuarial local control rate of parotid gland lesions after photon irradiation was 100%, and the survival rate was 65%. For minor salivary gland lesions, the 5-year actuarial local control was 78% and the survival rate with or without disease was 93%. All lesions were irradiated by accelerated hyperfractionated photons with twice-a-day fractions, 1.6 Gy per fraction, intermixed with various boost techniques, including electron beam, intraoral cone, interstitial implant, and/or submental photons, for a total of 65 to 70 Gy.

The Radiation Therapy Oncology Group (RTOG) in the United States and the Medical Research Council (MRC) in Great Britain sponsored a phase III study comparing the efficacy of fast-neutron radiotherapy versus conventional photon and/or electron radiotherapy for unresectable malignant salivary gland tumors. Patients with inoperable, recurrent, or unresectable malignant salivary gland tumors were randomly assigned to receive either neutron- or photon-based radiation therapy. The results of the initial report on the outcome of evaluable patients with minimum follow-up time of 2 years are presented in Table 21–3.[159]

After a total of 32 patients were entered into this study, it appeared that the group receiving fast-neutron radiotherapy had a significantly improved locoregional control rate along with a borderline improvement in survival, and the study was stopped earlier than planned for ethical reasons. In 1993, Laramore and associates published the final report on this study.[160] At 10-year follow-up, although there was still a statistically significant improvement in locoregional control for the neutron group (56% vs. 25%, $P = .009$), there was no improvement in survival (15% vs. 25%, $P = NS$). Distant metastases accounted for the majority of failures on the neutron arm, and locoregional failures accounted for the majority of failures on the photon arm. Although the incidence of morbidity graded "severe" was greater on the neutron arm, there was no significant difference in "life-threatening" complications.

A recent study of 75 patients with inoperable, recurrent, or incompletely resected ACC of the head and neck showed

TABLE 21–3 Neutron Versus Photon Therapy for Inoperable Salivary Gland Cancers

2-Year Follow-up	Neutron Therapy	Photon Therapy	P Value
Initial complete response	85%	33%	
Locoregional control	67%	17%	$P < .005$
2-Year survival	62%	25%	$P < .10$

Data from Griffin TW, Pajak TF, Laramore GE, et al: Neutron vs photon irradiation of inoperable salivary gland tumors: Results of an RTOG–MRC cooperative randomized study. Int J Radiat Oncol Biol Phys 15:1085–1090, 1988.

that fast-neutron radiotherapy provides higher local control rates than is provided by a mixed beam and photons. This advantage for neutrons in local control, however, was not translated into significant differences in survival because of a high incidence of distant metastasis, which occurred in 40% of these patients.[155] In another recent study of 72 patients with recurrent or gross residual ACC after surgery who had been treated with fast-neutron therapy, the recurrence-free survival was 83% after 1 year, 71% after 2 years, and 45% after 5 years.[154]

These data suggest that fast-neutron radiotherapy may be an effective treatment for patients with inoperable primary or recurrent malignant salivary gland tumors. It is hoped, therefore, that fast-neutron therapy will become more widely available for patients with unresectable salivary gland malignancy.

Chemotherapy

The poor outcome of patients with advanced, recurrent, or high-grade salivary gland cancers has prompted several investigators to explore the effectiveness of adjuvant chemotherapy in such cases.[161] Because a high percentage of patients with poor prognostic criteria die from their disease owing to systemic metastasis, it was hoped that the addition of adjuvant chemotherapy to standard treatment modalities would improve their survival. The data in the literature regarding the effectiveness of chemotherapy against salivary gland cancers are difficult to interpret. Most studies report a small number of patients, treated for different histologic types with various drug combinations, and include previously untreated patients along with those with recurrent disease.[85, 161]

In an effort to arrive at a rational basis for recommending specific drug regimens for specific histologic types of salivary gland cancers, Suen and Johns conducted a review of the literature and surveyed the experience of numerous institutions with chemotherapy for salivary gland malignancy.[162] A total of 85 cases of salivary gland cancers treated with chemotherapy were evaluated, and the overall response rate (complete and partial) was 42%. Although disease responded regardless of whether it was local, regional, or distant disease, there was a higher response rate with locoregional disease than with distant metastases.

Kaplan and colleagues reviewed 116 patients and found that adenocarcinomas responded best to a combination of cisplatin, doxorubicin, and 5-fluorouracil.[163] High-grade mucoepidermoid carcinoma may respond best to chemotherapeutic regimens that are effective against squamous cell carcinoma. Generally, combination therapy is more effective against cancer of the salivary glands than is single-drug treatment.[164] The most effective drug regimens included cisplatin, paclitaxel, doxorubicin, 5-fluorouracil, and epirubicin in different combinations.[165] In a recent phase II randomized trial comparing vinorelbine with vinorelbine plus cisplatin in patients with recurrent salivary gland malignancies, combination therapy resulted in better tumor control and improved median survival.[161]

Although salivary gland cancers show some response to various chemotherapeutic agents, these responses are rarely complete, are usually short-lived, and have not resulted in significant improvement in long-term survival.[166] A recent study indicated that the frequent expression of multidrug-resistant genes by carcinoma of the salivary glands might be responsible for the low response rates to conventional chemotherapy.[167] New drug combinations and high-dose chemotherapy with autologous bone marrow transplant are being explored in the treatment of advanced salivary gland cancer.[168] Before any conclusions can be made about the efficacy of chemotherapy in salivary gland malignancy, well-executed, multi-institutional, prospective, randomized clinical trials of specific drug regimens for specific histologic types are needed.

FACTORS INFLUENCING SURVIVAL

Clinical Factors

Stage

The stage of disease is probably the most significant factor in determining the outcome of cancers originating in the major[85, 152] or the minor[70, 169] salivary glands. Using a multivariate analysis of the outcome of 353 patients with minor salivary gland malignancy, Spiro and colleagues found that survival was significantly influenced by clinical stage and histologic grade, but the applicability of grading was limited to patients with MEC or adenocarcinoma.[170] Ten-year overall survival was 83%, 53%, 35%, and 24% for patients with stage I through stage IV, respectively.

With regard to ACC, Spiro and Huvos found that the stage of disease was much more significant than grade in predicting the outcome of treatment.[171] Cumulative 10-year survival was 75%, 43%, and 15% for stage I, stage II, and stages III and IV patients, respectively. Cause-specific survival at 10, 15, and 20 years is shown in Figure 21–20. The incidence of local recurrence after treatment was lower in stage I (23%) than in other stages (60%). Similarly, the incidence of regional metastasis was lower in stage I (19%) than in other stages (43%). Neither survival nor regional or distant metastases were predictable on the basis of tumor grade alone.[171]

Histology and Grade

The biologic behavior of malignant tumors of the salivary glands depends largely on the histologic type of malignancy.

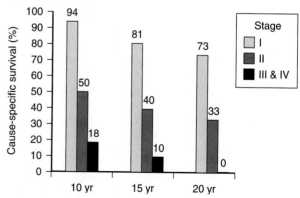

FIGURE 21–20 Effect of stage on survival of patients with adenoid cystic carcinoma.

TABLE 21-4 Effect of Histologic Grade of Mucoepidermoid Carcinoma on Clinical Outcome

Grade	Positive Margins	LN Metastasis	DNA Aneuploidy	Proliferative Fraction	Radiotherapy	Recurrence	Survival
Low	0%	0%	0%	5%	14%	0%	100%
Intermediate	44%	22%	13%	7%	35%	39%	70%
High	61%	72%	28%	13%	61%	61%	22%

LN, lymph node.
Adapted from Hicks MJ, el-Naggar AK, Flaitz CM, et al: Histocytologic grading of mucoepidermoid carcinoma of major salivary glands in prognosis and survival: A clinicopathologic and flow cytomertric investigation. Head Neck 17:89–95, 1995.

Squamous cell carcinoma, malignant mixed tumors, undifferentiated carcinoma, and salivary duct carcinoma are generally considered high-grade tumors and usually exhibit an aggressive biologic course, resulting in a poor outcome.[172] By contrast, acinic cell carcinoma and polymorphous low-grade adenocarcinoma are considered low-grade tumors with a more favorable prognosis.

ACC is generally considered a high-grade malignancy with a relentless tendency for local recurrence and ultimately a poor prognosis. However, the three histologic patterns of ACC may exhibit different biologic behaviors and, therefore, different outcomes. Generally, patients with the tubular pattern of ACC have a significantly better prognosis than do patients with the solid pattern.[71] Perzin and colleagues, reporting on the outcome of 62 patients with ACC, found that 75% of patients with no evidence of recurrence after treatment had the tubular pattern.[173] By contrast, all of the patients with the solid pattern experienced recurrent disease, and more than half of them died of disease. This tendency for a high incidence of local recurrence of patients with the solid pattern of ACC may have been related to the difficulty of achieving clear surgical margins in these patients. In the same study, none of the patients with solid pattern ACC had negative margins, but 13% of patients with the cribriform pattern and 43% of patients with the tubular pattern had clear surgical margins.[173]

Most authors agree that the outcome of MEC correlates highly with its grade. However, the histopathologic criteria most useful for grading MEC are still controversial. Auclair and coworkers proposed a grading system using certain histopathologic features and correlated them with clinical parameters and outcome in patients with intraoral MEC.[174] Histopathologic criteria that indicated high-grade behavior included an intracystic component of less than 20%, four or more mitotic figures per ten high-power fields, neural invasion, necrosis, and cellular anaplasia. The simultaneous assessment of these features showed improved prognostic correlation over individual parameters, and a quantitative grading system was devised using these features. Tumors with a point score of 0 to 4 were considered low grade, and none of 122 patients with scores in this range died of their tumor, although 9 had recurrences only and 3 had regional metastases. Point scores of 7 or above indicated highly aggressive behavior. Almost two thirds of patients with these high scores died of tumor. Most of these patients had local recurrences as well as regional metastases and distant metastases. Scores of 5 to 6 were considered intermediate between low grade and high grade.

Similarly, Hicks and associates described a three-tiered grading system for MEC of the major salivary glands.[97] Tumor size increased from 2.1 cm for low-grade tumors to 3.8 cm for high-grade tumors ($P = .01$). This grading system correlated well with clinical, pathologic, and flow cytometric factors that influenced the prognosis and overall survival of patients with MEC of the major salivary glands (Table 21–4).

Site

The primary site of origin of cancer of the salivary glands has a definite correlation with prognosis and outcome. Generally, cancers of the major salivary glands have a better prognosis than do those arising in the minor salivary glands.[87] Of all cancers arising from the minor salivary glands, those arising from the sinonasal tract tend to have the worst outcome.[70] Spiro and colleagues reported that the 10-year cure rate for patients with ACC of the parotid gland was 29%, but it was only 7% for those patients whose tumors originated from the sinonasal tract.[72]

The poor outcome of minor salivary gland cancers, particularly those of sinonasal origin, can be explained by several factors that have a detrimental impact on prognosis. First, cancers of the minor salivary glands tend to present at a more advanced *stage of disease*. For example, approximately 90% of cases of ACC of the nose and sinuses present with advanced-stage (III and IV) disease (Fig. 21–21). Second, carcinomas of the minor salivary glands have a higher incidence of *extension and fixation to contiguous structures* compared with tumors arising in the major salivary glands. This poses greater difficulty in achieving complete surgical resection with tumor-free margins.[84]

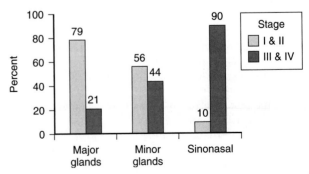

FIGURE 21–21 Stage of disease by site of origin in patients with adenoid cystic carcinoma.

Consequently, the incidence of local recurrence after treatment of cancer of the salivary gland is higher for sinonasal tumors (63%) than for other minor salivary gland tumors (54%) or major salivary gland tumors (32%).[72, 171] Third, tumors in the minor salivary glands of the oral cavity and paranasal sinuses tend to have a relatively high incidence of *bone involvement*. This is probably because of the immediate proximity of the mucoperiosteum of the palate and the sinonasal tract to the underlying bone. Bone involvement was present in approximately half of patients with ACC of the minor salivary glands.[72] Bone involvement has a significant negative impact on prognosis. The 10-year "cure" rate for patients without evidence of bone invasion was 32%, compared with 7% for patients with evidence of bone invasion.[72]

Lymph Node Metastasis

The presence of metastatic disease in the regional lymph nodes is generally considered a predictor of poor prognosis in patients with salivary gland malignancy.[85, 152] The 10- and 20-year survival rates of patients with nodal metastasis from ACC were only 38% and 8%, respectively, compared with 62% and 50%, respectively, in patients without evidence of regional disease in the lymph nodes.[171]

Surgical Margins

The presence or absence of tumor at the margins of surgical resection is considered by many to be the single most important factor influencing prognosis.[71, 152, 175] In one study of patients with ACC, 84% of patients with tumor-free margins of resection were alive with no evidence of disease, whereas only 17% of those who had residual tumor at the surgical margin were alive with no evidence of recurrence (Fig. 21–22).[173]

A NEGATIVE SURGICAL MARGINS

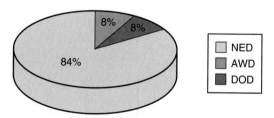

B POSITIVE SURGICAL MARGINS

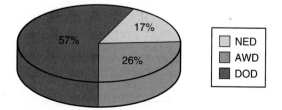

FIGURE 21–22 The outcomes of patients with adenoid cystic carcinoma according to whether surgical margins were (*A*) tumor-free or (*B*) positive for residual tumor. NED, No evidence of disease; AWD, alive with disease; DOD, dead of disease.

Although most studies agree that the presence of microscopic positive margins constitutes an adverse prognostic factor in patients with ACC, a study from the M.D. Anderson Cancer Center contends that local control is possible in a significant number of patients with positive margins treated with aggressive surgery and postoperative radiation therapy.[175] In patients with positive margins there was a trend toward better local control with increasing radiation dose. Crude control rates were 40% and 88% for doses of less than 56 Gy and 56 Gy or higher, respectively (*P* = .006). The authors concluded that excellent local control rates were obtained in this population with the use of surgery and postoperative radiotherapy, and they recommended a radiation dose of 66 Gy for patients with positive margins. Despite effective local therapy, failure due to distant metastatic disease remains a major problem in these patients, and good treatment to address this problem is lacking.[175]

Perineural Spread

Perineural spread (PNS) carries with it a poor prognosis in patients with squamous cell carcinoma of the head and neck.[83] Whether this is because of an inherently aggressive behavior of tumors with neurotropic tendency, or because of the difficulty of obtaining tumor-free margins of resection in these cases, is still unclear.[60] However, there is still considerable controversy about the prognostic significance of PNS in patients with ACC. The incidence of PNS in patients with ACC is overwhelmingly high and, as was previously mentioned, varies with the diligence of the pathologist in searching for and reporting this peculiar, and almost universal, neurotropism of ACC (see Fig. 21–14).[80] There have been conflicting reports in the literature regarding the prognostic significance of perineural spread in ACC. However, considerable evidence suggests that involvement of "major" or "named" nerves is a poor prognostic indicator.[70, 71, 85]

In a study of 198 patients with ACC treated at the M.D. Anderson Cancer Center, PNS was identified in 69% of patients.[175] Perineural invasion was an adverse prognostic factor only when a major (named) nerve was involved, which occurred in 28% of patients. The crude failure rates in patients with and without a major (named) nerve involved were 18% and 9%, respectively (*P* = .02).

Facial Nerve Paralysis

Eneroth reported facial nerve paralysis in 46 of 378 patients (12%) with cancer of the parotid gland.[176] All of the patients with facial nerve paralysis eventually died of their disease, and the average survival after the onset of paralysis was 2.7 years. The incidence of systemic metastasis in these patients was 77%. Similarly, Spiro and associates found evidence of facial nerve dysfunction in 43 of 288 patients (15%) with carcinoma of the parotid gland.[177] However, their study did not support Eneroth's assertion that the presence of facial nerve paralysis is invariably a sign of incurable cancer of the parotid gland. They reported a 5-year survival rate of only 14% in such patients. It is clear from these studies that, although facial nerve paralysis may not be associated with 100% mortality, it is still an indicator of a poor prognosis.

Pain

Patients with ACC who present with pain appear to have a less favorable outcome than do those presenting with an asymptomatic swelling. The 10-year "cure" rate was only 13% for patients presenting with a painful cancer, compared with 29% for those presenting with a painless swelling.[72] This may be so because the presence of pain may be an indication of local invasion to bone or sensory nerves, which carries a poorer prognosis.

Biologic Markers of Prognosis

Although certain clinical parameters such as disease stage, tumor histology and grade, site of origin, nodal metastasis, and perineural spread generally correlate with the prognosis of patients with cancer of the salivary glands, there is still a great deal of heterogeneity in outcome among patients with similar clinical parameters. The inability of clinical parameters to consistently predict the outcome of patients with cancer of the salivary glands has led to the recent extensive study of various biologic markers as predictors of prognosis in patients with cancer of the salivary glands.[178] These include a variety of tumor suppressor genes, oncogenes, growth factors, basement membrane proteins, extracellular matrix proteins, hormone receptors, cytokines, argyrophilic nucleolar organizer regions (AgNORs), and markers of cellular proliferation and ploidy.

Tumor Suppressor Genes and Oncogenes

Cancer is a disease of altered cellular genes. These altered genes, in turn, initiate or promote the malignant phenotype by inducing changes in key events involved in regulation of the cell cycle. Examples of such altered gene expression include inactivation of tumor suppressor genes and/or overexpression of oncogenes. Several such alterations have been investigated as potential prognostic indicators in patients with salivary gland cancers.

Point mutation of *TP53* (formerly known as *p53)*, a tumor suppressor gene, was associated with an increased likelihood of tumor recurrence in patients with ACC.[179] More recent studies emphasize the prognostic value of *TP53* alteration as an independent prognostic marker and its association with radiotherapy and chemotherapy resistance in patients with ACC.[180] *TP53* expression was detected in more than one third of patients with high-grade cancer of the salivary glands, and it has been implicated in carcinogenesis of tumors of salivary gland origin.[181] Loss of wild-type *TP53* and activation of *C-MYC* and *RAS p21* proto-oncogenes may play important roles in the malignant transformation of salivary gland pleomorphic adenoma.[182]

Another example of a tumor suppressor gene is *p27* (Kip1), a cyclin-dependent kinase inhibitor negatively that regulates the G1 phase progression of the cell cycle by binding to the cyclin E/cyclin-dependent kinase 2 complex. A recent study of the expression of *p27* in patients with MEC indicated its usefulness as a marker of tumor progression, aggressiveness, and prognosis. Significant correlation was found between low *p27* expression and tumors with high-grade, advanced T-stages, positive nodal status, and advanced clinical stages ($P = .001$). Multivariate analysis indicated that *p27* expression was a significant predictor of overall survival among these variables. Overall, patients with low *p27* expression showed poor prognosis.[183]

The tyrosine kinase receptor family, including the epidermal growth factor receptor (EGF-R), C-*ERBB2*, and more recently, C-*ERBB3*, has been recognized as having particular importance in many human malignancies.[184] Overexpression of C-*ERBB2*, an oncogene, was associated with advanced stage, a higher incidence of positive surgical margins, more frequent lymph node metastasis, and lower disease-free survival in patients with malignant tumors of the salivary glands.[185] Overexpression of C-*ERBB2* is also related to tumor differentiation and invasion in ACC.[184] Several other studies have confirmed that overexpression of C-*ERBB2* was significantly associated with aggressive tumor behavior, and it was found to be an independent prognostic factor is salivary carcinoma.[111, 186] Similarly, amplification of *HER2/NEU* expression correlated with shorter disease-free interval and poorer overall patient survival. Multivariate analysis showed that *HER2/NEU* immunostaining and amplification were markers of poor prognosis independent of histopathologic grade, tumor size, and involvement of regional lymph nodes.[187] Similar findings were reported for the H-*RAS* oncogene in patients with MEC.[34]

DNA Ploidy

Several studies have suggested a potentially important prognostic role for flow cytometric measurement of DNA content in salivary neoplasms. Significant statistical correlation between DNA content and tumor size, histologic grade, lymph node metastasis, and survival was found in patients with malignant tumors of the salivary glands.[188, 189] High-grade tumors such as undifferentiated carcinoma, adenocarcinoma, salivary duct carcinoma, squamous cell carcinoma, and carcinoma ex pleomorphic adenoma were more likely to have aneuploid DNA stem lines, and the survival time of patients with aneuploid tumors was considerably lower than for patients with diploid tumors.[190, 191] Aneuploid tumors are also more likely to be present with advanced disease stage; they have a higher rate of proliferation than diploid tumors and are more likely to recur after treatment.[192] DNA aneuploidy also closely correlates with *TP53* abnormalities.[191] These data emphasize the potential usefulness of DNA measurements as a prognostic indicator in patients with malignant tumors of the salivary glands.

Markers of Cellular Proliferation

Several markers of cellular proliferation were recently reported to bear prognostic significance in patients with cancer of the salivary glands.[193] The Ki-67 index, a marker of cellular proliferation, was found to be significantly higher in malignant than benign neoplasms of the salivary glands.[186] The Ki-67 index also correlated significantly with malignant tumor grade and patient survival.[194] Among patients with ACC, expression of Ki-67 was related to the morphologic type—the solid subtype had the highest frequency of Ki-67–positive cells. Because this subtype is recognized as the most aggressive of these tumors, Ki-67 may have the potential for providing an indication of the clinical behavior of ACC.[194]

The MIB 1 is a monoclonal antibody that recognizes the Ki-67 antigen in formalin-fixed, paraffin-embedded tumor tissue. High MIB 1 scores correlated with unfavorable outcome in patients with acinic cell carcinoma[195] and MEC.[196] Patients with MIB 1 scores higher than 10% frequently developed tumor recurrence or metastasis and had worse survival compared with those with lower MIB 1 scores. These data indicate that MIB 1 staining appears to be a significant prognostic factor in patients with acinic cell carcinoma and MEC.

Proliferating cell nuclear antigen (PCNA) is another marker of cellular proliferation that has been used to evaluate tumor growth potential in patients with malignant tumors of the salivary glands. In a recent study of patients with ACC, mean PCNA expression was higher in solid than in cribriform/tubular tumor areas, and high PCNA value was significantly correlated with shorter disease-free and overall survival.[197] Significant differences were also found in PCNA expression between low/intermediate-grade and high-grade MEC.[193, 198] These data suggest that PCNA may be a useful marker of tumor cell proliferation and that it correlates with the grade of malignant tumor found in the salivary gland.

Argyrophilic Nucleolar Organizer Regions

Several studies have found a positive correlation between the argyrophilic nucleolar organizer region (AgNOR) count and the aggressive clinical course of malignant salivary gland tumors.[191, 199] Vuhahula and colleagues measured AgNOR counts in 34 patients with ACC to determine (1) whether AgNOR count correlates with histologic grade and (2) whether AgNOR count can offer any additional prognostic advantage over histologic grading.[200] Patients were divided into two groups based on their outcomes. Group 1 consisted of 20 live patients without metastases, of whom 16 were free of disease, and group 2 comprised 14 patients with metastases, among whom 12 died of tumor. All patients from group 2 had mean AgNOR counts greater than 4, whereas 65% of patients from group 1 had mean AgNOR counts lower than 4. In addition, statistical analysis showed that the pooled mean AgNOR count of group 2 was significantly higher than that of group 1 ($P < .01$).[200] All unfavorable cases had high AgNOR counts regardless of histologic grade, suggesting that the metabolic alterations associated with the degree of malignancy of ACC may be partly portrayed by the AgNOR count, irrespective of histologic appearance. Cumulative survival rates of grade I tumors and of tumors with low AgNOR counts were better than those of grade III tumors and those with high AgNOR counts.[201]

Similarly, Yamamoto and colleagues found that AgNOR counts were lowest in the cribriform, intermediate in the trabecular, and highest in the solid patterns of ACC.[202] In cases with mixed histologic patterns, AgNOR staining appeared to be a useful technique for evaluation of the proliferative activity of each different histologic pattern area of ACC in the same tissue section. These studies show that AgNOR count exhibits the potential for identifying some aggressive ACCs that cannot be detected by histology alone,

and that it may be a useful supplementary method for prognostic evaluation of ACC.

Hormone Receptors

A variety of hormone receptors, including estrogen, progesterone, and androgen receptors, have been identified in and correlated with the clinical behavior of salivary gland tumors. Shick and coworkers confirmed the presence of progesterone receptors within normal and neoplastic salivary gland tissue and indicated that progesterone receptor expression may be of possible prognostic and therapeutic value in some patients with ACC.[203] Similar findings were reported concerning estrogen receptors.[204]

Because the morphology of salivary duct carcinoma (SDC) is remarkably similar to that of mammary ductal carcinoma, the question of whether these tumors also share common antigenic or hormonal features has been raised. Several studies from the University of Pittsburgh recently demonstrated that androgen receptor (AR)—a marker frequently detected in prostatic carcinoma—is expressed in more than 90% of cases of SDC, whereas two common breast carcinoma markers—estrogen and progesterone receptors (ERs and PRs)—are rarely expressed in these tumors.[107–109] This hormonal profile suggests that SDC, in contrast to its histologic similarity to ductal carcinoma of the breast, is immunophenotypically more related to prostatic carcinoma, and that antiandrogen therapy might be useful in patients with metastatic SDC.[108]

Basement Membrane and Extracellular Matrix Proteins

The hallmark of cancer is its ability for invasion and metastasis. Both tumor invasion and metastasis first involve attachment of tumor cells to and proteolysis of cellular basement membrane. This step is followed by proteolysis of extracellular matrix proteins and subsequent migration of tumor cells. Several basement membrane and extracellular matrix proteins such as collagen, laminin, and tenascin have been characterized in normal salivary gland tissue,[205, 206] and their level of expression has been correlated with prognosis in patients with malignant tumors of salivary gland origin. Laminin has been implicated in perineural invasion.

The expression of collagen type IV, a well-known basement membrane protein, was recently studied in 219 patients with tumors of the salivary glands.[207] Continuous and uninterrupted staining of the basal membrane with collagen IV antibody was significantly more frequent in benign than in malignant tumors of the salivary glands. Weak immunoreactivity for collagen IV was significantly ($P = .05$) associated with tumor recurrence in patients with malignant salivary gland tumors. Multivariate analysis showed that reduced collagen IV expression also correlated with advanced stage of disease. Intense collagen IV staining of the basal membrane was more frequent (35.9%) in patients who were alive, as compared with that (19.4%) in patients who died of salivary gland cancer ($P = .03$). Another recent study demonstrated that malignant tumors of the salivary glands have the ability to synthesize type IV collagenases, which plays an important role in degradation of collagen IV within the basement membrane.[208] These data indicate that the integrity of basement membrane proteins such as collagen IV may be an important barrier against invasion, and that destruction of this barrier by enzymatic degradation may be a crucial step in the development of metastasis.

Another important step in tissue invasion and metastasis is degradation of extracellular matrix proteins. Matrix metalloproteinases (MMPs) are a group of enzymes that are thought to play an important role in invasion and metastasis of various tumor types. Their effect is closely regulated by tissue inhibitors of metalloproteinases (TIMPs), which are produced by stromal cells to block the enzymatic activity of MMPs. There is evidence to suggest that the acquisition of metastatic ability by human salivary gland tumor cells is closely associated with increased secretion of several metalloproteinases, as well as decreased or altered TIMP-1 expression.[209]

Growth Factors

Transforming growth factor-β_1 (TGF-β_1) is a potent cytokine that affects growth inhibition of various cells and stimulates extracellular matrix production and angiogenesis. Loss of TGF-β receptor type II (TGF-β RII) expression has been related to tumor progression. In a recent study of patients with MEC, there was an inverse correlation between tumor grade and loss of expression of TGF-β RII. All low-grade MEC tumors yielded positive staining results, whereas only one case of intermediate-grade MEC had TGF-β RII expression, and no high-grade MEC showed TGF-β RII expression.[210] Conversely, TGF-α may play an important biologic role in promoting the growth of salivary gland ACC.[211]

◘ SUMMARY

Advances in molecular biology and genetics have provided new insights into the carcinogenesis and behavior of malignant tumors of the salivary glands. The WHO system provides a consistent taxonomy for tumors of the salivary glands, which may facilitate sharing of our experience with these relatively rare tumors. Clinical parameters such as advanced stage, high grade, nodal metastasis, positive margins, and perineural spread characterize patients with aggressive and potentially lethal tumors. The relatively high rate of failure to control the disease in these patients indicates the need for improvement in adjuvant therapy. It is hoped that better understanding of the molecular events associated with aggressive tumor behavior will provide the opportunity for development of targeted biologic therapy for "high-risk" patients with cancer of the salivary glands.

REFERENCES

1. Welton TS: Biographical brevities: Stensen's duct. Am J Surg 14:501, 1931.
2. Porter MJ, Wood SJ: Preservation of the great auricular nerve during parotidectomy. Clin Otolaryngol Allied Sci 22:251–253, 1997.
3. Debets JM, Munting JD: Parotidectomy for parotid tumours: 19-year experience from The Netherlands. Br J Surg 79:1159–1161, 1992.
4. Carlson GW: The salivary glands. Embryology, anatomy, and surgical applications. Surg Clin North Am 80:261–273, 2000.
5. Levin RJ, Bradley MK: Neuroectodermal antigens persist in benign and malignant salivary gland tumor cultures. Arch Otolaryngol Head Neck Surg 122:551–557 (discussion 557–558), 1996.
6. Dardick I: Mounting evidence against current histogenetic concepts for salivary gland tumorigenesis. Eur J Morphol 36:257–261, 1998.
7. Dardick I, Byard RW, Carnegie JA: A review of the proliferative capacity of major salivary glands and the relationship to current concepts of neoplasia in salivary glands. Oral Surg Oral Med Oral Patholy 69:53–67, 1990.
8. Dardick I, Burford-Mason AP: Current status of histogenetic and morphogenetic concepts of salivary gland tumorigenesis. Crit Rev Oral Biol Med 4:639–677, 1993.
9. Batsakis JG, Regezi JA: The pathology of head and neck tumors: Salivary glands, part 1. Head Neck Surg 1:59–68, 1978.
10. Batsakis JG, Regezi JA, Luna MA, et al: Histogenesis of salivary gland neoplasms: A postulate with prognostic implications. J Laryngol Otol 103:939–944, 1989.
11. Pammer J, Horvat R, Weninger W, et al: Expression of bcl-2 in salivary glands and salivary gland adenomas. A contribution to the reserve cell theory. Pathol Res Pract 191:35–41, 1995.
12. el-Naggar AK, Klijanienko J: Advances in clinical investigations of salivary gland tumorigenesis. Ann Pathol 19:19–22, 1999.
13. Land CE, Saku T, Hayashi Y, et al: Incidence of salivary gland tumors among atomic bomb survivors, 1950–1987. Evaluation of radiation-related risk. Radiat Res 146:28–36, 1996.
14. Spitz MR, Batsakis JG: Major salivary gland carcinoma. Descriptive epidemiology and survival of 498 patients. Arch Otolaryngol 110:45–49, 1984.
15. Modan B, Chetrit A, Alfandary E, et al: Increased risk of salivary gland tumors after low-dose irradiation. Laryngoscope 108:1095–1097, 1998.
16. Spitz MR, Sider JG, Newell GR, et al: Incidence of salivary gland cancer in the United States relative to ultraviolet radiation exposure. Head Neck Surg 10:305–308, 1988.
17. Chan JK, Yip TT, Tsang WY, et al: Specific association of Epstein-Barr virus with lymphoepithelial carcinoma among tumors and tumorlike lesions of the salivary gland. Arch Pathol Lab Med 118:994–997, 1994.
18. Tsai CC, Chen CL, Hsu HC: Expression of Epstein-Barr virus in carcinomas of major salivary glands: A strong association with lymphoepithelioma-like carcinoma. Hum Pathol 27:258–262, 1996.
19. Leung SY, Chung LP, Yuen ST, et al: Lymphoepithelial carcinoma of the salivary gland: In situ detection of Epstein-Barr virus. J Clin Pathol 48:1022–1027, 1995.
20. Nagao T, Ishida Y, Sugano I, et al: Epstein-Barr virus–associated undifferentiated carcinoma with lymphoid stroma of the salivary gland in Japanese patients. Comparison with benign lymphoepithelial lesion. Cancer 78:695–703, 1996.
21. Albeck H, Bentzen J, Ockelmann HH, et al: Familial clusters of nasopharyngeal carcinoma and salivary gland carcinomas in Greenland natives. Cancer 72:196–200, 1993.
22. Kuo T, Tsang NM: Salivary gland type nasopharyngeal carcinoma: A histologic, immunohistochemical, and Epstein-Barr virus study of 15 cases including a psammomatous mucoepidermoid carcinoma. Am J Surg Pathol 25:80–86, 2001.
23. Zheng W, Shu XO, Ji BT, et al: Diet and other risk factors for cancer of the salivary glands: A population-based case-control study. Int J Cancer 67:194–198, 1996.
24. Straif K, Weiland SK, Bungers M, et al: Exposure to nitrosamines and mortality from salivary gland cancer among rubber workers. Epidemiology 10:786–787, 1999.
25. Actis AB, Eynard AR: Influence of environmental and nutritional factors on salivary gland tumorigenesis with a special reference to dietary lipids. Eur J Clin Nutr 54:805–810, 2000.
26. Horn-Ross PL, Morrow M, Ljung BM: Menstrual and reproductive factors for salivary gland cancer risk in women. Epidemiology 10:528–530, 1999.
27. Pinkston JA, Cole P: Cigarette smoking and Warthin's tumor. Am J Epidemiol 144:183–187, 1996.
28. Johansen C, Boice J Jr, McLaughlin J, et al: Cellular telephones and cancer—a nationwide cohort study in Denmark. J Natl Cancer Inst 93:203–207, 2001.
29. Toida M, Balazs M, Mori T, et al: Analysis of genetic alterations in salivary gland tumors by comparative genomic hybridization. Cancer Genet Cytogenet 127:34–37, 2001.

30. el-Naggar AK, Hurr K, Kagan J, et al: Genotypic alterations in benign and malignant salivary gland tumors: Histogenetic and clinical implications. Am J Surg Pathol 21:691–697, 1997.

31. el-Naggar AK, Callender D, Coombes MM, et al: Molecular genetic alterations in carcinoma ex-pleomorphic adenoma: A putative progression model? Genes Chromosomes Cancer 27:162–168, 2000.

32. Johns MM 3rd, Westra WH, Califano JA, et al: Allelotype of salivary gland tumors. Cancer Res 56:1151–1154, 1996.

33. el-Naggar AK, Abdul-Karim FW, Hurr K, et al: Genetic alterations in acinic cell carcinoma of the parotid gland determined by microsatellite analysis. Cancer Genet Cytogenet 102:19–24, 1998.

34. Yoo J, Robinson RA: H-ras gene mutations in salivary gland mucoepidermoid carcinomas. Cancer 88:518–523, 2000.

35. Jeng YM, Lin CY, Hsu HC: Expression of the c-kit protein is associated with certain subtypes of salivary gland carcinoma. Cancer Lett 154:107–111, 2000.

36. Cerilli LA, Swartzbaugh JR, Saadut R, et al: Analysis of chromosome 9p21 deletion and p16 gene mutation in salivary gland carcinomas. Hum Pathol 30:1242–1246, 1999.

37. Nordkvist A, Roijer E, Bang G, et al: Expression and mutation patterns of p53 in benign and malignant salivary gland tumors. Int J Oncol 16:477–483, 2000.

38. el-Naggar AK, Lovell M, Killary A, et al: Trisomy 5 as the sole chromosomal abnormality in a primary mucoepidermoid carcinoma of the minor salivary gland. Cancer Genet Cytogenet 76:96–99, 1994.

39. Li X, Tsuji T, Wen S, et al: A fluorescence in situ hybridization (FISH) analysis with centromere-specific DNA probes of chromosomes 3 and 17 in pleomorphic adenomas and adenoid cystic carcinomas. J Oral Pathol Med 24:398–401, 1995.

40. Nordkvist A, Gustafsson H, Juberg-Ode M, et al: Recurrent rearrangements of 11q14-22 in mucoepidermoid carcinoma. Cancer Genet Cytogenet 74:77–83, 1994.

41. el-Naggar AK, Lovell M, Killary AM, et al: A mucoepidermoid carcinoma of minor salivary gland with t(11;19)(q21;p13.1) as the only karyotypic abnormality. Cancer Genet Cytogenet 87:29–33, 1996.

42. Nordkvist A, Mark J, Gustafsson H, et al: Non-random chromosome rearrangements in adenoid cystic carcinoma of the salivary glands. Genes Chromosomes Cancer 10:115–121, 1994.

43. Simpson RH: Classification of salivary gland tumours—a brief histopathological review. Histol Histopathol 10:737–746, 1995.

44. Seifert G, Sobin LH: The World Health Organization's Histological Classification of Salivary Gland Tumors. A commentary on the second edition. Cancer 70:379–385, 1992.

45. Seifert G: Histopathology of malignant salivary gland tumours. Eur J Cancer. Part B, Oral Oncol 28B:49–56, 1992.

46. Jessup JM, Menck HR, Winchester DP, et al: The National Cancer Data Base report on patterns of hospital reporting. Cancer 78:1829–1837, 1996.

47. Hoffman HT, Karnell LH, Robinson RA, et al: National Cancer Data Base report on cancer of the head and neck: Acinic cell carcinoma. Head Neck 21:297–309, 1999.

48. Spiro RH: Salivary neoplasms: Overview of a 35-year experience with 2,807 patients. Head Neck Surg 8:177–184, 1986.

49. Stewart CJ, MacKenzie K, McGarry GW, et al: Fine-needle aspiration cytology of salivary gland: A review of 341 cases. Diagn Cytopathol 22:139–146, 2000.

50. Michael CW, Hunter B: Interpretation of fine-needle aspirates processed by the ThinPrep technique: Cytologic artifacts and diagnostic pitfalls. Diagn Cytopathol 23:6–13, 2000.

51. Al-Khafaji BM, Afify AM: Salivary gland fine needle aspiration using the ThinPrep technique: Diagnostic accuracy, cytologic artifacts and pitfalls. Acta Cytol 45:567–574, 2001.

52. Jandu M, Webster K: The role of operator experience in fine needle aspiration cytology of head and neck masses. Int J Oral Maxillofac Surg 28:441–444, 1999.

53. Pitts DB, Hilsinger RL Jr, Karandy E, et al: Fine-needle aspiration in the diagnosis of salivary gland disorders in the community hospital setting. Arch Otolaryngol Head Neck Surg 118:479–482, 1992.

54. MacLeod CB, Frable WJ: Fine-needle aspiration biopsy of the salivary gland: Problem cases. Diagn Cytopathol 9:216–224 (discussion 224–225), 1993.

55. Feld R, Nazarian LN, Needleman L, et al: Clinical impact of sonographically guided biopsy of salivary gland masses and surrounding lymph nodes. Ear Nose Throat J 78:905, 908–912, 1999.

56. Heller KS, Dubner S, Chess Q, et al: Value of fine needle aspiration biopsy of salivary gland masses in clinical decision-making. Am J Surg 164:667–670, 1992.

57. Rabinov JD: Imaging of salivary gland pathology. Radiol Clin North Am 38:1047–1057, 2000.

58. Takashima S, Wang J, Takayama F, et al: Parotid masses: Prediction of malignancy using magnetization transfer and MR imaging findings. AJR Am J Roentgenol 176:1577–1584, 2001.

59. Kim KH, Sung MW, Yun JB, et al: The significance of CT scan or MRI in the evaluation of salivary gland tumors. Auris Nasus Larynx 25:397–402, 1998.

60. Hanna E, Janecka IP: Perineural spread in head and neck and skull base cancer. Crit Rev Neurosurg 4:109–115, 1994.

61. Martinoli C, Derchi LE, Solbiati L, et al: Color Doppler sonography of salivary glands. AJR Am J Roentgenol 163:933–941, 1994.

62. Bradley MJ, Durham LH, Lancer JM: The role of colour flow Doppler in the investigation of the salivary gland tumour. Clin Radiol 55:759–762, 2000.

63. Ajayi BA, Pugh ND, Carolan G, et al: Salivary gland tumours: Is colour Doppler imaging of added value in their preoperative assessment? Eur J Surg Oncol 18:463–468, 1992.

64. Keyes JW Jr, Harkness BA, Greven KM, et al: Salivary gland tumors: Pretherapy evaluation with PET. Radiology 192:99–102, 1994.

65. Keyes JW Jr, Watson NE Jr, Williams DW 3rd, et al: FDG PET in head and neck cancer. AJR Am J Roentgenol 169:1663–1669, 1997.

66. Lorain P, Robin C: Memoire sur deux nouvelles observations de tumeurs heteradeniques et sur la nature du tissu qui les compose. CR Soc Biol 209–221, 1854.

67. Billroth T: Die Cylindergeschwulst (cylindroma) in Untersuchungen uber die Entwicklung der Blutgerfarse, nebst Beobachtungen aus der Koniglichen chirurgischen Universitats-Kilink zu Berlin. In Reimer G (ed): Berlin, 1856, pp 1855–1869.

68. Dockerty MB, Mayo CW: Tumors of the submaxillary gland with special reference to mixed tumors. Surg Gynecol Obstet 74:1033–1045, 1942.

69. Foote FW, Frazell EL: Tumors of the major salivary glands. Cancer 6:1065–1133, 1953.

70. Khan AJ, DiGiovanna MP, Ross DA, et al: Adenoid cystic carcinoma: A retrospective clinical review. Int J Cancer 96:149–158, 2001.

71. Chummun S, McLean NR, Kelly CG, et al: Adenoid cystic carcinoma of the head and neck. Br J Plast Surg 54:476–480, 2001.

72. Spiro RH, Huvos AG, Strong EW: Adenoid cystic carcinoma of salivary origin. A clinicopathologic study of 242 cases. Am J Surg 128:512–520, 1974.

73. Toyoshima K, Kimura S, Cheng J, et al: High-molecular-weight fibronectin synthesized by adenoid cystic carcinoma cells of salivary gland origin. Jpn J Cancer Res 90:308–319, 1999.

74. Kimura S, Cheng J, Toyoshima K, et al: Basement membrane heparan sulfate proteoglycan (perlecan) synthesized by ACC3, adenoid cystic carcinoma cells of human salivary gland origin. J Biochem 125:406–413, 1999.

75. Kimura S, Cheng J, Ida H, et al: Perlecan (heparan sulfate proteoglycan) gene expression reflected in the characteristic histological architecture of salivary adenoid cystic carcinoma. Virchows Arch 437:122–128, 2000.

76. Irie T, Cheng J, Kimura S, et al: Intracellular transport of basement membrane-type heparan sulphate proteoglycan in adenoid cystic carcinoma cells of salivary gland origin: An immunoelectron microscopic study. Virchows Arch 433:41–48, 1998.

77. Renehan AG, Gleave EN, Slevin NJ, et al: Clinico-pathological and treatment-related factors influencing survival in parotid cancer. Br J Cancer 80:1296–1300, 1999.

78. Fordice J, Kershaw C, el-Naggar A, et al: Adenoid cystic carcinoma of the head and neck: Predictors of morbidity and mortality. Arch Otolaryngol Head Neck Surg 125:149–152, 1999.

79. Therkildsen MH, Reibel J, Schiodt T: Observer variability in histological malignancy grading of adenoid cystic carcinomas. APMIS 105:559–565, 1997.

80. Hutcheson JA, Vural E, Korourian S, et al: Neural cell adhesion molecule expression in adenoid cystic carcinoma of the head and neck. Laryngoscope 110:946–948, 2000.

81. Batsakis JG: Nerves and neurotropic carcinomas. Ann Otol Rhinol Laryngol 94:426–427, 1985.

82. Larson DL, Rodin AE, Roberts DK, et al: Perineural lymphatics: Myth or fact. Am J Surg 112:488–492, 1966.

83. Vural E, Hutcheson J, Korourian S, et al: Correlation of neural cell adhesion molecules with perineural spread of squamous cell carcinoma of the head and neck. Otolaryngol Head Neck Surg 122:717–720, 2000.

84. Pitman KT, Prokopakis EP, Aydogan B, et al: The role of skull base surgery for the treatment of adenoid cystic carcinoma of the sinonasal tract. Head Neck 21:402–407, 1999.

85. Hocwald E, Korkmaz H, Yoo GH, et al: Prognostic factors in major salivary gland cancer. Laryngoscope 111:1434–1439, 2001.

86. Regis De Brito Santos I, Kowalski LP, Cavalcante De Araujo V, et al: Multivariate analysis of risk factors for neck metastases in surgically treated parotid carcinomas. Arch Otolaryngol Head Neck Surg 127:56–60, 2001.

87. Prokopakis EP, Snyderman CH, Hanna EY, et al: Risk factors for local recurrence of adenoid cystic carcinoma: The role of postoperative radiation therapy. Am J Otolaryngol 20:281–286, 1999.

88. Iannetti G, Belli E, Marini Balestra F, et al: [Lymph node metastasis of adenoid cystic carcinoma]. Minerva Stomatol 50:85–89, 2001.

89. Jones AS, Hamilton JW, Rowley H, et al: Adenoid cystic carcinoma of the head and neck. Clin Otolaryngol Allied Sci 22:434–443, 1997.

90. Lopes MA, Santos GC, Kowalski LP: Multivariate survival analysis of 128 cases of oral cavity minor salivary gland carcinomas. Head Neck 20:699–706, 1998.

91. Le QT, Birdwell S, Terris DJ, et al: Postoperative irradiation of minor salivary gland malignancies of the head and neck. Radiother Oncol 52:165–171, 1999.

92. Anderson JN Jr, Beenken SW, Crowe R, et al: Prognostic factors in minor salivary gland cancer. Head Neck 17:480–486, 1995.

93. Spiro RH: Distant metastasis in adenoid cystic carcinoma of salivary origin. Am J Surg 174:495–498, 1997.

94. Conley J, Casler J: Data and statistics. In Casler CA (ed): Adenoid Cystic Cancer of the Head and Neck. New York, Thieme Medical Publishers, Inc, 1991, pp 21–25.

95. Pinkston JA, Cole P: Incidence rates of salivary gland tumors: Results from a population-based study. Otolaryngol Head Neck Surg 120:834–840, 1999.

96. Batsakis JG, Luna MA: Histopathologic grading of salivary gland neoplasms: I. Mucoepidermoid carcinomas. Ann Otol Rhinol Laryngol 99:835–838, 1990.

97. Hicks MJ, el-Naggar AK, Flaitz CM, et al: Histocytologic grading of mucoepidermoid carcinoma of major salivary glands in prognosis and survival: A clinicopathologic and flow cytometric investigation. Head Neck 17:89–95, 1995.

98. Brandwein MS, Ivanov K, Wallace DI, et al: Mucoepidermoid carcinoma: A clinicopathologic study of 80 patients with special reference to histological grading. Am J Surg Pathol 25:835–845, 2001.

99. Clode AL, Fonseca I, Santos JR, et al: Mucoepidermoid carcinoma of the salivary glands: A reappraisal of the influence of tumor differentiation on prognosis. J Surg Oncol 46:100–106, 1991.

100. Batsakis JG, Luna MA, el-Naggar AK: Histopathologic grading of salivary gland neoplasms: II. Acinic cell carcinomas. Ann Otol Rhinol Laryngol 99:929–933, 1990.

101. Timon CI, Dardick I: The importance of dedifferentiation in recurrent acinic cell carcinoma. J Laryngol Otol 115:639–644, 2001.

102. Olsen KD, Lewis JE: Carcinoma ex pleomorphic adenoma: A clinicopathologic review. Head Neck 23:705–712, 2001.

103. Lewis JE, Olsen KD, Sebo TJ: Carcinoma ex pleomorphic adenoma: Pathologic analysis of 73 cases. Hum Pathol 32:596–604, 2001.

104. Batsakis JG, el-Naggar AK, Luna MA: Epithelial-myoepithelial carcinoma of salivary glands. Ann Otol Rhinol Laryngol 101:540–542, 1992.

105. Cho KJ, el-Naggar AK, Ordonez NG, et al: Epithelial-myoepithelial carcinoma of salivary glands. A clinicopathologic, DNA flow cytometric, and immunohistochemical study of Ki-67 and HER-2/neu oncogene. Am J Clin Pathol 103:432–437, 1995.

106. Chetty R: Intercalated duct hyperplasia: Possible relationship to epithelial-myoepithelial carcinoma and hybrid tumours of salivary gland. Histopathology 37:260–263, 2000.

107. Fan CY, Melhem MF, Hosal AS, et al: Expression of androgen receptor, epidermal growth factor receptor, and transforming growth factor alpha in salivary duct carcinoma. Arch Otolaryngol Head Neck Surg 127:1075–1079, 2001.

108. Fan CY, Wang J, Barnes EL: Expression of androgen receptor and prostatic specific markers in salivary duct carcinoma: An immunohistochemical analysis of 13 cases and review of the literature. Am J Surg Pathol 24:579–586, 2000.

109. Kapadia SB, Barnes L: Expression of androgen receptor, gross cystic disease fluid protein, and CD44 in salivary duct carcinoma. Mod Pathol 11:1033–1038, 1998.

110. Lewis JE, McKinney BC, Weiland LH, et al: Salivary duct carcinoma. Clinicopathologic and immunohistochemical review of 26 cases. Cancer 77:223–230, 1996.

111. Felix A, el-Naggar AK, Press MF, et al: Prognostic significance of biomarkers (c-erbB-2, p53, proliferating cell nuclear antigen, and DNA content) in salivary duct carcinoma. Hum Pathol 27:561–566, 1996.

112. Epivatianos A, Dimitrakopoulos J, Trigonidis G: Intraoral salivary duct carcinoma: A clinicopathological study of four cases and review of the literature. Ann Dent 54:36–40, 1995.

113. Murrah VA, Batsakis JG: Salivary duct carcinoma. Ann Otol Rhinol Laryngol 103:244–247, 1994.

114. Batsakis JG, Pinkston GR, Luna MA, et al: Adenocarcinomas of the oral cavity: A clinicopathologic study of terminal duct carcinomas. J Laryngol Otol 97:825–835, 1983.

115. Vincent SD, Hammond HL, Finkelstein MW: Clinical and therapeutic features of polymorphous low-grade adenocarcinoma. Oral Surg Oral Med Oral Pathol 77:41–47, 1994.

116. Castle JT, Thompson LD, Frommelt RA, et al: Polymorphous low grade adenocarcinoma: A clinicopathologic study of 164 cases. Cancer 86:207–219, 1999.

117. Milchgrub S, Gnepp DR, Vuitch F, et al: Hyalinizing clear cell carcinoma of salivary gland. Am J Surg Pathol 18:74–82, 1994.

118. Batsakis JG, el-Naggar AK, Luna MA: Hyalinizing clear cell carcinoma of salivary origin. Ann Otol Rhinol Laryngol 103:746–748, 1994.

119. Batsakis JG, el-Naggar AK, Luna MA: "Adenocarcinoma, not otherwise specified": A diminishing group of salivary carcinomas. Ann Otol Rhinol Laryngol 101:102–104, 1992.

120. Taxy JB: Squamous carcinoma in a major salivary gland: A review of the diagnostic considerations. Arch Pathol Lab Med 125:740–745, 2001.

121. Fonseca I, Costa Rosa J, Felix A, et al: Simple mucin-type carbohydrate antigens (T, Tn and sialosyl-Tn) in mucoepidermoid carcinoma of the salivary glands. Histopathology 25:537–543, 1994.

122. Therkildsen MH, Mandel U, Christensen M, et al: Simple mucin-type Tn and sialosyl-Tn carbohydrate antigens in salivary gland carcinomas. Cancer 72:1147–1154, 1993.

123. Batsakis JG, McClatchey KD, Johns M, et al: Primary squamous cell carcinoma of the parotid gland. Arch Otolaryngol 102:355–357, 1976.

124. Shemen LJ, Huvos AG, Spiro RH: Squamous cell carcinoma of salivary gland origin. Head Neck Surg 9:235–240, 1987.

125. Ihrler S, Baretton GB, Menauer F, et al: Sjögren's syndrome and MALT lymphomas of salivary glands: A DNA-cytometric and interphase-cytogenetic study. Mod Pathol 13:4–12, 2000.

126. Hanna E, Wanamaker J, Adelstein D, et al: Extranodal lymphomas of the head and neck. A 20-year experience. Arch Otolaryngol Head Neck Surg 123:1318–1323, 1997.

127. Martin T, Weber JC, Levallois H, et al: Salivary gland lymphomas in patients with Sjögren's syndrome may frequently develop from rheumatoid factor B cells. Arthritis Rheum 43:908–916, 2000.

128. Jordan RC, Speight PM: Lymphoma in Sjögren's syndrome. From histopathology to molecular pathology. Oral Surg Oral Med Oral Pathol Oral Radiol Endod 81:308–320, 1996.

129. O'Brien CJ, McNeil EB, McMahon JD, et al: Incidence of cervical node involvement in metastatic cutaneous malignancy involving the parotid gland. Head Neck 23:744–748, 2001.

130. Pathak I, O'Brien CJ, Petersen-Schaeffer K, et al: Do nodal metastases from cutaneous melanoma of the head and neck follow a clinically predictable pattern? Head Neck 23:785–790, 2001.

131. Major Salivary Glands (Parotid, Submandibular, and Sublingual): AJCC Cancer Staging Manual, 5th ed. Philadelphia, Lippincott-Raven Publishers, 1997, pp 53–58.

132. Carinci F, Farina A, Pelucchi S, et al: Parotid gland carcinoma: 1987 and 1997 UICC T classifications compared for prognostic accuracy at 5 years. Eur Arch Otorhinolaryngol 258:150–154, 2001.

133. Numata T, Muto H, Shiba K, et al: Evaluation of the validity of the 1997 International Union Against Cancer TNM classification of major salivary gland carcinoma. Cancer 89:1664–1669, 2000.

134. Leonetti JP, Smith PG, Anand VK, et al: Subtotal petrosectomy in the management of advanced parotid neoplasms. Otolaryngol Head Neck Surg 108:270–276, 1993.

135. Weber RS, Byers RM, Petit B, et al: Submandibular gland tumors. Adverse histologic factors and therapeutic implications. Arch Otolaryngol Head Neck Surg 116:1055–1060, 1990.

136. Parsons JT, Mendenhall WM, Stringer SP, et al: Management of minor salivary gland carcinomas. Int J Radiat Oncol Biol Phys 35:443–454, 1996.

137. Sadeghi A, Tran LM, Mark R, et al: Minor salivary gland tumors of the head and neck: Treatment strategies and prognosis. Am J Clin Oncol 16:3–8, 1993.

138. Ferlito A, Shaha AR, Rinaldo A, et al: Management of clinically negative cervical lymph nodes in patients with malignant neoplasms of the parotid gland. ORL J Otorhinolaryngol Relat Spec 63:123–126, 2001.

139. Armstrong JG, Harrison LB, Thaler HT, et al: The indications for elective treatment of the neck in cancer of the major salivary glands. Cancer 69:615–619, 1992.

140. Rodriguez-Cuevas S, Labastida S, Baena L, et al: Risk of nodal metastases from malignant salivary gland tumors related to tumor size and grade of malignancy. Eur Arch Otorhinolaryngol 252:139–142, 1995.

141. Medina JE: Neck dissection in the treatment of cancer of major salivary glands. Otolaryngol Clin North Am 31:815–822, 1998.

142. Patel N, Har-El G, Rosenfeld R: Quality of life after great auricular nerve sacrifice during parotidectomy. Arch Otolaryngol Head Neck Surg 127:884–888, 2001.

143. Yu GY: Superficial parotidectomy through retrograde facial nerve dissection. J R Coll Surg Edinb 46:104–107, 2001.

144. Mehle ME, Kraus DH, Wood BG, et al: Facial nerve morbidity following parotid surgery for benign disease: The Cleveland Clinic Foundation experience. Laryngoscope 103:386–388, 1993.

145. Kuttner C, Berens A, Troger M, et al: [Frey syndrome after lateral parotidectomy. Follow-up and therapeutic outlook]. Mund Kiefer Gesichtschirurgie 5:144–149, 2001.

146. Olsen KD: Tumors and surgery of the parapharyngeal space. Laryngoscope 104:1–28, 1994.

147. Theriault C, Fitzpatrick PJ: Malignant parotid tumors. Prognostic factors and optimum treatment. Am J Clin Oncol 9:510–516, 1986.

148. Garden AS, Weber RS, Ang KK, et al: Postoperative radiation therapy for malignant tumors of minor salivary glands. Outcome and patterns of failure. Cancer 73:2563–2569, 1994.

149. Sakata K, Aoki Y, Karasawa K, et al: Radiation therapy for patients of malignant salivary gland tumors with positive surgical margins. Strahlenther Onkol 170:342–346, 1994.

150. Shingaki S, Ohtake K, Nomura T, et al: The role of radiotherapy in the management of salivary gland carcinomas. J Craniomaxillofac Surg 20:220–224, 1992.

151. Nutting CM, Rowbottom CG, Cosgrove VP, et al: Optimisation of radiotherapy for carcinoma of the parotid gland: A comparison of conventional, three-dimensional conformal, and intensity-modulated techniques. Radiother Oncol 60:163–172, 2001.

152. Tullio A, Marchetti C, Sesenna E, et al: Treatment of carcinoma of the parotid gland: The results of a multicenter study. J Oral Maxillofac Surg 59:263–270, 2001.

153. Hosokawa Y, Ohmori K, Kaneko M, et al: Analysis of adenoid cystic carcinoma treated by radiotherapy. Oral Surg Oral Med Oral Pathol 74:251–255, 1992.

154. Prott FJ, Micke O, Haverkamp U, et al: Results of fast neutron therapy of adenoid cystic carcinoma of the salivary glands. Anticancer Res 20:3743–3749, 2000.

155. Huber PE, Debus J, Latz D, et al: Radiotherapy for advanced adenoid cystic carcinoma: Neutrons, photons or mixed beam? Radiother Oncol 59:161–167, 2001.

156. Laramore GE: Fast neutron radiotherapy for inoperable salivary gland tumors: Is it the treatment of choice? Int J Radiat Oncol Biol Phys 13:1421–1423, 1987.

157. Buchholz TA, Laramore GE, Griffin BR, et al: The role of fast neutron radiation therapy in the management of advanced salivary gland malignant neoplasms. Cancer 69:2779–2788, 1992.

158. Wang CC, Goodman M: Photon irradiation of unresectable carcinomas of salivary glands. Int J Radiat Oncol Biol Phys 21:569–576, 1991.

159. Griffin TW, Pajak TF, Laramore GE, et al: Neutron vs photon irradiation of inoperable salivary gland tumors: Results of an RTOG-MRC cooperative randomized study. Int J Radiat Oncol Biol Phys 15:1085–1090, 1988.

160. Laramore GE, Krall JM, Griffin TW, et al: Neutron versus photon irradiation for unresectable salivary gland tumors: Final report of an RTOG-MRC randomized clinical trial. Radiation Therapy Oncology Group. Medical Research Council. Int J Radiat Oncol Biol Phys 27:235–240, 1993.

161. Airoldi M, Pedani F, Succo G, et al: Phase II randomized trial comparing vinorelbine versus vinorelbine plus cisplatin in patients with recurrent salivary gland malignancies. Cancer 91:541–547, 2001.

162. Suen JY, Johns ME: Chemotherapy for salivary gland cancer. Laryngoscope 92:235–239, 1982.

163. Kaplan MJ, Johns ME, Cantrell RW: Chemotherapy for salivary gland cancer. Otolaryngol Head Neck Surg 95:165–170, 1986.

164. Airoldi M, Brando V, Giordano C, et al: Chemotherapy for recurrent salivary gland malignancies: Experience of the ENT Department of Turin University. ORL J Otorhinolaryngol Relat Spec 56:105–111, 1994.

165. Airoldi M, Fornari G, Pedani F, et al: Paclitaxel and carboplatin for recurrent salivary gland malignancies. Anticancer Res 20:3781–3783, 2000.

166. Jones AS, Phillips DE, Cook JA, et al: A randomised phase II trial of epirubicin and 5-fluorouracil versus cisplatinum in the palliation of advanced and recurrent malignant tumour of the salivary glands. Br J Cancer 67:112–114, 1993.

167. Uematsu T, Hasegawa T, Hiraoka BY, et al: Multidrug resistance gene 1 expression in salivary gland adenocarcinomas and oral squamous-cell carcinomas. Int J Cancer 92:187–194, 2001.

168. Slichenmyer WJ, LeMaistre CF, Von Hoff DD: Response of metastatic adenoid cystic carcinoma and Merkel cell tumor to high-dose melphalan with autologous bone marrow transplantation. Invest New Drugs 10:45–48, 1992.

169. Vander Poorten VL, Balm AJ, Hilgers FJ, et al: Stage as major long term outcome predictor in minor salivary gland carcinoma. Cancer 89:1195–1204, 2000.

170. Spiro RH, Thaler HT, Hicks WF, et al: The importance of clinical staging of minor salivary gland carcinoma. Am J Surg 162:330–336, 1991.

171. Spiro RH, Huvos AG: Stage means more than grade in adenoid cystic carcinoma. Am J Surg 164:623–628, 1992.

172. Bradley PJ: Distant metastases from salivary gland cancer. ORL J Otorhinolaryngol Relat Spec 63:233–242, 2001.

173. Perzin KH, Gullane P, Clairmont AC: Adenoid cystic carcinomas arising in salivary glands: A correlation of histologic features and clinical course. Cancer 42:265–282, 1978.

174. Auclair PL, Goode RK, Ellis GL: Mucoepidermoid carcinoma of intraoral salivary glands. Evaluation and application of grading criteria in 143 cases. Cancer 69:2021–2030, 1992.

175. Garden AS, Weber RS, Morrison WH, et al: The influence of positive margins and nerve invasion in adenoid cystic carcinoma of the head and neck treated with surgery and radiation. Int J Radiat Oncol Biol Phys 32:619–626, 1995.

176. Eneroth CM: Facial nerve paralysis. A criterion of malignancy in parotid tumors. Arch Otolaryngol 95:300–304, 1972.

177. Spiro RH, Huvos AG, Strong EW: Cancer of the parotid gland. A clinicopathologic study of 288 primary cases. Am J Surg 130:452–459, 1975.

178. Pinto AE, Fonseca I, Martins C, et al: Objective biologic parameters and their clinical relevance in assessing salivary gland neoplasms. Adv Anat Pathol 7:294–306, 2000.

179. Papadaki H, Finkelstein SD, Kounelis S, et al: The role of p53 mutation and protein expression in primary and recurrent adenoid cystic carcinoma. Hum Pathol 27:567–572, 1996.

180. Preisegger KH, Beham A, Kopp S, et al: Prognostic impact of molecular analyses in adenoid cystic carcinomas of the salivary gland. Onkologie 24:273–277, 2001.

181. Mutoh H, Nagata H, Ohno K, et al: Analysis of the p53 gene in parotid gland cancers: A relatively high frequency of mutations in low-grade mucoepidermoid carcinomas. Int J Oncol 18:781–786, 2001.

182. Deguchi H, Hamano H, Hayashi Y: c-myc, ras p21 and p53 expression in pleomorphic adenoma and its malignant form of the human salivary glands. Acta Pathol Japon 43:413–422, 1993.

183. Choi CS, Choi G, Jung KY, et al: Low expression of p27(Kip1) in advanced mucoepidermoid carcinomas of head and neck. Head Neck 23:292–297, 2001.

184. Shintani S, Funayama T, Yoshihama Y, et al: Expression of c-erbB family gene products in adenoid cystic carcinoma of salivary glands: An immunohistochemical study. Anticancer Res 15:2623–2626, 1995.

185. Sugano S, Mukai K, Tsuda H, et al: Immunohistochemical study of c-erbB-2 oncoprotein overexpression in human major salivary gland carcinoma: An indicator of aggressiveness. Laryngoscope 102:923–927, 1992.

186. Giannoni C, el-Naggar AK, Ordonez NG, et al: c-erbB-2/neu oncogene and Ki-67 analysis in the assessment of palatal salivary gland neoplasms. Otolaryngol Head Neck Surg 112:391–398, 1995.

187. Press MF, Pike MC, Hung G, et al: Amplification and overexpression of HER-2/neu in carcinomas of the salivary gland: Correlation with poor prognosis. Cancer Res 54:5675–5682, 1994.

188. Franzen G, Nordgard S, Boysen M, et al: DNA content in adenoid cystic carcinomas. Head Neck 17:49–55, 1995.

189. Carrillo R, Batsakis JG, Weber R, et al: Salivary neoplasms of the palate: A flow cytometric and clinicopathological analysis. J Laryngol Otol 107:858–861, 1993.

190. Bang G, Donath K, Thoresen S, et al: DNA flow cytometry of reclassified subtypes of malignant salivary gland tumors. J Oral Pathol Med 23:291–297, 1994.

191. Ishii K, Nakajima T: Evaluation of malignant grade of salivary gland tumors: Studies by cytofluorometric nuclear DNA analysis, histochemistry for nucleolar organizer regions and immunohistochemistry for p53. Pathol Int 44:287–296, 1994.

192. Tytor M, Gemryd P, Wingren S, et al: Heterogeneity of salivary gland tumors studied by flow cytometry. Head Neck 15:514–521, 1993.

193. Hicks J, Flaitz C: Mucoepidermoid carcinoma of salivary glands in children and adolescents: Assessment of proliferation markers. Oral Oncol 36:454–460, 2000.

194. Yin HF, Okada N, Takagi M: Apoptosis and apoptotic-related factors in mucoepidermoid carcinoma of the oral minor salivary glands. Pathol Int 50:603–609, 2000.

195. Skalova A, Leivo I, Von Boguslawsky K, et al: Cell proliferation correlates with prognosis in acinic cell carcinomas of salivary gland origin. Immunohistochemical study of 30 cases using the MIB 1 antibody in formalin-fixed paraffin sections. J Pathol 173:13–21, 1994.

196. Skalova A, Lehtonen H, von Boguslawsky K, et al: Prognostic significance of cell proliferation in mucoepidermoid carcinomas of the salivary gland: Clinicopathological study using MIB 1 antibody in paraffin sections. Hum Pathol 25:929–935, 1994.

197. Cho KJ, Lee SS, Lee YS: Proliferating cell nuclear antigen and c-erbB-2 oncoprotein expression in adenoid cystic carcinomas of the salivary glands. Head Neck 21:414–419, 1999.

198. Cardoso WP, Denardin OV, Rapoport A, et al: Proliferating cell nuclear antigen expression in mucoepidermoid carcinoma of salivary glands. São Paulo Med J Rev Paul Med 118:69–74, 2000.

199. Epivatianos A, Trigonidis G: Salivary gland tumors studied by means of the AgNOR technique. Ann Dent 53:21–25, 1994.

200. Vuhahula EA, Nikai H, Ogawa I, et al: Prognostic value of argyrophilic nucleolar organizer regions (AgNOR) count in adenoid cystic carcinoma of salivary glands. Pathol Int 44:368–373, 1994.

201. Vuhahula EA, Nikai H, Ogawa I, et al: Correlation between argyrophilic nucleolar organizer region (AgNOR) counts and histologic grades with respect to biologic behavior of salivary adenoid cystic carcinoma. J Oral Pathol Med 24:437–442, 1995.

202. Yamamoto Y, Itoh T, Saka T, et al: Nucleolar organizer regions in adenoid cystic carcinoma of the salivary glands. Eur Arch Otorhinolaryngol 252:176–180, 1995.

203. Shick PC, Riordan GP, Foss RD: Estrogen and progesterone receptors in salivary gland adenoid cystic carcinoma. Oral Surg Oral Med Oral Pathol Oral Radiol Endod 80:440–444, 1995.

204. Ozono S, Onozuka M, Sato K, et al: Immunohistochemical localization of estradiol, progesterone, and progesterone receptor in human salivary glands and salivary adenoid cystic carcinomas. Cell Struct Funct 17:169–175, 1992.

205. Soini Y, Paakko P, Virtanen I, et al: Tenascin in salivary gland tumours. Virchows Arch A Pathol Anat Histopathol 421:217–222, 1992.

206. Skalova A, Leivo I: Basement membrane proteins in salivary gland tumours. Distribution of type IV collagen and laminin. Virchows Arch A Pathol Anat Histopathol 420:425–431, 1992.

207. Karja V, Syrjanen K, Syrjanen S: Collagen IV and tenascin immunoreactivity as prognostic determinant in benign and malignant salivary gland tumours. Acta Otolaryngol 115:569–575, 1995.

208. Soini Y, Autio-Harmainen H: Synthesis and degradation of basement membranes in benign and malignant salivary gland tumours. A study by in situ hybridization. J Pathol 170:291–296, 1993.

209. Azuma M, Tamatani T, Fukui K, et al: Role of plasminogen activators, metalloproteinases and the tissue inhibitor of metalloproteinase-1 in the metastatic process of human salivary-gland adenocarcinoma cells. Int J Cancer 54:669–676, 1993.

210. Dillard DG, Muller S, Cohen C, et al: High tumor grade in salivary gland mucoepidermoid carcinomas and loss of expression of transforming growth factor beta receptor type II. Arch Otolaryngol Head Neck Surg 127:683–686, 2001.

211. Chiang CP, Chen CH, Liu BY, et al: Expression of transforming growth factor-alpha in adenoid cystic carcinoma of the salivary gland. J Formos Med Assoc 100:471–477, 2001.

CHAPTER 22

Tumors of the Parapharyngeal Space

Eugene N. Myers

Jonas T. Johnson

Hugh D. Curtin

INTRODUCTION

Many head and neck surgeons state that a prime motive in choosing the discipline of head and neck surgery was fascination with anatomy. In many ways, the parapharyngeal space represents the ultimate example of how intimate knowledge of anatomy can facilitate diagnosis and is essential for proper management. Our objective in this chapter is to describe the anatomy of the parapharyngeal space (PPS); elaborate on patient evaluation based on history, physical findings, and imaging techniques; outline a plan of management; and present details of surgical technique.

ANATOMY

The PPS is a potential space invested by various layers of cervical fascia. The anatomic relationships of the PPS are complex. The PPS is commonly described as resembling an inverted triangle with its base at the base of the skull and the apex at the hyoid bone. The pharyngeal constrictor muscles and the oropharynx, including the palatine tonsil, form the medial wall of the PPS. The lateral wall of the PPS is the pterygoid muscles and the ascending ramus of the mandible.[1] The carotid sheath with its contents is in the posterior aspect of the PPS. For the sake of this discussion, we will include tumors arising from the contents of the carotid sheath as tumors of the PPS. The carotid sheath includes the carotid artery, internal jugular vein, and cranial nerves X, XI, and XII; the cervical sympathetic chain is located adjacent to the carotid sheath and may also, when involved by tumor, present as a mass in the PPS.

CLINICAL PRESENTATION

The signs and symptoms associated with tumors that arise in the PPS vary greatly and reflect the wide variety of pathology that may be encountered in this anatomic site (Table 22–1). Approximately 80% of parapharyngeal tumors are benign.

These tumors are frequently asymptomatic until they become very large.[2–5] Expansion of the tumor in the plane of least resistance usually results in medial displacement of the lateral pharyngeal wall and tonsil (Fig. 22–1). Alternatively, the mass may be found posterior or inferior to the angle of the mandible such as one would see in a mass in the neck or parotid. A more subtle finding is inferior displacement of the submandibular gland by a PPS tumor because the apex of the PPS is the submandibular triangle. Careful intraoral and cervical evaluation, including bimanual palpation, allows the clinician to formulate an initial impression of the extent of tumor.

The patient with a neurilemmoma arising from a cranial nerve may have an associated functional defect (e.g., vocal cord paralysis when the vagus nerve is affected). Benign lesions arising high in the PPS may rarely produce a jugular foramen syndrome. Thorough evaluation of the cranial nerves is necessary in every case. Malignancy may be accompanied by invasion of adjacent structures, pain, and functional compromise (e.g., trismus). Extension beyond the confines of the PPS to involve such structures as the infraorbital fissure, eustachian tube, or pterygomaxillary fossa is associated with a variety of symptoms that are predictable according to the anatomic structures existing in those areas.

Tumors of the PPS may be palpable in the parotid gland, the lateral neck, or both areas, as well as in the oropharynx. In patients in whom the tumor originates in the deep lobe of the parotid gland and passes through the relatively constricted area called *the stylomandibular tunnel* (Fig. 22–2), the mass will be seen in the oropharynx and palpated in the parotid gland.

Medial displacement of the wall of the oropharynx and the adjacent tonsil and soft palate may be associated with

TABLE 22–1 Symptoms of Tumors of the Parapharyngeal Space

Findings	Percentage of Patients
Neck mass	46
Pain	20
Dysphagia	13
Pharyngeal mass	9
Hoarseness	7
Foreign body sensation	6
Parotid mass	4
Otalgia	4
Trismus	2
Fatigue, malaise	2

Data from Carrau RL, Myers EN, Johnson JT: Management of tumors arising in the parapharyngeal space. Laryngoscope 100:583–589, 1990.

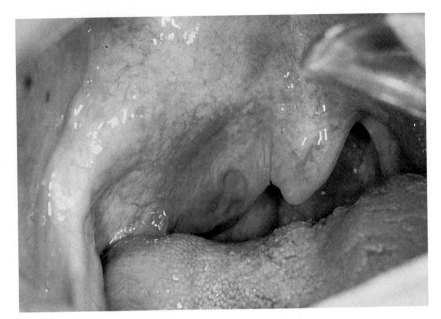

FIGURE 22–1 Intraoral examination demonstrates displacement of the palate and the superior pole of the tonsil.

dysarthria and dysphagia. The presence of trismus suggests infiltration into or pressure on the pterygoid muscles, or mechanical obstruction to excursion of the coronoid process of the mandible. Another presenting symptom may be an ill-fitting maxillary denture caused by displacement of the soft palate by tumor. Hearing loss resulting from middle ear effusion may be encountered when the cartilaginous portion of the eustachian tube is compressed by tumor. Obstructive sleep

apnea symptoms secondary to PPS lesions have been described. These symptoms include loud snoring, restless sleep, and daytime hypersomnolence from the airway encroachment secondary to palatal and tonsillar displacement from large tumors in the PPS (Fig. 22–3).

A significant proportion of asymptomatic tumors originating in the PPS are found incidentally on imaging studies (e.g., computed tomography [CT] and magnetic resonance imaging

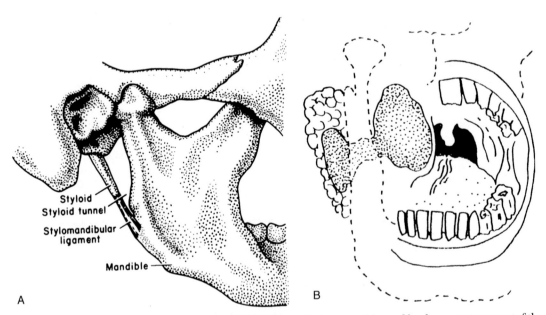

A

Styloid
Styloid tunnel
Stylomandibular
ligament
Mandible

B

FIGURE 22–2 *A,* Schematic drawing of the stylomandibular tunnel formed by the posterior aspect of the ascending ramus of the mandible, the skull base, and the stylomandibular ligament. (From Heeneman H, Johnson JT, Curtin HD, et al: The Parapharyngeal Space: Anatomy and Pathologic Conditions With Emphasis on Neurogenous Tumors, 2nd ed., Washington, DC, American Academy of Otolaryngology–Head and Neck Surgery Foundation, 1987.) *B,* Schematic drawing of the dumbbell tumor encountered when neoplastic degeneration of the deep lobe of the parotid passes through the stylomandibular tunnel.

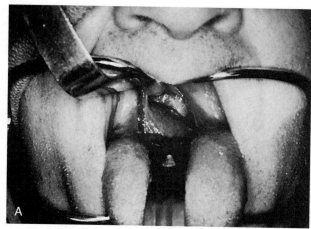
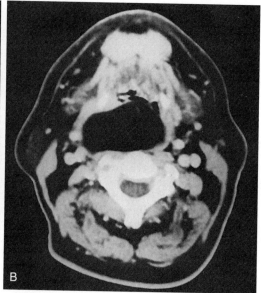

FIGURE 22–3 *A*, Oropharyngeal examination of a 54-year-old man demonstrates massive medial displacement of the oropharyngeal wall, which creates almost total pharyngeal obstruction. This man complained of snoring and symptoms of obstructive sleep apnea. *B*, CT scan demonstrates a massive lesion involving the parapharyngeal and retropharyngeal spaces. The density of this mass is characteristic of fat. A large lipoma was excised.

[MRI]) performed for other indications. Paraganglioma involving either the vagus or the carotid bifurcation is often first recognized as a mass in the neck. The classic description of the carotid body tumor is a mass that will move laterally but will not move cephalocaudad owing to fixation to the carotid artery. A bruit may occasionally be encountered.

DIAGNOSTIC CONSIDERATIONS

The most common tumors originating in the PPS arise either from salivary tissue of the deep lobe of the parotid gland or salivary gland rests, or from neuroectoderm associated with the cranial nerves, the cervical sympathetic chain, or the glomus bodies (chemoreceptors) adjacent to the cranial nerves and the bifurcation of the carotid artery (Table 22–2). Metastatic tumor may involve the lymphatics in the parapharyngeal space; however, metastases are encountered more commonly lateral to the carotid artery in the jugular chain of lymphatics or medially in the retropharyngeal space (node of

Rouvière). A wide variety of rare and unusual tumors may be initially interpreted as parapharyngeal in location, but modern imaging usually allows their distinction based on the site of origin (Table 22–3). For instance, sarcomatous lesions may develop in the maxilla or adjacent muscles and may expand into the parapharyngeal space.

Physical Examination

The physical examination should include careful inspection and palpation of the oropharynx and neck and assessment of the functional integrity of the cranial nerves.

Diagnostic Imaging

Imaging is the most important diagnostic step. Both MRI and CT provide excellent imaging of the parapharyngeal

TABLE 22–2 Histologic Diagnosis of Parapharyngeal Space Neoplasms (n = 77)

Diagnosis	No. of Patients (Percentage)
Pleomorphic adenoma	27 (36)
Carotid body tumor	15 (20)
Glomus vagale	7 (9)
Neurilemmoma	7 (9)
Neurofibroma	2 (3)
Meningioma	2 (3)
Metastatic tumor	2 (3)
Other	15 (20)

Data from Myers EN, Carrau RL: Tumors arising in the parapharyngeal space. Rev Bras Cir Cabeca Pescoco 18:6–12, 1994.

TABLE 22–3 Malignant Tumors of the Parapharyngeal Space (n = 33)

Tumor	No. of Patients
Carotid body tumor	2
Neurogenic sarcoma	2
Malignant mixed tumor	1
Adenoid cystic carcinoma	1
Neurofibrosarcoma	1
Leiomyosarcoma	1
Liposarcoma	1
Fibrosarcoma	1
Metastatic cancer of the thyroid	1
Malignant meningioma	21
Lymphoma	1

Data from Myers EN, Carrau RL: Tumors arising in the parapharyngeal space. Rev Bras Cir Cabeca Pescoco 18:6–12, 1994.

region. Although CT with contrast enhancement is an effective imaging study, many head and neck radiologists prefer MRI for this evaluation because it provides better definition of tissue planes.

The imaging characteristics of tumors originating in the parapharyngeal space can offer help in pinpointing the diagnosis with relative certainty, thus eliminating the need for biopsy. The effect of the lesion on the prestyloid fat, as well as the relationship of the lesion to several key landmarks, localizes the lesion into one of the two compartments of PPS, substantially limiting the possible diagnoses.

The fascia of the tensor veli palatini extends from the styloid process to the skull base and divides the PPS into prestyloid and poststyloid compartments (Figs. 22–4 and 22–5). Although the fascia itself cannot be reliably visualized on imaging, the effect of the fascia in dividing the prestyloid and poststyloid compartments helps in determination of the site of tumor origin. The prestyloid PPS is a potential space.

Under normal circumstances, it contains fat and a few small lymph nodes. The deep lobe of the parotid gland protrudes variably into the prestyloid compartment. The poststyloid PPS contains the carotid artery, the jugular vein, various cranial nerves, and the superior cervical ganglion.

Because tumor development depends on the types of tissues found normally in the PPS, the likely identity of a lesion depends primarily on the anatomic location of the tumor relative to the separating fascia. The majority of tumors found in the prestyloid compartment of the PPS (anterior to the fascia) arise from salivary gland tissue. Masses arising in the poststyloid PPS (posterior to the fascia) are almost entirely of neural origin. A majority of these tumors are paragangliomas, neuromas, or neurilemmomas.

Because location of origin is so important, imaging first attempts to determine if a lesion is in either the prestyloid or the poststyloid compartment. The key anatomic landmarks are the prestyloid fat, the medial pterygoid muscle, the carotid

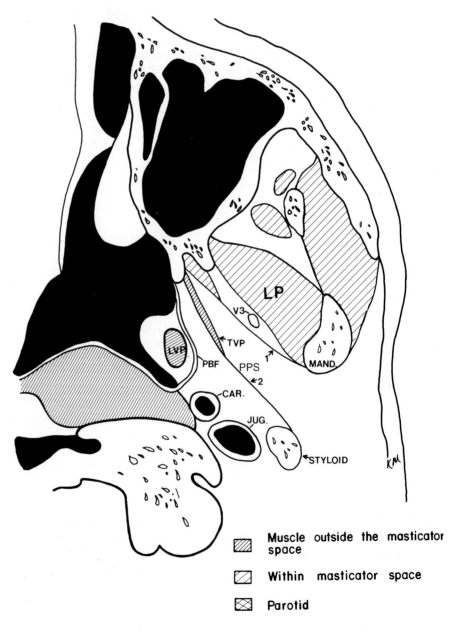

FIGURE 22–4 Axial section through the nasopharynx showing the important fascial layer compartmentalizing the parapharyngeal area. 1, Fascial layer representing fusion of the interpterygoid fascia with the fascia covering the medial pterygoid muscle. 2, Tensor veli palatini fascia, pharyngobasilar fascia (PBF), levator veli palatini (LVP), lateral pterygoid muscle (LP). The parotid gland passing through the stylomandibular tunnel would enter the prestyloid parapharyngeal space (PPS) between fascial planes 1 and 2. *Long arrow*, Pharyngeal recess; *short arrow*, torus tubarius; CAR, internal carotid artery; JUG, jugular vein; MAND, mandible; TVP, tensor veli palatini muscle. (From Curtin HD: Separation of the masticator space from the parapharyngeal space. Radiology 163:195, 1987.)

▨ **Muscle outside the masticator space**

▨ **Within masticator space**

▨ **Parotid**

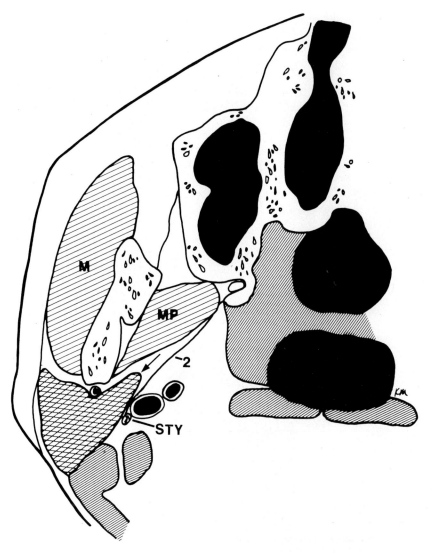

FIGURE 22–5 *Lower section* of parapharyngeal space. On this diagram, the parotid gland protrudes into the prestyloid parapharyngeal space. For key see Figure 22–4. *Arrow*, external carotid artery; MP, medial pterygoid muscle; M, masseter muscle; STY, styloid. (From Curtin HD: Separation of the masticator space from the parapharyngeal space. Radiology 163:195, 1987.)

artery, the posterior edge of the mandible, and the styloid process. Of these, the carotid artery and the styloid process are probably the most important (see Figs. 22–4 and 22–5).

A lesion in the prestyloid parapharyngeal space will be anterior to the carotid artery and posterior to the medial pterygoid muscle (Fig. 22–6). The fat of the prestyloid PPS is compressed along the medial aspect of the tumor. When these findings are present, the lesion is confidently localized in the prestyloid PPS.

Many prestyloid PPS tumors arise from the deep lobe of the parotid gland (Fig. 22–7). This relationship is easily noted on CT or MRI. In some cases, a fat plane exists between the parotid gland and the prestyloid PPS tumor. These lesions probably arise de novo from a salivary rest in the PPS.

Lesions in the poststyloid PPS almost always arise from the neural elements located posterior to the carotid artery (Fig. 22–8). Thus, they displace the carotid artery anteriorly. The carotid artery may be displaced slightly medially or laterally, but the lesion should not be anterior to the vessel. This finding becomes key in identification of lesions in the poststyloid PPS. If the lesion is of sufficient size to push

laterally, it will bulge behind the styloid process. The bulk of the lesion may be more anterior than the styloid process, but the lateral margin should point behind the styloid. The parapharyngeal fat is usually pushed anteriorly and laterally by a poststyloid PPS lesion.

Although determination of the precise anatomic site is the most important consideration, other imaging findings are important in further analysis of the lesion. Although most tumors arising in the prestyloid PPS are benign pleomorphic adenomas, some imaging findings may indicate that the lesion may be malignant. Pleomorphic adenoma characteristically has bright signal on T2-weighted MR imaging (T2WI) (Fig. 22–9). Dark areas on the T2WI are thought to indicate increased cellularity, and malignancy is considered somewhat more likely, although the finding is not specific. The margin of a pleomorphic adenoma is usually sharp at imaging, and irregularity or infiltration of contiguous soft tissues is considered suggestive of malignancy. If the margin is slightly lobulated (bosselated), pleomorphic adenoma is likely. Whenever a parotid lesion is identified, the fat pads around the facial nerve and along the course of the auriculotemporal nerve toward the trigeminal nerve

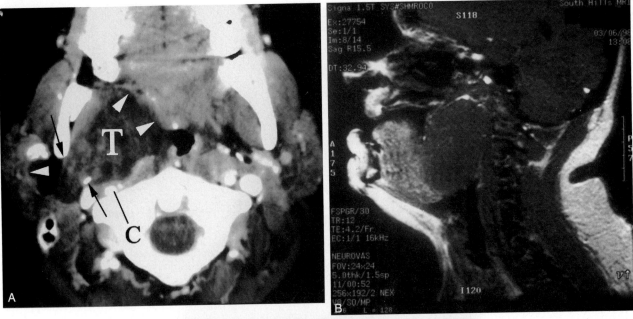

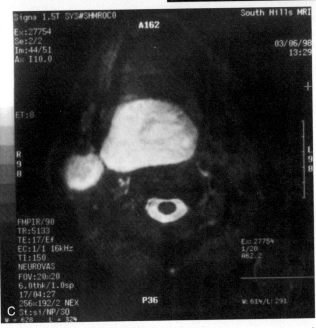

FIGURE 22–6 *A,* Axial CT. Axial section after intravenous contrast injection shows the tumor (T) filling the parapharyngeal space and squeezing through the stylomandibular tunnel *(between black arrows).* The margins of the lesion *(arrowheads)* can be clearly seen. The lateral extent pushes into the parotid, and the medial part causes a bulge in the pharyngeal wall. Note how the lesion is completely anterior to the carotid artery (C). *B,* This MR T1 sequence demonstrates a massive tumor of the prestyloid parapharyngeal space that appears to totally occlude the airway. The patient's clinical symptoms included symptoms of obstructive sleep apnea, as well as dysarthria and dysphagia. *C,* The same patient studied in the axial plane with a T2-weighted MRI further characterizes this massive tumor in the prestyloid parapharyngeal space, which is lobulated by the stylomandibular ligament.

in the masticator space are carefully examined (Fig. 22–10). Distortion or obliteration of the fat is a strong indicator of perineural spread and thus of malignancy. Usually, involvement of these nerves is suggested clinically.

Lesions in the poststyloid PPS are usually paragangliomas arising from the ganglion of the vagus nerve, or schwannomas related to the cranial nerves or superior

cervical ganglion. The demonstration of flow voids within the tumor indicates high vascularity, which is characteristic of paraganglioma (glomus vagale) (Fig. 22–11). Lack of flow voids suggests schwannoma. However, reports have indicated that flow voids may not be identified in small glomus tumors. Most schwannomas arising from the vagus nerve or other cranial nerves tend to push the internal carotid artery

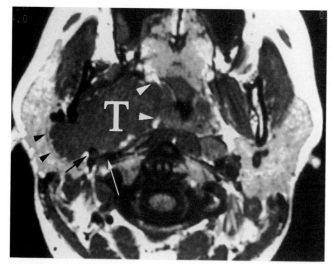

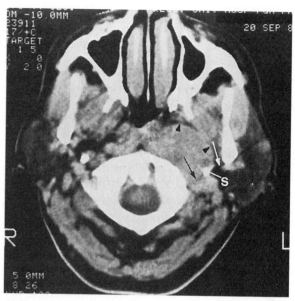

FIGURE 22–7 Precontrast MR axial T1-weighted image. The tumor (T) can be seen filling the prestyloid PPS and projecting through the stylomandibular tunnel into the parotid. The parapharyngeal fat (*white arrowheads*) is seen pushed medially. The facial nerve (*black arrowheads*) can be visualized as it passes along the lateral aspect of the tumor. The medial pterygoid muscle cannot be clearly differentiated from the tumor. The indentation caused by the styloid process is visualized, but the styloid process itself (*black arrow*) is poorly seen. The lesion remains anterior to the carotid artery (*white arrow*).

FIGURE 22–8 Paraganglioma in the poststyloid parapharyngeal space pushes the parapharyngeal fat anteriorly and laterally (*arrowheads*). The tumor tends to squeeze posterior (*black arrow*) to the styloid process (S). It does not go through the stylomandibular tunnel (*white arrow*).

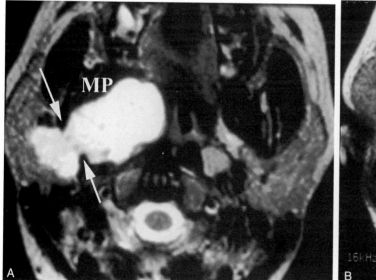

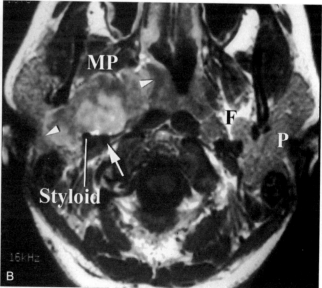

FIGURE 22–9 *A,* Axial T2-weighted image shows the tumor to have uniform high signal intensity or hyperintensity. The interface with the medial pterygoid (MP) is sharply defined. The stylomandibular tunnel (*between the white arrows*) causes a constriction on the central portion of the tumor. *B,* Axial T1-weighted postcontrast image. The margins of the lesion (*arrowheads*) push into the parotid and the parapharyngeal fat, making a clear separation between the tumor and the medial pterygoid muscle (MP). The carotid artery (*arrow*) is identified posterior to the tumor. Compare the appearance of the parotid gland (P) and the parapharyngeal (F) on the opposite side.

anteriorly and slightly medially (Fig. 22–12). Occasionally, the artery is pushed more laterally. In this case, the lesion may be arising from the sympathetic chain. A node of Rouvière may be identified as a mass medial to the artery (Fig. 22–13). However, if this node is abnormal enough to give the appearance of a mass, a primary lesion is almost always obvious.

The choice of initial imaging technique is somewhat controversial. Most radiologists prefer MRI because the location is almost always definable with the use of multiple sequences. The styloid process may not be as obvious as on CT but the carotid is usually seen; therefore, the site of origin can be determined. MRI also provides information regarding vascularity. Contrast is usually used, although it may not be necessary in all cases. CT is also excellent, but lesions may be difficult to see against the parotid gland tissue. This is particularly true with very fast CT scanners. After injection of contrast, there is a gradual increase in density as the contrast agent is accumulated in the tumor.[6] If imaging is done too early after the injection, there may not be sufficient difference between the appearance of the lesion and that of the gland parenchyma to allow identification of the margin. A delayed scan may increase conspicuousness as the tumor appears to become denser. This phenomenon can be avoided by injecting part of the contrast and then waiting for 5 or 10 minutes. The remaining contrast is then injected as the scan is performed so that vessels, particularly the internal carotid artery, can be confidently seen as well.

Most physicians feel that paraganglioma should be further evaluated with angiography. This is required if embolization is to be used as an adjuvant to surgery.

The need for other diagnostic procedures must reflect the physician's suspicions and concerns. For instance, fine-needle aspiration biopsy may be obtained; however, it is generally avoided when paraganglioma is suspected and may require CT or ultrasound guidance in these deeply seated tumors. The proximity of important neurovascular structures and of the overlying mandible makes fine-needle aspiration a challenge for most. Under many circumstances, it may be considered unnecessary.

We studied the degree of accuracy of imaging in a series of patients with PPS tumors.[5] CT scan accurately defined the position of the tumors relative to the styloid process in 96% (43/45) of the masses. The vascularity of the mass as seen on CT scan correlated with the angiographic findings (45/45). CT scan correctly assessed tumors of salivary gland origin in 88% (14/16) of cases, misdiagnosed a minor salivary gland tumor as being of parotid origin in 7%, and did not define the origin in another 7%. Angiography was performed for all vascular masses. It proved to be more specific than CT scan for the vascular lesions, yielding a correct diagnosis in 92% (23/25) of cases, whereas CT scan did not differentiate vascularized neurilemmomas, carotid body, and glomus vagale tumors in 30% (6/20).

In certain clinical situations, such as the multiple endocrine neoplasia (MEN) syndromes and the presence of paraganglioma, the finding of tachycardia, hypertension, or intermittent flushing should prompt evaluation of circulating catecholamines. This requires 24-hour urine collection for vanillylmandelic acid (VMA).

Fine-Needle Aspiration Biopsy

Fine-needle aspiration biopsy (FNAB) may contribute to the preoperative evaluation of PPS tumors. Aspiration may be easily undertaken in patients with tumor palpable in the neck. Deeply seated masses in the parapharyngeal space may be aspirated percutaneously under CT guidance.

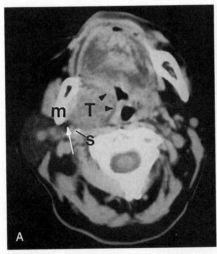
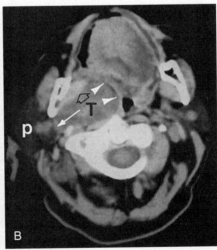

FIGURE 22–10 The patient presented with a bulge in the pharyngeal wall. *A*, Low slice shows the tumor (T) pushing the parapharyngeal fat medially (*arrowheads*). At this level, it does not protrude into the stylomandibular tunnel, and the tumor could be construed as arising from a salivary gland rest rather than the parotid gland. Note the small amount of fat (*arrow*) separating the tumor from the deep lobe of the parotid gland. m, mandible; s, styloid. *B*, Slightly higher-level slice shows the tumor (T) and its effect on the parapharyngeal fat (*arrowheads*). At this level, however, the tumor protrudes through the stylomandibular tunnel (*arrow*), revealing its origin from the deep lobe of the parotid gland. Note the distinction between tumor and the medial pterygoid muscle (*open arrow*). p, parotid.

Continued

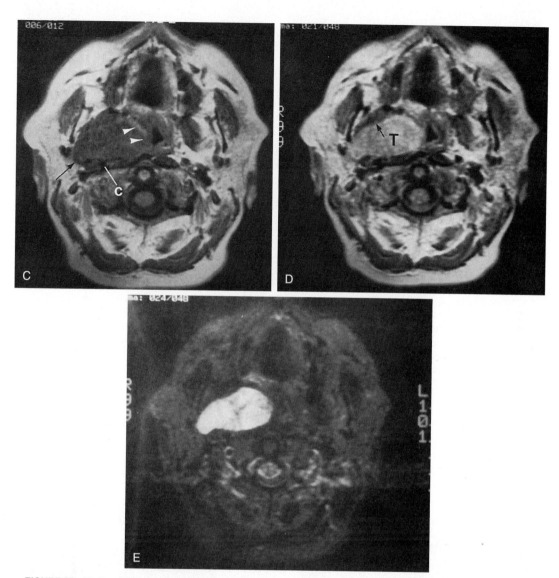

FIGURE 22–10, Cont'd *C,* T1-weighted image of the same tumor shows the tumor pushing parapharyngeal fat *(arrowheads)* medially. The tumor cannot be separated from the medial pterygoid muscle by this pulse sequence, but the lateral margin *(arrow)* is well seen. Note also the ease with which the carotid artery (c) is noted posterior to the lesion. *D,* Proton spin-density image. Early image of a T2-weighted sequence—long repetition time, short echo time—shows the tumor (T) in its relation to the medial pterygoid muscle *(arrow).* The lateral margin cannot be well defined. *E,* Late image of a T2-weighted sequence with long TR and long TE to maximize T2-weighting. The image is less pleasing but shows very distinctly the actual margins of the tumor.

FNAB is best avoided when paraganglioma is suspected because of the potential for bleeding. Whenever the FNAB produces results that do not match the clinical picture, the physician should be suspicious that a sampling error may have occurred. This serves as further indication for excision of the lesion and more complete histologic evaluation.

FNAB may be especially useful in patients with suspected malignant tumors (Fig. 22–14). When clinical findings such as pain, rapid growth, and fixation, together with radiographic evidence of bone destruction, suggest malignancy, the FNAB may aid in confirming the clinical impression and afford valuable information for treatment planning. Such information provides the surgeon the opportunity to better counsel the patient and family preoperatively.

◘ SPECIAL CONSIDERATIONS

Carotid Paraganglioma (Carotid Body Tumor)

Carotid body tumor is the most commonly encountered paraganglioma in the neck. These lesions characteristically originate in the bifurcation of the carotid artery. Angiography demonstrates the classic lyre sign (Fig. 22–15).

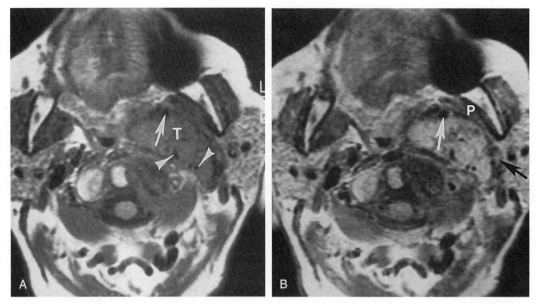

FIGURE 22–11 *A,* Axial T1-weighted image without gadolinium shows the tumor (T) pushing the carotid artery *(arrow)* anteriorly. Flow voids *(arrowheads)* are seen within the tumor, but the styloid process is not visible. *B,* Proton spin-density image shows higher signal within the tumor. The carotid artery *(white arrow)* is better seen, as are the flow voids. The mass is large enough to compress the medial pterygoid muscle (P). The styloid process cannot be clearly identified, but the styloid musculature *(black arrow)* can be identified. Because the tumor passes posterior to the styloid musculature, the location in the poststyloid parapharyngeal space is defined.

Some authors have advocated preoperative angiography and embolization of these lesions in an attempt to reduce intraoperative blood loss. Unfortunately, embolization may result in an intense inflammatory reaction, preventing the subadventitial dissection required for removal of the carotid body tumor. This may increase the risk of inadvertent entry into the carotid artery during tumor removal. Consequently, we do not recommend embolization of carotid body tumors preoperatively.

During removal of carotid paraganglioma, the tumor is mobilized in a subadventitial plane off the common carotid artery. In almost every case, the external carotid artery must

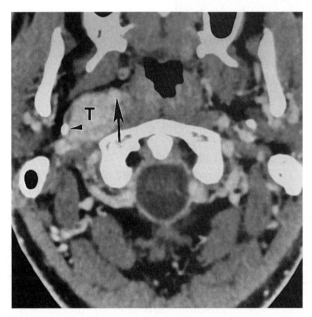

FIGURE 22–12 Glomus vagale tumor: CT with intravenous enhancement. The tumor (T) is seen pushing the carotid artery *(arrow)* anteriorly and medially. The lesion extends posterior to the styloid process *(arrowhead)*, indicating that it is in the poststyloid compartment.

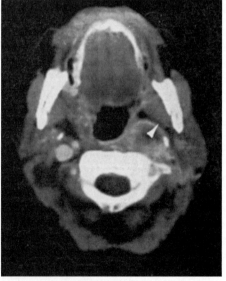

FIGURE 22–13 Metastatic carcinoma of the node of Rouvière. Lateral retropharyngeal node shows a typical poststyloid parapharyngeal mass pushing the parapharyngeal fat anteriorly and laterally *(arrowhead)*. The low-density center, however, strongly suggests metastatic carcinoma. (From Curtin HD: Separation of the masticator space from the parapharyngeal space. Radiology 163:195, 1987.)

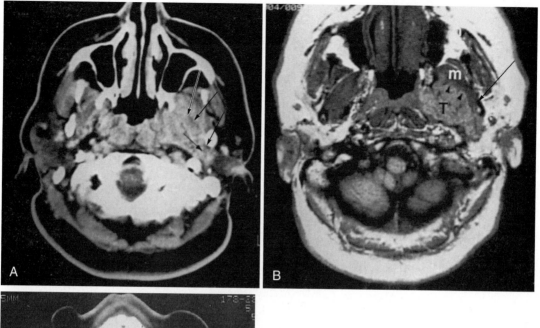

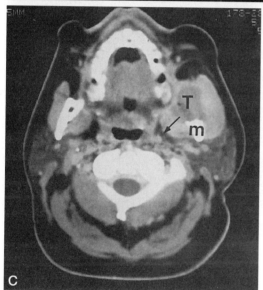

FIGURE 22–14 *A,* Metastatic thyroid carcinoma. The CT scan shows tumor in the parapharyngeal region protruding through the stylomandibular tunnel *(arrows).* The lesion cannot be separated from the medial pterygoid muscle. *B,* T1-weighted image of the same patient shows the tumor (T) with a very different signal intensity from that of the medial pterygoid muscle (m). The margin of the lesion with the muscle is irregular *(arrow),* indicating invasion. *C,* Carcinoma of the retromolar trigone extending into the masticator space with erosion of the mandible. The tumor is anterior and slightly lateral to the parapharyngeal fat. The parapharyngeal fat *(arrow)* is slightly compressed laterally. m, eroded mandible; T, tumor.

be divided as the tumor is "unwrapped" from the common and internal carotid arteries. This allows the surgeon to dissect the tumor off the internal carotid artery and to gain access to the deep extent of the tumor. Reconstruction of the external carotid artery is not required. Great care must be taken to mobilize and preserve the hypoglossal and vagus nerves early in this procedure. At best, these cranial nerves will be lying on the tumor. Sometimes, they actually seem to be embedded in the substance of the tumor. Invasion of the nerve is unusual. Although mobilization is usually possible, injury to the X and XII cranial nerves is always a risk.

The basic tenets of vascular surgery require proximal and distal control of the involved artery. Large carotid body tumors may make distal control of the internal carotid artery at the skull base either difficult or impossible. This possibility must be considered preoperatively. The relationship between the superior aspect of the tumor and the skull base

must be evaluated. Safe dissection requires that the surgeon have a minimum of space (about 1 cm) to effect distal vascular control of the internal carotid artery. In removing a large carotid body tumor in which there is no potential for distal control, preoperative angiography with balloon test occlusion and xenon evaluation of contralateral circulation is essential.[7] Under some circumstances, preoperative elective balloon occlusion of the carotid both proximal and distal to the lesion may be required to afford safe tumor removal. In one series, 5 of 9 patients with tumors larger than 5 cm required carotid ligation or resection and repair.[8] An alternative is to consider vascular reconstruction such as internal carotid artery to middle meningeal artery shunts. Failure to consider this and take the necessary steps preoperatively exposes the patient to the possibility of neurologic injury. Carotid paraganglioma, particularly occurring in the familial form (PGL 1) of the disease, may occasionally be associated with pheochromocytoma or may produce catecholamines.

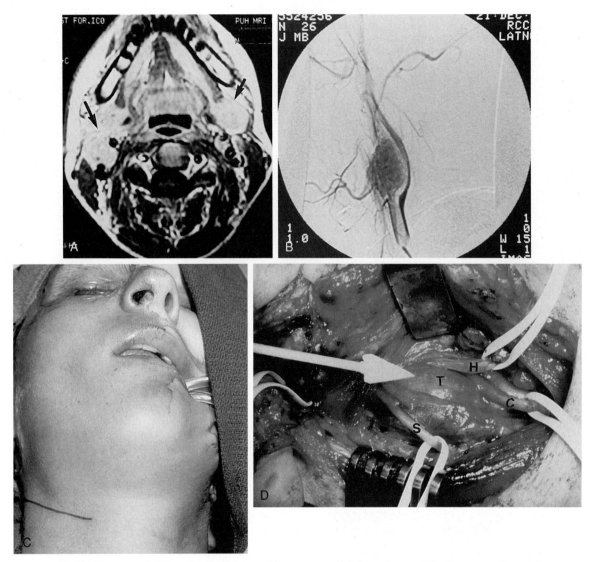

FIGURE 22–15 *A*, MRI scan of a 21-year-old woman with bilateral carotid body tumors (*arrows*). *B*, Angiogram of same patient demonstrates carotid body tumor. *C*, Incision placed in superior natural skinfold. *D*, The operative field, including the tumor (T). The carotid artery (C) and cranial nerves XI (S) and XII (H) have been identified; vessel loops are placed for safety.

Evaluation for urinary catecholamines should be undertaken preoperatively.

Vagal Paraganglioma

Most paragangliomas involving the vagus nerve present in the upper neck. They are fusiform. Contrast-enhanced imaging demonstrates the characteristic lesion with displacement of the internal carotid artery anteriorly and laterally (Fig. 22–16). This finding serves to distinguish the vagal paraganglioma from a carotid body tumor. The most common location is high in the PPS; however, we have observed these tumors anywhere along the vagus and recurrent laryngeal nerves.[9] On occasion, these lesions are very high in the neck, and resection of the mastoid tip or more of the temporal bone may be required to afford exposure at the cranial end.[10] These lesions

are less challenging than the carotid body tumor because the tumor is not attached to the carotid artery and because bleeding should not be excessive. Embolization preoperatively is not routinely necessary (Table 22–4).

Approximately 50% of patients with vagal paraganglioma present with vocal cord paralysis,[9] and 100% will have vocal cord paralysis after resection. We carry out immediate thyroplasty, which prevents aspiration and improves voice quality in most patients.[11] Solitary vagal paraganglioma rarely secretes catecholamines.

Hereditary Paraganglioma

Any patient with multiple paraganglioma or a family history of paraganglioma by definition falls into the category of the familial form of paraganglioma (PGL 1). Through

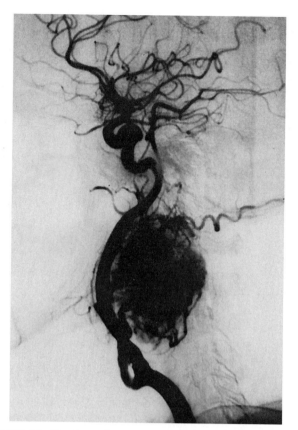

FIGURE 22–16 Carotid arteriography demonstrates a highly vascular lesion displacing the carotid artery anteriorly and laterally. This proved to be a glomus vagale tumor.

TABLE 22–5 Multiple Paraganglioma (n = 10)

Combination	No. of Patients
Vagal + carotid	4
Vagal + bilateral carotid	1
Vagal + vagal	1
Vagal + vagal + glomus	1
Vagal + carotid + tympanicum	1
Vagal + tympanicum	2

Data from Urquhart AC, Johnson JT, Myers EN, et al: Glomus vagale: Paraganglioma of the vagus nerve. Laryngoscope 104:440–445, 1991.

should undergo testing for the *PGL* gene. If a family member does not carry the gene, no further testing is necessary. Those who carry the gene should have an annual MRI of the head, neck, and abdomen.

In the setting of familial paraganglioma, bilateral carotid angiography may help in identification of occult tumors. The development of multiple paraganglioma has important clinical significance. In one series of 19 patients with vagal paraganglioma, 47% had a family history, and multiple paraganglioma was diagnosed in 53% (10 of 19) (Table 22–5). Of the patients with familial vagal paraganglioma, 89% (8 of 9) had multiple paraganglioma.

As noted, removal of vagal paraganglioma results in vocal cord paralysis in 100% of cases. Glossopharyngeal and hypoglossal nerve injury was encountered in 31%. The goal of treatment of paraganglioma is surgical excision. Carotid body tumors are present in 90% of patients with multiple paraganglioma.[13, 14] In some cases, multiple lesions may place both vagus nerves at risk. Many patients with bilateral vagal injury require tracheotomy because of airway obstruction. Unilateral vagal paragangliomas presenting with true vocal cord paralysis should be excised. Contralateral tumors may best be treated with irradiation to decrease the risk to the nerve and to prevent damage to the nerve through further tumor growth. In patients with bilateral carotid body tumors, a staged approach is indicated. The larger tumor is removed first. Subsequent assessment of cranial nerve function will help guide subsequent therapy. Some patients with bilateral carotid sinus denervation experience cardiovascular deregulation.[8] The presence of multiple paraganglioma emphasizes the need for lifelong follow-up.

The concern for malignant potential must be considered in patients with paraganglioma. There is no relation among mitotic activity, perineural or vascular invasion, and clinical course. Malignancy is diagnosed when metastatic deposits occur in lymph nodes or distant sites.[15, 16] It is estimated that malignancy may be encountered in approximately 10% of patients with hereditary paraganglioma. The presence of aneuploidy on flow cytometry has not been useful in predicting malignancy.

Functional paragangliomas that secrete vasoactive substances are unusual. Only four cases have been reported associated with vagal paraganglioma.[17] It has been suggested that functional paraganglioma may be more commonly encountered with hereditary syndrome, and the association of paraganglioma with pheochromocytoma in MEN 2B syndrome is well known. In the setting of elevated catecholamines with an unknown source, the meta-iodinated

genetic analysis of pedigrees of affected families, the pattern of inheritance of familial paraganglioma has been clarified and a gene linked to this disorder has been cloned and sequenced.[12] Therefore, we now have the mechanism by which to screen family members of affected individuals. Analysis of families carrying the *PGL 1* gene reveals germline mutations in the SDHD locus on chromosome 11q23. The *PGL 1* gene is inherited in an autosomal dominant fashion, with incomplete penetrance when transmitted through fathers. The disease does not occur in offspring when transmitted maternally. This inheritance pattern has been observed in all confirmed PGL 1 pedigrees and suggests that there is a sex-specific epigenetic modification consistent with genomic imprinting. We now suggest that the families of all patients with the diagnosis of paraganglioma

TABLE 22–4 Vagal Paragangliomas: Clinical Findings at Initial Presentation (n = 19)

Findings	No. of Patients
Neck mass	19
Vocal cord paralysis	9
Oropharyngeal swelling	3
Cervical adenopathy	0

Data from Urquhart AC, Johnson JT, Myers EN, et al: Glomus vagale: Paraganglioma of the vagus nerve. Laryngoscope 104:440–445, 1991.

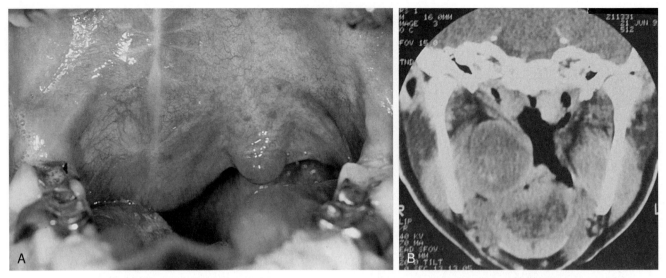

FIGURE 22–17 *A,* Neurilemmoma of the prestyloid PPS. Note the healed incision resulting from previous attempt at transoral excision elsewhere. *B,* CT scan appearance of neurilemmoma in the same patient.

benzylguanidine (MIBG) scan may help localize the secreting tumor.[17–19]

Neurilemmoma (Schwannoma)

Neurilemmoma (schwannoma) is a solitary tumor that may arise from the neuroectodermal sheath of a peripheral nerve.[20] Differentiating schwannoma from carotid body tumors may be difficult on CT scan alone. The presence of flow voids on contrast-enhanced CT suggests paraganglioma. Lack of flow voids suggests schwannoma; however, small paraganglioma may be similar. Angiography is often helpful in making the diagnosis because some neurilemmomas may be vascular on imaging; it is thought that the cell of origin for these lesions is the Schwann cell. In some cases, nerve fibers are draped over the schwannoma and do not pass directly through the lesion, so that it may be possible to dissect the nerve away from the lesion; however, temporary postoperative paresis is commonly encountered. Although recovery of function may be observed, in some cases the schwannoma develops from many smaller nerve fibers within the nerve and is inseparable from the nerve.

Neurilemmomas may demonstrate either an Antoni type A or a type B pattern.[21] Antoni type A describes a cellular pattern of elongated spindle cells. A palisading array of nuclei around a central mass of cytoplasm is called a *Verocay body.* Antoni type B describes the situation in which no distinctive pattern can be recognized and the cells are arranged in a loose myxoid matrix. Many tumors are composed of both patterns with intermittent degenerative and cystic changes. Pleomorphisms with irregular shapes and enlarged nuclei are common and do not imply malignancy.

Neurilemmomas are relatively uncommon in the parapharyngeal space (Fig. 22–17). Neurilemmoma originating from the superior cervical sympathetic ganglion removed by transection of the nerve allows no chance for recovery from Horner's syndrome. When the nerve is preserved intact following tumor removal, there is a chance for recovery. A malignant neurilemmoma (neurogenic sarcoma) is a rare tumor that accounts for approximately 5% of all head and neck sarcomas.[22, 23] Surgery is the treatment of choice but requires removal of the nerve of origin.

Neurofibroma

Neurofibromas are thought to result from Schwann cells. These lesions are most commonly subcutaneous; they may be multiple and are often associated with von Recklinghausen's disease. In contrast to neurilemmoma, the neurofibroma is not encapsulated and the nerve fibers are incorporated within the tumor. From a practical point of view, the nerve trunk may not be preserved during tumor removal.

Von Recklinghausen's Disease

The autosomal dominant disorder von Recklinghausen's disease occurs in 1 in 3000 births.[21]

Only 50% of cases have a positive family history. This suggests low penetrance of the gene. Five or more café au lait spots, characterized by light-brown cutaneous macules 1.5 cm or greater in diameter, is considered diagnostic.[24] Spina bifida, glioma, and other neurologic abnormalities may be observed. Cutaneous neurofibromas are the most common of these abnormalities. The cranial nerves may be affected. The optic and acoustic nerves are most commonly seen to be involved with neurofibromatosis type 2. Malignancy is less often encountered in patients with solitary neurofibroma than in those with von Recklinghausen's disease. Sarcoma is reported in 6% to 16% of patients with von Recklinghausen's disease.[25–27] Invasion of adjacent tissue or metastasis is the clearest indication of malignancy. Histologic criteria such as nuclear atypia and mitoses are less reliable. Some pathologists will not make a diagnosis of malignant neurofibroma unless the patient has von Recklinghausen's disease.

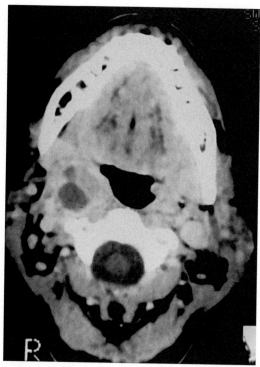

FIGURE 22–18 CT scan of patient with malignant schwannoma originating from superior cervical ganglion.

Malignant Fibromas

Malignancy occurs in about 10% of patients with von Recklinghausen's disease. Less commonly, malignant neurofibroma is encountered in patients with solitary neurofibroma. Invasion of adjacent tissue, or metastasis, is an indication of malignancy (Fig. 22–18). Other histologic criteria such as nuclear atypia and mitoses are less reliable. Malignant neurofibroma may be histologically indistinguishable from fibrosarcoma except for the relationship of the neurofibroma to a nerve trunk. Many pathologists will not make a diagnosis of malignant neurofibroma unless the patient has von Recklinghausen's disease.

◘ TREATMENT

The natural course of a disease is of foremost importance when treatment strategies are considered. Paragangliomas of the head and neck generally have an indolent growth pattern.[28] The progression of these tumors may lead to paralysis of cranial nerves. Some patients, particularly those with multiple paraganglioma, will die of diffuse metastasis.

Surgical intervention has greatly improved over the past decades. It is clear that surgery carries with it the potential for complications and adverse effects. For instance, removal of paraganglioma associated with the vagus nerve is associated with 100% incidence of permanent vocal cord paralysis. Modern phonosurgical techniques have rendered this a relatively limited problem.[11] Removal of paraganglioma involving the carotid bifurcation is associated with risk to the vagus and hypoglossal nerves and with a low but real risk of cerebrovascular accident. A large paraganglioma involving the jugular foramen may require a combined skull base approach, which places multiple cranial nerves (e.g., IX, X, XI, XII) at risk. Therefore, the risk of serious complications as a result of treatment remains an important factor in treatment decision making for individual patients and must be weighed against the natural course of these tumors.[28]

A recent article showed little benefit for surgery in paragangliomas occurring at the base of the skull.[29] In this series, all patients, regardless of whether they underwent surgery, had a life expectancy that was close to normal, whereas the group of patients who underwent surgery developed the greatest number of complications. For this reason, the authors became more cautious when performing surgery for vagal and glomus jugulare tumors and have acquired a large amount of follow-up imaging data.

Jansen and associates recently studied 48 untreated head and neck paragangliomas to calculate the tumor doubling times.[28] A large number of these patients had hereditary paragangliomas. Twenty-six patients studied had a total of 48 paragangliomas—20 of the carotid body, 17 of the vagal body, and 11 of the jugular tympanic bodies. The follow-up period ranged from 1 to 8 years with a median of 4.2 years. In 10 cases, the volume was unchanged, but in two tumors, a slight decrease in volume was estimated. A volume increase of greater than 20% was noted in 29 paragangliomas (60%), and these tumors were considered to be growing. The authors also observed that only 44% of the very small paragangliomas were growing compared with 75% of the tumors of intermediate size. The authors draw similarity to the clinical behavior of vestibular schwannomas (acoustic neuromas), which present similar problems with potential surgical complications. The authors conclude that the natural course of paragangliomas described in their study justifies a "watch and wait" policy for these tumors.

Radiation therapy has been used over the years for patients who either are old and firmly inoperable or do not wish to have surgery. Recently, Evenson and colleagues studied 15 patients with 23 paragangliomas (either carotid body or glomus vagale) who were treated with radiation therapy at the University of Florida between 1981 and 1995.[30] The local control rates at 10 years calculated by the Kaplan-Meier method were 96% for the overall group of 23 tumors, and 100% for the subset of 22 tumors that had not been previously irradiated. The 10-year cause-specific survival rate was 89% for all 15 patients, and 100% for the 14 patients who had received no previous radiation therapy. The authors concluded that irradiation offers a high probability of tumor control with relatively minimal risk for patients with carotid body and glomus vagale tumors. One must, however, look at these results in light of the paper by Jansen and coworkers, which indicates that many of these tumors would not have grown even if they had not been irradiated.[28] Therefore, one must be somewhat circumspect about the treatment of these patients with radiation therapy. One would think that these tumors, especially the smaller ones, may be monitored by imaging studies and irradiated only when growth is demonstrated.

Removal of neuromas and schwannomas that arise from the cervical sympathetic chain or cranial nerves is frequently, but not always, associated with permanent injury to the nerve of origin. Schwannomas may sometimes be dissected off the nerve with preservation of the main nerve trunk. Under this circumstance, some recovery of function may occur. Removal of prestyloid parapharyngeal space lesions is almost always indicated; however, procedures directed at these lesions often put the facial nerve at some risk.

Surgical Approach

The choice of surgical approach and subsequent technique for tumor removal necessarily reflects the anatomic location and suspected pathology. As always, previous experience and expert interpretation of the images are essential if success is to be attained.

Transoral Approach

A transoral/transmucosal approach has been reported for removal of small, isolated pleomorphic adenomas that originate from a minor salivary gland in the soft palate or lateral pharyngeal wall,[31] but it has the disadvantages of limited exposure and lack of opportunity to control the great vessels. Transoral/transmucosal biopsy or partial removal is not encouraged because this contaminates the pharyngeal mucosa and complicates subsequent removal.

Transcervical Submandibular Approach

The transcervical submandibular approach is ideally suited to tumors in the prestyloid parapharyngeal space that have no relationship to the parotid gland. This anatomic location is best confirmed by MRI or CT and suggests a neoplasm arising in the prestyloid PPS that is separated from the deep lobe of the parotid gland by an intact fat plane. A submandibular incision beginning at approximately the

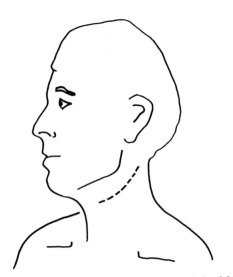

FIGURE 22–19 A horizontal incision in a normal skinfold allows exploration of the parapharyngeal space.

mastoid tip and carried in a natural horizontal skin crease to the lateral aspect of the larynx is developed (Fig. 22–19). Skin flaps are elevated for identification and preservation of the marginal branch of the facial nerve. The posterior border of the digastric muscle is identified, and the adjacent facial artery is divided and ligated. This allows the submandibular gland to be retracted anteriorly (Fig. 22–20). The parapharyngeal space is entered just anterior and deep to the posterior belly of the digastric muscle. Tumors are then dissected out bluntly and removed. The defect is drained and the wound closed.

Transcervical Transparotid Approach

A majority of tumors in the prestyloid PPS require formal identification and preservation of the main trunk of the facial nerve. These lesions are characterized by CT or MRI and usually represent pleomorphic adenomas arising in the deep lobe of the parotid gland. Some smaller tumors may lie just medial to the facial nerve. Others have deeply expanded into the PPS, displacing the palatine tonsil and lateral pharyngeal wall toward the midline.

A modified Blair incision is begun in the preauricular skin crease and is carried around the earlobe and then extended into a horizontal skin crease in the neck to the level of the submandibular gland (Fig. 22–21). The flaps are elevated as in parotidectomy. The external auditory canal, the anterior border of the sternocleidomastoid muscle, and the posterior belly of the digastric muscle are used as landmarks for identification of the main trunk of the facial nerve as it exits the stylomastoid foramen. The tumor is ordinarily identified just deep to the facial nerve (Fig. 22–22). The branches of the facial nerve are then identified and dissected off the capsule of the tumor. The submandibular gland is displaced as described previously. The tumor is then mobilized in a three-dimensional manner from the parotidectomy wound and the submandibular space and is removed. Retraction on the facial nerve must be done very gently to avoid temporary facial paresis. Transection of the stylomandibular ligament and anterior dislocation of the mandible may greatly increase exposure. The lateral lobe of the parotid gland may be pedicled anteriorly and replaced to effect a better cosmetic result. A suction drain is brought out through the skin posterior to the incision.

Transcervical Approach

The transcervical approach is used for excising tumors of the poststyloid space.[5] An incision is made in the most superior major skin crease of the neck. After the flaps have been elevated and the ramus mandibularis has been identified and protected, direct access to the poststyloid space is gained without the need to dissect the submandibular triangle. This has been ideally used in patients with paragangliomas and schwannomas. It also has the distinct advantage of providing excellent cosmesis.

Mandibulotomy Approach

An alternative approach to the poststyloid parapharyngeal space is to perform an anterior mandibulotomy.[32–34]

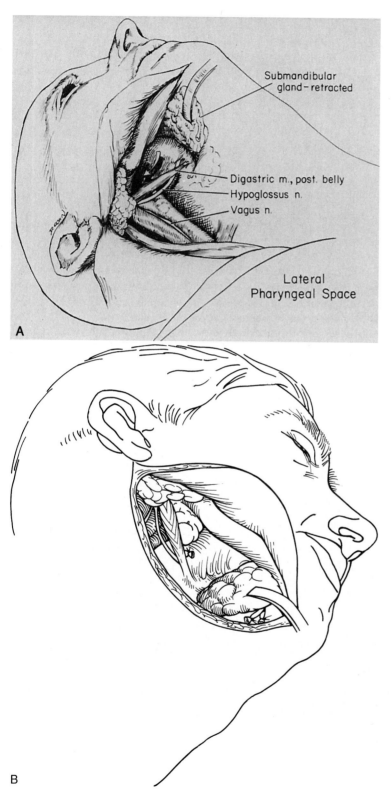

Submandibular
gland–retracted

Digastric m., post. belly
Hypoglossus n.
Vagus n.

Lateral
Pharyngeal Space

A

B

FIGURE 22–20 *A*, Artist's depiction of the PPS. The submandibular gland has been retracted anteriorly as the posterior belly of the digastric muscle is retracted inferiorly. (From Rabuzzi DD, Johnson JT: Diagnosis and Management of Deep Neck Infections. Washington, DC, American Academy of Otolaryngology–Head and Neck Surgery Foundation, 1976.) *B*, Following ligation of the external branch of the facial artery, the submandibular gland is retracted anteriorly; the parapharyngeal space tumor is visible just in front of the posterior belly of the digastric muscle. (From Myers EN, Carrau RL, Cass SP, et al [eds]: Operative Otolaryngology–Head and Neck Surgery. Philadelphia, WB Saunders, 1997.)

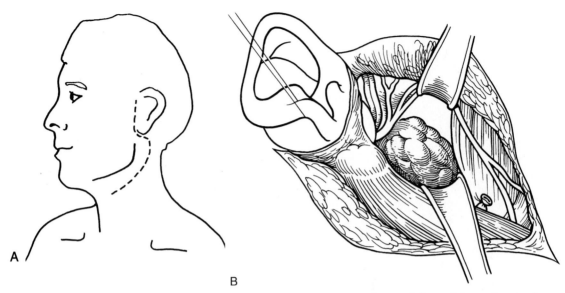

FIGURE 22-21 *A*, The horizontal submandibular incision is carried around the earlobe and up to the preauricular skin to afford exposure for superficial parotidectomy and simultaneous removal of a deep-lobe parotid tumor. *B*, Subsequent to superficial parotidectomy, the facial nerve can be elevated and protected while the deep-lobe tumor is removed. Note that the exposure is obtained just anterior to the posterior belly of the digastric muscle. (From Myers EN, Carrau RL, Cass SP, et al [eds]: Operative Otolaryngology–Head and Neck Surgery. Philadelphia, WB Saunders, 1997.)

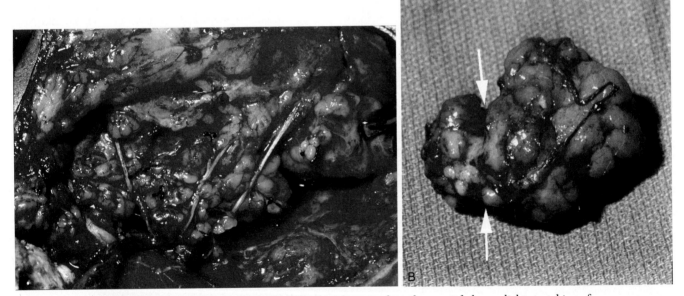

FIGURE 22-22 *A*, Surgical photograph. The lateral approach to the parotid shows slight stretching of the facial nerve. The tumor is not directly visible but is covered by a small amount of remaining parotid tissue. (Courtesy of Eugene Meyers, MD.) *B*, Photograph of a gross specimen shows the slightly lobulated surface as well as a constriction (*white arrows*) made by the stylomandibular tunnel. (Courtesy of Eugene Myers, MD.)

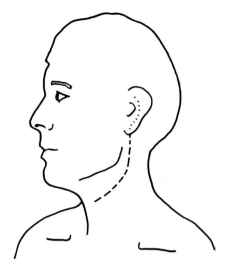

FIGURE 22–23 Transmastoid-transcervical excision of jugular bulb tumors may be done by employing a postauricular-cervical incision, which allows the surgeon to follow the facial nerve out of the mastoid, subsequent to which the mastoid tip can be taken down. Removal of the transverse process of the second cervical vertebra affords improved exposure to the vagus in this area.

The mucosa is then divided through the floor of the mouth, affording a direct but long approach to the poststyloid PPS. At the completion of the procedure, the mucosa of the floor of the mouth is closed, the osteotomy is repaired with a plating system, and a tracheotomy is carried out. We have not found this technique necessary for access to these tumors, and the morbidity involved rarely justifies the theoretical increased exposure.

Extended Approaches

A variety of approaches may be employed in performing more extended procedures. For instance, paragangliomas that extend into the jugular foramen would require a transmastoid approach to effect total removal (Fig. 22–23). Anterior transposition of the facial nerve out of the facial canal or division and repair of the facial nerve may be required as a necessary component of this approach.

Malignancies that involve the ascending ramus of the mandible or the posterior aspect of the maxilla might require a lateral approach, including resection of the mandible and infratemporal fossa dissection, or an anterior approach that includes maxillectomy. Comprehensive discussion of these specialized techniques is beyond the scope of this chapter.

◼ SUMMARY

Treatment of patients with tumors of the parapharyngeal space remains a very challenging area in head and neck surgery. New understanding of patterns of inheritance seen with hereditary paraganglioma offers the potential for improved screening of family members. Modern imaging, balloon occlusion testing, and xenon blood flow studies contribute to our ability to diagnosis and plan treatment. The evolution of surgical approaches to these tumors has contributed immeasurably to improved outcomes.

REFERENCES

1. Heeneman H, Johnson JT, Curtin HD, et al: The Parapharyngeal Space: Anatomy and Pathologic Conditions with Emphasis on Neurogenous Tumors, 2nd ed. Washington, DC, American Academy of Otolaryngology—Head and Neck Surgery Foundation, 1987.
2. Som PM, Biller HF, Lawson W, et al: Pharyngeal space masses: An updated protocol based upon 104 cases. Radiology 153:149–156, 1984.
3. Pensak ML, Gluckman JL, Shumrick K: Pharyngeal space tumors: An algorithm for evaluation and management. Laryngoscope 104: 1170–1173, 1994.
4. Olsen KD: Tumor and surgery of the parapharyngeal space. Laryngoscope 104(suppl 63):1–28, 1994.
5. Carrau RL, Myers EN, Johnson JT: Management of tumors arising in the parapharyngeal space. Laryngoscope 100:583–589, 1990.
6. Lev MH, Khanduja K, Morris PP, Curtin HD: Parotid pleomorphic adenomas: Delayed CT enhancement. AJNR Am J Neuroradiol 19:1835–1839, 1998.
7. De Vries EJ, Sekhar LN, Horton JA, et al: A new method to predict safe resection of the internal carotid artery. Laryngoscope 100:85–88, 1990.
8. Netterville JL, Reilly KM, Robertson D, et al: Carotid body tumors: A review of 30 patients with 46 tumors. Laryngoscope 105:115–126, 1995.
9. Urquhart AC, Johnson JT, Myers EN, et al: Glomus vagale: Paraganglioma of the vagus nerve. Laryngoscope 104:440–445, 1991.
10. Black FO, Myers EN, Parnes SM: Surgical management of vagal chemodectoma. Laryngoscope 87:1259, 1977.
11. Netterville JL, Jackson CG, Civantos F: Thyroplasty in the functional rehabilitation of neurotologic skull base surgery patients. Am J Otolaryngol 14:460–464, 1993.
12. Baysal BE, Ferrell RE, Willett-Brozick JE, et al: Mutations in SDHD, a mitochondrial complex II gene, in hereditary paraganglioma. Science 287:848–851, 2000.
13. Parkin J: Familial multiple glomus tumors and pheochromocytomas. Ann Otolaryngol 90:60–63, 1981.
14. Lawson W: Glomus bodies and tumors. NY State J Med 80: 1567–1577, 1980.
15. Hamberger CA, Hamberger CB, Wesall J, et al: Malignant catecholamine-producing tumor of the carotid body. Acta Pathol Microbiol Scand 69:489, 1967.
16. Strauss M, Nicholas GG, Abt AB, et al: Malignant catecholamine-secreting carotid body paraganglioma. Otolaryngol Head Neck Surg 91:315, 1983.
17. Karusseit VOL, Lodder JF: Functioning vagal body tumor. Br J Surg 74:1184–1185, 1987.
18. Sandler MD: The expanding role of MIBG in clinical medicine. J Nucl Med 29:1457–1459, 1988.
19. Carrau RL, Johnson JT, Myers EN: Management of tumors of the parapharyngeal space. Oncology 11:633–642, 1997.
20. Prasad S, Myers EN, Kamerer DB, et al: Neurilemmoma (schwannoma) of the facial nerve presenting as a parotid mass. Otolaryngol Head Neck Surg 108:76–79, 1993.
21. Kapadia SB: Tumors of the nervous system. In Barnes EL (ed): Surgical Pathology of the Head and Neck, 2nd ed. New York, Marcel Dekker, 2001, pp 787–888.
22. Hamza A, Fagan JJ, Weissman JL, et al: Neurilemmoma of the parapharyngeal space. Arch Otolaryngol Head Neck Surg 123: 622–626, 1997.
23. Conley J. Janecka IP: Neurilemmoma of the head and neck. Trans Am Acad Ophthalmol Otolaryngol Soc 80:459–464, 1975.
24. Fienman NL, Yakovac WC: Neurofibromatosis in childhood. J Pediatr 76:339, 1970.
25. Heard G: Malignant disease in von Recklinghausen's neurofibromatosis. Proc R Soc Med 56:402, 1963.
26. Holt JF, Wright EM: Radiologic features of neurofibromatosis. Radiology 51:647, 1948.

27. Preston FW, Walsh WS, Clarke TH: Cutaneous neurofibromatosis (von Recklinghausen's disease): Clinical manifestations and incidence of sarcoma in 61 male patients. Arch Surg 64:813, 1952.

28. Jansen JC, van den Berg R, Julper A, et al: Estimation of growth rate in patients with head and neck paraganglioma influences the treatment proposal. Cancer 88:2811–2816, 2000.

29. van der May AG, Frijns JH, Cornelisse CJ, et al: Does intervention improve the natural course of glomus tumors? A series of 106 patients seen in a 32-year period. Ann Otol Rhinol Laryngol 101:635–642, 1992.

30. Evenson LJ, Mendenhall WM, Parsons JT, Cassisi NJ: Radiotherapy in the management of chemodectomas of the carotid body and glomus vagale. Head Neck 20:609–613, 1998.

31. Goodwin WJ Jr, Chandler JR: Transoral excision of lateral parapharyngeal space tumors presenting intraorally. Laryngoscope 98:266–269, 1988.

32. Baker DC, Conley J: Treatment of massive deep lobe parotid tumors. Am J Surg 138:572–575, 1977.

33. Attia EL, Bentley KC, Head T, et al: A new external approach to the pterygomaxillary fossa and parapharyngeal space. Head Neck Surg 6:884–891, 1984.

34. Biller HF, Shugar JMA, Krespi YP: A new technique for wide-field exposure of the base of the skull. Arch Otolaryngol 107:698–802, 1981.

CHAPTER 23

Cancer of the Ear and Temporal Bone

Randall L. Breau
John L. Dornhoffer

INTRODUCTION

Malignant neoplasms involving the temporal bone are relatively rare, occurring in 1 in every 5000 to 1 in every 20,000 ear disorders.[1] These tumors may be broadly categorized into those involving the auricle and external auditory canal or temporal bone primarily, and those involving the temporal bone caused by local extension or distant spread. The most common malignancies in the first category are sun-induced basal and squamous cell carcinomas involving the auricle.[2–6] Malignancies arise less commonly from the external auditory canal, middle ear, and temporal bone and constitute a broad range of pathologic subtypes, including squamous cell carcinoma, basal cell carcinoma, melanoma, and various adenocarcinomas and sarcomas.[2] Temporal bone malignancies due to local extension from surrounding areas include those from the parotid gland, the temporomandibular joint, and the skin in the preauricular and postauricular regions.[3, 4, 7, 8] In addition, cancer of the nasopharynx may rarely extend up the eustachian tube into the middle ear space.[5, 9, 10] The temporal bone may also be involved with metastasis from tumors arising in more distant sites, including the breast, lung, kidney, and prostate.[11]

Malignant tumors of the ear and temporal bone often present in a subtle manner, which may delay diagnosis and present a significant diagnostic and therapeutic challenge. This chapter discusses the various histologic subtypes, with specific emphasis on preoperative planning and use of the multidisciplinary team approach in the treatment of these rare and complex tumors.

ANATOMY

The Auricle and External Auditory Canal

Although an in-depth discussion of temporal bone anatomy is beyond the scope of this chapter, certain anatomic relationships should be noted in a discussion of malignancies of the ear. Most malignancies of the temporal bone arise from the external ear and are related to sun exposure. The pinna and external canal in combination are considered to be the external ear. The pinna is composed of fibrocartilage that is enveloped by perichondrium and skin. This tissue tends to be tightly bound except at the attachment to the skull, where an additional loose alveolar tissue is found between the skin and the perichondrium. The lateral third of the external auditory canal is likewise composed of fibrocartilage and skin and is relatively insensitive to manipulation. The medial external auditory canal is bony and is lined by skin that is tightly adherent; it terminates at the skin-covered tympanic membrane. This area tends to be exquisitely sensitive.

Although this anatomic division of the external auditory canal may seem arbitrary, it is significant in the diagnosis and treatment of malignancies in this region. Skin adenexal structures, and tumors arising from them, predominate on the pinna and the lateral third of the external auditory canal. Furthermore, significant pain associated with a lesion of the external auditory canal suggests involvement of the bone of the medial canal. Finally, one must be acutely aware of potential preformed pathways in the external auditory canal that allow tumor spread anteriorly and along the skull base. The fissures of Santorini, found in the cartilage of the lateral external auditory canal, provide a potential pathway for tumor spread into the parotid gland, and a bony dehiscence known as the foramen of Huschke is frequently present in the medial portion of the external canal, allowing potential tumor spread to the temporomandibular joint and the skull base. The lymphatics of the external ear drain to the preauricular nodes of the parotid gland, the mastoid, and the subdigastric lymph nodes, which ultimately drain into the jugular chain of lymph nodes.

The Middle Ear

The anatomy of the middle ear is well known from a functional aspect and from the surgical management of otitis media; however, it is conceptually different from an oncologic perspective. Primary malignancies of the middle ear and mastoid are very rare, with most tumors in this region extending from the external ear. From this standpoint, the middle ear represents a potential space, or buffer, between the external ear and structures on its medial wall.

The tympanic membrane and mastoid cortex are lateral; the otic capsule, facial nerve, and great vessels are medial; and the eustachian tube is anterior. The mucosa of the middle ear is cuboidal epithelium, interspersed with secretory cells.

Adjacent Anatomy

An anatomic knowledge of adjacent structures is likewise essential in the surgical management of temporal bone malignancies. The sternocleidomastoid and digastric muscles attach to the tip of the mastoid process. The jugular vein and cranial nerves IX, X, and XI pass through the jugular foramen, which is located medial to these muscles. Medial to the jugular foramen is the styloid process. The carotid artery enters the temporal bone through the carotid canal just medial to the styloid process and anterior to the jugular foramen. Cranial nerve VII exits the stylomastoid foramen just anterior to the digastric notch and courses anteriorly through the parotid gland (Fig. 23–1). Anterior to

the lateral external auditory canal is the parotid gland, and more medially are the temporomandibular joint, the bony external auditory canal, and the carotid artery at the level of the middle ear (Fig. 23–2). Surgical extirpation of these structures can be extremely difficult, making anterior lesions some of the most dangerous to treat. The middle fossa of the skull, located superiorly, is a challenging area, not so much for its anatomic complexity but because of its close proximity to the middle ear and external auditory canal. The tegmen tympani, typically very thin (<1 mm), is found in the region of the epitympanum and mastoid and offers little barrier to intracranial tumor spread once bony erosion occurs superiorly in the external canal. Posteriorly and inferiorly are found the mastoid process and, further posteriorly, the sigmoid sinus. This area is well known to otologists and serves as an "anatomic buffer" to the posterior fossa. Because of this buffer, posterior lesions frequently offer a reasonable surgical margin for tumor removal with preservation of function. The otic capsule, facial nerve,

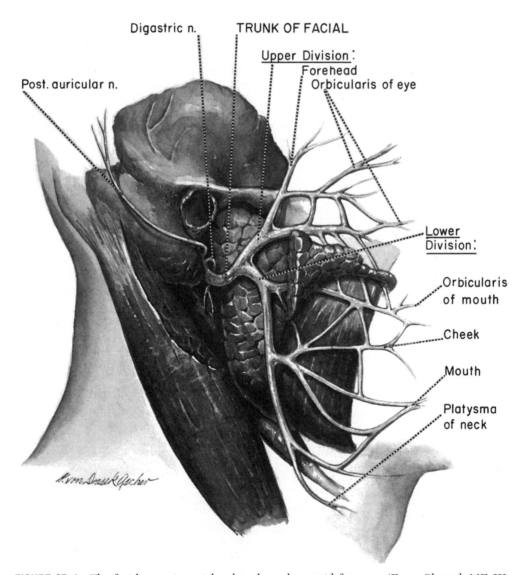

FIGURE 23–1 The facial nerve is peripheral to the stylomastoid foramen. (From Glassock ME III, Shambaugh GE Jr: Surgery of the Ear, 4th ed. Philadelphia, WB Saunders, 1990.)

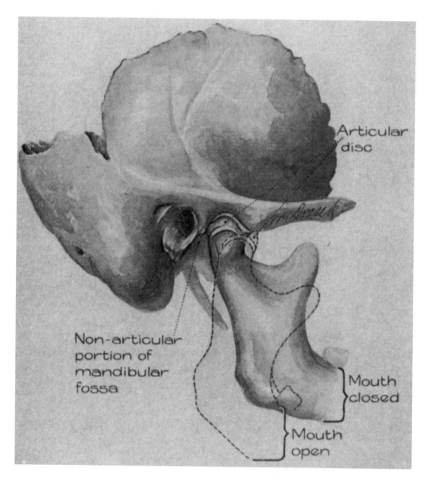

FIGURE 23–2 Mandibular joint closed and open in relation to the osseous meatus. (From Glassock ME III, Shambaugh GE Jr: Surgery of the Ear, 4th ed. Philadelphia, WB Saunders, 1990.)

jugular bulb, and carotid artery are medial. Although the otic capsule is itself a buffer to tumor spread and can be sacrificed with the facial nerve as part of the surgical margin, anterior involvement of the carotid artery and eustachian tube tends toward a poor prognosis.

PATHOLOGY

Primary Cancers of the Auricle

Neoplasms of the auricle represent 50% to 70% of all malignancies of the ear,[2, 12] with those spreading to the temporal bone representing 20% of all malignancies of the temporal bone.[1, 2, 12] These neoplasms usually occur in the fifth or sixth decade of life and are much more common among men,[4] which is likely a result of greater occupational exposure among men (e.g., farming). Excessive sun exposure is the most significant risk factor, with a history of frostbite also mentioned as a possible cause.[2, 4]

Opinions vary as to the most common histologic subtype for cancer of the auricle. A review of multiple series totaling 780 patients reports that 55% of malignancies of the auricle were squamous cell and 40% were basal cell carcinoma.[13] Other series have reported a higher incidence of melanoma or basal cell carcinoma in this subset of patients.[1, 4] The helix is the most frequent site for squamous cell carcinoma of the auricle, but other sites may also be involved, including the retroauricular sulcus, antihelix, tragus, concha, lobule, and antitragus.[14, 15] In contrast to squamous cell carcinoma, basal cell carcinoma infrequently involves the helix or lateral aspect of the auricle. The most common locations for basal cell carcinoma on or around the pinna are believed to be the postauricular, retroauricular, and preauricular areas.

Primary Cancers of the External Canal

Squamous cell carcinoma is the most common malignant tumor involving the external auditory canal, with several series reporting the incidence at 60% or greater.[3] It is more common among females, with an incidence of 2:1 over males.[3] The cause of squamous cell carcinoma of the external auditory canal is unknown. Exposure to ultraviolet (UV) radiation is an unlikely cause owing to the lack of sun exposure in this area. Some have suggested that recurrent or chronic ear infections may play a significant causative role in these malignancies.[3] Approximately half of patients with cancer of the external auditory canal and middle ear have a history of chronic or recurrent ear infections with otorrhea.[16–21] Lodge and associates suggested that chronic otitis might promote the development of cancer of the external auditory cancer in a manner analogous to the development of squamous cell carcinoma of the skin adjacent to draining sinuses, which results from chronic osteomyelitis (Marjolin's ulcers).[22] Some authors suggested exposure to aflatoxin, a product of *Aspergillus* species, as an etiologic factor; exposure to ionizing radiation has also been implicated in a small number of cases of squamous cell carcinoma involving the temporal bone.[23, 24]

Adenomatous malignancies of the external auditory canal are much less common, with studies reporting the incidence at approximately 20%.[4] Most series suggest that adenoid cystic carcinoma is the most common malignancy of glandular origin found in the external auditory canal.[4, 25–28] Even though the derivation of these tumors is unclear, Pulec suggested that they arise from ceruminous glands or ducts.[27] Microscopically, the neoplastic epithelial elements contain little cytoplasm and possess regular nuclei. The cells may take on varied arrangements, including cords, festoons, solid nests, or glandular elements. Extreme variations can be seen in the character of the interstitial stroma. Four distinct tumor patterns have been described—cribriform or classic, tubuloglandular, solid cellular, and hyaline or cylindromatous. Both sexes are equally affected by this tumor, with a mean age of presentation in the 40s.[15]

Adenomas and pleomorphic adenomas are benign tumors that may also arise in the external auditory canal. Adenocarcinomas are distinguished from adenomas by the degree of histologic invasion and may range from well-differentiated to poorly differentiated tumors. Other neoplasms occur more rarely, with melanoma having the highest incidence of these remaining primary tumors of the external auditory canal.[4]

Primary Cancers of the Middle Ear

Neoplasms of the middle ear have no sex predilection and have a much wider and younger age distribution than do external canal or auricular cancers. These usually present during the fourth decade of life; however, 20% of cases occur in patients younger than 20 years of age, and 16% of those cases occur in children younger than 10 years of age.[4] Squamous cell carcinomas account for a majority of these neoplasms and may range from well-differentiated to poorly differentiated types. Well-differentiated cancers demonstrate less nuclear atypia, with keratin pearls easily found throughout. Poorly differentiated cancer may be difficult to diagnose and may require special immunologic stains. The cause of these malignancies is unclear but is thought to be similar to factors involved in cancer of the external auditory canal. Although squamous cell carcinoma accounts for a majority of the neoplasms involving the middle ear in adults, sarcomas such as rhabdomyosarcoma are largely responsible for the cases found in younger patients. In fact, 10% of all cases of rhabdomyosarcoma occur in the ear.[29]

Secondary Neoplasms

Tumors may erode into the temporal bone from surrounding sites. These include tumors of the parotid gland (either by direct extension or by perineural invasion), temporomandibular joint, and skin in the preauricular and postauricular regions.[3, 4, 7, 8] In addition, in rare cases, nasopharyngeal carcinoma may extend up the eustachian tube into the middle ear space or may involve the temporal bone by direct extension.[5, 9, 10] The World Health Organization has classified nasopharyngeal carcinoma into three groups—squamous cell carcinoma (keratinizing squamous cell carcinoma), nonkeratinizing carcinoma, and undifferentiated carcinoma. From microscopic appearance, the first and third categories are descriptively correct. The second category includes carcinomas that do not yet produce keratin and are not always undifferentiated.[30, 31]

Chordomas are dysontogenetic neoplasms originating from the embryonic notochord that may also involve the temporal bone secondarily. These tumors occur most often in patients between the ages of 20 and 40 years, are more common among men than women, and typically involve the head and neck. Grossly, the tumor is lobulated, partially translucent, mucoid, and often nonencapsulated. Histologically, there are no absolute features of chordomas; however, the following four findings are fairly consistent: (1) The overall arrangement of cells in the neoplasm is lobular; (2) the cells tend to grow in cords, in irregular bands, or in pseudoacinar form; (3) a large amount of mucinous matrix is seen; and (4) large physaliphorous and vacuolated cells are present.[15]

Metastatic Neoplasms

Metastatic disease involving the temporal bone is uncommon and usually results from hematogenous spread of the primary tumor. Berlinger and colleagues reported the five routes of metastatic tumor spread to the temporal bone as (1) an isolated metastasis from a distinct primary tumor, (2) a direct extension from an original primary tumor, (3) meningeal carcinomatosis, (4) a leptomeningeal extension from an intracranial primary tumor, and (5) a leukemic or lymphomatous infiltration.[32] Proctor and Lindsay reported that the marrow of the petrosa is capable of filtering out tumor cells circulating in the bloodstream, which leads to metastatic deposits in this region.[33] In a review of 165 cases of cancer metastatic to the temporal bone, the most common primary sites were breast (29%), lung (11%), prostate (8%), unknown primary (8%), and kidney (6%).[3, 11]

A study by Nelson and Hinojosa reported data on 60 temporal bones from 33 patients with metastasis to the temporal bone.[34] They found that specific metastatic tumor location in the temporal bone was dependent on the mode of malignant spread. Metastasis due to hematogenous spread commonly involved the petrous apex; tumors that metastasized to the meninges involved the temporal bone by invasion of the internal auditory canal; and direct extension of tumors of the head and neck to the temporal bone most often involved the petrous apex and the foramen lacerum.[34] Schuknecht and associates noted that direct neoplastic invasion occurred among potential clefts and anatomic plains or within natural passages, such as the eustachian tube, the carotid canal, and the internal auditory canals.[35] Schuknecht and coworkers[35] and El Fiky and Paparella[36] found that metastatic lesions tended to be histologically less differentiated than the primary tumor. Metastasis to the external auditory canal has also been described in rare instances.[37]

INCIDENCE

Cancer of the temporal bone is a relatively rare disease, present in approximately 1 in 5000 to 1 in 20,000 ear disorders.[1] The age-adjusted yearly incidence is approximately 1 in 1,000,000 for women and 0.8 in 1,000,000 for men.[38] In several large series, approximately 60% to 70% of malignancies of the ear involved the auricle, 20% to 30% involved the external auditory canal, and 10% involved the middle ear and mastoid.[4, 6]

CLINICAL PRESENTATION

Primary Cancers of the Temporal Bone

The specific clinical presentation of cancer of the temporal bone depends on the site of the primary. Squamous cell carcinoma of the auricle usually appears as an ulcerative lesion with significant surrounding actinic changes that are prone to bleeding. Pain becomes a more common presenting symptom once bone or cartilage is involved. Basal cell carcinoma of the auricle may present as either a nodular lesion or plaque. These lesions tend to be firm and thick, compared with surrounding normal skin, and are relatively nontender.

Cancer of the external auditory canal and middle ear often presents with otalgia associated with sanguineous drainage. The lesion is frequently granular in appearance, although it may present as an ulcer in the skin reaching to the periosteum of the bony portion of the canal. These lesions are often confused with otitis externa; therefore, a high level of suspicion should be maintained and a biopsy performed if the patient fails to respond to medical management, or if there is any doubt as to the nature of the lesion.[39] A review of the literature on the frequency of presenting signs and symptoms in a combined population of 442 patients with cancer of the external auditory canal and temporal bone reported that otorrhea and otalgia were the most common presenting symptoms (Table 23–1).[3] The quality of the pain was described as chronic, dull, and deep-seated. Other less common presenting symptoms included hearing loss (29%), facial palsy (16%), and vertigo (15%). A majority of the patients (approximately 82%) had squamous cell carcinoma.

Metastases or Secondary Involvement of the Temporal Bone

The diagnosis of nasopharyngeal carcinoma secondarily involving the temporal bone usually occurs late in the disease because patients remain asymptomatic until the tumor grows to significant proportions. In fact, the tumor is often diagnosed after the patient discovers a metastatic lymph node in the neck. Another potential symptom is the presence of otitis media with effusion.

Review of the literature indicates that there are no consistent initial otologic symptoms of metastasis to the temporal bone.[40] A majority of reported cases indicate that otologic symptoms usually arise late in the course of the disease.[15, 34–36, 41, 42] Maddox, in a review of 29 reported cases of metastases to the temporal bone, noted that hearing loss was the most common presenting symptom, followed by otalgia, facial paralysis, periauricular swelling, otorrhea, and aural mass.[43] Schuknecht and coworkers reported that conductive and sensorineural hearing loss can occur.[35] They also noted that the bone of the otic capsule is quite resistant to invasion by neoplasm and that involvement of the inner ear by metastatic growth is uncommon. To help in identification of lesions metastatic to the temporal bone, Maddox suggested a symptom triad: otalgia, facial paresis, and preauricular swelling in the presence of an intact tympanic membrane.[43]

STAGING SYSTEMS

Staging of cancer of the temporal bone is difficult, and no single staging system is currently accepted by either the Union International Contre le Cancer (UICC) or the American Joint Committee on Cancer (AJCC). Several staging systems have been proposed, each with its advantages and disadvantages.

In 1985, Stell and McCormick proposed a staging system for cancer involving the external auditory canal and middle ear, based on their experience with 49 patients.[39] A subsequent revision was proposed in 1991 by Clark and associates after they observed a favorable outcome in several patients who had spread of cancer to the temporomandibular joint.[44] This staging system has the advantage of including all histologic subtypes and all sites of origin within the temporal bone while also considering the overall condition of the patient.[2] Spector published a prospective treatment plan for 34 patients with cancer of the external auditory canal who had been staged into four groups based on whether the cancer was limited to the external auditory canal, superficially invasive, deeply invasive, or beyond the temporal bone.[45] These patients all received adjuvant radiation therapy. Survival was 100% for disease limited to the external auditory canal (n = 7), 100% for superficial invasion (n = 3), 70% for deep invasion (n = 10), and 65% for tumors extending beyond the temporal bone (n = 14).[45] Pensak and colleages reported a series of patients with multiple histologic types whose staging was based on radiologic and intraoperative observation.[46] Recently, Manolidis and coworkers detailed 30 squamous cell carcinomas and basal cell carcinomas in their review of temporal bone malignancies.[47] Stage I tumors were confined to the external auditory canal, with higher stages having varying degrees of extension outside the external auditory canal.

Arriaga and associates proposed another staging system (Pittsburgh Staging System) for squamous cell carcinoma of

TABLE 23-1 Presenting Complaints in Tumors of the Temporal Bone

Presenting Complaint	Percent of Patients
Pain	60
Chronic otitis	60
Sanguineous otorrhea	40
Facial paralysis	35
Hearing loss and tinnitus	20
Palsy of other cranial nerves	10
Vertigo	10

the external auditory canal based on preoperative clinical and computed tomographic (CT) findings (Table 23–2).[16, 48] This staging system offers several advantages, including the use of imaging studies for the initial staging of the tumor. Early-stage lesions are differentiated by the amount of bone erosion (partial or full thickness) or involvement of soft tissue (<0.5 cm or ≥0.5 cm), and later-stage lesions are differentiated by the amount of bone erosion or extension outside of the external auditory canal. A recent study by Moody and colleagues provides evidence that validates this staging system.[49] Their retrospective case review of 32 patients demonstrated that 2-year survival data directly correlated with the staging system, with the 2-year survival rates for primary squamous cell carcinoma of the temporal bone reported as follows: T1 lesions—100%, T2 lesions—80%, T3 lesions—50%, and T4 lesions—7%. Even though the Pittsburgh Staging System has its advantages, it can be cumbersome owing to difficulty in assessing partial versus complete bone erosion and 0.5-cm soft tissue extension. In addition, a separate retrospective review noted that survival rates for early disease (T1 and T2 tumors) were the same (86%) when the Pittsburgh classification was used.[50]

Recently, a modification of the Pittsburgh Staging System was proposed for early external auditory canal lesions (Table 23–3).[51] This modification was initiated by a study involving 31 patients treated at the University of Arkansas for Medical Sciences. The cancers were of different histologic subtypes and had various origins in the temporal bone. The location of the treated lesions in relation to the external auditory canal was carefully examined in all 31 patients. Cancer involving the anterior canal wall had the worst

TABLE 23-3   University of Arkansas for Medical Sciences Staging System

T Status

T1	Tumor limited to posterior membranous EAC
T2a	Tumor involving anterior membranous EAC
T2b	Tumor limited to posterior EAC with bone erosion
T3	Tumor involving anterior EAC with bone erosion
	Parotid, TMJ involvement
	Invasion of bony labyrinth, mastoid, and middle ear
	Facial nerve involvement
T4	Involvement of the dura, carotid artery, and petrous apex

EAC, external auditory canal, TMJ, temporomandibular joint.
From Breau RL, Gardner EK, Dornhoffer JL: Cancer of the external auditory canal and temporal bone. Curr Opin Oncol (in press).

prognosis; of the six patients whose disease recurred, five had lesions that involved this location of the external auditory canal. Three patients in this study have died of distant disease, and all of these patients had lesions that involved the anterior canal wall. This modification places more emphasis on the site of disease and less on the size of the primary tumor or degree of bony invasion, which can often be difficult to determine on CT scan. This is consistent with the access of these tumors to the parotid gland and associated lymphatics through well-described anatomic pathways. This site also allows access to the temporomandibular joint, surrounding soft tissues, and dura. Posterior canal wall lesions have limited access to soft tissues or lymphatic pathways and are usually cleared effectively by standard otologic procedures.

TABLE 23-2   University of Pittsburgh TNM Staging System Proposed for the External Auditory Canal

T Status

T1	Tumor limited to the external auditory canal without bony erosion or evidence of soft tissue extension
T2	Tumor with limited external auditory canal bony erosion (not full-thickness), or radiographic finding consistent with limited (<0.5 cm) soft tissue involvement
T3	Tumor eroding the osseous external auditory canal (full-thickness) with limited (<0.5 cm) soft tissue involvement, or tumor involving middle ear and/or mastoid, or patients presenting with facial paralysis
T4	Tumor eroding the cochlea, petrous apex, medial wall of middle ear, carotid canal, jugular foramen, or dura, or with extensive (≥0.5 cm) soft tissue involvement

N Status

Involvement of lymph nodes is a poor prognostic finding and automatically places the patient in an advanced stage (i.e., stage III [T1, N1] or stage IV [T2, 3, and 4, N1] disease)

M Status

Distant metastasis indicates a very poor prognosis and immediately places a patient in the stage IV category

From Arriaga M, Curtin H, Takahashi H, et al: Staging proposal for external auditory meatus carcinoma based on preoperative clinical examination and computed tomography findings. Ann Otol Rhinol Laryngol 99:714, 1990.

PREOPERATIVE EVALUATION

Careful preoperative planning is necessary in all cases of cancer of the temporal bone. This is important not only for the successful treatment of these lesions but also for the preoperative education of the patient and for obtaining informed consent. As always, a careful history and physical examination are paramount before treatment is begun, particularly because the presenting symptoms differ depending on the site of the primary tumor. Usually, the patient presents with pain in the ear associated with sanguineous drainage. The lesion is frequently granular, although it may present as an ulcer in the skin reaching to the periosteum of the bony portion of the canal. During careful evaluation of the lesion, particular attention should be directed to its medial extent to assess for possible involvement of the middle ear. This lesion is often confused with otitis externa; therefore, a high level of suspicion should be maintained and a biopsy should be performed if the patient fails to respond to medical management, or if there is any doubt as to the nature of the lesion.[12]

A complete examination of the head and neck must be performed. Weakness or paralysis of the facial nerve points to direct involvement of the nerve or perineural invasion (adenoid cystic carcinoma or squamous cell carcinoma) and also allows the surgeon to plan for an intraoperative nerve

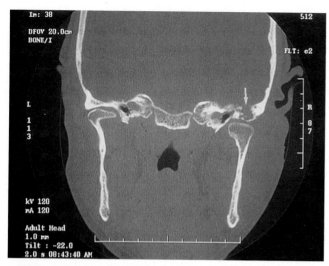

FIGURE 23–3 CT scan demonstrating erosion of the tegmen (*arrow*).

graft that uses the greater auricular or sural nerve. The nerves of the jugular foramen, including IX, X, and XI, may also be involved and should be carefully evaluated. The parotid gland is a frequent site of tumor involvement, either by direct extension of the tumor from the external auditory canal anteriorly or by metastasis to the intraparotid and paraparotid lymph nodes. The neck should also be evaluated for metastatic disease, especially in level II. The presence of trismus suggests involvement of the temporomandibular joint and therefore the need for its treatment or resection.

An audiogram is obtained preoperatively in all cases to evaluate the hearing in both ears. A fine-cut (1.5-mm) CT scan through the temporal bone is needed to assess the presence or absence of bone destruction and to determine the extent of the tumor (Fig. 23–3). An adequate preoperative biopsy is necessary in all cases to confirm the diagnosis.

In specific situations, selected studies, including magnetic resonance imaging (MRI), are necessary and helpful in both the preoperative planning and the treatment of these lesions. The first situation involves erosion of bone in the superior external auditory canal, as noted on CT scan, with specific attention directed at the dura of the middle fossa. The second situation involves erosion of the bone in the anterior external auditory canal. The extent of disease spread into the temporomandibular joint and parotid tissue is very difficult to determine clinically and should be assessed by imaging studies. Finally, if extensive involvement of the mastoid or middle ear with bone erosion is appreciated on CT, an MRI is obtained to assess involvement of the posterior fossa dura, the sigmoid sinus, and the carotid artery. Magnetic resonance angiogram or balloon occlusion studies are also obtained if involvement of the carotid artery is identified or suspected on any of the previous diagnostic studies.

SURGICAL MANAGEMENT

The approach to treatment of cancer of the auricle depends on both the pathologic diagnosis and the extent of disease.

Small lesions can be excised with frozen section control of margins and reconstruction using standard reconstructive techniques. Total auriculectomy is frequently necessary in large lesions with significant involvement of the cartilage and in those with extensive involvement of the postauricular sulcus. Attempts to preserve the superior aspect of the auricle are discouraged because this interferes with the proper construction of a prosthesis.

The team approach to dealing with these cancers has proved to be most effective. A head and neck surgeon, an otologist/neuro-otologist, and occasionally a neurosurgeon are needed for proper resection of these lesions. A surgeon with microvascular experience may also be necessary if additional reconstruction is required.

Controversy still exists as to the proper treatment of these rare cancers. The major obstacle in answering these questions and assessing outcomes has been the rarity of the lesions encountered. Most series evaluating squamous cell carcinoma of the temporal bone are case studies without control subjects; therefore, careful compiling of these studies is required if they are to be of help in determination of proper treatment guidelines.[52]

Among the controversies that exist in the treatment of these challenging tumors are the efficacy of piecemeal resection when compared with standard en bloc resection and the extent of surgery necessary in lesions confined to the external auditory canal. Analysis of series dealing with squamous cell carcinoma of the temporal bone has revealed no statistically significant difference in survival between mastoidectomy (50% 5-year survival), lateral resection of the temporal bone (48.6% 5-year survival), and subtotal resection of the temporal bone (50% 5-year survival) when disease was confined to the external canal. These data seem to allow for less of an en bloc resection with no compromise in survival, but caution needs to be used in making this statement because of the small number of patients in this series and the lack of uniformity in the patient population.[52]

When disease extends into the middle ear, the survival of patients treated with subtotal resection of the temporal bone (41.7% 5-year survival) appeared to be better than for those treated with lateral resection of the temporal bone (28.6% 5-year survival) or mastoidectomy (17.1% 5-year survival). Even though this difference was not statistically significant, it appears that surgery more extensive than lateral resection of the temporal bone can possibly prolong survival.[52] The value of total resection of the temporal bone when tumor involves the petrous apex remains unclear because of the limited number of cases. As a result, no statistically significant benefit of complete resection of the temporal bone over subtotal resection of the temporal bone has been demonstrated. Resection of dura, brain parenchyma, or the internal carotid artery also remains controversial because of the small numbers of patients reported; further study is required.

Although most surgeons recommend adjuvant radiation therapy for advanced lesions, treatment with adjuvant radiation therapy of early-stage lesions remains in question. In most studies of patients with disease confined to the external auditory canal, patients received postoperative radiation, precluding analysis of the data. However, no statistically significant difference in survival was seen between patients treated with lateral resection of the temporal bone and radiation therapy (48% 5-year survival) or with lateral resection of the temporal bone alone (44.4% 5-year survival). Analysis of patients with middle ear or greater involvement fails to validate the use of radiation therapy. This could be so because of the small number of patients in this study, which precluded statistical analysis, or it may be the result of the widespread use of radiation therapy in all patients with advanced lesions.[52]

The following discussion represents our current treatment protocol for temporal bone malignancies. The current modified Arkansas Staging System is used for classification (see Table 23–3).

T1 Lesions

T1 lesions with isolated involvement of the posterior canal without erosion require a classic core resection. This can be performed through an endaural or postauricular approach, depending on the size of the lesion and the width of the

external auditory canal. Skin incisions are made at the level of the tragus and concha and are carried to the underlying bone. Medial incisions are made at the level of the annulus but lateral to the tympanic membrane. This "core" of tissue is then removed, and margins are assessed. For posterior lesions, the tragus is usually left in place, with the plane of dissection between the skin and the perichondrium. The bony external auditory canal is typically drilled posteriorly down to the level of the mastoid air cells and anteriorly down to the level of the temporomandibular joint, leaving a thin layer of bone over each. A thin full-thickness skin graft is placed over the bone, and an appropriate dressing of Silastic sheeting and ear packing is placed (Fig. 23–4). This typically is removed 1 week postoperatively.

T2a Lesions

T2a lesions involving the anterior canal without erosion require a core resection with resection of the tragus. A superficial parotidectomy may be included, depending on

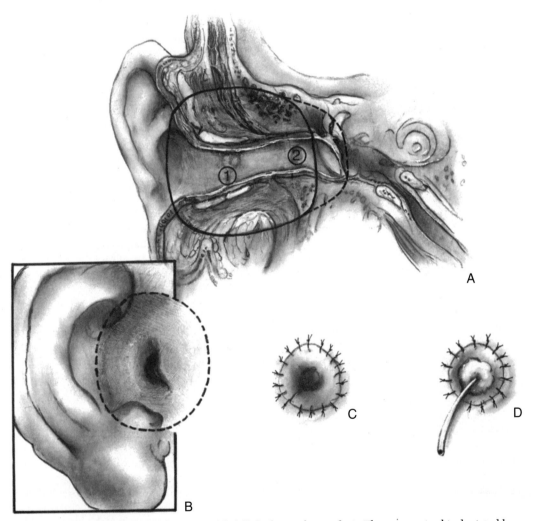

FIGURE 23–4 Endaural core resection with full-thickness skin graft. *A*, The area excised is depicted by the solid line for a lesion located in the cartilaginous external auditory canal (1). 2 represents the body canal. *B*, An incision is made surrounding the external auditory canal. *C*, Split-thickness skin graft in place. *D*, Packing placed to support the graft. (From Loré JM Jr: An Atlas of Head and Neck Surgery, 3rd ed. Philadelphia, WB Saunders, 1988.)

the extent of the disease as well as the histology. The same technique described earlier is used, with a few notable modifications. In this situation, the tragus is removed en bloc with the core resection of the external auditory canal and parotid tissue. After the incisions for the core resection have been made, as described previously, a standard preauricular parotid incision is made, except that instead of coursing anterior to the tragus, the incision connects with the core resection superiorly at the incisura and inferiorly below the tragus. A thin full-thickness skin graft is used in the reconstruction.

T2b Lesions

T2b lesions involving the posterior canal with erosion of the bony external auditory canal require resection of the skin and cartilage of the posterior concha (meatoplasty) and resection of the bony canal. If the lesion is only posterior, the skin of the anterior canal can be left intact in some cases when negative margins are obtained. We have found that we are able to preserve the hearing mechanism and avoid a classic superficial or lateral temporal bone resection in lesions isolated to the posterior canal. These procedures are quite similar to the classic modified radical mastoid surgeries familiar to the otologic surgeon. A postauricular skin incision is connected to incisions made previously in the external auditory canal, similar to those for core resection. A complete mastoidectomy is performed, the facial recess is opened, and the posterior canal wall is thinned so that the annulus can be visualized through the bone. The level of resection of the posterior canal depends on the extent of the lesion. If the lesion is lateral, it is possible to drill through the bony canal lateral to the annulus with en bloc removal of the external auditory canal and lesion. This technique, similar to a classic "Bondy" canal-down mastoidectomy, offers the possibility of preserving the tympanic membrane and hearing mechanism (Fig. 23–5).

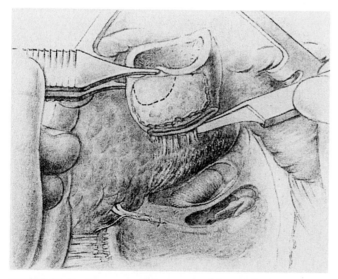

FIGURE 23–5 Resection of the ear canal lateral to the tympanic membrane, thereby preserving the hearing mechanism. (From Naumann HH, Jahrsdoefer RA, Helms J: Surgery for tumors of the auditory canal. In Head and Neck Surgery, vol. 2: The Ear. New York, Thieme, 1996, p 161.)

If the lesion extends significantly into the bony external auditory canal, the ossicular chain is disarticulated and the tympanic membrane, malleus, and incus are removed lateral to the facial nerve (Fig. 23–6). This differs from classic lateral resection of the temporal bone, however, in that the anterior tympanic membrane and annulus are maintained, allowing reconstruction of the drum and ossicular chain using either a type 3 mechanism or a prosthesis. This is very similar to the modified radical mastoidectomy used for cholesteatoma, differing only in that the canal wall and lesion are removed en bloc in an oncologic fashion, avoiding tumor spillage. The cavity created with this technique can be quite large owing to the normal aeration of the mastoid seen in this group of patients, compared with those with chronic otitis. Several patients have needed mastoid obliteration surgery several years after the primary surgery when it had been believed that the malignancy was eradicated. To avoid masking a recurrence, primary obliteration is not performed.

T3 Lesions

T3 lesions involving the anterior external auditory canal with erosion of the bone require a typical lateral superficial temporal bone resection (Fig. 23–7). A postauricular skin incision is used, and a complete mastoidectomy is performed. The facial recess is opened widely, and the incus is disarticulated. Superiorly, the zygomatic cell system is followed with the drill until the temporomandibular joint is encountered. Inferiorly, the chorda tympani nerve is sacrificed and an extended facial recess approach is performed, with drilling proceeding forward until the temporomandibular joint is encountered. With either the drill or the chisel, the incisions are connected medial to the annulus, just lateral to the eustachian tube. As a result, all tissue lateral to and including the tympanic membrane is resected. This is performed in continuity with the parotidectomy, including the deep lobe and possibly the temporomandibular joint if these structures are involved.

Options for reconstruction depend on whether the helix itself is involved by the malignancy. If the helix is not involved, a wide meatoplasty with split-thickness skin graft is performed. If the helix is involved and resected, a temporalis flap is rotated into the defect, with obliteration of the canal and placement of a split-thickness skin graft. If the tumor extends through the tympanic membrane to involve the medial wall of the middle ear and/or mastoid, a subtotal temporal bone resection with piecemeal removal is performed. After the lateral temporal bone resection has been completed, the otic capsule, along with all bone between the carotid artery and sigmoid sinus including the tegmen tympani, is removed with the drill. If the facial nerve is not involved, it is transposed superiorly. If it is involved, it is resected and a sural nerve graft is interposed.

T4 Lesions

T4 lesions involving the dura, carotid, or petrous apex require a multidisciplinary approach and are quite challenging. Although this treatment is controversial, it may prolong survival compared with the "piecemeal" removal described earlier. Once the tumor involves the petrous apex, an en bloc

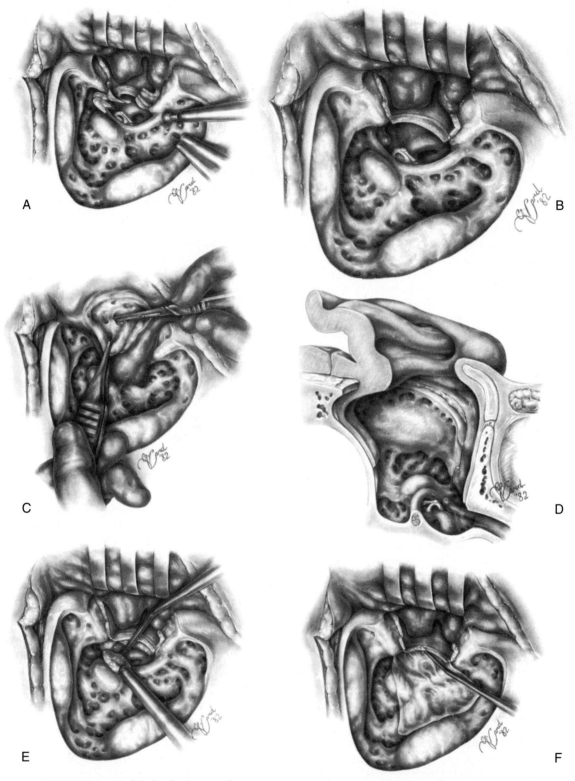

FIGURE 23–6 Modified radical mastoidectomy preserving the anterior annulus with reconstruction of the tympanic membrane. *A,* The posterior external auditory canal (EAC) must be lowered to the facial nerve. *B,* The anterosuperior EAC and mastoid top must be drilled to create a confluent middle cap and mastoid. *C,* Meatoplasty is performed. *D,* Superior and interior medial incisions are performed to create a posterior Korner's flap. *E,* The middle ear is packed with gelatin sponge. *F,* The graft is placed meatal to the annulus anteriorly and over the facial ridge posteriorly. (From Jackson CG, et al: Open mastoid procedures: Contemporary indications and surgical technique. Laryngoscope 95:1037, 1985.)

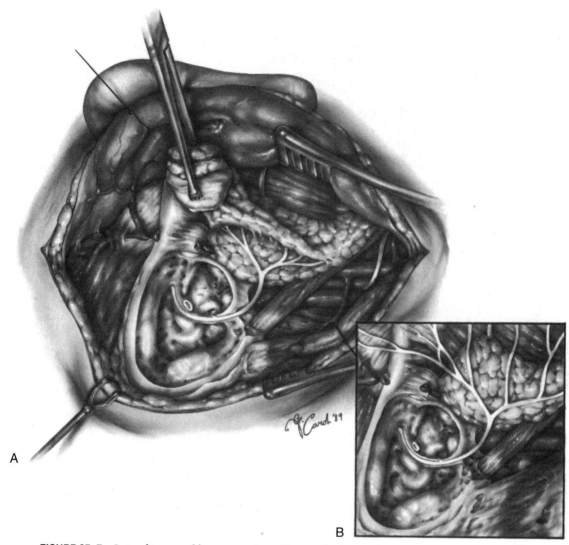

FIGURE 23–7 Lateral temporal bone resection with superfical parotidectomy. *A,* The external auditory canal and the tympanic membrane have been mobilized from the temporal bone. *B,* Superfical parotidectomy is completed for an en bloc resection. (From Glassock ME III, Shambaugh GE Jr: *Surgery of the Ear,* 4th ed. Philadelphia, WB Saunders, 1990.)

total resection of the temporal bone can be used to achieve total extirpation of the tumor (Fig. 23–8). Invasion by cancer of the dura mater, brain parenchyma, and internal carotid artery portends a poor prognosis, and the value of resection of these structures is unclear because prospective studies are lacking. If the dura is involved, it is resected and patched. At this point, management of the carotid artery is variable and depends on the patient's overall medical condition, as well as on radiologic studies such as the balloon occlusion test to assess the risks involved with resection of the internal carotid artery. The choice of removal of the internal carotid artery in patients with potential internal carotid artery involvement is controversial, but results have not been promising.[52]

ADJUVANT THERAPY

Adjuvant therapy is considered in all patients. Postoperative adjuvant radiation therapy is necessary in patients with

regional adenopathy or perineural/neural involvement and in those cases with close or positive margins. Often, large tumors are difficult to resect in an en bloc fashion, making piecemeal resection more advantageous. Adjuvant radiation therapy is provided in these patients.

RECONSTRUCTION

As with all malignancies in the head and neck, treatment of these complex problems not only features the surgical extirpation of the malignancies but requires reconstruction of the resulting defects. Efforts are made to enhance both the functional and the cosmetic aspects of reconstruction. If the facial nerve is resected, a cable graft involving the greater auricular or sural nerve is used. Frozen section must be used to exclude perineural or direct nerve involvement in the proximal and distal ends of the facial nerve. Care must also be taken to exclude

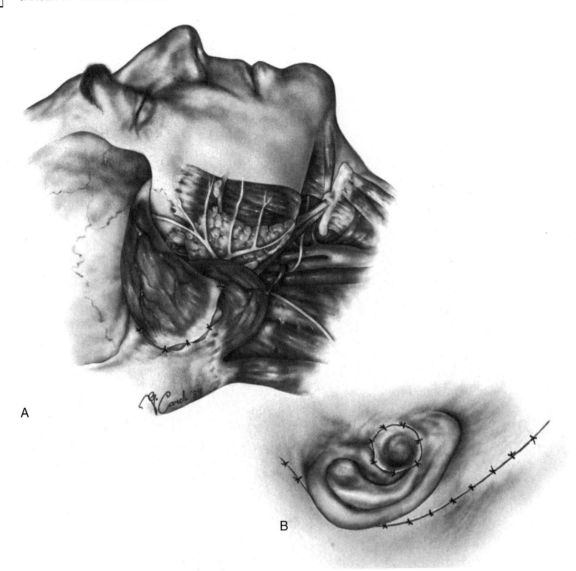

FIGURE 23–8 Total resection of the temporal bone with removal of the ascending ramus of the mandible and partial parotidectmy. *A,* Subtotal resection of the temporal bone with exposure of the middle fossa dura, major neurovascular structures, and parotid gland. *B,* Appearance following removal of the specimen demonstrating exposure of the carotid artery and obliteration of the eustachian tube. (From Glassock ME III, Shambaugh GE Jr: Surgery of the Ear, 4th ed. Philadelphia, WB Saunders, 1990.)

involvement of the greater auricular nerve if it is near the tumor.

For patients in whom reconstruction of the facial nerve is not possible, shortening of the lid, placement of a gold weight, and a brow lift may be performed, depending on the needs of the individual patient. The patient can also be offered a static sling to improve both function and cosmesis in the postoperative period, once the final cosmetic/functional outcome is known.

Coverage of the defect with vascularized skin and muscle is extremely important. The most important consideration is coverage of all exposed bone to help prevent postoperative complications, particularly osteoradionecrosis. The temporalis flap is also an excellent source of vascularized tissue in these defects. For larger defects, especially those involving extensive loss of tissue anterior to the external auditory

canal, multiple flaps, including myocutaneous and free flaps, may be used (Fig. 23–9). Each method has its merits and disadvantages, and the patient's needs are individualized. Additional aesthetic improvements can be performed for those patients requiring a total auriculectomy. Reconstructive options include osseointegrated implants and prosthetic ear replacement, with excellent cosmetic results (Fig. 23–10). The preservation of the tragus can further camouflage this area in selected patients.

◼ REHABILITATION

Auditory rehabilitation of patients with malignancies of the temporal bone can be quite challenging. Surgical intervention in this group of patients involves removal of the

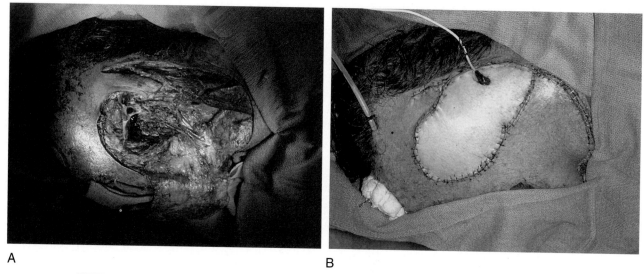

FIGURE 23–9 *A,* Postsurgical defect with extensive loss of skin and tissue. *B,* Reconstruction using rectus free flap.

external auditory canal and middle ear mechanism, resulting in significant conductive hearing loss. When auriculectomy is also performed, conventional hearing aids are very difficult, if not impossible, to use. Several options are available, depending on the patient's perceived difficulty with the unilateral hearing loss and the anatomic situation remaining after surgical intervention. If the ear canal and helix are present, the options are second-stage reconstructive surgery, conventional hearing aids, and cross-type hearing aids.

If the helix and the external auditory canal are not present, as in the case of a total or a lateral temporal bone resection, the options are much more limited. One option that has just become available in the United States is the Bone-Anchored Hearing Aid (BAHA).[22] This system works through integration of a titanium implant with a percutaneous attachment to which the hearing aid attaches. The osseointegrated implant can easily be placed in a postauricular area,

approximately 5 to 6 cm behind the external auditory canal, during surgery under local anesthesia in an outpatient setting. The patient's hearing should not be worse than 45 dB for the cochlear function, but the degree of conductive hearing loss added to this bone threshold is of no significance with this device.[23] Resulting sound perception has been reported to be excellent and to compare favorably with conventional hearing aids.[24]

◻ CONCLUSION

Cancer involving the ear and temporal bone is a relatively rare and often misdiagnosed disease. A high index of suspicion must be maintained for the diagnosis to be made as early in the disease as possible. Although the use of piecemeal resection and the need for postoperative radiation therapy in early-stage lesions are still in question, increased

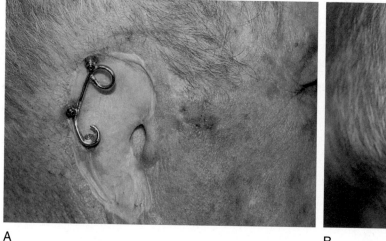
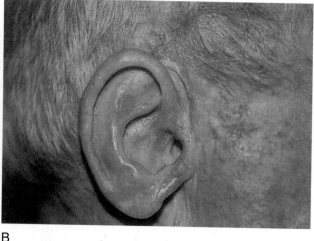

FIGURE 23–10 Osseous integrated implants *(A)* and prosthetic ear *(B)* in a patient following auriculectomy.

cure rates, improved functional results, and decreased postoperative complications can be obtained by careful preoperative planning and the use of a multidisciplinary team approach.

REFERENCES

1. Lewis JS: Surgical management of tumors of the middle ear and mastoid. J Laryngol Otol 97:299, 1983.
2. Koriwchak M: Temporal bone cancer. Am J Otolaryngol 14:623, 1993.
3. Kuhel WI, Hume CR, Selesnick SH: Cancer of the external auditory canal and temporal bone. Otolaryngol Clin North Am 29:827, 1996.
4. Conley J, Schuller K: Malignancies of the ear. Laryngoscope 86:1147, 1976.
5. Lederman J: Malignant tumors of the ear. J Laryngol 79:85, 1965.
6. Lewis JS: Cancer of the ear. A report of 150 cases. Laryngoscope 70:551, 1960.
7. Goodwin WJ, Jesse RH: Malignant neoplasms of the external auditory canal and temporal bone. Arch Otolaryngol 106:675, 1980.
8. Lewis JS: Temporal bone resection: Review of 100 cases. Arch Otolaryngol 101:23, 1975.
9. Lewis JS: Cancer of the ear. CA Cancer Clin 37:78, 1987.
10. Passe G: Primary carcinoma of the eustachian tube. J Laryngol Otol 62:314, 1948.
11. Cumberworth VL, Friedmann I, Glover GW: Late metastasis of breast carcinoma to the external auditory canal. J Laryngol Otol 108:808, 1994.
12. Arriaga M, Hirsch B, Kammerer D, et al: Squamous cell carcinoma of the external auditory meatus (canal). Otolaryngol Head Neck Surg 101:330, 1989.
13. Bumsted RM, Ceilley RI, Panje WR, et al: Auricular malignant neoplasms: When is chemotherapy (Mohs' technique) necessary? Arch Otolaryngol 107:721, 1981.
14. Huriez C, Lebeurre R, Lepere B: Etude de 126 tumeurs ariculaires malignés observées en 9 ans a la clinique dermatologic universitaire de Lille. Bull Soc Fr Dermatol Syphiligr 69:886, 1962.
15. Ross DA, Sasaki CT: Cancer of the ear and temporal bone. In Myers E, Suen JY (eds): Cancer of the Head and Neck, 3rd ed. Philadelphia, WB Saunders, 1996, pp 586–597.
16. Austin JR, Stewart KL, Fawzi N: Squamous cell carcinoma of the external auditory canal: Therapeutic prognosis based on a proposed staging system. Arch Otolaryngol Head Neck Surg 120:1228, 1994.
17. Hahn SS, Kim JA, Goodchild N, et al: Carcinoma of the middle ear and external auditory canal. Int J Radiat Oncol Biol Phys 9:1003, 1983.
18. Johns ME, Headington JT: Squamous cell carcinoma of the external auditory canal. Arch Otolaryngol 100:45, 1974.
19. Lederman J: Malignant tumors of the ear. J Laryngol 79:85, 1965.
20. Paaske PB, Witten J, Schwer S, et al: Results in treatment of carcinoma of the external auditory canal and middle ear. Cancer 59:156, 1987.
21. Phelps PD, Lloyd GA: The radiology of carcinoma of the ear. Br J Radiol 54:103, 1981.
22. Lodge WO, Jones HW, Smith MN: Malignant tumors of the temporal bone. Arch Otolaryngol 61:535, 1955.
23. Arena S, Keen M: Carcinoma of the middle ear and temporal bone. Am J Otol 9:351, 1988.
24. Beal DD, Linday J, Ward PH: Radiation induced carcinoma of the temporal bone. Arch Otolaryngol 81:9, 1965.
25. Hyams VJ: Pathology of tumors of the ear. In Thawley S, Panje W (eds): Comprehensive Management of Head and Neck Tumors. Philadelphia, WB Saunders, 1987, pp 168–180.
26. Perzin KH, Gullane P, Conley J: Adenoid cystic carcinoma involving the external auditory canal: A clinicopathologic study of 16 cases. Cancer 50:2873, 1982.
27. Pulec JL: Glandular tumors of the external auditory canal. Laryngoscope 87:1601, 1977.
28. Wetli CV, Pardo V, Millard M, et al: Tumors of ceruminous glands. Cancer 29:1169, 1972.
29. Wiener ES: Head and neck rhabdomyosarcoma. Semin Pediatr Surg 3:203, 1994.
30. Weiland LH: Nasopharyngeal carcinoma. In Barnes L (ed): Surgical Pathology of the Head and Neck, vol 1. New York, Marcel Dekker, Inc, 1985, pp 453–466.
31. Shanmugaratnam K, Sobin L: Histological typing of upper respiratory tract tumors. International Histologic Typing of Tumors, No. 19. Geneva, WHO, 1978.
32. Berlinger NT, Koutroupas S, Adams G, et al: Patterns of involvement of the temporal bone in metastatic and systemic malignancy. Laryngoscope 11:171, 1980.
33. Proctor B, Lindsay JR: Tumors involving the petrous pyramid of the temporal bone. Arch Otolaryngol 46:180, 1947.
34. Nelson EG, Hinojosa R: Histopathology of metastatic temporal bone tumors. Arch Otolaryngol Head Neck Surg 117:189, 1991.
35. Schuknecht HT, Allam AM, Murakami Y: Pathology of secondary malignant tumors of the temporal bone. Ann Otol Rhinol Laryngol 77:5, 1968.
36. El Fiky FM, Paparella NM: A metastatic glomus jugulare tumor. Am J Otol 5:197, 1984.
37. Crabtree JA, Britton BH, Pierce MK: Carcinoma of the external auditory canal. Laryngoscope 86:405, 1976.
38. Morton RP, Stell PM, Derrick PPO: Epidemiology of cancer of the middle ear cleft. Cancer 53:1612, 1984.
39. Stell PM, McCormick MS: Carcinoma of the external auditory meatus and middle ear: Prognostic factors and a suggested staging system. J Laryngol Otol 99:847, 1985.
40. Ruah CB, Bohigian RK, Vincent ME, et al: Metastatic sigmoid adenocarcinoma to the temporal bone. Otolaryngol Head Neck Surg 97:500, 1987.
41. Saldanha CB, Bennett JD, Evans JN, et al: Metastasis to the temporal bone, secondary to carcinoma of the bladder. J Laryngol Otol 103:599, 1989.
42. Jahn AF, Farkashidy J, Berman JM: Metastatic tumors in the temporal bone: A pathophysiologic study. J Otolaryngol 8:85, 1979.
43. Maddox HE: Metastatic tumors of the temporal bone. Ann Otol Rhinol Laryngol 76:149, 1967.
44. Clark LJ, Narula AA, Morgan DA, et al: Squamous carcinoma of the temporal bone: A revised staging. J Laryngol Otol 105:346, 1991.
45. Spector JG: Management of temporal bone carcinomas: A therapeutic analysis of two groups of patients and long-term follow-up. Otolaryngol Head Neck Surg 104:58, 1991.
46. Pensak ML, Gleich LL, Gluckman JL, et al: Temporal bone carcinoma: Contemporary perspectives in the skull base surgical era. Laryngoscope 106:1234, 1996.
47. Manolidis S, Pappas D, Von Doersten P, et al: Temporal bone and lateral skull base malignancy: Experience and results with 81 patients. Am J Otol 19:S1, 1998.
48. Arriaga M, Curtin H, Takahashi H, et al: Staging proposal for external auditory meatus carcinoma based on preoperative clinical examination and computed tomography findings. Ann Otol Rhinol Laryngol 99:714, 1990.
49. Moody SA, Hirsch BE, Myers EN: Squamous cell carcinoma of the external auditory canal: An evaluation of a staging system. Am J Otol 21:582, 2000.
50. Pfreundner L, Schwager K, Willner J, et al: Carcinoma of the external auditory canal and middle ear. Int J Radiat Oncol Biol Phys 44:777, 1999.
51. Breau RL, Gardner EK, Dornhoffer JL: Cancer of the external auditory canal and temporal bone. Curr Opin Oncol 4:76, 2002.
52. Janecka IP, Kapadia S, Moncuso A, et al: Surgical management of temporal bone cancer. In Harrison LB, Sessions RB, Hong WK (eds): Head and Neck Cancer: A Multidisciplinary Approach. Philadelphia, Lippincott-Raven, 1999, pp 749–776.

CHAPTER 24

Cancer of the Head and Neck in the Pediatric Population

Kenneth R. Whittemore, Jr.
Michael J. Cunningham

◐ INTRODUCTION

Cancer ranks second only to trauma as the principal cause of mortality in children from ages 1 through 14 years, accounting for more than 1500 childhood deaths annually.[1] An estimated 5% to 10% of primary malignant tumors in children originate in the head and neck, and one in four malignant lesions have eventual manifestations in the head and neck region.[2–8] The care of children with cervicofacial malignancies presents a unique challenge owing to potential adverse effects of both the disease process and the treatments employed on critical developing head and neck structures. A team approach is essential, and the overall rarity of many of these malignancies mandates referral to a center that specializes in the management of pediatric cancer.

Benign Lesions

A vast majority of head and neck neoplasms in children are benign. Included in this group are vasoformative lesions such as hemangiomas and vascular malformations, nasopharyngeal angiofibromas, papillomas, neurofibromas and schwannomas, craniopharyngiomas, epidermoids, dermoids, teratomas, nasal gliomas, fibro-osseous lesions, odontogenic tumors, and pilomatricomas. Most investigators would also include the diverse clinicopathologic variants of Langerhans cell histiocytosis.[9] Such benign lesions are of differential diagnostic value in that the clinical presentation of these lesions may mimic that of cervicofacial malignancies.

Malignant Lesions

Several extensive reviews of pediatric head and neck malignancies have been published,[3–8, 10–12] of which the largest, a 28-year review from the University of Pittsburgh, lists 411 childhood cases (Table 24–1). Excluding neoplasms of the central nervous system and retinoblastomas, lymphoma—particularly Hodgkin's lymphoma—is the predominant malignancy of childhood that presents in the area of the head and neck. Soft tissue sarcoma, specifically rhabdomyosarcoma, and well-differentiated thyroid carcinoma constitute the next most common groups. The most striking observation made in these series is the rarity of head and neck epidermoid carcinoma in children compared with adults. Nasopharyngeal carcinoma is the major epithelial malignancy in children. Mucoepidermoid carcinoma is the most common malignancy of the salivary glands.[11] Neuroblastomas and germ cell neoplasms may arise primarily or may present initially as metastases within this region.

An age-specific presentation pattern (Table 24–2) has also been noted. Malignant teratomas are primarily congenital lesions. Neuroblastomas tend to occur in infants and very young children. The sarcomatous neoplasms span the entire pediatric age range from infancy to young adulthood, with the majority of rhabdomyosarcomas occurring in children of preschool age. The non-Hodgkin's lymphomas similarly demonstrate a broad age range, with a predominant clustering noted in school-age children. Hodgkin's lymphoma usually occurs in early adolescence and rarely in children younger than 5 years.[11] Thyroid carcinoma, nasopharyngeal carcinoma, and salivary gland neoplasms all occur predominantly in adolescence.[13–15]

The neck is the most common anatomic site of presentation (Table 24–3). The oropharynx and nasopharynx, orbit, salivary glands, face and scalp, and auricular region follow in descending order of frequency. Certain clinical features of solid cervicofacial masses increase the likelihood of a malignant cause; these features include rapid growth, presentation in the neonatal period, fixation to surrounding structures, and size greater than 3 cm in diameter.[16] Other medical or historical information that may predispose a child to the development of malignancy includes a family history of childhood cancer, previous exposure to radiation, and immunosuppression secondary to medications or an underlying medical condition.[13, 14]

In a child with a suspected head and neck cancer, a thorough medical and family history should be obtained, and a complete head and neck examination is required. On occasion, examination under general anesthesia may be necessary because of either lack of patient cooperativity or the anatomic location of the mass. A systemic evaluation may also be warranted, including hematologic or radiographic studies and consultation with other specialties, the specifics of which are dictated by the suspected diagnosis based on anatomic location or confirmational biopsy.

Treatment of childhood malignancies is dictated by the histopathology and stage of disease. A multispecialty team approach is often required because many cancers are

TABLE 24-1 Histopathologic Features of 411 Pediatric Head and Neck Malignancies

Pathologic Diagnosis and Histopathologic Subtype*	Subtotal	No. of Children	Percentage of Total
Hodgkin's lymphoma (HL)		131	32
Nodular sclerosing	63		
Mixed cellularity	28		
Lymphocyte predominance	15		
Both nodular sclerosis and mixed cellularity	12		
Paragranuloma	6		
Granuloma	3		
Unclassified	3		
Lymphocyte depletion	2		
Non-Hodgkin's lymphoma (NHL)		117	28.5
Lymphoblastic	59		
Lymphocytic, poorly differentiated	20		
Undifferentiated, Burkitt's	14		
Histiocytic	12		
Undifferentiated, non-Burkitt's	8		
Mixed lymphocytic-histiocytic	2		
Unclassified	2		
Rhabdomyosarcoma (RMS)		53	13
Embryonal	46		
Alveolar	4		
Unclassified	3		
Other sarcomas		19	4.5
Mesenchymal chondrosarcoma	3		
Ewing's sarcoma	4		
Fibrosarcoma	2		
Malignant fibrohistiocytoma	2		
Synovial sarcoma	2		
Neurogenous sarcoma	1		
Chondromyxoid sarcoma	2		
Osteogenic sarcoma	2		
Unclassified	1		
Thyroid carcinoma (TC)		38	9
Papillary adenocarcinoma	21		
Mixed papillary–follicular	11		
Follicular adenocarcinoma	4		
Medullary carcinoma	1		
Mixed medullary and papillary	1		
Nasopharyngeal carcinoma (NPC)		18	4.5
Squamous cell carcinoma	6		
Undifferentiated carcinoma	8		
Nonkeratinizing carcinoma	4		
Neuroblastoma		20	5
Salivary gland malignancies (SGMs)		10	2
Mucoepidermoid carcinoma	7		
Adenocarcinoma	3		
Malignant teratoma		3	1
Other uncommon tumors		2	0.05
Squamous cell carcinoma of the skin	1		
Parathyroid adenoma	1		
Totals		411	100

*Histopathologic subtype classifications used are as follows: HL, Rye classification and Jackson and Parker classification[31, 32]; NHL, modified Rappaport classification[78, 80]; RMS, Intergroup Rhabdomyosarcoma Study classification[136]; NPC, World Health Organization classification[394]; TC and SGM, standard tumor nomenclature.
Data from University of Pittsburgh, Children's and Eye and Ear Hospitals, 1965 to 1993.

treated with multimodality therapy.[17, 18] Lesion-specific management is discussed in the sections that follow.

LYMPHOMAS

Hodgkin's Lymphoma

Hodgkin's lymphoma (HL) is a malignancy of the lymphoreticular system that most often affects adolescents and young adults. HL is uncommon in preadolescent children and is rarely seen in children younger than 5 years. Boys are affected twice as frequently as girls.[19, 20] Potential causative associations exist between HL and previous Epstein-Barr virus infection,[21] and between the mixed cellularity and lymphocyte depleted variants of HL and immunosuppression secondary to human immunodeficiency virus (HIV).[22]

Clinical Presentation

HL arises within lymph nodes in more than 90% of childhood cases. Extranodal primary sites are rare, but systemic

TABLE 24-2 Age Distribution of 411 Children with Head and Neck Malignancies

Malignancy	Average Age (yr)	Age Range (yr)
Malignant teratoma	—	NB
Neuroblastoma	1.9	NB–5
Rhabdomyosarcoma	6.4	NB–17
Non-Hodgkin's lymphoma	8.0	2–18
Other sarcomas	8.1	NB–18
Hodgkin's lymphoma	11.8	4–18
Thyroid carcinoma	12.4	6–18
Nasopharyngeal carcinoma	14.4	9–18
Salivary gland malignancies	15.2	7–18

NB, newborn.
From University of Pittsburgh, Children's and Eye and Ear Hospitals, 1965 to 1993.

involvement does occur with progression of the disease. The spleen is the most common extranodal site for HL, with the liver and lymph nodes in the abdomen and retroperitoneum also being common sites.[23, 24] The typical patient with HL presents with asymmetrical, firm, and nontender cervical or supraclavicular lymphadenopathy (Fig. 24–1). Waldeyer's ring is rarely involved in HL.[25] Mediastinal lymph node involvement is common, particularly in association with right supraclavicular cervical disease.[19, 20, 26, 27] Obstruction of the superior vena cava or tracheobronchial tree may occur as a complication of mediastinal adenopathy. Pulmonary involvement is often due to extranodal spread from contiguous mediastinal and hilar lymph nodes.[28] In contrast, bone and bone marrow involvement arises from hematogenous spread.[29] One third of children with HL have nonspecific systemic symptoms at the time of presentation; these so-called B-symptoms include unexplained fever, night sweats, weight loss, weakness, anorexia, and pruritus.[20, 26]

Pathology

HL is distinguished morphologically from non-Hodgkin's lymphoma by the diagnostic presence of Reed-Sternberg cells. Reed-Sternberg cells are binucleate or multinucleate

TABLE 24-3 Anatomic Locations of 411 Pediatric Head and Neck Malignancies

Site	Pathologic Diagnosis	Subtotal	No. of Children	Percentage of Total
Neck			286	70
	Hodgkin's lymphoma	131		
	Non-Hodgkin's lymphoma	78		
	Thyroid carcinoma	38		
	Neuroblastoma	20*		
	Rhabdomyosarcoma	5		
	Other sarcomas	10		
	Teratoma	3		
	Parathyroid adenoma	1		
Oronasopharynx			71	17
	Non-Hodgkin's lymphoma	33		
	Nasopharyngeal carcinoma	18		
	Rhabdomyosarcoma	18		
	Fibrohistiocytoma	2		
Orbit/paranasal sinuses			21	5
	Rhabdomyosarcoma	19		
	Chondrosarcoma	2		
Parotid			14	3
	Mucoepidermoid carcinoma	5		
	Non-Hodgkin's lymphoma	5		
	Adenocarcinoma	2		
	Rhabdomyosarcoma	2		
Facial region			10	2.5
	Rhabdomyosarcoma	3		
	Synovial sarcoma	2		
	Osteogenic sarcoma	2		
	Chondrosarcoma	2		
	Non-Hodgkin's lymphoma	1		
Ear/temporal bone			6	1.5
	Rhabdomyosarcoma	5		
	Squamous cell carcinoma	1		
Tongue			3	1.0
	Mucoepidermoid carcinoma	2		
	Adenocarcinoma	1		
Totals			411	100

*Fifteen neuroblastomas were likely cervical metastases from the abdomen.
From University of Pittsburgh, Children's and Eye and Ear Hospitals, 1965 to 1993.

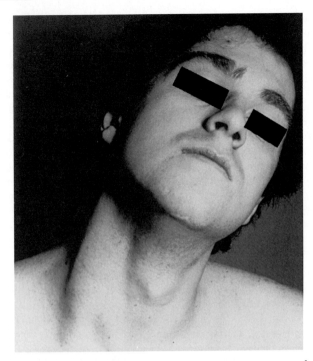

FIGURE 24-1 Hodgkin's lymphoma occurring as a mass in the right neck of a 17-year-old boy.

TABLE 24-4 REAL Classification

Types	Subtypes
Nodular lymphocytic predominant Hodgkin's lymphoma (NLPHL)	
"Classic" Hodgkin's lymphoma	Lymphocyte-rich
	Nodular sclerosis
	Mixed cellularity
	Lymphocyte depletion

Adapted from Harris N: Hodgkin's lymphomas: Classification, diagnosis, and grading. Semin Hematol 36:220, 1999; and Harris NL, Jaffe ES, Stein H, et al: A revised European-American classification of lymphoid neoplasms: A proposal from the International Lymphoma Study Group. Blood 84:1361, 1994.

giant cells with a clear halo zone around the nucleolus; they are suspected to be of B-cell lineage.[26, 30] The histogenesis is unknown, but the Reed-Sternberg cell represents the common malignant component of the diverse histopathologic HL subtypes.[27] The historically used Rye classification system recognizes four such subtypes: (1) lymphocyte predominance, (2) nodular sclerosis, (3) mixed cellularity, and (4) lymphocyte depletion.[31–33] Overall, about two thirds of children have nodular sclerosis HL at the time of presentation; the lymphocyte predominance and mixed cellularity subtypes are relatively more common in children 10 years of age and younger.[20, 32]

These histopathologic HL subtypes have prognostic implications.[27] Lymphocyte predominant HL has the most favorable prognosis, with poorer survival (in prognostic order) associated with nodular sclerosis, mixed cellularity, and lymphocyte depleted HL.[27] The more recent REAL (Revised European-American Lymphoid) classification separates HL into classic HL and nodular lymphocyte predominant HL (NLPHL) (Table 24–4).[34, 35] This system is based on the observation that NLPHL is clinically less aggressive than the other subtypes that constitute classic HL, with NLPHL having a decreased incidence of B-symptoms and mediastinal involvement, as well as typically presenting at an earlier stage.[34]

Diagnosis and Staging

A vast majority of patients with cervicofacial HL have disease at presentation outside of the head and neck region. Diagnosis is established by lymph node biopsy. Although fine-needle aspiration biopsy has been used to diagnose HL by the identification of Reed-Sternberg cells,[36] open

excisional biopsy is recommended in newly diagnosed cases for adequate tissue sampling.

It is essential that the full extent of the disease be defined in each patient before specific treatment is instituted. The Ann Arbor staging system, or a modification thereof, is presently in use (refer to Lymphoma chapter). The Ann Arbor staging system recognizes the fact that HL spreads via lymphatics in a contiguous fashion and can involve extralymphatic sites. The involvement of extranodal sites in HL is designated by E. The presence or absence of B-symptoms is designated by B or A, respectively.

Clinical staging includes history, physical examination, radiographic studies, and laboratory tests other than biopsy. Chest radiography with anteroposterior and lateral views may be required for the assessment of airway patency; masses that occupy more than one third of the thoracic diameter are associated with a poor prognosis.[37, 38] Computed tomography (CT) of the neck and chest is additionally important for assessment of mediastinal lymphadenopathy readily missed on plain films.[39] CT of the abdomen and pelvis is not a substitute for laparotomy because it has a sensitivity of only 40% in detecting abdominal adenopathy.[40] Abdominal-pelvic CT, however, does allow for the preoperative identification of suspicious nodal areas, helps in the determination of radiotherapy treatment ports, and provides a baseline for comparative assessment of response to treatment.[24] Positron emission tomography (PET) or magnetic resonance imaging (MRI) appears to be more accurate than CT in determining HL involvement of bone marrow or extranodal sites.[41, 42]

Pathologic staging of HL may involve a number of procedures and studies. The gold standard for determining intra-abdominal involvement has been exploratory laparotomy. Laparotomy is not necessary for children with stage IV disease because these children generally require chemotherapy.[20] In patients with clinical stage I, II, or III disease, in which the identification of intra-abdominal disease would change the therapeutic plan, exploratory laparotomy has historically been part of the routine pretreatment evaluation.[24] Laparotomy is now done less frequently owing to alternative imaging modalities previously mentioned, as well as to the fact that systemic therapy is more readily used for early-stage disease.[43]

In all patients, the pathologic stage differs from the clinical stage in 40% to 50% of patients when surgical staging is performed; in 20% to 30%, the clinical stage is advanced, and in 10% to 20%, it is lessened.[44] In a study of 133 children who underwent clinical staging, 28% experienced a change in stage after laparotomy, with stages in 10 declining and those in 27 increasing in severity.[45] PET scanning has also been found to alter the stage of disease in HL patients; most are upstaged based on CT, bone scanning, bone marrow biopsy, and laparotomy findings.[46] Bone marrow biopsy is typically reserved for patients with clinical stage III or IV disease, B-symptoms, or recurrent disease[26]; the histologic documentation of bone marrow involvement denotes pathologic stage IV disease.[47]

Treatment

The treatment of HL varies according to stage. Radiation therapy with or without chemotherapy may be used for patients with stage IA or IIA disease.[26, 43, 48] Patients with stage I disease with affected lymph nodes located in the upper neck may be treated with focal radiation with limited margins.[49] Chemotherapy is given in addition to radiotherapy in some institutions to patients with stage IIA disease owing to a high relapse rate in those with extensive mediastinal involvement.[50] Total nodal irradiation is one therapeutic choice for patients with stage IB or IIB disease.[48] Localized radiotherapy supplemented with chemotherapy, however, appears to offer the same therapeutic advantages of total nodal irradiation without the deleterious adverse effects.[51] Stage IIIA patients are treated with a combination regimen of extended-field radiation and chemotherapy. Patients with advanced stage IIIB or IV disease are treated with chemotherapy with or without the use of adjuvant radiation therapy.[52] Stem cell transplant with high-dose chemotherapy is an option in patients with relapsing HL.[52]

A majority of children, even those with low-stage disease, are likely to receive multimodality therapy; precise pathologic staging is therefore less critical, thereby obviating the need for laparotomy.[53] Low-dose radiotherapy combined with chemotherapy has been shown to be effective and to lessen growth impairment in treated children.[51] Management protocols are also different for children who have attained full growth versus those who are still growing, because the standard, high-dose, broad-field radiation therapy used for HL can lead to considerable long-term growth effects in children and young adolescents. Low-dose radiotherapy (<2500 cGy) combined with multiagent chemotherapy is recommended for children who have stage IA, IB, IIA, IIB, or IIIA$_1$ disease, who are still growing, who have bulky disease, or who have extranodal lesions.[20] Children of a similar age with stages IIIA$_2$, IIIB, IVA, or IVB disease are treated with a more prolonged course of chemotherapy in combination with low-dose total lymphoid irradiation.[20] More traditional protocols are used in adolescents and young adults who have obtained full growth.

Prognosis

With current treatments, more than 90% of all patients with HL, regardless of stage, initially achieve complete remission. Prolonged remission and cure are achieved in approximately 90% of patients with early stage I or II

disease and in 35% to 60% of those with advanced stage III or IV disease.[20, 54]

The long-term survival of patients successfully cured of HL has created additional concerns. Radiation therapy during the formative years of development has resulted in growth arrest in addition to hypothyroidism, sterility, and pulmonary fibrosis.[14, 55] Sepsis is a risk in patients who undergo splenectomy; therefore, vaccination for encapsulated organisms is recommended. All HL survivors, particularly those treated with both chemotherapy and radiation, also have an increased future incidence of second malignancies, specifically of the thyroid gland, breast, lung, gastrointestinal tract, and hematologic system, including acute nonlymphoblastic leukemia and non-Hodgkin's lymphoma.[53, 56–59] Such complications can be minimized through precise and proper selection of initial HL therapy.[60] Studies are under way to determine which patients can be treated with reductions in radiation dose and field size as well as tailored chemotherapy without jeopardizing treatment and long-term survival.[61]

Non-Hodgkin's Lymphoma

Non-Hodgkin's lymphoma (NHL) designates a heterogeneous group of solid primary neoplasms of the lymphoreticular system. In children, NHL occurs most commonly between the ages of 2 and 12 years, although the incidence increases with age.[62] There is a two- to threefold male predilection.[62–64] Immunodeficiency disorders, both acquired owing to immunosuppressive therapy or immunodeficiency syndrome (AIDS), and congenital such as X-linked lymphoproliferative disease, ataxia-telangectasia, or Wiskott-Aldrich syndrome, predispose to the development of NHL.[62, 65–70] High-grade B-cell lymphoma is actually designated as an AIDS-defining illness in patients with HIV infection.[71]

Clinical Presentation

The clinical features of NHL reflect the site of origin of the primary tumor and the extent of local and systemic disease. Asymptomatic lymphadenopathy is the initial presentation in the majority of patients.[72] Cervical, particularly supraclavicular, nodes are most commonly involved. Inguinal, axillary, and generalized nodal presentations are less frequent. Deep cervical lymph node involvement may masquerade as a deep neck abscess. Associated anterior mediastinal adenopathy may occur in up to one fourth of pediatric cases[62]; these children can have secondary superior vena cava syndrome, dyspnea due to airway compression, or pleural effusion.

NHL is more likely to present in the mediastinum, abdomen, and head and neck in children than in adults.[62, 65, 73, 74] Extranodal head and neck sites of origin (Fig. 24–2) include the oronasopharynx, nose and paranasal sinuses, orbit, larynx, trachea, and parotid and thyroid glands.[75–77] Waldeyer's ring involvement by NHL is particularly common.[6] The early detection of NHL involving Waldeyer's ring may be difficult because it may mimic benign adenotonsillar hypertrophy. A biopsy is warranted if there is tonsillar asymmetry, discoloration, or evidence of systemic symptoms. Diagnosis of NHL of the nose and

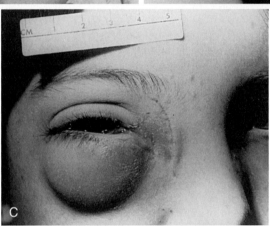

FIGURE 24–2 *A,* A 7-year-old child with non-Hodgkin's lymphoma of the nasopharynx who presented with otitis media with effusion and nasal obstruction. *B,* Lateral radiograph reveals complete soft tissue obstruction of the nasopharynx *(arrows). C,* The orbit is another common extranodal site of origin of non-Hodgkin's lymphoma.

paranasal sinuses requires a high index of suspicion, use of CT imaging, and surgical biopsy.[78]

Constitutional signs and symptoms correlate with advanced disease and include fever, weight loss, malaise, pancytopenia resulting from bone marrow infiltration, and neurologic manifestations. Among children with NHL, two thirds have metastatic disease.[62] In contradistinction to adults, children have a tendency toward leukemic transformation, hematogenous dissemination, and central nervous system (CNS) involvement.[63] Acute lymphoblastic leukemia is particularly prevalent in children with lymphoblastic lymphoma.[62]

Pathology

Childhood NHL differs from adult NHL in its typical diffuse rather than nodular histologic presentation and its greater likelihood of being composed of prognostically unfavorable cell types. The Rappaport histopathologic classification is traditionally used for NHL staging. Although confusing and controversial, it historically has proved useful for the prognosis and management of NHL.[79, 80] The development of immunologic markers for lymphocytic subtypes has led to changes in NHL classification.[81] Such immunologic typing allows separation of NHL into categories of B-cell, T-cell, and true histiocytic origins; the B- and T-cell lymphomas can be further subdivided based on morphologic appearance and the degree of lymphocytic transformation.[82]

In an attempt to combine histopathologic and immunologic classification systems, the Non-Hodgkin's Lymphoma Pathologic Classification Project developed a classification scheme that groups NHLs according to their natural histories and responsiveness to therapy (refer to Lymphoma chapter).[83] Such groups, however, represent a spectrum of disease, and new subgroups have been identified that do not fit well even into this classification scheme.[64] The REAL system has more recently been proposed.[35] The REAL system recognizes the complex histopathologic diversity of NHL and attempts to classify lymphomas according to histopathologic appearance and immunohistochemistry.

Diagnosis and Staging

The pathologic examination of tissue is necessary for the diagnosis of NHL; such tissue is best obtained by excisional biopsy, although fine-needle aspiration has been used for the diagnosis of NHL.[84]

The Ann Arbor staging classification used for HL has also historically been applied to patients with NHL. Alternative staging systems that account for the characteristic extranodal presentations and the tendency toward hematogenous dissemination in childhood NHL have also been proposed.[62, 85–87] The staging of nasal and paranasal sinus NHL is particularly problematic.[78]

The staging of NHL requires a comprehensive history and physical examination; serologic studies such as complete blood count, electrolytes, serum lactate dehydrogenase (LDH) concentration, and HIV testing; a chest radiograph; a bone scan; a bone marrow biopsy; and a cerebrospinal fluid (CSF) analysis. Abdominal, pelvic, and chest CT with contrast, gallium scanning, and ultrasound may additionally be necessary to assess extent of disease. Whole body hybrid PET scanning may be an adjuvant to CT scanning.[88] Laparotomy is not a routine procedure in the staging of NHL.[89]

Treatment and Prognosis

Other than confirmatory biopsy, surgery plays little additional role in NHL treatment. Surgical debulking may be indicated in selected cases of aerodigestive tract compression; the reduction of tumor load may also lower the risk that tumor lysis syndrome will develop.[90] The mainstay of treatment for all stages of NHL is chemotherapy. The use of chemotherapy recognizes the fact that NHL disseminates hematogenously and thus requires systemic treatment. Radiation therapy is used as an alternative to surgical debulking when tumor reduction is emergently required to relieve symptoms of tumor compression. Radiation therapy may also be used in the setting of CNS NHL involvement, in addition to intrathecal chemotherapy.

For stages I and II disease, chemotherapy results in a 5-year event-free survival of 85% to 95%.[62] The specific chemotherapeutic regimens used and the duration of treatment depend on the histopathology. Cyclophosphamide, vincristine, and prednisone are most commonly employed; the use of additional agents is variable. Given the excellent prognosis, current efforts are directed toward reducing the long-term deleterious effects of treatment without compromising efficacy.

For stages III and IV disease, the particular chemotherapy regimen employed again depends on the histopathology of the disease. The treatment of advanced lymphoblastic lymphoma is based on the same chemotherapeutic regimen used for acute lymphoblastic leukemia.[91–95] The phases of treatment of advanced lymphoblastic lymphoma include induction, consolidation, and continuation, with a long-term event-free survival of 65% to 75%.[62] Treatment of advanced lymphoblastic lymphoma consists of a multitude of agents given over 15 to 32 months. Advanced-stage large cell lymphoma is treated with a variety of different agents and protocols. Within the large cell lymphomas, there appears to be a better response among B-cell tumors than T-cell tumors.[96, 97]

Among patients with CNS involvement, most receive prophylactic intrathecal chemotherapy when there is no obvious involvement of the head and neck.[62] In a pediatric series of nasal and paranasal sinus lymphomas, chemotherapy with or without irradiation remains the mainstay of treatment.[78]

Prognosis is associated with stage, and children with CNS disease at the time of presentation do particularly poorly.[63, 98] Factors that have been shown to have prognostic importance include the maximum diameter of the largest tumor mass, the specific extranodal sites of involvement, the tumor proliferation rate, the immunologic characteristics of the lymphoma, the patient's performance status, and the serum LDH.[64, 65, 87] Concurrent lymphadenopathy, poor response to radiotherapy, dissemination of disease during treatment, and histiocytic lymphocytic histology predict a poor prognosis.[31, 78, 99] Patients who relapse do particularly poorly. Bone marrow transplantation may be used in patients who fail to achieve a second remission.

Burkitt's Lymphoma

Burkitt's lymphoma (BL) is an NHL that deserves special attention owing to its distinct epidemiologic and clinical features. It almost exclusively affects children. Epidemiologic differences separate BL into endemic African and nonendemic or sporadic American types. The male-to-female ratio in endemic BL is 2:1, although when the jaw is involved, the ratio is 3:1.[100] The male-to-female ratio in sporadic BL is 3:1.[100] The median age of patients with endemic BL is 6 years, compared with 19 years in patients with sporadic BL.[100] The limited geographic distribution of African BL suggests an infectious, specifically Epstein-Barr virus (EBV), etiology. Almost all patients with African BL demonstrate high antibody titers to EBV determinant antigens, and 80% to 95% of their tumor cells contain copies of the EBV DNA genome; in contrast, only 15% to 20% of patients with the sporadic American type of BL demonstrate this serologic and histopathologic EBV association.[100–102] There is notably a 1000-fold increase in the incidence of BL among patients with acquired immunodeficiency.[103] Another factor found to be associated with BL is the deregulation of the proto-oncogene *C-MYC*, which results from a genetic translocation.[100]

Clinical Presentation

The typical presentation of endemic African-type BL is that of mandibular involvement, which occurs in 58% of cases.[100] Mandibular involvement is rare in sporadic American-type BL, with an incidence of only 7%.[100] The head and neck is involved in approximately one fourth of patients with American-type BL. Asymptomatic cervical lymph node enlargement is most common; nasopharyngeal and oropharyngeal lymphoid involvement are also reported.[104] More than 90% of patients with American-type BL have abdominal involvement at presentation, typically of mesenteric lymph node or ileocecal lymph node origin.[100] The bone marrow and CNS are frequent sites of relapse. Burkitt's lymphoma has rapid proliferative potential, and tumors may quickly reach a large size. Rapid diagnosis, staging, and treatment are advocated.

Pathology

The diagnostic histopathologic pattern of BL is a diffuse proliferation of uniform, undifferentiated cells that contain small, noncleaved nuclei and a discrete rim of amphophilic cytoplasm.[31, 105] The presence of large macrophages interspersed among neoplastic cells, the so-called starry sky pattern, is highly characteristic but not pathognomonic of BL.

Diagnosis and Staging

Staging evaluation is similar to that employed in other NHLs. A greater emphasis is placed on CT scanning for localization of abdominal and head and neck masses. Gallium scans and serum LDH levels are useful for quantitating tumor burden and monitoring patients following treatment.[101] When BL presents in the head and neck, biopsy followed by abdominal CT is advocated.[106] Isolated intra-abdominal disease may require laparotomy for a tissue diagnosis; alternatively, cytologic diagnosis by either image-guided fine-needle aspiration of a mass or examination of ascitic fluid is possible.[107] Two clinical staging systems are currently in use for BL (Table 24–5). Both systems are based on the premise that the anatomic sites of predilection of BL do not conform readily to the conventional Ann Arbor NHL staging classification.[101, 104]

Treatment

Chemotherapy is the treatment of choice for BL; the most common agents used are cyclophosphamide, vincristine, and prednisone.[74, 101] Surgical intervention is typically limited to biopsy, as was mentioned earlier. Emergent surgical intervention may be required for intestinal obstruction owing to abdominal BL involvement.[108] Surgical excision is generally not attempted unless 90% of the tumor burden can be removed, and even this is questioned if such surgery or the complications thereof will delay the initiation of chemotherapy.[100, 106, 107] Radiation therapy has no established treatment role owing to the rapid proliferative growth of this tumor and its generally poor irradiation response.[100] Prophylactic intrathecal methotrexate is added in an attempt to decrease CNS relapse rates.[101]

Prognosis

Three- to 5-year event-free survival is 85% to 95% for limited disease (stages I and II) and 75% to 85% for advanced disease (stages III and IV).[22] Relapse rates are lower and survival rates are significantly higher in patients with a smaller tumor burden at presentation.[109] Children younger than 12 years of age have a better prognosis. High anti-EBV antigen titers in patients with American BL appear to be associated with a more favorable prognosis.[104] Initial CNS or bone marrow involvement does not worsen the prognosis in endemic BL; conversely, in sporadic BL, they portend a poor prognosis.[100]

SOFT TISSUE SARCOMAS

Rhabdomyosarcoma

Rhabdomyosarcoma is the most common soft tissue malignancy in the pediatric age group, accounting for 50% to 70% of all childhood sarcomas.[12, 110–113] Approximately 35% to 40% of pediatric rhabdomyosarcomas occur in the head and neck.[114] More than 50% of patients are younger than 6 years of age at diagnosis.[115] There is no apparent sex predilection. Rhabdomyosarcoma is four times more common in white children than in any other racial group.[116]

Clinical Presentation

Within the head and neck region, the most common sites of origin, in descending order of frequency, are the orbit, the nasopharynx, the middle ear mastoid region, and the sinonasal cavities.[117] Rhabdomyosarcomas of the head and neck can be classified as orbital, parameningeal, and nonparameningeal.[118, 119] Orbital rhabdomyosarcoma is the most frequent neoplasm of the orbit in children; rapidly progressive, unilateral proptosis in a child younger than 10 years is the typical presentation.[120] Parameningeal sites include the nasopharynx, paranasal sinuses, middle ear, and infratemporal fossa.[121] Rhabdomyosarcoma of the nasopharynx presents in an insidious fashion with unilateral otitis media, rhinorrhea, and nasal obstruction; a delay in diagnosis of several months after onset of symptoms is common.[122] Rhabdomyosarcoma of the paranasal sinuses may have manifestations analogous to either nasopharyngeal or orbital rhabdomyosarcoma; headache and pain are common symptoms and are often mistaken for sinusitis. Patients with rhabdomyosarcoma of the ear typically have unilateral otorrhea and a hemorrhagic, soft tissue mass in the external auditory meatus, middle ear, or both. An initial misdiagnosis of otitis media or otitis externa is often made.[123] Approximately

TABLE 24–5 Staging Classifications of Burkitt's Lymphoma

Stage*	Extent of Tumor
A	Single extra-abdominal site
B	Multiple extra-abdominal sites
C	Intra-abdominal tumor
D	Intra-abdominal tumor with involvement of multiple extra-abdominal sites
AR	Stage C but with >90% of tumor surgically resected

Stage†	Extent of Tumor
I	Single tumor mass: Extra-abdominal (IA) or abdominal (IB)
II	Two separate tumor masses either above or below the diaphragm
III	More than two separate tumor masses above and below the diaphragm
IV	Pleural effusion, ascites, or involvement of central nervous system or bone marrow

*From Ziegler JL: Burkitt's lymphoma. N Engl J Med 305:735, 1981.
†From Kapadia S: Hematologic diseases: Malignant lymphomas, leukemias, plasma cell dyscrasias, histiocytosis X, and reactive lymph node lesions. In Barnes L (ed): Surgical Pathology of the Head and Neck. New York, Marcel Dekker, 1985, p 1065.

50% of patients with aural rhabdomyosarcoma have neurologic findings at the time of diagnosis, with the facial nerve most commonly involved.[124, 125] Multiple cranial nerve palsies suggest skull base or CNS involvement from nasopharyngeal or sinonasal rhabdomyosarcoma.[115, 126]

Rhabdomyosarcoma metastasizes by both lymphatic and hematogenous routes.[110, 127, 128] The incidence of cervical lymph node metastases varies with the primary site; such metastases are particularly rare with orbital rhabdomyosarcoma. In the Intergroup Rhabdomyosarcoma Studies (IRS) I and II, no patients with orbital primary lesions presented with clinically positive neck nodes, whereas 8% of patients with other primary tumors had metastatic adenopathy.[129] Common sites of hematogenous metastatic disease are the lung, bone, and bone marrow. About 13% of patients with nonorbital rhabdomyosarcoma of the head and neck present with distant metastases.[130]

Pathology

Rhabdomyosarcoma appears grossly as a tan, firm mass that infiltrates into surrounding tissues.[115] Histopathologically, rhabdomyosarcoma consists of a variety of different subtypes—embryonal, alveolar, botryoid, spindle cell, and undifferentiated sarcoma.[131, 132] Embryonal is the most common subtype (54%) found within the head and neck; the cervicofacial rates of other histopathologic subtypes are 18.5% (alveolar), 6.5% (undifferentiated), and 4.5% (botryoid).[118] Embryonal rhabdomyosarcoma is characterized by small round cells with dark nuclei, mitotic figures, and occasional striations in a loose myxoid background. Botryoid rhabdomyosarcoma is actually a variant of embryonal that occurs in open cavities; the so-called sarcoma botryoid is polypoid, resembling a bunch of grapes.

Diagnosis and Staging

Biopsy is necessary for the diagnosis of rhabdomyosarcoma of the head and neck. Physical examination should focus on evaluating the extent of local disease as well as detecting regional and distant spread. Patients with head and neck rhabdomyosarcoma should have CT and/or MRI of the head, neck, and skull base to assess for local extension; lumbar puncture with CSF cytologic examination should also be performed (Fig. 24–3).[127, 133, 134] Skeletal survey, bone scan, and bone marrow biopsy are necessary for a complete systemic evaluation.

Treatment of rhabdomyosarcoma is determined by primary site and stage of disease. Within the head and neck, primary lesion size, local invasiveness, and regional and distant metastases have prognostic significance.[129, 135] The IRS have developed a clinical staging system (Table 24–6) based on extent of disease (localized, regional, or systemic) and whether complete excision of locoregional disease is accomplished.[136] A problem with this staging system is the fact that resectability and hence the stage of disease vary among institutions. An alternative staging system uses clinical tumor, nodes, and metastases (TNM) for staging but emphasizes local invasiveness as opposed to size criteria in determination of tumor (T) stage (Table 24–7).[137, 138]

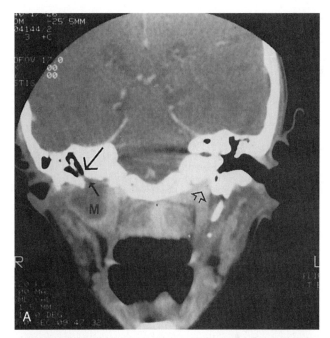

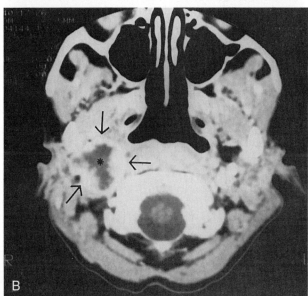

FIGURE 24–3 Axial and coronal CT scans demonstrate a rhabdomyosarcoma in the poststyloid compartment of the right parapharyngeal space in a 13-year-old girl. *A,* The mass (M) erodes the osseous margins of the jugular bulb *(short solid arrow)* and extends into the middle ear *(long arrow).* The normal left jugular bulb *(open arrowhead)* is demonstrated for comparison. *B,* The capsule-like periphery of the lesion *(arrows)* surrounds a low-density center *(asterisk),* suggesting necrosis within the mass.

Treatment

Through its multiple clinical trials, the IRS has established the superiority of multimodality therapy (including surgery, radiotherapy, and chemotherapy) over single-modality therapy in the treatment of rhabdomyosarcoma. Surgical excision is indicated when no excessive morbidity will result and when excision of the primary tumor will

TABLE 24-6 Staging of Rhabdomyosarcoma According to the Intergroup Rhabdomyosarcoma Study

Group	Description
Group I	Localized disease with tumor completely resected and regional nodes not affected Confined to muscle or organ of origin Contiguous involvement—infiltration outside the muscle or organ of origin
Group II	Localized disease with microscopic residual disease, or regional disease with no residual or with microscopic residual disease Grossly resected tumor with microscopic residual disease (nodes negative) Regional tumor completely resected (nodes positive or negative) Regional disease with involved nodes grossly resected but with evidence of microscopic residual disease
Group III	Incomplete resection or biopsy with gross residual disease
Group IV	Metastatic disease present at onset

From Barnes L: Tumors and tumorlike lesions of the soft tissues. In Barnes L (ed): Surgical Pathology of the Head and Neck. New York, Marcel Dekker, 1985, p 796.

permit either the elimination of postoperative irradiation or a reduction in dose. This is particularly true of many of the nonorbital and nonparameningeal head and neck sites,[139, 140] and it may apply to some tumors classified as

TABLE 24-7 TNM Classification of Rhabdomyosarcoma Modified by the IRS

Stage	Site	T	Size	N	M
I	Orbit, head, and neck, excluding parameningeal sites, genitourinary but not bladder or prostate	T1 or T2	A or B	Any N	M0
II	Bladder, prostate, T1 or T2 extremity, cranial and parameningeal sites, other	T1 or T2	A	N0 or Nx	M0
III	Bladder, prostate, T1 or T2 extremity, cranial and parameningeal sites, other	T1 or T2	A B	N1 Any N	M0 M0
IV	All	T1 or T2	A or B	N0 or N1	M1

Where TNM and the size of the tumor are defined as:
T1 is confined to the site of origin
T2 has extension or fixation to surrounding structures
A is a tumor ≤ 5 cm
B is a tumor > 5 cm
N0 is no clinically involved lymph nodes
N1 is regionally involved lymph nodes
Nx is clinical status of lymph nodes unknown
M0 is no distant metastasis
M1 is metastasis present

Adapted from Pappo AS, Shapiro DN, Crist WM: Biology and therapy of pediatric rhabdomyosarcoma. J Clin Oncol 13:2123, 1995.

parameningeal, such as those in the occiput and the infratemporal fossa.[119] When only partial tumor resection is possible or the tumor is orbital, initial surgery is limited to biopsy. Biopsy alone of orbital rhabdomyosarcoma is advocated because combined radiation and chemotherapy result in excellent long-term survival with limited morbidity.[130, 140, 141] Surgical exploration and biopsy may also be used to determine if a tumor has partially or completely responded to therapy.[118]

When rhabdomyosarcoma of the head and neck is not completely resectable, radiation therapy is commonly required. Radiation therapy is indicated for groups II, III, and IV tumors. Such radiotherapy is directed at the primary site and employs wide portals determined by the extent of tumor on pretreatment clinical and radiographic examination.[113, 142] In IRS-IV, there was no improvement in survival when a hyperfractionated protocol was used, as compared with conventional radiation therapy.[118]

Almost all patients with head and neck rhabdomyosarcoma receive systemic chemotherapy. Such chemotherapy is given postoperatively to patients with small resectable lesions. Several cycles of preoperative chemotherapy may be necessary as initial treatment for patients with larger lesions to decrease tumor volume before local treatment is started. The exact protocol chosen varies primarily with the stage of disease.[113, 143–145] IRS-V is designed to examine the use of various chemotherapeutic protocols in patients with higher-risk nonmetastatic disease, such as those with alveolar and undifferentiated disease, stage II/III disease, and group III embryonal disease.[118]

Patients with a clinically negative neck require no treatment other than chemotherapy. Children with a clinically positive neck benefit from neck dissection, with the addition of radiation therapy for those with multiple positive nodes.[136]

Prognosis

Before the IRS, 5-year survival for rhabdomyosarcoma of the head and neck, all sites considered, ranged from 8% to 20%; average survival was 15 months for orbital rhabdomyosarcoma, 7 to 12 months for middle ear mastoid rhabdomyosarcoma, and 17 months for rhabdomyosarcoma arising in the soft tissues of the face and the neck.[117] In IRS-I, the 3-year relapse-free survival rates increased to 91% for orbital primary disease, 46% for parameningeal (middle ear mastoid, sinonasal, nasopharyngeal, and infratemporal fossa) primary disease, and 75% for other head and neck sites.[130]

The IRS has demonstrated increasingly improved 3-year survival rates.[12, 136, 146–149] These gains are most evident in patients with gross residual tumor after surgery with no distant metastases.[149] Children with tumors in favorable sites, including the orbit and nonparameningeal areas of the head and neck, have an excellent prognosis.[136, 148, 150] Ongoing analysis of the IRS protocols suggests that the primary site is a more important prognostic factor than the histologic subtype.[149, 151] An equally important prognostic variable is response to treatment, because those who never achieve complete response do not survive.[152]

In IRS-I, two groups of patients did particularly poorly—those with distant metastases (group IV) and those with evidence of base of skull and CNS extension from parameningeal primary sites (group III). Survival in these groups was typically less than 12 months.[145] The meninges proved to be the most common site of tumor recurrence.[130] These observations led to protocol changes in IRS-II, in which an attempt was made to protect the CNS in high-risk patients with parameningeal disease by the addition of prophylactic cranial irradiation and intrathecal triple-drug therapy. This approach has proved efficacious.[153]

The 5-year survival rates in IRS-I and -II were 55% and 63%, respectively.[154] IRS-III and -IV had an improved 5-year survival of 71%.[154] The 5-year relapse-free survival in IRS-II was 82% to 88% for group I, 68% to 90% for group II, 67% to 79% for group III, and only 37% to 40% for group IV patients.[155] Improvements in IRS-III are reflected in group III patients whose 3-year survival increased to 80%.[113] On the other hand, in IRS-IV, it is patients with nonmetastatic disease whose 3-year failure-free and disease-free survival rates increased to 77% and 80%, respectively.[143]

Of importance to otolaryngologists is the prognosis of patients with middle ear rhabdomyosarcoma. Such patients have a comparatively better prognosis than do those with other parameningeal sites, with an overall 3-year survival of 88% when the multimodality therapeutic protocols of IRS-III and -IV are used.[147] Patients with rhabdomyosarcoma of the middle ear tend to present with favorable prognostic factors such as embryonal histology, age younger than 10 years old, and a low incidence of cervical metastases (14%).[147]

Overall favorable prognostic factors include specific primary sites such as the orbit, nonparameningeal head and neck, and genitourinary system; grossly resected disease; embryonal and botryoid histology; tumor size smaller than 5 cm; age younger than 10 years; and absence of metastatic disease.[154] Historically, individuals who are free of recurrence 2 years after treatment have been considered cured.[156] This long-term prognosis of rhabdomyosarcoma may have to be more guarded because late recurrences have been reported.[157, 158]

IRS-V divides patients into low-, intermediate-, and high-risk groups based on stage of disease, group, site, size, age, histology, presence of metastases, and lymph node involvement.[154] Patients are categorized according to their presenting characteristics and are then assigned a particular treatment regimen that includes variable chemotherapeutic protocols with or without radiation therapy. Both the botryoid variant of embryonal rhabdomyosarcoma and the spindle cell rhabdomyosarcoma have a favorable prognosis. Alveolar and undifferentiated rhabdomyosarcoma have a poor prognosis.[131, 132] Embryonal rhabdomyosarcoma has an intermediate prognosis. A major goal of IRS-V is to achieve improved control of disease with minimal morbidity.

Soft Tissue Sarcomas Other Than Rhabdomyosarcoma

Soft tissue sarcomas other than rhabdomyosarcoma (NRMS) account for 3% of malignant neoplasms in children younger than 15 years.[110] A bimodal age distribution curve with one peak in children younger than 5 years and the other peak in adolescence is characteristic of almost all soft tissue sarcomas.[159] The soft tissue sarcomas of infants and young children occur primarily in the head and neck region, whereas lesions in adolescents predominantly arise in the trunk and extremities. NRMSs arising within the head and neck include fibrosarcoma, synovial sarcoma, neurofibrosarcoma (malignant schwannoma), hemangiopericytoma, chondrosarcoma, and extraosseous Ewing's sarcoma. Children with von Recklinghausen's neurofibromatosis are at particular risk for developing neurofibrosarcomas.

Soft tissue sarcomas typically present as firm, enlarging masses in a variety of head and neck locations (Figs. 24–4 and 24–5). Because of their relative rarity, the study of NRMSs and the development of treatment regimens require multi-institution collaboration. In general, when possible, complete surgical excision without excessive morbidity is advocated, as is a multimodality therapeutic approach similar to that used in the treatment of rhabdomyosarcoma.[160–163] Chemotherapy and radiation therapy are generally reserved for NRMSs that are not completely resected.[164] In the treatment of NRMSs outside the head and neck region, when a pathologically confirmed surgical margin of greater than 1 cm can be obtained, the risk of local recurrence is reduced independent of tumor grade; when the margin is less than 1 cm, the use of postoperative radiation is efficacious.[165] This is an important observation because a 1-cm margin is often difficult to obtain in the surgical management of head and neck NRMSs.

Prognostic factors of NRMS of the head and neck include primary site, extent of disease, tumor grade, and disease bulk. NRMSs of the oral cavity or oropharynx have a particularly favorable prognosis.[164]

Fibrosarcoma

Fibrosarcoma accounts for 11% of soft tissue sarcomas, with the majority of cases occurring within the first 6 months of life.[110, 166, 167] Fifteen percent to 20% of fibrosarcomas occur in the head and neck region, predominantly in infants and young children.[159] Fibrosarcomas occur mostly in the extremities in adolescent patients.

Fibrosarcomas consist of uniform, small spindle or round cells arranged in a fascicular fashion; mitosis and necrosis may be present.[115] Documentation of local infiltration is used to distinguish well-differentiated fibrosarcoma from nonmalignant juvenile fibromatosis; this distinction can be difficult (see Fig. 24–5).[117, 168] The cause of fibrosarcoma in children is speculative.[169] Fibrosarcoma may occur in the setting of previous radiation therapy.[170]

Common sites of fibrosarcoma in the head and neck include the neck, oral cavity, scalp, auriculoparotid region, nose and paranasal sinuses, larynx, face, cheek, and hypopharynx.[117] A slowly enlarging, painless, firm mass is the typical presentation of a fibrosarcoma. Symptoms result from local extension and pressure on surrounding structures. Fibrosarcoma of the tracheobronchial airway may present with recurrent pneumonia, stridor, chronic cough, and hemoptysis.[171, 172] Fibrosarcoma is unique among the soft tissue sarcomas in that metastatic disease in infants and young children is infrequent. Lymph node metastases occur in fewer than 10% of patients.[173] Likewise, metastases to

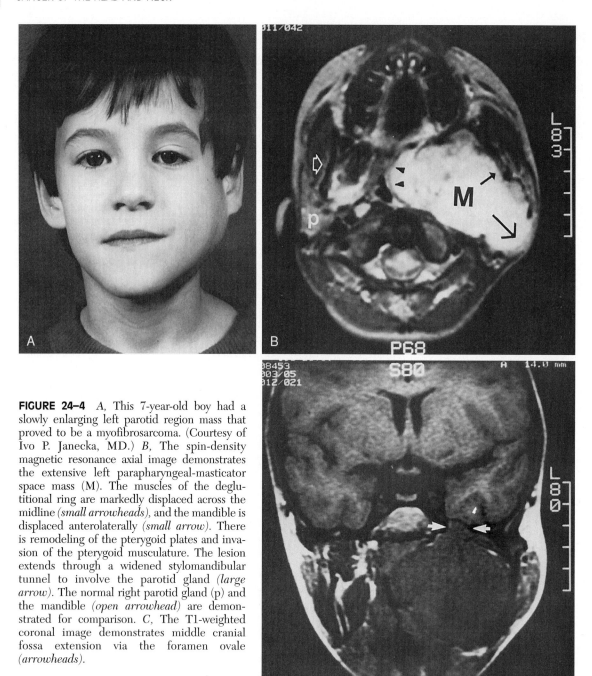

FIGURE 24–4 *A*, This 7-year-old boy had a slowly enlarging left parotid region mass that proved to be a myofibrosarcoma. (Courtesy of Ivo P. Janecka, MD.) *B*, The spin-density magnetic resonance axial image demonstrates the extensive left parapharyngeal-masticator space mass (M). The muscles of the deglutitional ring are markedly displaced across the midline *(small arrowheads)*, and the mandible is displaced anterolaterally *(small arrow)*. There is remodeling of the pterygoid plates and invasion of the pterygoid musculature. The lesion extends through a widened stylomandibular tunnel to involve the parotid gland *(large arrow)*. The normal right parotid gland (p) and the mandible *(open arrowhead)* are demonstrated for comparison. *C*, The T1-weighted coronal image demonstrates middle cranial fossa extension via the foramen ovale *(arrowheads)*.

lung and bone are reported in less than 10% of patients younger than 10 years; this figure increases to 50% in patients older than 15 years.[174, 175] Plain radiographs may reveal a soft tissue density associated with bone destruction. CT of the head and neck is important in assessing for base of skull erosion and intracranial extension.[176]

Therapy is directed at local disease control. Complete surgical excision is advocated when possible, although maintenance of function at the expense of incompletely resected disease may be necessary in head and neck disease. When resection is incomplete, local radiation therapy is used. Adjuvant chemotherapy is of uncertain value and is not employed routinely because of the low incidence of distant metastases.[160] Preoperative chemotherapy has been used to decrease the size of the tumor in an attempt to increase the likelihood of resectability and to assess a tumor's responsiveness to chemotherapy regimens that can be used in the postsurgical adjuvant setting.[168] The 5-year survival of infants and young children with fibrosarcoma is 80% to 90%.[169, 174]

Desmoid Fibromatosis

Desmoid fibromatosis (DF) is a rare benign tumor that can arise within the cervicofacial region. Approximately 10% of cases of extra-abdominal DF occur in the head and

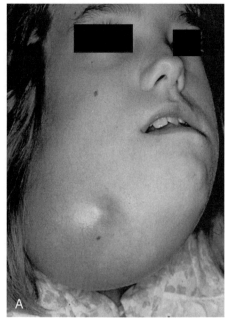
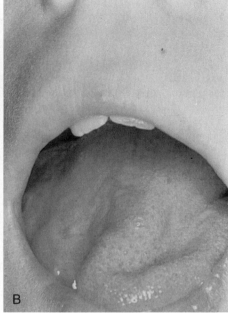
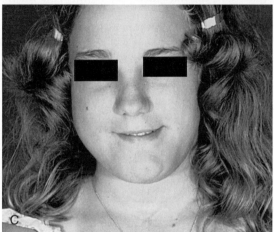

FIGURE 24–5 *A,* A child with fibrosarcoma involving the neck and oral cavity. *B,* Intraoral view. *C,* Appearance 2 years after excision of the tumor.

neck,[177] with the supraclavicular fossa being the most common site.[178] DF is characterized by local aggressiveness and a high recurrence rate after resection. Gardner's syndrome, pregnancy, estrogen exposure, trauma, and familial adenomatous polyposis have been associated with DF.

DF most often presents as an asymptomatic neck mass; potential symptomatic complaints include pain, radiculopathy, and upper extremity weakness.[178] The gross appearance of DF is that of a firm, tan mass; microscopic characteristics include fascicles of spindle fibroblasts in a myxoid background.[177]

The initial workup of a child suspected of having DF should include inquiry about previous trauma or any medical or historical information that may predispose to the development of malignancy. Head and neck examination to assess the extent of the lesion and the possible involvement of cranial nerves is important for preoperative planning. Similarly, imaging, including CT and/or MRI, should be obtained. Open biopsy or core needle biopsy is often needed for diagnosis.[178]

The standard treatment for DF of the head and neck is surgical excision. Multiple staged procedures are sometimes required. Given its potential local invasiveness, involvement of critical structures is possible and needs to be considered in preoperative planning. In cases of advanced disease not amenable to surgical intervention, radiation and chemotherapy have been used.[179–182] Also, because of the local aggressiveness, there is a high incidence of recurrence after resection, particularly in patients with positive margins.[183] Recurrence rates in the head and neck vary between 24% and 62%.[178, 184, 185] Despite this, the prognosis is adequate. In a study of 21 patients with head and neck fibromatosis, 18 patients were disease free and none had died of the disease at a mean follow-up of 54 months.[178]

Neurofibrosarcoma (Malignant Schwannoma)

Neurofibrosarcoma is a malignant tumor of neural sheath origin that accounts for 3% of childhood soft tissue sarcomas.[110] Neurofibrosarcomas are the malignant counterpart of neurofibromas.[186] Children with von Recklinghausen's neurofibromatosis are at increased risk for malignant transformation, with 5% to 16% of these children developing neurofibrosarcoma.[187]

Approximately 10% of all neurofibrosarcomas occur in the cervicofacial region, particularly in the neck. Such lesions arise from the cranial nerves, cervical plexus, or sympathetic chain.[117] The common presentation is an enlarging cervical mass with associated neuromuscular symptoms such as pain, paresthesias, dysphonia, dysphagia, muscle fasciculations, facial nerve dysfunction, or muscle weakness.[188] Radiologic imaging by CT or MRI is required for determination of the extent of local lesion involvement.

Surgical excision is advocated when possible. Local recurrence and pulmonary metastases are common. There may be a benefit of adjuvant radiotherapy and multiagent chemotherapy in accordance with IRS protocols.[133] Radiation contributes to local control of stage II patients; however, no chemotherapy regimen that results in acceptable disease-free survival rates in patients with advanced disease has emerged.[153, 189] Patients with extensive local disease or distant metastases do poorly despite aggressive multimodality therapy; cure rates are highest among patients with completely resectable disease.[110, 153, 189] Malignant schwannomas arising in patients with von Recklinghausen's disease are particularly aggressive. The 5-year survival for this group of patients is 15% to 30%, compared with 27% to 75% for patients whose tumors are not associated with von Recklinghausen's disease.[117]

Synovial Sarcoma

Synovial sarcomas account for 5% of pediatric soft tissue sarcomas.[110] Synovial sarcoma has a female predominance.[190] Synovial sarcomas primarily arise in the extremities, with fewer than 50 cases reported in the head and neck.[117, 190, 191] Synovial sarcoma is thought to arise from synovioblastic differentiation of mesenchymal stem cells; this explains the presence of synovial sarcomas in head and neck sites with no normal synovial structures.[192]

Grossly, synovial sarcomas appear well defined with a pseudocapsule. When sectioned, there may be areas of calcification. The most common histopathologic type of synovial sarcoma contains both epithelial and spindle cells and is called *biphasic*.[115]

Synovial sarcoma has been reported in the larynx, pharynx, tongue, tonsils, and orofacial soft tissues.[192] Synovial sarcoma commonly presents in the neck as a firm, gradually enlarging, parapharyngeal or retropharyngeal mass that becomes symptomatic by compromising contiguous structures. Radiographically, synovial sarcomas appear as soft tissue masses, usually without adjacent bone erosion. Imaging of synovial sarcoma by CT and MRI may reveal a homogeneous, well-demarcated mass, occasionally with multiple foci of calcification (Fig. 24–6).[193]

Treatment of local disease includes the widest possible surgical excision followed by radiation therapy.[194] A retrospective review of patients with synovial sarcoma not limited to the head and neck suggested an improved survival with adjuvant radiation therapy, even with complete resection.[195] Local recurrence and metastases to lymph nodes, bone marrow, and lung occur in approximately half of patients.[192] Five-year survival rates following surgical and radiation treatment alone approximate 50%; children with small, localized lesions have the best outcome.[117, 196] Because of the poor prognosis associated with distant (particularly lung) metastases, multimodality treatment regimens similar to those used for rhabdomyosarcoma are advocated in the treatment of synovial sarcoma, although the benefit of such adjuvant chemotherapy is uncertain.[195, 197] A study that used both radiation and chemotherapy after surgical resection of synovial sarcoma not limited to the head and neck led to a 5-year survival of 74%.[190]

Hemangiopericytoma

Hemangiopericytomas account for 3% of childhood soft tissue sarcomas.[110] Approximately 10% to 15% of hemangiopericytomas are seen in the pediatric age group.[198, 199] Two types of childhood hemangiopericytomas are recognized. Congenital or infantile hemangiopericytomas occur within the first year of life and follow a benign course despite malignant histopathologic characteristics.[200, 201] When hemangiopericytomas occur in children older than 1 year, they behave similarly to those in the adult population, with a malignancy rate of 20% to 35%.[198]

Hemangiopericytomas arise from Zimmermann's pericytes, cells that lie external to the reticulin sheath of capillaries. Microscopically, they consist of uniform round or spindle-shaped cells associated with a vascular background. Special stains reveal a reticulin pattern that distinguishes hemangiopericytomas from hemangiosarcomas and other vascular soft tissue tumors.[117] Histopathologic characteristics suggestive of malignancy include hemorrhage, calcifications, necrosis, and an increased mitotic rate.[200] Infantile hemangiopericytomas are more often multilobulated than are adult cases.

The nasal cavity and paranasal sinuses are the most common head and neck locations for hemangiopericytomas; less frequent sites include the orbital region, parotid gland, and neck.[195] The most common site in the oral cavity is the tongue.[202] Sinonasal hemangiopericytomas may occur as a polypoid mass causing nasal obstruction and epistaxis. The characteristic presentation in other locations is that of a slowly enlarging, painless mass of firm, fibrous consistency. Hemangiopericytomas have been diagnosed in utero by ultrasound.[203]

Wide local excision is the therapy of choice because hemangiopericytomas are not well encapsulated.[200] Infantile hemangiopericytoma is rarely associated with local recurrence or the development of metastatic disease; thus, adjuvant therapy is not necessary. However, adjuvant chemotherapy is advocated for the treatment of hemangiopericytoma in all other age groups.[204] Radiation therapy, in combination with chemotherapy, is also used in cases of unresectable or incompletely resectable local disease.[205]

Local recurrence and lung metastases characterize hemangiopericytoma of all sites, including the head and neck.[199, 206] The small number of childhood cases does not allow for age-specific survival figures. The overall survival at 5 years in adult series varies between 50% and 70%.[199, 206]

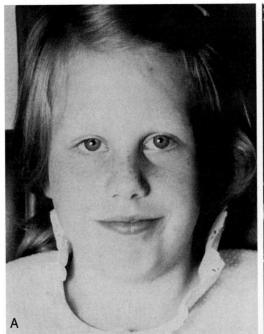

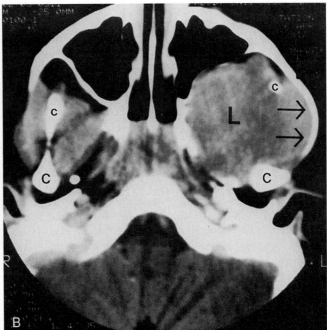

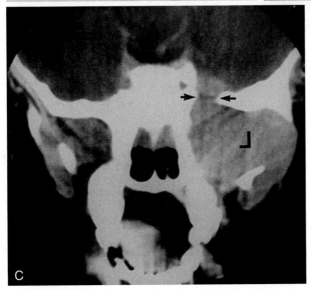

FIGURE 24–6 *A*, This 8-year-old girl presented with a 3-month history of left cheek swelling. *B*, CT axial scan demonstrates a large infratemporal fossa lesion (L) that bows the zygomatic bone outward *(arrows)*. Note the displacement of the coronoid (c) and condylar (C) processes on the left compared with the normal right side. *C*, Coronal view reveals enlargement of the foramen rotundum *(arrowheads)* with extension of the lesion into the middle cranial fossa. Biopsy of the mass revealed a synovial sarcoma.

Patients with unresectable local disease or metastatic disease at the time of presentation do poorly.

Extraosseous Ewing's Sarcoma

Extraosseous Ewing's sarcoma (EES), also called primitive neuroectodermal tumor, is a soft tissue malignancy identical histologically to Ewing's sarcoma of bone. The specific cell of origin is suspected to be a primitive mesenchymal stem cell.[207, 208] Histologic differentiation of EES from undifferentiated embryonal rhabdomyosarcoma may be difficult. The histopathologic appearance is that of small round cells without structural differentiation.[209]

A majority of individuals with EES are younger than 30 years of age.[210] The mean age of presentation is 15 years.[211] In the head and neck, EES often arises in the soft tissues adjacent to the cervical spine, such as in the scalp and paraspinal muscles.[211–213] Symptoms may include pain, tenderness, and neurologic disturbances related to cord compression, in addition to a palpable mass.[214] Vertebrae adjacent to EES may show periosteal thickening and new bone formation on radiographic evaluation.[215]

Multimodality regimens used in the treatment of rhabdomyosarcoma[216] and osseous Ewing's sarcoma[217] are used to treat both adults and children with EES.[211] The IRS protocol has been applied principally in the head and neck region. The IRS-I reported a 65% disease-free survival for EES patients treated by surgical excision with or without radiotherapy and chemotherapy.[218] A disease-free survival of 64% and good local control results of 82% were found in 11 patients treated with a combination of high-dose radiation and chemotherapy.[219] In a study of 24 patients treated with multimodality therapy with a 5-year survival of 61%, favorable prognostic factors included age older than 16 years and the ability to undergo a surgical resection, either complete or partial.[211] The most important prognostic factor for children with EES is the absence of metastatic disease at diagnosis.[211]

BONE SARCOMAS

Bone sarcomas represent approximately 5% of all malignant tumors in children. Osteosarcoma is the most common, accounting for approximately 60% of pediatric bone tumors, with Ewing's sarcoma, chondrosarcoma, malignant fibrous histiocytoma, and other rare tumors constituting the remaining 40%.[220, 221] In a review of 663 bone sarcomas in children, 4.5% occurred in the head and neck.[220] The most common sites were the mandible and the maxilla; an evident mass and focal pain are the most common sign and symptom, respectively.[220] Radiographic evaluation typically reveals a lytic lesion with varying degrees of contrast enhancement.

Osteosarcoma

Osteosarcoma is the most common bone sarcoma, with an incidence of 5.6 per million in children younger than 15 years of age; as such, osteosarcoma accounts for 2.6% of all pediatric malignant tumors.[220] Approximately 7% to 16% of osteosarcomas occur in the head and neck. Factors predisposing to the development of osteosarcoma include previous radiation therapy, Paget's disease, fibrous dysplasia, and hereditary retinoblastoma.[221, 222] In one study, 8 of 28 patients with osteosarcoma of the head and neck had previous radiation therapy to the eventual site of tumor occurrence.[220] The common sites of involvement are the mandible (38%), maxilla (23%), and orbit (15%).[221, 222] Primary occurrence at the base of the skull, cervical spine, or soft tissues is rare.

Osteosarcoma of the head and neck appears at a later age than that of the extremities. The typical presentation is that of pain with the subsequent appearance of a mass as the tumor expands through the bone cortex. Symmetrical widening of the periodontal ligament involving one or more teeth may be evident.[223] Radiographic findings vary, and lesions can appear either sclerotic or lytic. Osseous destruction is best seen on CT; MRI is additionally useful in demonstrating characteristic amorphous calcium deposits in the soft tissue.

The most frequent site of metastatic disease is the lung; bone metastases are also common. Approximately 20% of patients present with clinically detectable metastases at the time of diagnosis.[224] Micrometastases are presumably even more common, given the high likelihood of recurrence when solely local treatment with surgery and/or radiation therapy is employed. Metastatic evaluation should include chest radiograph, chest CT, and bone scan, as well as serum alkaline phosphate and lactate levels.

Multimodality therapy is used in osteosarcoma. Surgical excision is important in treatment because chemotherapy alone cannot eliminate gross disease. Multiagent chemotherapy is required, even if there is no clinically documented metastatic disease, because of the high likelihood of micrometastases. Agents used include doxorubicin, methotrexate, ifosfamide, and cisplatin.[225] Osteosarcoma is generally considered radioresistant; radiotherapy may occasionally be used in the setting of unresectable primary disease. Negative prognostic factors include incomplete surgical excision and systemic metastases at presentation.[220, 224]

Ewing's Sarcoma

Ewing's sarcoma is a small cell tumor that occurs primarily during the first three decades of life and is rare in the head and neck.[226–228] It is the second most common bone sarcoma in children. There is a 2:1 male-to-female predominance. Unlike osteosarcoma, Ewing's sarcoma is not associated with previous radiation exposure. Approximately 95% of patients have a translocation between chromosome 22 and either chromosome 11 or 21.[225]

A majority of Ewing's sarcoma lesions within the head and neck involve the mandible, skull, maxilla, and cervical spine. Most patients present with pain and localized swelling.[229] Systemic symptoms can include fever, anemia, and weight loss. There may be an associated leukocytosis and an increased erythrocyte sedimentation rate. These signs and symptoms herald metastatic disease involving the bone marrow. Although the medullary cavity appears to be the site of origin of Ewing's sarcomas, even in early stages of the disease, the bone cortex may be eroded by a friable, hemorrhagic mass. Cervical lymph node involvement is uncommon. The most common sites of distant metastases are the lung, other bones, the bone marrow, and the central nervous system.

Radiologic evaluation of the primary site includes CT and MRI analysis to evaluate the extent of disease and to determine the proper site for diagnostic biopsy. The usual appearance of Ewing's sarcoma on plain radiographs is that of a lytic or mottled pattern of bone destruction with poorly defined margins, a so-called onion skin appearance. Chest radiography and lung CT scan, bone scan, and bone marrow aspiration with biopsy are necessary to evaluate for metastatic disease.

The principal modality used for local treatment of Ewing's sarcoma of the head and neck is radiation therapy. Surgical resection may be selectively used for some mandibular lesions. Multiagent chemotherapy is essential in the treatment of Ewing's sarcoma owing to the high risk of microscopic metastases.[225]

Following multimodality therapy, long-term survival in patients with localized disease is 50% to 70%, decreasing to 19% to 30% for patients with metastatic disease.[225] Head and neck lesions are generally considered favorable sites, with the possible exception of the cervical spine and the maxilla.[228, 230] A large extraosseous mass, the presence of systemic symptoms, age older than 17 years, and an increased LDH level are associated with a poor prognosis.[228–233] Although patients with multiple bony metastases at diagnosis continue to have a poor outcome, aggressive treatment, including ablative chemotherapy and radiation therapy followed by autologous bone marrow transplant, can improve their survival rates.[234–236]

Chondrosarcoma

Chondrosarcomas are rare lesions, with 4.6% of pediatric cases occurring in the head and neck.[237] A 27-year review at the Armed Forces Institute of Pathology identified only 14 cases of pediatric chondrosarcoma of the head and neck.[237] Although most chondrosarcomas occur as isolated lesions, there is an increased risk of chondrosarcoma development with preexisting conditions such as enchondroma, exostosis, juxtacortical chondroma, Maffucci's syndrome, chondromyxoid fibroma, chondroblastoma, Paget's disease, previous intravenous Thorotrast contrast use, and previous local radiation.[238, 239]

Chondrosarcomas are slow-growing but locally aggressive neoplasms with a propensity for local recurrence. The most commonly involved head and neck sites include the maxilla, skull base, sinonasal tract, and mandible.[238, 240–242] Patients with laryngeal chondrosarcoma typically do not present until the sixth to seventh decades of life.[243, 244] Metastases are rare. Presenting symptoms depend on the location of the tumor and include nasal obstruction, sinusitis, epistaxis, pain, visual changes, and hoarseness, in addition to a local mass.[237] Standard radiographs reveal an osteolytic defect with expansion and local bone resorption and a ground glass appearance. CT reveals a mass with scalloped borders with calcification.

The primary treatment for chondrosarcoma is surgery. If an adequate resection margin can be obtained, the local control rate is good.[238, 241, 245] A beneficial effect of postoperative radiation therapy in cases of unresectable disease or inadequate surgical margins is suggested by analyses of chondrosarcomas at all body sites.[246, 247–251] Chemotherapy has also been used in some cases.

The survival rate of pediatric patients with head and neck chondrosarcomas approximates 50%; important prognostic factors include site of lesion and adequacy of surgical resection.[238, 252] In a study of 14 children, high histologic grade was not deemed an unfavorable prognostic factor.[237]

Additional Sarcomas

Additional sarcomatous neoplasms of the head and neck region in children include malignant hemangioendothelioma, leiomyosarcoma, liposarcoma, alveolar soft part sarcoma, and malignant fibrous histiocytoma.[110, 117, 167, 253] The use of surgery and radiation therapy to control local disease along with the administration of systemic chemotherapy to prevent metastases appears applicable to these rare lesions as well, particularly those of high histologic grade.

◻ NEUROECTODERMAL TUMORS

Neuroblastoma

Neuroblastoma accounts for 10% of all pediatric malignancies and is the most common malignancy among infants younger than 1 year.[15, 254, 255] Ninety percent of neuroblastomas occur in children younger than 10 years, with birth to 5 years representing the usual age range.[256] Neuroblastoma ranks second to leukemia in infant malignancy-related mortality and accounts for 15% of all cancer deaths in children.[257] There is a slight male predominance.

Clinical Presentation

Neuroblastoma primarily arises within the abdomen and thorax.[258] The adrenal gland is the most common site of origin; additional sites include the sympathetic chain in the retroperitoneum, the posterior mediastinum, and cervical regions. Only 1% to 4% of all neuroblastomas are primary cervical lesions.[258, 259] Metastatic disease to the head and neck from sites below the diaphragm is more common than primary cervical disease and must be excluded. Patients with primary cervical neuroblastoma typically present with a firm lateral neck mass. Signs and symptoms typically result from local extension of the disease and may include Horner's syndrome, respiratory distress, or feeding difficulties secondary to tracheal and esophageal involvement. Cranial neuropathies may result from skull base involvement, and other neurologic sequelae may result from a tumor's passing through the neural foramina into the spinal canal. Heterochromia has been associated with neuroblastoma and is thought to reflect anomalies of neural crest cell derivation.[260]

Spread to regional lymphatics can be documented in approximately 35% of patients who present with apparent isolated primary disease.[254] Children younger than 1 year are less likely (25%) to have disseminated disease than are older children (68%).[254] Common sites of distant disease include lung, bone, central nervous system, liver, and skin. Metastases to cervical lymph nodes, skull, orbit, and jaw are particularly common (Fig. 24–7).[259]

Pathology

The diagnosis of a neuroblastoma is typically made on histopathologic examination. Neuroblastomas fall into the category of small, round, blue cell tumors that also includes

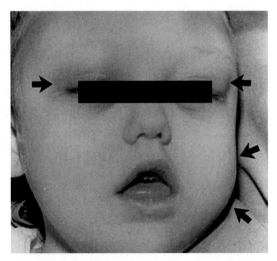

FIGURE 24–7 Neuroblastoma typically originates in sites below the diaphragm and commonly metastasizes to the skull and facial bones (*arrows*).

Ewing's sarcoma, rhabdomyosarcoma, NHL, small cell carcinoma, and primitive neuroectodermal tumor. The precursor cells of neuroblastoma are of neural crest origin from undifferentiated cells of the sympathetic nervous system.[261] The cells are small and round with a high nuclear-to-cytoplasmic ratio and may form rosettes. Electron microscopy and immunohistochemistry are typically necessary for diagnosis.[262] Histopathologic classification schemes to look at the amount of stroma, the mitotic rate, and differentiation of the tumor have been devised in an attempt to determine prognostic factors.[263, 264]

Diagnosis and Staging

A special diagnostic feature of neuroblastoma is the finding of elevated catecholamine levels in the urine. The substance usually measured is vanillylmandelic acid (VMA); the most accurate determination requires a 24-hour urine collection. Approximately 90% to 95% of patients will have elevated levels of catecholamines.[254]

Patients with neuroblastoma of the head and neck should have imaging with CT, MRI, or both for evaluation of tumor extent, with particular attention to the skull base. Because most cases of neuroblastoma of the head and neck are not primary tumors but rather metastatic, further workup should be performed to look for an intra-abdominal primary tumor. Imaging of the abdomen may include CT or MRI. A screening chest radiograph, with follow-up chest CT if there is suggestion of pulmonary involvement, should be performed in all patients. Other studies include skeletal evaluation with bone radiographs and scintigraphy and bilateral iliac crest bone marrow biopsies. Newer diagnostic procedures include body scanning with [^{131}I]-metaiodobenzylguanidine (MIBG), an agent taken up by neuroblasts, for detection of metastases.[265]

A number of molecular neuroblastoma markers have been found with possible prognostic implications; these include N-*MYC* proto-oncogene, tumor ploidy, deletion of chromosome 1p, and expression of the TRK gene.[254, 257, 266–271] The N-*MYC* proto-oncogene, which is found in 20% to 25% of neuroblastomas, is associated with increased tumor aggressiveness.[254] Stratification of patients into risk groups can be based, in part, on these molecular markers. Fine-needle aspiration has been used to obtain tissue for examination of molecular markers.[272]

The current staging of neuroblastoma takes into account the status of the lymph nodes and whether there is residual disease after surgical resection. Regional lymph node sampling is recommended at the time of the initial surgical procedure.[273] The staging system proposed by the International Neuroblastoma Staging System (INSS) Committee is shown in Table 24–8.

Treatment

The treatment of neuroblastoma may be surgical excision alone or surgery in combination with chemotherapy or, less likely, with radiotherapy. Complete excision without gross morbidity is the primary treatment of localized cervical neuroblastoma.[274] Surgical findings such as tumor resectability and involvement of regional lymph nodes are important in

TABLE 24–8 International Neuroblastoma Staging System

Stage	Description
Stage I	Local tumor confined to the area of origin Complete resection with or without microscopic residual disease Ipsilateral and contralateral lymph nodes without tumor
Stage IIa	Unilateral with complete or incomplete gross resection Ipsilateral and contralateral lymph nodes without tumor
Stage IIb	Unilateral with complete or incomplete gross resection Ipsilateral node with tumor and contralateral node without tumor
Stage III	Tumor extending across the midline with or without regional lymph node involvement Unilateral tumor with contralateral lymph node involvement Midline tumor with bilateral lymph node involvement
Stage IV	Dissemination of tumor to distant lymph nodes, bone marrow, or other organs, except as defined in Stage IVs
Stage IVs	Localized primary tumor as defined in stage I or II, with disseminated disease to the liver, skin, or bone marrow

Adapted from Castleberry RP: Biology and treatment of neuroblastoma. Pediatr Clin North Am 44:919, 1997.

INSS staging. The role of radiation therapy is not well defined, and it is generally avoided in children owing to the subsequent high incidence of secondary malignancies, particularly thyroid carcinoma, when used in the head and neck region. Multiagent chemotherapy is indicated if incomplete resection of a primary neck neuroblastoma is not possible, or if the cervical disease represents metastasis to the head and neck.[275] Current regimens include combinations of cyclophosphamide, ifosfamide, doxorubicin, etoposide, and either cisplatin or carboplatin.[254]

The treatment protocol may be dictated by a risk assessment based on age, N-*MYC* proto-oncogene status, histology, and tumor ploidy, dividing patients into low-, intermediate-, and high-risk groups.[254] Patients in the low-risk group are often treated with surgery alone, with chemotherapy reserved for recurrent disease. Intermediate-risk patients are treated at the outset with a combination of surgery and chemotherapy. High-risk patients have a poor prognosis and, in addition to surgery and chemotherapy, may be candidates for investigative therapies such as autologous bone marrow transplant, intraoperative radiation therapy, and immunotherapy with viral vectors.[276, 277]

Prognosis

The prognosis in neuroblastoma is influenced by age, stage, histologic grade, a variety of molecular characteristics, serum ferritin level, and primary tumor site.[254, 257, 265–271, 278, 279] Infants younger than 1 year can generally be cured regardless of their disease stage, whereas older patients with advanced disease have a poor prognosis. It seems clear that, for young patients with resectable disease, complete excision offers the best chance for cure, with 90% or better survival in those younger than 1 year. Primary neuroblastoma of the head and neck has a better prognosis than that of other sites, which is also attributable to presentation at an earlier stage.[275] For all patients with stage I, II, or IVs disease (see Table 24–8), the 3-year survival is 75% to 90%; metastatic stage IVs disease tends to resolve spontaneously in children younger than 1 year of age.[207, 280] For children younger than 1 year of age with stage III or IV disease, the survival is 80% to 90%.[254] Patients who are older than 1 year with stage III and IV disease have decreased survival rates of 50% and 15%, respectively.

Melanotic Neuroectodermal Tumor of Infancy

Approximately 95% of melanotic neuroectodermal tumors of infancy (MNTI) occur in patients younger than 1 year of age,[281] with an average age at presentation of 4 months.[282] There is no apparent sex predilection. Although it is typically a benign tumor, its local aggressiveness in the young patient population warrants discussion. There is a reported malignancy rate of 2% to 3% in MNTI.[281, 283]

Clinical Presentation

Typically, MNTI presents as a rapidly growing, painless, blue-black mass arising predominantly in the premaxilla (80% of reported cases) (Fig. 24–8).[284] Affected children may manifest nasal obstruction or feeding difficulties. Other reported sites of occurrence in the head and neck include the mandible, anterior fontanelle, temporal bone, calvarium, and brain.[285] Presentation outside the head and neck region is rare.[281]

Pathology

Neural crest cells are thought to be the cells of origin of MNTI. Grossly, the cut surface of the tumor is black. Histopathology reveals two cell populations—one group of small, nonpigmented cells in solid nests and another group of large, epithelioid cells containing melanin.[286] These cells are contained within a dense fibrous stroma. Immunohistochemistry is helpful in distinguishing MNTI from retinoblastoma, neuroblastoma, melanoma, and primitive neuroectodermal tumor. It is not possible to predict which tumors will behave in a malignant fashion based on pathology.

Diagnosis

The diagnosis of MNTI can generally be suspected based on clinical examination and radiographic findings. CT is the study of choice (see Fig. 24–8) and usually demonstrates a lytic, expansile lesion with surrounding reactive bone.[285] MRI is comparatively better at distinguishing the extent of the tumor into surrounding soft tissues.[285] Definite diagnosis requires histopathologic examination; fine-needle aspiration has been used preoperatively to diagnose MNTI.[287]

Treatment

Treatment is complete surgical excision, often via a partial maxillectomy in premaxilla lesions. The local recurrence rate is 10% to 15%.[281, 283, 284, 288] The tumor is often multifocal, which contributes to recurrence. The prognosis is very favorable when the tumor is completely excised.

◻ THYROID CARCINOMA

Carcinoma of the thyroid gland occurs in patients 19 years of age or younger, with a reported annual incidence rate of one case per million per year in the United States.[289]

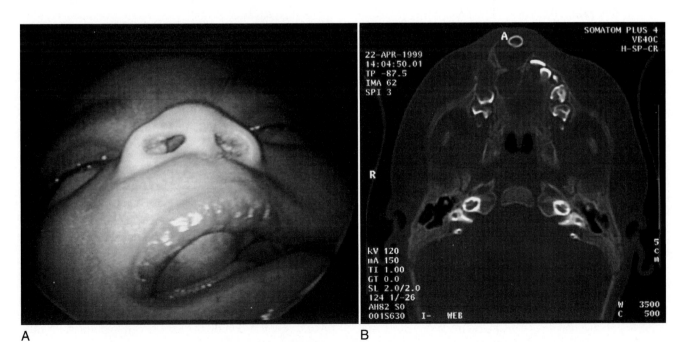

A   B

FIGURE 24–8   *A,* An infant with a neuroectodermal tumor of infancy of the right premaxilla. *B,* An axial CT scan demonstrates a 2.5 × 2-cm expansile, multiloculated cystic mass involving the superior alveolar ridge of the right maxilla.

Thyroid carcinoma represents 1.5% of all tumors that appear before age 15 years and 7% of all tumors of the head and neck in childhood.[290] Although increased incidence is demonstrated at puberty, thyroid carcinoma can present at any age and has even been reported in the neonatal period.[291] The average age of nonadult patients with thyroid carcinoma is 14 years[292]; in this population, the male-to-female ratio approximates 1:1.3.[292]

An increased incidence of thyroid carcinoma in children who had been exposed to radiation therapy was noted during the years 1945 to 1975[293, 294]; this finding led to the discontinuation of the use of radiation therapy for treatment of benign disease. Childhood exposure to radiation, however, continues to occur in certain environmental and clinical situations. For example, children who were exposed to radiation in Chernobyl have demonstrated a 62-fold increased risk of developing well-differentiated thyroid carcinoma.[295] Exposure to radiation in the setting of therapy for childhood malignancies also increases the risk of developing thyroid carcinoma; there are reports of secondary thyroid carcinomas arising in children treated with radiation therapy for both HL and acute lymphoblastic leukemia.[296–298]

Clinical Presentation

The most common presentation of thyroid cancer in children is an asymptomatic neck mass in the anterior or lateral neck (Fig. 24–9).[292, 299] History and clinical examination findings that increase suspicion of malignancy include previous exposure to radiation, family history of thyroid malignancy, hoarseness, dysphagia, fixation of the mass, rapid growth, or the presence of cervical adenopathy.[300–302] Palpable cervical lymph node metastases are present in 60% to 80% of pediatric patients at the time of initial evaluation.[292] Systemic metastases to lung and bone at presentation are also common, with rates of 15% and 5%, respectively.[303] In cases of familial medullary carcinoma associated with multiple endocrine neoplasia (MEN) syndrome, symptoms due to pheochromocytoma or hyperparathyroidism may also occur.[304] Familial medullary thyroid carcinoma rarely occurs without other associated endocrine involvement.

Pathology

Malignancies of the thyroid gland include but are not limited to papillary, follicular, medullary, anaplastic, and undifferentiated carcinomas. Papillary and follicular carcinoma are categorized as well-differentiated thyroid carcinomas. In children, papillary carcinoma constitutes between 69% and 94% of thyroid carcinomas, depending on the series reviewed; follicular carcinoma accounts for up to 29% of cases.[292] Anaplastic and undifferentiated carcinomas are comparatively rare.

The diagnosis of papillary carcinoma may be made cytopathlogically on fine-needle aspiration. Nuclear features of papillary carcinoma include nuclear grooves, the presence of pseudoinclusions, and enlarged prominent nuclei.[305] An intraoperative diagnosis can also be made on frozen section. The diagnosis of papillary carcinoma, however, is most definitively established on permanent histopathologic examination. The diagnosis of follicular carcinoma requires the

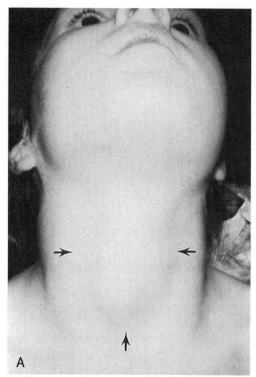

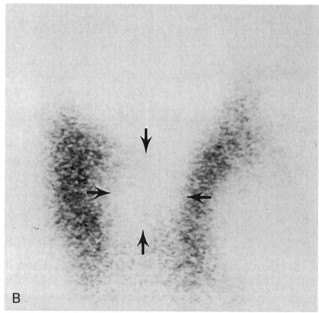

FIGURE 24–9 *A,* A firm, mobile mass in the anterior neck is the common presentation of thyroid carcinoma *(arrows)* in this 10-year-old girl. *B,* Thyroid scan demonstrates a cold nodule *(arrows).*

documentation of capsular or vascular invasion on permanent histopathology. Medullary thyroid carcinoma (MTC) is a malignancy of C-cells and is the only malignancy of the thyroid associated with amyloid; C-cell hyperplasia is often associated with MTC.

At least 30% to 50% of cases of MTC are familial, either isolated or associated with MEN types 2A and 2B.[306]

Diagnosis

The incidence of thyroid nodules in the pediatric population ranges from 0.2% to 2.0%, and the rate of malignancy in a solitary nodule ranges between 14% and 40%.[299, 301, 307, 308] The initial evaluation of a child or adolescent with a thyroid mass involves a history inquiring about risk factors for thyroid carcinoma and a physical examination assessing the consistency of the mass, the presence of cervical adenopathy, or vocal fold paralysis, any of which may suggest malignancy.

Laboratory evaluation is typically of limited differential diagnostic value because thyroxine (T_4), triiodothyronine (T_3), and thyroid-stimulating hormone (TSH) levels are nearly always normal in thyroid carcinoma.[309] Elevation of antithyroid and antimicrosomal antibody titers may suggest an inflammatory component, but these measurements alone cannot rule out malignancy.[300, 309]

In patients with MTC, baseline calcitonin levels are often elevated, and such levels increase further after stimulation by pentagastrin or calcium. These provocative tests may be used to screen family members for occult MTC. Screening at-risk patients with a family history of MEN can be performed to specifically look for mutation of the *ret* proto-oncogene found to be associated with MEN 2A.[310] Essentially all patients with MEN 2 syndrome develop MTC.[310–312]

Plain film radiography is of little benefit in assessing thyroid lesions but may demonstrate asymptomatic pulmonary metastases. Ultrasound examination is helpful in evaluating the size, position, and multiplicity of thyroid lesions, in determining their cystic or solid character, in identifying associated cervical adenopathy, and in directing fine-needle aspiration biopsy. Although a lesion with a cystic appearance on sonography generally indicates benign disease, malignant lesions on occasion can also have a cystic echogenic appearance; thus sonography alone cannot rule out carcinoma.[313]

Thyroid scanning using technetium or ^{123}I is a diagnostic technique used to evaluate solid thyroid nodules in children by determining the functional status of a thyroid nodule. Although most malignancies are "cold" (nonfunctional), this finding alone is not diagnostic of malignancy; biopsy for histopathologic examination is still warranted.[314] Similarly, although a "hot" or "warm" (functional) nodule is unlikely to be malignant, the high rate of malignancy in the pediatric population suggests that open surgical biopsy should be considered for all solid nodules in children.[305, 307, 320] Therefore, the use of radioactive thyroid scanning is discouraged in the evaluation of pediatric patients suspected of having a thyroid cancer. Some vary the approach to warm and hot nodules, depending on the presence or absence of antithyroid antibodies, the response to thyroxine suppression therapy, or the needle aspiration cytologic findings.[315]

Fine-needle aspiration of thyroid nodules has been performed in the pediatric population with a reported accuracy between 80% and 85% and a 90% specificity.[300, 316, 317] There are a few reported false-negative cases for thyroid carcinoma on fine-needle aspiration with a subsequent positive histopathologic diagnosis of carcinoma.[300, 316] These cases suggest that when fine-needle aspiration suggests benign disease and no additional tissue biopsy is planned, such patients require close follow-up.[320]

Treatment

As has been stated earlier, a majority of thyroid malignancies in children are papillary carcinoma. The specific histopathologic diagnosis may or may not be known preoperatively, depending on the results of the initial evaluation. When the diagnosis is uncertain, the initial surgical treatment should be limited to thyroid lobectomy. The use of frozen section diagnosis to guide further surgical management is controversial because some thyroid lesions are difficult to diagnose on frozen section analysis. In particular, the distinction between follicular adenoma and follicular carcinoma depends on documentation of capsular or vascular invasion best seen on permanent histology. Whenever intraoperative frozen section diagnosis is uncertain, further surgery should be deferred pending final histopathologic examination results.

Controversy regarding the surgical treatment of well-differentiated thyroid carcinoma in children concerns the extent of surgery. In a patient with a single focus of papillary carcinoma without metastases, partial, total, or near-total thyroidectomy is an option.[302] One of the sequelae of total thyroidectomy is the need for lifelong thyroid hormone replacement; there is also an inherent increased risk of the development of temporary or permanent hypocalcemia and bilateral recurrent laryngeal nerve injury. The higher incidence of multicentricity of thyroid cancer in children, however, argues on behalf of performing a total thyroidectomy.

The ablation of metastatic or residual disease by radioactive iodine therapy is also more successful following near-total or total thyroidectomy. Near-total thyroidectomy plus ablation of remaining thyroid tissue with ^{131}I has achieved excellent results while minimizing hypoparathyroidism.[318] Total thyroidectomy is indicated in patients with documented bilobar disease, regional or distant metastases, or gross carcinomatous infiltration into local tissues.

Elective lymph node dissection in the absence of regional nodal metastases is not warranted.[318, 319] Modified neck dissection is advocated when palpable cervical nodes are present. Classic radical neck dissection should be used only when there is gross extranodal extension of disease, given the fact that the presence of cervical disease does not reduce survival. Extensive surgery may be necessary with sacrifice of the trachea, esophagus, or recurrent laryngeal nerve when extensive invasion by tumor has occurred.

Residual functioning thyroid tissue makes it difficult to follow thyroglobulin levels or total body imaging with radioactive iodine tracer in evaluation for recurrent disease.[320] The goals of ^{131}I therapy are ablation of remaining thyroid tissue and treatment of residual tumor. The effective use of postoperative ^{131}I therapy requires previous near-total thyroidectomy.[321] The dose of ^{131}I needed to ablate any residual thyroid tissue in the neck depends largely on the size of the thyroid remnant. Because the prognosis in children with well-differentiated thyroid carcinoma is excellent, the benefits of ^{131}I therapy are debatable. Adverse effects of high-dose ^{131}I therapy include nausea, emesis, sialadenitis, lung fibrosis when extensive pulmonary metastases are present, temporary bone marrow suppression, and reversible spermatogenic damage.[14, 322] There is also a potentially increased risk of secondary malignancy, including salivary gland cancer, melanoma, and both acute and chronic leukemia.[314, 323] Given these observations, the initial postoperative use of ^{131}I therapy in pediatric patients is often limited to those with extensive locoregional disease that is unresectable or those with distant metastasis at presentation.[323] Subsequent ablation with high doses of ^{131}I remains a therapeutic option if late recurrence or metastases occur.

Postoperatively, all patients receive thyroxine to maintain a euthyroid state and thus suppress TSH. TSH is thought to have a growth-promoting effect on well-differentiated thyroid cancers.[324] T_4 is usually used for suppressive therapy rather than T_3 because of its longer half-life (1 week vs. 1 day). The exception to this rule is in the treatment of patients receiving ^{131}I therapy; the shorter half-life of T_3 is desirable here.[325] The role of thyroid hormone as a therapeutic agent remains controversial; the best results have been obtained in young patients.[326–328]

Treatment of MTC is total thyroidectomy with central node dissection when there is no clinically appreciable lymphadenopathy.[312, 329] Of note, there are a greater number of C-cells, the cells of origin of MTC, located in the upper pole of the thyroid; thus, complete removal of the superior pole is essential. MTC patients with suspected cervical lymph node metastases at presentation should undergo a regional lymph node dissection that may be unilateral or bilateral, depending on the location of disease. Mediastinal dissection is necessary in the setting of disease in the mediastinum. Adjuvant ^{131}I radiotherapy is of debatable benefit.[330]

Prognosis

Children with well-differentiated papillary and follicular thyroid carcinoma have a better prognosis than adults despite the comparatively increased incidence of cervical and distant metastases at presentation. Survival rates are generally greater than 90%.[314, 331] In a literature review of 540 pediatric patients with well-differentiated thyroid carcinoma, only 13 died of disease over a follow-up period of 12 to 33 years.[292]

In contrast to papillary and follicular thyroid carcinoma, the prognosis for children with MTC has a greater relationship to initial clinical presentation. At-risk patients, diagnosed by screening, do better than patients who present with an already existent neck mass.[332] Metastatic disease at presentation is a particularly poor prognostic factor.[314] Patients with MTC associated with MEN syndrome have a slightly better prognosis than those in whom MTC occurs sporadically.[311] The cause-specific mortality of patients with familial MTC at 18 years is 7%, compared with 23% for sporadic MTC; this difference may be secondary to earlier detection in the familial group.[311] MTC associated with MEN 2B occurs at an earlier age and is more aggressive than that associated with MEN 2A.[311, 312] For example, the incidence of cervical lymph node metastasis is 10% in patients with MEN 2A–associated MTC and 30% in patients with MEN 2B–associated MTC.[311] Given that more advanced disease worsens the prognosis in MTC and that essentially all patients with MEN 2 syndrome develop MTC, early genetic screening of at-risk children followed by prophylactic total thyroidectomy in those with positive screening is advocated.[312] Of note, MTC associated with MEN 2B has been diagnosed in a patient as young as 6 months of age.[332] Calcitonin levels may rise in patients with recurrent MTC and should be monitored after MTC surgical therapy. Children with a history of previous radiation exposure should undergo careful physical examination of the thyroid, cervical lymph nodes, and salivary glands at least every 2 years. Performance of a thyroid scan at initial evaluation is a consideration.

THYROGLOSSAL DUCT CYST CARCINOMA

Carcinoma arising in a thyroglossal duct cyst (TDCC) is an extremely rare disorder, with a rate of 1% in all removed specimens. The most common TDCC malignancy is papillary thyroid carcinoma[333–337]; follicular carcinoma, mixed papillary-follicular carcinoma, and squamous cell carcinoma have also been documented.[336, 338–340] A vast majority of TDCC cases occur in adults, with sporadic reports in the pediatric population.[341] Most TDCCs are found incidentally after surgical excision. A predominant solid component on preoperative ultrasonographic evaluation of a thyroglossal duct cyst should arouse suspicion. There are reports of fine-needle aspiration biopsy diagnosing papillary TDCC.[341]

The treatment for thyroid carcinoma arising in a thyroglossal duct cyst is typically en bloc resection via the Sistrunk procedure. This is adequate surgical management if histologically normal ectopic thyroid follicles can be found in the cyst, if the tumor does extend beyond the capsule, and if no cervical nodes are present. The rate of synchronous lesions in the thyroid gland is 11% to 27%.[335, 341] Postoperative thyroid hormone maintenance is recommended as suppression therapy. Total thyroidectomy and modified neck dissection, followed by ^{131}I ablation and hormone maintenance therapy, are indicated only if there is cervical metastatic disease. If invasion into surrounding musculature is present in the absence of cervical lymphadenopathy, the recommended therapy is a Sistrunk procedure with total thyroidectomy alone, followed by ablation and hormone suppression. An argument can be made for routinely performing total thyroidectomy in all children with TDCC to allow good long-term follow-up with thyroid scans.[335] Serial serum thyroglobulin screening may also identify possible recurrence.[335] The long-term behavior of these tumors has not been well defined.[342]

PARATHYROID CARCINOMA

Parathyroid carcinoma (PTC) is extremely rare and accounts for just 0.005% of malignancies in all ages.[343] The few reported cases of PTC in the pediatric population have principally occurred in adolescents.[344] Information on the clinical presentation, diagnostic evaluation, and therapy of

PTC is based on the adult population, given the paucity of cases in children. There may be a small female preponderance, but no predilection has been found based on race, ethnicity, or geographic location.[343] Familial hyperparathyroidism secondary to MEN syndrome is a risk factor for the development of PTC.[345] See Chapter 20 (Tumors of the Parathyroid Glands) for a more thorough discussion.

◘ CANCER OF THE SALIVARY GLANDS

Malignant neoplasms of the salivary glands in children are rare. A pathology review of 10,000 salivary gland lesions by the Armed Forces Institute revealed 54 malignancies in the pediatric age group.[346] Other major oncologic institutions have compiled individual totals of only 10 to 25 malignant salivary gland cases in young patients.[347–350] Most malignant neoplasms occur in older children and adolescents.[351, 352] There is an increased incidence of mucoepidermoid carcinoma in patients exposed to radiation therapy, as seen, for example, in patients treated with cranial irradiation for acute lymphocytic leukemia.[353]

Clinical Presentation

A vast majority of malignant tumors of salivary gland origin in children arise in the parotid gland; malignant tumors of the submandibular gland and the minor salivary glands are comparatively very rare.[350, 354, 355] The typical presentation of a parotid neoplasm in a child is an asymptomatic, firm mass in the preauricular facial region (Fig. 24–10). Rapid growth, facial weakness, pain, and associated cervical lymphadenopathy are all signs of possible malignancy. Excluding hemangiomas and lymphangiomas, approximately 50% of reported salivary gland tumors in children are malignant[347]; when vascular lesions are included, the comparative rate of malignancy decreases to 30%.[347] If one considers infectious and inflammatory lesions, this rate drops further to 4% to 16%.[356–358]

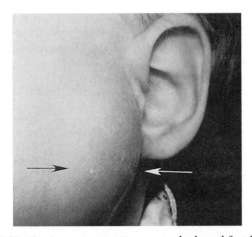

FIGURE 24–10 An asymptomatic mass in the lateral facial region (*arrows*) is the most common presentation of a salivary gland neoplasm in children.

Pathology

The World Health Organization (WHO) classifies malignancies of the salivary glands into 18 carcinoma and lymphoma subcategories[359] and further separates such lesions into high-grade and low-grade malignancies. The most common low-grade tumors include grade I mucoepidermoid carcinoma and acinic cell carcinoma. High-grade tumors include grade III mucoepidermoid carcinoma, undifferentiated carcinoma, carcinoma ex pleomorphic adenoma, and salivary duct carcinoma. Mucoepidermoid carcinoma is graded I through III depending on the histologic appearance; grade II mucoepidermoid carcinoma is considered intermediate grade. Adenocarcinoma also varies from low to high grade depending on the cytoarchitecture.[360]

The distribution of malignant salivary gland neoplasms in children is similar to that in the adult population, although the relative frequency of the various histologic types varies. Grade I mucoepidermoid carcinoma is the most common salivary gland malignancy in young patients.[361] The incidence of undifferentiated carcinoma is higher in children. Adenocarcinomas, acinic cell carcinomas, adenoid cystic carcinomas, and malignant mixed tumors occur less commonly. Salivary gland presentations of sarcomatous and lymphoid malignancies are infrequent. Cases of lymphoma in the salivary glands have been reported in the pediatric population, although a majority are reported in adults.[362] Pleomorphic adenoma is the most common benign nonvascular neoplasm in children.[363]

Diagnosis

Because a high percentage of childhood salivary gland tumors are malignant, histologic examination of all firm salivary gland masses is warranted. Fine-needle aspiration with cytologic diagnosis, as used in adults, is potentially applicable to children.[364] In an adult population, the sensitivity for fine-needle aspiration diagnosis of benign and malignant salivary gland lesions approximates 97% and 87%, respectively, with an overall specificity of 100%[365]; similar statistics for the pediatric population are not available. Caution is advised as to the use of fine-needle aspiration of salivary gland tumors in children because reports of false-negatives for malignant lesions do exist.[366] Also, associated hemorrhage or inflammatory response may prevent accurate histopathologic diagnosis of resected small tumors.

Incisional biopsy of parotid tumors is generally not recommended because of the risk of facial nerve injury; the exception is a clinically unresectable lesion for which diagnostic biopsy alone is needed.[367] Under most circumstances, excisional biopsy is preferred. This entails a superficial parotidectomy with preservation of the facial nerve for parotid lesions, or total excision of the submandibular gland for submandibular gland lesions.[347]

Imaging studies, including CT or MRI, are useful in evaluating a mass in the salivary gland. Such radiographic studies can help distinguish between lesions of the gland parenchyma and periglandular nodal disease. CT scans may delineate widening of bony foramina, suggesting cranial nerve involvement. MRI imaging is useful for determining surrounding soft tissue involvement and tumor extent.

Chest radiographs may demonstrate pulmonary metastases, especially in the setting of adenoid cystic carcinoma.

The TNM staging system is used for malignancies of the major salivary glands (see Chapter 21, Malignant Tumors of the Salivary Glands).[368] Given that the staging system depends on tumor extent, preoperative evaluation by imaging is recommended.

Treatment

For low-grade malignancies of the superficial parotid lobe or submandibular gland, surgical resection by means of superficial parotidectomy or submandibular gland excision alone may prove to be adequate treatment. Deep lobe and high-grade parotid tumors require total parotidectomy. Facial nerve resection is performed only if there is clinical or anatomic evidence of nerve involvement by malignancy—never on the basis of tumor histopathology.[349] When resection of the nerve is necessary, immediate facial reanimation by means of primary anastomosis, free nerve graft, muscle transfer procedures, or a combination of these procedures is advocated.[369]

Modified neck dissection is indicated in patients with salivary gland malignancy and a clinically positive neck. The role of neck dissection in the N0 neck is more controversial and is dictated by the risk of occult microscopic disease based on histopathology, tumor grade, tumor stage, and facial nerve involvement.[370] Patients with high-grade malignancies, advanced T-stage, and facial nerve involvement have an increased risk of lymph node metastasis.[371–373]

The use of adjuvant radiation therapy varies. Histopathologic findings such as nerve invasion, extraglandular extension of tumor, or metastatic adenopathy are indications for postoperative radiation therapy at some centers.[349, 374] Other institutions restrict the use of radiation therapy to specific histopathologies such as adenoid cystic carcinoma or high-grade mucoepidermoid carcinoma, or reserve its use for the management of recurrent disease, regardless of histopathologic findings.[349] Radiation therapy in the setting of positive surgical margins may afford improvement in local control and survival if reexcision is not possible.[375]

Chemotherapy is typically limited to palliative use, as adjuvant therapy in the treatment of high-grade salivary gland cancer, and in patients with recurrent disease.[376, 377] Both single-agent and multiagent chemotherapy in recurrent salivary gland cancer have shown promise for palliation of pain and control of local disease but fail to improve survival; multiagent therapy appears more efficacious.[376] The combination of cyclophosphamide, doxorubicin, and cisplatin is the most extensively studied chemotherapeutic regimen.[378] Cisplatin has shown particular promise in the treatment of adenoid cystic carcinoma.[379, 380] Salivary gland involvement by rhabdomyosarcoma is treated with a combination of surgery, radiotherapy, and chemotherapy, as dictated by the IRS protcols.[381]

Prognosis

The survival of children with salivary gland malignancy is chiefly determined by histopathologic findings.[349] Children with low-grade malignancies such as grade I or II mucoepidermoid carcinoma, well-differentiated adenocarcinoma, and acinic cell carcinoma tend to do well. The prognosis for children with mucoepidermoid and acinic cell carcinomas is particularly good, with 5-year survival rates of greater than 90%.[355, 369, 382] The 5-year mortality rate in patients with mucoepidermoid carcinoma is grade dependent, with figures of 0%, 30%, and 78% for grades I, II, and III, respectively.[372, 383] Children with high-grade malignancies such as grade III mucoepidermoid carcinoma, poorly differentiated adenocarcinoma, and undifferentiated tumors do poorly. The 5-year survival rates for patients with undifferentiated and squamous cell carcinoma are lower than 10%.[361] Survival rates for patients with adenoid cystic carcinoma are difficult to assess because recurrences can occur well after the standard 5-year follow-up.

In general, poor prognosis is predicted by facial nerve involvement, positive surgical margins, tumor fixation, a painful ulcerative mass, nodal disease, and recurrent disease.[361, 375] TNM stage is predictive of survival, although staging is confounded by histopathology because patients with high-grade malignancies most often present with higher-stage disease.[361] Patients presenting with malignancy in the submandibular gland with fixation have a particularly poor prognosis.[361]

■ NASOPHARYNGEAL CARCINOMA

Nasopharyngeal carcinoma (NPC) is rare in childhood, with an overall incidence of less than one case per year in most reviews.[6–8, 384] Despite this rarity, NPC accounts for one third of childhood nasopharyngeal malignancies; rhabdomyosarcoma and NHL account for the remainder.[385–388] NPC is generally found in older children, with a reported average age range of 10 to 14 years.[387, 388] There appears to be a 2:1 predilection for males compared with females and an increased incidence among black teenagers.[389–391]

Clinical Presentation

A majority of children with NPC have metastatic disease in the neck at the time of presentation; most present with lymphadenopathy rather than nasal obstruction.[384, 385, 387, 392, 393] The superior deep cervical lymph nodes are most often involved. Unilateral otitis media, rhinorrhea, and nasal obstruction symptoms are additional common manifestations. Cranial nerve neuropathies, headache, and facial pain suggest skull base involvement. The most common cranial nerve involved is the abducens nerve; such patients present with diplopia.[387] Nasopharyngeal rhabdomyosarcoma and NPC are difficult to distinguish clinically; two suggestive features are that NPC presents in an older age group and more frequently with cervical metastases.[387]

Pathology

NPC originates from the epithelial cells of the nasopharynx. The WHO original classification (1978) classified NPC into three groups—type 1, keratinizing squamous cell carcinoma; type 2, nonkeratinizing carcinoma; and type 3, undifferentiated carcinoma.[394] The more recent classification

(1991) by the WHO includes squamous cell carcinoma, nonkeratinizing differentiated carcinoma, and nonkeratinizing undifferentiated carcinoma as corresponding substitutes for the old types I, II, and III, respectively.[394] Almost all NPC in young patients is of the nonkeratinizing undifferentiated subtype. Histopathologic distinction of NPC from rhabdomyosarcoma, diffuse large cell lymphoma, olfactory neuroblastoma, and melanoma can sometimes be difficult; immunohistochemistry can be of significant help.[395]

There is a relationship between both nonkeratinizing differentiated and undifferentiated NPC but not squamous cell carcinoma with EBV exposure. A cause-and-effect relationship between EBV and NPC, however, has not been proved.[396] EBV antibody titers usually correlate with tumor burden and decrease with successful therapy. Rising titers during NPC therapy portend a poor prognosis; conversely, a decrease in the titer during the first 12 months of treatment is a good prognostic indicator.[397] Because titers tend to increase before the appearance of recurrent disease, they are a useful indicator of disease activity (see Chapter 11, Cancer of the Nasopharynx, for more detailed information).[398]

Diagnosis

Examination and biopsy of the NPC are required for diagnosis. CT or MRI allows evaluation of tumor extension with respect to the skull base and central nervous system, provides information about parapharyngeal extension and retropharyngeal adenopathy, and stages the remainder of the cervical lymph nodes. Systemic evaluation is directed toward ruling out hematogenous metastases, particularly to bone, lung, and liver.[393] CT of the chest and abdomen, radionuclide bone scanning, and liver enzyme assays may be performed if there is a high index of suspicion for metastatic disease. Baseline EBV serology may be useful in following the disease.

Staging of NPC has been revised in the TNM classification system.[368] The revised TNM classification system has been found to have improved prognostic significance compared with the older system.[399]

Treatment

The primary treatment modality of NPC is radiation therapy to the nasopharynx and to the neck bilaterally in anticipation of nodal metastases. Adjuvant chemotherapy is often added because patients treated with radiation therapy who fail treatment do so typically because of metastatic disease.[400] A prospective study, not limited to children, comparing radiotherapy alone with radiotherapy and chemotherapy in patients with stage III or IV disease showed improved survival in patients receiving combination therapy.[401] Retrospective studies assessing adjuvant chemotherapy in children with NPC suggest improved survival.[402] Because most children present with advanced disease, combined chemotherapy and radiation therapy has become the standard of care in this age group.

Surgery is generally reserved for obtaining tissue for diagnosis and for salvage therapy when appropriate. Neck dissection is indicated when there is isolated residual/recurrent cervical disease following radiotherapy.[403] Surgical excision of recurrent nasopharyngeal disease may be performed by various craniofacial approaches depending on tumor extent (see Chapter 11).[403]

Prognosis

Patients with stage I through III disease are considered to have early disease, with an overall 5-year survival rate of 75%.[399] The 5-year survival rate for stages IVA, IVB, and IVC are 48%, 74%, and 0%, respectively. Advanced tumor (T) stage portends a poor prognosis. Advanced nodal disease (N3) is surprisingly not a poor prognostic factor, as reflected in the 74% 5-year survival in patients with stage IVB disease who have an N3 neck.[399] Patients with systemic distant metastases do particularly poorly.

■ MELANOMA

Melanoma accounts for less than 1% of malignancies in children and is particularly rare in children younger than 12 years.[404–406] Melanoma can occur sporadically or in the setting of predisposing familial or congenital conditions. A familial occurrence of melanoma in patients with dysplastic nevus syndrome has been recognized.[407–409] Local transformation of giant congenital nevi into melanoma can occur; therefore, excision of giant congenital nevi early in life is recommended.[410, 411] A congenital form of generalized metastatic melanoma has also been described.[412] Patients with a family history of melanoma, xeroderma pigmentosum, or dysplastic nevi are at additional risk for developing melanoma.[413]

Clinical Presentation

Melanoma of the head and neck in children is most commonly found on the cheek, with other sites of predilection being the forehead, nose, scalp, and neck.[414] Characteristics of a pigmented lesion that should raise suspicion of melanoma include bleeding, change in size, change in color, irregular border, or itching. Asymptomatic lesions may be detected on routine physical examination. Regional lymph node metastases may occur; the incidence of such increases with increasing tumor thickness.[415] Disseminated systemic melanoma is unusual outside of infancy.

Pathology

The specific types of melanoma include superficial spreading, nodular, desmoplastic, lentigo maligna, and mucosal. The distinction between a benign pigmented lesion and melanoma requires histopathologic examination. Melanoma is characterized by the presence of proliferating atypical melanocytes and has a radial or a vertical growth phase or both. If a lesion has only radial growth and no vertical growth, the chance at cure after local excision is nearly 100%. The vertical growth phase or deep extension of melanoma has been described by both histopathology (Clark's level) and absolute measured thickness (Breslow depth).

Tumor thickness has been correlated with recurrence and survival.[416, 417]

Diagnosis

The procedure of choice for removal of a pigmented lesion is a full-thickness excisional biopsy. Once a diagnosis of melanoma has been made, the subsequent workup is directed toward identifying regional or systemic metastases. Distant disease particularly involves liver, bone, viscera, and the central nervous system. When the lesion is less than 0.75 mm thick, the likelihood of metastasis is small, and there is an excellent chance for cure with wide local excision alone. When the thickness is greater than 0.75 mm, the rate of metastasis increases, and the performance of a sentinel node biopsy may be warranted. Sentinel node biopsy has been used in both adults and children with melanoma. The presence of a positive biopsy may warrant a regional lymphadenectomy and is associated with an increased incidence of distant disease. CT and liver enzyme assays are useful for screening for distant disease.

Treatment

The biologic behavior of melanoma appears to be identical in all age groups, with the exception that juveniles have a shorter disease-free interval; therapy is therefore similar in adults and children[406, 413] (see Chapter 8, Melanoma of the Head and Neck).

Wide local excision of the lesion is the treatment of choice for melanoma. A prospective randomized study has shown that melanomas that are less than 2 mm thick, and especially those that are less than 1 mm thick, can be excised with a margin of 1 cm without increasing the risk of local recurrence or affecting patient survival. For thicker melanomas, a wider margin of no more than 3 cm is recommended.[418, 419] Superficial parotidectomy, modified neck dissection, or both are indicated when regional periauricular, parotid, or cervical metastases are present.[420, 421] Regional lymphadenectomy for the presence of palpable disease or a positive sentinel node biopsy improves locoregional control and is recommended even in the presence of distant disease. The role of surveillance neck dissection on an elective basis in the absence of palpable adenopathy is controversial.[406, 423] A prospective study examining the role of elective neck dissection in the setting of patients with N0 necks found an improved 5-year survival for primary lesions with thickness between 1 mm and 2 mm.[423] The use of adjuvant radiotherapy is discussed in Chapter 8.

Immunotherapy, including interleukin 2, harvested tumor-infiltrating cells, and interferon α 2b, has been used in the setting of advanced disease.[424, 425] The chemotherapeutic agent dacarbazine has been used alone or in combination with immunotherapeutic regimens or other chemotherapeutic agents with limited success.[426, 427]

Prognosis

Survival rates for children with melanoma, all sites considered, approximate 40% to 50%.[405, 406] Survival varies, depending principally on the anatomic location of disease, the presence or absence of regional metastases, and, at least in older children, the depth of invasion of the primary lesion.[428] Additional poor prognostic factors of the primary lesion include ulceration, higher mitotic rate, microscopic satellites, vascular invasion, and absence of tumor-infiltrating lymphocytes.[429] Patients with regional metastatic disease have an increased incidence of distant metastatic disease of 70% to 90%; the 5-year survival in these patients is very poor, at 10% to 20%.[430]

◨ SQUAMOUS CELL CARCINOMA

Cutaneous squamous cell carcinoma in children is rare. Risk factors for the development of cutaneous squamous cell carcinoma can be either acquired or congenital. Acquired risks include exposure to ultraviolet light, radiation therapy, and immunosuppression secondary to infection or medication.[431] Squamous cell carcinoma may arise in burn scars.[432] Predisposing conditions that increase the risk of squamous cell carcinoma include xeroderma pigmentosum and albinism. [413, 431] Xeroderma pigmentosum is an autosomal recessive condition in which a defective DNA repair mechanism makes the patient extremely susceptible to the carcinogenic effects of ultraviolet radiation; multiple skin cancers occur in sun-exposed areas. The principles of management of cutaneous squamous cell carcinoma are the same as in the adult population.

Squamous cell carcinoma of the aerodigestive tract in the pediatric population is extremely rare. Principally, the larynx has been involved in cases of previous irradiation for treatment of laryngeal juvenile respiratory papillomatosis. [433] There is an association of squamous cell carcinoma of the aerodigestive tract with immunosuppression and Fanconi's anemia.[434–438] Management is identical to that in the adult population.

◨ BASAL CELL CARCINOMA

Cutaneous basal cell carcinoma is rare in children, with only sporadic isolated cases reported in the head and neck region.[439, 440] An increased incidence in patients with xeroderma pigmentosum and nevus sebaceous is noted.[413] Multiple basal cell carcinomas may also occur in childhood in association with odontogenic cysts and other skeletal, dermatologic, and soft tissue anomalies in the inherited nevoid basal cell carcinoma syndrome.[440–443] The nevi in this syndrome usually do not become malignant until after the first decade of life. In children, radiation-associated basal cell carcinomas generally have occurred in patients treated for acute lymphoblastic leukemia or Hodgkin's lymphoma. Surgical excision is the treatment of choice for basal cell carcinoma.

◨ TERATOMA

Teratoma is a germ cell tumor found particularly in neonates, with an incidence of 1 in 4000 births.[444] Most teratomas are benign, with an overall malignancy rate of 20%, varying greatly depending on the primary site.[445] Approximately 5% of head and neck teratomas contain malignant elements; such are rare in neonates and occur primarily in adults.[446] Other malignant germ cell tumors include germinomas, embryonal carcinomas, yolk sac carcinomas, and choriocarcinomas.

Clinical Presentation

Lesions in the head and neck region account for approximately 5% of all benign and malignant germ cell neoplasms[447]; common sites include the neck, oropharynx, nasopharynx, orbit, and paranasal sinuses.[446, 449–452] Oropharyngeal and nasopharyngeal teratomas occur almost exclusively in neonates and young infants. Teratomas have a predilection for the oropharynx.[450] Orbital teratomas also typically present at birth with proptosis. Germ cell tumors have rarely been reported in the larynx.[451] The ovaries, testes, anterior mediastinum, retroperitoneum, and sacrococcygeal region are the most common noncervicofacial primary sites.

Even though the vast majority of pediatric cervical teratomas are histologically benign, morbidity and mortality are significant.[448] Secondary respiratory distress and feeding difficulties are common (Fig. 24–11).[452] Infants with large cervical teratomas have an increased incidence of polyhydramnios, prematurity, and stillbirth.

Pathology

Histologically, teratomas are composed of ectodermal, mesodermal, and endodermal components. Depending on the degree of differentiation of the components, teratomas are classified as mature or immature. A predominance of immature elements portends a poorer prognosis and may suggest malignancy.[453] This, however, is not true in the neonatal age group. Teratoma secretion of alpha-fetoprotein and beta human chorionic gonadotropin has implications regarding postoperative monitoring.

Treatment

The treatment of teratomas is surgical excision. Because malignant degeneration in head and neck teratomas among children is so rare, much of the experience in the therapy of pediatric germ cell malignancies has been achieved in treating these lesions in gonadal and other extragonadal locations. Therapy consists of surgical resection, if possible, followed by a prolonged course of multidrug chemotherapy. Patients with unresectable or residual disease also receive radiation to the primary site.[445, 449, 454] Metastasis from childhood teratomas is rare, although it has been reported.[449, 455] When systemic metastases are present, multiagent chemotherapy and surgical resection are advocated. Salvage chemotherapy is used in the setting of recurrent disease.[453]

Prognosis

Almost all patients demonstrate an initial response to therapy. After surgical resection of immature teratomas, the 3-year survival is 93%.[453] Orbital teratomas have an

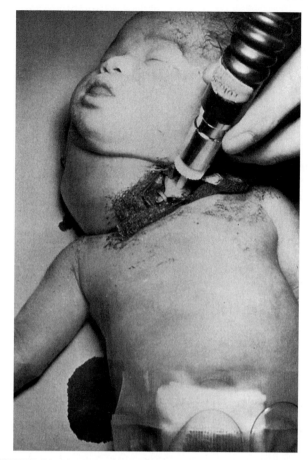

FIGURE 24–11 Respiratory distress requiring airway management occurs secondary to tracheal compression by large cervical teratomas. The teratoma in this newborn demonstrated actual tracheal invasion and histopathologic evidence of malignancy. (Courtesy of Sylvan Stool, MD.)

excellent prognosis after orbital exenteration.[448] In the setting of malignant teratoma, the 2-year disease-free survival is approximately 50%.[444, 449]

Regardless of the histopathology of the tumor, all patients should be followed for possible recurrence. Oropharyngeal and nasopharyngeal teratomas may require follow-up endoscopic examinations. Radiologic follow-up by means of CT or MRI is typically appropriate.[456] The tumor-secreted products alpha-fetoprotein and beta human chorionic gonadotropin can also be monitored.

◼ SUMMARY

The typical presentation of head and neck cancer in the pediatric age group is the appearance of an asymptomatic mass. Although reactive cervical lymphadenopathy, congenital lesions, and benign neoplasms are comparatively more common in the pediatric population, a noninflammatory firm neck mass in a child should be considered malignant until proven otherwise.

The early recognition of malignancies of the head and neck requires knowledge of historical factors suspected to increase the risk of malignancy in a child. These include a family history of childhood cancer, a previous primary neoplasm, a known systemic predisposition to cancer, and previous exposure to radiation therapy or to carcinogenic or immunosuppressive drugs.[13, 14]

A child suspected of having cancer in the head and neck requires a complete otolaryngologic and systemic evaluation. During the physical examination, attention should be directed to the abdomen and axillary and inguinal areas because the head and neck lesion may be one manifestation of a generalized process. The importance of a thorough otolaryngologic examination is underscored by the observation that one of every six children with a malignant neck mass has a primary oral or nasopharyngeal lesion.

Both the histopathologic diagnosis and the stage of the disease dictate the treatment of cancer of the head and neck in the pediatric age group. Coordination of treatment requires the interaction of pediatric specialists and support services. Radiation therapy and multidrug chemotherapy are presently the two primary treatment modalities for lymphoid and sarcomatous pediatric neoplasms. Surgical resection remains the primary treatment of glandular neoplasms and continues to have a primary therapeutic role for those mesenchymal tumors that are accessible to complete excision. Surgery remains a necessity in the treatment of all malignant lesions, for initial diagnosis and for staging purposes. Surgical intervention may additionally be required for debulking and salvage procedures, airway maintenance, and follow-up endoscopic or operative examinations.

REFERENCES

1. Landis SH, Murray T, Bolden S, et al: Cancer statistics, 1999. CA Cancer J Clin 49:8, 1999.
2. Sutow W, Montague E: Pediatric tumors. In MacComb W, Fletcher G (eds): Cancer of the Head and Neck. Baltimore, Williams & Wilkins, 1967, p 428.
3. Brugère J: Tumours of head and neck. In Bloom HJG, Lemerle J, Neidhardt MK, et al (eds): Cancer in Children: Clinical Management. Berlin, Springer-Verlag, 1975.
4. Sutow W, Lindberg R, Gehan E, et al: Three-year relapse-free survival rates in childhood rhabdomyosarcoma of the head and neck. Cancer 49:2217, 1982.
5. Rapidis AD, Economidis J, Goumas PD, et al: Tumours of the head and neck in children: A clinicopathological analysis of 1,007 cases. J Craniomaxillofac Surg 16:279, 1988.
6. Conley J: Tumors of the head and neck in children. In Conley J (ed): Concepts in Head and Neck Surgery. New York, Grune & Stratton, 1970.
7. Jaffe B: Pediatric head and neck tumors: A study of 178 cases. Laryngoscope 83:1644, 1973.
8. Cunningham MJ, Myers EN, Bluestone CD: Malignant tumors of head and neck in children: A 20 year review. Int J Pediatr Otorhinolaryngol 13:279, 1987.
9. Quraishi MS, Blayney AW, Walker D, et al: Langerhans' cell histiocytosis: Head and neck manifestations in children. Head Neck 17:226, 1995.
10. Sutow W: Cancer of the head and neck in children. JAMA 199:414, 1964.
11. Josephson GD, Wohl D: Malignant tumors of the head and neck in children. Curr Opin Otolaryngol Head Neck 7:61, 1999.
12. Crist WM, Kun LE: Common solid tumors of childhood. N Engl J Med 324:461, 1991.
13. Mulvihill JJ: Childhood cancer, the environment, and heredity. In Pizzo PA, Poplack DG (eds): Principles and Practice of Pediatric Oncology, 2nd ed. Philadelphia, JB Lippincott, 1993, p 11.
14. Meadows A, Silber J: Delayed consequences of therapy for childhood cancer. CA Cancer J Clin 35:271, 1985.
15. Silverberg E, Lubera J: Cancer statistics, 1987. CA Cancer J Clin 37:2, 1987.
16. McGuirt WF: The neck mass: A diagnostic and therapeutic approach. In: Johnson JT, Blitzer A, Ossoff RH, et al (eds): Instructional Courses. St. Louis, Mosby–Year Book, 1990, p 107.
17. Herrera JM, Krebs A, Harris P, et al: Childhood tumors. Surg Clin North Am 80:747, 2000.
18. Raney RB Jr, Handler SD: Management of neoplasms of the head and neck in children. II. Malignant tumors. Head Neck Surg 3:500, 1981.
19. Moran E, Ultmann JE: Clinical features and course of Hodgkin's disease. Clin Haematol 3:91, 1974.
20. Leventhal BG, Donaldson SS: Hodgkin's disease. In Pizzo PA, Poplack DG (eds): Principles and Practice of Pediatric Oncology, 2nd ed. Philadelphia, JB Lippincott, 1993, chap 24.
21. Alexander FE, Jarrett RF, Lawrence D, et al: Risk factor for Hodgkin's disease by Epstein-Barr virus (EBV) status: Prior infection by EBV and other agents. Br J Cancer 82:1117, 2000.
22. Frisch M, Biggar RJ, Engels EA, et al: Association of cancer with AIDS-related immunosuppression in adults. JAMA 285:1736, 2001.
23. Gladstein E, Guersney J, Rosenberg S, Kaplan H: The value of laparotomy and splenectomy in the staging of Hodgkin's disease. Cancer 24:709, 1969.
24. Gladstein E, Trueblood H, Enright L, et al: Surgical staging of abdominal involvement in unselected patients with Hodgkin's disease. Radiology 97:425, 1970.
25. Moghe GM, Borges AM, Soman CS, et al: Hodgkin's disease involving Waldeyer's ring: A study of four cases. Leuk Lymphoma 41:151, 2001.
26. Hudson MM, Donaldson SS: Hodgkin's disease. Pediatr Clin North Am 44:891, 1997.
27. DeVita V Jr, Hellman S: Hodgkin's disease and non-Hodgkin's lymphomas. In DeVita V Jr, Hellman S, Rosenberg S (eds): Cancer: Principles and Practice of Oncology. Philadelphia, JB Lippincott, 1982.
28. Fuller L, Madoc-Jones H, Gamble J, et al: New assessment of the prognostic significance of histopathology in Hodgkin's disease for laparotomy—negative stage I and stage II patients. Cancer 39:2174, 1977.
29. Mauch P, Larson D, Osteen R, et al: Prognostic factors for positive surgical staging in patients with Hodgkin's disease. J Clin Oncol 8:257, 1990.
30. Chan WC: The Reed-Sternberg cell in classical Hodgkin's disease. Hematol Oncol 19:1, 2001.
31. Kapadia S: Hematologic diseases: Malignant lymphomas, leukemias, plasma cell dyscrasias, histiocytosis X, and reactive lymph node lesions. In Barnes L (ed): Surgical Pathology of the Head and Neck. New York, Marcel Dekker, 1985.
32. Lukes R, Craver L, Hall T, et al: Report of the Nomenclature Committee. Cancer Res 26:1311, 1966.
33. Colby T, Hoppe R, Warnke R: Hodgkin's disease: A clinicopathologic study of 659 cases. Cancer 49:1848, 1981.
34. Harris N: Hodgkin's lymphomas: Classification, diagnosis, and grading. Semin Hematol 36:220, 1999.
35. Harris NL, Jaffe ES, Stein H, et al: A revised European-American classification of lymphoid neoplasms: A proposal from the International Lymphoma Study Group. Blood 84:1361, 1994.
36. Chieng DC, Cangiarella JF, Symmans WF, et al: Fine-needle aspiration cytology of Hodgkin disease: A study of 89 cases with emphasis on false negative cases. Cancer 93:52, 2001.
37. Roskos RR, Evans RC, Gilchrist GS, et al: Prognostic significance of mediastinal mass in childhood Hodgkin's disease. Cancer Treat Rep 66:961, 1982.
38. Robinson B, Kingston J, Nogueira-Costa R, et al: Chemotherapy and irradiation in childhood Hodgkin's disease. Arch Dis Child 59:1162, 1984.
39. Rostock RA, Siegelman SS, Lenhard RE, et al: Thoracic CT scanning for mediastinal Hodgkin's disease: Results and therapeutic implications. Int J Radiat Oncol Biol Phys 9:1451, 1983.
40. Baker LL, Parker BR, Donaldson SS, et al: Staging of Hodgkin's disease in children: Comparison of CT and lymphography with laparotomy. Am J Roentgenol 154:1251, 1990.
41. Bangerter M, Griesshammer M, Bergmann L: Progress in medical imaging of lymphoma and Hodgkin's disease. Curr Opin Oncol 11:339, 1999.

42. Weidmann E, Baican B, Hertel A, et al: Positron emission tomography (PET) for staging and evaluation of response to treatment in patients with Hodgkin's disease. Leuk Lymphoma 34:545, 1999.
43. Potter R: Paediatric Hodgkin's disease. Eur J Cancer 35:1466, 1999.
44. Jones S: Importance of staging in Hodgkin's disease. Semin Oncol 7:126, 1980.
45. Russell KJ, Donaldson SS, Cox RS, et al: Childhood Hodgkin's disease: Patterns of relapse. J Clin Oncol 2:80, 1984.
46. Bangerter M, Moog F, Buchmann I, et al: Whole-body 2-[18F]-fluoro-2-deoxy-D-glucose positron emission tomography (FDG-PET) for accurate staging of Hodgkin's disease. Ann Oncol 9:1117, 1998.
47. O'Carroll D, McKenna R, Brunning R: Bone marrow manifestations of Hodgkin's disease. Cancer 33:1717, 1976.
48. Hoppe R: Radiation therapy in the treatment of Hodgkin's disease. Semin Oncol 7:144, 1980.
49. Lange BJ: Hodgkin's disease. In D'Angio GJ, Sinniah D, Meadows AT, et al (eds): Practical Pediatric Oncology. New York, John Wiley & Sons, 1992.
50. Mauch P, Goodman R, Hellman S: The significance of mediastinal involvement in early stage Hodgkin's disease. Cancer 42:1039, 1978.
51. Donaldson SS, Link MP: Combined modality treatment with low-dose radiation and MOPP chemotherapy for children with Hodgkin's disease. J Clin Oncol 5:742, 1987.
52. Tesch H, Sieber M, Diehl V, et al: Treatment of advanced stage Hodgkin's disease. Oncology 60:101, 2001.
53. Kaldor JM, Day NE, Clarke A, et al: Leukemia following Hodgkin's disease. N Engl J Med 322:7, 1990.
54. Rosenberg SA, Kaplan HS: The evolution and summary results of the Stanford randomized clinical trials of the management of Hodgkin's disease: 1962–1984. Int J Radiat Oncol Biol Phys 11:5, 1985.
55. Green DM: Long-term Complications of Therapy for Cancer in Childhood and Adolescence. Baltimore, The Johns Hopkins University Press, 1989.
56. Swerdlow AJ, Barber JA, Vaughan-Hudson G, et al: Risk of second malignancy after Hodgkin's disease in a collaborative British cohort: The relation to age at treatment. J Clin Oncol 18:498, 2000.
57. Van Leeuwen FE, Klokman WJ, van't Veer MB, et al: Long-term risk of second malignancy in survivors of Hodgkin's disease treated during adolescence or young adulthood. J Clin Oncol 18:487, 2000.
58. DeVita V Jr: The consequences of the chemotherapy of Hodgkin's disease: The Tenth David A. Karnofsky Memorial Lecture. Cancer 47:1, 1981.
59. Urba WJ, Longo DL: Hodgkin's disease. N Engl J Med 326:678, 1992.
60. DeVita VT Jr, Hubbard SM: Hodgkin's disease. N Engl J Med 328:560, 1993.
61. Pastore G, Magnani C, Verdecchia A, et al: Survival of childhood lymphomas in Europe, 1978–1992: A report from the EUROCARE study. Eur J Cancer 37:703, 2001.
62. Sandlund JT, Downing JR, Crist WM: Non-Hodgkin's lymphoma in childhood. N Engl J Med 334:1238, 1996.
63. Wollner N: Non-Hodgkin's lymphoma in children. Pediatr Clin 23:371, 1976.
64. Armitage JO: Treatment of non-Hodgkin's lymphoma. N Engl J Med 328:1023, 1993.
65. Magrath I: Malignant non-Hodgkin's lymphomas in children. In Pizzo PA, Poplack DG (eds): Principles and Practice of Pediatric Oncology. Philadelphia, JB Lippincott, 1993, chap 23.
66. Taylor AMR, Metcalfe JA, Thick J, et al: Leukemia and lymphoma in ataxia telangiectasia. Blood 87:423, 1996.
67. Ellaurie M, Wiznia A, Bernstein L, et al: Lymphoma in pediatric HIV infection. Pediatr Res 25:150A, 1989 (abstract).
68. Gatti R, Good R: Occurrence of malignancy in immunodeficiency diseases. Cancer 28:89, 1971.
69. Beral V, Peterman T, Berkelman R, et al: AIDS-associated non-Hodgkin's lymphoma. Lancet 337:805, 1991.
70. Kaplan LD, Abrams DI, Feigal E, et al: AIDS-associated non-Hodgkin's lymphoma in San Francisco. JAMA 261:719, 1989.
71. Ziegler JL, Beckstead JA, Volderding PA, et al: Non-Hodgkin's lymphoma in 50 homosexual men. N Engl J Med 311:565, 1984.
72. Jones S: Clinical features and course of non-Hodgkin's lymphoma. Clin Haematol 3:131, 1974.
73. Sandlund JT, Hutchison RE, Crist WM: Non-Hodgkin's lymphoma. In Fernbach DJ, Viette TJ (eds): Clinical Pediatric Oncology, 4th ed. St. Louis: Mosby–Year Book, 1991, chap 18, p 335.
74. Murphy SB, Fairclough DL, Hutchison RE, et al: Non-Hodgkin's lymphoma of childhood: An analysis of the histology, staging, and response to treatment of 338 cases at a single institution. J Clin Oncol 7:186, 1989.
75. Cobleigh MA, Kennedy JL: Non-Hodgkin's lymphomas of the upper aerodigestive tract and salivary glands. Otol Clin North Am 19:685, 1986.
76. Weisberger EC, Davidson DD: Unusual presentations of lymphoma of the head and neck in childhood. Laryngoscope 100:337, 1990.
77. Cohen SR, Thompson JW, Siegel SE: Non-Hodgkin's lymphoma of the larynx in children. Ann Otol Rhinol Laryngol 96:357, 1987.
78. Bumpous JM, Martin DS, Curran P, et al: Non-Hodgkin's lymphoma of the nose and paranasal sinuses in the pediatric population. Ann Otol Rhinol Laryngol 103:294, 1994.
79. Jones SE, Fuks Z, Bull M, et al: Non-Hodgkin's lymphomas. IV. Clinicopathologic correlation in 405 cases. Cancer 31:806, 1973.
80. Peters MV: The need for a new clinical classification in Hodgkin's disease. Cancer Res 31:1713, 1971.
81. Lukes R, Collins R: Immunologic characterization of human malignant lymphomas. Cancer 34:1488, 1974.
82. Howard D, Batsakis J: Non-Hodgkin's lymphomas: Contemporary classification and correlates. Ann Otol Rhinol Laryngol 94:326, 1985.
83. The Non-Hodgkin's Lymphoma Pathologic Classification Project: National Cancer Institute sponsored study of classifications of non-Hodgkin's lymphomas. Summary and description of a working formulation for clinical usage. Cancer 49:2112, 1982.
84. Katz RL: Cytologic diagnosis of leukemia and lymphoma. Values and limitations. Clin Lab Med 11:469, 1991.
85. Murphy S: Childhood non-Hodgkin's lymphoma. N Engl J Med 299:1446, 1978.
86. Link MP, Donaldson SS, Berard CW, et al: Results of treatment of childhood localized non-Hodgkin's lymphoma with combination chemotherapy with or without radiotherapy. N Engl J Med 322:1169, 1990.
87. Shipp MA, Harrington DP, Anderson JR, et al: A predictive model for aggressive non-Hodgkin's lymphoma. N Engl J Med 329:987, 1993.
88. Tatsumi M, Kitayama H, Sugahara H, et al: Whole-body hybrid pet with (18) f-fdg in the staging of non-Hodgkin's lymphoma. J Nucl Med 42:601, 2001.
89. Chabner B, Fisher R, Young R, et al: Staging of non-Hodgkin's lymphoma. Semin Oncol 7:285, 1980.
90. Janus C, Edwards BK, Sariban E, et al: Surgical resection and limited chemotherapy for abdominal undifferentiated lymphomas. Cancer Treat Rep 68:599, 1984.
91. Anderson JR, Jenkin RD, Wilson SF, et al: Long-term follow-up of patients treated with COMP or LSA$_2$L$_2$ therapy for childhood non-Hodgkin's lymphoma: A report of CCG-551 from the children's cancer group. J Clin Oncol 11:1024, 1993.
92. Dahl GV, Rivera G, Pui CH, et al: A novel treatment of childhood lymphoblastic non-Hodgkin's lymphoma: Early and intermittent use of teniposide plus cytarabine. Blood 66:1110, 1985.
93. Patte C, Kalifa C, Flamant F, et al: Results of the LMT81 protocol, a modified LSA$_2$L$_2$ protocol with high dose methotrexate, on 84 children with non-B-cell (lymphoblastic) lymphoma. Med Pediatr Oncol 20:105, 1992.
94. Wollner N, Burchenal JH, Lieberman PH, et al: Non-Hodgkin's lymphoma in children: A comparative study of two modalities of therapy. Cancer 37:123, 1976.
95. Tubergen DG, Krailo MD, Meadows AT, et al: Comparison of treatment regimens for pediatric lymphoblastic non-Hodgkin's lymphoma: A children's cancer group study. J Clin Oncol 13:1368, 1995.
96. Hutchison RE, Berard CW, Shuster JJ, et al: B-cell lineage confers a favorable outcome among children and adolescents with large-cell lymphoma: A pediatric oncology group study. J Clin Oncol 13:2023, 1995.
97. Reiter A, Schrappe M, Parwaresch R, et al: Non-Hodgkin's lymphomas of childhood and adolescence: Results of a treatment stratified for biologic subtypes and stage-A report of the Berlin-Frankfurt-Munster group. J Clin Oncol 13:359, 1995.
98. Finlay JL, Bunin NJ, Sinniah D: Non-Hodgkin's lymphoma. In D'Angio GJ, Sinniah D, Meadows AT, et al (eds): Practical Pediatric Oncology. New York, John Wiley & Sons, 1992.
99. Murphy SB: Classification, staging, and end results of childhood non-Hodgkin's lymphomas: Dissimilarities from lymphoma in adults. Semin Oncol 7:332, 1980.

100. Magrath IT: African Burkitt's lymphoma: History, biology, clinical features and treatment. Am J Pediatr Hematol Oncol 13:322, 1991.
101. Ziegler J: Burkitt's lymphoma. N Engl J Med 305:735, 1981.
102. Kearns D, Smith R, Pitcock J: Burkitt's lymphoma. Int J Pediatr Otorhinolaryngol 12:73, 1986.
103. Beral V, Peterman T, Berkelman R, et al: AIDS-associated non-Hodgkin's lymphoma. Lancet 337:805, 1991.
104. Levine P, Komarciu L, Connely R, et al: The American Burkitt's lymphoma registry: Eight years' experience. Cancer 49:1016, 1982.
105. Burkitt D, O'Conner G: Malignant lymphoma in African children. I. A clinical syndrome. Cancer 14:258, 1961.
106. Stein JE, Schwenn MR, Jacir NN, et al: Surgical restraint in Burkitt's lymphoma in children. J Pediatr Surg 26:1273, 1991.
107. Miron I, Frappaz D, Brunat-Mentigny M, et al: Initial management of advanced Burkitt lymphoma in children: Is there still a place for surgery? Pediatr Hematol Oncol 14:555, 1997.
108. Kemeny M, Magrath I, Brennan M: The role of surgery in the management of American Burkitt's lymphoma. Ann Surg 196:82, 1982.
109. Magrath I, Lee Y, Anderson T, et al: Prognostic factors in Burkitt's lymphoma: Importance of total tumor burden. Cancer 45:1507, 1980.
110. Miser J, Pizzo P: Soft tissue sarcomas in childhood. Pediatr Clin North Am 32:779, 1985.
111. MacArthur CJ, McGill TJI, Healy GB: Pediatric head and neck rhabdomyosarcoma. Clin Pediatr 31:66, 1992.
112. Donaldson SS: Rhabdomyosarcoma: Contemporary status and future directions. Arch Surg 124:1015, 1989.
113. Mandell LR: Ongoing process in the treatment of childhood rhabdomyosarcoma. Oncology 7:71, 1993.
114. Newton WA, Soule EH, Hamoudi AB, et al: Histopathology of childhood sarcomas. Intergroup Rhabdomyosarcoma Studies I and II: Clinicopathologic correlation. J Clin Oncol 6:67, 1988.
115. Keel SB, Rosenberg AE: Soft tissue pathology of the head and neck. In Pilch BZ (ed): Head and Neck Surgical Pathology. Philadelphia, Lippincott Williams & Wilkins, 2001, pp 389–437.
116. McGill T: Rhabdomyosarcoma of the head and neck: An update. Otolaryngol Clin North Am 22:631, 1989.
117. Barnes L: Tumors and tumorlike lesions of the soft tissues. In Barnes L (ed): Surgical Pathology of the Head and Neck. New York, Marcel Dekker, 1985.
118. Crist W, Gehan EA, Ragab AH, et al: The third intergroup rhabdomyosarcoma study. J Clin Oncol 13:610, 1995.
119. Daya H, Chan HSL, Sirkin W, et al: Pediatric rhabdomyosarcoma of the head and neck: Is there a place for surgical management? Arch Otolaryngol Head Neck Surg 126:468, 2000.
120. Knowles D, Jacobiec F, Jones I: Rhabdomyosarcoma. In Jones I, Jacobiec F (eds): Diseases of the Orbit. Hagerstown, Md, Harper & Row, 1979.
121. Weiner ES: Head and neck rhabdomyosarcoma. Semin Pediatr Surg 3:203, 1994.
122. Canalis R, Jenkins H, Hemenway W, et al: Nasopharyngeal rhabdomyosarcoma: A clinical perspective. Arch Otolaryngol 104:122, 1978.
123. Schwartz R, Movassaghi N, Marion E: Rhabdomyosarcoma of the middle ear: A wolf in sheep's clothing. Pediatrics 65:1131, 1980.
124. Dehner L, Chen K: Primary tumors of the external and middle ear. A clinicopathologic study of embryonal rhabdomyosarcoma. Arch Otolaryngol 104:399, 1978.
125. Leviton A, Davidson R, Gilles F: Neurologic manifestations of embryonal rhabdomyosarcoma of the middle ear cleft. J Pediatr 80:596, 1972.
126. Fleischer A, Koslow M, Rovit R: Neurological manifestations of primary rhabdomyosarcoma of the head and neck in children. J Neurosurg 43:207, 1975.
127. Flamant F, Luboinski B, Couanet D, et al: Rhabdomyosarcoma in children: Clinical symptoms, diagnosis, and staging. In Maurer HM, Ruymann FB, Pochedly C (eds): Rhabdomyosarcoma and Related Tumors in Children and Adolescents. Boca Raton, Fla, CRC Press, 1991, chapter 4.
128. Garnsey LA, Gehan EA: Prognostic factors in rhabdomyosarcoma. In Maurer HM, Ruymann FB, Pochedly C (eds): Rhabdomyosarcoma and Related Tumors in Children and Adolescents. Boca Raton, Fla, CRC Press, 1991, chapter 6.
129. Lawrence W Jr, Hays DM, Heyn R, et al: Lymphatic metastases with childhood rhabdomyosarcoma: A report from the Intergroup Rhabdomyosarcoma Study. Cancer 60:910, 1987.
130. Sutow W, Lindberg R, Gehan E, et al: Three-year relapse-free survival rates in childhood rhabdomyosarcoma of the head and neck. Cancer 49:2217, 1982.
131. Asmar L, Gehan EA, Newton WA, et al: Agreement among and within groups of pathologists in the classification of rhabdomyosarcoma and related childhood sarcomas. Cancer 74:2579, 1994.
132. Pappo AS, Shapiro DN, Crist WM, et al: Biology and therapy of pediatric rhabdomyosarcoma. J Clin Oncol 13:2123, 1995.
133. Raney R Jr, Zimmerman R, Bilaniuk L, et al: Management of craniofacial sarcoma in childhood assisted by computed tomography. Int J Radiat Oncol Biol Phys 5:529, 1979.
134. Das Narla L, Walsh JW: Diagnostic imaging in rhabdomyosarcoma. In Maurer HM, Ruymann FB, Pochedly C (eds): Rhabdomyosarcoma and Related Tumors in Children and Adolescents. Boca Raton, Fla, CRC Press, 1991, chapter 5.
135. Kraus DH, Saenz C, Gollamudi S, et al: Pediatric rhabdomyosarcoma of the head and neck. Am J Surg 174:556, 1997.
136. Maurer H, Moon T, Donaldson M, et al: The Intergroup Rhabdomyosarcoma Study: A preliminary report. Cancer 40:2015, 1977.
137. Donaldson S, Belli J: A rational clinical staging system for childhood rhabdomyosarcoma. J Clin Oncol 2:135, 1984.
138. Pedrick T, Donaldson S, Cox R: Rhabdomyosarcoma: The Stanford experience using a TMN staging system. J Clin Oncol 4:370, 1986.
139. Wharam M, Foulkes M, Lawrence W Jr, et al: Soft tissue sarcoma of the head and neck in childhood: Nonorbital and nonparameningeal sites. Cancer 53:1016, 1984.
140. Wharam MD, Beltangady MS, Heyn RM, et al: Pediatric orofacial and laryngopharyngeal rhabdomyosarcoma. Arch Otolaryngol Head Neck Surg 113:1225, 1987.
141. Anderson GJ, Tom LWC, Womer RB, et al: Rhabdomyosarcoma of the head and neck in children. Arch Otolaryngol Head Neck Surg 116:428, 1990.
142. Tefft M, Lindberg R, Gehan E: Radiation therapy combined with systemic chemotherapy of rhabdomyosarcoma in children: Local control in patients enrolled in the Intergroup Rhabdomyosarcoma Study. Natl Cancer Inst Monogr 56:75, 1981.
143. Crist WM, Anderson JR, Meza JL, et al: Intergroup rhabdomyosarcoma study IV: Results for patients with nonmetastatic disease. J Clin Oncol 19:3091, 2001.
144. Raney RB Jr, Tefft M, Hays DM, et al: Rhabdomyosarcoma and the undifferentiated sarcomas. In Pizzo PA, Poplack DG (eds): Principles and Practice of Pediatric Oncology, 2nd ed. Philadelphia, JB Lippincott, 1993, chapter 32.
145. Maurer H, Donaldson M, Gehan E: The Intergroup Rhabdomyosarcoma Study: Update, November 1978. Natl Cancer Inst Monogr 56:61, 1981.
146. Maurer H: The Intergroup Rhabdomyosarcoma Study II: Objective and study design. J Pediatr Surg 15:371, 1980.
147. Hawkins DS, Anderson JR, Paidas CN, et al: Improved outcome for patients with middle ear rhabdomyosarcoma: A children's oncology group study. J Clin Oncol 19:3073, 2001.
148. Crist WM, Garnsey L, Gehan E, et al: Evidence of "stage shift" in IRS studies? J Clin Oncol 8:1768, 1990.
149. Crist WM, Garnsey L, Beltangady MS, et al: Prognosis in children with rhabdomyosarcoma: A report of the Intergroup Rhabdomyosarcoma Studies I and II. J Clin Oncol 8:443, 1990.
150. Raney R Jr, Hays DM, Tefft M, et al: Rhabdomyosarcoma and the undifferentiated sarcoma. In Pizzo PA, Poplack DG (eds): Principles and Practice of Pediatric Oncology, 2nd ed. Philadelphia, JB Lippincott, 1989.
151. Rodary C, Rey A, Olive D, et al: Prognostic factors in 281 children with non-metastatic rhabdomyosarcoma (RMS) at diagnosis. Med Pediatr Oncol 16:71, 1988.
152. Treuner J, Suder J, Keim M, et al: The predictive value of initial cytostatic response in primary unresectable rhabdomyosarcoma in children. Acta Oncol 28:67, 1989.
153. Raney R Jr, Tefft M, Newton W, et al: Improved prognosis with intensive treatment of children with cranial soft tissue sarcomas arising in nonorbital parameningeal sites: A report from the Intergroup Rhabdomyosarcoma Study II. Cancer 59:147, 1987.

154. Raney RB, Anderson JR, Barr FG, et al: Rhabdomyosarcoma and undifferentiated sarcoma in the first two decades of life: A selective review of Intergroup Rhabdomyosarcoma Study Group experience and rationale for Intergroup Rhabdomyosarcoma Study V. Am J Pediatr Hematol Oncol 23:215, 2001.

155. Maurer H, Foulkes M, Gehan E: Intergroup Rhabdomyosarcoma Study (IRS)-II: Preliminary report. Proc Am Soc Clin Oncol 2:70, 1983.

156. Raney R Jr, Crist W, Maurer H, et al: Prognosis of children with soft tissue sarcoma who relapse after achieving a complete response: A report from the Intergroup Rhabdomyosarcoma Study I. Cancer 52:44, 1983.

157. Wight RG, Harris SC, Shortland JR, et al: Rhabdomyosarcoma of the nasopharynx: A case with recurrence of tumour after 20 years. J Laryngol Otol 102:1182, 1988.

158. Wei W: Rhabdomyosarcoma of the soft palate: A case of late relapse. J Laryngol Otol 99:1029, 1985.

159. Chabalko J, Creagan E, Fraumeni J Jr: Epidemiology of selected sarcomas in children. J Natl Cancer Inst 53:675, 1974.

160. Jenkin D, Sonley M: Soft tissue sarcomas in the young: Medical treatment advances in perspective. Cancer 46:621, 1980.

161. Eavey RD, Janfaza P, Chapman PH, et al: Skull base dumbbell tumor: Surgical experience with two adolescents. Ann Otol Rhinol Laryngol 101:939, 1992.

162. Sanroman JF, De Hoyo A Jr, Diaz FJ, et al: Sarcomas of the head and neck. Br J Oral Maxillofac Surg 30:115, 1992.

163. Wanebo HJ, Koness RJ, MacFarlane JK, et al: Head and neck sarcoma: Report of the Head and Neck Sarcoma Registry. Head Neck 14:1, 1991.

164. Nasri S, Mark RJ, Sercarz JA, et al: Pediatric sarcomas of the head and neck other than rhabdomyosarcoma. Am J Otolaryngol 16:165, 1995.

165. Blakely ML, Spurbeck WW, Pappo AS, et al: The impact of margin resection on the outcome in pediatric nonrhabdomyosarcoma soft tissue sarcomas. J Pediatr Surg 34:672, 1999.

166. Palumbo JS, Zwerdling T: Soft tissue sarcomas of infancy. Semin Perinatol 23:299, 1999.

167. Miser JS, Triche TJ, Pritchard DJ, et al: The other soft tissue sarcomas of childhood. In Pizzo PA, Poplack DG (eds): Principles and Practice of Pediatric Oncology, 2nd ed. Philadelphia, JB Lippincott, 1993, chapter 34.

168. Beck JC, Devaney KO, Weatherly RA, et al: Pediatric myofibromatosis of the head and neck. Arch Otolaryngol Head Neck 125:39, 1999.

169. Soule E, Pritchard D: Fibrosarcoma in infants and children: A review of 110 cases. Cancer 40:1711, 1977.

170. Wexler H, Helman LJ: Pediatric soft tissue sarcomas. CA Cancer J Clin 44:211, 1994.

171. Postovsky S, Peleg H, Ben-Itzhak O, et al: Fibrosarcoma of the trachea in a child: Case report and review of the literature. Am J Otolaryngol 20:332, 1999.

172. Picard E, Udassin R, Ramu N, et al: Pulmonary fibrosarcoma in childhood: A fiberoptic bronchoscopic diagnosis and review of the literature. Pediatr Pulmonol 27:347, 1999.

173. Swain RE, Sessions DG, Ogura JH: Fibrosarcoma of the head and neck: A clinical analysis of 40 cases. Ann Otol Rhinol Laryngol 83:439, 1974.

174. Cheung E, Enzinger F: Infantile fibrosarcoma. Cancer 38:729, 1976.

175. Stout AP: Fibrosarcoma in infants and children. Cancer 15:1028, 1962.

176. Littman P, Raney B, Zimmerman R, et al: Soft-tissue sarcomas of the head and neck in children. Int J Radiat Oncol Biol Phys 9:1367, 1983.

177. Keel SB, Rosenberg AE: Soft tissue pathology of the head and neck. In Pilch BZ (ed): Head and Neck Surgical Pathology. Philadelphia, Lippincott Williams & Wilkins, 2001, pp 389–437.

178. Hoos A, Lewis JJ, Marshall JU, et al: Desmoid tumors of the head and neck—a clinical study of a rare entity. Head Neck 22:814, 2000.

179. Merchant TE, Nguyen D, Walter AW, et al: Long-term results with radiation therapy for pediatric desmoid tumors. Int J Radiat Oncol Biol Phys 47:1267, 2000.

180. Jelinek JA, Stelzer KJ, Conrad E, et al: The efficacy of radiotherapy as postoperative treatment for desmoid tumors. Int J Radiat Oncol Biol Phys 50:121, 2001.

181. Kamath SS, Parsons JT, Marcus RB, et al: Radiotherapy for local control of aggressive fibromatosis. Int J Radiat Oncol Biol Phys 36:325, 1996.

182. Azzarelli G, Gronchi A, Bertulli R, et al: Low-dose chemotherapy with methotrexate and vinblastine for patients with advanced aggressive fibromatosis. Cancer 92:1259, 2001.

183. Faulkner LB, Hajdu SI, Kher U, et al: Pediatric desmoid tumor: Retrospective analysis of 63 cases. J Clin Oncol 13:2813, 1995.

184. Fasching MC, Saleh J, Woods JE: Desmoid tumors of the head and neck. Am J Surg 156:327, 1988.

185. Masson KM, Soule EH: Desmoid tumors of the head and neck. Am J Surg 112:615, 1966.

186. Gooder P, Farrington T: Extracranial neurilemmomata of the head and neck. J Laryngol Otol 94:243, 1980.

187. Glover TW, Stein CK, Legius E, et al: Molecular and cytogenetic analysis of tumors in von Recklinghausen neurofibromatosis. Genes Chromosomes Cancer 3:62, 1991.

188. deCampora E, Radici M, deCampora L: Neurogenic tumors of the head and neck in children. Int J Pediatr Otolaryngol 49:S231, 1999.

189. Treuner J, Gross U, Maas E, et al: Results of the treatment of malignant schwannoma: A report from the German soft tissue sarcoma group (CWS). Med Pediatr Oncol 19:399, 1991.

190. Ladenstein R, Treuner J, Koscielniak E, et al: Synovial sarcoma of childhood and adolescence: Report of the German CES-81 study. Cancer 71:3647, 1993.

191. Moore D, Berke G: Synovial sarcoma of the head and neck. Arch Otolaryngol Head Neck Surg 113:311, 1987.

192. Barnes L, Peel R: Soft tissue tumors with special emphasis on the head and neck. Orlando, Fla, American Society of Clinical Pathologist Workshop No. 1074, October 1986.

193. Rangheard AS, Vanel D, Viala J, et al: Synovial sarcoma of the head and neck: CT and MR imaging findings of eight patients. Am J Neuroradiol 22:851, 2001.

194. Carson J, Harwood A, Cummings B: The place of radiotherapy in the treatment of synovial sarcoma. Int J Radiat Oncol Biol Phys 7:49, 1981.

195. Andrassy RJ, Okcu MF, Despa S, et al: Synovial sarcoma in children: Surgical lessons from a single institution and review of the literature. J Am Coll Surg 192:305, 2001.

196. Roth SA, Enzinger FM, Tannenbaum M: Synovial sarcoma of the neck: A follow-up study of 24 cases. Cancer 35:1243, 1975.

197. Spillane AJ, A'Hern R, Judson IR, et al: Synovial sarcoma: A clinicopathologic, staging, and prognostic assessment. J Clin Oncol 18:3794, 2000.

198. Kauffman S, Stout A: Hemangiopericytoma in children. Cancer 13:695, 1960.

199. Atkinson J, Mahour G, Isaacs H Jr, et al: Hemangiopericytoma in infants and children: A report of six patients. Am J Surg 148:372, 1984.

200. Enzinger F, Smith B: Hemangiopericytoma: An analysis of 106 cases. Hum Pathol 7:61, 1976.

201. Cohen J, Landon G, Byers R: Pathologic quiz case 1. Arch Otolaryngol Head Neck Surg 113:562, 1987.

202. Hasson O, Kirsch G, Lustmann J: Hemangiopericytoma of the tongue in an 11-year-old girl: Case report and literature review. Pediatr Dent 16:49, 1994.

203. Gotte K, Hormann K, Schmoll J, et al: Congenital nasal hemangiopericytoma: Intrauterine, intraoperative and histologic findings. Laryngoscope 108:589, 1999.

204. Ortega J, Finklestein J, Isaacs H Jr, et al: Chemotherapy of malignant hemangiopericytoma of childhood. Cancer 27:730, 1971.

205. Mira J, Chu F, Fortiner J: The role of radiotherapy in management of malignant hemangiopericytoma. Cancer 39:1254, 1977.

206. Backwinkel K, Diddams J: Hemangiopericytoma: Report of a case and comprehensive review of the literature. Cancer 25:896, 1970.

207. Variend S: Small cell tumors in childhood: A review. J Pathol 145:1, 1984.

208. Dickman PS, Triche TJ: Extraosseous Ewing's sarcoma versus primitive rhabdomyosarcoma: Diagnostic criteria and clinical correlation. Hum Pathol 17:881, 1986.

209. Boor A, Jurkovic I, Friedmann I, et al: Extraskeletal Ewing's sarcoma of the nose. J Laryngol Otol 115:74, 2001.

210. Angervall L, Enzinger F: Extraskeletal neoplasms resembling Ewing's sarcoma. Cancer 36:240, 1975.

211. Ahmad R, Mayol BR, Davis M, et al: Extraskeletal Ewing's sarcoma. Cancer 85:725, 1999.

212. Chao TK, Chang YL, Sheen TS: Extraskeletal Ewing's sarcoma of the scalp. J Laryngol Otol 114:73, 2000.

213. Gustafson R, Maragos N, Reiman H: Extraskeletal Ewing's sarcoma occurring as a mass in the neck. Otolaryngol Head Neck Surg 90:491, 1982.

214. Wilkins RM, Pritchard DJ, Burgert EO, et al: Ewing's sarcoma of bone: Experience with 140 patients. Cancer 58:2551, 1986.

215. Tefft M, Vawter G, Mitus A: Paravertebral "round cell" tumors in children. Radiology 92:1501, 1969.

216. Soule E, Newton W Jr, Moon T: Extraskeletal Ewing's sarcoma: A preliminary review of 26 cases encountered in the Intergroup Rhabdomyosarcoma Study. Cancer 42:259, 1978.

217. Rosen G, Caparros B, Mosende C, et al: Curability of Ewing's sarcoma and considerations for future therapeutic trials. Cancer 41:888, 1978.

218. Shimada H, Newton WA Jr, Soule EH, et al: Pathologic features of extraosseous Ewing's sarcoma: A report from the Intergroup Rhabdomyosarcoma Study. Hum Pathol 19:442, 1988.

219. Kinsella TJ, Loeffler JS, Fraass JS, et al: Extremity preservation by combined modality therapy in sarcomas of the hand and foot: An analysis of local control, disease free survival and functional result. Int J Radiat Oncol Biol Phys 9:1115, 1983.

220. Daw NC, Mahmoud HH, Meyer WH, et al: Bone sarcomas of the head and neck in children: The St. Jude Children's Research Hospital experience. Cancer 88:2172, 2000.

221. Young JL Jr, Miller RW: Incidence of malignant tumors in US children. J Pediatr 86:254, 1975.

222. Dahlin DC: Bone Tumors: General Aspects and Data on 6221 Cases, 3rd ed. Springfield, Illinois, Charles C Thomas, 1978.

223. Oda D, Bavisotto LM, Schmidt RA, et al: Head and neck osteosarcoma at the University of Washington. Head Neck 19:513, 1997.

224. Gardner DG, Mills DM: The widened periodontal ligament of osteosarcoma of the jaws. Oral Surg 41:652, 1976.

225. Meyers PA, Gorlick R: Osteosarcoma. Pediatr Clin North Am 44:973, 1997.

226. Arndt CAS, Crist WM: Common musculoskeletal tumors of childhood and adolescence. N Engl J Med 341:344, 1999.

227. Womer RB: The cellular biology of bone tumors. Clin Orthop 262:12, 1991.

228. Simmons WB, Haggerty HS, Ngan B, et al: Alveolar soft part sarcoma of the head and neck: A disease of children and young adults. Int J Pediatr Otolaryngol 17:139, 1989.

229. Mamede RM, Mello FV, Barbieri J: Prognosis of Ewing's sarcoma of the head and neck. Otolaryngol Head Neck Surg 102:650, 1990.

230. Siegal GP, Oliver WR, Reinus WR, et al: Primary Ewing's sarcoma involving the bones of the head and neck. Cancer 60:2829, 1987.

231. Grier HE: The Ewing family of tumors: Ewing's sarcoma and primitive neuroectodermal tumors. Pediatr Clin North Am 44:991, 1997.

232. Jurgens H, Exner U, Gadner H, et al: Multidisciplinary treatment of primary Ewing's sarcoma of bone: A 6-year experience of a European cooperative trial. Cancer 61:23, 1988.

233. Marcus RB Jr, Million RR: The effect of primary tumor size on the prognosis of Ewing's sarcomas. Int J Radiat Oncol Biol Phys 10:88, 1984. Abstract 24.

234. Mendenhall CM, Marcus RB Jr, Enneking WF, et al: The prognostic significance of soft tissue extension in Ewing's sarcoma. Cancer 51:913, 1983.

235. Marcus RB Jr, Graham-Pole JR, Springfield DS, et al: High-risk Ewing's sarcoma: End-intensification using autologous bone marrow transplantation. Int J Radiat Oncol Biol Phys 15:53, 1988.

236. Miser JS, Kinsella TJ, Triche TJ, et al: Preliminary results of treatment of Ewing's sarcoma of bone in children and young adults: Six months of intensive combined modality therapy without maintenance. J Clin Oncol 6:484, 1988.

237. Gadwall SR, Fanburg-Smith JC, Gannon FH, et al: Primary chondrosarcoma of the head and neck in pediatric patients: A clinicopathologic study of 14 cases with a review of the literature. Cancer 88:2181, 2000.

238. Burkey BB, Hoffman HT, Baker SR, et al: Chondrosarcoma of the head and neck. Laryngoscope 100:1301, 1990.

239. Spjut J, Dorfman H, Fechner R, et al: Atlas of Tumor Pathology, fascicle 5. Washington, DC, Armed Forces Institute of Pathology, 1971, p 84.

240. Webber PA, Hussain SS, Radcliffe GJ: Cartilaginous neoplasms of the head and neck. J Laryngol Otol 100:615, 1986.

241. Fu Y, Perzin KH: Non-epithelial tumors of the nasal cavity, paranasal sinuses, and nasopharynx: A clinicopathologic study. III. Cartilaginous tumors. Cancer 34:453, 1974.

242. Meyer C, Hauck KW, Gonzalez C: Chondrosarcoma of the facial skeleton in a child. Otolaryngol Head Neck Surg 101:591, 1991.

243. Rinaldo A, Howard DJ, Ferlito A: Laryngeal chondrosarcoma: A 24-year experience at the Royal National Throat, Nose and Ear Hospital Acta Otolaryngol 120:680, 2000.

244. Ferlito A, Nicolai P, Montaguti A, et al: Chondrosarcoma of the larynx: Review of the literature and report of three cases. Am J Otolaryngol 5:350, 1984.

245. Finn DG, Goepfert H, Batsakis JG: Chondrosarcoma of the head and neck. Laryngoscope 94:1539, 1984.

246. Harwood AR: Radiology of chondrosarcoma of bone. Cancer 45:2769, 1980.

247. Harwood AR, Cummings BJ, Fitzpatrick PJ: Radiotherapy for unusual tumors of the head and neck. J Otolaryngol 13:391, 1984.

248. Krochak R, Harwood A, Cummings B, et al: Results of radical radiation for chondrosarcoma of bone. Radiother Oncol 1:109, 1983.

249. McNaney D, Lindberg R, Ayala A, et al: Fifteen year radiotherapy experience with chondrosarcoma of bone. Int J Radiat Oncol Biol Phys 8:187, 1982.

250. Falconer MA, Bailey IC, Cuchen L: Surgical treatment of chordoma and chondroma of the skull base. J Neurosurg 29:261, 1968.

251. Heffelfinger MJ, Dahlin DC, MacCarty CS, et al: Chordomas and cartilaginous tumors at the skull base. Cancer 32:410, 1973.

252. Evans HL, Ayala AG, Romsdahl MM: Prognostic factors in chondrosarcoma of bone. Cancer 40:818, 1977.

253. Restrepo J, Handler S, Saull S, et al: Malignant fibrous histiocytoma. Otolaryngol Head Neck Surg 96:362, 1987.

254. Castleberry RP: Biology and treatment of neuroblastoma. Pediatr Clin North Am 44:919, 1997.

255. Myer CM III, Mortelliti AJ, Yank GA, et al: Malignant and benign tumors of the head and neck in children. In Smith JD, Bumstead RM (eds): Pediatric Facial Plastic and Reconstructive Surgery. New York, Raven, 1993.

256. Evans A, D'Angio G, Koop C: Diagnosis and treatment of neuroblastoma. Pediatr Clin North Am 23:161, 1976.

257. Maris JM, Matthay KK: Molecular biology of neuroblastoma. J Clin Oncol 17:2264, 1999.

258. Neuroblastoma. In Pizzo PA, Poplack DG (eds): Principles and Practice of Pediatric Oncology, 2nd ed. Philadelphia, JB Lippincott, 1993, p 746.

259. Brown R, Syzmula N, Lore J: Neuroblastoma of the head and neck. Arch Otolaryngol 104:395, 1978.

260. Jaffe N, Cassady R, Filler R, et al: Heterochromia and Horner's syndrome associated with cervical and mediastinal neuroblastoma. J Pediatr 87:75, 1975.

261. Barnes L, Peel R, Verbin R: Tumors of the nervous system. In Barnes L (ed): Surgical Pathology of the Head and Neck. New York, Marcel Dekker, 1985.

262. Weir MM: Cytopathology of the eye, orbit, jaws, oral cavity, and sinonasal tract. In Pilch BZ (ed): Head and Neck Surgical Pathology. Philadelphia, Lippincott Williams & Wilkins, 2001, pp 663–685.

263. Shimada H, Ambros IM, Dehner LP, et al: The International Pathology Classification (the Shimada System). Cancer 86:364, 1999.

264. Joshi VV, Cantor AB, Altshuler G, et al: Age-linked prognostic categorization based on a new histologic grading system of neuroblastomas. A clinicopathologic study of 211 cases from the Pediatric Oncology Group. Cancer 69:2197, 1992.

265. MacEwan AJ, Wyeth P, Ackery D: Radioiodinated iodobenzylguanidines for diagnosis and therapy. Int J Radiat Appl Instrum [A] 37:765, 1986.

266. Alvardo CS, London WB, Look AT, et al: Natural history and biology of stage A neuroblastoma: A pediatric oncology group study. J Pediatr Hematol Oncol 22:197, 2000.

267. Bown N, Cotterill S, Lastowska M, et al: Gain of chromosome arm 17q and adverse outcome in patients with neuroblastoma. N Engl J Med 340:1954, 1999.

268. Castleberry RP: Predicting outcome in neuroblastoma. N Engl J Med 340:1992, 1999.

269. Ambros IM, Zellner A, Roald B, et al: Role of ploidy, chromosome 1p, and Schwann cells in the maturation of neuroblastoma. N Engl J Med 334:1505, 1996.

270. Seeger C, Brodeur GM, Sather H, et al: Association of multiple copies of the N-myc oncogene with rapid progression of neuroblastoma. N Engl J Med 313:1111, 1985.

271. Nakagawara A, Arima-Nakagawara M, Scavarda NJ, et al: Association between high levels of expression of the TRK gene and favorable outcomes in human neuroblastoma. N Engl J Med 328:847, 1993.

272. Frostad B, Martinsson T, Tani E, et al: The use of fine-needle aspiration cytology in the molecular characterization of neuroblastoma in children. Cancer Cytopathol 87:60, 1999.

273. Contador MP, Johnston S, Smith EI, et al: Lymph node sampling in localized neuroblastoma: A Pediatric Oncology Group Study. J Pediatr Surg 34:967, 1999.

274. Cushing B, Slovis T, Philippart A, et al: A rational approach to cervical neuroblastoma. Cancer 50:785, 1982.

275. Carlsen N, Schroeder H, Bro P, et al: Neuroblastoma treated at the four major oncologic clinics in Denmark 1943–1980: An evaluation of 180 cases. Med Pediatr Oncol 13:180, 1985.

276. Brenner MK, Heslop H, Krance R, et al: Phase I study of chemokine and cytokine gene-modified autologous neuroblastoma cells for treatment of relapsed/refractory neuroblastoma using an adenoviral vector. Hum Gene Ther 11:1477, 2000.

277. Hass-Kogan Da, Fisch BM, Wara WM, et al: Intraoperative radiation therapy for high risk pediatric neuroblastoma. Int J Radiat Oncol Biol Phys 47:985, 2000.

278. Evans A, D'Angio G, Propert K, et al: Prognostic factors in neuroblastoma. Cancer 59:1853, 1987.

279. Stephenson SR, Cook BA, Mease AD, et al: The prognostic significance of age and pattern of metastases in stage IV-S neuroblastoma. Cancer 58:372, 1986.

280. Breslow N, McCann B: Statistical estimation of prognosis for children with neuroblastoma. Cancer Res 31:2098, 1971.

281. Cutler LS, Chaudhry AP, Topazian R: Melanotic neuroectodermal tumor of infancy: An ultrastructural study, literature review, and reevaluation. Cancer 48:257, 1981.

282. Kaya S, Unal OF, Sarac S, et al: Melanotic neuroectodermal tumor of infancy: Report of two cases and review of literature. Int J Pediatr Otorhinolaryngol 52:169, 2000.

283. Dehner LP, Sibley BK, Sauk JJ, et al: Malignant melanotic neuroectodermal tumor of infancy: A clinical, pathologic, ultrastructural and tissue culture study. Cancer 43:1389, 1979.

284. Batsakis JG: Melanotic neuroectodermal tumor of infancy. Ann Otol Rhinol Laryngol 96:128, 1987.

285. Mirich DR, Blaser SI, Harwood-Nash DC, et al: Melanotic neuroectodermal tumor of infancy: Clinical, radiologic, and pathologic findings in five cases. Am J Neuroradiol 12:689, 1991.

286. Nielsen GP, O'Connell JX, Rosenberg AE: Pathology of selected diseases affecting the bones and joints of the head and neck. In Pilch BZ (ed): Head and Neck Surgical Pathology. Philadelphia, Lippincott Williams & Wilkins, 2001, pp 438–475.

287. Galera-Ruiz H, Gomez-Angel D, Vasquez-Ramirez FJ, et al: Fine-needle aspiration in the pre-operative diagnosis of melanotic neuroectodermal tumor of infancy. J Laryngol Otol 113:581, 1999.

288. Crockett DM, McGill TJ, Healy GB, et al: Melanotic neuroectodermal tumor of infancy. Otolaryngol Head Neck Surg 96:194, 1987.

289. Stiller CA: International variations in the incidence of childhood carcinoma. Cancer Epidemiol Biomarkers Prev 3:305, 1994.

290. Anderson A, Bergdhal L, Boquist L: Thyroid carcinoma in children. Am J Surg 43:159, 1977.

291. Winship T, Rosvoll R: Childhood thyroid carcinoma. Cancer 14:734, 1961.

292. Feinmesser R, Lubin E, Segal K, et al: Carcinoma of the thyroid in children—a review. J Pediatr Endocrinol Metab 10:561, 1997.

293. Clark D: Association of irradiation with cancer of the thyroid in children and adolescents. JAMA 159:1007, 1955.

294. Favus M, Schneider A, Stachura M, et al: Thyroid cancer occurring as a later consequence of head and neck irradiation: Evaluation of 1056 patients. N Engl J Med 294:1019, 1976.

295. Nikkiforo Y, Gnepp DR: Pediatric thyroid cancer after the Chernobyl disaster: Pathomorphologic study of 84 cases (1991–1992) from the Republic of Belarus. Cancer 74:748, 1994.

296. Nygaard R, Garwicz S, Haldorsen T, et al: Second malignant neoplasms in patients treated for childhood leukemia. Acta Pediatr Scand 80:1220, 1991.

297. Black P, Straaten A, Gutjahr P: Secondary thyroid carcinoma after treatment for childhood cancer. Med Pediatr Oncol 31:91, 1998.

298. Sankila R, Garwicz S, Dollner H, et al: Risk of subsequent malignant neoplasm among 1,641 Hodgkin's disease patients diagnosed in childhood and adolescence: A population based cohort study in the five Nordic countries. J Clin Oncol 14:1442, 1996.

299. Hung BW: Nodular thyroid disease and thyroid cancer. Pediatr Ann 21:50, 1992.

300. Lugo-Vicente H, Ortiz VN, Irizarry H, et al: Pediatric thyroid nodules: Management in the era of fine needle aspiration. J Pediatr Surg 33:1302, 1998.

301. Hung BW, August GP, Randolph JG, et al: Solitary thyroid nodules in children and adolescents. J Pediatr Surg 17:225, 1982.

302. DeKeyser L, Van Herle A: Differentiated thyroid cancer in children. Head Neck Surg 8:100, 1985.

303. Exelby P, Frazell E: Carcinoma of the thyroid in children. Surg Clin North Am 49:249, 1969.

304. Keiser H, Beaven M, Doppman J: Sipple's syndrome: Medullary thyroid carcinoma, pheochromocytoma and parathyroid disease. Ann Intern Med 78:561, 1973.

305. Faquin WC: Cytopathology of the thyroid gland. In Pilch BZ (ed): Head and Neck Surgical Pathology. Philadelphia, Lippincott Williams & Wilkins, 2001, pp 686–700.

306. Root AW, Diamond FB, Duncan JA, et al: Ectopic and entopic peptide hormone secreting neoplasms of childhood. Adv Pediatr 32:369–415, 1985.

307. Rallison ML, Dobyns BM, Heating FR, et al: Thyroid nodularity in children. JAMA 233:1069, 1975.

308. Kirkland RT, Kirkland JL, Rosenberg HS, et al: Solitary thyroid nodules in 30 children and report of a child with a thyroid abscess. Pediatrics 51:85, 1973.

309. Ashcraft M, Van Herle A: Management of thyroid nodules: I. History and physical examination, blood tests, x-ray tests, and ultrasonography. Head Neck Surg 3:216, 1981.

310. Shimotake T, Iwai N, Inoue K, et al: Germline mutations of the RET proto-oncogene in pedigree with MEN type 2A: DNA analysis and its implications for pediatric surgery. J Pediatr Surg 31:779, 1996.

311. O'Rordain DS, O'Brien T, Weaver AL, et al: Medullary thyroid carcinoma in multiple endocrine neoplasia types 2A and 2B. Surgery 116:1017, 1994.

312. Lallier M, St-Vil D, Giroux M, et al: Prophylactic thyroidectomy for medullary thyroid carcinoma in gene carriers of MEN 2 syndrome. J Pediatr Surg 33:846, 1998.

313. Garcia CJ, Daneman A, Thorner P, et al: Sonography of multinodular thyroid gland in children and adolescents. Am J Dis Child 146:811, 1992.

314. LaQuaglia MP, Telander RL: Differentiated medullary thyroid cancer in childhood and adolescence. Semin Pediatr Surg 6:42, 1997.

315. Newman KD: The current management of thyroid tumors in children. Eur J Med 2:691, 1993.

316. Raab SS, Silverman JF, Elsheikh TM, et al: Pediatric thyroid nodules: Disease demographics and clinical management by fine-needle aspiration biopsy. Pediatrics 95:46, 1995.

317. Khurana KK, Labrador E, Izquierdo R, et al: The role of fine-needle aspiration biopsy in the management of thyroid nodules in children, adolescents and young adults: A multi-institutional study. Thyroid 9:383, 1999.

318. Goepfert H, Dichtel W, Samaan N: Thyroid cancer in children and teenagers. Arch Otolaryngol 110:72, 1984.

319. Segal K, Sidi J, Levy R, et al: Thyroid carcinoma in children and adolescents. Ann Otol Rhinol Laryngol 94:346, 1985.

320. Ashcraft M, Van Herle A: Management of thyroid nodules: II. Scanning techniques, thyroid suppressive therapy, and fine needle aspiration. Head Neck Surg 3:297, 1981.

321. Sisson G: Applying the radioactive eraser: I-131 to ablate normal thyroid tissue in patients from whom thyroid cancer has been resected. J Nucl Med 24:743, 1983.

322. Rose RG, Kelsey MP: Radioactive iodine in the diagnosis and treatment of thyroid cancer. Cancer 16:896, 1963.

323. Yeh SDJ, LaQuaglia M: [131]I therapy for pediatric thyroid cancer. Semin Pediatr Surg 6:128, 1997.

324. Clark O, Castner B: Thyrotropin receptors in normal and neoplastic human thyroid tissue. Surgery 85:624, 1979.

325. Clark OH: TSH suppression in the management of thyroid nodules and thyroid cancer. World J Surg 5:39, 1981.

326. Crile G Jr: Treatment of carcinomas of the thyroid. In Young S, Inman DR (eds): Thyroid Neoplasia. London, Academic Press, 1968.

327. Block GE: An appraisal of the hormonal control of carcinoma of the thyroid gland. Surg Gynecol Obstet 132:289, 1971.

328. Simpson WJ, Panzarella T, Carruthers JS, et al: Papillary and follicular thyroid cancer: Impact of treatment in 1578 patients. Int J Radiat Oncol Biol Phys 14:1063, 1988.

329. Geiger JD, Thompson NW: Thyroid tumors in children. Otolaryngol Clin North Am 29:711, 1996.

330. Corwin T: Medullary carcinoma of the thyroid. Surg Gynecol Obstet 138:453, 1974.

331. Withers E, Rosenfeld L, O'Neill J, et al: Long-term experience with childhood thyroid carcinoma. J Pediatr Surg 14:332, 1979.

332. Telander R, Moir CR: Medullary thyroid carcinoma in children. Semin Pediatr Surg 3:188, 1994.

333. Topf P, Fried MP, Strome M: Vagaries of thyroglossal duct cysts. Laryngoscope 98:740, 1988.

334. LaRouere MJ, Drake AF, Baker SR, et al: Evaluation and management of a carcinoma arising in a thyroglossal duct cyst. Am J Otolaryngol 8:351, 1987.

335. McNicoll MP, Hawkins DB, England K, et al: Papillary carcinoma arising in a thyroglossal duct cyst. Otolaryngol Head Neck Surg 99:50, 1988.

336. Androulakis M, Johnson JT, Wagner RL: Thyroglossal duct and second branchial cleft anomalies in adults. Ear Nose Throat J 69:318, 1990.

337. Trail ML, Zeringue GP, Chicola JP: Carcinoma in thyroglossal duct remnants. Laryngoscope 87:1685, 1977.

338. Hanna E: Squamous cell carcinoma in a thyroglossal duct cyst (TGDC): Clinical presentation, diagnosis, and management. Am J Otolaryngol 17:353, 1996.

339. Deshpande A, Bobhate SK: Squamous cell carcinoma in thyroglossal duct cyst. J Laryngol Otol 109:1001, 1995.

340. Trail ML, Zeringue GP, Chicola JP: Carcinoma in thyroglossal duct remnants. Laryngoscope 87:1685, 1977.

341. Kennedy TL, Whitaker M, Wadih G: Thyroglossal duct carcinoma: A rational approach to management. Laryngoscope 108:1154, 1998.

342. Allard HB: The thyroglossal duct cyst. Head Neck Surg 5:134, 1982.

343. Hundahl SA, Fleming ID, Fremgen AM, et al: Two hundred eighty six cases of parathyroid carcinoma treated in the U.S. between 1985–1995. Cancer 86:538, 1999.

344. Meier DE, Snyder WH III, Dickson BA, et al: Parathyroid carcinoma in a child. J Pediatr Surg 34:606, 1999.

345. Wassif WS, Moniz CF, Friedman E, et al: Familial isolated hyperparathyroidism: A distinct genetic entity with an increased risk of parathyroid cancer. J Clin Encodrinol Metab 77:1485, 1993.

346. Krolls S, Trodahl J, Boyers R: Salivary gland lesions in children: A survey of 430 cases. Cancer 30:459, 1972.

347. Schuller D, McCabe B: Salivary gland neoplasms in children. Otolaryngol Clin North Am 10:399, 1977.

348. Dahlqvist A, Ostberg Y: Malignant salivary tumors in children. Acta Otolaryngol 94:175, 1982.

349. Byers R, Piorkowski R, Luna M: Malignant parotid tumors in patients under 20 years of age. Arch Otolaryngol 110:232, 1984.

350. Baker S, Malone B: Salivary gland malignancies in children. Cancer 55:1730, 1985.

351. Vawter G, Tefft M: Congenital tumors of the parotid gland. Arch Pathol 82:242, 1966.

352. Hendrick J: Mucoepidermoid carcinoma of the parotid gland in a 1-year-old child. Am J Surg 108:907, 1964.

353. Rogers DA, Rao BN, Bowman L, et al: Primary malignancy of the salivary gland in children. J Pediatr Surg 29:44, 1994.

354. Winslow C, Batuello S, Chan KC: Pediatric mucoepidermoid carcinoma of the minor salivary gland. Ear Nose Throat J 77:390, 1998.

355. Castro E, Huvos A, Strong E, et al: Tumors of the major salivary glands in children. Cancer 29:312, 1972.

356. Chong GC, Beahrs OH, Chen MLC, et al: Management of parotid gland tumors in infants and children. Mayo Clin Proc 50:279, 1975.

357. Canacho AE, Goodman ML, Eavey RD: Pathologic correlation of the unknown solid parotid mass in children. Otolaryngol Head Neck Surg 101:566, 1989.

358. Orvidas LJ, Kasperbauer JL, Lewis JE, et al: Pediatric parotid masses. Arch Otolaryngol Head Neck 126:177, 2000.

359. Seifert G, Sobin LH: The World Health Organization's histologic classification of salivary gland tumors. Cancer 70:379, 1992.

360. Luna MA: Salivary glands. In Pilch BZ (ed): Head and Neck Surgical Pathology. Philadelphia, Lippincott Williams & Wilkins, 2001, pp 284–349.

361. Friedman M, Levin B, Grybauskas V, et al: Malignant tumors of the major salivary glands. Otolaryngol Clin North Am 19:625, 1986.

362. Colby TV, Dorfman RF: Malignant lymphomas involving the salivary glands. Pathol Annu 14:3071, 1979.

363. Malone B, Baker S: Benign pleomorphic adenomas in children. Ann Otol Rhinol Laryngol 93:210, 1984.

364. Sismanis A, Strong M, Merriam J: Fine needle aspiration biopsy diagnosis of neck masses. Otolaryngol Clin North Am 13:421, 1980.

365. Stewart CJ, MacKenzie K, McGarry GW, et al: Fine-needle aspiration cytology of salivary gland: A review of 341 cases. Diagn Cytopathol 22:139, 2000.

366. Eisenhut CC, King DE, Nelson WA, et al: Fine-needle biopsy of pediatric lesions: A three year study in an outpatient biopsy clinic. Diagn Cytopathol 14:43, 1996.

367. Eneroth C, Hamberger C: Principles of treatment of different types of parotid tumors. Laryngoscope 84:1732, 1974.

368. Head and neck sites. In AJCC Cancer Staging Manual, 5th ed. Philadelphia, Lippincott-Raven, 1997.

369. Conley J, Tinsley P Jr: Treatment and prognosis of mucoepidermoid carcinoma in the pediatric age group. Arch Otolaryngol 111:322, 1985.

370. Medina JE: Neck dissection in the treatment of major salivary glands. Otolaryngol Clin North Am 31:815, 1998.

371. Armstrong JG, Harrison LB, Thaler HT, et al: The indications for elective treatment of the neck in cancer of the major salivary glands. Cancer 69:615, 1992.

372. Frankenthaler RF, Byers RM, Luna MA, et al: Predicting occult lymph node metastasis in parotid cancer. Arch Otolaryngol Head Neck Surg 119:517, 1993.

373. Frankenthaler RA, Luna MA, Lee SS, et al: Prognostic variables in parotid gland cancer. Arch Otolaryngol Head Neck Surg 117:1251, 1991.

374. Callender DL, Frankenthaler RA, Luna MA, et al: Salivary gland neoplasms in children. Arch Otolaryngol Head Neck Surg 118:472, 1992.

375. Tran L, Sadeghi A, Hanson D, et al: Major salivary gland tumors: Treatment results and prognostic factors. Laryngoscope 96:1139, 1986.

376. Airoldi M, Brando V, Giordano C, et al: Chemotherapy for recurrent salivary gland malignancies: Experience of the ENT department of Turin University. ORL J Otorhinolaryngol Relat Spec 56:105, 1994.

377. Suen J, Johns M: Chemotherapy for salivary gland cancer. Laryngoscope 92:235, 1982.

378. Johns ME, Goldsmith MM: Incidence, diagnosis and classification of salivary gland tumors. Oncology 3:45, 1989.

379. Licetra L, Marchini S, Spinazze S, et al: Cisplatin in advanced salivary gland carcinoma: A Phase II study of 25 patients. Cancer 68:1874, 1991.

380. Sessions RB, Lehane DE, Smith RJ, et al: Intra-arterial cisplatin treatment of adenoid cystic carcinoma. Arch Otolaryngol 108:221, 1982.

381. Daou R, Schloss M: Childhood rhabdomyosarcoma of the head and neck: Two case reports on salivary glandular and paraglandular involvement. J Otolaryngol 11:52, 1982.

382. Levine S, Postic W: Acinic cell carcinoma of the parotid gland in children. Int J Pediatr Otorhinolaryngol 11:281, 1986.

383. Hicks MJ, El-Naggar AK, Byers RB, et al: Prognostic factors in mucoepidermoid carcinomas of major salivary glands: A clinicopathologic and flow cytometric study. Oral Oncol Eur J Cancer 30B:329, 1994.

384. Fernandez C, Cangir A, Samaan N, et al: Nasopharyngeal carcinoma in children. Cancer 37:2787, 1976.

385. Fearon B, Forte V, Brama I: Malignant nasopharyngeal tumors in children. Laryngoscope 100:470, 1990.
386. Bleichner JC, Ragsdale B, Hartmann DP, et al: Nasopharyngeal malignancies in children. Ear Nose Throat J 66:148, 1987.
387. Tom LWC, Anderson GJ, Womer RB, et al: Nasopharyngeal malignancies in children. Laryngoscope 102:509, 1992.
388. Deutsh M, Mercado R, Parsons JA: Cancer of the nasopharynx in children. Cancer 41:1128, 1978.
389. Green MH, Fraumeni JF, Hoover R: Nasopharyngeal cancer among young people in the United States: Racial variations by cell type. J Natl Cancer Inst 58:1267, 1977.
390. Easton JM, Levine PH, Hyams VJ: Nasopharyngeal carcinoma in the United States: A pathologic study of 177 US and 30 foreign cases. Arch Otolaryngol 106:88, 1980.
391. Ingersoll L, Woo SY, Donaldson S, et al: Nasopharyngeal carcinoma in the young: A combined M.D. Anderson and Stanford experience. Oncol Biol Phys 19:881, 1990.
392. Singh W: Nasopharyngeal carcinoma in Caucasian children: a 25 year study. J Laryngol Otol 101:1248, 1987.
393. Snow J: Carcinoma of the nasopharynx in children. Ann Otol 84:817, 1974.
394. Shanmugaratnam K, Sobin LH: International Histologic Classification of Tumours, No. 19: Histological Typing of Upper Respiratory Tract Tumours. Geneva, World Health Organization, 1978.
395. Pilch BZ: The nasopharynx and Waldeyer's ring. In Pilch BZ (ed): Head and Neck Surgical Pathology. Philadelphia, Lippincott Williams & Wilkins, 2001, pp 157–194.
396. Pearson G, Weiland L, Neel H, et al: Application of Epstein-Barr (EBV) serology to the diagnosis of North American nasopharyngeal carcinoma. Cancer 51:260, 1983.
397. Halprin J, Scott AL, Jacobson LJ, et al: Enzyme-linked immunosorbent assay of antibodies to Epstein-Barr virus nuclear and early antigens in patients with infectious mononucleosis and nasopharyngeal carcinoma. Ann Intern Med 104:331, 1986.
398. Naegele RF, Champion J, Murphy S, et al: Nasopharyngeal carcinoma in American children: Epstein-Barr virus–specific antibody titer and prognosis. Int J Cancer 29:209, 1982.
399. Tatsumi-Tamori A, Yoshizaki T, Miwa T, et al: Clinical evaluation of staging system for nasopharyngeal carcinoma: Comparison of fourth and fifth editions of UICC TNM classification. Ann Otol Rhinol Laryngol 109:1125, 2000.
400. Jenkin RD, Anderson JR, Jereb B, et al: Nasopharyngeal carcinoma— a retrospective review of patients less than thirty years of age: A report from Children's Cancer Study Group. Cancer 47:360, 1981.
401. Al-sarraf M, LeBlanc M, Giri PG, et al: Chemoradiotherapy versus radiotherapy in patients with advanced nasopharyngeal cancer: Phase III randomized intergroup study 0099. J Clin Oncol 16:1310, 1998.
402. Kim TH, McLaren N, Alvarado CS, et al: Adjuvant chemotherapy for advanced nasopharyngeal carcinoma in childhood. Cancer 63:1922, 1989.
403. Wei WI: Nasopharyngeal cancer: Current status of management: A New York Head and Neck Society lecture. Arch Otolaryngol Head Neck 127:766, 2001.
404. Makin GWJ, Eden OB, Lashford LS, et al: Leptomeningeal melanoma in childhood. Cancer 86:878, 1999.
405. Boddie A Jr, Smith J Jr, McBride C: Malignant melanoma in children and young adults: Effect of diagnostic criteria on staging and end results. South Med J 71:1074, 1978.
406. Fisher SR, Reintgen DS, Seigler HF: Juvenile malignant melanoma of the head and neck. Laryngoscope 98:184, 1988.
407. Greene MH, Clark WH Jr, Tucker MA, et al: Acquired precursors of cutaneous malignant melanoma: The familial dysplastic nevus syndrome. N Engl J Med 10:91, 1985.
408. Greene MH, Clark WH Jr, Tucker MA, et al: High risk of malignant melanoma in melanoma-prone families with dysplastic nevi. Ann Intern Med 102:458, 1985.
409. Kopf AW, Hellman LJ, Rogers GS, et al: Familial malignant melanoma. JAMA 256:1915, 1986.
410. Sasson M, Mallory SB: Malignant primary skin tumors in children. Curr Opin Pediatr 8:372, 1996.
411. Smith J Jr: Problems related to pigmented nevi and melanoma in children. Cancer Bull 24:22, 1972.
412. Skov-Jensen T, Hastrup J, Lambrethsen S: Malignant melanoma in children. Cancer 19:620–626, 1966.
413. Sutow W, Montague E: Pediatric tumors. In MacComb W, Fletcher G (eds): Cancer of the Head and Neck. Baltimore, Williams & Wilkins, 1967.
414. Shannon E, Samuel Y, Adler A, et al: Malignant melanoma of the head and neck in children: Review of the literature and report of a case. Arch Otolaryngol 102:244, 1976.
415. Rao BN, Hayes FA, Prat CB, et al: Malignant melanoma in children: Its management and prognosis. J Pediatr Surg 25:198, 1990.
416. Clark WH Jr, Ainsworth AM, Bernandino EA, et al: The developmental biology of primary human malignant melanomas. Semin Oncol 2:83, 1975.
417. Koh HK: Cutaneous melanoma. N Engl J Med 325:171, 1991.
418. Veronesi U, Cascinelli N, Adamus J, et al: Thin stage I primary cutaneous malignant melanoma. Comparison of excision with margins of 1 or 3 cm. N Engl J Med 318:1159, 1988.
419. Ho VC, Sober AJ: Therapy for cutaneous melanoma: An update. J Am Acad Dermatol 22:159, 1990.
420. Mahre E: Malignant melanoma in children. Arch Pathol Microbiol Scand 59:184, 1963.
421. Byers R, Smith J Jr, Russell N, et al: Malignant melanoma of the external ear. Am J Surg 140:518, 1980.
422. Balch CM, Cascinelli N, Milton GW, et al: Elective lymph node dissection pros and cons. In Balch CM, Milton GW (eds): Cutaneous Melanoma: Clinical Management and Clinical Results Worldwide. Philadelphia, JB Lippincott, 1985.
423. Balch CC, Soong SJ, Bartolucci AA, et al: Efficacy of an elective regional lymph node dissection of 1 to 4 mm thick melanomas for patients 60 years of age or younger. Ann Surg 224:255, 1996.
424. Kirkwood JM, Strawderman MH, Ernstoff MS, et al: Interferon alfa-2b adjuvant therapy of high-risk resected cutaneous melanoma: The Eastern Cooperative Oncology Group Trial EST 1684. J Clin Oncol 14:7, 1996.
425. Ceballos PI, Ruiz-Maldonadeo R, Mihm MC: Melanoma in children. N Engl J Med 332:656, 1995.
426. Philip PA, Flaherty LE: Biochemotherapy for melanoma. Curr Oncol Rep 2:314, 2000.
427. Sileni C, Nortilli R, Aversa SM, et al: Phase II randomized study of dacarbazine, carmustine, cisplatin and tamoxifen versus dacarbazine alone in advanced melanoma patients. Melanoma Res 11:189, 2001.
428. Pratt CB, Palmer MK, Thatcher M, et al: Malignant melanoma in children and adolescents. Cancer 47:392, 1981.
429. Duncan LM: Dermatopathology of the head and neck. In Pilch BZ (ed): Head and Neck Surgical Pathology. Philadelphia, Lippincott Williams & Wilkins, 2001, pp 534–617.
430. Clevens RA, Johnson TM, Wolf GT: Management of head and neck melanoma. In Cummings CW, Fredrickson JM, Harker LA, et al (eds): Otolaryngology—Head and Neck Surgery. St. Louis, Mosby, 1998.
431. Sasson M, Mallory SB: Malignant primary skin tumors in children. Curr Opin Pediatr 8:372, 1996.
432. Novick M, Gard DA, Hardy SB, et al: Burn scar carcinoma: A report and analysis of 46 cases. J Trauma 17:809, 1977.
433. McQuirt WF, Little JP: Laryngeal cancer in children and adolescents. Otolaryngol Clin North Am 30:207, 1997.
434. Clark R, Rosen I, Laperriere N: Malignant tumors of the head and neck in a young population. Am J Surg 144:459, 1982.
435. Lee YW, Gisser SD: Squamous cell carcinoma of the tongue in a 9 year renal transplant survivor: A case report with a discussion of the risk of development of epithelial carcinoma in renal transplant survivors. Cancer 41:1, 1978.
436. Bradford CR, Hoffman HT, Wolf GT, et al: Squamous carcinoma of the head and neck in organ transplant recipients: Possible role of oncogenic viruses. Laryngoscope 100:190, 1990.
437. Morehead JM, Parsons DS, McMahon DP: Squamous cell carcinoma of the tongue occurring as a subsequent malignancy in a 12-year-old acute leukemia survivor. Int J Pediatr Otorhinolaryngol 26:89, 1993.
438. Kennedy AW, Hart WR: Multiple squamous-cell carcinoma in Fanconi's anemia. Cancer 50:811, 1982.
439. Bhatia P, Gupta O, Samant H, et al: Juvenile epithelial malignancy of head and neck. J Otolaryngol 6:208, 1977.
440. Comstock J, Hansen RC, Korc A: Basal cell carcinoma in a 12-year-old boy. Pediatrics 86:460, 1990.
441. Lesueur BW, Silvis NG, Hansen RC: Basal cell carcinoma in children. Arch Dermatol 136:370, 2000.

442. Gorlin R, Goltz R: Multiple nevoid basal-cell epithelioma, jaw cysts and bifid rib: A syndrome. N Engl J Med 292:908, 1960.

443. Southwick GJ, Schwartz RA: The basal-cell nevus syndrome: Disasters occurring among a series of 36 patients. Cancer 44:2294, 1979.

444. Holt G, Holt J, Weaver R: Dermoids and teratomas of the head and neck. Ear Nose Throat J 58:520, 1979.

445. Grosfeld J, Billmire D: Teratomas in infancy and childhood. Curr Probl Cancer 9:1, 1985.

446. Azizkhan RG, Haase GM, Applebaum H, et al: Diagnosis, management, and outcome of cervicofacial teratomas in neonates: A children's cancer group study. Pediatr Surg 30:312, 1995.

447. Lack EE: Extragonadal germ cell tumors of the head and neck region: Review of 16 cases. Hum Pathol 16:56, 1985.

448. Gnepp D: Teratoid neoplasms of the head and neck. In Barnes L (ed): Surgical Pathology of the Head and Neck. New York, Marcel Dekker, 1985.

449. Stephenson JA, Mayland DM, Kun LE, et al: Malignant germ cell tumors of the head and neck in childhood. Laryngoscope 99: 732, 1989.

450. Gonzalez-Crussi F: Extragonadal teratomas. In Atlas of Tumor Pathology (series 2, fascicle 18). Washington, DC, Armed Forces Institute of Pathology, 1982.

451. Ohlms LA, McGill T, Healy GB: Malignant laryngeal tumors in children: A 15-year experience with four patients. Ann Otol Rhinol Laryngol 103:686, 1994.

452. Hawkins D, Park R: Teratoma of the pharynx and neck. Ann Otol Rhinol Laryngol 81:848, 1972.

453. Marina N, Cushing B, Giller R, et al: Complete surgical excision in effective treatment for children with immature teratomas with or without malignant elements: A pediatric oncology group/children's cancer group intergroup study. J Clin Oncol 17:2137, 1999.

454. Brodeur GM, Howarth CB, Pratt CB, et al: Malignant germ cell tumors in 57 children and adolescents. Cancer 48:1890, 1981.

455. Touran T, Applebaum H, Frost DB, et al: Congenital metastatic cervical teratoma: Diagnostic and management considerations. J Pediatr Surg 24:21, 1989.

456. April MM, Ward RF, Garelick JM: Diagnosis, management, and follow-up of congenital head and neck teratomas. Laryngoscope 108:1398, 1998.

CHAPTER 25

Cancer of the Head and Neck in HIV-Infected Patients

Bhuvanesh Singh

Ashutosh Kacker

◧ INTRODUCTION

The course of human history has been molded by many infectious diseases, including the "black death" of the bubonic plague and the "great white death" of tuberculosis. Currently, acquired immunodeficiency syndrome (AIDS) is exerting a profound influence internationally on social, political, and medical institutions.

The origin of AIDS has been traced to Africa, where its existence was demonstrated in stored sera from the 1950s.[1] However, it was not until 1981 that AIDS was reported in the medical literature as a distinct clinical entity.[2, 3] The AIDS epidemic evolved in the United States; the development of heterosexual and blood-borne transmission implied an infectious agent as the cause. Subsequently, new risk groups for AIDS emerged, included Haitians, intravenous drug abusers (IVDAs), blood transfusion recipients, sexual partners of infected persons, and children born to infected mothers. By 1982, evidence was clear that the sexual route of transmission was predominant.[4]

In 1983, French and American investigators identified a retrovirus as the cause of AIDS.[5, 6] Montagnier from the Pasteur Institute named this virus lymphadenopathy-associated virus (LAV); Gallo at the National Institutes of Health (NIH) named it human T-cell lymphotropic virus type III (HTLV-III). After much debate, the neutral term *human immunodeficiency virus (HIV)* was agreed on. As further characterization of this virus emerged, the development of screening tests resulted, including the enzyme-linked immunosorbent assay (ELISA) and the Western blot (WB) analysis, the combination of which yields a 99% sensitivity for the detection of HIV infection. Screening for HIV was instituted in 1985 as a routine practice in blood banks.[7] This led to a reduction in transmission of the virus through blood and blood products to about 1 in 153,000 transfusions.[8] In addition, although no cure or universally effective protective measures exist, the use of condoms and other modifications of sexual behaviors have slowly changed the spectrum of those infected by HIV.

AIDS has brought a myriad of challenges to the scientific and medical communities. Aside from the numerous scientific issues that remain unresolved, the social and economic difficulties of the epidemic, on a worldwide basis, have become one of the greatest challenges of modern times. More than 40 million people are currently infected with HIV. In this worldwide setting of economic stress and human suffering, the scientific community has made remarkable strides in our ability to understand the biologic nature of HIV and tailor the treatment.[8, 9] The treatment of HIV-infected patients has changed remarkably since early 1996, when more potent agents became available and were used in combination therapy. The development and use of highly active antiretroviral therapy (HAART) has been associated with a significant increase in survival rates and a decrease in opportunistic infections.[10] HAART involves the use of two or more antiretroviral agents from the following three groups: (1) nucleoside reverse transcriptase inhibitors (e.g., AZT [zidovudine]), (2) non-nucleoside reverse transcriptase inhibitors (e.g., efavirenz), and (3) protease inhibitors (e.g., nelfinavir).

Aside from opportunistic infections, the immune dysregulation caused by HIV is associated with a significant increase in the development of various malignant diseases. In HIV-positive patients, the cancers currently considered AIDS-defining in the United States include Kaposi's sarcoma (KS), lymphoma, and cervical cancer. Most of the malignancies seen in HIV-positive individuals have been associated with an underlying viral infection, such as human herpesvirus-8, Epstein-Barr virus, or human papilloma virus. The interplay of these viral infections with the abnormal immunologic and cytokine milieus induced by HIV has allowed us to understand some of the mechanisms of malignant disease in these individuals.

Furthermore, the prolonged survival of HIV-infected patients after use of HAART has changed the natural history of some of these malignancies. The introduction of highly active antiretroviral therapy has had a dramatic impact on the morbidity and mortality of individuals living with HIV. HAART has reduced the incidences of several AIDS-defining malignancies. The incidences of KS and primary central nervous system lymphoma (PCNSL) have dropped precipitously since the introduction of HAART. Systemic non-Hodgkin's lymphoma (NHL) appears to be declining in incidence as well, but to a lesser degree than KS and PCNSL. However, the incidence of invasive cervical carcinoma has not significantly changed in the HAART era. The impact of HAART on the epidemiology of other HIV-associated malignancies, including Hodgkin's disease and anal carcinoma, remains unclear. However, prolonged survival has also provided an opportunity for the development of additional cancers, which appear to be statistically increased in HIV-infected individuals.[10–13]

NATURAL COURSE OF HIV INFECTION

To understand AIDS and the processes that accompany it, an understanding of the natural course of HIV infection is necessary. Two forms of HIV virus have been identified. HIV-1 occurs predominantly in central Africa, Europe, and the United States, and HIV-2 occurs in West Africa.[14] Although these two viruses differ in the primary nucleotide sequence by about 55%, they have the same cellular interactions and can produce similar clinical manifestations.[14] In addition, there is sufficient homology between these two types to allow the detection of 90% of HIV-2–infected patients with the use of screening tests for HIV-1.

Infection with HIV occurs through person-to-person transmission of infectious viral particles. Although infectious viral particles have been reported in tears, middle ear secretions, saliva, and urine, they appear to be present in sufficient quantities to transmit infection only in semen, vaginal secretions, serum, and cerebrospinal fluid (CSF). Of these, CSF contains the highest concentration of infectious particles (10 to 1000/mL), followed by serum (10 to 50/mL) and semen (10 to 50/mL).[15–17]

Regardless of the subtype of the virus or mode of transmission, infection by HIV begins with the attachment of the virus to the membrane of the host cell. This attachment is facilitated by the presence of a receptor on the cell membrane (mainly CD4), for which the virus has a tropism.[18] The CD4 receptor is abundant on the membrane of T-helper lymphocytes, but it is also present in other cell types, including lymphocytes, macrophages, promyelocytes, cutaneous Langerhans cells, brain cells, and bowel epithelium.

Once attached, the virus releases into the cytoplasm its RNA genome, which contains reverse transcriptase, leaving its capsid behind. Reverse transcriptase forms circular DNA, which enters the nucleus and becomes incorporated into the host cell genome. Subsequently the virus may remain latent for long periods, producing the proteins necessary for viral replication only when activated.[19]

The natural course of HIV infection is described in the Centers for Disease Control and Prevention (CDC) staging system, in which AIDS is the endpoint of a longstanding infection (Table 25–1). Progression of HIV infection is influenced by a variety of factors, including age and preinfection medical status, and is generally correlated with a decline in CD4 lymphocytes. Stage I patients display an acute retroviral syndrome, a brief mononucleosis-like illness with or without central nervous system (CNS) involvement, which typically lasts 1 to 2 weeks. CD4 counts are normal (500 to 1000+/mm³) in these persons. An immune response toward HIV is activated during this stage, leading to seroconversion. Immunofluorescent assay for immunoglobulin M (IgM) can be detected within 2 weeks of onset of the acute viral illness. ELISA and WB analysis detect antibodies 6 to 12 weeks after resolution of the illness.[20, 21]

TABLE 25–1 Centers for Disease Control and Prevention Classification of HIV Infection

Stage	Manifestation	CD4 counts
Stage I	Acute infection—mononucleosis-like syndrome	Normal
Stage II	Asymptomatic infection	500+/mm³
Stage III	Persistent generalized lymphadenopathy	100–500/mm³
Stage IV	Other diseases Subgroup A—constitutional disease Subgroup B—neurologic disease Subgroup C—secondary infectious diseases Subgroup D—secondary cancers Subgroup E—other conditions	<200/mm³

Following the acute illness, the virus enters a latent period, which can last longer than 10 years. Patients in this group are asymptomatic with regard to HIV infection and belong to stage II in the CDC classification. However, these patients may display clinical and laboratory abnormalities, such as immune thrombocytopenic purpura and declining CD4 counts. When persistent generalized lymphadenopathy develops, patients are classified as being in stage III. Stages II and III are usually associated with CD4 counts of 500/mm³ or greater. However, as chronic or recurrent infections begin to develop in these patients, the CD4 count usually declines to the 100 to 500/mm³ range. Ultimately, full-blown AIDS or CDC stage IV disease develops and is defined by the occurrence of any of the criteria established by the CDC. It is in this stage that CD4 counts fall to below 200/mm³ and patients are predisposed to developing many opportunistic processes.

Although several factors have been investigated, the only consistent predictor of survival is the CD4 count. Its decline coincides with progression along the CDC stages, as well as the development of opportunistic processes. The time required for the decline does not appear to be as important as the CD4 count itself. Manifestations of HIV infection become prominent and clinical deterioration becomes obvious with CD4 counts below 150/mm³. Death is common among patients with CD4 counts below 50/mm³ and is usually related to infectious processes.

Since the advent of combined antiretroviral therapy in 1996, substantial decreases in HIV-related morbidity and mortality have been observed in the United States and other developed countries. To assess the effects on overall survival of specific AIDS-defining illnesses, survival among persons with AIDS in New York City before and after the introduction of combination therapy was investigated. Overall cumulative survival at 24 months increased from 43% among persons with AIDS diagnosed during 1990 to 1995, to 76% for those diagnosed from 1996 to 1998.[22]

MALIGNANCIES IN HIV INFECTION

The presence of HIV infection is related to an increase in the incidences of many benign and malignant neoplasms. Among the reasons for this increase are immune dysfunction and viral oncogenicity. Antineoplastic immunosurveillance

TABLE 25-2 Alterations in Head and Neck Malignancies in HIV-Infected Patients

Process	Age	Incidence	Location	Changes	Treatment
KS	Younger	Increased°	Cutaneous/oral	More aggressive; increased frequency	Depending on site, high recurrence
NHL	Younger	Increased	CNS/lymphatics	More aggressive; increased frequency	Modified or supplemented chemotherapy
HL	Between peaks	Unchanged	Lymphatics	Increased stage III/IV	Modified or supplemented chemotherapy
SCC	<45 yr	Increased in young	Larynx/oral cavity	Increased T3/T4; increased stage III/IV	Surgery/radiation therapy
Cutaneous SCC	Younger	Increased	More aggressive		Wide local excision or radiation therapy
Cutaneous BCC	Younger	Decreased	Increased trunk involvement		All modalities equally effective
Malignant melanoma		Decreased		Majority with Clark's level V disease	Surgery
Plasmacytoma			Gingiva/scalp	More aggressive	Modified or supplemented chemotherapy

CNS, central nervous system; KS, Kaposi's sarcoma; NHL, non-Hodgkin's lymphoma; HL, Hodgkin's lymphoma; SCC, squamous cell carcinoma; BCC, basal cell carcinoma.
°Decreased with the advent of highly active antiretroviral treatment (HAART).

is abnormal in HIV-infected patients. HIV not only invades T-lymphocytes of the CD4 type but also infects macrophages and B-lymphocyte elements. In addition, although natural killer cells have not been shown to be directly infected by HIV, their function is hampered in HIV-infected patients.[23,24] This leads to a profound immunodeficiency that affects both cellular and humoral immunity, resulting in increased carcinogenesis.

The higher incidence of neoplasms in HIV-infected patients cannot be explained by immunosuppression alone. For example, KS is 300 times more common among HIV-infected patients than among other immunocompromised groups. Carcinogenesis in the presence of HIV infection is further promoted by the disruption of the normal balance of cell proliferation and differentiation caused by the abnormal elaboration of growth factors and chronic antigenic stimulation, especially by viruses known to be oncogenic. In addition, HIV belongs to the lentivirus subfamily of retroviruses, which have been directly implicated as carcinogens. Although this ability has yet to be proved, some studies have implied that HIV is a direct oncogenic agent. Accordingly, the increase in the rate of neoplasia seen in HIV-infected patients is greater than that seen in other immunocompromised populations.

TABLE 25-3 Cancers in HIV-Infected Patients

AIDS defining (Stage IV, Subgroup D)
Kaposi's sarcoma
Squamous cell carcinoma
Non-Hodgkin's lymphoma
Carcinoma of cervix

Non–AIDS defining
Skin neoplasms
  Squamous cell carcinoma
  Basal cell carcinoma
  Malignant melanoma
Lymphoid neoplasms
  Hodgkin's lymphoma
  Plasma cell malignancies

HIV infection not only alters the incidence of many neoplastic processes but also affects the site of disease, clinical course, and management (Table 25-2). The malignancies that show the greatest increase in incidence, namely KS, high-grade NHL, and cervical carcinoma, are considered AIDS-defining neoplasms that account for more than 95% of neoplasms in HIV-infected patients. Other neoplastic processes are markedly changed by HIV infection but do not show sufficient prevalence to be considered AIDS-defining by the CDC. However, as the epidemic evolves, additional neoplasms will inevitably be added to the CDC's definition of AIDS (Table 25-3).

Many AIDS-associated neoplastic processes have manifestations in the head and neck region. The most common benign neoplasms occurring in the head and neck region include persistent generalized lymphadenopathy, benign lymphoepithelial lesions of the parotid, and hyperplasia of Waldeyer's ring structures. KS and NHL are the most common malignant neoplasms. Other malignant processes occurring in this region include (1) cutaneous malignancies, such as squamous cell carcinoma (SCC), basal cell carcinoma, and malignant melanoma, and (2) lymphatic malignancies, such as Hodgkin's lymphoma and plasma cell tumors. The classic head and neck manifestations, course, and management of these neoplasms have been altered by the presence of HIV infection. An understanding of these changes is a prerequisite if the clinician is to provide adequate treatment (Table 25-4).

MANAGEMENT ISSUES IN HIV-INFECTED PATIENTS

The management of malignancies in HIV-infected patients is complicated by the presence of many confounding factors. First, many physicians are reluctant to treat HIV-infected patients. Second, there is the risk for transmission of infection to the caregiver. Third, many conditions mimic malignancy,

TABLE 25-4 Estimated Risk of Various Malignancies Among Persons With AIDS Compared With the General U.S. Population

Strongly related to immune deficiency	
Kaposi's sarcoma	73,000
Homosexual men	106,000
Nonhomosexual men	13,000
Women	Unknown
Leiomyosarcoma	10,000
Non-Hodgkin's lymphoma	
Children	1,203
Adults	165
Hodgkin's disease	7.6
Possibly related to immune deficiency	
Multiple myeloma	4.5
Seminoma	2.9
Brain cancer	3.5
Anal cancer	31.7
Squamous cell conjunctival cancer	13.0
Lip cancer	4.1
Weak or no relationship to immune deficiency	
Cervical cancer, invasive	2.9
Nonseminoma male germ cell	1.5
Lung adenocarcinoma	2.5
Lung nonadenocarcinoma	1.2
Melanoma	1.1
Lymphoid leukemia	1.4
Myeloid leukemia	3.0
Insufficient data	
Nonmelanoma skin cancer	5.4
Hepatocellular carcinoma	Undefined
Penile cancer	Undefined
Vaginal and vulvar cancer	Undefined

From Goedert JJ: The epidemiology of acquired immunodeficiency syndrome malignancies. Semin Oncol 27:390–401, 2000.

making early diagnosis and treatment difficult. Finally, the standard protocols used in the treatment of cancers are not transferable to HIV-infected patients. Moreover, many treatment modalities are accompanied by the development of adverse effects and complications in HIV-infected patients and therefore must be modified.

The development of cancer is generally is associated with the stigma of terminal illness; although this stigma is slowly being overcome with the advent and perfection of new therapies, it is intensified in patients with HIV infection. This stigma is so intense and ingrained that even physicians tend to view the development of cancer in HIV-infected patients as a terminal event. It must be kept in mind that some patients with HIV infection survive for longer than 10 years, outliving the natural course of cancer in many cases. Accordingly, treatment, including surgery, should be undertaken in all HIV-infected patients, so long as the treatment does not hasten demise.

Universal Precautions

The risk for the transmission of HIV infection to the caregiver has also been a factor that limits the care of HIV-infected patients. However, this risk can be minimized with the use of universal precautions and should not influence therapeutic decisions. Thirty-seven confirmed cases and 145 suspected cases of HIV transmission to health care providers have been reported in the literature.[25–28] Of these, 84% were associated with parenteral exposure to contaminated blood or bodily fluids, mainly by needlestick injury. It is important to note that seroconversion after needlestick injury is rare. In a review of 14 studies on needlestick injury to health care workers, 6 of 2042 events of HIV exposure (0.3%) were associated with seroconversion, as compared with hepatitis B virus, which is transmitted in 9% to 30% of cases of exposure.[25, 29, 30] Furthermore, the overall risk of transmission is related to the object associated with the exposure, as well as to the depth and amount of infected matter injected. Hollow needles filled with infected fluids are the most contagious source of exposure, with injury by suture needles and scalpels carrying a much lower risk.

A great deal of attention has been given to the risk of exposure for surgeons. However, that risk may have been overstated. The relative incidence of exposure for surgeons has been reported as approximately 2.5 per 100 procedures, based on observation studies. At this rate, even with a 30% prevalence of HIV infection in population undergoing surgery, a surgeon performing 500 procedures per year has a 0.001% yearly risk for acquiring HIV infection (given a 0.3% rate of transmission).[31] This risk can be further minimized with the use of appropriate precautions.[32]

Guidelines for universal blood and body fluid precautions have been established by the CDC.[33] These guidelines have been mandated by the Occupational Safety and Health Administration (OSHA) and adopted as standard policy for nearly all hospitals in the United States.[34] The most important guidelines include the routine use of gloves and their removal after each contact. Hand washing before and after each contact should also be routine. This helps to reduce the risks of infection and transmission in cases in which the gloves were not an absolute barrier. In addition, masks should be worn, especially when prolonged contact with coughing patients is anticipated (e.g., during endoscopy). Furthermore, gowns should be worn when soiling of clothing is anticipated. Finally, the use of protective eyewear is mandatory in cases where the splashing or aerosolization of body fluids is anticipated.

The proper handling of sharp instruments is key to reducing exposure to HIV for the health care worker. Needles, scalpels, or other sharp instruments should be disposed of immediately after completion of use. In addition, recapping of needles should be avoided because it is responsible for the majority of needlestick injuries. If recapping is absolutely necessary, the sheath should be laid on the table, rather than held in the hand, while the needle is reinserted.

In the operating room, in addition to standard universal precautions, the interactions between the members of the operative team should be modifed. Most important, the passing of sharp instruments should be done with a "no touch" technique, in which the instruments are laid on an instrument pad or Mayo stand for passage between operating team members.[35] In addition, all sharp instruments should be removed from the field when not in use. Where possible, surgical techniques should be modified to exclude the use of sharp instruments.

The use of double gloving, water-impermeable boots and gowns, and face shields may further reduce risk of exposure.

In addition, changing gloves during surgical procedures lasting longer than 4 hours may be of benefit because puncture rates rise to 40% for these procedures. Finally, the most important protective measures are good communication among operating room personnel and meticulous surgical technique to minimize accidental exposures.

Problems With the Treatment of AIDS-Associated Neoplasms

The treatment of HIV-related malignancies is complicated by many other factors. These include adverse effects associated with treatment, difficulties in wound healing, and the risks of exposure for operating room personnel. Moreover, the benefit of aggressive therapy for neoplasia in patients with advanced forms of AIDS is in question because in most cases, mortality is probably not dependent on tumor-related factors. More important, aggressive therapy may lead to an earlier demise in patients with AIDS. Accordingly, the planning of therapeutic intervention, in addition to standard concerns, should take into account HIV-related factors. Finally, any antineoplastic therapy of HIV-infected patients should be supplemented with antiviral and anti-*Pneumocystis* therapy.

Surgical therapy may also present problems. These patients have profound wound-healing impairments at many different levels. A diminished ability to control bacterial infection in surgical wounds is seen in HIV-infected patients. Studies on healing of anal surgical wounds in HIV-infected patients show significant delays in healing in stage IV patients.[36] Furthermore, experimental studies show that depletion of T-cells causes decreased collagen deposition and wound-breaking strength because of its effect on fibroblast activity.[37]

Nutritional status is also an important factor in wound healing, as well as in cancer survival in general.[38, 39] Nutritional deficiencies in AIDS have been recognized since the 1970s in Africa as "slim disease."[40] These deficiencies are worsened by the presence of diarrhea, wasting syndrome, multiple infections, and the neoplastic processes seen in HIV-infected patients. Proteins, micronutrients (including zinc), and vitamins necessary for wound healing are commonly depleted in HIV-infected patients.[41–43] Accordingly, nutritional support should be started preoperatively and continued during the postoperative period in this patient population.

Nonsurgical antineoplastic interventions are also adversely affected by the presence of HIV infection. Radiation therapy to mucosal sites has been associated with a severe mucositis that causes pain, ulceration, and occasionally severe airway-compromising edema. Using antifungal and antiherpetic medications and decreasing the fractions and total amount of radiation delivered limit the development of mucositis.

Several studies show that standard-dose chemotherapy decreases overall survival in HIV patients through the intensified immunosuppression associated with the use of many chemotherapeutic agents. Accordingly, these therapeutic modalities must be modified in patients with HIV infection. These modifications may include dose reductions, shorter durations of therapy, and the use of bone marrow stimulators.

Mimics of Malignancy

Infection with the HIV virus is associated with the development of many benign and infectious processes that can mimic malignancies. Lymphoid tissue hyperplasia in Waldeyer's ring, chronic ulcerations and hairy leukoplakia in the oral cavity, cystic lesions of the parotid gland, and persistent cervical lymphadenopathy are a few examples. An understanding of these processes may facilitate differentiation from malignant disease (Table 25–5).

Persistent Generalized Lymphadenopathy

Persistent generalized lymphadenopathy (PGL) is defined as the presence of unexplained lymphadenopathy in two or more extrainguinal sites for longer than 3 months. The presence of PGL was reported as early as 1979 in homosexual patients; it now occurs in as many as 70% of HIV-infected patients.[44, 45] PGL usually develops early in the course of HIV infection. Its presence defines CDC stage III disease, but its prognostic significance has been questioned.[46] Some authors have shown an increased rate—a 29% incidence in 5 years—of progression to AIDS in patients with PGL. This incidence is increased to 50% in the presence of other infections.[47, 48]

Clinically, the lymph nodes in patients with PGL are soft and nontender, ranging from 1 to 5 cm.[49] Axillary lymph nodes are the most common site of involvement (reported in 99% of cases). The head and neck region is the second most common site of extrainguinal involvement. The most frequent head and neck site is the posterior cervical region (86% of patients). Other sites for PGL include preauricular (51%), postauricular (47%), submandibular (37%), submental (36%), supraclavicular (26%), and jugular lymph nodes (17%).[44, 52] This nodal distribution is different from that seen in both NHL and SCC (Table 25–6).

It is important that the different pathologic forms of this process be recognized to allow its differentiation from malignant disease. First, a follicular hyperplasia involving the nodal cortex, paracortex, and medullary structures is seen, along with an increase in the number and size of lymphatic follicles.[44, 45, 50] Progression to a mixed follicular hyperplasia and involution is the next stage. It is followed by a stage of lymphocyte depletion. The final stage is that of follicular involution.[50]

TABLE 25-5 Mimics of Malignancy in HIV-Infected Patients

Oral cavity
Oral hairy leukoplakia
Chronic ulcerations: Cytomegalovirus, herpesvirus, aphthae

Pharynx
Waldeyer's ring hyperplasia
Chronic ulcerations: Cytomegalovirus, herpesvirus, aphthae

Larynx
Human papilloma virus–associated lesions
Infectious processes: Tuberculosis, fungi

Neck
Progressive generalized lymphadenopathy
Tuberculosis

TABLE 25-6 Characterization of Lymphatic Disease in HIV-Infected Patients

	Progressive Generalized Lymphadenopathy	Isolated Cervical Tuberculosis	Non-Hodgkin's Lymphoma	Kaposis's Sarcoma	Squamous Cell Carcinoma
No. of lesions	Multiple	Multiple	Multiple	Usually single	Usually localized
Primary site	Posterior triangle	Anterior traingle	Jugular	Anterior triangle	Jugular
No. of lymphatic regions	Multiple	Single	Varied	Single	Localizing
Growth	Indolent	Rapid	Rapid	Indolent	Rapid
Associated symptoms	Rare	Frequent	Occasional	Rare	Rare
Consistency	Soft	Varied	Soft	Varied	Firm
Concurrent non-lymphatic disease	Rare	Rare	Common	Common	Usual

The need and indications for cervical lymph node biopsy are debatable. Most authors agree that nodes that are localized, asymmetrical, and larger than 3 cm should be biopsied. Acute enlargement, constitutional symptoms, and suspicious laboratory findings are other possible indications for biopsy. Biopsy may serve as a therapeutic tool to allay fears of malignancy when other diagnostic measures remain uncertain.[49, 51, 52] Fine-needle aspiration (FNA) biopsy is excellent for initial evaluation. Open biopsy should be done in cases in which FNA is nondiagnostic.

Multicentric Castleman's Disease

Multicentric Castleman's disease (MCD) is a heterogeneous lymphoproliferative disorder characterized by systemic symptoms, generalized lymphadenopathy, hepatosplenomegaly, proteinuria, and rash. MCD is associated with human herpesvirus-8/KS–associated herpesvirus.[53]

Nasopharyngeal Tissue Enlargement

Waldeyer's ring, especially the nasopharyngeal lymphoid tissue, can be affected by the same pathologic processes that affect PGL (Fig. 25–1).[54] Although involvement of the nasopharynx with PGL is less common than the involvement of other head and neck sites, symptoms are more common because of the spatial limitations.[55] The need for biopsy, because of the increased risks of NHL and SCC, has been debated.[56] Biopsy of nasopharyngeal lesions should be performed when there is evidence of ulceration, rapid growth, and asymmetrical involvement.

Lymphoepithelial Cyst of Parotid Gland

In the presence of HIV infection, lymphoepithelial cysts (LECs) of the parotid are common. Since Ryan and colleagues[57] called attention to the parotid as a possible site of expression for HIV infection in 1985, a review of the literature revealed 102 cases of LEC in HIV-infected patients, accounting for 87% of all parotid lesions in the reviewed series.[58] LEC presents as a unilateral or bilateral parotid enlargement, occasionally causing mild tenderness or Sjögren's syndrome–like symptoms, such as xerostomia.[49] Palpation reveals multinodular lesions, ranging in size from a few millimeters to several centimeters (Fig. 25–2). In contrast, cystic lesions of the parotid gland were rare findings before the onset of the AIDS epidemic. They accounted for

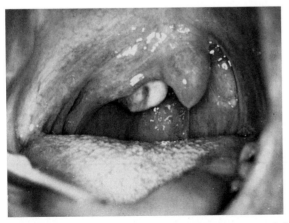

FIGURE 25–1 Nasopharyngeal tissue enlargement causing deflection of the soft palate and projecting below it.

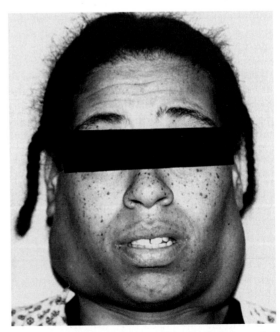

FIGURE 25–2 Bilateral lymphoepithelial cysts of the parotid glands.

5% of all salivary gland tumors, a majority of which were cystic components of neoplasms.[59]

Aggressive surgical management of these lesions is not required because LEC does not affect overall survival in these patients. However, the possibility of malignancy, especially with lymphoma, must be kept in mind.[60] Facial nerve involvement, rapid growth of the lesion, firmness of the lesion, or extension of the lesion to the nerve warrants further examination of the LEC in HIV-infected patients. FNA is an excellent diagnostic method. Cytologic examination of LEC shows colloid fluid that contains heterogeneous lymphoid and epithelial cells. If FNA of a highly suspicious lesion is nondiagnostic, open biopsy should be performed. Biopsy specimens in LEC show the presence of lymphoid hyperplasia, germinal center formation, and lymphoid infiltration of the parotid parenchyma with myoepithelial cyst or island formation.[61]

Computed tomography (CT) or magnetic resonance imaging (MRI) may be helpful. The LEC appears on CT as a multiloculated cystic lesion (Fig. 25–3). MRI shows multiple cysts that have a low signal intensity on T1-weighted images and a high intensity on T2-weighted images.[62] Variations of these parameters, especially in the presence of a solid lesion, are suspicious for malignancy.

Infectious Mimics of Malignancy

Infectious processes may also masquerade as malignancy in the presence of HIV infection. Chronic oral ulcerations can occur as a consequence of herpes simplex virus (HSV) or cytomegalovirus (CMV) infection. Lesions caused by HSV are usually 0.5 to 3.0 cm in diameter, show deep ulceration, are painful, and usually persist for weeks to months.[63] CMV-associated lesions are much less common and have manifestations similar to those of HSV lesions.[64] The most common

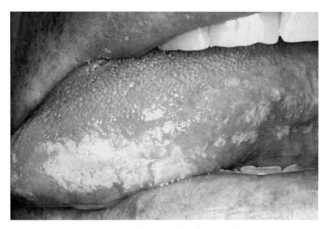

FIGURE 25–4   Oral hairy leukoplakia of the tongue.

sites of involvement are the palate and buccal mucosa. Major aphthous ulcers are also a frequent cause of chronic oral ulcers.[65] Most commonly, they involve the labial and buccal mucosa, tongue, and soft palate. In contrast, oral ulcerations associated with SCC most commonly involve the floor of the mouth.

In addition, exophytic growths may be caused by Epstein-Barr virus (EBV) infection in the form of oral hairy leukoplakia in the mouth and pharynx (Fig. 25–4). Oral hairy leukoplakia occurs in 5% to 25% of HIV-infected patients and presents as whitish, filiform lesions on the lateral aspect of the tongue.[66] It can also involve the floor of the mouth and the buccal and labial regions. Histologically, keratin and parakeratin projections, hyperparakeratosis, and hyperplasia of prickle cells are noted.

Tuberculosis (TB) may also cause ulceration and mass lesions involving the oral cavity, pharynx, and larynx, as well as the neck.[67, 68] Furthermore, isolated forms of TB in the head and neck region are the most difficult to diagnose and differentiate from malignancy. Often, the purified protein derivative (PPD) skin test is negative, further complicating the diagnosis. Neck nodal involvement is by far the most common site for this process, the characteristics of which are detailed in Table 25–6. In addition to cytologic examination, the FNA specimen should be examined for the detection of acid-fast bacilli. In the presence of advanced disease (CDC stage IV), the smear examination is sufficient for diagnosing the presence of TB infection in the majority of cases, thereby allowing for early detection.[69]

Infection with human papilloma virus (HPV) is most common in homosexual patients with HIV infection. This virus can cause papillomas, verruca vulgaris, condyloma acuminatum, and focal epithelial hyperplasia.[70] Involvement may occur anywhere along the upper aerodigestive tract, especially the oral cavity, and often mimics malignancy. These lesions are frequently painful and may cause problems with mastication, swallowing, and phonation. Because many patients with head and neck HPV lesions have concurrent anogenital involvement, HPV infection should be suspected if both regions are involved. However, in selected cases, biopsy may be required to rule out malignancies, such as verrucous carcinoma.

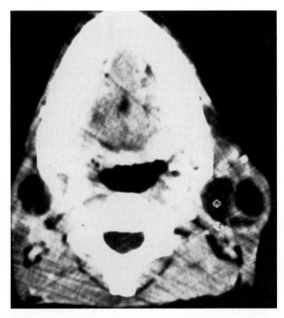

FIGURE 25–3   CT scan showing bilateral lymphoepithelial cysts with multiloculation.

■ MALIGNANT NEOPLASMS

Kaposi's Sarcoma

KS was the first malignancy to be described in association with HIV infection and is the most common malignancy seen in this patient population. At the onset of the AIDS epidemic, KS was seen in 35% to 40% of patients. However, the incidence declined to 14% by 1990.[71] KS has also dropped from being the second most common opportunistic process to the fourth, behind *Pneumocystis carinii* infection, HIV-associated wasting syndrome, and *Candida* infection. However, even though the overall incidence of KS has declined, its numbers are increasing overall, paralleling the increase in the number of HIV-infected patients.

Before AIDS, KS occurred in three distinct epidemiologic forms: (1) classic, (2) African or endemic, and (3) iatrogenically induced. The classic type was first described by Moritz Kaposi in 1872. It occurs predominantly in elderly males of European descent and accounts for 0.06% of cancers overall.[72] The more aggressive African subtype was recognized in the 1950s.[73] It has the same male predominance and usually responds well to therapy. The African subtype was much more common, accounting for 4% to 10% of all cancers in endemic regions. The iatrogenically induced variant was first seen in the 1960s in patients undergoing immunosuppression for organ transplantation.[74] It occurs in 6% of all transplant patients and has a lesser degree of male predominance, along with an excellent response to therapy.[75]

Pathogenesis

Although a great deal has been learned since the start of the AIDS epidemic, the reasons for the development of KS and its true course in HIV-infected patients remain obscure. An aberration of the immune system is a characteristic that seems central to the development of all forms of KS. The importance of immune dysfunction in the development of KS is best illustrated in the iatrogenic form of KS, which shows spontaneous regression of lesions after discontinuation of immunotherapy in as many as 84% of cases.[76]

However, the degree of immunosuppression does not correlate with an increase in the incidence of KS. In addition, and because KS is 300 times more common among HIV-infected than among chemically immunosuppressed patients,[77] many authors have speculated that a second, unidentified agent may act as an initiating or cofactor in the development of KS.[78] KS occurs in 36% of homosexual men with AIDS, 10.4% of Haitians with AIDS, 4.3% of IVDAs with AIDS, 1.9% of transfusion recipients with AIDS, and 1.9% of hemophiliac patients with AIDS.[79] Furthermore, in the United States, 95% of all cases of KS have occurred in homosexual men with AIDS.[80] The higher incidence of KS seen in patients acquiring HIV infection by sexual contact suggests that this agent may be sexually transmitted.[81]

AIDS-KS in the United States occurs predominantly, but not exclusively, among homosexual men. The risk of KS is strongly associated with numerous male homosexual partners. This and other similar findings prompted searches for a sexually transmissible "KS agent," culminating in the discovery in 1994 by Yuan Chang, Patrick Moore, and their colleagues of a previously unknown herpesvirus, called Kaposi's sarcoma–associated herpesvirus or human herpesvirus-8 (HHV-8). HHV-8 has numerous genes capable of deregulating mitosis, interrupting apoptosis (programmed cell death), increasing angiogenesis, and blocking presentation of antigenic epitopes. KS has significantly declined with the advent of HAART from 61 to 20 per 1000 person-years.[10, 11]

Clinical Presentation

KS in AIDS typically presents as a macular discoloration that has a multifocal origin. The lesions are usually red to violaceous but occasionally can be whitish and nonpigmented. AIDS-KS lesions show no defined growth pattern. They may change to nodulopapular lesions, remain static, or show spontaneous regression.[82, 83]

Although KS lesions can occur in almost any area of the body, before the AIDS epidemic they rarely involved the head and neck region.[84, 85] Involvement of this region occurred in only 14% of patients with classic KS, most of whom had disseminated disease. Head and neck involvement was especially rare in both the African and the iatrogenic variants. In AIDS patients, however, the incidence of KS involving this region is reported to be as high as 40% to 67%.[86–88]

In the head and neck region, cutaneous lesions predominate.[89] The most common sites of cutaneous involvement are the nasal region, postauricular region, scalp, and neck. The nasal region is a unique location for lesions in patients with AIDS-KS, occurring in 20% of patients (Fig. 25–5). Cutaneous lesions have an obvious cosmetic significance for infected persons, but they are rarely symptomatic. Nonetheless, a small number of patients (5%) with cutaneous head and neck involvement may develop pruritus, pain, or ulceration.

Mucosal lesions are reported as the most common site of head and neck involvement in some studies.[90] The principal site of mucosal involvement is the oral cavity. In the oral cavity, the hard palate, gingiva, buccal mucosa, dorsum of the tongue, and oropharynx are primarily involved. Involvement of the conjunctiva, nasal mucosa, pharynx, larynx, and esophagus has been reported but is less common (Figs. 25–6 and 25–7). Mucosal lesions are more likely than cutaneous lesions to be associated with symptoms. About 29% of mucosal lesions produce symptoms, most of which are caused by ulceration or local mass effect. Specifically, oral lesions cause

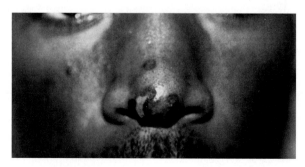

FIGURE 25–5 Kaposi's sarcoma of the nasal tip.

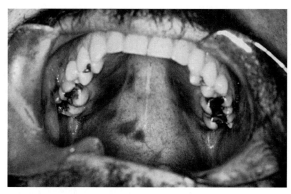

FIGURE 25–6 Kaposi's sarcoma of the hard palate.

symptoms in as many as 27% to 33% of patients.[91] Pain, ulceration, bleeding, dysfunctional mastication, and instability of teeth are most commonly described.[92] Involvement of the nasal mucosa and pharynx can cause facial pain, nasal congestion, dyspnea, dysphagia, odynophagia, dysphonia, and hoarseness.[93] Laryngeal lesions can cause hoarseness, dysphonia, dyspnea, and cough.[94] Moreover, laryngeal lesions, although rare, are more likely to require therapeutic intervention and to affect overall prognosis.

Lesions in deeper structures of the head and neck are rarely detected clinically. However, lymph node involvement is reported to be as high as 47% in patients with AIDS-KS in autopsy studies, compared with 13% detected in patients while alive.[95] This difference can be accounted for by the relatively large number of causes for lymph node enlargement in HIV-infected patients, combined with the indolent nature of KS involving these structures, causing physicians to disregard the presence of KS in asymptomatic lymphadenopathy. Other reported sites of deep structure involvement include the parotid gland and the masseter muscle.[91, 96] Involvement of these structures is rarely symptomatic, but symptoms such as facial edema, xerostomia, and pain have been reported.

KS in the upper respiratory tract or lungs often causes symptoms that prompt otolaryngologic consultation. As many as 85% of patients with pulmonary lesions develop some

degree of shortness of breath, cough, dyspnea, or hemoptysis.[97] These lesions can be difficult to diagnose and are often life threatening. All patients with pulmonary involvement have lesions that are visible on external examination. Accordingly, KS should be on the differential diagnosis of causes of pulmonary symptoms in AIDS patients with visible cutaneous or mucosal lesions.

The evaluation of patients known to have KS should focus on the cutaneous and mucosal surfaces in the head and neck. Patients who are symptomatic require further scrutiny. The presence of dyspnea or hoarseness is a certain indication for fiberoptic laryngoscopy. Shortness of breath, cough, or hemoptysis in combination with a normal head and neck examination necessitates a radiographic examination of the chest or bronchoscopy or both. The anatomic sites and sizes of the lesion should be documented for future comparison.[98]

Diagnosis

Although the differential diagnosis of KS lesions is broad, the diagnosis of KS in AIDS can be accepted based on characteristic appearance. Biopsy is rarely necessary. Suspicious cervical nodes in a patient with KS need not be biopsied unless this is the only involved site. However, if the diagnosis is questionable or treatment is contemplated, pathologic confirmation of KS should be obtained. Optimal pathologic diagnosis requires a 3- to 4-cm biopsy specimen that crosses the border between normal and involved regions. Biopsy of cutaneous lesions is rarely associated with bleeding. However, biopsy of mucosal lesions may cause severe bleeding. Accordingly, appropriate measures to control bleeding should be available when biopsy is performed, especially for pharyngeal, laryngeal, and endobronchial lesions.

Prognosis and Staging

The primary cause of death in HIV-infected patients is opportunistic infectious processes (CDC stage IV), which lead to 90% of fatalities. Remaining fatalities (10%) are caused by lymphoma, KS, gastrointestinal bleeding, suicide, or other noninfectious processes.[99] Accordingly, survival is related to the presence or absence of opportunistic infections. A mortality rate of 55% to 60% is seen in patients with opportunistic infections (with or without KS). However, patients with KS alone have a mortality rate of only 20% to 25%.[100, 101]

The CDC stage at the time of development of opportunistic infections is an important prognostic indicator, with a 6-month mortality of 27% for stage I or II patients, 42% for stage III patients, and 72% for stage IV patients. This concept is further supported by the fact that HIV-infected patients with CD4 counts greater than 300/mm³ have a median survival of 32 months, as compared with patients with counts 300/mm³ or less, who have less than a 24-month survival.[102] The occurrence of systemic symptoms has been associated with a median survival of less than 14 months. With head and neck lesions, survival is most often influenced by non–KS-related factors. In the small number of deaths directly attributed to KS, pulmonary or laryngeal involvement is most often encountered.[103]

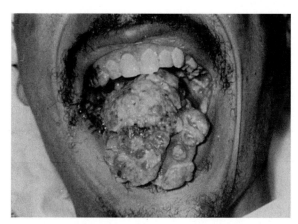

FIGURE 25–7 Kaposi's sarcoma of the tongue.

Treatment

The development and use of HAART has been associated with a significant decrease in the incidence of AIDS-KS. Guidelines for the treatment of patients with AIDS-KS are not well established and are based on a limited clinical experience. Because treatment with agents effective for other subtypes of KS has not proved to be as efficacious in AIDS-KS, therapy must be adapted to each clinical situation. Currently used modalities include surgery, chemotherapy, radiotherapy, and immunotherapy. Although the response to these modalities is good, recurrence is common and adverse effects are often severe.

A majority of patients with AIDS-KS of the head and neck do not require therapeutic intervention because the presence of KS does not influence their overall prognosis. Accordingly, therapy is best reserved for symptomatic lesions or for limited cosmetic purposes. Localized cutaneous lesions are effectively treated with radiotherapy, which is easily delivered and is essentially devoid of adverse effects. An excellent response is noted, with palliation of lesions in the range of 50% to 75%, although skin discoloration may remain after treatment.[92]

The injection of intralesional vinblastine in the treatment of oral mucosal lesions may be of some benefit in the temporary alleviation of symptoms. Injection of 0.1 to 0.2 mg of vinblastine to the depth of the lesions is well tolerated and is devoid of systemic adverse effects.[90]

However, because KS seen in association with AIDS is frequently disseminated, systemic therapy is often necessary. Currently available chemotherapeutic agents are associated with systemic adverse effects that may be severe. Immunosuppression is a feature that makes chemotherapy especially dangerous in AIDS patients. Immunosuppression is noted in patients with AIDS-KS who experience an increased incidence of opportunistic infections with chemotherapy. Accordingly, patients should be carefully selected for chemotherapeutic intervention. In general, single-agent therapy is best for patients with severe immunosuppression, those who cannot tolerate combination therapy, and those requiring palliation of tumor-related symptoms.[104]

A wide variety of chemotherapeutic agents has been used in the treatment of AIDS-KS, as part of both single and combination regimens.[105] These agents include bleomycin, doxorubicin (Adriamycin), teniposide, etoposide, methotrexate, vincristine (Oncovin), and vinblastine.[95, 106–110] Vincristine, with a response rate as high as 80%, is slowly emerging as the chemotherapeutic agent of choice in the treatment of AIDS-KS.[95, 111] Additionally, this agent does not cause myelosuppression, which could limit treatment in many patients.

In widely disseminated disease, cytotoxic or multiple-agent therapy must be employed. However, treatment is often limited by the development of myelosuppression. In addition, the use of antiviral agents with combination therapy may further reduce the duration of treatment.[112] The combination of doxorubicin, vincristine, and bleomycin, with a response rate of 79% in these cases, is recommended.[113] This chemotherapeutic regimen is reported to cause a lesser degree of myelosuppression and is better tolerated.

Finally, many noncytotoxic forms of therapy for AIDS-KS are being investigated, including interferons, retinoids, antiestrogens, and cytokines.[114–118] Of these, only interferon-α is in wide clinical use.[119] This agent allows for objective responses of approximately 30%, which can be sustained with the administration of long-term maintenance therapy.[116] Interferon-α has proved most effective in patients with high CD4 counts who do not have systemic or group B symptoms, and in those with opportunistic infections.[120] Furthermore, therapeutic synergy is reported with the use of zidovudine (AZT), which allows antiretroviral chemotherapy to proceed along with the treatment of KS.[121–123]

Non-Hodgkin's Lymphoma

Lymphoma is a process that results from the malignant proliferation of cells normally found within lymphoid tissue. It was first described by Thomas Hodgkin in 1832 and is classified as Hodgkin's type or non-Hodgkin's type by the pathologic presence or absence of Reed-Sternberg–type giant cells (Table 25–7).[124, 125]

NHL is the most common type of lymphoma overall. NHLs are neoplasms of monoclonal origin that vary in their malignant potential. They are especially common among immunosuppressed patients, including those with HIV infection. NHLs account for up to half of malignancies seen in primary immunodeficiency disorders and 14% of those seen in chemically immunosuppressed patients.[126, 127] The incidence of these neoplasms in immunosuppressed transplant patients is 30 to 50 times greater than in the general population and is similar to the magnitude of increase seen in

TABLE 25–7 Risk of Non-Hodgkin's Lymphoma Among Persons With AIDS

Working Group Formulation	Observed	Expected	Relative Risk
High grade			
Diffuse, immunoblastic	11	0.183	627
Lymphoblastic	4	0.095	42
Undifferentiated Burkitt's	38	0.173	220
Subtotal	157	0.451	348
Intermediate grade			
Diffuse, large cell	142	0.934	145
Diffuse mixed	10	0.186	54
Diffuse, small cell	6	0.209	29
Follicular, large cell	2	0.093	21
Subtotal	160	1.422	113
Low grade			
Follicular, mixed small cleaved and large cell	1	0.156	6
Follicular, small cleaved	1	0.337	3
Small lymphocytic	8	0.214	37
Subtotal	10	0.707	14
Otherwise specified	6	0.240	25
Not otherwise specified	183	0.315	580
Total	516	3.137	165

From Cote TR, Biggar RJ, Rosenberg PS, et al: Non-Hodgkin's lymphoma among people with AIDS: Incidence, presentation and public health burden. AIDS/Cancer Study Group. Int J Cancer 73:645–650, 1997.

HIV-infected patients.[128] The coexistence of immunosuppression alters the course of NHL, affecting its presentation, location, and aggressiveness. However, unlike KS, the natural course of NHL is similar in all immunocompromised groups, including those with AIDS.

Since the first description in 1982 of NHL in association with HIV infection, its incidence has risen sharply; it is now the second most common malignancy in AIDS,[129] and its incidence continues to increase. As survival in the general population of HIV-infected patients is becoming more prolonged, there is a 30% incidence of the development of NHL in patients who survive longer than 3 years with the use of antiretroviral chemotherapy.[130] The development of intermediate- or high-grade B-cell lymphomas in a patient infected by HIV is considered an AIDS-defining process.[131] These tumors are responsible for the advancement of HIV infection to full-blown AIDS in 2.5% to 5.0% of patients, and they develop in 10% to 12% of patients during the course of infection.[132, 133]

Pathogenesis

The role of viruses in the development of neoplasia is well elucidated. Viral agents, namely EBV and HTLV-I, have been implicated in the development of immunologic malignancies.[134] EBV infection is etiologic in cases of Burkitt's lymphoma in Africa; its presence is documented in 100% of cases.[135] It is also responsible for the development of B-cell NHL in immunosuppressed patients without HIV infection.[136] However, the role of EBV in the development of NHL in HIV-infected patients has been debated.

Increased anti-EBV titers and rates of oral hairy leukoplakia, as well as isolation of the EBV genome in lymphoma cells, support the association of NHL and EBV in HIV-infected patients.[137–139] In addition, in cases of progressive generalized lymphadenopathy, there is a greater likelihood for the development of NHL when EBV is identified than when EBV is not identified.[140] Furthermore, cytometric evaluation of lymphoma DNA infected by EBV has showed that infection by EBV took place before clonal expansion, suggesting that infection plays an etiologic role.[141]

Unlike in other immunocompromised groups, in which EBV has been found universally in cases of NHL, EBV has been isolated in only 20% to 70% of AIDS-associated NHLs, leading to the assumption that EBV is not the only agent promoting the development of these lesions.[142–144] Some authors report that EBV has a limited ability to immortalize B-cells, leading to a polyclonal proliferation. A second agent, such as a chromosomal derangement that leads to the presence of an oncogene, may be responsible for monoclonal malignant transformation.[145] Two studies have suggested that HIV itself may be the second agent in NHL development.[146, 147] These studies have shown both the development of lymphoma and the presence of the HIV genome in lymphoma cells of infected patients.

Clinical Presentation and Diagnosis

Classically, NHL has been described as a disease of adults in their fifth to sixth decades of life with an equal female-to-male ratio.[148] However, in the presence of HIV infection, a lower age group is affected (30 to 40 years of age), which is mirrored by the ages of patients who develop HIV infection.[149] Similarly, the large male predominance reported in these patients is similar to that for patients with HIV infection. The reported male-to-female ratio is 19:1, in contrast to the pre-HIV era, when a 1.5:1 ratio prevailed. Furthermore, the development of NHL usually accompanies marked immunosuppression, as documented by an inverted T4/T8 ratio and a CD4 count below 200/mm³ in the majority of patients.[150–152] This level of immunosuppression is typical of patients in CDC stage IV of HIV infection.

Before AIDS, lymphadenopathy alone marked the presentation in 24% of patients with NHL. Another 43% of patients had lymphadenopathy in conjunction with extranodal disease. Similarly, lymphatic involvement is overshadowed by the presence of extralymphatic disease in patients with HIV infection. Extralymphatic involvement occurs in 82% of cases overall and in the absence of lymphatic involvement in 31% of cases.[150, 153] The most common site of extralymphatic involvement is the CNS; this occurs in 26% to 33% of cases. Other reported sites of extralymphatic NHL are the bone marrow in 3% to 24%, the liver in 3% to 22%, the lung in 1% to 9%, and intraoral or anorectal tissue in 1% to 14% of patients.[144, 150–152, 154–156]

In non–HIV-infected patients, extranodal disease of the head and neck region usually involves the structures of Waldeyer's ring, especially the tonsils.[157] Outside Waldeyer's ring, the nose and paranasal sinuses are most often involved.[158] Head and neck involvement is also common in patients with HIV infection, with 36% of patients developing NHL in this region before the diagnosis of AIDS. However, in the presence of HIV infection, the most common site of head and neck involvement is the CNS. Patients with CNS involvement usually present with nonspecific cognitive symptoms or focal neurologic deficits (including cranial nerve palsies) or both.[159, 160] Headache and seizures are relatively rare. However, these symptoms can occur with a variety of AIDS-associated conditions, including toxoplasmosis, progressive multifocal leukoencephalopathy, and cryptococcosis.[161–163]

The definitive diagnosis of CNS lymphoma is based on CT scanning.[164] The classic appearance of a contrast-enhancing lesion with mass effect and surrounding edema is suggestive of NHL (Fig. 25–8). Toxoplasmosis, which has an identical appearance on CT, must be ruled out. Generally, patients with elevated *Toxoplasma* species titers in the presence of a suspicious CNS lesion can be treated empirically for toxoplasmosis for 2 weeks. If no response is detected on CT scan after 2 weeks, a brain biopsy is indicated. Lumbar puncture can be performed, if it is not contraindicated by CT findings, to help diagnose toxoplasmic encephalitis in complicated cases.[165] Cytologic examination of the CSF is rarely diagnostic of lymphoma.[166, 167] Nonetheless, cytology should be routinely requested for all CSF specimens.

Other extranodal head and neck sites in HIV-associated NHL include, in order of frequency, the facial bones, skin, paranasal sinuses, larynx, Waldeyer's ring, and orbit.[168] Symptoms are often nonspecific and related to the anatomic region of occurrence. Systemic, or group B, symptoms are present in the majority of patients and can easily lead to the suspicion of an infectious process. However, diagnosis can generally be obtained by various biopsy techniques, along

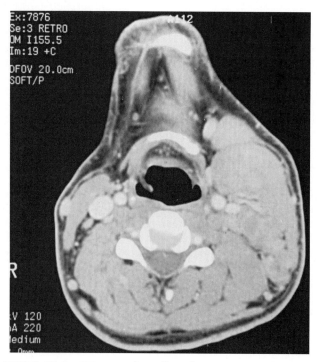

FIGURE 25–8 CT scan of rapidly enlarging mass, a biopsy of which revealed non-Hodgkin's lymphoma.

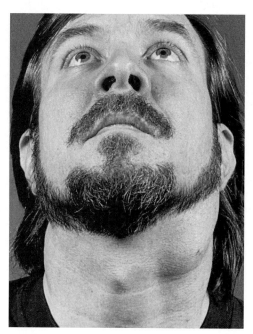

FIGURE 25–9 Non-Hodgkin's lymphoma in a cervical node.

with the application of endoscopy or nasopharyngoscopy in selected cases.

The cervical nodes are the most common site for head and neck involvement of NHL in HIV-infected patients.[147] Nodal NHL generally presents as an asymptomatic, enlarging mass that only rarely causes compressive symptoms. A majority of these lesions show capsular invasion with involvement of surrounding tissues. Diagnosis of cervical disease requires a high level of suspicion, FNA, and open biopsy if the diagnosis is not obtainable by other methods. At the time of open biopsy, an excisional biopsy of the largest, lowest lymph node in the affected chain should be performed to maximize diagnostic potential (Fig. 25–9).[169]

Staging and Prognosis

Most NHLs (74%), regardless of association, are either stage III or stage IV at the time of presentation. Accordingly, their staging and prognosis are not related to the Ann Arbor staging system, but rather to a working formulation established by the American Cancer Society. Based on this working formulation, NHL is categorized into three groups based on its malignant potential. These prognostic groups include low-, intermediate-, and high-grade lymphomas.

The distribution of patients along this pathologic grading is altered in HIV infection. In a review of 591 cases reported in the literature, a majority of patients presented with either high-grade (65%) or intermediate-grade lymphoma (33%); only 1% of cases were of low grade. The small noncleaved (35%) and the large cell immunoblastic (31%) are the most common types of high-grade lymphoma. The diffuse large cell type accounts for the vast majority of intermediate-grade

lymphomas. In sharp contrast are non–HIV-infected patients, in whom low-grade lymphomas account for 25% to 35% and high-grade disease is seen in only 10% of cases.[170, 171]

In the pre-AIDS era, the 5-year survival of patients with low-grade lymphomas was 50% to 70%; rates of 35% to 45% were seen for intermediate-grade NHL, and 23% to 32% for high-grade NHL. However, in the presence of HIV infection, survival is diminished across the board. Survival is especially influenced by the presence of CNS involvement.[172] Without treatment, CNS involvement with NHL is associated with a survival period of less than 1 month. Other poor prognostic indicators in patients with AIDS-associated NHL include CD4 counts below 200/mm^3, bone marrow involvement, and the presence of concurrent opportunistic infection.[173] Even with treatment, increase in survival is only a few months, and death is often associated with the development of opportunistic infections.

Treatment

The standard treatment for NHL has for many years included the use of chemotherapy. However, the generation of immunosuppression by the therapeutic regimen has limited its effectiveness. Although a 33% to 57% response rate has been reported with the use of intensive multidrug chemotherapy, survival has been uniformly poor, owing mainly to an increased incidence and aggressiveness of opportunistic infections.[174] These results are worsened if chemotherapy is intensified.[175] In addition, planned therapeutic dosages cannot be delivered in the majority of cases owing to the development of cytopenias.[176, 177] Accordingly, two alternative therapeutic regimens are being developed.

The first regimen uses lower doses of antineoplastic agents, and the second uses hematopoietic growth factor (HPF) in combination with a standard or higher-dose chemotherapeutic regimen.

The use of HPF has been reported to reduce the myelosuppression associated with chemotherapy.[177] This modality has resulted in reduced neutropenia. Although the response rate and survival among control and HPF-treated patients were the same in one study (response rate 67% and survival 8.0 to 11.4 months), the data suggest that increased intensity of chemotherapy may be better tolerated with the addition of HPF, which may allow an increased response and survival.[177]

The use of lower doses of chemotherapy has been reported to improve survival and decrease the risk for the development of opportunistic processes.[178] One such study reported using reduced doses of cyclophosphamide and doxorubicin in a regimen of m-BACOD (methotrexate, bleomycin, Adriamycin, cyclophosphamide, Oncovin, and dexamethasone), allowing for a 42% complete response rate, with lower associated toxicity.[178] In another study in which reduced m-BACOD was used, the response rate was found to be 51%, with a complete response in 46%. Overall survival was increased to 6.5 months for treated patients, with those showing complete response surviving to 15 months.[178] CNS involvement with NHL is difficult to treat. Attempts at therapy have included radiation therapy, which has increased survival by only a few months; death related to opportunistic infections occurs in the majority of cases.[179, 180]

Hodgkin's Disease

Hodgkin's disease (HD) is a process that was first described in association with AIDS in 1985.[181] Unlike NHL, the incidence of HD is not altered in association with immunodeficiency, including that associated with AIDS.[182] However, its presentation, course, and prognosis are dramatically altered by the presence of HIV infection. HD usually develops early in the course of HIV infection, preceding the onset of significant immunosuppression. Studies report a near-normal T4/T8 ratio and T-cell counts greater than 200/mm^3 at the onset of HD.[73, 152, 183]

In 114 cases reported in the literature, HD lesions occurred in patients averaging 32 years of age, with the majority of patients between 30 and 45 years of age.[73] In contrast, the incidence of HD in patients without HIV infection is bimodal, occurring in patients under 30 and older than 45 years of age. A study from King's County Hospital Center in Brooklyn, New York, revealed that advanced-stage disease (stage III/IV) was diagnosed in 80% of HIV-infected patients compared with 45% of noninfected patients.[184]

This process is unusually aggressive in the presence of HIV infection. A majority of patients (84%) present with either stage III or stage IV disease, compared with 40% of non–HIV-infected patients.[73] In addition, unlike HD not associated with AIDS, extranodal disease is common, occurring in 61% of patients with coexistent HIV infection. Bone marrow involvement, a poor prognostic indicator, occurs in 41% of HIV-infected patients, far outnumbering the 3.5% that was reported before AIDS. Other extranodal sites of HD include the liver (31%) and spleen (38%).[73]

HD accounts for only 5.0% to 8.6% of all lymphomas involving the head and neck region in HIV-infected patients.[147] Lymph node involvement is most common. Lymphatic disease generally presents with asymptomatic, rapid enlargement. However, extranodal disease involving the head and neck region has been reported in the tonsils and tongue.[152, 183]

Clinical Presentation

A majority of patients with HIV-associated HD present with group B symptoms (90%).[73] However, in many cases, systemic symptoms are secondary to HIV-related factors, rather than to the presence of HD, making their presence of limited usefulness as prognostic indicators. In addition, the presence of coexistent PGL in 57% of patients further complicates efforts at staging. It appears that the CD4 count and the presence of opportunistic infections play significant roles in terms of survival and are more important considerations than established staging methods in planning treatment and determining prognosis.

Prognosis and Treatment

Compared with the classic form of HD, there appears to be an increase in histologic types that show poorer prognosis, with mixed cellularity and lymphocyte-depleted forms making up 57% of cases.[73] The increase in prognostically poor histologic forms occurs at the expense of the nodular sclerosis type, the incidence of which is decreased to 29%. In addition, a unique variant of NHL has been reported in HIV-infected patients. This variant is characterized by the presence of fibrohistiocytoid stromal cells but is yet to be fully defined.

The survival of patients with coexistent HD and HIV infection has been poor, ranging from 7 to 15 months. Attempts at therapy using established regimens, including MOPP (nitrogen mustard, Oncovin, procarbazine, and prednisone), ABVD (Adriamycin, bleomycin, vinblastine, and dacarbazine), ABV, or combined or alternating dosing of MOPP and ABVD, have been successful in producing complete responders in 30% to 58% of cases, but they have not influenced long-term survival. Problems with therapy have been similar to those encountered in NHL, with a large number of patients developing opportunistic infections that lead to death. Accordingly, less aggressive forms of chemotherapy are also being explored for HD.

Squamous Cell Carcinoma

Although no studies to date have reported an increase in the incidence of head and neck SCC in HIV-infected patients, significant changes in the course of SCC have been brought about by the presence of HIV infection. A majority of patients with AIDS-related SCC of the head and neck are younger than 45 years of age (82%), accounting for 21% of cases of SCC in this age group.[185] Furthermore, less than 1% of patients older than 45 years of age have concomitant HIV infection. In our study, all patients with SCC along with HIV infection also had a significant history of alcohol, intravenous drug, or tobacco use.[185]

Clinical Presentation and Diagnosis

The most common site for SCC in HIV-infected patients is the larynx (62.5%), followed by the oral cavity (12%).[186] The oropharynx, nasopharynx, and parotid are less commonly involved. This is unlike SCC in the younger population without HIV infection, in whom involvement of the oral cavity and pharynx is most common.[187, 188] In addition, a majority of patients with SCC and HIV infection present with advanced local disease (79% with T3 or T4 tumors), with all patients having stage III and IV tumors at presentation.[185] Because advanced SCC of the upper aerodigestive tract shows a high tendency for lymph node metastasis, with a greater than 50% risk reported for T3 and T4 lesions, it is especially important that neck disease be evaluated in all HIV-infected patients.[189, 190] However, the evaluation of cervical metastasis is complicated by the multiple causes of lymphatic enlargement in HIV infection, leading to a clinical overestimation of nodal disease in 36% of cases.[185]

Although enlargement of jugulodigastric and submandibular nodes to greater than 1.5 cm in diameter and of other cervical nodes to greater than 1.0 cm has traditionally been associated with metastatic disease in 80% of patients, nodal size is not of value in the determination of metastasis in the presence of HIV infection. Rapid, localized enlargement remains the only consistent indicator of metastasis. CT or MRI has been reported to have a limited ability to delineate metastatic disease. Accordingly, the most accurate method for the evaluation of lymphatic disease is neck dissection. Selective neck dissections can be contemplated for smaller tumors; modified-radical or radical dissection should be performed for advanced local disease.

Treatment and Prognosis

The results of treatment of upper aerodigestive tract SCC in HIV-infected patients are disappointing.[185] Even with the use of multimodality therapy, poor survival is typical. Overall tumor-related survival of 57% at 1 year and 32% at 2 years is significantly less than the respective 74% and 59% rates seen in non–HIV-infected SCC patients. Moreover, death may be precipitated through the administration of therapeutic measures by acceleration of the development of opportunistic infections. Accordingly, it is important that prophylactic therapy (especially against *P. carinii* pneumonia) be administered while HIV-infected patients with SCC are being treated.

Epithelial Neoplasms

Basal Cell and Squamous Cell Carcinomas

Immunosuppression has been shown to be associated with the development of epithelial malignancies in transplant patients.[191–193] SCC is the most common of these malignancies, followed by basal cell carcinoma (BCC) and malignant melanoma (MM). Moreover, the 15:1 ratio of SCC to BCC reported for immunosuppressed transplant patients is in sharp contrast to the 1:3 to 5 ratio seen in the normal population.[194, 195] The course of epithelial malignancies in HIV-infected patients is different from that in both the normal and immunosuppressed transplant population.

Although the ratio of SCC to BCC in HIV-infected patients (1:6.7 to 8.3) remains comparable to that in the normal population, the presentation, location, and course of these lesions resemble those of transplant patients. BCC accounts for the majority of epithelial neoplasms seen in HIV-infected patients. It usually presents as a small, pearly-bordered papule or nodule with telangiectases and a tendency to show enlargement and central ulceration. Unlike in the normal population, in whom the head and neck region is involved in 85% of cases, BCC in HIV-infected patients most commonly involves the trunk, with the head and neck involved in only 29% of cases.[196] In addition, patients with HIV infection tend to develop BCC at a younger age, with 54% of cases occurring in patients younger than 40 years of age, compared with the 5% incidence in the normal population.[196]

Furthermore, BCC displays a greater aggressiveness in HIV-infected patients than in patients not infected with HIV, even though a majority of cases (67%) are accounted for by the less aggressive superficial subtype that makes up 9% to 11% of cases in the normal population.[197, 198] Early metastasis of BCC in HIV-infected patients has been reported but is unusual for these tumors.[199, 200] However, BCC in HIV-infected patients shows the same response to therapy as in patients without HIV infection. The overall recurrence rate after therapy was 3%, regardless of whether curettage and electrodesiccation, excision, liquid nitrogen cryotherapy, radiation therapy, or Mohs' micrographic surgery was used.[201]

Although the incidence of cutaneous SCC in HIV-infected patients is high, this increase is not as great as the 37-fold increase in incidence seen in transplant patients. The course of SCC in HIV-infected patients resembles that seen in transplant patients. A greater prevalence occurs in the younger population, along with markedly greater aggressiveness. The head and neck region is the most common site for cutaneous SCC in HIV-infected patients, accounting for 47% of cases.[201] These tumors generally present as non-healing ulcers with raised borders and marked induration, showing a tendency for multicentricity and early metastasis. Treatment in these patients is best accomplished by surgical excision because curettage and electrodesiccation is associated with a high recurrence rate.[196]

Malignant Melanoma

Whereas immunosuppressed patients have a threefold to sixfold increased risk for the development of MM relative to nonimmunosuppressed individuals,[202] MM remains rare in HIV-infected patients.[203–205] Nonetheless, authors have suggested a higher incidence of these neoplasms in HIV-infected patients than in non–HIV-infected individuals. In a prospective study of 1000 HIV-infected patients, 4 developed MM, far outnumbering the 4 to 13 cases per 100,000 expected for the non–HIV-infected population.[206]

MM in the presence of HIV infection displays increased aggressiveness, showing deeper invasion at the time of presentation, with the majority of patients presenting with Clark level V involvement.[207] In addition, multicentricity and metastasis are common among these patients, making the overall prognosis poor.[208–210] Head and neck involvement is less common than in the general population, with a compensatory increase in trunk disease. The ideal treatment of MM in association with HIV infection remains to be delineated. However, wide excision with removal of involved lymphatics is the best modality in patients who can tolerate surgery.

Plasma Cell Malignancies

Myeloma, being a neoplasm of B-cells, can be viewed as a form of NHL. However, myeloma differs from NHL by the fact that it is made up of differentiated B-cells that have the ability to produce immunoglobulins. Authors speculate that an increase in the incidence of both solitary (plasmacytomas) and multiple myelomas occurs in association with HIV infection. The presence of EBV DNA has been detected in the genome of plasma cell malignancy in an HIV-infected patient, implying that these tumors have a pathogenesis similar to that of NHL. This supports the theory and increased occurrence of plasma cell malignancies, paralleling the increase in B-cell lymphomas.[211] However, these assertions have yet to be proved owing to the relatively small number of cases involved.

A younger population is affected by these neoplasms (30 to 40 years of age) as compared with non–HIV-infected patients (50 to 60 years of age).[212–214] In addition, plasma cell tumors have an aggressive course in the presence of HIV infection. There is an increased incidence of extramedullary disease as compared with the normal population, with the gingiva and skull being the areas most often involved in the head and neck region (Figs. 25–10 and 25–11).[215, 216]

Response to therapy appears inconsistent. Although some authors have reported good response to chemotherapy, radiation therapy has failed to control disease in most cases.[217, 218] In two reports, disease progression could not be halted by radiation therapy or chemotherapy; death resulted from treatment in one case. Elevated levels of lactate dehydrogenase were noted in both cases of unresponsive plasmacytoma and may be a poor prognostic indicator in patients with HIV-associated plasma cell malignancies.[219, 220] Currently, most authors recommend the use of supplemented or modified chemotherapy, similar to that used in the treatment of NHL, for treating plasma cell tumors in HIV-infected patients.[221]

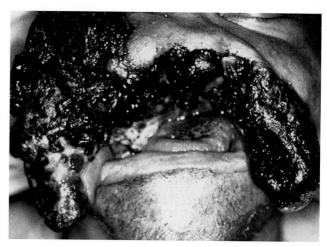

FIGURE 25–11 Progression of the lesion shown in Figure 25–10, which has replaced most of the midface.

Cancers Among Children With AIDS

With more and more children being infected with HIV, a pattern has emerged. NHL is the most common neoplasm seen in children with AIDS, with B-cell lineage being the predominant subtype. The gastrointestinal system and the CNS are common extranodal sites of involvement. Other neoplasms include Hodgkin's disease, mucosa-associated lymphoid tissue (MALT) lymphomas, KS, and leiomyosarcomas.

◻ HIV AND THYROID FUNCTION AND DISEASE

Hypothyroidism as indicated by elevated basal thyroid-stimulating hormone (TSH) and abnormal thyrotropin-releasing hormone (TRH) response is common among HIV-infected children and may contribute to failure of growth in these children. Replacement therapy has resulted in correction of abnormal TSH and improvement in growth.[222]

Subclinical infections of the thyroid gland are also common among HIV-positive patients. In a prospective autopsy study of the thyroid in 100 patients in Brazil who died of complications from AIDS, a wide range of bacterial, fungal, viral, and neoplastic disorders were observed. *Mycobacterium tuberculosis* was recorded in 23% of patients, cytomegalovirus in 17%, *Cryptococcus* in 5%, *Mycobacterium avium* in 5%, *Pneumocystis* in 4%, and other bacteria or fungi in 7%. KS was recorded in 2% of patients and occult papillary carcinoma in 4%.[223]

◻ PALLIATIVE THERAPY FOR HIV PATIENTS WITH INCURABLE CANCER

A distinct group of patients with HIV infection develop incurable cancer or advanced AIDS, precluding cure. Many physicians regard these patients as terminal, and because of

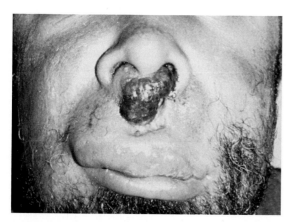

FIGURE 25–10 Plasmacytoma eroding into the maxilla.

this, they have a tendency to think that nothing can be done. Nevertheless, it is especially important that therapy be provided to these patients, albeit with noncurative intent. Lessons learned in the treatment of terminal cancer can be directly applied to the management of these patients, with some modifications. Goals of therapy include palliation of symptoms, assistance with daily functioning, and most important, psychosocial support. Moreover, any therapeutic intervention must take into account the anticipated course of disease and is best provided by a team of physicians working in conjunction with the efforts of family members. The efforts of this team should be coordinated toward a single goal, namely, the efficient and humane management of the process of dying.

The psychological stresses accompanying HIV infection can be devastating. Coupled with the presence of incurable cancer, depression is all but inevitable. Psychological support is invariably necessary and should be started early by the family and primary physician, as well as by the otolaryngologist–head and neck surgeon, the infectious disease specialist, and the clinical psychologist. This support may also serve to assist patients as they progress through the stages of dying, including denial and isolation, anger, bargaining, depression, and finally, acceptance.[224] Furthermore, not only the patient but also family members who may be devastated by the patient's affliction should be counseled and treated.

As long as possible, independence should be encouraged and outpatient management provided.[225] When hospitalization is required, the hospital setting should be modified to create a homelike environment through the incorporation of familiar objects. During this time, positive aspects of bodily function should be stressed, along with the limitations of negative aspects, including diseased or infected organs and unpleasant symptoms. In addition, patients should be allowed to continue certain habits with moderation, including smoking and alcohol use.

A symptomatic approach to treatment should be initiated early, especially for the control of pain, nausea, and depression.[226] The development of these symptoms should be anticipated and appropriate pharmacologic interventions provided. Administration of therapy should be sufficient to eliminate and prevent the recurrence of the targeted symptom.

More important, in patients with HIV infection along with cancer, each symptom may signify the development of a life-limiting underlying process, especially opportunistic infectious diseases, which are the single most common cause of death in AIDS patients. Accordingly, each symptom must be investigated and treatment of the underlying cause provided along with palliation. Finally, diagnostic testing should be limited to tests that will improve management of the process of dying; needless testing should be avoided.

It is more difficult to treat those you cannot cure than those you can. However, both types of treatment are equally important. It is important to continue to provide support and care and not give the patient a feeling of abandonment or hopelessness. It is the physician's role to assist patients through the process of dying so that it occurs with as much dignity and as little discomfort as possible.

REFERENCES

1. Nahmias AJ, Weiss J, Yao X, et al: Evidence of human infection with an HTLV-III/LAV-like virus in Central Africa 1959. Lancet 1:127–128, 1986.
2. Kaposi's sarcoma and *Pneumocystis* pneumonia among homosexual men—New York City and California. MMWR Morb Mortal Wkly Rep 30:305–308, 1981.
3. *Pneumocystis* pneumonia—Los Angeles. MMWR Morb Mortal Wkly Rep 30:250–252, 1981.
4. Sorvino D, Lucente FE: Acquired immunodeficiency syndrome—the epidemic. Otolaryngol Clin North Am 25:1147–1158, 1992.
5. Gallo R, Salahuddin S, Popoviv M, et al: Frequent detection and isolation of cytopathic retrovirus (HTLV-III) from patients with AIDS and at risk for AIDS. Science 224:500–503, 1984.
6. Barre-Sinoussi F, Nugeyre M, Dauguet C, et al: Isolation of a T-lymphocyte retrovirus from a patient at risk for acquired immune deficiency syndrome. Science 220:868–871, 1983.
7. Viele MK, Donegan EA: Rational use of blood and blood components. Otolaryngol Clin North Am 25:1321–1339, 1993.
8. Goedert JJ: The epidemiology of acquired immunodeficiency syndrome malignancies. Semin Oncol 27:390–401, 2000.
9. Cote TR, Biggar RJ, Rosenberg PS, et al: Non-Hodgkin's lymphoma among people with AIDS: Incidence, presentation and public health burden. AIDS/Cancer Study Group. Int J Cancer 73:645–650, 1997.
10. Tashima KT, Flanigan TP: Antiretroviral therapy in the year 2000. Infect Dis Clin North Am 14:827–849, 2000.
11. Cannon M, Cesarman E: Kaposi's sarcoma–associated herpes virus and acquired immunodeficiency syndrome–related malignancy. Semin Oncol 27:409–419, 2000.
12. Gates AE, Kaplan LD: AIDS malignancies in the era of highly active antiretroviral therapy. Oncology (Huntingt) 16:657–665, 2002.
13. Boshoff C, Weiss R: AIDS-related malignancies. Nat Rev Cancer 2:373–382, 2002.
14. Guyader M, Emerman M, Sonigo P, et al: Genome organization and transactivation of human immunodeficiency virus type 2. Nature 326:662–669, 1987.
15. Levy JA: The human immunodeficiency virus and its pathogenesis. In Sande MA, Volberding PA (eds): The Medical Management of AIDS. Philadelphia, WB Saunders, 1988, pp 3–17.
16. Sooy CD, Gerberding JL, Kaplan MJ: The risk for otolaryngologists who treat patients with AIDS and AIDS virus infection: Report of a study in progress. Laryngoscope 97:430–434, 1987.
17. Levy JA, Kaminsky LS, Morrow WJW, et al: Infection by the retrovirus associated with the acquired immunodeficiency syndrome. Ann Intern Med 103:694–699, 1985.
18. Stein BS, Gowda SD, Lifson JD, et al: pH-Independent HIV entry into CD4 positive T-cells via virus envelope fusion to the plasma membrane. Cell 49:659–668, 1987.
19. Zurlo JJ: The human immunodeficiency virus. Basic concepts of infection and host response. Otolaryngol Clin North Am 25: 1159–1181, 1992.
20. Bartlett JA: Current and future treatment of HIV infection. Oncology 4:19–26, 1990.
21. Tindall B, Cooper DA: Primary HIV infection: Host responses and intervention strategies. AIDS 5:1–14, 1991.
22. Fordyce EJ, Singh TP, Nash D, et al: Survival rates in NYC in the era of combination ART. J Acquir Immune Defic Syndr 30:111–118, 2002.
23. Bonavida B, Katz J, Gottlieb M: Mechanism of defective NK cell activity in patients with acquired immunodeficiency syndrome (AIDS) and AIDS-related complex. I. Defective trigger on NK cells for NKCF production by target cells, and partial restoration by IL-2. J Immunol 137:1977–1984, 1986.
24. Creemers PC, Stark DF, Boyko WJ: Evaluation of natural killer cell activity in patients with persistent generalized lymphadenopathy and acquired immunodeficiency syndrome. Clin Immunol Immunopathol 36:141–150, 1985.
25. Henderson DK, Fahey BJ, Willy M, et al: Risk of occupational transmission of human immunodeficiency virus type 1 (HIV-1) associated with clinical exposures. Ann Intern Med 113:740–746, 1990.
26. McCray E, The Cooperative Needlestick Surveillance Group: Occupational risk of the acquired immunodeficiency syndrome among health care workers. N Engl J Med 314:1127–1132, 1986.

27. Update: Human immunodeficiency virus infection in health care workers exposed to blood and infected patients. MMWR Morb Mortal Wkly Rep 36:85–89, 1987.

28. Update: Universal precautions for prevention of transmission of human immunodeficiency virus, hepatitis B virus and other blood borne pathogens in the health care setting. MMWR Morb Mortal Wkly Rep 37:377–388, 1988.

29. Public Health Service inter-agency guidelines for screening donors of blood, plasma, organs, tissue and semen for evidence of hepatitis B and hepatitis C. MMWR Morb Mortal Wkly Rep 40:1–17, 1991.

30. Osguthrope JD: Occupational human immunodeficiency virus exposure. Risks to the health care worker. Otolaryngol Clin North Am 25:1341–1353, 1992.

31. Bartlett JG: HIV infection and surgeons. Curr Probl Surg 29:197–280, 1992.

32. Wong ES, Stotka JL, Chinchilli VM, et al: Are universal precautions effective in reducing the number of occupational exposures among health care workers? JAMA 265:1123–1128, 1991.

33. Guidelines for the prevention of human immunodeficiency virus and hepatitis-B virus to healthcare and public safety workers. MMWR Morb Mortal Wkly Rep 38:3–37, 1989.

34. Enforcement Procedure for Occupational Exposure to Hepatitis B virus (HBV) and Human Immunodeficiency virus (HIV). Washington, DC, US Department of Labor, OSHA Instruction CPL 2-2.44B, February 27, 1990.

35. Lucente FE: Impact of the acquired immunodeficiency syndrome epidemic on the practice of laryngology. Ann Otol Rhinol Laryngol 102:1–24, 1993.

36. Burke EC, Orloff SL, Freise CE, et al: Wound healing after anorectal surgery in human immunodeficiency virus—infected patients. Arch Surg 126:1267–1271, 1991.

37. Peterson JM, Barbul A, Breslin RJ, et al: Significance of T-lymphocytes in wound healing. Surgery 102:300–305, 1987.

38. Schilling JA: Wound healing. Surg Clin North Am 56:859–874, 1976.

39. Vlock DR: Immunologic aspects of head and neck cancer. Clinical and laboratory correlates. Hematol Oncol Clin North Am 5:797–820, 1991.

40. Serwadda D, Sewankambo NK, Carswell JW, et al: Slim disease: A new disease in Uganda and its association with HTLV-III infection. Lancet 2:849–852, 1985.

41. Keusch GT, Thea DM: Malnutrition in AIDS. Med Clin North Am 77:795–814, 1993.

42. Gray RH: Similarities between AIDS and PCM. Am J Public Health 73:1332, 1983.

43. Fabris N, Mocchegiani E, Galli M, et al: AIDS, zinc deficiency, and thymic hormone failure. JAMA 259:839–840, 1988.

44. Abrams DI, Lewis BJ, Beckstead JH, et al: Persistent diffuse lymphadenopathy in homosexual men: End point or prodrome? Ann Intern Med 100:801–808, 1984.

45. Metroka CE, Cunningham-Rundles S, Pollack MS, et al: Generalized lymphadenopathy in homosexual men. Ann Intern Med 99:585–591, 1983.

46. Osmond D, Chaisson R, Moss A, et al: Lymphadenopathy in asymptomatic patients seropositive for HIV. N Engl J Med 317:246, 1987.

47. Kaplan JE, Spira TJ, Fishbein DB, et al: Lymphadenopathy syndrome in homosexual men. JAMA 257:335–337, 1987.

48. Mather-Wagh U, Mildvan D, Senie RT: Follow-up at 4 1/2 years on homosexual men with generalized lymphadenopathy. N Engl J Med 313:1542–1543, 1985.

49. Davidson BJ, Morris MS, Kornblut AD, et al: Lymphadenopathy in the HIV-seropositive patient. Ear Nose Throat J 69:478–486, 1990.

50. Turner RR, Levine AM, Gill PS, et al: Progressive histopathologic abnormalities in persistent generalized lymphadenopathy syndrome. Am J Surg Pathol 11:625–632, 1987.

51. Lee KC, Cheung SW: Evaluation of the neck mass in human immunodeficiency virus infected patients. Otolaryngol Clin North Am 25:1287–1305, 1992.

52. Abrams DI: AIDS-related lymphadenopathy: The role of biopsy. J Clin Oncol 4:126–127, 1986.

53. Saif MW: Castleman disease in an HIV-infected patient with Kaposi sarcoma. AIDS Read 11:572–576, 2001.

54. Barzan L, Carbone A, Saracchini S, et al: Nasopharyngeal lymphatic tissue hypertrophy in HIV-infected patients. Lancet 1:42–43, 1989.

55. Tami TA, Wawrose SF: Diseases of the nose and paranasal sinuses in human immunodeficiency virus–infected population. Otolaryngol Clin North Am 25:1199–1210, 1992.

56. Stern JC, Lin P, Lucente FE: Benign nasopharyngeal masses and human immunodeficiency virus infection. Arch Otolaryngol Head Neck Surg 116:206–208, 1990.

57. Ryan JR, Ioachim HL, Marmer J, et al: Acquired immunodeficiency syndrome–related lymphadenopathies presenting in the salivary lymph nodes. Arch Otolaryngol Head Neck Surg 111:554–556, 1985.

58. Huang RD, Pearlman S, Freidman WH, et al: Benign cystic vs. solid lesions of the parotid gland in HIV patients. Head Neck 13:522–527, 1991.

59. Hoffman E: Branchial cysts within the parotid gland. Ann Surg 152:290–295, 1960.

60. Fishleder A, Tubbs R, Hesse B, et al: Uniform detection of immunoglobin-gene rearrangements in benign lymphoepithelial lesions. N Engl J Med 316:1118–1121, 1987.

61. Finfer MD, Schinella RA, Rothstein SG, et al: Cystic parotid lesions in patients at risk for the acquired immunodeficiency syndrome. Arch Otolaryngol Head Neck Surg 114:1290–1294, 1988.

62. Shugar JM, Som PM, Jacobson AL, et al: Multicentric parotid cysts and cervical lymphadenopathy in AIDS patients. A newly recognized entity. CT and MR manifestations. Laryngoscope 98:772–775, 1988.

63. Quinnan GV, Masur H, Rook AH, et al: Herpes virus infections in the acquired immunodeficiency syndrome. JAMA 252:72–77, 1984.

64. Kanas RJ, Jensen JL, Abrams AM, et al: Oral mucosal cytomegalovirus as a manifestation of the acquired immune deficiency syndrome. Oral Surg Oral Med Oral Pathol 64:183–189, 1987.

65. Phelan JA, Eisig S, Freedman PD, et al: Major aphthous-like ulcers in patients with AIDS. Oral Surg Oral Med Oral Pathol 71:68–72, 1991.

66. Scully C, Laskaris G, Pindborg J, et al: Oral manifestations of HIV infection and their management. I. More common lesions. Oral Med Oral Surg Oral Pathol 71:158–166, 1991.

67. Dodaro J, Singh B, Har-El G, et al: Mimics of laryngeal carcinoma in patients with AIDS. Presented at the American Laryngological, Rhinological, and Otological Society, Eastern Section Meeting, Pittsburgh, Pennsylvania, January 28, 1995.

68. Singh B, Balwally AN, Nash M, et al: Laryngeal tuberculosis in HIV-infected patients: A difficult diagnosis. Laryngoscope 106:1238–1240, 1996.

69. Singh B, Balwally AN, Har-El G, et al: Isolated cervical tuberculosis in patients with HIV infection. Presented at the American Academy of Otolaryngology-Head and Neck Surgery Annual Meeting, Pittsburgh, Pennsylvania, September 20, 1994.

70. Dichtel WJ: Oral manifestations of human immunodeficiency virus infection. Otolaryngol Clin North Am 25:1211–1226, 1992.

71. Freidman-Klein AE, Saltzman BR: Clinical manifestations of classical, endemic African and epidemic AIDS-associated Kaposi's sarcoma. J Am Acad Dermatol 22:1237–1250, 1990.

72. Kaposi M: Classics in oncology. Idiopathic multiple pigmented sarcoma of skin. Cancer 32:342–347, 1982.

73. Safai B, Diaz B, Schwartz J: Malignant neoplasms associated with human immunodeficiency virus infection. CA Cancer J Clin 42:74–95, 1992.

74. Harwood AR, Osoba D, Hofstader SL, et al: Kaposi's sarcoma in recipients of renal transplants. Am J Med 67:759–765, 1984.

75. Penn I: Kaposi's sarcoma in organ transplant patients. Report of 20 cases. Transplantation 27:8–11, 1979.

76. Brooks JJ: Kaposi's sarcoma: A reversible hyperplasia. Lancet 2:1309–1311, 1986.

77. Beral V, Paterman TA, Berkelman RL, et al: Kaposi's sarcoma among persons with AIDS: A sexually transmitted infection? Lancet 335:123–128, 1990.

78. Siegal B, Levinton-Kriss S, Schiffner A, et al: Kaposi's sarcoma in immunosuppression. Possibly the result of a dual virus infection. Cancer 65:492–498, 1990.

79. Haverkos HW, Drotman DP, Morgan M: Prevalence of Kaposi's sarcoma among patients with AIDS. N Engl J Med 312:1518, 1985.

80. Revision of the case definition of acquired immune deficiency syndrome for national reporting—United States. MMWR Morb Mortal Wkly Rep 34:373–375, 1985.

81. Sarid R, Olsen SJ, Moore PS. Kaposi's sarcoma–associated herpesvirus: Epidemiology, virology, and molecular biology. Adv Virus Res 52:139–232, 1999.

82. Friedman-Klein AE, Saltzman BR, Cao Y, et al: Kaposi's sarcoma in an HIV-negative homosexual male. Lancet 335:168–169, 1990.

83. Safai B, Good RA: Kaposi's sarcoma: A review and recent developments. Clin Bull 10:62–69, 1990.

84. Harawi SJ, O'Hara CL: Pathology and Pathophysiology of AIDS- and HIV-Related Diseases. St Louis, Mosby-Year Book, 1989, pp 83–134.

85. Gnepp DR, Chandler W, Hyams V: Primary Kaposi's sarcoma of the head and neck. Ann Intern Med 100:107–114, 1984.

86. Marcusen D, Sooy CD: The otolaryngologic and head and neck manifestations of acquired immune deficiency syndrome (AIDS). Laryngoscope 95:401–405, 1985.

87. Abemayor E, Calcaterra TC: Kaposi's sarcoma and community acquired immune deficiency syndrome. An update with emphasis on its head and neck manifestations. Arch Otolaryngol 109:536–542, 1983.

88. Stafford SD, Herdman RCD, Forster S, et al: Kaposi's sarcoma of the head and neck in patients with AIDS. J Laryngol Otol 103:379–382, 1989.

89. Singh B, Har-El G, Lucente FE: Kaposi's sarcoma of the head and neck in patients with acquired immunodeficiency syndrome. Otolaryngol Head Neck Surg 111:618–624, 1994.

90. Epstein JB, Scully C: HIV infection: Clinical features and treatment of 36 homosexual men with Kaposi's sarcoma. Oral Surg Oral Med Oral Pathol 71:38–41, 1991.

91. Ficarra G, Berson AM, Silverman S, et al: Kaposi's sarcoma of the oral cavity: A study of 134 patients with a review of the pathogenesis, epidemiology, clinical aspects and treatment. Oral Surg Oral Med Oral Pathol 66:543–550, 1988.

92. Spittle MF: Diagnosis and treatment of Kaposi's sarcoma. J Antimicrob Chemother 23:127–135, 1989.

93. Emery CD, Wall SD, Federle MP, et al: Pharyngeal Kaposi's sarcoma in patients with AIDS. Am J Radiol 147:919–922, 1986.

94. Levy FE, Tansek KM: AIDS-associated Kaposi's sarcoma of the larynx. Ear Nose Throat J 69:177, 181–184, 1990.

95. Safai B, Johnson KG, Myskowski PL, et al: The natural history of Kaposi's sarcoma in the acquired immunodeficiency syndrome. Ann Intern Med 103:744–750, 1985.

96. Yeh C-K, Fox PC, Fox CH, et al: Kaposi's sarcoma of the parotid gland in acquired immunodeficiency syndrome. Oral Surg Oral Med Oral Pathol 67:308–312, 1989.

97. Gill PS, Bisher A, Colletti P, et al: Pulmonary Kaposi's sarcoma: Clinical findings and results of therapy. Am J Med 87:57–61, 1989.

98. Edinburgh KJ, Jasmer RM, Huang L, et al: Multiple pulmonary nodes in AIDS: Usefulness of CT in distinguishing among potential causes. Radiology 214:427–432, 2000.

99. Kovacs JA, Masur H: Opportunistic Infections. In AIDS: Etiology, Diagnosis, Treatment and Prevention, 2nd ed. Philadelphia, JB Lippincott, 1988, pp 199–225.

100. Longo DL, Steis G, Lane HC, et al: Malignancies in AIDS patients: Natural history, treatment strategies, and preliminary results. Ann N Y Acad Sci 437:421–430, 1985.

101. Update: AIDS—Europe. MMWR Morb Mortal Wkly Rep 35:35–46, 1986.

102. Chachoua A, Krigel R, Lafleur F, et al: Prognostic factors and staging classification of patients with epidemic Kaposi's sarcoma. J Clin Oncol 7:744–750, 1989.

103. Moskowitz L, Hensley GT, Chan JC, et al: Immediate causes of death in acquired immunodeficiency syndrome. Arch Pathol Lab Med 109:735–738, 1985.

104. Lilenbaum RC, Ratner L: Systemic treatment of Kaposi's sarcoma: Current status and future directions. AIDS 8:141–151, 1994.

105. Groopman JE: Biology and therapy of epidemic Kaposi's sarcoma. Cancer 58:633–637, 1987.

106. Volberding P, Abrams DI, Conant M, et al: Vinblastine therapy for Kaposi's sarcoma in the acquired immune deficiency syndrome. Ann Intern Med 103:335–338, 1985.

107. Mintzer D, Real FX, Jovino L, et al: Treatment of Kaposi's sarcoma and thrombocytopenia with vincristine in patients with acquired immune deficiency syndrome. Ann Intern Med 102:200–202, 1985.

108. Laubenstein LJ, Krigel RL, Odajnyk CM, et al: Treatment of epidemic Kaposi's sarcoma with etoposide or a combination of doxorubicin, bleomycin, and vinblastine. J Clin Oncol 2:1115–1120, 1984.

109. Schwartsmann G, Sprinz E, Kronfeld M, et al: Phase II study of teniposide in patients with AIDS-related Kaposi's sarcoma. Eur J Cancer 27:1637–1639, 1991.

110. Lassoued K, Clauvel JP, Katlama C, et al: Treatment of acquired immunodeficiency syndrome–related Kaposi's sarcoma with bleomycin as a single agent. Cancer 66:1869–1872, 1990.

111. Mintzer DM, Real FX, Jovino L, et al: Treatment of Kaposi's sarcoma and thrombocytopenia with vincristine in patients with acquired immunodeficiency syndrome. Ann Intern Med 102:200–202, 1985.

112. Brunt AM, Goodman AG, Philips RH, et al: The safety of intravenous chemotherapy and zidovudine when treating epidemic Kaposi's sarcoma. AIDS 3:457–460, 1989.

113. Gill PS, Rarick MU, Byron E, et al: Advanced acquired immune deficiency syndrome–related Kaposi's sarcoma. Results of pilot studies using combination chemotherapy. Cancer 65:1074–1078, 1990.

114. Pluda JM, Parkinson DR, Feigalal E, et al: Non-cytotoxic approaches to the treatment of HIV-associated Kaposi's sarcoma. Oncology 7:25–33, 1993.

115. Krown SE: Interferon and other biologic agents for the treatment of Kaposi's sarcoma. Hematol Oncol Clin North Am 5:311–322, 1991.

116. Krigel RL, Padavic SK, Rudolph AR, et al: Exacerbation of epidemic Kaposi's sarcoma with the combination of interleukin-2 and beta-interferon: Results of a phase 2 study. J Biol Response Mod 8:359–365, 1989.

117. Gagliario A, Collins DC: Inhibition of oncogenesis by anti-estrogens. Cancer Res 53:533–535, 1993.

118. Von Roenn J, Von Gunten C, Mullane M, et al: All-trans retinoic acid (TRA) in the treatment of AIDS-related Kaposi's sarcoma: A phase II study. Illinois Cancer Center Study (abstract). Proc Am Soc Clin Oncol 12:51–59, 1993.

119. Mitsuyasu RT: Interferon-alpha in the treatment of AIDS-related Kaposi's sarcoma. Br J Haematol 79:s69–s73, 1991.

120. Evans LM, Itri LM, Campion M, et al: Interferon-alpha-2a in the treatment of acquired immune deficiency-related Kaposi's sarcoma. J Immunother 10:39–50, 1991.

121. Kovacs JA, Deyton L, Davy R, et al: Combined zidovudine and interferon-alpha therapy in patients with Kaposi's sarcoma and acquired immunodeficiency syndrome (AIDS). Ann Intern Med 111:280–287, 1989.

122. Krown SE, Gold JWM, Niedwiecki D, et al: Interferon-alpha with zidovudine: Safety, tolerance, and clinical virologic effects in patients with Kaposi's sarcoma associated with the acquired immune deficiency syndrome (AIDS). Ann Intern Med 112:812–821, 1990.

123. Fischl MA, Uttamchandani RB, Resnick L, et al: A Phase I study of recombinant human interferon-alpha-2a or human lymphoblastoid interferon alpha-n1 and concomitant zidovudine in patients with AIDS-related Kaposi's sarcoma. J Acquir Immune Defic Syndr 4:1–10, 1991.

124. Hodgkin T: On some morbid appearances of the absorbent glands and spleen. Med Chir Trans 17:68–114, 1832.

125. Seif GS, Spriggs AI: Chromosomal changes in Hodgkin's disease. J Natl Cancer Inst 39:557–570, 1967.

126. Kersey JH, Spector BD, Good RA: Primary immunodeficiency diseases and cancer: The immunodeficiency-cancer registry. Int J Cancer 12:333–347, 1973.

127. Penn I: The occurrence of malignant tumors in immunocompromised states. Prog Allergy 37:259–300, 1986.

128. Beral V, Peterman T, Berkelman R, et al: AIDS-associated non-Hodgkin lymphoma. Lancet 337:805–809, 1991.

129. Doll DC, List AF: Burkitt's lymphoma in a homosexual (letter). Lancet 1:1026–1027, 1982.

130. Opportunistic non-Hodgkin's lymphoma among severely immuno-compromised HIV-infected patients surviving for prolonged periods on anti-retroviral therapy—United States. MMWR Morb Mortal Wkly Rep 40:591–600, 1991.

131. Revision of CDC surveillance case definition for the acquired immunodeficiency syndrome. MMWR Morb Mortal Wkly Rep 36:1s–15s, 1987.

132. Kaplan LD, Abrams DI, Feigal E, et al: AIDS-associated non-Hodgkin's lymphoma in San Francisco. JAMA 261:719–724, 1989.

133. Levine AM: Acquired immunodeficiency syndrome–related lymphoma. Blood 80:8–20, 1992.

134. Purtilo DT, Stevenson M: Lymphotrophic viruses as etiologic agents of lymphoma. Hematol Oncol Clin North Am 5:901–923, 1991.

135. Kieff E, Dambaugh T, Hummel M, et al: Epstein Barr virus transformation and replication. Adv Viral Oncol 3:133–182, 1983.

136. Hanto DW, Gajl-Peczalska KJ, Fizzera G, et al: Epstein Barr virus (EBV) induced polyclonal and monoclonal B-cell lymphoproliferative diseases occurring after renal transplantation: Clinical, pathologic, and virologic findings and implications for therapy. Ann Surg 198:356–369, 1983.

137. Lane HC, Fauci AS: Immunologic abnormalities in acquired immunodeficiency syndrome. Ann Rev Immunol 3:477–500, 1985.

138. Greenspan JS, Greenspan D, Lennette ET, et al: Replication of EBV within epithelial cells of oral "hairy" leukoplakia, an AIDS associated lesion. N Engl J Med 313:1564–1571, 1985.

139. Belton CM, Eversole LR: Oral hairy leukoplakia: Ultrastructural features. J Oral Pathol 15:493–499, 1986.

140. Shibata D, Weiss LM, Nathwani BN, et al: Epstein-Barr virus in benign lymph node biopsies from individuals infected with the human immunodeficiency virus is associated with the concurrent or subsequent development of non-Hodgkin's lymphoma. Blood 77:1527–1533, 1991.

141. Neri A, Barrigia F, Inghirami G, et al: Epstein Barr virus infection preceded clonal expansion in Burkitt's and acquired immunodeficiency syndrome–associated lymphoma. Blood 77:1092–1095, 1991.

142. Ernberg I, Altiok E: The role of Epstein-Barr virus in lymphomas of HIV carriers. APMIS 8:58–61, 1989.

143. Subar M, Neri A, Inghirami G, et al: Frequent c-*myc* oncogene activation and infrequent presence of Epstein-Barr virus genome in AIDS-associated lymphoma. Blood 72:667–671, 1988.

144. Hamilton-Dutoit SJ, Pallesen G, Franzmann MB, et al: AIDS-related lymphoma: Histopathology, immunophenotype, and association with Epstein-Barr virus as demonstrated by in situ nucleic acid hybridization. Am J Pathol 138:149–163, 1991.

145. Yarchoan R, Redfield RR, Broder S: Mechanisms of B-cell activation in patients with acquired immunodeficiency syndrome and related disorders. Contribution of antibody-producing B cells, of Epstein-Barr virus infected B cells, and immunoglobin production induced by human T cell lymphotrophic virus, type III/lymphadenopathy associated virus. J Clin Invest 78:439–447, 1986.

146. Laurence J, Astrin SM: Human immunodeficiency virus induction of malignant transformation in human B lymphocytes. Proc Natl Acad Sci USA 88:7635–7639, 1991.

147. Finn D: Lymphoma of the head and neck and acquired immunodeficiency syndrome: Clinical investigation and immunohistochemical study. Laryngoscope 105:1–18, 1995.

148. Cotran RS, Kumar V, Robbins SL (eds): Robbins Pathologic Basis of Disease, 4th ed. Philadelphia, WB Saunders, 1989, pp 703–754.

149. Non-Hodgkin's Lymphoma Pathologic Classification Project: National Cancer Institute sponsored study of classifications of non-Hodgkin's lymphomas: Summary and descriptions of a working formulation for clinical usage. Cancer 49:2112–2135, 1982.

150. Biggar RJ: AIDS-related cancers in the era of highly active antiretroviral therapy. Oncology 15:439–448; discussion 448–449, 2001.

151. Lowenthal DA, Straus DJ, Campbell SW, et al: AIDS-related lymphoid neoplasia: The Memorial Hospital experience. Cancer 61:2325–2337, 1988.

152. Knowles DM, Chamulak GA, Subar M, et al: Lymphoid neoplasia associated with the acquired immune deficiency syndrome (AIDS). The New York University Medical Center experience with 105 patients (1981–1986). Ann Intern Med 108:744–753, 1988.

153. Pluda JM, Broder S, Yarchoan R: Therapy of AIDS and AIDS-associated neoplasms. Cancer Chemother Biol Response Mod 13:404–439, 1992.

154. Ioachim HL, Dorsett B, Cronin W, et al: Acquired immunodeficiency syndrome–associated lymphomas: Clinical, pathologic, immunologic, and viral characteristics of 111 cases. Hum Pathol 22:659–673, 1991.

155. Raphael M, Gentilhomme O, Tulliez M, et al: Histopathological features of high-grade non-Hodgkin's lymphoma in acquired immunodeficiency syndrome. Arch Pathol Lab Med 115:15–20, 1991.

156. Monfardini S, Tirelli U, Vaccher E, et al: Malignant lymphoma in patients with or at risk for AIDS: A report of 50 cases observed in Italy. Cancer Detect Prev 12:237–241, 1988.

157. Wong D, Fuller L, Butler J, et al: Extranodal non-Hodgkin's lymphoma of the head and neck. Am J Radiol 123:471–481, 1975.

158. Brugere J, Schlieng M, Gerard-Merchant R, et al: Non-Hodgkin's malignant lymphoma of the upper digestive and respiratory tracts: Natural history and results of radiotherapy. Br J Cancer 31:435–440, 1975.

159. Remick SC, Diamond C, Migliozzi JA, et al: Primary central nervous system lymphoma in patients with and without the acquired immune deficiency syndrome: A retrospective analysis and review of the literature. Medicine 69:345–360, 1990.

160. Rosenblum M, Levy ML, Bredesen DE: Primary central nervous system lymphomas in patients with AIDS. Ann Neurol 23:S13–S16, 1988.

161. Zuger A, Louie E, Holzman RS, et al: Cryptococcal disease in patients with the acquired immunodeficiency syndrome. Ann Intern Med 104:234–240, 1986.

162. Berger JR, Moskowitz L, Fischl M, et al: Neurologic disease as the presenting manifestation of acquired immunodeficiency syndrome. South Med J 80:683–686, 1987.

163. Price RW, Brew B: Management of the neurologic complications of HIV infection and AIDS. In Sande MA, Volberding PA (eds): The Medical Management of AIDS. Philadelphia, WB Saunders, 1988, pp 111–126.

164. Goldstein JD, Zeifer B, Chao C, et al: CT appearance of primary central nervous system lymphoma in patients with acquired immunodeficiency syndrome. J Comput Assist Tomogr 15:39–44, 1991.

165. Levy LM, Bredesen DE, Rosenblum ML: Neurological manifestations of the acquired immunodeficiency syndrome (AIDS): Experience at UCSF and review of the literature. J Neurosurg 62:475–495, 1985.

166. Li CY, Witzig TE, Phyliky RL, et al: Diagnosis of B-cell non-Hodgkin's lymphoma of the central nervous system by immunohistochemical analysis of cerebrospinal fluid lymphocytes. Cancer 57:737–744, 1986.

167. Murray K, Kun L, Cox J: Primary malignant lymphoma of the central nervous system: Results of treatment of 11 cases and review of the literature. J Neurosurg 65:600–607, 1986.

168. Leess FR, Kessler DJ, Mickel RA: Non-Hodgkin's lymphoma of the head and neck in patients with AIDS. Arch Otolaryngol Head Neck Surg 113:1104–1106, 1987.

169. Cobleigh MA, Kennedy JL: Non-Hodgkin's lymphomas of the upper aerodigestive tract and salivary glands. Otolaryngol Clin North Am 19:685–710, 1986.

170. Rosenberg SA, Berard CW, Brown BW, et al: National Cancer Institute sponsored study of non-Hodgkin's lymphomas: Summary and description of a working formulation for clinical usage. Cancer 49:2112–2135, 1982.

171. Gallagher CJ, Gregory WM, Jones AE, et al: Follicular lymphoma: Prognostic factors for response and survival. J Clin Oncol 4:1470–1480, 1986.

172. Remick SC, Diamond C, Migliozzi JA, et al: Primary central nervous system lymphoma in patients with and without the acquired immunodeficiency syndrome: A retrospective analysis and review of the literature. Medicine (Baltimore) 69:345–360, 1990.

173. Levine AM, Loureiro C, Sullivan-Halley J, et al: HIV positive high or intermediate grade lymphomas: Prognostic factors related to survival (abstract). Blood 72:247a, 1988.

174. Broder S, Karp JE: The expanding challenge of HIV associated malignancies. CA Cancer Clin J 42:69–73, 1992.

175. Gill PS, Levine AM, Krailo M, et al: AIDS-related malignant lymphoma: Results of prospective treatment trials. J Clin Oncol 5:1322–1328, 1987.

176. Kaplan LD: AIDS-associated lymphoma. Infect Dis Clin North Am 2:525–532, 1988.

177. Kaplan LD, Kahn JO, Crowe S, et al: Clinical and virological effects of recombinant granulocyte-macrophage colony-stimulating factor in patients receiving chemotherapy for human immunodeficiency virus–associated non-Hodgkin's lymphoma: Results of a randomized trial. J Clin Oncol 9:929–940, 1991.

178. Levine AM, Wernz JC, Kaplan LD, et al: Low dose chemotherapy with CNS prophylaxis and zidovudine maintenance for AIDS related lymphoma: Follow-up data from a multi-institutional trial (abstract). Blood 74:897a, 1989.

179. Formenti SC, Gill PS, Lean E, et al: Primary central nervous system lymphoma in AIDS: Results of radiation therapy. Cancer 63:1101–1107, 1989.

180. Goldstein JD, Dickson DW, Moser FG, et al: Primary central nervous system lymphoma in acquired immunodeficiency syndrome: A clinical and pathological study, with results of treatment with radiation. Cancer 67:2756–2765, 1991.

181. Schoeppel SL, Hoppe RT, Dorfman RF, et al: Hodgkin's disease in homosexual men with generalized lymphadenopathy. Ann Intern Med 102:68–70, 1985.

182. Bernstein L, Levin D, Menck H, et al: AIDS-related secular trends in cancer in Los Angeles County men: A comparison by marital status. Cancer Res 49:466–470, 1989.

183. Ames ED, Conjalka MS, Goldberg AF, et al: Hodgkin's disease in AIDS: Twenty-three new cases and a review of the literature. Hematol Oncol Clin North Am 5:343–356, 1991.

184. Poluri A, Shah KG, Carew JF, et al: Hodgkin's disease of the head and neck in human immunodeficiency virus–infected patients. Am J Otolaryngol 23:12–16, 2002.

185. Singh B, Balwally AN, Shaha AR, et al: Upper aerodigestive tract squamous cell carcinoma. The human immunodeficiency virus connection. Arch Otolaryngol Head Neck Surg 122:639–643, 944, 1996.

186. Roland JT, Rothstein SG, Mittal KR, et al: Squamous cell carcinoma in HIV-positive patients under 45. Laryngoscope 103:509–511, 1993.

187. Clark RM, Rosen IB, Laperriere NJ: Malignant tumors of the head and neck in a young population. Am J Surg 144:459–462, 1982.

188. Mendez P, Maves MD, Panje WR: Squamous cell carcinoma of the head and neck in patients under 40 years of age. Arch Otolaryngol 111:762–764, 1985.

189. Lindberg R: Distribution of cervical lymph node metastasis from squamous cell carcinoma of the upper respiratory and digestive tracts. Cancer 29:1446–1449, 1972.

190. Shah JP, Medina JE, Shaha AR: Cervical lymph node metastasis. Curr Probl Surg 30:1–335, 1993.

191. Penn I: Immunosuppression and skin cancer. Clin Plast Surg 7: 361–368, 1980.

192. Gupta AK, Cardella CJ, Naberman HF: Cutaneous malignant neoplasms in patients with renal transplant. Arch Dermatol 12:1288–1293, 1986.

193. Maize JE: Skin cancer in immunosuppressed patients. JAMA 237: 1857–1858, 1977.

194. Barr BB, Benton EC, McLaren K, et al: Human papillomavirus infection and skin cancer in renal allograft recipients. Lancet 1:124–129, 1989.

195. Scotto J, Fears T, Fraumeni J: Incidence of nonmelanomatous skin cancer in the United States. Washington, DC, U.S. Dept of Health and Human Services, Publication No. (NIH)83–2433, 1983.

196. Smith KJ, Skelton HG, Yeager J, et al: Cutaneous neoplasms in a military population of HIV-1–positive patients. J Am Acad Dermatol 29:400–406, 1993.

197. Sitz KV, Keppen M, Johnson DF: Metastatic basal cell carcinoma in acquired immunodeficiency syndrome–related complex. JAMA 257:340–343, 1987.

198. Hruza GJ, Snow SN: Basal cell carcinoma in a patient with acquired immunodeficiency syndrome: Treatment with Moh's micrographic surgery fixed-tissue technique. J Dermatol Surg Oncol 15: 545–551, 1989.

199. Fisher BK, Warner LC: Cutaneous manifestations of acquired immunodeficiency syndrome: Update 1987. Int J Dermatol 26: 615–630, 1987.

200. Myskowski PL, Straus DJ, Safai B: Lymphoma and other HIV associated malignancies. J Am Acad Dermatol 22:1253–1260, 1990.

201. Lobo DV, Chu PC, Grekin RC, et al: Nonmelanoma skin cancers and infection with human immunodeficiency virus. Arch Dermatol 128:623–627, 1992.

202. Greene MH, Young TI, Clark WH Jr: Malignant melanoma in renal transplant recipients. Lancet 1:1196–1199, 1981.

203. Van Ginkel CJW, Tjon Lim Sang R, Blauwgeers JLG, et al: Multiple primary malignant melanomas in an HIV infected man. J Am Acad Dermatol 24:284–285, 1991.

204. Krause W, Mittag H, Gieler U, et al: A case of malignant melanoma in a man seropositive for human immunodeficiency virus. Arch Dermatol 123:867–868, 1987.

205. Gupta S, Imam A: Malignant melanoma in a homosexual man with HTLV-III/LAV exposure. Am J Med 82:1027–1030, 1987.

206. Rasokat H, Steigleder GK, Bendick C, et al: Malignes Melanom und HIV-Infektion. Z Hautkr 64:581–587, 1989.

207. Rivers JK, Kopf AW, Postel AH: Malignant melanoma in a man seropositive for human immunodeficiency virus. J Am Acad Dermatol 20:1127–1128, 1989.

208. McGregor JM, Newell M, Ross J, et al: Cutaneous malignant melanoma and human immunodeficiency virus infection: A report of three cases. Br J Dermatol 126:519, 1992.

209. Tindall B, Finlayson R, Mutimer K, et al: Malignant melanoma associated with human immunodeficiency virus infection in three homosexual men. J Am Acad Dermatol 20:587–591, 1989.

210. Cockerell CJ, Freidman-Klein AE: Skin manifestations of HIV infection. Prim Care 16:621–644, 1989.

211. Voelkerding KV, Sandhaus LM, Kim HC, et al: Plasma cell malignancy in the acquired immune deficiency syndrome. Association with Epstein-Barr virus. Am J Clin Pathol 92:222–228, 1989.

212. Pizarro A, Gamallo C, Sanchez-Munoz JF, et al: Extramedullary plasmacytoma and AIDS-related Kaposi's sarcoma. J Am Acad Dermatol 30:797–800, 1994.

213. Bataille R: Localized plasmacytomas. Clin Hematol 11:113–122, 1982.

214. Meis JM, Butler JJ, Osborne BM, et al: Solitary plasmacytomas of the bone and extramedullary plasmacytomas: A clinicopathologic and immunohistochemical study. Cancer 59:1475–1485, 1987.

215. Gastaut J, Quilichini R, Horchowski N, et al: Localized extramedullary plasmacytomas (LEP) and HIV (abstract). In IV International Conference on AIDS Program and Abstract Book, vol 2, 1988, p 327.

216. Karnad AB, Martin AW, Koh HK, et al: Nonsecretory multiple myeloma in a 26-year-old man with acquired immunodeficiency syndrome, presenting with multiple extramedullary plasmacytomas and osteolytic bone disease. Am J Hematol 32:305–310, 1989.

217. Gold JE, Schwam ML, Castella A, et al: Malignant plasma cell tumors in human immunodeficiency virus–infected patients. Cancer 66: 363–368, 1990.

218. Finn DG: Lymphoma of the head and neck and acquired immunodeficiency syndrome: Clinical investigation and immunohistological study. Laryngoscope 105:1–18, 1995.

219. Barlogie B, Smallwood L, Smith TL, et al: High serum levels of lactic dehydrogenase identify a high-grade lymphoma-like myeloma. Ann Intern Med 110:521–525, 1989.

220. Dimopoulos MA, Barlogie B, Smith TL, et al: High serum lactate dehydrogenase level as a marker for drug resistance and short survival in multiple myeloma. Ann Intern Med 115:831–935, 1991.

221. Gold JE: Plasma cell tumors and the acquired immune deficiency syndrome (letter). Am J Hematol 34:234, 1990.

222. Rana S, Nunlee-Bland G, Valyasevi R, et al: Thyroid dysfunction in HIV-infected children: Is L-thyroxine therapy beneficial? Pediatr AIDS HIV Infect 7:424–428, 1996.

223. Basilio-De-Oliveira CA: Infectious and neoplastic disorders of the thyroid in AIDS patients: An autopsy study. Braz J Infect Dis 4:67–75, 2000.

224. Kubler-Ross E: On Death and Dying. New York, Macmillan, 1969.

225. Lucente FE: Treatment of head-and-neck carcinoma with noncurative intent. Am J Otolaryngol 15:99–102, 1994.

226. Walsh TD: An overview of palliative care in cancer and AIDS. Oncology 5:7–11, 1991.

CHAPTER 26

Lymphomas Presenting in the Head and Neck: Current Issues in Diagnosis and Management

Maria A. Rodriguez

INTRODUCTION

Lymphomas are a heterogeneous group of lymphoproliferative disorders that are broadly subclassified as Hodgkin's lymphoma and non-Hodgkin's lymphomas.[1] Under the current classification system, the non-Hodgkin's lymphomas are further subcategorized as B-cell and T-cell disorders. These diseases present most frequently with lymphadenopathy and often involve the head and neck region. Hodgkin's lymphomas very rarely present with extranodal disease, whereas non-Hodgkin's lymphomas may present with extranodal masses as their primary disease presentation. The gastrointestinal (GI) tract is the most frequent site of extranodal disease, followed by other nonlymphatic sites in the head and neck region.

Lymphomas, as a whole, are both chemosensitive and radiation-sensitive tumors and thus constitute a group of malignancies that may be curable. Distinction of lymphomas from carcinomas and other malignancies is therefore critical in treatment planning. The objective of this chapter is to review the clinical presentation, diagnostic methods, staging, and treatment of this group of diseases with emphasis on patient treatment when presentation includes localized lymph node or extranodal disease in the head and neck region.

CLINICAL PRESENTATION

Lymphoma most often presents as a painless nodal mass. These masses may become painful if the rate of growth of the lymphoma is rapid, causing central necrosis of the lymph nodes. This is most often seen in lymphomas such as Burkitt's or lymphoblastic lymphoma but sometimes may also be a manifestation of certain aggressive large cell lymphomas. Hodgkin's disease rarely presents in extranodal sites in the head and neck area (Table 26–1). Non-Hodgkin's lymphoma, however, often presents with extranodal disease in Waldeyer's ring.[2] The tonsil and the nasopharynx are the most common sites in this area to be involved by disease. Symptoms related to presentation include a sore throat, globus sensation, dysphagia, and hearing loss secondary to otitis media. Patients with disease in the nasal cavity and paranasal sinuses, which are the second most common extranodal sites in the head and neck region, can present with symptoms and signs of nasal obstruction, sinusitis, bloody drainage, or pain. Less frequent sites of involvement include the thyroid gland, the orbit, and the parotid gland. Classic systemic symptoms of lymphoma include fever, night sweats, and weight loss, but relatively few patients with truly localized presentations in the head and neck area manifest these constitutional symptoms.

IMMUNOHISTOLOGIC CLASSIFICATION

Lymphomas are currently classified by the internationally recognized World Health Organization system, which is derived from the Revised European-American Lymphoid (REAL) malignancy classification. This current system of classification divides the lymphomas into three broad categories: (1) Hodgkin's lymphoma, (2) B-cell disorders, and (3) T-cell disorders (Table 26–2).

Hodgkin's Lymphoma

Hodgkin's lymphoma is now recognized to be a disorder of B-lymphocytes, although it is subcategorized separately

TABLE 26-1 Clinical Features of Lymphomas

Hodgkin's	Non-Hodgkin's
Lymph nodes are involved in an anatomic contiguous pattern	Noncontiguous lymph node involvement is common
Extranodal disease is rare	Extranodal disease is common; most frequent sites of involvement include gastrointestinal tract, Waldeyer's ring, testes, bone marrow, and liver
Localized or contiguous nodal disease is common	Localized nodal disease is rare

TABLE 26-2 Revised European-American Lymphoma (REAL) Classification

B-Cell Neoplasms

I. °Precursor B-cell neoplasms: Precursor B-lymphoblastic leukemia or lymphoma
II. Peripheral B-cell neoplasms
    1. B-cell chronic lymphocytic leukemia or prolymphocytic leukemia or small lymphocytic leukemia
    2. Lymphoplasmacytoid lymphoma or immunocytoma
    °3. Mantle cell lymphoma
    4. Follicular center lymphoma; follicular provisional grades: 1, small cell; 2, mixed; 3, large cell°; provisional subtype: Diffuse, predominantly small cell type
    5. Marginal zone B-cell lymphoma, extranodal (MALT type ± monocytoid B-cells), provisional subtype: Nodal (monocytoid B-cells)
    6. Provisional entity: Splenic marginal zone lymphoma (± villous lymphocytes)
    7. Hairy cell leukemia
    8. Plasmacytoma or plasma cell myeloma
    °9. Diffuse, large B-cell lymphoma subtype: Primary mediastinal B-cell lymphoma
    °10. Burkitt's lymphoma
    °11. Provisional entity: High-grade B-cell lymphoma, Burkitt's-like

T-Cell and Putative NK-Cell Neoplasms

I. °Precursor T-cell neoplasms: Precursor T-lymphoblastic lymphoma or leukemia
II. Peripheral T-cell and NK-cell neoplasms
    1. T-cell chronic lymphocytic leukemia or prolymphocytic leukemia
    2. Large granular lymphocyte leukemia: T-cell type, NK-cell type
    3. Mycosis fungoides or Sézary syndrome
    °4. Peripheral T-cell lymphomas, unspecified
    °5. Angioimmunoblastic T-cell lymphoma
    °6. Angiocentric lymphoma
    °7. Intestinal T-cell lymphoma (± enteropathy associated)
    °8. Adult T-cell leukemia or lymphoma
    °9. Anaplastic large cell lymphoma, CD30+, T- and null-cell types
    °10. Provisional entity: Anaplastic large cell lymphoma, Hodgkin's-like

Hodgkin's Disease

  I. Lymphocyte predominance
  II. Nodular sclerosis
  III. Mixed cellularity
  IV. Lymphocyte depletion
  V. Provisional entity: Lymphocyte-rich classic Hodgkin's disease

---

°Clinically aggressive non-Hodgkin's lymphoma.
MALT, mucosa-associated lymphoid tissue; NK, natural killer.

owing to its unique immunohistology and clinical behavior. Histologically, Hodgkin's lymphoma classically shows a marked pleomorphic lymphoproliferative reaction, giving it an appearance distinct from the more monomorphic appearance of the non-Hodgkin's lymphoma.[3] Evidence for the histogenesis of this disease comes from cytogenetic and molecular genetic data that demonstrate immunoglobulin gene rearrangements in Reed-Sternberg cell–enriched isolates from lymph node biopsies.[4, 5] Cytogenetics demonstrates frequent abnormalities of chromosome 14, the chromosome that (1) contains the heavy chain immunoglobulin genes and (2) is most often rearranged in B-cell non-Hodgkin's lymphoma.[6, 7] The pattern of surface antigen expression in Hodgkin's disease, however, is different from that in B-cell disorders, with one exception. The behavior

and phenotypic expression of lymphocyte-predominant Hodgkin's disease are similar to those of indolent B-cell disorders.

Non-Hodgkin's Lymphomas: B-Cell and T-Cell Disorders

Histology

Lymphomas are described according to two primary histologic features of the lymphoid tissue: (1) *architectural pattern*—the lymph node may retain the follicular pattern of the normal lymphoid follicles, or this pattern may be completely erased with the malignant lymphocytes seen in a diffuse pattern, and (2) *cell type*—the lymphocytes may be of various sizes from small to large, or cell sizes may be mixed; also, they may exhibit certain nuclear characteristics that may be described as cleaved or noncleaved, with various degrees of chromatin density.

Immunochemistry

The most common lymphomas, which are of B-cell origin, constitute approximately 75% to 80% of all lymphomas. T-cell lymphomas account for 10% to 15%, and Hodgkin's lymphoma is noted in fewer than 10% of all lymphomas. Immunohistochemical markers that aid in the diagnosis of B-cell lymphoma include expression of the light chain kappa or lambda on the cell surface or in the cytoplasm, expression of heavy chains in the cytoplasm, and expression of pan-B-cell markers on the cell surface (Table 26-3). T-cell lymphomas express either mature T-cell antigen markers, such as T-helper or T-suppressor antigen, or T-cell differentiation markers.

Clinical Behavior: Indolent Versus Aggressive

Both B- and T-cell lymphomas may be either indolent or aggressive in their behavior. The definitions of *indolent* and *aggressive* rest on the expected survival of patients at 5 years. Members of an international study group looked at the frequency of the various subtypes of lymphoma according to the REAL classification and the clinical course.[8] They designated two groups according to survival. Indolent lymphomas have a 50% or better life expectancy at 5 years, and aggressive lymphomas have less than a 50% survival rate.

Although indolent lymphomas are anticipated to have the longest median survival, they are almost uniformly incurable, unless limited to localized stage of disease in lymph node areas. Remissions are readily obtained with a number of chemotherapeutic and immunotherapeutic modalities. However, indolent lymphomas tend to recur until they become completely refractory to therapy and are ultimately fatal. Aggressive lymphomas, on the other hand, are potentially curable with chemotherapy, although the expected fraction of cured patients varies depending on the stage of disease at presentation and the patient's risk score. The most widely recognized system of risk score is the International Prognostic Index, which takes into account primarily clinical features of the illness (Table 26-4).[9] A large body of evidence, however, indicates that many other biologic factors play a role in the behavior of the

TABLE 26-3 Immunophenotypic Profile of the More Common Lymphomas

	CD20	CD5	CD3	CD23	CD10	FMC7	CD30	Leu ML
B CLL/small lymphocytic	+	+	−	+	−	−	−	−
Mantle cell	+	+	−	−	−	+	−	−
Follicular	+	−	−	−	+	−	−	−
Immunocytoma	+	−	−	−	−	+	−	−
Marginal zone	+	−	−	+/−	−	+	−	−
T-cell	−	+	+	−	−	−	−	−
"B" large cell	+	−°	−	−	+/−	−	−	−
Hodgkin's	−°	−	−	−	−	−	+	+

°Rarely (+).
B CLL, B-cell chronic lymphocytic leukemia.

lymphomas, although these are not currently incorporated into any formal risk prognosis system. T-cell lymphomas in general may have a worse prognosis than B-cell lymphomas.[10–12]

ETIOLOGY

The underlying etiology of lymphoma, as with most malignancies, is not known. However, a number of factors may be associated with these disorders. Exposure to certain environmental toxins or irradiation, for example, may be implicated. Exposure to various organic substances, such as phenoxy acids, chlorophenols, dioxins, and benzenes, has been found to have some correlation with increased incidence of lymphoma.[13, 14] Occupations in which exposure to these agents may occur are associated with a higher-than-normal risk for lymphoma; these include woodworking industries, agriculture, rubber and petrochemical industries, and dry cleaning occupations.

Survivors of the Nagasaki and Hiroshima nuclear blasts have been studied for long-term health effects of irradiation. Lymphomas have occurred at an increased rate, but the age of onset is much later than that of leukemia, with the average time of onset for lymphomas being approximately 20 years after exposure.[15] Data from participants in the U.S. nuclear test "Smoky" show no significant increase in risk for lymphoma, although one study of Mormon families living near the Nevada test site has revealed a small but significant increase in the incidence of lymphomas.[16, 17]

In addition to environmental factors, infection may cause or predispose the host to lymphoma. The one bacterial

TABLE 26-4 5-Year Survival Rate (%) According to International Prognostic Index Risk

Risk Group	Number of Risk Factors*	All Patients (n = 2031)	Age ≤ 60	Age > 60
Low	0 or 1	73	83	56
Low intermediate	2	51	69	44
High intermediate	3	43	46	37
High	4 or 5	26	32	21

*One risk point awarded for each of the following factors at presentation: Age > 60 years; lactate dehydrogenase > normal; Ann Arbor stage III/IV; patient not fully ambulatory (Eastern Cooperative Oncology Group performance status 2 or more); 2 or more extranodal sites of disease.

infection that seems causally related to lymphoma is that caused by the *Helicobacter pylori* bacterium, which is linked to mucosa-associated lymphoid tissue (MALT) lymphoma in the stomach.[18] Epstein-Barr virus (EBV) has been implicated in the development of B-cell lymphomas in immune-compromised hosts and has been implicated in some patients with Hodgkin's disease or Burkitt's lymphoma. Immunosuppressed patients for whom an increased incidence of lymphoma is known include organ transplant recipients receiving prolonged immunosuppressive therapy, individuals with congenital combined immunodeficiency syndrome, and those with acquired immunodeficiency syndrome (AIDS).[19–25] EBV is a B-lymphocyte tropic virus that immortalizes the lymphocytes it infects. In a normal host, the T-lymphocyte–mediated immune system controls and checks the growth and proliferation of the infected B-lymphocyte pools. If the T-lymphocyte immune system is impaired, as is the case in the immunosuppressed conditions discussed previously, the proliferation of B-lymphocytes is uncontrolled, and what clinically manifests is a lymphadenopathy that appears to be polyclonal but that eventually becomes monoclonal as one of the B-lymphocyte clones becomes overtly malignant in behavior.[22]

EBV was originally isolated, in fact, from lymphomas of African children that had the clinically distinct presentation of a mass in the jaw and a histologically distinct appearance as well.[23] Initially described by Burkitt, these lymphomas are now known to be of B-cell origin. In the United States, however, a majority of cases of Burkitt's lymphoma, and indeed most cases of B-cell lymphoma other than the immunocompromised situations described here, do not manifest in any consistent manner the presence of EBV in the tumor cells. The nasal cavity lymphomas of T-cell/natural killer (NK)-cell subtype, on the other hand, are nearly always positive for EBV.[24–26]

In humans, the only virus that has been clearly shown to be the causative agent of a lymphoma is the retrovirus designated as human T-cell lymphotropic virus (HTLV-I).[27] This virus causes a T-lymphocyte malignancy that can be aggressive and fatal. This entity is rare in the United States but common in Japan, and it presents with leukemic and lymphomatous disease.[28] The HTLV-I virus, which was originally isolated from a patient in the United States, is an RNA retrovirus unique to humans.[29]

Finally, other unknown mechanisms of an immune nature may underlie the onset of lymphomas. An increased incidence of non-Hodgkin's lymphoma has been noted in diseases of disordered immunity, such as rheumatoid arthritis, celiac disease, and Sjögren's syndrome. Lymphomas of the thyroid arise most frequently in patients with a history of Hashimoto's thyroiditis or with the histologic findings of Hashimoto's thyroiditis at diagnosis of a lymphoma. Whether viruses also play a role in secondary lymphomas in these illnesses is not known.[30–34]

EPIDEMIOLOGY

The descriptions of epidemiology in this section refer to the population in the United States. The incidence of lymphoma has been increasing over the past 5 decades.[35] Although lymphomas account for less than 10% of all malignancies, they have a significant effect on health care in that they are one of the leading causes of cancer death in adolescents and young adults.

Hodgkin's lymphoma has a bimodal incidence curve, with the first peak occurring in teenagers to young adults, and the second peak noted in middle-aged adults (50 to 60 years old). There is a higher frequency among males than females. The incidence of non-Hodgkin's lymphomas rises steadily with age.[36] The distribution of histologies tends to be aggressive (high-grade, such as lymphoblastic and Burkitt's types) in children and adolescents, but indolent low-grade lymphoma tends to be more frequent among elderly adults (60 to 80 years old). A slightly higher incidence has been reported among males compared with females. The reported average age for Hodgkin's disease is 32 years, and for non-Hodgkin's lymphomas 42 years, thus leading to the ranking of lymphomas as fourth in total person-years of life lost among all the cancer deaths in the United States.

DIAGNOSTIC EVALUATION

Fine-Needle Aspiration

When a patient presents with a lesion in the head and neck region that is suspected to be lymphoma, a needle aspiration is useful in distinguishing a lymphoma from a carcinoma or other malignant process. Information that can be obtained from the cytologic specimen includes the phenotype (B or T), which is determined by either immunohistochemical studies or flow cytometric studies. In addition, if the sample is sufficiently large, cytogenetic studies may be obtained from a fine-needle aspiration specimen, along with molecular studies.[37] There are limitations, however, to the diagnostic capability of fine-needle aspiration. Because the classification of lymphomas also relies on the histologic pattern of the malignancy in the lymph node, a surgical biopsy specimen is necessary, particularly in the diagnosis of follicular lymphoma, and is *essential* for diagnosing Hodgkin's lymphoma. Fine-needle aspiration may also miss the diagnosis of lymphoma in cases in which a concurrent reactive hyperplasia may occur as a response to the lymphoma in the lymph node, or it may incorrectly suggest lymphoma in cases of benign conditions such as infectious mononucleosis in which individual cells may appear aberrant.

Biopsy

Biopsy of a representative lymph node is still the optimal diagnostic procedure for establishing the initial diagnosis and appropriate classification of lymphomas and is supported by National Comprehensive Cancer Network (NCCN) guidelines.[38] Optimal selection and handling of lymph nodes remain as recommended by Larson and colleagues.[39] The surgeon should select a biopsy site representative of the disease process. In cases in which more than one lymph node area is involved, the lymph node area with the most representative lymph nodes should be selected. Certain lymph node areas such as the parotid region and the submandibular area may not be representative of the malignancy because chronic inflammation may occur in these areas.

When an appropriate lymph node has been selected, the entire lymph node should be removed in one piece and its capsule maintained intact. It is important to handle the lymph node gently during surgery to avoid crush artifact, which makes diagnosis difficult. Biopsies of the tonsil, base of the tongue, and nasopharynx are done in the same manner as biopsy in squamous cell carcinoma. The pathologist should also be made aware that lymphoma is suspected in the case. It is important that the tissue be placed in a saline solution and transferred as quickly as possible to the laboratory. This prevents dehydration and distortion of the lymph node. The pathologist is responsible for technical factors as well. It is necessary that excellent sections of the lymph node be obtained so that the cytologic features of individual cells can be appreciated, because the nuclear characteristics of cells also play an important part in the determination of subclassification.

Electron Microscopy

In cases in which the lymphoma may be anaplastic, and differentiation among lymphoma, anaplastic carcinoma, and another malignant process is not clear with the use of the diagnostic tools discussed previously, electron microscopy may be helpful. The presence of desmosomes distinguishes lymphoma from a malignancy of epithelial origin. The finding of melanosomes confirms the diagnosis of a melanoma, and identification of neuroendocrine granules excludes the diagnosis of lymphoma.[40]

Immunohistochemical Studies

As has been mentioned previously, immunohistochemical studies are used in subdividing lymphomas according to their lineage, that is, B- or T-cell origin. Immunohistochemical studies may also be useful in distinguishing Hodgkin's lymphoma from other classifications of non-Hodgkin's lymphoma that can be confused with Hodgkin's lymphoma. The markers that are most useful in the identification of the most common subtypes of lymphoma are outlined in Table 26–3. In cases in which the diagnosis of lymphoma is also in question, additional surface marker studies such as keratin, mucin stain, or S100 may also be useful in excluding squamous cell carcinoma, adenocarcinoma, and melanoma, respectively.

TABLE 26-5 Distinct Chromosomal Translocations in Lymphoma

Cytogenetic Abnormality	Oncogenes	Histologic Subtype
t(8; 14) (q24; q32)	*myc*	Burkitt's or Burkitt's-like lymphoma
t(14; 18) (q32; q21)	BCL2	Follicular lymphomas; some large cell lymphomas
t(11; 14) (q13; q32)	BCL1 (cyclin D1)	Mantle cell lymphoma
t(1; 14) (p22; q32)	BCL10	Marginal zone lymphomas (MALT)
t(2; 5) (p23; q35)	ALK1	Anaplastic large cell lymphomas

Cytogenetics

Lymphomas are characterized by certain recurrent characteristic nonrandom chromosomal changes that tend to exhibit specific patterns according to the histologic subtype of the lymphoma (Table 26–5).[41, 42] Burkitt's lymphoma and small noncleaved cell lymphoma are characterized by translocations involving chromosome 8, at a point at which the *myc* oncogene resides in the long arm of chromosome 8.[41] These translocations are reciprocal with the respective chromosomes for either the heavy chain immunoglobulin gene (chromosome 14) or the kappa and lambda light chain immunoglobulin genes (chromosomes 2 and 22, respectively). Follicular lymphomas are characterized by translocations that involve the heavy chain immunoglobulin gene on chromosome 14 and the region of the BCL2 gene on chromosome 18. Abnormalities involving the long arm of chromosome 14 (14q) are in fact the most frequent chromosomal abnormalities noted in lymphomas. Lymphomas of T-cell lineage most often have abnormalities involving a segment of the long arm of chromosome 14, where some of the loci encoding the T-cell receptor gene reside.[43]

Molecular Studies

Although cytogenetics provides evidence of certain repeated or reproducible chromosomal changes, the methodology of cytogenetics is applicable only to situations in which evaluable metaphases are available, which occurs in approximately half of the samples studied. Further refinement of cytogenetic techniques involves the use of molecular DNA probes to look for specific chromosomal patterns of rearrangement with the use of DNA extracted from tumor samples. This methodology is most useful in lymphoid malignancies. Early in the development of lymphoid cells, stem cells commit to a T-cell or a B-cell lineage by undergoing gene rearrangements. Each cell thus has a specific genetic rearrangement of either the immunoglobulin or the T-cell receptor genes. Malignant processes are clonal, that is, their origin can be traced to a single cell. Thus, all cells in a given lymphoid tumor should have the same pattern of gene rearrangement and thus a specific imprint for that rearranged gene. Probes for the immunoglobulin genes can be routinely used to ascertain whether there is a clonal rearrangement for the immunoglobulin

genes; similarly, probes for the T-cell receptor gene can be used to ascertain clonal T-cell rearrangement.[41–46] This may be useful in cases in which marker studies are uninterpretable, or in neoplasms that are histologically undifferentiated and do not express immunoglobulin or mature T-cell receptors on their cell surface or in the cytoplasm. It may also be useful in the detection of small populations of malignant cells in tumors with a high proportion of reactive normal lymphocytes.

Staging

The staging evaluation of a patient with lymphoma begins with a good physical examination. Close attention should be paid to all areas of peripheral lymph node concentration, notably the cervical, supraclavicular, infraclavicular, axillary, epitrochlear, inguinal, and femoral regions. Attention should also be paid to the abdomen for detection of possible splenomegaly. Patients who present with primary lesions in the head and neck region should have a thorough head and neck examination.

The Ann Arbor Classification System is currently the most widely used system for staging lymphomas (Table 26–6).[47] This system was originally designed to stage Hodgkin's disease, which is a malignancy that tends to spread in a pattern of anatomic contiguity. The system thus serves very well as a prognostic indicator of disease outcome in Hodgkin's disease. It has several limitations, however, in the staging of non-Hodgkin's lymphomas, which do not necessarily follow the same pattern of dissemination as is seen in Hodgkin's disease. The Ann Arbor system, for example, does not take into account the size of the primary lesions. Several investigators have noted that the size of the tumor mass does have major prognostic significance in terms of the outcome of non-Hodgkin's lymphomas.[48–50] The inadequacies of the Ann Arbor system for staging non-Hodgkin's lymphoma are widely recognized, and experts in lymphoma who met in Lugano at an international meeting proposed a new risk classification system (see Table 26–4) that is currently widely used.[51]

In addition to routine laboratory studies, a bone marrow biopsy should be performed to exclude involvement of the marrow by lymphoma, which is more prevalent among the

TABLE 26-6 Ann Arbor Staging Classification for Hodgkin's Disease

Stage I	Involvement of a single lymph node region (I), or a single extralymphatic organ or site (I_E)
Stage II	Involvement of two or more lymph node regions on the same side of the diaphragm (II), or localized involvement of an extralymphatic organ or site (II_E)
Stage III	Involvement of lymph node regions on both sides of the diaphragam (III), or localized involvement of an extralymphatic organ or site (III_E) or spleen (III_S) or both (III_{SE})
Stage IV	Diffuse or disseminated involvement of one or more extralymphatic organs with or without associated lymph node involvement
A	Asymptomatic
B	Fever, sweats, weight loss > 10% of body weight

low-grade lymphomas and is more common in non-Hodgkin's lymphomas than in Hodgkin's disease. Markers on lymphocytes in the bone marrow and the peripheral blood are also helpful for patients with low-grade lymphoma in that many of these patients may already have circulating malignant cells. In addition, serum protein electrophoresis may be useful, particularly in patients with low-grade lymphomas.

Radiographic studies should include a computed tomographic (CT) scan of the head and neck or magnetic resonance imaging (MRI), as well as routine CT scans of the chest, abdomen, and pelvis. In patients whose primary lesions present in the oropharynx, an upper GI series may also be helpful because these patients may have additional lesions throughout their mucosa in the GI tract. The presentation of multiple mucosal lesions throughout the GI tract that have small lymphocytic histology and are associated with *H. pylori* is unique to the MALT lymphomas recognized first by Isaacson and associates as a unique clinico-pathologic entity.[52-57]

Positron emission tomography (PET) for staging and evaluation of patients with malignancy has been evolving over the past decade. The use of radioactive isotope and PET as a method of imaging head and neck cancers has been proposed for some time.[58] The currently applied radioactive tracer for imaging of lymphomas is ^{18}F fluorodeoxyglucose (^{18}FDG) because an increase in the metabolism of glucose in Hodgkin's and non-Hodgkin's lymphomas has been documented.[59-61] It has been proposed as a method of staging and evaluating treatment response in both disorders. However, PET is limited in that its sensitivity to inflammatory changes is high; therefore, false-positivity clouds its diagnostic specificity.[62] This is particularly true with extranodal disease sites, but false-positivity can also occur in nodal sites such as the thymus in rebound.[63] In the head and neck area, inflammatory sites in the sinuses and the oral cavity could also cloud the specificity of staging. After treatment, the presence of residual PET sites should not be blindly accepted as an indication of residual active disease because false-positive residual uptake has been documented in clinical trials. If it is absolutely critical for treatment decision making, histology should be obtained after therapy at sites of residual uptake to confirm persistent active disease. The newly developed fusion technology for CT scans and PET imaging will likely improve on the specificity and application of this procedure. Its greatest usefulness may lie in the planning of radiation ports.

TREATMENT

Indolent Lymphomas

Lymphomas localized to the head and neck region fall into the staging category of I or II in the Ann Arbor staging system, with or without local extension into extranodal tissues (extension into extranodal tissues is designated by the letter *E*). Indolent lymphomas present infrequently with localized disease. Because of this feature, few studies exclusively address the management of Ann Arbor stage I and II lymphomas of low-grade histology. Further limitations

result from the fact that approximately 80% of patients with these histologies who present with clinical stage I or II disease are shown on laparotomy to have microscopically positive lymph nodes in the abdomen.[64, 65] Thus, the outcome of treatment strategies in various studies may not be entirely comparable when staging studies are not comparable. Nevertheless, despite the limitations, several published studies seem to indicate that radiotherapy alone may cure approximately 50% of these patients.[66-69]

The usefulness of chemotherapy added to radiotherapy for these patients is not clear. Several studies have addressed this question using cytoxan, vincristine, and prednisone (CVP) as the chemotherapy regimen. The best-designed study is that of Monfardini and colleagues, who studied a small number of laparotomy-staged patients (26 total) with low-grade histologies who were randomly assigned to receive irradiation or combined treatment.[70] A difference in survival was noted at 5 years (93% vs. 62%), favoring the combined approach, but this did not reach statistical significance, probably owing to the small numbers, nor was a significant difference in disease-free survival noted. Other studies have shown differences in disease-free survival but no difference in survival or no difference in any parameters at all.[71-74] Because irradiation cures only half of these patients, the question still remains whether the remaining half could be helped by adjuvant chemotherapy.

Lymphomas in the Parotid Gland

Sjögren's syndrome is associated with an increased risk of lymphoid malignancy, particularly in the parotid glands and the conjunctiva. The classic lymphoma associated with Sjögren's syndrome is of the MALT subtype.[75] These lymphomas are of B-cell type and are often indolent, that is, they are characterized by a slow course of progression.[76] They are exquisitely sensitive to radiation. Involved field radiation can be curative in patients with localized disease. More recent trials of treatment with anti-CD20 monoclonal antibodies indicate that this treatment may also be highly effective. When a patient presents with a mass in the parotid, it is important that other sites be carefully examined to rule out additional sites of disease. Additional lesions in the conjunctiva, skin, gastrointestinal tract, and respiratory tract may be found in association with lymphoma in the parotid gland. Lesions of MALT lymphoma outside of the stomach are usually not associated with *H. pylori*; hence, treatment with antibiotics is not appropriate. However, rare cases of lymphoma in the parotid gland associated with *H. pylori* have been reported.[77]

Aggressive Lymphomas

In large cell lymphomas, which constitute the majority of cases that present in the head and neck, the usefulness of chemotherapy in obtaining cure is clear. Miller and Jones[78] and Cabanillas[79] established that chemotherapy alone, with the CHOP (cyclophosphamide, doxorubicin, vincristine, and prednisone) regimen, could be curative for stage I and II large cell lymphomas. Radiotherapy alone had been the mainstay of treatment for these disorders until curative combination chemotherapies were developed. For localized (stage I and II) aggressive lymphomas, published studies have shown overall excellent results when the patient is treated with chemoradiation. Complete response rates are in the order of 90%, and 5-year disease-free survival figures are in the range of 70% to 80%.[80–84] Furthermore, using combined chemoradiotherapy, Connors and associates have shown that the use of a limited number of chemotherapy cycles (three treatments of CHOP) is as effective as more extensive chemotherapy (six to eight cycles).[81] It should be noted that Connors' series included mostly favorable patients, that is, patients with low lactate dehydrogenase (LDH), no systemic symptoms, and small tumor masses. Nevertheless, the results indicated that for many stage I/II patients, limited chemotherapy and irradiation could be curative.

Longo and colleagues, from the National Cancer Institute, also published results in 49 stage I intermediate-grade lymphoma patients, of whom 18 had disease localized to the head and neck. The patients were treated with four cycles of ProMACE-MOPP (prednisone, methotrexate, doxorubicin, cyclophosphamide, etoposide, nitrogen mustard, procarbazine), a more intensive and complex chemotherapy combination than CHOP, followed by radiotherapy.[84] Follow-up in these patients was much shorter than in previous studies, with a median of 42 months. The complete response rate was 96%, and none of the patients had relapsed at the time of publication (100% disease-free survival). The patients, again, overall had favorable presentations, with only three cases showing an elevated LDH level. Overall, stage I patients do very well even with CHOP-based treatments, and it is in stage II patients that relapses are more commonly seen.

A large randomized Southwest Oncology Group (SWOG) trial published by Miller and coworkers showed better outcome for patients with limited stage I/II disease who were treated with three cycles of CHOP, followed by radiation therapy, when compared with eight cycles of CHOP without radiation.[85] However, longer follow-up has shown less favorable outcome for stage II patients. Hence, stage II patients may require more extensive chemotherapy than three cycles of CHOP. In elderly patients, the addition of rituximab (a monoclonal antibody targeted against the pan-B-CD20 antigen) to CHOP improves survival.[86]

Hence, future studies will likely address the benefit of monoclonal antibodies in limited-stage disease as well. Burkitt's lymphoma and lymphoblastic lymphoma indisputably must be treated with aggressive chemotherapy regimens.[87–89] They rarely present with localized head and neck nodal or extranodal disease but may include neck disease as part of a more extensive systemic disease presentation. The rate of growth of these lymphomas is extremely rapid, with doubling times of days, and lymph node masses in the neck may grow to become airway management problems. Patients who are diagnosed with these histologic findings should be considered to have an acutely critical illness and should be referred immediately for chemotherapy.

EBV and Aggressive Lymphomas: Special Cases

Lethal midline granuloma is a term previously applied to a clinical entity characterized by relentless ulcerative destruction of the nose and deep midfacial structures. It can be confused with other diseases, including infection (e.g., granulomatous reactions to syphilis, fungal infections, or tuberculosis), Wegener's granulomatosis, other vasculitic entities, and nonlymphoid neoplasms.[90] Today, it is recognized that this disorder is actually a lymphoma of NK/T-cell origin.[91] Histologically, it is characterized by necrosis and therefore may be difficult to diagnose on a single biopsy. Often, these patients require multiple biopsies before a definitive diagnosis is made. Also characteristic of this disease is that angiocentric tumor involvement may be evident, and EBV or its proteins are usually detected in the malignant cells.[92, 93] The angiocentric histology is an independent predictor of shorter disease-specific and overall survival for patients with this disorder. Other important prognostic factors include high LDH and high β_2-microglobulin levels. The therapeutic intervention that appears to have the most established benefit for this disease is radiation. The combination of chemotherapy and radiation has been reported to have possible additive benefit.

Patients with immune deficiency, either secondary to post-transplant immune suppression or due to human immunodeficiency virus (HIV) infection, may have lymphoproliferative disorders also presenting in the oral cavity, nodes, or salivary glands. These disorders, however, may have an initial polyclonal presentation, appearing to be merely inflammatory.[94, 95] When the proliferation evolves to a monoclonal state, the disorder can be much more aggressive. In the case of post-transplant lymphoproliferative disorder (PTLD), the disorders in the polyclonal phase may respond to withdrawal of immune suppressants.[95] If the disorder progresses to a monoclonal large cell B-cell disorder, the anti-CD20 monoclonal antibody rituximab has been reported to be effective in achieving remissions. Combined-modality treatment with chemotherapy and radiation can also be effective, particularly for localized tumor lesions, although it is associated with an anticipated risk of infection.

Although patients with AIDS related to HIV infection may also present with polyclonal lymphoproliferative disorders, most often the disorders are monoclonal.[96] In addition, although PTLDs are almost always associated with EBV infection in tumor tissues, only half of AIDS-related lymphomas (ARLs) are EBV positive.[97] The immunohistologic subtypes of ARL range from T-cell to large B-cell lymphomas, as well as the more recently described plasmablastic lymphomas of the oral cavity.[98] The latter are clinically aggressive and are immunologically characterized by the lack of B- or T-cell markers but with positive plasma cell specific markers such as CD79a.

The current use of triple antiretroviral therapy for HIV infection has improved both the quality and duration of life for patients. If the virus is controlled, HIV-associated lymphomas can be treated aggressively, appropriate to the histology of the lymphoma.[99] The outcome of aggressive chemoradiation management depends in part on the patient's T-cell function and other comorbid conditions. Prognostic indicators identified in HIV-related aggressive lymphomas include not only lymphoma-related factors such as histologic subtype but also age, CD4 count, level of LDH, other intercurrent infections, and marrow reserve.[100]

SUMMARY

The lymphomas are a diverse group of lymphoid malignancies with variable clinical manifestations. The incidence of lymphomas in the United States is rising, and their effects on mortality in the young and in productive adults are important. Their prognosis varies according to both the extent of disease at treatment and the immunohistologic subclassification. Because the immunohistologic classification plays a critical and important role in the treatment decisions of patients, appropriate diagnostic procedures are essential. The most important diagnostic step still remains surgical excision; the success of the pathologist in appropriately diagnosing the disease rests in part on the technical skill of the surgeon in removing and handling the surgical specimen. Increasingly sophisticated methodologies have been developed in recent years that aid in the diagnosis and differentiation of lymphomas from other malignancies. These range from immunohistochemical markers to cytogenetics and molecular genetic techniques, which allow us to distinguish the origin of the lymphocytes to T- or B-cell lineage and may allow exclusion of nonlymphoid neoplasms in cases in which the cells are highly anaplastic and the cell of primary origin is not histologically evident.

Current controversy exists in the management of stage I/II lymphomas. For low-grade lymphomas, the issue is whether chemotherapy adds any benefit to irradiation. Chemotherapy plays a critical role in the cure of aggressive lymphomas, and the controversy centers more around the additive role of irradiation and monoclonal antibodies. Finally, the Ann Arbor system of classification is useful as a prognostic tool and for therapeutic planning in Hodgkin's disease, but it has shortcomings for the staging of non-Hodgkin's lymphomas. It is hoped that new risk classification systems that incorporate various factors of prognostic importance, including the genetic profile of the tumors, will aid us in tailoring treatments more appropriately to the anticipated prognosis of the disease, with less aggressive treatment for those whose outlook is excellent and, conversely, with new aggressive approaches for those who cannot be cured with current treatment strategies.

REFERENCES

1. DeVita V, Jaffe ES, Mauch P, et al: Lymphocytic lymphomas. In DeVita VT, Hellman S, Rosenbert SA (eds): Cancer: Principles and Practice of Oncology, 3rd ed. Philadelphia, JB Lippincott, 1993, pp 1741–1798.
2. Jacobs C, Weiss L, Hoppe RT: The management of extranodal head and neck lymphomas. Arch Otolaryngol Head Neck Surg 112:654–658, 1986.
3. Lukes RJ, Butler JJ: The pathology and nomenclature of Hodgkin's disease. Cancer Res 26:1063–1083, 1966.
4. Frizzera G: The distinction of Hodgkin's disease from anaplastic large cell lymphoma. Semin Diagn Pathol 9:291–296, 1992.
5. Weiss LM, Stickler JG, Hu E, et al: Immunoglobulin gene rearrangements in Hodgkin's disease. Hum Pathol 17:1009–1014, 1986.
6. Stein H, Hansman ML, Lennert K, et al: Reed-Sternberg and Hodgkin cells in lymphocyte predominant Hodgkin's disease of nodular subtype contain J chain. Am J Clin Pathol 86:292–297, 1986.
7. Cabanillas F, Pathak S, Trujillo J, et al: Cytogenetic features of Hodgkin's disease suggest possible origin from a lymphocyte. Blood 71:1615–1617, 1988.

8. Non-Hodgkin's Lymphoma Pathologic Classification Project: National Cancer Institute sponsored study of classification of non-Hodgkin's lymphomas: Summary and description of a working formulation for clinical usage. Cancer 40:2112–2135, 1982.
9. Harris NL, Jaffe ES, Stein H, et al: A revised European-American classification of lymphoid neoplasms: A proposal from the International Lymphoma Study Group. Blood 84:1361–1392, 1994.
10. Lippman SM, Miller TP, Spier CM, et al: The prognostic significance of the immunotype in diffuse large-cell lymphoma: A comparative study of the T-cell and B-cell phenotype. Blood 72:436–441, 1988.
11. Armitage JO, Vose JH, Linder J, et al: Clinical significance of immunophenotype in diffuse aggressive non-Hodgkin's lymphoma. J Clin Oncol 7:1783–1790, 1989.
12. Coiffier B, Brousse N, Peuchmaur M, et al: Peripheral T-cell lymphomas have a worse prognosis than B-cell lymphomas: A prospective study of 361 immunophenotyped patients treated with the LNH-84 regimen. Ann Oncol 1:45–50, 1990.
13. Hardell L, Eriksson M, Lennet P, et al: Malignant lymphoma and exposure to chemicals, especially organic solvents, chlorophenols and phenoxy acids. A case control study. Br J Cancer 43:169–171, 1981.
14. Olsson H, Brandt L: Risk of non-Hodgkin's lymphoma among men occupationally exposed to organic solvents. Scand J Work Environ Health 14:246–251, 1988.
15. Finch SC: Leukaemia and lymphoma in atomic bomb survivors. In Boice JD, Fraumeni JF (eds): Radiation Carcinogenesis: Epidemiology and Biological Significance. New York, Raven Press, 1984, pp 37–44.
16. Johnson CJ: Cancer incidence in an area of radioactive fallout downwind from the Nevada test site. JAMA 251:230–236, 1984.
17. Caldwell GG, Kelley D, Zack M, et al: Mortality and cancer frequency among military nuclear test (Smoky) participants, 1957 through 1979. JAMA 250:620–624, 1983.
18. Hanto DW, Frizzera G, Purtillo DT, et al: Clinical spectrum of lymphoproliferative disorders in renal transplant recipients and evidence of the role of Epstein-Barr virus. Cancer Res 41:4253–4261, 1981.
19. Hanto D, Birkenbach M, Frizzera G, et al: Confirmation of the heterogeneity of post-transplant Epstein-Barr virus-associated B-cell proliferations by immunoglobulin gene rearrangement analysis. Transplantation 47:458–462, 1989.
20. Filipovich A, Mathur A, Kamat D, et al: Primary immunodeficiencies: Genetic risk factors for lymphoma. Cancer Res 52:5465–5467, 1992.
21. Shibata D, Weiss L, Hernandez A, et al: Epstein-Barr virus-associated non-Hodgkin's lymphoma in patients infected with the human immunodeficiency virus. Blood 81:2102–2109, 1993.
22. Robinson JC: Diffuse polyclonal B-cell lymphoma during primary infection with Epstein-Barr virus. N Engl J Med 302:1293–1297, 1980.
23. Epstein MA, Achong BG, Barr YM: Virus particles in cultures of lymphoblasts from Burkitt's lymphoma. Lancet 1:702–703, 1964.
24. Ambinder RF, Browning PJ, Lorenzana I, et al: Epstein-Barr virus and childhood Hodgkin's disease in Honduras and the United States. Blood 81:462–467, 1993.
25. Borisch B, Henning I, Laeng R, et al: Association of the subtype 2 of the Epstein-Barr virus with T-cell non-Hodgkin's lymphoma of the midline granuloma type. Blood 82:858–864, 1993.
26. Kanavaros P, Less MC, Briere J, et al: Nasal T-cell lymphoma: A clinicopathologic entity associated with peculiar phenotype and with Epstein-Barr virus. Blood 81:2688–2695, 1993.
27. Waldmann TA: Human T-cell lymphotropic virus type 1-associated adult T-cell leukemia. JAMA 73:731–737, 1995.
28. Yamaguci K: Human T-lymphotropic virus type I in Japan. Lancet 243:213–216, 1994.
29. Poiesz BJ, Ruscetti FW, Gagdar AF, et al: Detection and isolation of type C retrovirus particles from fresh and cultured lymphocytes of a patient with cutaneous T-cell lymphoma. Proc Natl Acad Sci U S A 77:7415–7419, 1980.
30. Bernard SM, Cartwright RA, Darwin CM, et al: A possible association between multiple sclerosis and lymphoma/leukemia. Br J Haematol 65:122–123, 1987.
31. Holm LE, Blomgren H, Lowhmage T: Cancer risk in patients with chronic lymphocytic thyroiditis. N Engl J Med 312:601–604, 1985.
32. Isomaki HA, Hakulinen T, Joutsenlahti U: Excess risk of lymphoma, leukemia, and myeloma in patients with rheumatoid arthritis. J Chron Dis 31:691–696, 1978.
33. Cooper BT, Holmes GKT, Cooke WT: Lymphoma risk in coeliac disease of later life. Disgestion 23:89–92, 1982.

34. Swinson CM, Coles EC, Slavin G, et al: Coeliac disease and malignancy. Lancet 1:111–115, 1983.

35. Palackdharry CS: The epidemiology of non-Hodgkin's lymphoma: Why the increased incidence? Oncology 8:67–73, 1994.

36. Raber M: Clinical applications of flow cytometry. Oncology 2:35–39, 1988.

37. Ordonez NG: Application of immunocytochemistry in the diagnosis of poorly differentiated neoplasms and tumors of unknown origin. Cancer Bull 41:142–151, 1989.

38. Sneige N, Dekmezian R, Katz R, et al: Morphologic and immunocytochemical evaluation of 220 fine needle aspirates of malignant lymphoma and lymphoid hyperplasia. Acta Cytol 34:311–322, 1990.

39. Larson DL, Robbins KT, Butler JJ: Lymphoma of the head and neck: A diagnostic dilemma. Am J Surg 148:433–437, 1984.

40. MacKay B, Ordonez NG: Poorly differentiated neoplasms and tumors of unknown origin. In Fer MF, Greco FA, Oldham RK (eds): The Role of the Pathologist in the Evaluation of Poorly Differentiated Tumors and Metastatic Tumors of Unknown Origin. Orlando, Fla, Grune & Stratton, 1986, pp 3–73.

41. LeBeau M: Chromosomal abnormalities in non-Hodgkin's lymphomas. Semin Oncol 17:20–29, 1990.

42. Cabanillas F, Pathak S, Trujillo J, et al: Frequent nonrandom chromosome abnormalities in 27 patients with untreated large cell lymphoma and immunoblastic lymphoma. Cancer Res 48:5557–5564, 1988.

43. Sadamori N, Kusano M, Nishimo K, et al: Abnormalities of chromosome 14 at 14q11 in Japanese patients with adult T-cell leukemia. Cancer Genet Cytogenet 17:279–282, 1985.

44. Arnold A, Cossmann J, Bakhshi A, et al: Immunoglobulin gene rearrangements as unique clonal markers in human lymphoid neoplasms. N Engl J Med 309:1593–1599, 1983.

45. Greisser H, Tkachuk D, Reis MD, et al: Gene rearrangements and translocations in lymphoproliferative diseases. Blood 73:1402–1415, 1989.

46. Trainor KJ, Brisco MJ, Wan JH, et al: Gene rearrangement in B- and T-lymphoproliferative diseases detected by the polymerase chain reaction. Blood 78:192–196, 1991.

47. Carbone PP, Kaplan HS, Musshoff K, et al: Report of the committee on Hodgkin's disease staging. Cancer Res 31:1860–1861, 1971.

48. Kong JS, Fuller LM, Butler JJ, et al: Stages I and II non-Hodgkin's lymphomas of Waldeyer's ring and the neck. Am J Clin Oncol 7:629–639, 1984.

49. Jagannath S, Velasquez WS, Tucker SL, et al: Tumor burden assessment and its implications for a prognostic model in advanced diffuse large cell lymphoma. J Clin Oncol 4:859–865, 1986.

50. MacKintosh JF, Cowan RA, Jones M, et al: Prognostic factors in stage I and II high and intermediate grade non-Hodgkin's lymphoma. Eur J Cancer Clin Oncol 24:1617–1622, 1988.

51. Shipp MA, Harrington DP, Anderson JR, et al: A predictive model for aggressive NHL: The international non-Hodgkin's lymphoma prognostic factors project. N Engl J Med 329:987–994, 1993.

52. Rodriguez J, Cabanillas F, McLaughlin P, et al: A proposal for a simple staging system for intermediate grade lymphoma and immunoblastic lymphoma based on the "tumor score." Ann Oncol 3:711–717, 1992.

53. American Joint Committee on Cancer: Handbook for Staging of Cancer, 4th ed. Philadelphia, JB Lippincott, 1993.

54. Swan F Jr, Velasquez WS, Tucker S, et al: A new serologic staging system for large-cell lymphomas based on initial beta-2-microglobulin and lactate dehydrogenase levels. J Clin Oncol 7:1518–1527, 1989.

55. Isaacson PG, Spencer F: Malignant lymphoma of mucosa associated lymphoid tissue. In Habeshaw JA, Lauder I (eds): Malignant Lymphomas. Edinburgh, Churchill Livingstone, 1988, pp 179–200.

56. Roggero E, Zucca E, Pinotti G, et al: Eradication of Helicobacter pylori infection in primary low-grade gastric lymphoma of mucosa-associated lymphoid tissue. Ann Intern Med 122:767–769, 1995.

57. Wotherspoon AC, Doglioni C, Isaacson PG: Low grade gastric B-cell lymphoma of mucosa-associated lymphoid tissue (MALT): A multifocal disease. Histopathology 20:29–34, 1992.

58. Leskinen-Kallio S, Nagren K, Lehikoinen P, et al: Carbon-11-methionine and PET is an effective method to image head and neck cancer. J Nucl Med 33: 691–695, 1992.

59. Lapela M, Leskinen S, Minn HRI, et al: Increased glucose metabolism in untreated non-Hodgkin's lymphoma: A study of positron emission tomography with fluorine-18-fluorodeoxyglucose. Blood 86:3522–3527, 1995.

60. Moog F, Bangerter M, Deiderichs C, et al: Lymphoma: Role of 2-deoxy-2-(F-18) fluoro-D-glucose (FDG) PET in nodal staging. Radiology 203:795–800, 1997.

61. Hoh CK, Glaspy J, Rosen P, et al: Whole-body FDG-PET imaging for staging of Hodgkin's disease and lymphoma. J Nucl Med 38:343–348, 1997.

62. Weidman E, Baican B, Hertel A, et al: Positron emission tomography (PET) for staging and evaluation of response to treatment in patients with Hodgkin's disease. Leuk Lymphoma 34:545–551, 1999.

63. Weinblatt ME, Zanzi I, Belakhlef A, et al: False-positive FDG-PET imaging of the thymus in a child with Hodgkin's disease. J Nucl Med 38:888–900, 1997.

64. Goffinett DR, Warnke R, Dunnick NR, et al: Clinical and surgical (laparotomy) evaluation of patients with non-Hodgkin's lymphoma. Cancer Treat Rep 61:981–992, 1977.

65. Chabner BA, Johnson RE, Young RC, et al: Sequential nonsurgical and surgical staging of non-Hodgkin's lymphoma. Ann Intern Med 85:149–154, 1976.

66. Chen MG, Prosnitz LR, Gonzalez-Serva A, et al: Results of radiotherapy in control of stage I and II non-Hodgkin's lymphoma. Cancer 43:1245–1254, 1979.

67. Paryani SB, Hoppe RT, Cox RS, et al: Analysis of non-Hodgkin's lymphoma with nodular and favorable histologies, stages I and II. Cancer 52:2300–2307, 1983.

68. Bush RS, Gospodarowicz M: Malignant lymphomas: Etiology, immunology, pathology, treatment. In Rosenberg SA, Kaplan HS (eds): The Place of Radiation Therapy in the Management of Localized Non-Hodgkin's Lymphoma. New York, Academic Press, 1982, pp 485–502.

69. Gospodarowicz MK, Bush RS, Brown TC, et al: Prognostic factors in nodular lymphomas: A multivariate analysis based on the Princess Margaret Hospital experience. Int J Radiat Oncol Biol Phys 10:489–497, 1984.

70. Monfardini S, Banfi A, Bonadonna G, et al: Improved 5 year survival after combined radiotherapy-chemotherapy for stage I–II non-Hodgkin's lymphoma. Int J Radiat Oncol Biol Phys 6:125–134, 1980.

71. McLaughlin P, Fuller LM, Velasquez WS, et al: Stage I–II follicular lymphoma. Cancer 58:1596–1602, 1986.

72. Carde P, Burgers JMV, Van Glabbeke M, et al: Combined radiotherapy-chemotherapy for early stages of non-Hodgkin's lymphoma: The 1975-1980 EORTC controlled lymphoma trial. Radiother Oncol 2:301–312, 1984.

73. Bron D, Strychmans P: Role of chemotherapy for localized non-Hodgkin's lymphomas? Eur J Cancer Clin Oncol 23:459–463, 1987.

74. Soubeyrah P, Eghbali F, Bonichon JM, et al: Localized follicular lymphomas: Prognosis and survival of stages I and II in a retrospective series of 103 patients. Radiother Oncol 13:91–98, 1988.

75. Isaacson PG, Spencer J: Malignant lymphoma of mucosa-associated lymphoid tissue. Histopathology 11:445–462, 1987.

76. Sung SS, Seibani K, Fishleder A, et al: Monocytoid B-cell lymphoma in patients with Sjögren's syndrome: A clinico-pathological study of 13 patients. Hum Pathol 22:422–427, 1991.

77. Nishimura M, Miyajima S, Okada N: Salivary gland MALT lymphoma associated with Helicobacter pylori infection in a patient with Sjögren's syndrome. J Dermatol 27:450–452, 2000.

78. Miller TP, Jones SE: Initial chemotherapy for clinically localized lymphomas of unfavorable histology. Blood 62:413–418, 1984.

79. Cabanillas F: Chemotherapy as definitive treatment of stage I–II large cell and diffuse mixed lymphomas. Hematol Oncol 3:25–31, 1985.

80. Longo DL: Combined modality therapy for localized aggressive lymphoma: Enough or too much? J Clin Oncol 7:1179–1181, 1989.

81. Connors JM, Klimo P, Fairey RN, et al: Brief chemotherapy and involved field radiation therapy for limited stage aggressive histology lymphoma. Ann Intern Med 107:25–30, 1987.

82. Mauch P, Leonard R, Skarin A, et al: Improved survival following combined radiation therapy and chemotherapy for unfavorable prognosis stage I–II non-Hodgkin's lymphomas. J Clin Oncol 3:1301–1308, 1985.

83. Jones SE, Miller TP, Connors JM: Long term follow-up and analysis for prognostic factors for patients with limited stage diffuse large cell lymphoma treated with initial chemotherapy with or without adjuvant radiotherapy. J Clin Oncol 7:1186–1191, 1989.

84. Longo DL, Glatstein E, Duffey PL, et al: Treatment of localized aggressive lymphomas with combination chemotherapy followed by involved field radiation therapy. J Clin Oncol 7:1295–1302, 1989.

85. Miller TP, Dahlberg S, Cassady JR, et al: Chemotherapy alone compared with chemotherapy plus radiotherapy for localized intermediate- and high-grade non-Hodgkin's lymphoma. N Engl J Med 339:21–26, 1998.

86. Coiffer B, LePage E, Briere J, et al: CHOP chemotherapy plus rituximab compared with CHOP alone in elderly patients with diffuse large B-cell lymphoma. N Engl J Med 346:235, 2002.

87. Slater DE, Mertlesmann R, Doziner B, et al: Lymphoblastic lymphoma in adults. J Clin Oncol 4:57–67, 1986.

88. Bernstein JI, Coleman NC, Strickler JG, et al: Combined modality therapy for adults with small non-cleaved cell lymphoma (Burkitt's and non-Burkitt's types). J Clin Oncol 4:847–858, 1986.

89. Lopez TL, Hagemeister FB, McLaughlin P, et al: Small non-cleaved cell lymphoma in adults: Superior results for stages I-III disease. J Clin Oncol 8:615–622, 1990.

90. Aviles A, Rodriguez L, Guzman R, et al: Angiocentric T-cell lymphoma of the nose, paranasal sinuses, and hard palate. Hematol Oncol 10:141–145, 1992.

91. Jaffe ES, Chan JKC, Ho FCS, et al: Report on the workshop on nasal and related extranodal angiocentric T/natural killer cell lymphomas: Definitions, differential diagnosis and epidemiology. Am J Surg Pathol 20:103–110, 1996.

92. Kanavaros P, Lescs MC, Gaulard P, et al: Nasal T-cell lymphoma: A clinicopathologic entity associated with peculiar phenotype and with Epstein-Barr virus. Blood 81:2688–2692, 1993.

93. Pallesen G, Hamilton Dutoit SJ, Zhou X: The association of Epstein-Barr virus (EBV) with T-cell lymphoproliferations and Hodgkin's disease: Two new developments in the EBV field. Adv Cancer Res 62:179–183, 1993.

94. Helsper J, Formenti S, Levine A: Initial manifestation of acquired immune deficiency syndrome in the head and neck. Am J Surg 152:403–407, 1986.

95. Shapiro A, Shechtman F, Guida R, et al: Head and neck lymphoma in patients with the acquired immune deficiency syndrome. Otolaryngol Head Neck Surg 106:253–258, 1992.

96. Young L, Alfieri C, Hennessy K, et al: Expression of Epstein-Barr virus transformation-associated genes in tissues of patients with EBV lymphoproliferative disease. N Engl J Med 321:1080–1085, 1989.

97. Shiramizu B, Herndier B, Meeker T, et al: Molecular and immunophenotypic characterization of AIDS-associated, Epstein-Barr virus-negative, polyclonal lymphoma. J Clin Oncol 10:383–389, 1992.

98. Rossi G, Donisi A, Casari S, et al: The international prognostic index can be used as a guide to treatment decisions regarding patients with human immunodeficiency virus-related systemic non-Hodgkin's lymphoma. Cancer 86:2391–2397, 1999.

99. Carbone A, Gaidano G, Gloghini A, et al: AIDS-related plasmablastic lymphomas of the oral cavity and jaws: A diagnostic dilemma. Ann Otol Rhinol Laryngol 108:95–99, 1999.

100. Hagemeister FB, Khetan R, Allen P, et al: Stage, serum LDH, and performance status predict disease progression and survival in HIV-associated lymphomas. Ann Oncol 5:541–546, 1994.

CHAPTER 27

Unusual Tumors

James Y. Suen
Emre A. Vural
Milton Waner

INTRODUCTION

This chapter summarizes some unusual head and neck lesions and tumors. The malignant tumors discussed in this chapter are the less frequently encountered neoplasms, which are usually presented as case reports or small case series in the head and neck literature. We have compiled the data provided by previously published experiences for the purpose of summarizing the management of these unusual tumors.

Hemangiomas and vascular malformations of the head and neck are also discussed in this chapter. Despite their benign histopathologic appearance, these tumors may be quite aggressive and locally destructive. Some of these tumors can cause life-threatening conditions, and the management of these neoplasms may be challenging for head and neck surgeons.

LIPOSARCOMA

Liposarcomas are malignant soft tissue tumors originating from adipose tissue. Liposarcomas in the head and neck (HNLs) are uncommon, accounting for only 1% of all head and neck sarcomas and 3% to 5% of all liposarcomas.[1-3] Because of its rare occurrence, published experience about HNL is usually based on case reports with or without a review of the literature. Therefore, it is difficult for the head and neck surgeon to implement a comprehensive treatment plan for the patient with HNL.

Epidemiology

HNL can be diagnosed at any age between 6 months and 90 years; however, a majority of cases occur between the fourth and sixth decades.[1, 4] HNL is more common among men, with an approximate male-to-female ratio of 2:1.[1, 4, 5] It has been diagnosed in many anatomic locations in the head and neck region, including the tongue,[6, 7] floor of the mouth,[8] soft palate,[9] lip,[10] buccal mucosa,[11] larynx,[2, 13-15] hypopharynx,[16-18] maxilla,[19, 20] scalp,[21] parapharyngeal space,[22] retropharyngeal space,[23, 24] temporal bone,[25] parotid,[26] neck,[27-29] orbit,[30] and cheek.[31] Theoretically, HNL can originate from any location in the head and neck. Although liposarcomas arising from lipomas have been reported, almost all liposarcomas are considered as having arisen de novo.[32] There are reported cases of liposarcoma in the literature that occurred following irradiation and trauma, but the evidence is not strong enough to eliminate the chance of coincidence in these cases.[25, 32, 33]

Clinical Presentation

Symptoms in HNL vary according to the size and site of the tumor. Because the face, neck, and larynx/hypopharynx are the most common sites of origin for HNL, patients usually present with a slowly growing, painless mass in the head and neck region, or with upper aerodigestive tract symptoms, such as dysphagia, dysphonia, and airway obstruction caused by the mechanical effects of the tumor.[1, 34] Most laryngeal liposarcomas are supraglottic, and most hypopharyngeal liposarcomas originate from the pyriform sinus.[5, 34-36]

Diagnosis

Methods of diagnosis, imaging, and biopsy for HNL do not differ substantially from those for other tumors in the head and neck. Computed tomography (CT) and magnetic resonance imaging (MRI) are useful imaging modalities for determining the extent of tumor. Tissue biopsy is the most important diagnostic tool because fine-needle aspiration biopsy may not be sufficient for making the diagnosis, especially in well-differentiated tumors that might be confused with lipomas or other soft tissue tumors (e.g., neurofibroma, mesenchymoma, or angiofibrolipoma).[6, 37] Although immunohistochemical staining is commonly positive for vimentin and S-100 staining, findings are non-specific for liposarcomas.[36]

Classification

Histopathologic classification of liposarcomas is of utmost importance because their biologic behavior is directly related to the tumor subtype. Therefore, consultation with a pathologist who has extensive experience with soft tissue tumors is critical to the successful management of patients with these tumors. There are five different histopathologic variants of liposarcoma: well-differentiated, myxoid, round cell, pleomorphic, and dedifferentiated subtypes (Table 27–1). Well-differentiated liposarcomas are

TABLE 27–1 Histopathologic Variants of Liposarcoma

Well-differentiated
   Lipoma-like
   Sclerosing
Myxoid
Round cell
Pleomorphic
Dedifferentiated

further divided into two subgroups, namely, lipoma-like and sclerosing.[32] Myxoid liposarcoma is the most commonly encountered subtype of HNL; of the well-differentiated sclerosing type, upper aerodigestive tract liposarcomas are most common.[2, 5, 36] These two subtypes have similarly high 5-year survival rates: 85% to 100% for well-differentiated tumors, and 71% to 95% for myxoid tumors.[1, 32] In contrast, pleomorphic and round cell liposarcomas have approximately 20% 5-year survival rates, with a high propensity for distant metastases, especially to the lungs and the bones.[5, 35]

Treatment and Prognosis

The preferred treatment for HNL is wide local excision with negative margins. Well-differentiated liposarcomas can be misdiagnosed as lipomas, and resultant inadequate excision results in recurrence. This is especially true for the liposarcomas located in the larynx and hypopharynx, where the surgeons might be more conservative in their resection with the goal of minimizing patient morbidity. However, it has been reported that patients who have undergone radical excision for laryngeal lesions (i.e., total or supraglottic laryngectomy) never had a recurrence, and conservative simple local excision resulted in multiple recurrences.[2, 34] Therefore, wide excision with negative margins is advocated, even for well-differentiated or myxoid tumors. Previous reviews on HNL revealed 50% to 55% overall recurrence rates over an average period of 3.9 years; however, 80% to 95% of these recurrences were in patients who underwent simple or incomplete initial excision. In contrast, the recurrence rate for complete wide local or radical excision was only 8% to 16%.[35, 36]

As with all sarcomas of the head and neck, HNL rarely metastasizes to regional lymph nodes.[5, 34] Nodal involvement in HNL was given as 0% in a recent review.[36] Therefore, neck dissection is not recommended, unless the lymph nodes are clinically positive.[34, 36] Almost all reported metastatic disease for HNL is related to cases with poorly differentiated variants of liposarcoma.[5, 35, 36] Well-differentiated HNLs rarely metastasize, and death is rare for patients with this variant, even in cases with multiple recurrences.[34, 36] The role of adjuvant radiation treatment and chemotherapy in HNL is unclear; however, these treatments may be useful in patients with extensive or metastatic disease.[38]

◘ CHONDROSARCOMA

Epidemiology

Chondrosarcomas are cartilage-forming malignant mesenchymal tumors that account for 8% of all head and neck

sarcomas and only 0.1% of all head and neck malignancies.[39, 40] Three percent to 12% of all chondrosarcomas occur in the head and neck region.[41, 42] Although chondrosarcoma usually arises from either cartilage- or bone-derived chondroid precursors, it may also arise from primitive mesenchymal cells in tissues where cartilage is not present.[40] Its cause is unknown despite proposed etiologic factors such as trauma, previous exposure to irradiation, beryllium, asbestos, aluminum, Teflon, iron, or radioactive isotopes.[40, 43]

Although 12% to 38% of chondrosarcomas develop secondary to a previous condition such as solitary or multiple exostoses, Ollier's disease, Mafucci's syndrome, Paget's disease, and fibrous dysplasia, most are sporadic lesions without any known causative factor.[40, 44] Some secondary chondrosarcomas have also been reported to be associated with certain malignant conditions such as osteosarcoma, malignant melanoma, leukemia, and fibrosarcoma.[40] Sites that are reported to be involved with this tumor include the nasal septum,[41, 45] sphenoid sinus,[46] larynx,[43, 47–50] maxilla,[51, 52] mandible,[53] external auditory canal,[54] temporal bone,[55] temporomandibular joint,[56] parapharyngeal space,[57] skull base,[58–61] trachea,[62] hyoid,[63] nasopharynx,[64] and hard palate.[65]

Although chondrosarcoma is the most commonly encountered sarcoma of the larynx, accounting for 75% of all laryngeal sarcomas, the craniofacial skeleton is the more common site of occurrence of this tumor type.[40, 66] According to a recent study that reviewed head and neck chondrosarcoma based on information from the National Cancer Database, the median age for this tumor is reported to be 51 years with a slight male preponderance (54.5%). However, the age and sex distribution for chondrosarcoma of the head and neck differs according to the site. Patients older than 50 years of age represent most of the laryngotracheal cases (90%); only 38% of this age group had tumors of the facial skeleton.[40] A large proportion of patients with laryngotracheal chondrosarcoma were males (77%), and 65% of patients with sinonasal tumors were females.[42, 66]

Classification

Chondrosarcomas are classified in five different histopathologic categories, including conventional, myxoid, mesenchymal, clear cell, and dedifferentiated tumors. More than 80% of chondrosarcomas are of the conventional type; clear cell and dedifferentiated variants are extremely rare. More than 90% of conventional tumors are of low grade, and 70% of these are early tumors. This may somewhat explain the fact that head and neck chondrosarcoma has the best prognosis among all chondrosarcomas and among all head and neck sarcomas.[67] Mesenchymal and myxoid variants are relatively rare, constituting 11% and 9% of all tumors, respectively.[40] In contrast to conventional tumors, most mesenchymal tumors occur in patients between 10 and 30 years of age and show equal sex distribution. Almost 70% of mesenchymal tumors are of high grade, and they represent extensive lesions with poorer survival rates when compared with the conventional subtype.[40, 68]

Regional and distant metastases are rare in chondrosarcomas of the head and neck. Koch and associates reported that 88% of chondrosarcomas of the head and neck are confined to the primary site without any regional or distant metastases; the proportions of regional and distant metastases at the time of diagnosis were reported to be 6% and 7%, respectively.[40] However, no patients with regional or distant metastases were reported in three other published series on chondrosarcomas of the head and neck.[42, 66, 69] If distant metastasis occurs, it is almost exclusively located in the bones or the lungs.

Clinical Presentation and Diagnosis

Although the clinical findings are not specific for this tumor type, and a wide variety of symptoms (depending on the site and size of the lesion) could be part of the clinical picture, most patients present with a mass in the head and neck region or with airway symptoms. Definitive diagnosis requires tissue sampling, although chondrosarcomas can easily be confused with some other tumors such as chordoma, chondroid chordoma, and chondroblastic osteosarcoma. If the tissue biopsy does not contain any cartilaginous component of the tumor, it may also be difficult to differentiate this tumor from hemangiopericytoma, anaplastic carcinoma, rhabdomyosarcoma, synovial sarcoma, and especially Ewing's sarcoma–peripheral neuroectodermal tumor.[44] Therefore, consultation with an experienced pathologist is essential before the most appropriate treatment plan is selected. Both CT and MRI are useful imaging modalities for determining the extent of tumor. Because calcifications are seen in 75% to 80% of chondrosarcomas, observation of this finding may suggest the diagnosis. MRI usually shows a mass with an intermediate signal density on T1-weighted and an increased signal density on T2-weighted images.[70]

Treatment and Prognosis

Recommended treatment for chondrosarcoma of the head and neck is wide excision with negative margins. Elective neck dissection is not recommended in the absence of clinically positive cervical nodes because regional metastasis is rare. Although the overall recurrence rate has been reported to be almost 40% to 50%, most recurrences follow conservative or subtotal resection.[40, 66] Because a majority of chondrosarcomas of the head and neck are of low grade and histopathologic dedifferentiation is not common even in the presence of multiple recurrences, patients with recurrent disease can be treated with salvage surgery without compromising survival.[66, 71]

Overall survival for patients with chondrosarcoma was reported to be 78% to 90% at 5 years, and 64% to 81% at 10 years, with most patients dying from local failure (especially from intracranial spread and airway compromise).[40, 42, 66] Even patients with distant metastases had a 72% 5-year survival rate.[40] Five-year and 10-year disease-specific survival rates for head and neck chondrosarcoma were reported to be 87% and 71%, respectively.[40] These relatively high survival rates are probably due to the low histopathologic grade of most head and neck chondrosarcomas. The 5-year disease-specific survival rate for low-grade tumors was reported to be 93% and was 67% for high-grade tumors.[40]

Adjuvant or therapeutic radiation treatment is usually reserved for patients with extensive or high-grade lesions, patients with tumors with unfavorable histopathology (mesenchymal, dedifferentiated), those with inoperable or unresectable tumors, patients with positive resection margins, and those with recurrent tumor.[42] The recommended dose for radiation treatment is 6000 to 7000 cGy, delivered in 30 to 35 fractions.[42] Chemotherapy has no known role in the treatment of chondrosarcoma; however, it can be used with the intent of palliation in selected cases.[72]

◘ LEIOMYOSARCOMA

Epidemiology

Leiomyosarcoma is a malignant tumor arising from smooth muscle; it most commonly occurs in the uterus, the gastrointestinal tract, and the retroperitoneal area. It represents only 5% to 6% of all soft tissue sarcomas, and only 3% to 4% of this is tumor localized in the head and neck region.[73] Therefore, accumulated experience about the management of leiomyosarcoma of the head and neck (HNLe) also depends on case reports and literature reviews, as seen in other sarcomas of the head and neck. The low incidence of this tumor in the head and neck region is attributed to the scarcity of smooth muscle in this area, which is limited to vessel walls, erector pili muscle of the hair follicles, esophagus, and the posterior wall of the trachea.[74, 75] Although most leiomyosarcomas of the head and neck originate from these structures, it has also been proposed that some of these tumors might originate from undifferentiated mesenchymal cells.[76] A few reports in the literature suggest that radiation treatment or chemotherapy is a causative factor for the development of leiomyosarcoma, but there is not enough evidence to support these theories.[77–80]

HNLe can be diagnosed in patients of any age; however, most patients with this diagnosis who have been reported in the literature are in their fifth or sixth decade.[73, 74, 76, 81, 82] It seems that there is no sex predilection for this tumor (various ratios have been published that suggest equal distribution). The most common site for HNLe is the oral cavity (22%), followed by sinonasal tract (19%) and skin (17%).[73]

Clinical Presentation and Diagnosis

Clinical symptoms are usually site-specific, and patients most commonly present with a painless mass of the oral cavity or skin tumors; nasal obstruction and epistaxis for sinonasal tract tumors; and hoarseness, stridor, and dyspnea for laryngeal tumors. Macroscopically, HNLe presents as a polypoid or pedunculated, rubbery or firm, gray-tan or pink-colored mass.[76] Three subtypes of leiomyosarcoma have been described based on light microscopic findings, namely, conventional, vascular, and epithelioid.[73] Diagnostic imaging findings on CT and MRI are not specific for leiomyosarcoma and usually reveal a soft tissue mass.[83] Definitive diagnosis of leiomyosarcoma is made with tissue biopsy and immunohistochemical studies. α-Smooth muscle actin staining might be necessary because differentiation of leiomyosarcoma from fibrosarcoma, malignant schwannoma, and spindle cell carcinoma can be difficult in some cases. It has been reported that 86% to 89% of leiomyosarcomas are positive for α-smooth muscle actin in immunostaining.[76, 84] γ-Smooth muscle isoactin gene expression determination with polymerase chain reaction is promising in differentiating benign smooth muscle tumors from malignant ones.[85]

Treatment and Prognosis

Although drawing conclusions about the treatment and outcome of HNLe based on the limited reported experience is extremely difficult, the generally accepted treatment for this tumor is wide local excision with negative margins. Involvement of the cervical lymph nodes is not common in HNLe and accounts for only 10% to 15% of cases.[86] Therefore, neck dissection is usually not recommended in the absence of clinically positive cervical lymph nodes. Reported experience with radiation treatment and chemotherapy is limited and not promising.[76, 81]

Recurrence rates are variable, depending on the site of the tumor. They have been reported as 42% for oral cavity and skin lesions, 70% for paranasal sinus tumors, and 25% for tumors of the larynx.[73] Interestingly, no recurrences were reported for tumors confined to the nasal cavity.[76] Distant metastasis—primarily to the lungs and bones—occurred in 38% of patients with tumors of the oral cavity, in 17% of those with tumors of the sinonasal tract, and in 16% of those with tumors of the esophagus.[73, 86] Although subcutaneous leiomyosarcomas have a 50% to 60% rate of recurrence and a 33% to 53% rate of metastasis, superficial cutaneous counterparts rarely recur or metastasize.[87, 88] Overall survival rates are variable with an average of 50%; however, follow-up periods reported in the literature rarely approach 5 years.[73, 74, 76]

◗ SPINDLE CELL CARCINOMA (CARCINOSARCOMA, PSEUDOSARCOMA)

Spindle cell carcinoma (SpCC) is a malignant biphasic tumor that has also been referred to by names such as pseudosarcoma, carcinosarcoma, sarcomatoid carcinoma, pleomorphic carcinoma, metaplastic carcinoma, and collision tumor. Histopathologically, SpCC consists of a squamous cell carcinoma with a spindle cell component; there are four different categories of tumors, namely, squamous cell carcinoma with reactive or desmoplastic stroma, spindle cell squamous carcinoma, carcinosarcoma, and collision tumor.[89] These subtypes are potentially separable only by electron microscopy or immunohistochemistry.

Epidemiology

SpCC of the head and neck usually involves males, with a median age of 60 to 70.[90–94] The reported percentage of females involved with this tumor in the literature ranges from 0% to 22%.[90–94] Smoking, poor oral hygiene, alcohol use, and exposure to ionizing irradiation have all been considered as predisposing factors for SpCC of the head and neck.[90, 94, 95] Most common sites of origin for this tumor

appear to be the larynx, oral cavity, and hypopharynx; however, paranasal sinuses, nasal cavity, esophagus, nasopharynx, tonsil, skin, and parotid involvement have also been reported.[91, 95–103]

Controversy is noted in the literature about the outcomes of patients who have this tumor, according to primary site. Some authors believe that tumors originating from extralaryngeal sites, especially the sinonasal tract, have the worst prognosis.[95, 96] Batsakis reported an overall death rate of 76% for sinonasal SpCC, while tumors of the larynx had a 34% mortality rate.[95] However, some authors have indicated that tumors of the larynx behave more aggressively than their extralaryngeal counterparts, with a 39% versus a 53% 5-year disease-free survival rate.[91] Although it is difficult to draw a conclusion about the outcomes of SpCC of the head and neck according to the site of origin, tumors primarily arising from skin with their low overall mortality rate of 11% do not seem as aggressive as those in other head and neck subsites.[103]

Another controversy about this tumor is whether the gross morphologic appearance at initial presentation affects the outcome. About 80% of SpCC of the head and neck presents as a firm, pink, polypoid or pedunculated mass, with or without superficial ulceration.[94] Remaining tumors are usually infiltrative, ulcerative, and/or sessile lesions. Several authors have related a better prognosis with those tumors, which are more exophytic in appearance; others have proposed that the extent of the tumor, not its gross appearance, is the more important prognostic indicator.[92, 104] The possibly improved prognosis for polypoid tumors could be attributed to the fact that clear margins can be obtained more easily in patients with polypoid lesions.[96, 105]

Prognosis

Tumor stage is an important prognostic indicator for SpCC in that T1–T2 tumors have better reported overall 5-year survival rates than do T3–T4 tumors.[91] The reported regional metastasis rate of SpCC varies between 0% and 24% in the literature, and the metastatic component of this biphasic tumor can be epidermoid, spindle cell, or a combination of these.[91, 92, 95, 105] Regional metastasis is correlated with worse prognosis.[93, 104] An analysis of 21 previously reported patients with SpCC metastatic to the neck showed only one survivor at the end of 3 years.[104] Another study revealed a 75% cure rate in a group of patients with SpCC who had negative surgical margins and no cervical nodal involvement.[105] Overall 3-year mortality rates for SpCC vary between 29% and 45%.[91, 94–96]

Treatment

Generally accepted treatment of SpCC is wide local excision with negative margins. The presence of clinically positive cervical lymph nodes is an absolute indication for neck dissection. Some authors suggest neck dissection for supraglottic, extensive glottic, and hypopharyngeal tumors, regardless of cervical nodal status.[104] The role of primary or adjuvant radiation therapy in the treatment of SpCC is unclear. It has been reported that 5-year disease-specific survival rates for primarily irradiated T1 and T2 laryngeal

SpCC were not different from those for similarly staged squamous cell carcinoma.[90] Although several authors consider SpCC a radioresistant tumor, radiotherapy might be useful for sinonasal tract tumors, in cases with positive surgical margins, and in patients who cannot tolerate surgical excision for other reasons.[91, 104] The role of chemotherapy in the management of this tumor has not been clearly defined; however, a bladder SpCC controlled with combined gemcitabine and cisplatin treatment has been reported.[106]

ANGIOSARCOMA

Epidemiology

Angiosarcomas are rare malignant tumors composed of vascular endothelial cells that can originate from either blood vessels or lymphatic vessels. Angiosarcomas account for only 1% to 3% of all soft tissue sarcomas.[125] Although these tumors are rare in the head and neck region, almost 50% of angiosarcomas occur in this area.[126] Angiosarcomas account for only 10% to 15% of all soft tissue sarcomas of the head and neck.[67, 127] They are seen in males 3 to 4 times more frequently than in females, with a median age of 61 to 67.[127–129] Although trauma, previous irradiation, and longstanding lymphedema have all been thought of as etiologic factors, its cause is unknown.[125, 126] The scalp and facial skin are the most common sites of origin for this tumor; however, it has also been reported to arise in the nasopharynx, nose, paranasal sinuses, oral cavity, submandibular gland, middle ear, temporal bone, orbit, mandible, larynx, and thyroid.[125, 127]

Clinical Presentation and Diagnosis

Angiosarcomas usually present as solitary or multiple bruiselike macules with ill-defined margins; they may be confused with vascular malformations or other skin conditions, which typically leads to delay in diagnosis. Most tumors are usually asymptomatic even after the tumors have become deeply infiltrative; however, some tumors present as indurated, nodular, or ulcerative lesions with or without bleeding.[125–129]

Diagnosis is made with biopsy, but immunohistochemical staining might be necessary in differentiating this tumor, especially from hemangiopericytoma.[125]

Treatment and Prognosis

Wide local excision with negative margins seems to be the best treatment modality for well-circumscribed and solitary tumors. However, this may be difficult to achieve, given that these tumors may spread extensively through the soft tissues of the face and scalp. Adjuvant radiation treatment may improve survival.[129] Tumors with ill-defined margins may benefit from radiation with or without surgical excision. Local recurrence and distant metastasis—especially to the lungs—are frequent, regardless of the treatment modality. The overall 5-year survival rate for angiosarcoma has been reported to be 22% to 26%.[127, 129]

EXTRAMEDULLARY PLASMACYTOMA

Extramedullary plasmacytoma (EMP) is a form of plasma cell neoplasm characterized by monoclonal neoplastic proliferation of plasma cells in a location outside of the bone. Other types of plasma cell neoplasms include multiple myeloma, plasma cell leukemia, and solitary plasmacytoma of bone. The latter is usually considered to be a form fruste of multiple myeloma because 35% to 85% of these cases progress to multiple myeloma. Multiple myeloma is the disseminated, infiltrating, and most common form of plasma cell neoplasms.[107, 111] EMP accounts for only 10% of all plasma cell neoplasms, but it is the most commonly encountered form of plasma cell neoplasm in head and neck region.[108] Almost 80% to 90% of all EMPs occur in submucosal areas of the head and neck; however, they account for less than 1% of all head and neck tumors.[109–111] EMPs of the head and neck are usually submucosal, well-localized, locally destructive, and solitary soft tissue tumors composed of dense, homogeneous infiltrate of monoclonal plasma cells. Approximately 10% of these tumors have multiple sites of involvement.[107]

EMP can be confused with benign reactive plasmacytosis, undifferentiated carcinoma, non-Hodgkin's lymphoma, malignant melanoma, and esthesioneuroblastoma.[108] Although transformation to multiple myeloma is not commonly seen as in solitary plasmacytoma of bone, it has been reported that 10% to 32% of these lesions convert to multiple myeloma, usually within 2 years of diagnosis.[108, 112] Unfortunately, this conversion cannot be predicted and may occur as late as 22 to 36 years following the initial diagnosis.[112] Therefore, lifelong follow-up of patients with EMP is mandatory.[108, 112]

Epidemiology

EMP affects males more than females, with a percentage varying between 65% and 85% male patients; usually, patients are diagnosed in their fifth to seventh decades of life.[108, 111, 113] The most common site of involvement in the head and neck region is the sinonasal tract (i.e., the nasal cavity, paranasal sinuses, nasopharynx), which accounts for 55% to 71% of cases.[108, 113] Other reported sites of involvement include the larynx, parotid gland, submandibular gland, thyroid gland, hyoid bone, middle ear cavity and mastoid, skull base, mandible, tonsils, palate, trachea, buccal mucosa, orbit, skin, and cervical lymph nodes.[108, 111, 114–123]

Clinical Presentation

EMP usually presents as a soft tissue mass. The symptoms are not specific to this tumor. Rather, they are usually related to the size and site of the lesion. Because the most common site of involvement is the sinonasal tract, the most commonly encountered symptoms are nasal obstruction and epistaxis.[108] Airway and digestive tract symptoms such as dysphonia, dyspnea, and dysphagia may also occur owing to mechanical obstruction.

Diagnosis

CT and MRI are helpful diagnostic tools in defining the exact location and extent of the tumor. However, CT and MRI findings are not specific and usually reveal a soft tissue mass. Definitive diagnosis of EMP depends on adequate tissue sampling, and this can be performed successfully most of the time because the tumor is usually accessible for an endoscopic or an open biopsy. In most cases, fine-needle aspiration (FNA) fails to obtain an adequate tissue sample for immunohistochemical analysis. The classic FNA finding of EMP is a cluster of plasma cells, which may be difficult or impossible to differentiate from other inflammatory and reactive conditions.[108] However, FNA may be helpful in ruling out other tumors such as squamous cell carcinoma. It can also be used as a diagnostic tool to identify local or regional recurrence in follow-up of patients with a previously proven and treated EMP.[108, 111] Immunohistochemical staining necessitates fresh tissue samples and reveals the monoclonal nature of the plasma cells, producing either lambda or kappa light chain.[108] Additional diagnostic studies such as urinalysis (for Bence Jones protein), serum protein electrophoresis, bone marrow examination, and skeletal survey should also be performed to rule out multiple myeloma.

EMP is staged according to the extent of the tumor. Stage I represents tumors confined to one anatomic site, stage II corresponds to tumors with local extension or regional metastasis, and stage III represents tumors with distant metastatic spread.[107]

Treatment and Prognosis

EMP is generally considered to be a radiosensitive tumor, and the radiation treatment seems as effective as surgical excision. Local control can be achieved through radiation treatment alone as the primary treatment modality in 75% to 80% of cases.[108, 111] Radiation doses of 45 to 60 Gy delivered as daily fractions of 1.75 to 2 Gy are recommended for EMP of the head and neck.[108]

The 5-year survival rate with radiation alone has been reported to be as high as 69%, with a disease-free survival of 63%.[124] Surgery can be reserved for limited tumors, which can be resected with negative margins without giving the patient a significant morbidity, or can be performed in salvage of the radiation failures. Regional metastasis occurs in 15% to 20% of cases; however, it does not seem to affect the prognosis.[112] Local recurrence rates following radiation or surgery have been reported as 6% to 10%.[111] Neck dissection is indicated in cases with regional metastasis. Prognosis is good, with more than 70% of patients having a 10-year disease-free survival rate.[111, 112] Chemotherapy, especially melphalan and cyclophosphamide, can be administered in cases with disseminated disease.[112]

◼ CONGENITAL VASCULAR LESIONS

For years, the terminology for congenital vascular lesions was confusing, until Mulliken and Glowacki presented a classification based on their clinical and biologic behavior.[130]

TABLE 27-2 Congenital Vascular Lesions

Hemangiomas
Vascular malformations
Capillary
Venular
Venous
Lymphatic
Mixed
Arteriovenous
Venous-lymphatic

They recognized two entirely distinct groups of congenital vascular lesions—hemangiomas and vascular malformations (Table 27–2). Knowledge of this classification facilitates the correct diagnosis of these lesions, leading to appropriate, individualized treatment.

Hemangiomas

Hemangiomas are usually not obvious at birth, but most appear during the first month of life. They are most commonly found in the head and neck, and they start as flat, erythematous macules. They proliferate rapidly during the first year of life, then reach a plateau and stabilize for variable periods. Following the stable phase, there is usually complete involution, which may take up to 12 years.

Hemangiomas are the most common tumor of infancy, and they are more common among females.[130, 131] They can be classified as superficial (cutaneous), deep (subcutaneous), or mixed (compound). Histologic features include tubules of plump, proliferating, endothelial cells surrounding narrow vessels and an abundance of mast cells.

In 2001, North and associates[132] reported that true hemangiomas had four immunohistochemical markers, which were identical to placental tissue and unlike any other tissue tested. The markers are glutamine transferase (Glut 1), merrosine, Lewis Y antigen, and Fc gamma receptor II. This leads to the hypothesis that hemangiomas are seeded from the placenta during embryonic development. Research is being directed toward this hypothesis, and if substantiated, it could lead to new methods of diagnosis and treatment. Glut 1 is now considered a reliable immunohistochemical marker for hemangiomas.

Another vascular lesion that is seen at birth and appears to be a hemangioma is fairly large at birth and begins to involute within the first few weeks of life. This lesion is called a rapidly involuting childhood hemangioma (RICH) (Fig. 27–1). It is not a true hemangioma in that it does not test positive for Glut 1.

All hemangiomas proliferate during the first year of life. The timing and rate may vary. The proliferative phase usually begins at 6 to 12 weeks and can lead to rapid enlargement. During this phase, complications are not uncommon and should be anticipated and appropriately treated. Complications include (1) ulceration, bleeding, or scarring; (2) visual axis obstruction with deprivation, amblyopia, and blindness (Fig. 27–2); (3) airway obstruction from laryngotracheal involvement; (4) high-output cardiac failure, which is rare and usually incipient and persists even during the earlier phases of involution (it may be associated with a

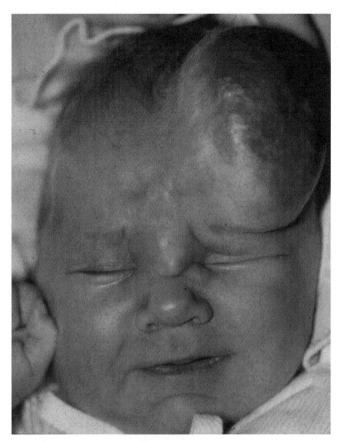

FIGURE 27–1 Newborn child with a rapid involuting childhood hemangioma. It began involuting within the first weeks of life.

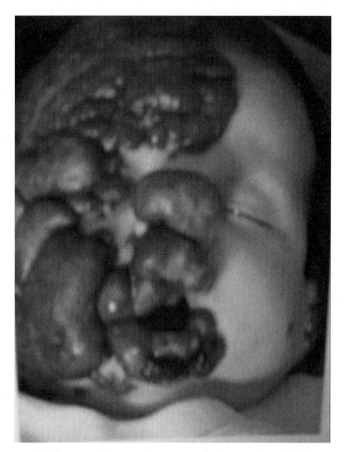

FIGURE 27–2 Patient with extensive hemangiomas obstructing the vision and nasal airway. This child was treated with high-dose steroids and vincristine with excellent results.

single large hemangioma or multiple lesions and is potentially fatal); and (5) Kasabach-Merritt syndrome.

In the past, Kasabach-Merritt syndrome had been considered to be associated with hemangiomas; however, it has been shown to be caused by kaposiform hemangioendothelioma (KHE).[134] Kasabach-Merritt syndrome results from platelet sequestration and destruction within the lesions, resulting in a consumptive coagulopathy. If the syndrome is left untreated, profound thrombocytopenia results and a generalized bleeding disorder develops. Kasabach-Merritt syndrome is usually clinically evident within the first few weeks of life; hallmark features include edema and ecchymoses surrounding a rapidly proliferating lesion (Fig. 27–3). Histologic features include infiltrative sheets and nodules of endothelial cells with islands of dilated lymphatic-type vessels. North and Waner have found that with the use of a triple stain technique, a mixed lymphatic and endothelial component can be identified (unpublished data). This syndrome is fatal in up to 60% of cases. Early recognition and treatment are essential for survival.

Toward the end of the first year of life hemangiomas stop proliferating, and involution follows over the next 2 to 12 years. The lesion feels softer and more compressible, and eventually shrinkage becomes evident. In superficial lesions, the color changes from a bright red to a more dusky purple and in some areas disappears completely. The

histologic correlate of involution is a progressive flattening of the endothelial cells until an endpoint of flat, inactive cells surrounding ectatic, thin-walled vessels, not dissimilar to capillaries. As the lesion shrinks, the number of vessels diminishes, and they are replaced by fibrofatty tissue. The

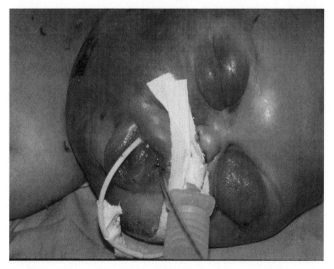

FIGURE 27–3 This child had Kasabach-Merritt syndrome with extensive edema and ecchymosis. This baby died after several weeks of treatment with no response.

rate of involution is extremely variable. In general, the more rapid the rate of involution, the more complete it is. Sequelae from hemangiomas include the residuum and consist of fibrofatty changes and telangiectasia on the surface. About 60% of all patients require some type of corrective surgery.[135]

Diagnosis

The diagnosis of a hemangioma is usually obvious from the history and physical examination. With known immuno-histochemical markers, a biopsy can confirm the diagnosis but is rarely necessary. Radiographic studies such as CT and MRI scans can be useful in determining the extent of the lesion.

On MRI, hemangiomas are high-flow, solid tissue lesions of intermediate intensity on T1-weighted images, and of high intensity on T2-weighted images. Flow voids are usually seen in T1- and T2-weighted images, and these lesions enhance with gadolinium (Fig. 27–4).

Arteriograms are not usually indicated unless intervention is planned, such as surgical resection or embolization procedures.

Treatment

Traditional treatment for hemangiomas is expectant because of the likelihood of involution, unless there is significant potential for a complication to develop. If one of the complications mentioned previously is present, supportive or curative treatment is indicated. We are more aggressive with respect to treatment because we feel there are

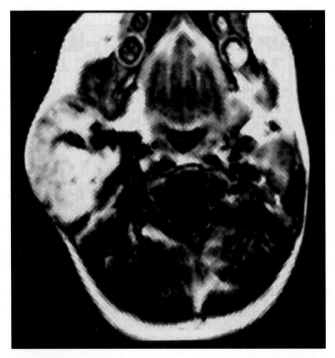

FIGURE 27–4 MRI of a parotid hemangioma with high intensity on T1-weighted images, which can enhance more notably with gadolinium. Notice high flow voids within the lesion.

significant psychosocial factors involved with the large, extensive hemangiomas that can take years to involute, and because technologic advances allow treatment with minimum risks or complications.

MEDICAL TREATMENT

It should be stressed that the medical treatment discussed here is useful only during proliferation and is not effective during involution.

Cutaneous or Superficial Hemangiomas. For cutaneous or superficial hemangiomas, laser photocoagulation can be very effective. Treatment with a pulsed dye laser has been found to be effective in flat, macular lesions.[136–138] With the use of a 7-mm spot size, a 595-nm wavelength, and dynamic cooling, the entire lesion should be treated with between 10 and 12 J/cm^2 to an endpoint of uniform purplish-gray discoloration. This may require several pulses over the same area during one treatment. Treatment should commence at the earliest sign of the lesion and should be repeated at 4- to 6-week intervals until the lesion has been completely eliminated.[131, 136, 138]

Subcutaneous or Deep Hemangiomas. Subcutaneous or deep hemangiomas will not respond to a flash lamp pumped dye laser. Some centers in Europe have used an interstitial neodymium:yttrium-aluminum-garnet (Nd:YAG) laser, which can result in some shrinkage but requires a general anesthetic and special equipment, causes significant scarring, and can injure adjacent nerves.

Segmental Hemangiomas. Hemangiomas that are growing rapidly and causing problems should be treated initially with steroids. Steroids are very effective during the proliferative phase, and response is dose-dependent. For segmental involvement, oral prednisone is the treatment of choice. A dose of 4 to 6 mg/kg/day is recommended for a period of 4 to 6 weeks and is tapered over another 2 to 4 weeks. A significant response is seen in more than 75% of children.[139] Rebound proliferation occurs within a few days of completion of this course in 40% of patients. A second course, after a rest of several weeks, may be tried if the initial response was good. If proliferation should recur, a daily maintenance dose of between 0.75 and 1 mg/kg body weight may then be considered. A pediatrician should be involved with this treatment because steroids can cause significant adverse effects.

Focal Hemangiomas. Focal or isolated hemangiomas can be treated with intralesional steroids. The use of intra-lesional steroids was first described in 1970 by Azzolini and Nouvenne, who felt that they would eliminate systemic adverse effects.[140] The injection must be carefully performed because the steroids cause significant atrophy of any tissue around the hemangioma. The recommended dose of intralesional steroids is a mixture of 1 mL of 40 mg triamcinolone/mL and 1 mL of 6 mg betamethasone/mL. One to 2 mL of this mixture can be injected into the hemangioma, with care taken to distribute the steroids evenly and stay within the lesion. An initial response rate of up to 80% has been noted. A second or third injection may be necessary between 6 and 8 weeks later.

Other Medical Treatments. Vincristine has been found to be very effective for hemangiomas that are not responding to routine treatments, but it is an off-label use of this drug. The dose of vincristine for hemangiomas is 1.5 mg/m² intravenously weekly for 6 weeks. For children weighing less than 10 kg, the dose is 0.05 mg/kg intravenously weekly (M. Waner, unpublished observations). It may be necessary to repeat the treatment in cases of rebound.

Interferon α 2a has been recommended for hemangiomas because of its antiangiogenic effect. We discourage the use of interferon because there is significant potential for neurologic complications such as spastic diplegia of the extremities, which is usually permanent and disabling.[141, 142] At present, there are other good options, so we do not recommend the use of interferon for hemangiomas.

SURGICAL RESECTION

Surgical resection is also an option and can be selected during either proliferation or involution. For a localized lesion that is rapidly expanding, surgery can be a safe and effective option. Many of these lesions act as a skin expander that can facilitate primary closure after resection. Also, the rapid expansion often compresses surrounding tissue and results in an identifiable border around the lesion. With careful dissection, a relatively bloodless plane can be found, and with the use of a bipolar cautery, monopolar cautery, or Shaw thermal scalpel, these lesions can be removed safely with very little blood loss. Resection must be completed during the proliferative phase, or the residual lesion will continue to proliferate.

During involution, it is not as crucial that the entire lesion be removed because small areas left behind will eventually involute completely. Large involuting hemangiomas can take years to involute, and because of the psychosocial effects that often occur, resection should be considered. There are also many hemangiomas of the lips and nose that should be resected because of the facial deformities that occur and the unwanted attention and ridicule that can result if they are left untreated (Fig. 27–5).[143] These can be easy to remove, with dramatic results noted immediately.

Untreated hemangiomas involving the skin commonly leave atrophic scars and telangiectases. The atrophic scars can respond well to skin resurfacing with an erbium:yttrium-aluminum-garnet (Er:YAG) laser, and the telangiectasia can be treated with a flash lamp pumped dye laser. Residual fibrofatty tissue that is a problem should be excised.

Vascular Malformations

Vascular malformations are frequently called hemangiomas, but their pathogenesis is distinct. They are true developmental anomalies, and although they are always present at birth, they may not be apparent.[130] They do not proliferate, nor do they involute; instead, they usually undergo a slow, steady hypertrophy. This hypertrophy is believed to be a result of progressive dilatation of preformed vascular channels. It is primarily the size of the vascular channels and not the number that causes the hypertrophy. Periods of rapid enlargement may occur, frequently around puberty and other periods of hormonal modulation such as pregnancy. Infection may result in sudden enlargement of a lymphatic malformation, especially during infancy, which can be confused with a hemangioma. With antibiotic

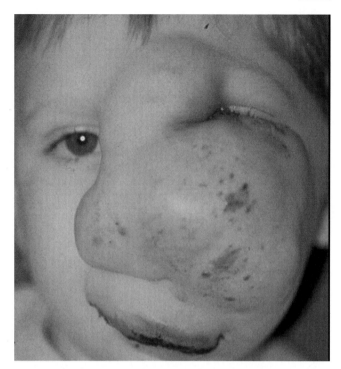

FIGURE 27–5 This hemangioma is in the involuting stage but would take years to resolve. This patient is a candidate for surgical reduction of the mass lesion.

treatment, the enlargement may resolve to the preinfection size. Arteriovenous malformations may change rapidly owing to high flow with shunting, making them potentially very destructive.

Vascular malformations are classified in accordance with their vascular content.[130] The following subtypes are described:

- Capillary malformations
- Venular malformations (port wine stains)
- Venous malformations
- Lymphatic malformations
- Mixed malformations
  - Arteriovenous malformations
  - Venous-lymphatic malformations

The malformations that will be discussed in this chapter are venous, lymphatic, and mixed malformations. These vascular malformations are tumorlike and can be very destructive, similar to malignancies.

Venous Malformations

CLINICAL PRESENTATION

Venous malformations can occur anywhere in the head and neck. They commonly involve the tongue, palate, pharynx, larynx, and soft tissues of the face and neck (Fig. 27–6). They may be isolated with well-delineated borders and can be resected totally, or they may be very diffuse and almost impossible to remove completely. They grow as the patient grows. Venous malformations are soft, compressible, and nontender. With the patient in the Trendelenburg position, these lesions enlarge by engorgement and become much

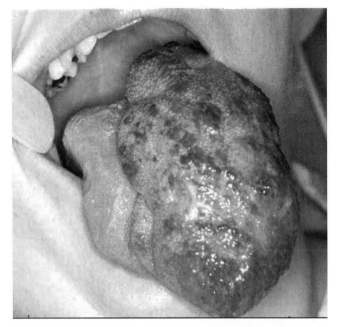

FIGURE 27–6 Patient with extensive venous malformation of only one side with compression of the tongue on the opposite side. Numerous physicians had told her never to have surgery.

more obvious. They usually show bluish discoloration, depending on their proximity to the skin or mucosa. There is no pulsation, thrill, or bruit.

DIAGNOSIS

MRI is the best imaging study, and it can delineate the lesion well. Phleboliths are commonly found within the malformation, especially in adults, and can be seen on the MRI or CT scan. Venous malformations are low-flow lesions, isointense with muscle on T1-weighted images, and very intense on T2-weighted images (Fig. 27–7). The phleboliths appear as low-intensity punctate areas in T2-weighted images and as calcifications on CT scans.

Arteriograms are neither helpful nor recommended with venous malformations because there are no major arterial feeders.

TREATMENT

Treatment for venous malformations depends on the site and extent and the capabilities of the treating physician. The choices are laser photocoagulation, sclerotherapy, surgical resection, and a combination of these. Some venous malformations may not be curable and should be treated for symptom relief.

Malformations that involve mucosal surfaces can be treated with an Nd:YAG laser.[144] The power settings vary between 20 to 30 watts at a 0.3- to 0.5-second duration; because the very thin covering over the venous malformation may rupture at the higher settings, it is worthwhile to do a test application. The laser is applied in a polka dot pattern with about 2 to 3 mm of space between spots. A whitish spot should appear on the surface where the laser hits (Fig. 27–8). Because of the low blood flow involved, firm pressure for a few minutes usually stops the bleeding.

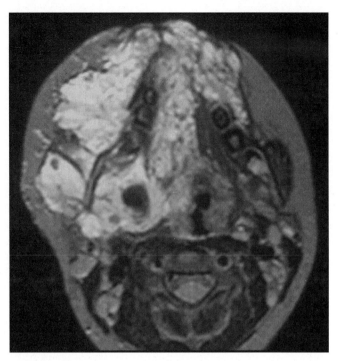

FIGURE 27–7 MRI of an extensive venous malformation. It is very intense on T2-weighted images. There are several rounded, low-intensity areas representing phleboliths.

For very large, extensive lesions, two separate treatments given about 8 weeks apart may be required for satisfactory shrinkage to be obtained. Initial shrinkage can be dramatic but is only temporary.

In the past the Nd:YAG laser was not recommended for skin surfaces because significant absorption by the melanin

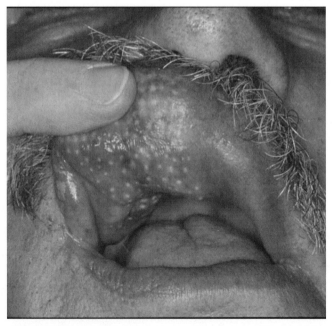

FIGURE 27–8 Patient with venous malformation of the upper lip and oral cavity being treated with YAG laser. The whitish spots on the surface represent the YAG laser treatment sites.

in skin can result in skin damage, ulceration, and sloughs with scarring. Newer technology uses surface cooling to protect the skin from injury. Because mucosa has little melanin, the epithelial surface is not damaged very much, and it heals very nicely.

Sclerotherapy using sodium tetradecol or pure alcohol has been used successfully to clot areas of the malformation, but the result is temporary and the procedure must be done under general anesthesia, carries significant risks, and can be very painful. Sclerotherapy can also be used as an adjunct a few days before surgical resection. However, because only a limited amount of sclerosing agent can be injected in one setting, if the lesion is quite large sclerotherapy may not be beneficial before surgery.

Surgery should be considered, especially if MRI shows the venous malformation to have a defined border and to be accessible. When the mass is totally resected, surgery can be curative. However, any residual lesion may expand over time. Venous malformation surgery involving the face is more complicated, because the facial nerve can be very difficult to dissect without significant injury. The surgeon must be willing to spend the 4 to 6 hours needed to identify, dissect, and preserve the facial nerve.

Involvement of the tongue is common, and if the tongue is symptomatic it should be treated. If MRI shows the venous malformation to have a definable margin, resection should be considered. If the lesion seems to involve only one side of the tongue, it frequently can be resected with a hemiglossectomy and the tongue reconstructed (Fig. 27–9). If diffuse involvement is present, Nd:YAG laser treatments can significantly reduce the size of the malformation and can improve symptoms (Fig. 27–10).[144] Two treatments given 6 to 8 weeks apart may be required for satisfactory shrinkage to be obtained. The venous malformation will reexpand within 1 or 2 years, and additional laser treatments will be required.

For venous malformations that cannot be resected, the clinician must stress to patients that they should sleep with the head elevated at an incline of at least 45 degrees for the rest of their lives. Significant venous distention of these vessels occurs over the years as a result of supine positioning.

Lymphatic Malformations

All lymphatic malformations are present at birth, but they may not become apparent until the first or second year of life. The growth is usually slow and steady and commensurate with the growth of the child, although sudden or rapid expansion may result from infection, trauma, or hormonal changes.

CLINICAL PRESENTATION

Lymphatic malformations may be superficial, deep, or both. They may be cystic or diffuse with interstitial involvement, and they can be described as macrocystic, microcystic, or mixed.

Macrocystic lymphatic malformations include the cystic hygromas. These tend to be more localized, are found most often in the neck and the parotid area, and are more likely to be cured with treatment. The macrocystic lymphatic malformations are usually obviously cystic and may be extremely large.

Microcystic lymphatic malformations are diffuse and infiltrate into surrounding structures from the mucosal surface to the deep tissues. Microcystic lymphatic malformations may not be life threatening but may cause significant deformity. They rarely involve the skin in the head and neck; rather, they usually involve the mucosa and appear as multiple tiny, clear vesicles on the mucosal surface. Because of the superficial location, some of the vesicles have blood mixed within them from trauma, which may confuse the diagnosis. Beneath the vesicular areas, the tissue is enlarged and hypertrophied. The adjacent tissues such as the mandible may become hypertrophied, causing dental abnormalities and occlusive problems. These lesions frequently enlarge rapidly during the first few years of life when patients contract upper respiratory tract infections, but with prompt antibiotic treatment they shrink to their original size within a week or two. Large microcystic lymphatic malformations continue to grow over time, and growth spurts may occur with infection, hormonal changes such as puberty and pregnancy, and trauma. Aspiration reveals a straw-colored fluid with lymphocytes and no epithelial tissue, whereas branchial cleft cysts contain cholesterol and epithelial debris.

The mixed type includes both types of findings, and the cysts are usually not very large.

Longstanding lymphatic malformations cause hypertrophy of the involved tissues and include the mandible, often resulting in malocclusion (Fig. 27–11). The pharynx may be involved, causing airway obstruction and requiring a tracheotomy. The larynx is seldom involved.

DIAGNOSIS

The diagnosis is made by history and physical examination and can be confirmed by MRI. The MRI findings are very similar to those of venous malformations, with a few exceptions. They do not have phleboliths, and occasionally, fluid-fluid levels are seen. They are isointense with muscle on T1-weighted images and are hyperintense on T2-weighted images (Fig. 27–12).

TREATMENT AND PROGNOSIS

Macrocystic lymphatic malformations are treated by surgical excision or sclerosis. Because they can be extremely large, their treatment can be urgent. An experienced surgeon can excise them easily, but adequate exposure is needed, and the nerves and major vessels involved with the lesion must be preserved. Usually, there is a distinct capsule that must be followed, and the surgeon must take care not to break the capsule. The neurovascular structures can be dissected away from the capsule. When macrocystic lesions are removed completely, they can be cured.

Another acceptable method of treating these large macrocystic lesions is with a sclerosing agent. The drug with the most success is OK 432.[145, 146] This drug is a lyophilized incubation mixture of low virulent SU strain type III, Group A Strep P with Pen G.K. Enough data are available from multiple studies to verify its effectiveness and safety, but the drug is not yet approved by the Federal Drug Administration in the United States.

Microcystic lesions and the mixed types are much more difficult to treat because of their locations in the head and

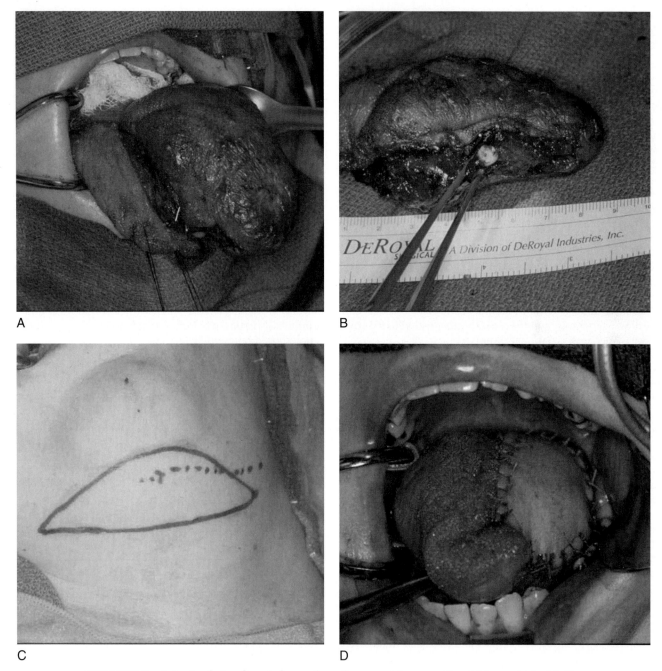

A

B

C

D

FIGURE 27–9 *A,* Lesion being dissected away from the normal tongue with a fairly good identifiable plane. *B,* A phlebolith after surgical excision, which is seen only in venous malformations. *C,* Submental flap based on submental artery for reconstruction of the tongue. *D,* Submental flap has been carried into the oral cavity and used to reconstruct the tongue.

neck. Most of these involve the mucosal surfaces of the oral cavity, oropharynx, and hypopharynx and the soft tissues of the face and neck, where they are very infiltrative and cannot be removed without removal of much of the involved normal tissues.

Microcystic lesions that involve the mucosa of the oral cavity can be treated with lasers. The vesicular lesions on the surface can be treated with the CO_2 laser, followed by use of an Nd:YAG laser to treat the deeper portion under the surface. The settings of the Nd:YAG laser are between 20 and 30 watts of power delivered at a 0.3- to 0.5-second exposure

time. The penetration of this laser is from 5 to 8 mm deep. The contraction obtained with treatment can be significant (Fig. 27–13), and a second treatment about 2 months later causes a much greater shrinkage. However, this treatment is only a temporizing solution because the malformation will recur and will need further treatment 1 to 2 years later. When the Nd:YAG laser is used on a large surface, there may be significant edema of the tongue and throat, which may last for several weeks. Steroids, antibiotics, and elevation can be used to decrease the edema. Patients may not be able to close the mouth for several days because of the

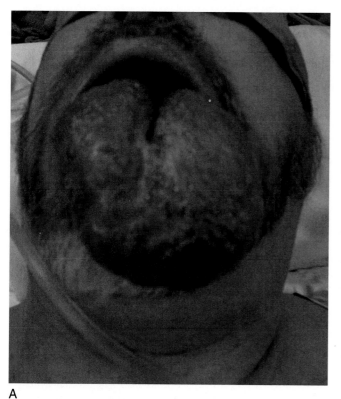

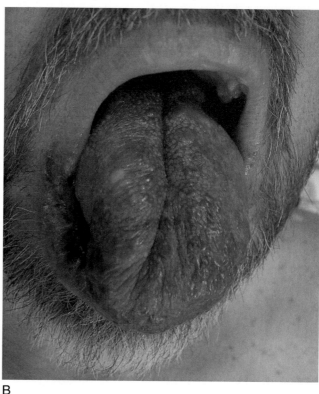

A   B

FIGURE 27–10 *A*, Patient with extensive venous malformation before treatment with a YAG laser. *B*, Patient 2 months after second treatment with YAG laser.

edema of the tongue. However, tracheotomy is rarely required.

Large microcystic malformations can also be treated surgically, but with great difficulty, primarily because of the presence of the facial nerve and lingual and hypoglossal nerves, which must be identified and preserved. The surgeon must be prepared to spend hours identifying and preserving these nerves, then removing the adjacent involved tissue.

OK 432 is not effective for microcystic lymphatic malformations, probably because of the numerous septations that prevent contact with other spaces.

Mixed Malformations

LYMPHATIC-VENOUS MALFORMATIONS

There are some true mixed lymphatic and venous malformations. The venous portion may be resectable, whereas the lymphatic portion may be too diffuse to remove without major tissue loss and disabilities. These mixed types usually are the microcystic type. These will continue to grow with time; the venous portion may need to be resected because of the extensive size that can be reached if left untreated.

ARTERIOVENOUS MALFORMATIONS

Arteriovenous malformations (AVMs) are congenital lesions that are present at birth but may not become apparent

until years later.[130] Most become clinically apparent before the age of 30. Previous reports of patients being diagnosed after the age of 50 are most likely cases of misdiagnosis; these malformations probably are venous malformations.

An AVM is an abnormal congenital communication between arteries and veins. These communications consist

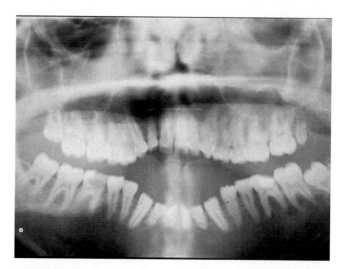

FIGURE 27–11 Panorex of a patient with lymphatic malformation, showing significant malocclusion (open bite) from hypertrophy of the mandible.

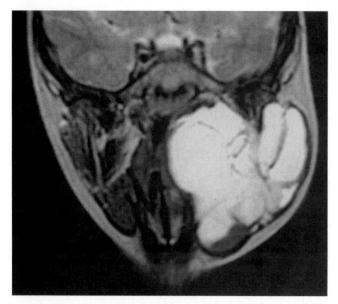

FIGURE 27–12 MRI of lymphatic malformation, which is hyperintense on T2-weighted images. This shows a multiseptated macrocystic lymphatic malformation. (Courtesy of Dr. Charles James.)

of multiple microfistulous tracts, called the nidus. Histologically, the nidus shows a heterogeneous mixture of vessel types, including tortuous arteries and dilated veins with thickened walls and intimal changes, dispersed within a complex background of numerous smaller arteries and veins, as well as arterioles, capillaries, and venules. Areas of capillary proliferation presumably represent a reaction to the altered hemodynamics of the lesion. The underlying abnormality appears to be an absence of precapillary sphincters. Arteriovenous shunting occurs across this capillary bed, and over time, the lesion is extended by recruitment of adjacent capillary beds as well as by hypertrophy of the feeding arteries and capillaries and dilation of the draining veins. The AVM expands through hemodynamic changes that result from the shunting of the blood. For years, the AVMs may be low-flow lesions, and change or expansion occurs slowly. They eventually become high-flow lesions and the expansion becomes very rapid, causing many problems. AVMs can be life threatening because of the destructive changes to the involved tissues and the potential for severe bleeding. Therefore, their behavior can be described as locally "malignant," and they require prompt and effective treatment.

An AVM is different from an arteriovenous fistula, which consists of only one or two fistulous tracts and is acquired as the result of trauma. The arteriovenous fistula is much easier to treat.

Diagnosis. AVMs manifest themselves at different ages, but almost all are obvious by 30 years of age. The ones that become high flow before the age of 1 year are very destructive and can result in death if not controlled. They can be confused with hemangiomas but will not respond to steroids or vincristine and do not involute spontaneously, as hemangiomas do. AVMs will have a capillary blush overlying them,

which looks like a port wine stain. There may be a fibrotic change on the overlying skin, which is the result of ischemia and a "steal" syndrome because the AVM shunts blood from the skin to the nidus (Fig. 27–14). There is always a strong pulsation to the mass, and a palpable thrill may be felt over the mass. Dilated tortuous veins are commonly noted. Skeletal overgrowth or hypertrophy of adjacent soft tissue may result from the increased blood supply. In advanced disease, there is skin involvement with ulcerations and bleeding (Fig. 27–15). Involvement of the tongue usually results in hypertrophy, ulcerations, and bleeding. It is extremely difficult to determine the extent of the AVM because of the enlargement of the feeding vessels and the draining veins, which may not be part of the nidus but are the result of the hemodynamic changes resulting from the malformation.

MRI can be helpful and demonstrates vessels with high-flow voids in a serpiginous pattern seen in both T1- and T2-weighted images. An arteriogram is the best radiographic test for diagnosing and delineating an AVM, but delineating the location and extent of the lesion can still be difficult (Fig. 27–16). CT scan is not very helpful for the diagnosis or delineation of the full extent of these lesions.

Treatment. Of all the vascular malformations, the AVM is the most difficult to manage. The only chance for cure is complete resection of the AVM. The nidus must be completely removed because any residuum will result in a recurrence. Determining the location of the nidus margin may be difficult because of all the reactive vessels that enlarge from the shunting over time. Frozen sections may be helpful but require a pathologist experienced in vascular lesions. One test that is helpful is compression of the remaining tissues with a finger or instrument to look for a "rebound" phenomenon. This rebound is seen as rapid refilling of the tissue and is usually a sign of residual disease.

Surgical resection requires considerable experience in control of bleeding with the use of several methods, such as monopolar and bipolar electrocautery, hemoclips, and manual compression. One of the major challenges during surgery is to preserve major nerves in the middle of the nidus. Generally, the experience of a head and neck cancer surgeon who is used to major ablative procedures and doing major reconstruction is required. Surgical resection of an AVM should never be undertaken lightly. Once the diagnosis has been made, resection should not be delayed, because the AVM only becomes larger with time and requires even more extensive tissue removal.

Surgical ligation alone of the feeder vessels is ineffective after a few days or weeks because a new blood supply develops rapidly. Also, ligation compromises the ability of the surgeon to embolize the lesion in the future.

Embolization alone should be performed primarily for emergency situations such as acute bleeding and unresectable lesions. It is only a temporary solution, lasting days to weeks and occasionally months. This procedure should be performed by an experienced interventional radiologist. The best use of embolization is in combination with surgery. We recommend that an arteriogram be done 1 to 3 days before surgery and that the malformation be embolized during that procedure.

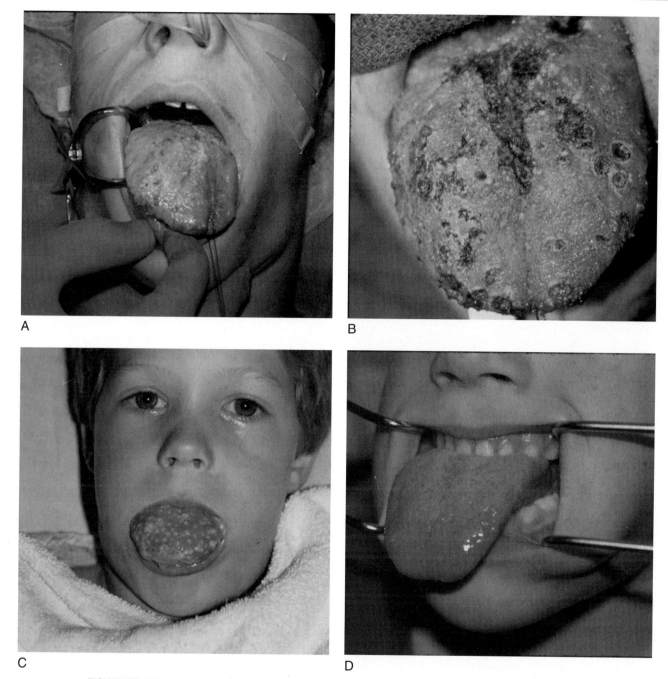

FIGURE 27–13 *A*, Extensive lymphatic malformation of the tongue before treatment. *B*, CO_2 laser was used to remove these vesicular lesions down to the level of the muscle. *C*, Polka-dot white spots from the YAG laser treatment, with significant edema days after laser treatment, *D*, Six months after second laser treatment.

Sclerotherapy is recommended in some AVMs that are unresectable. The primary sclerotic agent used is pure alcohol. These procedures can have significant complications, such as pain, swelling, and injuries to nerves, and should be performed by an experienced interventional radiologist.

The vascular blush overlying AVMs may reveal primary involvement of the skin or may represent secondary changes from the high flow of blood through the nidus. It may also represent a true port wine stain. Treatment varies according

to the cause. True involvement of the skin by the AVM will require resection of the involved skin because the AVM will continue to enlarge and cause problems. If the blush is believed to be secondary to the high blood flow beneath it, it can be left alone during surgery and may eventually diminish. If it is a true port wine stain, it can be treated with lasers.

It is extremely important for the clinician to understand the classification and natural history of these congenital vascular lesions so that the diagnosis can be made and the

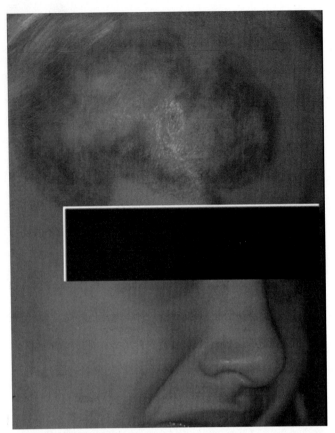

FIGURE 27–14 An AV malformation with ischemia of the skin from a "steal" syndrome. The supraorbital artery feeder vessel is noticeable in the upper eyelid.

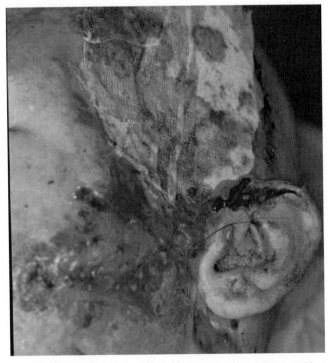

FIGURE 27–15 Patient with recurrent and advanced AV malformations with extensive ulceration and bleeding. He had been treated with multiple embolization procedures.

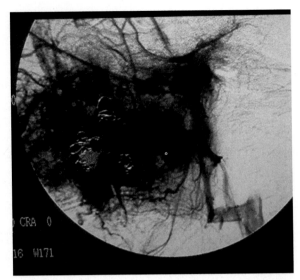

FIGURE 27–16 An arteriogram of a young child with extensive AV malformations of the maxillary sinus and skull base. Multiple coils are seen from previous embolization procedures.

proper treatment selected. These lesions certainly act like tumors and have many malignant properties.

REFERENCES

1. Golledge J, Fisher C, Rhys-Evans PH: Head and neck liposarcoma. Cancer 76:1051–1058, 1995.
2. Esclamado RM, Disher MJ, Ditto JL, et al: Laryngeal liposarcoma. Arch Otolaryngol Head Neck Surg 120:422–426, 1994.
3. Torosian MH, Friedrich C, Godbold J, et al: Soft-tissue sarcoma: Initial characteristics and prognostic factors in patients with and without metastatic disease. Semin Surg Oncol 4:13–19, 1988.
4. McCulloch TM, Makielski KH, McNutt MA: Head and neck liposarcoma. A histopathologic reevaluation of reported cases. Arch Otolaryngol Head Neck Surg 118:1045–1049, 1992.
5. Yueh B, Bassewitz HL, Eisele DW: Retropharyngeal liposarcoma. Am J Otolaryngol 16:331–340, 1995.
6. Saddik M, Oldring DJ, Mourad WA: Liposarcoma of the base of tongue and tonsillar fossa: A possibly underdiagnosed neoplasm. Arch Pathol Lab Med 120:292–295, 1996.
7. Larson DL, Cohn AM, Estrada RG: Liposarcoma of the tongue. J Otolaryngol 5:410–414, 1976.
8. Baden E, Newman R: Liposarcoma of the oropharyngeal region. Review of the literature and report of two cases. Oral Surg Oral Med Oral Pathol 44:889–902, 1977.
9. Saunders JG, Jaques DA, Casterline PF, et al: Liposarcomas of the head and neck: A review of the literature and addition of four cases. Cancer 43:162–168, 1979.
10. Sauk JJ: Liposarcoma of the head and neck. J Oral Surg 29:38–40, 1975.
11. Ramon Y, Horowitz Y, Oberman M, et al: Liposarcoma of the buccal mucosa. Int J Oral Surg 6:226, 1977.
12. Brauchle RW, Farhood AI, Pereira KD: Well-differentiated liposarcoma of the epiglottis. J Laryngol Otol 115:593–595, 2001.
13. Hurtado JF, Lopez JJ, Aranda FI, et al: Primary liposarcoma of the larynx. Case report and literature review. Ann Otol Rhinol Laryngol 103:315–317, 1994.
14. Gaynor EB, Raghausan U, Weisbrot IM: Primary myxoid liposarcoma of the larynx. Otolaryngol Head Neck Surg 92:476–480, 1984.
15. Meis JM, Mackay B, Goepfert H: Liposarcoma of the larynx. Arch Otolaryngol Head Neck Surg 112:1289–1292, 1986.

16. Fahmy FF, Osborne J, Khalil HS, et al: Well-differentiated liposarcoma of the hypopharynx. J Laryngol Otol 112:880–882, 1998.
17. Nofal F, Thomas M: Liposarcoma in the pharynx. J Laryngol Otol 103:1080–1082, 1989.
18. Reed JM, Vick EG: Hypopharyngeal liposarcoma. Otolaryngol Head Neck Surg 114:499–500, 1996.
19. Adkins WY Jr, Putney FJ, Kreutner A, et al: Liposarcoma of the maxilla. Otolaryngology 860:710–713, 1978.
20. Friedman JL, Bistritz JI, Robinson MJ: Pleomorphic liposarcoma of the pterygomandibular space involving the maxilla. Oral Surg Oral Med Oral Pathol Oral Radiol Endod 79:488–491, 1995.
21. Kessler A, Berenholz L, Eviatar E, et al: Liposarcoma of the scalp: A case report and review of the literature. Otolaryngol Head Neck Surg 117:412–414, 1997.
22. Fagan JJ, Myers EN, Barnes L: A parapharyngeal myxoid liposarcoma. J Laryngol Otol 113:179–182, 1999.
23. Menown IB, Liew SH, Napier SS, et al: Retro-pharyngeal liposarcoma. J Laryngol Otol 106:469–471, 1992.
24. Prince ME, Nasser JG, Fung BR, et al: Liposarcoma of the retropharyngeal space: Review of the literature. J Otolaryngol 26:139–142, 1997.
25. Coatesworth AP, Martin-Hirsch DP, MacDonald A: Post-irradiation liposarcoma of the temporal bone. J Laryngol Otol 110:779–781, 1996.
26. Jones JK, Baker HW: Liposarcoma of the parotid gland: Report of a case. Arch Otolaryngol 106:497–499, 1980.
27. Kaplan R, Bratcher GO, Freeman D, et al: Liposarcoma of the neck. Report of a case. Laryngoscope 91:1375–1378, 1981.
28. Stoller FM, Davies DG: Liposarcoma of the neck. Arch Otolaryngol 88:419–422, 1968.
29. Morse MA, Bossen E, D'Amico TA, et al: Myxoid liposarcoma of the supraclavicular fossa. Chest 117:1518–1520, 2000.
30. Favrot SR, Ridley MB, Older JJ, et al: Orbital liposarcoma. Otolaryngol Head Neck Surg 111:111–115, 1994.
31. Ruacan S, Onerci M, Gedikoglu G, et al: Liposarcoma of the cheek: Report of a case. J Oral Pathol Med 22:46–47, 1993.
32. Barnes L: Tumors and tumor-like lesions of the soft tissues. In Surgical Pathology of the Head and Neck. New York, Marcel Dekker, 2001, pp 974–979.
33. Griem KL, Robb PK, Caldarelli DD, et al: Radiation-induced sarcoma of the thyroid. Arch Otolaryngol Head Neck Surg 115:991–993, 1989.
34. Wenig BM, Heffner DK: Liposarcomas of the larynx and hypopharynx: A clinicopathologic study of eight new cases and a review of the literature. Laryngoscope 105:747–756, 1995.
35. McCulloch TM, Makielski KH, McNutt MA: Head and neck liposarcoma. A histopathologic reevaluation of reported cases. Arch Otolaryngol Head Neck Surg 118:1045–1049, 1992.
36. Mandell DL, Brandwein MS, Woo P, et al: Upper aerodigestive tract liposarcoma: Report on four cases and literature review. Laryngoscope 109:1245–1252, 1999.
37. Collins BT, Gossner G, Martin DS, et al: Fine needle aspiration biopsy of well-differentiated liposarcoma of the neck in a young female. A case report. Acta Cytol 43:452–456, 1999.
38. Farr HW: Soft part sarcomas of the head and neck. Semin Oncol 8:185–189, 1981.
39. Mark RJ, Tran LM, Sercarz JA, et al: Chondrosarcoma of the head and neck: The UCLA experience, 1955–1988. Am J Clin Oncol 16:232–237, 1993.
40. Koch BB, Karnell LH, Hoffman HT, et al: National cancer database report on chondrosarcoma of the head and neck. Head Neck 22:408–425, 2000.
41. Downey TJ, Clark SK, Moore DW: Chondrosarcoma of the nasal septum. Otolaryngol Head Neck Surg 125:98–100, 2001.
42. Burkey BB, Hoffman HT, Baker SR, et al: Chondrosarcoma of the head and neck. Laryngoscope 100:1301–1305, 1990.
43. Bough ID Jr, Chiles PJ, Fratalli MA, et al: Laryngeal chondrosarcoma: Two unusual cases. Am J Otolaryngol 16:126–131, 1995.
44. Barnes L: Diseases of the bones and joints. In Surgical Pathology of the Head and Neck. New York, Marcel Dekker, 2001, pp 1142–1146.
45. Blotta P, Carinci F, Pelucchi S, et al: Chondrosarcoma of the nasal septum. Ann Otol Rhinol Laryngol 110:202–204, 2001.
46. Bates GJ, Herdman RC: Chondrosarcoma of the sphenoid—a case report and review. J Laryngol Otol 102:727–729, 1988.
47. Said S, Civantos F, Whiteman M, et al: Clear cell chondrosarcoma of the larynx. Otolaryngol Head Neck Surg 125:107–108, 2001.
48. Uygur K, Tuz M, Dogru H, et al: Chondrosarcoma of the thyroid cartilage. J Laryngol Otol 115:507–509, 2001.
49. Friedlander PL, Lyons GD: Chondrosarcoma of the larynx. Otolaryngol Head Neck Surg 122:617, 2000.
50. LeJeune FE Jr, Van Horn HW 3rd, Farr GH: Chondrosarcoma of the larynx: Excision of massive recurrence. Ann Otol Rhinol Laryngol 91:392–394, 1982.
51. Chidambaram A, Sanville P: Mesenchymal chondrosarcoma of the maxilla. J Laryngol Otol 114:536–539, 2000.
52. Selz PA, Konrad HR, Woolbright E: Chondrosarcoma of the maxilla: A case report and review. Otolaryngol Head Neck Surg 116:399–400, 1997.
53. Ozkul H, Kayhan FT, Kiyak E, et al: Pathologic quiz case 1. Chondrosarcoma of the mandible. Arch Otolaryngol Head Neck Surg 121:694–696, 1995.
54. Worley GA, Wareing MJ, Sergeant RJ: Myxoid chondrosarcoma of the external auditory meatus. J Laryngol Otol 113:742–743, 1999.
55. Reid CB, Fagan PA, Turner J: Low-grade myxoid chondrosarcoma of the temporal bone: Differential diagnosis and report of two cases. Am J Otol 15:419–422, 1994.
56. Batra PS, Estrem SA, Zitsch RP, et al: Chondrosarcoma of the temporomandibular joint. Otolaryngol Head Neck Surg 120:951–954, 1999.
57. Okabe Y, Shibutani K, Nishimura T, et al: Chondrosarcoma of the parapharyngeal space. J Laryngol Otol 105:484–486, 1991.
58. Lau DP, Wharton SB, Antoun NM, et al: Chondrosarcoma of the petrous apex. Dilemmas in diagnosis and treatment. J Laryngol Otol 111:368–371, 1997.
59. Donaldson DR, Myers LL, Diaz-Ordaz E, et al: Pathologic quiz case 2. Chondrosarcoma of the jugular foramen. Arch Otolaryngol Head Neck Surg 125:229–230, 1999.
60. Harvey SA, Wiet RJ, Kazan R: Chondrosarcoma of the jugular foramen. Am J Otol 15:257–263, 1994.
61. Gay I, Elidan J, Kopolovic J: Chondrosarcoma at the skull base. Ann Otol Rhinol Laryngol 90:53–55, 1981.
62. Farrell ML, Gluckman JL, Biddinger P: Tracheal chondrosarcoma: A case report. Head Neck 20:568–572, 1998.
63. Greer JA Jr, Devine KD, Dahlin DC: Gardner's syndrome and chondrosarcoma of the hyoid bone. Arch Otolaryngol 103:425–427, 1977.
64. Singh D, Seth HN: Chondrosarcoma of the nasopharynx. Report of a case with a follow-up of ten years. Ann Otol Rhinol Laryngol 81:230–234, 1972.
65. Gregoriades G: Chondrosarcoma of the hard palate. J Laryngol Otol 86:513–518, 1972.
66. Lewis JE, Olsen KD, Inwards CY: Cartilaginous tumors of the larynx: Clinicopathologic review of 47 cases. Ann Otol Rhinol Laryngol 106:94–100, 1997.
67. Wanebo HJ, Koness RJ, MacFarlane JK, et al: Head and neck sarcoma: Report of the Head and Neck Sarcoma Registry. Society of Head and Neck Surgeons Committee on Research. Head Neck 14:1–7, 1992.
68. Huvos AG, Marcove RC: Chondrosarcoma in the young: A clinicopathologic analysis of 79 patients younger than 21 years of age. Am J Surg Pathol 11:930–942, 1987.
69. Thome R, Thome DC, de la Cortina RA: Long-term follow-up of cartilaginous tumors of the larynx. Otolaryngol Head Neck Surg 124:634–640, 2001.
70. Mishell JH, Schild JA, Mafee MF: Chondrosarcoma of the larynx. Diagnosis with magnetic resonance imaging and computed tomography. Arch Otolaryngol Head Neck Surg 116:1338–1341, 1990.
71. Lavertu P, Tucker HM: Chondrosarcoma of the larynx. Case report and management philosophy. Ann Otol Rhinol Laryngol 93:452–456, 1984.
72. Finn DG, Goepfert H, Batsakis JG: Chondrosarcoma of the head and neck. Laryngoscope 94:1539–1544, 1984.
73. Barnes L: Tumors and tumor-like lesions of the soft tissues. In Surgical Pathology of the Head and Neck. New York, Marcel Dekker, 2001, pp 979–984.
74. Paczona R, Jori J, Tiszlavicz L, et al: Leiomyosarcoma of the larynx. Review of the literature and report of two cases. Ann Otol Rhinol Laryngol 108:677–682, 1999.
75. Wadhwa AK, Gallivan H, O'Hara BJ, et al: Leiomyosarcoma of the larynx: Diagnosis aided by advances in immunohistochemical staining. Ear Nose Throat J 79:42–46, 2000.

76. Kuruvilla A, Wenig BM, Humphrey DM, et al: Leiomyosarcoma of the sinonasal tract. A clinicopathologic study of nine cases. Arch Otolaryngol Head Neck Surg 116:1278–1286, 1990.

77. Font RL, Jurco S III, Brechner RJ: Postradiation leiomyosarcoma of the orbit complicating bilateral retinoblastoma. Arch Ophthalmol 101:1557–1561, 1983.

78. Seo IS, Clark SA, McGovern FD, et al: Leiomyosarcoma of the urinary bladder 13 years after cyclophosphamide therapy for Hodgkin's disease. Cancer 55:1597–1603, 1985.

79. Fujii H, Barnes L, Johnson JT, et al: Post-radiation primary intranodal leiomyosarcoma. J Laryngol Otol 109:80–83, 1995.

80. Lalwani AK, Kaplan MJ: Paranasal sinus leiomyosarcoma after cyclophosphamide and irradiation. Otolaryngol Head Neck Surg 103:1039–1042, 1990.

81. Cocks H, Quraishi M, Morgan D, et al: Leiomyosarcoma of the larynx. Otolaryngol Head Neck Surg 121:643–646, 1999.

82. Batra PS, Kern RC, Pelzer HJ, et al: Leiomyosarcoma of the sinonasal tract: Report of a case. Otolaryngol Head Neck Surg 125:663–664, 2001.

83. Patel SC, Silbergleit R, Talati SJ: Sarcomas of the head and neck. Top Magn Reson Imaging 10:362–375, 1999.

84. de Saint Aubain Somerhausen N, Fletcher CD: Leiomyosarcoma of soft tissue in children: Clinicopathologic analysis of 20 cases. Am J Surg Pathol 23:755–763, 1999.

85. Trzyna W, McHugh M, McCue P, et al: Molecular determination of the malignant potential of smooth muscle neoplasms. Cancer 80:211–217, 1997.

86. Thomas S, McGuff HS, Otto RA: Leiomyosarcoma of the larynx. Case report. Ann Otol Rhinol Laryngol 108:794–796, 1999.

87. Kaddu S, Beham A, Cerroni L, et al: Cutaneous leiomyosarcoma. Am J Surg Pathol 21:979–987, 1997.

88. Fields JP, Helwig EB: Leiomyosarcoma of the skin and subcutaneous tissue. Cancer 47:156–169, 1981.

89. Barnes L: Larynx, hypopharynx and esophagus. In Surgical Pathology of the Head and Neck. New York, Marcel Dekker, 2001, pp 174–181.

90. Ballo MT, Garden AS, El-Naggar AK, et al: Radiation therapy for early stage (T1-T2) sarcomatoid carcinoma of true vocal cords: Outcomes and patterns of failure. Laryngoscope 108:760–763, 1998.

91. Berthelet E, Shenouda G, Black MJ, et al: Sarcomatoid carcinoma of the head and neck. Am J Surg 168:455–458, 1994.

92. Randall G, Alonso WA, Ogura JH: Spindle cell carcinoma (pseudosarcoma) of the larynx. Arch Otolaryngol 101:63–66, 1975.

93. Giordano AM, Ewing S, Adams G, et al: Laryngeal pseudosarcoma. Laryngoscope 93:735–740, 1983.

94. Olsen KD, Lewis JE, Suman VJ: Spindle cell carcinoma of the larynx and hypopharynx. Otolaryngol Head Neck Surg 116:47–52, 1997.

95. Batsakis JG: Pseudosarcoma of the mucous membranes in the head and neck. J Laryngol Otol 95:311–316, 1981.

96. Leventon GS, Evans HL: Sarcomatoid squamous cell carcinoma of the mucous membranes of the head and neck. A clinicopathologic study of 20 cases. Cancer 48:994–1003, 1981.

97. Shindo ML, Stanley RB, Kiyabu MT: Carcinosarcoma of the nasal cavity and paranasal sinuses. Head Neck 12:516–519, 1990.

98. Hafiz MA, Mira J, Toker C: Postirrdaiation carcinosarcoma of the nasal cavity. Otolaryngol Head Neck Surg 97:319–321, 1987.

99. Nofal F: Spindle cell carcinoma of the nasopharynx. J Laryngol Otol 97:1057–1063, 1983.

100. Mankodi RC, Shah RM: Tonsillar pseudosarcoma. J Postgrad Med 26:147–148, 1980.

101. Ishibishi T, Hojo H: Spindle cell carcinoma of the parotid gland. J Laryngol Otol 109:683–686, 1995.

102. John DG, Cross SS, Lewis MS: Pseudosarcoma of the esophagus. J Laryngol Otol 102:954–958, 1988.

103. Patel NK, McKee PH, Smith NP, et al: Primary metaplastic carcinoma (carcinosarcoma) of the skin. A clinicopathologic study of four cases and review of the literature. Am J Dermatopathol 19:363–372, 1997.

104. Lambert PR, Ward PH, Berci G: Pseudosarcoma of the larynx. Arch Otolaryngol 106:700–708, 1980.

105. Friedel W, Chambers RG, Atkins JP: Pseudosarcomas of the pharynx and larynx. Arch Otolaryngol 102:286–290, 1976.

106. Froehner M, Gaertner HJ, Manseck A, et al: Durable complete remission of metastatic sarcomatoid carcinoma of the bladder with cisplatin and gemcitabine in an 80 year-old man. Urology (online) 58:799, 2001.

107. Kinney MC, Swerdlow SH: Hematopoietic and lymphoid disorders. In Barnes L (ed): Surgical Pathology of the Head and Neck. New York, Marcel Dekker, 2001, pp 1323–1326.

108. Miller FR, Lavertu P, Wanamaker JR, et al: Plasmacytomas of the head and neck. Otolaryngol Head Neck Surg 119:614–618, 1998.

109. Weissman JL, Myers JN, Kapadia SB: Extramedullary plasmacytoma of the larynx. Am J Otolaryngol 14:128–131, 1993.

110. Kapadia SB, Desui U, Cheng VS: Extramedullary plasmacytoma of the head and neck: A clinicopathologic study of 20 cases. Medicine (Baltimore) 61:317–329, 1982.

111. Wax MK, Yun KJ, Omar RA: Extramedullary plasmacytomas of the head and neck. Otolaryngol Head Neck Surg 109:877–885, 1993.

112. Sulzner SE, Amdur RJ, Weider DJ: Extramedullary plasmacytoma of the head and neck. Am J Otolaryngol 19:203–208, 1998.

113. Hotz MA, Schwaab G, Bosq J, et al: Extramedullary solitary plasmacytoma of the head and neck. A clinicopathological study. Ann Otol Rhinol Laryngol 108:495–500, 1999.

114. Welsh J, Westra WH, Eisele D, et al: Solitary plasmacytoma of the epiglottis: A case report and review of the literature. J Laryngol Otol 112:174–176, 1998.

115. Mochimatsu I, Tsukuda M, Sawaki S, et al: Extramedullary plasmacytoma of the larynx. J Laryngol Otol 107:1049–1051, 1993.

116. Rothfield RE, Johnson JT, Stavrides A: Extramedullary plasmacytoma of the parotid. Head Neck 12:352–354, 1990.

117. Goel S, Moorjani V, Kulkarni P, et al: Plasmacytoma of the hyoid. J Laryngol Otol 108:604–606, 1994.

118. Panosian MS, Roberts JK: Plasmacytoma of the middle ear and mastoid. Am J Otol 15:264–267, 1994.

119. Marais J, Brookes GB, Lee CC: Solitary plasmacytoma of the skull base. Ann Otol Rhinol Laryngol 101:665–668, 1992.

120. Burns JA, Lezzoni JC, Reibel JF, et al: Extensive extramedullary amyloid-rich plasmacytoma of the mandible. Otolaryngol Head Neck Surg 120:937–939, 1999.

121. Hanna EYN, Lavertu P, Tucker HM, et al: Bilateral extramedullary plasmacytomas of the palatine tonsils: A case report. Otolaryngol Head Neck Surg 103:1024–1027, 1990.

122. Seoane J, De la Cruz A, Pomareda M, et al: Primary extramedullary plasmacytoma of the palate. Otolaryngol Head Neck Surg 120:530, 1999.

123. Logan PM, Miller RR, Muller NL: Solitary tracheal plasmacytoma: Computed tomography and pathological findings. Can Assoc Radiol J 46:125–126, 1995.

124. Kotner LM, Wang CC: Plasmacytoma of the upper air and food passages. Cancer 45:2983–2986, 1980.

125. Barnes L: Tumors and tumor-like lesions of the soft tissues In Surgical Pathology of the Head and Neck. New York, Marcel Dekker, 2001, pp 991–995.

126. Fedok FG, Levin RJ, Maloney ME, et al: Angiosacoma: Current review. Am J Otolaryngol 20:223–231, 1999.

127. Aust MR, Olsen KD, Lewis JE, et al: Angiosarcomas of the head and neck: Clinical and pathological characteristics. Ann Otol Rhinol Laryngol 106:943–951, 1997.

128. Panje WR, Mpran WJ, Bostwick DG, et al: Angiosarcoma of the head and neck: Review of 11 cases. Laryngoscope 96:1381–1384, 1986.

129. Mark RJ, Tran LM, Sercarz J, et al: Angiosarcoma of the head and neck. The UCLA experience 1955 through 1990. Arch Otolaryngol Head Neck Surg 119:973–978, 1993.

130. Mulliken JB, Glowacki J: Hemangiomas and vascular malformations in infants and children: A classification based on endothelial characteristics. Plast Reconstr Surg 69:412–422, 1982.

131. Holmdahl K: Cutaneous hemangiomas in premature and mature infants. Acta Paediatr 44:370, 1955.

132. North PE, Waner M, Mizeracki A, et al: A unique microvascular phenotype shared by juvenile hemangiomas and human placentas. Arch Dermatol 137:559–570, 2001.

133. North PE, Waner M, James CA, et al: Congenital non-progressive hemangioma, a distinct clinicopathologic entity unlike infantile hemangioma. Arch Dermatol 137:1607–1620, 2001.

134. Enjolras O, Wassef M, Mazoyer E, et al: Infants with Kasabach-Merritt syndrome do not have "true" hemangiomas. J Pediatr 130:631–640, 1997.

135. Fin MD, Glowacki J, Mulliken JB: Congenital vascular lesions: Clinical applications of a new classification. J Pediatr Surg 18:894, 1983.

136. Waner M, Suen JY, Dinehart S, et al: Laser photocoagulation of superficial proliferating hemangiomas. J Dermatol Surg/Oncol 20:1–4, 1994.

137. Ashinoff R, Geronemus RG: Capillary hemangiomas and treatment with the flashlamp pumped dye laser. Arch Dermatol 127:202–205, 1991.

138. Garden JM, Bakus AD, Paller AS: Treatment of cutaneous hemangiomas by the flashlamp pumped pulsed dye laser: Prospective analysis. J Pediatr 4:555–560, 1992.

139. Enjolras O, Riche MD, Merland JJ, et al: Management of alarming hemangiomas in infancy: A review of 25 cases. Pediatrics 85:491–498, 1990.

140. Azzolini A, Nouvenne R: Nuove prospettive nella terapia degli angiomi immaturi dell infanzia, 115 lesion: Trattate can infiltraziona. Intralesionali di triamcinolone acetonide. Acta Biomed 41:51, 1970.

141. Mulliken J, Boon L, Takahashi K, et al: Pharmocologic therapy for endangering hemangiomas. Current Opinion in Dermatology, 2nd ed. Philadelphia, Lippincott Williams & Wilkins, 1995, pp 109–113.

142. Vesikari T, Nuutila A, Cantell K: Neurologic sequelae following interferon therapy of juvenile laryngeal papilloma. Acta Paediatr Scand 77:619–622, 1988.

143. Waner M, Suen JY: Advances in the management of congenital vascular lesions of the head and neck. Adv Otolaryngol 10:31–54, 1996.

144. Suen JY, Waner M: Treatment of oral cavity vascular malformations using the Nd:YAG laser. Arch Otolaryngol Head Neck Surg 115:1329–1333, 1989.

145. Ogita S, Tsuto T, Deguchi E, et al: OK-432 therapy for unresectable lymphangiomas in children. J Pediatr Surg 26:263–270, 1991.

146. Ogita S, Tsuto T, Nakamura K, et al: OK-432 therapy for lymphangioma in children: Why and how does it work? J Pediatr Surg 31:477–480, 1996.

Reconstruction of Major Defects in the Head and Neck Following Cancer Surgery

Steven H. Sloan

Keith E. Blackwell

Jeffrey R. Harris

Eric M. Genden

Mark L. Urken

◼ INTRODUCTION

Contemporary management of cancer of the head and neck is the product of the continued application of new oncologic and reconstructive techniques. Patient survival and functional rehabilitation have improved since the mid-1940s, before which orthovoltage radiation was the mainstay of treatment of cancer of the head and neck. With the introduction of safer anesthesia and new techniques of radical surgery, wide resection of primary cancers of the upper aerodigestive tract and in-continuity neck dissection of regional metastases resulted in improved cure rates. Thereafter, advances in radiation therapy led to the introduction of "combined therapy." As an accepted trade-off for improved survival rates, this aggressive approach often resulted in prolonged hospitalization, major functional and cosmetic deficits, and in many cases, social isolation, as well as the inability to maintain gainful employment.

The development of reconstructive techniques for head and neck surgery did not progress at the same pace as combined therapy for eradication of cancer of the head and neck. In fact, most authors either failed to acknowledge the issue of reconstruction or deemed it unnecessary. Hayes Martin,[1] the father of modern head and neck surgery, wrote:

> Excessive or too frequent resort[ing] to more complicated and technical procedures, such as skin graft for pharyngeal defects, skin graft of the tongue or buccal surface, . . . bone grafts in mandibular defects, and particularly nerve grafts for [seventh cranial] nerve defects, is not characteristic of the mature or resourceful surgeon.

Before 1963, most oral and pharyngeal defects were closed primarily, reconstructed with random-pattern skin flaps (such as the nape-of-neck flap), or reconstructed with tubed, pedicled flaps of skin from the trunk. These flaps rarely matched the tissue requirements of the defect. Furthermore, such repairs were unpredictable and frequently resulted in flap necrosis, salivary fistula, bone or carotid artery exposure, or other complications that led to prolonged hospitalization or the patient's death.

Previously limited ability of surgeons to resurface mucosal defects of the head and neck improved with the description of the forehead flap by McGregor[2] in 1963 and the deltopectoral flap by Bakamjian[3] in 1965. These well-vascularized, axial-pattern skin flaps permitted more reliable closure of oral and pharyngeal defects at the time of ablative surgery. Although these reconstructive techniques permitted extensive resection to be performed more safely, their limitations soon became apparent. The limited arc of rotation frequently necessitated multistaged delayed procedures and prolonged hospitalization. The need to perform skin grafts for all but the smallest donor defects contributed to suboptimal aesthetic results. Furthermore, the limitations of the transferred tissue in restoration of function frequently led to permanent impairment of deglutition, articulation, and mastication. Despite their drawbacks, the forehead and deltopectoral flaps were the mainstays of soft tissue reconstruction of head and neck defects for nearly two decades. These flaps also played an important role in improving our understanding of cutaneous circulation, which expedited the search for better techniques.

The rehabilitation of patients with cancer of the head and neck has been revolutionized since the mid-1970s by the development of advanced reconstructive techniques. Pedicled myocutaneous flaps and free-tissue transfers have allowed reliable and safe one-stage reconstruction of defects of the upper aerodigestive tract in the primary setting. In the late 1970s and early 1980s, the pedicled pectoralis major myocutaneous flap was popularized and became the predominant method used in reconstruction of the head and neck. Other regional flaps, such as the trapezius and latissimus dorsi flaps, were described for reconstruction of the head and neck. As clinical experience accumulated, the limitations of pedicled flaps for some reconstructive problems became apparent. These include the limited lengths of the pedicle and arcs of rotation, excessive bulk, and donor site morbidities. In addition, the inability of surgeons to reliably transfer vascularized bone for mandibular reconstruction stimulated the search for alternative techniques.

A new approach to transferring tissue became available in 1973 with the advent of microvascular surgery. Subsequently, free-tissue transfer rapidly evolved from a reconstructive "last resort" into a preferred method for a variety of complex head and neck defects. As new donor sites were discovered and microsurgical techniques were refined, the advantages of free-tissue transfer for certain reconstructive problems became apparent. These advantages include the following: (1) superior vascularity of the tissues, resulting in improved tissue survival and wound healing in unfavorable recipient beds; (2) freedom from a limited arc of rotation and length of the vascular pedicle; (3) greater availability, variety, and versatility of donor tissue, which allows more efficient use of functionally similar tissue; and (4) presence of donor sites that are less morbid and conspicuous.

Surgeons who perform ablative procedures are now able to perform more extensive resections while knowing that the available reconstructive procedures can successfully close the defect in the primary setting and provide the cancer patient with the best opportunity for a rapid functional and cosmetic rehabilitation. A good example of the interplay between reconstructive and ablative surgery is seen in cases affecting the region of the cranial base, where vital structures such as the brain and carotid artery can be reliably covered and protected with well-vascularized tissue. This ability has been critical to the advancement of the emerging discipline of cranial base surgery. Despite longer and more technically demanding procedures, the success rate of microvascular free-tissue transfers to the head and neck region has been reported to be greater than 90%.[4, 5] Consequently, free-tissue transfer has become an essential part of the comprehensive management of many surgical defects in the head and neck.

This chapter presents our approach to the various problems of head and neck reconstruction. Available techniques, indications for clinical application, and functional and aesthetic issues are discussed. Although skin grafts and local flaps are effective for the resurfacing of small mucosal and cutaneous defects, reconstruction of larger defects usually requires tissue from regional or distant sites. This chapter addresses the latter techniques.

Successful reconstruction requires accurate preoperative assessment and formulation of an individualized treatment plan. Careful consideration of a variety of factors is essential, the most important of these factors being the nature of the head and neck defect. Other important considerations include the following: (1) specific histologic features of the tumor, clinical stage, and associated prognosis; (2) age, sex, body habitus, and associated health problems of the patient; (3) available flap donor sites; (4) compliance, expectations, and psychosocial needs of the patient; and (5) clinical experience and skills of the surgeon. Consequently, a rigid "cookbook," algorithm-based approach for reconstruction of the head and neck is ill-advised. Superior results are seen when the reconstructive team has a wide range of options, which permits the reconstruction to be customized to the individual patient, based on careful consideration of all pertinent tumor- and patient-related factors.

◼ GOALS OF RECONSTRUCTION

The primary goal of head and neck cancer treatment is to effect a cure or significant palliation. In addition, every effort should be made to restore the patient to the premorbid level of functioning and quality of life. Despite advances in other therapeutic modalities, this frequently requires radical surgical ablation of the primary site and removal of regional nodal metastases. Except in rare cases, some form of reconstruction is necessary. No reconstructive procedure, however elaborately or creatively conceived, should preempt adequate tumor resection, nor should such a plan be rigidly adhered to if events during the ablation dictate that an alternative approach will result in a preferred outcome.

Successful reconstruction of defects in the head and neck requires that the surgeon define the nature of the defect and appreciate the functional and aesthetic capacities of the ablated tissues in order to replace them with an appropriate substitute. Optimal results usually require reconstruction with tissues that duplicate the appearance and function of the resected tissue. The tissues required to achieve these goals may include the following: (1) epithelium, to resurface a mucosal or skin defect; (2) muscle, to restore motion or bulk; and (3) cartilage or bone, to provide skeletal support. Less frequently, tissues such as fascia and fat may be required for static suspension or for contour restoration. Complex defects of the head and neck, such as those resulting from oromandibular and cranial base resections, may necessitate reconstruction with a composite flap. It is in such cases that microvascular free-tissue transfer has been most widely used.

The first priority in reconstruction of defects in the head and neck should be safety. It is essential to prevent life-threatening complications, such as carotid blowout, overwhelming aspiration, or cerebrospinal fluid (CSF) leak and subsequent meningitis, after resection of the cranial base. The next priority is to return the upper aerodigestive tract to a functional state. Restoration of oral competence, deglutition, and articulation is the objective of oromandibular reconstruction. Maintaining mobility of the tongue, palatal closure, and pharyngeal continuity is the specific reconstructive challenge in these patients. Restoration of functional mastication is a lesser priority, but it frequently can be achieved after resection of the mandible and maxilla. Advances in dental prosthetics and the ability of surgeons to reliably transfer vascularized bone have been essential in this regard.

Traditionally, aesthetic rehabilitation has been a lesser priority in patients with head and neck cancer. Surgeons should be sensitive to the impact of physical appearance on the patient's sense of well-being and to the patient's ability to reintegrate into previous occupational and social environments. Reconstruction with local tissue is preferred for cutaneous defects because skin adjacent to the defect provides the optimal match in color and texture. If local tissue is unavailable, the skin quality of potential flaps to be transferred from regional or distant donor sites should be considered. Similarly, when maintenance of bulk in the flap is aesthetically important, the progressive atrophy of denervated muscle should be anticipated. The use of innervated muscle or well-vascularized subcutaneous fat may provide a more effective long-term result. Aesthetic units should be managed as a total entity when possible, especially in resurfacing of defects of the cheek, nose, lips, forehead, and less critically, the neck. To maximize the aesthetic result in the patient with head and neck cancer, adjunctive procedures, such as scar revision and flap recontouring, can be performed subsequent to the initial reconstructive effort. In other cases, aesthetics are relatively unimportant and functional concerns are paramount. Defects of the oral cavity and oropharynx, especially those involving the tongue and palate, frequently require more elaborate techniques for the restoration of effective articulation and deglutition. Maintenance of a patent pharyngoesophageal segment and restoration of velopharyngeal competence are vital functional outcomes. Smaller defects and those in functionally less essential areas may be closed primarily or resurfaced with a skin graft with good preservation of function.

PREOPERATIVE PLANNING AND TIMING OF RECONSTRUCTION

Comprehensive management of the patient with cancer of the head and neck begins with thorough preoperative planning. This should involve multiple disciplines. Patients with cancer typically present with numerous comorbidities and risk factors, including cardiac, pulmonary, cerebrovascular, and hepatic disease. Malnutrition and general debilitation secondary to the disease process or to previous surgery, radiation, or chemotherapy are common. A thoroughly performed initial office visit provides an evaluation of these risk factors and an assessment of the extent of the tumor, estimation of the probable extent of resection, and consideration of reconstructive possibilities. Endoscopic examination under anesthesia, as a separate procedure, is extremely valuable in most cases.

The anticipated defect should be classified according to its rigid, soft tissue, and neurologic components. Consideration of the functional region encompassed by the deficit is of far greater importance than a description of the total area or volume of tissue involved. The possible need for coverage of the carotid artery or dura is discussed. If free-tissue transfer is contemplated, potential donor sites and recipient vessels should be evaluated to assess their suitability. Based on all available information, a reconstructive plan is formulated. A second, and even a third, "fallback" option should be available in the event that the initial plan proves to be unfeasible or fails during the immediate postoperative period.

Most head and neck reconstructive procedures are optimally performed in one stage at the time of ablation. Primary reconstruction should be extensive and virtually all-encompassing. Optimal conditions for reconstruction are present at the completion of tumor resection: (1) The defect is widely exposed; (2) bone and soft tissue requirements are readily and accurately assessed; and (3) potential recipient vessels for microvascular anastomoses, if indicated, are already dissected. Furthermore, surgical margins can be cleared by frozen section pathologic analysis, which permits definitive wound repair. This approach avoids the problems associated with delayed reconstruction, including fibrosis of remaining muscles and contraction of other soft tissues within the wound bed. Consequently, primary reconstruction has been shown to provide superior functional and aesthetic results when compared with delayed reconstruction. In addition, the attitude of patients undergoing primary reconstruction is greatly improved when maximal form and function are restored promptly.

Certain reconstructive procedures of the head and neck, however, should be performed in a staged or delayed manner. Multistaged repair of complex nasal and auricular defects is an example. In this instance, one should plan to perform the fewest number of procedures necessary to obtain superior results in the shortest possible time. In cases in which tumor-free margins are in question, reconstruction should be delayed until permanent pathologic confirmation is made. Frequently, the functional and cosmetic results of an elaborate reconstructive effort can be maximized by subsequent revisions. These secondary procedures may include scar revision, flap debulking, and placement of endosteal dental implants for oromandibular rehabilitation.

RECONSTRUCTIVE OPTIONS

In general, the least complex method that provides a safe reconstruction while restoring form and function to the region should be selected. The reconstructive surgeon should first consider primary closure or the use of a skin graft, which is most expedient for small defects. Larger defects usually require alternative methods, such as local or regional flaps. The effect of regional tissue on the form and function of the reconstructed area must be assessed in a critical fashion to determine whether the use of a free flap from a distant site would provide a better result. This logical progression from simple to more complex techniques provides a systematic approach for evaluating whether a given technique satisfies the functional and cosmetic requirements of each head and neck defect. Each step in this approach is governed by the clinical experience and judgment of the reconstructive surgeon.

Local Flaps

Local flaps are effective reconstructive alternatives for certain small to medium-sized defects of the face, neck, and upper aerodigestive tract. When used judiciously, local tissue transfer is aesthetically and functionally superior to the use of more elaborate and potentially morbid regional or distant free flaps. The use of tissue adjacent to the defect often provides the best match of skin in terms of its color and texture. Furthermore, morbidity is usually limited to an additional scar for closure of the donor defect.

The size and location of the defect and the properties of the available local tissue help to determine whether a local flap is an appropriate reconstructive method. The vascular supply of each local flap is unique and dictates the amount of tissue that can be reliably transferred. In this regard, local flaps are classified according to their vascular supply. The vascular pattern can be axial or random, depending on whether a direct cutaneous artery and vein course along the long axis of the flap.

Alternatively, local flaps can be classified according to the way in which they are transferred (e.g., rotated, advanced) and the tissues within them (e.g., skin, muscle, or mucosa). Nasal and lip defects are optimally reconstructed with local muscle-skin flaps, such as forehead, nasolabial, Abbé-Estlander, and Karapandzic flaps. Similarly, small intraoral defects can be closed with palatal, tongue, and buccal mucosal flaps.[6] More detailed description of the various local flaps is beyond the scope of this chapter.

Regional Flaps

The reconstruction of large defects in the head and neck frequently requires transfer of tissues from adjacent regions, such as the chest and back. Pedicled regional flaps have been used extensively to provide closure of large defects in the neck, face, scalp, oral cavity, and pharynx. Regional flaps can be classified as fasciocutaneous, such as the deltopectoral flap, or as muscle or myocutaneous, such as the pectoralis major, trapezius, and latissimus dorsi flaps. Most regional flap procedures can be performed in one stage. However, a delay may be instituted to more reliably increase the overall size of the flap.

The selection of a specific regional flap depends on the location and size of the defect and the intrinsic properties of the regional flap. For most cutaneous defects of the neck, the thin, supple quality of the deltopectoral flap is preferable to the bulkiness of most myocutaneous flaps. However, for coverage of the carotid artery or reconstruction of a large oropharyngeal defect, the additional bulk and reliable vascular supply of a myocutaneous flap are advantageous. The location of the defect may not be suitable for a regional flap owing to the limited arc of rotation. Only the pedicled latissimus dorsi and lower island trapezius flaps have an extensive arc of rotation for use in large defects of the scalp.

Deltopectoral Flap

The medially based deltopectoral flap was described and extensively applied to head and neck reconstruction by Bakamjian[7] in the mid-1960s. It became the primary method of resurfacing cutaneous and mucosal defects until the late 1970s, when the pectoralis myocutaneous flap was popularized. The deltopectoral flap is an axial-pattern fasciocutaneous flap of the upper chest that is based on the second and third perforating branches of the internal mammary artery. Harvesting the flap is technically easy. The superior incision is made through skin, subcutaneous fat, and pectoral fascia just below and parallel to the clavicle. An inferior incision extends along the fourth or fifth intercostal space, parallel to the upper incision. The distolateral extent of the flap is determined by the location of the defect relative to the rotational length of the flap. The flap is elevated in a subfascial plane from lateral to medial and is transposed to the recipient site. One-stage transfer can be reliably performed provided the flap does not extend much beyond the deltopectoral groove. If greater flap length is desirable, a delay procedure is often necessary to incorporate a random portion of skin over the deltoid muscle.

The deltopectoral flap is primarily used for resurfacing cutaneous defects of the neck. The introduction of other regional or distant tissue transfer has limited the role of the deltopectoral flap for facial, oral, and pharyngeal reconstruction. The reasons for this limitation include the following: (1) unreliability of the flap's distal, random portion; (2) lack of the bulk that is beneficial for many defects; and (3) the requirement, in most cases, for a skin graft to close the donor defect. Nonetheless, it remains a useful tool for selected reconstructive needs.

Myocutaneous Flaps

Head and neck surgery was revolutionized in the late 1970s by the introduction of regional myocutaneous flaps. These axially based flaps have segmental vascular pedicles that enter the deep surface of the muscle, course longitudinally, and send perforating branches through the muscle and subcutaneous tissue to the overlying skin. This arrangement provides a large amount of well-vascularized tissue and has allowed single-stage reconstruction of almost any defect in the head and neck, from the pharyngoesophagus to the skull base. Furthermore, the donor site on the chest or back can nearly always be closed primarily.

Despite their widespread use, regional myocutaneous flaps have disadvantages. In defects that require thin, pliable skin, the excess bulk of a myocutaneous flap may lead to a less than optimal result. Regional myocutaneous flaps have a limited length, skin paddle size, and arc of rotation. The sacrifice of a regional muscle to provide a vascular supply to the overlying skin may result in some degree of functional disability as well as in moderate distortion of the anterior chest or back.

PECTORALIS MAJOR FLAP

Among the regional myocutaneous flaps, the pectoralis major flap (Fig. 28–1) has by far enjoyed the greatest popularity and versatility in head and neck reconstruction. Although initially described for chest wall reconstruction, it was first popularized for head and neck reconstruction by Baek and associates[8] and Ariyan[9] in 1979. Owing to its reliability, versatility, and ease of harvesting, it rapidly replaced most preexisting reconstructive techniques. Although it has undergone numerous modifications and its shortcomings have been described, it is still considered the "workhorse" flap for head and neck reconstruction.

The pectoralis major muscle is a thick, triangular muscle that acts to adduct and medially rotate the arm. Its primary vascular supply is from the pectoral branch of the thoracoacromial artery, with a lesser contribution from the lateral thoracic artery. The pectoralis major myocutaneous flap has been applied to most major head and neck defects since the late 1970s. When first introduced, it was used primarily for reconstruction of mucosal defects of the oral cavity and pharynx and cutaneous defects of the neck. Following transposition, the pectoralis major muscle provides protection of the great vessels as well as obliteration of the dead space after mediastinal dissection (Fig. 28–2). Numerous modifications to overcome certain flap limitations have been described. Through the design of two independent skin paddles, full-thickness defects of the cheek and pharynx can be closed. An osteomyocutaneous flap for mandible reconstruction has also been described, but this application has

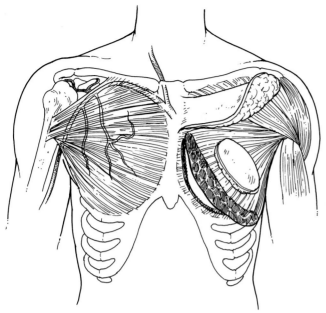

FIGURE 28–1 The pectoralis myocutaneous flap receives its primary blood supply from the pectoral branch of the thoracoacromial artery, which arises from the second portion of the auxillary artery. A lesser and more variable contribution is made by the lateral thoracic artery. If the need for the future regional tissue transfer is anticipated, a deltopectoral flap can be delayed concurrent with harvesting of the pectoralis myocutaneous flap. During flap elevation, care should be taken to preserve the perforating branches of the internal mammary artery that supplies the deltopectoral flap by not dissecting in the 2-cm zone lateral to the sternum in the second and third intercostal spaces.

been superseded by the use of vascularized, bone-containing free flaps.

The pectoralis major myocutaneous flap is extremely reliable, as indicated by a low incidence of reported complications. The incidence of total flap necrosis has been reported as 1% to 3%.[10] The incidence of partial flap necrosis, as high as 30% in some series, is probably related to the degree of caudal extension of the skin paddle over the rectus sheath. Depending on the patient's body habitus, the pectoralis flap may be less reliable for more cephalic defects of the face, scalp, and pharynx. Furthermore, the effect of gravity on the bulky pectoralis major muscle may be detrimental, especially when the flap is placed in an unfavorable recipient bed or when a patient is at risk for compromised wound healing. Donor site complications, such as hematoma and wound dehiscence, are rare.

TRAPEZIUS FLAPS

The trapezius muscle is a broad, thin, triangular muscle that covers most of the upper back and posterior neck. The muscle arises from the occipital bone, the ligamentum nuchae, and the spinous processes of the seven cervical and twelve thoracic vertebrae. These fibers insert on the lateral clavicle, the acromium, and the spine of the scapula. The muscle is innervated by the spinal accessory nerve, and it elevates and suspends the shoulder girdle and rotates the scapula.

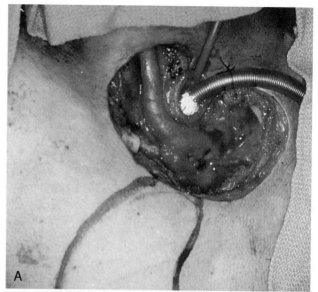

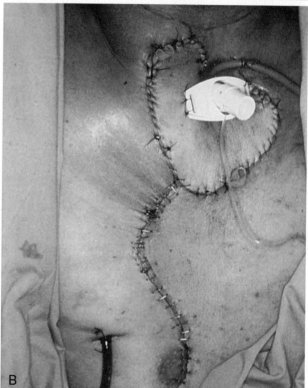

FIGURE 28–2 *A,* Surgical defect that resulted from resection of peristomal recurrence of squamous cell carcinoma of the larynx. The resection included the sternum and clavicular heads and resulted in exposure of the aortic arch, innominate artery, and branchiocephalic vein. *B,* The mediastinal defect has been reconstructed using a right pectoralis major myocutaneous flap. The pectoralis muscle has been used to cover the great vessels, and a semilunar-shaped skin paddle has been used to replace the peristomal skin defect. The chest donor site has been closed primarily.

The vascular supply of the trapezius muscle is more complex and variable than that of the other regional myocutaneous flaps used for reconstruction in the head and neck. The dominant blood supply is from the transverse cervical artery, which consists of a superficial branch and a deep branch. The deep branch of the transverse cervical artery is also known as the dorsal scapular artery. Lesser contributions from the occipital artery and the posterior intercostal perforators are present.

Of the three distinct trapezius flaps (Fig. 28–3), the superior trapezius flap[11] is the most reliable. Based on the posterior intercostal perforating arteries, it is used primarily for protection of the carotid artery and for the resurfacing of lateral cervical cutaneous defects (Fig. 28–4). The lateral island trapezius flap[12] is based on the transverse cervical artery. It can reach the anterior neck, oral cavity, and pharynx in some cases, but its arc of rotation is frequently limited by the unfavorable vascular anatomy of the transverse cervical system in the posterior triangle of the neck. The lower island flap[13] is the most versatile of the three trapezius myocutaneous flaps. The skin paddle is designed over the inferior third of the trapezius muscle, between the vertebrae and the scapula. The superior arc of rotation of this flap permits reliable closure of defects in the posterior neck, temporal bone, and scalp. Less frequently, it has been used for reconstruction in the oral cavity and pharynx. The major disadvantage of the lower island flap is

the necessity to place the patient in the lateral decubitus position.

LATISSIMUS DORSI FLAP

When all pedicled myocutaneous flaps are considered, the latissimus dorsi flap (Fig. 28–5) has the largest potential skin area (25 × 40 cm) available for transfer to the head and neck.[14–17] Two separate cutaneous paddles may be designed based on the intramuscular bifurcation of the thoracodorsal vascular pedicle for reconstruction of through-and-through defects. The functional disability that results from the transfer of the latissimus dorsi muscle is reportedly less than that resulting from the use of either the pectoralis or the trapezius muscle.[18] This flap is frequently transferred as a free flap, and details relevant to the anatomy, surgical technique, and clinical application of the latissimus dorsi flap are discussed further in the following section on the subscapular system of free flaps.

Microvascular Free-Tissue Transfer

Reconstructive surgery was revolutionized in 1973 when Daniel and Taylor[19] performed the first successful free groin

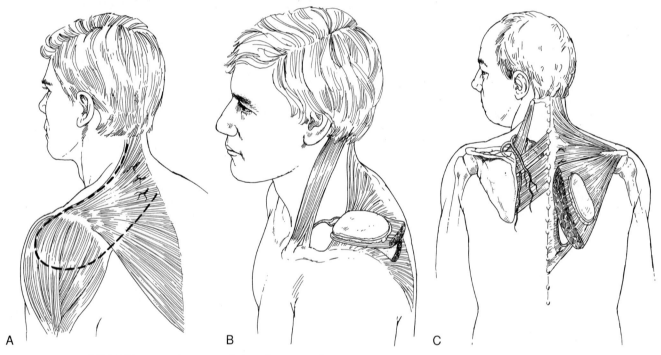

FIGURE 28–3 *A,* The superiorly based trapezius flap receives its primary blood supply from paraspinous perforators, with a lesser contribution from the occipital artery. Unlike other trapezius flaps that are based on branches of the transverse cervical artery, the superior trapezius flap may be used after previous radical neck dissection. *B,* The skin paddle of the lateral island trapezius flap is centered over the lateral aspect of the cephalic portion of the trapezius muscle, near its insertion into the distal third of the clavicle. Before the skin paddle is incised, the transverse cervical artery and vein should be dissected to ascertain that the pedicle anatomy is favorable. *C,* The lower island trapezius flap is supplied by the distal ramifications of the transverse cervical artery. The upper portion of the caudal trapezius muscle is supplied by the superficial branch of the transverse cervical artery, which runs superficial to the levator scapulae and rhomboid muscles. The most inferior portion of the trapezius muscle is supplied by the dorsal scapular artery, which enters the undersurface of the trapezius muscle after traveling deep to the levator scapulae and rhomboid minor muscles. Distal skin paddles are most reliable when the dorsal scapular artery is included in the flap. This frequently requires inclusion of a 2-cm cuff of rhomboid muscle around the pedicle to achieve an adequate arc of rotation.

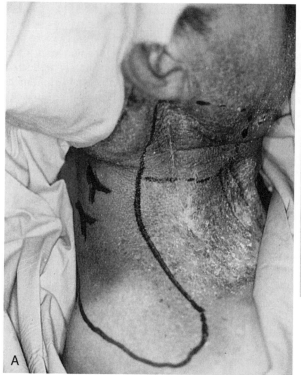

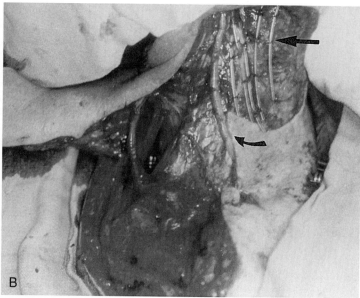

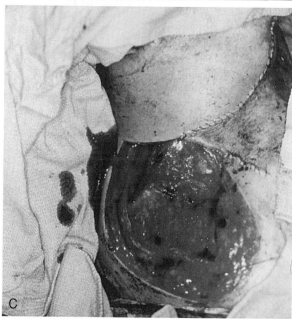

FIGURE 28–4 *A,* Recurrent right cervical metastatic squamous cell carcinoma after previous radical neck dissection and external beam radiotherapy. Fixation to the carotid artery and involvement of the skin adjacent to the angle of the mandible have occurred. A superior trapezius flap, based on paraspinous perforators, is outlined for reconstruction of the anticipated defect. The distal aspect of the flap can be reliably extended distal to the acromion. Sacrifice of the transverse cervical artery during the previous neck dissection acts as an effective delay procedure for the superior trapezius flap. *B,* An intraoperative photograph of the surgical defect shows a saphenous vein graft (*curved arrow*) for carotid artery replacement, and iridium-192 afterloading catheters (*straight arrow*) for delivery of interstitial radiotherapy. The trapezius flap has been elevated temporarily folded posteriorly. *C,* The trapezius flap has been transposed anteriorly to provide coverage of the carotid artery graft. The anterior limit of the arc of rotation is the midline of the neck. The resulting donor site defect on the shoulder will be resurfaced with a skin graft.

flap by performing a vascular anastomosis with the use of an operating microscope. Soon after this report, free-tissue transfer was applied to oral and pharyngoesophageal reconstruction. However, there was initial skepticism regarding the application of these novel techniques to the head and neck. Arguments that were used against the use of free flaps included the following: (1) surgical time was increased, (2) special skills and equipment were needed, and (3) most defects could be closed with pedicled myocutaneous flaps.

Since the mid-1970s, microvascular surgery has grown tremendously. Vast experience in a variety of surgical specialties has proved not only its reliability but also its superior

ability to restore function and aesthetics to certain head and neck defects. Free-tissue transfers have been used for one-stage reconstruction of virtually all major defects in the head and neck. A 93% to 96% success rate has been reported in large series of free-tissue transfers.[20, 21] Furthermore, mounting clinical evidence suggests that free-tissue transfers provide a higher level of functional recovery relative to that seen with other techniques. Consequently, free-tissue transfer has become an essential part of the comprehensive management of cancer of the head and neck.

Of the large variety of benefits of free-tissue transfer, one of the most important is the superior blood supply that

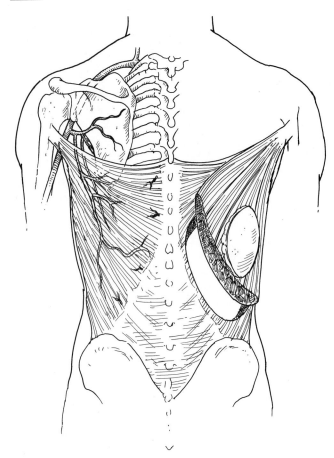

FIGURE 28–5 The pedicled latissimus dorsi myocutaneous flap receives its blood supply from the thoracodorsal artery, which arises from the subscapular axis. Paraspinous perforators to the latissimus dorsi muscle are transected during flap elevation. Transection of the thoracodorsal nerve causes predictable atrophy of the muscle component of the flap.

maximizes tissue survival and wound healing in unfavorable, contaminated head and neck recipient sites. The second major benefit relates to the freedom of being able to inset a free flap without being restricted to a limited vascular pedicle, as is common with the use of pedicled flaps. The skin islands of the pedicled pectoralis, trapezius, and latissimus flaps are often transferred from the distal and least vascular portions of the territory for use in resurfacing the defect. Free-tissue transfers are more efficient in that the most reliable portion of the flap can be placed into the defect without placement of the bulk of the muscle carrier.

Another advantage of free flaps is the greater variety and versatility of donor sites. No longer is the surgeon limited to the use of tissue that is adjacent to the defect. Although adjacent donor sites may be available, distant donor sites frequently possess qualities better suited to reconstructive needs. Reconstruction of floor-of-the-mouth and anterior mandibular defects illustrates this point. Although the pectoralis muscle and rib can be used, the marginal blood supply of the rib and the poor quality of bone prevent functional restoration of the mandible. Osteocutaneous donor sites, such as the iliac crest, fibula, and scapula, have largely overcome these tissue deficiencies. Furthermore, free-tissue

transfers permit the harvesting of multiple tissue paddles based on a single vascular pedicle. Similarly, free-tissue transfers can be designed to replace the ablated tissues more precisely than can the tissues from adjacent regional donor sites.

In select situations, free flaps are absolutely indicated and provide a distinct advantage in the reestablishment of form and function to the recipient site. In primary osseous restoration of the mandible, the use of free flaps containing vascularized bone is the most reliable reconstructive method. Reconstruction of complex defects in the cranial base in an unfavorable recipient bed with exposure of the dura or the carotid artery invariably requires microvascular free-tissue transfer. Complex, three-dimensional midface defects that require bone with both internal and external epithelial lining are best reconstructed with the use of free flaps. In addition, free-tissue transfer is now considered the method of choice for the reconstruction of select circumferential pharyngoesophageal defects.

In other major defects of the head and neck, free-tissue transfer may be more advantageous than local and regional pedicled flaps. For example, in soft tissue reconstruction, the bulk and pliability of the transferred tissue are of primary concern in the reestablishment of contour and function. The geometry of the defect may require a unique flap design that dictates selection of a particular donor site. For example, through-and-through defects of the pharynx or oral cavity are ideally reconstructed with a flap that has two independent skin paddles. Certain recipient sites, in particular the scalp and cranial base, may be beyond the reach of most regional flaps. Even if a regional myocutaneous flap reaches the defect, the effect of gravity on the pedicle may place additional tension on a tenuous suture line.

The disadvantages of free-tissue transfer arise from the complexity of the technique and the increased surgical time required. As with regional pedicled flaps, the color and contour of free flaps in certain cases may not exactly match those of the recipient site. Microvascular tissue transfers are labor-intensive, often requiring two surgical teams and a cooperative multidisciplinary effort. If patients are poor surgical risks, more expedient and less complex techniques that use regional flaps offer safer reconstructive alternatives.

The morbidity associated with borrowing tissue from a given site must be critically evaluated in each patient. For example, the distortion and donor site scar associated with the use of the pectoralis flap may be aesthetically unacceptable to many women. In other patients with advanced and recurrent cancer, reconstructive options that use regional pedicled flaps have already been exhausted. Finally, the accessibility of the donor site for a simultaneous two-team approach should be considered during the decision-making process to help reduce operative time.

It is essential that the characteristics of various free-tissue transfer approaches be carefully considered. Several anatomic areas, including the groin, abdomen, back, and extremities, provide reliable fasciocutaneous, musculocutaneous, and osteomusculocutaneous tissues. Each donor site has inherent advantages and disadvantages in terms of specific texture, color, contour, hair-bearing characteristics, length and size of the vascular pedicle, and potential for sensory and motor reinnervation. For vascularized, bone-containing free flaps, the amount of bone stock available and the flexibility of the soft tissue component in relation to the bone are important considerations. The morbidity of the donor site following free-flap harvest must also be taken into account.

Fasciocutaneous Free Flaps

Fasciocutaneous free flaps provide a segment of skin and subcutaneous fat of variable size and thickness for reconstruction of a wide variety of frequently encountered defects. Flaps commonly used for head and neck reconstruction include (1) the radial forearm flap, (2) the lateral arm flap, (3) the anterolateral thigh flap, (4) the lateral thigh flap, and (5) the scapular and parascapular flaps. The pliability of these flaps allows for precise anatomic restoration of resected tissue during oromandibular and pharyngeal reconstruction. The radial forearm, lateral arm, anterolateral thigh, and lateral thigh flaps have the potential for sensory reinnervation, which may be helpful for the rehabilitation of mastication and deglutition in head and neck cancer patients. Because adipose tissue within revascularized flaps does not atrophy, fasciocutaneous flaps allow for precise and permanent restoration of contour deformities. In addition, scapular skin and parascapular skin have favorable texture and color for the reconstruction of facial and cervical cutaneous defects.

RADIAL FOREARM FLAP

The radial forearm free flap (Fig. 28–6), or Chinese flap, is a fasciocutaneous flap that is harvested from the volar aspect of the forearm. It is based on the radial artery and its venae comitantes, or the subcutaneous veins of the forearm. It provides a large amount of thin, pliable skin that has the potential for sensory reinnervation via the antebrachial cutaneous nerves. Consequently, it has become the free-tissue transfer of choice for the resurfacing of oral cavity and oropharyngeal defects.[22] It has also gained considerable popularity for reconstruction of the hypopharynx and cervical esophagus. In select situations, it has also been used to resurface the scalp and a variety of areas of the face, including the cheek, nose, chin, and forehead.

The radial forearm flap has numerous advantages:

1. It provides a large amount of relatively thin, often hairless, skin that can be folded on itself to conform to nearly any mucosal or cutaneous defect.
2. It has a long vascular pedicle and vessels of large size, facilitating dissection and revascularization.
3. Sensation can be restored to the skin paddle by the incorporation of the medial or lateral antebrachial cutaneous nerves.[23, 24]
4. The donor site permits simultaneous two-team harvest and dissection under tourniquet control.
5. An abundant amount of subcutaneous fat can be left attached to the vascular pedicle, either for protection of the great vessels and the flap's vascular pedicle or for augmentation of contour deformities, such as those seen after radical neck dissection.
6. The radial forearm flap can also be used as an osteocutaneous free flap because a 10- to 12-cm long bone segment encompassing 40% of the circumference of the radius can be harvested with the skin paddle.[25]

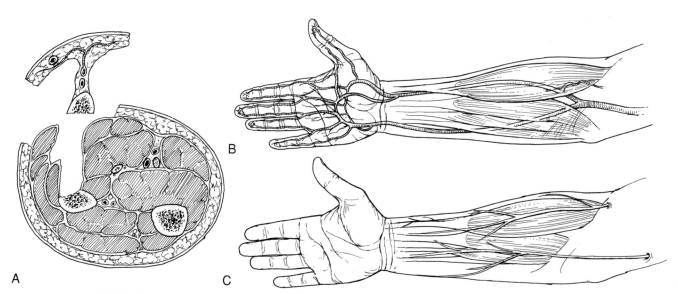

FIGURE 28–6 *A,* Cross-sectional anatomy of the forearm shows septocutaneous perforators of the radial artery, which travels in the intermuscular septum between the flexor carpi radialis and the brachioradialis muscles and supplies the skin paddle of the radial forearm flap. An osteofasciocutaneous flap containing up to 40% of the radius bone can be harvested based on periosteal perforators. *B,* The radial artery terminates in the deep palmar arch of the hand, which supplies circulation to the thumb and the index finger. Adequate collateral circulation via the deep palmar branch of the ulnar artery must be established preoperatively with the use of Allen's test to determine the safety of sacrificing the radial artery. *C,* Depending on the location from which the skin paddle is harvested, sensory reinnervation of the radial forearm flap can be accomplished by anastomosing either the lateral or medial antebrachial cutaneous nerves to appropriate recipient nerves in the head and neck.

However, when used as an osteocutaneous flap for mandibular or maxillary reconstruction, the limited bone stock restricts the potential for functional dental restoration. In addition, the incidence of pathologic fracture of the residual radius is unacceptably high. Consequently, we reserve its use for soft tissue reconstruction only.

The disadvantages of the radial forearm free flap are primarily aesthetic. Unless extremely small, the forearm donor defect requires skin grafting and can be unsightly. In addition, the color and texture match to facial skin is only fair. A potentially devastating complication of the radial forearm flap is vascular compromise of the hand. This occurs when a lack of collateral circulation through the distal branches of the ulnar artery results from sacrifice of the radial artery. To avoid this complication, a preoperative Allen's test is essential to assess the circulation of the hand. Other complications include numbness of the hand as a result of trauma to the superficial branches of the radial nerve and exposure of the forearm tendons as a result of incomplete healing of the skin graft over the donor defect.

LATERAL ARM FLAP

The lateral arm flap (Fig. 28–7) was first described by Song and colleagues[26] in 1982. Although this flap is harvested most frequently as a fasciocutaneous flap, it can also be raised with a monocortical segment of vascularized humerus, triceps tendon, or brachialis muscle. Alternatively, the flap can be deepithelialized and used as a vascularized fascia-fat flap for soft tissue augmentation. The lateral arm flap is supplied by the posterior radial collateral artery (PRCA), which is the terminal branch of the profunda brachii artery. The PRCA usually has a diameter of 1.5 to 2.0 mm and travels within the lateral intermuscular septum of the arm. Dye injection studies indicate that the PRCA supplies a cutaneous paddle that varies from 8 × 10 cm to 14 × 15 cm. The width of skin that is harvested with the lateral arm flap is usually limited to 6 to 8 cm, which is the largest cutaneous defect that can be closed primarily. The PRCA is accompanied by two venae comitantes, which usually fuse proximally into a single vein with an average diameter of 2.5 mm. Less commonly, the venous drainage of the lateral arm flap is based on the subcutaneous cephalic vein.[27]

In the head and neck region, the lateral arm flap has been used most frequently for facial and intraoral reconstruction.[28, 29] For soft tissue augmentation, it provides a flap of skin that is of intermediate thickness relative to the thin radial forearm flap and the thicker anterolateral thigh, lateral thigh, or scapular system flap. Two sensory nerves are harvested with the lateral arm flap. The posterior cutaneous nerve of the arm supplies the skin paddle of the flap and therefore can be used for sensory reinnervation. The posterior cutaneous

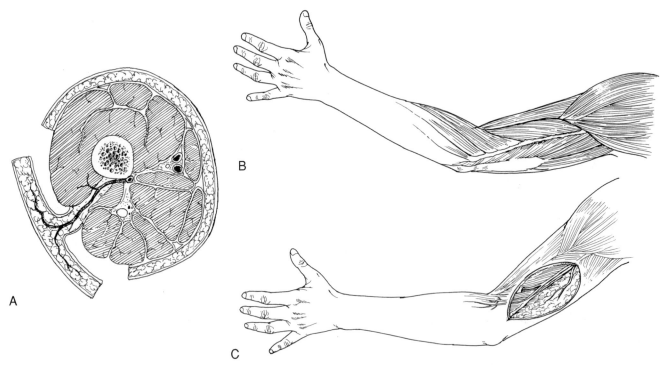

FIGURE 28–7 *A*, Cross-sectional anatomy of the arm shows the neurovascular pedicle of the lateral arm flap lying near the lateral cortex of the humerus. The skin paddle of the lateral arm flap is supplied by terminal branches of the posterior radial collateral artery and vein, located in the lateral intermuscular septum of the arm. *B*, The lateral intermuscular septum of the arm, between the brachialis and triceps brachii muscles, lies parallel and 2 cm posterior to a line connecting two palpable landmarks—the deltoid insertion and the lateral epicondyle of the humerus. *C*, An anterior approach to flap elevation reveals two nerves that can be harvested with the lateral arm flap. The posterior cutaneous nerve of the arm supplies sensation to the skin paddle of the flap, whereas the posterior cutaneous nerve of the forearm can be used as a vascularized interposition nerve graft.

nerve of the forearm passes through the intermuscular septum on its way to the posterior lateral forearm and can be used as a vascularized interposition nerve graft.

The lateral arm flap has several advantages over other fasciocutaneous flaps commonly employed in head and neck reconstruction. Unlike with the radial forearm flap, which requires harvesting of the radial artery, harvesting of the PRCA with the lateral arm flap entails no risk for limb ischemia, and the donor site rarely requires a skin graft, which yields improved cosmetic results. Unlike the scapular fasciocutaneous flap, the lateral arm flap may be harvested with the patient in the supine position, which allows two surgical teams to operate simultaneously.

Relative disadvantages of the lateral arm flap include a linear scar on the lateral aspect of the arm and anesthesia of the forearm as a result of transection of the posterior cutaneous forearm nerve. Dissection of the vascular pedicle of the lateral arm flap can be more tedious than harvesting procedures for the radial forearm or scapular fasciocutaneous flaps. This pedicle has an average length of 8 to 10 cm, which limits its application to certain head and neck defects.

ANTEROLATERAL THIGH FLAP

The anterolateral thigh flap (Fig. 28–8) is a fasciocutaneous flap that is harvested from the anterior thigh in the area overlying the septum between the rectus femoris and the vastus lateralis muscles. It is based on the descending branch of the lateral circumflex artery and its venae comitantes. The lateral circumflex artery arises from the profunda femoris artery in the majority of patients, or less commonly as a direct branch of the femoral artery.[30] The vascular pedicle can be up to 15 cm in length with large-diameter vessels. Primary closure of the donor site can often be achieved, even following the harvest of large skin paddles. Sensory reinnervation is possible with incorporation of the lateral cutaneous nerve of the thigh. It has become quite popular for use in head and neck reconstruction.[31, 32]

The anterolateral thigh flap is often used in situations in which the lateral thigh flap would be considered, including

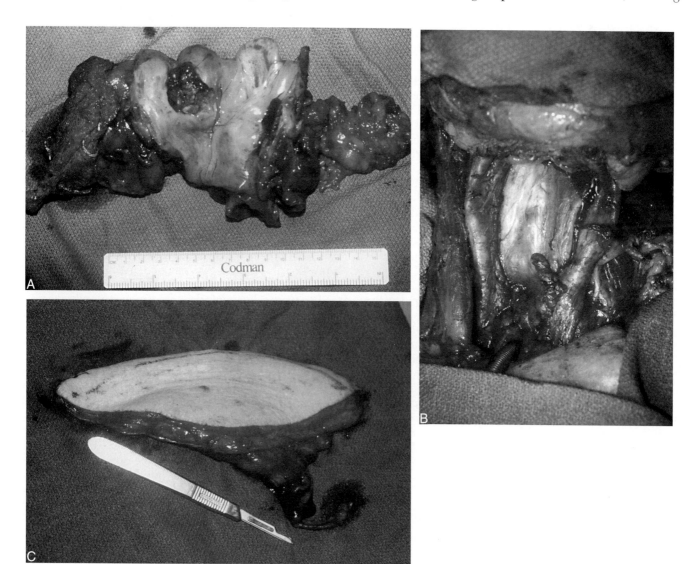

FIGURE 28–8 *A,* Advanced cancer of the laryngopharynx, *B,* Defect left by resection of laryngopharyngeal cancer. *C,* Anterolateral thigh flap.

pharyngoesophageal defects or other large mucosal defects. Its advantages include a large area of skin for harvest and a relatively straightforward dissection with minimal donor site morbidity. Its location allows for an easy two-team approach, and no special positioning is required.

Disadvantages of this flap include excessive flap thickness in obese patients, the potential for hair-bearing skin in men, and the necessity to take a cuff of vastus lateralis muscle in 60% of patients in whom the skin is supplied by perforators that traverse the muscle rather than by a pure septocutaneous route.[33]

LATERAL THIGH FLAP

The lateral thigh flap is a moderately thick fasciocutaneous flap, first described by Baek[34] in 1983. Its vascular supply is from septocutaneous branches of the third perforator of the profunda femoris artery and vein, which travel within the intermuscular septum separating the anterior and posterior muscle compartments of the lateral thigh. The vascular pedicle extends 8 to 15 cm and contains large-caliber vessels that measure 2 to 4 mm in diameter. The skin paddle has the potential for sensory reinnervation through incorporation of the lateral femoral cutaneous nerve.

The lateral thigh flap has been used primarily for pharyngoesophageal reconstruction, but it can be used to resurface any mucosal or cutaneous defect in the head and neck. The primary advantage of this flap is its relative lack of donor site morbidity. Flaps up to 25 × 14 cm can be harvested and the donor site can still be closed primarily. In addition, its location allows simultaneous two-team surgery without patient repositioning.

The major disadvantage of the lateral thigh flap is the tedious and more challenging dissection required to harvest the flap, especially in very muscular and very obese patients. Anomalies of the vascular pedicle do exist and need to be anticipated. Other potential disadvantages include a hair-bearing skin paddle in some males and a thick proximal flap in obese patients with "saddlebags."

Myocutaneous Free Flaps

Myocutaneous free flaps are a versatile reconstructive tool for the head and neck surgeon because they provide bulky tissue with reliable vascularity to the overlying skin and offer distinct advantages over regional myocutaneous flaps, namely a greater versatility in design. Their use is most appropriate for the reconstruction of extensive defects of the tongue, scalp, skull base, and paranasal sinuses, and of any other defect that requires a large amount of soft tissue. In addition, free muscle flaps can be reinnervated for reanimation of the paralyzed face. The most commonly used musculocutaneous free flaps include (1) rectus abdominis, (2) latissimus dorsi (see under The Scapular System of Flaps), (3) gracilis, (4) fibula, and (5) iliac crest.

RECTUS ABDOMINIS FLAP

The rectus abdominis flap (Fig. 28–9) is one of the most versatile and commonly performed free-tissue transfers in head and neck reconstruction.[35] It is used frequently when bulky soft tissue is required for reconstruction of large skull base, total glossectomy, and orbitomaxillary defects. The flap most commonly is designed as a myocutaneous flap with

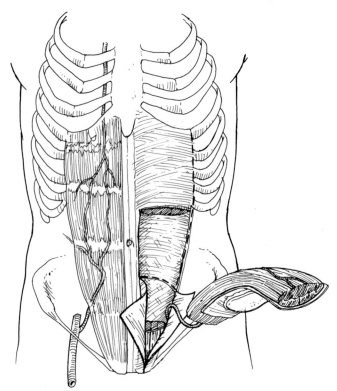

FIGURE 28–9 The primary blood supply to the rectus abdominis muscle is derived from the deep superior epigastric artery and the deep inferior epigastric artery, which anastomose with each other between the costal margin and the umbilicus. Musculocutaneous perforators are most frequently found in the periumbilical region. The inferior rectus abdominis free flap can be harvested, including a segment of vascularized anterior rectus sheath. The posterior rectus sheath becomes attenuated inferior to the arcuate line, so the anterior rectus sheath should be preserved below this landmark to lessen the risk of postoperative ventral hernia formation.

a variable amount of skin and subcutaneous fat. Alternatively, a myofascial or muscle flap can be harvested when a cutaneous paddle is not necessary or would be excessively bulky.

The rectus abdominis flap offers numerous advantages:

1. Its vascular pedicle—the deep inferior epigastric artery and vein—is long and of large diameter.
2. It can be harvested rapidly with the patient in the supine position, allowing a two-team approach.
3. A large amount of tissue can be harvested and primary closure of the donor defect can still be achieved.
4. The rich vascularity of the abdominal wall allows great flexibility in the design of the paddles. Multiple skin paddles of varying thickness, based on the periumbilical perforating vessels, can be designed for use in the reconstruction of complex three-dimensional defects. The skin paddles can be oriented in a transverse, a vertical, or an oblique direction.
5. Donor site morbidity is minimal, so long as the rectus fascia is repaired to prevent ventral hernia formation.
6. The durable anterior rectus fascial sheath and tendinous inscriptions facilitate suture placement during insetting of the flap. This allows for watertight closure and dead space obliteration, which are critical in the oral cavity and in reconstruction of the cranial base.[36]

The major potential disadvantage of the rectus free flap is its excessive bulk, especially in obese patients. This can be corrected by subsequent debulking procedures or by intraoperative modification of the flap's design. An alternative solution is to harvest the muscle alone or in combination with a variable thickness of subcutaneous tissue. A skin graft can be placed to resurface the muscle if necessary. In any case, postoperative atrophy of the muscle layer should be anticipated. Another disadvantage of the rectus muscle is its segmental nerve supply, which prevents effective sensory or motor reinnervation. The poor color match of abdominal skin is apparent when cutaneous defects of the face, scalp, or neck are resurfaced.

GRACILIS FLAP

The gracilis muscle and myocutaneous flaps (Fig. 28–10) have primarily been used for soft tissue coverage in the trunk and extremities,[37] but this donor site also has applications in the head and neck. The gracilis muscle is favored by many surgeons who perform free-tissue transfer for facial reanimation because the muscle's individual fascicular territories allow the use of smaller muscle units for restoration of specific facial movements. It can also be used as an innervated myocutaneous flap for tongue reconstruction or for radical parotidectomy defects when the mimetic facial muscles are resected or cannot be reinnervated.[38, 39]

Vascularized, bone-containing free flaps have revolutionized the reconstruction of segmental mandibular and palatomaxillary defects by reliably restoring continuity of bone and soft tissue in the primary setting and have recently been applied to palatomaxillary defects. The iliac crest, scapula, and fibula all provide vascularized bone of adequate stock to replace the resected segment. All have advantages, limitations, and donor site morbidities and are thus used in different circumstances. The most important differences relate to the quality, quantity, and reliability of the soft tissue component of the composite flap. Other essential differences include (1) the potential for osseointegration of the bone component,[40, 41] (2) the length and caliber of the vascular pedicle, (3) the ease of positioning, harvesting, and insetting of the flap, and (4) the potential complications and functional deficits associated with the sacrifice of bone and adjacent soft tissue at the donor site.

FIBULA FLAP

The free revascularized fibula bone flap (Fig. 28–11) was first described by Taylor and coworkers[42] in 1975 for long bone reconstruction after trauma or cancer surgery. Since Hidalgo[43] reported its use for mandible reconstruction in 1989, the osteocutaneous fibula flap has enjoyed great popularity in head and neck reconstruction. Its principal attribute is the exceptional length of bone it provides, making it the only bone-containing free flap that is adequate for total or subtotal mandibular reconstruction. Up to 25 cm of fibula bone can be harvested in the adult male, and the rich periosteal blood supply of the fibula allows the creation of multiple osteotomies for precise contouring of the neomandible without compromise of bone viability. The thick bicortical bone accepts plates and screws for secure fixation and osseointegrated implants for dental rehabilitation. The donor site location allows simultaneous two-team harvest with the patient in the supine position. Furthermore, sensory reinnervation of the skin paddle is possible through incorporation of the lateral sural nerve into the flap design. More recently, the fibula free flap has been applied to palatomaxillary reconstruction.[44]

The main disadvantage of the fibula free flap is the limitation imposed by its soft tissue component. Fasciocutaneous and musculocutaneous perforators of the peroneal artery supply the skin over the lateral calf and permit the harvest of a composite osteocutaneous flap. However, the poor arc of rotation of the skin island relative to the bone and its unpredictable pattern of vascularity limit its application to soft tissue reconstruction. Although methods to increase the reliability of the skin paddle have been described,[45] extensive composite oromandibular defects should be reconstructed with an alternative flap, such as the scapula osteocutaneous free flap or the internal oblique–iliac crest composite free flap. Alternatively, a bone-containing

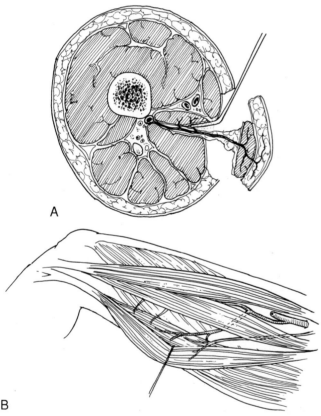

A

B

FIGURE 28–10 *A*, Cross-sectional anatomy of the thigh shows the adductor branch of the profunda femoris artery supplying the gracilis myocutaneous flap. The vascular pedicle to the gracilis runs between the adductor longus muscle anteriorly and the adductor magnus muscle posteriorly. It supplies the skin of the medial thigh through a dominant musculocutaneous perforator that enters the skin at a point 8 to 10 cm inferior to the pubic tubercle. *B*, Medial view of the thigh shows the medial femoral circumflex artery, which can serve as a secondary vascular pedicle, entering the gracilis flap. The anterior division of the obturator nerve supplies motor innervation to the gracilis muscle and enters the muscle cephalic to the vascular pedicle. The fascicular branching pattern of the obturator nerve allows the gracilis muscle to be separated into at least two functional motor units for the purpose of facial reanimation.

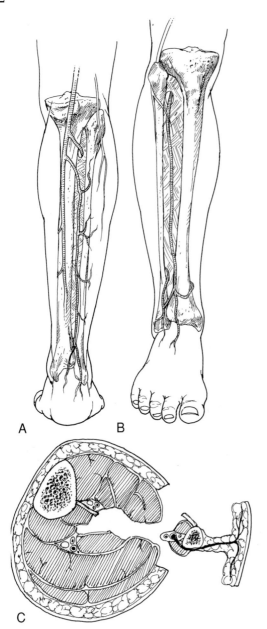

FIGURE 28–11 *A*, Vascular supply to the lower leg, posterior view. The popliteal artery bifurcates to form the posterior tibial artery and the peroneal artery. The posterior tibial artery commonly provides the dominant contribution to the plantar vascular arch of the foot. The peroneal artery supplies a single medullary branch and numerous periosteal branches to the fibula. The lateral sural cutaneous nerve, which is a branch of the common peroneal nerve, can be used for sensory reinnervation of the skin paddle harvested with the fibular osteocutaneous flap. *B*, Vascular supply to the lower leg, anterior view. The anterior tibial artery, which pierces the superior aspect of the interosseous membrane, commonly provides the dominant contribution to the dorsal vascular arch of the foot. The common peroneal nerve is most susceptible to injury superiorly, where it winds around the neck of the fibula. *C*, Cross-sectional anatomy of the lower leg shows the fibular osteocutaneous free flap harvested with its peroneal vascular pedicle. Perforators to the skin may take either a septocutaneous or a musculocutaneous course. Therefore, a cuff of flexor hallucis longus and soleus muscles should be harvested adjacent to the perforating vessels.

free flap can be used in combination with a separate fasciocutaneous free flap or a regional pedicled flap. The presence of atherosclerosis or congenital vascular anomalies of the lower extremity may contraindicate the harvest of the fibula free flap owing to poor collateral circulation to the foot. A preoperative angiogram should be performed to delineate these abnormalities.

The donor site morbidity associated with the fibula osteocutaneous flap is minimal. The two potential complications are injury to the peroneal nerve, which results in footdrop, and instability of the knee or ankle joints. Both of these morbidities can be avoided provided that the proximal and distal 6 to 8 cm of fibula bone is preserved. A plaster splint is applied for 5 to 7 days after surgery, and ambulation is resumed soon thereafter. Most patients are left with an aesthetically acceptable linear scar on the lateral leg.

In summary, the osseous and composite osteocutaneous fibula flaps are valuable additions to the available composite flaps used for oromandibular and palatomaxillary reconstruction. The donor site provides the largest length of available bone with limited functional impairment relative to other bone donor sites. As an osseous flap, it is ideal for subtotal and total mandibular reconstruction. Its application as an osteocutaneous flap, however, is restricted by limitations imposed by the skin paddle.

ILIAC CREST FLAP

The large amount of bone available from the ileum has made it a popular source for nonvascularized bone grafts, corticocancellous chips, and more recently, vascularized bone transfer (Fig. 28–12). The advantages of the ileum as a donor site are numerous. They include (1) the thick bicortical bone stock, which facilitates dental prosthetic rehabilitation with osseointegrated implants; (2) the ability of the donor site scar to be well hidden by conventional undergarments; and (3) the ease of flap harvest by a separate surgical team with the patient in a supine position. In addition, the anterior ileum is similar in shape to the native hemimandible. A total of 14 to 16 cm of bone can be harvested and osteotomies can be made in the outer cortex to reconstruct hemimandibular or angle-to-angle defects. Furthermore, depending on the soft tissue needs of the patient, the iliac crest free flap can be harvested as an osseous flap, an osteocutaneous flap, or a tripartite osteomyocutaneous flap when used in combination with the internal oblique muscle. The iliac crest free flap with the internal oblique muscle has been applied to palatomaxillary reconstruction with good results, allowing placement of osseointegrated implants and closure of the palate with the use of the soft tissue components.[46]

Although the ileum has several vascular contributions, Swartz and associates[47] and Taylor and colleagues[48] demonstrated the dominance of the deep circumflex iliac artery (DCIA) and vein when describing the osteocutaneous flap. The skin paddle extends superior to and lateral from the anterior superior iliac spine and is supplied by muscular perforators that are located along the medial aspect of the ileum. The integrity of circulation to the skin requires harvest of a large skin paddle for these perforators to be reliably incorporated. Furthermore, the bulkiness, limited pliability, and restricted mobility of the skin paddle relative

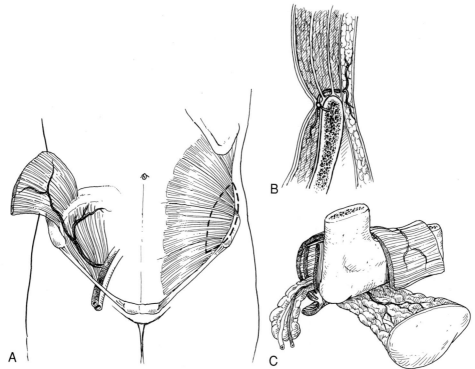

FIGURE 28–12 *A,* The deep circumflex iliac artery (DCIA) and vein (DCIV) arise from the external iliac vessels, a few centimeters superior to the inguinal ligament. They run superiorly and laterally to the anterior superior iliac spine, where the ascending branch is given off to the internal oblique muscle. The distal DCIA and DCIV continue in a curvilinear course along the inner cortex of the iliac crest, giving off endosteal and periosteal branches to the bone and musculocutaneous perforators to the overlying skin. *B,* Cross-sectional anatomy shows that the musculocutaneous perforators pierce all three layers of the abdominal wall musculature to reach the skin. A 2-cm cuff of these muscles should be harvested along the medial aspect of the iliac bone to preserve the cutaneous perforators. *C,* The tripartite iliac crest–internal oblique osteomusculocutaneous flap is oriented for reconstruction of a through-and-through right mandibulectomy defect. The internal oblique muscle is transposed over the bone to reconstruct the floor of mouth and alveolar ridge. The skin paddle is inset externally to replace the cutaneous defect.

to the bone limit the use of the osteocutaneous flap for reconstruction of complicated composite defects.

Ramasastry and coworkers[49] first described the internal oblique muscle flap for reconstruction of the extremity after identifying the ascending branch of the DCIA as the primary blood supply to the internal oblique muscle. A tripartite iliac crest–internal oblique flap was subsequently developed that permitted the simultaneous transfer of two independent soft tissue flaps with the iliac bone. Urken and others[50, 51] popularized the use of this flap for oromandibular reconstruction in 1989 (Fig. 28–13). The highly mobile, thin, and well-vascularized internal oblique muscle can be used to resurface oral cavity and pharyngeal mucosal defects. Similarly, a portion of the muscle is used to cover the bone graft and reconstruction plate. Skin grafting of the internal oblique muscle is unnecessary because the well-vascularized flap rapidly becomes covered by mucosa. The denervated muscle subsequently undergoes atrophy and provides a thin, well-vascularized, and immobile tissue layer over the mandible. The skin paddle is used to reconstruct associated cutaneous defects or is incorporated into a cervical suture line to act as an external monitor of flap viability.[52]

The iliac crest free flap has been applied to the reconstruction of a variety of other head and neck defects. Salibian and colleagues[53] reported the use of the iliac crest osteocutaneous flap for reconstruction of the anterior mandible in association with total or subtotal glossectomy defects. In this instance, the iliac bone is placed transversely in the floor of the mouth to support the skin paddle, which is used to reconstruct the tongue. Excellent long-term maintenance of the height of the neotongue has been reported with this flap design. The iliac crest free flap has also been used for reconstruction of skull base and maxillectomy defects.[54]

The harvest of the iliac crest free flap involves a considerable amount of dissection. Because most of the lower abdominal wall muscles and part of the inguinal ligament are divided, ventral hernia formation is a significant potential risk. Meticulous closure of the donor site, including the use of Marlex mesh for select cases, helps to minimize this risk. During both the harvesting and the closure, the surgeon must pay careful attention to neighboring structures, including the femoral nerve and the intraperitoneal contents. The patient experiences postoperative hip pain and weakness, but this generally subsides after several weeks. Despite these

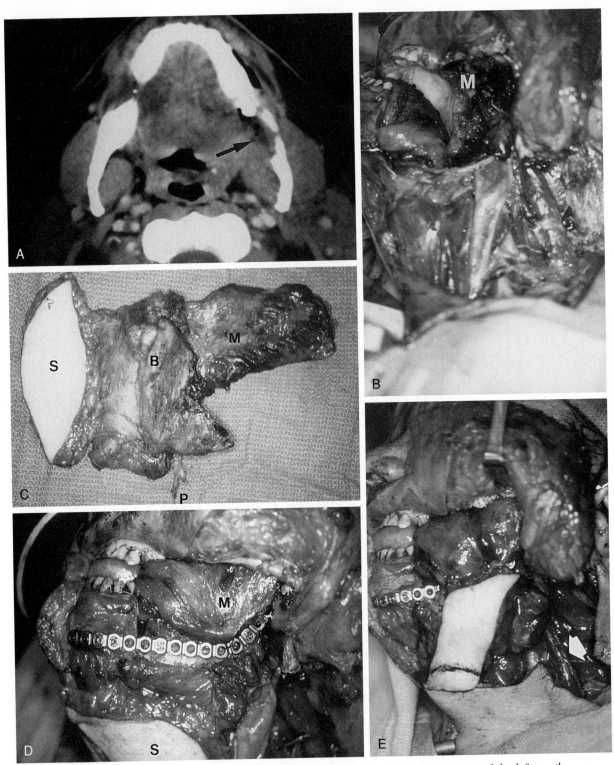

FIGURE 28–13 *A,* Axial computed tomography shows a T4 squamous cell carcinoma of the left tonsil invading the left mandibular angle and ramus (*arrow*). *B,* An intraoperative photograph shows the defect that resulted from resection. The defect classification is bone: B, R; soft tissue: B, SP^H,PH^L; neurologic: N^L, N^{IA} (see Tables 28–1 and 28–2, Fig. 28–16) and also includes resection of the left posterior maxillary infrastructure (M). *C,* The tripartite iliac crest–internal oblique free flap, based on the deep circumflex iliac vascular pedicle (P), contains vascularized bone (B) and two separate soft tissue components—the internal oblique muscle (M) and the segment of skin (S) with subcutaneous fat. *D,* The iliac bone flap has been secured to a contoured reconstruction plate. The internal oblique muscle (M) has been folded into the oral cavity along the medial aspect of the iliac bone and is then redraped over the reconstructed alveolar ridge. The skin paddle (S) of the flap lies in the submandibular fossa. *E,* A small portion of the skin paddle is incorporated into a cervical suture line to serve as a clinical monitor of flap circulation during the postoperative period. The portion of the skin flap superior to the inked line will be deepithelialized and used to restore subcutaneous contour to the region of the resected masseter muscle. The deep circumflex iliac vascular pedicle (*arrow*) has been anastomosed to the transverse cervical artery and the external jugular vein.

potential donor site problems, extensive clinical experience with the iliac crest free flap has demonstrated its reliability in achieving functional oromandibular reconstruction for even the most complex composite mandibulectomy defects.

The Scapular System of Flaps

Flaps based on the distal ramifications of the subscapular artery provide a wide array of available tissue for head and neck reconstruction (Fig. 28–14). These flaps include the scapular and parascapular fascial or fasciocutaneous free flaps, the lateral or medial scapular osteocutaneous free flaps, the serratus anterior flap, the latissimus dorsi muscle or myocutaneous flap, the latissimus dorsi–rib flap, and the serratus anterior–rib flap.[55–58]

The subscapular artery most frequently arises from the third portion of the axillary artery. This vessel is 3 to 4 mm in diameter and passes inferiorly and posteriorly through the axilla for an average distance of 2.2 cm before branching into the circumflex scapular artery and the thoracodorsal artery.[59] The circumflex scapular artery passes posteriorly through a muscular triangle bounded by the teres major, the teres minor, and the long head of the triceps. The overall length of the circumflex scapular artery is 4 to 8 cm. Periosteal branches supply the lateral border of the scapula, and 10 to 14 cm of lateral scapular border may be harvested based on these branches. The straight segment of bone may be osteotomized and contoured for mandible reconstruction.[60] An additional 3 to 4 cm of bone may be taken at the tip of the scapula to allow for reconstruction of the angle of the mandible without an osteotomy. The two terminal branches of the circumflex scapular artery are the transverse and descending cutaneous branches, on which the scapular and parascapular skin paddles, respectively, are based.[61] Preservation of the fascial attachments between the distal scapular skin flap and the underlying bone allows for harvest of the thin medial scapular bone as an osteocutaneous flap for reconstruction of the orbital floor or palate.[62]

After its takeoff from the subscapular artery, the thoracodorsal artery descends along the surface of the serratus muscle for a distance of 9 cm before entering the latissimus dorsi muscle. The latissimus dorsi muscle may be harvested as a pedicled or free muscle flap, a myocutaneous flap, or an osteomyocutaneous flap incorporating a segment of rib. The

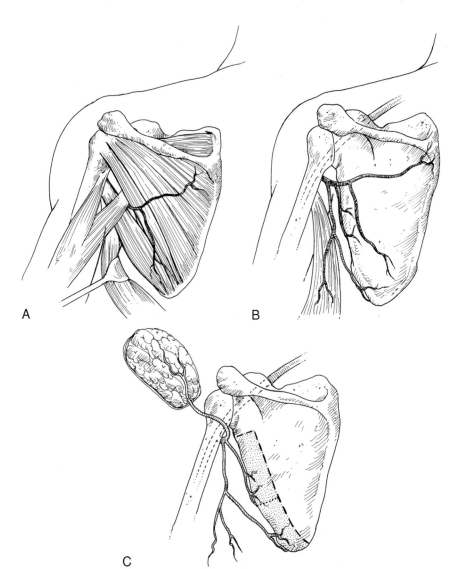

FIGURE 28–14 *A*, The circumflex scapular artery (CSA), which arises from the subscapular artery, emerges through the triangular space of the posterior axilla, bounded by teres minor, teres major, and the long head of the triceps. A horizontally oriented scapular skin paddle can be harvested based on the transverse branch of the CSA, whereas an obliquely oriented parascapular skin flap can be centered over the descending branch of the CSA. *B*, With the overlying muscles removed, the remaining branches of the subscapular axis are seen. Periosteal branches to the lateral scapular border arise from the CSA and from the angular branch of the thoracodorsal artery (TDA). The TDA gives off additional branches to the latissimus dorsi and serratus anterior muscles. *C*, Periosteal branches of the subscapular system arising from the CSA and TDA allow for the harvesting of two segments of lateral scapular bone separated by a 15-cm arc of rotation.

thoracodorsal artery is consistently accompanied by the thoracodorsal vein and the thoracodorsal nerve, which is the motor nerve to the latissimus dorsi muscle. This neurovascular pedicle has been used to provide reinnervated muscle for total glossectomy reconstruction and facial nerve rehabilitation.

Prior to its entry into the latissimus dorsi muscle, the thoracodorsal artery gives off two ramifications of clinical interest. One to three branches supply the serratus anterior muscle. The lower third of this muscle can be harvested with or without a segment of rib as a pedicled or free flap. Preservation of the superior portion of the serratus muscle prevents postoperative winging of the scapula. The angular branch arises from the thoracodorsal vessels or the branch to the serratus anterior and supplies the periosteum of the tip of the scapula. Dissection and inclusion of this branch allows for up to 8 cm of scapular tip to be harvested independently from a separate lateral scapular bone flap based on the circumflex scapular artery. This permits the transfer of two separate scapular bone segments based on a single subscapular vascular pedicle and separated by a 13- to 15-cm arc of rotation.[63]

The scapular system of flaps has been used for a wide variety of head and neck reconstructive problems. The scapular and parascapular flaps have been employed as osteocutaneous flaps for reconstruction of oromandibular and orbitomaxillary defects,[64, 65] whereas fasciocutaneous flaps have been found to be useful for augmentation of a variety of congenital and acquired facial cutaneous and contour deficiencies.[66–68] The serratus anterior muscle flap has been used for augmentation of small to moderate soft tissue defects, and when harvested with the inferior fascicle of the long thoracic nerve, it has been used for reanimation of the paralyzed eyelid and oral commissure. The latissimus dorsi flap has been used for reconstruction of a wide variety of oromandibular, pharyngoesophageal, midface, craniotemporal, and craniofacial defects.[69] Several skin, bone, and muscle flaps can be harvested on a single subscapular vascular pedicle, creating the so-called megaflap (Fig. 28–15).[70] Up to 875 cm² of tissue has been reported to be transferred on a single pedicle with the use of this technique. Separate arcs of rotation around the periosteal, transverse cutaneous, and descending cutaneous branches of the circumflex scapular artery and the muscular and angular branches of the thoracodorsal artery provide for extreme flexibility in the use of this flap for reconstruction of extensive and complex head and neck wounds.[71]

The major disadvantage of the scapular system of flaps arises from the lateral decubitus surgical position required for flap harvest. This position frequently requires intraoperative repositioning of the patient and precludes simultaneous head and neck ablative surgery. Both the iliac crest and the fibula provide better bone stock for mandibular reconstruction with regard to length of available bone and width of bone to support an implant-borne dental prosthesis. In addition, the cutaneous paddles of the scapular, parascapular, and latissimus dorsi flaps are not amenable to sensory reinnervation. Scapulohumeral rotation can be significantly limited after the lateral scapular osteocutaneous flap is harvested. Postoperatively, patients should have immobilization of the shoulder for 5 days followed by

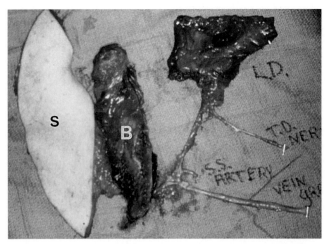

FIGURE 28–15 The subscapular (S.S.) system "megaflap" includes a scapular fasciocutaneous paddle (S), a vascularized segment of lateral scapular border (B), and a portion of the latissimus dorsi muscle (L.D.). The thoracodorsal nerve (T.D.) has been included because latissimus dorsi reinnervation will serve to preserve muscle volume after flap transfer. A saphenous vein graft has been used to increase the length of the venous pedicle.

physical therapy consisting of gradually increased range-of-motion exercises.

◘ OROMANDIBULAR RECONSTRUCTION

The goals of reconstruction following ablative surgery for cancer of the oral cavity are to restore oral function and to preserve facial aesthetics. Functional parameters such as articulation, mastication, deglutition, oral competence, and airway protection play a significant role in postoperative quality of life. Despite recent advances in reconstructive surgery, achievement of these goals remains a complex endeavor. The technical challenges are numerous and are compounded by the need to operate in a contaminated field.

Classification of composite defects is a critical initial step in achieving a successful reconstruction of the oral cavity. Stratification of these defects should account for the status of bone, soft tissue, and neurologic structures in this region.[72] The mandible can be divided into various segments based on a number of factors, including the functional impairment that results from disruption of the muscles of mastication and the suprahyoid muscles that insert into the mandible and participate in laryngeal suspension and elevation (Fig. 28–16). The complexity associated with reconstruction of specific structures, such as the condyle and temporomandibular joint, should also be reflected in the classification scheme.

The classification of soft tissue defects is more complex owing to the highly specialized and dynamic nature of the oral lining and muscles (Table 28–1). Because of the critical importance of the tongue in oral function, glossectomy defects should be analyzed carefully. The mobile tongue should be distinguished from the base of the tongue, and the extent of tissue loss should be quantified. Denervated

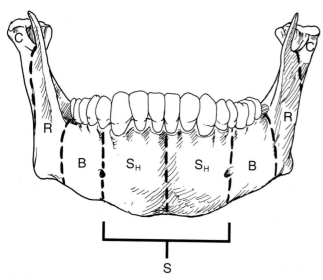

FIGURE 28–16 Classification of segmental defects of the mandible. S, symphysis; S$_H$, hemisymphysis; B, body; R, ramus; C, condyle.

tongue should be distinguished from functional tongue tissue. Adjacent soft tissue defects are defined, including those involving the palate, pharynx, floor of mouth, lips, and buccal mucosa. External cutaneous defects of the cheek, chin, and neck must also be addressed. Neurologic deficits involving the hypoglossal, lingual, facial, and inferior

TABLE 28–1 Classification of Soft Tissue Defects in the Oral Cavity

Defect	Abbreviation
Mucosa	
Labial	L
Buccal	B
Soft palate	SP
Hemi	SP^H
Total	SP^T
Floor of mouth	FOM
Anterior	FOM^A
Lateral	FOM^L
Pharynx	PH
Lateral	PH^L
Posterior	PH^P
Tongue	
Mobile	T^M
One quarter	T$^M_{1/4}$
One half	T$^M_{1/2}$
Three quarters	T$^M_{3/4}$
Nonfunctional	T$^M_{NF}$
Tongue base	T^B
One quarter	T$^B_{1/4}$
One half	T$^B_{1/2}$
Three quarters	T$^B_{3/4}$
Nonfunctional	T$^B_{NF}$
Total glossectomy	T^G
Cutaneous defects	C
Cheek	C^{CH}
Neck	C^N
Mentum	C^M
Lips	C^L
Upper	C^{UL}
Lower (1/4, 1/2, 3/4, total)	C^{LL}

TABLE 28–2 Classification of Neurologic Defects

Defect	Abbreviation
Nerve	
Hypoglossal	N^H
Lingual	N^L
Facial	N^F
Inferior alveolar	N^{IA}
Bilateral defects	N^B

alveolar nerves must be specified (Table 28–2). Although it is always attractive to try to simplify the classification of such defects, the complexity of the oral anatomy as well as the degree of detail that can be restored to these anatomic regions demands an equally detailed description. Furthermore, the condition of the remaining tissues must be considered. A heavily irradiated or densely scarred recipient bed generally requires well-vascularized tissue for reconstruction.

Reconstruction of the Mandible

The number of approaches that have been applied to the restoration of mandibular continuity attests to the complexity of the problem.[73–76] Two major criticisms of mandibular reconstruction in the past were the high failure rate of primary reconstruction and the inability of patients whose mandibles were restored to wear dentures that allowed them to effectively chew. Prior to the availability of vascularized bone grafts, the low success rate of mandibular restoration with free bone grafts and alloplastic materials discouraged primary reconstruction.[77] Avascular mandibular substitutes, which relied on neovascularization and creeping substitution, were prone to infection and extrusion. In contrast, vascularized bone grafts undergo primary healing even in unfavorable recipient beds,[78] and success rates of oromandibular reconstruction using vascularized bone–containing free flaps now approach 96%.[79] Endosteal dental implants, which function as tooth root analogues, have provided a solution to the problem of denture instability and poor retention (Fig. 28–17). This form of dental rehabilitation can provide superior functional results as documented by the testing of bite force and chewing performance.[80–82]

The iliac crest, scapula, and fibula composite flaps are the most commonly used vascularized bone–containing free flaps for restoration of mandibular continuity.[83–88] Each of these composite flaps differs with respect to (1) the quality and quantity of available bone and soft tissue; (2) the length, caliber, and reliability of the vascular pedicle; (3) donor site morbidity; and (4) the feasibility of a simultaneous two-team approach. When appropriately applied, all three flaps can allow predictable bony and soft tissue restoration of complex oral cavity defects. There is no single composite flap that satisfies the needs of all patients. It is therefore incumbent on the reconstructive surgeon to be familiar with all three donor sites to optimize the rehabilitation of each patient. Careful flap selection may allow for improved functional and aesthetic results, with more rapid reintegration of the patient into society.

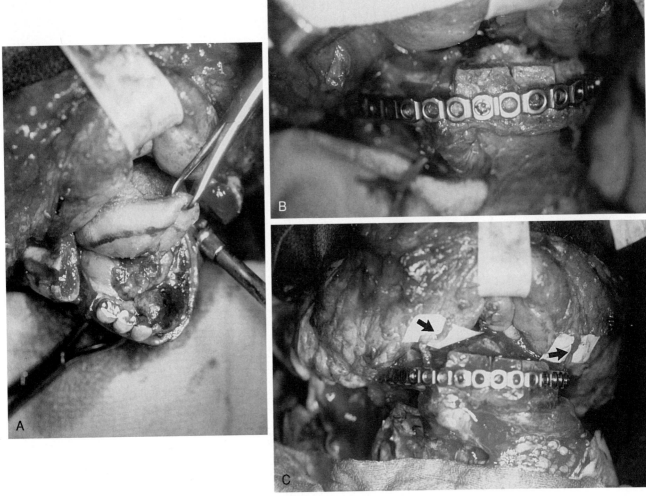

FIGURE 28–17 *A,* A T4 squamous cell carcinoma involving the anterior floor of mouth and ventral tongue, exposed after elevation of a visor flap. The defect classification is bone: S; soft tissue: FOM^A, T$^M_{1/4}$; nerve: N^{IAB} (see Tables 28–1 and 28–2, Fig. 28–16). *B,* The mandibulectomy defect has been reconstructed with the use of an iliac crest composite free flap. The anterior mandibular contour has been reconstructed by making multiple osteotomies in the iliac bone. *C,* The lower lip has been reinnervated by lateral femoral cutaneous nerve cable grafts between the inferior alveolar and mental nerves bilaterally (*arrows*).

Continued

Soft Tissue Reconstruction

The restoration of tongue function is both the most critical factor and the most challenging problem in the rehabilitation of oral cancer patients. A small resection of the mobile tongue may be closed primarily with minimal disturbance of function. When a defect of the tongue extends into the adjacent floor of the mouth, reconstruction with a redundant split-thickness skin graft helps to prevent tethering of the tongue. Local flaps of buccal, palatal, or lingual mucosa have been used to reconstruct small to medium defects of the tongue. These procedures may, however, result in reduced mobility of the tongue.

Larger defects that involve at least one half of the mobile tongue cause a greater degree of oral dysfunction. Patients who have undergone resection of the entire tongue or who are left with a denervated tongue remnant have the greatest

difficulty with articulation, deglutition, and protection of the airway. Decisions regarding the management of the larynx to prevent overwhelming aspiration are based on a variety of factors, including age, pulmonary reserve, and motivation of the patient. In these cases, it is critical that the mobility of the residual tongue be preserved by the use of redundant, thin, pliable tissue and that the reconstruction of the mobile tongue and adjacent defects of the floor of the mouth be compartmentalized to ensure separation of the root of the tongue from the lingual surface of the mandible. The pliability and rich vascularity of the radial forearm flap afford the flexibility in design that makes this flap an ideal source of tissue for customized reconstruction of many oral cavity defects (Fig. 28–18).[89] A considerable amount of vascularized fat can be harvested with the radial forearm flap when bulk is necessary to achieve contact between the neotongue and the palate or pharyngeal wall. Furthermore, sensation

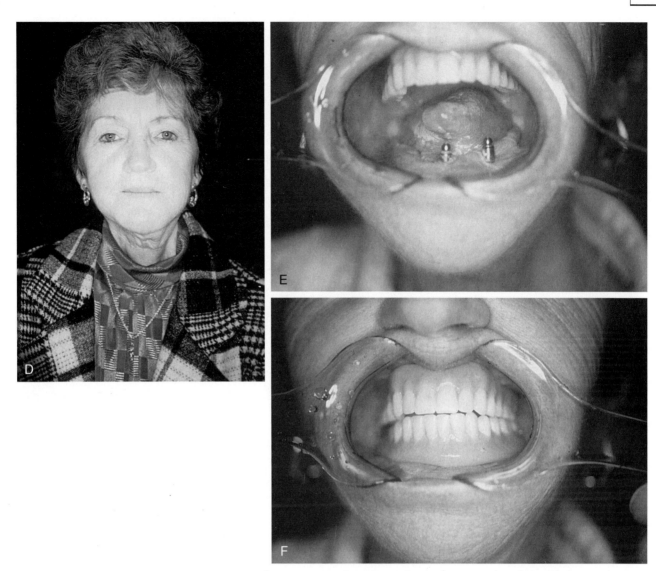

FIGURE 28–17, cont'd *D*, A 9-month postoperative frontal view shows restoration of good mandibular contour. *E*, Intraoral view shows two endosteal dental implants placed within the reconstructed segment of mandible. *F*, A prosthesis-borne lower denture is shown in place. This type of denture has greater stability and retention than a soft tissue–borne denture.

to the skin paddle of the forearm flap can be restored by anastomosis of the antebrachial cutaneous nerves to appropriate recipient nerves in the head and neck.

For mandible-sparing total glossectomy defects, it is desirable to reconstruct the neotongue with sufficient bulk consisting of adipose tissue rather than denervated muscle, with the goal of achieving long-term tongue-to-palate contact. Regional myocutaneous flaps tend to atrophy and sag over time owing to the effects of denervation and gravity on the muscle pedicle. Free myocutaneous flaps, including rectus abdominis and latissimus dorsi flaps, may provide superior long-term results. Free flaps can be directly sutured to the mandible or muscles of mastication to support the position of the skin paddle and to combat the long-term effects of gravity. Motor reinnervation achieved with the use of the stump of the hypoglossal nerve helps to maintain the bulk of the transferred muscle, although meaningful movement of the neotongue has not been adequately

documented. Another parameter to consider in the physiologic reconstruction of total glossectomy defects involves sensory reinnervation to assist with control of the food bolus. Bulkier, sensate fasciocutaneous free flaps, such as lateral thigh and lateral arm flaps, may be helpful in this regard.

A variety of reconstructive options are available for total or near-total glossectomy defects associated with segmental mandibulectomy. For lateral defects, a mandibular reconstruction plate can be used in conjunction with a soft tissue free flap (Fig. 28–19). However, we have noted an incidence of delayed external plate extrusion with this technique that approaches 30% when patients are followed for longer than 12 months. For reconstruction of anterior mandibulectomy defects, the composite iliac crest flap is inset with the bone in a horizontal position to support the accompanying skin paddle, which is used intraorally to replace the tongue.[90]

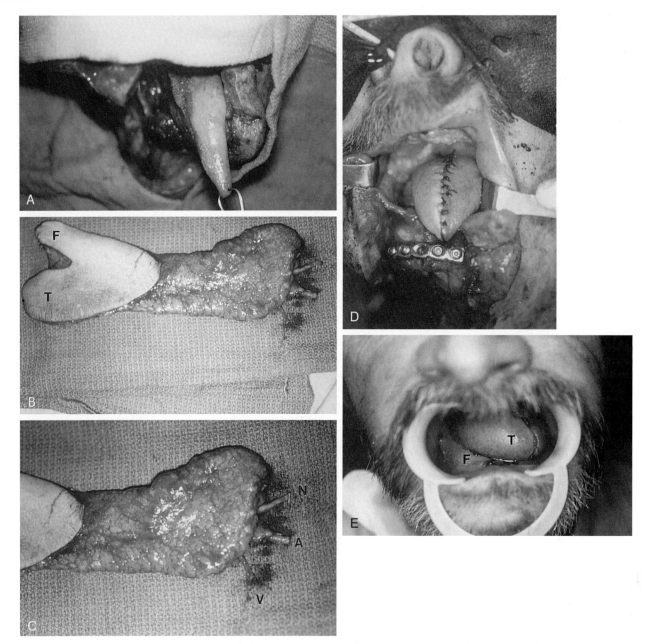

FIGURE 28–18 *A,* A right partial glossectomy defect is shown after resection of squamous cell carcinoma, approached through a midline mandibulotomy. Defect classification is soft tissue: FOM^{LA}, $T^M_{1/2}$; nerve: N^L (see Tables 28–1 and 28–2). *B,* A bilobed neurofasciocutaneous radial forearm flap has been harvested, which includes separate skin segments for reconstruction of the tongue (T) and the floor of the mouth (F). A segment of vascularized subcutaneous tissue has been harvested proximal to the skin paddle. This fat will serve to protect the great vessel and the vascular pedicle from salivary contamination and to restore cervical contour after modified radical neck dissection. *C,* Close-up view of the pedicle shows the radial artery (A), the cephalic vein (V), and the lateral antebrachial cutaneous nerve (N). *D,* An intraoperative photograph shows the forearm flap after being inset. The mandibulotomy has been closed with a reconstruction plate. *E,* A 6-week postoperative view shows restoration of the sulcus between the reconstructed tongue (T) and the floor of mouth (F) with preservation of tongue mobility.

For larger or more complex soft tissue defects associated with segmental mandibulectomy, a single composite free flap may be inadequate to meet reconstructive needs. Of the scapula, fibula, and iliac crest osteocutaneous free flaps, only the scapular skin paddle has a sufficient degree of mobility relative to the position of the bone component to allow for reconstruction of the complex sulcular anatomy of the oral cavity. However, the scapular skin flap is relatively thick and is not amenable to sensory reinnervation. The skin paddle of the fibula free flap is amenable to sensory reinnervation with the use of the lateral sural cutaneous flap. However, this skin flap has an unpredictable vascularity and

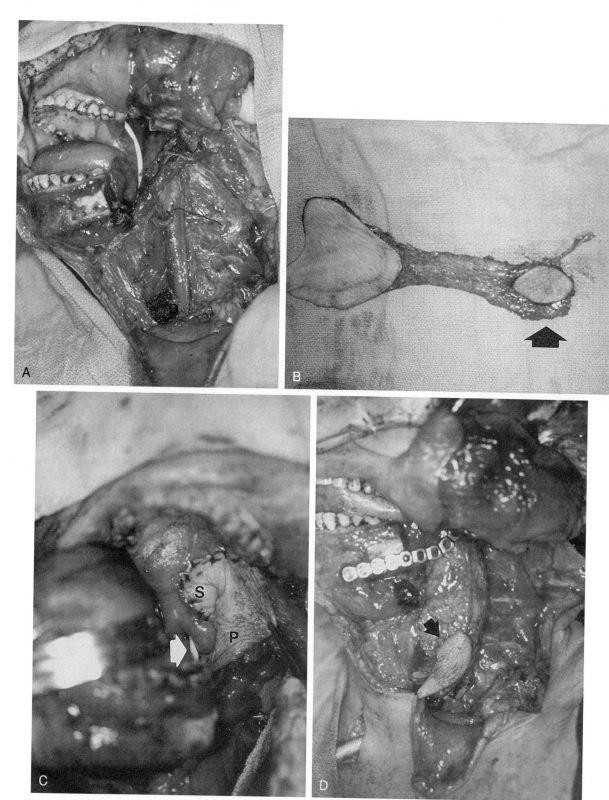

FIGURE 28–19 *A,* A composite resection defect that resulted from resection of a left tonsillar squamous cell carcinoma. Defect classification is bone: R; soft tissue: B, SP^H, FOM^L, PH^L, T$^B_{1/2}$; neurologic: N^L, N^{IA} (see Tables 28–1 and 28–2, Fig. 28–16). *B,* A bilobed radial forearm flap is harvested for reconstruction of the complex oropharyngeal anatomy. A proximal skin paddle (*arrow*) is included to serve as a monitor of postoperative flap perfusion. *C,* The forearm flap is inset into the soft tissue defect. The thin, pliable forearm flap is folded on itself to reconstitute both the oropharyngeal and nasopharyngeal surfaces of the soft palate (S) and the posterior pharyngeal wall (P). The nasogastric tube (*white arrow*) is visible adjacent to the uvula. *D,* The lateral mandibulectomy defect is reconstituted using a titanium hollow-screw reconstruction plate. The forearm flap pedicle is brought into the neck through the space medial to the plate. The proximal skin monitor (*arrow*) is incorporated into the neck incision. The subcutaneous fat of the forearm flap has been draped over the great vessels and separates the vascular pedicle from the oropharyngeal suture line.

a limited arc of rotation with respect to the underlying bone. The skin paddle of the iliac crest composite flap is excessively bulky for intraoral application in obese patients and is not amenable to sensory reinnervation. In this situation, a fasciocutaneous or musculocutaneous free flap combined with a vascularized, bone-containing free flap allows for more precise duplication of normal oral anatomy and physiology.

When mandibulectomy is performed concurrent with significant glossectomy, pharyngectomy, or soft palate resection, radial forearm and lateral arm neurosensory free flaps have been used successfully in conjunction with a vascularized, bone-containing free flap.[91–93]

Despite reconstructive efforts, virtually all patients who undergo major resection of the oral cavity and oropharynx have some degree of dysarthria, dysphagia, and sometimes, aspiration. Although many patients achieve adequate compensation, some have prolonged disability. Adjunctive procedures should be performed to facilitate postoperative deglutition when indicated. These procedures include laryngeal suspension, cricopharyngeal myotomy, and tubed epiglottic laryngoplasty. Speech and swallowing therapy is helpful to maximize the ultimate success of the reconstructive effort.

◘ PALATOMAXILLARY RECONSTRUCTION

With recognition of the functional and aesthetic success gained in mandibular reconstruction, attention has turned to functional restoration of palatomaxillary defects. The goals of reconstruction of palatomaxillary defects are to restore the form of the midfacial area while preserving the function of the palatomaxillary complex. The functional roles of this complex include the provision of an occlusal surface and support for the globe, and the creation of a patent nasal airway. Functional dental rehabilitation is a critical goal that can be achieved through the application of dental implant technology. Numerous techniques, including prosthetic devices, local flaps, regional flaps, and more recently, free-tissue transfer, have been applied to the restoration of these complex defects.

Prostheses have been the most popular method of rehabilitation for many palatomaxillary defects. The advantages of prosthetic rehabilitation include a rapid return to function, simplification of the surgical aspects of reconstruction, and facilitated direct visualization of the surgical site by removal of the prosthesis, especially in the edentulous patient, for oncologic monitoring. Considerations when the use of a tissue-borne prosthesis is planned include the size of the defect, remaining dentition for stabilization of the prosthesis, and availability and location of surrounding bone if an osseointegrated implant system is to be used to fix the prosthesis in position.

Although still the most popular form of restoration of most palatomaxillary defects, prosthetic management has significant drawbacks. Instability of the prosthesis, poor separation of the oral and nasal cavities, patient discomfort, malodor due to stasis of secretions, and daily cleaning and maintenance are genuine concerns associated with prosthetic rehabilitation. Consideration of these problems has led to the investigation of alternative methods of rehabilitation. Recently, free-tissue transfer has become a reliable method of optimizing rehabilitation of the patient with a palatomaxillary defect.[94]

Small defects that involve the hard palate and a minimal amount of the tooth-bearing alveolus may be rehabilitated with either a prosthesis or soft tissue reconstruction. Prostheses placed in these defects are usually very stable and well tolerated. However, some patients may have difficulty with the daily prosthetic hygiene required or may simply be unhappy with the effort required to maintain the prosthesis. Numerous techniques for soft tissue reconstruction of this area have been described, including temporalis muscle flaps, buccal mucosal flaps, and the palatal island flap.[95] Free-tissue transfers have also recently been applied to these defects.

For reconstruction of small to medium-sized defects of the hard palate and maxillary alveolus, our choice is the palatal island flap.[96] In cases of larger defects that cannot be covered effectively by the palatal island flap, or when the patient has had previous irradiation that precludes local tissue transfer, the radial forearm flap provides a reliable and functional closure.

Larger defects resulting from the classic maxillectomy, including the hemipalatectomy defect, are common, and their ideal reconstruction is controversial.[97, 98] Alternatives include prosthetic management, soft tissue reconstruction using pedicled or free-tissue transfer, vascularized soft tissue with free bone grafts, and free-tissue transfer of vascularized bone. Prosthetic management of these defects is challenging, especially in the edentulous patient. The remaining dental arch and palate may be insufficient to adequately support a prosthetic device, leading to instability and poor separation of the nose and mouth. Free-flap soft tissue reconstruction with or without bone grafts provides an option for these patients. However, restoration of dentition is difficult, and dentures tend to have poor stability owing to a reduced gingivobuccal sulcus and palatal arch. Free-flap reconstruction with vascularized bone has been reported with good results. Free-bone transfer allows the greatest chance of functional dental restoration with osseointegrated implants. Free flaps from the scapula, fibula, and iliac crest have been described for this purpose. The scapula free flap provides the greatest degree of soft tissue mobility, but the bone stock is occasionally too limited for placement of implants.[99] The fibula free flap provides a large amount of bone that is adequate for implant placement.[100] Limitations include a frequent requirement for vein grafts to reach cervical vessels, limited soft tissue mobility, and difficulty in providing adequate form to the orbital rim and zygomatic body.

The iliac crest flap with the internal oblique muscle has recently been described for palatomaxillary reconstruction.[101] The composite flap provides the greatest amount of bone stock for reconstruction of defects with a large vertical component, including the zygoma and the orbital floor. In addition, the internal oblique muscle, with its axial pattern blood supply in up to 80% of cases, affords the necessary mobility to achieve both palatal and nasal closure. The relatively short vascular pedicle can pose a challenge for flap revascularization. However, cephalad dissection of the facial artery and vein can usually circumvent the necessity for introduction of vein grafts.

Large anterior defects of the palate, including both canine teeth, or total palatal defects leave little support for a prosthesis. A large tipping force is applied when the anterior teeth are used to bite into food, and this translates to difficulty in using a prosthesis that cannot be adequately supported by remaining tissue. Free flaps containing vascularized bone, as discussed earlier, allow placement of implants and securing of an implant-borne prosthesis, which maximizes stability and retention.

◼ PHARYNGOESOPHAGEAL RECONSTRUCTION

The ideal method for reconstruction of the hypopharynx and cervical esophagus after resection of locally advanced malignancy is an immediate, single-stage technique with low morbidity that allows for rapid restoration of function. Formulation of these goals recognizes the fact that despite advances in surgical techniques, radiation therapy, and adjuvant chemotherapy, the 5-year survival for patients with stage III and IV carcinomas arising in this region is on the order of 10% to 30%; any intervention should therefore be considered palliative. Methods employed for pharyngoesophageal reconstruction include local skin flaps, regional skin flaps, regional myocutaneous flaps, visceral pedicled flaps (including gastric pullup and colon interposition), and microvascular free flaps.[102, 103]

Local and Regional Skin Flaps

The earliest methods of pharyngoesophageal reconstruction employed local and regional skin flaps. In the 1940s, Wookey[104] popularized the staged repair of pharyngolaryngectomy defects using laterally based cervical skin flaps. In the 1960s, Bakamjian[105] described the use of the tubed deltopectoral flap, which became the standard method of pharyngoesophageal reconstruction until the advent of myocutaneous flaps in the late 1970s. These techniques resulted in a relatively high rate of distal anastomotic stricture, and most patients required three or four staged procedures over a period of several months before a patent pharyngoesophageal segment was achieved. This prolonged therapy is disadvantageous in a patient population with a limited life expectancy.

Myocutaneous Flaps

The pectoralis major and trapezius myocutaneous flaps gained popularity for pharyngoesophageal reconstruction in the late 1970s and early 1980s. These two flaps were superior to the deltopectoral flaps in that they allowed transfer of large amounts of skin without delay, potentially allowing for single-stage reconstruction. However, the regional myocutaneous flaps tended to have excessive bulk, which hindered tubing of the cutaneous paddle. Pharyngocutaneous fistulas were common sequelae of attempts to reconstruct circumferential defects, particularly when lesions had been irradiated. The development of a fistula often led to prolonged hospitalization, delayed oral nutrition, and stricture formation long-term. In attempts to overcome these difficulties, staged reconstructions employing skin-grafted pectoralis major muscle flaps and the creation of controlled pharyngostomes were attempted. However, these modifications eliminated the advantages of single-stage reconstruction of myocutaneous flaps over previous methods of pharyngoesophageal reconstruction.

Visceral Pedicled Flaps

Colon Interposition

The application of large intestine for esophageal reconstruction has consisted primarily of the interposition of pedicled segments of right or left colon. Whereas some surgeons prefer the right colon for its isoperistaltic orientation after interposition, most prefer the left colon for its more reliable blood supply. Colon interposition has fallen into disfavor, as published reports have documented a 45% incidence of major medical complications, a 25% incidence of reconstructive complications (including organ necrosis, fistula formation, and stricture), and an overall perioperative mortality of 20%. Over time, the transferred colon usually becomes distended, contributing to postoperative dysphagia. Colon interposition is now generally reserved for patients who have undergone previous gastric surgery or who have portal hypertension, in which cases gastric transposition is not possible. Colon also can be brought through the substernal mediastinum to serve as a bypass conduit in cases of unresectable thoracic esophageal cancer and caustic esophageal stricture, where periesophageal fibrosis significantly increases the risk of thoracic esophagectomy.[106]

Gastric Transposition

Ong and Lee reported the first cases of pharyngogastric anastomosis in 1960.[107] This method became widely used for pharyngoesophageal reconstruction after Orringer and Sloan[108] popularized the blunt esophagectomy technique in 1978. The primary advantage of gastric transposition is that it allows for reliable one-stage reconstruction with a single enteric anastomosis. The entire esophagus is removed in cases of advanced hypopharyngeal carcinoma, in which distal submucosal tumor spread and synchronous esophageal primaries are of concern. Gastric transposition, which is pedicled on the right gastric and gastroepiploic vessels, is extremely reliable, with an incidence of organ necrosis of only 3%. The overall success rate for swallowing exceeds 80%, and institution of oral alimentation is generally accomplished in 7 to 12 days. Many patients are able to achieve neoesophageal speech because negative intrathoracic pressure facilitates injection of air into the mediastinal portion of the gastric pouch.

The combined abdominal, thoracic, and cervical surgery of gastric pullup contributes significantly to overall morbidity. In the modern era, the rate of major perioperative complications is 50%, and the operative mortality remains on the order of 10%. The most common long-term complication is reflux, which is symptomatic in 20% of patients undergoing pharyngogastric anastomosis. This problem complicates gastric transposition in patients undergoing laryngeal preservation, in that life-threatening aspiration can result. Careful patient selection is critical so that suitable candidates for a gastric pullup procedure are selected, especially with regard to cardiopulmonary disease, and perioperative morbidity and mortality are limited.[109, 110]

Microvascular Free Flaps

Gastro-omental Free Flap

Hiebert and Cummings[111] reported the first successful case of pharyngoesophageal reconstruction using a segment of revascularized gastric antrum in 1961. Since that time, the gastro-omental flap (Fig. 28–20) has been employed for a variety of head and neck reconstructive needs.

The gastro-omental flap is pedicled on the right gastroepiploic artery and vein, which arise from the celiac trunk via the gastroduodenal artery and vein. These vessels

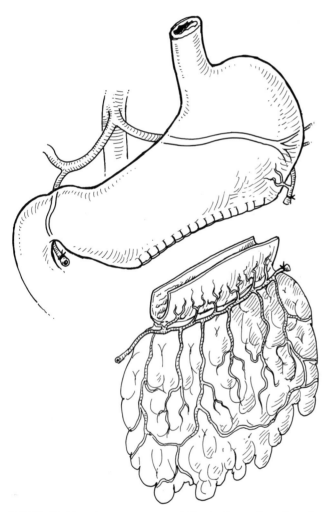

FIGURE 28–20 The gastro-omental flap is shown, based on the right gastroepiploic vascular pedicle. Harvesting a segment of gastric mucosa from a region distant to the pylorus lengthens the vascular pedicle and reduces the risk of gastric outlet obstruction. A variable number of descending branches of the gastroepiploic artery supply the adjacent greater omentum.

commonly have a proximal diameter of 2 to 3 mm, and it is possible to achieve a total pedicle length of 30 cm. The right gastroepiploic artery passes along the greater curvature of the stomach, supplying the adjacent gastric mucosa via several short gastric arteries. Several additional branches descend from the right gastroepiploic artery to supply the omentum, a mesothelium-lined trabecular sheath that drapes over the transverse colon.

A 10×10-cm segment of gastric mucosa from the greater curvature can be harvested for the purpose of reconstructing pharyngoesophageal mucosal defects. A tubed segment of gastric mucosa can be harvested very rapidly with an enteric stapling device and then opened at each end to achieve a suitable epithelium-lined tube. Omentum is frequently harvested with the flap to provide carotid artery protection after concurrent neck dissection or protection of the mediastinal contents when a mediastinal dissection is performed.[112] The inclusion of omentum with the tubed gastric mucosal flap is particularly useful for overcoming impaired wound healing in patients who have undergone previous radiotherapy with or without chemotherapy. Alternatively, omentum alone can be harvested after division and ligation of the short gastric arteries. The omental free flap has been used to reconstruct extensive soft tissue defects of the calvarium and scalp in conjunction with a skin graft.[113] Omental free flaps are also useful for cases requiring subcutaneous soft tissue augmentation (e.g., hemifacial microsomia, Romberg's hemifacial atrophy, facial contour deficiencies resulting from tumor ablation), dura or carotid artery coverage, and revascularization of areas of osteoradionecrosis.[114–118]

The chief advantage of the gastro-omental flap is that it provides ample pliable soft tissue that closely approximates native pharyngeal mucosa. The long vascular pedicle can reach more remote recipient vessels, including those in the contralateral neck or ipsilateral axilla. The secretory capacity of the gastric mucosa has been helpful in controlling the symptoms of xerostomia in patients who have received previous radiation therapy. During the first postoperative 7 to 10 days, mucus production is copious, and patients with retained larynges often require airway protection with a cuffed tracheotomy tube. Gastric mucosal rugae quickly flatten after transfer, and patients have fewer problems with halitosis than do patients undergoing jejunal transposition for pharyngoesophageal reconstruction, in which food sometimes becomes lodged within the circular folds of the transferred jejunum. Omentum contains a rich lymphatic network, and omental transfer has been used to treat various forms of chronic lymphedema, although clinical experience with omental flaps for treatment of head and neck lymphedema has been disappointing.[119] Experimental evidence suggests that omentum possesses special qualities that promote the formation of fibrous tissue ingrowth, capillary ingrowth, encapsulation of infarcted tissue, and hemostasis, making it suitable for reconstruction of previously irradiated or contaminated surgical defects.[120, 121]

Disadvantages of the gastro-omental flap include the need for two surgical teams and the morbidity related to laparotomy. Previous gastric surgery is a contraindication to surgery, and adhesions related to previous abdominal surgery or peritonitis may make dissection of the omentum more difficult. Gastrointestinal obstruction is a potential complication and may be caused by pyloric spasm or stenosis, volvulus, or adhesion formation.

Jejunal Free Flap

The jejunal free flap (Fig. 28–21) has become a popular technique for reconstruction in patients who require circumferential pharyngectomy or laryngopharyngectomy with preservation of the cervical esophagus.[122–124] During flap harvest, a segment of jejunum that is supplied by a single vascular arcade is selected by transillumination of the mesentery. The pedicle is dissected proximally to its origin from the superior mesenteric vessels. An appropriate length of small bowel is then divided, but perfusion of the flap by its arcade is maintained until the recipient site has been prepared. Subsequently, the flap is transferred to the head and neck, where it is placed in an isoperistaltic orientation.

Superior and inferior enteric anastomoses are performed in an end-to-end fashion. Whereas the inferior jejunoesophageal anastomosis sometimes is amenable to stapled closure, this technique appears to be associated with increased risk of subsequent stricture formation. The superior enteric anastomosis between the jejunum and the pharynx is often carried out after the antimesenteric border of the jejunum is incised for a distance of 2 to 4 cm, to enlarge the graft lumen and to provide a more suitable size match with the upper resection margin. Microvascular anastomosis is carried out after selection of appropriate recipient vessels in

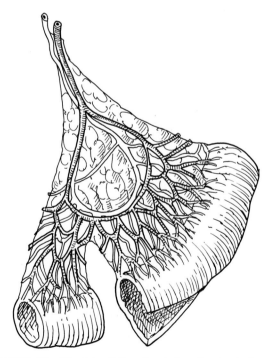

FIGURE 28–21 The jejunal free flap is based on a single mesenteric vascular arcade. A small segment of jejunum is externalized to serve as a monitor of the circulation when a buried jejunal flap is used for pharyngoesophageal reconstruction. The jejunal segment can be opened along the antimesenteric border to increase the size of the lumen of the graft.

the neck. Exteriorization of a portion of jejunal mucosa allows for postoperative monitoring through assessment of flap color, peristalsis, and the quality of mucosal bleeding. The external monitor is left in place during the first postoperative week, when the risk of flap failure is highest, after which the mesentery to the monitor is divided and the exteriorized segment of jejunum is removed.

Free jejunal autografts and pedicled gastric transpositions are currently the most commonly employed methods for circumferential pharyngoesophageal reconstruction.[125, 126] Jejunal free flaps have been used after laryngopharyngectomy, esophagectomy with laryngeal preservation, wide field resection of stomal recurrences, and pharyngoesophagectomy for chronic pharyngoesophagocutaneous fistulas. For noncircumferential defects, jejunal autografts can be opened along the antimesenteric border and used as patch grafts for a wide variety of oral and pharyngeal reconstructions.

Perioperative mortality in patients undergoing pharyngoesophageal reconstruction by jejunal autotransplantation is approximately 4%. Acute graft failure occurs in 9% of patients, typically within 72 hours of surgery. Graft failure has been reported as late as 18 months postoperatively. This implies that jejunal autografts are never truly integrated into the surrounding tissues by neovascularization, presumably because of the relatively impermeable jejunal serosa. Pharyngocutaneous fistulas develop in approximately 18% of patients undergoing jejunal free flaps; two thirds of such fistulas heal spontaneously. The most common late complication is stricture formation, which occurs in approximately 20% of patients. Overall, approximately 80% of patients are able to maintain their weight on oral feedings alone after undergoing pharyngoesophageal reconstruction by a jejunal free flap.[127]

Jejunal autografts have several advantages over other methods of pharyngoesophageal reconstruction. They allow for immediate, single-stage reconstruction, which shortens time to oral alimentation and length of hospitalization compared with those necessitated by cutaneous and myocutaneous flap reconstructions. Jejunal mucus production is beneficial to patients with xerostomia secondary to previous radiation therapy. Compared with patients undergoing gastric pullup, perioperative morbidity and mortality are less because there is no violation of the thorax. Also, jejunal autografts easily reach the nasopharynx without the excessive anastomotic tension and mucosal ischemia that can occur after gastric pullup.[128]

Disadvantages of free jejunal autografts are apparent. A successful outcome depends on the results of two microvascular and three enteric anastomoses, which require expertise in both microvascular surgical techniques and gastrointestinal surgery. The inferior pharyngeal anastomosis may be difficult to perform in cases in which tumor extends into the thoracic esophagus. Many authors feel that the peristaltic contractions of transplanted jejunum are not coordinated with the swallowing mechanism, and that these contractions may therefore contribute to postoperative dysphagia. However, the motor activity of jejunal autografts decreases over time after transplantation, and functionally, they become inert conduits. One of the major criticisms of jejunal free flaps has been their failure to enable adequate neoesophageal speech after laryngectomy. However, other reports document successful speech rehabilitation with the use of autoinsufflation and tracheojejunal fistulas.[129, 130]

Fasciocutaneous Free Flaps

The radial forearm,[131, 132] lateral arm, lateral thigh, anterolateral thigh, and scapular and parascapular fasciocutaneous free flaps can be inset as tubed, skin-lined flaps for reconstruction of circumferential pharyngoesophageal defects (Fig. 28–22). The rectus abdominis musculocutaneous free flap can be harvested with only a small cuff of muscle in the periumbilical region and used in a similar fashion in thin patients. The primary advantage of tubed fasciocutaneous free flaps is that they allow for one-stage pharyngoesophageal reconstruction while greatly limiting the potential donor site morbidity associated with a laparotomy for harvest of all forms of visceral flaps. All aforementioned fasciocutaneous flaps, with the exception of the scapular and parascapular flaps, allow for simultaneous cancer ablation and flap harvest, thus decreasing operative time. Creation of a 2- to 3-cm wedge extension at the distal margin of the flap produces a triangular skin extension that can be inset into a longitudinal cut made in the end of the distal esophageal stump. This "wedge-and-slot" technique disrupts the annular distal anastomosis and may help to prevent distal stricture formation. The radial forearm, lateral arm, and lateral thigh flaps have the additional advantage of being sensate flaps.

A relative disadvantage of fasciocutaneous free flaps includes the need for a longer suture line to create a tubed flap. In addition, all of the previously mentioned flaps, with the exception of the radial forearm flap, can be excessively bulky in obese patients, and all of the above donor sites may transfer hair-bearing skin in male patients. The latter concern is obviated in patients who are to receive postoperative radiation therapy, which will destroy hair follicles within the transferred tissue.

■ CHEEK RECONSTRUCTION

Soft Tissue Reconstruction

Large defects of the cheek provide a significant challenge for the reconstructive surgeon. The exposure of this portion of the face and the ability of the eye to detect even the mildest of asymmetries place great demands on the reconstructive surgeon to achieve a favorable cosmetic result. The goals of reconstruction include a cosmetically favorable result with good color and texture match for the skin, as well as symmetrical-appearing form. For extensive lesions involving the deeper structures, attention must be given to both function and cosmesis, with attention to rehabilitation of the facial nerve paralysis that often results from resections in this area.

For smaller lesions of the cheek not amenable to primary closure, local flaps are the reconstructive method of choice. These provide an excellent match for both color and texture. Flap design should take into consideration tension on nearby structures such as the lip or periorbital area, camouflaging of incisions, and adequacy of blood supply to the flap. Consideration should be given to the aesthetic units of the cheek in achieving an optimal result.

Larger defects of the cheek may require a regional flap for closure. The cervicofacial flap is the most popular flap for reconstruction of extensive cheek defects. It can provide a large area of skin by borrowing tissue from the adjacent cervical region. The color and texture match is excellent and donor site morbidity is minimal. However, previous surgery in the area may compromise vascular supply to the flap and lead to an increased risk of necrosis. Defects that are of considerable surface area or depth may not be best served by the cervicofacial flap owing to limitations with size and bulk. In these situations, other regional flaps, such as the posterior scalping flap or the submental flap, or free-tissue transfer should be considered. Ablative procedures that require facial nerve sacrifice may also require more extensive treatment, including the use of interposition nerve grafts or even innervated muscle transfer, or temporalis muscle transposition when the mimetic muscles are resected as well.

Posterior Scalping Flap

The posterior scalping flap is an excellent option for reconstruction of the cheek defect that cannot be closed with other techniques owing to the size of the defect or previous surgery. It was first described by Arena in 1977 as an extension of the retroauricular temporal flap that had been reported by Washio several years earlier.[133, 134] It is a two-stage flap that provides a large area of non–hair-bearing skin from the nape of neck area using the scalp as a vascular carrier (Fig. 28–23). The flap is elevated in a subfascial plane over the splenius capitus and trapezius muscle to the level of the superior nuchal line, at which point the dissection transitions to a plane deep to the galea. The blood supply to the flap is from the superficial temporal, supraorbital, and supratrochlear arteries. The skin at the inferior end of the flap is then sutured into the defect, and at 3 to 4 weeks, the pedicle is divided and the scalp replaced to its original site.

The advantages of this flap include a large area of non–hair-bearing skin that has an excellent color and texture match for facial defects. The donor site is well camouflaged, especially in women with longer hair. Disadvantages include the necessity for a two-stage procedure and the requirement for a skin graft on the posterior neck.

Submental Island Flap

The submental island flap provides a vascularized flap of regional tissue for reconstruction of cheek defects. It was first described by Martin in 1993[135] and was further popularized by Gullane and associates in 1997.[135a] The blood supply to the flap is provided by the submental artery. The submental artery runs superficial to the mylohyoid muscle and either superficial or deep to the anterior digastric muscle. Elevation of the flap is performed after a skin paddle is designed with its anterior margin running parallel to the lower border of the mandible. The width of the flap may extend from the midbody or angle of the mandible on one side to that of the other. The inferior incision is determined by a pinch test to assess the limits of primary closure.

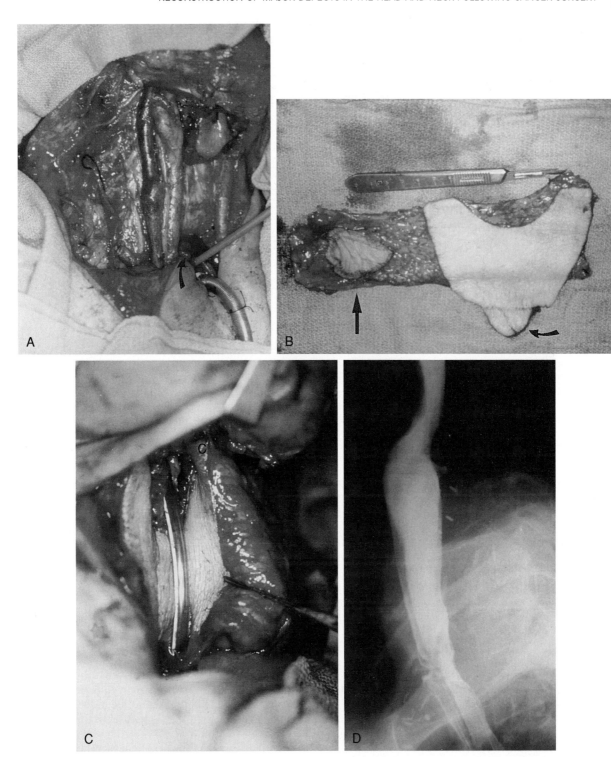

FIGURE 28–22 *A*, A patient with a circumferential defect extending from the base of the tongue to the cervical esophagus (*arrow*) after total laryngopharyngectomy. *B*, A radial forearm free flap is harvested for pharyngoesophageal reconstruction. The wide portion of the shield-shaped distal skin paddle will be inset into the proximal enteric anastomosis. The wedge-shaped extension at the narrow end of the flap (*curved arrow*) will be inset into a vertical incision in the cervical esophageal remnant to disrupt the annular anastomosis and prevent distal stricture formation. The proximal forearm skin paddle (*straight arrow*) will be exteriorized to serve as a monitor of perfusion for the buried portion of the flap. *C*, An intraoperative photograph shows insetting of the forearm flap. The proximal and distal enteric anastomoses have been completed, and a nasogastric tube has been placed through the lumen of the reconstructed hypopharynx. The flap will be tubed to complete the reconstruction. *D*, A lateral projection cervical esophagram obtained 4 months postoperatively demonstrates patency of the reconstructed hypopharyngeal segment.

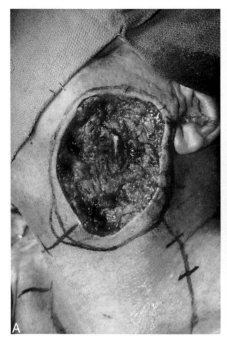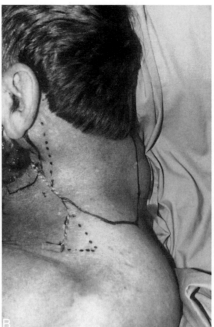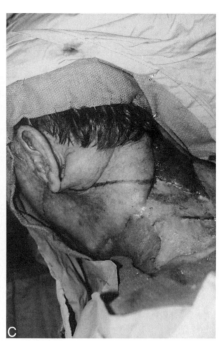

FIGURE 28–23 *A*, A left cheek defect has been created following Mohs' surgery for a Merkel cell carcinoma. A reexcision of the bed and perimeter tissues is outlined, along with an ipsilateral lymph node dissection. *B*, A reconstruction of this defect is outlined with a posterior scalping flap transferring a significant amount of tissue from the suboccipital nape of neck region, with incisions extending up the postauricular sulcus and along the midline of the scalp. Nerve grafts were placed in order to bridge the gap in the facial nerve defect. *C*, Following a requisite period of time for neovascularization, the posterior scalp flap is returned in order to resurface the defect over the occiput.

Elevation contralateral to the pedicle side is performed deep to the platysma and superficial to the anterior digastric muscle. The ipsilateral anterior digastric is included in the dissection to ensure preservation of the vascular pedicle.

Advantages of this flap include its matching skin color for facial skin defects, the relative lack of donor site morbidity, and its location, which is in the field of the ablative defect.[136] Disadvantages include the hair-bearing quality of the skin in males. Oncologic principles must be considered in view of the fact that this donor site includes tissue from the level I cervical nodal group.[137]

Rehabilitation of the Paralyzed Face

The mimetic facial muscles are innervated by the motor fibers of the seventh cranial nerve. Impulses originate in the cerebral cortex, synapse in the pontine facial nuclei, and then pass through the temporal bone and parotid gland to the periphery. Tumor involvement or surgical resection of neurons anywhere along this pathway can result in facial paralysis. Articulation, oral competence, and eye protection are compromised. Facial symmetry and expression are lost, introducing a potentially devastating functional, social, and emotional disability.

Facial nerve rehabilitation after major head and neck cancer surgery continues to be one of the most difficult challenges of reconstructive surgery. Both the surgeon and the patient must accept the fact that no surgical technique can fully restore normal facial function and appearance. Nonetheless, successful reanimation with partial restoration of function can usually be accomplished with either one or more surgical procedures.

Facial nerve rehabilitation after resection of cancer of the head and neck has evolved considerably over the past 25 years, since the introduction of microneural and microvascular techniques. Rehabilitation of facial paralysis encompasses four basic goals: The first is to achieve ocular and oral sphincter competence. The second is to attain facial symmetry at rest. The third is to obtain symmetrical voluntary facial movement. The fourth and ultimate goal is to restore involuntary mimetic facial expression. Ideally, the techniques used to achieve these goals should result in minimal donor site morbidity.

Each patient with cancer of the head and neck who requires facial nerve resection is unique; therefore, the approach to rehabilitation should be individualized. Careful analysis of the patient's deficits and timely intervention are the keys to a successful result. The specific technique or techniques used depend on many factors, including the degree and site of neural injury, the physiologic status of the proximal and distal nerve and facial muscles, and the patient's prognosis and general medical condition. In addition, the desires, expectations, and motivations of the patient need to be considered when the rehabilitative effort is planned.

The procedures used for the rehabilitation of the paralyzed face can be categorized as either static or dynamic. Generally, immediate, dynamic methods (with neural reconstitution or muscle transfer) are preferable to static or delayed methods. An exception to this rule is the case of facial paralysis that occurs in an elderly patient with a poor prognosis. In this situation, static procedures, such as a fascial sling or a gold weight implant, can reliably restore oral and ocular competence, thus preventing morbid complications. In other circumstances, such as when a facial nerve–sparing resection causes neurapraxia, medical therapy and observation may be all that is indicated. Protection of the eye is the main priority of therapy while the facial nerve recovers.

Dynamic Procedures

Dynamic procedures are of four types and are listed in ascending order of their ability to provide an ideal functional and cosmetic result: (1) direct nerve repair; (2) interposition nerve grafting; (3) nerve substitution procedures; and (4) muscle transfer procedures.

Direct Nerve Repair. Direct nerve repair, or neurorrhaphy, is indicated when the facial nerve is transected, or when a small segment is resected and can be reapproximated without tension at the suture line. Neurorrhaphy, which requires the presence of a proximal and distal nerve stump and viable muscle, is the procedure most likely to reestablish mimetic control of the face. The key to successful neural repair is the atraumatic, precise, and tension-free approximation of the nerve stumps. We prefer to place two to four epineural 9–0 or 10–0 nylon sutures with the use of an operating microscope. Optimal results are obtained when the repair is performed at the time of tumor resection, but good results can occur when neurorrhaphy is performed within 1 year of injury. Although some degree of weakness and abnormal movement is always present after direct nerve repair, facial tone and symmetry are improved. Ninety-five percent of appropriately selected patients can expect some return of motion.

Interposition Nerve Grafting. An interposition nerve graft is indicated when neural tissue is deficient after facial

nerve sacrifice and nerve-rerouting procedures are unable to provide a tension-free direct nerve repair (Fig. 28–24). This technique is most commonly performed after radical parotidectomy or temporal bone resection with facial nerve sacrifice. Similar to direct nerve repair, it requires the presence of proximal and distal nerve stumps, as well as viable facial mimetic muscles. The extent of facial nerve resection is determined intraoperatively based on the location, clinical stage, and histologic characteristics of the tumor. Interposition nerve grafts can be designed to bridge specific defects. For example, following a radical parotidectomy, the availability of several peripheral nerve branches may require the use of a nerve graft with multiple branches. If it is feasible oncologically, the zygomatic, buccal, and marginal mandibular branches should be grafted preferentially to rehabilitate the eye, midface, and oral commissure.

The greater auricular nerve and the sural nerve are the most commonly used donor nerves for facial nerve interposition grafting. The greater auricular nerve provides great adaptability and convenience in that it is frequently already exposed in the surgical field and is easily identified and dissected. Usually, an 8- to 10-cm graft with two or three branches of adequate diameter can be obtained. The major drawbacks to using the greater auricular nerve are its limited length and possible absence due to surgical excision in cases of tumor proximity. The sural nerve is preferred by some surgeons for various reasons, including (1) its greater length (up to 28 cm); (2) its location in the leg, which allows simultaneous harvesting of the graft and preparation of the recipient bed; and (3) its more favorable neural-to-connective tissue ratio, which is thought to provide superior reinnervation. The sural nerve is found posterior to the lateral malleolus and can be exposed by making serial "stair-step" horizontal incisions or a single curvilinear incision upward along the posterolateral leg. The medial antebrachial cutaneous nerve of the forearm has become popular as an

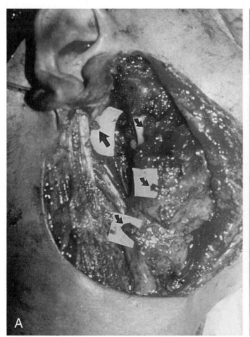
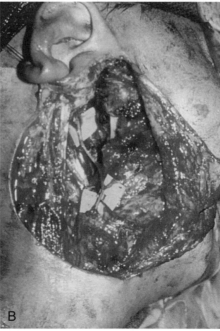

FIGURE 28–24 *A*, A total parotidectomy defect resulting from resection of adenoid of cystic carcinoma. The proximal stump (*large arrow*) and the distal branches (*small curved arrows*) of the facial nerve were found to be free of tumor on frozen section analysis. *B*, The continuity of the marginal mandibular and buccal branches of the facial nerve has been restored using a great auricular nerve cable graft. The paralyzed eyelid has been rehabilitated separately with the use of a gold weight to limit postoperative synkinesis.

alternative donor site for the bridging of long facial nerve defects.[138]

The ultimate success or failure of interposition nerve grafting is dependent on a variety of factors, the most critical of which is the interval between nerve interruption and repair. Although the best results are obtained when the grafting is performed immediately, acceptable results can be obtained up to 1 year from the time of injury. Other factors may also impact on the success of the procedure.

Nerve Substitution Procedures. When the proximal stump of the facial nerve is not available for grafting, nerve substitution techniques, such as a hypoglossal-facial nerve crossover, are appropriate.[139]

Muscle Transfer Procedures. Dynamic muscle transfer techniques are primarily used for the rehabilitation of long-standing facial paralysis and concomitant atrophy of the facial muscles as a result of prolonged lack of neural input. This occurs approximately 2 years after complete denervation and is represented by electrical silence on electromyography (EMG). In addition, patients with parotid, facial, or oral cavity tumors that require facial muscle resection may benefit from these techniques. In these cases, a local or distant muscle is transferred to portions of the face. The temporalis and masseter muscles are the most commonly used local muscles; such transfers make use of an intact trigeminal innervation. Alternatively, muscle from distant sites can be transferred with the use of microneurovascular techniques.[140] The gracilis and latissimus dorsi muscles are popular donor sites for this purpose.[141] In cases in which the ipsilateral facial nerve is not available for proximal anastomosis, distant muscle transfer must be preceded by placement of a cross–facial nerve graft.[142, 143]

Static Procedures

Static procedures, such as fascial slings, can provide immediate symmetry at rest but do not restore facial movement. They are effective alternatives in patients who are not candidates for dynamic nerve or muscle reanimation procedures. Included are patients with limited life expectancies and those who are unwilling to undergo more extensive surgery. Particular attention must be given to the protection of the paralyzed eyelid. In patients forgoing dynamic techniques and in those in whom dynamic techniques may eventually restore eye closure via reinnervation of the orbicularis oculi muscle, temporary measures to prevent corneal desiccation include use of ocular lubricants, eyelid-tightening procedures, and use of prosthetic implants, such as eyelid gold weights and palpebral springs.[144–146]

◘ RECONSTRUCTION OF DEFECTS OF THE CRANIAL BASE

Collaborative efforts among neurosurgeons, neurotologists, and head and neck surgeons have recently opened new frontiers in the removal of benign and malignant tumors of the cranial base. Contributions in related fields, including diagnostic and interventional radiology, anesthesiology, and radiation oncology, have also helped to revolutionize the management of skull base tumors. Similarly, modern reconstructive methods have had a major impact on the ability of physicians to successfully manage lesions that were considered untreatable just 20 years ago. Until the advent of modern reconstructive techniques and the ability of surgeons to reliably transfer vascularized tissue to this region, removal of tumors from the cranial base could not be performed safely. Our inability to protect the brain and subarachnoid space from the contaminated upper aerodigestive tract left the patient at an unacceptably high risk of CSF leak and ascending infection, often with a disastrous outcome.

In approaching reconstruction in a systematic fashion, classification of defects of the cranial base is essential. Traditionally, defects of the cranial base have been classified by site of involvement into anterior, middle, or posterior defects, and they arbitrarily have been subclassified by size into small, medium, and large defects. This simplified classification scheme does not accurately describe the complex reconstructive problems that are currently encountered. Urken and associates[147] have proposed a classification scheme that includes seven major defect categories (Table 28–3): (1) dura, (2) bone, (3) cutaneous, (4) mucosal, (5) cavity, (6) neurologic, and (7) carotid artery. The status of each of these categories has a significant impact on reconstruction of the cranial base, including selection of the reconstructive method, flap design, and method of insetting. Patient factors that may affect outcome include age, intercurrent illnesses, Karnofsky performance status, and

TABLE 28-3 Classification of Skull Base Defects

Defect	Abbreviation
Dura	Intact (D_I) Primary repair (D_R) Patch graft (D_G)
Mucosa	Nasal-nasopharyngeal (M_N) Oral-oropharyngeal (M_O) Sphenoid (M_S)
Skin	Scalp (S_S) Forehead (S_F) Midface (S_M) Lower face (S_L) Neck (S_N) Auricle (S_A)
Bone	Calvarium (B_C) Zygoma (B_Z) Palate (B_P) Mandible (B_M) Orbital floor (B_O) Temporal (B_T)
Cavities	Maxillary (C_M) Orbital (C_O) Infratemporal (C_I)
Neurologic	Facial (N_F) Lingual (N_L) Glossopharyngeal (N_G) Vagus (N_V) Accessory (N_A) Hypoglossal (N_H)
Carotid artery	Intact (A_I) Ligated (A_L) Grafted (A_G)

previous treatment interventions, particularly surgery or radiation therapy.

The basic goals of reconstruction are to seal the CSF within the intradural space, to provide coverage of exposed vital structures (including the dura and carotid artery), and to replace lost tissue in ways that are as cosmetically acceptable as possible. These goals can be achieved by the use of a variety of techniques, depending on the complexity of the defect. Reconstructive methods currently available include (1) primary wound closure and nonvascularized tissue grafts, (2) local tissue flaps, (3) regional pedicled flaps, and (4) distant flaps.[148–150]

Nonvascularized tissue grafts are used in conjunction with primary wound closure for reconstruction of limited defects in noncontaminated, nonirradiated beds. Repair of the dura is achieved by primary closure, dura homografts, or autogenous fascia grafts, such as temporalis fascia or tensor fasciae latae. Repair of dural defects may be augmented with the use of fibrin glue in areas where sutures are difficult to place, including the sphenoid sinus and jugular foramen. Abdominal fat grafts are used to bolster dural repair sites and to restore contour. Large defects of the skull are repaired with autogenous bone grafts, usually split rib or parietal calvarium.[151]

Local flaps employed for lateral and posterior skull base reconstruction include the temporalis muscle flap and the temporoparietal fascial flap (Fig. 28–25). The temporoparietal fascia is the superior extension of the subcutaneous musculoaponeurotic system, lying just deep to the subdermal fat and hair follicles. This axial pattern fascial flap is based on the superficial temporal vessels. It can be reliably harvested almost to the midline, having an overall length of approximately 10 cm.[152] The temporalis muscle flap, based on the deep temporal branches of the internal maxillary artery, has a much shorter arc of rotation.

Pericranial and galeopericranial flaps are based anteriorly on branches of the supraorbital and supratrochlear vessels or laterally on the superficial temporal artery. The thin, pliable, anteriorly based pericranial flap is frequently employed for reconstruction of anterior craniofacial defects and will reliably reach as far posterior as the planum sphenoidale and clivus. The thicker combined galeopericranial flap is useful for reconstruction of larger defects, or when the vascularity of the pericranium is questionable. Dissection of the galeopericranial flap requires separation of the galea from the overlying skin in a plane immediately deep to the hair follicles, which increases the risk of scalp necrosis and alopecia. Permanent anesthesia of the forehead and loss of frontalis muscle function are common consequences of these techniques.[153, 154]

Regional pedicled flaps employed for reconstruction of the cranial base include the pectoralis, latissimus dorsi, and trapezius flaps. The pectoralis myocutaneous flap, which has been a "workhorse" flap for oropharyngeal reconstruction, has limited application in cranial base surgery. Extension of the cutaneous paddle inferior to the sixth rib is associated with an increased risk of distal flap necrosis. Therefore, the pectoralis flap does not reliably extend above the level of the tragus unless the skin paddle is delayed or the vascular pedicle is exteriorized. In both cases, a two-stage reconstruction may be necessary. After release of its tendinous insertion

into the humerus, the pedicled latissimus dorsi flap easily reaches the vertex of the skull. Because of the large amount of tissue available for transfer, this flap is useful for reconstruction of massive scalp defects. The lower island trapezius flap is probably the most useful pedicled regional flap for reconstruction of the cranial base, and it is used frequently for reconstruction of temporal bone defects accompanied by auriculectomy (Fig. 28–26). However, both the

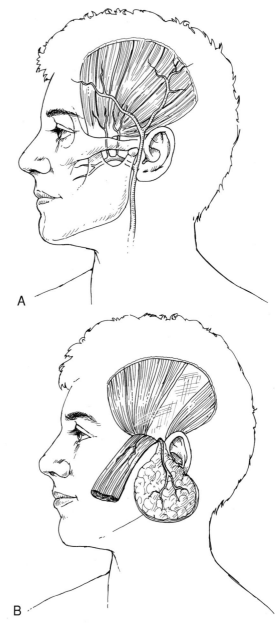

FIGURE 28–25 *A,* The vascular supply of the temporoparietal fascia and temporalis muscle flaps is based on the terminal branches of the external carotid artery. The temporoparietal fascia is supplied by the superficial temporal artery, whereas the temporalis muscle is supplied by the anterior and posterior deep temporal branches of the internal maxillary artery. *B,* The temporoparietal fascia flap and temporalis muscle flap are shown after elevation. The central third of the temporalis muscle has been harvested with the technique used for reanimation of the paralyzed eyelid or oral commissure.

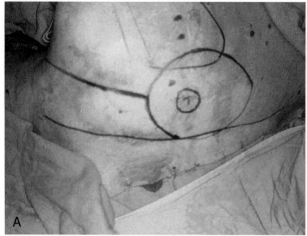
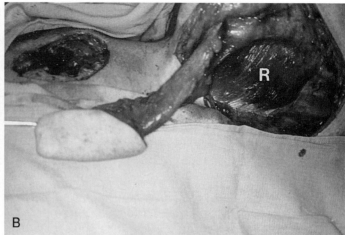
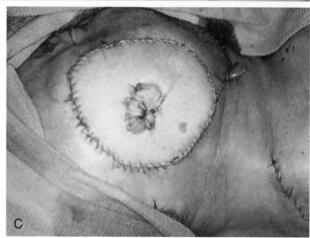

FIGURE 28–26 *A,* A lower island trapezius flap is designed for reconstruction of a lateral skull base defect resulting from resection of an auricular basal cell carcinoma. The defect classification is $D_IS_{A, M, S}B_TA_I$ (see Table 28–3). The skin paddle of the flap is placed between the vertebrae and the medial border of the scapula. *B,* The lower island trapezius flap has been elevated. Preservation of the rhomboid major and minor muscles (R), which lie deep in the trapezius muscles, serves to prevent postoperative winging of the scapula. *C,* The trapezius flap has been inset into the soft tissue defect. The flap has been perforated in its midportion to reconstruct the external auditory canal.

latissimus dorsi flap and the lower island trapezius flap may require intraoperative repositioning of the patient.

Extensive defects of the cranial base in unfavorable recipient tissue beds require the use of microvascular free-tissue transfer. The rectus abdominis muscle flap has been the most popular reconstructive option for this purpose (Fig. 28–27).[155] It provides an ample volume of muscle to protect the intracranial contents or the carotid artery from exposed pharyngeal or paranasal sinus cavities, and skin can be included to replace lost cutaneous tissue or to serve as a clinical monitor of the vascularity of the underlying muscle during the postoperative period. The superior portion of the anterior rectus sheath can be incorporated as a vascularized fascial graft for dura replacement, and the long vascular pedicle frequently reaches cervical recipient vessels without the use of vein grafts. Other microvascular flaps that have been used for reconstruction of the cranial base include the latissimus dorsi, radial forearm, scapular, parascapular, greater omentum, and tensor fascia lata free flaps.[156]

FUTURE CHALLENGES AND NEW DIRECTIONS IN HEAD AND NECK RECONSTRUCTION

Over the past several decades, reconstruction of the head and neck has dramatically changed. The introduction of microvascular free-flap reconstruction by Seidenberg in 1959 marked the beginning of a new era of reconstruction of defects in the head and neck.[157] Subsequently, an evolution in technology and technique has enhanced the reliability of free-tissue transfer and solved many of the most difficult challenges of the reconstructive surgeon. Free-tissue transfer has become a valuable tool for reconstruction of the pharyngoesophageal segment, mandible, and cranial base; however, the reconstruction of complex organ systems such as the larynx, trachea, and tongue remains an unsolved problem.

Although partial defects of the larynx, trachea, and tongue are well managed with pedicled and free-flap reconstruction, current reconstructive methods are limited in their ability to provide adequate function for patients who have sustained near-total or total organ ablation. Each of these organs is highly specialized, and achieving an acceptable level of rehabilitation with autologous tissue reconstruction remains a problem. Transplantation may offer the opportunity to regain this function without the morbidity associated with the donor site defect of a free-tissue transfer.

Transplantation within the head and neck is not a new concept; however, until recently, previous experimental work in this area has yielded only marginal results. This has largely been the result of (1) the toxic adverse effects associated with nonspecific immunosuppression and (2) a poor understanding of the immunobiology of these organ systems.

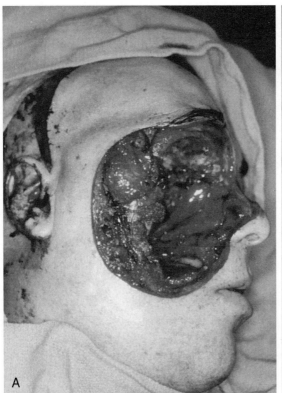

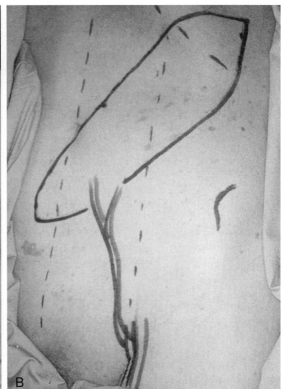

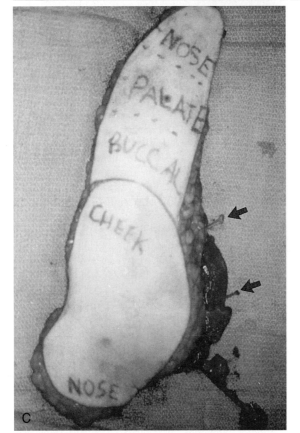

FIGURE 28–27 *A,* Large right orbitomaxillary defect resulting from resection of advanced maxillary sinus adenoid cystic carcinoma. The defect classification is $D_I M_{NOS} S_M B_{CZPO} C_{MQI} N_{FL} A_I$ (see Table 28–3). *B,* A left thoracoumbilical rectus abdominis myocutaneous flap is designed, based on the deep inferior epigastric vessels. *C,* The rectus flap is shown after harvest. Various components of skin paddle are marked as they will be oriented during insetting to seal the exposed dura and infratemporal fossa from the adjacent cavities and external cutaneous defect. Transitional zones located between the nasal and palatal skin and between the buccal and cheek skin will be deepithelialized. The segmental innervation of the rectus muscle (*arrows*) is apparent.

Continued

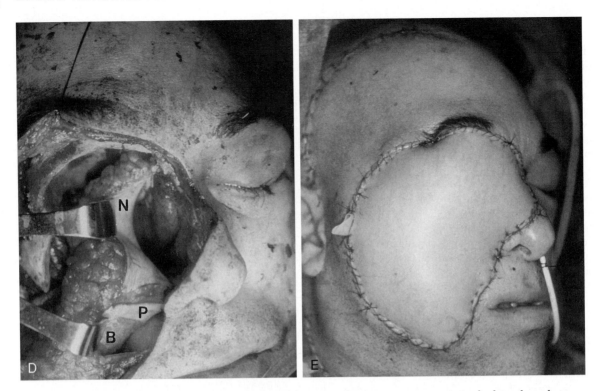

FIGURE 28–27, cont'd *D,* The distal portion of the rectus flap is inset to reconstitute the lateral nasal wall (N), palate (P), and buccal mucosa (B). *E,* The postoperative appearance shows the proximal portion of rectus skin paddle reconstituting the cutaneous defect of the cheek, orbit, and nose.

Over the past several years, great strides have been made in the development of new, highly selective forms of immunosuppression that expose the patient to a decreased risk of toxicity. As a result, investigators have raised questions regarding the feasibility of transplantation within the head and neck. Experimental success with transplantation of the trachea, larynx, and tongue has shown that transplantation of these organ systems is possible, and recent clinical success with laryngeal transplantation is encouraging as head and neck reconstruction embarks upon this new era.[158–161]

Physiologic reconstruction of the tongue remains challenging. The tongue is a complex organ composed of secretory glands, the end organs for taste and touch, and muscles oriented in a fashion that provides a wide array of voluntary and involuntary movements. Three critical components constitute reconstruction of the tongue: restoration of a mucosal surface, restoration of sensation, and restoration of coordinated motor activity. With the use of available methods, mucosal secretory function can be restored by the transfer of segments of jejunum or stomach. Neurosensory free flaps appear to be effective in restoration of the sensory modalities of pain, temperature, and two-point discrimination.[162, 163] Restoration of coordinated tongue motion is a more difficult goal to achieve. The tongue is composed of four paired extrinsic muscles and a complex, interlacing network of intrinsic muscles that work in a concerted fashion to change the position and shape of the organ during articulation, mastication, and deglutition. Even if the technical challenges of reinnervated free muscle transfer are overcome, finding a donor site to provide this wide array of movements remains a formidable challenge.[164]

Future advances in biomedical engineering promise to make significant contributions, with clinical application in the foreseeable future. The development of new, reliable technologies for monitoring microsurgical free-tissue transfers would greatly simplify the postoperative care of patients undergoing free-flap reconstruction of the head and neck. The rate of thrombosis after microvascular anastomosis is on the order of 5% to 15%, and successful salvage after anastomotic failure depends on the timely detection of impaired flap perfusion and rapid surgical intervention. More rapid detection of anastomotic failure translates into earlier intervention and a greater likelihood of successful salvage. Although several methods for the detection of anastomotic failure have undergone clinical trial (Table 28–4), clinical evaluation of bleeding, capillary refill, and color remains the most reliable method of assessing flap viability. Unfortunately, this is labor intensive and requires considerable observer experience.[165–167] Application of implantable

TABLE 28–4 Available Monitoring Devices for the Assessment of Free Flap Viability

Transcutaneous PO_2 monitoring
Surface temperature monitoring
Implantable thermocouple probe
Dermofluorometry
Surface Doppler ultrasonography
Laser Doppler flowmetry
Intravenous fluorescein
Photoplethysmography
Electrical impedance plethysmography

microcatheters that continuously monitor interstitial oxygen tension, carbon dioxide tension, and pH may provide a method for objective assessment of flap viability that is not dependent on observer expertise.

Recent research has led to the development of new and innovative approaches to reconstructive surgery. Distraction osteogenesis allows for replacement of segmental bone defects with the use of adjacent autogenous bone. A modified external fixator device is used to gradually advance a periosteum-lined bone transport disc across a segmental bone gap, which fills the defect through the process of tension-induced osteogenesis. This method was originally developed in a long bone model[168, 169] but has been applied for treatment of human mandibular defects.[170] The continuing discovery and clinical application of growth factors may lead to the development of new techniques for in situ growth of lost tissues. For instance, bone morphogenic protein is a glycoprotein isolated from demineralized bone matrix that acts as an osteoinductive agent, causing fibroblasts to differentiate into osteoblastic cells. In animal models, this substance has been used to induce new bone formation within soft tissue flaps, creating customized composite flaps.[171]

Although the prevention and cure of head and neck cancer remain the primary goals of physicians who treat this disease, advances in reconstruction have provided and will continue to provide a better quality of life for patients. In many cases, innovations in reconstruction have provided to surgeons the freedom to pursue new and more aggressive ablative surgical procedures. If the next 10 years bring advances to this discipline comparable to those that have been accomplished over the past decade, then the treatment of head and neck cancer will be radically different during the first decade of the 21st century, and the quality of life of patients with cancer of the head and neck will be significantly improved.

REFERENCES

1. Martin H: Surgery of Head and Neck Tumors. New York, Harper & Row, 1964.
2. McGregor IA: The temporal flap in intra-oral cancer: Its use in repairing the post-excisional defect. Br J Plast Surg 16:318, 1963.
3. Bakamjian VY: A two-stage method for pharyngoesophageal reconstruction with a primary pectoral skin flap. Plast Reconstr Surg 36:173, 1965.
4. Urken ML, Buchbinder D, Weinberg H, et al: Microvascular free flaps in head and neck reconstruction: Report of 200 cases and review of complications. Arch Otolaryngol Head Neck Surg 120:633, 1994.
5. Urken ML: Composite free flaps in oromandibular reconstruction: Review of the literature. Arch Otolaryngol Head Neck Surg 117:724, 1991.
6. Komisar A, Lawson W: A compendium of intraoral flaps. Head Neck Surg 8:91, 1985.
7. Bakamjian VY: A two-stage method for pharyngoesophageal reconstruction with a primary pectoral skin flap. Plast Reconstr Surg 36:173, 1965.
8. Baek S, Biller HF, Krespi YP, et al: The pectoralis major myocutaneous island flap for reconstruction of the head and neck. Head Neck Surg 1:293, 1979.
9. Ariyan S: The pectoralis major myocutaneous flap. Plast Reconstr Surg 63:73, 1979.
10. Baek S, Lawson W, Biller HF: An analysis of 133 pectoralis major myocutaneous flaps. Plast Reconstr Surg 69:460, 1982.
11. Aviv JE, Urken ML, Lawson W, et al: The superior trapezius myocutaneous flap in head and neck reconstruction. Arch Otolaryngol Head Neck Surg 118:702, 1992.
12. Netterville JL, Panje WR, Maves MD: The trapezius myocutaneous flap: Dependability and limitations. Arch Otolaryngol Head Neck Surg 113:271, 1987.
13. Urken ML, Buchbinder D, Weinberg H, et al: Primary placement of osseointegrated implants in microvascular mandibular reconstruction. Arch Otolaryngol Head Neck Surg 101:56, 1989.
14. Barton FE, Spicer TE, Byrd HS: Head and neck reconstruction with the latissimus dorsi myocutaneous flap: Anatomic observations and report of 60 cases. Plast Reconstr Surg 71:199, 1983.
15. Maves MD, Panje WR, Shagets FW: Extended latissimus dorsi myocutaneous flap reconstruction of major head and neck defects. Otolaryngol Head Neck Surg 92:551, 1984.
16. Quillen CG: Latissimus dorsi myocutaneous flaps in head and neck reconstruction. Plast Reconstr Surg 63:664, 1979.
17. Schuller DE: Latissimus dorsi myocutaneous flap for massive facial defects. Arch Otolaryngol 108:414, 1982.
18. Maves MD, Panje WR, Shagets FW: Extended latissimus dorsi myocutaneous flap reconstruction of major head and neck defects. Otolaryngol Head Neck Surg 92:551, 1984.
19. Daniel RK, Taylor GI: Distant transfer of an island flap by microvascular anastomosis. Plast Reconstr Surg 52:111, 1973.
20. Urken ML, Buchbinder D, Weinberg H, et al: Microvascular free flaps in head and neck reconstruction: Report of 200 cases and review of complications. Arch Otolaryngol Head Neck Surg 120:633, 1994.
21. Urken ML, Biller HF: A new bilobed design for the sensate radial forearm flap to preserve tongue mobility following significant glossectomy. Arch Otolaryngol Head Neck Surg 120:26, 1994.
22. Soutar DS, Scheker LR, Tanner NS, et al: The radial forearm flap: A versatile method for intra-oral reconstruction. Br J Plast Surg 36:1, 1983.
23. Boyd B, Mulholland S, Gullane P, et al: Reinnervated lateral antebrachial cutaneous neurosome flaps in oral reconstruction: Are we making sense? Plast Reconstr Surg 93:1350, 1994.
24. Urken ML, Weinberg H, Vickery C, et al: The neurofasciocutaneous radial forearm flap in head and neck reconstruction: A preliminary report. Laryngoscope 100:101, 1990.
25. Soutar DS, Widdowson WP: Immediate reconstruction of the mandible using a revascularized segment of radius. Head Neck Surg 8:232, 1986.
26. Song R, Song Y, Yu Y, et al: The upper arm free flap. Clin Plast Surg 9:27, 1982.
27. Yousif NJ, Warren R, Matloub HS, et al: The lateral arm fascial free flap: Its anatomy and use in reconstruction. Plast Reconstr Surg 86:1138, 1990.
28. Katsaros J, Tan E, Zoltie N, et al: Further experience with the lateral arm free flap. Plast Reconstr Surg 87:902, 1991.
29. Sullivan MJ, Carroll WR, Kuriloff DB: Lateral arm free flap in head and neck reconstruction. Arch Otolaryngol Head Neck Surg 118:1095, 1992.
30. Pribaz JJ, Orgill DP, Epstein MD, et al: Anterolateral thigh free flap. Ann Plast Surg 34:585, 1995.
31. Kimura N, Satoh K: Consideration of a thin flap as an entity and clinical applications of the anterolateral thigh flap. Plast Reconstr Surg 97:985, 1996.
32. Koshima I, Fukuda H, Yamamoto H, et al: Free thin anterolateral thigh flaps for reconstruction of head and neck defects. Plast Reconstr Surg 92:421, 1993.
33. Xu DA, Zong SZ, Kong JM, et al: Applied anatomy of the anterolateral femoral free flap. Plast Reconstr Surg 82:305, 1988.
34. Baek S: Two new cutaneous free flaps: The medial and lateral thigh flaps. Plast Reconstr Surg 71:354, 1983.
35. Urken ML, Turk JB, Weinberg H: The rectus abdominis free flap in head and neck reconstruction. Arch Otolaryngol Head Neck Surg 117:857, 1991.
36. Meland NB, Fisher J, Irons GB, et al: Experience with 80 rectus abdominis free-tissue transfers. Plast Reconstr Surg 83:481, 1989.
37. Yousif NJ, Matloub HS, Kolachalam R, et al: The transverse gracilis musculocutaneous flap. Ann Plast Surg 29:482, 1992.
38. Harii K, Ohmori K: Free gracilis muscle transplantation with microneurovascular anastomoses for the treatment of facial paralysis. Plast Reconstr Surg 57:133, 1976.
39. Manktelow RT, Zuker RM: Muscle transplantation by fascicular territory. Plast Reconstr Surg 73:751, 1984.

40. Moscoso J, Keller J, Genden E, et al: Vascularized bone flaps in oromandibular reconstruction: A comparative anatomic study from various donor sites to assess suitability for endosseous dental implants. Arch Otolaryngol Head Neck Surg 120:36, 1994.

41. Frodel J, Funk J, Capper DT, et al: Osseointegrated implants: A comparative study of bone thickness in four vascularized bone flaps. Plast Reconstr Surg 92:449, 1993.

42. Taylor GI, Miller GH, Ham FJ: The free vascularized bone graft: Clinical extension of microvascular techniques. Plast Reconstr Surg 55:533, 1975.

43. Hidalgo DA: Free fibula flap: A new method of mandible reconstruction. Plast Reconstr Surg 84:71, 1989.

44. Schusterman MA, Reece GP, Miller MJ: Osseous free flaps for orbit and midface reconstruction. Am J Surg 166:341, 1993.

45. Schusterman MA, Reece GP, Miller MJ, et al: The osteocutaneous free fibula flap: Is the skin paddle reliable? Plast Reconstr Surg 90:787, 1992.

46. Brown SJ. Deep circumflex iliac artery free flap with internal oblique muscle as a new method of immediate reconstruction of maxillectomy defect. Head Neck 18:412, 1996.

47. Swartz WM, Battis JC, Newton ED, et al: The osteocutaneous scapular flap for mandibular and maxillary reconstruction. Plast Reconstr Surg 77:530, 1986.

48. Taylor GI, Miller GH, Ham FJ: The free vascularized bone graft: Clinical extension of microvascular techniques. Plast Reconstr Surg 55:533, 1975.

49. Ramasastry SS, Tucker JB, Swartz WM, et al: Internal oblique muscle flap: An anatomic and clinical study. Plast Reconstr Surg 73:721, 1984.

50. Urken ML, Vickery C, Weinberg H, et al: The internal oblique-iliac crest osseomyocutaneous free flap in head and neck reconstruction. J Reconstr Microsurg 5:203, 1989.

51. Urken ML, Vickery C, Weinberg H, et al: The internal oblique-iliac crest osseomyocutaneous free flap in oromandibular reconstruction: Report of 20 cases. Arch Otolaryngol Head Neck Surg 115:339, 1989.

52. Urken ML, Vickery C, Weinberg H, et al: The internal oblique–iliac crest osseomyocutaneous free flap in composite defects of the oral cavity involving bone, skin, mucosa. Laryngoscope 101:257, 1991.

53. Salibian AH, Allison GR, Rappaport I, et al: Total and subtotal glossectomy: Function after microvascular reconstruction. Plast Reconstr Surg 85:513, 1990.

54. Shenaq SM: Reconstruction of complex cranial and craniofacial defects utilizing iliac crest–internal oblique microsurgical free flap. Microsurgery 9:154, 1988.

55. Barwick WJ, Goodkind DJ, Scrafin D: The free scapular flap. Plast Reconstr Surg 69:779, 1982.

56. Maruyama Y, Urita Y, Ohnishi K: Rib–latissimus dorsi osteomyocutaneous flap in reconstruction of a mandibular defect. Br J Plast Surg 38:234, 1985.

57. Schmidt DR, Robson MC: One-stage composite reconstruction using the latissimus myo-osteocutaneous free flap. Am J Surg 144:470, 1982.

58. Whitney TM, Buncke HJ, Alpert BS, et al: The serratus anterior free-muscle flap: Experience with 100 consecutive cases. Plast Reconstr Surg 86:481, 1990.

59. Rowsell AR, Davies DM, Taylor GI: The anatomy of the subscapular-thoracodorsal arterial system: Study of 100 cadaver dissections. Br J Plast Surg 37:574, 1984.

60. Baker SR, Sullivan MJ: Osteocutaneous free scapular flap for one stage mandibular reconstruction. Arch Otolaryngol Head Neck Surg 114:267, 1988.

61. Dos Santos LF: The vascular anatomy and dissection of the free scapular flap. Plast Reconstr Surg 73:599, 1984.

62. Thoma A, Archibald S, Payk I, et al: The free medial scapular osteofasciocutaneous flap for head and neck reconstruction. Br J Plast Surg 44:477, 1991.

63. Coleman JJ, Sultan MR: The bipedicled osteocutaneous scapula flap: A new subscapular system free flap. Plast Reconstr Surg 87:682, 1991.

64. Sullivan MJ, Baker SR, Crompton R, et al: Free scapular osteocutaneous flap for mandibular reconstruction. Arch Otolaryngol Head Neck Surg 115:1334, 1989.

65. Swartz WM, Battis JC, Newton ED, et al: The osteocutaneous scapular flap for mandibular and maxillary reconstruction. Plast Reconstr Surg 77:530, 1986.

66. Chandrasekhar B, Lorant JA, Terz JJ: Parascapular free flaps for head and neck reconstruction. Am J Surg 160:450, 1990.

67. Sullivan MJ, Carroll WR, Baker SR: The cutaneous scapular free flap in head and neck reconstruction. Arch Otolaryngol Head Neck Surg 116:600, 1990.

68. Upton J, Albin RE, Mulliken JB, et al: The use of scapular and para-scapular flaps for cheek reconstruction. Plast Reconstr Surg 90:959, 1992.

69. Baker SR: Closure of large orbito-maxillary defects with free latissimus dorsi myocutaneous flaps. Head Neck Surg 6:828, 1984.

70. Aviv JE, Urken ML, Vickery C, et al: The combined latissimus dorsi–scapular free flap in head and neck reconstruction. Arch Otolaryngol Head Neck Surg 117:1242, 1991.

71. Urken ML, Bridger AG, Zur KB, et al: The scapular osteofasciocutaneous flap: A 12-year experience. Arch Otolaryngol Head Neck Surg 127:862, 2001.

72. Urken ML, Weinberg H, Vickery C, et al: Oromandibular reconstruction using microvascular composite free flaps: Report of 71 cases and a new classification scheme for bony, soft-tissue, and neurologic defects. Arch Otolaryngol Head Neck Surg 117:733, 1991.

73. Disher MJ, Esclamando RM, Sullivan MJ: Indications for the AO plate with a myocutaneous flap instead of revascularized tissue transfer for mandibular reconstruction. Laryngoscope 103:1264, 1993.

74. Marx RE: Mandibular reconstruction. J Oral Maxillofac Surg 51:466, 1993.

75. Raveh J, Stitch H, Sutter F, et al: Use of the titanium-coated hollow screw and reconstruction plate system for bridging lower jaw defects. J Oral Maxillofac Surg 42:281, 1984.

76. Urken ML: Composite free flaps in oromandibular reconstruction: Review of the literature. Arch Otolaryngol Head Neck Surg 117:724, 1991.

77. Lawson W, Loscalzo L, Baek S, et al: Experience with immediate and delayed mandibular reconstruction. Laryngoscope 92:5, 1982.

78. Mirante JP, Urken ML, Aviv JE, et al: Resistance to osteoradionecrosis in vascularized bone. Laryngoscope 103:1168, 1993.

79. Urken ML: Composite free flaps in oromandibular reconstruction: Review of the literature. Arch Otolaryngol Head Neck Surg 117:724, 1991.

80. Komisar A: The functional result of mandibular reconstruction. Laryngoscope 85:364, 1990.

81. Urken ML, Buchbinder D, Weinberg H, et al: Primary placement of osseointegrated implants in microvascular mandibular reconstruction. Arch Otolaryngol Head Neck Surg 101:56, 1989.

82. Urken ML, Buchbinder D, Weinberg H, et al: Functional evaluation following microvascular oromandibular reconstruction of the oral cancer patient: A comparative study of reconstructed and non-reconstructed patients. Laryngoscope 101:935, 1991.

83. Baker SR, Sullivan MJ: Osteocutaneous free scapular flap for one stage mandibular reconstruction. Arch Otolaryngol Head Neck Surg 114:267, 1988.

84. Hidalgo DA: Free fibula flap: A new method of mandible reconstruction. Plast Reconstr Surg 84:71, 1989.

85. Kuriloff DB, Sullivan MJ: Mandibular reconstruction using vascularized bone grafts. Otolaryngol Clin North Am 24:1391, 1991.

86. Sullivan MJ, Baker SR, Crompton R, et al: Free scapular osteocutaneous flap for mandibular reconstruction. Arch Otolaryngol Head Neck Surg 115:1334, 1989.

87. Urken ML: Composite free flaps in oromandibular reconstruction: Review of the literature. Arch Otolaryngol Head Neck Surg 117:724, 1991.

88. Urken ML, Vickery C, Weinberg H, et al: The internal oblique–iliac crest osseomyocutaneous free flap in head and neck reconstruction. J Reconstr Microsurg 5:203, 1989.

89. Urken ML, Biller HF: A new bilobed design for the sensate radial forearm flap to preserve tongue mobility following significant glossectomy. Arch Otolaryngol Head Neck Surg 120:26, 1994.

90. Urken ML, Vickery C, Weinberg H, et al: The internal oblique–iliac crest osseomyocutaneous free flap in oromandibular reconstruction: Report of 20 cases. Arch Otolaryngol Head Neck Surg 115:339, 1989.

91. Nakatsuka T, Harii K, Yamada A, et al: Dual free flap transfer using forearm flap for mandibular reconstruction. Head Neck Surg 14:452, 1992.

92. Sanger JR, Matloub HS, Yousif J: Sequential connection of flaps: A logical approach to customized mandibular reconstruction. Am J Surg 160:402, 1990.

93. Urken ML, Weinberg H, Vickery C, et al: The combined sensate radial forearm and iliac crest free flaps for reconstruction of significant glossectomy-mandibulectomy defects. Laryngoscope 102:543, 1992.

94. Okay DJ, Genden E, Buchbinder D, et al: Prosthodontic guidelines for surgical reconstruction of the maxilla: A classification system of defects. J Prosthet Dent 86:352, 2001.

95. Komisar A, Lawson W: A compendium of intraoral flaps. Head Neck Surg 8:91, 1985.

96. Genden EM, Lee BB, Urken ML: The palatal island flap for reconstruction of palatal and retromolar trigone defects revisited. Arch Otolaryngol Head Neck Surg 127:837, 2001.

97. Brown SJ: Deep circumflex iliac artery free flap with internal oblique muscle as a new method of immediate reconstruction of maxillectomy defect. Head Neck 18:412, 1996.

98. Funk G, Laurenzo JF, Valentino J, et al: Free tissue transfer reconstruction of midfacial and cranio-orbito-facial defects. Arch Otolaryngol Head Neck Surg 121:293, 1995.

99. Funk G, Laurenzo JF, Valentino J, et al: Free tissue transfer reconstruction of midfacial and cranio-orbito-facial defects. Arch Otolaryngol Head Neck Surg 121:293, 1995.

100. Schusterman MA, Reece GP, Miller MJ: Osseous free flaps for orbit and midface reconstruction. Am J Surg 166:341, 1993.

101. Genden EM, Wallace D, Buchbinder D, et al: Iliac crest internal oblique osteomusculocutaneous free flap reconstruction of the postablative palatomaxillary defect. Arch Otolaryngol Head Neck Surg 127:854, 2001.

102. Shangold LM, Urken ML, Lawson W: Jejunal transplantation for pharyngoesophageal reconstruction. Otolaryngol Clin North Am 24:1321, 1991.

103. Surkin MI, Lawson W, Biller HF: Analysis of the methods of pharyngoesophageal reconstruction. Head Neck Surg 6:953, 1984.

104. Wookey H: The surgical treatment of carcinoma of the pharynx and upper esophagus. Surg Gynecol Obstet 75:449, 1942.

105. Bakamjian VY: A two-stage method for pharyngoesophageal reconstruction with a primary pectoral skin flap. Plast Reconstr Surg 36:173, 1965.

106. Surkin MI, Lawson W, Biller HF: Analysis of the methods of pharyngoesophageal reconstruction. Head Neck Surg 6:953, 1984.

107. Ong GB, Lee TC: Pharyngogastric anastomosis after esophagopharyngectomy for carcinoma of the hypopharynx and cervical esophagus. Br J Surg 48:193, 1960.

108. Orringer MB, Sloan H: Esophagectomy without thoracotomy. J Thorac Cardiovasc Surg 76:643, 1978.

109. Gullane P, Havas T, Patterson A, et al: Pharyngeal reconstruction: Current controversies. J Otolaryngol 16:169, 1987.

110. Spiro RH, Bains MS, Shah JP, et al: Gastric transposition for head and neck cancer: A critical update. Am J Surg 162:348, 1991.

111. Hiebert CA, Cummings G: Successful replacement of the cervical esophagus by transplantation and revascularization of a free graft of gastric antrum. Ann Surg 154:103, 1961.

112. Baudet J: Reconstruction of the pharyngeal wall by free transfer of the greater omentum and stomach. Int J Microsurg 1:53, 1979.

113. McLean DH, Buncke HJ: Autotransplant of omentum to a large scalp defect, with microsurgical revascularization. Plast Reconstr Surg 49:268, 1972.

114. Goldsmith HS, Beattie EJ: Carotid artery protection by pedicled omental wrapping. Surg Gynecol Obstet 130:57, 1970.

115. Harii K: Clinical application of free omental flap transfer. Clin Plast Surg 5:273, 1978.

116. Moran WJ, Panje WR: The free greater omental flap for treatment of mandibular osteoradionecrosis. Arch Otolaryngol Head Neck Surg 113:425, 1987.

117. Netterville JL, Civantos FJ: Defect reconstruction following neurotologic skull base surgery. Laryngoscope 103:55, 1993.

118. Upton J, Mulliken JB, Hicks PD, et al: Restoration of facial contour using free vascularized omental transfer. Plast Reconstr Surg 66:560, 1980.

119. Harii K: Clinical application of free omental flap transfer. Clin Plast Surg 5:273, 1978.

120. Panje WR, Little AG, Moran WJ, et al: Immediate free gastro-omental flap reconstruction of the mouth and throat. Ann Otol Rhinol Laryngol 96:15, 1987.

121. Panje WR, Pitcock JK, Vargish T: Free omental flap reconstruction of complicated head and neck wounds. Otolaryngol Head Neck Surg 100:588, 1989.

122. Carlson GW, Schusterman MA, Guillamondegui OM: Total reconstruction of the hypopharynx and cervical esophagus: A 20-year experience. Ann Plast Surg 29:408, 1992.

123. Fisher SR, Cameron R, Hoyt DJ, et al: Free jejunal interposition graft for reconstruction of the esophagus. Head Neck Surg 12:126, 1990.

124. Seidenberg BS, Rosenak ES, Hurwitt ES, et al: Immediate reconstruction of the cervical esophagus by a revascularized isolated jejunal segment. Ann Surg 149:162, 1959.

125. Coleman JJ, Sultan MR: The bipedicled osteocutaneous scapula flap: A new subscapular system free flap. Plast Reconstr Surg 87:682, 1991.

126. Gullane P, Havas T, Patterson A, et al: Pharyngeal reconstruction: Current controversies. J Otolaryngol 16:169, 1987.

127. Shangold LM, Urken ML, Lawson W: Jejunal transplantation for pharyngoesophageal reconstruction. Otolaryngol Clin North Am 24:1321, 1991.

128. Schusterman MA, Shestak K, deVries EJ, et al: Reconstruction of the cervical esophagus: Free jejunal transfer versus gastric pull-up. Plast Reconstr Surg 85:16, 1990.

129. Shangold LM, Urken ML, Lawson W: Jejunal transplantation for pharyngoesophageal reconstruction. Otolaryngol Clin North Am 24:1321, 1991.

130. Ziesmann M, Boyd B, Manktelow RT, et al: Speaking jejunum after laryngopharyngectomy with neoglottic and neopharyngeal reconstruction. Am J Surg 158:321, 1989.

131. Harii K, Ebihara S, Ono I, et al: Pharyngoesophageal reconstruction using a fabricated forearm free flap. Plast Reconstr Surg 75:463, 1985.

132. Hiebert CA, Cummings G: Successful replacement of the cervical esophagus by transplantation and revascularization of a free graft of gastric antrum. Ann Surg 154:103, 1961.

133. Arena S: The posterior scalping flap. Laryngoscope 137:98, 1977.

134. Mandell DL, Genden EM, Biller HF, et al: Posterior scalping flap revisited. Arch Otolaryngol Head Neck Surg 126:303, 2000.

135. Martin D, Pascal JF, Baudet J, et al: The submental island flap: A new donor site. Anatomy and clinical application as a free or pedicled flap. Plast Reconstr Surg 92:867, 1993.

135a. Curran AJ, Neligan P, Gullane PJ: Submental artery island flap. Laryngoscope 107(11 pt 1):1545, 1997.

136. Pistre V, Pellissier P, Martin D, et al: Ten years of experience with the submental flap. Plast Reconstr Surg 108:1576, 2001.

137. Vural E, Suen JY: The submental island flap in head and neck reconstruction. Head Neck 22:572, 2000.

138. Netterville JL, Civantos FJ: Defect reconstruction following neurotologic skull base surgery. Laryngoscope 103:55, 1993.

139. Conley J, Baker DC: Hypoglossal-facial nerve anastomoses for reanimation of the paralyzed face. Plast Reconstr Surg 63:63, 1979.

140. Aviv JE, Urken ML: Management of the paralyzed face with microneurovascular free muscle transfer. Arch Otolaryngol Head Neck Surg 118:90, 1992.

141. Harii K, Ohmori K: Free gracilis muscle transplantation with microneurovascular anastomoses for the treatment of facial paralysis. Plast Reconstr Surg 57:133, 1976.

142. Anderl H: Reconstruction of the face through cross-facial nerve transplantation in facial paralysis. Chir Plast 2:17, 1973.

143. O'Brien BM, Franklin JD, Morrison WA: Cross-facial nerve grafts and microneurovascular free muscle transfer for long-established facial paralysis. Br J Plast Surg 33:202, 1980.

144. Jobe RP: A technique for lid loading in the management of lagophthalmos in facial palsy. Plast Reconstr Surg 53:29, 1974.

145. Levine RE, House WF, Hitselberger WE: Ocular complications of seventh nerve paralysis and management with the palpebral sling. Am J Opthalmol 73:219, 1972.

146. Smellie GD: Restoration of the blinking reflex in facial paralysis by a simple lid load operation. Br J Plast Surg 19:279, 1966.

147. Urken ML, Catalano PJ, Post K, et al: Free tissue transfer for skull base reconstruction: Analysis of complications and a classification scheme for defining skull base defects. Arch Otolaryngol Head Neck Surg 119:1318, 1993.

148. Baker SR: Surgical reconstruction after extensive skull base surgery. Otolaryngol Clin North Am 17:591, 1984.

149. Jackson GC, Netterville JL, Glasscock ME, et al: Defect reconstruction and cerebrospinal fluid management in neurotologic skull base tumors with intracranial extension. Laryngoscope 102:1205, 1992.

150. Schuller DE, Goodman JH, Miller CA: Reconstruction of the skull base. Laryngoscope 94:1359, 1984.

151. Netterville JL, Civantos FJ: Defect reconstruction following neurotologic skull base surgery. Laryngoscope 103:55, 1993.

152. Cheney ML, Vavares MA, Nadol JB: The temporoparietal fascia flap in head and neck reconstruction. Arch Otolaryngol Head Neck Surg 119:618, 1993.

153. Price JC, Loury M, Carson B, et al: The pericranial flap for reconstruction of anterior skull base defects. Laryngoscope 98:1159, 1988.

154. Snyderman CH, Janecka IV, Sekhar LN, et al: Anterior cranial base reconstruction: Role of galeal and pericranial flaps. Laryngoscope 100:607, 1990.

155. Jones NF, Sekhar LN, Schramm VL: Free rectus abdominis muscle flap reconstruction of the middle and posterior cranial base. Plast Reconstr Surg 78:471, 1986.

156. Urken ML, Catalano PJ, Post K, et al: Free tissue transfer for skull base reconstruction: Analysis of complications and a classification scheme for defining skull base defects. Arch Otolaryngol Head Neck Surg 119:1318, 1993.

157. Seidenberg BS, Rosenak ES, Hurwitt ES, et al: Immediate reconstruction of the cervical esophagus by a revascularized isolated jejunal segment. Ann Surg 149:162, 1959.

158. Daniel RK, Taylor GI: Distant transfer of an island flap by microvascular anastomosis. Plast Reconstr Surg 52:111, 1973.

159. Haughey BH, Beggs JC, Bong J, et al: Microneurovascular allotransplantation of the canine tongue. Laryngoscope 109:1461, 1999.

160. Strome M, Wu J, Strome S, et al: A comparison of preservation techniques in a vascularized rat laryngeal transplant model. Laryngoscope 104:666, 1994.

161. Strome M, Stein J, Eclamado R, et al: Laryngeal transplantation and 40-month follow-up. N Engl J Med 344:1676, 2001.

162. Boyd B, Mulholland S, Gullane P, et al: Reinnervated lateral antebrachial cutaneous neurosome flaps in oral reconstruction: Are we making sense? Plast Reconstr Surg 93:1350, 1994.

163. Urken ML, Weinberg H, Vickery C, et al: The neurofasciocutaneous radial forearm flap in head and neck reconstruction: A preliminary report. Laryngoscope 100:101, 1990.

164. Urken ML, Moscoso JF, Lawson W, et al: A systematic approach to functional reconstruction of the oral cavity following partial and total glossectomy. Arch Otolaryngol Head Neck Surg 120:589, 1994.

165. Jones BM: Monitors for the cutaneous microcirculation. Plast Reconstr Surg 73:843, 1984.

166. Jones NF: Intraoperative and postoperative monitoring of microsurgical free tissue transfers. Clin Plast Surg 19:783, 1989.

167. Neligan PC: Monitoring techniques for the detection of flow failure in the postoperative period. Microsurgery 14:162, 1993.

168. Ilizarov GA: The tension-stress effect on the genesis and growth of tissues: I. The influence of stability of fixation and soft-tissue preservation. Clin Orthop 238:249, 1989.

169. Ilizarov GA: The tension-stress effect on the genesis and growth of tissues: II. The influence of the rate and frequency of distraction. Clin Orthop 239:263, 1989.

170. McCarthy JG, Schreiber J, Karp N, et al: Lengthening the human mandible by gradual distraction. Plast Reconstr Surg 89:1, 1992.

171. Khouri RK, Koudsi B, Reddi H: Tissue transformation into bone in vivo: A potential practical application. JAMA 266:1953, 1991.

Oral Rehabilitation of Patients With Head and Neck Cancer

Mark S. Chambers

James C. Lemon

Jack W. Martin

Adam S. Garden

Béla B. Toth

◻ INTRODUCTION

Optimal care of patients with cancer requires the combined efforts of a team of health care providers whose collective goal is not only to ensure the well-being of patients during treatment but also to cure patients of malignant disease. In most patients with cancer, problems in the oral cavity mirror those in the general population—moderate to advanced periodontal disease, poorly restored dentition, and soft tissue pathologies associated with tobacco use, alcohol use, nutritional neglect, general hygiene neglect, or a combination of these factors.[1, 2] Evaluation, treatment, and prevention of any oral and dental preexisting disease are important aspects of the overall treatment outcome for patients with cancer.[1, 2] In addition, patients undergoing aggressive anticancer treatment encounter preventable, if not treatable, oral mucosal and dental sequelae that could produce morbid events.[3] Complications vary with each patient, depending on the individual's oral and dental status, the type of malignancy, and the therapeutic approach.[4] Common and frequent treatment-limiting problems, such as mucositis, infection, and bleeding, can be minimized and in some cases eliminated, if evaluated and treated early by an involved, trained prosthodontic team. Early dental intervention can decrease inpatient days by reducing sites of oral infection and can decrease risk factors for oral complications (e.g., osteoradionecrosis [ORN]). In some cases, ablated structures can be replaced immediately with prostheses that restore function and aesthetics.

Now more than ever before, treating physicians have a medical, legal, and fiscal responsibility to ensure that patients receiving head and neck surgery, radiation therapy, chemotherapy, or regimens involving a combination of these treatments first receive a thorough, systematic oral examination.[1, 4] Additionally, physicians have placed a major emphasis on the prevention of malignancies through the identification and control of factors such as tobacco use and alcohol consumption, which are associated with carcinogenic tissue changes.[5–10] Chemopreventive agents such as synthetic retinoids (e.g., 13-*cis*-retinoic acid) have been successful in reversing oral leukoplakic lesions before malignant transformation.[9, 11]

Over the past several decades, care of complex cases of advanced head and neck cancer has involved multidisciplinary teamwork with important contributions from head and neck surgeons, radiation therapists, medical oncologists, reconstruction plastic surgeons, prosthodontists, speech therapists, and nutritionists. Over the past decade, discovery of the cellular changes associated with the development of cancer in humans has resulted in improved techniques for diagnosing and treating malignant disease.[5] Today, the treatment of patients with head and neck cancer consists primarily of surgery, radiation therapy, and chemotherapy, or some combination thereof. The primary goal of treatment is to thoroughly obliterate the local disease while maximizing function, cosmesis, and quality of life. Restoring function and aesthetics and reducing post-treatment sequelae are the secondary aims.[12–15]

Toward these ends, team effort between the head and neck surgeon, prosthodontist, and reconstructive surgeon should be fostered. Planning and preparation for rehabilitation should be coordinated by the responsible specialists before the surgical procedure. Miscommunication or lack of communication between the surgeon and the maxillofacial prosthodontist can cause post-treatment complications associated with the rehabilitation of patients with head and neck disease.[12, 13] Maxillofacial prosthodontics is the branch of dentistry concerned with the prosthetic rehabilitation of intraoral and extraoral structures that have been affected by disease, injury, surgery, or congenital malformation.[14] Patients should be referred to the maxillofacial prosthodontist as early as possible in their treatment workup for the evaluation of oral/dental status and for discussion of the treatment options of prosthetic rehabilitation. The primary surgeon can then integrate results of this evaluation into the overall treatment plan.

This chapter describes for oral care practitioners the scope and integration of oral oncology concepts in the treatment of patients with cancer. The chapter also addresses general and specific aspects of oral complications arising from radiation therapy and chemotherapy and outlines practical approaches for preventing, recognizing, and treating the oral sequelae associated with such therapy. Finally, this chapter presents current concepts regarding oral and facial prosthetic rehabilitation and oncologic principles associated with the care of patients with head and neck cancer.

GENERAL CONSIDERATIONS

An oral and dental consultation before chemotherapy, radiation therapy, or head and neck surgery is extremely important in the oral management of patients with cancer.[1, 16–21]

Oral complications associated with cancer therapy can be classified into several general types—stomatitis, infection, bleeding, mucositis, pain, loss of function, and xerostomia.[22] In most cases, preexisting conditions strongly influence the development and persistence of these complications in the oral cavity. Such complications arise primarily in three anatomic sites—the mucosa, periodontium, and teeth.[4]

Complications arising during cancer therapy may result either from treatment or from the malignant disease process (e.g., chemotherapeutic complications related to myelosuppression or immunosuppression, or direct cytotoxic effects of chemical agents on oral tissues). For patients receiving a tumor-ablative procedure involving the oral cavity, the treating physician should aim to control oral and dental problems during the recovery phase and before adjunct therapy. As part of the immediate postsurgical planning, the oral cavity should be prepared for appropriate prosthetic rehabilitation to correct postsurgical deficits. If radiation therapy or chemotherapy or both are planned, the treating physician should be aware that the resultant oral complications may be devastating; furthermore, the degree and type of oral sequelae may affect the patient's compliance with or continuance of cancer treatment.[23–26]

Radiation therapy may directly damage oral mucosa, salivary glands, bone, or oral musculature, resulting in xerostomia, infection, ORN, trismus, dermatitis, extensive dental caries, abnormal bone development, and alteration in taste acuity.[1, 17, 27, 28] Because preexisting oral disease may increase the risk of severe oral complications, a thorough oral and dental examination before cancer therapy is essential.[17, 25, 29, 30]

A head and neck evaluation, an oral and dental clinical examination, and an intraoral radiologic evaluation all should be performed during the initial visit. Selected dental radiographs are essential in evaluating potential areas of infection that are not obvious on clinical examination (e.g., periodontal-periapical tooth disease, residual cysts, and impacted or partially erupted exfoliating teeth). In addition, the dental oncologist or prosthodontist should gather and record the patient's history of present illness, past medical and dental history, social history, review of systems, current medications, and adverse drug reactions, as well as the anticipated cancer treatment plan. From this information, the prosthodontist can plan oral treatment to control immediate needs. However, treatment of disease must always take priority over treatment of complications.[1, 31]

Prosthodontists should communicate with the treating physicians to be aware of the diagnosis and staging of malignant disease, the goals of proposed therapy, the patient's prognosis, the type and dose of therapy to be administered, and the timing of treatment. If radiation therapy is to be used in the head and neck area, the prosthodontist must know the volume of tissue to be irradiated, the treatment schedule, the dosimetry, the fractionation scheme, the method of administration (e.g., external beam radiation therapy or brachytherapy), the type of energy (e.g., photon, electron, or mixed beam), and the total dose to be administered.[16, 18, 32–36]

Prosthodontists should educate patients using tobacco, alcohol, or illicit drugs on the physical effects of these agents and explain their possible impact on the malignant disease process.[37, 38] In addition, the treatment team should immediately discourage further use of these substances and should provide information on cessation programs. The nutritional status of patients should be assessed, and counseling should be provided, if needed, to enable patients to avoid debilitation, delayed wound healing, and increased susceptibility to dental caries.[27, 28, 39–41]

The prosthodontist's initial examination and early treatment of the patient are directed at documenting and reversing any preexisting acute or chronic pathologic conditions—such as dental abscesses, advanced periodontal disease, dental calculus causing gingivitis, partially erupted teeth with the potential for pericoronitis, or soft tissue tooth trauma—that may be factors in the treating physician's selection of an overall cancer treatment strategy.[1, 22] Even if the planned cancer treatment is not toxic to the mucosa and is not myelosuppressive (e.g., hormonal therapy), the potential for infection remains. Additionally, the cancer may eventually progress, necessitating prompt and aggressive therapy; hence, the patient's oral and dental status should be optimal to ensure minimal predictable complications. The periodontal status and degree of tooth decay are evaluated during the initial examination, as are the patient's ability and initiative to maintain optimal oral hygiene.[42] Patients must modify their oral care and hygiene techniques, if possible, to minimize mucosal and gingival complications that are associated with their specific treatment.[42–44] One major objective of oral hygiene is to reduce and control the formation of plaque, a proteinaceous, adherent, bacteria-laden debris material, on teeth and soft tissue. Plaque can be colonized by normal flora and by opportunistic pathogenic organisms, and its accumulation can lead to several harmful conditions, including gingivitis and periodontal disease, the latter of which occurs when calculus formation induces the pathologic loss of supporting soft tissue and bone.[4] Caries is another adverse condition resulting from increased caries-forming organisms and is in itself an important consideration in patients with drug- or radiation-induced xerostomia due to potential pulpal involvement and subsequent periapical abscess formation.[4, 42, 45]

Oral surgery, definitive or intermediate restorations, and oral prophylactic procedures may be performed quickly and safely, if needed, under local dental anesthesia, intravenous sedation or general anesthesia, or a combination of both to expeditiously remove acutely and chronically infected tissue. The prosthodontist must review the patient's medical and hematologic status with the treating oncologist before initiating any such dental treatment.[46]

Prophylactic periodontal procedures and scaling and root planing may be necessary before or during cancer treatment to reduce the oral bacterial load. Daily plaque removal procedures should be emphasized, including brushing with fluoride toothpaste and flossing. Oral hygiene procedures may require modification during cancer therapy—for instance, using an exceptionally soft-bristled toothbrush. The daily use of topically applied fluorides (e.g., 0.4% stannous fluoride, 1.0% sodium fluoride, or 5000 ppm sodium fluoride) and sodium bicarbonate or chlorhexidine gluconate mouth rinses may be beneficial to the patient in reducing microbial and fungal contamination.[47] The prescribed mouth rinse should be carefully selected because some ingredients, such as alcohol and phenol, are caustic to oral mucosal tissues. Customized soft trays for fluoride application should be constructed for patients undergoing head and neck radiation therapy and should be used throughout the period of external beam radiation therapy and thereafter.[1, 45]

Oral treatment plans should be designed to correct restoration overhangs, rough or sharp edges on teeth, and any other defects likely to cause soft tissue irritation.[1, 48] Patients should be instructed to avoid abrasive foods likely to traumatize soft tissues. Ill-fitting intraoral prostheses should not be worn during cancer therapy. Dental implants should be carefully assessed, and their removal should be considered if maintenance of peri-implant health cannot be reasonably anticipated, or if integration is poor; the implants should not be removed if such surgery would be performed less than 2 weeks before the initiation of cancer therapy.[49–51]

Any potential source of oral infection should be identified and eliminated. Findings of periapical disease, questionable periodontal disease, unrestorable teeth with advanced caries, supererupted teeth, and possibly unopposed dentition should be considered for extraction. Endodontic therapy is a viable alternative for pulpally necrosed dentition, provided that the treatment can be expeditiously performed before the initiation of cancer therapy.[21, 45] To ensure exposed bone coverage and adequate wound healing, extractions should be performed 2 to 3 weeks before initiation of cancer therapy.[24, 52–55] Extractions and associated alveoloplasty should be performed as atraumatically as possible and should include smoothing sharp surrounding hard tissue, providing appropriate irrigation, and attempting primary closure to promote rapid healing.[21, 55] However, ORN can occur in areas in which teeth were extracted before, during, or after radiation therapy.[55–57] Sufficient healing time is critical, particularly before radiation therapy is initiated. In general, periodontal surgical procedures should be avoided because prolonged healing and meticulous oral hygiene are needed for the desired results to be achieved.

Patients receiving myelosuppressive or immunosuppressive drugs can develop post-treatment oral or systemic infections, such as viruses (e.g., herpes simplex virus [HSV]), fungi (e.g., candidiasis), or Gram-positive or -negative microorganisms believed to have originated in the oral cavity.[58, 59] As a result, some oncology centers perform microbiologic cultures to assess HSV antibody titers, fungal activity, and microbes with appropriate sensitivity testing as part of the protocol for all oral-related toxicity from cancer therapy. In cases of a positive titer, prophylactic use of an antiviral agent such as acyclovir, an antifungal agent such as nystatin, or an antimicrobial agent such as clindamycin is common.[60–62]

The following sections describe methods of integrating dental and oral treatment into specific oncologic therapies.

ORAL AND DENTAL ANATOMY

Head and neck surgeons should have a thorough knowledge of the oral and dental anatomy to enable accurate communication with the prosthodontist who is responsible for the patient's rehabilitation. For example, it is important to know which teeth will be removed as part of the surgical procedure so the prosthodontist can plan and fabricate an immediate or postoperative prosthesis. The universal numbering system of teeth should be used for this purpose. In this system, teeth are sequentially numbered in the adult from 1 to 32, starting with the right maxillary third molar, going to the left maxillary third molar, then continuing with the opposing left mandibular third molar and finishing with the right mandibular third molar (Fig. 29–1).[63]

Anatomic landmarks important in prosthetic rehabilitation in the edentulous maxillary and mandibular arches are shown in Figure 29–2. In the maxilla, the tuberosity, alveolar ridge, and hard palate are the major supporting tissues for a prosthesis. In comparison, the mandibular landmarks of importance are the alveolar ridge, retromolar pad, and buccal shelf. Preserving, enhancing, or reconstructing these tissues is important for support and retention of a prosthesis. Periodontally healthy teeth in the dentate patient are, of course, essential for prosthesis retention and support. Conservation of the supporting tissues, consistent with disease removal, should be a priority.[64]

ORAL AND DENTAL EVALUATION

Oral and dental evaluation by the surgeon should be part of the routine head and neck examination. The surgeon should be able to recognize acute or chronic pathologic conditions related to the dentition or supporting structures, such as advanced periodontal disease, gross dental caries, tissue irritation from poorly fitting prostheses, and poor oral hygiene.[65] Gross caries, plaque, and calculus formation on teeth indicate poor oral hygiene and possibly periodontal disease (Fig. 29–3). Oral and dental disease should be noted by the surgeon.[66] The patient should then be referred to the maxillofacial prosthodontist for evaluation and appropriate treatment.

The initial oral-dental examination by the dentist will confirm any preexisting acute and chronic oral pathologic conditions (e.g., dental abscesses, teeth with advanced periodontal disease, or dental calculus causing gingivitis).[65] The dental clinician will obtain appropriate diagnostic radiographs as indicated or requested. The more common diagnostic radiographs used in an oral-dental examination are panoramic, periapical, bitewing, and occlusal radiographs (Fig. 29–4). A panoramic radiograph gives an overall topographic picture of the dentition, maxilla, mandible, sinuses, nasal cavity, and temporomandibular joints.[67, 68] These radiographs may be of diagnostic value to the surgeon (i.e., in diagnosis of bony invasion of the maxilla or mandible by tumor) and are easily obtained in most dental offices.

The dentition is evaluated with respect to its periodontal, restorative, and hygiene status. The dentist should also determine the ability of the patient to maintain oral hygiene after the cancer treatment. Every effort should be made to

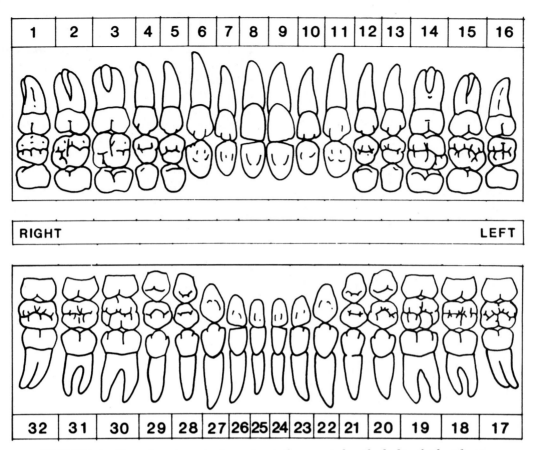

FIGURE 29–1 The universal numbering system is the accepted method of tooth identification.

eradicate before treatment any areas of infection associated with the dentition. Unrestorable teeth can be removed at the time of the ablative surgery (Fig. 29–5). Teeth should not be removed indiscriminately because of their significance to function and their potential to support and retain a prosthesis. Impressions of the maxilla, mandible, or external facial structures are made at the time of initial evaluation. Casts obtained from these impressions may be helpful in fabricating surgical prostheses if they are needed. Patients are instructed in physical therapy and oral hygiene methods that will play an important part in the postoperative rehabilitation period. Pertinent findings associated with the oral and dental examination are then presented at the combined treatment planning session.[69, 70] Stone casts obtained from impressions of the maxillas and mandible during the initial dental visit may be useful if an intraoral or an extraoral surgical prosthesis or both are required (e.g., a surgical obturator for a patient who has undergone a maxillectomy) (Fig. 29–6).[71] Teeth with a poor or questionable prognosis should be identified and extracted before or at the time of the primary ablative surgery.

◻ GENERAL SURGICAL PRINCIPLES

Patients who receive radiation therapy of the head and neck area involving the major salivary glands usually experience reduced saliva flow (i.e., salivary hypofunction or xerostomia) and increased susceptibility to dental caries and oral infection. Clinically, the severity of the morbidity depends on the radiation dose, volume of tissue treated, and age of the patient when treated.[65] These patients should be placed on a fluoride regimen; numerous studies have shown that fluoride reduces radiation-induced decay of teeth if used in a systematic, predictable manner.[72, 73] Caries is in itself an important consideration in patients with drug- or radiation-induced xerostomia (Fig. 29–7).[65, 74] Reducing the potential for dental infection while maintaining optimal oral health can significantly decrease the chances of ORN in a patient who receives radiation therapy or of a septic condition in a patient who receives chemotherapy.[72, 75, 76] The surgeon should understand the importance of this concept and ensure, at follow-up visits, that the patient is being compliant.

Meticulous oral, dental, and prosthetic hygiene is encouraged as soon as possible after head and neck surgery.[74] In general, patients are hesitant about starting oral and dental hygiene postoperatively because of a fear that the surgery site will be disturbed. Routine oral and dental hygiene can be initiated 2 weeks following surgery. In the immediate postoperative period, within a 2-week period, oral care may be limited to oral lavage and rinses.[65, 72, 74]

Postoperative physical therapy is an additional consideration in rehabilitation, and suitable techniques can be discussed and explained to the patient before surgery and

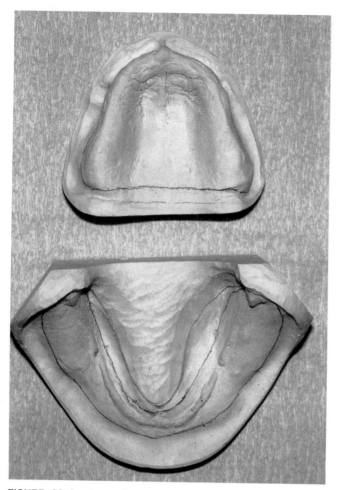

FIGURE 29–2 Areas that may support prostheses should be conserved, consistent with disease removal. In the maxilla, these areas include the tuberosity, alveolar ridge, and hard palate. In the mandible, the areas are the retromolar pad, alveolar ridge, and buccal shelf.

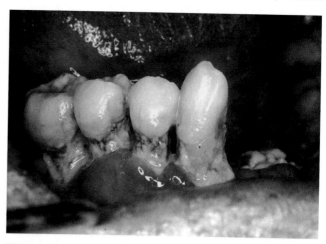

FIGURE 29–3 Gross caries, plaque, and calculus formation indicate poor oral hygiene and should be noted in the primary medical evaluation. Mobile teeth indicate bone loss and periodontal disease.

reinforced postoperatively. Such therapy can maintain the oral opening and allow the patient better access to the surgical defect and to the remaining oral cavity.[74, 77, 78] Simple opening exercises using wooden tongue blades or the fingers may be effective in restoring normal opening after surgery (Fig. 29–8). In more complex cases, electrotherapy, ultrasound, and other advanced techniques may need to be implemented by a physical therapist.[72, 78]

☐ RADIATION THERAPY

More than 80% of patients diagnosed with head and neck cancer receive a course of radiation therapy as a component of therapy.[1, 79] Many small or early-stage tumors of the head and neck region can be treated with radiation alone; more advanced disease often requires a combination of therapies. If surgery is a component of the management strategy for an advanced cancer, radiation may be sequenced so that it is administered either before or after the surgical procedure. Chemotherapy is also used for patients with advanced disease and is delivered in a neoadjuvant (induction) or

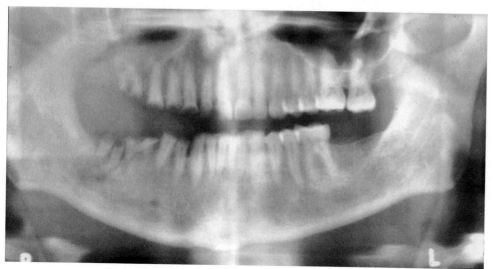

FIGURE 29–4 A panoramic radiograph is a valuable diagnostic aid that gives an overall topography of the dentition, maxillas, mandible, sinuses, and related structures. Note the broken teeth, rampant caries, and periapical abscesses of this patient, who has received head and neck radiation therapy and has developed multiple oral complications.

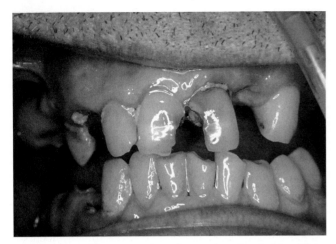

FIGURE 29–5 This patient has obvious dental pathology. These teeth should be removed at the time of the primary ablative procedure.

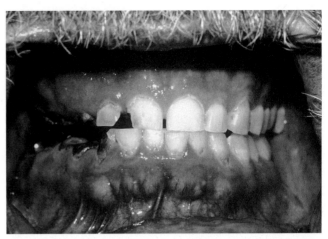

FIGURE 29–7 Radiation-induced xerostomia can result in rapid onset and progression of rampant dental caries, and ultimately may result in osteoradionecrosis (same patient as seen in Figure 29–4).

adjuvant setting. More recently, studies have revealed that administering chemotherapy concurrently with radiation therapy can improve the therapeutic ratio, resulting in improvement in disease control and survival rates.[9–11, 79]

Before a patient receives radiation therapy, the target volume and the surrounding unaffected structures must be defined. The target volume can consist of gross tumor and potential sites of microscopic extension, as well as a volume of tissue to allow for variations in daily patient setup. These volumes are determined by physical examination and by diagnostic imaging techniques such as radiographic and radionuclide studies, magnetic resonance imaging (MRI), and computed tomography (CT). Treatment planning starts with a simulation—a procedure that is implemented with

the use of a special radiographic unit that can reproduce the geometric conditions of a patient on the radiation therapy machine.[36] During simulation, the patient is usually placed in the treatment (i.e., supine) position. Patients are immobilized, usually with a thermoplastic mask, to ensure that the treatment position can be reproduced (Fig. 29–9). Following immobilization, the treatment fields are delineated with the assistance of fluoroscopy and diagnostic radiographs. A CT scan for dosimetry is provided as part of the treatment planning session (Fig. 29–10). The target volume is determined, and normal structures are localized. Treatment portals are designed and verified radiographically. The physician prescribes the tumor dose (including fractionation schedules) and, in cooperation with a physicist and a dosimetrist, calculates doses, computes beams, and generates isodose curves.[36] Treatment is implemented by the radiation therapy technician under the direct supervision of the treating physician and in consultation with the physicist. Periodically, localization films are used and doses on the charts are verified. Tumor response and the patient's tolerance of the radiation treatment are routinely evaluated.

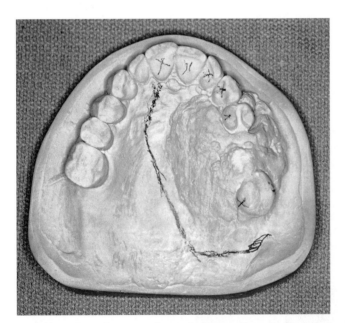

FIGURE 29–6 The cast obtained during the initial dental examination can be used to fabricate the surgical prosthesis. The surgeon has outlined the planned resection across the hard palate. Note that a portion of the premaxilla is retained to increase support of the prosthesis.

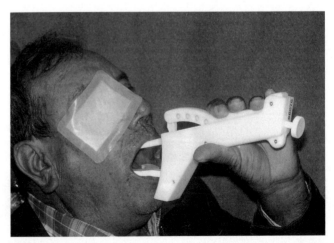

FIGURE 29–8 Physical therapy may be helpful for maintaining the oral opening. A Therabite oral opening device will stretch fibrotic tissues during healing and radiation therapy.

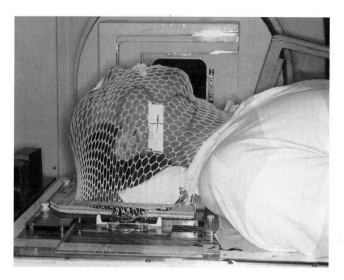

FIGURE 29–9 A thermoplastic mask is used for head and neck repeatable positioning and for immobilizing the head during external beam radiation treatment.

Oral Complications From Radiation Therapy

A healthy oral status before radiation therapy reduces the risk of complications from therapeutic administration of ionizing radiation to the head and neck. These consequences can be categorized as either acute (e.g., mucositis, infectious stomatitis, alteration of taste or smell acuity, dermatitis, pain, inflammation, and difficulty swallowing) or chronic (e.g., xerostomia, caries, abnormal development, fibrosis, trismus, photosensitivity, ORN, and pain).[1, 37, 45] The severity of treatment-induced morbidity depends on multiple factors, such as radiation dose, energy source, volume of tissue treated, pretreatment performance status, and pretreatment periodontal condition.[55] The irradiated tissue is susceptible to dermatitis and mucositis, which are often accompanied by salivary gland hypofunction, dysgeusia, dysphagia, odynophagia, hypovascularity of soft and hard tissues, fibrosis, or trismus.[1, 22, 54, 55] Widespread oral melanotic hyperpigmentation and hypopigmentation have been reported. Developmental abnormalities of the dentition and jaws may occur in children undergoing head and neck radiation therapy.[80–82] In patients of all ages, altered tissues within the volume of tissue radiated are highly susceptible to infectious processes, especially with fungal organisms such as *Candida albicans* or other *Candida* species; bacterial infections, especially streptococci and staphylococci; and viral infections, especially HSV.[59]

Mucositis

Oral mucositis generally occurs 5 to 7 days after initiation of external beam radiation therapy. Oral mucosal changes depend on fractionation, energy source, total dose of radiation, and oral and dental status (Fig. 29–11).[55] When an electron beam is used with high-energy photon beams in the treatment of deep lesions, the mucosal reactions on the side

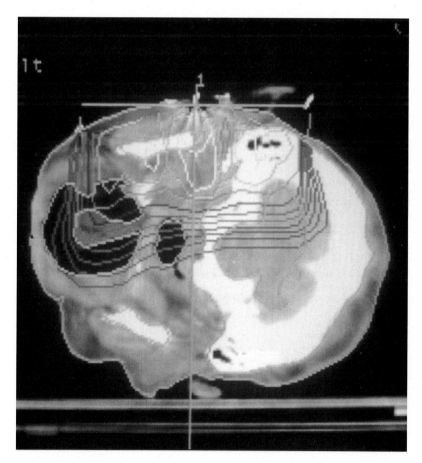

FIGURE 29–10 A computed tomography scan is used for dosimetry purposes in the radiation treatment planning session.

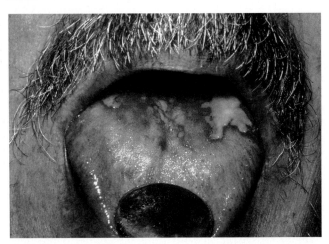

FIGURE 29–11 Radiation-induced mucositis on the lateral tongue is secondary to backscattering from a gold dental restoration.

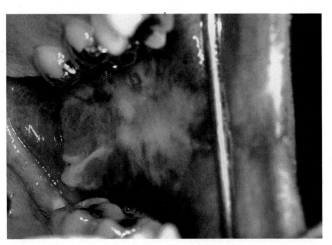

FIGURE 29–12 Radiation-induced mucositis is exacerbated by an alcohol-containing mouth rinse.

of the entering beam may consist of patchy or confluent exudate, whereas the contralateral side may show only erythema. Conventional daily dosing causes the rate of destruction of the basal cell layer to exceed the proliferation of new cells.

During the course of radiation therapy, the mucosa becomes thin as a result of direct cell death and the sloughing off of rapidly replicating epithelial cells.[36, 83] Subepithelial edema can provoke an epithelial breakdown. By the end of treatment, diffuse erythema, ulceration, spontaneous bleeding, and white or yellow pseudomembrane formation may be present.[84] Late radiation-induced changes in the oral mucosa are thought to be due primarily to damage of the microvasculature and the connective tissue. Telangiectasia, occlusion of capillaries, thickening of blood vessel walls (lack of tonus), and increased hyaline and fibrous deposition contribute to thin, atrophic, and relatively avascular mucous membranes.[79, 83] Such changes predispose the patient to hypersensitivity to trauma, infection of the oral mucosa, and delayed wound healing, particularly after minor surgical procedures.[1] Dental hygiene procedures may cause an increased risk of infection or chronic ulceration.[4, 23, 37]

The grade of oral mucositis can be partially controlled by elimination of all secondary sources of irritation, such as alcohol, smoking, coarse or hot foods, alcohol- or phenol-containing mouth rinses, and sodium products that can further dehydrate oral tissues (Fig. 29–12).[21, 84] Treatment of mucositis typically consists of palliative pain reduction therapy. Physicians have advocated several agents for topical use, including benzydamine hydrochloride, allopurinol, sucralfate suspension, kamillosan, povidone-iodine, antacids, sodium bicarbonate, local anesthetic agents (such as lidocaine hydrochloride), chlorhexidine gluconate, oral suspension of prostaglandin E_2, and aloe vera with the active ingredient acemannan.[84–89] Unfortunately, very few clinical trials have examined these substances, and the results have shown only moderate clinical efficacy.[3, 10, 16, 25, 82] Many physicians recommend that mouth rinses containing alcohol, phenolics, or astringents be avoided owing to the potential of such agents to dehydrate the mucosa and increase oral discomfort.[1, 45, 55, 82]

Gingival tissues are sensitive to radiation therapy, and increased gingival recession may occur without signs or symptoms of periodontal inflammation.[23] This recession may be due to the hypovascularity induced by the radiation and to the marked reduction of the quality and quantity of salivary secretions following irradiation.[90–92] There is evidence that a limited amount of gingival revascularization may occur over time, provided that the total radiation dosage delivered was relatively low.[35]

Superinfection

Good oral hygiene is essential to improving oral comfort and reducing the risk of oral contamination. Bacterial, fungal, and viral infections can occur as superinfections with mucositis but are less likely to induce septicemia in patients undergoing radiation therapy than in patients receiving chemotherapy, particularly because radiation therapy induces fewer pancytopenic effects than does chemotherapy.[1] However, patients receiving a concurrent regimen of radiation therapy and chemotherapy may be at greater risk of infectious mucositis than are patients treated with either therapy alone.

With fungal infections, such as oral candidiasis, the pathogenes can be invasive, refractory to treatment, and potentially systemically disseminated.[59, 82] Candidiasis can manifest as pseudomembranous, hyperplastic, or atrophic (erythematous) oral lesions.[25, 59] The sites most frequently affected are the tongue, buccal mucosa, hard or soft palate, and commissure labiorum oris (i.e., angular cheilitis) (Fig. 29–13). Diagnosis of candidiasis is based on an exclusion of therapy-related toxicity and a clinical evaluation that includes fungal cultures or visualization of organisms using potassium hydroxide stain or Gram stain.[1, 93, 94] After the diagnosis has been confirmed, treatment consists of topical antifungal agents such as nystatin oral suspension or clotrimazole troches, depending on the degree of xerostomia.[27, 53, 59] Patients with unresponsive or disseminated candidiasis may require systemic therapy, such as with ketoconazole, fluconazole, itraconazole, amphotericin B (liposomal), or a combination of antimicrobials with antifungal therapy.[27, 59]

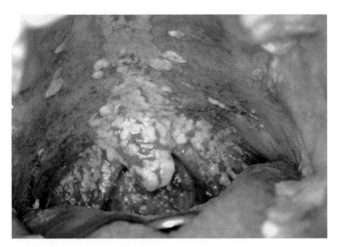

FIGURE 29–13 Oral candidiasis infection, culture positive, is present in a patient undergoing head and neck radiation therapy involving the major salivary gland tissues.

Osteoradionecrosis

Radiation can permanently destroy cellular elements of bone and thus limit the potential for wound maintenance and the ability to heal after infection or trauma (e.g., dental extraction, alveoloplasty).[95, 96] Further, the risk of complications following trauma or oral surgical procedures in an irradiated field can be highly significant, depending on a predetermined threshold of irradiation, and can result in ORN (Fig. 29–14).[54, 55, 57, 96] For these reasons, elective oral surgical procedures, such as extractions or soft tissue surgery, are contraindicated within an irradiated field owing to the potential for treatment-induced hypovascularity, hypocellularity, and hypoxia.[1] However, nonsurgical dental procedures that can safely be performed include routine restorative procedures and oral prophylaxis, radiography, and endodontic and prosthodontic procedures.[1, 37, 45]

Optimal oral health must be maintained during and after radiation therapy. However, to avoid soft tissue injury during the postradiation healing period, patients must curtail all but the most basic oral hygiene procedures (i.e., tooth brushing, flossing, and fluoride therapy). Conventional oral physical therapy (i.e., oral opening exercises) can be performed during and after radiation therapy, especially if the pterygoid regions are involved in the radiation treatment fields, which results in increased fibrosis of masticatory musculature and trismus.[25, 78, 98] Trismus is a challenging problem that may prove to be irreversible (Fig. 29–15). Therefore, patients should be encouraged to perform mouth stretching exercises before, during, and after radiation therapy.[1, 16, 78, 93] Oral opening exercises using opening devices may be needed. In addition to these exercises, other supportive care adjuncts may include nutritional counseling and smoking cessation therapy.

If oral or periodontal surgical intervention is required after radiation therapy, the clinician should discuss with the treating radiation therapist the volume of tissue irradiated and specific treatment parameters and should request a copy of the simulation or port films and a treatment summary.

Preoperative hyperbaric oxygen (HBO) therapy administered after radiation therapy may increase the potential for wound healing while minimizing the risk of ORN by promoting angiogenesis and osteogenesis.[76, 98, 99] HBO therapy should be used as an adjunct to debridement (sequestrectomy), wound care, parenteral antibiotics (as dictated by bone culture results), and composite bone and muscle grafts by free-tissue transfer (subject to the availability of personnel with the requisite microvascular skills).[98, 99] Benefits of HBO therapy include improved wound healing in infected ischemic tissue, osteoclastic stimulation, the restoration of normal defense mechanisms responsible for bacterial killing, and the direct killing of anaerobes. Antibiotics are chosen on the basis of macrodilution or microdilution sensitivity testing. During HBO therapy, it is important that edema be reduced and that the associated diffusion barrier be altered while adequate tissue oxygenation is maintained.[99, 100]

HBO therapy is time-consuming and expensive and must be performed in an accredited wound care center. However, compared with postradiation oral surgical treatment consisting of radical debridement and reconstruction, HBO treatment can be cost-effective. HBO also may preclude the need for jaw amputation, large resection, or microvascular surgery.

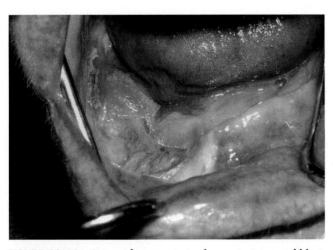

FIGURE 29–14 Osteoradionecrosis in the posterior mandible is secondary to trauma.

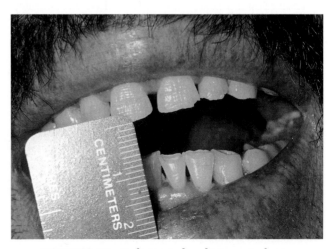

FIGURE 29–15 Radiation-induced trismus is shown.

To augment overall oral wound healing, prosthodontists usually prescribe the Marx protocol, consisting of 20 preoperative HBO treatments followed by 10 postoperative treatments.[76, 100] This prescription may be altered by increasing the number of HBO treatments, as decided by the treatment team, to maximize the wound-healing capacity of the patient.

Following initial recovery from radiation effects, nonsurgical periodontal therapy, usually with prophylactic antibiotic coverage, is appropriate for treatment of the periodontium within the irradiated field. It is important after radiation therapy that dental caries or traumatic dental injury that could lead to pathosis be detected and treated. However, ORN can occur spontaneously if healing of wounds caused by trauma or infection is compromised.[101, 102]

If postradiation extractions are necessary, HBO therapy, along with a specific oral care regimen, is indicated to augment wound healing. In such cases, tissues should be managed gently, and antibiotic coverage is required. Local anesthetics containing epinephrine should be avoided, when possible, to prevent further vascular constriction.[21] Workers have reported successful placement of endosseous implants in irradiated fields with a pretreatment regimen of HBO therapy.[103] However, there are also reports of initiation of ORN by such elective surgical intervention.[101–103]

Dental Caries

Dental caries is a common postradiation morbid sequela that is often exacerbated by xerostomia (see Fig. 29–7). Radiation of major salivary glands leads to qualitative and quantitative changes in salivary secretions,[1, 92, 104] thus increasing plaque and mucoid debris accumulation, reducing the salivary pH, and reducing the buffering capacity of saliva.[91] These conditions create a cariogenic oral environment, particularly in patients ingesting a diet high in carbohydrates or sucrose.

Some workers have attributed the pathogenicity of radiation therapy administered to salivary glands to the atrophic effects of this treatment on the secretory cells of the glands.[92] Others have attributed salivary gland dysfunction to the direct effects of radiation on the vascular and connective tissues of the glands.[92, 104] Saliva is a complex bodily fluid that consists of multiple small organic molecules, electrolytes, and immunoglobulins that defend the oral cavity from contamination and promote healing. Salivary hypofunction can increase the risk for dental caries, compromise mucosal integrity, and impair chewing and swallowing functions.[1] Therefore, when the salivary glands are within the radiation field, the risk of irreversible damage due to the cytotoxic effects of the radiation is eminent, as are the clinical manifestations of xerostomia. Even low-dose total body irradiation and mantle field treatment (as used in the treatment of Hodgkin's disease or lymphoma) may induce varying degrees of salivary hypofunction.[35, 104] Dryness of the mucosal tissues may increase susceptibility to oral infections and lead to difficulty in chewing, swallowing, and speaking.[57, 92] Susceptibility to caries is not limited to the dentition within the volume of tissue irradiated.

An effective combination of oral hygiene, frequent dental follow-up examinations, and appropriate prophylactic treatment procedures consisting of flossing, tooth brushing,

and fluoride therapy is essential to caries prevention. A daily fluoride program can decrease postradiation dentinal hypersensitivity, remineralize cavitated enamel matrices, and, more importantly, inhibit caries-forming organisms.[1, 55]

Fluoride treatment should consist of a daily application of 0.4% stannous fluoride or 1.1% sodium fluoride applied to the dentition using a brush-on technique or gel-filled trays (i.e., fluoride carriers) (Fig. 29–16).[1, 55, 90, 91] Compared with sodium fluoride, stannous fluoride is slightly more acidic, but its uptake into the enamel matrices is four times greater.[1, 55]

In adults with xerostomia, fluoride leaches out of the enamel within 24 hours; thus, the fluoride regimen must be performed daily for optimal protection. The most efficient method of fluoride application is the use of a custom-made polypropylene fluoride carrier that completely covers, and extends slightly beyond, the tooth surface.[55] Patients fill the carriers with fluoride gel and place them onto the dentition daily for 10 minutes.[1, 55] Patients who receive low doses of radiation and who are expected to have a slight degree of xerostomia can use a toothbrush to apply the fluoride gel.[105] Sensitivity and pain are common adverse effects of fluoride and may necessitate a change in the fluoride concentration or the method of application.

Xerostomia

Radiation therapy can transiently or permanently decrease salivary flow. In a study of patients followed for up to 25 years after radiation therapy, Liu and coworkers found that, compared with a nonirradiated group, patients who received bilateral ionizing radiation therapy involving the major salivary gland tissue exhibited, over time, mean decreases of 81% in stimulated and 78% in unstimulated salivary flow.[104] Patients who received unilateral radiation therapy involving only one parotid and one submandibular gland experienced mean decreases of 60% in stimulated and 51% in unstimulated salivary flow.[104] Patients who underwent cervical with supraclavicular radiation therapy (i.e., mantle field treatment) experienced mean decreases of 43% in stimulated and 32% in unstimulated salivary flow.[104]

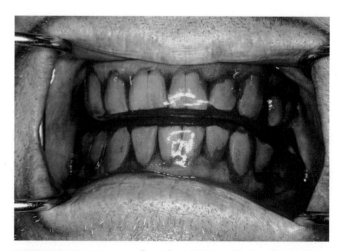

FIGURE 29–16 Stannous fluoride 0.4% is applied to the dentition with custom-made polypropylene carriers.

Radiation-induced reductions in salivary flow are worrisome because saliva protects the oral mucosa from dehydration and assists in the mechanical lavage of food and microbial debris from the oral cavity.[92] To avoid oral infections and to reduce the mucositis that may arise from radiation therapy, patients must frequently rinse the oral cavity to reduce oral microorganisms and to maintain mucosal hydration. Such oral lavage can be performed by rinsing with a solution of 1 teaspoon of sodium bicarbonate dissolved in 1 quart of water several times each day to alkalinize the oral cavity and keep the oral and oropharyngeal tissues moist.[1, 37]

The traditional treatment for radiation-induced xerostomia and mucositis is inadequate because no salivary substitute for patients with these conditions can replicate natural salivary mucin and protective salivary components.[48, 55] Mouth rinses, saliva substitutes, and gustatory stimulants are frequently abandoned by patients treated with head and neck radiation therapy. Such patients should be encouraged to increase their intake of water, decrease their intake of acidic and carbonated beverages, and decrease their intake of sodium during treatment. Sialagogue therapy, such as with cholinergic agonists (e.g., pilocarpine hydrochloride), has been shown to provide clinically significant relief of symptoms of postradiation xerostomia.[106, 107] Other rinses reported to decrease oral discomfort related to xerostomia or mucositis contain cytokines (e.g., granulocyte-macrophage colony-stimulating factor [GM-CSF], keratinocyte growth factor, transforming growth factor-β_3), interleukin 11 (IL-11), oral glutamine, amifostine, aloe vera derivatives, or antibiotics.[108–121] These rinses may be less irritating and more effective in reducing the symptoms of therapy-induced oral complications.[85–89] When administered intravenously during radiation therapy, amifostine, a free radical scavenger, has been shown to diminish the toxic effects of irradiation on salivary glands.[1]

Intensity-Modulated Radiation Therapy

One recent advance in radiation therapy has been the introduction of CT. CT images can be transferred to target planning computers to define tumor volumes and normal tissues for the development of radiation beam arrangements.[122] The process, known as three-dimensional conformal radiation therapy, enables a higher dose to be directed at the tumor while minimizing the effects on normal tissue. Another new technology in radiation oncology is intensity-modulated radiation therapy (IMRT), a technique that delivers radiation more precisely to the tumor while sparing the surrounding normal tissues.[123] IMRT also allows inverse planning and computer-controlled radiation deposition and normal tissue avoidance—new concepts that represent marked improvements over the conventional trial-and-error approach.[123] IMRT has wide application in most aspects of radiation oncology because of its abilities to create multiple targets and multiple avoidance structures, to treat different targets simultaneously at different doses, and to weight targets and avoidance structures according to their vital importance. Therefore, the IMRT is an approach to conformal therapy in which high-dose radiation is administered to target volumes while low-dose radiation is delivered

to sensitive structures. With certain head and neck treatment schedules, IMRT may reduce the total dose to major salivary glands, thus mitigating postradiation-induced xerostomia.

If these guidelines are followed, healthy oral tissues can be maintained following radiation therapy. Achievement of this goal depends not only on careful oral planning but also on the patient's cooperation and compliance.

Special Considerations for Head and Neck Irradiation

Radiation therapy is cytotoxic—that is, it permanently impairs the healing capability of the treated tissue volume. For this reason, most authors of articles concerned with prosthodontic rehabilitation of previously irradiated patients advise the prosthodontist to obtain radiation treatment details.[124–127] The geometry of the treatment volume, energy source, total dose, and daily fraction are the most desirable details. In some instances, this information may not be available directly from the treating radiation therapist; however, careful examination of the patient, together with information the patient can provide, usually suffices for the experienced maxillofacial prosthodontist. Certain dramatic characteristics are evident in patients who have previously received therapeutic radiation; for example, the skin within the treatment area is often permanently hyperpigmented, epilation is particularly noticeable on men, and the skin texture is often almost infantile. Telangiectatic changes are common in previously irradiated skin and mucosa. If major salivary glandular tissue was within the irradiated tissue volume, xerostomia is very apparent.

As has been mentioned previously, the maxillofacial prosthodontist or oncologic dentist, as a member of the treatment team, should have the opportunity to evaluate the patient before any definitive radiation therapy is given. Potential dental complications, such as irregular bony contours, severe bony undercuts, pathologic conditions of soft or hard tissue, or decayed teeth, can often be treated at the time of the definitive surgical procedure. However, the dental treatment plan must be discussed with the entire treatment team. It is the dental specialist's responsibility to present a realistic dental plan that takes into consideration the patient's prognosis and the areas of the oral cavity to be treated but that does not unnecessarily delay cancer therapy.

Extraction of Troublesome Teeth

The following guidelines are used to identify potentially troublesome teeth for extraction before radiation therapy and thus to minimize the risk of ORN. Teeth within the irradiation tissue volume that demonstrate moderate or severe periodontal disease, advanced caries, or periapical pathologic conditions are particularly in need of extraction. Also, impacted teeth, unopposed teeth, and teeth that would, if not extracted, oppose a segment of a resected jaw or complicate future prosthodontic rehabilitation should be extracted.[128] In addition, healthy teeth may need to be extracted if the patient is clinically judged to be unable to maintain adequate oral hygiene following radiation therapy. Radiologic observation is the most important diagnostic tool in diagnosing impacted teeth, intrabony cysts, or other hard tissue disease.

Oral Hygiene Protocol

The evaluation appointment is the ideal time for presenting to the patient an oral hygiene protocol designed to minimize or prevent complications associated with radiation therapy to the paranasal sinuses and neck. Because radiation therapy involving the major salivary glands produces a permanent xerostomia that results in dramatic susceptibility to dental caries, the patient must be placed on a proven regimen of fluoride therapy.[55, 91, 129–133] Oral hygiene procedures designed to reduce plaque and oral flora must also be instituted. Because the effects of radiation are permanent, the patient must plan to continue this protocol throughout his or her life.

Obturator Prosthesis

Postmaxillectomy radiation therapy is usually begun approximately 4 to 6 weeks after the surgical procedure. During the intervening healing period, the prosthodontist repeatedly modifies the surgical obturator to compensate for changes in tissue contour. Thus, if the healing time is adequate for irradiation to begin, soft tissue conditioners can be replaced with hard, polished acrylic resin. Tissue conditioners are unsuitable for contacting treated tissues during irradiation owing to their surface irregularities, porosity, and hydrophobic nature.

If possible, the interim obturator worn during the period of radiation therapy should be designed to have little contact with the surgical margins of the defect, merely covering the antrum rather than entering it. This design permits the unobstructed swelling of the treated tissues that results from radiation-induced mucositis, and it minimizes the risk that the obturator will perforate the mucosa and expose bone.

Meticulous oral hygiene, involving frequent oral and antral irrigations with a very dilute sodium bicarbonate solution together with repeated cleanings of the obturator prosthesis, is necessary to minimize mucositis and infection during the treatment period. An artificial saliva substitute to replace lost salivary lubrication can be soothing to the inflamed mucosa. Topical anesthetic agents, chewing gum containing aspirin, and commercial mouthwashes containing anesthetics should be avoided. These agents are themselves additional irritants to already irritated irradiated tissues. The anesthetic effect can also increase the risk of aspiration if such agents are swallowed.

Although every consideration must be given to the aesthetic, physiologic, and psychological comforts of patients during the period of radiation therapy, the risk of additional tissue damage from continuous wearing of the obturator prosthesis usually grossly exceeds its benefits, even when patient follow-up is provided daily. In our clinic, patients are advised to wear the obturator only when necessary, primarily during meals or for short periods of social contact during the day, but certainly never during sleep. Occasionally, even very limited use of a prosthesis during the irradiation period results in a tissue reaction so severe that the obturator cannot be worn. The patient may then have to rely on a moist gauze pack to obturate the defect until the treatment-induced mucositis has subsided.

Radiation Stents

When neck metastasis is not a consideration, custom-made radiation stents should be used to depress the mandible and tongue beyond the radiation field, thus minimizing radiation to tissues not at risk or not diseased (e.g., in patients with maxillary sinus cancer or nasal cancer) (Fig. 29–17). In contrast, the tongue-depressing/mouth-opening radiation device can be fabricated to position the oral tongue and mandible into the field of radiation treatment for repeatable positioning of the oral cavity and tongue during external beam treatment (Fig. 29–18).[134] This approach, along with an aquaplast mask, allows for a therapy of exactness and thus eliminates error caused by head or mouth movement. Such stents are relatively simple to fabricate and can be supplied by the maxillofacial prosthodontist.[134, 135] If dental support of this specialty is not available, the radiation therapist or the radiation staff can fabricate a simple device with a tongue blade (composed of Lucite) and a large cork held together with tape. However, this measure is not strongly advocated.

Circumstances necessitating irradiation of the cervical lymphatics or perioral tissues require a modification in the stent design for protection of the oral tongue. Replacing the horizontal tongue blade portion with an inclined ramp and placing the ventral tongue on the ramp thus permits the tongue to be positioned posterior to the primary treatment field (Fig. 29–19). When the neck is treated, the tongue is placed on the ramp and is thus positioned superior to the neck fields.

A further modification of the basic stent design is required if a maxillectomy, a procedure that results in an oroantral

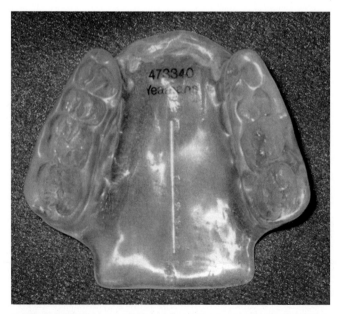

FIGURE 29–17 A methylmethacrylate custom-made radiation therapy stent is designed to depress the mandible and tongue inferiorly out of the volume of tissue to be irradiated (soft palate cancer).

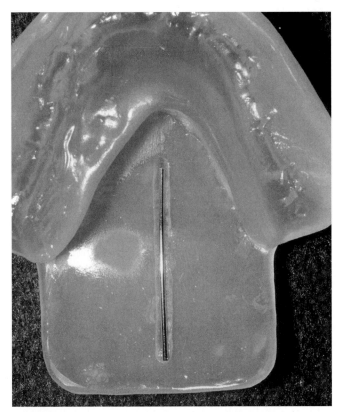

FIGURE 29–18 A custom-fabricated stent contains a piece of orthodontic wire to delineate the dorsum of the tongue on the simulator and port radiographs.

communication, has been performed (Fig. 29–20). Incorporation of a cradlelike modification into the stent design allows a water-filled latex balloon bolus (Faultless Balloon Rubber Co., Ashland, Ohio) to be supported within the surgical defect, thus eliminating the air gap.[134] This device, along with placement of a tissue-equivalent material in the defect, permits a more homogeneous energy distribution.

Patients who undergo radiation involving a unilateral treatment field benefit from a unilateral radiation device (Fig. 29–21). The device, known as a parotid stent, deviates the tongue and associated tissues to the contralateral side, thus reducing treatment-related morbidity to the contralateral tissues. A Lipowitz alloy is added to the unilateral radiation stent for added protection when the treated tissue volume receives electron beam energy or combined electron/photon energy weighted 4:1. A shielding alloy can potentiate a forward scattering effect during external beam radiation therapy if photon energy is exclusively used; this will involve the anatomic area in which a radiation device is used.

Prosthetic Rehabilitation After Radiation Therapy

The primary concern of the prosthodontist in fabricating a prosthesis for a patient who has undergone irradiation of the head and neck is the risk of traumatizing extremely friable tissue. In addition to adhering rigidly to proven prosthodontic principles, the prosthodontist must exercise special caution in designing the prosthesis to avoid causing trauma to tissues previously subjected to surgery or irradiation. Ideally, portions of the obturator that are adjacent to surgical margins should be fabricated of acrylic resin to permit easy adjustment. Tooth gingival margins should be avoided, and all surfaces in contact with tissue must be thoroughly polished to minimize the exposure of these tissues to plaque buildup on the prosthesis.

Prosthodontic rehabilitation for patients who have received radiation therapy requires that the prosthodontist pay particular attention to detail. Irradiated tissues do not necessarily become less sensitive with time and can readily change in contour. Follow-up of these patients must include a regular recall schedule for evaluation and possible prosthesis adjustment or modification.

A problem frequently encountered after maxillectomy by a patient who has had postsurgical radiation therapy is a definite decrease in intermaxillary distance. This reduction

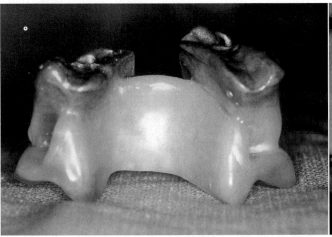

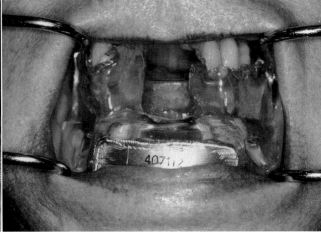

A   B

FIGURE 29–19 *A,* Posterior superior aspect of an intraoral (wax pattern) illustrates the inclined ramp design. The tongue is elevated by an inclined ramp to a position superior to the cervical treatment fields. *B,* The radiation stent in place with ramp design, as shown in Figure 29–19*A.*

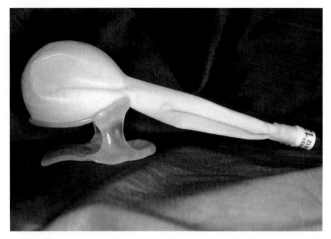

FIGURE 29–20 Lateral aspect of an intraoral stent illustrates the cradle support for the balloon water bolus (tissue equivalent) that is placed into a maxillectomy defect. The balloon is fitted with a No. 12 French catheter to facilitate the injection of water

of the oral opening can be prevented by instituting, in the immediate postsurgical period, a physical therapy program designed to overcome surgically induced fibrosis. Because surgically traumatized muscle fibers are extremely susceptible to radiation-induced fibrosis, a near-normal intermaxillary opening is not attainable unless it is achieved by the time radiation therapy begins. Radiation, to the degree necessary to be cancerocidal, also produces changes in the capillaries and arterioles, thereby further reducing an already surgically reduced blood supply to the muscles of mastication. Failure to treat this problem after radiation therapy results in continuing progressive muscle fibrosis and a further decrease in oral opening.

▣ CHEMOTHERAPY

Today, most patients with cancer receive chemotherapy as a single- or multiple-drug regimen, either alone or in combination with other therapies.[79, 136–139] The duration of treatment ranges from several months to years, depending

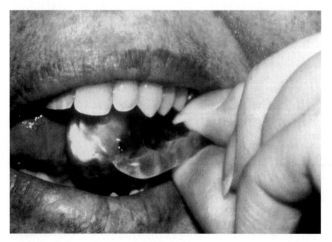

FIGURE 29–21 Unilateral radiation stent (parotid stent) contains a Lipowitz shielding alloy.

on how long the therapy remains effective or how long the patient can tolerate it. Because chemotherapeutic agents damage mitotically active normal tissue cells or multiplying tumor cells, chemotherapy often induces toxicity in the hematopoietic cells, skin, and aerodigestive tract.[37, 79] Such toxicity may cause treatment-induced complications in the oral cavity, especially if myelosuppression has occurred. Many of the sequelae of chemotherapy are similar to those induced by radiation therapy, but sometimes they are more episodic in relation to the chemotherapy regimen owing to the dosing schedule or agents administered.

Oral Complications From Chemotherapy

Treating oral conditions resulting from chemotherapy is interesting and challenging for the dental practitioner. The medical team often experiences anxiety over precipitating oral problems during therapy, and patients, after reading the literature addressing the sequelae of chemotherapy, are sometimes overtly fearful of the complications (e.g., fear that brushing the gingival tissues can result in a septic condition).[1, 37, 140] Thus, a regular regimen of dental visits and good hygiene practices is replaced with suboptimal oral care practices.

Acute oral conditions detected during the oral and dental evaluation of patients with cancer must be treated before chemotherapy if the patient's health or hematologic values permit or, if not, when the opportunity arises between treatment cycles and an appropriate performance status has been established. Chronic problems should not go unattended but should be treated strategically as the patient continues with chemotherapy.[37] Through appropriate coordination, acute problems can be treated promptly. If left untreated, chronic conditions may become acute at a time when the patient's physical well-being or hematologic parameters will not allow oral treatment intervention.

Dental practitioners must not lose sight of the long-term medical and oncologic goals for patients with cancer; additionally, they must not implement elaborate restorative plans or treat periodontal conditions that would have a guarded prognosis in patients without cancer.[139] During oncologic therapy, the treatment plan for patients with cancer should be simple, practical, and functional in relation to the patient's oral or dental health and should not be in the realm of cosmetic dentistry, fixed prosthodontics, or advanced periodontal therapy.[37, 141] Dental specialists face an almost overwhelming temptation to give aesthetic possibilities undue consideration while failing to recognize the difficulty patients face in coping with their cancer diagnosis and undergoing drug therapies that have serious adverse effects.[1, 37, 45]

Oral Infection

Even before chemotherapy commences, individual malignancies can predispose individuals to infectious risks, with neoplastic processes of either bone marrow or lymphoid tissue (i.e., lymphoma) having the greater potential for infection.[142, 143] The risk of infection further increases after treatment has started and is compounded for patients at more advanced stages of the therapeutic regimen or with more advanced stages of disease.[37]

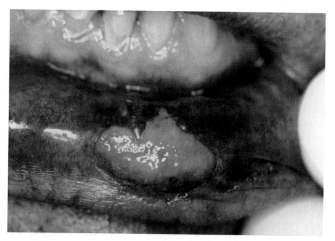

FIGURE 29–22 Patient with chemotherapy-induced pancytopenia has traumatized labial tissues caused by eating, resulting in a septic condition.

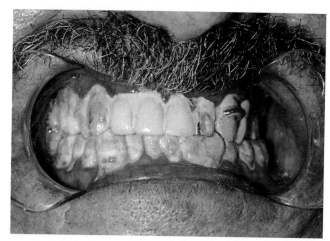

FIGURE 29–23 Patient undergoing chemotherapy with poor oral hygiene has heavy calculus and plaque.

Oncologic therapy designed to control or cure disease and to prolong survival can severely weaken the immune system, creating excellent conditions for infection to develop locally or to become a septic focus.[144, 145] Despite major preventive practices such as prophylactic antibiotics; various isolation techniques such as protected environments; and treatments such as immunologic leukocyte growth factors, the immune system is still immensely impaired by both the malignancy and the therapeutic regimen used to control infection. Even more challenging is the potential or presence of an existing infection that can be manifested by a broad spectrum of clinical signs and symptoms owing to a severely impaired immune response or the common use of prophylactic rather than therapeutic antibiotic, antifungal, or antiviral agents during treatment. Oral complications associated with cancer and its therapy have been well documented and are broadly categorized as infection, mucositis, or bleeding problems (Fig. 29–22).[23, 146]

Malignancy coupled with aggressive chemotherapeutic regimens profoundly compromises the immune system, leading to multiple serious infections with varying potential to involve the oral cavity. Empirical use of prophylactic antimicrobial agents may substantially lower the risk of infection of the oral cavity and alter the presenting signs and symptoms of infection during chemotherapy.[37] Oncologic physicians and treatment centers vary in their treatment philosophies on the use of such anti-infectious agents. The dentoalveolar complex should be thoroughly evaluated for microbial reservoirs or sanctuaries (e.g., plaque, calculus, or periodontal pockets), and these infectious foci should be eliminated before the start of chemotherapy (Fig. 29–23).[23, 37] A compromised periodontal status presents a risk of infection.[147, 148] Clinically, however, the risk of infection depends on multiple interacting factors, such as oral hygiene, immunomyelosuppressive status, chemotherapeutic agents used, prophylactic or therapeutic antimicrobial agents used, and the degree of periodontal disease.

ORAL CARE

To minimize the risks of oral infection, it is important that simple and practical guidelines be developed for maintaining oral health and for diagnosing, preventing, and treating oral-periodontal infection during therapy.[1, 37] Patients with cancer should make regular dental visits for overall dental and periodontal assessment. Patients receiving chemotherapy can undergo a dental cleaning provided that they meet the following hematologic conditions: First, an absolute neutrophil count of approximately $1000/mm^3$ (white blood cell count times percent neutrophils equals the absolute neutrophil count), a level at which the risk of developing an infection is minimal; and second, a platelet count above $50,000/mm^3$ with a normal coagulation profile.[149] The administration of prophylactic antibiotics is essential owing to the induced bacteremia, immunocompromised status, and potential for hypofunctioning white blood cells introduced by chemotherapy. The American Heart Association recommends that a viable antibiotic regimen to prevent subacute bacterial endocarditis be administered before periodontal procedures.[150, 151] The second dose should be given 6 to 8 hours after the loading dose.

Patients with an uninfected dentition and good periodontal health do not pose a treatment challenge, nor do patients with advanced periodontal disease that mandates immediate surgical intervention. However, patients with increased loss of attachment from resultant bone loss with root exposure or periodontal pocket formation pose a treatment dilemma.[37] Patients in whom the gingival loss parallels the bone loss and in whom pocket depth is normal can be treated with regular periodontal care and maintenance. Extraction should be considered only for patients with pathologic mobility of dentition or with a fulminant periapical abscess.[1, 37]

Patients with moderate to advanced periodontal disease present a greater challenge and would, under usual circumstances, receive instructions for infection prophylaxis and dental hygiene, as well as surgical correction. However, the feasibility of such comprehensive therapy during chemotherapy can be limited by several factors, including performance status, type of malignant disease, cycling of chemotherapy, and hematologic competence. The clinician should strive to provide a thorough scaling and to encourage maintenance through exceptional plaque control (i.e., tooth brushing, flossing, and use of chlorhexidine gluconate).[37, 152, 153]

To reduce the risk of septic foci, extractions should be considered for patients with any exacerbated acute periodontal infection. This oral surgical correction should be performed at the appropriate time in the treatment cycle or when the patient's cancer is in complete remission. If chemotherapy is on hold, oral-periodontal surgery could be considered provided that the hematologic status is appropriate. The prosthodontist must discuss with the treating medical oncologist the patient's oral status, treatment plan, and contraindications to surgical intervention, as well as the appropriate timing of oral treatment intervention.[37, 79, 136]

PERIODONTAL CARE

Tooth brushing and flossing should be the standard of dental care for patients who routinely brush and floss. However, as in the general population, many patients with cancer either do not floss or floss only infrequently. Thus, clinicians either may instruct patients to floss or may stress brushing techniques only. If the clinician identifies an area in which food continually lodges, the patient should be encouraged to floss the area to reduce the risk of gingival inflammation.[45]

Patients who floss regularly are instructed to modify the flossing technique in certain clinical situations: First, patients are instructed to floss gently when the lining of the oral cavity starts to become sensitive to thermal changes or food substances, indicating mucosal thinning due to suppressive effects of chemotherapy on the normally proliferative epithelium.[84] Second, patients are instructed to floss only to the gingiva when the platelet count is below 50,000/mm³. This technique removes most of the debris from this area.[37]

Tooth brushing is imperative for plaque control. The patient should be instructed to brush after each meal. In certain clinical situations, such as increased mucosal sensitivity to food or thermal changes, increased sensitivity to toothbrush bristles, irritation of the gingival tissues by the toothbrush, or profound thrombocytopenia (<20,000/mm³), patients should change from a soft to an ultrasoft-bristled or sensitive-bristled toothbrush.[1, 37, 45, 59]

In controlling plaque accumulation, it is important that the risk of gingival inflammation be minimized, along with the oral bacterial load and the potential for infection.[154] Along with routine brushing and flossing, rinsing with chlorhexidine gluconate should be initiated when patients begin chemotherapy. Such rinsing is an adjunct to ideal oral-periodontal care and can also be used when indications arise, such as oral mucosal changes secondary to chemotherapy and subsequent increased soft tissue sensitivity.[37, 152, 153] Patients undergoing chemotherapy should be encouraged to rinse with a dilute saline and sodium bicarbonate solution (5%) to reduce adherent mucoid debris on oral soft tissues, to lubricate oral mucosal and oropharyngeal tissues, and to elevate the pH of oral fluids.[45] Patients who experience nausea and anorexia should be encouraged to rinse with the sodium bicarbonate and salt water solution several times throughout the day to reduce oral acidity and minimize the mucosal insult.[155, 156]

Another challenge cancer patients face is the risk of local infection or septicemia associated with dental implants. If an implant with its restorative component poses a risk of infection for patients under normal circumstances, this risk

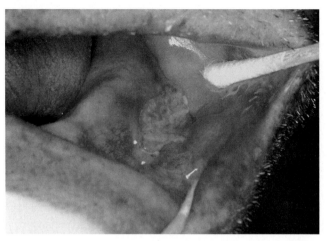

FIGURE 29–24 Patient undergoing chemotherapy has ill-fitting prostheses, causing multiple pressure and frictional ulcerations.

will be intensified during chemotherapy. Interventional antibiotics and aggressive hygiene have limited ability to control infection caused by a poorly integrated endosseous implant, whereas a well-integrated implant should not pose problems if its integrity is maintained with effective dental hygiene practices.[49–51]

Aggressive anticancer therapy severely undermines the integrity of the mucosal epithelium of the oral cavity. In addition, the oral cavity is a focused area for trauma from teeth, denture prostheses, and hot or cold dietary substances.[4] Many patients are at risk for infection from resident microflora or opportunistic pathogens sequestered in sanctuary areas (Fig. 29–24). Furthermore, cancer patients share with the general population common problems of the oral cavity, such as poor hygiene, poorly maintained dentition, periodontal disease, and prostheses in poor repair, as well as the associated mucosal disease.[37] With all these interactive injurious influences in such close proximity, even small alterations in the area could cause a problem. Each course of chemotherapy introduces this threat of oral complication, and the risk of developing complications with subsequent courses increases as local or systematic resistance is challenged. Appropriate evaluation of the oral cavity and correction of existing oral and dental pathology can minimize, and in some cases eliminate, treatment-limiting toxicities such as mucositis, oral infections, and bleeding that necessitate chemotherapy dose reduction or termination.[4, 79, 157]

Mucositis

The oral mucosal response to chemotherapy is varied and unpredictable. Some patients undergo the most aggressive treatment regimens with no problems; others experience increased mucosal sensitivity to food and thermal changes due to the thinning of the mucosal epithelium. However, some patients develop profound ulcerative wounds that may (or may not) be associated with the cycling of chemotherapy. These soft tissue mucosal reactions can confuse treating physicians, leading to inappropriate local oral treatment parameters and substantially influencing whether chemotherapy is continued.

DIAGNOSIS

Oral mucosal reactions must be identified as either stomatitis or mucositis; the distinction determines the treatment and provides insight into the overall effectiveness of the chemotherapeutic regimen.[1, 37, 43, 45] A diagnosis of oral stomatitis should be made when the integrity of the mouth has been altered by traumatic events, such as a coarse diet, an ill-fitting denture prosthesis, or infectious agents (i.e., viral, bacterial, and fungal). In contrast, a diagnosis of oral mucositis should be reserved for oral tissue changes that are the direct cytotoxic effects of chemotherapy (Fig. 29–25). All other factors must be ruled out before a condition is diagnosed as mucositis. An incorrect diagnosis of mucositis could cause unnecessary delay, reduction in dose, or complete discontinuance of effective chemotherapy. Incorrect mucosal assessment can also lead to improper care and treatment and thus to the persistence of the mucosal disease.[37] This problem can be further compounded by superinfection, pain, decreased nutritional intake, bleeding, or a focus for sepsis, effects that increase the treatment morbidity, treatment costs, length of hospital stay, need for additional antibiotic therapy, and need for parenteral nutritional support. Stomatitis is preventable, and the condition can be corrected or significantly modified with antimicrobial or dental therapy, such as correction of a plunger cusp causing frictional irritation of the lateral tongue and subsequent ulceration and marked discomfort.

ETIOLOGY AND PROGRESSION

Patients vary considerably in their tolerance of various chemotherapy agents and the development of mucositis. Chemotherapeutic agents (e.g., antimetabolites, antibiotics, alkylating agents, and vinca alkaloids) known to produce mucositis may not produce a mucosal reaction when given at the appropriate dose and duration, whereas other agents not known to produce mucositis, if given at an intensified dose or for a sufficient duration, can produce mucosal toxicity, thus necessitating dose reduction.[22, 84, 158]

Mucositis, the most common acute complication of chemotherapy, has a specific, defined mechanism of

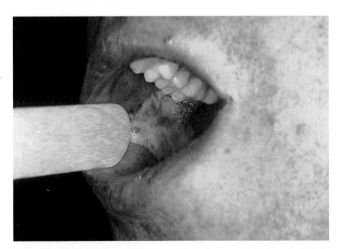

FIGURE 29–25 Chemotherapy-induced mucositis (grade III by WHO classification) is shown.

progression: mucosal erythema progresses to oral sensitivity and then to mucosal denudation.[3, 22, 84, 158] Several grading scales for oral mucositis have been developed to assess the severity of the mucosal reaction during each course of chemotherapy. These grading scales allow the clinician to prescribe appropriate preventive or therapeutic measures to treat mucosal situations after chemotherapy or during subsequent treatment courses. Grading scales range from the simple to the complex.[23, 159–162]

In cases of appropriately diagnosed mucositis, the emergence of mucosal toxicity would be expected to coincide with the administration of chemotherapy. However, mucosal HSV infections occurring early in the chemotherapy cycle can mimic mucositis. Failure to collect diagnostic cultures with each mucosal reaction can lead to a misdiagnosis of mucositis, in which case the infection goes untreated.[163–167] Culturing at this early stage of therapy is essential for differentiating mucositis from infectious stomatitis, which can be caused by a bacterial, fungal, or viral agent and which is usually associated with low hematologic values (i.e., the nadir).[1, 37] Oral mucosal infectious agents must be correctly identified and treated because the loss of mucosal integrity creates a portal of entry for systemic infection in immunocompromised patients.[146]

CHEMOTHERAPEUTIC AGENTS ASSOCIATED WITH MUCOSITIS

Chemotherapy-induced pancytopenia, combined with mucositis, can cause oral infection and bleeding events. Severe thrombocytopenia (platelets < 20,000/mm³) and neutropenia (neutrophils < 500/mm³) may be present despite normal-appearing oral mucosa. Serious complications, such as hemorrhagic diathesis or sepsis, can occur if hematologic parameters are not considered in the treatment of the oral cavity. Thus, clinicians should conduct a benefit-versus-risk analysis of the intended therapy and should thoroughly assess the hematologic values before each treatment intervention. Treatment guidelines based on such assessments have been established.[1, 3, 23, 37, 157]

Drug-related mucositis can be severe, with onset occurring within 7 days after initiation of chemotherapy and with duration varying from several days to weeks. Compared with single-agent therapy, combination drug therapy or chemoradiation therapy is more likely to induce intensified mucosal morbidity. Maximal myelosuppression can induce thrombocytopenia, thereby causing gingivitis and gingival bleeding.

Drugs most frequently associated with mucositis and myelosuppression include cytoxan, etoposide, cyclophosphamide, doxorubicin, dactinomycin, daunorubicin, 5-fluorouracil, bleomycin, melphalan, and methotrexate.[3, 16, 25, 32, 79, 82, 136, 139, 156] Chemotherapy is usually administered over 3 to 5 days, and recovery intervals of 21 to 28 days are usually provided between chemotherapeutic sessions.[37, 141] Drug-induced myelosuppression renders patients susceptible to hemorrhage and increased infectious potential.[156]

TREATMENT

Unlike the approach to oral stomatitis, effective therapy for oral mucositis has not been standardized. All interventional agents are aimed at either the prevention and reduction or the palliation of toxicity caused by chemotherapy.

The many agents used vary widely in their mechanisms of action.[158] In cases of mucositis that can be controlled, chemotherapeutic agents, alone or in combination regimens with mucositis medication, are escalated to higher doses to achieve the ultimate goal of cure of cancer. Gingival hemorrhage can usually be controlled by local measures such as the application of pressure, cool water, periodontal dressings, topical thrombin, gelatin sponges, oxidized cellulose, prefabricated stents lined with a hemostatic agent, or tranexamic acid.[1] Persistent hemorrhage may require platelet support.[16, 21, 37]

ANTIBIOTICS AND DIET

As was previously mentioned, any emergent oral treatment given while patients undergo myelosuppressive chemotherapy requires prophylactic antibiotic coverage, and all patients with in-dwelling central venous catheters require prophylactic antibiotic coverage for procedures likely to induce bacteremia.[45] The prosthodontist should consult with the patient's treating oncologist for selection of the most appropriate antibiotic.

Although grossly overlooked, diet profoundly influences the stability of the oral tissues and can cause mucosal problems when a patient is undergoing chemotherapy.[1, 136] During the myelosuppressive phase of therapy or when the mucosa is thinned owing to chemotherapy, the diet should consist of nontraumatizing soft foods that cannot puncture, abrade, or otherwise damage the compromised mucosal epithelium. Hard or abrasive food items can lead to increased pain, infection, or bleeding episodes.

PATIENTS AT HIGHER RISK

Although all patients with cancer who are undergoing chemotherapy are at risk for oral complications, the risk is greater in some patients than in others, depending primarily on the type of malignancy and the aggressiveness of the cancer treatment. Patients with hematologic malignancies (e.g., leukemia and lymphoma) have a greater risk than do patients with solid tumors (e.g., oral cancer, lung cancer, and sarcomas) because the protective elements that maintain bodily homeostasis are part of the malignant process of hematologic malignancies.[79, 136] Additional aggressive therapy that is given cyclically or that allows hematologic recovery before the start of the next chemotherapeutic cycle further increases the risk of oral complications in these patients.

Viral reactivity may lead to severe oral or disseminated infection during periods of myeloimmunosuppression. In particular, HSV infections are often associated with severe, painful, and prolonged ulcerations atypical of those found in immunocompetent hosts (Fig. 29–26).[26, 163–166] Suspected HSV lesions should be treated with antiviral agents such as acyclovir administered orally or intravenously and should be managed as described earlier for irradiated patients. The diagnosis should be established with the use of viral cultures, direct immunofluorescence, or other rapid diagnostic tests, as well as histologic assessment of the lesions.[26, 163–167]

Bacterial infection following chemotherapy can cause localized mucosal lesions, sialoadenitis, periodontal abscesses, pericoronitis, or acute necrotizing ulcerative gingivitis.[37, 139]

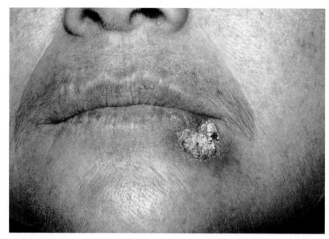

FIGURE 29–26 Culture-positive herpes simplex virus oral infection is treated with antiviral systemic and topical medications.

Because systemic infection is a serious complication in neutropenic patients, constant vigilance must be maintained to prevent or manage oral infection of any type.[1, 11, 37, 45] Oral infection should be treated with selected antibiotic combinations (broad-spectrum antibiotics), including an agent effective against anaerobic Gram-negative bacilli such as *Pseudomonas* species, *Klebsiella* species, or enterobacteria, which are often found in the oral cavity of immunocompromised individuals.[37, 45, 139] Oral microbial culture testing should be used to ensure antibiotic sensitivity and resistance selection and to assist in identification of causative organisms.[37]

◻ PROSTHETICS FOR INTRAORAL AND LOWER FACE DEFECTS

Presurgical Evaluation

Prosthetic rehabilitation of intraoral and facial defects following the surgical removal of tumors from the nasal and paranasal sinus areas begins during initial treatment planning. The modalities needed to cure the disease are considered first, but when postoperative loss of function and appearance are anticipated, rehabilitative factors must also be addressed. The dental evaluation determines how well the patient's presenting dental condition can contribute to the prosthetic rehabilitation and how much of the dentition must be altered to prevent post-therapy problems.

The need for psychiatric or psychological counseling may or may not be recognized at the time of treatment planning.[136] However, some patients who acquire orofacial defects as a consequence of surgery may benefit from psychological counseling during their rehabilitation. Dealing with cancer of any kind is very stressful. The additional loss of normal appearance and loss of ability to speak, eat, and control oral fluids are especially traumatic, both to patients and to their families. Until he or she has accepted a prosthesis, a patient cannot resume normal function in the community. Consequently, there is a recognizable need for a clinical psychologist and/or a social worker on the rehabilitation team.

In patients with head and neck cancer, removable prostheses are sometimes needed to replace surgically removed anatomy.[65, 77] There are usually three phases of prosthetic rehabilitation—surgical, interim, and definitive. Each phase includes the fabrication or modification of a prosthesis. These phases may span several months to a year. Initially, surgical and interim prostheses may require frequent adjustments while tissues are healing.[71] Such prostheses are used to immediately restore oral contour and function after a maxillectomy. A common problem associated with maxillary obturator prostheses is the leakage of fluids around the prostheses and through the nose. Speech and swallowing may also be compromised. In most of these cases, such problems can be corrected during the immediate postoperative period.

Surgical Procedures That Enhance Prosthetic Rehabilitation

Maxilla

Lesions of the maxillary sinus, hard palate, and oral alveoli may leave the patient with significant postoperative speech and swallowing problems. These problems can be reduced or eliminated by careful cooperative planning by the surgeon and dentist. The dental cast obtained at the initial dental visit can be used in discussion of the surgical procedure with the surgeon and in fabrication of the surgical prosthesis.

Following are some of the most common surgical principles that can be incorporated into a maxillectomy procedure to improve prosthetic rehabilitation:

1. Make the alveolar cuts through the socket of an extracted tooth (or an edentulous space) in a dentate patient to prevent iatrogenic bone loss and to ensure the longevity of the tooth next to this cut.[72]
2. When making the palatal cut, spare as much of the premaxilla as possible. The premaxilla is very important for support and retention of a prosthesis (Fig. 29–27). If the cancer is located in the anterior region of the sinus, it may be possible to spare the maxillary tuberosity on the defect side and thus further increase prosthetic support.
3. As a general rule, place a split-thickness skin graft (STSG) in the maxillary defect.[168] The STSG provides an excellent scar tissue band for retention of the prosthesis; it decreases mucus secretion and crust formation in the ablated sinus, making it easier for the patient to maintain hygiene of this area (Fig. 29–28).
4. If the palatal mucosa is not affected by disease, it can be retained and wrapped around the midline portion of the palatal cut.
5. Remove the inferior and middle turbinates to allow extension of the prosthesis into the defect area (Fig. 29–29). If the turbinates are not removed, they often become irritated by the prosthesis.[72]
6. Consider removing the mandibular molars on the side of the maxillectomy; they can become a hygiene problem and are essentially nonfunctional after a maxillectomy.
7. If possible, perform the maxillectomy intraorally to eliminate the need for the Weber-Fergusson facial incision that is generally used to gain access for the maxillectomy. Intraoral maxillectomy also makes manipulation of the lip and cheek easier for the dentist and patient during postoperative prosthetic procedures.[64, 65, 71, 168]
8. Place a surgical obturator prosthesis to restore the oral contour for immediate function and postoperative

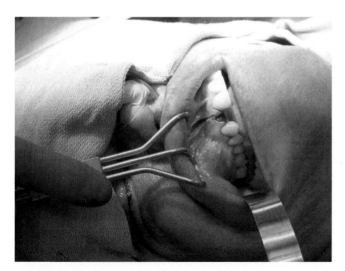

FIGURE 29–27 The maxillectomy incision is made through the socket of tooth 7, with a portion of the premaxilla retained. Some surgeons routinely make a midline incision between teeth 8 and 9, reducing the amount of supporting tissue.

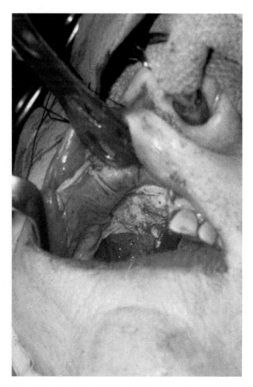

FIGURE 29–28 Lining the maxillary defect with split-thickness skin grafts makes hygiene of the defect easier. Note that the surgical packing has been placed intraorally before placement of the surgical obturator.

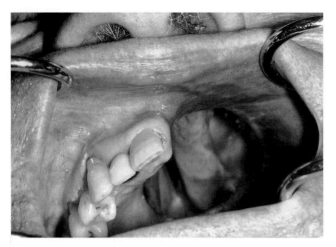

FIGURE 29–29 Proper extension of the prosthesis into the defect is impeded by the turbinate and nasal septum, reducing retention of the prosthesis. The border seal of the defect is compromised, causing leakage of food and liquids into the nasal cavity.

aesthetics. This prosthesis will support the surgical packing and can be fixated to the remaining teeth with surgical wire or retained with a bone screw in an edentulous patient (Fig. 29–30). An obturator may negate the use of a nasogastric tube and decrease the time of rehabilitation postoperatively; it will maintain proper lip and cheek support during healing, helping to reduce the contracture of scar tissue. When the surgical packing has been removed (usually within 3 to 5 days of the procedure), the surgical obturator can be converted into an interim prosthesis. Use of a surgical prosthesis can also improve the patient's mental outlook.[64, 71, 168]

Some clinicians have suggested that maxillary defects should be closed completely with the use of free-tissue grafts.[169] This method occludes the surgical defect but may preclude prosthetic rehabilitation. Complete closure is an excellent alternative for patients who do not desire a prosthesis after maxillectomy and who do not require observation for recurrent disease (e.g., those with trauma or congenital defects).

Complete closure of a maxillectomy defect with soft tissue flaps is uncommon among patients with cancer because the surgical site in such patients must be observed for recurrence of the disease and because complete closure does not favor prosthesis placement and may even make prosthesis placement impossible.[170] Closing a defect may be indicated, however, in a patient who cannot tolerate a prosthesis or in a patient who has lost a portion of the maxilla to benign disease or trauma. Free-tissue transfer with bone that can reestablish a functional alveolar ridge for prosthesis support would be particularly desirable in patients who have received a total maxillectomy; continuing work in this area holds promise for restoration of function to these patients.[171]

Although an STSG remains the preferred means of repairing a maxillectomy defect, other tissue-equivalent materials are being examined (e.g., AlloDerm grafting material, LifeCell Corp., Branchburg, New Jersey). This skin graft provides a sturdy tissue base that is resistant to abrasive force and that can support a prosthesis.[74, 168] A secondary and beneficial function is that the STSG decreases the amount of nasal mucus, which in turn limits the amount of crusting in the defect and thus makes oral hygiene easier for the patient to maintain (Fig. 29–31). This skin graft may also reduce contraction of the facial tissues during healing.

To ensure minimum morbidity and hospitalization and a rapid recovery, the best possible surgical obturator should be made available at the time of surgery. Doing so requires that the maxillofacial prosthodontist be given sufficient time before surgery to see the patient, to determine with the surgeon the extent of surgery, and to make the surgical obturator. The sophistication and quality of the prosthesis are proportionate to the time available for developing it.

Prosthetic rehabilitation of maxillectomy patients is managed in three distinct stages. The first is the surgical stage, which begins at the time of the ablative procedure,

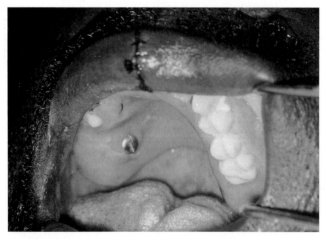

FIGURE 29–30 The surgical obturator is retained with a bone screw. The surgical obturator, which maintains stent and graft placement, is removed 5 to 7 days after surgery, and an interim obturator prosthesis is placed.

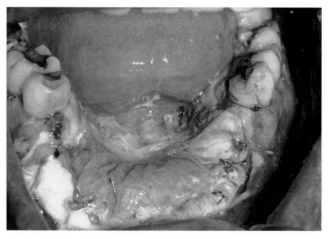

FIGURE 29–31 Split-thickness skin grafts placed during the primary surgical procedure separate the floor of the mouth from the labial mucosa, allowing the remaining alveolus to be used for support of a prosthesis.

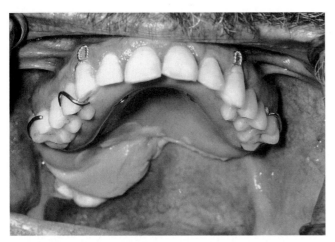

FIGURE 29–32 Surgical phase of intraoral postmaxillectomy rehabilitation begins with placement of the surgical obturator. This prosthesis immediately restores the contour of the hard palate and can be retained with screws or wire.

with the placement of the surgical packing and the surgical obturator (Fig. 29–32). The surgical obturator may or may not have teeth, depending on the situation. It is usually retained by screws or wires in the edentulous patient and by interdental wire in the dentate patient. It remains in place for approximately 5 to 7 days. The purpose of this prosthesis is to reestablish the oral contours and make it possible for the patient to start a liquid diet almost immediately postoperatively. The surgical obturator frequently precludes the placement of a nasogastric tube. It is sometimes possible to modify an existing maxillary removable partial denture or complete denture to be used as a surgical obturator.[14, 172] Before the surgical prosthesis is placed, packing material is inserted into the defect to maintain hemostasis and to immobilize a skin graft.

At the second stage, interim obturation, the surgical obturator and packing are removed (Fig. 29–33). The surgical obturator, or a new prosthesis made from postoperative impressions, is modified with a soft intermediate dental material to reestablish the contour of the oral cavity. The patient is counseled and coached, if necessary, to reinforce oral hygiene and physical therapy procedures. This stage is the most demanding because of the soft tissue changes caused by healing. An average of 12 to 14 appointments over the next 3 months can be expected.[173] During this time, the patient's progress is monitored, and the prosthesis is modified to conform to these changes. Leakage around the prosthesis is to be expected. This usually improves as the obturator is modified and the patient learns to use the prosthesis. Speech and swallowing functions should approach normal during the interim phase of rehabilitation.

The third stage, definitive obturation, is usually initiated after the patient has completed all modalities of treatment and the maxillary hard and soft tissues have healed (Fig. 29–34). This period can vary from 3 months to longer than a year after the maxillectomy procedure.[173]

Information given to the patient regarding prosthetic rehabilitation must be tempered by the experience and judgment of the clinicians. Questions and issues concerning the diagnosis and prognosis of the disease should be referred to the primary surgeon in charge of the patient's overall care. This information can be given to the patient by the dentist or surgeon to ensure the patient's overall satisfaction with the rehabilitation. The patient should also be informed of any variables beyond the control of the clinician that may compromise an ideal result. Members of the treatment team should never lead the patient to believe and expect that the maxillofacial prosthodontist will be able to completely restore original appearance and function.

The surgical defect can be rinsed and cleaned following pack removal with the use of a gravity irrigation system (Oral Irrigation Kit, Mentor Corporation, Health Care Products, Santa Barbara, Calif) consisting of a holding tank and hose with a plastic nozzle.[174] Powered lavage systems, such as the Water Pik (Teledyne Dental, Buffalo, New York) and the SurgiLav 201 (Stryker Co., Kalamazoo, Mich), can also be used and are commercially available for patient use. After the surgical obturator and packing are removed, the patient is instructed to use the irrigation system to rinse three times

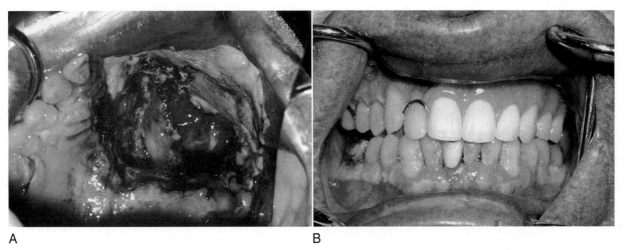

A   B

FIGURE 29–33 *A,* Interim phase begins with removal of the surgical obturator and placement of an interim prosthesis. *B,* The interim prosthesis is modified as needed to conform to the changes caused by healing, as seen in Figure 29–33A.

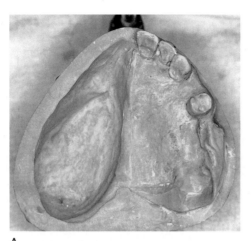

A

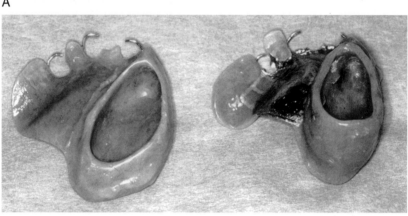

B

FIGURE 29–34 The definitive phase begins when the defect stabilizes. The definitive prosthesis maximizes stability, support, and function. *A*, A stone cast of a maxillectomy defect. *B*, The interim *(left)* and definitive *(right)* prostheses. The definitive prosthesis has a metal framework.

a day with a saline solution (Fig. 29–35). This solution is made by adding 1 tsp of salt and 1 tsp of sodium bicarbonate to 16 oz of water. The irrigation system must provide enough pressure to ensure that the prepared saline rinse reaches all parts of the surgical defect. (Because there are some concerns that the patient may injure the surgical defect and skin graft if a

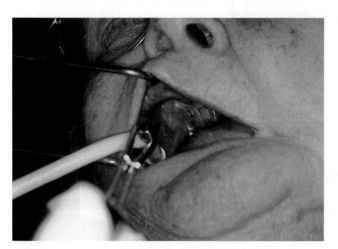

FIGURE 29–35 Oral irrigation of a maxillectomy defect. The patient is advised to rinse the oral cavity and defect three times a day.

power-spray lavage system is used during the initial healing period of the first 3 weeks, the patient should be instructed in the proper use of the lavage system.)

Routine dental hygiene (i.e., tooth brushing and flossing) should be resumed when the surgical pack is removed. Because most patients are apprehensive about resuming tooth brushing and flossing owing to concerns that doing so may harm the surgical site, patients must be specifically instructed to begin oral hygiene. Oral hygiene is one of the most important aspects of postoperative care and cannot be stressed too much.

During the fourth week of postoperative healing, rinsing with a 1:1 dilution of 3% hydrogen peroxide in water can be added to the routine. This mixture is helpful in loosening dried crust and debris in the surgical defect before the patient rinses with the salt and sodium bicarbonate mix. A piece of gauze measuring 4 in. × 4 in. or a washcloth can be wrapped around the index finger and used to clean the skin graft portion of the defect. Ora-Swab (Sage Products, Crystal Lake, Ill), a sponge-tipped applicator, may also be used for this purpose. After the surgical site has been cleaned, the entire oral cavity, including the tongue, cheek, and remaining hard palate, should be rinsed.

The use of commercial and prescription mouth rinses during the initial healing period is discouraged because the alcohol and phenol in these products may irritate the tissues. These products may also irritate the oral tissues in patients who have received chemotherapy or irradiation as adjunctive treatment.[174, 175]

The extent of decreased oral opening, loss of innervation, and facial deformity secondary to maxillectomy vary according to the extent of surgery and adjunctive treatments such as radiation therapy and chemotherapy. If the maxillectomy has been confined to the alveolus and hard palate and has been done through an intraoral approach, postoperative revisions of the obturator can be done with relative ease. However, when a more aggressive approach is required, such as a Weber-Fergusson incision and resection of the orbit, zygoma, and pterygoid muscles, the loss of oral opening and facial deformity can be more severe and can make difficult postoperative revision of the obturator prosthesis.

When the clinician anticipates these problems, oral opening exercises should be initiated as soon as the patient can tolerate them. In dentate patients, wooden tongue blades can be inserted between the posterior teeth in sequence until maximum relaxed opening is obtained (see Fig. 29–8). Opening is then increased by inserting another tongue blade between the aforementioned blades until another increment in the size of the opening is obtained. This opening is maintained for several minutes to allow the forming scar tissue to stretch. Tongue blades are sequentially added until a pain threshold is reached.

Besides tongue blades, several other devices can be used for oral opening exercises. Some devices, such as the Dynamic Bite Opener, can be custom-made for the patient. Another commercial device, the Therabite mouth opener (Therabite Co., Bryn Mawr, Penn), is a handheld device that has two cushioned intraoral plates separating the maxillas from the mandible upon engagement of a spring-retained trigger. Clinicians must instruct patients in the proper use of each device to ensure that teeth do not incur orthodontic movement or damage.

The edentulous patient can use the fingers, placed between the maxillary and mandibular ridges, to forcefully stretch the mouth open. Oral opening exercises can be combined with extraoral palpation and stretching of the cheek and upper lip to keep the tissues as pliable as possible during healing. Patients with an intraoral scar band should be instructed to stretch this tissue by digital massage. During the first 4 weeks, the patient is instructed to do these exercises three or four times a day (15 minutes each session). Oral opening measurements should be recorded during each clinic visit to help both the clinician and the patient measure the progress of these exercises. If there is no improvement, more advanced means of physical therapy should be instituted by a trained physical therapist. Even with excellent results, these patient exercises should be continued for at least 1 year with the knowledge that they may need to be extended indefinitely. When an oral opening of less than 10 mm anteriorly results, even simple oral hygiene may be impossible. For this reason, mandibular posterior teeth that are unopposed and on the defect side should be considered for extraction during the primary surgical procedure. If a patient has a sudden loss of oral opening, one should immediately suspect and rule out recurrence of disease. Infection can also cause loss of oral opening.[100, 176]

Soft Palate

When the soft palate is involved in the surgical procedure, the surgeon must consider whether the remaining soft palate will be functional. It is easier to rehabilitate a patient's speech and swallowing if the entire soft palate is removed (Fig. 29–36).[72] If the remaining portion of the soft palate is nonfunctional, rehabilitation can be difficult or even impossible (Fig. 29–37). Sometimes, a thin strip of soft palate can be useful for prosthesis retention in a patient with limited supporting tissue.[64, 77]

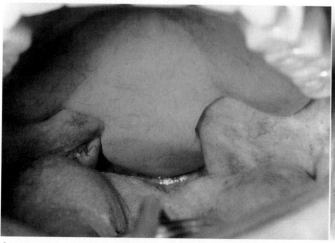
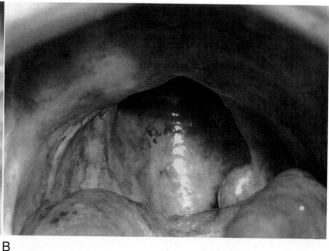

A   B

FIGURE 29–36 *A,* Definitive obturator prosthesis in a patient with a soft palate resection. *B,* The tissue located posteriorly near the palatal extension of the prosthesis is the posterior pharyngeal wall, which moves in speech and swallowing and compensates for the missing soft palate by closing the nasal cavity during function.

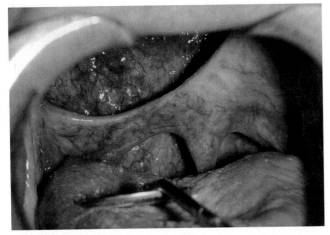

FIGURE 29–37 Surgeons are taught to maintain tissue when possible, but a nonfunctional soft palate can make prosthetic rehabilitation challenging.

Primary irradiation of the soft palate may cause palatal incompetency resulting from fibrosis and tumor necrosis. Patients with an irradiated soft palate may regurgitate liquid and food through the nose and may have speech impairment.[72] In this situation, prosthetic rehabilitation may be impossible because of poor access to the oral pharynx.

Mandible

Free-tissue transfer has revolutionized mandibular reconstruction because of its predictable results, even in cases of radiation therapy plus mandibulectomy. To repair mandibulectomy defects, three types of osseous free-tissue transfer have frequently been used—scapular, iliac crest, and fibular. Each type of transfer includes the overlying muscle, soft tissue, and skin. The fibular graft appears to be the most adaptable graft for rehabilitation because this graft supplies the length and quality of bone to repair any defect of the mandible (Fig. 29–38).[177] The fibular graft is an excellent choice for dental implant placement and support of a prosthesis.

Most patients who have had mandibular reconstruction present with an inadequate vestibular depth, a bulky load-bearing tissue base over the reconstructed alveolar ridge, and physiologic characteristics that are insufficient for adequate retention and support of a prosthesis. Two procedures routinely used to correct these problems are vestibuloplasty (with placement of an STSG) and placement of dental implants.[72, 77]

Patients with a mandibular neoplasm may need surgical stents, arch bars, or both to reposition the mandibular segments properly before surgical reconstruction. If the normal association of the mandibular segments with the glenoid fossa and maxilla is not maintained, prosthetic rehabilitation may be limited or even impossible. The maxillary teeth opposing the mandibular reconstruction may need to be removed to prevent trauma to bone and soft tissue flaps. When reconstruction is not indicated in a patient who has had a mandibulectomy, removal of the condyle and ramus on the affected side prevents migration of these structures toward the maxilla. Such movement may adversely affect prosthetic rehabilitation.

Marginal mandibulectomies (alveolectomies) can be reconstructed primarily with an STSG. Skin grafts are important because they provide a sound tissue base for a prosthesis and also separate the floor of the mouth from the buccal mucosa (see Fig. 29–31). When the tongue, the floor of the mouth, or both are sutured to the buccal or labial mucosa,

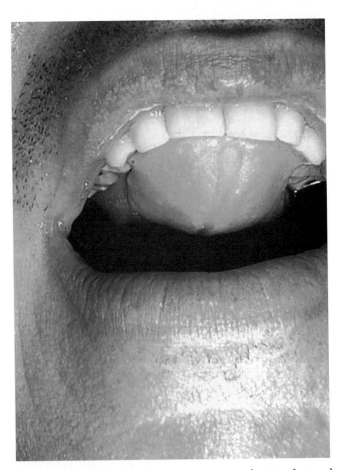

FIGURE 29–39 The palatal augmentation prosthesis is designed to lower the palate to the remaining or reconstructed tongue for function in speech and swallowing. A speech pathologist's assistance in fabricating this prosthesis optimizes results.

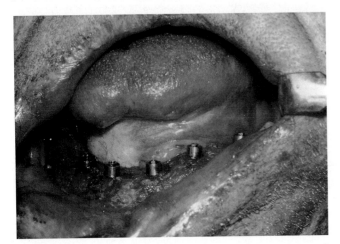

FIGURE 29–38 The patient after hemimandibulectomy with reconstruction using a fibula graft.

prosthetic rehabilitation is limited and may be impossible.[77] As with the maxilla, conservation of the supporting tissue in the mandible, consistent with removal of disease, is important.

Tongue

Speech and swallowing dysfunction are common problems in patients after glossectomy. Palatal augmentation prostheses that are approximated to the maxilla conform to postoperative tongue movements and help to normalize speech and swallowing (Fig. 29–39).

Tongue prostheses can be fabricated, but in general, they have poor function and are not readily accepted by patients. Several types of flaps can be used to restore the tongue; although nonfunctional, they reduce space in the oral cavity and make prosthesis fabrication easier and more effective.[178, 179]

◘ PROSTHETICS FOR MIDFACE DEFECTS

Presurgical Evaluation

Surgical defects of the midface in patients with head and neck cancer are the most difficult to restore. Rehabilitation is directly influenced by the ablative and reconstructive efforts of the surgical team (Fig. 29–40). The reconstructive surgeon has several options, but if the defect is to be restored prosthetically, the surgeon should consult with the maxillofacial prosthodontist both preoperatively and intraoperatively to optimize areas of support and retention. This type of communication can directly affect the timing, cost, and overall success of the prosthetic rehabilitation.[69] The result should be a facial prosthesis designed for comfort, easy placement and removal, hygiene, and pleasing aesthetics.

Following examination and surgical planning by the head and neck surgeon, the patient should be referred to the maxillofacial prosthodontist for an initial examination and discussion of all possible rehabilitative outcomes.[69] This presurgical counseling should be adapted to the needs of the patient and should allow the patient and family members to ask questions and to view examples of facial defects and prosthetic restoration. Most often, patients are concerned about time (i.e., when work on the prosthesis will begin or how long it will take to make the prosthesis), aesthetic effects, the cost of the prosthesis, and the associated supplies that will be needed to attach and maintain the prosthesis.

Preoperative photographs and presurgical facial impressions may be made to record facial features (Fig. 29–41).

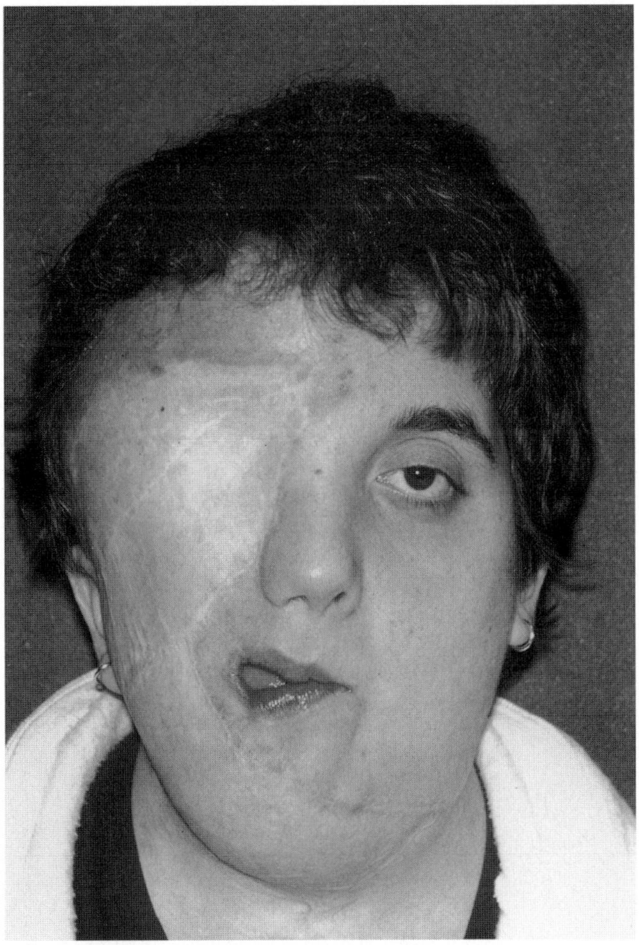

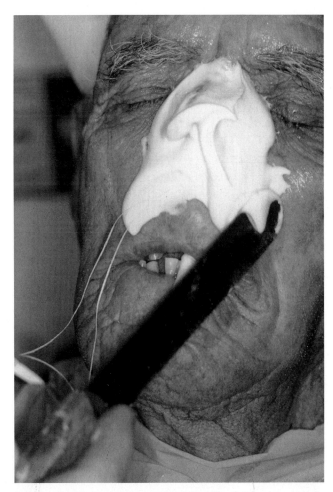

FIGURE 29–40 Overcontoured free flap is used to repair the orbital defect. This flap will require revision before prosthetic rehabilitation is provided.

FIGURE 29–41 Impression making (moulage) of a patient who has had a rhinectomy and requires a nasal prosthesis.

Facial contours following surgery can then be more accurately reproduced and made cosmetically acceptable to the patient. On occasion, the presurgical casts will be used in fabricating a surgical prosthesis to be placed after the ablative procedure.

Surgical Preparation

Classification of surgical defects of the midface is difficult owing to the numerous combinations that exist. Historically, midface defects have been defined as those confined to the middle third of the face (i.e., the nose, orbit, cheek, or upper lip) that communicate with intraoral maxillary defects.[180] Some combination defects are classified by size, that is, small, medium, or large. In the following sections, midface defects are broadly classified into those of the nose, orbit, and surrounding tissues.

Nose

Malignancies involving the nose sometimes require complete or partial rhinectomy. In such cases, nasal reconstruction with local flaps, when supporting structures such as nasal bones and the anterior nasal spine remain, has produced excellent results (Fig. 29–42). However, when these structures are removed during ablative surgery, reconstruction may be compromised. When a prosthesis is the treatment of choice, surgical preparation of the defect becomes the most important issue in the success of the prosthesis.[15, 181, 182]

Saving even a portion of the nasal bone allows vertical support for the prosthesis and, if necessary, for eyeglasses. Reducing the profile of the distal end of the nasal bone allows a prosthesis to be overlaid without increasing nasal projection. This procedure also gives the clinician greater control in determining the final dimensions of the nasal prosthesis, which may need to be decreased to avoid unfavorable alteration of lip contours following rhinectomy. Unsupported tissue tags, such as a remnant of the alae, should be resected (Fig. 29–43).[180, 181] The borders of the resection and any exposed bone, such as the nasal bone or the anterior nasal spine, should be lined with an STSG because skin grafts over these bones not only provide tissue for support and retention of a prosthesis but also help reduce secretions.[181] The use of an STSG in this setting is better than healing by second intention or direct suturing of the remaining skin to the mucosa; these techniques produce marked distortion of the midfacial contours. Secretions may also be controlled

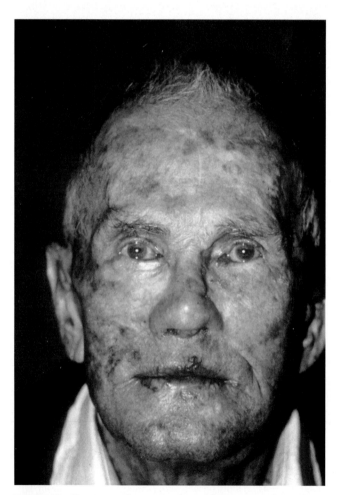

FIGURE 29–42 Surgical reconstruction of the nose with good cosmetic results.

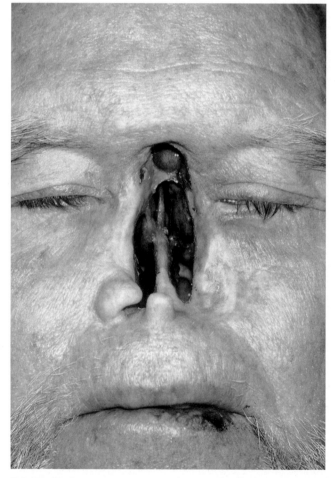

FIGURE 29–43 A tissue tag compromises the final prosthesis and functional results.

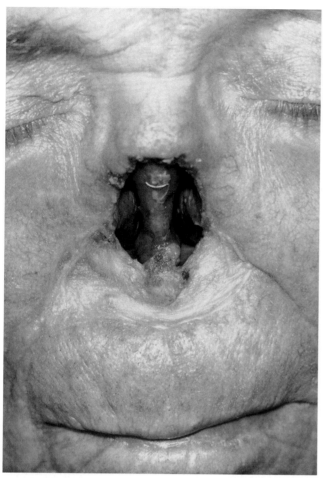

FIGURE 29–44 A reduced nasal septum is shown. Note that the skin graft on the lower aspect creates a dam for controlling secretions.

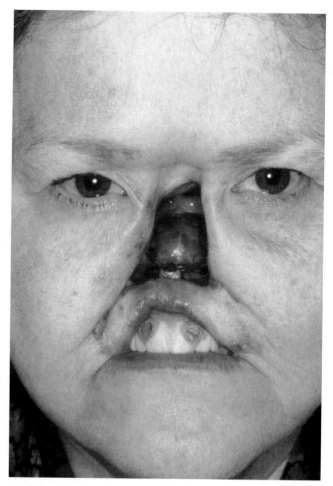

FIGURE 29–45 Postoperative contracture of the upper lip can result in superior migration and exposure of the anterior dentition.

by creation of a dam or roll of tissue at the inferior portion of the nasal defect (Fig. 29–44). If the septum remains, the anterior border should be reduced to increase the space for a properly contoured prosthesis. Contracture of the graft at the periphery of the surgical site decreases the amount of muscular action during facial movements (e.g., smiling and eating) and makes the prosthesis more stable.

When the surgical site is closed, every attempt should be made not to position the upper lip in a more superior position.[182] Following a rhinectomy procedure, the upper lip tends to contract superiorly despite the surgeon's efforts to maintain a normal intraoperative position. When this contraction occurs, the lip is everted and raised to expose the anterior dentition or prosthesis. However, with preservation of the nasal spine, the superior lip attachments remain in a normal position (Fig. 29–45).

When the defect extends laterally from the nose to include the orbit or soft tissues of the cheek, surgical preparation is even more important (Fig. 29–46). Once an orbital exenteration has been initiated, the entire contents of the globe and extraocular muscles should be removed.[181] Removal of the upper and lower eyelids is recommended to provide better access to the bony orbit. The eyebrows, however, should be left intact and in normal position. All sharp areas

of marginal bone should be smoothed. Reconstruction of the inferior orbital rim or cheek region can then provide support for facial tissue and possible future implant sites. Finally, an STSG should be attached to all exposed bone and periosteum.

Orbit

In a total orbital exenteration, several surgical considerations can improve prosthetic rehabilitation. The eyelid should be resected while the position of the eyebrow is maintained. Any sharp or rough bony margins should be smoothed and rounded. If possible, the infraorbital bony margin is reconstructed. An STSG is placed to the depth of the defect, covering any exposed bone; hence, hygiene is easier for the patient. This STSG also allows the prosthesis to be extended into the defect for greater orientation and stability (Fig. 29–47).[183]

Nose and Orbit

The combination of nasal, orbital, and zygomatic resection can lead to larger defects that are best aesthetically

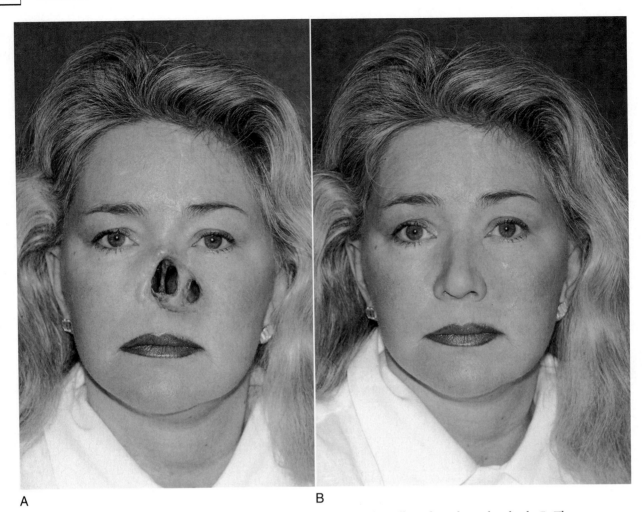

A   B

FIGURE 29–46 *A,* Frontal view of a nasal defect extending laterally and involving the cheek. *B,* The definitive nasal prosthesis is in place in the patient shown in Figure 29–46*A.*

restored with a prosthesis.[180, 181] Some large defects, besides violating the nasal and orbital cavities, may violate the maxillary sinus through any of its bony walls. If the sinus has been violated, the violated wall should be resected to open the sinus cavity for prosthetic access. This pyramidal cavity can afford considerable support for secure placement of a prosthesis.[181, 184] The respiratory mucosa should be replaced with an STSG to provide support for the prosthesis and to prevent future polyp formation in the sinus (Fig. 29–48).[181]

The interior of a surgical defect can be recruited to mechanically augment the retention of a prosthesis. Close communication between the surgeon and the prosthodontist then becomes critical. As the defect becomes larger (i.e., approaches the medial canthal regions of the eyes) or involves intraoral components, surface adhesion becomes limited; in turn, mechanical augmentation becomes more important.[181] The interlocking pieces of a combination prosthesis enable many tissue surfaces in the surgical site to be used; in contrast, a single-piece prosthesis cannot take full advantage of the opposing retentive regions available in the surgical site.

Often, a portion of the hard palate is resected with midface tumors. In such cases, an intraoral prosthesis is required to restore speech and deglutition.[15] A stable intraoral prosthesis can also augment retention of a facial prosthesis. This goal is achieved by placing the facial portion of the prosthesis into properly and surgically prepared anatomic recesses within the midface defect and mechanically connecting the intraoral and facial prostheses (Figs. 29–49 through 29–52). Intraoral and extraoral prostheses can support and retain each other if attachments that anchor one prosthesis to the other are included in each. One common attachment is the magnet.[184, 185] In some cases, however, the forehead is the only stable structure that can be used to retain a prosthesis (Fig. 29–53).[186] In that case, a headplate can be fabricated to help intraoral and extraoral attachments support and retain the prosthesis.

A large defect of the midface may be reconstructed by microvascular transfer of tissue, effectively eliminating an external cavity. However, if a patient desires a prosthesis after this type of reconstruction, the flap should be positioned to allow adequate space for development of proper contours of

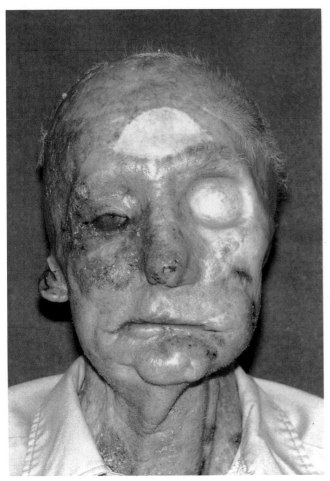

FIGURE 29–47 Orbital exenteration is reconstructed with a split-thickness skin graft. This graft allows extension of the prosthesis into the defect, improving retention and support.

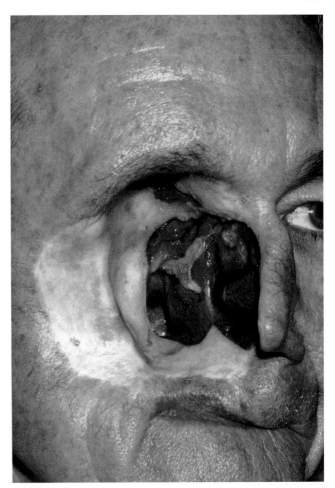

FIGURE 29–48 A split-thickness skin graft in the maxillary sinus is shown.

the prosthesis (Fig. 29–54). Negative flap contours generally produce a better aesthetic result.

Ear

As with the nose, surgeries of the ear can vary from subtotal resection to a total auriculectomy. It is easier to develop a prosthesis to replace the complete ear than to develop a prosthesis to replace a part of the ear. With a total ear replacement, the maxillofacial prosthodontist has more freedom to determine the shape, size, and location of the prosthesis. The recipient area should be flat or concave; convexities from excessive tissue bulk can hamper aesthetic results. Skin devoid of hair provides a good adhesive base; an STSG is even better. Tissue pockets assist in the orientation and stability of the prosthesis and allow the margins to extend in a 0-degree emergence profile.[183]

If tissue can be spared, the tragus is the first choice because it is a separate landmark that is not easily displaced.[183] The tragus allows the anterior margin of the prosthesis to be hidden behind the posterior flexure. Hair, the angle of the helical rim, or both provide posterior margin concealment. The inferior half of the soft tissue pinna is of little or no use. The

lobe of the auricle lacks cartilaginous support and therefore is normally drawn down and away from the head. This effect is difficult to capture in an impression, and bilateral symmetry usually cannot be achieved. The lobe margin is difficult to maintain and can be a problem when the patient attempts to insert or place the prosthesis. The superior half of the auricle has better cartilaginous support yet tends to distort postsurgically. This distortion is accentuated when the residual auricle is rotated and used to close the defect. Preserving a portion of the root of the helix provides a good landmark and support for eyeglasses. This area may help later in vertical support of the prosthesis. The anterior superior helical rim should remain if possible. Posterior regions may be grafted (Fig. 29–55).

Lip

When the ablative procedure includes the upper lip, a decision needs to be made as to the lip's reconstruction.[180, 181] In most cases, lip reconstruction by itself will not improve the function or aesthetics of a midface prosthesis. If more than half of the lip is involved with disease, resection of the remaining portion is indicated for several reasons (Fig. 29–56).

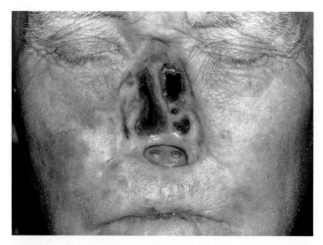

FIGURE 29–49 Frontal view of a midface with an intraoral and an extraoral defect of the patient shown in Figure 29–48.

First, if less than half of the lip remains, primary closure will reduce oral opening and limit access to the oral cavity for fabrication of an intraoral prosthesis (Fig. 29–57). Second, conserving a thin band of upper lip tissue that lacks muscle tone poses a management problem because this remaining band of tissue can become fibrotic, position itself posteriorly and superiorly in relation to other facial structures, and in

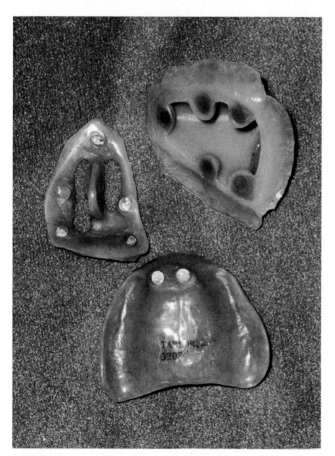

FIGURE 29–50 Intraoral and extraoral framework (acrylic resin) components of the facial prosthesis used in the patient in Figure 29–48 is shown here.

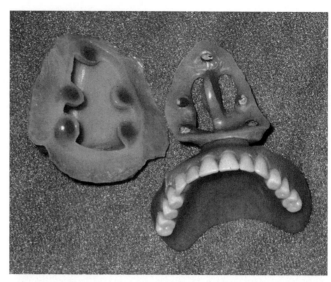

FIGURE 29–51 Framework components are engaged by magnets. Note the interior view of the nasal prosthesis, illustrating the location of the magnets.

turn hamper prosthetic management of the lip and intraoral rehabilitation. Therefore, whenever possible, nonfunctional upper lip tissue should be removed so that prosthetic rehabilitation of this area can restore sufficient function and aesthetics.[77]

In summary, several surgical techniques can enhance the recipient tissue bed for prosthetic rehabilitation. It is understood that the foremost concern of the treating surgeon is the elimination of disease, with potential modification of the surgical plan to accommodate prosthetic considerations. The general principles of ablative and reconstructive surgery are as follows: (1) Smooth all bony margins at the conclusion of the resection. (2) Place an STSG on exposed bone or periosteum not covered with free tissue or a pedicled flap. (3) Remove unsupported tissue tags. (4) Avoid overbulking the surgical site when placing free-tissue transfer flaps or pedicled flaps. (5) Match graft tissue to the tissue surrounding

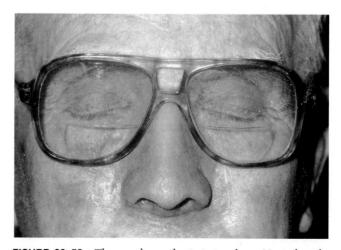

FIGURE 29–52 The nasal prosthesis is in place. Note that the eyeglasses help conceal the margins of the prosthesis.

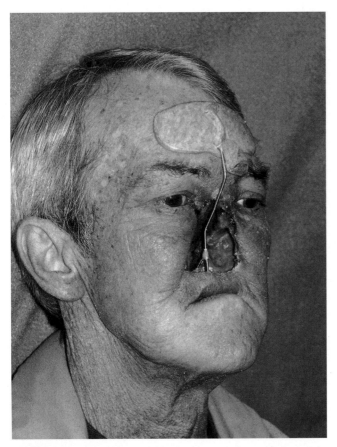

FIGURE 29–53 A forehead plate is used to retain and position the intraoral and facial prostheses.

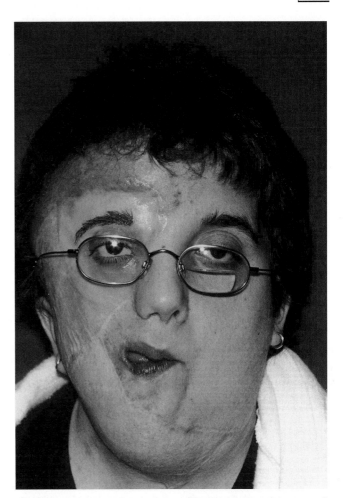

FIGURE 29–54 Aesthetically compromised prosthetic result created by a convex orbital flap in the patient shown in Figure 29–40.

the recipient bed. Any advantage gained at the time of surgery will reduce the time involved in the rehabilitation phase and will improve the final results.

The success of a future maxillofacial prosthesis can be greatly enhanced by careful presurgical evaluation and communication between the patient, surgeon, and prosthodontist.[69] Physically and psychologically preparing the patient to receive a prosthesis postoperatively is thus one of the most important aspects of treatment. Prosthetic replacement of missing facial tissues has several advantages over surgical reconstruction. The process allows for periodic evaluation and cleaning of the surgical site and is an alternative to surgery in unsuitable candidates. The fabrication process is relatively short, and unlike the surgeon, the dental clinician has complete control of the color, shape, and position of the prosthesis. Disadvantages include possible irritation of the tissue site, the need for periodic remakes, and the need to rely on adhesives or some form of retention. Furthermore, the patient may view the prosthesis as a mask and not as part of his or her body.

OSSEOINTEGRATED IMPLANTS AND FREE-TISSUE TRANSFER

Implants can vastly improve the retention and stability of a facial prosthesis. The surgeon and maxillofacial prosthodontist

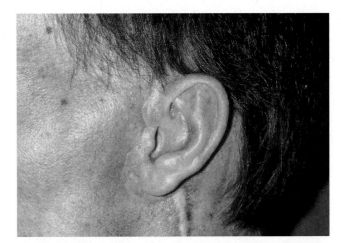

FIGURE 29–55 A complete ear prosthesis is in place and is retained by adhesive. Note that the tragus was preserved and hides the margins of the prosthesis anteriorly. The prosthesis can be worn for 3 to 4 days at a time before removal and cleaning are needed.

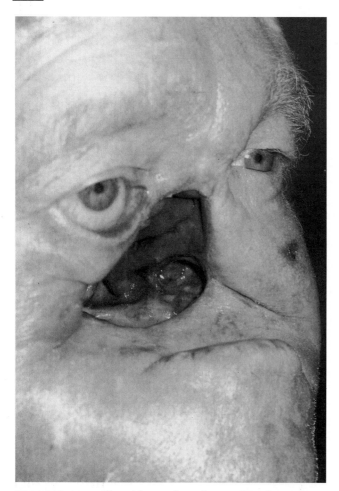

FIGURE 29–56 A flaccid lip resulting from midfacial surgery can hinder prosthetic rehabilitation.

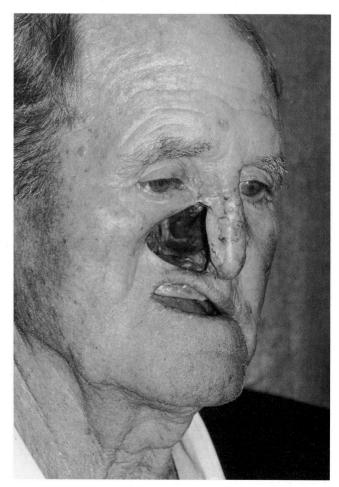

FIGURE 29–57 Primary closure of the lip can compromise function and aesthetics in the patient shown in Figure 29–56.

should participate in a presurgical planning session to determine the number, type, and positioning of implants in the defect. Three or four implants are required for most midface defects.[70] Suitable recipient sites are the zygomatic buttress, the supraorbital rim, the horizontal part of the hard palate, and the vomer. A free-tissue transfer flap composed of bone, muscle, associated soft tissue, and skin can be removed from a donor site and, through microvascular surgery, can be used to restore supporting tissues resected during cancer ablative surgery of the head and neck (Figs. 29–58 and 29–59).[177] Microvascular techniques can also be used to create or improve sites for implant placement.

A variety of implant systems are available, and each has its own characteristics. Most of these systems have similar placement and restoration procedures that are usually done in two stages. Stage 1 is the surgical placement of the implant in the recipient bone. The surgical sites are prepared in bone by techniques designed to prevent soft and hard tissue damage at the cellular level.[70] Initially, the soft tissue is reflected to expose the bone. The recipient site of the bone may need to be flattened to provide proper surface adaptation of the implant. An air-driven, slow-speed handpiece (15 to 20 rpm) with copious amounts of irrigation is then used in preparing the recipient site and preventing overheating of the bone.[70] Implant sites are enlarged in small

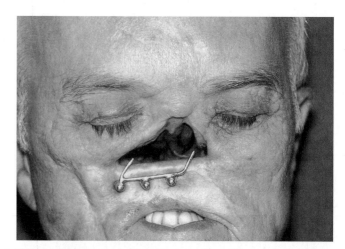

FIGURE 29–58 Postsurgical view of a patient with midface reconstruction using free-tissue microvascular transfer following total rhinectomy and maxillectomy. Note the three endosseous implants and the bar-clip system used to retain the facial prosthesis.

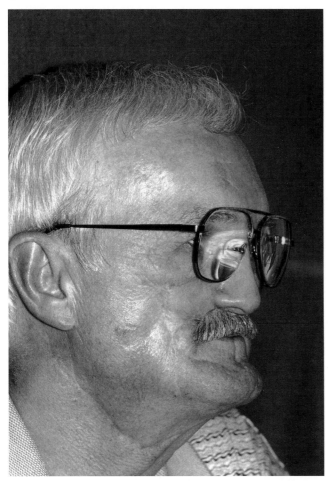

FIGURE 29–59 The definitive facial prosthesis of the patient in Figure 29–58. A moustache was added to conceal the discrepancy of the upper lip.

increments with the use of increasingly larger burrs and are then tapped to receive the threaded implants. Following placement of the implant, a healing cap or cover screw is placed, and the surgical site is readapted by primary closure of the tissue flap. The implants are not disturbed for 3 to 4 months to allow for osseointegration. Following this period, stage 2 can be initiated. The implants are uncovered and the abutments placed. An abutment is positioned onto the implant and secured in place to allow for interlocking attachments that will connect and support an overlying prosthesis.

When fabricating the facial prosthesis, several retentive elements can be placed (i.e., bar and clips, magnets, and simple ball attachments) on the implants for retention and support. The choice of attachment system depends on the needs of the individual patient.

▢ CONCLUSIONS

The oral cavity should be thoroughly evaluated in all patients diagnosed with cancer, as well as in patients undergoing chemotherapy or radiation therapy to the head and neck region. Preventing and treating the oral complications

of cancer and its therapy are important responsibilities of the dental oncologist or maxillofacial prosthodontist, and anticipating primary and secondary mucosal insults and recognizing oral complications promptly in this setting can decrease the incidence of such complications or ameliorate their morbid adverse effects. By fostering communication and compliance among the multidisciplinary team, the prosthodontist can ensure the quality of preventive and prosthetic treatment, as well as maintenance care, for patients with head and neck cancer.

REFERENCES

1. Chambers MS, Toth BB, Martin JW, et al: Oral and dental management of the cancer patient: Prevention and treatment of complications. Support Care Cancer 3:168–175, 1995.
2. King GE, Toth BB, Fleming TJ: Oral dental care of the cancer patient. Texas Dent J 105:10–11, 1988.
3. National Institutes of Health: Consensus Development Conference Statement: Oral complications of cancer therapies: Diagnosis, prevention, and treatment. J Am Dent Assoc 119:179–183, 1989.
4. Toth BB, Martin JW, Fleming TJ: Oral and dental care associated with cancer therapy. Cancer Bull 43:397–402, 1991.
5. Chambers MS, Jacob RF: How carcinogens cause cancer. Tex Dent J June:13–19, 1994.
6. Rankin KV, Jones DL: Oral Health in Cancer Therapy: A Guide for Health Care Professionals. Austin, Texas, Texas Cancer Council, 1999.
7. Gritz ER: Cigarette smoking: The need for action by health professionals. CA Cancer J Clin 38:194–212, 1988.
8. Holmstrup P, Pindborg JJ: Oral mucosal lesions in smokeless tobacco users. CA Cancer J Clin 38:230–235, 1988.
9. Lamey PJ: Management options in potentially malignant and malignant oral epithelial lesions. Community Dent Health 10:53–62, 1993.
10. Peterson DE, D'Ambrosio JA: Nonsurgical management of head and neck cancer patients. Dent Clin North Am 38:425–445, 1994.
11. Toth BB, Martin JW, Chambers MS, et al: Oral cancer, leukoplakia, and chemoprevention. Oral Dis Update 3:8–9, 1997.
12. Andres C: Survey of materials used in extraoral maxillofacial prosthetics. In Setcos JC (ed): Transactions of The Academy of Dental Materials: Proceedings of Conference on Materials Research in Maxillofacial Prosthetics, vol 5, 1992, pp 25–40.
13. Barnhart GW: A new material and technique in the art of somatoprosthesis. J Dent Res 39:836–844, 1960.
14. Beumer JP, Curtis TA, Firtell DN: Maxillofacial Rehabilitation. St. Louis, CV Mosby, 1979, pp 333–334.
15. Beumer JP, Kurrasch M, Kagawa T: Prosthetic restoration of oral defects secondary to surgical removal of oral defects secondary to surgical removal of oral neoplasms. Calif Dent Assoc J 10:47–54, 1982.
16. Hurst PS: Dental considerations in management of head and neck cancer. Otolaryngol Clin North Am 18:573–603, 1985.
17. Lockhart PB, Clark J: Pretherapy dental status of patients with malignant conditions of the head and neck. Oral Surg Oral Med Oral Pathol 77:236–241, 1994.
18. Marciani RD, Ownby HE: Treating patients before and after irradiation. J Am Dent Assoc 123:108–112, 1992.
19. Niehaus CS, Meiller TF, Peterson DE, et al: Oral complications in children during cancer therapy. Cancer Nurs 10:15–20, 1987.
20. Peters E, Monopoli M, Woo SB, et al: Assessment of the need for treatment of postendodontic asymptomatic periapical radiolucencies in bone marrow transplant recipients. Oral Surg Oral Med Oral Pathol 76:45–48, 1993.
21. Wescott WB: Dental management of patients being treated for oral cancer. Calif Dental Assoc J 13:42–47, 1985.
22. Toth BB, Fleming TJ: Oral care for the patient with cancer. Highlights Antineoplastic Drugs 8:27–35, 1990.
23. Toth BB, Martin JW, Fleming TJ: Oral complications associated with cancer therapy: An M.D. Anderson Cancer Center experience. J Clin Periodontol 17:508–515, 1990.
24. Morton ME, Simpson W: The management of osteoradionecrosis of the jaws. Br J Oral Maxillofac Surg 24:332–341, 1986.

25. Morton M, Roberts H: Oral cancer and precancer: After-care and terminal care. Br Dent J 168:283–287, 1990.

26. Poland J: Prevention and treatment of oral complications in the cancer patient. Oncology 5:45–62, 1991.

27. American Dental Association: Head and Neck Cancer Patients Receiving Radiation Therapy. Chicago, American Dental Association, 1989, pp 1–30.

28. Semba SE, Mealey BL, Hallmon WW: The head and neck radiotherapy patient. Part 1. Oral manifestations of radiation therapy. Compend Contin Educ Dent 15:250–261, 1994.

29. Ghalichebaf M, DeBiase CB, Stookey GK: A new technique for the fabrication of fluoride carriers in patients receiving radiotherapy to the head and neck. Compend Contin Educ Dent 15:470–476, 1994.

30. Shrout MK: Managing patients undergoing radiation. J Am Dent Assoc 122:69–70,72, 1991.

31. Lingeman RE, Singer MJ: Evaluation of the patient with head and neck cancer. In Suen JY, Myers EN (eds): Cancer of the Head and Neck. New York, Churchill Livingstone, 1981, pp 15–16.

32. Allard WF, el-Akkad S, Chatmas JC: Obtaining pre-radiation therapy dental clearance. J Am Dent Assoc 124:88–91, 1993.

33. Kluth EV, Jain PR, Stuchell RN, et al: A study of factors contributing to the development of osteoradionecrosis of the jaws. J Prosthet Dent 59:194–201, 1988.

34. Lowe O: Pretreatment dental assessment and management of patients undergoing head and neck irradiation. Clin Prev Dent 8:24–30, 1986.

35. Markitziu A, Zafiropoulos G, Tsalikis L, et al: Gingival health and salivary function in head and neck-irradiated patients. A five year follow up. Oral Surg Oral Med Oral Pathol 73:427–433, 1992.

36. Brady LW, Day JL, Tapley ND: Clinical Applications of Electron Beam Therapy. In Perez CA, Brady LW (eds): Principles and Practices of Radiation Oncology. Philadelphia, Lippincott, 1987, pp 199–212.

37. Toth BB, Chambers MS, Fleming TJ, et al: Minimizing oral complications of cancer treatment. Oncology 9:851–858, 1995.

38. Hays GL, Lippman SM, Flaitz CM, et al: Co-carcinogenesis and field cancerization: Oral lesions offer first signs. J Am Dent Assoc 126:47–51, 1995.

39. Dwyer JT, Efstathion A, Palmer C, et al: Nutritional support in treatment of oral carcinomas. Nutr Rev 49:332–337, 1991.

40. Guo CB, Ma DQ, Zhang KH: Applicability of the general nutritional status score to patients with oral and maxillofacial malignancies. Int J Oral Maxillofac Surg 23:167–169, 1994.

41. McAndrew PG: Oral cancer and precancer: Treatment. Br Dent J 168:191–198, 1990.

42. Lindquist SF, Hickey AJ, Drane JB: Effects of oral hygiene on stomatitis in patients receiving cancer chemotherapy. J Prosthet Dent 40:312–314, 1978.

43. Jackson KC, Chambers MS: Management of oral complications in palliative care. J Pharm Care Pain Symptom Control 8:143–161, 2000.

44. Epstein J, Ransier A, Lunn R: Enhancing the effect of oral hygiene with the use of a foam brush with chlorohexidine. Oral Surg Oral Med Oral Pathol Oral Radiol Endod 77:242–247, 1994.

45. Toth BB, Chambers MS, Fleming TJ: Prevention and management of oral complications associated with cancer therapies: Radiotherapy/chemotherapy. Texas Dent J 113:23–29, 1996.

46. King GE, Lemon JC, Martin JW: Multidisciplinary teamwork in the treatment and rehabilitation of the head and neck cancer patient. Tex Dent J June:9–12, 1992.

47. Ciancio S: Expanded and future uses of mouthrinses. J Am Dent Assoc 125:29S–32S, 1994.

48. Engelmeier RL: A dental protocol for patients receiving radiation therapy for cancer of the head and neck. Spec Care Dentist 7:54–58, 1987.

49. Karr RA, Kramer DC, Toth BB: Dental implants and chemotherapy complications. J Prosthet Dent 67:683–687, 1992.

50. Sager RD, Theis RM: Dental implants placed in a patient with multiple myeloma: Report of a case. J Am Dent Assoc 121:699–701, 1990.

51. Vassos DM: Dental implant treatment in a severely compromised (irradiated) patient. J Oral Implantol 18:142–147, 1992.

52. Makkonen TA, Kiminki A, Makkonen TK, et al: Dental extractions in relation to radiation therapy of 224 patients. Int J Oral Maxillofac Surg 16:56–64, 1987.

53. Peterson DE: Dental care for the cancer patient. Compend Contin Educ Dent 4:115–120, 1983.

54. Marciani R, Ownby H: Osteoradionecrosis of the jaws. J Oral Maxillofac Surg 4:218–223, 1986.

55. Fleming TJ: Oral tissue changes of radiation-oncology and their management. Dent Clin North Am 34:223–237, 1990.

56. McDermott IG, Rosenberg SW: Overdentures for the irradiated patient. J Prosthet Dent 51:314–317, 1984.

57. Schweiger JW: Oral complications following radiation therapy: A five-year retrospective report. J Prosthet Dent 58:78–82, 1987.

58. Chambers MS, Lyzak WS, Martin JW, et al: Oral complications associated with aspergillosis in patients with a hematological malignancy: Presentation and treatment. Oral Surg Oral Med Oral Pathol Oral Radiol Endod 79:559–563, 1995.

59. Toth BB, Martin JW, Chambers MS, et al: Oral candidiasis: A morbid sequela of anticancer therapy. Texas Dent J 115:24–29, 1998.

60. Dreizen S, McCredie KB, Bodey GP, et al: Mucocutaneous herpetic infections during cancer chemotherapy. Postgrad Med 84:181–188, 1988.

61. Wade JC, Newton B, McLaren C, et al: Intravenous acyclovir to treat mucocutaneous herpes simplex virus infection after marrow transplantation: A double blind study. Ann Intern Med 96:265–269, 1982.

62. Whitley RJ, Blum MR, Barton N, et al: Pharmacokinetics of acyclovir in humans following intravenous administration. A model for the development of parenteral antivirals. Am J Med 73:165–171, 1982.

63. Fuller JL, Deneky GE: Concise Dental Anatomy and Morphology, 2nd ed. Chicago, Year Book Medical Publishers, 1984, p 9.

64. Beumer JP, Curtis TA: Restoration of acquired hard palate defects. In Maxillofacial Rehabilitation: Prosthodontic and Surgical Considerations. St. Louis, CV Mosby, 1979, p 188.

65. Chambers MS, Toth BB, Martin JW, et al: Oral and dental management of the cancer patient: Prevention and treatment of complications. Support Care Cancer 3:168–175, 1995.

66. Lingeman RE, Singer MJ: Evaluation of the patient with head and neck cancer. In Sven JY, Myers EN (eds): Cancer of the Head and Neck. New York, Churchill Livingstone, 1981, p 15.

67. Langland OE, Langlais RP, Morris CR: Principles and Practice of Panoramic Radiology. Philadelphia, WB Saunders, 1982.

68. Blaschbe DP, Osborn AG: The mandible and teeth. In Bergeron RT, Osborn AG, San PM (eds): Head and Neck Imaging. St. Louis, CV Mosby, 1984, p 279.

69. King GE, Lemon JC, Martin JW: Multidisciplinary teamwork in the treatment and rehabilitation of the head and neck cancer patient. Tex Dent J 109:9–12, 1992.

70. King GE, Martin JW, Lemon JC, et al: Maxillofacial prosthetic rehabilitation combined with plastic and reconstructive surgery. M.D. Anderson Oncology Case Reports & Review 8:1–11, 1993.

71. Martin JW, Jacob RF, Larson DL, et al: Surgical stents for the head and neck cancer patient. Head Neck Surg 7:44, 1984.

72. Martin JW, Lemon JC, King GE: Maxillofacial restoration after tumor ablation. Clin Plast Surg 21:87–96, 1994.

73. Fleming TJ: Oral tissue changes of radiation-oncology and their management. Dent Clin North Am 34:233–237, 1990.

74. Martin JW, Austin JR, Chambers MS, et al: Postoperative care of the maxillectomy patient. ORL Head Neck Nurs 12:15–20, 1994.

75. King GE, Jacob RFK, Martin JW: Oral and dental rehabilitation. In Johns ME (ed): Complications in Otolaryngology Head and Neck Surgery. Philadelphia, BC Decker, 1986, p 131.

76. Marx RE, Johnson R: Studies in the radiobiology of osteoradionecrosis and their clinical significance. Oral Surg Oral Med Oral Pathol Oral Radiol Endod 64:379–390, 1987.

77. Lemon JC, Martin JW, Jacob RF: Prosthetic rehabilitation. In Weber RS, Miller MJ, Goepfert H (eds): Basal and Squamous Cell Skin Cancers of the Head and Neck. Philadelphia, Williams & Wilkins, 1996, pp 305–312.

78. Barrett NV, Martin JW, Jacob RF, et al: Physical therapy techniques in the treatment of the head and neck patient. J Prosthet Dent 59:343, 1988.

79. Fleming ID, Brady LW, Mieszkalski GB, et al: Basis for major current therapies for cancer. In Murphy GP, Lawrence W, Lenhard RE (eds): American Cancer Society Textbook of Clinical Oncology, 2nd ed. Atlanta, American Cancer Society, 1995, pp 96–134.

80. Dahllöf G, Krekmanova L, Kopp S, et al: Craniomandibular dysfunction in children treated with total-body irradiation and bone marrow transplantation. Acta Odontol Scand 52:99–105, 1994.

81. Dury DC, Roberts NW, Miser JS, et al: Dental root agenesis secondary to irradiation therapy in a case of rhabdomyosarcoma of the middle ear. Oral Surg Oral Med Oral Pathol 57:595–599, 1984.

82. Fleming P: Dental management of the pediatric oncology patient. Curr Opin Dent 1:577–582, 1991.

83. Sonis S, Clark J: Prevention and management of oral mucositis induced by antineoplastic therapy. Oncology 5:11–18, 1991.

84. Borowski B, Benhamou E, Pico JL, et al: Prevention of oral mucositis in patients treated with high-dose chemotherapy and bone marrow transplantation: A randomized controlled trial comparing two protocols of dental care. Eur J Cancer B Oral Oncol 30B:93–97, 1994.

85. Pfeiffer P, Madsen EL, Hansen O: Effect of prophylactic sucralfate suspension on stomatitis induced by cancer chemotherapy. A randomized, double-blind cross-over study. Acta Oncol 29:171–173, 1990.

86. Loprinzi CL, Cianflone SG, Dose AM: A controlled evaluation of an allopurinol mouthwash as prophylaxis against 5-fluorouracil-induced stomatitis. Cancer 65:1879–1882, 1990.

87. Wadleigh RZG, Redman RS, Graham ML: Vitamin E in the treatment of chemotherapy-induced mucositis. Am J Med 92:481–484, 1992.

88. Mills EE: The modifying effects of beta-carotene on radiation- and chemotherapy-induced oral mucositis. Br J Cancer 57:416–417, 1988.

89. Gordon B, Spadinger A, Hodges E: Effect of granulocyte-macrophage colony-stimulating factor on oral mucositis after hematopoietic stem-cell transplantation. J Clin Oncol 12:1917–1922, 1994.

90. Toljanic JA, Saunders VW Jr: Radiation therapy and management of the irradiated patient. J Prosthet Dent 52:852–858, 1984.

91. Keene HJ, Fleming TJ: Prevalence of caries-associated microflora after radiotherapy in patients with cancer of the head and neck. Oral Surg Oral Med Oral Pathol Oral Radiol Endod 64:421–426, 1987.

92. Mandel ID: The role of saliva in maintaining oral homeostasis. J Am Dent Assoc 119:298–303, 1989.

93. Mealey BL, Semba SE, Hallmon WW: The head and neck radiotherapy patient. Part 2. Management of oral complications. Compend Contin Educ Dent 15:442–458, 1994.

94. Samaranayake LP, MacFarlane TW, Lamey PJ, et al: A comparison of oral rinse and imprint sampling techniques for the detection of yeast, coliform and *Staphylococcus aureus* carriage in the oral cavity. J Oral Pathol 15:386–388, 1986.

95. Beumer J, Silverman S Jr, Benak SB Jr: Hard and soft tissue necrosis following radiation therapy for oral cancer. J Prosthet Dent 27:640–644, 1972.

96. Epstein JB, Giuseppe R, Wong FL: Osteoradionecrosis: Study of the relationship of dental extractions in patients receiving radiotherapy. Head Neck Surg 10:48–54, 1987.

97. Rocabardo M, Johnston BE Jr, Blakney MG: Physical therapy and dentistry: An overview. J Craniomandib Pract 1:46–49, 1983.

98. Farmer JC, Shelton PL, Angelillo JF: Treatment of radiation induced tissue injury by hyperbaric oxygen. Ann Otolaryngol 87:707–715, 1978.

99. Mansfield MJ, Sanders DW, Heimbach RD: Hyperbaric oxygen as an adjunct in the treatment of osteoradionecrosis of the mandible. J Oral Surg 39:585–589, 1981.

100. Marx RE, Johnson RP, Kline SN: Prevention of osteoradionecrosis: A randomized prospective clinical trial of hyperbaric oxygen versus penicillin. J Am Dent Assoc 111:49–54, 1985.

101. McClure D, Barker G, Barker B, et al: Oral management of the cancer patient. Part II. Oral complications of radiation therapy. Compend Contin Educ Dent 8:88–92, 1987.

102. Epstein JB, Wong FLW, Stevenson-Moore P: Osteoradionecrosis: Clinical experience and a proposal for classification. J Oral Maxillofac Surg 45:104–110, 1987.

103. Granström G, Jacobsson M, Tjellström A: Titanium implants in irradiated tissues: Benefits from hyperbaric oxygen. Int J Oral Maxillofac Implants 7:15–25, 1992.

104. Liu RP, Fleming TJ, Toth BB: Salivary flow rates in patients with head and neck cancer 0.5 to 25 years after radiotherapy. Oral Surg Oral Med Oral Pathol Oral Radiol Endod 70:724–729, 1990.

105. Keene HJ, Fleming TJ, Toth BB: Cariogenic microflora in patients with Hodgkin's disease before and after mantle field radiotherapy. Oral Surg Oral Med Oral Pathol 78:577–581, 1994.

106. Johnson JT, Feretti GA, Nethery WJ, et al: Oral pilocarpine for post-irradiation xerostomia in patients with head and neck cancer. N Engl J Med 329:390–395, 1993.

107. LeVeque FG, Montgomery M, Potter D, et al: A multicenter, randomized, double-blind, placebo-controlled, dose-titration study of oral pilocarpine for treatment of radiation-induced xerostomia in head and neck cancer patients. J Clin Oncol 11:1124–1131, 1993.

108. Makkonen TA, Minn H, Jekunen A, et al: Granulocyte macrophage-colony stimulating factor (GM-CSF) and sucralfate in prevention of radiation-induced mucositis: A prospective randomized study. Int J Radiat Oncol Biol Phys 46:525–534, 2000.

109. Schneider SB: Filgrastim (r-metHuG-CSF) and its potential use in the reduction of radiation-induced oropharyngeal mucositis: An interim look at a randomized, double-blind, placebo-controlled trial. Cytokines Cell Mol Ther 5:175–180, 1999.

110. Wagner W, Alfrink M, Haus U, et al: Treatment of irradiation-induced mucositis with growth factors (rhGM-CSF) in patients with head and neck cancer. Anticancer Res 19:799–803, 1999.

111. Crawford J: Reduction of oral mucositis by filgrastim (r-metHuG-CSF) in patients receiving chemotherapy. Cytokines Cell Mol Ther 5: 187–193, 1999.

112. Rosso M, Blasi G, Gherlone E, et al: Effect of granulocyte-macrophage colony-stimulating factor on prevention of mucositis in head and neck cancer patients treated with chemo-radiotherapy. J Chemother 9:382–385, 1997.

113. Dorr W, Noack R, Spekl K, et al: Modification of oral mucositis by keratinocyte growth factor: Single radiation exposure. Int J Radiat Biol 77:341–347, 2001.

114. Sonis ST, Van Vugt AG, Brien JP, et al: Transforming growth factor-beta 3 mediated modulation of cell cycling and attenuation of 5-fluorouracil induced mucositis. Oral Oncol 33:47–54, 1997.

115. Sonis ST, Peterson RL, Edwards LJ, et al: Defining mechanisms of action of interleukin-11 on the progression of radiation-induced oral mucositis in hamsters. Oral Oncol 36:373–381, 2000.

116. Huang EY, Leung SW, Wang CJ, et al: Oral glutamine to alleviate radiation-induced oral mucositis: A pilot randomized trial. Int J Radiat Oncol Biol Phys 46:535–539, 2000.

117. Cockerham MB, Weinberger BB, Lerchie SB: Oral glutamine for the prevention of oral mucositis associated with high-dose paclitaxel and melphalan for autologous bone marrow transplantation. Ann Pharmacother 34:300–303, 2000.

118. Brizel DM, Wasserman TH, Henke M, et al: Phase III randomized trial of amifostine as a radioprotector in head and neck cancer. J Clin Oncol 18:3339–3345, 2000.

119. Grotz KA, Wüstenbert R, Kohnen B, et al: Prophylaxis of radiogenic sialadenitis and mucositis by coumarin/troxerutine in patients with head and neck cancer—a prospective, randomized, placebo-controlled, double-blind study. Br J Oral Maxfac Surg 39:34–39, 2001.

120. Ripamonti C, Zecca E, Brunelli C, et al: A randomized, controlled clinical trial to evaluate the effects of zinc sulfate on cancer patients with taste alterations caused by head and neck irradiation. Cancer 82:1938–1945, 1998.

121. Hanson WR: Protection from radiation-induced oral mucositis by a mouth rinse containing the prostaglandin E1 analog, misoprostol: A placebo-controlled, double-blind clinical trial. Adv Exp Med Biol 400:811–818, 1997.

122. Low DA, Chao KS, Mutic S: Quality assurance of serial tomotherapy, for head and neck patient treatment. Int J Radiat Oncol Biol Phys 42:681–689, 1998.

123. Teh BS, Woo SY, Butler EB: Intensity modulated radiation therapy (IMRT): A new promising technology in radiation oncology. Oncologist 4:433–442, 1999.

124. Chalian VA, Drane JB, Standish SM: Maxillofacial Prosthetics, Multidisciplinary Practice. Baltimore, Williams & Wilkins, 1971, pp 178–207.

125. Matalon V: Evaluation of radiotherapists' reports for treatment of prosthodontic patients after irradiation. J Prosthet Dent 38:446, 1977.

126. Rahn AO, Boucher LJ: Maxillofacial Prosthetics, Principles and Concepts. Philadelphia, WB Saunders, 1950, pp 31–82.

127. Rahn AO, Drane JB: Dental aspects of the problems, care and treatment of the irradiated oral cancer patient. J Am Dent Assoc 74:957, 1967.

128. Fleming TJ: Dental care of cancer patients receiving radiotherapy to the head and neck. Cancer Bull 34:63, 1982.

129. Brown LR, Dreizen S, Handler S, et al: The effect of radiation-induced xerostomia on human oral microflora. J Dent Res 54:740, 1975.

130. Dreizen S, Brown LR, Handler S, et al: Radiation-induced xerostomia in cancer patients: Effects on salivary and serum electrolytes. Cancer 38:273, 1976.

131. Dreizen S, Daly TE, Drane JB: Oral complications of cancer radiotherapy. Postgrad Med J 61:85, 1977.

132. Shannon IL, Starke EN, Wescott WB: Effect of radiotherapy on whole saliva flow. J Dent Res 56:693, 1977.

133. Shannon IL, Tradahl JN, Starke EN: Radiosensitivity of the human parotid gland. Proc Soc Exp Biol Med 157:50, 1978.

134. Kaanders JH, Fleming TJ, Ang KK, et al: Devices valuable in head and neck radiotherapy. Int J Radiat Oncol Biol Phys 23:639–645, 1992.

135. Köstler WJ, Hejna M, Wenzel C, et al: Oral mucositis complicating chemotherapy and/or radiotherapy: Options for prevention and treatment. CA Cancer J Clin 51:290–315, 2001.

136. Lenhard RE, Lawrence W, McKenna RJ: General approach to the patient. In Murphy GP, Lawrence W, Lenhard RE (eds): American Cancer Society Textbook of Clinical Oncology, 2nd ed. Atlanta, American Cancer Society, 1995, pp 64–74.

137. Bakemeier RF, Oazi R: Basic concepts of cancer chemotherapy and principles of medical oncology. In Rubin P (ed): Clinical Oncology: A Multidisciplinary Approach for Physicians and Students, 7th ed. Philadelphia, WB Saunders, 1993, pp 105–116.

138. Krakoff IH: Cancer chemotherapeutic and biologic agents. CA Cancer J Clin 41:264–278, 1991.

139. Rosenberg SW: Oral care of chemotherapy patients. Dent Clin North Am 34:239–250, 1990.

140. Nikoskelainen J: Oral infections related to radiation and immunosuppressive therapy. J Clin Periodontol 17:504–507, 1990.

141. Karr RA, Kramer DC: You can treat the chemotherapy patient. Tex Dent J 109:15–20, 1992.

142. Sickles EA, Greene WH, Wiernik PH: Clinical presentation of infection in granulocytopenic patients. Arch Intern Med 135:715–719, 1975.

143. Weinshel EL, Peterson BA: Hodgkin's disease. CA Cancer J Clin 43:325–346, 1993.

144. Greenberg MS, Cohen SG, McKitrick JC: The oral flora as a source of septicemia in patients with acute leukemia. Oral Surg Oral Med Oral Pathol Oral Radiol Endod 315:1501–1505, 1986.

145. Hickey AJ, Toth BB, Lindquist SF: Effects of intravenous hyperalimentation and oral care on the development of oral stomatitis during cancer chemotherapy. J Prosthet Dent 47:188–193, 1982.

146. Meurman JH, Pyrhönen S, Teerenhovi L, et al: Oral sources of septicaemia in patients with malignancies. Oral Oncol 33:389–397, 1997.

147. Overholser CD, Peterson DE, Williams LT, et al: Periodontal infection of patients with acute nonlymphocyte leukemia: Prevalence of acute exacerbations. Arch Intern Med 42:551–554, 1982.

148. Peterson DE, Minah GE, Overholser CD: Microbiology of acute periodontal infection in myelosuppressed cancer patients. J Clin Oncol 5:1461–1468, 1987.

149. Bodey GP: Quantitative relationship between circulating leukocytes and infection in patients with acute leukemia. Ann Intern Med 64:328–340, 1966.

150. Dajani AS, Taubert KA, Wilson W, et al: Prevention of Bacterial Endocarditis: Recommendations by the American Heart Association. Dallas, Lippincott, July 1997, pp 96, 358–366.

151. Everett ED, Hirschmann JV: Transient bacteremia and endocarditis prophylaxis—a review. Medicine 56:61–77, 1977.

152. Epstein JB, Vickars L, Spinelli J, et al: Efficacy of chlorhexidine and nystatin rinses in prevention of oral complications in leukemia and bone marrow transplantation. Oral Surg Oral Med Oral Pathol 73:682–689, 1992.

153. Feretti GA, Ash RC, Brown AT, et al: Chlorhexidine for prophylaxis against oral infections and associated complications in patients receiving bone marrow transplants. J Am Dent Assoc 114:461–467, 1987.

154. Lefkoff MA, Beck FM, Horton JE: The effectiveness of a disposable tooth cleansing device on plaque. J Periodontol 66:218–221, 1995.

155. Pizzo PA: Management of fever in patients with cancer and treatment-induced neutropenia. N Engl J Med 328:1323–1332, 1993.

156. Drugs of choice for cancer chemotherapy. Med Lett 37:25–32, 1995.

157. Toth BB, Frame RT: Dental oncology: The management of disease and treatment-related oral/dental complications associated with chemotherapy. Curr Probl Cancer 7:7–35, 1983.

158. Sonis ST: Mucositis as a biological process: A new hypothesis for the development of chemotherapy-induced stomatotoxicity. Oral Oncol 34:39–43, 1998.

159. Schubert MM, Williams BE, Lloid ME, et al: Clinical assessment scale for the rating of oral mucosal changes associated with bone marrow transplantation: Development of an oral mucositis index. Cancer 69:2469–2477, 1992.

160. Parulekar W, Mackenzie R, Bjarnason G, et al: Scoring oral mucositis. Oral Oncol 34:63–71, 1998.

161. Seto BG, Kim M, Wolinsky L, et al: Oral mucositis in patients undergoing bone marrow transplantation. Oral Surg Oral Med Oral Pathol 60:493–507, 1985.

162. Sonis ST, Eilers JP, Epstein JB, et al: Validation of a new scoring system for the assessment of clinical trial research of oral mucositis induced by radiation or chemotherapy. Cancer 85:2103–2113, 1999.

163. Tang ITL, Shepp DH: Herpes simplex virus infection in cancer patients: Prevention and treatment. Oncology 6:101–109, 1992.

164. Greenberg MS: Oral herpes simplex infections in patients with leukemia. J Am Dent Assoc 114:483–486, 1987.

165. MacPhail LA, Hilton JF, Heinic GS, et al: Direct immunofluorescence vs. culture for detecting HSV in oral ulcers: A comparison. J Am Dent Assoc 126:74–78, 1995.

166. Montgomery MT, Redding SW, LeMaistre CF: The incidence of oral herpes simplex virus infection in patients undergoing cancer chemotherapy. Oral Surg Oral Med Oral Pathol 61:238–242, 1986.

167. Flaitz CM, Hammond HL: The immunoperoxidase method for the rapid diagnosis of intraoral herpes simplex virus infection in patients receiving bone marrow transplants. Spec Care Dent 8:82–85, 1988.

168. Teichgraeber J, Larson DL, Castaneda O, et al: Skin grafts in intraoral reconstruction: A new stenting method. Arch Otolaryngol Head Neck Surg 101:463, 1984.

169. Cordeiro PG, Wolfe SA: The temporalis muscle flap revisited on its centennial: Advantages, newer uses, and disadvantages. Plast Reconstr Surg 98:980–987, 1996.

170. Sisson GA, Becker SP: Cancer of the nasal cavity and paranasal sinuses. In Suen JY, Myers EN (eds): Cancer of the Head and Neck. New York, Churchill Livingstone, 1981, pp 242–279.

171. Swartz WM, Banis JC, Newton D, et al: The osteocutaneous scapular flap for mandibular and maxillary reconstruction. Plast Reconstr Surg 77:530, 1986.

172. Desjardins RP: Early rehabilitative management of the maxillectomy patient. J Prosthet Dent 38:311–338, 1977.

173. King GE, Chambers MS, Martin JW: Patient appointments during interim obturation: Is it cost-effective? J Prosthod 4:168–172, 1995.

174. Krugmen M, Beumer J: Maxillectomy cavity care with a pulsating stream irrigator. Eye Ear Nose Throat Mon 54:104, 1975.

175. Hammond J: Dental care of the edentulous patient after resection of the maxilla. Br Dent J 120:591, 1966.

176. Kottke FJ, Stillwell GK, Lehmann JF: Krusen's Handbook of Physical Medicine and Rehabilitation, 3rd ed. Philadelphia, WB Saunders, 1982, pp 102–123.

177. Schusterman MA, Reece GP, Miller MJ, et al: The osteocutaneous free fibula flap: Is the skin paddle reliable? Plast Reconstr Surg 90: 787, 1992.

178. Godoy AJ, Perez DG, Lemon JC, et al: Rehabilitation of a patient with limited oral opening following glossectomy. Int J Prosthod 4: 70–74, 1991.

179. Cantor R, Curtis T: Prosthetic management of edentulous mandibulectomy patients. Part II: Clinical procedures. J Prosthet Dent 25:546, 1971.

180. Marunick MT, Harrison R, Beumer J: Prosthodontic rehabilitation of midfacial defects. J Prosthet Dent 54:553–560, 1985.

181. Martin JW, Lemon JC: Prosthetic rehabilitation. In Bailey BJ (ed): Head and Neck Surgery—Otolaryngology. Philadelphia, JB Lippincott, 1993, pp 1431–1438.

182. Parr GR, Goldman BM, Rahn AO: Maxillofacial prosthetic principles in the surgical planning for facial defects. J Prosthet Dent 46:323, 1981.

183. Martin JW, Lemon JC, King GE: Oral and facial restoration after reconstruction. In Kroll S (ed): Reconstructive Plastic Surgery for Cancer. St. Louis, Mosby, 1996, pp 130–138.

184. Javid J: The use of magnets in a maxillofacial prosthesis. J Prosthet Dent 25:234, 1971.

185. Udagama A, King GE: Mechanically retained facial prostheses: Helpful or harmful? J Prosthet Dent 49:85, 1983.

186. Martin JW, Lemon JC, Jacobsen ML, et al: Extraoral retention of an obturator prosthesis. J Prosthodont 1:65–68, 1992.

CHAPTER 30

Nursing Care

Mary Ann Horn
Jenny W. Badley

INTRODUCTION

Nursing care of the head and neck cancer patient can be one of the most difficult and challenging, yet possibly one of the most rewarding, arenas of holistic nursing care delivery. The scope of this nursing practice area is bounded only by the individual nurse's imagination and interest.

As humans, we rely on the socialization of face-to-face contact, dialogue with those in our surrounding environment, sharing a meal with family or friends, and the most basic functions of an intact airway. By the very nature of the disease, those who suffer from head and neck cancer are affected in those most vital areas of their existence—where they breathe, where they communicate, where they take in nourishment, and where they identify themselves as individuals. "... It is considered by many to be the most dreaded site for cancer to occur, as both the disease and treatment cannot be hidden from view."[1]

This area of nursing abounds with opportunities for creativity and self-expression in providing a constant, assuring atmosphere as well as excellent nursing care for the patient with head and neck cancer. Advances in surgical as well as nonsurgical treatment of patients with cancer of the head and neck continue to improve cure rates and to enhance quality of life through improved function and cosmesis. For nurses, knowledge of head and neck anatomy and function, disease process, treatment modalities, medications and their adverse effects, and signs of complications is integral to the care of these patients. The head and neck oncology nurse has the task of teaching, intervening when necessary, and fostering return of independent function to the highest degree possible. The care provided must reflect an attitude of compassion without pity, optimism without false hope, and support without dependence.[2]

PATIENT ASSESSMENT AND DIAGNOSIS

The first contact with the patient who has cancer of the head and neck can often be the most crucial. The individual presents either with a confirmed diagnosis of cancer of the head and neck or with suspicious signs and symptoms of the disease. This is a time of great stress for the patient, family, and significant others. An astute practitioner will be aware of this when eliciting a history from the patient. Clear facts regarding the chief complaint, the onset of symptoms, and any other related information are pivotal in facilitating an accurate and speedy diagnosis.

The patient must be questioned regarding risk factors and medical, surgical, and social history, as well as allergies. Data regarding medications the patient takes must extend to over-the-counter medications, herbal medications, and alternative and health food regimens. During this time, spiritual and cultural attitudes may be revealed.[3]

Important information regarding dysphagia, odynophagia, weight loss, and difficulty breathing must be assessed. Pain and its properties (location, onset, precipitating factors, relieving factors, quality, and duration) can afford a great number of clues about the patient's diagnosis. Attitudes toward pain vary greatly among individuals. Another risk factor is the use of tobacco, alcohol, and illicit drugs. A nonjudgmental attitude fosters accuracy in this area of history taking. The patient, if possible, should be the primary source of information, but the family or significant others may contribute, and previously acquired data can be supplied by the referring physician.

The physical examination during the initial visit must be thorough. The overall appearance of the head and neck region is noted, as are skin lesions, obvious deformities, or visible lymphadenopathy. The function of the cranial nerves must also be assessed. The ears, nose, oral cavity, oropharynx, hypopharynx, larynx, and neck are assessed. In addition, the physician must use a flexible or rigid nasopharyngoscope to visualize the nasal cavity, nasopharynx, oropharynx, hypopharynx, and larynx. Explanation of the rationale and technique of these procedures can alleviate the patient's anxiety.[4] If topical decongestants or anesthetics are used, allergies to these substances must be assessed. The patient should be made aware of the numbness associated with use of a topical anesthetic.

After the initial examination has been completed, it is usually necessary to obtain a biopsy for histologic or cytologic diagnosis of any noted suspicious areas. A fine-needle aspiration biopsy may be performed in patients with a palpable mass in the neck. Tumors arising in the oral cavity are readily accessible, and the biopsy can be done in the office with the patient under local anesthesia with the use of cup forceps or punch biopsy. Patients with a tumor in the larynx or hypopharynx require endoscopy and biopsy performed under general anesthesia. Patients with cancer of the head and neck usually undergo a panendoscopy and biopsy before the surgical resection is begun. This is a combination of laryngoscopy, esophagoscopy, and in select cases, bronchoscopy.

It is necessary for the clinician to thoroughly evaluate the tumor, as well as its extension to other surrounding structures, and to detect the presence of second primary tumors in the upper aerodigestive tract. Nonpalpable tumors noted on radiographic studies may require image-guided biopsy. Complete evaluation of the patient's disease status will probably include other diagnostic procedures such as computed tomographic (CT) scans of the head, neck, and chest; magnetic resonance imaging (MRI); barium swallow studies; pulmonary function studies; Panorex radiograph; bone scans; angiography; and laboratory evaluations. These are ordered at the physician's discretion to assess the extent of the lesions, metastatic disease, involvement of the mandible, or vascularity of the lesion. The patient's subjective symptoms may alert the clinician to possible areas of metastasis that require further evaluation.

Because most tumors of the head and neck spread by direct extension or spread regionally to the cervical lymph nodes, a full metastatic evaluation is not warranted unless the patient exhibits symptoms suggestive of metastasis. Chest radiographs are performed routinely as part of the baseline medical evaluation to rule out a second primary tumor in the lung or metastasis. If no evidence of disease is detected, further evaluation may not be necessary. During this phase of the patient's treatment, it is crucial for health care professionals to remember that lack of diagnosis can be the single most anxiety-provoking aspect of the entire cancer experience. Oftentimes, patients express relief even when the diagnosis is proved to be cancer because the known entity is perceived to be much easier to deal with than the stress of not knowing the actual diagnosis.

◘ TREATMENT CHOICES AND PSYCHOLOGICAL PREPARATION

Treatments for head and neck cancer have seen great strides in recent years. The prospects of cure with surgery, radiation, combined chemotherapy, or a combination of any of these modalities are on the rise. In addition to standard therapy, the efficacy of many novel treatments is being investigated in patients with cancer of the head and neck. The multitude of treatment choices can be very confusing to the patient.[1]

After diagnosis, the physician will explain to the patient the nature and extent of the disease; various treatment options will be discussed, and the optimal treatment strategy will be recommended. The nurse can reiterate therapy recommendations, reinforce the physician's rationale, and answer questions for the patient or significant others.

If the primary choice for definitive treatment is surgery, the patient enters the preoperative phase of treatment. In this phase, the nurse plays a major role in physical and psychological preparation of the patient. The psychological preparation of the patient is integrated with all aspects of care provided from the moment the patient is first seen by the health care team. The primary area of concern to patients and families is usually the diagnosis of cancer. The

patient may also bring to the preoperative experience preconceived notions, hearsay information, or negative past experiences of family members. Accurate information is of ultimate importance. The health care team must work with the patient and significant others to help each one understand and cope with the diagnosis. Hope must be encouraged and balanced with realistic expectations.

In addition to the diagnosis of cancer, there may be great concern regarding the treatment modality selected. Fears of mutilation, pain, loss of control, and death are associated with all forms of cancer therapy, and these fears must be handled on an individual basis. Loss of normal communication skills, fear of not being able to eat regular food, altered body image, and problems of sexuality are other sources of anxiety for the patient and family. Techniques for communication after surgery must be reviewed with the patient. Initially, every effort is made to anticipate the patient's needs. During the postoperative period, communication by writing is encouraged. If the patient is illiterate, flash cards can be developed, or the patient can use a communication picture board to indicate needs. Even with permanent loss of voice, alternative methods of communication are available to the patient.[5]

Alterations in body image and sexuality may be an area of concern to both the patient and the significant other. During the preoperative phase, most patients are concerned about "surviving the operation and eliminating the cancer." Consequently, fear of body image alteration is usually not expressed until after surgery. Changes in appearance occur as a consequence of many head and neck cancer operations. It must be emphasized to the patient that every possible rehabilitative measure will be provided to minimize the change but that removing the cancer is the primary goal.[6] Explanations about the extent of surgical resection may also be helpful in minimizing fears. Reinforcement should be offered to the patient and partner regarding appearance and the ability to function sexually. By displaying affection, the partner can do much to alleviate the fear expressed by the patient. Special counseling may be necessary to help the patient and the partner cope with this problem.[7]

◘ MULTIDISCIPLINARY TEAM REFERRALS

Referrals to other members of the health care team are made during the preoperative period. This allows the patient and family to incorporate information and possible body and lifestyle changes in a more controlled manner.

In addition to the patient's physician, other professionals may be asked to assist the patient. Included in the team are the nurse specialist, audiologist, speech pathologist, occupational therapist, physical therapist, social worker, maxillofacial prosthodontist, nutritionist, radiation oncologist, medical oncologist, internal medicine physician, plastic reconstructive surgeon, and gastrointestinal surgeon. It is the physician's responsibility to determine which services should be consulted so that maximum benefit can be provided to the patient. The nurse specialist usually coordinates these services and assesses the patient's needs, both physical and psychosocial.

The audiologist is consulted to assess the patient's ability to hear. This is done to rule out hearing loss that could interfere with the patient's ability to communicate postoperatively. Tumors causing eustachian tube dysfunction, such as tumors of the nasopharynx and palate, can cause middle ear effusion and conductive hearing loss. Tumors involving the temporal bone or the skull base can invade the eighth cranial nerve and result in sensorineural hearing loss. Surgery, radiation, and chemotherapy may result in additional hearing loss, further downgrading the patient's ability to achieve effective communication.

The speech-language pathologist is a vital member of the head and neck team. These individuals provide diagnostic testing and therapy for patients with swallowing disorders, as well as speech rehabilitation and exercises for patients with speaking deficits. Information regarding tracheoesophageal prosthesis is offered when appropriate; if it is determined that the patient is a candidate for the procedure, it may be done at the time of the laryngectomy. Intensive teaching and therapy are required for each patient during the entire perioperative and rehabilitation periods.

The assistance of the maxillofacial prosthodontist is crucial. Special intraoral appliances that facilitate speech and swallowing are fabricated. Preoperative impressions are required if an appliance is needed in the immediate postoperative period. For patients requiring radiation therapy, a thorough dental evaluation and treatment or removal of carious teeth will be necessary before treatment is initiated. Instructions for long-term care, including fluoride treatment, are provided. The facial prosthetics team is consulted for patients undergoing orbital exenteration, rhinectomy, or other ablative surgery requiring aesthetic rehabilitation. This skill is highly technical and requires much empathy and sensitivity to provide the patient with the best possible result.

The social worker will perform a patient/family psychosocial assessment in the preoperative period. During the assessment, discharge planning will begin. Discussions of where the patient will go following hospitalization, who will be available to assist the patient, employment concerns, and financial concerns must occur early in the treatment process.

The occupational or physical therapist is consulted for patients undergoing neck dissection. The spinal accessory nerve is often stretched or even sacrificed if it is involved with tumor. Special exercises taught by the therapist are required to maintain maximal range of motion and muscle strength. Occasionally, it is necessary that the patient wear a clavicle brace to prevent pain associated with shoulder drop.

For patients who need assistance with strengthening or progressive ambulation, physical therapy is beneficial. Patients having mandibular reconstruction with fibular free grafts must also be given instructions by physical therapists in non-weightbearing ambulation. This allows the affected limb adequate healing time.

In addition to symptoms of pain and difficulty in swallowing, the patient may exhibit substantial weight loss before diagnosis. A nutritional assessment performed by the nursing staff or a nutritionist should be completed early in the hospital period. Daily weight, anthropometric measurements, blood evaluation measurements, and calorie and protein intake recordings should be kept routinely for all patients. The nutritionist interacts directly with the patient and family but must also participate in patient care conferences to update the health care team on the patient's progress.

Radiation oncologists, internists, general surgeons, plastic and reconstructive surgeons, neurosurgeons, gastroenterologists, and medical oncologists are consulted when their expertise is needed. Plastic surgeons and general surgeons are extensively integrated into the team for reconstruction as well as placement of gastrostomy tubes or central venous ports.

▣ SURGICAL TREATMENT

Preoperative Preparation

The nurse is important in organizing the preoperative testing procedures and coordinating schedules to ease travel time and stress for the patient. When the patient has decided, on the advice of the physician, to undergo surgery, time is of a premium in most cases. Ongoing explanations and reinforcement in teaching can be the most reassuring factor in the surgical preparation. Use of models, handouts, and diagrams, as well as hands-on illustrations of medical supplies, are of great value to the patient, especially those who learn best visually. Written instructions are essential because the patient and family are overloaded with new information at this time. Seeing the physician draw the anatomic alteration can be helpful for the patient to fully understand the planned procedure. Often, a visit from a patient who has undergone a similar procedure can be invaluable to the patient. The nurse must be sensitive to the patient's needs and to what level of information brings the most comfort to him or her regarding the surgery ahead. Hands-on contact with drains, feeding tubes, actual tracheotomy tubes, and dressing supplies can remove the "mystique" and fear associated with these trappings of the planned procedure.

A brief description of the schedule of the hospitalization period will help the patient and family understand the need for the intensive care unit, overnight recovery observation, and the planned length of stay. The patient must also be educated regarding anesthesia, admission the morning of surgery, medications to be taken, preoperative consults, and the hospital rules that apply to family and visitors. Knowing the rationale for these aspects can take much of the confusion out of preoperative planning. Information regarding discharge and postdischarge care is also presented at this time, as are plans for supplies, equipment, and medical provider companies.

The single most important aspect of preoperative preparation is providing patients with contact information, should they have any questions or concerns. This is a crucial link for the patient once he or she leaves the medical facility. If the patient has the comfort and confidence of reestablishing a connection to a key person, his or her ability to cope with the difficulties associated with treatment, as well as to accept the plans ahead, will improve. This is an excellent time to reassure the patient that even though pain is expected, pain relief is a priority. Often just knowing that this is a priority to the health care team will allay fears and decrease actual postoperative pain levels. Clarification of pain level and characteristics is valuable at this time. The patient should know that in many cases, the level of pain usually is less severe after the tumor has been removed. Establishing a form of communication in the event the patient may not be able to communicate verbally is necessary at this time. Assurances should be given to the patient and the family that message boards, writing tablets, or other means of communication will be available for him or her postoperatively to convey his or her needs.

Briefing the patient on nursing procedures is helpful and can be reinforced by nurses in the preoperative, intraoperative, and postoperative specialty areas if possible. The family and significant others should be given general time frames for the procedure, recovery, hospitalization, and rehabilitation, but flexibility in schedules should be urged. Every individual behaves differently. Soliciting questions from the patient and family will assure them that their needs are recognized and will be met by the entire health care staff as the operative experience progresses.

Postoperative Phase

The nature of many surgical procedures used in treating cancer of the head and neck requires that the patient may be kept in an intensive care setting postoperatively. Extensive surgical resections and microvascular tissue transfers and the presence of a tracheotomy warrant close, one-on-one, high-level medical and nursing care in the immediate postoperative period. Airway management is the first priority, and the patient may be on the ventilator for the first 12 to 36 hours. Risk factors that are responsible for cancer of the head and neck can also increase the risk of postoperative cardiac, vascular, pulmonary, renal, or hepatic complications. Wound care, oral care, tracheotomy care, fluid and electrolyte management, and pain control must be optimized and stabilized in the immediate postoperative period. It is essential that the nurse-clinician have an extensive knowledge of the operative procedures performed. Only through understanding of the surgical procedure can comprehensive holistic care be provided. By understanding these procedures, the nurse may then confidently take medical intervention one step farther, that is, to include education, psychosocial support, and empathy, which are necessary for the provision of competent nursing care.

Airway Management

The most important and demanding aspect of nursing care of patients undergoing head and neck surgery is management of the airway. Many patients undergoing head and neck surgery require a tracheotomy to avoid airway obstruction from postoperative edema or other anatomic alterations. Positioning the head of the patient's bed at 30 to 45 degrees is the first step in managing the airway of the postsurgical patient with or without a tracheotomy. This elevation eases the process of air exchange and minimizes postoperative edema, which may contribute to airway obstruction.

A tracheotomy tube with a high volume–low pressure cuff is usually used during the postoperative period. The inflatable cuff protects the airway from aspiration of secretions and provides a seal between the tube and the trachea for assisted or controlled ventilation. If the cuff is increased to an abnormally high pressure, necrosis of the tracheal mucosa may occur. Careful observation is required to monitor the inflation pressure of the cuff. Deflating the cuff is recommended when the risk of aspiration is minimal.

The type of tracheotomy tube used will vary according to the physician's preference, institutional guidelines, and the physique of the individual patient. Anatomic differences such as a short, thick neck can present special circumstances that require a specialized tracheotomy tube that is longer than usual. Nonstandard tracheotomy tubes require a special order from the manufacturer with the measurements taken before or at the time of the surgical procedure, which is very impractical. Operating rooms should have a supply of tubes that have an adjustable neck plate so that the length of the tube can be adjusted to the neck of the patient (Fig. 30–1).

Most tracheotomy tubes have three parts—an inner cannula, an outer cannula, and an obturator. The obturator is placed into the outer cannula to provide a smooth tip as the outer cannula is introduced into the patient's tracheotomy site. Once proper placement has been achieved, the obturator is removed and the outer cannula is left in place and secured by suturing the neck plate to the skin (Fig. 30–2). The inner cannula is placed inside the outer cannula. Some tracheotomy tubes have a disposable inner cannula that may be replaced according to institutional guidelines. If bulky or pressure dressings are used over the neck, the inner cannula must have a flap to prevent occlusion of the tube by the dressing.

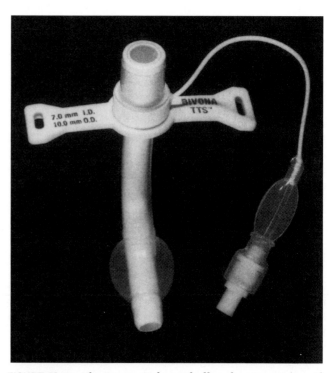

FIGURE 30–1 The Bivona Tight to Shaff tracheostomy tube with cuff inflated.

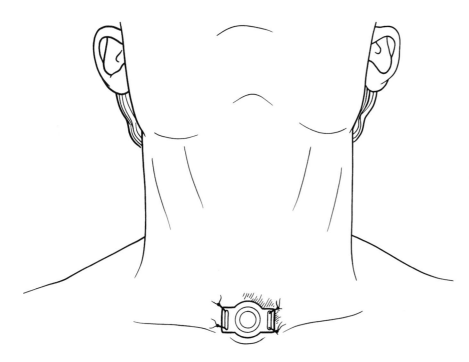

FIGURE 30–2 The neck plate of the tracheostomy tube is sutured to the skin to avoid the use of tapes. (From Myers EN: Tracheostomy. In Myers EN, Carrau RL, Cass SP, et al [eds]: Operative Otolaryngology–Head and Neck Surgery. Philadelphia, WB Saunders, 1997, pp 575–585.)

In the patient with a tracheotomy tube, the single most important postsurgical step is to keep the airway clear of secretions. The patient should be encouraged to cough and breathe deeply every 1 to 2 hours. Coughing clears the airway and also expands the lungs to prevent atelectasis and pneumonia. If the patient has a decreased coughing effort or thickened secretions resulting in ineffective cough, the trachea must be suctioned frequently.

The following equipment is needed to suction a patient's airway: a 14F suction catheter, a wall-mounted or portable suction unit that applies 40 to 60 mm Hg of pressure, and a container filled with sterile water. Suction to the trachea should be applied only upon withdrawal of the catheter, the catheter should be rotated as it is withdrawn, and suction should be applied for no longer than 10 seconds before the patient is allowed to breathe. Irrigating the tracheotomy tube with normal saline will thin secretions and make them more easily removable. Routine instillation of saline every 4 hours is helpful in preventing mucus plugs in patients with a double-cannula tracheotomy tube; this is done every 1 to 2 hours in patients with a single-cannula tracheotomy tube (a tube without an inner cannula). Care should be taken when suctioning not to traumatize the trachea because this will result in bleeding. Gentle suctioning of the oral and nasal cavities may also be performed to clear secretions, but a different catheter should be used. Approximately 3 days after the tracheotomy has been performed, the physician may change the patient's cannula from a cuffed to a cuffless one. This tube exerts less pressure on the tracheal mucosa, is easier to manage, and provides the patient with the ability to speak. This is important, especially if the tracheotomy tube will be used over a long term and the patient will be discharged home with the cannula in place.

The inner cannula of the tracheotomy tube should be removed for cleaning every 2 to 4 hours to maintain the patency of the airway. The tracheotomy tube is cleaned with a solution of hydrogen peroxide and water and a nylon-bristle brush. A specialized tracheotomy tube brush may be used, or the patient may use a brush such as is used to clean baby bottle nipples. After the inner cannula has been soaked and thoroughly cleaned with the tracheotomy tube brush, it is replaced within the outer cannula. The inner cannula should be securely locked into place to prevent dislodging when the patient coughs. The collar of the outer cannula and the skin around the tracheotomy are cleaned with hydrogen peroxide and cotton-tipped applicators to loosen any crust. If the patient has a neck dressing, it may not be possible to clean around the outer cannula until the neck dressing has been removed. The area is then rinsed well with water or saline to prevent skin irritation from the peroxide. A thin coat of antibiotic ointment may be applied to the surrounding skin and the collar of the tracheotomy tube to help maintain hygiene of the tube. Neomycin compounds can cause inflammation of the skin in some patients and should be avoided. A dry gauze sponge or a special tracheotomy dressing may be used under the collar of the tracheotomy tube to prevent irritation from the tube and tracheal secretions. This dressing must be changed frequently to prevent skin irritation from the moisture in the dressing. An alternative is to avoid placement of a dressing. This prevents the accumulation of secretions in the dressing that may irritate the skin. Tracheotomy ties are used to secure the cannula and prevent it from sliding out of the trachea. The ties must be loose enough to allow entry of the fingertips under them, thereby avoiding excessive pressure and facilitating cleaning of the skin beneath the tube collar. Ties should be changed when soiled. New ties should be secured before the soiled ties are removed to prevent dislodging of the tube, which may precipitate an airway emergency.

The initial removal of the entire tracheotomy cannula (both inner and outer) is the responsibility of the physician.

Future changes by the nursing team depend on the hospital policy and the individual physician's preference.

Tracheostoma covering is necessary to provide filtering, humidification, and cosmesis for the patient. Various covers may be used, including crocheted covers, commercially made foam rubber shields, turtleneck sweaters or shirts, or specially created beaded or jeweled shields.[8]

Humidification in the tracheotomy patient is essential to prevent mucus plugging of the tracheotomy tube. A humidified tracheotomy collar or bedside humidifier usually provides adequate humidification. Normal saline drops or sprays can be used three or four times a day to increase humidification. The center of the stoma cover can be moistened with water to add humidification to the air.

When the patient has recovered postoperatively to the point that he or she can readily visualize the tracheotomy site, the nurse should begin teaching tracheotomy care to the patient. The patient can be taught to clean the inner cannula as well as the skin around the tracheostoma. If the patient has had a laryngectomy and a tracheostoma tube is required, instructions for changing and cleaning the entire tube can be given after the tube is removed the first time for cleaning.

Teaching the patient tracheotomy suction techniques varies according to patient needs, physician preference, and hospital policy. Professional health care workers should perform the tracheal suctioning because trauma to the tracheal mucosa may occur. At discharge, most patients are managing their secretions adequately and do not need home suctioning. It is important to emphasize to the patient the necessity of deep breathing, coughing techniques, and proper humidification to maintain a clear airway. The patient may feel more comfortable having a suction machine at home for emergency use in the case of a mucus plug or thick secretion that he or she is unable to mobilize by coughing.

When the physician has determined that postoperative edema has subsided to the point that the patient no longer needs the tracheotomy cannula, it is removed and the stoma is allowed to close. The site does not require suture or closure, so gauze dressing is used for the first few days. The patient is instructed to apply pressure over the site when talking, swallowing, or coughing to prevent air and secretions from coming through the stoma and blocking closure.

Wound Care

Wound care requiring close observation and immediate action is imperative in the immediate postoperative phase to prevent complications. The wound of the head and neck patient consists of a surgical incision on the skin and often an intraoral and/or a pharyngeal incision.

DRAINAGE

One responsibility of the nurse postoperatively is to check the drain for adequate drainage. The amount of drainage may vary depending on the surgical procedure and the number of catheters inserted. For example, approximately 100 to 150 mL of sanguineous drainage is expected during the first 24 hours following radical neck dissection. A daily decrease in the amount of drainage is anticipated, with a change to serous drainage within 48 hours. The drainage

catheters must remain patent to prevent accumulation of fluid under the skin flap. Neck drains may be aspirated every 4 to 6 hours with the use of a blunt-tipped needle or angiocatheter. In addition, the tubing can be "milked" to remove any clots adherent to the catheters. The physician should be notified if the drainage becomes milky or contains particulate matter, which would imply a chylous or a salivary leak.

The first 24 to 72 hours is critical in monitoring the amount and consistency of the drainage to assess early for any possible postoperative complications. The drainage should be measured and recorded according to hospital policy, with a total given once every 24-hour period. The drain will be removed when drainage is minimal.

An opening in the skin that results from wound infection known as a *fistula* presents a complicated nursing care challenge. Nursing care of the fistula consists of physical cleaning of the wound, as well as psychological reassurance to the patient, who often becomes depressed because of the prolonged hospitalization and increased care requirements.

WOUND COMPLICATIONS

Possible wound complications that may occur in the head and neck patient include hematoma and seroma formation, loss of flap viability, infection with or without a salivary leak, chylous fistula, and carotid rupture. These complications can occur at any time in the postoperative period, but the first 24 to 72 hours is the most crucial time.

Hematoma and Seroma. An increase in the amount of bloody drainage, edema of the neck, sudden tightness of the neck dressing, or excessive bruising or ecchymosis of the skin of the neck and upper chest should alert the nurse to the development of a hematoma. An increase in the amount of serous drainage, edema, and tightness of the neck dressing may indicate a seroma. If a patient does not have a tracheotomy and a hematoma does develop, the patient should be watched closely for any signs of airway distress.

Fistula. The nurse should also observe the patient for signs of a chylous fistula. A chylous fistula is the result of a lymphatic leak (usually from the thoracic duct on the left side). The wound drainage may appear opaque or milky after the patient is fed if a chylous fistula is present. Fluid and electrolyte imbalances can occur in the presence of a chyle leak; therefore, monitoring of the laboratory data is essential. A low-fat diet is used to help decrease production of chyle.

Rupture of the Carotid Artery. Rupture of the carotid artery is a life-threatening emergency that can occur at any time during the postoperative period from hours, days, to weeks after surgery. Carotid artery rupture is usually the result of wound breakdown, fistula formation, necrosis, or loss of cervical skin flap and exposure of the vessel. The first warning signal may be a small trickle of blood. The nurse who acts rapidly in response to this sentinel bleeding can prevent a fatal outcome. The surgeon should be notified immediately. Precautions that should be taken in the patient who has the potential for a carotid artery rupture include close monitoring, current typing and cross-matching of blood, and keeping some supplies and equipment at the bedside, such as gloves, heavy gauze pads, hemostats, IV administration set with solution, cut-down tray, suture set, and a cuffed tracheotomy tube. If carotid artery rupture occurs, the nurse should apply firm pressure to the bleeding site, inflate the cuff of the tracheotomy tube, suction the trachea as needed, start an IV line or increase the fluid rate of the present IV line, remain with the patient, and call for assistance. If the patient is in a terminal state and a do-not-resuscitate (DNR) order has been documented, no effort should be made to resuscitate the patient.[9]

DRESSING

Depending on physician preference, neck pressure dressings may be applied after surgery to prevent collection of fluid, which might interfere with wound healing. The dressing requires close observation for excess drainage. The dressing should be tight enough to help keep the skin flap flat but loose enough to prevent airway compromise in the patient without a tracheotomy or to prevent a choking feeling in the patient with a tracheotomy. The tightness of the dressing can be checked by placing two fingers under its edge. If the fingers fit with minimal difficulty, the dressing is adequate.

Neck dressings are usually removed 24 hours after postoperative drains have been discontinued. After the neck dressing has been removed, the suture line is cleaned with hydrogen peroxide and water, and a thin coat of antibiotic ointment is applied twice a day (Fig. 30–3).

POSITIONING

Proper positioning of the patient after head and neck surgery is essential to prevent edema of the face and neck. The head of the bed should be elevated at least 45 degrees, and the patient should avoid sleeping on the operative side. The patient's input and output should be monitored to rule out fluid overload, which could increase facial edema. Also, if a dressing is excessively tight, the edges may have to be cut to help decrease facial edema.

FLAP VIABILITY

Flap viability is another important aspect of nursing care in the postoperative period in patients who had an anteriorly

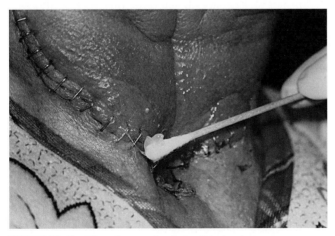

FIGURE 30–3 Wound care: Apply antibiotic ointment to suture line.

based regional, pedicle, or free-flap reconstruction. Dressings usually are not used in these patients, as they may compromise the circulation and cause excessive pressure on the flap. The patient is positioned with the head at 30 to 45 degrees and rotated toward the flap site. Tracheotomy ties are avoided, and the tracheotomy tube is sutured to the skin to eliminate pressure on a flap caused by the ties. Other items avoided are down-ties and humidification collars. If needed, humidification collars should be applied loosely or pinned to clothing. It is imperative that close observation of drain patency be maintained to prevent accumulation of fluid under the flap and constriction of the blood supply. Frequent monitoring of the flap for color, temperature, edema, and drainage is imperative for early detection of decreased flap viability. Often, a laser Doppler monitor is used in the first 24 to 72 hours to rapidly detect any circulation problems in the flap.[10]

DONOR SITES

If a split-thickness skin graft is used as a reconstructive method, the nurse must monitor the recipient and donor sites. Care of the recipient site involves keeping the edges clean and reinforcing the dressing as indicated. This can be difficult if dressing packs known as bolsters are sutured over the graft for the first 5 postoperative days. The bolster places pressure on the skin graft, enabling it to adhere to the new tissue bed. This immobilization of the skin graft to the underlying recipient tissue is essential to the development of new vascularity within the skin graft. The bolster is usually removed on the fifth postoperative day.

Dressings applied to the skin graft donor site vary according to physician choice but include (1) clear, translucent types that remain over the area until the donor site has healed and (2) supra-absorbent types that remain over the area for 7 days. A gauze dressing is not suggested because the epithelial cells grow into the gauze, and removal is painful and causes bleeding. A heat lamp may be used to promote drying of some types of dressings and should be used according to hospital policy and physician choice. Use of a heat lamp should be monitored closely and should not exceed 20-minute intervals two or three times a day. It is important to keep the heat lamp positioned at least 24 to 30 inches from the patient to prevent accidental burns.

Other Complications. Patients who have undergone a combination craniofacial resection and lateral rhinotomy for removal of sinonasal tumors should be monitored for additional complications, including cerebrospinal fluid leak and neurologic changes. Continuous nasal drainage should be reported to the physician. The patient should be instructed to avoid blowing the nose, sneezing with the mouth closed, lifting more than 5 pounds, and straining during bowel movements. A stool softener should be given routinely. Saline nasal spray should be used two or three times daily to soften crusting and facilitate removal. Only an experienced physician should examine and debride the nasal cavity, as inexpert care could damage the reconstructive flap or cause a cerebrospinal fluid leak. A neurologic examination to assess cognitive changes should be done every 4 to 8 hours for 1 or 2 days postoperatively. Heavy sedation should be avoided to ease the assessment of these changes.

Flap Donor Site Care

In some patients, a large flap consisting of skin and muscle or of skin, muscle, and bone is needed to reconstruct an area after excision of tumor. Microvascular free flaps are harvested from a donor site and transferred with their own nutrient blood vessels for microvascular anastomosis with blood vessels at the recipient site. This procedure may be done with a second surgeon who is experienced in free-flap reconstruction. Forearm, fibula, rectus abdominis, latissimus dorsi, and jejunum are often used for reconstruction of the pharynx, the mandible, and esophageal defects. Large lesions excised from the pharyngeal wall sometimes require a relatively large, thin, and pliable tissue for reconstruction. The radial forearm flap is often selected for this reconstruction. If more bulk is required, the surgeon may choose rectus abdominis or latissimus dorsi muscle. The fibula or scapula may be used in bony reconstruction of mandibular defects. Reconstruction of circumferential defects of the pharynx is usually done with the use of a jejunum microvascular free flap.[10]

When a free flap is used, nursing care issues relate to the donor and recipient sites. Patients requiring a forearm flap must have the donor arm in a splint for 3 weeks, with daily dressing changes after 5 days. This prevents the tendon under the donor site from flexing and forcing the skin graft used to cover the donor site area away from the healing wound. Depending on physician preference, dressing changes may consist of general cleaning of the graft edges with either half-strength peroxide and water or normal saline. Xeroform gauze or antibiotic ointment may be placed over the edges of the graft and covered with 4 × 4 dressings. The area is usually covered with a light gauze wrap, and the splint is replaced. The hand is monitored for signs of edema, decreased circulation, or permanent stiffness of the hand and fingers.

Patients receiving fibula free flaps also require immobilization of the donor site. The patient is not allowed weight-bearing on the affected limb for 10 to 14 days and is maintained in an ankle-foot or leg splint for 6 weeks. Wound care to the graft covering the donor site is also necessary. It is done in a fashion similar to the care of the forearm flap and also begins approximately on postoperative day 5.

Jejunal flaps require abdominal surgery for harvesting; this procedure is done by a combination approach with a head and neck surgeon, a general surgeon, and often a plastic and reconstructive surgeon. In these patients, astute observation for signs of possible bowel obstruction or gastrointestinal complications is imperative. A loop of jejunum is normally left outside the neck wound as a sentinel loop to monitor motion, color, and secretions of this segment as signs of flap viability. The physician is notified immediately if the loop becomes cyanotic or motionless. If secretions are noted from the jejunum, a colostomy pouch may be used to maintain moisture and provide a route for observation. The jejunal loop is removed at the bedside with the use of local anesthetic when flap viability is no longer a concern postoperatively.[10]

Patients requiring rectus abdominis or latissimus dorsi flaps will have drains at the donor site. This donor site is normally closed primarily, with no requirement for skin grafts. Care of the donor site should focus on drain maintenance, wound care, and pain control.

The single most important postoperative nursing care activity in the free-flap patient is monitoring of viability of the flap. This is done not only with the physical examination but also with the use of the laser Doppler. The physician should specify postoperatively the optimal range of normal Doppler readings, and the nurse should monitor the Doppler every 30 minutes to 1 hour for any change. Most often, the free-flap patient is in an intensive care unit for the first 24 to 72 hours. This aids in close monitoring of flap viability and quick notification of the physician if any problems in the flap occur. It is very important that clinicians quickly take action to prevent loss of the flap if any compromise in perfusion occurs.[11]

Wound Care Technique

Wound-cleaning techniques vary according to the location of the wound and physician preference. Cleaning solutions that may be used include hydrogen peroxide, Dakin's solution, or antibiotic solutions. Plain or iodoform gauze dressing may be used to pack the wound, or wet-to-dry dressings may be preferred to assist in debridement of the area. External pressure dressings are often applied after cleaning, and it is important that dressing changes under sterile technique using the solutions ordered by the physician be performed in a timely manner to promote proper wound healing. The goal of fistula care is to promote healing from inside the wound outward.

If increased drainage is aggravating the fistula, the patient may be given an anticholinergic medication such as glycopyrrolate to decrease secretions. A feeding tube may also need to be inserted, if not already present, to prevent contamination of the area and promote healing. If the patient has a stoma, a cuffed tracheotomy tube may be placed to prevent aspiration of secretions from the fistula. If there are signs of cellulitis or deep neck infection, the patient usually is given antibiotics according to the results of bacterial culture and sensitivity.

The physician may debride the wound to remove necrotic debris and promote wound healing. This may be done at the bedside or in the operating room. The patient should be medicated with the prescribed analgesic before the procedure to promote comfort.

Well-vascularized flaps may be required to cover the wound if healing does not occur in a timely fashion. Psychosocial support is needed if an additional surgical procedure is required. The stress of a postoperative infection, an additional surgical procedure, and possible physical changes caused by a fistula can be devastating to the patient.

The patient with a fistula can often be managed at home by a home health nurse or by a family member who has been trained in proper wound care. This helps to minimize the number of hospital days, which can be an important mental boost for the patient. The role of the nurse is to instruct the patient and family in wound care technique and to discharge the patient with adequate cleaning and dressing supplies. Support of the patient's family and the home health nurse by telephone is also a nursing responsibility.

Shoulder Care

Patients undergoing neck dissection may require sacrifice or mobilization of the spinal accessory nerve for adequate removal of lymph nodes at risk of, or involved by, metastasis. Postoperatively, the patient may experience temporary or permanent shoulder dysfunction. The nursing role is to administer analgesics promptly on request and instruct the patient to support his or her arm and shoulder with pillows when in bed or in a chair. The arms should also be supported against the patient's body or in a sling during ambulation. An occupational or physical therapist is often needed to prescribe exercises to strengthen the affected shoulder. A clavicle brace may also be necessary for the patient who experiences persistent pain secondary to shoulder drop. The nurse's role is to encourage and assist the patient in performing exercises after instruction by an occupational therapist and to emphasize the importance of continuing the exercises at home.

Mouth Care

The patient requires mouth care following intraoral surgery. The physician orders irrigation or power spray to be given for 1 or 2 days postoperatively. The goals of irrigation include (1) to maintain hygiene in the surgical area, (2) to stimulate the blood supply, (3) to decrease edema, and (4) to prevent or resolve infection. The technique of irrigation varies with the institution. Oral care should be provided four times daily. Commonly used solutions include table salt and baking soda, hydrogen peroxide and water or saline, and antibiotic solutions. Irrigation may be performed with the use of an elongated catheter and syringe, an irrigating catheter and bag, a Water Pik, or a power spray system. The nurse should ensure that the chosen technique reaches the oral defect or incision line, that low-pressure settings are used with a Water Pik or power sprayer, that damage to suture lines or skin grafts is avoided, and that the patient is educated about the method of irrigation that will be continued at discharge. The nurse should also observe for wound dehiscence or infection during irrigation.[12]

Nutrition

Enteral Feeding

Proper nutrition is essential for healing. This is usually achieved by enteral feeding through a nasogastric or gastrostomy feeding tube. The methods of delivery include bolus, syringe, and mechanical pump feedings. The tube feed formula is given at room temperature to prevent abdominal cramping and diarrhea. The patient should be fed in a sitting position and should remain upright for 1 to 2 hours after feeding is complete. The advantage of a gastrostomy tube is that it is less visible and allows a freer lifestyle if tube feeding is to be given over the long term. It also does not clog as easily and therefore promotes a more versatile diet. Simplified placement procedures such as percutaneous endoscopic gastrostomy (PEG) have decreased risk and have made gastrostomy tubes more readily available and desirable for patients.

Regardless of the type of feeding tube used, the following nursing measures should be taken: (1) Evaluate placement of the tube before administering the feeding; (2) check for residual food from the previous feeding by aspirating stomach contents; (3) place the patient in a sitting position; (4) administer the feeding at room temperature and slowly to prevent bloating and diarrhea; (5) observe for aspiration from regurgitated feedings, which can be prevented by inflating the cuff of the tracheotomy tube (if one is present) before, during, and after feeding, and check for proper positioning of the patient; and (6) follow the feeding with 50 to 100 mL of water to rinse the tube and prevent high sodium syndrome. The nurse should also clean around the tube and change tape, ties, or dressings daily according to institutional guidelines.

Various types of diets are available for the patient who is receiving tube feeding. Consultation with a nutritionist before feeding will provide a diet with adequate calorie and protein content for wound healing. Many commercial products provide total protein and calorie intake in a small volume. Blenderized and liquid foods may be more cost-effective, but care should be taken to evaluate that adequate nutrition is received to promote healing. Commercial products are available for the lactose intolerant patient.

Oral Feeding

Oral feeding may be difficult because of extensive surgical changes, nerve deficits, and previous treatments with radiation and chemotherapy. Many methods can be used to facilitate resumption of oral intake, such as the use of a straw, a syringe with a catheter attached to allow food to be injected farther into the oropharynx, spoon feeding, tilting of the head, use of thicker liquids or carbonated beverages, or supraglottic swallowing. A speech pathologist or a swallowing team and modified barium swallow may be needed to evaluate and manage patients who have extreme difficulty with swallowing, or if aspiration occurs with oral intake.

The nurse is responsible for (1) obtaining a nutritional assessment, including information regarding food allergy, intolerance, and dislikes; (2) setting realistic goals and emphasizing the importance of nutrition and swallowing exercises; (3) weighing the patient daily; (4) maintaining an accurate intake and output record; (5) encouraging the patient to eat small, frequent meals; and (6) reinforcing the importance of persistence in attempting to swallow even if failure occurs.[13]

Patients who have had partial laryngectomy procedures or surgery of the pharynx or base of the tongue are especially prone to swallowing difficulty and aspiration. Careful positioning of the patient for swallowing exercises that strengthen the larynx, for the supraglottic swallow, or for a combination of these may be required to avoid aspiration. The nurse and speech pathologist must work closely together to support and reinforce the teaching of swallowing techniques and exercises to the patient.

▣ FOLLOW-UP CARE

Physical Care

As with most oncology treatment modalities, long-term ongoing care of patients with cancer of the head and neck by the physician, the nurse-specialist, and other members of the health care team is mandated. Frequent clinic visits, rehabilitative care, and home health support are standard. The nurse acts as a liaison to facilitate this ongoing physical care. The patient must be monitored in the posthospitalization phase for progression of healing, weight maintenance, and return to function. This is a critical period of communication between the patient and the physician, nurse-specialist, home health nurse, and clinic staff. The patient and family must be able to recognize signs and symptoms of late wound infection, pulmonary complications, and nutritional compromise. Pain control may require ongoing management even after discharge. As time progresses and the patient continues to regain strength, rehabilitate, and do well, the chance for complications decreases. It is important to remember that the patient may be preparing for additional treatment at this time. After successful healing, radiation and/or chemotherapy may be needed. The nurse can reinforce the rationale and explanation of the procedure for any adjuvant therapy that the physician may order. Coordination of consultations and treatment schedules is a great help to an already stressed patient and family. Assurances of support and a reminder of the goals and time limits of therapy may also be helpful for the patient.

Emotional Care

It is perhaps at this time that the magnitude of the diagnosis begins to have an impact on the head and neck cancer patient. Body image, loss of function, and impaired livelihood all take their toll on the patient and his or her significant others. Depression may be a part of the postoperative sequelae. The nurse may be the first to note this in dealing with the patient postoperatively. Referrals to mental health professionals as well as suggestions for support groups and mentors can prove invaluable. Antidepressants and/or sleep medications can aid the patient on a short-term basis. The constancy of care, both physical and emotional at this time, can be paramount to the patient's outcome.

Recurrent Disease

The reality of head and neck cancer is that despite the best efforts of the surgeon, medical oncologist, radiation oncologist, nursing staff, and ancillary support teams, the cancer may recur. This may take place locally, regionally, or in the form of distant metastasis. The diagnostic process may begin anew if a recurrence is noted, and this may only add to the sense of defeat and foreboding the patient may feel. Realistic expectations on the part of the physician and support staff must be conveyed. This may be a time of new decisions regarding conventional versus experimental

treatment, or whether to receive any treatment at all. The astute nurse aids the patient in gathering and assimilating this new information to make critical informed decisions. The patient and his family must be assured that there are no "wrong decisions" for continuing care. Smoking and alcohol cessation programs should be encouraged by the physician in an effect to prevent recurrence.

End-of-Life Issues

When the patient with head and neck cancer is considered to have incurable disease, this affords the nurse-specialist the opportunity to perform nursing care at the purest holistic level. Besides physical support of the dying patient, referrals for hospice care either in the patient's home or in a hospice facility may be needed. The nurse can be guardian for the patient's quality of life. Together with the family, the nurse can assess pain control and level of consciousness and family needs and can ease the physical, emotional, and spiritual burdens for the dying patient and loved ones. At no other time are the advocacy and caring support of the nurse as valuable to the patient.

REFERENCES

1. Hickey M: The challenges of postoperative radiotherapy for postsurgical head and neck patients. In Perspectives: Recovery Strategies from the OR to Home, vol 3, no 2. Burlington, Vermont, Saxe Healthcare Communications, 2002.
2. Rice DH, Spiro RH: Current Concepts in Head and Neck Cancer. Washington, DC, The American Cancer Society, 1989.
3. Fink RM, Gates RA: Oncology Nursing Secrets. Philadelphia, Hanley & Belfus, 1997.
4. Brill EL, Kilts DF: Foundations for Nursing. New York, Appleton-Century-Crofts, 1980, p 425.
5. Dropkin MJ: Coping with disfigurement and dysfunction after head and neck cancer surgery: A conceptual framework. Semin Oncol Nurs 5:3, 1989.
6. Droughton ML, Verbic M: Body image reintegration after head and neck surgery. J Soc Otorhinolaryngol Head Neck Nurse 6:19–23, 1988.
7. Body image disturbance. In Practice Guidelines for Otorhinolaryngology—Head and Neck Nursing. New Smyrna Beach, Florida, Society of Otorhinolaryngology Head and Neck Nurses, 1994.
8. Lockhart JS, Troff JL, Artim LS: Total laryngectomy and radical neck dissection. AORN J 55:2, 1992.
9. Society of Otolaryngology and Head and Neck Nurses. Carotid artery rupture. In Practice Guidelines for Otolaryngology—Head and Neck Nursing. New Smyrna Beach, Florida, Society of Otolaryngology and Head and Neck Nurses, 1994.
10. Westlake C: Commitment to function: Microsurgical flaps. Plast Surg Nurs 11:3, 1991.
11. Maksud DP: Nursing management of patients following combined free flap mandible reconstruction. Plast Surg Nurs 12:95–105, 1992.
12. Sigler BA, Schuring LT: Ear, Nose, and Throat Disorders. St. Louis, Mosby—Year Book, 1993, pp 41–43, 222–259.
13. Bryce JC: Aspiration: Causes, consequences, and prevention. ORL Head Neck Nurse 13:2, 1995.

CHAPTER 31

General Principles of Radiation Therapy for Cancer of the Head and Neck

K. Kian Ang

Luka Milas

Almon S. Shiu

◧ INTRODUCTION

Radiation oncology is a medical specialty that focuses predominantly on the treatment of neoplastic diseases with the use of ionizing radiation given either alone or in combination with surgery, chemotherapy, or both. Anecdotal uses of ionizing radiation for treating various diseases started very shortly after the discovery of x-rays by Wilhelm Conrad Röntgen in 1895 and the isolation of radium by Marie and Pierre Curie in 1898.

Fractionation in Radiotherapy, edited by Thames and Hendry,[1] is an excellent reference for readers interested in the history of the specialty. Briefly, one of the first documented uses of x-ray therapy was by a Viennese dermatologist, Leopold Freund, to treat a hairy nevus with the use of the very low dose x-ray tube, which became available in 1896, only 1 year after Röntgen's discovery. Without a rudimentary understanding of how radiation affected living tissues, it was used primarily, often by dermatologists and surgeons, as a form of cautery in the beginning of the 20th century. During the first two decades, high single radiation doses were generally given, which caused sloughing of tissue and led to morbid sequelae. Such casual application of radiation caused a general skepticism about its usefulness as a therapeutic modality. From about 1920, there was a swing toward fractionated treatment in Paris, Zurich, and Vienna, based on the pioneering clinical work of Regaud, Coutard, Schwarz, Holzknecht, and others and on results of experimental studies of the sterilization of testicles in the grasshopper and the rabbit. The field of radiation therapy then evolved, first in combination with diagnostic radiology, and thereafter growing into a separate specialty at varying rates in different countries.

Refinement of radiotherapy techniques and regimens thus occurred empirically during the first half of the 20th century. The invention of the telecobalt therapy unit and later of linear accelerators that produced higher-energy photons and electrons that penetrate more deeply brought the specialty a big step forward. Subsequently, progress in the understanding of the mechanisms of radiation effects at the cellular level and factors governing tissue response to radiation led to the design of more biologically sound regimens that had been subjected to clinical testing. A large number of phase III clinical trials conducted by many cooperative groups, starting from the late 1970s, have identified three altered fractionation schedules that yield better therapeutic benefit than the standard 2-gray (Gy) fraction radiation regimen commonly used in the United States.

In its current state, radiation therapy plays an important role in the treatment of cancer of the head and neck. For most early-stage cancers of the head and neck, radiation therapy is as effective as surgery in curing the disease but is in general better in preserving the structural integrity and function of organs. Therefore, the choice of treatment in individual patients mostly depends on the expertise of the medical team, underlying medical conditions of patients, individual preferences, and the anticipated morbidity. For intermediate-stage carcinomas, many oncologists prefer radiotherapy to surgery for better functional and aesthetic outcomes and based on the experience that many surgically treated patients may need postoperative radiotherapy because of the presence of adverse surgical-pathologic features. For locally advanced cancers of the head and neck, radiotherapy is frequently given as an adjunct to surgery to yield maximal locoregional tumor control. These two modalities are complementary: surgical resection of gross tumor eliminates the most common source of radiation failure, and radiotherapy sterilizes microscopic tumor spread beyond surgical section margins, which is the main cause of recurrence after surgery.

Recently, however, the combination of radiation with chemotherapy has gained popularity in the nonsurgical treatment of locally advanced cancer of the head and neck because many randomized trials have showed that several such combined regimens improved overall survival and/or organ preservation rates over radiation alone.

Recent advances in radiation physics and in computer and imaging technology have dramatically improved the sophistication in planning and delivery of radiotherapy, enabling more precise tumor volume delineation and targeting, which leads to increased efficacy by dose escalation and reduced toxicity through avoidance of normal tissue. In parallel, increasing insight into the molecular processes of malignant transformation and the mechanisms governing cellular radiation sensitivity is leading to the development of specific molecular targeted radiation sensitization of tumors. There is little doubt that creative combinations of precision delivery of radiation with molecular target–driven radiation sensitization will be conceived in the foreseeable future, resulting in further improvement in tumor control and quality of life.

This chapter presents a brief overview of the basic principles and terminology of radiation therapy for clinicians who have no formal training in radiation oncology. It begins with the basics of radiation physics and elementary radiation biology, that is, mode of cell killing, kinetics of tissue response to radiation, tumor control and normal tissue complication probability, and choice of dose fractionation. Also included is an introduction to conformal radiotherapy as well as an explanation of the rationales of combined treatment and molecular targeted radiation sensitization. In addition, this chapter provides an overview of the history and advances made in radiation oncology and a description of some of the directions of current research. More detailed descriptions of biology, physics, and clinical applications are available in radiation oncology textbooks such as those edited by Hall,[2] Gunderson and associates,[3] and Perez and colleagues.[4]

◼ BASIC RADIATION PHYSICS

External Beam Radiation

Electromagnetic Radiation

High-energy x-rays or gamma (γ)-rays are used most often in clinical radiotherapy. X-rays and γ-rays have similar physical and biologic properties but differ in how they are produced and in their tissue penetration characteristics (see later and Fig. 31–1A). X-rays are generated in linear accelerators (linacs), which accelerate electrons to high energy and direct them to hit a metal target, usually made of tungsten, thereby converting part of the kinetic energy (energy of motion) of the electrons into x-rays. In contrast, γ-rays are emitted by fission of radioactive isotopes. Because of a higher dose rate and perceived radiation safety advantages, most modern radiotherapy centers primarily use high-energy x-rays produced by linacs. The energy of x-rays is specified by MV (megavolt or million volt) to reflect the fact that a continuum of energies is produced; the number (e.g., 6 MV) refers to the maximum energy of the spectrum.

X-rays or γ-rays, visible light, radio waves, radar, and radiant heat are all electromagnetic radiations traveling at the same velocity (c), but they differ greatly in their wavelength (λ) and hence in the corresponding frequency (ν), in that the velocity of the electromagnetic wave is the product of its wavelength and frequency ($c = \lambda \times \nu$). For example, the wavelengths of typical x-rays, visible light, and radio waves are approximately 10^{-8} cm, 10^{-5} cm, and 300 m, respectively.

Alternatively, x-rays can be thought of as a stream of photons, each containing an amount of energy equal to hν (where h is known as Planck's constant).[5] Therefore, radiation with short wavelength, such as x-rays, has a high frequency; hence the energy per photon is large. The concept of photon energy is important in radiotherapy because the biologic effects of ionizing radiation on cells and tissues result from absorption of such photon energies.

Particle Radiation

Because of attractive depth-dose distribution characteristics, electron beams (Fig. 31–1B) have found wide application in external radiotherapy, and protons are being tested in a small number of centers around the world. Neutron irradiation was studied because of its different biologic properties, but this study has been largely abandoned because of very limited usefulness except perhaps for unresectable or recurrent salivary gland cancers.[6] Other types of radiation such as α-particles, negative π mesons, and heavy charged ions have been tested in specialized centers and hence are not addressed here.

Electrons are small, negatively charged particles that can be accelerated to a specific high energy, namely, up to 50 MeV (million electron volts), by means of a linear accelerator. In the electron mode of linac operation, the electron beam is directed to strike an electron-scattering foil instead of a tungsten target so that the beam is spread and uniform electron fluence is yielded across the treatment portal. The higher the energy of the electron beam, the more deeply it penetrates into tissue (see Fig. 31–1B).

Protons are positively charged particles that have a mass about 1835 times greater than that of electrons but have essentially the same radiobiologic properties as conventional electron or photon beams. Because of the heavier mass, more complex and expensive equipment (e.g., cyclotron or synchrotron) is needed to accelerate protons to clinically useful energies.[7] However, because of the greater flexibility of modulating proton beams such as to generate dose distribution to better conform to the depth and shape of the target volume (Fig. 31–1C), proton therapy has advantages for use in irradiating tumors located close to critical organs, such as choroidal melanomas and skull base chordomas and sarcomas. To what extent the slightly better physical dose distribution of proton therapy over that of conformal photon therapy will translate to clinical benefit in terms of improved therapeutic ratio in more common neoplasms remains to be critically assessed. The number of currently operational proton facilities is quite small (about 16 centers worldwide), but several centers are planning to build hospital-based proton facilities to test the value of proton therapy.

Interaction of Radiation With Living Tissues

Absorption of the energy of electromagnetic or particle radiation in the body produces a minimal amount of heat and, more importantly, ionizations that lead to a variety of biologic effects.[8] The type of physical interaction between radiation and tissues depends on several variables, including the energy and type of radiation and the composition of the tissue at the interaction site.

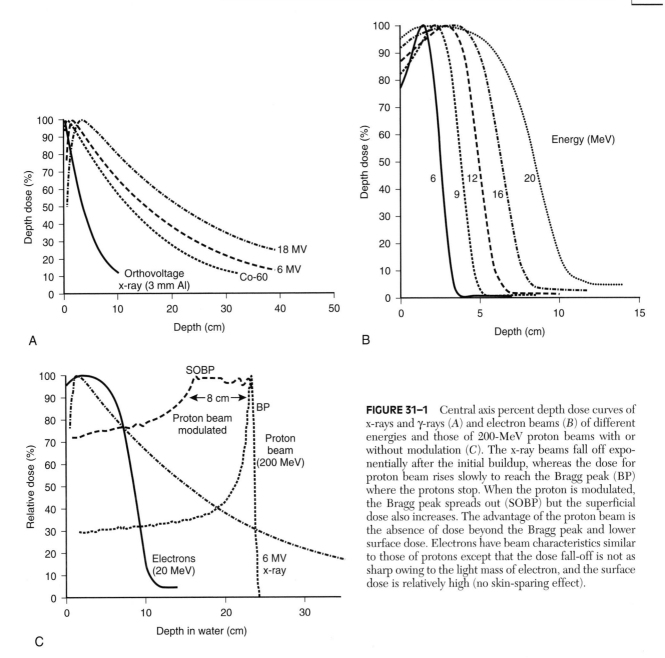

FIGURE 31–1 Central axis percent depth dose curves of x-rays and γ-rays (*A*) and electron beams (*B*) of different energies and those of 200-MeV proton beams with or without modulation (*C*). The x-ray beams fall off exponentially after the initial buildup, whereas the dose for proton beam rises slowly to reach the Bragg peak (BP) where the protons stop. When the proton is modulated, the Bragg peak spreads out (SOBP) but the superficial dose also increases. The advantage of the proton beam is the absence of dose beyond the Bragg peak and lower surface dose. Electrons have beam characteristics similar to those of protons except that the dose fall-off is not as sharp owing to the light mass of electron, and the surface dose is relatively high (no skin-sparing effect).

Electromagnetic Radiation

X-ray or γ-ray photons within the energy range normally used in radiotherapy (up to 10 MV) interact with atoms within tissues mainly through three mechanisms: Compton scattering, photoelectric effect, and pair production.

In the most common mode of interaction, referred to as *Compton scattering,* each incident photon interacts with a loosely bound electron at the outer shell of an atom, which produces a Compton (or recoil) electron and a scattered photon of lower energy. The proportion of the photon energy transferred to the Compton electron increases with increasing energy of the original photon. High-energy photons thus produce high-energy recoil electrons. The direction of both the recoil electron and the scattered photon is also dependent on the photon energy of the original beam, with high-energy photons giving rise to recoil electrons and

scattered photons predominantly moving in the forward direction. Consequently, high-energy photons produce little backscatter, or radiation scattered back toward the surface, and thus provide significant skin sparing, compared with lower-energy (orthovoltage or superficial) x-rays.

As the original photon beam is gradually attenuated and scattered by this Compton effect, progressively lower energy photons are produced, and eventually, the sufficiently low-energy photons (10 to 50 kilo-electron volts [keV]) transfer all their remaining energy to inner electrons of atoms, resulting in ejection of these electrons. This phenomenon is referred to as the *photoelectric effect.* The photoelectrons are ejected predominantly at right angles to the direction of the incident photon and have a very limited range in tissue; the secondary ionizations they cause produce local biologic damage. The photoelectric effect, unlike the Compton effect, varies strongly with the atomic number (Z) of scattering material (approximately expressed as Z^3). The selective attenuation of photons via this effect is the basis for diagnostic x-rays to distinguish elements of different atomic number, such as bone and soft tissue.

Pair production refers to the annihilation of a photon, resulting in production of an electron-positron pair in the strong electromagnetic field of an atomic nucleus. The electron induces secondary ionization as described earlier, and the positron soon combines with an electron in the medium and annihilates with production of a pair of photons, each with energy of 0.51 MeV. Thus this process has threshold energy of 1.02 MeV and accounts for about 28% of the total energy absorption for a 10-MV photon.

Other absorption processes can take place at higher energies, but these are not of concern here.

Particle Radiation

Electrons entering tissues undergo either elastic or inelastic collision with electrons or atoms of the absorbing material in a proportion dependent on several variables, including electron energy and tissue composition. An elastic collision can be thought of as a collision of billiard balls, wherein the kinetic energy (energy of motion) after the collision is the same as before, except it is now shared by two or more particles. With inelastic collision, however, the sums of the kinetic energies before and after the collision are not equal. In the billiard ball analogy, an inelastic collision represents a scenario in which one of the balls is broken or chipped in a collision, with some of the original kinetic energy being used to "break" the chip away. Unlike with billiard balls, the charged electrons must merely come close to each other so that their electric fields can interact; they need not actually collide for these phenomena to occur.

The elastic interaction among electrons is one means of transferring energy and producing ionization by removing one outer electron from neutral atoms. Because the binding energy of an outer electron in most elements in tissue is small, this scattering process continues, leaving a track of ionization and biologic damage in its way, until all of the electrons have expended their energy. Elastic interaction can occur between an electron and a nucleus of an atom; in this process, the electron converts some of its energy to a γ-ray photon and a reduced energy electron that is available for secondary ionization. The γ-ray photon generated through bremsstrahlung may or may not undergo any secondary interaction before leaving the body.

Absorbed Dose

The absorbed radiation dose is defined as the ratio between the average amount of energy (E) deposited in a small volume with mass (M). The older unit of absorbed dose was the rad, which corresponds to 100 ergs of energy deposited in 1 gram of material. More recently, an international commission changed the standard unit to a *gray (Gy)*,[9] which represents 1 joule of energy deposited in a kilogram of material. Numerically, a dose in gray is equivalent to a dose in rad multiplied by a factor of 100 (i.e., 1 Gy = 100 rad). Therefore, one centigray (cGy), a frequently quoted unit, is equivalent to one rad. For an equivalent absorbed dose, megavoltage photons and electrons produce similar biologic effects.

The absorbed dose at a particular point in an irradiated medium is often referred to as the *depth dose*. The ratio of this depth dose to the dose at a reference depth (usually the depth of maximum dose, D_{max}) along the central axis, multiplied by 100%, represents the central axis percent depth dose: $\%DD = D/D_{max} \times 100\%$. The percent depth dose varies with radiation quality, field size, source to skin distance (SSD), properties of the medium, and depth from skin surface and thickness of the tissue distal to the point of interest.

The variation of percent depth dose with photon energy and depth is shown in Figure 31–1A. With the exception of orthovoltage or superficial x-rays, the percent depth dose exhibits an initial rise (referred to as *the buildup region*) with depth until the maximum dose (D_{max}) is reached. The characteristics of the dose buildup region (a result of forward scattering of primary and secondary electrons until an equilibrium is reached) provide a measure of skin-sparing effect of the beam (allowing delivery of a greater radiation dose at depth for a given skin reaction). This skin sparing is more pronounced with high-energy photon beams but can be lost when material such as clothing or other blocks are present to intercept the beam within a few centimeters of the patient. It is also clear from Figure 31–1A that the percent depth dose falls less rapidly with depth for higher-energy radiation. For treatment of cancer of the head and neck, for instance, the use of very high energy photons may result in underdosage of superficially located target volumes.

Electron beams are valuable for radiation treatment because their depth of penetration varies with the energy, and beyond the 80% depth line, the dose falls off rather sharply (see Fig. 31–1B). This characteristic allows, for example, irradiation of posterior neck nodes that overlie the spinal cord with minimum dose contribution to this critical organ. Because electron beams have less skin-sparing effect than photons, the full course of radiotherapy is rarely given with electron beams alone. However, photon and electron beams are often combined for the treatment of cancer of the head and neck.

◼ ELEMENTARY RADIATION BIOLOGY

Radiation Cell Killing

Ionizing radiation delivered to cells or tissues initiates a chain of events that vary according to the energy and type of radiation, as discussed earlier. The energy deposited is converted into secondary electrons that break chemical bonds either directly or indirectly via the production of free radicals (e.g., hydroxyl radicals formed by interaction between radiation and intracellular water molecules) and thereby initiate biologic effects. Sparsely ionizing radiations, such as x-rays or γ-rays, induce damage mainly (about 70%) through indirect effects, whereas densely ionizing radiations, such as neutrons and α-particles, cause damage primarily through direct effects. Although ionizing radiation can affect tissue through many mechanisms, depending on the size of the dose, cell killing is the major effect in the therapeutic dose range. Lethally injured cells die in two distinct ways, that is, by mitotic death or by apoptosis.

In *mitotic (reproductive) death,* which is generally considered the dominant mode of cell killing, cells die when they attempt to divide. However, depending largely on the radiation dose, the doomed cells may die either at the first postirradiation division or after they have undergone a limited number of seemingly normal divisions. At a clinically relevant dose of 2 Gy, for example, irradiated cells may appear morphologically and metabolically and functionally intact; they typically complete two or three apparently successful divisions before undergoing classic necrotic changes characterized by cell swelling, dissolution of organized cellular structures, and rupture of cell membranes. Cells that survive radiation, in contrast, retain their reproductive function, namely, their capacity for sustained proliferation, that is, the forming of colonies analogous to those formed by bacteria. This ability is commonly measured with a clonogenic cell survival assay, in which a given number of single cells, plated on suitable growth medium, are exposed to varying doses of radiation, and the fraction that retains its ability to grow into visible colonies is counted (Fig. 31–2).

At a molecular level, DNA molecules, the genetic apparatus residing in the cell nucleus, are the critical targets of injury in which radiation causes different types of lesions. Single-strand breaks (SSBs) are the most frequent lesions, but they are readily repaired and are of little significance in cell killing by ionizing radiation. Although much less frequent than SSBs, double-strand breaks (DSBs) and chromosomal aberrations, which occur in association with or as a result of DSBs, are generally considered to be the main molecular events causing mitotic cell death.

Cell death by *apoptosis* after radiation is more variable among tissues but in general occurs less frequently than mitotic cell killing. Like mitosis, the term *apoptosis* comes from the Greek, denoting "falling of leaves from trees." Radiation-induced apoptosis is not usually linked to cell division. Radiobiologists have known apoptosis for decades under the term *interphase death,* which occurs preferentially in certain cell types, including some classes of lymphocytes and spermatogonia. Unlike mitotic death, interphase death usually occurs within hours of radiation exposure and typically is already observable after lower radiation doses. Apoptosis is an active mode of cell death characterized by distinctive biochemical and morphologic features, which include endonuclease activation, chromatin condensation, and margination, along with cellular shrinkage and fragmentation. The affected cells shrink in volume and detach from neighboring cells, then fragment into a cluster of membrane-bound apoptotic bodies that, in tissues, are phagocytosed by adjacent cells or macrophages (Fig. 31–3). At a biochemical level, endonucleases are activated and cleave DNA into nucleosomal pieces of 180 to 200 base pairs. These produce a characteristic "ladder" pattern on gel electrophoresis. Another enzyme, *transglutaminase,* causes protein cross-linking, which primarily affects cellular membrane by preventing leakage of cytoplasmic content.

Intensive research on apoptosis during the past decade has established its importance in many biologic processes. As a normal, physiologic mechanism of cell deletion, for example, apoptosis is involved in embryonic development, metamorphosis, hormone-dependent tissue growth and atrophy, maturation of lymphocytes, removal of self-reactive immune cells, tumor development and growth, and so forth. Apoptosis is genetically controlled by products of many genes, both proapoptotic (e.g., p53 [TP53] and BAX) and antiapoptotic (e.g., BCL2) genes. Because of its physiologic

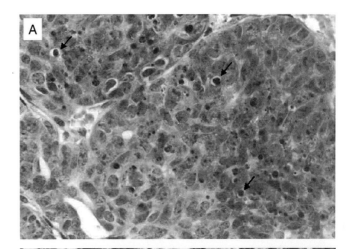

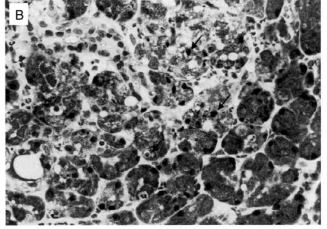

FIGURE 31–3 Histologic features of apoptosis in a mouse mammary carcinoma (A) and salivary gland of monkeys (B). Tissues were irradiated with 15 Gy of γ-rays in a single exposure and were sampled 4 hours later for histologic analysis. *Arrows* depict some apoptotic cells.

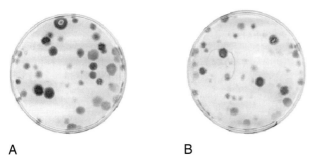

A   B

FIGURE 31–2 Number of colonies formed after plating of 100 cells without irradiation (A), or plating of 3200 cells exposed to a single dose of 6 Gy (B).

role and tight genetic regulation, apoptosis is frequently referred to as "programmed cell death."

Apoptosis plays an important role in determining the responses of some tumors and normal tissues to radiotherapy, chemotherapy, and their combination. Some tumor types such as lymphomas and seminomas are very susceptible to this form of radiation-induced cell death. Experimental studies with rodent tumors have shown that about one third of solid tumors respond to radiation by apoptosis.

Both reproductive death and apoptosis are dependent on radiation dose but have different dose-response features. The former is an exponential function of radiation dose, whereas the latter appears to be most conspicuous at between 1.5 and 5 Gy. It should be noted that serous cells of salivary and lacrimal glands are particularly sensitive to radiation-induced apoptosis, which explains the rapid onset of xerostomia and xerophthalmia after administration of even modest radiation doses.

Radiation Effects on Cell Kinetics

In addition to inflicting injury that leads to cell lethality by mitotic or apoptotic death, radiation perturbs progression of surviving cells through the division cycle. In general, cellular progression through the division cycle is rigidly orchestrated by two families of proteins—cyclins and cyclin-dependent kinases (CDK or CDC) operating in rigidly controlled sequence. Briefly, cyclin D1 associates with CDK4 and CDK6 and regulates the transition of cells through the G1 phase before cyclin E binds CDK2 during the late G1 phase to govern the entry of cells into S-phase. Then, cyclin A attaches to CDK2 during the S-phase, and finally, cyclin B binds CDC2 to control the entry of cells into mitosis. The activation of kinases by cyclins is regulated by a number of proteins. For example, p21 or p27 can inhibit CDK2 activation by cyclin E and thereby influence the G1/S transition.

Radiation affects the expression of both cyclins and cyclin-dependent kinases. This effect is most pronounced at the early part of the G1 phase and at the G1/S boundary, resulting in a net delay in cellular progression through the division cycle. The duration of such mitotic delay depends on radiation dose, dose rate, cell type, and cell position in the division cycle. The delay, for example, is longer with increasing radiation dose.

Radiation Effects on Tissue Structure and Function

Although most normal tissues can tolerate varying moderate radiation doses without losing structural integrity or function, distinct radiation-induced tissue injuries occur when critical numbers of clonogenic cells are killed, because mature cells lost through the normal physiologic wear-and-tear process can no longer be adequately replenished. The timing of damage manifestation, however, depends largely on the organizational structure and kinetics of cellular turnover of tissues and varies widely among tissues. For practical purposes, tissue damage is commonly referred to as *acute*, *subacute*, or *late response*.

In general, tissues having hierarchical organization (type H), that is, a small number of slowly proliferating stem cells

that produce a highly rapidly proliferative compartment of progenitor cells that then differentiate into mature, non-proliferating functional cells, manifest radiation injury *acutely* (i.e., usually within days or a few weeks after initiation of irradiation). Examples in the head and neck area include the mucosa and the skin. In these tissues, irradiation depletes both stem cell and progenitor cell compartments, but the differentiated cells can maintain tissue function until they are depleted through normal physiologic wear and tear. Consequently, radiation injury appears at a rather predictable time determined by the life span of the mature cells. Patchy mucositis, for example, begins to manifest by the third week of conventionally fractionated radiotherapy. These tissues, however, recover essentially all of their functions when a sufficient number of stem cells survives to reconstitute depleted cell compartments.

Subacute injury manifests several months after radiation in tissues that have a longer cell turnover time than mucosa and skin and is in general reversible. Examples in the head and neck area include Lhermitte's syndrome (electric shock sensation induced mostly by flexion of the head), somnolence, and subacute pneumonitis after irradiation of the spinal cord, brain, and lung, respectively.

Late responses occur in tissues composed of functional parenchymal cells with very low cell turnover rates that retain the flexibility to regain reproductive function in the event of tissue loss, hence referred to as flexible (type F) tissues. Examples of such tissues in the head and neck region include bone, soft tissue, and nervous system and endocrine tissues. The late responses manifest many months or years after radiation, and their time of onset depends to some degree on radiation dose. Such injuries also tend to increase in severity over time as a result of an "avalanche" phenomenon; that is, the first wave of cell death recruits other doomed cells into proliferation, which then die while attempting to divide, leading to progressive massive cell depletion and severe functional failure. Typical late complications of concern include fibrosis of the neck, trismus, necrosis of soft tissue and bone, and the dreaded myelopathy. Clinical radiation regimens have mostly been designed to minimize these types of late complications.

Radiation Dose-Response Curves

Because radiation energy deposition and infliction of chemical injury is a random process, radiation cell killing is exponential as a function of dose; that is, doubling the dose that reduces the survival rate to 50% diminishes the survival rate to 25%, and tripling the dose decreases it to 12.5%, and so forth. Therefore, it has become customary for *radiation survival curves* to be plotted on semilogarithmic coordinates with the surviving fraction on the logarithmic ordinate and the radiation dose on the linear abscissa (Fig. 31–4A). An exponential function comes out as a straight line in such a plot, the slope of which represents the mean lethal dose (D_0) which is the dose that would have been sufficient to kill all the cells in the population should each lethal lesion hit each individual cell. However, because of the random distribution, 100 lethal lesions inflicting a population of 100 equally sensitive cells result, on average, in about 37 cells receiving zero, 37 receiving one, 18 receiving two,

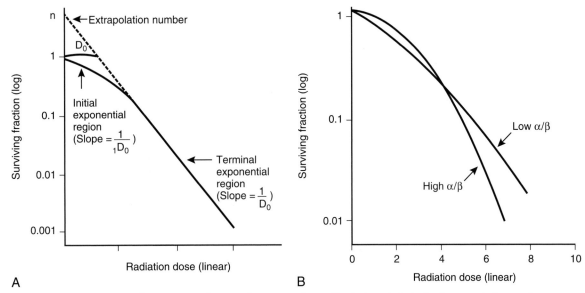

FIGURE 31–4 Radiation survival curves for mammalian cells. *A*, A typical single-dose survival curve has a "shoulder" followed by a terminal exponential region. The slope of the terminal region is defined by $1/D_0$ (D_0 is specified in the text). The "shoulder" consists of an initial exponential region, with the slope of $1/_1D_0$, followed by a downward-bending portion that merges with the terminal exponential region. The terms *n* (extrapolation number) and D_0 (quasithreshold dose) are derived by extrapolating the terminal exponential region to the zero dose axis and the 100% cell survival level, respectively. These two parameters determine the width of the "shoulder," which correlates with the amount of cellular repair from sublethal radiation damage (SLD). *B*, Representative cell survival curves for acutely responding tissues characterized by a high α/β ratio and for late-responding tissues characterized by a low α/β ratio. Radiation dose fractions smaller than the dose where the two curves intersect will preferentially spare the late-responding tissues.

6 receiving three, and an occasional 1 receiving even four or five lethal lesions (Poisson statistics). Therefore, the mean lethal dose kills on the average 63% of the cells in a given population (i.e., reduces survival to 37%), and each additional dose of D_0 reduces cell survival to 37% of the previous level.

The exponential dose-response relationship was first demonstrated in bacteria but later was also shown in mammalian cells, with the exception of the low-dose region in which the slope was initially shallower but curved downward (referred to as *the shoulder*) over the range of the first few Gy (see Fig. 31–4A). Within the shoulder region, the efficiency of cell killing increases progressively until it reaches the final exponential slope. The shoulder region is of greatest interest in radiotherapy because it corresponds to the range of fractional doses of commonly used radiotherapy regimens.

Several biophysical models, such as the accumulation of sublethal radiation damage and the saturation of cellular repair mechanisms, were proposed to explain the shoulder of the dose-survival curve. Similarly, a number of mathematical models were put forward to describe the shape of the cell survival curve, among which the *linear-quadratic model* has gained popularity because it is simple and yields generally a better fit with experimental data. According to this model, there are two components of cell killing—one proportional to the dose (αD; linear) and the other proportional to the square of the dose (βD^2; quadratic). The net surviving fraction (SF) of a cell population to a given dose can be computed with the equation $SF = e^{-(\alpha D + \beta D^2)}$. The linear component represents cell killing by single-hit mechanisms (causing irreparable damage), and the quadratic component represents cell killing by double-hit mechanisms (causing reparable damage). The dose at which the linear and quadratic components are equal is the ratio of α/β.

The ratio of α/β describes the shape of the shoulder region of the survival curve. A high ratio of α/β exemplifies a curve in the shoulder region that has a steep initial slope and a small curvature, whereas a low α/β ratio typifies a curve in the shoulder region that has a shallow initial slope and a larger curvature (Fig. 31–4B). The size of the shoulder is characterized by the absolute values of α and β and varies considerably among different cell types; this may be affected by other factors such as cell-cycle position, whether the cells are in contact with each other at the time of irradiation, and so forth.

When radiation dose is fractionated, allowing several hours to elapse between individual doses, the shoulder region reappears after each dose increment because cells are able to repair sublethal injury during the interval. Consequently, equal doses of radiation produce equal decrements in cell survival, and the cumulative dose-survival curve appears as a simple exponential straight line on a semilogarithmic plot (Fig. 31–5). The slope of the fractionated radiation survival curve, called *effective D_0 [$D_{0(eff)}$]*, is always shallower than that of a single-dose exposure and is dependent on the dose per fraction. It becomes progressively shallower as the dose per fraction decreases until all

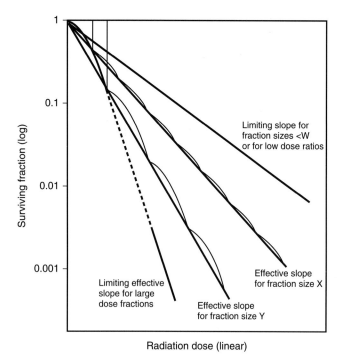

FIGURE 31–5 Survival curves of fractionated radiation delivered in equal doses per fraction separated by time interval, allowing complete repair from SLD to elapse. The curves become exponential as a function of radiation dose. The slope of each curve is defined by the respective "effective" D_0 [$D_{0(eff)}$] for a particular fraction size. The $D_{0(eff)}$ can never exceed $_1D_0$, because this denotes single-hit killing that results from irreparable damage.

cell killing results from single-hit (α type) events. The surviving fraction of the total dose (D) can be computed with the equation $S = e^{-D/Do(eff)}$ wherein the value of $D_{0(eff)}$ is in the range of 2.5 to 5.0 Gy for the commonly used 2 Gy per fraction clinical regimen.

Factors Affecting Radiation Sensitivity

Besides repair of sublethal injury and the reappearance of the shoulder (illustrated in the dose-response curve section), many factors affect the sensitivity of normal and malignant cells and the responses of normal tissues and tumors to radiation. The impact of a few major factors is briefly described because of their relevance to fractionated radiation.

Oxygen Status

Molecular oxygen is the most potent modulator of cellular radiosensitivity. Its effect was noted close to a century ago through the observation that interference with the blood supply to the irradiated area reduced the intensity of erythema. However, the full recognition of its importance in tissue response to radiation began in the early 1950s. Oxygen affects radiosensitivity by altering how cells process radiation-induced free radicals that break chemical bonds. When present, oxygen reacts with free radicals, producing irreparable chemical changes in key molecules and leading

to cell lethality. Therefore, it is said that molecular oxygen "fixes" labile radiation injury, a process that takes place within milliseconds of irradiation. In the absence of oxygen (hypoxia), many of these chemical lesions are repaired, which increases the resistance of cells to radiation cell killing.

The oxygen effect increases with its concentration, with the maximum change in radiosensitivity occurring in the range of 0 to 20 mm Hg (beyond this, further increase has little effect). The magnitude of oxygen effect is called the oxygen enhancement ratio (OER), which has a maximal value of 2.5 to 3 for most mammalian cells. There is some evidence showing that the OER may be lower for small doses per fraction or low-dose-rate irradiation.

Many solid tumors contain radioresistant hypoxic cells because of deficient or aberrant neoangiogenesis. Because oxygen diffusion distance is rather limited, cells situated more than 100 to 150 μm away from vascular capillaries remain hypoxic for long periods (*chronic hypoxia*). This is in contrast to *acute hypoxia*, which results from temporary closure of tumor blood vessels. Recent work has showed that the presence of hypoxia in head and neck carcinomas, detected by oxygen probe measurements, is associated with poorer outcome.[10–12]

Cell Age in the Division Cycle

Mammalian cells exhibit significant variation in radiosensitivity as they move through the division cycle, as can be demonstrated with the use of synchronized cell populations. Generally, cells in late G2 or mitosis are most sensitive, whereas those in late S are most radioresistant. Cells in late G1 and early S-phase exhibit intermediate radiosensitivity. Cells having a long G1 phase tend to show a peak of resistance in early G1. The relative magnitude of this variability, for example, is demonstrated by an in vitro study on V-79 cells exposed to 2 Gy, showing that the most resistant late S-phase cells under well-oxygenated conditions had higher survival than did the most sensitive G2/M phase cells under hypoxic conditions.[2]

Type of Radiation

Different types of radiation induce different densities of ionization or energy deposition per unit length of track, called linear energy transfer (LET). X-rays and γ-rays, electrons, and protons are low-LET radiation because they produce sparse density of ionization. In contrast, neutrons and heavy nuclei produce dense ionization and are referred to as high-LET radiation. High-LET radiation, gray for gray, produces stronger biologic effect than does low-LET radiation because it kills cells primarily by an irreparable single-hit mechanism. Therefore, compared with low-LET radiation, the shape of the radiation dose-survival curve of high-LET radiation has a smaller or no shoulder and a steeper terminal slope. Consequently, there is much less sparing effect of dose fractionation; hence, the relative biologic effect (RBE) of high-LET irradiation increases with decreasing dose per fraction. In addition, cell killing by high-LET radiation is less dependent on oxygen or on the position of cells in the cell cycle.

Biologic Basis of Dose Fractionation

Fractionated radiotherapy has gradually replaced single-dose exposure since 1920, mostly on the basis of clinical experience. However, the scientific rationale for dose fractionation was not understood until a while later. The four well-known biologic processes underlying dose fractionation are repair of sublethal damage, redistribution, regeneration, and reoxygenation, the so-called four R's of radiotherapy.

Repair of Sublethal Damage

As was mentioned earlier, the reappearance of the shoulder when radiation dose is fractionated reflects the ability of cells to recover from damage that does not directly cause lethality. The repair capacity, however, varies among cells and tissues, and is consistently greater in late-responding than in rapidly reacting tissues. The cell survival curves of late-responding tissues are characterized by small α/β ratios, whereas those of rapidly reacting tissues have large α/β ratios. The clinical implication is that decreasing dose per fraction will result in greater sparing of late-responding tissues, which is usually dose-limiting in radiotherapy. Recognition of this phenomenon underlies the birth of the hyperfractionated radiotherapy regimen (see under Clinical Radiobiology—Altered Fractionation).

Redistribution

Cells vary considerably in their radiosensitivity as they move through the division cycle. In initially asynchronous cell populations, the first radiation dose preferentially kills cells in sensitive phases. Consequently, cells surviving the first dose tend to be partially synchronized in more resistant phases. However, these cells will resume their progression through the division cycle into more radiosensitive phases, resulting in a net sensitization to the next dose fraction. The magnitude of this phenomenon is proportional to the cell proliferation kinetics. It takes place mainly in tissues with moderate to rapid cell turnover, such as acutely reacting normal tissues and tumors, and is negligible in late-responding normal tissues. Therefore, redistribution results generally in a net gain in the therapeutic ratio between tumor control and late normal tissue injury.

Regeneration (Repopulation)

Depletion of cells by radiation, partial surgical resection, or any cytotoxic agent, in both normal and neoplastic tissues, triggers a regenerative response by speeding up clonogenic proliferation rate, a process called *regenerative response* or *accelerated repopulation,* resulting in a net increase in cell production. The time of onset and kinetics of regeneration vary greatly among tissues, and the magnitude depends on the number of surviving cells retaining their proliferative capacity. Acutely responding tissues with rapid cell turnover in which cell depletion occurs rapidly exhibit early onset of regenerative response. Although it is beneficial in terms of reducing normal tissue injury, regeneration in tumors reduces the likelihood for cure. When the regenerative potential of the tumor exceeds that of the critical, acute-reacting normal tissue, such as occurs in a subset of head and neck carcinomas, therapeutic gain results from shortening the course of radiotherapy (accelerated fractionation; see also under Clinical Radiobiology—Altered Fractionation).

Reoxygenation

As has been discussed briefly, the presence of hypoxic cells in most solid tumors and their relative radiation resistance are major causes of tumor radiation resistance. Ample experimental data show that during a course of fractionated radiation, the oxygen status of originally hypoxic cells may gradually improve before subsequent doses are given. This process, called *reoxygenation,* may result from a number of mechanisms. For example, the preferential elimination of more radiosensitive, oxygenated cells increases oxygen availability to surviving hypoxic cells and also lowers the interstitial pressure on microvessels within a tumor, resulting in improved tumor microcirculation and oxygen supply. In addition, tumor shrinkage and active tumor cell migration bring previously hypoxic microregions closer to blood vessels.

A number of clinical observations suggest that reoxygenation takes place in human tumor, although its magnitude is not exactly known. For example, many human tumors are cured by doses of radiation that would be inconsistent with the presence of a significant number of hypoxic tumor cells. More direct evidence for tumor reoxygenation occurring during fractionated radiation has recently been provided by measurements of tumor Po_2 during radiotherapy.[12]

Tumor Control Probability

Sigmoid Tumor Control Probability Curves

Because a single surviving clonogen (a cell capable of sustained proliferation) is able to cause tumor regrowth (recurrence), permanent tumor control does not occur until the last clonogen is killed by radiation or cytotoxic drug or is removed by surgery. In terms of radiation, although increasing the dose delivered to a given tumor progressively decreases the number of surviving tumor clonogens (and thus the tumor size), the probability for permanent local control remains at 0% up to a dose that reduces the number of surviving clonogens to one. An incremental dose above this threshold, however, causes the tumor control probability (TCP) to jump straight up from 0% to 100% upon elimination of the last surviving clonogen.

Because cell killing is a random process (see under Radiation Dose-Response Curves), the shape of the TCP curve for a series of tumors with identical features is sigmoid above the threshold dose because there will be a Poisson distribution of numbers of surviving clonogens per tumor (Fig. 31–6A). Poisson statistics correlate the TCP with cell survival by the formula $P_{control} = e^{-(M \times SF)}$, where M is the initial clonogen number (depending on the size and clonogen density of the tumor) and SF is the surviving fraction (determined by the intrinsic clonogen radiosensitivity and radiation dose, D, where $SF = e^{-(\alpha D + \beta D^2)}$). For example, if a dose reduced the clonogen survival in a series of identical

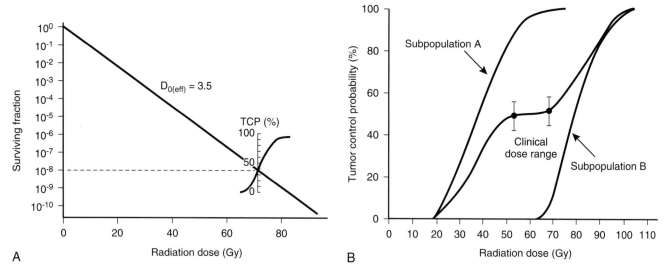

FIGURE 31–6 *A,* The relationship between $D_{0(eff)}$ of fractionated radiation and the tumor control probability (TCP). *B,* The effect of tumor heterogeneity on tumor control dose-response relationship using the example of two equal subpopulations of tumors, which differ substantially in radiocurability. Under this condition, even accurately defined control probability rates would show no significant dose-response relationship in the clinical dose range.

tumors to an average of one per tumor, 37% of tumors would result in no survivors, 37% in one, 18% in two, and 8% in three or even more surviving clonogens. As a result, the local control rate would be 37% (i.e., e^{-1}) instead of 0%. Correspondingly, doses that reduce the clonogen survival to averages of 2.3 and 0.1 per tumor would yield 10% ($e^{-2.3}$) and 90% ($e^{-0.1}$) tumor control rates, respectively (see under Radiation Dose-Response Curves).

Slope of the Tumor Control Probability Curve

For a homogeneous population of tumors, the slope of the sigmoid TCP curve is relatively steep, that is, TCP increases rapidly over a small dose range. However, any variability in tumor clonogen number or other radiobiologic property governing response will flatten the TCP curve. This is because subsets of tumors, each with a steep dose-response function, may be separated by some distance on the dose axis, and when analysis is done of the group as a whole, the observed segment of the composite dose-response curve will be shallow or even flat (Fig. 31–6*B*). Within such dose ranges, no dose-response relationship for tumor control exists for the population as a whole. Such heterogeneity combined with patient selection biases and variability in dose prescription and radiotherapy technique can make it difficult or improbable to demonstrate dose-response relationships from a retrospective analysis of clinical data. It is important to remember, however, that the probability of controlling individual tumors by radiotherapy is dose-dependent; therefore, cure of the most curable subsets of tumors will be most affected when radiation dose is reduced, unless the existing level of tumor control is very high or very low. Because of the sigmoid shape of the TCP curve, little change in tumor control probability with dose is to be expected toward the high and low ends of the curve even with a uniform group of tumors.

Effect of Combined-Modality Therapy on Tumor Control Probability

In a series of identical tumors containing, for example, 10^7 initial number of clonogens, a radiation dose that reduces the clonogen survival rate to 10^{-7} (i.e., on average one surviving clonogen per tumor) would yield a 37% cure rate. With other factors being equal, a 10-fold increase in clonogenic cell killing (e.g., by administering radiosensitizing chemotherapy concurrently) would reduce surviving clonogens from an average of 1 to 0.1 per tumor and, thereby, would increase the local control rate from 37% (e^{-1}) to 90% ($e^{-0.1}$). Similarly, a 10-fold reduction in clonogen number before radiotherapy, such as by surgical debulking of 90% of the tumor volume, would theoretically achieve the same effect. The actual benefit derived from debulking surgery is in general smaller than this arithmetic product because the remaining clonogens would proliferate, likely at an accelerated rate (regenerative response), during the interval between surgery and commencement of postoperative radiotherapy. Three clonogenic cell doublings occurring during the interval (resulting in an 8-fold increase in the clonogenic cell number) would almost completely eliminate the effect of surgical debulking. This is the reason that a long interval between surgery and postoperative radiotherapy leads to a poorer outcome, as demonstrated by the data from a recently completed prospective trial.[13]

Accelerated repopulation is thought to account for the detrimental effect of split-course radiotherapy and the lack of therapeutic benefit resulting from induction or neoadjuvant chemotherapy, in spite of the high initial complete and partial response rates, in cancer of the head and neck. According to the scenario presented in the preceding paragraph, without adjustments in the radiation dose, one clonogenic cell doubling taking place during the interruption would reduce the TCP from 37% (e^{-1}) to about 14% (e^{-2}), and two divisions would diminish the TCP further to approximately 2% (e^{-4}).

The shallower slopes of human tumor TCP curves reduce the magnitudes of changes illustrated previously. Nevertheless, these general principles are valid for individual tumors, and all efforts should be taken to apply them properly to maximize therapeutic outcome.

Normal Tissue Complication Probability

Because of exponential cell killing, normal tissue complication probability (NTCP) curves also have sigmoid shape above a threshold dose. However, the NTCP curves have much steeper slopes than do TCP curves because there is much less heterogeneity among normal tissue cells. Therefore, above an 80% to 85% TCP, increasing the radiation dose would generally increase normal tissue complications to a greater extent than it would improve tumor control. NTCP curves for various normal tissues have been generated from experimental animal models. Detailed dose-response data for late normal tissue complications in humans are not available because radiation oncologists have been conservative in prescribing radiation doses to avoid the severe complications that affect quality of life.

The tolerance doses published earlier, such as a 5% probability of complications occurring within 5 years (TD5/5) and a 50% probability of complications occurring within 5 years (TD50/5), have been generated mostly based on clinical impressions.[14, 15] However, revised and perhaps more accurate dose-response estimates for various normal tissues, compiled through a Late Effects of Normal Tissues (LENT) Consensus Conference held in August of 1992, were published in a special issue of the *International Journal of Radiation Oncology, Biology, and Physics* in March of 1995.

◼ ADVANCES IN RADIATION ONCOLOGY

Cancer of the head and neck is the subject of intensive laboratory and clinical investigations. Because of the ease of clinical assessment and a relatively low incidence of systemic dissemination, head and neck cancers are good models for testing the efficacy of new therapeutic concepts, such as radiation fractionation regimens and combined treatment modalities, that are aimed at improving the locoregional control rate. A vast majority of the clinical radiobiology research on altered fractionation and the combination of radiation and chemotherapy, for example, has been conducted on patients with advanced head and neck cancers.

Clinical Radiobiology—Altered Fractionation

Advancement in radiobiologic concepts has led to the development of two classes of new fractionation schedules, referred to as *hyperfractionation* schedules and *accelerated fractionation* schedules.[16] Hyperfractionation exploits the difference in fractionation sensitivity between tumors and normal tissues that manifest late morbidity. As is illustrated in Figure 31–7, most tumor and acutely reacting normal tissue responses to fractionated radiation are less sensitive to changes in dose per fraction, particularly below 2 Gy, than are those of late-responding normal tissues. This difference

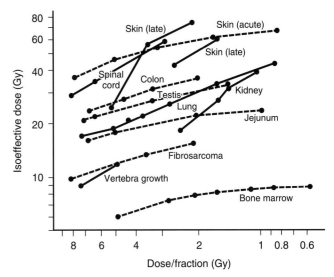

FIGURE 31–7 Isoeffect curves (total doses inducing an equal biologic effect vs dose per fraction) for acutely (*dashed lines*) and late-responding (*solid lines*) tissues. The curves for late effects are steeper than those for acute reactions, indicating that as the dose per fraction is reduced, higher total dose of radiation is needed to inflict the same magnitude of damage.[73]

can be exploited to increase the total radiation dose through a hyperfractionation schedule, that is, by giving two or more small dose fractions on each treatment day but keeping the overall treatment time conventional or slightly reduced. The use of smaller fractions increases the tolerance of late-reacting tissues such that the total radiation dose can be increased by about 10% to 15% without worsening of late complications. In contrast, accelerated fractionations attempt to reduce tumor proliferation, which is a major cause of radiotherapy failure.

These radiobiologic concepts have undergone intensive testing in patients with cancer of the head and neck during the past two and a half decades. The published results of the first 10 completed phase III clinical trials have been reviewed and discussed.[17] The updated results of large randomized trials[18–20] are briefly summarized in Table 31–1 to illustrate that rational application of radiobiologic principles gained from laboratory studies can improve radiotherapy outcomes. In aggregate, trials with sufficient follow-up data addressing hyperfractionation show a moderate (10% to 15%) but consistent improvement in local control. The incidence of late toxicity associated with a 10% to 15% total dose increment delivered in smaller than standard fraction sizes, twice a day, was within the range observed with conventional fractionation schedules, although none of the studies was designed to test equivalence of late morbidity. These data support the experimental finding of the existence of differential sensitivity to radiation dose fractionation between human tumors and late-responding normal tissues.

The collective results of accelerated fractionation trials show that tumor clonogen repopulation is indeed a major cause of failure to cure head and neck carcinomas by fractionated radiotherapy, and therefore that shortening of overall treatment time can increase tumor control rate (see Table 31–1). However, an overall time reduction of more than 1.5 weeks without a decrease in the total dose induces

TABLE 31-1 Phase III Trials Addressing Altered Fractionation in Patients With Head and Neck Cancer

Tumor Site and Stage	No. of Pts	d (Gy)	n and Ti (h)	D (Gy)	T	Tumor Response	Complications	Authors
Oropharynx. T2–3N0–1	356	1.15	2 (6–8)	80.5	7 w	5-yr LRC: 59% vs. 40% ($P=.02$)	More acute mucositis with HF	Horiot et al, 1992[18]
		2.0	1	70.0	7 w	Improved local control of T3 tumors	No difference in late complication rate	
Various sites. T3–4N0 or any TN⁺	331	1.45	2	58.0	4 w	5-yr LRC: 45% vs. 37% ($P=.01$)	More acute mucositis with HF	Cummings et al, 2000[19]
		2.55	1	51.0	4 w	5-yr OS: 40% vs. 30% ($P=.01$)	5-yr grade III–IV late toxicity: 8% vs. 14% ($P=.31$)	
Various sites. Stages III–IV, selected stage II	1073	1.20	2 (≥6)	81.6	7 w	LRC: Higher with HF and AF-CB ($P=.045$ and .05)	More acute mucositis with all altered fractionations	Fu et al, 2000[20]
		1.60	2 (≥6)	67.2	6 w	DFS: Strong trend in favor of HF and CB ($P=.067$ and .054)	No difference in late complication rate	
		1.8°	1–2 (≥6)	72.0	6 w			
		2.0	1	70.0	7 w			
All sites and all stages	1485	2.0	1	68.0	6 w	5-yr LRC: 66% vs. 57% ($P=.01$)	More acute mucositis with HF	Overgaard et al, 2000[21]
		2.0	1	68.0	7 w	5-yr DFS: 72% vs. 65% ($P=.04$)	No difference in late complication rate	
Larynx. T1–3N0	395	2.0	1	66.0	6.5 w	LRC: Higher with AF ($P=.03$)	More acute reactions with HF	Hliniak et al, 2000[22]
		2.0	1–2 (≥6)	66.0	5.5 w		No difference in late complications except for telangiectasia	
All sites. Oropharynx— 75%; T4—70%	268	2.0	2	~63	3 w	2-yr LRC: 58% vs. 34% ($P <.01$)	Grades III and IV mucositis: 83% vs. 28% ($P <.01$). Similar late toxicity	Bourhis et al, 2000[23]
		2.0	1	70	7 w			

°Boost given in 1.5 Gy per fraction.

AF, accelerated fractionation; CB, concomitant boost; d, dose per fraction; D, total dose, DFS, disease-free survival; h, hours; HF, hyperfraction; LRC, locoregional control; n, number of fractions per day; OS, overall survival; Pts, patients; T, overall treatment time; Ti, time interval between fractions; yr, year; w, weeks.

intolerable acute mucosal toxicity,[21, 22] and delivery of more than 2 fractions per day can cause a higher incidence of late toxicity.[23] Table 31–1 shows the results of four accelerated fractionation regimens that yield improvement in tumor control without demonstrable increased late toxicity. These are the concomitant boost,[20] six fractions per week,[24, 25] and very accelerated[26] regimens. Similar to hyperfractionation, the average magnitude of improvement in locoregional control is on the order of 10% to 15%.

Conformal Radiotherapy

Computed tomography (CT)-based two-dimensional (2-D) systems are widely used in the planning and delivery of radiation therapy. Many technologic advances have progressively made radiation delivery more practical and accurate and more sophisticated. A few examples are presented.

Progress in the engineering of medical linear accelerators, such as the introduction of the computer-operated multileaf collimator (MLC), enables flexible portal shaping and modification (e.g., the use of field-in-field technique) during a single radiation session. This technique is useful in achieving the desired dose distribution within the target volume. Figure 31–8 shows the dose distributions at the midsagittal plane from the primary large opposed lateral fields. Without beam modulation, the dose gradients, plotted in 5% increments, varied from 95% (cold spot) to 115% (hot spot) relative to the isocenter (see Fig. 31–8A). With new linacs, it is relatively easy to adjust collimator leafs to progressively block off the hot spot regions (see Fig. 31–8B to F) to yield a more homogeneous dose distribution, as can be accomplished with a more cumbersome missing tissue compensator.[27] The same procedure can be applied to the off–spinal cord and conedown boost portals to yield homogeneous composite dose distribution through the axial, sagittal, and coronal planes, as shown in Figure 31–9. The magnitude of dose fall-off within the portal and the desired dose homogeneity determine the required number of field-in-field segments. The advantage of this method is the ease with which the segments can be visually determined.

Advances in beam intensity modification and in radiation planning–dosimetry technology, along with improvements in the accuracy of tumor delineation through progress in diagnostic imaging methodology, have introduced a new era of high-precision radiation therapy. The new technology has made it possible to deliver high radiation doses in three-dimensional (3-D) volumes that conform to the shape of the tumor and involved nodes, thereby reducing the dose administered to normal tissues. In general terms, such high-precision radiation delivery is therefore referred to as three-dimensional conformal radiotherapy (3-D CRT), or simply as conformal radiotherapy.[28–31] Conformal radiotherapy has the prospect of improving the therapeutic index of

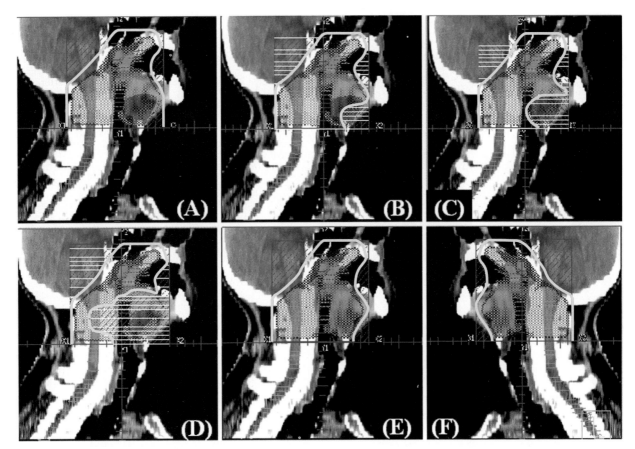

FIGURE 31–8 Distribution of radiation dose across the midsagittal plane (plotted in 5% gradients) of the initial large opposed lateral portals encompassing the primary tumor and upper cervical nodal basins. Without beam modulation, the dose distribution varies from 95% (blue colorwash) to 115% (dark sky-blue colorwash) (A). With the use of MLC leaves (*white lines*) to shield the 115% isodose line from the right lateral field (B), the 110% line from the left lateral field (C), and finally the 105% line from the right portal (D) yields a dose distribution on the central plane to within 5% of the primary prescribed dose (E and F).

radiotherapy in two ways. First, for patients with early- or intermediate-stage tumors with a relatively high probability of cure, the emphasis on normal tissue avoidance without compromise of tumor coverage would decrease morbidity and thus improve quality of life. Second, for patients with advanced neoplasms, it offers the possibility of escalating radiation dose to the tumor, which leads to improvement in tumor control probability, without overdose of normal tissues.

Briefly, conformal radiotherapy can be delivered through two techniques—through the use of geometric field shaping alone, or by the combination of field shaping with modulation of the intensity of fluence across the portal. The latter, referred to as intensity-modulated radiation therapy (IMRT), has gained popularity because of its practicality.

The improved precision in radiation delivery demands better command of head and neck anatomy and the natural history of cancer, including routes of contiguous and lymphatic spread, to avoid geographic miss. Planning of conformal radiotherapy begins with careful delineation of the macroscopic or gross tumor volume (GTV) and regions with the likelihood of harboring microscopic disease through contiguous or lymphatic spread (referred to as clinical target volume [CTV]), requiring elective radiation and outlining of the normal tissues to be spared whenever possible. Then, safety margins are added around the CTV to generate the planning target volume (PTV) to compensate for inaccuracies in beam and patient setup and the effects of organ, tumor, and patient movement. Subsequently, the number and shape of portals and the beam intensity pattern are generated with the use of computer optimization techniques. Figure 31–10 shows an example of a plan for the treatment of carcinoma of the right tonsil extending to the soft palate, to deliver a minimum of 66 Gy to the GTV and 54 Gy to the CTV while limiting the dose to the superficial parotid lobes to less than 30 Gy. About 25% to 30% of clinical radiotherapy cases require concave dose distributions to avoid a critical organ, which is difficult to achieve without IMRT.

Combination of Radiation With Cytotoxic Agents

Combining radiation with chemotherapy to improve tumor control, organ preservation, and survival rates has been the subject of intensive investigation in various cancers

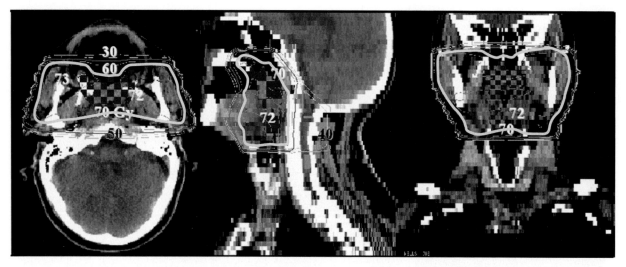

FIGURE 31–9 The composite dose distribution in the transverse, sagittal, and coronal planes.

during the past several decades. Typically, cytotoxic agents have been given before (referred to as induction or neoadjuvant chemotherapy), after (referred to as adjuvant chemotherapy), or concurrently with radiation. A very large number of phase I and II studies have been conducted, mostly to test regimens that evolved empirically rather than those designed based on mechanisms of interaction. To date, only a fraction of regimens investigated have undergone proper evaluation in randomized clinical trials.

The Meta-analysis of Chemotherapy on Head and Neck Cancer Collaborative Group[32] undertook the most extensive meta-analysis of phase III trials conducted between 1965 and 1993 to compare locoregional treatment with and without chemotherapy.[32] The data of 63 randomized trials, including 5 unpublished series and 6 series reported in abstracts only, enrolling a total of 10,741 patients, were updated and analyzed. The investigators noted a marked heterogeneity among the trials with regard to tumor and patient characteristics, therapy regimen, and follow-up, which complicates analysis and data interpretation. Nonetheless, they found that chemotherapy yielded an overall hazard ratio of death of 0.9 (95% confidence interval [CI] = 0.85–0.94, P <.0001), corresponding to an absolute survival benefit of 4 percentage points both at 2 years (from 50% to 54%) and at 5 years (from 32% to 36%).

Analysis by the mode of combined therapy revealed no significant benefit resulting from neoadjuvant (induction) and adjuvant chemotherapy, which were associated with 2% (P = .10) and 1% (P = .75) higher absolute survival at 5 years, respectively. The regenerative response of tumor clonogen as the potential explanation for the lack of efficacy of neoadjuvant chemotherapy is described under Tumor Control Probability, above. In contrast to the disappointing results of induction chemotherapy, concurrent chemoradiation produced an 8% overall increase in 5-year absolute survival (P <.0001), but considerable heterogeneity was found between trials.

The results of recently completed randomized trials enrolling predominantly patients with non-nasopharyngeal carcinomas[33–37] confirm the survival benefit as found through meta-analyses. Analysis of the pattern of relapse

and iatrogenic toxicity also provided useful direction for further refinement of combined therapy. The trial of a French cooperative group (GORTEC), for example, showed that the combination of radiation with carboplatin and fluorouracil yielded a significantly higher actuarial 3-year survival rate than was attained with radiation alone (51% vs. 31%, P = .02).[35] This survival advantage was found to result from an improvement in locoregional disease control (3-year actuarial rate: 66% vs. 42%, P = .03) and not from a reduction in the frequency of distant metastases (11% vs. 11%) or a change in the intercurrent disease–related mortality (19% vs. 13%). The trial of a German cooperative group yielded identical findings.[34] This observation suggests that concurrent chemotherapy may act mainly through sensitization of tumor cells to radiation cell killing.

With longer patient follow-up, however, evidence has also emerged showing that improvement in survival with concurrent radiation and chemotherapy has been achieved at the expense of increased late toxicity, mainly fibrosis and dysphagia leading to feeding tube dependency. The updated GORTEC data,[38] for example, show that the addition of carboplatin and fluorouracil to radiation improved the 5-year survival from 16% to 23% (P = .05) but also increased the grade III to IV late complication rate from 32% to 49% (P = .02).

Targeted Combined-Modality Therapy

The results of current combined therapy presented earlier show that there is still substantial room to refine therapy for patients with cancer of the head and neck. Some improvement is expected to result from a more thoughtful integration of currently available modalities. For example, a judicious application of conformal radiotherapy, which enables a more precise physical targeting of tumor and thereby reduces the volume of normal tissues exposed to high radiation dose, in combination with chemotherapy is expected to reduce some of the long-term morbidity. The flexibility of conformal radiotherapy in tailoring the dose distribution to irregular or horseshoe-shaped tumors and in escalating the radiation dose to the gross disease while

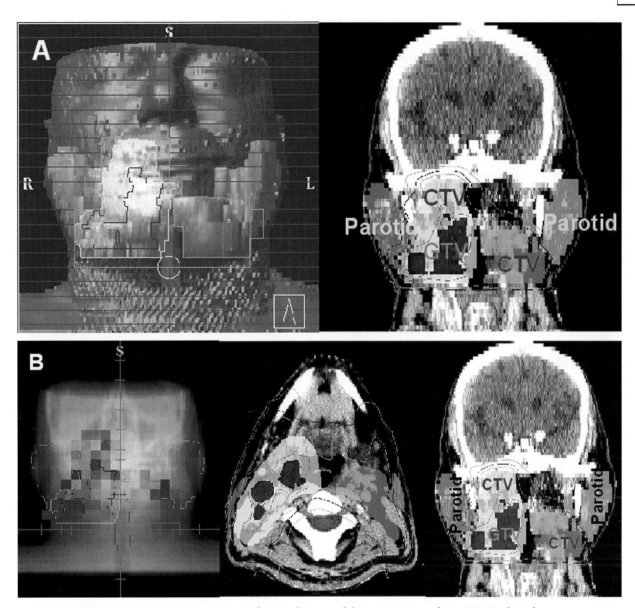

FIGURE 31–10 *A*, Beam-eye view and coronal image of the gross tumor volume (GTV), clinical target volume (CTV), parotid glands, and spinal cord of a patient with an intermediate oropharyngeal carcinoma. *B*, Intensity = modulated beam delivery and the distribution of radiation dose. The tumor receives a minimum of 66 Gy, regions at risk of harboring microscopic disease receive 54 Gy, and the superficial lobe of the contralateral parotid gland receives less than 30 Gy.

avoiding critical structures has the prospect of increasing tumor control rate in some patients. Many clinical trials testing these principles are under way, and final results will become available in the next few years.

The limitation of current standard therapy also motivates the search for novel strategies for selective enhancement of tumor response. Improving insight into the biology of normal and neoplastic tissues has begun to generate exciting innovative research ideas. Comprehensive review of this refreshing and rapidly growing field is beyond the scope of this chapter; however, a couple of examples of biologic targeting, e.g., modulation of epidermal growth factor receptor (EGFR) and cyclooxygenase-2 (COX-2), are presented.

EGFR is a transmembrane glycoprotein with intracytoplasmic tyrosine kinase activity. On ligand binding, such as with epidermal growth factor (EGF) or transforming growth factor-α (TGF-α), EGFR is phosphorylated and initiates transduction signals that regulate cell division, proliferation, differentiation, and death,[39, 40] all of which play important roles in malignant cellular transformation and tumor response to therapy. This receptor, tyrosine kinase, has attracted the attention of head and neck oncologists since the emergence of data showing that a majority of head and neck carcinomas have elevated levels of EGFR, and that EGFR overexpression is associated with poorer therapy outcome.[41, 42] In parallel, many in vitro experimental studies have yielded evidence linking EGFR with cellular resistance to cytotoxic drugs[40, 43–46] or radiation.[47, 48] Our own study of murine tumors with a wide range of EGFR expressions in vivo, for example, shows that higher EGFR-expressing tumors had a lower propensity for radiation-induced apoptosis and a lower tumor cure rate.[49]

These experimental findings have induced enthusiasm for the development of approaches targeting EGFR over-expression. Strategies that are in various stages of development include blockade of the extracellular receptor domain,[50–56] inhibition of intracellular tyrosine kinase activity (reviewed by Fry[57] and Noonberg and associates[58]), inhibition of receptor production by antisense approaches,[52, 59] and expression of a truncated dominant-negative EGFR mutant.[60] Of these strategies, antibody against EGFR, C225, has been most extensively investigated. Our initial in vivo study was designed to assess the impact of EGFR blockade by C225 on the response of a high EGFR-expressing tumor, A431 carcinoma, to radiation.[53] This work revealed that C225 given alone (in one or three doses) had minimal effects on tumor growth, but when administered in conjunction with radiation, it substantially enhanced tumor response, that is, by factors of 1.59 and 3.62 for one dose and three doses of C225, respectively (Fig. 31–11). Histologic examination revealed that C225 plus radiation induced striking central tumor necrosis, associated with hemorrhage and vascular thrombosis, increased tumor cell differentiation, and reduced tumor angiogenesis. This study thus showed that C225 enhances tumor response to radiation through multiple mechanisms that may involve direct and indirect actions on tumor cell survival.[53] Subsequent studies have revealed that C225 given with radiation also increased tumor cure probability, that is, decreased the median tumor control dose (TCD_{50}) by a factor of 1.92 in A431 xenograft.[54]

A phase III trial to test the role of C225 in combination with radiotherapy in the treatment of stages III and IV head and neck carcinomas activated in late 1999 is nearing completion of patient accrual. The results of this prospective study will likely be available by the end of 2003.

Cyclooxygenase catalyzes the conversion of arachidonic acid to prostaglandins, which regulate critical physiologic functions (e.g., blood clotting, nerve growth and development, wound healing, renal function, blood vessel tone, and immune response) and cellular responses (e.g., adhesion, differentiation, and mitogenesis) in humans. COX-1 displays the characteristics of a "housekeeping" gene[61] and is constitutively expressed in almost all tissues to regulate production of prostaglandins (PGs) that are important for homeostatic functions, such as maintaining the integrity of the gastric mucosa, mediating normal platelet function, and regulating renal blood flow.[62] On the other hand, COX-2 is the product of an "immediate-early" gene that is rapidly inducible and tightly regulated. COX-2 expression is highly restricted under normal circumstances but is upregulated by a variety of conditions and agents such as inflammatory stimuli, cytokines, growth factors, and tumor promoters.[63, 64]

An increasing body of data shows that COX-2 and PGs coregulate tumor growth and dissemination. Even before the discovery of COX-2 a decade ago, it was known that malignant tumors often produce excessive quantities of PGs, which were associated with more aggressive biologic behavior.[65–68] Recent immunohistochemical analyses have revealed that COX-2 is overexpressed in a variety of human cancers, including head and neck, lung, colon, breast, and pancreas.[69] Therefore, the discovery of selective COX-2 inhibitors has inspired many investigators to test their efficacy in cancer treatment.

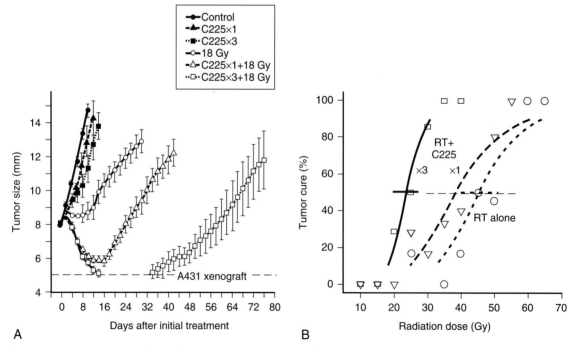

FIGURE 31–11 *A*, Effects of anti-EGFR antibody (C225) on radiation response of A431 xenograft. The curves (*left to right*) represent the growth of tumors receiving no treatment (control), C225×1, C225×3, 18 Gy, C225×1 + 18 Gy, and C225×3 + 18 Gy. *B*, Effects of C225 on radiocurability of A431. The curves (*right to left*) represent dose response for radiation (RT) alone (□), RT+C225×1 (∇), and RT+C225×3 (○). (Modified from Milas and associates[53] and Nasu and colleagues.[54])

One of our experimental studies, for example, addressed the effects of SC-'236, a selective COX-2 inhibitor, on tumor and normal tissue radiation response in rodent models.[70] This work revealed that SC-'236 by itself had little effect on the growth kinetics of a fibrosarcoma (FSA) but, when given in combination with radiation, it significantly prolonged the regrowth delay (enhancement factor, 2.14) and reduced the median tumor control dose (TCD_{50}) by a factor of 1.87; it did not, however, substantially alter the radiation-induced damage to jejunal crypts nor the development of late leg contracture. Further analyses showed that SC-'236 did not potentiate radiation-induced apoptosis but inhibited angiogenesis, and that enhancement of tumor response was associated with a decrease in tumor prostaglandin E_2 (PGE_2) levels. Two other experiments showed that SC-'236 greatly enhanced the tumor response of the NFSA murine sarcoma (Fig. 31–12)[71] and the human U251 glioma xenograft[72] in nude mice. Many clinical trials addressing the role of COX-2 inhibitors in the treatment of cancer of the lung, uterine cervix, pancreas, and other sites have been launched based on the results of these experimental studies.

SUMMARY

Enormous research efforts have been directed toward investigating the biology, treatment, and prevention of cancer. Such long-term investment in cancer research has finally begun to turn the tide against the majority of neoplasms as the death rate from all cancers in the United States (after rising continuously from the inception of record keeping) for the first time fell by 2.6% between 1991 and 1995.[73] Most of this decrease in the mortality rate was observed in patients younger than age 65.

Research on head and neck carcinomas has been exciting and rewarding during the past few decades. This is reflected in the enthusiasm associated with enrolling patients into large-scale, cooperative group clinical trials testing, for example, combinations of radiation and chemotherapy and biologically sound fractionation regimens. It is pleasing to learn that the highest decline in the cancer mortality rate (9.6%) has occurred in patients with cancer of the head and neck, irrespective of age.[73] Unfortunately, with longer follow-up of patients enrolled in randomized trials addressing combined-modality therapy, we begin to realize that this reduction in mortality rate is achieved too often at the cost of increased toxicity, particularly when cytotoxic agents are given concurrently with radiation therapy. However, recent advances in radiation oncology have generated a great deal of optimism as novel strategies for improving quality of life and survival rates are being developed for clinical testing.

Technical innovations in radiation therapy planning and delivery have significantly improved the precision of radiation treatment, which will at least reduce the toxicity of combined therapy and perhaps improve tumor control in some specific sites by allowing radiation dose escalation. Advances in radiobiologic insight are leading to conception of molecular targeted approaches for selectively sensitizing tumors to radiation.

There is little doubt that the pace of discovery will increase over the years to come. For example, it is reasonable to envision the not-too-distant availability of improved methods for anatomic and biologic tumor imaging and for characterizing the genetic profiles of cancers that can depict their individual virulence, predict therapy response, and guide treatment selection. Such progress will hopefully result in further reduction in the mortality rate of patients with cancer of the head and neck.

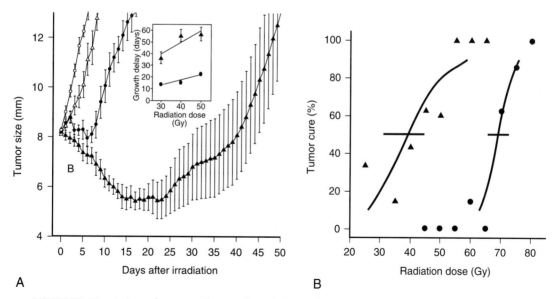

FIGURE 31–12 *A*, Growth curves of tumor (*from left to right*) receiving no treatment, 6 mg/kg SC-'236, 30 Gy, and SC-'236 + 30 Gy. The *insert* shows the absolute (*bottom*) and normalized (*top*) regrowth delay as a function of radiation dose. *B*, Local control curves of tumors treated with single doses of radiation with (▲) or without (●) SC-'236. SC-'236 enhanced the tumor control probability by a factor of 1.77. (Modified from Milas and coworkers.[71])

REFERENCES

1. Thames HD, Hendry JH: Fractionation in Radiotherapy. London, Taylor & Francis, 1987.
2. Hall EJ: Radiobiology for the Radiologist, 5th ed. Philadelphia, Lippincott Williams & Wilkins, 2000.
3. Gunderson LL, Tepper JE: Clinical Radiation Oncology. New York, Churchill Livingstone, 2000.
4. Perez CA, Brady LW: Principles and Practice of Radiation Oncology, 3rd ed. Philadelphia, Lippincott-Raven, 1998.
5. Evans RD: Radius of nuclei. In Evans RD (ed): The Atomic Nucleus. New York, McGraw-Hill, 1955, pp 49–50.
6. Douglas JG, Lee S, Laramore GE, et al: Neutron radiotherapy for the treatment of locally advanced major salivary gland tumors. Head Neck 21:255–263, 1999.
7. Wilson RR: Radiological use of fast protons. Radiology 47:487–491, 1946.
8. Johns HE, Cunningham JR: The Physics of Radiology. Springfield, Charles C Thomas, 1983.
9. Wyckoff HO, Allisy A, Linden K: The new special names of SI units in the field of ionizing radiations. Acta Radiol Ther Phys Biol 14:590–591, 1975.
10. Höckel M, Knoop C, Schlenger K, et al: Intratumoral pO2 predicts survival in advanced cancer of the uterine cervix. Radiother Oncol 26:45–50, 1993.
11. Nordsmark M, Overgaard M, Overgaard J: Pretreatment oxygenation predicts radiation response in advanced squamous cell carcinoma of the head and neck. Radiother Oncol 41:31–39, 1996.
12. Brizel DM, Sibley GS, Prosnitz LR, et al: Tumor hypoxia adversely affects the prognosis of carcinoma of the head and neck. Int Radiat Oncol Biol Phys 38:285–289, 1997.
13. Ang KK, Trotti A, Brown BW, et al: Randomized trial addressing risk features and time factors of surgery plus radiotherapy in advanced head and neck cancer. Int J Radiat Oncol Biol Phys 51:571–578, 2001.
14. Rubin P, Cassarett GW: Clinical Radiation Pathology. Philadelphia, WB Saunders, 1968.
15. Emami B, Lyman J, Brown A, et al: Tolerance of normal tissue to therapeutic irradiation. Int Radiat Oncol Biol Phys 21:109–122, 1991.
16. Thames HD, Withers HR, Peters LJ, et al: Changes in early and late radiation responses with altered dose fractionation: Implications for dose-survival relationships. Int J Radiat Oncol Biol Phys 8:219–226, 1982.
17. Ang K: Altered Fractionation in Head and Neck Cancer. Semin Radiat Oncol 8:230–236, 1998.
18. Horiot JC, LeFur RN, Guyen T, et al: Hyperfractionation versus conventional fractionation in oropharyngeal carcinoma: Final analysis of a randomized trial of the EORTC cooperative group of radiotherapy. Radiother Oncol 25:231–241, 1992.
19. Cummings B, O'Sullivan B, Keane T, et al: 5-year results of a 4 week/twice daily radiation schedule—the Toronto Trial. Radiother Oncol 56:S8, 2000.
20. Fu KK, Pajak TF, Trotti A, et al: A radiation therapy oncology group (RTOG) phase III randomized study to compare hyperfractionation and two variants of accelerated fractionation to standard fractionation radiotherapy for head and neck squamous cell carcinomas: First report of RTOG 9003. Int J Radiat Oncol Biol Phys 48:7–16, 2000.
21. Jackson SM, Weir LM, Hay JH, et al: A randomised trial of accelerated versus conventional radiotherapy in head and neck cancer. Radiother Oncol 43:39–46, 1997.
22. Skladowski K, Maciejewski J, Golen M, et al: Randomized clinical trial on 7-day continuous accelerated irradiation (CAIR) of head and neck cancer—report on 3-year tumor control and normal tissue toxicity. Radiother Oncol 55:93–102, 2000.
23. Horiot JC, Bontemps P, van den Bogaert V, et al: Accelerated fractionation (AF) compared to conventional fractionation (CF) improved head and neck cancers: Results of the EROTC 22851 randomized trial. Radiother Oncol 44:111–121, 1997.
24. Overgaard J, Hansen HS, Grau C, et al: The DAHANCA 6 and 7 trial. A randomized multicenter study of 5 versus 6 fractions per week of conventional radiotherapy of squamous cell carcinoma (scc) of the head and neck. Radiother Oncol 56:S4, 2000.
25. Hliniak A, Gwiazdowska B, Szutkowski Z, et al: Radiotherapy of laryngeal cancer. The estimation of the therapeutic gain and the enhancement of toxicity by the one-week shortening of the treatment time. Results of the randomized phase III multicenter trial. Radiother Oncol 56:S5, 2000.
26. Bourhis J, Lapeyre M, Tortochaux J, et al: Very accelerated versus conventional radiotherapy in HNSCC: Results of the GORTEC 94-02 randomized trial. Int J Radiat Oncol Biol Phys 48:S111, 2000.
27. Tyburski LL, Kestin L, Yan D, et al: An efficient method to improve dose uniformity of tangential breast radiotherapy using multiple MLC segments. Int Radiat Oncol Biol Phys 45:423, 1999.
28. Simpson JR, Purdy JA, Manolis JM, et al: Three-dimensional treatment planning considerations for prostate cancer. Int Radiat Oncol Biol Phys 21:243–252, 1991.
29. Altschuler MD, Powlis WD, Censor Y: Teletherapy treatment planning with physician requirements included in the calculation: 1. Concepts and methodology. In Paliwal BR, Herbert DE, Orton CG (eds): Optimization of Cancer Radiotherapy. New York, American Institute of Physics, 1984, pp 443–452.
30. Galvin JM, Smith AR, Moeller RD, et al: Evaluation of multileaf collimator design for a photon beam. Int Radiat Oncol Biol Phys 23:789–801, 1992.
31. Powlis WD, Smith AR, Cheng E, et al: Initiation of multi-leaf collimator conformal radiation therapy. Int Radiat Oncol Biol Phys 25:171–179, 1993.
32. Pignon JP, Bourhis J, Domenge C, et al: Chemotherapy added to locoregional treatment for head and neck squamous-cell carcinoma: Three meta-analyses of updated individual data. Lancet 355:949–955, 2000.
33. Brizel DM, Albers ME, Fisher SR, et al: Hyperfractionated irradiation with or without concurrent chemotherapy for locally advanced head and neck cancer. N Engl J Med 338:1798–1804, 1998.
34. Wendt TG, Grabenbauer GG, Rodel CM, et al: Simultaneous radiochemotherapy versus radiotherapy alone in advanced head and neck cancer: A randomized multicenter study. J Clin Oncol 16:1318–1324, 1998.
35. Calais G, Alfonsi M, Bardet E, et al: Randomized trial of radiation therapy versus concomitant chemotherapy and radiation therapy for advanced-stage oropharynx carcinoma. J Natl Cancer Inst 91:2081–2086, 1999.
36. Adelstein DJ, Adams GL, Li Y, et al: A phase III comparison of standard radiation therapy (RT) versus RT plus concurrent cisplatin (DDP) versus split-course RT plus concurrent DDP and 5-fluorouracil (5FU) in patients with unresectable squamous cell head and neck cancer (SCHNC): An intergroup study [abstract]. Proc ASCO 19:411a, 2000.
37. Bernier J, Domenge C, Eschwege F, et al: Chemo-radiotherapy, as compared to radiotherapy alone, significantly increases disease-free and overall survival in head and neck cancer patients after surgery: Results of EORTC phase III trial 22931. Int J Radiat Oncol Biol Phys 51:1, 2001.
38. Calais G, Alfonsi M, Bardet E, et al: Radiation alone (RT) versus RT with concomitant chemotherapy (CT) in stages III and IV oropharynx carcinoma. Final results of the 94-01 GORTEC randomized study. Int Radiat Oncol Biol Phys 51:1, 2001.
39. Salomon DS, Brandt R, Ciardiello R, et al: Epidermal growth factor-related peptides and their receptors in human malignancies. Crit Rev Oncol Hematol 19:183–232, 1995.
40. Mendelsohn J, Fan Z: Epidermal growth factor receptor family and chemosensitization. J Natl Cancer Inst 89:341–343, 1997.
41. Maurizi M, Almadori G, Ferrandina G, et al: Prognostic significance of epidermal growth factor receptor in laryngeal squamous cell carcinoma. Br J Cancer 74:1253–1257, 1996.
42. Grandis J, Melhem M, Gooding W, et al: Levels of TGF-α and EGFR protein in head and neck squamous cell carcinoma and patient survival. J Natl Cancer Inst 90:824–832, 1998.
43. Dickstein BN, Wosikowski K, Bates S: Increased resistance to cytotoxic agents in ZR75B human breast cancer cells transfected with epidermal growth factor receptor. Mol Cell Endocrinol 110:205–211, 1995.
44. Hancock MC, Langton BC, Chan T, et al: A monoclonal antibody against the c-erbB-2 protein enhances the cytotoxicity of cis-diamminedichloroplatinum against human breast and ovarian tumor cell lines. Cancer Res 51:4575–4580, 1991.

45. Pietras RJ, Fendly BM, Chazin VR, et al: Antibody to HER-2/neu receptor blocks DNA repair after cisplatin in human breast and ovarian cancer cells. Oncogene 9:1829–1838, 1994.

46. Baselga J, Norton L, Albanell, et al: Recombinant humanized anti-HER2 antibody (Herceptin™) enhances the antitumor activity of paclitaxel and doxorubicin against HER2/neu overexpressing human breast cancer xenografts. Cancer Res 58:2825–2831, 1998.

47. Balaban N, Moni J, Shannon M, et al: The effect of ionizing radiation on signal transduction: Antibodies to EGF receptor sensitize A431 cells to radiation. Biochim Biophys Acta 1314:147–156, 1996.

48. Sheridan MT, O'Dwyer T, Seymour CB, et al: Potential indicators of radiosensitivity in squamous cell carcinoma of the head and neck. Radiat Oncol Invest 5:180–186, 1997.

49. Akimoto T, Hunter NR, Buchmiller L, et al: Inverse relationship between epidermal growth factor receptor expression and radio-curability of murine carcinomas. Clin Cancer Res 5:437–443, 1999.

50. Goldstein NI, Prewett M, Zuklys K, et al: Biological efficacy of a chimeric antibody to the epidermal growth factor receptor in a human tumor xenograft model. Clin Cancer Res 1:1311–1318, 1995.

51. Hoffmann T, Hafner D, Ballo H, et al: Antitumor activity of anti-epidermal growth factor receptor monoclonal antibodies and cisplatin in ten human head and neck squamous cell carcinoma lines. Anticancer Res 17:4419–4425, 1997.

52. Grandis JR, Chakraborty A, Melhem MF, et al: Inhibition of epidermal growth factor receptor gene expression and function decreases proliferation of head and neck squamous carcinoma but not normal mucosal epithelial cells. Oncogene 15:409–416, 1997.

53. Milas L, Mason K, Hunter N, et al: In vivo enhancement of tumor radioresponse by C225 antiepidermal growth factor receptor antibody. Clin Cancer Res 6:701–708, 2000.

54. Nasu S, Ang KK, Fan Z, et al: C225 antiepidermal growth factor receptor antibody enhances tumor radiocurability. Int J Radiat Oncol Biol Phys 51:474–477, 2001.

55. Huang SM, Harari PM: Modulation of radiation response after epidermal growth factor receptor blockade in squamous cell carcinomas: Inhibition of damage repair, cell cycle kinetics, and tumor angiogenesis. Clin Cancer Res 6:2166–2174, 2000.

56. Shin DM, Donato NJ, Perez-Soler R, et al: Epidermal growth factor receptor-targeted therapy with C225 and cisplatin in patients with head and neck cancer. Clin Cancer Res 7:1204–1213, 2001.

57. Fry DW: Inhibition of the epidermal growth factor receptor family of tyrosine kinases as an approach to cancer chemotherapy: Progression from reversible to irreversible inhibitors. Pharmacol Ther 82:207–218, 1999.

58. Noonberg SB, Benz CC: Tyrosine kinase inhibitors targeted to the epidermal growth factor receptor subfamily. Drugs 59:753–767, 2000.

59. He Y, Zeng Q, Drenning SD, et al: Inhibition of human squamous cell carcinoma growth in vivo by epidermal growth factor receptor antisense RNA transcribed from the U6 promoter. J Natl Cancer Inst 90:1080–1087, 1998.

60. Contessa JN, Reardon DB, Todd D, et al: The inducible expression of dominant-negative epidermal growth factor receptor-CD533 results in radiosensitization of human mammary carcinoma cells. Clin Cancer Res 5:405–411, 1999.

61. Xie W, Chipman JG, Robertson DL, et al: Expression of a mitogen-responsive gene encoding prostaglandin synthase is regulated by mRNA splicing. Proc Natl Acad Sci USA 88:2692–2696, 1991.

62. Vane J, Botting R: The future of NSAID therapy: Selective COX-2 inhibitors. Int J Clin Pathol 54:7–9, 2000.

63. Eberhart CE, Coffey RJ, Radhika A, et al: Up-regulation of cyclooxygenase 2 gene expression in human colorectal adenomas and adenocarcinomas. Gastroenterology 107:1183–1188, 1994.

64. Jones MK, Wang H, Peskar BM, et al: Inhibition of angiogenesis by nonsteroidal anti-inflammatory drugs: Insight into mechanisms and implications for cancer growth and ulcer healing. Nature Med 5:1418–1423, 1999.

65. Rigas B, Goldman IS, Levine L: Altered eicosanoid levels in human colon cancer. J Lab Clin Med 122:518–523, 1993.

66. Bennett A: Survival time after surgery is inversely related to amounts of prostaglandin extracted from human breast cancer. Br J Pharmacol 66:451, 1979.

67. Furuta Y, Hall E, Sanduja S, et al: Prostaglandin production by murine tumors as a predictor for therapeutic response to indomethacin. Cancer Res 48:3002–3007, 1988.

68. Tang D, Honn KV: Eicosanoids and tumor cell metastasis. In Harris J, Braun DP (eds): Prostaglandin Inhibitors in Tumor Immunology and Immunotherapy. Boca Raton, CRC, 1994, pp 73–108.

69. Koki A, Leahy KM, Masferrer JL: Potential utility of COX-2 inhibitors in chemoprevention and chemotherapy. Expert Opin Invest Drugs 8:1623–1638, 1999.

70. Kishi K, Petersen S, Petersen C, et al: Preferential enhancement of tumor radioresponse by a cyclooxygenase-2 inhibitor. Cancer Res 60:1326–1331, 2000.

71. Milas L, Kishi K, Hunter N, et al: Enhancement of tumor response to gamma-radiation by an inhibitor of cyclooxygenase-2 enzyme. J Natl Cancer Inst 91:1501–1504, 1999.

72. Petersen C, Petersen S, Milas L, et al: Human glioma cell radiosensitization by a selective COX-2 inhibitor. Clin Cancer Res 6:2513–2520, 2000.

73. The nation's investment in cancer research. Report from the National Cancer Institute, 1998.

CHAPTER 32

Chemoprevention

Vassiliki A. Papadimitrakopoulou
Waun Ki Hong

◘ INTRODUCTION

Epithelial carcinogenesis is a multiyear, multipath disease of progressive genetic and associated tissue damage. In the case of head and neck squamous cell carcinoma (SCCHN), this process is closely linked to the widely accepted risk factors of tobacco smoking[1,2] and alcohol use and is manifested in the head and neck region by the presence of multiple premalignant lesions that are synchronous and metachronous to the presence of squamous cell cancer. This process can potentially be interrupted, reversed, or modulated.

SCCHN, the most common epithelial malignancy arising in the upper aerodigestive tract, is an important public health problem, accounting for approximately 40,100 new cancer cases and 12,000 cancer deaths annually in the United States[3] and 500,000 cases annually worldwide.[4] Although SCCHN accounts for only 3% to 4% of all cancers in the United States, the adverse effect of SCCHN on health quality can be dramatic. In many developing countries, the increasing prevalence of SCCHN has had a dramatic effect on public health.[5] Unfortunately, despite multimodality treatment efforts (including surgery, radiation therapy, and chemotherapy), all of which have been associated with substantial morbidity to patients, the overall survival rates for these cancers (approximately 45%) have only marginally improved over the past 3 decades.[6] The main reasons for treatment failure are the development of second primary cancers in patients with early-stage disease (stages I and II) and the development of local recurrence and metastasis for patients with advanced SCCHN.[7] There is a constant and continuing risk (from 2.7% to 4% per year) of second primary tumor (i.e., aerodigestive tumors) formation each year following initial treatment.[8] The probability of a second malignancy arising within 5 years after the initial tumor presentation can reach 22%,[9] and patients who develop a second malignancy have only a 25% 5-year survival rate.[10] These troubling data demonstrate the need for new approaches to both enhance primary disease control and prevent primary and second primary cancers.[6,11]

Chemoprevention, the use of drugs or other agents to inhibit, delay, or reverse carcinogenesis, is recognized as a very promising and important area in cancer research.[12,13] The dismal prognosis for most patients with cancer of the head and neck who are diagnosed at advanced stages is one of the reasons why chemoprevention is gaining in priority among research approaches in this area. Major clinical and laboratory advances have been made in the area of chemoprevention and, recently, in understanding of the molecular biology of head and neck carcinogenesis.

This chapter reviews the status of chemoprevention of cancer of the head and neck.

◘ EPIDEMIOLOGY OF CANCER

It has been estimated that dietary and smoking habits contribute to at least 70% of all deaths from cancer.[14] The astounding figures of tobacco use worldwide (1 billion smokers and 600 million chewers) and in the United States (44 million current smokers, 44 million former smokers, and 12 million chewers[15]) underscore the urgent need for new prevention strategies, in addition to continued smoking cessation efforts, to control tobacco-related cancers of the head and neck.[16,17]

Although the role of tobacco and alcohol consumption in the etiology of SCCHN is well accepted, the genetic predisposition and alterations that lead to cancer of the head and neck are incompletely understood. In fact, although more than 90% of patients with SCCHN have a history of tobacco and alcohol use, a vast majority of individuals who smoke and drink do not develop SCCHN. The tendency of the upper aerodigestive tract epithelium to undergo transformation in certain patients and not others when exposed to these agents probably reflects genetic alterations in the regional mucosa. These alterations are the subject of studies in both molecular epidemiology and molecular genetics.

One of the methods developed to assess an individual's genetic sensitivity to environmental carcinogens is the mutagen sensitivity assay.[1,2] This assay quantifies bleomycin-induced chromosome breaks in cultured peripheral blood lymphocytes and is thought to reflect the sensitivity of cells to clastogenic (DNA break–inducing) carcinogens and their ability to repair resultant DNA damage.[17] Two case-control studies have assessed the ability of the mutagen sensitivity assay to indicate the risk of primary cancer of the head and neck. The first study included 75 cancer patients and 108 controls (healthy subjects).[18] The second study included 108 cancer patients and 108 controls.[19] Both studies found mutagen sensitivity (defined as greater than a 0.8 chromosomal break per cell after in vitro exposure to bleomycin) to be a significant independent risk factor for cancer of the head and neck, and both found an interactive effect between smoking and mutagen sensitivity in increasing the risk of SCCHN. The odds ratios for cancer of the head and neck in the second, larger case-control study were 3.2 (95% confidence interval [CI] = 0.5–18.7) for mutagen sensitivity, 8.1 (1.7–37.8) for smoking, and 23.0 (5.0–106.0) for both.[19]

Bleomycin-induced mutagen sensitivity in patients with cancer of the head and neck may involve specific chromosomes. Chromosomes 3 and 7 have the highest frequency of bleomycin-induced breaks,[20] and specific sites with the highest rates of bleomycin-induced breaks have been identified on chromosomes 3 (3p21, 3q21) and 7 (7q22, 7q32). Studies of mutagen sensitivity with the mutagen benzo(a)pyrene diol epoxide (BPDE), which is more etiologically appropriate for smoking-induced cancers, have also suggested that high values for BPDE-induced chromatid breaks per cell in lymphocytes are an independent risk factor for SCCHN.[21] Moreover, subjects with sensitivity to both BPDE and bleomycin were at a 19.2-fold increased risk of cancer compared with those who were not sensitive to either agent.[22] Studies concentrating on the role of independent genes in susceptibility to tobacco-related cancers have suggested that low expression of genes such as *hMLH1* and *hGTBP/hMSH6* (which have been implicated in DNA repair capacity) is associated with an increased risk of cancer of the head and neck.[23] Other studies have identified the carcinogen-metabolizing gene *glutathione-S-transferase (GST)M1* and *GSTT1* null phenotypes as independent risk factors for SCCHN.[24]

Risk factors for the development of secondary primary cancers (SPCs) in patients with cancer of the head and neck are similar to those for development of primary cancer. Most retrospective studies found higher SPC rates for patients who continue to smoke after diagnosis of the primary cancer.[2]

The overall annual SPC rates range from 1.2% to 4.7% in retrospective studies, and this rate appears to be constant (i.e., the risk does not appear to decrease over time). In prospective studies,[17] however, these rates ranged from 4% to 7%. Similar to the findings in primary SCCHN, a prospective study of 278 patients with cancer of the head and neck demonstrated that mutagen hypersensitivity (more than 1.0 break per cell) occurred in 44% of patients and was associated with a 2.67 relative risk of SPC development.[25] The mean number of chromatid breaks per cell for patients who developed SPCs was 1.17 compared with 0.98 break per cell for those who did not develop SPCs (*P* = .04). These findings were confirmed by a second study,[26] which found a higher mean number of breaks per cell for patients developing SPCs than for patients who did not (1.20 vs. 0.96, *P* = .025).

BIOLOGY OF CARCINOGENESIS OF THE HEAD AND NECK

SCCHN is thought to arise from the transformation of the genetic material of normal cells, followed by successive genetic alterations in a multistep fashion. The process leads to clonal evolution of progeny cells with a proliferative advantage,[27] induced by field-wide exposure to tobacco carcinogens.[28] According to this theory, tumors grow by the process of clonal evolution driven by mutations, by which multiple "hits" (mutations) on a cell are needed for cancer to develop.[29] These two biologic concepts are clinically translated into multifocal, unsynchronized premalignant and malignant lesions. Identification of early genetic alterations in the tissue before cancer formation would enhance our understanding of the biology of squamous epithelial carcinogenesis and aid in the design of novel systemic approaches to stopping or reversing the process of carcinogenesis.

CHEMOPREVENTION

Chemoprevention is the use of drugs or other agents to halt or reverse carcinogenesis through reregulation of growth and differentiation and possibly elimination of genetically and phenotypically aberrant clones.[12, 13] Chemoprevention studies in cancer of the upper aerodigestive tract are based on these fundamental premises and the identification of molecular genetic and biologic cellular changes. These alterations represent biomarkers of the carcinogenesis process and ultimately, if validated, could serve as intermediate endpoints for these studies.

When cancer incidence is used as the ultimate endpoint in chemoprevention trials, many subjects and long periods of follow-up are needed, thus limiting the number, doses, and schedules of agents tested and the possible knowledge to be gained regarding mechanisms of carcinogenesis. Biomarkers that could ultimately be used as intermediates are being developed to address these feasibility problems in chemoprevention trials.[30, 31] Molecular genetic studies have increased our understanding of the head and neck tumorigenesis process and are described in the chapter that addresses the molecular aspects of pathogenesis of head and neck cancer (see Chapter 2). The use of molecular methods in cell line and human tissue studies has led to the discovery of genetic alterations in premalignant and malignant epithelial cells. These alterations include activation of oncogene products that positively stimulate growth and inactivation of tumor suppressor genes, leading to unchecked neoplastic cell growth. Certain genetic alterations provide cells with a growth advantage, allowing unregulated cell growth (clonal expansion) to occur. The sequence of gene changes is less critical to clonal evolution and carcinogenesis than is the specific set of genes that is altered.

Great efforts are being made to develop effective new strategies to control many deadly epithelial cancers, including cancer of the head and neck. One relatively new and promising approach is cancer chemoprevention—the use of specific agents to stop carcinogenesis and prevent the development of invasive cancer.[32] This field of clinical investigation emerged from laboratory and epidemiologic studies indicating the presence of thousands of potential inhibitors of carcinogenesis. The basic concepts of field carcinogenesis and multistep carcinogenesis (reviewed earlier) underlie the expanding field of chemoprevention. The clinical premise of chemoprevention is that carcinogenesis in early (premalignant) stages is reversible, a concept supported by preclinical and epidemiologic data. Chemoprevention studies in cancer of the head and neck have been directed at the reversal of premalignant lesions and the prevention of SPCs.

Retinoids

To date, more than 2000 agents from more than 20 chemical classes have been shown in preclinical studies to have chemopreventive activity. A few of these, including β-carotene, alpha-tocopherol, and selenium, have been tested clinically in the head and neck. Retinoids, however, are by far the best-studied class of chemopreventive agents.[12, 32–34]

The retinoid class includes more than 3000 natural derivatives and synthetic analogues of vitamin A.[12, 32–35] Naturally occurring retinoids include retinol, retinal, retinyl esters, and all-trans-retinoic acid, and their metabolites (e.g., 13-cis-retinoic acid [13cRA] and 9-cis-retinoic acid). In animal model studies, retinoids have suppressed carcinogenesis at many epithelial sites, including the breast, bladder, lung, cervix, skin, prostate, and head and neck. Clinical retinoid trials have achieved significant chemopreventive activity in the lung, skin, cervix, bladder, ovary, and head and neck.[12, 32, 33]

Retinoids have potent effects on premalignant and malignant cell growth, differentiation, and apoptosis in many human systems,[12, 32–39] apparently modulating gene expression to achieve these effects. The major advance in understanding of the molecular mechanism of retinoid action and how retinoids affect gene expression was the discovery of nuclear retinoid receptors.[40] Nuclear retinoid receptors are ligand-activated DNA-binding proteins that modulate gene transcription by interacting with response elements in the promoter regions of specific genes. Current data suggest that the various receptor subtypes have distinct functions and different retinoid binding affinity patterns and are distributed in different tissues.[41] Retinoic acid receptors (RARs) were the first class of nuclear retinoid receptors to be discovered. Three RARs have been identified: RAR-α, RAR-β, and RAR-γ.[41] The RARs were discovered because of their sequence homology (which is strongest in the DNA-binding domain) with the steroid receptor family.

Retinoid-X receptors (RXRs) were the second class of nuclear retinoic acid receptors to be discovered, and three RXR subtypes also have been identified—α, β, and γ.[41]

Trials in Premalignant Oral Lesions

Many characteristics of a premalignant lesion of the oral cavity make it an excellent system for the study of chemoprevention in humans.[7, 8, 42–46] First, it is well described and is associated with cancer of the oral cavity. Leukoplakia is found near oral cancer tissue in as many as 100% of cases in some series (median rate from all published series, 30% to 40%). These premalignant lesions are associated with the long-term development of cancer in 10% to 20% of patients overall. This association (transformation rate) doubles in high-risk dysplastic lesions.[47] Up to 30% to 40% of premalignant lesions regress spontaneously, although rarely completely. The variable natural history of leukoplakia, especially its substantial spontaneous regression rates, underscores the need for randomization in clinical chemoprevention trials in this disorder.

The second major research attribute of this system is that the oral cavity and oropharynx are easily and noninvasively monitored, in contrast to the colon and lung, which require invasive procedures (e.g., colonoscopy and bronchoscopy) to monitor the carcinogenic process. The ease of access for observation of leukoplakia and repeat biopsies has led to frequent incorporation of intermediate biomarker studies within leukoplakia trials.

The third and perhaps most important attribute of this model system is the implication for other epithelial cancers of the aerodigestive tract. Premalignant lesions in the oral cavity are biologically and etiologically (through tobacco exposure) similar to carcinogenesis throughout the aerodigestive tract. Chemoprevention studies for premalignant lesions in the oral cavity have contributed to the design of a retinoid trial (discussed in detail later) that significantly suppressed SPCs in patients with cancer of the head and neck.

Although high-risk dysplastic lesions account for only 10% to 20% of all premalignant lesions of the oral cavity, these percentages translate into hundreds of thousands of cases worldwide. A substantial percentage of patients with dysplasia are not amenable to surgical[8] or other[48] local therapies because of diffuse multiple precancerous foci resulting from the field carcinogenic process. Therefore, a systemic intervention such as chemoprevention is necessary for control of high-risk lesions. No standard systemic approach now exists.

Retinoid Trials

Chemoprevention trials in oral premalignancy initially were reported in the late 1950s.[12, 16, 32–34, 39, 49] These early trials often focused on the use of systemic or topical vitamin A. Subsequent trials have explored the efficacy of other retinoids. To date, more than 400 patients with leukoplakia have been treated with eight different retinoids in prospective studies. The activity of retinoids in these settings has been thoroughly established by significant response rates in each of the five randomized retinoid trials conducted to date.[50–54] Dose-related mucocutaneous toxicity has been the major adverse effect encountered in these trials.

The first study of synthetic retinoids in oral leukoplakia was reported in 1978 by Koch.[49] Seventy-five patients with leukoplakia (with or without epithelial dysplasia) were treated with all-trans-retinoic acid, 13cRA, or etretinate. The study design included an 8-week induction phase followed by a lower dose maintenance period. Induction response rates for the three synthetics were 59%, 87%, and 91%, respectively. After follow-up of 2 to 6 years, 43%, 45%, and 51% of patients, respectively, remained in prolonged remission.

Five randomized trials have tested four different retinoids: 13cRA (in two trials), natural vitamin A, and two retinamides.[50–54] Three of these trials were primary lesion therapy trials and two were maintenance trials, that is, trials with either a retinoid induction phase or excision of the lesion followed by maintenance retinoid therapy.

The first randomized trial was conducted by Hong and coworkers.[50] They evaluated 13cRA in 44 patients with oral leukoplakia. Patients were randomly assigned to receive either high-dose 13cRA (2 mg/kg per day) or placebo for 3 months, after which they were followed off-treatment for 6 months. Complete or partial remissions occurred in 16 of the 24 patients in the 13cRA arm. Only 2 of the 20 patients on placebo responded (P = .0002). Thirteen of the 24 13cRA patients had histopathologic improvement, compared with only 2 of the 20 patients receiving placebo. More than half of the responding patients had relapse in the follow-up portion of the trial, typically within 2 or 3 months after therapy had ended. Cheilitis and/or skin dryness/peeling occurred in 19 of 24 patients (79%), conjunctivitis in 13 of 24 (54%), and hypertriglyceridemia in 17 of 24 (71%) receiving 13cRA. Two of the 24 13cRA patients were unable to complete the study because of toxicity.

This study clearly demonstrated the efficacy of 13cRA in the treatment of oral leukoplakia, but it also revealed several problems. Relapses off treatment were frequent, which indicated the need for maintenance therapy. Although 2 mg/kg per day was tolerable for a short time, it seemed unlikely that this dose could be given for long periods. Furthermore, although the premalignant lesion (oral leukoplakia) was reversed, this relatively small, short-term trial did not ascertain whether reversal of the premalignant lesion is associated with a decreased risk of eventual cancer development.

These problems were addressed by a follow-up trial[53] designed to evaluate the long-term maintenance of retinoid response in oral premalignancy. Maintenance consisted of 9 months of either low-dose 13cRA (0.5 mg/kg per day) or β-carotene following induction with 3 months of high-dose 13cRA (1.5 mg/kg per day). At the end of induction therapy, 66 patients could be evaluated; 59 had either remission or stable disease and were randomly assigned to receive either β-carotene or 13cRA. During maintenance, only 2 of the 24 patients (8%) in the retinoid group showed cancer progression, whereas 16 of the 29 patients (55%) receiving β-carotene showed progression (P < .001).

Retinoid intervention in human oral carcinogenesis provides an excellent model for the study of intermediate endpoint biomarkers in chemoprevention.[55, 56] Retinoid chemopreventive activity in oral premalignancy is well established and so provides a strong context for comparative evaluations of phenotypic and genotypic biomarkers of carcinogenesis. Several recently reported clinical laboratory translational studies were included in the maintenance trial of 13cRA. Translation work based on premalignant lesion biopsies from these chemoprevention trials has focused on studies of chromosome polysomy and TP53 expression. Chromosome polysomy (defined as the presence of three or more copies of the chromosome), a crude description of genetic damage and instability, was associated with increased risk of cancer development,[57, 58] a finding confirmed by more recent studies by Sudbo and associates showing that DNA content (tetraploidy and aneuploidy) in oral leukoplakia lesions appeared to be a strong predictor of malignant transformation.[59] Another important finding of the translational studies tied into the clinical chemoprevention trial was that TP53 protein accumulation is associated with retinoid resistance.[60, 61] Similarly, loss of heterozygosity at 3p and 9p21, which has been frequently observed in oral premalignant lesions and is closely associated with their phenotype and clinical behavior,[62, 63] was found by Mao and colleagues to predict cancer development.[64] The most striking findings, however, concern RAR-β loss in oral carcinogenesis and reversal of the process by 13cRA.[65] Xu and coworkers[66] developed a nonradioactive in situ hybridization method to study RAR-mRNA and RXR-mRNA expression in vivo in resection specimens in patients with cancer of the head and neck. They observed a selective and progressive loss of RAR-β (the RAR-β gene is located on chromosome 3p) in 56% of dysplastic lesions and 35% of invasive lesions, and they suggested that loss of RAR-β is an early event in head and neck carcinogenesis.

Following up on these findings in cancer of the head and neck, Lotan and associates[65] studied RAR expression in the 13cRA maintenance trial within the oral premalignancy model. Again, the expression of only one receptor, RAR-β, was lost (in 60% of oral premalignant lesions), compared with no loss in control normal oral tissue (P = .005). One of the major mechanisms for loss of RAR-β appears to be methylation of the gene promoter.[67] Another major finding of the study of Lotan and coworkers was the striking upregulation by 13cRA of RAR-β expression in premalignant oral lesions (from expression in 40% of lesions before to 90% after treatment, P < .0001).

RAR-β expression is progressively lost in head and neck carcinogenesis and is significantly upregulated in vivo by high-dose 13cRA. These features make RAR-β an excellent candidate for potential intermediate endpoint biomarker studies within the retinoid-oral premalignancy system.[55, 56]

Another randomized response induction trial tested N-4-(hydroxycarbophenyl) retinamide.[52] Patients received either the retinamide (40 mg/day orally and 40 mg/day topically) or placebo for 4 months. Major responses occurred in 27 of the 31 patients on treatment (87.1%), including several complete remissions. Only 5 of the 30 patients on placebo (16.7%) had major responses. Toxicity was minimal, consisting of minor elevations of serum transaminase in two patients. No data on skin toxicity were reported.

The third primary lesion therapy trial, conducted by Stich and colleagues,[51] evaluated the effects of vitamin A in 65 patients (tobacco users or betel nut chewers) with oral leukoplakia in India. Thirty participants were randomly assigned to receive 100,000 IU of vitamin A twice weekly, and 35 were assigned to placebo. Little change in their oral tobacco use habits was noted during the study. Compliance was excellent in patients who completed the trial because medication was administered under nursing supervision. Even so, effects could be evaluated in only 21 of the 30 patients receiving vitamin A, and the authors do not explain why. Among these 21 patients, 12 (57.1%) had complete remissions (partial responses were not reported), and no patient's cancer progressed during treatment. Among the 33 subjects receiving placebo, only 1 (3.0%) had a complete remission, and cancer progressed in 7 (21.2%).

The second randomized maintenance trial[54, 68] evaluated 170 patients randomly assigned to receive either fenretinide (200 mg/day) or no intervention (control) for 1 year following laser resection of oral leukoplakia. To date, local relapses or new lesions have occurred in 25 (29%) of the 86 patients in the placebo control arm, compounded with an 18% failure rate (15/84) in the fenretinide group (P = .01). More than half of the fenretinide arm failures occurred after the 1-year intervention. This fenretinide result is consistent with the earlier 13cRA maintenance result.[53] Toxicity has been minimal (Table 32–1).

TABLE 32-1 Chemoprevention Trials in Oral Premalignancy and Laryngeal Premalignancy

Investigator(s)	Agent(s)	No. of Patients	Results
Hong et al, 1986[50]	13cRA at 1–2 mg/kg/day for 3 mo vs. placebo	44	Positive
Stich et al, 1988[70]	β-Carotene + retinol (100,000 IU/wk) (180 mg/wk) vs. placebo	103	Positive
Stich et al, 1988[51]	Vitamin A (200,000 IU/wk) orally for 6 mo vs. placebo	64	Positive
Han et al, 1990[52]	4-HCR (40 mg/day) vs. placebo	61	Positive
Lippman et al, 1993[53]	13cRA (1.5 mg/kg/day) for 3 mo followed by 13cRA (0.5 mg/kg per day) for 9 mo vs. β-carotene (30 mg/day) for 9 mo	70	Positive
Chiesa et al, 1993[54]	4-HPR (200 mg/day) for 52 wk vs. placebo	153	Positive
Zaridze et al, 1993[78]	β-Carotene (40 mg/day) + retinol (100,000 IU/wk) + vitamin E (80 mg/wk) vs. placebo	675	Positive
Papadimitrakopoulou et al, 1999[82]	13cRA (100 mg/m²/day), alpha-tocopherol 1200 IU/day, interferon + 3 MU/SC m² biweekly for 12 mo	36	Positive for laryngeal lesions

13cRA, 13-*cis*-retinoic acid; 4-HCR, 4(hydroxycarbophenyl) retinamide; 4-HPR, 4-N-(4-hydroxyphenyl) retinamide.

Nonretinoid Trials

Seven nonrandomized trials have tested β-carotene in oral leukoplakia.[16, 69–74] The rationale for studying this agent includes β-carotene's strong supportive epidemiologic data in squamous cell carcinoma of the lung—its antioxidant structure, provitamin A activity in vivo, lack of acute clinical toxicity, low expense, and wide availability. Many differences—in patient groups (smokers and snuff and betel nut users), in response and evaluation criteria, and in β-carotene preparations, doses, schedules, and durations—occurred among these trials. Widely varying 3-month response rates (ranging from 22% to 71%) had an inverse relationship to dose (ranging from 30 to 120 mg/day).[16, 69–74] In 1994, the value of β-carotene in tobacco-related carcinogenesis was seriously questioned by the results of a phase III study[75] of this agent in nearly 30,000 smokers. This trial reported a significant increase in lung cancer incidence (the primary trial endpoint) in the smokers receiving β-carotene.

Vitamin E, a nontoxic lipid phase antioxidant under intensive general study in chemoprevention, has undergone one trial in oral leukoplakia.[76] Trial results suggested drug activity with minimal toxicity,[76, 77] supporting positive epidemiologic data on vitamin E in the prevention of cancer of the head and neck.

Combinations of naturally occurring chemopreventive agents have also been clinically tested. A study performed in Uzbekistan found a significant decrease in the prevalence odds ratio of oral leukoplakia to 62% in subjects given a combination of retinal (100,000 IU), β-carotene, and vitamin E compared with results for those given only riboflavin or a combination of riboflavin, retinal, β-carotene, and vitamin E.[78]

Another agent tested in oral leukoplakia is Bowman-Birk inhibitor concentrate (BBIC), a soybean-derived serine protease inhibitor with both trypsin and chymotrypsin inhibitory activities, which prevents development of malignancy in a large number of animal model systems.[79] In a phase II trial in 32 subjects, BBIC taken orally for 1 month resulted in a 31% response rate and decreases in protease activity measured in oral mucosal cells.[80]

Advanced Premalignant Lesions

Advanced premalignant lesions of the upper aerodigestive tract described as moderate to severe dysplasia are associated with a well-defined risk of progressively invasive cancer, with the risk ranging from 36% to 50% as described in series specific to lesions in the oral cavity and larynx.[47, 81] Advanced premalignant lesions in the oral cavity are resistant to single-agent retinoid chemoprevention; to provide a chemoprevention strategy for this high-risk group, a combination of interferon-α, alpha-tocopherol, and 13-cRA was evaluated.[82] The study found that this combination was active in preventing progression of laryngeal lesions but not oral lesions. After 12 months of treatment, laryngeal sites showed a 50% complete histologic response rate, and oral cavity sites showed no complete responses. Based on these findings and the fact that molecular genetic alterations in the form of 9p21 loss persisted in post-treatment specimens despite evidence of complete histologic response,[83] a new study addressing exclusively laryngeal dysplasia that incorporated a year of induction with the same regimen and 2 years of maintenance with fenretinide or placebo has been designed, and the results are eagerly awaited.

Trials to Prevent Second Primary Cancers

As was mentioned earlier, patients who have "cured" primary head and neck cancer are at very high risk of developing an SPC.[7, 84, 85] Three prospective studies[85–88] that have been conducted in this area detected annual SPC rates of 4% to 7%. SPCs associated with cancer of the head and neck disperse in a characteristic pattern: More than 70% to 80% occur within the aerodigestive tract (head and neck, lung, and esophagus). Surgical and cytotoxic (local and systemic) approaches do not eliminate or ameliorate the field, or multifocal, carcinogenic process.[6, 11, 69]

Accumulated data from retrospective and prospective studies indicate that the annual 4% to 7% SPC rate in patients surviving cancer of the head and neck is constant; these patients' risk of developing SPCs will not improve over time. Therefore, the cumulative incidence of SPCs is greatest in patients with early-stage cancer of the head and neck, who survive the longest after definitive primary treatment. Advanced diagnostic techniques, supportive care, and treatment of primary cancers will improve survival among patients with all types of cancer of the upper aerodigestive tract and lung and thus will increase the overall impact of SPCs.

On the basis of positive retinoid data in oral leukoplakia and the lack of effective adjuvant therapy in the prevention

TABLE 32-2 Randomized Chemoprevention Trials in Patients With SCCHN to Prevent Second Primary Tumors

Investigator(s)	Patient Population	No. of Patients	Median Follow-up (mo)	Agent(s)	Results
Hong et al, 1990[86] Benner et al, 1994[87]	SCCHN	103	54	13cRA (50–100 mg/m²) for 12 mo vs. placebo	Positive
Bolla et al, 1994[88]	SCCHN	316	41	Etretinate (50 mg/day) for 1 mo followed by 25 mg/day for 24 mo vs. placebo	No difference
EUROSCAN 2000[91]	SCCHN/ NSCLC	2592	49	1) Retinyl palmitate (300,000 IU/daily for 1 yr) followed by 150,000 IU for a 2nd yr 2) N-Acetylcysteine 600 mg/daily for 2 yr 3) Both 4) Neither	No difference in SPT rate, event- free survival, or overall survival among the four arms
Khuri et al, 2001 (HNSP trial)[89]	SCCHN	1191	36	13cRA 30 mg/day for 3 yr vs. placebo	Final results pending. SPT current, former, never-smokers (4.2%, 3.2%, 1.9% current vs. never-smokers, P = .018)

SCCHN, squamous cell carcinoma of the head and neck; NSCLC, non–small cell lung cancer; 13cRA, 13-cis-retinoic acid; SPT, second primary tumor.

of primary recurrence or SPCs, Hong and colleagues[86] designed an adjuvant chemoprevention trial of high-dose 13cRA in patients with cancer of the head and neck (Table 32–2). After definitive local therapy with radiotherapy, surgery, or both, 103 patients were randomly assigned to receive either 13cRA or placebo for 12 months. The major trial endpoints were recurrence of the primary disease, development of an SPC (of a different histologic type or at a site farther than 2 cm from the previous disease, or occurring more than 3 years after initial diagnosis), and survival.

The first report of this trial included a median follow-up of 32 months; only 2 of the 51 patients receiving 13cRA developed an SPC, whereas 12 of the 49 patients receiving placebo developed an SPC (P = .005). As with retinoids in other preclinical and clinical carcinogenesis systems, the effect of the retinoid on annual overall SPC incidence has decreased over time after completion of the 12 months' intervention. A later report[87] updating results of this trial (after a median follow-up of 55 months) indicates that seven patients in the retinoid group developed SPCs compared with 16 patients in the placebo arm (14% vs. 31%, P = .04). A subset analysis of only SPCs within the high-risk tobacco-exposed field of the head and neck, lung, and esophagus showed a chemopreventive effect that persisted at the same level of significance as earlier overall results. This long-lasting retinoid activity is unprecedented in previously reported clinical or preclinical retinoid carcinogenesis studies.

Although SPCs were significantly reduced in the retinoid arm, survival in the retinoid arm compared with that in the placebo arm was not significantly improved. Several factors may have contributed to this lack of survival benefit: (1) similar primary recurrence rates in the two arms, (2) relatively small study sample size, (3) high toxicity-related dropout in the retinoid arm, and (4) early detection and definitive local

therapy of SPCs in this closely monitored prospective trial. This last factor applies mostly to the placebo arm because it had a much higher rate of SPCs.

On the basis of the positive findings of the trial by Hong and colleagues,[86] the National Cancer Institute sponsored the largest chemoprevention trial in head and neck cancer to date (NCI C91-002), in which patients were prospectively randomly assigned to low-dose 13cRA or placebo for 3 years. This trial was closed to accrual in June of 1999 with more than 1200 participants. An interim analysis found annual secondary primary tumor rates in active, former, and never-smokers of 5.1%, 4.1%, and 3%, respectively (P = .06 for active smokers vs. never-smokers).[89] Treatment results are eagerly awaited.

The synthetic retinoid etretinate was tested in 1994 in a French trial[88] designed to prevent SPCs following definitive treatment of squamous cell carcinoma of the oral cavity or oropharynx. Patients were randomly assigned to receive either placebo or etretinate (50 mg/day for 1 month followed by 25 mg/day for 24 months). SPCs were not reduced in the retinoid group. SPC and primary recurrence rates were equivalent in both study arms.

Although the results were negative, this prospective French trial did confirm other prospective trial data[85–88] showing a high rate of SPCs associated with cancer of the head and neck. Twenty-four percent of the French patients experienced SPCs within a median follow-up of 41 months. Seventy-nine percent of these SPCs developed in the head and neck, lung, or esophagus, a pattern that is consistent with the field carcinogenesis concept. The most important difference between this trial[88] and the earlier trial[86, 87] relates to the varying mechanistic and pharmacologic properties of the two retinoids studied.[39] In addition, the French report provided few details regarding tobacco and alcohol

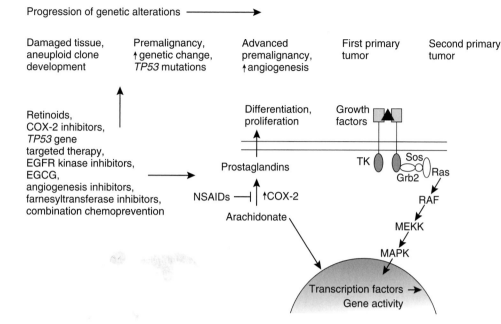

Progression of genetic alterations ⟶

Damaged tissue, aneuploid clone development

Premalignancy, ↑genetic change, *TP53* mutations

Advanced premalignancy, ↑angiogenesis

First primary tumor

Second primary tumor

Retinoids, COX-2 inhibitors, *TP53* gene targeted therapy, EGFR kinase inhibitors, EGCG, angiogenesis inhibitors, farnesyltransferase inhibitors, combination chemoprevention

Differentiation, proliferation

Growth factors

Prostaglandins

NSAIDs —|↑COX-2

TK

Sos
Grb2 Ras

RAF

MEKK

MAPK

Arachidonate

Transcription factors ⟶
Gene activity

FIGURE 32–1 Integration of molecularly targeted agents in head and neck cancer chemoprevention. COX-2, cyclooxygenase-2; EGFR, epidermal growth factor receptor; NSAIDS, nonsteroidal anti-inflammatory drugs; TK, tyrosine kinase.

usage, study adherence, or toxicity, making interpretation difficult.

Based on a report by Pastorino and coworkers[90] in 1993 that adjuvant high-dose retinyl palmitate in stage I non–small cell lung cancer resulted in annual SPC rates of 3.1% in the retinoid arm and 4.8% in the no-treatment control arm, the EUROSCAN trial[91] was designed. This phase III study compared the efficacy of retinyl palmitate and/or N-acetylcysteine in secondary tumor prevention after resection of a primary cancer of the head and neck or lung and found no benefit in patients with cancer of the head and neck in terms of survival, event-free survival, or secondary primary cancers.

Several large, randomized trials were done in various parts of the world to determine the efficacy of retinoids in preventing SPCs in the head and neck and the lung.[7, 17, 92] Nevertheless, problems with retinoid toxicity and the need for long-term therapy suggest that other new chemopreventive approaches also are needed. Future agents for use in preventing cancer of the head and neck most likely will be selected from new agent studies in the oral premalignancy

system (Table 32–3, Fig. 32–1). Current study in these two areas involves intervention targeted toward *TP53* abnormalities, selective cyclooxygenase (COX)-2 inhibitors, epidermal growth factor receptor (EGFR) kinase inhibitors, and farnesyl transferase inhibitors.

◧ SUMMARY

Head and neck carcinogenesis is a multistep, field-wide process involving accumulation of genetic damage in the tissue at risk. This process is potentially reversible or can be halted through the use of natural or synthetic agents. Encouraging activity has been documented with retinoids, and continued investigation focused on agents targeting specific signaling pathways or clearly identified genetic events in the process holds promise for the future. Efforts to better understand the molecular pathogenesis of head and neck cancer are clearly warranted to guide these efforts and, along with innovative smoking cessation and prevention strategies, should lead to prevention of cancer of the head and neck.

TABLE 32-3 New Agents in Head and Neck Chemoprevention

Nonsteroidal anti-inflamatory agents
• Nonselective (ketorolac trial in OPLs)
• Selective COX-2 inhibitors (celecoxib trial in OPLs in progress)
p53 targeting therapy
• ONYX-015 virus (clinical trial in oral dysplasia in progress)
• Adenovirus *p53* gene therapy (clinical trial in OPLs planned)
EGFR tyrosine kinase inhibitors (clinical trial in OPLs planned)
Farnesyl-transferase inhibitors (clinical trial for SPT prevention planned)
GTE (clinical trial in oral premalignant lesions planned)

OPLs, oral premalignant lesions; COX-2, cyclooxygenase-2; EGFR, epidermal growth factor receptor; SPT, second primary tumor; GTE, green tea extract.

REFERENCES

1. Spitz MR: Epidemiology and risk factors for head and neck cancer. Semin Oncol 21:281, 1994.
2. Lippman SM, Spitz M, Trizna Z, et al: Epidemiology, biology, and chemoprevention of aerodigestive cancer. Cancer 74:2719, 1994.
3. Greenlee RT, Hill-Harmon MB, Murray T, et al: Cancer statistics. CA Cancer J Clin 51:15, 2001.
4. Mashberg A: Re: Oral cavity cancer in non-users of tobacco. J Natl Cancer Inst 85:1525, 1993.
5. Boyle P, Macfarlane GJ, Zheng T, et al: Recent advances in epidemiology of head and neck cancer. Curr Opin Oncol 4:471, 1992.
6. Vokes EE, Weichselbaum RR, Lippman SM, et al: Head and neck cancer. N Engl J Med 328:184, 1993.
7. Lippman SM, Hong WK: Second malignant tumors in head and neck squamous cell carcinoma: The overshadowing threat for patients with early-stage disease. Int J Radiat Oncol Biol Phys 17:691, 1989.

8. Jovanovic A, van der Tol IG, Kostense PJ, et al: Second respiratory and upper digestive tract cancer following oral squamous cell carcinoma. Eur J Cancer 30B:225, 1994.

9. Dhooge IJ, De Vos M, Van Cauwenberge PB: Multiple primary malignant tumors in patients with head and neck cancer: Results of a prospective study and future perspectives. Laryngoscope 108:250, 1998.

10. Larson JT, Adams GL, Fattah HA: Survival statistics for multiple primaries in head and neck cancer. Otolaryngol Head Neck Surg 103:14, 1990.

11. Hong WK, Lippman SM, Wolf GT: Recent advances in head and neck cancer—larynx preservation and cancer chemoprevention: The Seventeenth Annual Richard and Hinda Rosenthal Foundation Award Lecture. Cancer Res 53:5113, 1993.

12. Lippman SM, Benner SE, Hong WK: Cancer chemoprevention. J Clin Oncol 12:851, 1994.

13. Hong WK, Sporn MB: Recent advances in chemoprevention of cancer. Science 278:1073, 1997.

14. Castigliano SG: Influence of continued smoking on the incidence of second primary cancers involving mouth, pharynx, and larynx. J Am Dent Assoc 77:580, 1968.

15. Parker SL, Tong T, Bolden S, et al: Cancer statistics, 1996. CA Cancer J Clin 46:5, 1996.

16. Lippman SM, Hong WK: Retinoid chemoprevention of upper aerodigestive tract carcinogenesis [review]. Important Adv Oncol 93, 1992.

17. Lippman SM, Spitz MR, Huber MH, et al: Strategies for chemoprevention study of premalignancy and second primary tumors in the head and neck. Curr Opin Oncol 7:234, 1995.

18. Spitz MR, Fueger JJ, Beddingfield NA, et al: Chromosome sensitivity to bleomycin-induced mutagenesis, an independent risk factor for upper aerodigestive tract cancers. Cancer Res 49:4626, 1989.

19. Spitz MR, Fueger JJ, Halabi S, et al: Mutagen sensitivity in upper aerodigestive tract cancer: A case-control analysis. Cancer Epidemiol Biomarkers Prev 2:329, 1993.

20. Dave BJ, Hsu TC, Hong WK, et al: Non-random distribution of mutagen-induced chromosome breaks in lymphocytes of patients with different malignancies. Int J Oncol 733, 1994.

21. Wang LE, Sturgis EM, Eicher SA, et al: Mutagen sensitivity to benzo(a)pyrene diol epoxide and the risk of squamous cell carcinoma of the head and neck. Clin Cancer Res 4:1773, 1998.

22. Wu X, Gu J, Hong WK, et al: Benzo[a]pyrene diol epoxide and bleomycin sensitivity and susceptibility to cancer of upper aerodigestive tract. J Natl Cancer Inst 90:1393, 1998.

23. Wei Q, Eicher SA, Guan Y, et al: Reduced expression of hMLH1 and hGTBP/hMSH6: A risk factor for head and neck cancer. Cancer Epidemiol Biomarkers Prev 7:309, 1998.

24. Cheng L, Sturgis EM, Eicher SA, et al: Glutathione-S-transferase polymorphisms and risk of squamous-cell carcinoma of the head and neck. Int J Cancer 84:220, 1999.

25. Spitz MR, Hoque A, Trizna Z, et al: Mutagen sensitivity as a risk factor for second malignant tumors following malignancies of the upper aerodigestive tract. J Natl Cancer Inst 86:1681, 1994.

26. Cloos J, Braakhuis BJ, Steen I, et al: Increased mutagen sensitivity in head-and-neck squamous-cell carcinoma patients, particularly those with multiple primary tumors. Int J Cancer 56:816, 1994.

27. Vogelstein B, Kinzler KW: The multistep nature of cancer. Trends Genet 9:138, 1993.

28. Slaughter DP, Southwick HW, Smejkal W: "Field cancerization" in oral statified squamous epithelium. Clinical implications of multicentric origin. Cancer 6:963, 1953.

29. Califano J, van der Riet P, Westra W, et al: Genetic progression model for head and neck cancer: Implications for field cancerization. Cancer Res 56:2488, 1996.

30. Zelen M: Are primary cancer prevention trials feasible? J Natl Cancer Inst 80:1442, 1988.

31. Schatzkin A, Freedman LS, Schiffman MH, et al: Validation of intermediate end points in cancer research. J Natl Cancer Inst 82:1746, 1990.

32. Lippman SM, Benner SE, Hong WK: The chemoprevention of cancer. In Weed DL (ed): Cancer Prevention and Control. New York, Marcel Dekker, 1995, p 329.

33. Sporn MB, Lippman SM: Chemoprevention of cancer. In Bast RC Jr (ed): Cancer Medicine, 4th ed. Baltimore, William & Wilkins, 1997, p 495.

34. Lippman SM, Kessler JF, Meyskens FLJ: Retinoids as preventive and therapeutic anticancer agents (Part II). Cancer Treat Rep 71:493, 1987.

35. Mangelsdorf DJ, Umesono K, Evans RM: The retinoid receptors. In Goodman DS (ed): The Retinoids. New York, Raven Press, 1994, p 319.

36. Zhang LX, Mills KJ, Dawson MI, et al: Evidence for the involvement of retinoic acid receptor RAR alpha-dependent signaling pathway in the induction of tissue transglutaminase and apoptosis by retinoids. J Biol Chem 270:6022, 1995.

37. Delia D, Aiello A, Formelli F, et al: Regulation of apoptosis induced by the retinoid N-(4-hydroxyphenyl) retinamide and effect of deregulated bcl-2. Blood 85:359, 1995.

38. Lotan R, Dawson MI, Zou CC, et al: Enhanced efficacy of combinations of retinoic acid- and retinoid X receptor-selective retinoids and alpha-interferon in inhibition of cervical carcinoma cell proliferation. Cancer Res 55:232, 1995.

39. Mayne ST, Lippman SM: Retinoids and carotenoids. In DeVita VT Jr, Hellman J, Rosenberg SA (eds): Cancer: Principles and Practice of Oncology, 6th ed. Philadelphia, JB Lippincott, 2001.

40. Mangelsdorf DJ, Ong ES, Dyck JA, et al: Nuclear receptor that identifies a novel retinoic acid response pathway. Nature 345:224, 1990.

41. Leid M, Kastner P, Chambon P: Multiplicity generates diversity in the retinoic acid signalling pathways. Trends Biochem Sci 17:427, 1992.

42. Ozanne B, Richards CS, Hendler F, et al: Over-expression of the EGF receptor is a hallmark of squamous cell carcinomas. J Pathol 149:9, 1986.

43. Maxwell SA, Sacks PG, Gutterman JU, et al: Epidermal growth factor receptor protein-tyrosine kinase activity in human cell lines established from squamous carcinomas of the head and neck. Cancer Res 49:1130, 1989.

44. Kawamoto T, Takahashi K, Nishi M, et al: Quantitative assay of epidermal growth factor receptor in human squamous cell carcinomas of the oral region by an avidin-biotin method. Jpn J Cancer Res 82:403, 1991.

45. Grandis JR, Tweardy DJ: Elevated levels of transforming growth factor alpha and epidermal growth factor receptor messenger RNA are early markers of carcinogenesis in head and neck cancer. Cancer Res 53:3579, 1993.

46. Ishitoya J, Toriyama M, Oguchi N, et al: Gene amplification and over-expression of EGF receptor in squamous cell carcinomas of the head and neck. Br J Cancer 59:559, 1989.

47. Silverman SJ, Gorsky M, Lozada F: Oral leukoplakia and malignant transformation. A follow-up study of 257 patients. Cancer 53:563, 1984.

48. Eisbruch A, Blick M, Lee JS, et al: Analysis of the epidermal growth factor receptor gene in fresh human head and neck tumors. Cancer Res 47:3603, 1987.

49. Koch HF: Biochemical treatment of precancerous oral lesions: The effectiveness of various analogues of retinoic acid. J Maxillofac Surg 6:59, 1978.

50. Hong WK, Endicott J, Itri LM, et al: 13-Cis-retinoic acid in the treatment of oral leukoplakia. N Engl J Med 315:1501, 1986.

51. Stich HF, Hornby AP, Mathew B, et al: Response of oral leukoplakias to the administration of vitamin A. Cancer Lett 40:93, 1988.

52. Han J, Jiao L, Lu Y, et al: Evaluation of N-4-(hydroxycarbophenyl) retinamide as a cancer prevention agent and as a cancer chemotherapeutic agent. In Vivo 4:153, 1990.

53. Lippman SM, Batsakis JG, Toth BB, et al: Comparison of low-dose isotretinoin with beta carotene to prevent oral carcinogenesis. N Engl J Med 328:15, 1993.

54. Chiesa F, Tradati N, Marazza M, et al: Fenretinide (4-HPR) in chemoprevention of oral leukoplakia. J Cell Biochem Suppl 17F:255, 1993.

55. Hong WK, Lippman SM, Hittelman WN, et al: Retinoid chemoprevention of aerodigestive cancer: From basic research to the clinic. Clin Cancer Res 1:677, 1995.

56. Lippman SM, Lee JS, Lotan R, et al: Biomarkers as intermediate end points in chemoprevention trials. J Natl Cancer Inst 82:555, 1990.

57. Lee JS, Kim SY, Hong WK, et al: Detection of chromosomal polysomy in oral leukoplakia, a premalignant lesion. J Natl Cancer Inst 85:1951, 1993.

58. Kim HJ, Lee JS, Shin DM, et al: Chromosomal instability, p53 expression, and retinoid response in oral premalignancy [abstract]. Proc Am Soc Clin Oncol 14:81, 1995.

59. Sudbo J, Kildal W, Risberg B, et al: DNA content as a prognostic marker in patients with oral leukoplakia. N Engl J Med 344:1270, 2001.

60. Lippman S, Shin D, Lee J, et al: p53 and retinoid chemoprevention of oral carcinogenesis. Cancer Res 55:16, 1995.
61. Shin DM, Xu XC, Lippman SM, et al: Accumulation of p53 protein and retinoic acid receptor beta in retinoid chemoprevention. Clin Cancer Res 3:875, 1997.
62. Partridge M, Pateromichelakis S, Phillips E, et al: A case-control study confirms that microsatellite assay can identify patients at risk of developing oral squamous cell carcinoma within a field of cancerization. Cancer Res 60:3893, 2000.
63. Rosin MP, Cheng X, Poh C, et al: Use of allelic loss to predict malignant risk for low-grade oral epithelial dysplasia. Clin Cancer Res 6:357, 2000.
64. Mao L, Lee JS, Fan YH, et al: Frequent microsatellite alterations at chromosomes 9p21 and 3p14 in oral premalignant lesions and their value in cancer risk assessment. Nat Med 2:682, 1996.
65. Lotan R, Xu XC, Lippman SM, et al: Suppression of retinoic acid receptor-beta in premalignant oral lesions and its up-regulation by isotretinoin. N Engl J Med 332:1405, 1995.
66. Xu XC, Ro JY, Lee JS, et al: Differential expression of nuclear retinoid receptors in normal, premalignant, and malignant head and neck tissues. Cancer Res 54:3580, 1994.
67. Widschwendter M, Berger J, Hermann M, et al: Methylation and silencing of the retinoic acid receptor-beta2 gene in breast cancer. J Natl Cancer Inst 92:826, 2000.
68. De Palo G, Veronesi U, Marubini E, et al: Controlled clinical trials with fenretinide in breast cancer, basal cell carcinoma and oral leukoplakia. J Cell Biochem 22:11, 1995.
69. Epstein JB, Wong FL, Millner A, et al: Topical bleomycin treatment of oral leukoplakia: A randomized double-blind clinical trial. Head Neck 16:539, 1994.
70. Stich HF, Rosin MP, Hornby AP, et al: Remission of oral leukoplakias and micronuclei in tobacco/betel quid chewers treated with beta-carotene and with beta-carotene plus vitamin A. Int J Cancer 42:195, 1988.
71. Garewal HS, Meyskens FLJ, Killen D, et al: Response of oral leukoplakia to beta-carotene. J Clin Oncol 8:1715, 1990.
72. Malaker K, Anderson BJ, Beecroft WA, et al: Management of oral mucosal dysplasia with beta-carotene retinoic acid: A pilot cross-over study. Cancer Detect Prev 15:335, 1991.
73. Toma S, Benso S, Albanese E, et al: Response of oral leukoplakia to β-carotene treatment. In Pennington Symposium, Vitamins and Cancer Prevention. Baton Rouge, Louisiana State University Press, 1991, p 222.
74. Garewal HS, Pitcock J, Friedman S, et al: Beta-carotene in oral leukoplakia [abstract]. Proc Am Soc Clin Oncol 11:141, 1992.
75. Anonymous: The effect of vitamin E and beta carotene on the incidence of lung cancer and other cancers in male smokers. The Alpha-Tocopherol, Beta Carotene Cancer Prevention Study Group. N Engl J Med 330:1029, 1994.
76. Benner SE, Winn RJ, Lippman SM, et al: Regression of oral leukoplakia with alpha-tocopherol: A community clinical oncology program chemoprevention study. J Natl Cancer Inst 85:44, 1993.
77. Benner SE, Wargovich MJ, Lippman SM, et al: Reduction in oral mucosa micronuclei frequency following alpha-tocopherol treatment of oral leukoplakia. Cancer Epidemiol Biomarkers Prev 3:73, 1994.
78. Zaridze D, Evstifeeva T, Boyle P: Chemoprevention of oral leukoplakia and chronic esophagitis in an area of high incidence of oral and esophageal cancer. Ann Epidemiol 3:225, 1993.
79. Messadi DV, Billings P, Shklar G, et al: Inhibition of oral carcinogenesis by a protease inhibitor. J Natl Cancer Inst 76:447, 1986.
80. Armstrong WB, Kennedy AR, Wan XS, et al: Clinical modulation of oral leukoplakia and protease activity by Bowman-Birk inhibitor concentrate in a phase IIa chemoprevention trial. Clin Cancer Res 6:4684, 2000.
81. Blackwell KE, Calcaterra TC, Fu YS: Laryngeal dysplasia: Epidemiology and treatment outcome. Ann Otol Rhinol Laryngol 104:596, 1995.
82. Papadimitrakopoulou VA, Clayman GL, Shin DM, et al: Biochemoprevention for dysplastic lesions of the upper aerodigestive tract. Arch Otolaryngol Head Neck Surg 125:1083, 1999.
83. Mao L, El-Naggar AK, Papadimitrakopoulou V, et al: Phenotype and genotype of advanced premalignant head and neck lesions after chemopreventive therapy. J Natl Cancer Inst 90:1545, 1998.
84. Lippman SM, Hong WK: Not yet standard: Retinoids versus second primary tumors. J Clin Oncol 11:1204, 1993.
85. Vikram B: Changing patterns of failure in advanced head and neck cancer. Arch Otolaryngol Head Neck Surg 110:564, 1984.
86. Hong WK, Lippman SM, Itri LM, et al: Prevention of second primary tumors with isotretinoin in squamous-cell carcinoma of the head and neck. N Engl J Med 323:795, 1990.
87. Benner SE, Pajak TF, Lippman SM, et al: Prevention of second primary tumors with isotretinoin in patients with squamous cell carcinoma of the head and neck: Long-term follow-up. J Natl Cancer Inst 86:140, 1994.
88. Bolla M, Lefur R, Ton Van J, et al: Prevention of second primary tumours with etretinate in squamous cell carcinoma of the oral cavity and oropharynx. Results of a multicentric double-blind randomised study. Eur J Cancer 30A:767, 1994.
89. Khuri FR, Kim ES, Lee JJ, et al: The impact of smoking status, disease stage, and index tumor site on second primary tumor incidence and tumor recurrence in the head and neck retinoid chemoprevention trial. Cancer Epidemiol Biomarkers Prev 10:823, 2001.
90. Pastorino U, Infante M, Maioli M, et al: Adjuvant treatment of stage I lung cancer with high-dose vitamin A. J Clin Oncol 11:1216, 1993.
91. van Zandwijk N, Dalesio O, Pastorino U, et al: EUROSCAN, a randomized trial of vitamin A and N-acetylcysteine in patients with head and neck cancer or lung cancer. For the European Organization for Research and Treatment of Cancer Head and Neck and Lung Cancer Cooperative Groups. J Natl Cancer Inst 92:977, 2000.
92. Benner SE, Pajak TF, Stetz J, et al: Toxicity of isotretinoin in a chemoprevention trial to prevent second primary tumors following head and neck cancer. J Natl Cancer Inst 86:1799, 1994.

CHAPTER 33

Chemotherapy in the Treatment of Cancer of the Head and Neck

Cathy Eng

Everett E. Vokes

INTRODUCTION

Although cancer of the head and neck represents only 5% of all newly diagnosed malignancies in the United States, it remains one of the most challenging to treat. The term *cancer of the head and neck* comprises a heterogeneous group of malignancies extending from the lips to the cervical esophagus, with squamous cell carcinoma (SCC) representing the most prevalent histology. At initial presentation, more than two thirds of patients have locally advanced disease (American Joint Committee on Cancer [AJCC] stage III or IV). Patients with SCC of the head and neck (SCCHN) often have a history of chronic tobacco and alcohol use, which has a well-defined relationship with cancer of the head and neck. Consequently, the treatment approach must take into account preexisting related comorbidities, including malnutrition and substance abuse, with acute and chronic sequelae that may develop following the primary treatment modalities of surgery, radiation therapy, and chemotherapy.

Following initial therapy, disease recurrence may manifest itself locally at the primary site, regionally with lymph node involvement, or distantly with metastases. A majority of patients with SCCHN are also at risk of developing a second primary cancer (SPC) of the aerodigestive tract. The term *field cancerization* was initially introduced by Slaughter in the early 1950s to denote how chronic carcinogenic insults to the aerodigestive tract give origin to multiple independent foci of premalignant and malignant lesions.[1] Therefore, despite treatment with curative intent, a person's risk of developing a second malignancy remains 3% to 5% annually.[2] It is estimated that 10% to 40% of patients with cancer of the head and neck will develop second primary cancers.[3] A large retrospective study of more than 9000 patients determined that the risk of developing an SPC was 9.4%.[4] Approximately half of diagnosed metachronous tumors (developing longer than 6 months after the initial diagnosis of the primary cancer) occurred within 31 months of the primary cancer. The mean time between the first and a second primary cancer was 45 months. Similar findings were reported in a retrospective study of 3436 patients with SCC, with a 9.1% risk of SPC and a median time of onset of 36 months.[5]

The risk of developing an SPC is influenced by the degree of alcohol and tobacco consumption, with the risk of SPC decreasing after 5 years of smoking cessation.[6] Hence, patient education before, during, and after treatment should be reinforced. The creation of novel agents to combat the development of cancer of the head and neck and the continued problem of recurrent disease remains a challenge in the field of medical oncology.

The role of chemotherapy in the treatment of cancer of the head and neck has advanced significantly over the past 2 decades. Cytotoxic chemotherapy was initially used only for palliation in the treatment of cancer of the head and neck. However, the objectives of chemotherapy in this field have dramatically changed. The roles of chemotherapy now include radiation sensitization and chemoprevention. This chapter reviews the general background of cancer of the head and neck and the role of chemotherapy in its management.

EPIDEMIOLOGY

Globally, cancer of the head and neck is believed to have affected more than 630,000 men and 227,000 women in the year 1999 alone, resulting in 9% of all cancer-related deaths.[7] Overall, incidence of oral and pharyngeal cancer is increasing in developing countries and in southern and Eastern Europe.[8] An estimated 37,200 new cases of cancer of the head and neck will be diagnosed in the United States, resulting in approximately 11,000 deaths in the year 2003.[9] From 1973 to 1997, an 11.5% decrease in the incidence of oral cavity and pharyngeal cancer and a 17.8% decrease in the incidence of laryngeal cancer was manifested, with a corresponding decrease in mortality of 30.4% and 12.3%, respectively (SEER Database 1973–1997).[9a] Overall, a steady decline has occurred primarily in white males, with a small increase in oral cavity and pharyngeal cancers among black males. Although the incidence of cancer of the oral cavity and pharynx is decreasing in females of all races, the incidence of cancer of the larynx continues to rise.

Development of cancer of the head and neck can be attributed to numerous factors but is commonly associated with tobacco and alcohol consumption (in 75% of patients with cancer of the oral cavity and pharynx).[10] Tobacco and alcohol are independently carcinogenic, and their combination has a synergistic effect rather than an additive effect.[10] Other identified risk factors include environmental viral exposures such as Epstein-Barr virus (EBV) and human papilloma virus (HPV).

The impact of geographic variation can be seen classically in nasopharyngeal cancer, which is an uncommon entity in the United States (0.4 cases per 100,000) but occurs frequently in Asia (26 cases per 100,000). It is associated with EBV exposure. However, EBV exposure is not unique to patients with nasopharyngeal cancer, indicating that there are other unidentified cofactors. Diverse cultural influences such as the chewing of betel nut quid in the Philippines and in India have been determined to increase by almost eightfold the risk for cancers of the oral cavity and oropharynx.[11]

INTRODUCTION OF CHEMOTHERAPY

The primary modality of treatment for early-stage disease (AJCC stage I/II) is surgery and/or radiation therapy. Previously, these treatment methods also applied to patients with locally advanced disease (AJCC stage III/IV) if it was found to be resectable. Patients with cancer judged to be unresectable were offered radiation therapy only, with complete response rates of less than 30%.[12] Treatment failure commonly occurred within the first 2 years, indicating that surgery and/or radiation therapy could not solely eradicate the cancer cells. Hence, novel treatment methods or adjuncts continue to be investigated to provide advances in this complex field.

PALLIATIVE TREATMENT FOR RECURRENT AND METASTATIC DISEASE

Cytotoxic Single Agents

Chemotherapy was initially used in the palliative care of patients with recurrent or metastatic disease. If left untreated, their survival rate is dismal, with a median survival of 4 months.[13] Effective single chemotherapy agents in recurrent and metastatic head and neck cancer are listed in Table 33–1.

Cisplatin. Review of the literature identifies cisplatin as the only chemotherapy agent evaluated in a randomized phase III trial in comparison with best supportive care; it provided an extension in overall survival of approximately 10 weeks.[14] Standard regimens have evaluated cisplatin 100 mg/m^2 every 21 to 28 days.[15, 16] However, systemic treatment with cisplatin may be difficult to tolerate, with potential adverse reactions of emetogenicity (vomiting), electrolyte disturbance, nephrotoxicity, peripheral neuropathy, and ototoxicity.

Carboplatin. The platinum analogue carboplatin is associated with reduced nephrotoxicity and emetogenicity but is infrequently used as a palliative single agent.[17] However, carboplatin has been extensively examined in combination regimens. A National Cancer Institute (NCI)–sponsored study is currently examining the third-generation platinum analogue oxaliplatin in the palliative treatment setting. Other single agents with known clinical activity include methotrexate, ifosfamide, 5-fluorouracil (5-FU), bleomycin, and the taxanes.

Methotrexate and Edatrexate. Methotrexate is an antifolate that was initially considered the standard for palliative treatment owing to its ease of administration and moderate associated toxicities. Methotrexate provided variable response rates ranging from 10% to 40% with a short median duration of response.[16, 18–20] Several characteristics of methotrexate qualify it as an ideal palliative agent, but its inability to have a significant impact on duration of response or overall survival requires further evaluation of other chemotherapy agents. Its structural analogue, edatrexate, demonstrated promising preclinical activity and was believed to be superior to methotrexate with similar associated toxicities. However, phase II and III studies of edatrexate were less than favorable in large multicenter trials.[20]

Ifosfamide. The efficacy of ifosfamide has been investigated in the palliative care setting. Ifosfamide is a synthetic analogue of cyclophosphamide. Table 33–1 reveals the diversified schedules that have been attempted when ifosfamide is used, with variable response rates.[19, 21–24] The administration of ifosfamide may be cumbersome, requiring a 24-hour intravenous infusion and the infusion of mesna for effective metabolic clearance.

5-Fluorouracil. 5-FU is given primarily by continuous infusion for 4 to 5 days every 3 weeks.[15, 25] A single-institution retrospective analysis observed a response rate of 31% with bolus infusion of 5-FU.[26] Primary toxicities that have been encountered with 5-FU on both continuous infusion and bolus schedules are palmar-plantar erythrodysesthesia (hand-foot syndrome), mucositis, myelosuppression, and diarrhea. Investigators have attempted to alter the metabolism of 5-FU through biochemical modulation by using hydroxyurea (Hydrea), phosphonacetyl-L-aspartate (PALA), interferon-α, and methotrexate to improve its efficacy.

Paclitaxel and Docetaxel. Members of the taxoid class, paclitaxel (Taxol) and docetaxel (Taxotere), have a distinct mechanism. Paclitaxel functions to promote the assembly of microtubules from tubulin dimers and to stabilize microtubules by preventing depolymerization, resulting in mitotic arrest at the G2/M phase and subsequent apoptosis (programmed cell death).[27] This cytotoxic agent was originally discovered in 1971 and is derived from the Pacific yew tree, *Taxus baccata*. Paclitaxel is formulated in Cremophor (polyoxyethlated castor oil), resulting in severe hypersensitivity reactions in 2% to 4% of patients. Additional adverse events that have been reported include urticaria, angioedema, dyspnea, hypotension, and anaphylaxis. All patients require premedication with corticosteroids, diphenhydramine, and H$_2$-antagonists to prevent adverse reactions.

A variety of infusion schedules have been evaluated to determine the optimal method of administering paclitaxel without compromising efficacy (see Table 33–1).[28–31] The

TABLE 33-1 Single-Agent Studies

Chemotherapy	Author	Phase of Trial	Dose	Overall Response Rate (%)	Median Survival (weeks)
Cisplatin	Morton et al, 1985[14]	III	100 mg/m^2 q 28 days	13.3	NA
	Campbell et al, 1987[16]	III	100 mg/m^2 q 28 days	40	37
	Jacobs et al, 1992[15]	III	100 mg/m^2 q 21 days	17	40
Carboplatin	Eisenberger et al, 1986[17]	I	60–80 mg/m^2 daily (days 1–5) q 28–35 days	26	18
Bleomycin	Morton et al, 1985[14]	III	15 mg/m^2 (days 1–5)	13.6	NA
Methotrexate	Campbell et al, 1987[16]	III	40 mg/m^2 q 14 days	19	11
	Eisenberger et al, 1989[17]	III	40 mg/m^2/week	25	24
	Forastiere et al, 1992[18]	III	40 mg/m^2/week	10	22
	Schornagel et al, 1995[20]	III	40 mg/m^2/week	16	24
5-Fluorouracil	Tapazoglou et al, 1986[25]	II	1 g/m^2 continuous infusion (days 1–4 or days 1–5) q 21 days	72	28
	Jacobs et al, 1992[15]	III	1 g/m^2 continuous infusion (days 1–4) q 21 days	13	23
Ifosfamide	Cervellino et al, 1991[21]	II	3.5 g/m^2/day (days 1–5) q 28 days	42.7	44
	Buesa et al, 1991[22]	II	5–6.25 g/m^2/day	28	27
	Huber, 1996[23]	II	2 g/m^2/day for 4 days	25.8	27
	Sandler et al, 1998[24]	II	1.5 g/m^2/day (days 1–5) q 21 days	4.3	16
Paclitaxel	Smith et al, 1995[28]	II	250 mg/m^2 (24-hr infusion) q 21 days	35	NA
	Gebbia et al, 1996[29]	II	175 mg/m^2 (3-hr infusion) q 21 days	20	NA
	Forastiere et al, 1998[31]	II	250 mg/m^2 (24-hr infusion) q 21 days	40	38
	Mickiewicz et al, 1998[30]	II	200 mg/m^2 (1-hr infusion) q 21 days	36	NA
Docetaxel	Dreyfuss et al, 1996[34]	II	100 mg/m^2 q 21 days	42	35
	Couteau et al, 1999[35]	II	100 mg/m^2 q 21 days	21	27
Vinorelbine	Saxman et al, 1998[41]	II	30 mg/m^2 weekly	7.5	20
	Degardin et al, 1998[40]	II	30 mg/m^2 weekly	14	32
Irinotecan (CPT-11)	Murphy et al, 1999[42]	II	125 mg/m^2 q 21 days	30	NA

NA, not available.

European Organization for Research and Treatment of Cancer (EORTC) completed a three-arm randomized phase II trial comparing weekly methotrexate with two different schedules of paclitaxel (3-hour and 24-hour infusions).[32] The response rates were 18%, 11%, and 23%, respectively, with median survival of 6.3 months, 5.4 months, and 6.1 months, respectively. Significant toxicities were encountered in the 24-hour paclitaxel infusion arm. Based on the toxicity profile and minimal response (fewer than 7 responses in each arm), the trial was closed early. Paclitaxel continues to be evaluated in both single-agent and combination chemotherapy treatment regimens. Response rates have varied from 20% to 40% in the recurrent or metastatic disease setting. Peripheral neuropathy and myelosuppression are the primary treatment-limiting toxicities.

The semisynthetic taxane docetaxel has a mechanism of action similar to paclitaxel's in promoting microtubule stabilization. Unlike paclitaxel, however, docetaxel does not alter the number of protofilaments in the bound microtubules, and it prevents formation of the centrosome rather than affecting the mitotic spindle. In vitro studies have determined docetaxel to be 100-fold more potent than paclitaxel in BCL2 phosphorylation, further modulating apoptosis.[33]

Traditional schedules of docetaxel in the treatment of cancer of the head and neck have been administered at 100 mg/m^2 every 21 days with response rates of 20% to 40%. Dreyfuss and colleagues examined single-agent docetaxel in chemotherapy-naïve patients with locoregional and metastatic SCCHN.[34] Docetaxel was determined to be active and safe, with an overall response rate of 42%. A similar French study provided an overall response rate of 20.8%.[35] These two studies differ in their patient populations, with the majority of patients in the French study (73.9%) having metastatic disease. Principal toxicities of docetaxel include leukopenia, asthenia, peripheral edema, peripheral neuropathy, and hypersensitivity reactions. Docetaxel continues to be evaluated in palliative, induction, and concurrent radiation treatment settings.[36, 37]

Gemcitabine, Vinorelbine, and Irinotecan. Other active single agents include gemcitabine, vinorelbine (Navelbine), and irinotecan (CPT-11, Camptosar). Gemcitabine is a synthetic pyrimidine antimetabolite with both cytotoxic and radiosensitizing properties. Early phase I studies established a recommended phase II dose of 1000 mg/m^2 for 3 of 4 weeks. An EORTC multicenter phase II trial in advanced and/or recurrent head and neck cancer established a modest overall response rate of 13%, with primary toxicities including fatigue and grade I/II elevated liver enzymes.[38] Gemcitabine continues to be investigated in combination with other chemotherapy agents and as an adjunct to radiation therapy.[39]

The semisynthetic vinca alkaloid vinorelbine disrupts microtubule assembly, resulting in mitotic arrest. Vinorelbine is commonly administered at 30 mg/m^2 weekly. Overall response rates in the recurrent and advanced disease setting have been less than promising at 7.5% to 14%.[40, 41] Common toxicities encountered when vinorelbine is administered include myelosuppression, constipation, asthenia, and peripheral neuropathy.

Irinotecan is a topoisomerase I inhibitor with activity in several tumor cell lines, including non–small cell lung carcinoma, colon cancer, pancreatic cancer, and SCCHN. Investigators at Vanderbilt University examined CPT-11 (125 mg/m^2) given weekly for 4 weeks, every 6 weeks, to previously untreated patients with metastatic and/or recurrent cancer of the head and neck. Preliminary analysis revealed an overall response rate (ORR) of 30%.[42] Despite a favorable response, frequent toxicities such as vomiting, diarrhea, neutropenia, and infection resulted in 60% of patients receiving a dose reduction. Other topoisomerase I inhibitors have been evaluated in the palliative care setting but have proved ineffective.[43, 44]

Combination Cytotoxic Chemotherapy Regimens

Combination chemotherapy regimens in recurrent and metastatic cancer of the head and neck have provided superior response rates in comparison with each respective single agent but have not demonstrated an improvement in survival.

Combination Chemotherapy With Cisplatin/5-FU

Several randomized clinical trials have provided conclusive evidence for the superiority of cisplatin/5-FU (PF) as the standard in this patient population.[15, 18, 45, 46] The primary method of administration for this doublet regimen is cisplatin 100 mg/m^2 on day 1 and continuous-infusion 5-FU 1 g/m^2 on days 1 to 4 or 5.

A large phase III randomized trial of combined PF versus each respective agent was initiated by Jacobs and associates; an improved overall response rate was determined for this doublet regimen at 32% (P = .035) versus cisplatin (17%) versus 5-FU (13%) in advanced head and neck cancer.[15] The median time to progression of approximately 2 months for the combination (P = .023) was less than satisfactory. The median survival in all three arms was approximately 5.7 months (P = .489). Although the combination of cisplatin/5-FU was deemed to be superior in response, this was at the expense of increased grade III/IV vomiting (35%) in comparison with the single-agent arm of cisplatin (18%, P = .02).

A large randomized phase III trial conducted by the Southwest Oncology Group (SWOG) determined that the response rates of cisplatin/5-FU (32%) and carboplatin/5-FU (21%) exceeded that of single-agent methotrexate (10%).[18] Forastiere and colleagues randomly assigned 272 patients with SCC to one of three arms: (1) cisplatin (100 mg/m^2)/continuous-infusion 5-FU (1000 mg/m^2/day, days 1 to 4) repeated every 21 days; (2) carboplatin (300 mg/m^2)/continuous-infusion 5-FU (1000 mg/m^2/day, days 1 to 4) repeated every 28 days; and (3) methotrexate (40 mg/m^2 weekly).[18] Although the combined chemotherapy arms clearly had an improved response when compared with methotrexate, median survival was found to be equivalent in all 3 arms.

Various methods of enhancing the cytotoxicity of chemotherapy agents have been explored, including the use of interferon-α. In vitro studies of interferon-α have revealed enhanced cytotoxic effects of 5-FU when administered in combination. Based on this premise, investigators examined the combination of cisplatin/5-FU/interferon-α in a pilot trial.[47] An overall response rate of 30% was seen. A larger phase III trial of PF with randomization to interferon-α was pursued in patients with cancer of the head and neck who had a poor prognosis.[48] After completion of the study, no statistical difference in response rate or median survival benefit could be ascertained. Increased toxicities of anorexia, fever, leukopenia, and thrombocytopenia were noted to occur in the interferon-α arm.

Unfortunately, these and other phase III trials have been unable to establish an improved benefit in survival when a combined regimen is used, and increased toxicity is often noted. A critical drawback to several of the earlier studies was the consideration of response rather than overall survival in the setting of recurrent or metastatic disease as the primary endpoint. Moreover, a majority of studies failed to determine the impact of treatment on quality of life, an important consideration in patients with a poor prognosis. Clinical investigators in cancer of the head and neck have recently recognized quality of life as an important facet in the success of clinical trials, and they continue to evaluate the impact of both acute and chronic sequelae.

Combination Chemotherapy With the Taxanes

DOCETAXEL (TAXOTERE)/PLATINUM COMBINATIONS

Novel combinations incorporating the taxanes have been initiated and continue to be evaluated. Previously, several phase II clinical trials have examined the benefits of docetaxel combined with cisplatin or 5-FU. The EORTC investigated the combination of docetaxel (100 mg/m^2)/cisplatin (75 mg/m^2) every 21 days in taxane-naïve patients.[49] Forty-one patients were eligible for treatment, and 31 patients were evaluated for response. The median number of chemotherapy cycles received was four in this novel combination. A favorable ORR of 53.7% was determined on an intent-to-treat analysis (14.6% complete remission [CR], 39% partial remission [PR]), with a median duration of response of 18 months and a median survival at 1 year of 50%. A majority of the adverse events noted were primarily hematologic, resulting in anemia (98%) and leukopenia (79%). Asthenia developed in 47% of patients with this combination regimen and is a known frequent toxicity associated with docetaxel. The favorable response rate in this combination setting may be a result of the minority of patients (six total) with distant metastatic disease. However, the encouraging response rate and duration of response require that this novel taxane combination be considered in the primary treatment of locally advanced disease. A Japanese study using a lower dose of docetaxel (60 mg/m^2) had similar findings for the combination of docetaxel/cisplatin with an ORR of 42.4%.[50]

DOCETAXEL/5-FLUOROURACIL COMBINATIONS

A second phase II trial was initiated in a small group of 17 patients with recurrent or metastatic SCCHN.[51] Patients received docetaxel (70 mg/m^2, day 1)/5-FU (800 mg/m^2, days 1 to 5) every 28 days. This clinical trial was terminated after the first-stage interim analysis failed to demonstrate a response in fewer than 5 patients (ORR = 24%). Common grade III/IV toxicities noted to occur in this suboptimal combination included neutropenia (24%) and mucositis (26%). Median duration of response was 3 months.

In contrast, a larger study of 54 patients examined a similar combination of docetaxel (75 mg/m^2, day 1)/5-FU (1000 mg/m^2/day, days 1 to 5) given every 21 days. A dose reduction in 5-FU (750 mg/m^2/day) was required as a result of grade III/IV neutropenia (65%) and mucositis (30%).[52] At the conclusion of the study, 44 patients were evaluated for response, resulting in 4 CR (9%), 11 PR (25%), and 15 stable disease (SD) (34%), for an ORR of 34%.

DOCETAXEL TRIPLET REGIMENS

Other investigators have attempted to evaluate the triplet combination of docetaxel and cisplatin/5-FU in these poor-prognosis patients. A European study provided preliminary results of the combination of docetaxel (80 mg/m^2, day 1), cisplatin (40 mg/m^2, days 1 and 2), and continuous-infusion 5-FU (750 mg/m^2/day, days 1 to 3) in 19 patients with recurrent or advanced head and neck cancer, concluding an overall response rate of 44% with acceptable toxicity.[53]

The oral fluoropyrimidine capecitabine (Xeloda) is selectively activated by thymidine phosphorylase, consequently prolonging the half-life of 5-FU. Therefore, it is thought that its administration may mimic continuous-infusion 5-FU. A single-institution small-cohort phase I/II study in patients with advanced solid tumors has been completed. Patients received docetaxel/cisplatin and capecitabine (2 to 3 g/m^2/day in two divided doses, days 1 to 4) every 3 to 4 weeks.[54] Overall, this triplet regimen provided disappointing results, with a PR in one of ten head and neck cancer patients after a preliminary analysis.

PACLITAXEL (TAXOL)/PLATINUM COMBINATIONS

Numerous studies have combined paclitaxel with cisplatin in the setting of recurrent cancer of the head and neck, resulting in a wide range of response rates from 30% to 70%. Both high- and low-dose paclitaxel combinations have been created to determine if a dose-response relationship exists for 24-hour infusion of paclitaxel. The myelosuppressive effects of paclitaxel often require hematologic support with granulocyte colony-stimulating factor (G-CSF) if high doses are to be administered.

The Eastern Cooperative Oncology Group (ECOG) conducted a randomized phase III study in 210 patients of high doses of paclitaxel (200 mg/m^2 over 24 hours) and cisplatin (75 mg/m^2)/G-CSF versus low-dose paclitaxel (135 mg/m^2 over 24 hours) and cisplatin (75 mg/m^2) in patients with unresectable, recurrent, or metastatic head and neck cancer.[55] No significant difference in response could be determined (35% vs. 36%, respectively). Profound grade III/IV granulocytopenia developed in both the high- and low-dose paclitaxel arms (70% and 78%, respectively). Each arm of this randomized study resulted in an unacceptable death rate of 10%. Consequently, neither of these combination regimens is recommended for continued evaluation. Furthermore, a dose-response relationship on this schedule was not found.

Investigators at Loyola University Medical Center completed a single-institution trial in patients with cancer of the head and neck to evaluate the palliative effects of carboplatin and paclitaxel, a standard regimen in the treatment of advanced NSCLC.[56] Thirty-seven chemotherapy-naïve patients received paclitaxel (200 mg/m^2 over 3 hours) and carboplatin (area under the concentration-time curve [AUC] = 6) every 21 days. Patients were allowed to receive G-CSF at the discretion of the treating physician for hematologic support. A majority of patients had distant disease involvement (19% distant disease only, 43% locoregional and distant disease). Based on an intent-to-treat analysis, the overall response rate was 27% (1 CR, 9 PR, 6 SD). The median survival of all patients was 4.9 months, with a median survival of 12.9 months in patients who demonstrated an initial response. Patients with distant disease only fared significantly better, with an ORR of 43% and median survival of 15.7 months.

To determine if the taxanes could provide superior benefit in comparison with the standard PF regimen for palliation, an Intergroup trial was initiated by ECOG and SWOG.[57] Nearly 200 patients with previously untreated metastatic or recurrent head and neck cancer were randomly assigned to PF or cisplatin/paclitaxel. No difference in overall survival (*P* = .22), response rate (*P* = .4), or quality of life was determined.

PACLITAXEL TRIPLET COMBINATIONS

Investigators at the University of Texas M.D. Anderson Cancer Center have conducted a clinical trial examining the triplet regimen (TIP) paclitaxel (175 mg/m^2), cisplatin (60 mg/m^2), ifosfamide (1000 mg/m^2, days 1 to 3), and mesna given every 21 to 28 days.[58] An ORR of 58% was established; 9 patients achieved a CR, and 6 of these patients (67%) remained disease free after a median follow-up of longer than 16 months. Disease site comparison established the improved response rate of patients with distant disease compared with patients with locoregional disease involvement (80% vs. 30%, respectively; *P* = .003). The primary adverse nonhematologic toxicity was peripheral neuropathy in almost half of the patients enrolled. Grades III to IV neutropenia occurred in 90% of patients; neutropenic fever occurred in 27% of patients. The role of the TIP regimen continues to be investigated toward the goal of organ preservation.

After efficacy and safety were demonstrated in recurrent and advanced cancer of the head and neck, a decision was made to undertake an analogous regimen of carboplatin/paclitaxel/ifosfamide (TIC).[59] The objective of this study was to maintain if not improve the response rate while decreasing the cumulative peripheral neuropathy that patients often experienced after receiving more than 4 cycles of the TIP regimen. Patients received the standard regimen of carboplatin (AUC = 6) and paclitaxel (175 mg/m^2), followed by ifosfamide (1000 mg/m^2, days 1 to 3) and mesna (600 mg/m^2, days 1 to 3) every 21 to 28 days. A majority of patients had received radiation therapy. An overall response rate of 59% (CR 17%) was determined in this study of patients with mostly recurrent locoregional disease (56% of patients).

◼ TREATMENT OF NEWLY DIAGNOSED DISEASE

The role of chemotherapy in the treatment of primary cancer of the head and neck is multifaceted. Its purpose is vast and may include radiosensitization, organ preservation, locoregional and distant control, and overall survival. The timing of administration results in induction (neoadjuvant), concomitant, or adjuvant therapy.

Concomitant Chemoradiotherapy

Concomitant chemoradiotherapy has been investigated over the past 4 decades as a primary treatment approach in locally advanced cancer of the head and neck. It is administered with the intent of curing locoregional disease and controlling the occurrence of distant disease. Theoretically, systemic control may be feasible if the dose of chemotherapy administered is equivalent to standard systemic doses when given in combination with radiotherapy. Chemotherapy should also act as a radiation sensitizer (is not directly cytotoxic but improves the tumoricidal activity of radiation) or as an enhancer (has direct cytotoxic properties and also improves the tumoricidal activity of radiation). Therefore, combined chemoradiotherapy provides potentially increased antitumor activity, often at the risk of substantial local toxicity.

Generally, radiation therapy is administered in two basic schedules: concomitant (simultaneous) or in an interrupted fashion (alternating or split-course schedule). The method of radiation delivery may also have an impact on treatment outcome and acute and chronic sequelae. The Radiation Therapy Oncology Group (RTOG) has completed a randomized phase III trial (RTOG 9003) in more than 1000 patients with locally advanced cancer of the head and neck.[60] The four arms were as follows: (1) standard radiotherapy, (2) hyperfractionated twice-daily radiotherapy, (3) accelerated fractionated twice-daily therapy, and (4) accelerated fractionated therapy with concomitant boost. After a median follow-up of 23 months, it was determined that hyperfractionated or accelerated radiation therapy with boost provided increased locoregional control and a trend toward improved disease-free survival in comparison with conventional radiation therapy. However, no improvement was noted in overall survival. Patients given accelerated split-course fractionation had outcomes similar to those who

had received conventional radiotherapy. Clinical investigators continue to incorporate accelerated fractionated, hyperfractionated, and intensity-modulated radiotherapy (IMRT) approaches in an attempt to maximize tumoricidal activity while minimizing associated toxicities.

Single-Agent Chemoradiation Trials

Initial studies examined single-agent chemotherapy with concomitant daily radiotherapy. Cytotoxic agents used in the palliative setting for recurrent or advanced disease have demonstrated single-agent activity when combined with radiation therapy. Frequently administered single agents include cisplatin, methotrexate, 5-FU, bleomycin, ifosfamide, and the taxanes. Several randomized studies have been completed, demonstrating the benefits of combined therapy in comparison with radiation therapy alone.

One of the most promising classic agents used with concomitant radiotherapy is 5-FU (Table 33–2). Lo and coworkers randomly assigned 136 patients with advanced oral cavity or oropharyngeal carcinoma to radiotherapy alone or radiotherapy combined with bolus 5-FU.[61] Patients with oral cavity tumors clearly demonstrated superior local control and survival.

Byfield demonstrated enhanced radiosensitization properties of 5-FU when administered continuously for at least 48 hours following radiation therapy.[62] Thus, the exposure time to 5-FU must exceed the doubling time of the tumor cell. The previously described 5-FU bolus study by Lo was informative and demonstrated efficacy. However, Byfield determined via in vitro studies that continued exposure to 5-FU (via continuous infusion rather than bolus) following radiation therapy would increase the doubling time of the tumor cell, providing superior radiosensitization. On the basis of this principle, a phase I/II pilot study was conducted to study the effects of dose-escalating continuous-infusion 5-FU (20 to 30 mg/kg in 5-mg/kg increments) over a 5-day period with four sequential daily fractions (2.5 Gy) on days 1 to 4, repeated every 14 days.[63] A complete response rate of 75% was attained in stage IV patients.

In a similar fashion, investigators at the University of Chicago have extensively investigated the activity of continuous-infusion 5-FU but have also chosen to examine the biomodulatory effects of hydroxyurea on 5-FU. Hydroxyurea is an oral agent that inhibits ribonucleotide diphosphate reductase, interfering with the synthesis of

TABLE 33–2 5-FU Concomitant Chemoradiotherapy Trials

Trial	n	Regimen	Results ORR (CR + PR)	DFS	OS
Lo et al, 1976[61]	136	Bolus 5-FU/daily XRT	—	49% (2-yr)	32% (5-yr)
		Daily XRT	—	18%	14%
Browman et al, 1994[68]	175	Infusional 5-FU (1.2 g/m²/day, weeks 1, 3)/daily XRT	68%	—	63% (2-yr)
		Daily XRT	56%	—	50%
Byfield et al, 1984[63]	18	Continuous infusion 5-FU/XRT	75% (stage IV)	—	—

CR, Complete remission; DFS, disease-free survival; 5-FU, 5-fluorouracil; ORR, overall response rate; OS, overall survival; PR, partial remission; XRT, radiation therapy.

DNA, specifically the S-phase of the cell cycle. Sinclair and associates have demonstrated in preclinical animal models that hydroxyurea may inhibit cells from leaving the G1 radiosensitive phase and entering the radioresistant S-phase.[64] Early studies have demonstrated little or no efficacy associated with the use of single-agent hydroxyurea.[65] It has received FDA approval for use in patients with cancer of the head and neck when administered concomitantly with radiotherapy based on promising results from earlier studies.[66]

The foundation for combining hydroxyurea and 5-FU is based on in vitro pharmacokinetics denoting modulation of 5-FU by the depletion of deoxyuridine monophosphate, a metabolic product of 5-FU. In turn, increased binding of 5-FU to thymidylate synthase augments the cytotoxicity of 5-FU. At the University of Chicago, biomodulation of 5-FU by hydroxyurea combined with concomitant radiation therapy (FHX) has provided the platform for the majority of our studies of patients with intermediate (AJCC stage II/III), locally advanced (AJCC stage III/IV), and recurrent cancer of the head and neck.

An initial study of 39 patients examined escalating doses of hydroxyurea (500 to 3000 mg/d in 500-mg/day increments), fixed doses of continuous-infusion 5-FU (800 mg/m²/day for days 1 to 5), and accelerated fractionated radiotherapy.[67] Each cycle was repeated every 14 days. A subset analysis of radiotherapy-naïve patients demonstrated favorable clinical response rates (71% CR, 29% PR) and time to progression of 14 months. Three patients experienced treatment failure locally. Minimal locoregional recurrence prompted continued investigation of hydroxyurea as an adjunct to 5-FU–based regimens at the University of Chicago.

Browman and colleagues randomly assigned 175 stage III or IV head and neck cancer patients to standard daily radiotherapy (total 66 cGy) with or without 72-hour infusion of 5-FU (1.2 g/m²) during weeks 1 and 3.[68] As expected, increased toxicity, including stomatitis ($P = .001$) and radiation dermatitis ($P = .03$), occurred in the chemoradiation arm. However, a trend toward improved overall survival ($P = .08$) and progression-free survival ($P = .06$) was demonstrated in the chemoradiotherapy arm. Superiority in median survival remains in the combined-modality arm after a follow-up of nearly 10 years (27 vs. 16 months).[69] The benefits of combined chemoradiation were greatest within the first 2.5 years.

Earlier studies of bleomycin examined potential synergistic activity in combination with radiotherapy. Two previous randomized studies involving more than 200 patients suggested improved locoregional control in the combined chemoradiation arm.[70, 71] However, the EORTC could not confirm benefit of response after completing a randomized study of conventional radiotherapy with or without single-agent bleomycin.[72] Only 64% of patients in the chemoradiation arm received the recommended dose, which may have contributed to the suboptimal response rate and survival time in the combined chemoradiation arm.

The platinum analogues, carboplatin and cisplatin, have a well-defined role in combination with radiation therapy. An early Intergroup trial of 371 patients compared conventional radiation therapy with combined low-dose weekly cisplatin (20 mg/m²) and conventional radiotherapy.[73] At the conclusion of the study, no statistical difference in complete response (34% for the concurrent modality vs. 30% in the radiation therapy alone arm) or overall survival was found. The final results of this study were never published.

A large phase III European study evaluated the benefits of concomitant cisplatin (100 mg/m², days 1, 22, and 43) with radiation therapy.[74] The study randomly assigned 334 patients to daily radiation therapy or chemoradiotherapy. After a median follow-up of 34 months, the 3-year disease-free survival ($P = .0096$), locoregional control ($P = .0014$), and time to progression ($P = .0016$) were superior in the chemoradiation therapy arm. It is too early to determine if the addition of chemotherapy has had an impact on the development of distant disease or second primary tumors, or if it offers a survival benefit.

Several studies have concluded that there is an advantage to platinum-based radiation therapy over radiation therapy alone, notably in the setting of nasopharyngeal carcinoma.[75, 76] Whether cisplatin is equivalent or superior to carboplatin as an adjunct to radiation therapy is unclear. Few randomized studies have addressed this issue. A recent Japanese study randomly assigned patients to cisplatin (4 mg/m² daily, weeks 1 to 4) or carboplatin (100 mg/m², day 1, weeks 1 to 4), with concomitant daily radiation therapy (65 Gy, 66 Gy for hypopharyngeal carcinoma).[77] No statistically significant difference was determined in 4-year overall survival (OS) or disease-free survival. Other potential chemosensitizing agents that remain largely investigational include the taxanes, gemcitabine, and irinotecan (Table 33–3).[78–82]

TABLE 33-3 Single Agent Chemoradiation Studies

Clinical Study	n	Regimen	Results
Jacobs et al, 1989[98]	26	Carboplatin (60–400 mg/m²)/daily radiotherapy	52% CR, 24% PR
Kamioner et al, 1993[79]	41	A: Carboplatin (100 mg/m² per week)/daily radiotherapy	55% CR
		B: Cisplatin (20 mg/m² per week)/daily radiotherapy	69% CR
Hesse et al, 2000[80]	6	Docetaxel (15 mg/m²)/daily radiotherapy	50% CR, 16% PR
Sunwoo et al, 2001[81]	33	Continuous infusion paclitaxel (105–120 mg/m², days 1–5)/daily radiotherapy	70% CR
Eisbruch et al, 2001[82]	29	Weekly gemcitabine (10–300 mg/m²)/daily radiotherapy	77%

CR, complete remission; PR, partial remission.

Platinum Therapy as the Standard of Care:
Nasopharyngeal Cancer

A landmark study by the RTOG provided justification for the continued consideration of concomitant chemoradiotherapy. Al-Sarraf and associates initiated a phase II study of cisplatin (100 mg/m², days 1, 22, and 42) and standard radiotherapy in 124 patients with locally advanced cancer of the head and neck.[76] An impressive CR of 70% was attained for all patients; a subset analysis of patients with nasopharyngeal carcinoma revealed an impressive CR of 89%. Comparison with historically matched controls revealed that the disease-free survival and overall survival were greater in the concomitant arm, thereby revolutionizing the standard treatment of nasopharyngeal cancer.[83] This trial provided the precedent for a large phase III Intergroup study of daily radiotherapy and cisplatin (100 mg/m², days 1, 22, and 43) followed by 3 cycles of adjuvant cisplatin (80 mg/m², day 1) and continuous-infusion 5-FU (1000 mg/m², days 1 to 4) every 28 days. Overall, superiority of treatment was seen in the concomitant chemoradiation therapy arm in comparison with radiotherapy alone, with a 3-year disease-free survival of 69% vs. 24% ($P < .001$) and a 3-year OS of 78% vs. 47% ($P = .005$), respectively.

Chicago investigators have determined a superior survival rate in a recent subset analysis using an induction regimen of PF/leucovorin/interferon-α (PFL-INF) followed by concomitant chemoradiotherapy with 5-FU/hydroxyurea.[84] Twenty-seven patients were determined to have locally advanced nasopharyngeal carcinoma. Following the completion of induction chemotherapy, a clinical response was seen in all patients treated (CR 52%, PR 46%). After a median follow-up of 51.5 months, 89% of these patients are alive and remain disease free.

A meta-analysis of six randomized trials evaluating chemoradiation therapy (induction, concomitant, and adjuvant) versus radiation therapy alone verified that the addition of chemotherapy to radiation therapy increased the disease-free survival by 37% at 2 years, 40% at 3 years, and 34% at 5 years. The addition of chemotherapy also conferred a 20% increase in OS at 2 years.[85]

In contrast, in a large single-institution study in Hong Kong, 240 patients were randomly assigned to radiation therapy or to two or three cycles of induction chemotherapy (cisplatin 60 mg/m² and epirubicin 110 mg/m²) followed by radiation therapy.[86] After a median follow-up of 71 months, the investigators determined no statistical benefit with induction chemotherapy in nodal relapse-free survival ($P = .13$), prevention of distant metastases ($P = .56$), or survival ($P = .55$).

Current investigative trials for the treatment of nasopharyngeal carcinoma continue to evaluate the taxane and platinum analogues, the alkylating agent mitomycin C, gemcitabine, and the topoisomerase I inhibitor epirubicin in various combinations.

Multiagent Chemoradiotherapy

After studies documented the success and feasibility of several single-agent chemoradiation regimens, the natural consideration was to consider the feasibility of multiagent

chemoradiation schedules. Given the effectiveness of the PF regimen in palliative therapy and the individual activity of each respective agent with radiation therapy, the PF regimen has become the classic multiagent chemoradiotherapy regimen.

The Eastern Cooperative Oncology Group (ECOG) completed a pilot study in 57 patients.[87] Patients received three courses of continuous-infusion 5-FU (days 1 to 4), cisplatin bolus (day 1), and split-course radiotherapy (weeks 1 to 3). On day 28, chemotherapy was repeated. Patients were then reevaluated. Patients with a CR or those patients with unresectable disease were treated again with chemoradiotherapy on weeks 9 to 12. Salvage surgery was offered to all patients with a PR, if resectable. A CR of 77% was achieved with a 4-year estimate of OS of 49%.

Adelstein and colleagues have since provided preliminary results of the PF regimen in patients with cancer of the oral cavity, oropharynx, and hypopharynx. Organ preservation served as the primary endpoint in the study.[88] Patients received hyperfractionated twice-daily radiotherapy and two courses of concomitant 5-FU (1000 mg/m²/day) and cisplatin (20 mg/m²/day), both given by continuous infusion. Patients were offered salvage surgery or neck dissection at the conclusion of the study. After a median follow-up of 26 months, the 2-year projected overall survival is 80%. This study revealed superior locoregional control at a rate of 90% as well as evidence of distant disease failure (19%). What was exemplary about this study was the lack of treatment breaks or dose reductions. Only one of 42 patients required a gastric tube for longer than 1 year, suggesting a benefit in terms of quality of life.

Several notable prospective randomized trials have since been completed in attempts to discern the absolute benefits of concomitant chemoradiotherapy in locoregional and distant disease control (Table 33–4).[89–93] In all, more than 70 randomized trials have compared radiation alone with chemoradiotherapy. Several of these studies involved small cohorts of patients. Hence, meta-analyses were created to assess a larger patient population and to help determine the absolute benefits of chemotherapy.[94, 95] The largest meta-analysis to date is the Meta-Analysis of Chemotherapy in Head and Neck Cancer (MACH-NC) study, which evaluated 63 trials with a total of 10,741 patients.[94] The type of chemotherapy administered was predominantly multiagent chemotherapy during induction and monotherapy treatment in the concomitant radiotherapy and adjuvant settings. No statistically significant benefit was associated with either induction or adjuvant treatment. Concomitant chemoradiotherapy provided an absolute benefit of 7% and 8% at 2 and 5 years ($P = .16$), with an overall benefit of 4%. The meta-analyses determined that concomitant chemoradiotherapy conferred an absolute benefit of 8% at 5 years. If our calculations are correct, for every 10,000 patients who receive chemotherapy, 800 patients remain alive at 5 years.

CURRENT MULTIAGENT INVESTIGATIVE APPROACHES

One of the largest studies to date examining three approaches to concomitant chemoradiotherapy was presented recently by members of the RTOG (9703) (Fig. 33–1).[96] When comparison was made with historical controls who

TABLE 33–4 Randomized Multi-Agent Chemoradiation vs. Radiation Alone

Collaborators	n	Location	Regimen	Results 3-yr OS	LCR
Merlano et al, 1996[93]	157	Oral cavity, oral pharynx, and larynx	A: Daily XRT B: Alternating schedule: cisplatin (20 mg/m²/day, days 1–5) and CIFU (200 mg/m²/day, days 1–5), weeks 1, 4, 7, 10/daily XRT, weeks 2–3, 5–6, and 8–9	10% (5-yr) 24%	32% 64%
Wendt et al, 1998[89]	298	Oropharynx, oral cavity, hypopharyngeal/larynx, and floor of mouth	A: 3 courses of hyperfractionated bid XRT (1.8 Gy/fraction, total 70.2 Gy) B: Day 2: Cisplatin (60 mg/m²)/5-FU (350 mg/m²)/ LV (50 mg/m²) followed by days 2–5: CIFU (350 mg/m²)/LV (100 mg/m²)/hyperfractionated XRT (1.8 Gy/fraction, total 70.2 Gy) throughout	24% 48% ($P < .0003$)	17% 36% ($P < .004$)
Brizel et al, 1998[92]	116	Squamous cell carcinoma, including the nasopharynx	A: Hyperfractionated bid radiotherapy (75 Gy) B: Hyperfractionated bid radiotherapy (70 Gy)/ cisplatin (12 mg/m²/day) and CIFU (600 mg/m²/day, days 1–5), weeks 1 and 6	34% 55% ($P = .07$)	44% 70% ($P = .01$)
Adelstein et al, 2000[91]	100	Excluding nasopharyngeal, paranasal, and salivary glands	A: Daily XRT (66–72 Gy) B: Daily XRT/CIFU (1000 mg/m²/day, days 1–4, 22–25)/cisplatin (20 mg/m²/day, days 1–4, 22–25)	48% (5-yr) 50%	45% 77%
Calais et al, 2001[90]	226	Oropharynx	A: Daily XRT (70 Gy) B: Daily XRT/carboplatin (70 mg/m²/day)/CIFU (600 mg/m²/day, days 1–4)—chemotherapy weeks 1, 4, 7 only	31% 51%	27% 53%

CIFU, continuous-infusion 5-fluorouracil; LCR, locoregional control; OS, overall survival; XRT, radiation therapy.

received radiation only, the estimated 1- and 2-year survival rates remained superior in the concomitant chemoradiotherapy trial, regardless of which arm was evaluated. Unsurpassed overall survival was also noted with multiagent chemoradiotherapy compared with RTOG 8117 (daily radiation therapy/cisplatin [100 mg/m², weeks 1, 4, and 7]).

Collaborating investigators with the University of Chicago continue to incorporate the biomodulatory agent, hydroxyurea, with 5-FU. After it was determined that the FHX regimen was reasonably well tolerated and feasible, we have sought to incorporate other cytotoxic agents into this combination. The goal is superior locoregional control without neglect of the possibility of distant disease. Therefore, full systemic doses of chemotherapy are used during radiation therapy. Innovative methods include replacing standard daily radiation therapy with hyperfractionated twice-daily radiotherapy when appropriate.

The first agent examined in combination with FHX was cisplatin (C-FHX). Recently, results were reported of a phase II study of 72 chemoradiation-naïve patients with stage III/IV disease.[97] After a median follow-up of 38 months, the 3-year locoregional control rate was 92%, distant disease control was 83%, and overall survival was 55%.

In a similar fashion, the effects of replacing cisplatin with paclitaxel (20 mg/m²/daily) (TFHX) were examined. At 3 years, the progression-free survival was 63%, locoregional control was 86%, systemic control was 79%, and overall survival was 60%.[98] A preliminary review of the data revealed effective locoregional control but ineffective distant disease control in 20% of our patients. These findings were confirmed in a recent analysis of 230 patients treated with previous regimens that used hyperfractionated concomitant FHX-based chemoradiotherapy; an unexpected pattern of distant failure was detected after a median

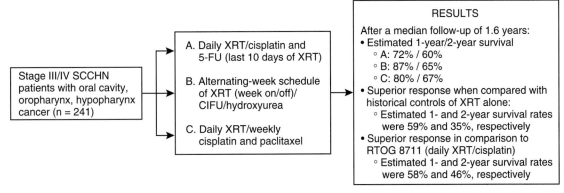

FIGURE 33–1 Schemata of RTOG 9703. (5-FU, 5-fluorouracil; CIFU, continuous-infusion FU; SCCHN, squamous cell carcinoma of the head and neck; XRT, radiation therapy.)

follow-up of 5 years.[99] A prognostic indicator for locoregional recurrence was T-stage (T4), with nodal distribution (N2c–N3) being the foremost predictor of distant disease involvement. Historically, the pattern of failure of combined chemoradiotherapy has been locoregional recurrence.

Hence, investigators at the University of Chicago have chosen to incorporate induction chemotherapy as a means of reducing micrometastatic disease. A phase II study of induction chemotherapy followed by intensive concomitant chemoradiotherapy is currently being conducted in locally advanced SCCHN. However, the investigators have chosen to evaluate the platinum analogue carboplatin rather than cisplatin because of carboplatin's improved toxicity profile. The current investigative approach is two cycles of carboplatin/paclitaxel followed by concomitant hyperfractionated twice-daily radiotherapy, with concomitant TFX and salvage surgery as deemed necessary. This is an ongoing trial with preliminary results to be reported shortly.

Induction Chemotherapy

Induction chemotherapy is administered in a sequential fashion before provision of definitive surgery and/or radiation therapy. The goal of induction therapy is to assist in both local and distant disease control. Locally, this is done by reducing overall tumor burden before definitive treatment, which ultimately allows organ preservation and function, and possibly improved quality of life. Distantly, the systemic effects of induction chemotherapy may prevent microscopic disease from disseminating, eventually promoting overall survival. A diagnosis of cancer of the larynx or of hypopharynx carcinoma will often provoke trepidation in the patient and the physician when the possibility of total laryngectomy is discussed, along with its associated physical and psychological sequelae, which undoubtedly have a profound impact on quality of life. A distinction in organ preservation and function should be delineated. If organ function is not preserved, then organ preservation has not fulfilled the intent of treatment, and quality of life may be adversely affected.

In achieving the desired goals of induction chemotherapy, combination treatment with platinum-based 5-FU has been the traditional approach based on its earlier success in recurrent and advanced disease. Review of the literature suggests that all studies incorporating induction chemotherapy have failed to provide locoregional control and do not provide a benefit in overall survival.

Collaborators at the University of Chicago and at Northwestern University Medical Center have integrated dual biomodulation during induction chemotherapy. The PFL-interferon regimen consisted of 3 cycles of interferon-α (2 MU/m^2 daily on days 1 to 6) and leucovorin (100 mg orally every 4 hours or 300 mg/m^2 continuous infusion during infusion of 5-FU), combined with cisplatin (100 mg/m^2, day 1)/5-FU (continuous-infusion 640 mg/m^2/day, days 1 to 5) (PFL-IFN), followed by 6 to 8 cycles of concomitant 5-FU/hydroxurea/daily radiation therapy (FHX).[100, 101] A majority of patients (66%) had high-risk stage IV (N2–N3) cancer of the larynx or pharynx. Sixty-six percent of patients had a clinical CR at the completion of induction chemotherapy. Salvage surgery was offered at the completion of

induction. At 5 years, the progression-free survival was 68% and the overall survival was 62%, with local failure in 25% of patients. Surgery was organ-preserving; only a single laryngectomy and no glossectomies were performed in primary management. This suggests that FHX may have provided the primary stimulus for effective cytotoxic therapy.

A recent subset analysis of 32 patients with cancer of the larynx revealed that a pathologic CR was achieved in 94% of patients at completion of the study.[102] After a median follow-up of 63 months, locoregional control was maintained in 78% of patients and voice preservation in 75%, and only two total laryngectomies were required. No patient experienced distant failure. The use of induction chemotherapy appears to have therapeutic benefit in laryngeal cancer and should be investigated further in clinical studies.

Three landmark phase III trials have established the benefits of induction chemotherapy in laryngeal preservation. The Veterans Affairs Laryngeal Study randomly assigned 332 patients with stage III or IV laryngeal carcinoma to receive three cycles of cisplatin/5-FU (PF) followed by conventional radiotherapy or laryngectomy followed by conventional radiotherapy.[103] Response was assessed after the completion of 2 cycles of chemotherapy. Patients with a PR received a third cycle of chemotherapy followed by radiotherapy. In contrast, nonresponders immediately underwent a laryngectomy followed by radiation therapy. An integral component of this study was salvage surgery, which was offered to all patients with residual disease at the completion of radiotherapy. After two cycles of induction, the ORR was 85% (31% CR, 54% PR). Histologic specimens were obtained in 103 patients at the completion of chemotherapy, validating a complete response in 88% of patients with a clinical CR; 45% of those presumed to have a clinical PR were confirmed histologically. Overall, 64% of patients had a histologically confirmed complete response. After a median follow-up of 33 months, the estimated 2-year survival was 68% in both treatment groups, and there was no difference in overall survival (P = .9846). However, preservation of the larynx was maintained in 64% of patients. Patterns of recurrence differed between the two groups, with increased locoregional disease failure (P = .0005) but decreased metastatic disease (P = .016) in the induction chemotherapy group. Although there was no significant difference in overall survival, this study demonstrates that induction chemotherapy is feasible in the setting of laryngeal carcinoma, allowing organ preservation without compromising overall survival. It should be noted that of the 166 patients on the chemotherapy arm, 120 patients (72%) had N0 or N1 disease.

Forastiere and colleagues have incorporated a radiation-only arm in a similar phase III Intergroup trial (R91-11) of 547 patients with stage III/IV laryngeal carcinoma.[104] Patients were randomly assigned to arm A: 3 cycles of induction chemotherapy of cisplatin/5-FU followed by daily radiation therapy; arm B: concurrent cisplatin (100 mg/m^2, days 1, 22, 43) and radiation therapy; or arm C: daily radiation therapy only (70 Gy). The primary endpoint was laryngeal preservation rather than overall survival. A preliminary analysis of laryngectomy-free survival at 2 years showed improvement in both chemotherapy arms A and B, but notably so in the concurrent chemotherapy arm (58% vs. 66%). No difference in overall survival could be ascertained in arm B or C in comparison with control arm A, although disease-free survival appeared to be favorable in both chemotherapy arms in comparison with radiation therapy only. Time to laryngectomy was superior in the concurrent chemotherapy arm in comparison with the induction arm (P = .0094). Hence, it can be concluded that despite variation in methods of treatment, neither has provided an advantage in overall survival. Nonetheless, the results from this trial suggest a prolonged disease-free survival and laryngectomy-free interval with the addition of chemotherapy to radiation therapy.[105]

The EORTC verified the benefits of organ preservation in a randomized phase III clinical trial in patients with stage III/IV cancer of the pyriform sinus or aryepiglottic folds.[106] One hundred ninety-four eligible patients were randomly assigned to immediate surgery followed by radiotherapy (94 patients) or induction chemotherapy (100 patients) with cisplatin (100 mg/m^2, day 1) and continuous-infusion 5-FU (1000 mg/m^2/day, days 1 to 5). An endoscopic examination was completed after each cycle. Patients with a CR or a PR following cycle 2 were offered a third cycle of chemotherapy. Unlike the Veterans Affairs Laryngeal Cancer Study, patients were required to achieve a CR before undergoing radiation therapy; patients with stable disease were offered salvage surgery followed by radiotherapy.

Induction chemotherapy resulted in a CR in 54% of patients at the primary site, and 51% of patients achieved a locoregional CR. Overall, induction chemotherapy provided fewer distant failures (P = .041) and an improved median survival (44 months) versus the surgical arm (25 months). Unfortunately, neither arm demonstrated superiority in the prevention of locoregional recurrence. Treatment with induction chemotherapy managed to preserve the larynx in 42% and 35% of patients evaluated for 3- and 5-year estimates of survival. This European study suggests that induction chemotherapy is a feasible alternative if organ preservation is desired without compromise of overall survival. However, it should be noted that only 31% of patients had N2/N3 disease, of which only 6% were N3. Furthermore, patients with N3 disease were eventually excluded from this trial because the first six patients failed to achieve a CR following induction.

Hence, induction chemotherapy fulfills the goal of laryngeal preservation as a primary endpoint but fails to fulfill the goals of improved locoregional recurrence and overall survival. Therefore, induction chemotherapy outside of a clinical trial cannot be justified except in the setting of organ preservation for laryngeal or hypopharyngeal disease.

Current Clinical Approaches of Induction Chemotherapy

The Dana Farber Cancer Institute has recently reported the maximal tolerated dose of cisplatin when given in combination with docetaxel and 5-FU as induction chemotherapy in patients with locally advanced head and neck cancer.[36] Patients received three cycles of docetaxel (75 mg/m^2, day 1), cisplatin (75 mg/m^2 or 100 mg/m^2) and continuous-infusion 5-FU (1000 mg/m^2 on days 1 to 4) repeated every 21 days, followed by hyperfractionated

radiotherapy and neck dissection for bulky disease. Empirical antibiotics were provided on days 5 to 15. If a PR was achieved following the completion of chemotherapy, patients underwent definitive therapy at the institution's discretion. Toxicities were similar at both dose levels, consisting of chemotherapy-induced electrolyte imbalance in 30% of patients and grade III/IV neutropenia in 95% of patients. Patients were considered evaluable for response if more than 2 cycles were completed. The overall clinical response rate was 94% (40% CR, 54% PR). Post-treatment biopsies were completed in 25 patients (58%). Ninety-two percent of patients with a primary site CR had a negative biopsy; 54% had a pathologically confirmed PR.

These investigators have recently provided an overview of four previous phase II trials of TPF-based induction chemotherapy trials involving more than 100 patients.[107] After a median follow-up of longer than 32 months, the ORR exceeded 90% in each individual trial. The 2-year survival exceeded 70%. An analysis of failure reveals that one third of the patients experienced recurrence, with the majority of patients having locoregional recurrence. These promising results have provided the basis for an ongoing randomized phase III trial comparing TPF with PF as induction chemotherapy, followed by sequential chemoradiotherapy with carboplatin. This trial could be criticized because of the lack of a chemoradiotherapy-only arm without induction. Therefore, it may be misconstrued that induction chemotherapy is standard treatment for locally advanced disease.

◼ REIRRADIATION FOR PATIENTS WITH LOCALLY RECURRENT CANCER

Patients with locoregional recurrence often have limited treatment options other than palliative chemotherapy. Consideration to reirradiate patients remains primarily investigational and is an aggressive method to combat recurrent disease in a previously irradiated field. Patients often have residual sequelae from their previous therapy, further complicating matters. Several single-agent treatments, combination chemotherapy regimens, and radiation schedules have been investigated with varied results (Table 33–5).[39, 108–112]

The RTOG has recently reported results of a multi-institutional phase II study (RTOG 9610) evaluating the effectiveness of four cycles of bolus 5-FU (300 mg/m^2)/hydroxyurea (1.5 g/m^2)/hyperfractionated twice-daily radiotherapy every other week.[111] Eighty-one patients were evaluable. Median survival was 8.1 months, and estimated 1- and 2-year survival rates were 41.7% and 16.2%, respectively.

A single-institution pilot study by the Mayo Clinic examined the activity of cisplatin (80 mg/m^2)/continuous-infusion 5-FU (1000 mg/m^2, days 1 to 4) with concomitant hyperfractionated twice-daily radiotherapy in patients with recurrent disease.[113] Patients went on to receive two more cycles of PF at the completion of radiation therapy. Median survival was 9 months, and estimated 1-year survival was 41%. Patients with recurrent cancer of the head and neck longer than 2 years after their original diagnosis fared better, with a median survival of 16 months. On the same note, the

TABLE 33-5 Clinical Trials of Reirradiation

Clinical Trial	N	Regimen	Results
Gandia et al, 1993[108]	33	CIFU/HU/daily XRT	40% CR, 15% PR
Hartsell et al, 1994[109]	21	Cisplatin/CIFU/daily XRT	48% CR, 24% PR
Haraf et al, 1996[110]	45	Cisplatin/CIFU/HU/hyperfractionated bid XRT	5 yr: 14.6% OS, 20% LRC
Haraf, 1997[a]	48	Paclitaxel/CIFU/HU/XRT (daily escalated to hyperfractionated bid XRT)	2 yr: 31% OS, 44% PFS, 59% LRC
Wheeler et al, 2001[111]	86	Bolus 5-FU/HU/hyperfractionated bid XRT RTOG 96-10	1-yr: 41.7% OS; 2-yr: 16.2% OS
Humerickhouse, 2000[112]	31	CPT-11/CIFU/HU/hyperfractionated bid XRT	Pending
Eng et al, 2001[39]	73	Paclitaxel/CIFU/HU/gemcitabine/hyperfractionated bid XRT	61% CR, 16% PR
RTOG 99-11	Pending	Paclitaxel/cisplatin/hyperfractionated bid XRT	Pending
University of Chicago ongoing studies	Pending	Tirapazemine/cisplatin/daily radiotherapy followed by hyperfractionated bid XRT with boost	Pending
	Pending	Bevacuzimab/CIFU/HU/daily XRT	Pending

[a]Haraf DF, Stenson K, List M, et al: Continuous infusion paclitaxel, 5-fluorouracil, and hydroxyurea with concomitant radiotherapy in patients with advanced or recurrent head and neck cancer. Semin Oncol 24(Suppl 2): S2–68, S2–71, 1997.
CIFU, continuous-infusion 5-fluorouracil; CR, complete remission; HU, hydroxyurea; LCR, locoregional control; OS, overall survival; PR, partial remission; XRT, radiation therapy.

University of Chicago has aggressively pursued intensive multiagent chemoradiotherapy with various regimens, demonstrating promising preliminary results. Additional studies are currently being conducted with the use of innovative agents.

◼ NOVEL APPROACHES

Despite the refinement of radiation techniques and the combined use of modern chemotherapy agents, new approaches are currently under way.

Intratumoral and Intra-arterial Administration

Other methods to deliver chemotherapy outside of traditional intravenous methods have been explored. One example is direct intra-arterial infusion of chemotherapy for locoregional disease to target the dominant blood supply of the targeted tumor. A phase I study by Robbins and colleagues assessed the maximum dose intensity of cisplatin by selective intra-arterial infusion.[114] Forty-two patients received escalating doses of intra-arterial infusion of cisplatin (160 to 200 mg/m^2). Approximately half of patients had been previously treated. Patients received sodium thiosulfate to neutralize the systemic toxicity of cisplatin. The maximal tolerated dose (MTD) was 150 mg/m^2 weekly for 4 weeks. The ORR was 86% for previously untreated patients and 62% for patients with recurrent disease. One drawback to the intra-arterial infusion technique is the risk of subcutaneous necrosis of the surrounding tissue.

The RTOG examined the feasibility of intra-arterial cisplatin and daily radiation therapy in 62 patients with stage IV SCCHN.[115] After a median follow-up of 18.4 months, the 2-year locoregional tumor control and overall survival rates were 62% and 58%, respectively.

Regine and colleagues examined the effects of hyperfractionated twice-daily radiation therapy with intra-arterial cisplatin (150 mg/m^2) in a small cohort of 24 patients.[116] After a median follow-up of 18 months, locoregional control was demonstrated in 14 patients (58%).

A phase I Japanese study examined intra-arterial carboplatin in locally advanced SCCHN and determined that daily carboplatin (20 mg/m^2, total dose 500 mg/m^2) and radiotherapy (50 to 60 Gy daily) was tolerable and feasible.[117] Patients were allowed to undergo salvage surgery after the completion of their treatment. After a median follow-up of 47 months, the locoregional control rate was 62%. Cancer of the oral tongue and the base of the tongue fared better with this technique with an improved local control rate of 82%.

A method of administration that may provide improved direct tumor penetration is intratumoral injection. PV701 is a live, attenuated oncolytic virus derived from a vaccine strain of Newcastle disease virus (NDV), an avian paramyxovirus. PV701 is a triple-plaque purified isolate of NDV. The virus is grown in specific-pathogen–free embryonated chicken eggs and purified from the allantoic fluid. Preclinical testing demonstrated a high degree of selectivity for killing a large and diverse panel of human cancer cells while sparing normal human cells. Consequently, clinical investigative studies were initiated.

A multicenter clinical trial of intravenous PV701 has been performed in the treatment of patients with advanced or recurrent solid tumors.[118] One CR (head and neck) and two PRs (colon and mesothelioma) were observed at higher doses, and six patients with diverse malignancies had measurable tumor reduction. The MTD was determined to be 12 billion plaque-forming units/m^2. A multi-institutional phase I study has since been initiated to determine the MTD of PV701 via intratumoral injection in patients with locally advanced HNSCC.

Molecular Targets

Epidermal Growth Factor Receptors

Recent investigative focus has been on aspects of signal transduction. Growth factor receptors have been recognized as promising potential cytostatic targets in tumor cell growth and survival. Overexpression of the epidermal growth factor receptor (EGFR) is recognized in more than 80% of SCCs.[119] Ligand binding of the extracellular domain results in homodimerization or heterodimerization, causing phosphorylation of the tyrosine kinase domain and leading to cell proliferation and activation. An inverse correlation may also exist between EGFR expression and radioresistance.[120] Administration of the chimeric monoclonal antibody against the EGFR IMC-C225 (cetuximab) has been shown to increase radiosensitization, decrease tumor cell line growth, and increase apoptosis (programmed cell death).[121]

C225 (CETUXIMAB)

Baselga and colleagues have provided results from their phase I study of C225 used alone (5, 20, 50, and 100 mg/m²) and in combination (IMC-C225 of 5 to 400 mg/m²) with cisplatin (60 mg/m² every 28 days) in patients with solid tumors overexpressing EGFR.[122] The use of the combination regimen was limited to head and neck or non–small cell lung carcinoma patients. The most frequent adverse events reported with C225 were flulike symptoms and an acneiform rash. Although response was not a primary endpoint, 11 of 19 patients (58%) had stable disease; two patients had a PR. Nine of 13 patients (69%) who had received more than 50 mg/m² of C225 achieved disease stabilization and received all 12 weeks of therapy.

An interesting companion study completed by Hong and colleagues evaluated the effectiveness of C225 in combination with cisplatin in cisplatin-refractory patients.[123] Patients with recurrent disease received two cycles of cisplatin. If there was evidence of stable disease or progression, patients went on to receive C225/cisplatin. An objective response of therapy was achieved in 21% of patients, and disease stability resulted in 58% of patients. It is unclear if similar results could be achieved with single-agent C225. The final results of this trial are pending.

Preclinical studies explored the interaction between C225 and radiation in human SCC cell lines.[124] Cells were treated with C225 alone, radiation alone, or C225 and radiation. The degree of cell proliferation was markedly inhibited with the combined treatment, regardless of the degree of EGFR overexpression. When the cell lines were assessed at 48 hours, the extent of apoptosis was greatest in the C225/radiation-treated cell line.

A phase I study of IMC-C225 (loading dose 100 to 500 mg/m²; weekly maintenance dose 100 to 250 mg/m²) with concomitant daily or hyperfractionated twice-daily radiotherapy was initiated.[125] A total of 15 patients were evaluated for response. All patients had an objective response; 13 patients had a CR (87%) and 2 patients had a PR. The median duration of response was 28 months. It should be noted that patient accrual included both chemoradiotherapy-naïve and recurrent disease patients. A randomized phase III trial is being undertaken at the University of Alabama in AJCC stage III/IV patients to compare radiation alone with C225/radiation (daily, hyperfractionated twice daily, or fractionated with concomitant boost).

Tyrosine Kinase Inhibitors

The oral agents OSI-774 and ZD1839 are selective EGFR tyrosine kinase antagonists that competitively prevent binding of ATP to the intracellular domain of the EGF receptor, causing inhibition of ligand-induced cell growth.

OSI-774

An initial phase I study evaluated the MTD of the daily administration of OSI-774 in patients with advanced solid malignancies not amenable to other therapy.[126] Several patients with epidermoid malignancies were noted to have response or prolonged disease stabilization. The recommended phase II dose for daily, continuous, uninterrupted OSI-774 is 150 mg/day. A multi-institutional phase II study of single-agent OSI-774 was initiated in the setting of recurrent and/or metastatic head and neck cancer.[127] All tumor specimens were examined by immunohistochemistry for EGFR expression. In a manner similar to cetuximab, adverse toxicities included an acneiform rash (72%), diarrhea, and fatigue. Preliminary analysis of 78 patients demonstrated a PR in 10 patients (5.6%). The impact of OSI-774 on quality of life will soon be reported.

ZD1839

Collaborators at the University of Illinois and the University of Chicago have extensive experience with the oral epidermal growth factor receptor tyrosine kinase inhibitor, ZD1839 (Iressa). A multi-institutional phase II study has recently been completed in patients refractory to standard treatment.[128] Patients received ZD1839 (500 mg orally twice daily) for 21 of every 28 days. Common adverse reactions included mild diarrhea and an acneiform rash. Preliminary results indicate a favorable toxicity profile and promising single-agent activity, with the majority of patients demonstrating prolonged stabilization of disease. Invariably, combination therapy with a cytotoxic agent increases overall survival and response rate. The natural progression of clinical investigation would be to consider the use of ZD1839 as an adjunct to combined chemoradiation therapy.

Angiogenesis

Angiogenesis is being extensively investigated. Angiogenesis is the process by which a tumor obtains its own vascular supply to facilitate independent cell growth and in turn cause metastatic disease. Vascular endothelial growth factor (VEGF), a protein associated with angiogenesis, is known to increase vascular permeability. Elevated VEGF levels have been implicated as a poor prognostic indicator of increased risk of recurrent disease and increased radioresistance.[129, 130]

Thalidomide

Thalidomide, a glutamic acid derivative, is an oral agent that is believed to inhibit angiogenesis. Preclinical animal models demonstrate an inhibitory effect of thalidomide on neovascularization of the basic fibroblast growth factor.[131] A single-agent phase II study of thalidomide (escalating doses of 200 to 1000 mg daily) was initiated in patients with recurrent or metastatic disease.[132] Thalidomide failed to demonstrate activity as a single agent in this heavily pre-treated population. Thalidomide continues to be investigated in hematologic and other solid tumor malignancies.

SU5416

SU5416 is a tyrosine kinase inhibitor of the VEGF Flk-1 receptor that has been directly linked with endothelial cell proliferation and angiogenesis.[133] To date, preliminary results evaluating single-agent SU5416 in solid organ tumors are disappointing.[134] However, in vivo studies suggest promising activity in hematologic malignancies.[135–137] Solid organ activity may be best seen in combination with cytotoxic agents. Investigators at Memorial Sloan-Kettering are examining the palliative effects of single-agent SU5416 in recurrent or advanced head and neck cancer. Collaborators in Ireland and at Cleveland Clinic and Case Western University are examining the potential activity of SU5416 combined with paclitaxel in recurrent and/or metastatic head and neck cancer. This trial continues to accrue; preliminary results are pending at this time.

Bevacizumab

The recombinant humanized monoclonal antibody against VEGF, bevacizumab, has been investigated in combination with chemotherapy for patients with advanced solid organ tumors.[138] Multiple phase II studies have determined evident activity in colon cancer, non–small cell lung cancer, and breast cancer.[139–141] Rare episodes of life-threatening pulmonary hemorrhage were attributed to bevacizumab when it was administered to patients with non–small cell lung cancer.[142] Risk factors that have been identified include squamous cell histology and centrally located lesions lying adjacent to major blood vessels. Given the similar histology between cancer of the lung and that of the head and neck, investigators at the University of Chicago have proceeded to investigate bevacizumab in a phase I dose escalation study with concomitant chemoradiotherapy for patients with recurrent cancer of the head and neck who may benefit from locoregional radiotherapy (see Table 33–5).

Inhibition of EGF and VEGF Receptors

Conceptually, inhibiting both the extracellular and the intracellular domains of tyrosine kinase may promote further tumoricidal activity. Eventual resistance to EGFR inhibitors has been well established but is largely due to an unknown mechanism. Previous in vitro studies have demonstrated upregulation of VEGF expression through activation of EGFR.[143] A correlation with resistance to anti-EGFR inhibitors and increased levels (twofold) of VEGF mRNA in epidermoid cell line strains has been established in in vivo studies.[144] Although VEGF levels were eventually downregulated in vitro by as much as 50% following administration of an EGFR inhibitor, resistant epidermoid cell lines continued to demonstrate two- and fourfold increased VEGF levels in comparison with the parent cell line. Hence, combined inhibition of both EGF and VEGF receptors should result theoretically in increased apoptosis, decreased cell proliferation, decreased vascular permeability, and improved cytostatic activity in comparison with its respective activity as a single agent.

Tumor Suppressor Gene Mutations

RAS: Farnesyl Transferase Inhibitors

Farnesyl transferase inhibitors are believed to target the oncoprotein *RAS*. A point mutation in *RAS* is associated with continuous activation of these oncoproteins, contributing to chemotherapy resistance and increased cell proliferation. This combination has the resultant effect of increasing the genetic instability of populations of cancer cells. Very few neoplastic diseases exist where a *RAS* mutation is not found, but it is not common in any one specific malignancy. The oral farnesyl transferase inhibitors BMS-24662, R115777, and SCH6636 are currently being investigated in phase I clinical trials of both solid tumors and SCCHN.[145, 146] Thus far, these agents appear to be tolerated well and have evident activity.

TP53: ONYX-015

Unique to ONYX-015 is its manner and vehicle of administration. ONYX-015 is a novel intratumoral selective adenovirus vector composed of the wild-type *TP53* gene with preferential replication in *TP53*-deficient cells, resulting in cell lysis. *TP53* serves to regulate the cell cycle by acting as a checkpoint to ensure appropriate cell replication and division. Therefore, its mutation has been implicated as an indicator of a poor prognosis in SCCHN.

In the recurrent disease setting, intratumoral ONYX-015 was combined with cisplatin/5-FU, resulting in improved overall response rates of 63% versus the standard regimen of cisplatin/5-FU at 37%.[147] A small study of 40 patients with disease refractory to conventional treatment received daily ONYX-015 alone or combined with hyperfractionated therapy.[148] Antitumor activity in both arms was modest (10% to 14%) and did not appear to be influenced by the schedule administered.

A multi-institutional trial evaluating the potential chemo-preventive properties of ONYX-015 as a mouthwash for patients with premalignant oral dysplasia is currently being conducted.[149]

Tumor Hypoxia and Radioresistance

The relationship between tumor hypoxia and resistance to radiation therapy has been well described and results in G1/S-phase arrest.[150] However, the cytotoxic effects of radiation therapy occur primarily in the G2/M phase. Hence, tumor hypoxia is an area of considerable interest. Early preclinical animal studies demonstrated the bioreductive alkylating agent mitomycin C to have selective cytotoxicity to hypoxic cells.[151] A phase III trial of 203 patients randomly assigned patients to daily radiotherapy or concomitant radiotherapy with mitomycin C.[152] After a median follow-up of longer than 10 years, locoregional control was found to be superior in concomitant chemoradiation therapy in comparison with radiation alone (70% vs. 51%, $P < .005$).[153]

Misonidazole

Danish investigators have examined the role of pure hypoxic cell radiosensitizers such as misonidazole and nimorazole in improving overall survival.[154, 155] Misonidazole failed to demonstrate an improvement in comparison with placebo, and it caused profound treatment-related peripheral neuropathy, preventing further investigation.

Tirapazamine

A highly investigated agent, tirapazamine is a hypoxia-selective compound onefold to twofold greater in strength than mitomycin C.[156] Its mechanism of action results in a one-electron reduction, inducing DNA double-strand breaks and cell death under hypoxic conditions. The free radical is oxidized back to the parent compound under aerobic conditions. In vitro and in vivo studies have demonstrated that tirapazamine is 40 to 300 times more effective under hypoxic conditions. In combination with a platinum compound, the cytotoxic effects may be equivalent to five times the dose of cisplatin without the actual toxicities that would be encountered.[157]

Rishchin and colleagues have recently reported results of a phase I trial of conventional fractionated radiotherapy with concurrent tirapazamine (290 mg/m^2), cisplatin (75 mg/m^2) weeks 1, 4, and 7, and tirapazamine alone (160 mg/m^2, thrice weekly weeks 2, 3, 5, and 6) in untreated stage IV head and neck cancer patients.[158] The cohort was small at 20 patients. Although survival was a secondary endpoint in this phase I study, after a median follow-up of 2.7 years, the 3-year OS was 69%, with a 3-year disease-free survival rate of 88%.

A multi-institutional study from Lee and colleagues evaluated the effects of tirapazamine with daily radiotherapy in patients with stage III/IV head and neck cancer.[159] The primary endpoint was locoregional control. Patients received concomitant tirapazamine (159 mg/m^2 three times weekly for 12 doses). Mild toxicities often encountered included muscle cramps (77%) and nausea/vomiting (62%). After a median follow-up of only 13 months, the actuarial 1- and 2-year locoregional control rates were 64% and 59%, respectively.

Investigators at Stanford University have conducted a phase II study examining the benefits of tirapazamine in a regimen of induction chemotherapy. Patients were randomly assigned to receive PF with or without tirapazamine during induction chemotherapy and concomitant chemoradiotherapy.[160] The induction regimen was composed of cisplatin (100 mg/m^2/day, days 1, 22) and continuous-infusion 5-FU (1000 mg/m^2, days 1 to 5, 22 to 26). Patients on the tirapazamine arm received a dose of 300 to 330 mg/m^2 (days 1, 22) followed by a concomitant chemoradiotherapy regimen of tirapazamine, cisplatin, and 5-FU. The most frequent toxicities were granulocytopenia and mucositis. The recommended dose of tirapazamine during induction chemotherapy is 300 mg/m^2, and 220 mg/m^2 during simultaneous chemoradiotherapy was determined to be feasible in this combination.

Taking into account the relationship between tumor hypoxia and radioresistance and the tolerability of tirapazamine, it is natural to consider its use in the treatment of recurrent head and neck cancer. The University of Chicago is currently collaborating with French investigators on a phase I trial of tirapazamine in previously irradiated patients (see Table 33–5). Patients will receive standard daily radiotherapy and tirapazamine (weeks 1 to 3) combined with cisplatin (weeks 3 and 5), converting to hyperfractionated radiotherapy with boost for weeks 4 to 6.

◼ SUMMARY

Treatment of cancer of the head and neck encompasses an array of different disease entities none less challenging than the other. Initially, treatment of the primary cancer is of the utmost concern, but the threat of a second primary cancer lingers despite treatment with curative intent. Whereas previous treatment regimens focused on the synergistic activity of cytotoxic chemotherapy and radiation therapy alone, current approaches are evaluating aspects of tumor biology that will result in focused treatment combinations to enhance tumoricidal activity.

REFERENCES

1. Slaughter DP, Southwick HW, Smejkal W: "Field cancerization" in oral stratified squamous epithelium: Clinical implications of multicentric origin. Cancer 6:963, 1953.
2. Khuri FR, Lee JJ, Winn RJ: Interim analysis of randomized chemoprevention trial of HNSCC. Proc Annu Meet Am Soc Clin Oncol 18:A1503, 1999.
3. Licciardello JT, Spitz MR, Hong WK: Multiple primary cancer in patients with cancer of the head and neck: Second cancer of the head and neck, esophagus, and lung. Int J Radiat Oncol Biol Phys 17:467–476, 1989.
4. Panosetti E, Luboinski B, Mamelle G, et al: Multiple synchronous and metachronous cancers of the upper aerodigestive tract: A nine-year study. Laryngoscope 99:1267–1273, 1989.
5. Jones AS, Morar P, Phillips DE, et al: Second primary tumors in patients with head and neck squamous cell carcinoma. Cancer 75:1343–1353, 1995.
6. Day GL, Blot WJ, Shore RE, et al: Second cancers following oral and pharyngeal cancer: Patients' characteristics and survival patterns. Eur J Cancer B Oral Oncol 30B:381–386, 1994.
7. Parkin DM, Pisani P, Ferlay J: Global cancer statistics. CA Cancer J Clin 49:33–64, 31, 1999.
8. Franceschi S, Bidoli E, Herrero R, et al: Comparison of cancers of the oral cavity and pharynx worldwide: Etiological clues. Oral Oncol 36:106–115, 2000.
9. Jemal A, Murray T, Samuels A, et al: Cancer statistics, 2003. CA Cancer J Clin 53:5–26, 2003.
9a. SEER: Surveillance, epidemiology and end results provided by NCI. SEER.cancer.gov.
10. Blot WJ, McLaughlin JK, Winn DM, et al: Smoking and drinking in relation to oral and pharyngeal cancer. Cancer Res 48:3282–3287, 1988.
11. Jussawalla DJ, Deshpande VA: Evaluation of cancer risk in tobacco chewers and smokers: An epidemiologic assessment. Cancer 28:244–252, 1971.
12. Eng C, Vokes EE: Combined modality strategies in the treatment of head and neck cancer. In Choy H (ed): Cancer Drug Discovery and Development Series: Chemoradiation in Cancer Therapy. Totowa, New Jersey, Humana Press, 2003, pp 145–174.

13. Kowalski LP, Carvalho AL: Influence of time delay and clinical upstaging in the prognosis of head and neck cancer. Oral Oncol 37:94–98, 2001.

14. Morton RP, Rugman F, Dorman EB, et al: Cisplatinum and bleomycin for advanced or recurrent squamous cell carcinoma of the head and neck: A randomised factorial phase III controlled trial. Cancer Chemother Pharmacol 15:283–289, 1985.

15. Jacobs C, Lyman G, Velez-Garcia E, et al: A phase III randomized study comparing cisplatin and fluorouracil as single agents and in combination for advanced squamous cell carcinoma of the head and neck. J Clin Oncol 10:257–263, 1992.

16. Campbell JB, Dorman EB, McCormick M, et al: A randomized phase III trial of cisplatinum, methotrexate, cisplatinum + methotrexate, and cisplatinum + 5-fluorouracil in end-stage head and neck cancer. Acta Otolaryngol 103:519–528, 1987.

17. Eisenberger M, Hornedo J, Silva H, et al: Carboplatin (NSC-241-240): An active platinum analog for the treatment of squamous-cell carcinoma of the head and neck. J Clin Oncol 4:1506–1509, 1986.

18. Forastiere AA, Metch B, Schuller DE, et al: Randomized comparison of cisplatin plus fluorouracil and carboplatin plus fluorouracil versus methotrexate in advanced squamous-cell carcinoma of the head and neck: A Southwest Oncology Group study. J Clin Oncol 10:1245–1251, 1992.

19. Eisenberger M, Krasnow S, Ellenberg S, et al: A comparison of carboplatin plus methotrexate versus methotrexate alone in patients with recurrent and metastatic head and neck cancer. J Clin Oncol 7:1341–1345, 1989.

20. Schornagel JH, Verweij J, de Mulder PH, et al: Randomized phase III trial of edatrexate versus methotrexate in patients with metastatic and/or recurrent squamous cell carcinoma of the head and neck: A European Organization for Research and Treatment of Cancer Head and Neck Cancer Cooperative Group study. J Clin Oncol 13:1649–1655, 1995.

21. Cervellino JC, Araujo CE, Pirisi C, et al: Ifosfamide and mesna for the treatment of advanced squamous cell head and neck cancer. A GET-LAC study. Oncology 48:89–92, 1991.

22. Buesa JM, Fernandez R, Esteban E, et al: Phase II trial of ifosfamide in recurrent and metastatic head and neck cancer. Ann Oncol 2:151–152, 1991.

23. Huber MH, Lippman SM, Benner SE, et al: A phase II study of ifosfamide in recurrent squamous cell carcinoma of the head and neck. Am J Clin Oncol 19:379–382, 1996.

24. Sandler A, Saxman S, Bandealy M, et al: Ifosfamide in the treatment of advanced or recurrent squamous cell carcinoma of the head and neck: A phase II Hoosier Oncology Group trial. Am J Clin Oncol 21:195–197, 1998.

25. Tapazoglou E, Kish J, Ensley J, et al: The activity of a single-agent 5-fluorouracil infusion in advanced and recurrent head and neck cancer. Cancer 57:1105–1109, 1986.

26. Amer MH, Al-Sarraf M, Vaitkevicius VK: Factors that affect response to chemotherapy and survival of patients with advanced head and neck cancer. Cancer 43:2202–2206, 1979.

27. Milross CG, Mason KA, Hunter NR, et al: Relationship of mitotic arrest and apoptosis to antitumor effect of paclitaxel. J Natl Cancer Inst 88:1308–1314, 1996.

28. Smith RE, Thornton DE, Allen J: A phase II trial of paclitaxel in squamous cell carcinoma of the head and neck with correlative laboratory studies. Semin Oncol 22:41–46, 1995.

29. Gebbia V, Testa A, Cannata G, et al: Single agent paclitaxel in advanced squamous cell head and neck carcinoma. Eur J Cancer 32A:901–902, 1996.

30. Mickiewicz E, Temperley G, Giglio R: Taxol (paclitaxel) 1-hour infusion in recurrent head and neck cancer patients. Proc Annu Meet Am Soc Clin 17:A1571, 1998.

31. Forastiere AA, Shank D, Neuberg D, et al: Final report of a phase II evaluation of paclitaxel in patients with advanced squamous cell carcinoma of the head and neck: An Eastern Cooperative Oncology Group trial (PA390). Cancer 82:2270–2274, 1998.

32. Vermorken J, Catimel G, Mulder PD, et al: Randomized phase II trial of weekly methotrexate (MTX) versus two schedules of triweekly paclitaxel (taxol) in patients with metastatic or recurrent squamous cell carcinoma of the head and neck (SCCHN). Proc Annu Meet Am Soc Clin Oncol 18:pA1527, 1997.

33. Hortobagyi GN: Recent progress in the clinical development of docetaxel (Taxotere). Semin Oncol 26:32–36, 1999.

34. Dreyfuss AI, Clark JR, Norris CM, et al: Docetaxel: An active drug for squamous cell carcinoma of the head and neck. J Clin Oncol 14:1672–1678, 1996.

35. Couteau C, Chouaki N, Leyvraz S, et al: A phase II study of docetaxel in patients with metastatic squamous cell carcinoma of the head and neck. Br J Cancer 81:457–462, 1999.

36. Posner MR, Glisson B, Frenette G, et al: Multicenter phase I-II trial of docetaxel, cisplatin, and fluorouracil induction chemotherapy for patients with locally advanced squamous cell cancer of the head and neck. J Clin Oncol 19:1096–1104, 2001.

37. Posner MR: Docetaxel in squamous cell cancer of the head and neck. Anticancer Drugs 12(suppl 1):S21–S24, 2001.

38. Catimel G, Vermorken JB, Clavel M, et al: A phase II study of gemcitabine (LY 188011) in patients with advanced squamous cell carcinoma of the head and neck. EORTC Early Clinical Trials Group. Ann Oncol 5:543–547, 1994.

39. Eng C, Haraf D, Stenson K, et al: Phase I study of concomitant chemoradiotherapy with gemcitabine (G), paclitaxel (T), and 5-fluorouracil (5-FU) with poor prognosis head and neck cancer patients. Lung Cancer 34(Suppl 1): Abstracts of the 2nd International Chicago Symposium on Malignancies of the Chest and Head and Neck. Chicago, Oct. 4–6, 2001.

40. Degardin M, Oliveira J, Geoffrois L, et al: An EORTC-ECSG phase II study of vinorelbine in patients with recurrent and/or metastatic squamous cell carcinoma of the head and neck. Ann Oncol 9:1103–1107, 1998.

41. Saxman S, Mann B, Canfield V, et al: A phase II trial of vinorelbine in patients with recurrent or metastatic squamous cell carcinoma of the head and neck. Am J Clin Oncol 21:398–400, 1998.

42. Murphy BA, Douglas S, Dang T: Phase II trial of irinotecan (CPT-11) in metastatic or recurrent squamous cell carcinoma of the head and neck. Proc Annu Meet Am Soc Clin Oncol 18:A1578, 1999.

43. Lad T, Rosen F, Sciortino D, et al: Phase II trial of aminocamptothecin (9-AC/DMA) in patients with advanced squamous cell head and neck cancer. Invest New Drugs 18:261–263, 2000.

44. Murphy BA, Leong T, Burkey B, et al: Lack of efficacy of topotecan in the treatment of metastatic or recurrent squamous carcinoma of the head and neck: An Eastern Cooperative Oncology Group Trial (E3393). Am J Clin Oncol 24:64–66, 2001.

45. Clavel M, Vermorken JB, Cognetti F, et al: Randomized comparison of cisplatin, methotrexate, bleomycin and vincristine (CABO) versus cisplatin and 5-fluorouracil (CF) versus cisplatin (C) in recurrent or metastatic squamous cell carcinoma of the head and neck. A phase III study of the EORTC Head and Neck Cancer Cooperative Group. Ann Oncol 5:521–526, 1994.

46. Amrein PC, Fabian RL: Treatment of recurrent head and neck cancer with cisplatin and 5-fluorouracil vs. the same plus bleomycin and methotrexate. Laryngoscope 102:901–906, 1992.

47. Bensmaine ME, Azli N, Domenge C, et al: Phase I-II trial of recombinant interferon alpha-2b with cisplatin and 5-fluorouracil in recurrent and/or metastatic carcinoma of head and neck. Am J Clin Oncol 19:249–254, 1996.

48. Schrijvers D, Johnson J, Jiminez U, et al: Phase III trial of modulation of cisplatin/fluorouracil chemotherapy by interferon alfa-2b in patients with recurrent or metastatic head and neck cancer. Head and Neck Interferon Cooperative Study Group. J Clin Oncol 16:1054–1059, 1998.

49. Schoffski P, Catimel G, Planting AS, et al: Docetaxel and cisplatin: An active regimen in patients with locally advanced, recurrent or metastatic squamous cell carcinoma of the head and neck. Results of a phase II study of the EORTC Early Clinical Studies Group. Ann Oncol 10:119–122, 1999.

50. Fujii H, Tsukuda M, Murakami S: Combination phase I-II study of taxotere (TXT) and cisplatin (CDDP) in patients with head and neck. Lung Cancer 34(Suppl 1): Abstracts of the 2nd International Chicago Symposium on Malignancies of the Chest and Head and Neck. Chicago, Oct. 4–6, 2001.

51. Colevas AD, Adak S, Amrein PC, et al: A phase II trial of palliative docetaxel plus 5-fluorouracil for squamous-cell cancer of the head and neck. Ann Oncol 11:535–539, 2000.

52. Filippi MH, Cupissol D, Calais G: A phase II study of docetaxel (taxotere) and 5-fluorouracil (5-FU) in metastatic or recurrent squamous cell carcinoma of the head and neck. Proc Annu Meet Am Soc Clin Oncol 18:A1552, 1999.

53. Janinis J, Papadakou M, Xidakis E: Combination chemotherapy with docetaxel, cisplatin, and 5-fluorouracil in previously treated patients with advanced/recurrent head and neck cancer: A phase II feasibility study. Am J clin Oncol 23:128–131, 2000.

54. Levy SG, Haddad RI, Echo DAV: A phase I study of taxotere (T), cisplatin (DDP), and escalating doses of xeloda (X) for recurrent, locally advanced, or metastatic solid tumors. Lung Cancer 34(Suppl 1): Abstracts of the 2nd International Chicago Symposium on Malignancies of the Chest and Head and Neck. Chicago, Oct. 4–6, 2001.

55. Forastiere A, Leong T, Rowisky E: Phase III comparison of high-dose paclitaxel + cisplatin + granulocyte colony-stimulating factor versus low-dose paclitaxel + cisplatin in advanced head and neck cancer: Eastern Cooperative Oncology Group study E1393. J Clin Oncol 19:1088–1095, 2001.

56. Clark JI, Hofmeister C, Choudury A: Phase II evaluation of paclitaxel in combination with carboplatin in advanced head and neck carcinoma. Cancer 92:2334–2340, 2001.

57. Murphy B, Li Y, Cella D: Phase III study comparing cisplatin (C) & 5-fluorouracil (F) versus cisplatin & paclitaxel (T) in metastatic/recurrent head & neck cancer. Proc Annu Meet Am Soc Clin Oncol 20:A894, 2001.

58. Shin DM, Glisson BS, Khuri FR, et al: Phase II trial of paclitaxel, ifosfamide, and cisplatin in patients with recurrent head and neck squamous cell carcinoma. J Clin Oncol 16:1325–1330, 1998.

59. Shin DM, Khuri FR, Glisson BS, et al: Phase II study of paclitaxel, ifosfamide, and carboplatin in patients with recurrent or metastatic head and neck squamous cell carcinoma. Cancer 91:1316–1323, 2001.

60. Fu KK, Pajak TF, Trotti A, et al: A Radiation Therapy Oncology Group (RTOG) phase III randomized study to compare hyperfractionation and two variants of accelerated fractionation to standard fractionation radiotherapy for head and neck squamous cell carcinomas: First report of RTOG 9003. Int J Radiat Oncol Biol Phys 48:7–16, 2000.

61. Lo TC, Wiley AL, Ansfield FJ, et al: Combined radiation therapy and 5-fluorouracil for advanced squamous cell carcinoma of the oral cavity and oropharynx: A randomized study. Am J Roentgenol 126:229–235, 1976.

62. Byfield JE, Calabro-Jones P, Klisak I, et al: Pharmacologic requirements for obtaining sensitization of human tumor cells in vitro to combined 5-fluorouracil or ftorafur and X rays. Int J Radiat Oncol Biol Phys 8:1923–1933, 1982.

63. Byfield JE, Sharp TR, Frankel SS, et al: Phase I and II trial of five-day infused 5-fluorouracil and radiation in advanced cancer of the head and neck. J Clin Oncol 2:406–413, 1984.

64. Sinclair WK: Hydroxyurea: Effects on Chinese hamster cells grown in culture. Cancer Res 27:297–308, 1967.

65. Hussey DH, Abrams JP: Combined therapy in advanced head and neck cancer: Hydroxyurea and radiotherapy. Prog Clin Cancer 6:79–86, 1975.

66. Richards GJ Jr, Chambers RG: Hydroxyurea in the treatment of neoplasms of the head and neck. A resurvey. Am J Surg 126:513–518, 1973.

67. Vokes EE, Haraf DJ, Panje WR, et al: Hydroxyurea with concomitant radiotherapy or locally advanced head and neck cancer. Semin Oncol 19:53–58, 1992.

68. Browman GP, Cripps C, Hodson DI, et al: Placebo-controlled randomized trial of infusional fluorouracil during standard radiotherapy in locally advanced head and neck cancer. J Clin Oncol 12:2648–2653, 1994.

69. Browman GP, Cripps C, Hodson DI: Placebo-controlled randomized trial of infusional fluorouracil during standard radiotherpay in locally advanced head and neck cancer, Author Update. Classic Papers Current Comments 4:625–630, 1999.

70. Shanta V, Krishnamurthi S: Combined bleomycin and radiotherapy in oral cancer. Clin Radiol 31:617–620, 1980.

71. Fu KK, Phillips TL, Silverberg IJ, et al: Combined radiotherapy and chemotherapy with bleomycin and methotrexate for advanced inoperable head and neck cancer: Update of a Northern California Oncology Group randomized trial. J Clin Oncol 5:1410–1418, 1987.

72. Eschwege F, Sancho-Garnier H, Gerard JP, et al: Ten-year results of randomized trial comparing radiotherapy and concomitant bleomycin to radiotherapy alone in epidermoid carcinomas of the oropharynx: Experience of the European Organization for Research and Treatment of Cancer. NCI Monogr 6:275–278, 1988.

73. Haselow RE, Warshaw MC, Oken MM, et al: Radiation alone versus radiation with weekly low dose cis-platinum in unresectable cancer of the head and neck. In Fee WE Jr, Johns ME (ed): Head and Neck Cancer. Philadelphia, BC Decker, 1980, pp 279–281.

74. Bernier J, Domenge C, Eschwege F: Chemo-radiotherapy, as compared to radiotherapy alone, significantly increases disease-free and overall survival in head and neck cancer patients after surgery: Results of EORTC phase III trial 22931. Int J Radiat Oncol Biol Phys 51:A1, 2001.

75. Bachaud JM, David JM, Boussin G, et al: Combined postoperative radiotherapy and weekly cisplatin infusion for locally advanced squamous cell carcinoma of the head and neck: Preliminary report of a randomized trial. Int J Radiat Oncol Biol Phys 20:243–246, 1991.

76. Al-Sarraf M, Pajak TF, Marcial VA, et al: Concurrent radiotherapy and chemotherapy with cisplatin in inoperable squamous cell carcinoma of the head and neck. An RTOG Study. Cancer 59:259–265, 1987.

77. Tsuchiya K, Nishioka T, Shirato H: A randomized trial of concomitant chemoradiotherapy for head-and-neck cancers: Cisplatin (CDDP) vs. carboplatin (CBDCA). Int J Radiat Oncol Biol Phys 51:S2215, 2001.

78. Jacobs MC, Eisenberger M, Oh MC, et al: Carboplatin (CBDCA) and radiotherapy for stage IV carcinoma of the head and neck: A phase I-II study. Int J Radiat Oncol Biol Phys 17:361–363, 1989.

79. Kamioner DH, Haddad E, Vallantin X: Carpoplatin-radiotherapy versus cisplatin-radiotherapy according to a concurrent schedule in advanced head and neck cancer; preliminary resutls of a randomized study (Meeting abstract). 4th Int Congress on Anticancer Chemotherapy. Feb. 2005, Paris, France.

80. Hesse K, Heinrich B, Zimmermann F, et al: Combined radio-chemotherapy with docetaxel in patients with unresectable locally advanced head and neck tumors. Strahlenther Onkol 176:67–72, 2000.

81. Sunwoo JB, Herscher LL, Kroog GS, et al: Concurrent paclitaxel and radiation in the treatment of locally advanced head and neck cancer. J Clin Oncol 19:800–811, 2001.

82. Eisbruch A, Shewach DS, Bradford CR: Radiation concurrent with gemcitabine for locally advanced head and neck cancer. J Clin Oncol 19:792–799, 2001.

83. Al-Sarraf M, Pajak TF, Cooper JS, et al: Chemo-radiotherapy in patients with locally advanced nasopharyngeal carcinoma: A Radiation Therapy Oncology Group study. J Clin Oncol 8:1342–1351, 1990.

84. Oh J, Vokes E, Kies M, et al: Induction chemotherapy followed by concomitant chemoradiotherpay in the treatment of locoregionally advanced nasopharyngeal cancer. Lung Cancer 34(Suppl 1): Abstracts of the 2nd International Chicago Symposium on Malignancies of the Chest and Head and Neck. Chicago, Oct. 4–6, 2001.

85. Huncharek M, Kupelnick B: Combined chemo/radiation versus radiation therapy alone in locally advanced nasopharyngeal carcinoma: Results of a meta-analysis of 1528 patients from six randomized trials. Lung Cancer 34(Suppl 1): Abstracts of the 2nd International Chicago Symposium on Malignancies of the Chest and Head and Neck. Chicago, Oct. 4–6, 2001.

86. Chua D, Sham J, Wei WI: Control of regional metastasis after induction chemotherapy and radiotherapy for nasopharyngeal carcinoma. Head Neck 24:350–360, 2002.

87. Adelstein DJ, Kalish LA, Adams GL, et al: Concurrent radiation therapy and chemotherapy for locally unresectable squamous cell head and neck cancer: An Eastern Cooperative Oncology Group pilot study. J Clin Oncol 11:2136–2142, 1993.

88. Adelstein DJ, Saxton JP, Lavertu P, et al: Maximizing local control and organ preservation in advanced squamous cell head and neck cancer (SCHNC) with hyperfractionated and concurrent chemotherapy. Proc Annu Meet Am Soc Clin Oncol 20:A893, 2001.

89. Wendt TG, Grabenbauer GG, Rodel CM, et al: Simultaneous radiochemotherapy versus radiotherapy alone in advanced head and neck cancer: A randomized multicenter study. J Clin Oncol 16:1318–1324, 1998.

90. Calais G, Alfonsi M, Bardet E: Radiation alone (RT) versus RT with concomitant chemotherapy (CT) in stages III or IV oropharynx carcinoma. Final results of the 94-01 GORTEC randomized study. Int J Radiat Oncol Biol Phys 51:A2, 2001.

91. Adelstein DJ, Lavertu P, Saxton JP, et al: Mature results of a phase III randomized trial comparing concurrent chemoradiotherapy with radiation therapy alone in patients with stage III and IV squamous cell carcinoma of the head and neck. Cancer 88:876–883, 2000.

92. Brizel DM, Albers ME, Fisher SR, et al: Hyperfractionated irradiation with or without concurrent chemotherapy for locally advanced head and neck cancer. N Engl J Med 338:1798–1804, 1998.

93. Merlano M, Benasso M, Corvo R, et al: Five-year update of a randomized trial of alternating radiotherapy and chemotherapy compared with radiotherapy alone in treatment of unresectable squamous cell carcinoma of the head and neck. J Natl Cancer Inst 88:583–589, 1996.

94. Pignon JP, Bourhis J, Domenge C, et al: Chemotherapy added to locoregional treatment for head and neck squamous-cell carcinoma: Three meta-analyses of updated individual data. MACH-NC Collaborative Group. Meta-Analysis of Chemotherapy on Head and Neck Cancer. Lancet 355:949–955, 2000.

95. Bourhis J, Pignon JP: Meta-analyses in head and neck squamous cell carcinoma. What is the role of chemotherapy? Hematol Oncol Clin North Am 13:769–775, 1999.

96. Garden AS, Pajak TF, Vokes E: Preliminary results of RTOG 9703—a phase II randomized trial of concurrent radiation (RT) and chemotherapy for advanced squamous cell carcinomas (SCC) of the head and neck. Proc Annu Meet Am Soc Clin Oncol 20:A891, 2001.

97. Vokes EE, Kies MS, Haraf DJ, et al: Concomitant chemoradiotherapy as primary therapy for locoregionally advanced head and neck cancer. J Clin Oncol 18:1652–1661, 2000.

98. Kies MS, Haraf DJ, Rosen F, et al: Concomitant infusional paclitaxel and fluorouracil, oral hydroxyurea, and hyperfractionated radiation for locally advanced squamous head and neck cancer. J Clin Oncol 19:1961–1969, 2001.

99. Brockstein B, Haraf DJ, Kies M, et al: Patterns of failure and risk factors for locoregional and distant metastases after intensive concomitant chemotherapy and hyperfractionated radiotherapy for head and neck cancer. Lung Cancer 34(Suppl 1): Abstracts of the 2nd International Chicago Symposium on Malignancies of the Chest and Head and Neck. Chicago, Oct. 4–6, 2001.

100. Vokes EE, Kies M, Haraf DJ, et al: Induction chemotherapy followed by concomitant chemoradiotherapy for advanced head and neck cancer: Impact on the natural history of the disease. J Clin Oncol 13:876–883, 1995.

101. Kies MS, Haraf DJ, Athanasiadis I, et al: Induction chemotherapy followed by concurrent chemoradiation for advanced head and neck cancer: Improved disease control and survival. J Clin Oncol 16:2715–2721, 1998.

102. Mantz CA, Vokes EE, Kies MS, et al: Sequential induction chemotherapy and concomitant chemoradiotherapy in the management of locoregionally advanced laryngeal cancer. Ann Oncol 12:343–347, 2001.

103. The Department of Veterans Affairs Laryngeal Cancer Study Group: Induction chemotherapy plus radiation compared with surgery plus radiation in patients with advanced laryngeal cancer. N Engl J Med 324:1685–1690, 1991.

104. Forastiere AA, Berkey B, Maor M: Phase III trial to preserve the larynx: Induction chemotherapy and radiotherapy versus concomitant chemoradiotherapy versus radiotherapy alone, Intergroup trial R91-11. Proc Annu Meet Am Soc Clin Oncol 20:4a, 2001.

105. Wolf G: Commentary: Phase III trial to preserve the larynx: Induction chemotherapy and radiotherapy versus concurrent chemotherapy and radiotherapy versus radiotherapy—Intergroup trial 91-11. J Clin Oncol 19:28s–31s, 2001.

106. Lefebvre JL, Chevalier D, Luboinski B, et al: Larynx preservation in pyriform sinus cancer: Preliminary results of a European Organization for Research and Treatment of Cancer phase III trial. EORTC Head and Neck Cancer Cooperative Group. J Natl Cancer Inst 88:890–899, 1996.

107. Haddad R, Tishler R, Busse P, et al: Taxotere, platinum, and 5-fluorouracil (TPF) based induction chemotherapy for locally advanced head and neck cancer: Long-term results and pattern of failure. Lung Cancer 34(Suppl 1): Abstracts of the 2nd International Chicago Symposium on Malignancies of the Chest and Head and Neck. Chicago, Oct. 4–6, 2001.

108. Gandia D, Wibault P, Guillot T, et al: Simultaneous chemoradiotherapy as salvage treatment in locoregional recurrences of squamous head and neck cancer. Head Neck 15:8–15, 1993.

109. Hartsell WF, Thomas CR, Murthy AK, et al: Pilot study for the evaluation of simultaneous cisplatin/5-fluorouracil infusion and limited radiation therapy in regionally recurrent head and neck cancer (EST P-C385). Am J Clin Oncol 17:338–343, 1994.

110. Haraf DJ, Weichselbaum RR, Vokes EE: Re-irradiation with concomitant chemotherapy of unresectable recurrent head and neck cancer: A potentially curable disease. Ann Oncol 7:913–918, 1996.

111. Wheeler RH, Harris J, Spencer S: RTOG 9610: Phase II study of reirradiation (RRT) with concurrent hydroxyurea (HU) and 5-fluorouracil (FU) in patients (pts) with recurrent squamous cell cancer of the head and neck: Survival results. Proc Annu Meet Am Soc Clin Oncol 20:A887, 2001.

112. Humerickhouse RA, Haraf D, Stenson K, et al: Phase I study of irinotecan (CPT-11), 5-FU, and hydroxyurea with radiation in recurrent or advanced head and neck cancer. Proc Annu Meet Am Soc Clin Oncol 19:A1650, 2001.

113. McLaughlin MP, Thomas C, Pearson B: Reirradiation with concurrent cisplatin/5-fluorouracil in patients with recurrent squamous cell carcinomas of the head and neck. Int J Radiat Oncol Biol Phys 51:A2223, 2001.

114. Robbins KT, Storniolo AM, Kerber C, et al: Phase I study of highly selective supradose cisplatin infusions for advanced head and neck cancer. J Clin Oncol 12:2113–2120, 1994.

115. Kumar P, Robbins K, Harris J: Intra-arterial (IA) cisplatin and radiation therapy (RT) is feasible in a multi-institutional setting for the treatment of stage IV-T4 head/neck (H/N) squamous cell carcinoma (SCCa): Initial results of Radiation Therapy Oncology Group (RTOG) trial 9615. Proc Annu Meet Am Soc Clin Oncol 20:A918, 2001.

116. Regine W, Valentino J, Arnold S: A phase II study of concomitant hyperfractionated radiation therapy and double-dose intra-arterial cisplatin for squamous cell carcinoma of the head and neck. Proc Annu Meet Am Soc Clin Oncol 20:A935, 2001.

117. Fuwa N, Ito Y, Matsumoto A, et al: A combination therapy of continuous superselective intraarterial carboplatin infusion and radiation therapy for locally advanced head and neck carcinoma. Phase I study. Cancer 89:2099–2105, 2000.

118. Pecora AL, Rizvi N, Cohen GI, et al: An intravenous phase I trial of a replication-competent virus, PV701, in the treatment of patients with advanced solid cancers. Proc Annu Meet Am Soc Clin Oncol 20:1009a, 2001.

119. Grandis JR, Melhem MF, Gooding WE, et al: Levels of TGF-alpha and EGFR protein in head and neck squamous cell carcinoma and patient survival. J Natl Cancer Inst 90:824–832, 1998.

120. Maurizi M, Almadori G, Ferrandina G, et al: Prognostic significance of epidermal growth factor receptor in laryngeal squamous cell carcinoma. Br J Cancer 74:1253–1257, 1996.

121. Huang SM, Bock JM, Harari PM: Epidermal growth factor receptor blockade with C225 modulates proliferation, apoptosis, and radiosensitivity in squamous cell carcinomas of the head and neck. Cancer Res 59:1935–1940, 1999.

122. Baselga J, Pfister D, Cooper MR, et al: Phase I studies of anti-epidermal growth factor receptor chimeric antibody C225 alone and in combination with cisplatin. J Clin Oncol 18:904–914, 2000.

123. Hong WK, Arquette M, Nabell L: Efficacy and safety of the epidermal growth factor antibody (EGFR) IMC-C225, in combination with cisplatin, in patients with recurrent squamous cell carcinoma of the head and neck (SCCHN) refractory to cisplatin containing therapy. Proc Annu Meet Am Soc Clin Oncol 20:A895, 2001.

124. Bonner JA, Raisch KP, Trummell HQ, et al: Enhanced apoptosis with combination C225/radiation treatment serves as the impetus for clinical investigation in head and neck cancers. J Clin Oncol 18:47S–53S, 2000.

125. Robert F, Ezekiel MP, Spencer SA, et al: Phase I study of anti–epidermal growth factor receptor antibody cetuximab in combination with radiation therapy in patients with advanced head and neck cancer. J Clin Oncol 19:3234–3243, 2001.

126. Hidalgo M, Siu LL, Nemunaitis J, et al: Phase I and pharmacologic study of OSI-774, an epidermal growth factor receptor tyrosine kinase inhibitor, in patients with advanced solid malignancies. J Clin Oncol 19:3267–3279, 2001.

127. Senzer NN, Soulieres D, Siu L, et al: Phase 2 evaluation of OSI-774, a potent oral antagonist of the EGFR-TK, in patients with advanced squamous cell carcinoma of the head and neck. Proc Annu Meet Am Soc Clin Oncol 20:A6, 2001.

128. Cohen EEW, Rosen F, Eng C, et al: Phase II study of ZD1839 (Iressa) in recurrent or metastatic squamous cell carcinoma of the head and neck cancer. Lung Cancer 34(Suppl 1): Abstracts of the 2nd International Chicago Symposium on Malignancies of the Chest and Head and Neck. Chicago, Oct. 4–6, 2001.

129. Geng L, Donnelly E, McMahon G, et al: Inhibition of vascular endothelial growth factor receptor signaling leads to reversal of tumor resistance to radiotherapy. Cancer Res 61:2413–2419, 2001.

130. Lee CG, Heijn M, di Tomaso E, et al: Anti-vascular endothelial growth factor treatment augments tumor radiation response under normoxic or hypoxic conditions. Cancer Res 60:5565–5570, 2000.

131. D'Amato RJ, Loughnan MS, Flynn E, et al: Thalidomide is an inhibitor of angiogenesis. Proc Natl Acad Sci USA 91:4082–4085, 1994.

132. Tseng JE, Glisson BS, Khuri FR: Phase II study of the antiangiogenesis agent thalidomide in recurrent or metastatic squamous cell carcinoma of the head and neck. Cancer 92:2364–2373, 2001.

133. Millauer B, Wizigmann-Voos S, Schnurch H, et al: High affinity VEGF binding and developmental expression suggest Flk-1 as a major regulator of vasculogenesis and angiogenesis. Cell 72:835–846, 1993.

134. Eng C, Kindler HL, Stadler WM: SU5416 in advanced colorectal cancer: A University of Chicago phase II consortium study. Proc Annu Meet Am Soc Clin Oncol 20:A2215, 2001.

135. Takamoto T, Sasaki M, Kuno T, et al: Flk-1 specific kinase inhibitor (SU5416) inhibited the growth of GS-9L glioma in rat brain and prolonged the survival. Kobe J Med Sci 47:181–191, 2001.

136. Smolich BD, Yuen HA, West KA, et al: The antiangiogenic protein kinase inhibitors SU5416 and SU6668 inhibit the SCF receptor (c-kit) in a human myeloid leukemia cell line and in acute myeloid leukemia blasts. Blood 97:1413–1421, 2001.

137. Fiedler WM, Tinnefeld H, Mende T, et al: A phase II study of SU5416 in c-kit positive AML. Proc Annu Meet Am Soc Clin Oncol 20:A1148, 2001.

138. Margolin K, Gordon MS, Holmgren E, et al: Phase Ib trial of intravenous recombinant humanized monoclonal antibody to vascular endothelial growth factor in combination with chemotherapy in patients with advanced cancer: Pharmacologic and long-term safety data. J Clin Oncol 19:851–856, 2001.

139. Sledge G, Miller K, Novotny W, et al: A phase II trial of single-agent rhumab VEGF (recombinant humanized monoclonal antibody to vascular endothelial cell growth factor) in patients with relapsed metastatic breast cancer. Proc Annu Meet Am Soc Clin Oncol 19:A5C, 2000.

140. DeVore RF, Fehrenbacher L, Herbst RS, et al: A randomized phase II trial comparing rhumab VEGF (recombinant humanized monoclonal antibody to vascular endothelial cell growth factor) plus carboplatin/paclitaxel (CP) to CP alone in patients with stage IIIB/IV NSCLC. Proc Annu Meet Am Soc Clin Oncol 19:A1896, 2000.

141. Bergsland EK, Fehrenbacher L, Novotny W, et al: Bevacizumab (BV) + chemotherapy (CT) may improve survival in metastatic colorectal cancer (MCRC) subjects with unfavorable prognostic indicators. Proc Annu Meet Am Soc Clin Oncol 20:A2247, 2001.

142. Novotny W, Holmgren E, Griffing S, et al: Identification of squamous cell histology and central, cavitary tumors as possible risk factors for pulmonary hemorrhage (PH) in patients with advanced NSCLC receiving bevacizumab (BV). Proc Annu Meet Am Soc Clin 20:A1318, 2001.

143. O-charoenrat P, Rhys-Evans P, Eccles SA: Expression of vascular endothelial growth factor family members in head and neck squamous cell carcinoma correlates with lymph node metastasis. Cancer 92:556–568, 2001.

144. Viloria-Petit A, Crombet T, Jothy S, et al: Acquired resistance to the antitumor effect of epidermal growth factor receptor-blocking antibodies in vivo: A role for altered tumor angiogenesis. Cancer Res 61:5090–5101, 2001.

145. Holden SN, Eckhardt SG, Fisher S: A phase I pharmacokinetic (PK) and biological study of the farnesyl transferase inhibitor (FTI) R115777 and capecitabine in patients (PTS) with advanced solid malignancies. Proc Annu Meet Am Soc Clin Oncol 20:A316, 2001.

146. Kim KB, Shin DM, Summey CC: Phase I study of farnesyl transferase inhibitor, BMS-214662, in solid tumors. Proc Annu Meet Am Soc Clin Oncol 20:313a, 2001.

147. Khuri FR, Nemunaitis J, Ganly I, et al: A controlled trial of intratumoral ONYX-015, a selectively replicating adenovirus, in combination with cisplatin and 5-fluorouracil in patients with recurrent head and neck cancer. Nat Med 6:879–885, 2000.

148. Nemunaitis J, Khuri F, Ganly I, et al: Phase II trial of intratumoral administration of ONYX-015, a replication-selective adenovirus, in patients with refractory head and neck cancer. J Clin Oncol 19:289–298, 2001.

149. Cohen EE, Papadimitrakopoulou VA, Silverman S, et al: A phase II trial of attenuated adenovirus, Onyx-015, as mouthwash therapy in premalignant oral dysplasia. Proc Annu Meet Am Soc Clin Oncol 20:A915, 2001.

150. Vaupel P, Kelleher DK, Hockel M: Oxygen status of malignant tumors: Pathogenesis of hypoxia and significance for tumor therapy. Semin Oncol 28:29–35, 2001.

151. Rockwell S: Use of hypoxia-directed drugs in the therapy of solid tumors. Semin Oncol 19:29–40, 1992.

152. Haffty BG, Son YH, Papac R, et al: Chemotherapy as an adjunct to radiation in the treatment of squamous cell carcinoma of the head and neck: Results of the Yale Mitomycin Randomized Trials. J Clin Oncol 15:268–276, 1997.

153. Haffty BG, Yung HS, Papac R, et al: Chemotherapy as adjunct to radiation in the treatment of squamous cell carcinoma of the head and neck: Results of the Yale Mitomycin Randomized Trials. Classic Papers Comments 4:631–640, 1999.

154. Overgaard J, Hansen HS, Andersen AP, et al: Misonidazole combined with split-course radiotherapy in the treatment of invasive carcinoma of larynx and pharynx: Report from the DAHANCA 2 study. Int J Radiat Oncol Biol Phys 16:1065–1068, 1989.

155. Overgaard J, Hansen HS, Overgaard M, et al: A randomized double-blind phase III study of nimorazole as a hypoxic radiosensitizer of primary radiotherapy in supraglottic larynx and pharynx carcinoma. Results of the Danish Head and Neck Cancer Study (DAHANCA) Protocol 5-85. Radiother Oncol 46:135–146, 1998.

156. Rowinsky EK: Novel radiation sensitizers targeting tissue hypoxia. Oncology (Huntingt) 13:61–70, 1999.

157. Dorie MJ, Brown JM: Tumor-specific, schedule-dependent interaction between tirapazamine (SR 4233) and cisplatin. Cancer Res 53:4633–4636, 1993.

158. Rischin D, Peters L, Hicks R, et al: Phase I trial of concurrent tirapazamine, cisplatin, and radiotherapy in patients with advanced head and neck cancer. J Clin Oncol 19:535–542, 2001.

159. Lee DJ, Trotti A, Spencer S, et al: Concurrent tirapazamine and radiotherapy for advanced head and neck carcinomas: A Phase II study. Int J Radiat Oncol Biol Phys 42:811–815, 1998.

160. Pinto HA, Le Q, Terris DJ: Toxicity of tirapazamine, cisplatin, & fluorouracil as induction chemotherapy & simultaneous chemoradiotherapy for organ preservation in head & neck cancer. Proceedings of the 11th NCI-EORTC-AACR Symposium on New Drugs in Cancer Therapy 6:312a, 2000.

CHAPTER 34

Immunotherapy of Cancer of the Head and Neck

Carter Van Waes

Erik S. Kass

also provide new approaches in the prevention of cancers in individuals at high risk.

INTRODUCTION

Squamous cell carcinoma of the head and neck (SCCHN) is the most prevalent cancer of the upper aerodigestive tract. Because of the site of origin, SCCHN and ablative therapies often result in impaired function of organs involved in communication, including voice, speech, smell, and taste. Further, despite advances in organ preservation surgery and chemoradiation therapy, there has been no improvement in overall survival of patients with SCCHN over the past 30 years, and more than half of these patients eventually die of aggressive local, regional, or distant disease. The development of effective biologic therapy for SCCHN that could eradicate abnormal cancer cells while preserving the structure and function of organs involved in communication and swallowing would be highly desirable. Further, development of biologic therapy against the microscopic deposits of cancer cells at local and distant sites that result in recurrence following treatment with current therapeutic modalities is needed to improve survival.

During the past century, increased knowledge and understanding of cellular and molecular immunology have led to continued progress toward the development of biologic treatment for cancer. Recombinant cytokines, antibodies, and immunomodulatory molecules that have biologic activity have been identified and developed. Clinical trials using immunomodulatory agents have resulted in regression or stabilization of disease in a small subset of patients with cancer. Viral and other DNA vectors have been developed, and studies of vector-based therapy without and with genes with biologic activity have been undertaken. It is hoped that the recent improvement in understanding of the mechanisms by which these aggressive cancers evade host immunity and promote tumorigenesis will lead to the development of more effective biologic therapies. Recently, investigators have gained an improved understanding of the molecular mechanisms underlying tumor development, angiogenesis, and spread, thereby expanding opportunities for biologic therapy. Agents that modulate immunologic and tumor-related mechanisms involved in the pathogenesis of SCCHN may

IMMUNOSURVEILLANCE

Ehrlich in 1909 and Burnet in 1970 are recognized for proposing that one function of the immune system may be to provide immunosurveillance against the development of cancer, through the capability of the immune system to recognize and eliminate abnormal cancer cells as "altered-self."[1, 2] Studies undertaken in animal models to find evidence for this hypothesis of immunosurveillance have provided evidence that thymus-deficient mice, which lack lymphocytes derived from the thymus (T-lymphocytes), are susceptible to an increased incidence of lymphoid cancers, particularly those induced by animal viruses that transform lymphocytes.[3] A similar increase in the development of malignancies of lymphatic origin has been observed in immunocompromised human patients, including those with hereditary immunodeficiency disorders, and in patients infected with Epstein-Barr virus (EBV) and human immunodeficiency virus (HIV). Although thymus-derived T-lymphocytes appear to play a role in resistance to virally induced lymphoid cancers, the evidence for immunosurveillance in epithelial cancers such as SCCHN is less compelling.

Indirect evidence for immunosurveillance against transformed epithelial cells has been obtained from studies of the tumorigenic potential in vivo of skin or oral keratinocytes transformed by carcinogens in vitro. A subset of transformed skin or oral keratinocytes that grow in immune-deficient mice has been found to regress when implanted in immune-competent animals, suggesting that at least some epithelial cancer cells can be recognized and eliminated by host immunity.[4, 5] In humans, development of SCCHNs involving the skin, lip, or upper aerodigestive tract has been reported in patients undergoing long-term immunosuppressive therapy following transplantation and in patients with acquired immunodeficiency syndrome (AIDS).[6] Additionally, a case of spontaneous remission (discovered at autopsy) in a patient with carcinoma of the larynx who underwent incomplete resection has been taken as evidence for potential immunity to SCCHN.[7] However, the low frequency with which immunodeficient animals or humans develop the most common epithelial cancers that result from hereditary, chemical, or physical carcinogenesis has been interpreted to indicate that immunosurveillance against cancer is not a primary function of the immune system.[3]

◻ TUMOR ANTIGENS AND IMMUNITY IN HEAD AND NECK SQUAMOUS CELL CARCINOMA

Despite the limited evidence for a natural immune resistance to the development of cancer, studies of experimental and human tumors have demonstrated that these cancers express antigens that can induce tumor rejection or regression. Complete surgical removal of some types of tumors in animals has revealed that these cancers can induce immunologic resistance to rechallenge with the same cancer, but not with cancers from other inbred animals that have an identical genetic background. Similarly, inbred animals immunized with attenuated or subtumorigenic doses of tumor cells can exhibit resistance to the same cancer but not to others.

These observations have led to the conclusion that many cancers express antigens that are specifically expressed by one tumor, but not by others; these have been called *tumor-specific antigens* (TSAs).[3] Most often, TSAs are the result of mutations that give rise to expression of a mutant form of an expressed protein. Another type of antigen commonly detected on cancer cells is the molecule that is shared or expressed on cancers from different animals or patients; these are called *tumor-associated antigens* (TAAs).[3] TAAs are molecules that are expressed more in tumors than in normal tissue. Molecular studies over the past decade have provided evidence that mutations occur and result in the altered expression of proteins in all cancers, providing potential tumor antigens that are recognizable as "altered-self." Both TSAs and TAAs have been shown in preclinical animal studies to induce immune-mediated regression of tumors.[3, 8] Several studies of vaccines developed against TAAs have been completed in patients with melanoma and have demonstrated immunogenicity and growth inhibition or regression in a small percentage of patients.[9] Several TAAs and TSAs have also been identified in SCCHN; a representative list is shown in Table 34–1.

TABLE 34–1 Antigens Detected in Squamous Cell Carcinoma

Antigen	Structure	Function
Tumor-associated antigens (TAAs)		
A9	Integrin α6β4	Laminin adhesion
E48	Ly6 Family	Cell-cell adhesion
U36	CD44v6	Cell-cell adhesion
CEA	Ig Family	Cell-cell adhesion?
Lewis(a)	Sialyl protein	Cell-cell adhesion?
TP53	TP53 family	DNA repair and apoptosis
Tumor-specific antigens (TSAs)		
Casp-8	Caspase	Apoptosis
6A1-1D7, SART	Leucine zipper	Transcription?
HLA-24 restricted antigen	KIAA0156	Unknown
EF2	Elongation factor	Protein synthesis

Tumor-Associated Antigens

Early examples of TAAs detected in SCCHN include the antigens detected by monoclonal antibodies, such as A9, E48, and U36. A9 antigen has been found to be highly expressed in most SCCHNs, while its expression in normal squamous epithelia has been restricted to the basal layer. A9 was identified as the integrin α6β4, a heterodimeric cell adhesion receptor for the extracellular matrix substance laminin.[10] Increased expression of A9 was found to be associated with poor prognosis in immunohistopathologic studies; thus, A9 may be a potentially useful marker for immunodiagnostic and prognostic use in vitro.[11] E48 and U36 are also antigens found to be highly expressed in SCCHN when compared with normal epithelia.[12] E48 was found to be a cell-surface molecule homologous to Ly-6 antigen ThB, which is a protein with evolutionary homology within the immunoglobulin superfamily. U36 was found to bind cell determinant 44 variant 6 (CD44v6). Ly-6 and CD44v6 have been reported to function in cell-cell adhesion. The E48 and U36 monoclonal antibodies have been coupled to radionuclides for diagnostic imaging and as candidates for radionuclide- and antibody-directed cell cytotoxic therapy in patients with SCCHN.[12]

SCCHN has recently been reported to express another TAA—carcinoembryonic antigen (CEA).[13] CEA is also an immunoglobulin superfamily cell-surface molecule that is expressed by embryonic and malignant epithelia. SCCHN lines that express CEA may be lysed by CEA-specific cytolytic T-lymphocytes (CTLs), making CEA a candidate TAA for immunotherapy in SCCHN.[13] CEA has been most widely studied in clinical immune vaccines in colon cancer, where it is highly expressed.[14] Although CEA TAAs lack mutations, T- and B-lymphocyte responses to these over-expressed molecules have been detected in animals and human subjects given investigational vaccines.[14]

The glycoantigen sialyl Lewis(a), which has been used as a target for human immunotherapy, has been detected in approximately 50% of SCCHNs,[15] but no clinical trials showing activity against squamous cell carcinoma (SCC) have been reported to date. The TP53 molecule, a 53-kD protein involved in DNA repair and programmed cell death, is over-expressed in normal or mutant form in more than 50% of SCCHNs and is a potential tumor antigen.[16] However, tumors from patients with SCCHN have been reported to lose expression of normal TP53, suggesting that immune responses against normal TP53 as a TAA may select for epitope loss variants.[17] Recently, a novel 100-kD antigen recognized by cytolytic T-lymphocytes has been detected in squamous cell carcinomas.[18]

The potential of TAA for vaccine development faces several limitations. Because of the lack of mutations in TAA, vaccination often requires hyperstimulation of the immune system with adjuvants. Responses have been detected but have rarely been shown to induce complete regression or remission in animals or patients with established tumors. Furthermore, because TAAs are expressed at low levels in some normal cells, an increased potential for initiation of autoimmune disease by immunostimulation exists. The potential for and seriousness of autoimmunity may differ significantly depending on the tissue distribution and function of the molecule.

Tumor-Specific Antigens

TSAs have been detected in a variety of human and murine cancers, and TSAs have been shown to arise from mutations in genes that are important to malignant phenotype.[19] A number of TSAs have been detected in SCCHN; a few of these have also been molecularly characterized (Table 34–1). Specific T-lymphocytes that react with SCCHN cells from the same patient have been detected by several investigators.[20–22] T-lymphocytes that can specifically recognize tumors have been used to identify antigenic peptides and to isolate cDNA clones that encode the mutant genes. Mandruzzato and associates reported the identification of a TSA in a patient with SCCHN arising from a mutation in the caspase 8 gene, one of the genes that mediates resistance of SCCHN to cell death by factors such as tumor necrosis factor and FAS ligand.[23] Shichijo and colleagues have identified several SCC antigenic peptide sequences from novel proteins and genes whose functions remain to be defined.[24] A mutant peptide from elongation factor 2 has been detected in SCC of the lung.[25] This mutation was not found in other SCCs studied. Elongation factor 2 is a molecule involved in protein synthesis.

The detection and identification of specific mutations in genes that are important to cell function and the malignant phenotype in SCC are consistent with results obtained in experimental animal studies.[19] However, although the identification of antigenic peptides in SCCHN offers the potential for development of specific immune therapy for individual patients or patients with the same mutations, use of TSAs for vaccines also faces obstacles. Both the expression of these mutations in individual patients and the labor-intensive requirements for vaccine development have thus far limited the development and use of TSA vaccines.

IMMUNE UNRESPONSIVENESS AND IMMUNE ESCAPE

There is now considerable evidence that tumors may escape immune detection and immune therapy through a variety of mechanisms. Tumors may lose or downregulate expression of antigens recognized by lymphocytes, but usually some antigens are retained.[19, 26] More often, a lack of immune responsiveness occurs as a result of underexpression or overexpression of other important immunomodulatory signals that affect antitumor immunity, resulting in immune unresponsiveness and escape. Understanding of the mechanisms of tumor immunity and escape may bring about improvement in the effectiveness of natural and therapeutically induced immunity to control the development of SCCHN and other cancers.

ANTIGEN PRESENTATION AND THE ROLE OF THE MAJOR HISTOCOMPATIBILITY COMPLEX AND COSTIMULATORY MOLECULES

Several important cellular and molecular signals that are required for the immune response to antigens expressed by

tumors and pathogens have been defined and are illustrated in Figure 34–1. One signal required for activation of lymphocyte responses is the presentation of antigen by cell-surface molecules of the major histocompatibility complex (MHC). Normal and malignant squamous cells usually express the class I type of MHC molecule, which is needed for presentation of antigens to cytolytic T-lymphocytes (CTLs). CTLs have been shown to be effective mediators of immune destruction and regression of tumors.[3] Downregulation of MHC class I molecule expression by tumor cells may be one mechanism by which tumors can escape immune recognition, and investigators have reported decreased MHC class I expression by SCCHN.[28] Class I and II MHC expression in SCCHN may be induced by interferon-γ (IFN-γ)[28]; therefore, this deficiency may be correctable by therapy with IFN-γ or cytokines such as interleukin 12 (IL-12) that induce IFN-γ production by T-helper 1 cells (see Fig. 34–1).

Antigen shed by tumor cells or given as a vaccine is also processed by antigen presenting cells (APCs) of the immune system, which include dendritic cells, Langerhans cells, and macrophages.[29] These cells may express antigen in the context of the class II type of MHC molecule. As illustrated in

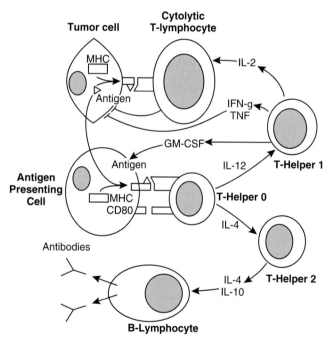

FIGURE 34–1 Cells and factors involved in the immune response to cancer. Tumor antigen is presented to cytolytic T-lymphocytes by major histocompatibility complex (MHC) molecules on the surfaces of tumor cells. Antigen is also shed and processed by antigen presenting cells, which present antigen to T-helper lymphocytes in the presence of MHC and the co-stimulatory molecule CD80. The T-helper 1 and cytolytic T-lymphocyte (CTL) responses needed for tumor cell killing are influenced by the presence of CD80 and IL-12; lack of CD80 and IL-4 may favor T-helper 2 and antibody responses. T-helper 1 cells produce the IL-2 needed to help CTL, along with interferon-γ (IFN-γ) and tumor necrosis factor (TNF), which can inhibit or kill tumor cells. Granulocyte-macrophage colony-stimulating factor (GM-CSF) promotes maturation and expression of MHC by antigen presenting cells.

Figure 34–1, MHC class II molecule presentation of antigen by APC can activate T-helper cells, which produce cytokines that are needed to help mount CTL and natural killer (NK) cell responses (cellular immunity), or B-cell synthesis of antibodies (humoral immunity).[29] The absence of MHC class II molecule expression by tumor cells and the lack of adequate APCs may be other mechanisms contributing to limited immune responsiveness to cancers, including SCCHN. Introduction of class II MHC molecule expression or induction of APCs that express MHC class II by expression or administration of granulocyte macrophage colony-stimulating factor (GM-CSF) has been reported to increase the immunogenicity of vaccines and tumor cells.[30, 31] However, SCCHNs have been shown to produce GM-CSF while growing progressively,[32] and several studies suggest that production of GM-CSF by established tumors may promote growth and immune unresponsiveness.[33] It will be important to determine if GM-CSF may have immunostimulatory effects when given together with purified antigens or nonviable tumor cell vaccines.[34]

A second costimulation signal provided by a cell determinant designated CD80 has been shown to be necessary for induction of immunity to antigens, including tumors such as SCC.[5, 34] Presentation of antigen in the absence of costimulation can result instead in a state of immune unresponsiveness, called *anergy*. Consistent with this, Thomas and associates found that oral keratinocytes transformed by carcinogen in vitro that retain CD80 may be rejected, and those that do not express CD80 grow progressively.[5, 35] Most human SCCHNs appear to lack CD80.[36] Gene therapy approaches have been developed to promote expression of CD80 and other costimulatory molecules; these are the subject of active preclinical and phase I clinical studies.[34]

T-HELPER CYTOKINES AND CYTOLYTIC T-LYMPHOCYTE RESPONSES

T-helper lymphocytes are thymus-derived cells that provide cytokine factors that assist activation and proliferation of a variety of cell types (see Fig. 34–1). T-helper 1 and T-helper 2 cells can produce a distinct repertoire of cytokines. T-helper 1 cells produce interleukin 2 (IL-2), IFN-γ, and tumor necrosis factor (TNF). T-helper 1 cells promote delayed-type hypersensitivity inflammatory responses, along with the CTL and NK cell immune responses necessary for tumor rejection.[3] T-helper 2 cells produce cytokines that help primarily B-cell responses, which produce antibody (humoral) immunity. Several studies have provided evidence that T-helper 1 responses decline, while T-helper 2 cytokines interleukin 4 (IL-4) and interleukin 10 (IL-10) and antibody responses are more strongly induced in animals and SCCHN patients bearing established tumors.[37–40] Antibody responses and immune complexes have been detected in patients with SCCHN, but these have been associated with poorer prognosis rather than protective immunity.[40] Furthermore, cytokine IL-4 produced by T-helper 2 lymphocytes may in fact promote proliferation of SCCHN,[39] and IL-10 may suppress the protective T-helper 1 and killer cell responses.[38]

Several strategies have been explored to promote protective T-helper 1–type responses. Because IL-2 has been shown to be necessary for CTL responses, it has been administered in preclinical and human studies.[3, 29] Preclinical studies in a lung SCC model have shown that the T-helper 1–inducing cytokine IL-12 can inhibit tumor growth.[41] Studies in an oral SCC model in mice have shown that interleukin-12 can promote rejection of oral SCC tumors and can stimulate CD4+ T-helper subset responses.[35] The protective IL-12 response was shown to be dependent on expression of the costimulatory molecule CD80 by tumor cells, as well as IFN-γ production by the host for immune rejection. IL-12 and IFN-γ in combination with costimulation may therefore be promising candidates for immune and biologic therapy of SCCHN.

NATURAL KILLER AND LYMPHOKINE-ACTIVATED KILLER CELL RESPONSES

NK cells and lymphokine-activated killer (LAK) cells that are also induced by the T-helper 1 cytokine IL-2 have been characterized.[42, 43] NK and LAK cells from patients have been expanded with the use of IL-2 and have been given along with IL-2 to patients with a variety of cancers. Response rates in large series have been limited to 5% to 12% of patients, but cases of tumor regression and prolonged remission in patients with melanoma and renal cell carcinoma have been reported.[44]

CLINICAL TRIALS OF IMMUNE THERAPY IN HEAD AND NECK SQUAMOUS CELL CARCINOMA

A variety of clinical trials using cytokine-, antibody-, and vector-based therapy have been completed and are the subject of continued investigation in patients with SCCHN (Table 34–2); details are provided in the following sections.

Cytokine-Based and Cellular Adoptive Therapy

Cellular immune deficiency is a consistent finding in patients with advanced cancer of the head and neck.[45] Recombinant cytokines and lymphocytes expanded ex vivo have been used in an effort to augment antitumor immune responses.[46] A study by Cortesina and colleagues, which employed perilymphatic injections of natural IL-2 for 10 days, demonstrated a clinical response in 13 of 20 patients with recurrent, inoperable SCCHN.[47] There were three complete responses, three partial responses, and seven minimal responses. However, despite these initial responses, the cancer uniformly recurred, and subsequent courses of IL-2 were poorly effective. No effects on NK or LAK activity were detected.[47]

Another approach attempted to increase tumor cytolytic activity by tumor-infiltrating lymphocytes (TILs) through local administration of recombinant IL-2 (rIL-2). In an Eastern Cooperative Oncology Group–sponsored phase IB

TABLE 34-2 Summary of Clinical Trials of Biologic Therapy in SCCHN

Therapy	Responses	Reference
Cytokine-based therapy		
Natural interleukin 2	13/20	47
Interleukin 2	2/36	48
Interleukin 2	0/14	49
Interleukin 2, cisplatin, 5-FU	16/30	50
Interleukin 2, interferon-alpha	5/14	51
Interleukin 2, interferon-alpha	2/11	52
Interferon-γ	3/8	65
Natural cytokine mixture (IRX-2)	8/15	70
Monoclonal antibody–based therapy		
186-Re-U36	3/13	81
C225, radiation	15/15	82
EMD 72000	0/9	83
Vector-based therapy		
ONYX-015	5/22 (necrosis)	88
ONYX-015	14% (complete)	89
ONYX-015	21% (complete)	90
ONYX-015, cisplatin, 5-FU	27%	91
ONYX-015, cisplatin, 5-FU	33%	92
Allovectin	1/69 (complete)	100
E1A	0%	101

5-FU, 5-fluorouracil.

trial, 36 patients with stage IV cancer of the head and neck received peritumoral and intranodal injections of escalating doses of rIL-2. Cytolytic activity of TILs isolated from post–rIL-2 tissue was increased against autologous tumor targets; however, there were only two partial clinical responses.[48] In a phase II study, intravenous bolus rIL-2 was administered in patients with recurrent/metastatic carcinoma of the nasopharynx (NPC). Fourteen patients with recurrent/metastatic NPC were entered into the study. No clinical responses and only one treatment-related death from acute myocardial infarction were noted. In short, single-modality intravenous bolus IL-2 was clinically ineffective in patients with NPC, although many patients had received previous therapy that could be potentially immunosuppressive.[49]

Most recently, a phase I pilot study of rIL-2 administration after cisplatin and 5-fluorouracil in 30 patients with advanced cancer of the head and neck showed an overall response rate of 53.3%, with eight complete responses and eight partial responses. It was impressive that the median complete response (CR) duration was 16.2 months.[50]

Currently, there are two phase I trials (IL-2 + IL-12, IL-2 + bryostatin) and one phase III trial studying the effects of IL-2 in head and neck cancer. The phase III trial is evaluating perilymphatic IL-2 administration in combination with radiotherapy.

A phase II study in patients with advanced cancer of the head and neck evaluated the efficacy of combination systemic rIL-2 and IFN-α and assessed laboratory correlates between tumor response and (1) tumor differentiation and (2) NK cell activation.[51] Five of fourteen patients responded; two had partial responses and three had transient responses (one complete and two partial, each lasting less than 4 weeks). Patients who responded had relatively less tumor burden and poorly differentiated metastases. No response was observed in those few individuals in whom natural immune function was only minimally enhanced by therapy. Major toxicity, including but not limited to fever, fatigue, and pulmonary compromise, allowed only 3 of 14 patients to complete three cycles of therapy. This preliminary phase II study shows that combination rIL-2/IFN-α therapy has clinical antitumor activity and that the level of NK cell activation and the degree of tumor differentiation may correlate with response.[51]

In another phase II study of these cytokines in 11 patients with recurrent cancer of the head and neck, two patients (18%) achieved a partial response. Toxic effects were substantial. Three of 11 patients experienced grade III hypotension, and three patients had grade III oliguria. Grade III fatigue was one of the most common reasons for withdrawal from the study. There were no deaths, and there was no need for intensive care monitoring. In view of the 18% response rate, additional investigation of biologic therapy in advanced cancer of the head and neck is warranted.[52] Several trials incorporating IFN-α alone[53] or as an adjuvant combined with retinoic acid and/or standard chemotherapeutic agents have been completed. Low response rates and frequent toxic events were reported.[54-61] In contrast, two recent phase II trials of patients receiving induction chemotherapy combined with IFN-α and concomitant chemoradiotherapy in the management of locoregionally advanced SCCHN demonstrated improved locoregional control and survival rates compared with more standard treatment approaches. It is important to note that there were significant treatment-related toxicities, including 6 deaths among the 93 patients enrolled in these trials.[62, 63]

A phase II adjuvant trial to prevent recurrence or second primary tumors with the use of 13-*cis*-retinoic acid, IFN-α, and alpha-tocopherol in locally advanced-stage head and neck cancer after definitive local treatment with surgery, radiotherapy, or both showed promising results. Thirty-eight (86%) of 44 patients completed the full 12-month treatment course. Median 1- and 2-year rates of overall survival were 98% and 91%, respectively, and rates of disease-free survival were 91% and 84%, respectively. Six patients did not complete treatment owing to intolerable toxicity or social problems. Toxicity generally was consistent with previous IFN-α and 13-*cis*-retinoic acid reports.[64]

Currently, phase I trials are investigating IFN-α in combination with standard chemotherapy in SCCHN. A pilot study is under way to look at the effects of intralesional IFN-α in SCCHN. A multi-institutional phase III randomized study of 13-*cis*-retinoic acid, IFN-α, and alpha-tocopherol (vs. no treatment) to prevent recurrence or second primary tumors in SCCHN patients has been initiated.

A phase I to II trial of recombinant human IFN-γ, given by means of a 24-hour infusion repeated weekly four times in eight patients with cancer of the head and neck, demonstrated that three patients had clinically measurable responses with minimal adverse effects.[65] Preclinical studies of the antitumor effects of IFN-γ in vitro and in murine models suggest that further clinical evaluation of this T-helper 1 cytokine is warranted.[66] Preclinical studies with another T-helper 1 cytokine—IL-12—have shown that it has potent antitumor properties.[67-69] Presently, three phase I trials are under way to look at IL-12 administration alone or in combination with IL-2 in SCCHN. In one of the trials, biodegradable microspheres are being employed as a delivery vehicle. In addition, a phase I trial combining Herceptin antibody directed against the *HER2/NEU* receptor in combination with IL-12 in patients with cancer of the head and neck is currently under way.

A natural cytokine mixture (IRX-2) in combination with cyclophosphamide, indomethacin, and zinc was evaluated in a phase II trial in patients with SCCHN. Eight of 15 patients responded clinically to the 21-day IRX-2 protocol, with one complete response and seven partial responses. IRX-2 immunotherapy induced lymphocyte mobilization and infiltration. Minimal toxic effects were observed, and overall survival may have been improved.[70]

In vitro studies have shown that treatment of mononuclear cells with high-dose human rIL-2 generates a population of LAK cells capable of lysing a variety of human cancer cells in culture in a non–MHC-restricted manner.[71] Preclinical and early clinical trials have shown LAK cells to have anticancer activity in vivo as well.[72] Similarly, TILs have been clonally expanded ex vivo in the presence of rIL-2 in an effort to enrich populations of MHC-restricted tumor-specific T-cells.[73] However, this approach has been largely unsuccessful in SCCHN owing to impaired proliferative responses to cytokine treatment and depressed cytotoxicity against different target cells compared with peripheral blood lymphocytes, despite attempts at sensitization with autologous tumor cells.

A pilot phase I study on the effect of locoregional injections of rIL-2 in association with LAK cells was performed in advanced, recurrent head and neck cancer patients. Fourteen patients were treated with autologous LAKs and rIL-2 given peritumorally. The total daily dose of rIL-2 was escalated from 2400 to 1.8×10^6 IU. Clinical evaluation was performed 30 days from the onset of therapy; there were three partial (95%, 66%, and 50% reduction) responses. These partial responses were found in patients with a tumor burden less than 20 cm². Cervical node metastasis did not respond to treatment. No significant adverse effects were reported.[74]

A nonrandomized phase I clinical trial was conducted to evaluate systemic adoptive T-cell immunotherapy in 17 patients with unresectable SCCHN. Patients were inoculated in the inguinal area with irradiated autologous tumor cells admixed with GM-CSF followed by three additional daily injections of GM-CSF at the vaccination site. Eight to 10 days later, the draining regional lymph nodes were harvested. Lymphocytes were activated ex vivo with staphylococcal enterotoxin A, expanded in IL-2, and infused into patients peripherally. Two patients did not receive T-cells owing to a limited immune response. The toxic effects of infusion were limited to grade II reactions in three treatments, with one patient requiring overnight hospitalization for fever and emesis. The median cell expansion factor was 37, and the median cell dose was 7.5×10^9, with T-cells being the predominant cell type. Three patients demonstrated stabilization of previously progressive disease. Two patients experienced favorable clinical courses after adoptive T-cell transfer, including one patient with no evidence of disease 4 years after surgical resection of a vertebral body metastasis.[75]

Additional studies employing intra-arterial LAK cell infusion at the tumor site have demonstrated limited clinical responses.[76, 77]

Antibody-Based Therapy

Several monoclonal antibodies with reactivity to SCCHN have been developed over the past 2 decades (A9, SCCA, E48, U36, CEA).[11–13, 78, 79] Of these, the monoclonal antibody U36 has shown the most promise for specific targeting of SCCHN.[80] A phase I study to evaluate the suitability of [186]RE-labeled chimeric Mab U36 ([186]RE-cMab U36) for radioimmunotherapy of SCCHN was recently completed. Dosage escalations of 11, 27, and 41 mCi/m² were employed, and tumor detection was monitored by gamma camera. The maximum tolerated dose was established at 27 mCi/m² in 13 patients with recurrent or metastatic disease, and administrations were well tolerated with reportedly excellent targeting of tumor. Myelotoxicity was the only toxicity observed, resulting in dose-limiting toxicity in two patients treated at the highest dose (41 mCi/m²). Two patients showed a marked reduction in tumor size, and another showed stable disease over 6 months.[81]

A number of monoclonal antibodies that have been approved by the U.S. Food and Drug Administration (FDA) for use in the diagnosis and treatment of cancer are under investigation in patients with SCCHN. A phase II/III trial evaluated the safety, pharmacokinetics, and efficacy of a chimeric anti–epidermal growth factor receptor monoclonal antibody, cetuximab (C225), in combination with radiation therapy (RT) in patients with advanced SCCHN. Sixteen patients were treated in a standard dose escalation procedure, with three patients entered into the study at each dose level. The most commonly reported adverse events were fever, transaminase elevation, asthenia, nausea, and skin toxicity (grade I or II in most patients). Skin toxicity outside of the RT field was not strictly dose dependent; however, grade II or higher events were observed in patients treated with higher dose regimens. There was one grade IV allergic reaction; however, most acute adverse effects (xerostomia, mucositis, and local skin toxicity) were associated with RT. All patients achieved an objective response (13 complete and 2 partial remissions), and neutralizing antibodies did not develop against cetuximab in any of the patients. This study demonstrated that cetuximab can be safely administered with RT.[82] Currently, patients with SCCHN are being accrued for a phase II trial and for two phase III trials with C225 in combination with either chemotherapy or RT.

In an open, uncontrolled phase I study, nine patients with stage III and IV SCCHN were treated with five doses of the humanized anti–epidermal growth factor receptor monoclonal antibody EMD 72000 in three consecutive ascending-dose groups. The following adverse events were reported: 5 events of toxicity grade III, 18 events of toxicity grade II, 66 events of toxicity grade I, and 38 events of toxicity grade 0. All adverse events of toxicity grade III were considered to be not related or only remotely related to EMD 72000. The most frequent drug–related adverse events were fever and a transient hepatic enzyme elevation. No objective clinical responses were reported. Overall, this trial demonstrated that EMD 72000 was well tolerated in patients with advanced SCCHN.[83] Most recently, the FDA has approved Herceptin (anti-c-erb-B2) for combined use with chemotherapy in the treatment of advanced breast cancer. Currently, several phase I and II trials are under way to evaluate the use of Herceptin in patients with solid tumors, including SCCHN.

Recently, two clinical trials were completed with anti-CEA monoclonal antibodies in patients with metastatic medullary thyroid carcinoma. In a phase I/II trial of 15 patients with metastatic medullary thyroid carcinoma treated with the radiolabeled bivalent fragment of anti-CEA monoclonal antibody MN-14 (^{131}I-MN-14F(ab)$_2$), myelosuppression was the only significant treatment-related dose-limiting toxicity. Antibodies developed in eight patients 2 to 6 weeks following treatment. Seven patients showed a reduction in serum levels of tumor markers by a median of 55%. One patient showed a dramatic improvement in mass effect on the airway caused by hypopharyngeal lesions, with a 45% reduction of overall tumor burden. Stable disease continued to be radiologically evident in 11 of 12 assessable patients for a period of 3+ to 26+ months. In summary, treatment with ^{131}I-MN-14F(ab)$_2$ was shown to be well tolerated, with evidence of antitumor activity. Humanized chimeric Mab fragments will be necessary in future trials with repeated dose schedules owing to development of human anti-murine antibody response.[84]

A radiolabeled human/murine chimeric monoclonal antibody (^{90}Y-cT84.66), with high affinity and specificity to CEA, was evaluated in a phase I trial of patients with metastatic CEA-producing malignancies, including medullary thyroid carcinoma. Although no major responses were observed, three patients demonstrated stable disease for a period of 3 to 27 months' duration, and two demonstrated a mixed response. A reduction in tumor size was observed with five tumor lesions. Radiolabeled ^{90}Y-cT84.66 was well tolerated, with reversible thrombocytopenia and leukopenia being the only dose-limiting adverse events. Thirteen patients developed an immune response to the antibody.[85] Future trials will focus on strategies to allow for higher dosing and the use of combined therapy with radiation-enhancing chemotherapy drugs. Further efforts to reduce immunogenicity through humanization of the antibody are also planned.

Vector-Based Biologic and Immunotherapy

Over the past decade, viral vectors that express genes targeting nonimmune and immune biologic mechanisms of cancer have been developed. Initial studies demonstrating the feasibility of using these viral vectors to infect SCCHN and other cancers have enabled the development and study of viral vectors that express genes encoding immunomodulatory molecules.

Several studies have been undertaken with ONYX-015, an adenovirus with a deletion of the *E1B* gene, which reportedly selectively replicates in and lyses *p53*-deficient cells.[86] *p53* abnormalities are detected in about 50% of SCCHNs. A phase I study of ONYX-015 was completed in 22 patients with recurrent head and neck cancer. The virus was administered by a single intratumoral injection. Treatment was well tolerated, with the main toxicity being grade I/II flulike symptoms. The highest dose administered (10^{11} plaque-forming units) did not cause any dose-limiting toxicity. Twenty-one of the 22 patients demonstrated an increase in neutralizing antibody to adenovirus. In situ hybridization showed viral replication in 4 of 22 patients treated, all of whom had mutant *p53* tumors. No objective responses were observed with the use of conventional response criteria; however, radiological evidence of tumor necrosis was seen at the site of viral injection in five patients. Of these five cases, four had mutant *p53* tumors. An additional eight patients had stable disease in the injected tumors, lasting from 4 to 8 weeks. These preliminary results show that intratumoral administration of ONYX-015 is feasible, well tolerated, and associated with biologic activity.[87]

Of note, a recently completed phase I trial of intravenous delivery of ONYX-015 in 10 patients with advanced carcinoma metastatic to the lung was also well tolerated at doses up to 2×10^{13} particles. Infection of metastatic pulmonary sites with ONYZ-015 showed subsequent intratumoral viral replication, suggesting feasibility of this approach.[88]

In a phase II trial of 40 patients with recurrent/relapsing SCCHN following previous conventional treatment, multiple intratumoral injections of ONYX-015 resulted in a complete response rate of 14%, a stable disease rate of 41%, and a progressive disease rate of 45%. Treatment-related toxicity included mild to moderate fever and pain at the injection site. Detectable circulating ONYX-015 genome in 41% of tested patients during the first week following administration of the virus was suggestive of intratumoral replication. This study demonstrated that multiple intralesional injections of ONYX-15 can be safely administered with evidence to suggest the presence of modest antitumoral activity.[89]

A second phase II trial of multiple intratumoral and peritumoral ONYX-015 injections in 37 patients with recurrent head and neck carcinoma showed evidence of selective infectivity of ONYX-015 in the tumor tissue of 7 of 11 patients but not in immediately adjacent normal tissue (0 of 11 patients; $P = .01$). In 21% of evaluable patients, significant tumor regression (>50%) occurred, whereas no toxicity to injected normal peritumoral tissues was demonstrated. Tissue destruction was also highly selective in that *p53* mutant tumors were significantly more likely to undergo ONYX-015–induced necrosis (7 of 12) than were *p53* wild-type tumors (0 of 7; $P = .017$). It is interesting to note that high neutralizing antiadenovirus antibody titers did not prevent infection and/or replication within tumors.[90]

Although ONYX-015 and chemotherapy have demonstrated antitumoral activity in patients with recurrent head and neck cancer, disease recurs rapidly with either therapy alone. Two recently completed phase II trials of a combination of intratumoral ONYX-015 injection with cisplatin and 5-fluorouracil in patients with recurrent SCCHN showed substantial objective responses, including a high proportion of complete responses (27% and 33%). In one of these studies, none of the responding tumors had progressed by 6 months, whereas all noninjected tumors treated with chemotherapy alone had progressed. In both trials, the toxic effects were acceptable. This novel treatment approach offers hope for patients with limited treatment alternatives and provides the foundation for a phase III clinical trial.

Currently, a phase I study of intra-arterial ONYX-015 is being conducted, as is a phase II trial of intratumoral ONYX-015 administration in combination with RT and chemotherapy.[91, 92] Plans for a phase III trial of ONYX-015 in patients with SCCHN are under way.[93]

In addition to adenoviral vectors, recombinant pox viruses are being employed to generate immune responses to tumor antigens in preclinical[94, 95] and clinical studies of solid tumors,[96, 97] and studies that include patients with SCCHN are currently under way. In a phase I trial, 18 patients with advanced solid tumors expressing CEA received recombinant vaccinia (rV)-CEA and recombinant avipox-CEA vaccinations. CEA-specific T-cell responses were seen without significant toxicity, and antibody production against CEA was observed in some of the treated patients. The treatment was well tolerated. Limited clinical activity was seen with the use of vaccines alone in this patient population with end-stage disease. Further trials are planned in patients with less advanced disease, in whom the vaccine could potentially have greater clinical activity.[98] A phase I trial employing fowlpox-CEA-TRICOM and rV-CEA-TRICOM in advanced solid tumors recently opened, and a second phase I trial of intralesional fowlpox-TRICOM is currently being conducted in patients with advanced SCCHN.

Allovectin-7 is a drug designed to produce expression of a foreign class I MHC protein (HLA-B7). The construct comprises a plasmid complementary DNA complexed with a cationic lipid.[99] A total of 69 patients were enrolled in three clinical trials—a single-center phase I trial followed by two multicenter phase II trials. In the phase I trial, nine patients with advanced SCCHN who had failed conventional therapy and did not express HLA-B7 were treated with Allovectin-7 by direct intratumoral injection. No toxic effects from the gene therapy were noted. Four patients demonstrated a partial response to treatment, evidenced by a gradual reduction in tumor size. Analysis of the biopsy specimens from two of the patients who responded to therapy demonstrated HLA-B7 expression. In subsequent trials, patients with advanced SCCHN received two biweekly intratumoral injections of Allovectin-7 followed by 4 weeks of observation. Treatment was repeated once in patients with stable or responding disease after the observation period had ended. Overall, treatment was well tolerated, with no grade III or IV drug-related toxic effects. Of 69 patients treated, 23 (33%) had stable disease or a partial response after the first cycle of treatment and proceeded to the second cycle. After the second cycle, six patients had stable disease, four had a partial response, and one had a complete response. Responses persisted for 21 to 106 weeks.[100] Further investigations are planned in patients with less advanced disease, in whom Allovectin-7 therapy could potentially improve patient survival. A multicenter phase II trial of Allovectin-7 in SCCHN patients is currently under way.

The *E1A* adenovirus gene functions as a tumor inhibitor gene that induces apoptosis of cancer cells. *E1A* also sensitizes cancer cells to chemotherapeutic drugs such as etoposide, cisplatin, and taxol. A phase I study was conducted of the *E1A* gene delivered by intratumoral injection as a lipid complex with 3-beta[*N*-(n',n'-dimethylaminoethane)-carbamoyl]-cholesterol/dioleoylphosphatidyl-ethanolamine (tgDCC-E1A). Nine patients with recurrent and unresectable head and neck cancer were enrolled. No dose-limiting toxicity was observed, and all patients tolerated the injections, although several experienced pain and bleeding at the injection site. A maximally tolerated dose was not reached in this study. *E1A* gene transfer was demonstrated in 14 of 15 tumor samples tested.[101]

OBSTACLES REMAINING

Besides the lack of appropriate signals for development of immunity, it is becoming increasingly clear that SCCHN produces factors that may have deleterious effects on the immune system. Young and coworkers have identified a subset of CD34+ inflammatory cells that inhibit immunity and are associated with aggressive growth.[102] Infiltration and activation of these cells appear to be stimulated by vascular endothelial growth factor and GM-CSF produced by SCCHN cells.[102, 103] Gastman and associates have shown that T-lymphocytes in patients with SCCHN undergo increased cell death in the peripheral blood and tumor environment, and this appears to result from the production of FAS ligand by SCCHN cells.[104] Duffey and Sunwoo and their colleagues have shown that inhibition of expression of these and other cytokine factors inhibits tumorigenesis of SCCHN xenografts in mice.[105, 106] These factors appear to have effects that promote blood supply (angiogenesis) to SCCs.[106]

FUTURE DIRECTIONS

Understanding the complex processes involved in antitumor immune responses and tumor evasion mechanisms is important for evaluating the limited effectiveness of clinical immunotherapy studies observed to date and for developing approaches for more effective immune and biologic therapy in the future. To optimize the likelihood that remaining obstacles will be overcome, future immunotherapeutic strategies must continue to take into account three fundamental goals: (1) The mechanisms of immune unresponsiveness need to be determined and strategies included that inhibit the effects of negative regulatory factors; (2) the host immune system should be maximally stimulated to specifically recognize and attack tumor cells without inducing unacceptable autoimmune toxicitiy; and (3) tumor cells should be maximally accessible for processing, and for recognition and attack by the immune system. The recent appreciation that many of the factors involved in immune modulation also promote tumor growth through non-immunologic mechanisms such as autocrine proliferation and angiogenesis may expand the opportunities for biologic therapy targeted against these mechanisms.

REFERENCES

1. Himmelweit B: The Collected Papers of Paul Ehrlich. Oxford, England, Pergamon Press, 1957.
2. Burnet FM: The concept of immunological surveillance. In Schwartz RS (ed): Progress in Experimental Tumor Research. Basel, Karger, 1970, p 1.

3. Schreiber HS: Tumor immunology. In Paul WE (ed): Fundamental Immunology, 3rd ed. New York, Raven Press, 1993, p 1143.

4. Collins JL, Patek PQ, Cohn M: *In vivo* surveillance of tumorigenic cells transformed *in vitro*. Nature 299:169, 1982.

5. Thomas GR, Chen Z, Oechsli MN, et al: Decreased expression of CD80 is a marker for increased tumorigenicity in a new murine model of oral squamous-cell carcinoma. Int J Cancer 82:377, 1999.

6. Penn I: Principles of tumor immunity: Immunocompetence and cancer. In De Vita VT, Hellman S, Rosenberg SA (eds): Biologic Therapy of Cancer. Philadelphia, JB Lippincott, 1995, p 103.

7. Levine MI, Reidbord HE, Busis SN: Carcinoma of the larynx: A case of apparent regression after inadequate therapy. Arch Otolaryngol 91:385, 1970.

8. Kawakami Y, Robbins PF: Biology of tumor antigens. In De Vita VT, Hellman S, Rosenberg SA (eds): Biologic Therapy of Cancer. Philadelphia: JB Lippincott, 1995, p 53.

9. Mastrangelo MJ, Maguire HC, Lattime EC, et al: Whole cell vaccines. In De Vita VT, Hellman S, Rosenberg SA (eds): Biologic Therapy of Cancer. Philadelphia, JB Lippincott, 1995, p 648.

10. Van Waes C, Kozarsky KF, Warren AB, et al: The A9 antigen associated with aggressive human squamous cell carcinoma has structural and functional similarity to the integrin alpha6/beta4. Cancer Res 51:2395, 1991.

11. Van Waes C, Carey TE: Overexpression of the A9 antigen/alpha 6 beta 4 integrin in head and neck cancer. Otolaryngol Clin North Am 25:111, 1992.

12. van Dongen GA, Brakenhoff RM, ten Brink CT, et al: Squamous cell carcinoma–associated antigens used in novel strategies for the detection and treatment of minimal residual head and neck cancer. Anticancer Res 16:2409, 1996.

13. Greiner JW, Kantor JA, Tsang KY, et al: Carcinoembryonic antigen as a target for specific immunotherapy of head and neck cancer. Cancer Res 62:5049, 2002.

14. Hodge JW: Carcinoembryonic antigen as a target for cancer vaccines. Cancer Immunol Immunother 43:127, 1996.

15. Makino K, Ogata T, Miyake H, et al: Expression of tumor-associated glycoantigen, sialyl Lewis(a), in human head and neck squamous cell carcinoma and its application to tumor immunotherapy. Jpn J Cancer Res 85:887, 1994.

16. Ropke M, Hald J, Guldberg P, et al: Spontaneous human squamous cell carcinomas are killed by a human cytotoxic T lymphocyte clone recognizing a wild-type p53-derived peptide. Proc Natl Acad Sci U S A 93:14704, 1996.

17. Hoffmann TK, Nakano K, Elder EM, et al: Generation of T cells specific for the wild-type sequence p53(264–272) peptide in cancer patients: Implications for immunoselection of epitope loss variants. J Immunol 165:5938, 2000.

18. Nakao M, Shichijo S, Imaizumi T, et al: Identification of a gene coding for a new squamous cell carcinoma antigen recognized by the CTL. J Immunol 164:2565, 2000.

19. Beck-Engeser GB, Monach PA, Mumberg D, et al: Point mutation in essential genes with loss or mutation of the second allele. Relevance to the retention of tumor-specific antigens. J Exp Med 194:285, 2001.

20. Yasumura S, Hirabayashi H, Schwartz DR, et al: Human cytotoxic T-cell lines with restricted specificity for squamous cell carcinoma of the head and neck. Cancer Res 53:1461, 1993.

21. Caignard A, Dietrich PY, Morand V, et al: Evidence for T-cell clonal expansion in a patient with squamous cell carcinoma of the head and neck. Cancer Res 54:1292, 1994.

22. Hald J, Rasmussen N, Claesson MH: Tumour-infiltrating lymphocytes mediate lysis of autologous squamous cell carcinomas of the head and neck. Cancer Immunol Immunother 41:243, 1995.

23. Mandruzzato S, Brasseur F, Andry G, et al: A CASP-8 mutation recognized by cytolytic T lymphocytes on a human head and neck carcinoma. J Exp Med 186:785, 1997.

24. Shichijo S, Nakao M, Imai Y, et al: A gene encoding antigenic peptides of human squamous cell carcinoma recognized by cytotoxic T lymphocytes. J Exp Med 187:277, 1998.

25. Hogan KT, Eisinger DP, Cupp SB 3rd, et al: The peptide recognized by HLA-A68.2-restricted, squamous cell carcinoma of the lung-specific cytotoxic T lymphocytes is derived from a mutated elongation factor 2 gene. Cancer Res 58:5144, 1998.

26. Van Waes C, Urban JL, Rothstein JL, et al: Highly malignant tumor variants retain tumor-specific antigens recognized by T helper cells. J Exp Med 164:1547, 1986.

27. Grandis JR, Falkner DM, Melhem MF, et al: Human leukocyte antigen class I allelic and haplotype loss in squamous cell carcinoma of the head and neck: Clinical and immunogenetic consequences. Clin Cancer Res 6:2794, 2000.

28. Arosarena OA, Baranwal S, Strome S, et al: Expression of major histocompatibility complex antigens in squamous cell carcinomas of the head and neck: Effects of interferon gene transfer. Otolaryngol Head Neck Surg 120:665, 1999.

29. Restifo NP, Wunderlich JR: Biology of cellular immune responses. In De Vita VT, Hellman S, Rosenberg SA (eds): Biologic Therapy of Cancer. Philadelphia, JB Lippincott, 1995, p 3.

30. Shedlock DJ, Weiner DB: DNA vaccination: Antigen presentation and the induction of immunity. J Leukoc Biol 68:793, 2000.

31. Kass E, Panicali DL, Mazzara G, et al: Granulocyte/macrophage-colony stimulating factor produced by recombinant avian poxviruses enriches the regional lymph nodes with antigen-presenting cells and acts as an immunoadjuvant. Cancer Res 61:206, 2001.

32. Chen Z, Malhotra PS, Thomas GR, et al: Expression of proinflammatory and proangiogenic cytokines in patients with head and neck cancer. Clin Cancer Res 5:1369, 1999.

33. Bronte V, Chappell DB, Apolloni E, et al: Unopposed production of granulocyte-macrophage colony-stimulating factor by tumors inhibits CD8+ T cell responses by dysregulating antigen-presenting cell maturation. J Immunol 162:5728, 1999.

34. Grosenbach DW, Barrientos JC, Schlom J, et al: Synergy of vaccine strategies to amplify antigen-specific immune responses and antitumor effects. Cancer Res 61:4497, 2001.

35. Thomas GR, Chen Z, Enamorado I, et al: IL-12- and IL-2-induced tumor regression in a new murine model of oral squamous-cell carcinoma is promoted by expression of the CD80 co-stimulatory molecule and interferon-gamma. Int J Cancer 86:368, 2000.

36. Lang S, Atarashi Y, Nishioka Y, et al: B7.1 on human carcinomas: Costimulation of T cells and enhanced tumor-induced T-cell death. Cell Immunol 201:132, 2000.

37. Ghosh P, Komschlies KL, Cippitelli M, et al: Gradual loss of T-helper 1 populations in spleen of mice during progressive tumor growth. J Natl Cancer Inst 87:1478, 1995.

38. Karcher J, Reisser C, Daniel V, et al: Cytokine expression of transforming growth factor-beta2 and interleukin-10 in squamous carcinomas of the head and neck. Comparison of tissue expression and serum levels. HNO 47:879, 1999.

39. Myers JN, Yasumura S, Suminami Y, et al: Growth stimulation of human head and neck squamous cell carcinoma cell lines by interleukin 4. Clin Cancer Res 2:127, 1996.

40. Vlock DR, Schantz SP, Fisher SG, et al: Clinical correlates of circulating immune complexes and antibody reactivity in squamous cell carcinoma of the head and neck. The Department of Veterans Affairs Laryngeal Cancer Study Group. J Clin Oncol 11:2427, 1993.

41. Myers JN, Mank-Seymour A, Zitvogel L, et al: Interleukin-12 gene therapy prevents establishment of SCC VII squamous cell carcinomas, inhibits tumor growth, and elicits long-term antitumor immunity in syngeneic C3H mice. Laryngoscope 108:261, 1998.

42. Whiteside TL, Vujanovic NL, Herberman RB: Natural killer cells and tumor therapy. Curr Top Microbiol Immunol 230:221, 1998.

43. Rosenberg SA: The development of new immunotherapies for the treatment of cancer using interleukin-2. A review. Ann Surg 208:121, 1988.

44. Rosenberg SA, Lotze MT, Yang JC, et al: Prospective randomized trial of high-dose interleukin-2 alone or in conjunction with lymphokine-activated killer cells for the treatment of patients with advanced cancer. J Natl Cancer Inst 85:622, 1993.

45. Cortesina G, De Stefani A, Sacchi M, et al: Immunomodulation therapy for squamous cell carcinoma of the head and neck. Head Neck 15:266, 1993.

46. Rosenberg SA, Packard BS, Aebersold PM, et al: Use of tumor-infiltrating lymphocytes and interleukin-2 in the immunotherapy of patients with metastatic melanoma. A preliminary report. N Engl J Med 319:1676, 1988.

47. Cortesina G, De Stefani A, Giovarelli M, et al: Treatment of recurrent squamous cell carcinoma of the head and neck with low doses of interleukin-2 injected perilymphatically. Cancer 62:2482, 1988.

48. Whiteside TL, Letessier E, Hirabayashi H, et al: Evidence for local and systemic activation of immune cells by peritumoral injections of interleukin 2 in patients with advanced squamous cell carcinoma of the head and neck. Cancer Res 53:5654, 1993.

49. Chi KH, Myers JN, Chow KC, et al: Phase II trial of systemic recombinant interleukin-2 in the treatment of refractory nasopharyngeal carcinoma. Oncology 60:110, 2001.

50. Airoldi M, De Stefani A, Marchionatti S, et al: Survival in patients with recurrent squamous cell head and neck carcinoma treated with bio-chemotherapy. Head Neck 23:298, 2001.

51. Schantz SP, Dimery I, Lippman SM, et al: A phase II study of interleukin-2 and interferon-alpha in head and neck cancer. Invest New Drugs 10:217, 1992.

52. Urba SG, Forastiere AA, Wolf GT, et al: Intensive recombinant interleukin-2 and alpha-interferon therapy in patients with advanced head and neck squamous carcinoma. Cancer 71:2326, 1993.

53. Vlock DR, Andersen J, Kalish LA, et al: Phase II trial of interferon-alpha in locally recurrent or metastatic squamous cell carcinoma of the head and neck: Immunological and clinical correlates. J Immunother Emphasis Tumor Immunol 19:433, 1996.

54. Voravud N, Lippman SM, Weber RS, et al: Phase II trial of 13-cis retinoic acid plus interferon-alpha in advanced squamous cell carcinoma of head and neck, refractory to chemotherapy. Invest New Drugs 11:57, 1993.

55. Roth AD, Abele R, Alberto P: 13-cis-retinoic acid plus interferon-alpha: A phase II clinical study in squamous cell carcinoma of the lung and the head and neck. Oncology 51:84, 1994.

56. Cascinu S, Del Ferro E, Ligi M, et al: Phase II trial of 13-cis-retinoic acid plus interferon-alpha in recurrent head and neck cancer. Oncology 51:84, 1994.

57. Cascinu S, Fedeli A, Luzi Fedeli S, et al: 5-Fluorouracil and interferon alpha 2b for recurrent or metastatic head and neck cancer. Br J Cancer 69:392, 1994.

58. Langer CJ, Schaebler D, Sauter E, et al: Phase II study of N-phosphonacetyl-L-aspartate, recombinant interferon-alpha, and fluorouracil infusion in advanced squamous cell carcinoma of the head and neck. Head Neck 20:385, 1998.

59. Schrijvers D, Johnson J, Jiminez U, et al: Phase III trial of modulation of cisplatin/fluorouracil chemotherapy by interferon alfa-2b in patients with recurrent or metastatic head and neck cancer. Head and Neck Interferon Cooperative Study Group. J Clin Oncol 16:1054, 1998.

60. Gravis G, Pech-Gourgh F, Viens P, et al: Phase II study of a combination of low-dose cisplatin with 13-cis-retinoic acid and interferon-alpha in patients with advanced head and neck squamous cell carcinoma. Anticancer Drugs 10:369, 1999.

61. Goncalves A, Camerlo J, Bun H, et al: Phase II study of a combination of cisplatin, all-trans-retinoic acid and interferon-alpha in squamous cell carcinoma: Clinical results and pharmacokinetics. Anticancer Res 21:1431, 2001.

62. Shin DM, Khuri FR, Murphy B, et al: Combined interferon-alfa, 13-cis-retinoic acid, and alpha-tocopherol in locally advanced head and neck squamous cell carcinoma: Novel bioadjuvant phase II trial. J Clin Oncol 19:3010, 2001.

63. Mantz CA, Vokes EE, Kies MS, et al: Sequential induction chemotherapy and concomitant chemoradiotherapy in the management of locoregionally advanced laryngeal cancer. Ann Oncol 12:343, 2001.

64. Mantz CA, Vokes EE, Stenson K, et al: Induction chemotherapy followed by concomitant chemoradiotherapy in the treatment of locoregionally advanced oropharyngeal cancer. Cancer J 7:140, 2001.

65. Richtsmeier WJ, Koch WM, McGuire WP, et al: Phase I–II study of advanced head and neck squamous cell carcinoma patients treated with recombinant human interferon gamma. Arch Otolaryngol Head Neck Surg 116:1271, 1990.

66. Baron S, Tyring SK, Fleischmann WR Jr, et al: The interferons. Mechanisms of action and clinical applications. JAMA 266:1375, 1991.

67. Rodolfo M, Colombo MP: Interleukin-12 as an adjuvant for cancer immunotherapy. Methods 19:114, 1999.

68. Kuriakose MA, Chen FA, Egilmez NK, et al: Interleukin-12 delivered by biodegradable microspheres promotes the antitumor activity of human peripheral blood lymphocytes in a human head and neck tumor xenograft/SCID mouse model. Head Neck 22:57, 2000.

69. Parmiani G, Rivoltini L, Andreola G, et al: Cytokines in cancer therapy. Immunol Lett 74:41, 2000.

70. Barrera JL, Verastegui E, Meneses A, et al: Combination immunotherapy of squamous cell carcinoma of the head and neck: A phase 2 trial. Arch Otolaryngol Head Neck Surg 126:345, 2000.

71. Rayner AA, Grimm EA, Lotze MT, et al: Lymphokine-activated killer (LAK) cell phenomenon. IV. Lysis by LAK cell clones of fresh human tumor cells from autologous and multiple allogeneic tumors. J Natl Cancer Inst 75:67, 1985.

72. Sussman JJ, Shu S, Sondak VK, et al: Activation of T lymphocytes for the adoptive immunotherapy of cancer. Ann Surg Oncol 1:296, 1994.

73. Rosenberg SA, Packard BS, Aebersold PM, et al: Use of tumor-infiltrating lymphocytes and interleukin-2 in the immunotherapy of patients with metastatic melanoma. A preliminary report. N Engl J Med 319:1676, 1988.

74. Squadrelli-Saraceno M, Rivoltini L, Cantu G, et al: Local adoptive immunotherapy of advanced head and neck tumors with LAK cells and interleukin-2. Tumori 76:566, 1990.

75. To WC, Wood BG, Krauss JC, et al: Systemic adoptive T-cell immunotherapy in recurrent and metastatic carcinoma of the head and neck: A phase 1 study. Arch Otolaryngol Head Neck Surg 126:1225, 2000.

76. Ikawa T, Eura M, Fukiage T, et al: Adoptive immunotherapy by intra-arterial infusion of ATLAK or Allo-TLAK cells in patients with head and neck cancer. Gan To Kagaku Ryoho 16:1438, 1989.

77. Sato M, Yoshida H, Kaji R, et al: Induction of bone formation in an adenoid cystic carcinoma of the maxillary sinus by adoptive immunotherapy involving intra-arterial injection of lymphokine-activated killer cells and recombinant interleukin-2 in combination with radiotherapy. J Biol Response Mod 9:329, 1990.

78. de Bree R, Roos JC, Quak JJ, et al: Radioimmunoscintigraphy and biodistribution of technetium-99m-labeled monoclonal antibody U36 in patients with head and neck cancer. Clin Cancer Res 1:591, 1995.

79. Cataltepe S, Gornstein ER, Schick C, et al: Co-expression of the squamous cell carcinoma antigens 1 and 2 in normal adult human tissues and squamous cell carcinomas. J Histochem Cytochem 48:113, 2000.

80. Colnot DR, Quak JJ, Roos JC, et al: Phase I therapy study of 186 Re-labeled chimeric monoclonal antibody U36 in patients with squamous cell carcinoma of the head and neck. J Nucl Med 41:1999, 2000.

81. Colnot DR, Quak JJ, Roos JC, et al: Radioimmunotherapy in patients with head and neck squamous cell carcinoma: Initial experience. Head Neck 23:559, 2001.

82. Robert F, Ezekiel MP, Spencer SA, et al: Phase I study of anti–epidermal growth factor receptor antibody cetuximab in combination with radiation therapy in patients with advanced head and neck cancer. J Clin Oncol 19:3234, 2001.

83. Bier H, Hoffmann T, Hauser U, et al: Clinical trial with escalating doses of the antiepidermal growth factor receptor humanized monoclonal antibody EMD 72 000 in patients with advanced squamous cell carcinoma of the larynx and hypopharynx. Cancer Chemother Pharmacol 47:519, 2001.

84. Juweid ME, Hajjar G, Swayne LC, et al: Phase I/II trial of (131)I-MN-14F(ab)2 anti–carcinoembryonic antigen monoclonal antibody in the treatment of patients with metastatic medullary thyroid carcinoma. Cancer 85:1828, 1999.

85. Wong JYC, Chu DZ, Yamauchi DM, et al: A phase I radioimmunotherapy trial evaluating 90 yttrium-labeled anti-carcinoembryonic antigen (CEA) chimeric T84.66 in patients with metastatic CEA-producing malignancies. Clin Cancer Res 6:3855, 2000.

86. Heise C, Sampson-Johannes A, Williams A, et al: ONYX-015, an E1B gene-attenuated adenovirus, causes tumor-specific cytolysis and antitumoral efficacy that can be augmented by standard chemotherapeutic agents. Nat Med 3:639, 1997.

87. Ganly I, Kirn D, Eckhardt SG, et al: A phase I study of Onyx-015, an E1B attenuated adenovirus, administered intratumorally to patients with recurrent head and neck cancer. Clin Cancer Res 6:798, 2000.

88. Nemunaitis J, Cunningham C, Buchanan A, et al: Intravenous infusion of a replication-selective adenovirus (ONYX-015) in cancer patients: Safety, feasibility and biological activity. Gene Ther 8:746, 2001.

89. Nemunaitis J, Khuri F, Ganly I, et al: Phase II trial of intratumoral administration of ONYX-015, a replication-selective adenovirus, in patients with refractory head and neck cancer. J Clin Oncol 19:289, 2001.

90. Nemunaitis J, Ganly I, Khuri F, et al: Selective replication and oncolysis in p53 mutant tumors with ONYX-015, an E1B-55kD gene-deleted adenovirus, in patients with advanced head and neck cancer: A phase II trial. Cancer Res 60:6359, 2000.

91. Khuri FR, Nemunaitis J, Ganly I, et al: A controlled trial of intratumoral ONYX-015, a selectively-replicating adenovirus, in combination with cisplatin and 5-fluorouracil in patients with recurrent head and neck cancer. Nat Med 6:879, 2000.

92. Lamont JP, Nemunaitis J, Kuhn JA, et al: A prospective phase II trial of ONYX-015 adenovirus and chemotherapy in recurrent squamous cell carcinoma of the head and neck (the Baylor experience). Ann Surg Oncol 7:588, 2000.

93. [No authors listed]: Onyx plans phase III trial of ONYX-015 for head & neck cancer. Oncologist 4:432, 1999.

94. Kass E, Parker J, Schlom J, et al: Comparative studies of the effects of recombinant GM-CSF and GM-CSF administered via a poxvirus to enhance the concentration of antigen-presenting cells in regional lymph nodes. Cytokine 12:960, 2000.

95. Kass E, Schlom J, Thompson J, et al: Induction of protective host immunity to carcinoembryonic antigen (CEA), a self-antigen in CEA transgenic mice, by immunizing with a recombinant vaccinia-CEA virus. Cancer Res 59:676, 1999.

96. Horig H, Lee DS, Conkright W, et al: Phase I clinical trial of a recombinant canarypoxvirus (ALVAC) vaccine expressing human carcinoembryonic antigen and the B7.1 co-stimulatory molecule. Cancer Immunol Immunother 49:504, 2000.

97. Marshall JL, Hawkins MJ, Tsang KY, et al: Phase I study in cancer patients of a replication-defective avipox recombinant vaccine that expresses human carcinoembryonic antigen. J Clin Oncol 17:332, 1999.

98. Marshall JL, Hoyer RJ, Toomey MA, et al: Phase I study in advanced cancer patients of a diversified prime-and-boost vaccination protocol using recombinant vaccinia virus and recombinant nonreplicating avipox virus to elicit anti-carcinoembryonic antigen immune responses. J Clin Oncol 18:3964, 2000.

99. Lew D, Parker SE, Latimer T, et al: Cancer gene therapy using plasmid DNA: Pharmacokinetic study of DNA following injection in mice. Hum Gene Ther 6:553, 1995.

100. Gleich LL, Gluckman JL, Nemunaitis J, et al: Clinical experience with HLA-B7 plasmid DNA/lipid complex in advanced squamous cell carcinoma of the head and neck. Arch Otolaryngol Head Neck Surg 127:775, 2001.

101. Yoo GH, Hung MC, Lopez-Berestein G, et al: Phase I trial of intratumoral liposome E1A gene therapy in patients with recurrent breast and head and neck cancer. Clin Cancer Res 7:1237, 2001.

102. Young MR, Petruzzelli GJ, Kolesiak K, et al: Human squamous cell carcinomas of the head and neck chemoattract immune suppressive CD34(+) progenitor cells. Hum Immunol 62:332, 2001.

103. Pak AS, Wright MA, Matthews JP, et al: Mechanisms of immune suppression in patients with head and neck cancer: Presence of CD34(+) cells which suppress immune functions within cancers that secrete granulocyte-macrophage colony-stimulating factor. Clin Cancer Res 1:95, 1995.

104. Gastman BR, Atarshi Y, Reichert TE, et al: Fas ligand is expressed on human squamous cell carcinomas of the head and neck, and it promotes apoptosis of T lymphocytes. Cancer Res 59:5356, 1999.

105. Duffey DC, Chen Z, Dong G, et al: Expression of a dominant-negative mutant inhibitor-kappaBalpha of nuclear factor-kappaB in human head and neck squamous cell carcinoma inhibits survival, proinflammatory cytokine expression, and tumor growth in vivo. Cancer Res 59:3468, 1999.

106. Sunwoo JB, Chen Z, Dong G, et al: Novel proteasome inhibitor PS-341 inhibits activation of nuclear factor-kappa B, cell survival, tumor growth, and angiogenesis in squamous cell carcinoma. Clin Cancer Res 7:1419, 2001.

CHAPTER 35

Rehabilitation of Swallowing and Speech in Head and Neck Surgery

Thomas Murry

Tamara Wasserman

Ricardo L. Carrau

◘ INTRODUCTION

The interrelated management of swallowing and speech disorders in patients with head and neck cancer dates back to more than 100 years ago when the first reported laryngectomy by Billroth and Gussenbauer in 1874 also included a report of fitting a patient with a pneumatic artificial larynx that introduced sound into the pharynx through a surgically created fistula.[1] The fistula aided the patient in communication, and it also reduced the propelling force associated with swallowing. Since that time, attention to swallowing and communication skills has increased dramatically with the advent of numerous surgical procedures to preserve voice and speech in patients after treatment of cancer of the head and neck.

The management of dysphagia began its modern era only recently in 1983 with the publication of Logemann's text on the evaluation and treatment of swallowing disorders.[2] Logemann outlined the rationale for fluoroscopic assessment of swallowing disorders and the protocol for identifying the disordered phases of swallowing. This functional evaluation using the modified barium swallow (MBS) assessment protocol is rooted in the early work of Barclay, who in 1930 reported on the use of fluoroscopy to identify normal swallowing behavior.[3] Many current surgical procedures as well as nonsurgical therapies, including radiation and combined chemoradiation, used in the management of patients with cancer of the head and neck disrupt the natural swallowing patterns or compound already existing problems of swallowing caused by the disease process. Moreover, these oncologic procedures contribute to voice changes such as hoarseness and weak voice, altered resonance, and disorders of speech articulation.[4, 5]

The oral cavity, pharynx, and larynx share the functions of channeling expiratory air flow and voice upward and outward and propelling food, liquids, and medications downward into the esophagus and stomach. Because of this shared passage, the speech-language pathologist (SLP) who is uniquely trained in the anatomy, physiology, and neurology of the head, neck, and upper aerodigestive tract is the ideal person to coordinate the preoperative and postoperative rehabilitation of voice, speech, and swallowing for patients with head and neck cancer. The otolaryngologist and the SLP maintain a close relationship during the rehabilitation period.

Over the past 125 years, speech, voice, and swallowing problems of patients with cancer of the larynx have been addressed extensively with esophageal speech, artificial and electronic larynges, and tracheoesophageal voice prostheses.[6] However, conservation surgery such as supracricoid partial laryngectomy and cricohyoidoepiglottopexy (CHEP),[7] as well as radiation and chemoradiation treatments for the management of cancer of the larynx,[8] have resulted in new challenges for the SLP in treating swallowing and speech disorders following these alternative oncologic treatments. The return of swallowing function after organ-preserving nonsurgical or conservation surgical treatment for cancers of the oral cavity or of the oropharynx requires a coordinated program of dysphagia management.[9] As these treatments are refined to improve chances for survival, patients' needs for speech and swallowing rehabilitation also increase if an optimal quality of life is to be achieved.[10, 11]

This chapter combines the issues of dysphagia rehabilitation and recovery of speech and voice in order to promote understanding of the complex problems and management alternatives associated with speech and swallowing disorders following treatment for cancer of the head and neck. Because aspiration often occurs in patients with advanced head and neck cancer, rehabilitation issues associated with speech, voice, and swallowing should be addressed early and aggressively to ensure maximal nutrition and communication before, during, and after treatments for head and neck cancer.[12]

Stenson and associates found that only 26 of 79 patients with stage III or IV head or neck cancer had normal swallowing function, highlighting the high incidence of swallowing disorders in the head and neck cancer population before treatment.[13] Measures of treatment efficacy[14–17] and treatment effectiveness[18] have shown that comprehensive management that begins before curative treatment maximizes recovery of swallowing function and improves quality of life following treatment for patients with cancer of the head and neck.

THE NORMAL SWALLOW

Phases of Swallowing

Normal swallowing comprises four physiologically distinct phases—the oral preparatory, oral, pharyngeal, and esophageal phases.[2] During the oral preparatory and oral phases, the food is prepared for ingestion. These two phases involve movements that are voluntary; the oral preparatory phase mainly comprises mastication, and the oral phase involves manipulation of the bolus and preparation for its transfer into the oropharynx. During the oral phase, the base of the tongue elevates to reach the soft palate, thus providing a mechanical barrier that impedes premature spillage into the pharynx before it is ready to receive the bolus. The complexity of the oral preparatory and oral phases is often underestimated; preparation of the bolus involves a complex interaction of the mastication apparatus, facial muscles, tongue, and oropharynx.[19] Although these two phases are considered "voluntary," the preparation of the bolus of food to an adequate consistency and size, through grinding of the teeth and the addition of saliva, is completed without a conscious effort. Additionally, during the oral preparatory and oral phases, afferent input from the oral cavity triggers reflexes in the pharynx and larynx that prepare the latter to receive the bolus of food.

At the end of the oral stage, the bolus of food is propelled to the oropharynx, and the pharyngeal phase is initiated. Radiographically, the onset of the pharyngeal phase is defined as the onset of hyoid elevation. Arrival of the bolus in the oropharynx triggers the swallowing reflex, resulting in elevation of the palate to open the pharyngeal introitus. Elevation of the palate also serves to seal off the nasopharynx, and the posterior motion of the base of the tongue actively transfers the bolus of food into the hypopharynx. Propulsion of the bolus through the hypopharynx is elicited by the contraction of the tongue against the pharyngeal walls ("tongue pump"). As the bolus is transferred into the pharynx, the suprahyoid muscles elevate the larynx anteriorly and superiorly. This laryngeal position is maintained throughout the pharyngeal phase; the hypopharynx is dilated to create a subatmospheric pressure (i.e., "hypopharyngeal suction") that further aids in transfer of the bolus. Laryngeal elevation is a also a key event in preventing aspiration by pressing the epiglottis upward and forward against the base of tongue, which helps in preventing spillage of the bolus into the larynx. Limitation of laryngeal elevation—for example, as caused by the tethering effects of a tracheotomy tube or by neuromuscular dysfunction of the suprahyoid and the strap muscles—may predispose the patient to aspiration.

During the pharyngeal phase, effective separation of the tracheobronchial tree from the pharyngoesophagus is achieved through the sphincteric mechanism of the larynx. True vocal fold adduction occurs at the midpoint of laryngeal elevation and is initiated by an afferent reflex, mediated by the superior laryngeal nerve (laryngeal closure reflex). Closure of the true vocal folds is rapidly followed by the sequential closure of the false vocal folds, aryepiglottic folds, and epiglottis. The glottis, however, is the main sphincter, and vocal fold adduction and abduction occur in synchrony with laryngeal ascent and descent. Laryngeal closure is followed by sequential contraction of the middle and inferior constrictor muscles and relaxation of the upper esophageal sphincter (UES) (mediated by the vagus nerve), which is then opened by anterosuperior displacement of the larynx. The pressure generated by the bolus also distends the UES. The pharyngeal wave is extremely rapid, and the bolus advances 5 to 10 cm per second with a pressure of 20 to 80 mm Hg. Once the bolus has passed into the esophagus, it is transferred into the stomach by vigorous peristaltic contractions.

The esophageal phase of swallowing is completely involuntary. A series of reflexes, including contraction of the UES, protects against retrograde aspiration into the airway. Gastric or esophageal distention, belching, or vomiting produces closure of the true vocal folds.

Central Control

Cortex

The motor cortex is involved with modulation of the motor output of the face, tongue, pharynx, and larynx (precentral gyrus). The primary somatosensory cortex plays a coordinating role via connections with the primary motor cortex.[20] Other areas such as the inferior frontal cortex, the supplementary motor area, and the superior and transverse gyri are also involved during normal swallowing. The thalamic area (i.e., subcortical) includes pathways with the cortex and with striae that may be important for sensory and motor integration.

Swallowing Center

Swallowing involves a coordinated sequence of events initiated by a "central pattern generator." The swallowing center responsible for this neural response includes nuclei for cranial nerves V (trigeminal nucleus), IX, X (nucleus solitarius, nucleus ambiguus), and XII (hypoglossal nucleus).[21] The swallowing center acts as a relay station in transmitting and coordinating efferent impulses to the different muscles of the face, masticatory apparatus, pharynx, larynx, and esophagus. Afferent impulses from different organs and/or muscles provide input that is important for coordinating the sequence of events and modulating the efferent (i.e., muscular) response.[22]

The "swallowing center" and lower cranial nerves may be affected by a variety of traumatic, infectious, vascular, and neoplastic conditions. In our experience, cerebrovascular accidents involving the posterior circulation, neoplasms, and cranial base surgery are the most common factors causing these conditions. A high vagal paralysis (i.e., site of lesion proximal or immediately distal to its exit at the cranial base) caused by direct injury to its nuclei or to the proximal nerve trunk produces the most significant deficits. Table 35–1 outlines the major effects of a high vagal neuropathy. Both

TABLE 35-1   Major Clinical Effects of a High Vagal Neuropathy

Defect	Effect	Defect	Effect
Velopalatine insufficiency	Hypernasal speech Nasal regurgitation Loss of pharyngeal pressure during swallow	UES dysfunction	"Pooling" of secretions Postprandial aspiration
Pharyngeal paralysis	Poor propulsion "Pooling" of food and/or secretions Postprandial aspiration	Esophageal dysfunction	Poor propulsion GER Postprandial aspiration (food, GE refluxate)
Laryngeal hemisparalysis/anesthesia	Vocal fold paralysis Loss of "laryngeal closure reflex" Dysphonia (short MPT) Ineffective cough/Valsalva Prandial penetration/aspiration		

GE, gastroesophageal; GER, gastroesophageal reflux; MPT, maximum phonation time; UES, upper esophageal sphincter.

upper esophageal and esophageal dysfunction may result, and swallowing is significantly compromised by both the motor and sensory insults.

Efferent (i.e., motor) branches of the vagus nerve supply the soft palate, inferior constrictor muscle, vocal fold, and cervical esophagus. Parasympathetic fibers have an inhibitory effect (i.e., relaxation) over the cricopharyngeal muscle, which constitutes the most critical part of the UES. Afferent fibers are responsible for sensory input from the entire laryngopharyngeal region and thus for the swallowing and laryngeal closure reflexes.

BOLUS PROPERTIES

The study of fluids and their physical properties, called *rheology*, is critical for understanding the nature of dysphagia management. The significance of bolus consistencies for swallowing is not completely understood. However, use of standard diets based on the texture, viscosity, density, and flow resistance of the bolus reduces inconsistencies in food preparation and contributes to proper nutrition in patients with swallowing disorders following treatment for cancer of the head and neck. Understanding of the flow time constants of various foods and liquids allows the clinical team to adjust the diet when early spillage or delayed swallow behaviors are identified during instrumental testing.

Several fundamental properties that impact swallowing function, including volume, viscosity, density, and texture, are discussed here to provide insight into how these parameters impact the assessment and management of patients with swallowing disorders.

Bolus Effects

Volume

As the bolus increases in volume, greater overlap occurs between the oral and pharyngeal phases of swallowing.[23] With increased volume, oral and laryngeal motion occurs earlier than with a smaller bolus. However, transit time does not appear to change as a function of volume.

Viscosity

Viscosity is the resistance to flow or alteration of the shape of a substance that occurs as a result of molecular cohesion. Thus, as viscosity increases, oral and pharyngeal transit times and the duration of pharyngeal constriction increase. Equally important, as viscosity increases, flow volume through the sphincters also increases.[24] Early postoperative swallowing should not be done with highly viscous materials when there is concern about postswallow aspiration.

Viscosity is the prime variable in the study of Newtonian fluids, which are fluids with a linear rate of flow.[25] Viscosity can be viewed as being proportional to the force required to move the fluid through an area. For example, whole milk has a higher viscosity than water when swallowed normally.

Density

Density refers to the compactness of a substance or the ratio of its mass to its volume. Highly dense food preparations delay oral and pharyngeal transit times and flow through the cricopharyngeus muscle. As fluids are added to a dense mixture, viscosity decreases and volume increases. For instance, mashed potatoes, when not mixed with milk, are very dense. When they are mixed with milk, density decreases and viscosity and volume increase. A patient who is complaining of dryness in the mouth may experience greater problems with dense food substances, such as pudding, rice, or certain bread products, than a person with normal salivary function. It should be pointed out that manometric studies have shown that pharyngeal constriction, strength, and duration do not increase with increased density.[26]

Texture

The texture of food and liquid refers to their composition. Commonly identified textures include nectar, puree, honey, sticky, soft, and mechanical soft. These terms remain primarily perceptual in that they may all have a wide range of viscosities and densities. Although density and viscosity

TABLE 35-2 Dysphagia Diets Based on Viscosity, Density, and Texture

Diet Stage	Bolus Consistencies
Level 1	Pureed food and thickened liquid—the most conservative level. This diet is used in patients with severe oral preparatory, oral phase, and pharyngeal dysphagia.
Level 2	Pureed and mechanically altered foods, plus thick or thickened liquids and very soft foods that require minimal chewing (e.g., cottage cheese, macaroni, pancakes with syrup). This diet is used in patients with deficits of the oral phase or with decreased pharyngeal peristalsis. This is also the most common diet for patients who are suspected of having or identified with aspiration. It is first used under therapeutic control; the patient is then advanced to independent intake when the clinician deems it safe to do so.
Level 3	Mechanically altered and soft foods with liquids allowed as tolerated. This diet is advised for individuals who are beginning to chew and to rehabilitate chewing and bolus propulsion.
Level 4	Soft foods and all liquids, avoiding rough or coarse foods. This diet usually precedes advancement to a regular diet.

can be altered by materials that thin and thicken, the texture of the bolus does not change drastically with added substances.

Bolus Effects and Dysphagia Diets

Based on the rheologic properties of foods and liquids, broad guidelines for dysphagia diets have been proposed.[27] These are presented in Table 35-2. Table 35-3 lists the manner in which bolus consistencies may be modified. Although modification is desirable in working toward maximal oral nutrition, modifications may cause misunderstanding in the reporting of testing results, either at the bedside or during instrumental evaluations. Thus, the need to use standard consistencies and volumes during assessment procedures must be recognized.

Cichere and colleagues recently identified viscosity shear rate profiles and found that standard barium has a rather high density.[28] When modified or mixed with other fluids such as milk, juice, or water, the properties of the barium

TABLE 35-3 Consistency Modifications Used to Change Viscosity, Density, or Texture of a Food or Liquid

Consistency	Effects
Thin or clear liquids: Water, broth, skim milk	Decreases viscosity Increases bolus flow
Thicker liquids: Whole milk	Reduces density of a bolus Decreases transit times
Thick liquids: Cream soups, milkshakes, nectars	Increases density and viscosity Reduces transit times May increase pooling in vallecula or pyriform sinus

may range from a thin liquid to a rather thick paste. Thus, without a clear indication of the type of barium in the barium mixture, the testing of swallowing with cinefluoroscopy can lead to significant misinformation. Recently, a product called Varibar has been introduced in an attempt to standardize barium mixtures.[29]

◼ COMPREHENSIVE EVALUATION OF SWALLOWING

The clinical presentation of swallowing disorders includes a variety of symptoms and findings that may reflect a primary problem of the aerodigestive tract or the manifestation of a systemic disease. Clinical evaluation is critical in helping the clinician to select the appropriate test or tests needed to determine the cause of the swallowing disorder, its severity, and associated prognosis so that therapy can be guided realistically. The clinical evaluation per se is not the optimal time for predicting aspiration in the head and neck cancer population, but it provides preliminary guidance for subsequent management.[30]

Clinical Evaluation

History

A differential diagnosis and a diagnostic algorithm are formulated based on the initial history and physical examination. Table 35-4 differentiates swallowing problems according to their origin. "Difficulty swallowing" does not mean the same thing for every patient or clinician. The clinician should ask the patient directly and review the records to elicit a history of pain or discomfort associated with swallowing or food getting "caught" in one place or another, and whether some foods or liquids are easier to swallow than others, as well as a history of choking, regurgitation, chronic cough, pneumonia, bronchitis, and cyanosis.[31-33] Kazandjian, Dikeman, and Adams initially outlined the critical aspects of the clinical presentation of the swallowing disorder.[34] Table 35-5 presents a comprehensive clinical history to be used for diagnosing or treating a swallowing disorder.

Symptoms suggesting that the swallowing disorder is associated with systemic disease or neoplasm include pain, fever, weight loss, sensation of a lump in the neck, drooling, nasal regurgitation, episodes of coughing, frequent clearing of the throat, heartburn, and gastroesophageal reflux disease.[35, 36] Equally important are changes in the patient's ability to communicate, especially changes in voice quality such as hoarseness or a wet, gurgling sound.[37]

Conditions that affect the neurologic system or the upper aerodigestive tract, such as cerebrovascular accident, diabetes, immunosuppression, sarcoidosis, amyloidosis, multiple sclerosis, myasthenia gravis, trauma, and previous surgery of the head and neck or esophagus, are relevant to the outcome of treating the swallowing disorder associated with cancer of the head and neck.[2, 38]

The clinical history may help in classification of the swallowing problem as either obstructive, due to narrowing by intrinsic or extrinsic space-occupying lesions; or

TABLE 35-4 Assessment of Swallowing Disorders Based on Origin

Origin	Feature to be Assessed
Neurologic system	Gait/balance
	Cranial nerves
	Motor function: Fine skills, strength, muscle bulk, coordination
	Deep tendon reflexes
Oral area	Oral continence:
	Lip pursing
	"Trumpeter" maneuver
	Drooling
	Buccal tone
	Gutters:
	Gingivobuccal
	Gingivolingual
	Tongue range of motion:
	Extends beyond lower lip
	Approximates gingivobuccal areas
	Can push against tongue blade
	Tongue sensation:
	Buccal tongue palate
Oropharynx/ nasopharynx	Motion of soft palate:
	Contact with posterior wall
	Symmetry of contact with lateral walls
	Sensation:
	Tongue blade/swab
	Cold laryngeal mirror
	Gag reflex
	Swallow reflex
Laryngopharynx	Hypopharynx, endolarynx:
	Quiet/forced reproduction
	Coughing
	Speaking
	Swallowing
	Retention of secretions in vallecula or hypopharynx
	Penetration/aspiration of secretions
	Motion (symmetry, range) of base of tongue, arytenoid, epiglottis, false vocal cords, true vocal cords (fixation vs. paralysis)
	Velopharyngeal closure:
	Lateral walls
	Velum
	Laryngeal closure reflex:
	Touch
	FEES-ST
	Voice quality:
	Whispering/weak
	Wet/gurgly
	MPT
	VPI: form sound /k/
	Laryngeal tenderness
	Laryngeal crepitus
	Laryngeal elevation
	Adenopathy
	Thyroid
	Other masses
	Scars
	Motion
	Range of motion
	Muscle mass
	Strength
	Rigidity/dystonia/spasticity

FEES-ST, fiberoptic endoscopic evaluation of swallowing with sensory testing; MPT, maximum phonation time; VPI, velopharyngeal insufficiency.

TABLE 35-5 Key Elements of the Clinical History Related to the Swallowing Disorder

Definition of the problem
  Drooling
  Sensation of food sticking or "getting caught"
  Choking, coughing during or after the swallow
  Pain/discomfort
  Reflux/regurgitation
  Problem related to specific food type or bolus consistency
Onset
  Postsurgical
  Cerebrovascular accident
  Other
Time elapsed from initiation of swallow to symptoms
  <2 seconds = pharyngeal
  >2 seconds = esophageal
Associated symptoms
Present and past illnesses
  Neuromuscular
  Neuroplasm
  Autoimmune
  Endocrine
  Infection
  Cardiopulmonary
Tracheotomy tube type/size
Surgical history
Trauma history (especially head and neck)
Medications
  Prescribed
  Over-the-counter
  Alternative medicines
Social history/habits
  Alcohol
  Tobacco
  Marijuana
  Cocaine
  Other
Family history
Review of systems

functional, having a neural, neuromuscular, or muscular origin. For example, a patient with an obstructive problem caused by a slow-growing neoplasm or a stricture usually presents with a history of progressive dysphagia to solids.[39] Conversely, a patient with neurogenic dysphagia initially presents with dysphagia to liquids, but a motility problem usually manifests dysphagia to both solids and liquids.[40] Degenerative diseases may be associated with dysphagia to solids and/or liquids, which is often accompanied by swallowing fatigue and changes in speech and voice.

The time difference between the initiation of the swallow and the onset of the swallowing problem may help to differentiate a pharyngeal from an esophageal problem. In normal individuals, pharyngeal swallow usually lasts less than 1 second; therefore, patients with problems at the pharyngeal level present symptoms that begin less than 2 seconds or longer after the initiation of the swallow; often multiple swallows are required to clear the bolus. Conversely, the esophageal phase usually lasts 3 to 4 seconds and may extend up to 20 seconds after initiation of the swallow; thus, problems that begin 2 seconds after the initiation of swallowing suggest an esophageal disorder. Although not pathognomonic, the longer the elapsed time between initiation of the swallow and the onset of symptoms, the more distal the site of the lesion. Symptoms such as reflux or heartburn also suggest the presence of an esophageal disorder. However, it should be noted that esophageal disease, especially that involving the lower esophageal sphincter, may refer pain, discomfort, or a sensation of a globus to the pharynx. In fact, one third of patients with carcinoma at the distal third of the esophagus experience referred symptoms to the pharynx.[41]

Physical Examination

A complete physical examination includes a neurologic evaluation of gait, balance, sensory and motor function of the extremities, deep tendon reflexes, and cranial nerves.

Observation and palpation of the thyroid notch during swallowing provides an estimate of laryngeal elevation and coordination of the pharyngeal swallow and may detect laryngotracheal deviation caused by displacement by a tumor. Palpation and examination of the neck may reveal tumors and may allow an estimation of the severity of spasticity or rigidity; limited range of motion is seen in patients with severe degenerative kyphosis or those with cerebral palsy.

Flexible laryngoscopy allows examination of the anatomy of the pharynx and larynx during quiet and forced respiration, coughing, speaking, and swallowing. Symmetry, coordination, and range of movement of the base of the tongue and pharyngeal walls should be noted as the endoscope is passed. Pooling of secretions or food residue in the vallecula or pyriform sinuses should also be noted. The laryngeal closure reflex may be tested by gently touching the epiglottis or aryepiglottic folds with the tip of the endoscope. This maneuver requires some experience in that the examiner should avoid eliciting a gag reflex or laryngospasm. This test is often deferred until the endoscopic examination and swallow assessment have been completed. Sensation of the vallecula and lateral pharyngeal walls also can be tested with this technique. Alternatively, a more objective measure of the laryngeal closure reflex and the sensory function of the upper aerodigestive tract can be obtained with the use of a flexible fiberoptic laryngoscope with sensory testing capability, as described by Aviv.[42] This test uses a specially designed instrument to deliver a pulse of air to the aryepiglottic fold or vocal fold and measures the threshold of response to the air pulse.

Functional Evaluation

Although clinical assessment may identify some patients with swallowing disorders, it has been shown that clinical assessment is not highly predictive of aspiration. A complete assessment of swallowing includes one or more instrumental tests following the bedside clinical assessment. Functional tests of swallowing, such as fiberoptic endoscopic evaluation of swallowing (FEES),[43] modified barium swallow (MBS),[44] and scintigraphy,[45] provide specific information regarding aspiration and focus on the physiologic aspects of the total swallow behavior. MBS and FEES provide diagnostic information because they assess the swallowing of the patient under a variety of circumstances, employing boluses with different consistencies and varying positions of the neck. These tests assist the clinician in planning a therapeutic protocol and identifying compensatory maneuvers, as well as in designing diet modifications to be used in the treatment of the swallowing disorder.

BEDSIDE CLINICAL EVALUATION

A bedside evaluation is usually performed by an SLP experienced in the diagnosis and management of swallowing disorders. Interpretation of the oral motor examination, assessment of cognitive status, and observations of actual swallows constitute the clinical experience. Rarely is the bedside swallow assessment the final procedure for determining if a patient can safely begin oral nutrition. Rather, it should be considered the first step in advancing the patient to oral nutrition.

MODIFIED BARIUM SWALLOW

The MBS is a multidisciplinary evaluation of the swallowing mechanism, usually performed by a radiologist in collaboration with the SLP. Candidates for a MBS include those patients presenting with dysphagia who have had a normal barium esophagram, those with postoperative swallowing dysfunction (following head and neck oncologic surgery), patients with neuromuscular problems (including cerebrovascular accident and other disorders of the central nervous system), and those who complain of unspecified difficulty swallowing.

MBS is the best way to evaluate the oral phase and the entire pharyngeal phase of swallowing. It provides detailed analysis of the coordination and timing of swallowing. Events that may cause dysphagia include abnormal movements of the tongue in forming the bolus and initiating deglutition, pooling of residual barium in the valleculae or pyriform sinuses, and aspiration of barium into the airway. MBS also provides information about the function of the upper esophageal sphincter.

Under fluoroscopic observation controlled by the radiologist, the patient ingests barium of varying consistencies under the direction of the SLP. The consistency of the barium is chosen to approximate the consistencies of food that a patient is likely to encounter in his or her daily diet. The initial consistency may be guided by the bedside evaluation. Preselected barium consistency as well as normal food coated with barium can be prepared to better approximate a normal meal.

Frontal and lateral views are obtained during the MBS with the patient standing or sitting. Figure 35–1A and B shows the frontal and lateral views typically seen in the MBS. Unlike the barium swallow, the MBS is purely dynamic; thus, it is recorded on videotape for review and may be used for patient education.

Entry of barium into the airway may be the most important information that the MBS can provide. The extent of aspiration, including the amount or percentage of bolus, and the most distal level of entry should be defined clearly. The terms *aspiration* and *penetration* are not standardized. To complicate matters further, the terms *glottic penetration* and *laryngeal penetration* have also been used. Therefore, it is preferable that the location of the barium that extends farthest into the airway (i.e., subglottic, glottic, trachea, bronchi, lungs) be described. This may be as subtle as a

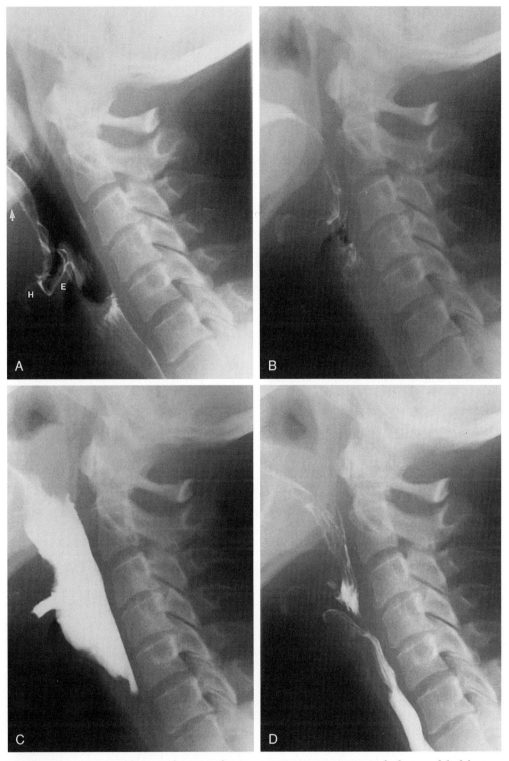

FIGURE 35–1 *A,* Lateral view of a normal patient in resting position just before modified barium swallow. Note the epiglottis (E) at the inferior edge of the mandible *(arrow)* and the position of the hyoid (H) relative to the mandible. The air-filled trachea is visualized. *B,* As the bolus approaches the oropharynx, the tongue is retracted and the velum has sealed the nasal cavity, as shown by modified barium swallow. Note the elevated position of the hyoid relative to the inferior edge of the mandible. *C,* During the swallow, the epiglottis is inverted with the hyoid and larynx fully elevated. The airway is closed. The head of the bolus is at the cricopharyngeal sphincter. *D,* The bolus has passed; the epiglottis remains inverted and the hyoid begins to descend. Immediately following the passage of the bolus into the esophagus, the larynx and hyoid return to the resting position shown in *A.*

coating of the laryngeal surface of the epiglottis or as obvious as gross aspiration of the barium into the lower tracheobronchial tree. As with the traditional barium swallow, reflux of barium into the nasopharynx should also be documented.

Observers should also note the patient's response to the aspiration, such as coughing or clearing of the throat, and the degree to which the barium is cleared out of the airway. "Silent" aspiration is defined as aspiration that fails to elicit a normal cough response. Silent aspiration cannot be detected during a clinical (bedside) swallowing examination, but it is readily apparent on the MBS. Abnormal motion of the epiglottis, diminished contractions of the pharyngeal constrictor muscles, and abnormal laryngeal elevation can all be identified on the MBS.

Fluoroscopic examination has been shown to be far more sensitive than a bedside swallowing study to even small amounts of aspiration. If barium enters the airway, the effectiveness of airway protective maneuvers and attempts to vary the consistency of the barium bolus can be assessed directly by viewing under fluoroscopy. Maneuvers include prompted coughing if the patient does not cough spontaneously, repeated swallowing to clear retained barium, neck flexion to propel the bolus into the esophagus, neck extension to allow gravity to assist in swallowing, various tilting and turning positions of the head, and the supraglottic swallow (inhale, hold breath, swallow, exhale) to close the larynx before swallowing. These are discussed more extensively in the following sections.

FIBEROPTIC ENDOSCOPIC EVALUATION OF SWALLOWING

The assessment of swallowing using FEES requires the passage of a flexible fiberoptic endoscope into the nares and over the velum to a position above the epiglottis.[43] Topical anesthesia is applied with the use of cotton-tipped applicators to avoid anesthetizing the pharynx. Velopalatine anatomy and function can be evaluated before the endoscope is passed into the oropharynx. Before liquid or food is offered to the patient, the examiner notes the anatomic structures and observes the functions of the velum (sustained phonation, repeating "coca-cola"), epiglottis, and larynx. After several "dry swallows" have been evaluated, specific amounts of liquids and varying food consistencies treated with food dye are viewed as they pass the pharynx and larynx. The quantity of retained secretions present in the vallecula and hypopharynx is also noted. Pharyngeal and laryngeal functions should be documented with different consistencies and amounts of bolus, along with various changes of the position of the head. The supraglottic swallow and chin tuck strategies may also be used to identify the possible causes of dysphagia. During the time of airway closure, the swallow cannot be visualized because the pharyngeal walls contract over the bolus, collapsing the lumen over the endoscope ("whiteout phase").

Monitoring of the bolus is possible only before and after the pharyngeal swallow. However, the bolus can be monitored as it enters into view from the oral cavity to the pharynx. The speed of the pharyngeal swallow, premature flow of food or liquid into the pharynx and larynx, and residual amounts of the bolus can all be visualized during this examination. Unlike with the MBS, the endoscope may remain in place for long periods of time, allowing the clinician to monitor the residual bolus and examine anatomic structures. Swallowing with the use of compensatory strategies and changes in neck position is easily accomplished while the endoscope is in place. FEES is more sensitive than MBS in detecting pooling of oropharyngeal secretions and subtle abnormalities of the palate, pharynx, and larynx; it provides better anatomic information than is revealed by the MBS (Fig. 35–2). It does not assess the oral phase and does not evaluate the upper esophageal sphincter or the esophageal phase of swallowing.

FEES may be particularly useful when a patient cannot be easily transported to a radiology unit, has a significant voice quality change, or has limited ability to follow directions.

A FEES may not be indicated for patients with extreme movement disorders, those who cannot tolerate the endoscopes, and those who have a history of bronchospasm or laryngospasm.

FEES-ST

Fiberoptic endoscopic evaluation of swallowing with sensory testing (FEES-ST) employs the standard FEES testing with the addition of sensory testing of the supraglottic mucosa to determine the presence of a sensory dysfunction in patients with dysphagia.[43, 46] For this test, an air pulse generator is used to send a pulse of air through a port in a specially designed flexible endoscope. Air pulses can be delivered to the supraglottic larynx and the hypopharynx. Sensory thresholds can then be determined by means of psychophysical testing methods.

SCINTIGRAPHY

Scintigraphy is typically performed in the nuclear medicine suite by trained personnel. When used to track movement of the bolus and to quantify the residual bolus in

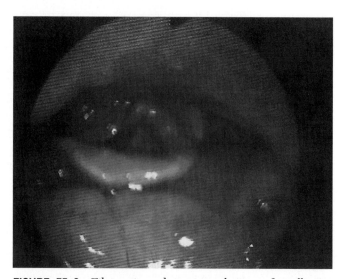

FIGURE 35–2 Fiberoptic endoscopic evaluation of swallowing (FEES). This patient's chief complaint was "food sticking in the throat." In this view, a portion of the bolus has reached the vallecula and is retained. The remainder of the bolus has passed into the esophagus. A trace of the bolus remains in the right pyriform sinus. The endoscope may remain in place until the bolus has cleared.

the oropharynx, pharynx, larynx, and trachea, this test is done by having the patient swallow a small amount of a radionuclide material (such as technetium-99m) combined with liquid or food. A special camera (gamma camera) records images of the organs of interest over time to reveal a quantitative image of the transit along with metabolic aspects.

Because there is no time limit for this testing, scintigraphy can be used to identify trace aspiration and to quantify the aspiration over short or long time periods (e.g., delayed "postprandial" or "reflux aspiration"). Scintigraphy can also be used to calculate the transit time and residual pooling of a bolus in patients suffering degenerative neuromuscular diseases, both before and after treatment.[45] Perhaps the strongest indication for the use of scintigraphy is in identifying those patients with reflux aspiration and those patients who, despite limited aspiration, have the ability to clear the aspirate quickly, as well as those in whom the aspirate does not reach the distal airways—thus revealing a subset of patients who may be fed by mouth.

Despite its objective quantitative analysis of aspiration, scintigraphy does not provide an adequate definition of the anatomy of the upper aerodigestive tract. Scintigraphy is also more costly than videofluorography or FEES. For these reasons, it is not used routinely.

ULTRASONOGRAPHY

Ultrasound uses high-frequency sounds (>2 MHz) from a transducer held or fixed in contact with skin to obtain a dynamic image of soft tissues. Because ultrasound does not penetrate bone, it is limited to the soft tissues of the oral cavity and parts of the oropharynx. Because it is noninvasive and does not require exposure to radiation, it is very useful in testing children, or when multiple swallows are required to make a diagnosis. The swallowing functions of the upper surface of the tongue, the intrinsic tongue muscles, and the soft tissue anatomy of the mouth are within the "view" of the transducer. Ultrasonography provides a method for studying tongue morphology and identifying lingual tumors, as well as a method for studying tongue movement and control of bolus in the oral preparatory and oral phases of swallowing.[47] Ultrasonography does not require the use of any special bolus or contrast (real food can be used). However, if dysphagia due to pharyngeal or laryngeal dysfunction is suspected, this technique offers little diagnostic or treatment information.

MAGNETIC RESONANCE IMAGING

High-speed magnetic resonance imaging (MRI), such as fast low-angle shot (FAST) or echoplanar imaging, has allowed a dynamic analysis of the pharyngeal phase of swallowing that was impossible with the use of conventional MRI.[48, 49] The pharynx, oral cavity, laryngeal lumen, and musculature can be evaluated during motion, allowing assessment of the swallowing mechanism.

During a FAST MRI, intravenous contrast is injected into the patient and the patient is given an oral contrast containing ferric ammonium sulfate as a food bolus substitute. Images are obtained as the bolus is moved from the oral cavity to the esophagus. This technique, however, can assess the activity of the oral cavity and pharynx only during short periods of time.

MRI has the advantage of not exposing the patient to radiation. However, the temporal and spatial resolution of MRI is inferior to that with videofluoroscopy; thus, images with poor resolution are produced. MRI is costly, and swallowing in the supine position may not reflect the true physiologic mechanism of swallowing.

Functional MRI to study swallowing is a technique that affords the clinician the opportunity to examine the functional roles of the cortical, subcortical, and brain stem areas in the control of swallowing. Thus, this procedure provides investigators with a tool that may enable a better understanding of the control of swallowing by the central nervous system.

Anatomic Evaluation

BARIUM SWALLOW AND COMPUTED TOMOGRAPHIC SCAN

Imaging techniques such as the barium swallow esophagram, the computed tomographic (CT) scan, and MRI are recommended when alterations of the anatomy are suspected. The esophagram provides an evaluation of the endoluminal anatomy, suggests extraluminal compression, and demonstrates the motility of the pharyngeal and esophageal tracts. It is important that the challenge of barium be relevant to the patient's symptomatology (e.g., difficulty swallowing solids vs. liquids, pills vs. bread). The barium swallow esophagram detects obstruction, such as that caused by neoplasms, strictures, webs, or achalasia, with high accuracy. CT scan or MRI provides exquisite definition of the anatomy within the head and neck region and the chest. These are usually reserved for identifying and staging neoplasms and vascular abnormalities/strokes and for detecting the presence of degenerative brain disease, such as multiple sclerosis.

DIRECT LARYNGOSCOPY/ESOPHAGOSCOPY

Endoscopy of the upper aerodigestive tract is recommended to rule out or biopsy a neoplasm. A direct endoscopy is recommended for patients with history of tobacco or alcohol abuse who are at high risk for the development of upper aerodigestive tract cancer.

OTHER

Electromyography. Electromyography ascertains the presence of specific nerve or neuromuscular unit deficits, such as vagal or recurrent laryngeal nerve paralysis. It establishes the presence of a systemic myopathy or a degenerative neuromuscular disease. When used for the diagnosis of vocal fold paralysis, it may also provide information regarding the prognosis for spontaneous recovery.[50] In addition, electromyography is used as a guide when botulinum toxin is injected into hyperkinetic muscles of the larynx, pharynx, or neck.

Flexible Esophagogastroduodenoscopy, 24-Hour pH-metry, or Manometry. These tests are used by the gastroenterologist for evaluating patients in whom neoplasms, motility disorders, or gastroesophageal reflux is suspected.

■ SURGERY OF THE CRANIAL BASE AS A CAUSE OF SWALLOWING DISORDERS

Depending on the location of the tumor, cranial base surgery may produce injuries or deficits of the lower cranial nerves or brain stem and/or mechanical displacement of the soft tissues of the upper aerodigestive tract, thereby leading to dysfunction of the mechanisms for speech, swallowing, and airway protection. Deficits that were caused by the neoplasm or by the extirpative oncologic surgery may be compounded by the reconstructive surgery, especially in patients who require reconstruction with soft tissue flaps, which are insensate and bulky. Therefore, patients who undergo surgery of the cranial base frequently require an enteral tube and/or tracheotomy to treat nutritional deficiencies and to help with tracheal toilette. These therapies, although effective on a temporary basis, ultimately cause further impairment of swallowing.

Deficits of the lower cranial nerves are a common presentation of tumors of the cranial base and are common sequelae or complications of surgery of the cranial base. Of utmost importance is the presence of a high vagal injury that produces ipsilateral laryngeal and pharyngeal anesthesia and paralysis (see Table 35–1). In addition, it produces paralysis of the ipsilateral soft palate and loss of vagally mediated relaxation of the cricopharyngeus muscle, thus resulting in discoordination in the relaxation of the muscle. These problems result in a very inefficient swallow that is associated with nasal regurgitation, retention of oral secretions and/or food in the paralyzed side of the pharynx, spillage into the laryngeal and/or tracheal airway (penetration/aspiration), and a weak voice and cough. Injury to lower cranial nerve IX or XII further compounds the deficit. Paralysis of the tongue impairs the oral phase of preparation and transport of the bolus. In the presence of a velopalatine paralysis, paralysis of the tongue can produce premature spillage of the bolus before the pharynx and larynx are prepared to receive it, leading to preprandial (i.e., before the swallow) aspiration. A weak or incompetent laryngeal sphincter allows aspiration of secretions during swallowing (i.e., prandial aspiration) and the aspiration of secretions or food that accumulate in the pharynx (i.e., postprandial aspiration). In addition to all of these deficits, a high vagal paralysis also causes discoordination of esophageal peristalsis and the lower esophageal sphincter.[51] This increases the likelihood of reflux, which in the presence of an incompetent larynx can lead to aspiration.

Deficits of the third division of the trigeminal nerve (cranial nerve V3) affect sensation of the ipsilateral tongue and floor of the mouth and buccal sulcus, thus leading to lack of awareness of residual food in the ipsilateral side of the mouth; such deficits can also produce a weakness or paralysis of the muscles of mastication.[52] A facial nerve deficit (cranial nerve VII) causes an incontinent oral sphincter (poor lip closure), which leads to drooling and retention of food and secretions in the gingival buccal sulcus, caused by the weakness of the muscle buccinator muscle.

Tumor or surgery in the infratemporal fossa or lateral cranial base can produce scarring of the pterygoid muscles or the temporalis muscle; temporomandibular joint disorder leading to trismus can also result. Significant trismus (<1.5 cm) impairs both eating and mastication.

■ MANAGEMENT OF SWALLOWING DISORDERS

Preoperative Treatment

The management of swallowing disorders ideally begins with treatment counseling, documentation of pretreatment dysfunction, prognostic assessment, and patient education. The purposes of counseling are to reduce the patient's fears about changes in voice, speech, or swallowing that might occur after surgery[53] and to apprise the patient of the resources available for rehabilitation. Counseling prepares the patient for what he or she may expect during hospitalization and when discharged to home and informs the patient of what changes will occur if radiotherapy is provided. This phase of treatment should not be compromised regardless of the changes in health care guidelines, scheduling conflicts, or lack of provider availability. The initial visit by the SLP should be scheduled immediately following the clinical diagnosis, and intervention should begin at that time.

Preoperative treatment information may predict the severity and duration of post-treatment dysfunction.[54] Stenson and coworkers found that patients with cancer of the hypopharynx and larynx had a higher degree of functional impairment than did those with cancer of the oropharynx.[13] Moreover, speech and voice disorders before surgery, radiation, or chemoradiation should also be documented so that realistic post-treatment communication expectations can be outlined and swallowing exercises that may help to prevent long-term disability can be initiated.

Surgical Treatment

The goals of surgical treatment are to enhance the compensatory mechanisms of the unaffected side and to improve the sphincteric function of the swallowing mechanism. In extreme cases, the surgery may be of a palliative nature and may separate the trachea from the esophagus to stop aspiration.

Vocal Fold Medialization

Medialization of the vocal fold may be achieved with injection or implantation of biocompatible materials.

VOCAL FOLD INJECTION

Injection of a paralyzed, weak, atrophic, or bowed true vocal fold (TVF) may be performed via direct laryngoscopy with the use of transoral or transcutaneous techniques, while the glottis is observed with a flexible laryngoscope or a mirror.[55] Transoral and transcutaneous injection may be done in the office. Injection lateral to the vocal fold may medialize a paralyzed vocal fold or may add bulk to a paretic or atrophic bowed TVF. Vocal fold medialization with the use of a lateral injection may achieve complete closure of a glottic gap; thus, swallowing efficiency and safety may be improved if there is normal sensation at the level of glottic closure.

Injection of the vocal fold has the advantage of avoiding open surgery. Although conceptually simple, a precise injection is technically demanding. The margin of error is small, and experience is required to achieve optimum results. Injection of the vocal fold may be complicated by hematoma, swelling, airway obstruction, and so forth. Contraindications for injection of the vocal fold include a compromised airway, coagulopathy, and a history of allergic reaction to the proposed injectable material.

Gelfoam, a mixture of gelatin powder in a buffered saline solution, may be injected as a temporary implant for vocal fold paralysis. Gelfoam is usually reabsorbed within 12 weeks, making Gelfoam injection of the vocal fold an excellent option when recovery of the vocal fold paralysis is likely.[56] Micronized acellular dermis may also be injected into the TVF as a long-term, if not permanent implant. Teflon, previously considered the gold standard for medialization of the TVF, has lost favor as an injectable material for the larynx, owing to the occurrence of Teflon granuloma, the availability of other materials, and the popularization of laryngeal framework surgery.

Injection of autologous fat has been advocated for the treatment of both voice and swallowing disorders. Its reabsorption is variable, thus making the final result somewhat unpredictable. During a typical injection, the vocal fold is overinjected to account for the initial reabsorption of fat, thus creating a convex free edge. This convexity causes early anterior contact and creates or increases a posterior gap, thereby increasing the risk of aspiration. We do not favor the use of fat unless it is used as a temporary implant and the initial overinjection is avoided.

LARYNGEAL FRAMEWORK SURGERY

Medialization Laryngoplasty. Medialization laryngoplasty for unilateral vocal fold paralysis, paresis, bowing, or atrophy requires the insertion of an implant between the ala of the thyroid cartilage and the vocal fold. Silicone, Gore-Tex, and hydroxyapatite implants are most commonly used as customized or premade implants to medialize the vocal fold.[57, 58] Indications for medialization of the paralyzed vocal fold include glottic incompetence secondary to unilateral vocal fold paralysis, sacrifice of or injury to cranial nerve X during cranial base surgery, incomplete glottic closure secondary to vocal fold paresis, atrophy, and selected traumatic or postsurgical defects.

Arytenoid Adduction/Arytenoid Medialization. The goal of the arytenoid adduction procedure is to place traction on the muscular process of the arytenoids, thereby imitating the action of the lateral cricoarytenoid muscle.[59] The arytenoid is rotated internally, displacing the vocal process medially and caudally, thereby adducting the vocal fold. Additionally, the arytenoid, which may be subluxated anteriorly, may be pulled back to a more anatomic position. The arytenoid adduction may correct the vocal fold foreshortening and often corrects the difference in TVF height.

Medialization of the arytenoid involves displacement of the arytenoids medially and posteriorly. The arytenoid cartilage is then sutured to the cricoid cartilage to maintain this

position. Arytenoid medialization corrects the difference in the vertical position of the TVFs and lengthens the paralyzed fold.

The techniques of arytenoid adduction and arytenoid medialization specifically address the posterior gap. Thus, both arytenoid adduction and arytenoid medialization are indicated to close the posterior gap in patients with unilateral paralysis of the vocal cord who have symptoms of significant glottic incompetence (breathy voice, aspiration, weak cough) and in whom flexible laryngoscopy reveals a unilateral laryngeal paralysis with a posterior gap during phonation and/or swallowing.

Cricopharyngeal Myotomy

Cricopharyngeal myotomy should be considered in patients with swallowing disorders associated with an incomplete relaxation of the UES, or when the UES has abnormal muscular contractions during the relaxation period.[60] Patients with paralysis of the vocal folds due to pathology of the brain stem or to vagus nerve lesions frequently have associated impairment of pharyngeal motor and sensory functions, which contribute to the swallowing impairment. In such patients, restoration of glottic closure may not be sufficient to correct the dysphagia and aspiration. In patients with unilateral pharyngeal paresis, pharyngeal propulsion is often inadequate to propel the bolus past the cricopharyngeal sphincter, which, in patients with high vagal defects, may lose its ability to relax for the passage of the food bolus owing to its bilateral innervation. This leads to pharyngeal pooling of the swallowed material and spillage over the arytenoids/aryepiglottic folds into the larynx (penetration). In the insensate larynx, it leads to postswallow aspiration. In such patients, cricopharyngeal myotomy is a useful adjunct to vocal fold medialization.

Our experience with the use of botulinum toxin for the treatment of UES hypertonicity using transcutaneous injection under electromyographic guidance or via rigid esophagoscopy (60 to 100 units of botulinum toxin A) shows that botulinum toxin A provides significant relaxation of the UES for up to 1 year. This technique is a feasible alternative for those patients with dysfunction of the UES not associated with fibrosis.

Palatopexy/Pharyngeal Flap

Acquired velopalatine incompetence can result from partial or complete loss of the soft palate or neurogenic dysfunction of the soft palate. Neurogenic dysfunction resulting in either unilateral or bilateral paralysis of the soft palate creates varying degrees of velopalatine incompetence. During the process of swallowing, velopalatine incompetence causes regurgitation of liquids, and rarely solids, into the nasopharynx/nasal cavity.

Unilateral palatal adhesion (palatopexy) is indicated for patients with symptomatic unilateral palatal paralysis. An adhesion is surgically created at the level of Passavant's ridge, a site of "normal" closure of the velopalatine valve. Even patients with very mild liquid reflux often exhibit a moderate to severe nasal quality to their speech, which dramatically improves with palatal adhesion. Alternatively, a pharyngeal flap may be used to correct the velopharyngeal incompetency.

Surgical Closure of the Larynx

Patients who continue to aspirate and develop pulmonary complications such as pneumonia or pneumonitis, despite the use of conservative measures and adjunctive surgical procedures, may require surgical closure of the larynx. The most common diagnoses of patients requiring a laryngotracheal separation are neurologic disorders such as cerebrovascular accidents (i.e., severe cognitive deficit) and end-stage neurodegenerative disorders such as amyotrophic lateral sclerosis, multiple sclerosis, and progressive supranuclear palsy.[61] Laryngotracheal diversion, known as the standard Lindeman procedure, involves the creation of an anastomosis between the subglottic trachea and the esophagus and a permanent stoma from the distal trachea. Laryngotracheal separation (modified Lindeman procedure) involves closure of the proximal subglottic trachea as a blind pouch and the creation of a permanent stoma from the distal trachea. This technique of laryngotracheal separation best meets the desired criteria of simplicity, reliability, and reversibility, compared with other procedures.

The presence of a high tracheotomy is a relative contraindication to a laryngotracheal separation. A high tracheotomy implies a short or absent proximal tracheal stump that presents a formidable challenge to collapse and close. Other techniques, such as a total laryngectomy or a laryngofissure with supraglottic closure, should be considered in these patients. A variety of glottic and supraglottic closures have been described. Multilayer closure of the supraglottis, with suturing of the epiglottis to the aryepiglottic folds and arytenoids and closing of the ventricular folds, is a reliable although technically demanding technique.

Adjunct Procedures

GASTROSTOMY/JEJUNOSTOMY

Percutaneous endoscopic gastrostomy (PEG), percutaneous endoscopic gastrojejunostomy (PEGJ), open gastrostomy, or jejunostomy provides an adequate route for feeding and hydration (temporary or permanent). It should be noted, however, that these enteral routes do not prevent aspiration because the patient can aspirate his or her own secretions. PEG and gastric-tubes are associated with gastroesophageal reflux that may also be aspirated.

TRACHEOTOMY

A tracheotomy provides an airway and permits suctioning of secretions. The presence of a tracheotomy does not enhance the ability of the patient to swallow; in fact, it results in greater swallowing dysfunction and aspiration owing to the tethering effect of the tracheotomy cannula that limits laryngeal elevation, to the loss of positive subglottic pressure during swallowing, and to the ineffective clearing of laryngeal or pharyngeal residue by coughing.

An expiratory valve (Passy-Muir) is a removable valve that opens to permit inhalation but closes during expiration to divert air flow through the larynx. A speaking valve has the advantage of increasing verbal communication and directing the air flow upward through the larynx to provide proprioceptive cues during swallowing. Vocal fold adduction is maximized because the buildup of subglottic air pressure aids in bolus propulsion.

Postoperative Treatment

The goals of postoperative treatment by the SLP are to achieve the recovery of speech and swallowing function and to improve overall quality of life. Patient education focuses on the changes that have altered the physiology of swallowing because of surgery or adjuvant therapy and the steps for recovery of function. Patients are also informed about swallowing maneuvers, exercises, and diet modifications that will be implemented to reduce the risk of aspiration. Patients with T3 and T4 cancer usually have significant deglutition and speech disorders. Logemann found that patients with oral cavity and pharyngeal cancer tend to have worse swallow function than patients with laryngeal cancer.[54] She suggests that the structures involved in these regions are responsible for bolus transit and clearance.

Following patient education, the bedside clinical assessment protocol, as described earlier, assesses the patient's readiness to participate in the recovery process. Patients who refuse to participate or who decline to communicate may require referral to a counselor for assessment of depression.

REHABILITATION

Rehabilitation of patients with cancer of the head and neck requires a multidisciplinary team approach that includes the surgeon, medical oncologist, radiation oncologist, maxillofacial prosthodontist, SLP, physical therapist, and oncology nurse.[53] The rehabilitation team coordinates treatment from the time of diagnosis to the completion of rehabilitation by way of tumor board meetings, planning conferences, and patient/family conferences. The SLP is a vital member of the team and is responsible for the evaluation, recommendations, and treatment of speech and swallowing disorders that are encountered in patients diagnosed with cancer of the head and neck. The goals of the SLP are to educate patients about their disorders, identify the safest diet, teach techniques to prevent aspiration, increase speech intelligibility, monitor progress during different phases of treatment, and report results of treatments to the management team.

Regardless of the primary choice of treatment—surgery, chemotherapy, and/or radiation—all have significant effects on speech, voice, or swallowing functions.[62]

To manage patients effectively, the SLP who has specialized training in speech and swallowing disorders must understand the critical components of the disease and how the disease affects communication and swallowing. The size, location, and extent of tumor must be identified so that possible treatments can be planned because each of these parameters directly affects speech and swallowing. The effects of radiotherapy, including xerostomia, mucositis, and tissue fibrosis, must be considered because they negatively affect swallowing and may also cause changes in the voice.[53] These issues must be addressed before the time of treatment and during the short- and long-term follow-up stages.

The reconstructive technique used following resection of the tumor also affects swallowing function.[54] Techniques using primary closure or split-thickness skin grafts tend to minimize dysphagia and speech impairments compared with reconstructive procedures that introduce tissue from other parts of the body.[13] The lack of adequate blood supply and nerve function usually limits motion as well as decreases sensation[54] and thus increases the possibility of poor oral, pharyngeal, or laryngeal control of secretions.

Each of these issues, as well as the need for assistance in the management of patients' environmental and social issues, underscores the need for a well-trained SLP to be integrated into the head and neck team. The team must be aware that goals for speech and swallowing change during the different phases of treatment and that the timing of an intervention may affect the outcome. For some patients with small lesions, speech and swallowing goals are met relatively early following primary treatment; for others (e.g., those with extended supraglottic laryngectomy), extensive rehabilitation may take 6 months or longer.[63] Unfortunately, in some cases, patients do not recover normal swallow function and may need additional surgery to manage aspiration or may require a permanent feeding tube to meet nutritional needs. Others with permanent speech disability, such as those who have undergone total glossectomy, may require additional nonoral communication devices.

Swallowing Dysfunctions Following Treatment of Head and Neck Cancer

Patients with cancer of the head and neck exhibit somewhat predictable patterns of dysphagia and dysarthria based on the critical components of the disease (location, extent, tumor size). The problems with swallowing are generally greater than those associated with communication.

Tracheotomy

Recently, swallowing therapy has become more specialized. Exercises specific to the impairment must be done if improvement is to be achieved. Carrau and Murry have identified specific head and neck swallowing impairments for which exercises may be used.[63] Murry and Carrau reported a series of exercises specific to the impairment being treated.[33] Many patients require a tracheotomy following surgery of the head and neck to manage secretions or to ensure an airway. The presence of a tracheotomy tube has been reported by some authors to change the biomechanics of swallowing by decreasing laryngeal elevation, thereby preventing adequate opening of the cricopharyngeal muscle.[64]

Dettelbach and associates have demonstrated that the use of a Passy-Muir valve is beneficial in decreasing aspiration in some patients.[65] Their study suggests that the lack of subglottic air pressure and glottic air flow after tracheotomy precipitates aspiration. A recent study examined eight patients with cancer of the head and neck and found that not all patients benefit from digital occlusion and that patients must be evaluated individually with videofluoroscopy.[66]

Recently, Naudo and colleagues presented functional outcomes of swallowing following decannulation. Naudo suggests that early removal of the tracheotomy tube is important for successful recovery of swallowing following surgery for supracricoid laryngectomy with cricohyoid-epiglottopexy (CHEP).[67]

Anterior/Lateral Tongue Resection

Resection of lesions of the tongue often disrupts manipulation and transfer of the bolus. The severity depends on the extent of resection, the mobility of the residual portion, and the type of reconstruction. The lack of lingual propulsion reduces swallowing efficiency in foods with higher viscosities.[68] In a recent study by Furia and coworkers, patients who underwent a partial glossectomy exhibited an increase in oral transit time for paste foods, stasis in the oral cavity, a reduction of anteroposterior propulsion of the tongue, and an increase in the number of deglutitions to clear the valleculae.[69]

The degree of surgical resection has a significant effect on the degree and duration of swallowing dysfunction. Patients with less than 50% resection of the tongue usually have temporary swallowing problems.[5, 70-73] Patients with greater than 50% resection experience more severe effects, such as decreased lingual propulsion and inadequate contact of the remaining tongue with the palate. With these patients, palatal augmentation with a palatal drop prosthesis may be required to reduce the volume in the oral cavity and to provide greater lingual contact with the palate.

Resection of lesions in the anterior oral cavity does not affect the pharyngeal stage of swallowing; however, if resection includes portions of the lateral pharyngeal wall, initiation of the pharyngeal swallow is delayed and weakened pharyngeal peristalsis causes residue that is often aspirated after the swallow is completed.[71] Rehabilitation efforts begin with the choice of safest consistency for oral feedings. During the postoperative stage, most patients benefit from lower-viscosity food choices such as broth or skim milk. Patients are taught maneuvers that will assist with bolus transfer. Range-of-motion exercises are practiced to achieve maximum movement from the remaining tongue.

Total Glossectomy

The tongue is a dynamic organ that is involved in the oral preparatory phase, the oral phase, and the beginning of the pharyngeal phase of swallowing. When patients undergo total glossectomy, all three phases of swallowing are affected.

Furia and associates used videofluoroscopy to examine eight patients who previously underwent total glossectomy with laryngeal preservation and reconstruction with a myocutaneous flap.[69] They found residue of the materials in the area of the valleculae, the pharynx, and the superior esophageal sphincter. Patients were able to clear occasional laryngeal penetration, and the risk of aspiration was eliminated with compensatory and airway protection maneuvers. These strategies included backward tilt of the head to allow gravity to assist in clearing residue in the oral cavity, multiple swallows to decrease stasis in the oropharynx, the supraglottic swallow maneuver to increase airway protection during and after the swallow, and the Mendelsohn maneuver to address the stasis in the superior esophageal sphincter. The Mendelsohn maneuver requires that the patient make successive attempts to elevate the larynx by repeatedly pushing the tongue anteriorly and superiorly toward the palate.

Anterior Floor of the Mouth

Resection of the anterior floor of the mouth creates oral dysphagia because of impaired range of motion of the tongue. Postoperative edema prevents adequate manipulation of the bolus and transfer of certain consistencies. Patients are taught to place the bolus posteriorly in the oral cavity to improve oral transit time. Postoperatively, foods may be restricted to a consistency that flows. Thin liquids can be easily aspirated before the swallow owing to loss of oral control; therefore, thickened liquids are usually the best choice for patients after this type of surgery.

Tonsil/Palatal

Disorders of speech and deglutition vary according to the site and extent of the palatal defect. Postoperatively, patients can experience nasal regurgitation, especially with thin liquids, and hypernasality is prominent during speech production owing to velopharyngeal incompetence. Large defects may require flap reconstruction; after the tissue has healed, a prosthodontist can begin fitting the patient with a dental prosthesis. Brown and colleagues have investigated the effects of reconstruction in this area and have reported that addition of the superiorly based pharyngeal flap to the radial forearm flap in soft palate reconstruction results in improved speech and swallowing.[72]

Resection of Tonsil/Base of the Tongue

The base of the tongue has been identified as an important generator of pressure for normal swallowing.[73] Following excision of the base of the tongue, propulsion of the bolus is reduced and pharyngeal residue is likely to increase. If a portion of the base of the tongue is resected, the efficiency of the swallow is impaired and the amount of pharyngeal residue will vary, but the patient remains at risk for aspiration after the swallow. Excision of the tonsil area can lead to a delay in initiation of the swallow during the pharyngeal phase, and patients may experience temporary difficulty with thin liquids. Thicker viscosities, such as pudding, usually cause a greater number of problems for patients because their ability to drive the bolus down the pharynx has diminished. The chin tuck strategy often benefits the patient because it expands the opening of the valleculae. Patients are most successful with a full liquid diet following surgery, which includes such items as cream soups and milkshakes.

Posterior Pharyngeal Wall

Resection of the posterior pharyngeal wall results in reduced pharyngeal transit, especially with a bolus of high viscosity. During normal swallowing, the pharyngeal wall makes contact with the base of the tongue, pharyngeal pressure builds, and a pharyngeal swallow is triggered. Contraction of the pharyngeal walls continues progressively down the pharynx to the upper esophageal sphincter. Pharyngeal transit normally takes 1 second or less, and when it is completed, very little residue is left in the pharynx. When the pharyngeal wall is resected, transit time usually increases and excessive residue is left.[73] In a study of 55 patients, Julieron and associates reported that swallow function had recovered within 16 days after resection of small tumors.[74] In a 1-year postoperative follow-up, the results showed that patients who had reconstruction with the myocutaneous flap experienced greater difficulty with swallowing than did those with a platysma or a free radial forearm flap. This suggests that bulky flaps may cause decreased sensation and may compromise swallowing function.

Following surgical resection for cancer of the pharynx, swallow assessment begins when the patient is able to tolerate deflation of the cuff, or after decannulation has occurred. Once the patient is able to properly manage secretions and does not require suctioning, the tracheotomy tube is capped for 24 hours, then removed if the patient does not experience shortness of breath. A liquid diet is often tried during the postoperative stage with patients who have small defects and is advanced as the patient tolerates. Rehabilitation focuses on base of tongue exercises, the "effortful" swallow, the Mendelsohn maneuver, and the supraglottic swallow.

Many patients with advanced cancer receive radiation following surgery. It has been reported that high-dose radiation to this region can cause serious complications, such as necrosis of the mucosa, laryngeal edema, and odynophagia, requiring tracheotomy and tube feedings.[75]

Supraglottic Laryngectomy

Anatomic changes following surgery of the supraglottic larynx result in the patient's dependence on voluntary airway protection measures while eating and drinking. Logemann found that patients treated with supraglottic laryngectomy exhibited aspiration problems before (a delayed reflex), during (decreased vocal fold adduction), and after the swallow (decreased pharyngeal peristalsis and decreased laryngeal elevation). Reduced vocal fold adduction and reduced laryngeal elevation were the two most prevalent problems. Treatment starts when the patient tolerates a speaking valve. Adduction exercises, base of tongue exercises, the Mendelsohn maneuver, and the pseudo-supraglottic swallow technique are taught during the early phases of rehabilitation.

Regardless of when the rehabilitation process starts (before or after decannulation), the patient is taught the supraglottic swallow technique to decrease the risk of aspiration. The goal of the supraglottic swallow is to enhance airway protection before and during the swallow.

The increased effort associated with using the supraglottic swallow tilts the arytenoids forward and brings whatever remains of the false vocal folds closer together to completely close the airway entrance above the true vocal folds.

Patients using the supraglottic swallow are started on a diet consisting of thickened liquids and pureed or soft foods. The supraglottic swallow can usually be mastered in 2 or 3 days if there are no postoperative complications. Thus, patients can be discharged on an oral diet. Most patients eventually return to a regular diet and no longer have to use compensatory strategies to protect the airway.

The extended supraglottic laryngectomy requires longer rehabilitation because additional structures have been resected, and swallowing function is compromised even further. Many of these patients have a difficult time achieving goals before discharge, especially those patients who have undergone resection of the base of the tongue. They require insertion of a feeding tube, either nasogastric or gastric. Over a period of time and with rehabilitation, feeding tubes are usually removed and patients return to an oral diet.

Supracricoid Laryngectomy

The supracricoid laryngectomy is a conservation procedure for selected cancer of the glottis and supraglottis and preserves voice and swallowing. This surgery includes resection of the true and false vocal folds, the paraglottic spaces bilaterally, and the thyroid cartilage but spares at least one arytenoid. Naudo and colleagues have studied the functional outcome of patients who had undergone supracricoid laryngectomy with CHEP and cricohyoidopexy (CHP).[67] The first attempt to remove the tracheotomy tube occurred on the third postoperative day. Normal swallowing was achieved by the end of the first year in 98.9% of those who underwent CHEP and in 91% of those who experienced CHP.

Factors increasing the risk of aspiration in patients following supracricoid laryngectomy include the following: (1) resection of arytenoid cartilage or the superior laryngeal nerve, (2) previous medical history of chronic obstructive pulmonary disease or diabetes mellitus, and (3) irradiation of patients preoperatively or postoperatively. Swallowing rehabilitation is required postoperatively; however, the timing of intervention remains controversial. Some clinicians prefer that the tracheotomy tube remain in place while oral feedings are initiated; others advocate early removal of the tracheotomy before oral feedings are introduced.[76]

Decannulation indicates that a patient is generally able to manage secretions. Removal of the tracheotomy tube also allows for better phonation and generally increased laryngeal elevation during the swallow.[77-79] The rehabilitation plan for swallowing is similar to that following a supraglottic laryngectomy. Patients are first taught to manage their secretions and then to use the supraglottic swallow technique to increase airway protection. Oral feedings monitored by the SLP are initiated with pureed foods and thickened liquids. Eventually, these patients resume an oral diet without the need for compensatory strategies.

Vertical Partial Laryngectomy

Patients usually experience minimal difficulty with swallowing following a standard hemilaryngectomy. This technique involves removal of one false vocal cord, one ventricle, and a true vocal fold and excludes the arytenoids. Occasionally, patients exhibit mild swallowing problems that

resolve soon after surgery. Postoperatively, these patients should be seen by the SLP to learn strategies that will minimize the risk of aspiration. Patients usually benefit from the chin tuck strategy and head rotation to the operated side to improve laryngeal closure.

Total Laryngectomy

After total laryngectomy, the trachea and esophagus are permanently separated; therefore, patients are not at risk for aspiration and do not require techniques to increase airway protection during swallowing. Postoperatively, patients receive nasogastric feedings, which begin when peristalsis has returned and continue until the patient is able to swallow saliva without odynophagia and relies on bedside suction for less than 50% of saliva clearance.[80] A liquid diet is initiated on or before postoperative day 7, and the nasogastric tube (if one has been used) is removed. However, patients with previous irradiation or those who have had a free-flap or gastric pullup should not begin an oral diet until a barium swallow has confirmed the integrity of the anastomosis. Reduced propulsion of the bolus results from lack of pharyngeal pressure. Postoperatively, liquids are chosen because they are easier to swallow and require less effort for propulsion. The diet is slowly advanced to pureed and soft foods for the first 2 weeks, and a normal diet is typically resumed 1 month after surgery.

Complications that may deter oral feedings include the development of a pharyngocutaneous fistula; the development of a neopharyngeal pouch, which some authors suggest leads to dysphagia in 10% to 40% of laryngectomy patients[81, 82]; a stricture at the distal end of the pharyngeal repair; and leakage around or through the tracheoesophageal puncture. Rehabilitation provided by the SLP is primarily for voice restoration. Preoperatively, the SLP should meet with the patient to review the options for voice restoration and to explain the environmental and social changes that occur after surgery.

Chemotherapy/Radiation Therapy

Radiation and chemotherapy may be used as primary treatment modalities or in conjunction with surgical resection. These treatments may control the spread of cancer but often leave the patient with adverse effects that create dysphagia or make existing swallowing problems worse. Complications with radiotherapy begin during the first few weeks of treatment and include xerostomia, taste dysfunction, and oral mucositis.[83] Patients often complain of sore lips and tongue, burning sensations, and ulcerations during the time of radiation treatment. Xerostomia can cause dysphagia with certain foods, especially those with a thicker viscosity, because the ability of the patient to propel the food to the oropharynx is delayed. In addition, the discomfort patients experience during radiotherapy may delay swallowing rehabilitation, and some of the gains made before radiotherapy may be temporarily lost. Lazaruz and coworkers reported that patients who had undergone radiotherapy presented with reduced movement of the tongue base, decreased laryngeal elevation, and decreased oropharyngeal efficiency.[84] If there is poor oropharyngeal efficiency, residue may remain in the pharynx and place the patient at risk for aspiration after the swallow.

Prolonged and debilitating abnormalities of swallowing function well beyond 1 year have been documented by Smith and associates.[11] In this study, pharyngeal transport dysfunction, epiglottic dysmotility, vallecular residue, laryngeal penetration, and/or aspiration were reported in all patients. The SLP should become involved during the pretreatment stage to prepare patients for the events to follow. Patients should understand the immediate adverse effects of radiation, as well as the possibility that they may develop more problems 1 year or longer after the completion of radiotherapy. Range-of-motion exercises should be implemented at least twice daily during radiotherapy treatment and for several months afterward to prevent trismus. Swallow rehabilitation should focus on the Mendelsohn maneuver, base of tongue exercises, swallowing maneuvers to increase airway protection, and diet modifications. Logemann and colleagues has reported less aspiration with irradiated patients who use the supraglottic swallow maneuver.[85]

Communication Following Head and Neck Surgery

Following surgery to one or more organs of the head or neck, communication may be impaired owing to problems of articulation, resonance, or voice. Articulation and resonance disorders arise from structural changes to the lips, tongue, palate, mandible, maxilla and velum, nasopharynx, and sinonasal cavities. Voice disorders result from anatomic and/or physiologic changes to the larynx and vocal folds.

Oral Cavity Cancer

The communication problems associated with oral cavity cancer depend on the type and extent of treatment. Nonsurgical management of oral cancer usually results in only minor impairments to articulation and little effect on overall speech intelligibility. Pauloski and coworkers found that the effects of radiation therapy on speech are less severe than on swallowing.[38] Tissue changes that lead to fibrosis may limit speed of movement and lingual, labial, and/or mandibular strength, as well as range of motion. Resultant speech limitations include articulatory imprecision and sound substitutions. With extensive speaking, rate of speech may be reduced and can become labored, thus interfering with the naturalness of speech.

Treatment may improve articulation and speech intelligibility. Logemann and associates demonstrated improved speech intelligibility with the use of range-of-motion exercises following oral and oropharyngeal tumor resection.[54] Treatment is more likely to be successful if it is started early, and it produces little change if it is started longer than 1 year after surgery or radiation.

Prosthetic management improves speech and articulation following surgical resection. Prosthetic management of soft palate defects is directed to separate oral and nasal cavities, increasing intraoral pressure and creating contact points for the tongue to improve precision of articulation. This results also in reduced nasal speech. Zaki has demonstrated excellent results with speech aids that extend postero-orally from the soft palate into the pharyngeal region.[86]

Hard palate defects treated prosthetically result in immediate separation of oral and nasal cavities, thus allowing for increased intraoral pressure and a greater number of contact points for the tongue.

Tongue Defects

Total glossectomy is a severe detriment to speech production. The tongue is responsible for articulation of more than two thirds of the English language. The patient with a total glossectomy can be treated with a mandibular tongue prosthesis.[86] The success of tongue rehabilitation depends on the presence of teeth to anchor the prosthesis. With proper dentition, the prosthesis can be anchored, and sounds such as /t, d, k, g, p, b/ can be articulated with improved precision. Leonard and Gillis reported significant improvement in both speech and swallowing when a prosthetic tongue was fitted properly in patients with total glossectomy.[87]

Partial glossectomy reconstruction consists of palatal augmentation or mandibular augmentation.[88] The augmentation prosthesis fills the void created by surgical excision.

Cancer of the Oropharynx

Treatment of cancer of the oropharyngeal or posterior oral cavity does not interfere significantly with speech when the base of the tongue is left intact.[89, 90] Nonetheless, a defect above the larynx and vocal folds will have an effect on the sound of the voice and may increase the perception of hoarseness or strain. Factors such as edema, structural defects, and postradiation stiffness affect the resonance of the oral cavity and may restrict base of tongue motion, thus distorting the /kg/ speech sounds. Extent of tumor, nerve function, and patient motivation all affect the degree of recovery of speech in patients with oropharyngeal cancer.

Cancer of the Larynx

SLPs have participated in the rehabilitation of speech and voice in laryngeal cancer patients. Three forms of voice production after total laryngectomy are available: Esophageal speech, electrolaryngeal speech, and tracheoesophageal speech.

Zanoff and colleagues[91] reported that about 25% of all laryngectomy patients achieve proficient esophageal speech. Electrolarynges are in common use, but they suffer in general from poor quality, sex difference confusion, and difficulty with placement in patients who have also undergone neck dissection.

New advances in the development of the electrolarynx include the ability to control the frequency of the vibratory sound source, thus altering the perceived pitch of the patient's alaryngeal voice. This has yielded some degree of perceived sex difference between male and female patients who underwent laryngectomy. In addition, devices such as the TruTone (Griffin Laboratories, Temecula, Calif) alter the frequency of the vibratory source, depending on the position of the tongue that allows for intraphase pitch modulation.

Another recent innovation in electrolaryngeal speech is the development of UltraVoice (UltraVoice Inc., Newtown Square, Penna). UltraVoice is an alaryngeal sound source that is placed on an upper denture or orthodontic retainer. The patient controls the volume and pitch of the voice with a handheld device. UltraVoice also offers a hands-free option for patients who have problems with motor control. The device is protected from saliva, food, and liquids by a flexible protective membrane. An orthodontist fits the device, and the patient is then trained by an SLP in its use.

Tracheoesophageal Speech

Tracheoesophageal speech has become the primary method of voice restoration following total laryngectomy.[6] This method of speech production has nearly eliminated the use of esophageal speech following total laryngectomy. Tracheoesophageal speech has been shown to be acoustically and perceptually more similar to laryngeal speech than is esophageal speech.[92, 93] Moreover, tracheoesophageal speakers can maintain greater volume over a longer period than can either esophageally or electrolaryngeally aided speakers.

Before the development of indwelling devices, patients using tracheoesophageal speech were fitted with traditional duckbill prostheses. The sole advantage of the duckbill was ease of placement. This allowed many patients to maintain the prosthesis without the aid of a physician and/or a speech pathologist. However, duckbills require frequent replacement owing to leakage of food/saliva into the trachea.

Current improvements to the original tracheoesophageal speech models include an indwelling tracheoesophageal speech device that is biflanged, self-retaining, and constructed of medical grade Silicon. The Blom-Singer prosthesis (In Health Technologies, Carpenteria, Calif) is a low-resistance device that can be inserted into the tracheoesophageal fistula at the time of the laryngectomy, or as a secondary procedure. As with other indwelling devices, it must be fitted and replaced by a qualified SLP. However, many patients clean and care for their own prosthesis to increase the length of time between replacements. The Provox (Atos Medical AB, Sweden) is a prosthesis that has increased useful expectancy over others. Van Weissenbruch and Albers reported the lifetime of the Provox to range from 3 months to over 2 years, with an average life of 5.4 months.[94]

Radiographic evaluation is becoming increasingly common to assess the function of the pharyngoesophageal segment to determine the prognosis for a patient's success with tracheoesophageal speech. Van As and coworkers proposed the use of videofluoroscopy as a means of evaluating the anatomic and morphologic characteristics of the neoglottis in relation to the perceptual evaluation of the tracheoesophageal voice.[95] In short, a good voice was highly correlated with the presence of a neoglottic bar during phonation. A normotonic or hypertonic neoglottis was related to the likelihood of yielding a good voice. In contrast, a hypotonic neoglottis was not found in any patients studied by van As and associates who were judged to have a good voice.

◨ SUMMARY

The management of dysphagia at the outset of the diagnosis of cancer of the head or neck has been shown to be unequivocally significant in the recovery process. Swallowing disorders are anticipated when key anatomic structures are removed or treated with radiation and/or chemotherapy. The critical valve—the vocal folds—provides the necessary protection against aspiration; therefore, examination of the larynx and vocal folds is an essential aspect of management of patients with head and neck tumors, as well as those with swallowing difficulty after a cerebrovascular accident or surgery that may lead to high vagal lesions.

The otolaryngologist and the SLP are the key managers of swallowing disorders. Surgical and nonsurgical methods of rehabilitation provide the patient with improved swallow function and enhanced quality of life and speed the recovery process. There is a growing body of evidence to support the need for short-term as well as long-term management of swallowing disorders caused by anatomic changes, tissue changes, such as fibrosis long after radiotherapy, and nutritional needs.

REFERENCES

1. Gussenbauer C: Veber cie Erste Durch The Billroth Am Menschen Ausgefhrte Kehlkopf-Exstirpation Und die Anwendung Eines Kunstlichen Kehlkopfses. Archiv fur Klinische Chirugie 17:334–356, 1874.
2. Logemann JA: Evaluation and Treatment of Swallowing Disorders. San Diego, Calif, Singular Publishing Group, 1983, pp 1–100.
3. Bachman A: Methodology in the radiographic examination of the larynx and hypopharynx. J Med 1155–1163, 1963.
4. Murry T, Bone R. Changes in voice production during radiotherapy for laryngeal cancer. J Speech Hear Dis 34:194–201, 1974.
5. Pauloski BR, Logemann JA, Rademaker AW, et al: Speech and swallow function after tonsil/base of tongue resection with primary closure. J Speech Hear Res 36:918–926, 1993.
6. Blom ED: Evolution of tracheoesophageal voice prosthesis. In Blom ED, Singer MI, Haymaker RC (eds): Tracheoesophageal Voice Respiration Following Total Laryngectomy. San Diego, Calif, Singular Publishing Group, 1998, pp 1–8.
7. Laccourreye H, Laccourreye O, Weinstein G, et al: Supracricoid laryngectomy with cricohyoidoepiglottopexy: A partial laryngeal procedure for glottic carcinoma. Ann Otol Rhinol Laryngol 99:421–426, 1990.
8. Murry T, Madasu R, Martin A, et al: Acute and chronic changes in swallowing and quality of life following intraarterial chemoradiation for organ preservation in patients with advanced head and neck cancer. Head Neck 20:31–37, 1998.
9. Wasserman T, Murry T, Johnson JT, et al: Management of swallowing in supraglottic and extended supraglottic laryngectomy patients. Otolaryngol Head Neck Surg (in press).
10. Samant S: Quality of life assessment in head and neck cancer. In Robbins KT, Murry T (eds): Head and Neck Cancer. San Diego, Calif, Singular Publishing Group, 1998, pp 131–133.
11. Smith RV, Kotz T, Beitter JJ, et al: Long-term swallowing problems after organ preservation therapy with concomitant radiation therapy and intravenous hydrosyurea. Arch Otolaryngol Head Neck Surg 126:384–389, 2000.
12. Logemann JA, Pauloski BR, Rademaker AW, et al: Speech and swallowing rehabilitation for head and neck cancer patients. Oncology 11:651–663, 1997.
13. Stenson KM, MacCracken E, List M, et al: Swallowing function in patients with head and neck cancer prior to treatment. Arch Otolaryngol Head Neck Surg 126:371–377, 2000.
14. Logemann JA: Speech language pathology: Moving toward the 21st century. Paper presented at the American Speech-Language-Hearing Association Annual Convention, November 1993, Anaheim, California.

15. Erlichman M: The role of speech language pathologists in the management of dysphagia. Health Technol Assess Rep 1:1, 1989.
16. Joint Commission on Accreditation of Hospitals: Physical Rehabilitation Services (RH): Accreditation Manual for Hospitals. Chicago, Joint Commission on Accreditation of Hospitals, 1998.
17. Health Insurance Association of America: Report on consumer and professional relations. Allied Health Relat 2:86, 1986.
18. Agency for Health Care Policy and Research: Diagnosis and treatment of swallowing disorders (dysphagia) in acute-care stroke patients: Evidence. Rep/Technol Assess 8:1–131, 1999.
19. Palmer JB, Rudin NJ, Gustavo L, et al: Coordination of mastication and swallowing. Dysphagia 7:187–200, 1992.
20. Martin RE, Sessle BJ: The role of the cerebral cortex in swallowing. Dysphagia 8:195–202, 1993.
21. Moiser K, Patel R, Liu WC, et al: Cortical representation of swallowing in normal adults: Functional implications. Laryngoscope 109:1417–1423, 1999.
22. Shaker R, Dodds WJ, Dantas RO, et al: Coordination of deglutitive glottic closure with oropharyngeal swallowing. Gastroenterology 98:1478–1484, 1990.
23. Dantas RO, Kern MK, Massey BT, et al: Effect of swallowed bolus variables on the oral and pharyngeal phases of swallowing. Am J Physiol 258:G675–G681, 1990.
24. Molseed L: Clinical evaluation of swallowing: The nutritionist's perspective. In Carrau RL, Murry T (eds): Comprehensive Management of Swallowing Disorders. San Diego, Calif, Singular Publishing Group, 1999, pp 60–69.
25. Li M, Brasseur JG, Kern MK, et al: Viscosity measurements of barium sulfate mixtures for use in motility studies of the pharynx and esophagus. Dysphagia 7:17–30, 1992.
26. Brasseur JC, Dodds WJ: Interpretation of intraluminal manometric measurements in terms of swallowing mechanics. Dysphagia 6:100–119, 1991.
27. Pandoe EM: Development of a multistage diet for dysphagia. J Am Diet Assoc 93:568–571, 1993.
28. Cichere JA, Hay G, Murdoch BE, et al. Videofluoroscopic fluids versus meal time fluids: Difference in viscosity and density made clear. J Med Speech Lang Pathol 5:203–215, 1997.
29. Varibar C: E-Z EM Incorporated, 717 Main Street, Westbury, NY 11590.
30. Splaingard M, Hutchins B, Sultan L: Aspiration in rehabilitation patients: Videofluoroscopic vs bedside clinical assessment. Arch Phys Med Rehabil 69:637–640, 1988.
31. Daniels SK, McAdam CP, Brailey K, et al: Clinical assessment of swallowing and prediction of dysphagia severity. Am J Speech Lang Pathol 6:617–623, 1997.
32. Cherney LR, Pannell JJ, Cantieri CA: Clinical evaluation of dysphagia in adults. In Cherney LR (ed): Clinical Management of Dysphagia in Adults and Children. Gaithersburg, Md, Aspen Publishers, 1994.
33. Murry T, Carrau RL: Clinical Manual for Swallowing Disorders. San Diego, Calif, Singular Publishing Group, 2001, pp 79–111.
34. Kazandjian MS, Dikeman KJ, Adams E: Communication management of the ventilator-dependent and tracheotomized patient. Paper presented at the Annual Convention of the American Speech-Language-Hearing Association, November 24, 1991, Atlanta, Georgia.
35. Koufman JA: The otolaryngologic manifestations of gastroesophageal reflux disease (GERD): A clinical investigation of 225 patients using ambulatory pH monitoring and an experimental investigation of the role of acid and pepsin in the development of laryngeal injury. Laryngoscope 101:1–78, 1991.
36. Shaker R, Ren J, Hogan WJ, et al: Glottal function during post prandial gastroesophageal reflux. Gastroenterology 104:A581, 1993.
37. Leder SB, Sasaki CT, Burrell MI: Fiberoptic endoscopic evaluation of dysphagia to identify silent aspiration. Dysphagia 13:19–21, 1998.
38. Pauloski BR, Logemann JA, Rademaker AW: Speech and swallowing function after oral and oral pharyngeal resections: One year follow-up. Head Neck 16:313–322, 1994.
39. Pou Am, Carrau RL, Eibling DE, et al: Laryngeal framework surgery for the management of high vagal lesions. Am J Otolarygol 19:1–8, 1998.
40. Crany MA: A direct intervention program for chronic neurogenic dysphagia secondary to brainstem stroke. Dysphagia 10:6–18, 1995.
41. Cunningham ET, Banich WJ, Jones B, et al: Vagal reflexes referred from the upper aerodigestive tract: An infrequently recognized cause of common cardiorespiratory response. Ann Intern Med 116:575–582, 1992.
42. Aviv JE: Sensory discrimination in the larynx and hypopharynx. Otolaryngol Head Neck Surg 116:331–337, 1997.
43. Langmore SE, Schatz K, Olsen N: Fiber-optic endoscopic examination of swallowing safety: A new procedure. Dysphagia 2:216–219, 1998.
44. Logeman JA: Role of the modified barium swallow in the management of patients with dysphagia. Otolaryngol Head Neck Surg 116:335–338, 1997.
45. Hamlet S, Choi J, Kumpuris T, et al: Quantifying aspiration in scintigraphic deglutition testing: Tissue attenuation effects. J Nucl Med 104:1159–1162, 1994.
46. Aviv JE, Sacco RL, Thompson J: Silent laryngopharyngeal sensory deficits after stroke. Ann Otol Rhinol Laryngol 106:87–93, 1997.
47. Sobin J, Nathanson A, Engstrom CF: Endoluminal ultrasonography: A new method to evaluate dysphagia. J Otolaryngol 58:105–109, 1996.
48. Suto Y, Kamba M, Kato T: Dynamic analysis of the pharynx during swallow using Turbo-FLASH magnetic resonance imaging combined with an oral positive contrast agent: A preliminary study (technical note). Br J Radiol 68:1099–1102, 1995.
49. Gilbert RJ, Daftary S, Woo P, et al: Echo-planner magnetic resonance imaging of deglutive vocal fold closure: Normal and pathologic patterns of displacement. Laryngoscope 106:568–572, 1996.
50. Min YB, Finnegan EM, Hoffman HT, et al: A preliminary study of the prognostic role of electromyography in laryngeal paralysis. Otolaryngol Head Neck Surg 111:770–775, 1994.
51. Netterville JL, Civantos FJ: Rehabilitation of cranial nerve deficits after neurotologic skull base surgery. Laryngoscope 103:45–54, 1993.
52. Miller AJ: Neurophysiological basis of swallowing. Dysphagia 1:91–100, 1986.
53. Lazarus CL: Management of swallowing disorders in head and neck cancer patients: Optional patterns of care. Semin Speech Lang 21: 293–307, 2000.
54. Logemann JA: Evaluation and Treatment of Swallowing Disorders, 2nd ed. Austin, Texas, Pro-Ed, 1998.
55. Rosen CA: Vocal fold injection. In Carrau RL, Murry T (eds): Comprehensive Management of Swallowing Disorders. San Diego, Calif, Singular Publishing Group, 1999, pp 285–290.
56. Schranm VL, May M, Lavorato AS: Gelfoam paste injection for vocal fold paralysis: Temporary rehabilitation of glottic incompetence. Laryngoscope 88:1268–1273, 1978.
57. Netterville JL, Jackson CG, Civantos F: Thyroplasty in the functional rehabilitation of neurotologic skull base surgery patients. Am J Otol 14:460–464, 1993.
58. Koufman JA, Isaacson G: Laryngoplastic phonosurgery. Otolaryngol Clin North Am 24:1151, 1991.
59. Kraus DH, Orilikoff RF, Rizk SS, et al: Arytenoid adduction as an adjunct to type I thyroplasty for unilateral vocal cord paralysis. Head Neck 1:52–59, 1999.
60. Woodson GE: Cricopharyngeal myotomy and arytenoid adduction in the management of combined laryngeal and pharyngeal paralysis. Otolaryngol Head Neck Surg 116:339–343, 1997.
61. Eibling DE, Bacon G, Snyderman CH: Surgical management of chronic aspiration. Adv Otolaryngol Head Neck Surg 6:93, 1992.
62. McConnel FMS, Pauloski BR, Logemann JA, et al: Functional results of primary closure vs flaps in oropharyngeal reconstruction: A prospective study of speech and swallowing. Arch Otolaryngol Head Neck Surg 124:625–630, 1998.
63. Murry T: Therapeutic intervention for swallowing disorders. In Carrau RL, Murry T (eds): Comprehensive Management of Swallowing Disorders. San Diego, Calif, Singular Publishing Group, 1999, pp 243–248.
64. Ebling DE, Diez Gross R: Subglottic air pressure: A key component of swallowing efficiency. Ann Otol Rhinol Laryngol 105:253–258, 1996.
65. Dettelbach MA, Gross RD, Mahlmann J, et al: The effect of the Passy-Muir Valve on aspiration patients with tracheostomy. Head Neck 17:297–302, 1995.
66. Logemann, JA, Pauloski BR, Colangelo L: Light digital occlusion of the tracheostomy tube: A pilot study of effects on aspiration and biomechanics of the swallow. Head Neck 20:52–57, 1998.

67. Naudo P, Laccourreye O, Weinsten G, et al: Functional outcome and prognosis factors after supracricoid partial layngectomy with cricohyoidopexy. Ann Otol Rhinol Laryngol 106:291–295, 1997.

68. McConnel FMS, Logemann JA, Rademaker AW, et al: Surgical variables affecting postoperative swallowing efficiency in oral cancer patients: A pilot study. Laryngoscope 104:87–90, 1994.

69. Furia CLB, Carrara-Angelis E, Martins NMS, et al: Video fluoroscopic evaluation after glossectomy. Arch Otolaryngol Head Neck Surg 126:378–383, 2000.

70. Conley JJ: Swallowing dysfunctions associated with radical surgery of the head and neck. AMA Arch Surg 80:602–612, 1960.

71. Hirano M, Kuroiwa Y, Tanaka S, et al: Dysphagia following various degrees of surgical resection for oral cancer. Ann Otol Rhinol Laryngol 101:138–141, 1992.

72. Brown JS, Zuydam AC, Jones DC, et al: Functional outcome in soft plate reconstruction using a radical forearm free flap in conjunction with a superiorly based pharyngeal flap. Head Neck 19:524–534, 1997.

73. Cerenko D, McConnel FMS, Jackson RT: Quantitative assessment of pharyngeal bolus driving forces. Otolaryngol Head Neck Surg 100:57–63, 1989.

74. Julieron M, Kolb F, Scwaab G, et al: Surgical management of posterior pharyngeal wall carcinomas: Functional and oncologic results. Head Neck 23:80–86, 2001.

75. Meoz-Mendez RT, Fletcher GH, Guillamondegui OM, et al: Analysis of the results of irradiation in the treatment of squamous cell carcinomas of the pharyngeal walls. Int J Radiat Oncol Biol Phys 4:579–585, 1978.

76. Pene F, Avedian V, Eschwwege F, et al: A retrospective study of 131 cases of carcinoma of the posterior pharyngeal wall. Cancer 42:2490–2493, 1978.

77. Logemann JA: Aspiration in head and neck surgical patients. Ann Otol Rhinol Laryngol 94:373–376, 1985.

78. Shah JP, Shaha AR, Spiro RH, et al: Carcinoma of the hypopharynx. Am J Surg 132:439–443, 1976.

79. Spiro RH, Kelly J, Vega AL, et al: Squamous carcinoma of the posterior pharyngeal wall. Am J Surg 160:420–423, 1990.

80. Ruiz CR: Policy for Speech and Swallowing Rehabilitation for Supracricoid Laryngectomy Patients. Department of Otorhinolaryngology/Speech Language Pathology. Philadelphia, University Hospital, 1993.

81. Galati LT, Myers EN: Pathophysiology of swallowing disorders: Laryngectomy. In Carrau RL, Murry T (eds): Comprehensive Management of Swallowing Disorders. San Diego, Calif, Singular Publishing Group, 1999, pp 147–154.

82. Kirchner JA, Scatliff JH: Disabilities resulting from healed salivary fistula. Arch Otolarngol 75:60–68, 1962.

83. Davis RV, Vincent ME, Shapshay SM, et al: The anatomy and complication of 'T' versus vertical closure for the hypopharynx after laryngectomy. Laryngoscope 93:16–22, 1962.

84. Lazaruz CL, Logemann JA, Pauloski BR, et al: Swallowing disorders in head and neck cancer patients treated with radiation therapy and adjunct chemotherapy. Laryngoscope 106:1157–1166, 1996.

85. Logemann JA, Pauloski BR, Rademaker AW, et al: Super-supraglottic swallow in irradiated head and neck cancer patients. Head Neck 19:535–540, 1997.

86. Zaki HS: Dental prosthetics. In Carrau RL, Murry T (eds): Comprehensive Management of Swallowing Disorders. San Diego, Calif, Singular Publishing Group 1999, pp 249–254.

87. Leonard R, Gillis R: Effects of a prosthetic tongue on vowel intelligibility and food management in a patient with total glossectomy. J Speech Hear Dis 47:25–29, 1982.

88. Hirano M, Kuroiwa Y, Tanaka S, et al: Dysphagia following various degrees of surgical resection for oral cancer. Ann Otol Rhino Laryngol 101:138–141, 1992.

89. Teichgraeber J, Bowman J, Goepfert H: Functional analysis of treatment of oral cavity cancer. Arch Otolaryngol Head Neck Cancer Surg 112:959–965, 1986.

90. Galati LT, Johnson JT: Surgery of the oral cavity, oropharynx and hypopharynx. In Carrau RL, Murry T (eds): Comprehensive Management of Swallowing Disorders. San Diego, Calif, Singular Publishing Group, 1999, pp 141–146.

91. Zanoff DJ, Wold D, Mantague JC Jr, et al: Tracheoesophageal speech: With and without tracheostoma valve. Laryngoscope 100:498–502, 1990.

92. Robbins J, Fisher HB, Blom ED, et al: A comparative acoustic study of normal, esophageal, and tracheoesophageal speech production. J Speech Hear Disord 49:202–210, 1984.

93. Debruyne F, Delaere P, Wouters J, et al: Acoustic analysis of tracheoesophageal versus oesophageal speech. J Laryngol Otol 108:325–328, 1994.

94. van Weissenbruch R, Albers FW: Vocal rehabilitation after total laryngectomy using the Provox voice prosthesis. Clin Otolaryngol 18:359–64, 1993.

95. van As CJ, Op de Coul BM, van den Hoogen FJ, et al: Quantitative videofluoroscopy: A new evaluation tool for tracheoesophageal voice production. Arch Otolaryngol Head Neck Surg 127:161–169, 2001.

CHAPTER 36

Supportive and Palliative Care

Ahmed Elsayem

Christina A. Meyers

Eduardo D. Bruera

◉ INTRODUCTION

Palliative care is a discipline that strives to alleviate the physical and psychological suffering of patients and their families and to allow them to express their maximum potential during the course of their illness.

Patients with cancer of the head and neck may suffer from severe symptoms, including pain, anorexia, fatigue, cachexia, dyspnea, and psychological distress. In addition, cancer treatments such as surgery, radiation, chemotherapy, and immunotherapy have adverse effects such as mucositis, neutropenia, infection, neurocognitive dysfunction, and psychological distress due to mutilating procedures. The purpose of this chapter is to discuss the assessment and management of these complex symptoms in patients with cancer of the head and neck at all stages of their disease.

◉ SIGNS AND SYMPTOMS ASSOCIATED WITH CANCER OF THE HEAD AND NECK

Cancer of the head and neck is frequently associated with many physical symptoms related to the cancer itself or to associated treatment. Surgery and radiation therapy are the main modes of treatment, although chemotherapy is frequently used.[1] Radiation therapy doses sufficient to produce tumor regression are associated with mucositis and xerostomia (dry mouth).[2] In addition, significant disfigurement and functional loss often accompany surgical interventions.[3] Many vital functions such as taste, speech, mastication, and swallowing can be affected.[4] Late effects of treatment, particularly radiation ports that include incidental brain exposure, may cause significant cognitive impairment.[5] Cancers of the head and neck are particularly problematic because of their impact on the airway and gastrointestinal tract, which results in significant compromise of breathing and nutrition. Table 36–1 describes the incidence of the most common symptoms of advanced cancer of the head and neck.

TABLE 36–1 Incidence of Common Signs and Symptoms of Advanced Head and Neck Cancer

Symptom	Approximate Percentage
Pain	79
Weight loss	79
Feeding difficulties	74
Dysphagia	74
Cough	66
Communication	53
Bleeding	47
Candida	47
Fistula	21
Aspiration	10

Modified from Forbes K: Palliative care in patients with cancer of the head and neck. Clin Otolaryngol 22:117, 1997.

Pain

Pain is a common symptom in this patient population. In most patients with advanced cancer, chronic pain is due to direct stimulation of afferent nerve structures by the primary or metastatic cancer. Pain associated with direct tumor involvement occurs in 65% to 85% of patients with advanced cancer.[6] Cancer therapy accounts for 15% to 25% of pain syndromes.[7] Pain syndromes are categorized as nociceptive or neuropathic. Nociceptive pain is further divided into somatic and visceral. For example, nociceptive pain related to cancer of the larynx or bony metastases results from activation of pain receptors in these tissues and organs. Neuropathic pain, such as trigeminal or glossopharyngeal neuralgia, results from direct injury to the peripheral or central nervous system. Somatic pain is usually localized and tender to pressure; neuropathic pain is often described as burning or shooting.[8]

Patients with advanced cancer often have chronic, constant pain intermittently punctuated by acute breakthrough pain. Patients may have acute pain following certain procedures, such as postoperative pain or radiation-induced mucositis. Incidental pain is usually acute and may be triggered by certain maneuvers such as swallowing, mastication, or speech.

Weight Loss

Cachexia-anorexia occurs in more than 80% of patients with advanced cancer and is a major factor contributing to morbidity and mortality.[9] Patients with cancer of the head and neck are particularly susceptible because of the effects of cancer and its treatment on eating, including altered taste and difficulty chewing and swallowing. Cachexia is characterized by weight loss, wasting, anorexia, and change in body image with resulting asthenia and psychological distress.

Fatigue

Fatigue is the most frequent symptom of advanced cancer.[10] It is characterized by unusual and profound tiredness after minimal effort, accompanied by an unpleasant sensation of generalized weakness. Cancer-related fatigue, unlike fatigue in a person who is not ill, does not respond to rest.

Psychological Distress

Patients with cancer of the head and neck face enormous psychological distress because of the structural and functional deficits associated with the cancer and its treatment. Facial disfigurement and loss of taste, speech, and sometimes sight result in altered body image, low self-esteem, and possibly depression.[11] Moreover, patients with cancer of the head and neck often have a history of chronic alcohol and tobacco use[12] accompanied by physical and neurocognitive disabilities.[13] It is estimated that 80% of patients with cancer of the head and neck have such a history, which may complicate their care and rehabilitation.[14]

◼ ASSESSMENT OF SIGNS AND SYMPTOMS

Pain

Deficient expertise among health care professionals in the use of assessment tools for pain and other symptoms is the main reason for poor management of symptoms.[15] Patient self-reporting should be the primary source of information for the measurement of symptoms. Observer ratings of symptom severity correlate poorly with patient ratings. Simple tools such as the visual analogue scale (VAS), numeric rating systems (NRSs), and verbal descriptor scales have proved to be effective and reproducible means of measuring pain and other symptoms.[16] Other scales include the Memorial Symptom Assessment Scale (MSAS)[17] and the well-validated M.D. Anderson Symptom Inventory, which is currently being validated in a number of different languages.[18] Pain in cancer patients is frequently complicated by a high level of distress.[19] The emotional suffering experienced by cancer patients manifests itself as fear, anxiety, and depression, which result in increased sensitivity to pain and other symptoms.[20] Therefore, a unidimensional approach to pain that considers 100% of the pain complaint as nociceptive may not address other treatable conditions, thus depriving the patient of appropriate additional therapies.

Assessment of pain should address the cause of the pain and should measure the intensity, onset, duration, location, character, and factors that aggravate and relieve it. One of the most widely used pain assessment systems is the Brief Pain Inventory,[21] which has also been translated and validated in a number of languages. Regular reporting in the patient's medical records of the patient's pain and other symptoms assists the team that is treating the patient in monitoring these symptoms and providing appropriate treatment. The Edmonton Symptom Assessment System (Fig. 36–1) graphically displays the most common symptoms reported among cancer patients.[22–23]

A positive history of alcoholism may be associated with a higher risk for the use of medications to cope with emotional distress.[26] Four-item questionnaires, although widely used, have been found to be insensitive tools for screening problem drinking.[24] Well-validated tools are available for quantifying alcohol use, both current and past,[25] although there are limitations to the accuracy of any self-report questionnaire about alcohol use. Some groups have found that a history of alcoholism is an independent prognostic factor for the development of opioid dose escalation and opioid-related neurotoxicity[26] and that such a history predisposes the patient to preexisting cognitive deficits.[27] However, other studies have found no increased pain reporting or use of higher analgesic doses in patients who screen positively for alcoholism.[24] Another study found that a history of alcoholism was not predictive of postoperative delirium in patients with cancer of the head and neck; age was the only significant predictor in this study.[28] Although patients with a significant alcohol history may need more frequent monitoring and counseling to achieve good pain control, a history of substance abuse or emotional problems is not an indication for limiting pain treatment.

Unfortunately, pharmacologic treatment of pain may lead to worsening of other symptoms such as opioid-related nausea, constipation, and delirium. Given the complexity of the interaction among the various physical and psychosocial domains, there is a growing acceptance that the assessment of pain in cancer patients requires a multidimensional approach.

Weight Loss

Weight loss is the main clinical finding in patients with cancer cachexia. In patients with cancer of the head and neck, this may result from local factors affecting food intake such as altered taste, smell, or swallowing. It may also be due to decreased appetite. A weight loss of 10% or more usually indicates moderately severe malnutrition.[29] The presence of edema, ascites, or pleural effusion may make the interpretation of weight loss difficult. Assessment of caloric intake can be made at the bedside by a nutritionist or a trained nurse. Anorexia is a major target of both nutritional and pharmacologic interventions.

Fatigue

Fatigue is often measured according to subjective assessment and functional capacity. Commonly used performance status scales, such as the Karnofsky Performance Scale and the Eastern Cooperative Oncology Group (ECOG) scale, do not adequately measure fatigue. It is preferable in both patient care and clinical research settings that a well-validated tool such as the Brief Fatigue Inventory be used.[30]

Referral Date:	Referring Physician:										
Date:											
Pain (0–10)*											
Fatigue (0–10)*											
Nausea (0–10)*											
Depression (0–10)*											
Anxiety (0–10)*											
Drowsiness (0–10)*											
Shortness of breath (0–10)*											
Appetite (0–10)*											
Sleep (0–10)*											
Feeling of well-being (0–10)*											
Mini Mental State Score (0–30)											
Assessment from: Pt/SO/HCP (If SO or HCP—use red ink)											
Total opioid MEDD: mg/day											
Staff initials (signature and title below)											

* 0 = No symptoms/ Best   10 = Worst Imaginable

FIGURE 36–1 Edmonton Symptom Assessment System. (From Bruera E, Kuehn N, Miller MJ, et al. The Edmonton Symptom Assessment System [ESAS]: A simple method for the assessment of palliative care patients. J Palliat Care 7:6-9, 1991.)

☐ MANAGEMENT OF SIGNS AND SYMPTOMS

Pain

Successful management of pain depends on the physician's ability to assess the patient and the pain, identify the pain syndrome, and formulate and discuss the treatment plan with the patient. A pharmacologic approach is the primary treatment provided for cancer pain. In more advanced and complex cases, in which suffering and psychological distress complicate pain perception, a multidisciplinary approach is required for effective pain management. The World Health Organization proposed a simple analgesics ladder for the pharmacologic management of cancer pain, which has been shown to be safe and effective. This ladder begins with simple nonopioid analgesics, proceeds to weak opioids, and then recommends strong opioids as the disease progresses and pain expression escalates. Most patients need opioids for the management of cancer pain. Patients should receive appropriate counseling and information regarding their pain, opioids, medication adverse effects, and the costs of treatment.

Nonopioid Analgesics

Acetaminophen or nonsteroidal anti-inflammatory drugs (NSAIDs) are effective analgesics for patients with mild cancer pain and can be combined with opioids such as codeine and oxycodone in patients with moderate to severe pain.[31] Acetaminophen does not inhibit prostaglandin synthesis or affect platelet function; therefore, it is widely used in the treatment of cancer pain, either alone or in combination with opioids such as codeine or oxycodone. The major

toxicity of acetaminophen is its hepatotoxic effect, which is dose related. Therefore, the cumulative daily dose should not exceed 4 g. The main limitations of NSAIDs include their relatively flat dose-response curves and associated gastrointestinal, renal, and bleeding adverse effects. These effects are related to the inhibition of the enzyme cyclooxygenase-1. A new generation of cyclooxygenase-2 inhibitors such as celecoxib and rofecoxib have a lower frequency of toxicity and are effective when used alone or in combination with opioids.

Opioids

Opioids remain the mainstay in the treatment of cancer pain. Opioids interrupt pain perception at different levels in the central nervous system. Table 36–2 summarizes the general principles that apply to opioid treatment of cancer pain.

ROUTES OF OPIOID DELIVERY

The oral route of opioid administration is preferable because it is safe, effective, and convenient and can be used in the home setting. However, 80% of patients taking oral opioids require an alternative route before death.[32] The intravenous route is more suitable for the immediate postoperative period and when the gastrointestinal route is not available because of concerns about wound healing, vomiting, dysphagia, or mucositis. Patient-controlled analgesia (PCA), administered with different types of pumps, is a widely used technique that has proved to be effective in the treatment of pain in hospitalized patients, especially during the postoperative period.[33] Although the overuse of medication by confused or psychologically impaired patients, particularly those with a history of addiction, is possible, this is easily handled by limiting the number of doses that can be

TABLE 36-2 Opioid Treatment of Cancer Pain

Administer around the clock.
Titrate doses individually. Allow extra doses for rescue analgesia.
Consider long-acting opioids when pain is better controlled.
Make oral route the first choice.
Educate patient regarding tolerance, adverse effects, and low risk of
  addiction.
Aggressively prevent nausea and constipation.
Consider adjuvant drugs to manage adverse effects or a specific
  pain syndrome.
Consider opioids as only one part of the total pain management plan.

administered over a given period of time. The subcutaneous route is a safe and effective mode of opioid delivery wherein opioids can be administered by the patient or a family member with the use of a preloaded syringe.[34] The rectal route is also safe and effective, but it is uncomfortable for many patients. The transdermal route (patch) is an effective alternative to the oral route and is more suitable for patients with stable pain complaints who need a relatively small dose of opioids. Drugs such as morphine and hydromorphone can be given safely through the transdermal route.

SPECIFIC OPIOIDS

Patients with cancer pain need to be maintained on opioids in such a way that a constant blood level of the drug can be provided. In addition, patients need to have access to rescue doses of opioid for episodes of pain exacerbation. Table 36–3 summarizes the opioids most frequently recommended for cancer pain.

Weak Opioids. Members of this group, including codeine and hydrocodone, tend to have a flat dose-response curve and are frequently associated with fewer restrictions for prescriptions. Codeine is frequently combined with acetaminophen or aspirin. Propoxyphene is not recommended for long-term use in cancer pain because it includes the active metabolite norpropoxyphene, which can cause confusion and hallucinations.

TABLE 36-3 Opioid Analgesics Most Frequently Recommended for Cancer Pain

Type of Opioid	Name of Opioid	Common Route	Equivalent Price ($)	Other Routes
Weak	Codeine°	PO	—	IV, SC
	Hydrocodone°	PO	—	—
Strong	Morphine	PO	1	IV, SC, Supp
	SR Morphine	PO	5	—
	Hydromorphone	PO	3	IV, SC, Supp
	Oxycodone	PO	3.6	SC°°
	SR Oxycodone	PO	6.5	—
	Fentanyl	TD	6.5	TM, IV
	Methadone	PO	0.15	IV, Supp
	Diamorphine°°	IV	—	SC

°Products may contain paracetamol. Make sure the daily paracetamol dose
  does not exceed 4 g.
°°Not available in the United State (available in Canada and the UK).
$,Approximate relative price when a daily dose equivalent to morphine
  100 mg by mouth is used.
PO, oral; IV, intravenous; SC, subcutaneous; Supp, suppository; TD,
  transdermal; TM, transmucosal; SR, slow release.

Strong Opioids. Morphine has been considered the strong opioid of choice. However, other opioid agonists such as hydromorphone and oxycodone exhibit similar properties. A typical starting dose of morphine is 5 to 10 mg every 4 hours in patients who have not taken opioids previously. The starting dose may not be sufficient, and relatively rapid titration may be needed, particularly if pain is severe. When the effective dose of short-acting morphine has been established, patients may be maintained on this preparation, or at this point a slow-release preparation may be administered every 12 or 24 hours. When a patient is switched from one opioid to another, or when one opioid is substituted for another, it is important for the clinician to calculate the equianalgesic dose of the previous opioid to determine the correct dose of the new opioid.

Hydromorphone is a semisynthetic derivative of morphine that is approximately five to six times more potent. It is well absorbed from the gastrointestinal tract. Usually, it is given as an immediate-release preparation every 4 hours, although in some countries such as Canada, slow-release preparations are available.

Methadone is a synthetic opioid with good bioavailability; it is inexpensive and less constipating than other opioids, making it a suitable drug for the treatment of chronic cancer pain. It has no active metabolites; therefore, it is particularly useful in patients with renal failure. However, methadone has a prolonged and unpredictable half-life and complex pharmacokinetics, making it relatively difficult to titrate. Currently, the practice of starting treatment with methadone should be limited to physicians who are experienced with its use.

Fentanyl is available as a transdermal patch with approximately 3 days' duration of action. A disadvantage of fentanyl is the difficulty associated with titrating the dose when a steady state is not reached.

Meperidine should not be used on a long-term basis for cancer pain because of the associated production of a neurotoxic metabolite, normeperidine, which can cause seizures and other central nervous system adverse effects.

OPIOID ADVERSE EFFECTS

A number of adverse effects are associated with the use of opioids for cancer pain. In most patients, these adverse effects can be managed easily through patient education, selection of the appropriate route of administration, and use of additional drugs such as antiemetics and laxatives. Table 36–4 summarizes the main adverse effects of opioids.

Sedation, constipation, and nausea are the most common adverse effects. Sedation and nausea usually improve spontaneously in about 3 days. Sedation can be exacerbated by coadministration of alcohol or benzodiazepines. If sedation persists, the administration of a psychostimulant such as methylphenidate may improve arousal during the day.[35] Nausea is caused by the opioid effect on the chemoreceptor trigger zone and by delayed gastric emptying. Antiemetics such as metoclopramide are effective against both mechanisms.

Constipation is the most common adverse effect of opioids. Opioids act at multiple sites in the gastrointestinal tract to decrease both peristalsis and intestinal secretions. Unlike sedation and nausea, tolerance to constipation develops very slowly. Therefore, patients will most likely require

TABLE 36-4 Common Adverse Effects of Opioids

Problem	Suggested Intervention
Sedation	May improve spontaneously with continued use. If it persists, consider psychostimulant (e.g., methylphenidate).
Nausea	Start metoclopramide 10 mg every 4 hours around the clock for 3 days, then as needed.
Constipation	Start laxative concomitantly (e.g., senna products). Titrate the dose.
Pruritus	Give antihistamine.
Cognitive slowing	Consider opioid rotation, improved hydration; review current psychoactive medications and educate family.
Respiratory depression	Reduce the opioid dose for mild depression. If moderate or severe, treat with opioid antagonists (e.g., naloxone).

regular laxative treatment for the duration of opioid therapy. A major myth is that constipation is a normal response to poor oral intake. Health care providers should be educated about the physiologic shedding of the lining of the gastrointestinal tract and bacterial proliferation in the colon, both of which contribute to the formation of stool.

Opioid-induced cognitive dysfunction can be a problematic adverse effect of opioids. A variety of opioids such as morphine, hydromorphone, and meperidine have active metabolites that can cause excessive sedation, cognitive slowing, hallucinations, delirium, and seizures. These active metabolites, such as morphine-3-glucuronide, bind to opioid receptors in the brain. The concentration of these metabolites is affected by opioid dose, length of treatment, dehydration, and renal failure. The first steps in treating neurotoxic adverse effects without compromising pain relief are to (1) change the type of opioid that is being administered (opioid rotation), (2) hydrate the patient to enhance excretion of the drug and its metabolites, and (3) provide appropriate support to the patient and the family. In rare cases in which severe agitation, hallucinations, or delusions develop, haloperidol may be required.

Rotation of opioids is a safe and reliable method of alleviating symptoms in patients who develop opioid-induced neurotoxicity, although the ideal alternative opioid has not been determined. If the patient is taking morphine, a trial of hydromorphone, oxycodone, or fentanyl is usually effective. The dose of the second opioid should be determined according to guidelines that determine an equianalgesic ratio.

Other less common adverse effects resulting from opioid use include sweating, pruritus, urinary retention, and pulmonary edema. Respiratory depression is a rare and serious complication of opioid use, especially when it occurs in patients with no previous history of opioid use who have not developed tolerance to the respiratory depressant effect of the drug.

Pain in Special Situations

Incidental Pain. Incidental pain is sudden and severe pain provoked by special maneuvers such as swallowing or movement. An increase in opioid dose during episodes of incidental pain may result in excessive sedation after the pain episode has subsided. In such cases, attempts should be made to increase the local control of pain with the use of techniques such as radiation therapy, orthopedic procedures, and neurosurgical procedures

Neuropathic Pain. Neuropathic pain is usually caused by damage to the nerves from direct tumor effect or its treatment. The pain can be burning or shooting. Neuropathic pain responds less to opioid therapy than does somatic or visceral pain, although it is generally alleviated by opioids to some degree. These patients frequently require the administration of adjuvant drugs in addition to opioids. The most commonly used drugs are tricyclic antidepressants, gabapentin, carbamazepine, clonazepam, baclofen, and corticosteroids.

Mucositis. Mucositis in patients with cancer of the head and neck usually results from the effects of chemotherapy, radiotherapy, or both. Pain is usually moderate in severity and the condition is self-limited in most cases, although rarely, pain can be severe and dose limiting. Mouth ulcers lead to dehydration from infection and decreased oral intake, especially among neutropenic patients receiving chemotherapy. Rehydration, local antiseptics, and oral opioids can frequently control the condition, although in severe cases, intravenous opioids may be required.

Nonpharmacologic Interventions. Some patients have severe pain that does not respond adequately to pharmacologic intervention; others develop intolerable toxicity. In these patients, adjuvant nonpharmacologic interventions should be considered (Table 36-5). Approaches such as transcutaneous nerve stimulation and physical therapy can be attempted in most patients because of their relatively limited adverse effects and low costs. Radiation therapy should be considered in patients with bony metastases. Single large fractions may be as effective as multiple fractions and may reduce the patient's discomfort as well as treatment costs.[36] In difficult pain syndromes, some neurosurgical and anesthesiologic procedures, such as cordotomy, rhizotomy, and different nerve blocks, may be helpful.

A number of psychological techniques can be very effective adjuvant treatments for enhancing pain control. These include relaxation therapy, cognitive therapy, biofeedback, and hypnosis.[37] These techniques can affect both the sensory aspects of pain and the psychological distress that many

TABLE 36-5 Nonpharmacologic Methods of Treating Cancer Pain

Radiotherapy
Neurosurgery
Orthopedic surgery
Anesthesiologic procedures
Physical therapy
Occupational therapy
Biofeedback
Cognitive-behavioral therapy
Hypnosis
Relaxation techniques
Transcutaneous electrical nerve stimulation (TENS)
Acupuncture

patients in pain experience. In addition, they tend to be of relatively low cost and free of adverse effects.

Cachexia-Anorexia

Until recently, cachexia was believed to be the result of an energy imbalance caused by the combination of increased energy consumption by the tumor and decreased energy intake due to tumor-related factors affecting the satiety center in the brain. Attempts to reverse cachexia associated with cancer by administering parenteral or enteral nutrients led to no significant improvement.[38] The emerging view of cachexia associated with cancer is summarized in Figure 36–2. A recent review describes the roles of cytokines such as tumor necrosis factor (TNF), interleukins 1 and 6 (IL-1, IL-6), and interferon-α. Long-term administration of these cytokines can cause many of the classic features of anorexia.[39]

Anorexia is the most frequent distressing symptom in patients with cachexia associated with cancer. Profound anorexia adds a nutritional deprivation component to the metabolic abnormalities. This deprivation is more severe in patients with dysphagia related to cancer of the head and neck. Anorexia is also worsened by nausea caused by tumor by-products, decreased gastric emptying, constipation, and pain medications. Moreover, patients with cancer of the head and neck can suffer from alterations of taste and smell that result in anorexia.

Management of Cachexia

One of the main challenges in the management of cachexia is defining a properly reasonable outcome for nutritional and pharmacologic interventions. A reasonable goal is to improve general comfort and ease the symptoms of anorexia, nausea, fatigue, and constipation.

NUTRITIONAL APPROACH

Nutritional counseling may help improve daily caloric intake in many patients; however, it is unlikely to reduce weight loss in most patients. Adequate counseling of patients and their families about the metabolic mechanism of cachexia helps to alleviate the anxiety of family members that their relatives are starving to death.

Parenteral nutrition has no advantages over enteral nutrition and is more expensive. Enteral nutrition is safer and can be administered at home. Patients with cancer of the head and neck who have dysphagia or difficulties with mastication or swallowing may benefit from gastrostomy tube placement. This tube may also be used for administration of medications.

PHARMACOLOGIC APPROACH

Table 36–6 summarizes the most useful drugs for the treatment of cancer cachexia. Promising research is under way to evaluate the possible beneficial effects of anticytokine therapies such as pentoxifylline, thalidomide, and melatonin. Moreover, molecular approaches using antisense strategies or antibodies to TNF and IL-6 have shown some promise in preclinical studies.[40, 41]

Fatigue

Cancer-related fatigue is characterized by persistent and unusual tiredness occurring after usual or minimal effort, accompanied by an unpleasant anticipatory sensation of generalized weakness that is not relieved by rest. The three main mechanisms associated with fatigue are direct tumor effects, tumor-induced by-products, and medical complications, including anemia, paraneoplastic syndromes, and chronic infection. Figure 36–3 depicts the major causes of fatigue.

The relationship between fatigue and cachexia is complex; most patients with advanced cancer experience both.

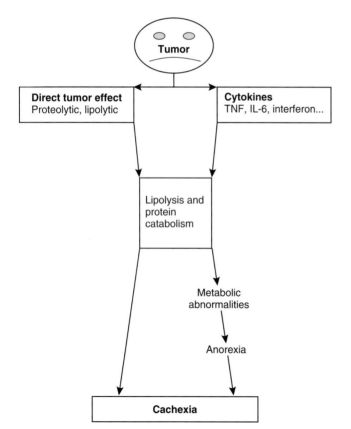

FIGURE 36–2 Mechanism of cachexia. TNF, tumor necrosis factor.

TABLE 36-6 Drugs Useful for Treatment of Cachexia

Drug	Comment
Metoclopramide	Most effective in patients with chronic nausea and autonomic failure, and those on opioids.
Corticosteroids	Effect is short-lived (up to 1 month). Suitable for advanced cancer. Significant adverse effects.
Megestrol acetate	Associated weight gain. Drug of first choice. Use associated with thromboembolism. Expensive.
Medroxyprogesterone acetate	Associated thromboembolic disease.

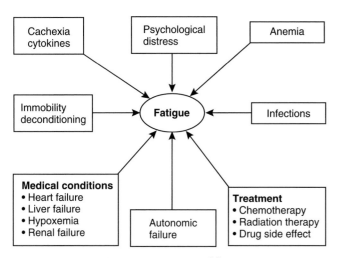

FIGURE 36–3 Causes of fatigue.

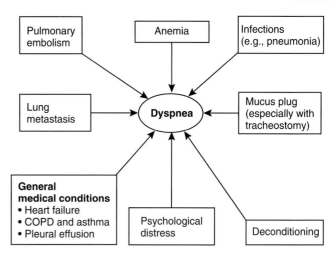

FIGURE 36–5 Causes of dyspnea in head and neck cancer. COPD, chronic obstructive pulmonary disease.

However, some patients with advanced cancer may have fatigue without malnutrition, whereas patients with conditions such as anorexia nervosa may experience severe malnutrition with no fatigue.

Management

Figure 36–4 presents a clinical approach to the management of fatigue. If specific causes can be identified, their correction will lead to significant improvement. General nonpharmacologic measures, such as adapting activities of daily living and providing physical therapy and occupational therapy, help in matching clinical function and symptom status with the expectations of patients and their families.[42] Counseling and appropriate pharmacotherapy may help patients in whom fatigue is exacerbated by an affective disorder such as anxiety or depression.

Dyspnea

Dyspnea has been defined as an uncomfortable awareness of breathing. It is an unpleasant subjective sensation and cannot be measured by any physical abnormalities.

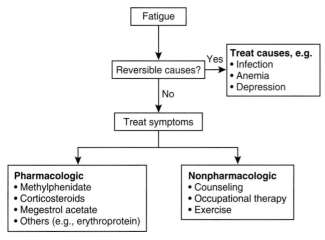

FIGURE 36–4 Algorithm for the management of fatigue.

Figure 36–5 summarizes the causes of dyspnea in cancer of the head and neck.

Patients with a tracheotomy have special problems related to accumulation of secretions and blockage of the stomal lumen due to enlargement of the tumor. The lumen can also be blocked during removal of the tracheotomy tube for cleaning. This can result in significant distress for the patient. In addition, the nursing staff often are stressed by caring for patients with tracheotomy.[43]

Many of the causes of dyspnea improve with treatment of the underlying condition, such as antibiotics for pneumonia, anticoagulation for pulmonary embolism, or blood transfusions for anemia. The symptoms of dyspnea are treated with oxygen, opioids, and behavioral strategies. Several randomized, controlled trials have shown that opioid therapy is beneficial for cancer dyspnea.[44] Corticosteroids are effective in the management of dyspnea associated with carcinomatous lymphangitis; they are frequently used in the management of superior vena cava syndrome.[44]

Delirium

Delirium is the most common neuropsychiatric disorder, affecting approximately 85% of patients with advanced cancer.[45] Patients with delirium experience a combination of cognitive dysfunction, fluctuating levels of consciousness, reversal of the sleep-wake cycle (insomnia and daytime sleepiness), hallucinations (especially visual and tactile hallucinations), delusions, and other perceptual abnormalities. The condition is frequently misdiagnosed by clinicians as anxiety or insomnia, which may lead to certain interventions that worsen the delirium, such as prescribing benzodiazepines. Hospitalized elderly patients are particularly at risk, and clinicians should maintain a high degree of vigilance when patients experience sudden alteration in mental status. Family members are particularly helpful in identifying early changes in cognitive function and mood.

Figure 36–6 highlights the causes of delirium in cancer patients. Common causes of delirium in cancer patients include infection, adjuvant medications (especially corticosteroids and opioids), and electrolyte imbalance. Delirium is

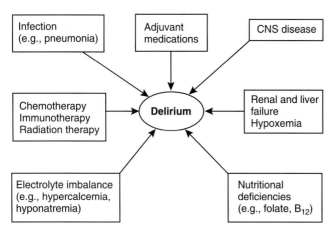

FIGURE 36–6 Causes of delirium in head and neck cancer.

classified according to psychomotor activity as hyperactive (agitated), hypoactive (hypoalert), or mixed.[46] The hyper-alert type of delirium is most common and tends to have the shortest duration and the best outcome.[47]

A detailed history is of utmost importance in the diagnosis of delirium. Simple bedside tests, such as the Mini-Mental State Examination,[48] may be useful for screening patients suspected of having frank delirium, although such brief tools are not helpful in patients with focal lesions or mild to moderate cognitive dysfunction.[49] In cases of suspected but mild cognitive dysfunction, neuropsychological assessment may be useful. Neuropsychological evaluations are also useful in differentiating organic from functional disorders and in identifying early dementia unrelated to cancer.

The most important interventions in the management of delirium are to remove any contributing medications, to use opioid rotation, and to treat any contributing underlying medical conditions. Haloperidol can be used for symptomatic management of delirium. In about two thirds of patients, delirium can be reversed and patients return to their baseline level of mental function.[50] Patients treated with haloperidol tend to have a shorter duration of this distressing state.[47]

SUMMARY

Patients with cancer of the head and neck suffer from multiple devastating physical and psychological symptoms. Pain, fatigue, cachexia, dyspnea, delirium, and psychological distress are precipitated by cancer and cancer treatment. These symptoms worsen the quality of life of patients with cancer of the head and neck and complicate their treatment. A history of alcoholism or poor psychosocial support may further complicate care. Multidimensional assessment of cancer-related symptoms is essential in helping to avoid complications, in providing early interventions, and in helping the patient and family cope better with the disease and its treatments. Palliative care, which can result in the provision of successful multidimensional care to patients with cancer of the head and neck and their families during the complete course of the disease, should be integrated early in the trajectory of the illness.

REFERENCES

1. Ganz P: Current issues in cancer rehabilitation. Cancer 65:742, 1990.
2. Beumer J, Curtis T, Harrison RE: Radiation therapy of the oral cavity: Sequel and management. Head Neck Surg 1:301, 1979.
3. Krause JH, Krause HJ, Fabian RL: Adaptation to surgery of head and neck cancer. Laryngoscope 99:789, 1989.
4. Million RR, Cassisi NJ, Clark JR: Cancer of head and neck. In Devita V, Hellman S, Rosenberg SA (eds): Cancer: Principles and Practices, 3rd ed. Philadelphia, JB Lippincott, 1989, pp 488–490.
5. Meyers CA, Geara F, Wong P, et al: Neurocognitive effects of therapeutic irradiation for base of skull tumors. Int J Radiat Oncol Biol Phys 46:51, 2000.
6. Foley KM: Pain syndromes in patients with cancer. In Bonica JJ, Ventafridda V (eds): Advances in Pain Research and Therapy. New York, Raven Press, 1979, pp 59–65.
7. Higginson IJ: Innovations in assessment: Epidemiology and assessment of pain in advanced cancer. In Jansen TS, Turner JA, Wiesenfield-Hallen Z (eds): Proceedings of the 8th World Congress on Pain, Progress in Pain Research and Management. Seattle, IASP Press, 1997, pp 707–716.
8. Nguyen P, Zekry H, Bruera E: Cancer pain assessment and palliative care management. Oncology 3:135, 2000.
9. Ma G, Alexandar HR: Prevalence and pathophysiology of cancer cachexia. In Bruera E, Portenoy RK (eds): Topics in Palliative Care, vol 2. New York, Oxford University Press, 1998, pp 91–129.
10. Neuenschwander H, Bruera E: Asthenia. In Doyle D, Hanks GWC, MacDonald N (eds): Oxford Textbook of Palliative Care, 2nd ed. New York, Oxford University Press, 1998, pp 573–581.
11. Breitbart W, Holland J: Psychological aspects of head and neck cancer. Semin Oncol 15:61, 1988.
12. Shedd DP: Cancer of the head and neck. In Holland JF, Frei E III (eds): Cancer Medicine, 2nd ed. Philadelphia, Lea & Febiger, 1982, pp 167–185.
13. Rothman K, Keller A: The effect of joint exposure to alcohol and tobacco on risk of cancer of the mouth and pharynx. J Chron Dis 25:711, 1972.
14. Deleyiannis FWB, Thomas DB, Vaughan TL, et al: Alcoholism: Independent predictor of survival in patients with head and neck cancer. J Natl Cancer Inst 88:542, 1996.
15. Lame F, Colleau SM, Brasseur L, et al: Multicenter study of cancer pain and its treatment in France. Br Med J 310:1034, 1995.
16. Price DD, MacGrath PA, Rafii A, et al: The validation of visual analogue scales as a ratio scale measurement for chronic and experimental pain. Pain 17:45, 1983.
17. Portnoy RK, Thaler HT, Kornblith AB, et al: The Memorial Symptom Assessment Scale: An instrument for the evaluation of symptom prevalence, characteristics and distress. Eur J Cancer 30A:1326, 1994.
18. Cleeland CS, Mendoza T, Wang XS, et al: Assessing symptom distress in cancer patients: The M.D. Anderson Symptom Inventory. Cancer 89:1634, 2000.
19. Allende S, Carvell HC: Mexico: Status of cancer pain and palliative care. J Pain Symptom Manage 12:118, 1996.
20. McCaffery M: Pain control, barriers to the use of available information. World Health Organization Expert Committee on Cancer Pain Relief and Active Supportive Care. Cancer 70:1438, 1992.
21. Cleeland CS: Measurement of pain by subjective report. In Chapman CR, Loeser JD (eds): Advances in Pain Research and Therapy, vol 12, Issues in Pain Measurement. New York, Academic Press, 1989, pp 391–403.
22. Chang VT, Hwang SS, Feurman M: Validation of the Edmonton Symptom Assessment Scale. Cancer 88:2164, 2000.
23. Bruera E, Moyano J, Seifert L, et al: The frequency of alcoholism among patients with pain due to terminal cancer. J Pain Symptom Manage 10:599, 1995.
24. Chow E, Connolly R, Wong R, et al: Use of the CAGE questionnaire for screening problem drinking in an out-patient palliative radiotherapy clinic. J Pain Symptom Manage 21:491, 2001.
25. Selzer ML, Vinokur A, van Rooijen L: A self-administered Short Michigan Alcoholism Screen Test (SMAST). J Stud Alcohol 36:117, 1875.
26. Bruera E, Scheller T, Wenk R, et al: A prospective multicenter assessment of the Edmonton staging system for cancer pain. J Pain Symptom Manage 10:348, 1995.

27. Parsons OA, Nixon SJ: Neurobehavioral sequelae of alcoholism. Neurol Clin 11:205, 1993.
28. Saleeba AK: Predictors of post surgery delirium in head and neck cancer patients [master's thesis]. University of Houston, Houston, TX, 1999.
29. Burman R, Chamberlain J: The assessment of the nutritional status, caloric intake, and appetite of patients with advanced cancer. In Bruera E, Higginson I (eds): Cachexia-Anorexia in Cancer Patients. Oxford, Oxford University Press, 1996, pp 83–93.
30. Mendoza TR, Wang XS, Cleeland CS, et al: The rapid assessment of fatigue severity in cancer patients: Use of the Brief Fatigue Inventory. Cancer 85:86, 1999.
31. American Pain Society: Principle of analgesic use in the treatment of acute pain and chronic cancer pain: A concise guide to medical practice. Skokie, IL, American Pain Society, 1992.
32. Fainsinger R, Bruera E, Miller MJ, et al: Symptom control during the last week of life on a palliative care unit. J Palliat Care 7:5, 1991.
33. Ripamonti C, Bruera E: Current status of patient-controlled analgesia in cancer patients. Oncology 11:373, 1997.
34. Ventafridda V, Spoldi E, Carceni A, et al: The importance of continuous SC morphine administration for cancer pain control. Pain Clin 1:47, 1986.
35. Bruera E, Brenneis C, Paterson A, et al: Use of methylphenidate as an adjuvant to narcotic analgesics in patients with advanced cancer. J Pain Symptom Manage 4:3, 1989.
36. Steenland E, Leer J, Houwelingen H, et al: The effect of a single fraction compared to multiple fractions on painful bone metastases: A global analysis of the Dutch Bone Metastasis study. Radiother Oncol 52:103, 1999.
37. Meyers CA: Psychologic management of cancer pain. Curr Rev Pain 1:126, 1997.
38. Klein S, Koretz RL: Nutrition support in patients with cancer. What do the data really show? Nutr Clin Pract 9:91, 1994.
39. Plata-Salaman CR: Cytokines and anorexia: A brief overview. Semin Oncol 25:64, 1998.
40. Eliaz R, Wallch D, Kost J: Long term protection against the effects of tumor necrosis factor by controlled delivery of the soluble p55-TNF receptor. Cytokine 8:482, 1996.
41. Kawamura I, Morishita R, Tomita N, et al: Intratumoral injection of oligonucleotides to the NF Kappa B binding site inhibits cachexia in a mouse tumor model. Gene Ther 6:91, 1999.
42. Neuenschwander H, Bruera E, Cavalli F: Matching the clinical function and symptom status with the expectations of patients with advanced cancer, their families, and health care workers. Support Care Cancer 4:252, 1997.
43. De Carle B: Tracheostomy care. Nursing Times 81:50,1985.
44. Walsh TD, West TS: Controlling symptoms in advanced cancer. Br Med J 296:477, 1988.
45. Breitbart W, Bruera E, Chochinov H, et al: National Cancer Institute of Canada workshop on symptom control and supportive care in patients with advanced cancer: Methodological and administrative issues. Neuropsychiatric syndromes and psychological symptoms in patients with advanced cancer. J Pain Symptom Manage 10:131, 1995.
46. Liptzin B, Levkoff SE: An empirical study of delirium subtypes. Br J Psychiatry 161:843, 1992.
47. Olofsson SM, Weitzner MA, Valentine AD, et al: A retrospective study of the psychiatric management and outcome of delirium in the cancer patient. Support Care Cancer 4:351, 1996.
48. Folstein MF, Folstein S, McHugh RR: "Mini-mental state," a practical method for grading the cognitive state of patients for the clinician. J Psychiatry Res 12:189, 1975.
49. Lezak MD: Neuropsychological Assessment, 3rd ed. New York, Oxford University Press, 1995.
50. Ingham J, Breitbart W: Epidemiology and clinical features of delirium. In Portenoy R, Bruera E (eds): Topics in Palliative Care. New York, Oxford University Press, 1997, pp 564–575.

CHAPTER 37

Quality of Life in Patients With Head and Neck Cancer

Ernest A. Weymuller, Jr.

Frederic F. W.-B. Deleyiannis

Bevan Yueh

INTRODUCTION

Why study quality of life (QOL) in head and neck cancer? Perhaps the dominant impetus is the disquieting truth that, when the traditional endpoints of survival and locoregional control are used, in many instances a significant difference between treatment options cannot be identified.[1] Additionally, some studies support the contention that QOL of patients undergoing treatment for head and neck cancer is worse than that of patients with more common cancers.[2, 3] It is thus important to understand the conceptual foundations related to QOL measures so that they may be properly applied both in selection of treatment and in design of new clinical trials.

Head and neck cancer and its treatment affect some of the most fundamental functions of life, including eating, communication, and social interaction. Treatment may consist of surgery, radiation, and/or chemotherapy and is often functionally and cosmetically devastating. Facial disfigurement, speech impediment, difficulty with swallowing and chewing, loss of taste, and shoulder pain are common consequences of treatment. These disabilities can alter self-esteem, limit activity and employment, and decrease social interaction with family and friends.

Disease-free survival, overall survival, and tumor response rates are the traditional outcome measures that have been used to judge the efficacy of treatment. Patients with stage I or II cancer of the head and neck generally have an 80% to 90% cure rate with minimal morbidity when managed by single-modality surgical treatment.[4] However, 5-year survival rates for patients with stage III and IV head and neck cancer are generally poor. Whether treatment is palliative or curative, the disability associated with treatment for advanced cancer often seems worse to the patient than the untreated cancer. For example, in his series of patients with stage IV head and neck cancer treated with curative or palliative intent, Burns reported that 42% of patients believed that "there was virtually no joy in life after treatment."[5] Gamba in his series of 66 patients treated surgically for advanced cancer of the head and neck without evidence of disease found that 18% of his subjects believed the disadvantages outweighed the advantages and that 30% believed the post-treatment difficulties were "too harsh."[6] In other words, the traditional outcome measures of treatment efficacy, such as tumor recurrence and survival time, are often meaningless to the patient. What matters is his or her ability to return to pre-illness function and psychosocial well-being.

Quality of life is the term used to describe the nontraditional outcome measures of functional status and psychosocial well-being. Especially in oncology, incorporation of QOL outcome measures to supplement standard clinical trial endpoints has recently increased.[7–9] QOL endpoints and assessment have been used in clinical trials for advanced colorectal cancer,[10] Hodgkin's disease,[11] advanced ovarian cancer,[12] lung cancer,[13] and chronic medical conditions such as hypertension, diabetes, and coronary artery disease.[14, 15] Furthermore, to promote the use of QOL outcome measures, both the National Institutes of Health and the National Cancer Institute sponsored workshops on QOL assessment in 1990, including the recent conference on "Measuring and Reporting Quality of Life in Head and Neck Cancer," sponsored by the National Institutes of Health, held in McLean, Virginia, in October 2002. This conference attracted an international audience representing quality of life researchers from 20 countries.[16, 17]

QOL research is not lacking in the head and neck literature. A number of articles provide reviews of previous QOL studies and highlight the need for further QOL research.[18, 19] Particularly helpful general reviews are the contributions from Ringash and Bezjak[20] and Long and associates.[21] Head and neck cancer QOL research has primarily consisted of descriptive, retrospective studies. However, this situation is changing. In 1993, Browman and colleagues used a QOL instrument to measure acute morbidity due to radiotherapy in a prospective, randomized study of concurrent 5-fluorouracil (5-FU) and radiotherapy in the treatment of advanced head and neck cancer.[22] Moreover, over the past few years, a number of general head and neck QOL questionnaires have been validated.[23, 24] Preliminary results indicate that these questionnaires are responsive to clinical change and could be incorporated into clinical trials.

This chapter has been written with a twofold purpose: first, to stress the importance of QOL assessment in the evaluation of treatment outcomes and rehabilitation needs, and second, to facilitate the design of future studies that will incorporate QOL measures. The following five questions will be answered:

1. What are the dimensions and the definition of QOL?
2. What general and disease-specific measures of QOL are available?
3. What research methodology may be used and what statistical criteria must be satisfied in the design of a head and neck cancer QOL instrument?
4. How has QOL assessment been used in head and neck cancer research?
5. What are the future uses and direction of QOL assessment?

◧ DEFINING THE CONCEPT AND THE CONTENT OF QUALITY OF LIFE

QOL is a multidimensional construct without a universally accepted definition. Ferrans and Powers define QOL as a "person's sense of well-being that stems from satisfaction or dissatisfaction with the areas of his life that are important to him."[25] According to Cella, QOL is a "patient's appraisal of and satisfaction with current level of functioning as compared to what they perceive to be possible or ideal."[26, 27] Crucial to any definition is the recognition that different people have different values that cause aspects of their lives to have different impacts on their QOL.[28] For example, a disease or treatment that would interfere with an individual's ability to work or to be active would have a more profound impact on the QOL of an individual who was employed and enjoyed exercising regularly than on the QOL of an individual who was retired and led a relatively sedentary life. It is also conceptually important to acknowledge that individual QOL varies over time according to a wide variety of extrinsic and intrinsic factors.[29]

An extraordinary range of components has been proposed to define the content of QOL. Aaronson stated that there are minimally four core dimensions of QOL: (1) functional status (i.e., activity level, vocational activity), (2) physical complaints (e.g., somatic sensations, disease symptoms, adverse effects), (3) psychological distress (e.g., anxiety, depression), and (4) social interactions (i.e., quality and quantity of relationships with significant others).[30, 31] Schipper and coworkers presented a similar classification of four dominant QOL domains: (1) vocation/activity, (2) affect/psychological state, (3) social interaction, and (4) somatic sensation.[32] Additional factors that have been proposed for inclusion in QOL assessment include financial/economic status, satisfaction with medical treatment, sexuality, spirituality, body image, sleep, and the ability to pursue personal leisure activities.

Health-related QOL should be differentiated conceptually from health status and overall QOL.[33] Health status refers to the functional, physical, and emotional effects of disease, whereas health-related QOL is a measure of how patients perceive and react to their health status. Overall QOL includes health-related QOL and non–health-related factors, such as family, friends, employment, and other life circumstances.

Existing assessments of QOL in patients with head and neck cancer have included a large variety of the components of QOL. Functional status and physical complaints are the most frequently used QOL dimensions. Questions frequently focus on concerns unique to head and neck cancer, such as difficulties with eating, swallowing, and speaking. Ability to return to work, interaction with others, and mood also receive particular attention. Two studies ask patients to rate the importance of QOL dimensions for the purpose of determining the relative value of each QOL domain.[34, 35]

◧ GENERAL VERSUS DISEASE-SPECIFIC QUALITY OF LIFE MEASURES

The increasing use of QOL assessment in clinical research has led to renewed discussion concerning the relative advantages of general and disease-specific QOL measures.[36] General measures, such as the Sickness Impact Profile (SIP), the Quality of Well-Being Scale, and the Medical Outcomes Study (MOS), summarize the general health status of an individual by asking detailed and numerous questions from a spectrum of the components of QOL (Table 37–1).[37–39] They are used for QOL assessment in a broad range of patients, particularly those with chronic disease. For example, the SIP has been used in patients who have rheumatoid arthritis,[40] cancer,[41] end-stage renal disease,[42] benign chronic pain,[43] and chronic obstructive pulmonary disease.[44] The principal advantage of general QOL measures is that they allow a comparison of results across different diseases.

Disease-specific health status consists of the physical symptoms, functional limitations, and emotional consequences of a particular disease. General health status includes the disease being studied and any clinically significant comorbidity. Clinically significant comorbidity can be defined as any concomitant ailment expected to have a physical, functional, or emotional impact. For patients who have head and neck cancer, health-related problems of alcoholism, such as pancreatitis, cirrhosis, or delirium tremens, or of smoking, such as lung cancer and chronic obstructive pulmonary disease, would be expected to have significant impact on general health status. Because a patient's general health status is an important determinant of treatment and prognosis, any interpretation of outcome should also include an analysis of comorbidity.[45, 46] Health-related QOL is a measure of how patients perceive and react to their disease-specific and/or general health status. Overall QOL includes not only health-related factors but also such nonmedical factors as employment, family, and friends.

Disease-specific measures are designed to assess specific diagnostic groups or patient populations. Specific questions are asked about clinical changes that clinicians think are important and detectable. For example, a cancer-specific measure should take into account that the patient has already been diagnosed with cancer and should distinguish functional states within this population. Disease-specific measures thus are often more responsive than general measures to changes in patient status over time but are less generalizable to other QOL studies. The Karnofsky

TABLE 37-1 Sickness Impact Profile Categories and Selected Items

Behavior Category	Selected Items*
1. Sleep and rest	I sit during much of the day.
	I sleep or nap during the day.
2. Eating	I am eating no food at all; nutrition is taken through tubes or intravenous fluids.
	I am eating special or different food.
3. Work	I am not working at all.
	I often act irritably toward my work associates.
4. Home management	I am not doing any of the maintenance or repair work around the house that I usually do.
	I am not doing heavy work around the house.
5. Recreation and pastimes	I am going out for entertainment less.
	I am not doing any of my usual physical recreation or activities.
6. Ambulation	I walk shorter distances or stop to rest often.
	I do not walk at all.
7. Mobility	I stay within one room.
	I stay away from home only for brief periods of time.
8. Body care and movement	I do not bathe myself at all, but I am bathed by someone else.
	I am very clumsy in body movements.
9. Social interactions	I am doing fewer social activities with groups of people.
	I isolate myself as much as I can from the rest of the family.
10. Alertness behavior	I have difficulty reasoning and solving problems, for example, making plans, making decisions, learning new things.
	I sometimes behave as if I were confused or disoriented in place or time, for example, where I am, who is around, directions, what day it is.
11. Emotional behavior	I laugh or cry suddenly.
	I act irritably and impatiently with myself, for example, talk badly about myself, swear at myself, blame myself for things that happen.
12. Communication	I am having trouble typing or writing.
	I do not speak clearly when I am under stress.

*Note: The complete questionnaire includes 136 items.
From Bergner M, Bobbitt RA, Carter WB, et al: The Sickness Impact Profile: Development and final revision of a health status measure. Med Care 19: 787–805, 1981.

Performance Status Rating Scale for cancer[47] and the New York Heart Association Functional Classification[48] are examples of disease-specific measures that have been used for decades.

To gain the advantages of both types of measures, investigators have recently synthesized both approaches into one measurement strategy, called *a modular approach to QOL assessment*.[30, 49] In this approach, a set of core disease-specific questions is supplemented by a set of site- or treatment-specific questions. The Functional Assessment of Cancer Therapy (FACT) and European Organization for Research and Treatment of Cancer (EORTC) scales are examples of

the modular approach.[35, 49] These instruments have a core cancer QOL measure with modules for different types of cancer, such as breast, lung, and head and neck cancer. General health questionnaires can be used concurrently with the core and modular questionnaires to obtain additional QOL information. As has been noted by Osaba, there is ample evidence "that some multidimensional measures of HQL (health-related QOL) may be more accurate predictors of survival than either KPS (Karnofsky Performance Status) or the Eastern Cooperative Oncology Group (ECOG) performance status."[50] If this is true, a disease-specific head and neck QOL assessment could be an important stratification variable for prospective randomized trials in head and neck cancer.

RESEARCH METHODOLOGY

QOL research originates from a long history of theoretical and methodological research in the social sciences, particularly in the assessment and quantification of subjective experience. The hesitancy to incorporate QOL outcome measures into clinical oncology trials originates partially from a lack of familiarity with this methodology. Several of the more salient methodological issues involved in the design or selection of QOL outcome measures address the following questions:

1. What should be measured?
2. Who should assess QOL?
3. When should QOL be measured and with what question time frame?
4. What are some of the considerations for response scales and the computation of an overall QOL score?

What Should Be Measured?

The scope of QOL inquiry is particularly important. Restrictions of measurement to functional status or physical complaints alone may fail to assess the impact of disease or treatment on a patient's entire life. However, more global measurements may fail to adequately assess dominant functional deficits or complaints. Investigators must strike some balance between the breadth of the domains of QOL and the depth of coverage within domains. If information concerning the impact of disease or treatment is limited, the assessment of a fairly large range of QOL domains may be necessary for characterizing QOL. However, if the expected difference due to treatment or disease is relatively small and difficult to detect, a more detailed instrument assessing only those domains that are uniquely affected by the disease or treatment may be more appropriate.

One of the most critical steps in QOL analysis is the matching of the research question with an appropriate QOL test instrument. Our experience at the University of Washington has demonstrated the inefficiency and inordinate costs of "across the board" QOL data collection.[51] Investigators will be best served by identifying a precise QOL question that addresses a specific head and neck site and then selecting a QOL instrument whose domains address the issues at hand.

What Is the Ideal Quality of Life Test?

In his text *Guide to Clinical Trials*, Spilker comments that "there are no ideal tests at present to evaluate quality of life."[52] A test that could become a gold standard would have the following characteristics:

1. Be rapid to complete.
2. Be reproducible.
3. Be valid either in a single patient population or across a large number of diseases.
4. Be widely accepted.
5. Not require excessive training of staff to administer.
6. Be easy to interpret.
7. Yield objective results.

The view of some researchers is that finding a test that meets all of these criteria is as difficult as finding the Holy Grail. It is an even greater challenge to devise a test that is applicable to patients in different national cultures.[52]

The conceptual formulation that has emerged, and that is gaining acceptance, defines QOL functionally in terms of patients' perception of performance in four areas—physical and occupational function, psychological state, social interaction, and somatic sensation. In this model, the patient serves as his or her own control, the comparisons being made against expectation of function.[53]

Spilker also notes that "the simplest classification of quality of life tests divides them into indexes, profiles, and batteries … An index is a test that *yields a single number* at its conclusion. It usually evaluates multiple domains and often tests multiple components of each domain. The test may include measures of the quantity as well as the quality of life."[54]

Functional disability scales (which are discussed as a subset of QOL assessment by Spilker) are more strictly used for the periodic assessment of physical disabilities. Increasingly, clinicians and researchers need reliable and validated measures of functional disability to measure clinical progress, evaluate programs, and establish appropriate eligibility for social and insurance programs.[55]

The inclusion of a global question in the process of QOL analysis is an important adjunct. According to Spilker, "Some authors and tests focus on objective criteria to define and measure quality of life, whereas others stress the measurement of subjective aspects of this concept. Using both approaches is best."[56]

Which type of instrument should be used (general vs. disease-specific) for a particular study becomes clarified once the researcher has decided on the necessary spectrum and depth of QOL domains. Pilot studies will aid in determination of the appropriate instrument. Instead of creating an instrument de novo, Cella recommends supplementing an existing instrument with relevant and specific items that are not included in the existing instrument.[27]

Cultural and Language Specificity

As has been noted, a number of head and neck disease–specific QOL instruments have been validated and used to support clinical research. As QOL investigation becomes more internationally recognized, it will be increasingly important for clinicians to understand that the QOL instruments that have been validated in a particular language or culture cannot be extrapolated to another simply by translation. Translated versions of existing QOL instruments must undergo rigorous methodological evaluation when transposed to a new language or culture.

Who Should Assess Quality of Life?

Data concerning QOL can be obtained from patient self-report or from others such as health care providers or persons close to the patient, such as friends or family members. In oncology trials, it has historically been the physician who has graded the performance status of the patient. However, several studies have documented the poor inter-physician reliability of performance scores obtained from physician-based observations, and perhaps more importantly, the low level of agreement between scores from patients' self-ratings and ratings determined by physicians.[57, 58] Consequently, current opinion endorses patient self-report, either from an interview or through a questionnaire completed by the patient, as the more reliable and valid source of QOL information.

Self-administered questionnaires should be designed in such a way that questions can be answered by individuals with varying educational backgrounds. Their use excludes patients who cannot read or write because of either educational or health reasons. They are frequently used in large trials in which training and deploying interviewers is not feasible. One potential disadvantage is the potential misinterpretation of the significance of incorrectly answered or inadequately completed questionnaires. The researcher is unable to determine if this is the result of a random error of omission or of bias resulting from the patient's unwillingness to provide certain information.

The principal advantage of interviewer-administered questionnaires is that there is less restriction on who can be interviewed and what can be asked. Anderson and colleagues also report that interviewer-administered questionnaires are less likely to underreport dysfunction than are self-administered questionnaires.[59] To avoid vague answers, the interviewer should ask specific and detailed questions instead of open-ended questions. The main disadvantage of interviewer-administered questionnaires is that the quality of the data is highly interviewer dependent. Possible areas of bias include the interviewer's level of training and preconceptions about the data, as well as age, sex, and race. If additional persons must be employed as interviewers, interviewer-administered questionnaires can be financially more costly than self-administered questionnaires.

When Should Quality of Life Be Measured and With What Question Time Frame?

Specific assessment times are determined primarily by the natural history of the disease, the characteristics of treatment, and the purpose of QOL assessment in a particular study. Cella suggests QOL measurement at four points during the course of treatment and follow-up: (1) immediately before treatment, (2) in the middle of treatment, (3) at the end of successful treatment, or at the point when the patient is considered to be nonresponsive to treatment, and

(4) at 6-month follow-up after time point 3.[27] In clinical trials in which the primary interest is the short-term or acute effects of treatment (i.e., the toxic effects of chemotherapy and/or radiotherapy during consecutive treatment cycles), more frequent QOL assessment may be appropriate. QOL assessment at more distant time points would be necessary to measure the long-term effects of successful or palliative treatment, for example, to determine the late complications of radiotherapy.

Researchers have employed a spectrum of time frames for QOL questions, primarily ranging from "at this moment" to 1 month. If the time frame is too long or is not specified, patients may be confused as to which period they should report. For example, if a patient was asked to describe his or her activity level during the 1-month period following chemotherapy, the patient might describe only the immediate effects of the chemotherapeutic drugs, such as nausea and vomiting, and not the beneficial effects of the chemotherapy on his or her primary cancer that enabled return to work 3 weeks after completion of therapy. Thus, it may be essential to limit the time frame to a relatively short period for interpretable and comparable responses to be obtained.

It is also important to consider the cost of QOL studies before embarking on a longitudinal project. In discussing clinical trials to evaluate QOL, Spilker indicates, "Implicit in this strategy is the large volume of data that flows from a quality of life study. Several variables are measured at each encounter and patients are followed for a considerable time. In addition to the usual clinical information, several items of quality of life data will be collected. This has clear workload implications."[60]

We have found this statement to be painfully accurate. In order to pursue QOL data for longitudinal analysis, one must be committed to thorough data collection and must account for the attendant costs. Collection of data at the University of Washington for 4 years generated costs in excess of $250,000 in personnel salary alone.

Although longitudinal studies may be the ideal model, some QOL issues can be effectively addressed with less expense and in a shorter time frame. Cross-sectional analysis describes the technique used to study a cohort of patients at a particular juncture (before or after treatment). Examples include the work of Terrell and associates, who evaluated QOL outcomes in survivors of the VA Laryngeal Trial,[61] and of Rogers and colleagues, who examined QOL in long-term survivors after surgery for oral cancer.[62] Cross-sectional analysis has significant limitations; in particular, it addresses only survivors, thus failing to evaluate the subset of patients who are likely to have the worst QOL (those who die from recurrent head and neck cancer). Nevertheless, cross-sectional studies are efficient and can provide useful information as long as the limitations of the technique are recognized.

What Are Some of the Considerations for Response Scales and for the Computation of an Overall QOL Score?

The two principal response scales are Likert-type scales and visual analogue scales (Table 37–2). Likert scales use

TABLE 37-2 Questionnaire Response and Importance Scales

a. Circle one number:

Not at all	A little bit	Somewhat	Quite a bit	Very much
0	1	2	3	4

b. Mark the appropriate position on the line:

No pain _____ Extreme pain
                    (10 cm)

c. Mark the appropriate position on the line:

No pain _____ Extreme pain

| 0 | | 1 | | 2 | | 3 | | 4 |

d. Circle one number:

How important is your physical well-being to your QOL?

Not at all   0   1   2   3   4   5   Very much

a. Likert-type scale. b. Visual analogue scale. c. Hybrid scale. d. Importance scale.

categorical data and present patients with a set of ordinal items from which they choose the item that best describes their experience. Visual analogue scales typically are 10-cm lines with descriptive anchors at the ends. The anchors represent polar responses. Patients are instructed to answer questions by making a mark on the scoring line at the point that best represents their response. A hybrid scale combines the 10-cm line and descriptive anchors of the visual analogue with the categorical guides of the Likert scale. Visual analogue and hybrid scales theoretically offer patients an increased number of responses and consequently may more closely approximate patients' true level of functioning. However, many investigators favor the Likert scale because the level of abstraction required by Likert scales is less than that required by visual analogue and hybrid scales. For example, in a prospective, randomized trial comparing QOL of patients receiving two different treatment programs for advanced, metastatic, non–small cell lung cancer, Ganz and coworkers reported that even after receiving oral and written instructions, patients still incorrectly marked the hybrid scale of the Functional Living Index—Cancer, a cancer-specific QOL measure.[63]

Overall QOL scores are computed in one of two principal ways: individual items are summed, or individual items are summed after being adjusted by a relative weight. In the latter format, item response scores are typically adjusted by an importance scale. For each item, patients are requested to indicate its importance to them on a Likert scale. The importance score is then used to calculate a unique patient-specific score for each item. This score is often the product of the response score and the importance score. The rationale behind this adjustment is that satisfaction with important domains of QOL has a greater influence on overall QOL than does dissatisfaction with relatively unimportant domains.

Importance Weighting

We favor the opinion of Spilker—"Another limitation of health status questionnaires is the unresolvable issue of whether each item should be equally weighted. From a clinical perspective, not all activities of daily living are equal for a patient, and the technology of deriving weights leaves the clinician dissatisfied …"[64] How does one weight the individual domain scores so as to arrive at a reasonable overall QOL score? At the present time, no studies have resolved this issue. It may be that the relative weightings of QOL domain scores are themselves variable over time, and hence not amenable to fixed weighting. Many researchers are now more confident in the use of QOL subscores as probes (not as diagnostics) and suggest that an assessment of QOL may include both an overall score, as defined precisely for the instruments being used, and component subscores. From an analytic point of view, this makes it possible for the clinician to begin to dissect component factors of quality of life and the variable impact that treatment may have on each.[60]

Our conclusion is that importance weighting may add a level of complexity that is generally not worth the trouble because we do not believe that the process of weighting is well defined or appropriate in most settings. When specific research inquiry warrants importance weighting, it is reasonable to ask the patient how he or she would weight the importance of a particular domain. This technique was used by Deleyiannis and associates in an analysis of postlaryngectomy QOL.[65]

▨ STATISTICAL CRITERIA FOR JUDGING QUALITY OF LIFE QUESTIONNAIRES

Once a questionnaire has been designed and deemed acceptable by patients, it must satisfy the statistical criteria of validity, reliability, and responsiveness before it is accepted for general use.

As an instrument is being developed, the researcher must consider whether it will ultimately be accepted by the patients for whom it is intended. Acceptance is defined as a patient's willingness to complete a specific instrument (i.e., questionnaire, interview), or the patient's preference for one instrument compared with another. Factors that influence acceptability include the ease and speed with which the instrument can be completed and the general health of the patient. For example, people with cancer may feel too ill to concentrate on lengthy, complicated forms.

Validity

Validity refers to the ability of an instrument to assess what it was designed to measure. There are three main types of validity: construct, content, and criterion validity.[66] Construct validity refers to how a particular instrument relates to previous expectations or theory. Content validity indicates the internal validity of the items of the questionnaire and their role in the overall goal of the questionnaire. Criterion validity is a comparison between the outcome results obtained with an accepted gold standard and the new QOL questionnaire being studied. In QOL research, there is not a consensus that a single QOL measure is the gold standard.

Generally, QOL questionnaires that are lengthier and cover more aspects of QOL are considered more valid.

Validity is statistically evaluated by examining the association between the study questionnaire and other similar measures completed at the same time. Relatively high correlation coefficients are expected for convergent validity. There is no accepted rule for the degree of correlation that is required for a test to be considered valid, but a coefficient of correlation (i.e., Pearson product-moment correlation coefficient) greater than 0.7 is regarded as strongly valid.[67] To confirm the validity of the computed QOL score, investigators can also ask patients to give a global rating (a single score) for overall QOL.

Reliability

Reliability indicates whether a measuring instrument would repeatedly produce the same results when applied to the same person under the same circumstances. It indicates the reproducibility of data and is established by test-retest results. In clinical trials, QOL measures must have a high degree of reliability to ensure that any observed change is due to the treatment and not to variation in the responses given to QOL questions. A variety of statistical test values, such as correlation coefficients, kappa values, and standard deviations of repeated measurements, can be used to indicate reliability.[68, 69] Similar to validity, a QOL measure with a coefficient of correlation greater than 0.7 is considered to be strongly reliable.

Responsiveness

Responsiveness measures the ability of a questionnaire to detect clinical change over time and after clinical intervention. Therefore, responsiveness is proportionate to the change in scores determined from a particular questionnaire before, during, and after treatment. A highly responsive QOL instrument can detect small changes in QOL. An overall QOL score ought to a have logical relation to specific oncologic stage. For example, a patient with stage I cancer ought to have a significantly higher disease-specific QOL score than a patient with stage IV cancer. It is also important that a questionnaire be sensitive to detect changes in QOL within an oncologic stage. For example, two patients with an identical oral cancer site and stage who have received identical treatment may perceive their QOL differently. This difference might be attributed to such differences as the patients' pretreatment medical or psychiatric status, treatment-induced complications, and ability to return to pretreatment employment.

▨ CANCER-SPECIFIC QUALITY OF LIFE QUESTIONNAIRES

General Cancer Questionnaires

Numerous valid and reliable QOL measures have been developed in oncology. The Karnofsky, ECOG, and American Joint Committee on Cancer (AJCC) Performance Scales are the three most widely used measures (Table 37–3).[47, 70, 71]

Karnofsky Performance Status Rating Scale. In 1949, the Karnofsky Performance Status Rating Scale was

TABLE 37-3 The Eastern Cooperative Oncology Group (ECOG), Karnofsky, and AJCC Performance Scales of the Host (H)

Performance	ECOG Scale	Karnofsky Scale (%)	AJCC
Normal activity	0	90–100	H0
Symptomatic but ambulatory; cares for self	1	70–80	H1
Ambulatory more than 50% of time; occasionally needs assistance	2	50–60	H2
Ambulatory 50% or less of time; nursing care needed	3	30–40	H3
Bedridden; may need hospitalization	4	10–20	H4

TABLE 37-4 Questions Asked in the Functional Living Index—Cancer

1. Most people experience some feelings of depression at times. Rate how often you feel these feelings.
2. How well are you coping with your everyday stress?
3. How much time do you spend thinking about your illness?
4. Rate your ability to maintain your usual recreation or leisure activities.
5. Has nausea affected your daily functioning?
6. How well do you feel today?
7. Do you feel well enough to make a meal or do minor household repairs today?
8. Rate the degree to which the cancer has imposed a hardship on those closest to you over the past 2 weeks.
9. Rate how often you feel discouraged about your life.
10. Rate your satisfaction with your work and your jobs around the house in the past month.
11. How uncomfortable do you feel today?
12. Rate, in your opinion, how disruptive your cancer has been to those closest to you over the past 2 weeks.
13. How much is the pain or discomfort interfering with your daily activities?
14. Rate the degree to which your cancer has imposed a hardship on you (personally) over the past 2 weeks.
15. How many of your usual household tasks are you able to complete?
16. Rate how willing you have been to see and spend time with those closest to you over the past 2 weeks.
17. How much nausea have you had in the past 2 weeks?
18. Rate the degree to which you are frightened of the future.
19. Rate how willing you were to see and spend time with friends over the past 2 weeks.
20. How much of your pain or discomfort over the past 2 weeks was related to cancer?
21. Rate your confidence in your prescribed course of treatment.
22. How well do you appear today?

From Schipper H, Clinch J, McMurray A, et al: Measuring the Quality of Life of Cancer Patients: The Functional Living Index—Cancer: Development and Validation. J Clin Oncol 2: 472–483, 1984.

developed to assess the physical well-being of cancer patients receiving chemotherapeutic agents. The scale is physician-administered and is thus based on the physician's subjective determination of the adjustment of the patient to the disease and its treatment effects. It offers little in assessing the patient's own perception of his or her QOL. The scale consists of 10 different levels that describe the functional status of the patient. For example, a score of 100 is assigned to a patient who is "normal" or free of symptoms, whereas a score of 0 is assigned when a patient is dead. The scale is graded by factors of 10 (i.e., 0, 10, 20, ... , 100). The large steps between levels and the crudeness of the scale have proved to make it unresponsive to subtle differences in the psychosocial and functional status of patients. Several studies have found its reliability to be as high as .89 with good validity, whereas other studies have questioned these conclusions.[57, 58]

ECOG Performance Scale. The ECOG scale, like the Karnofsky Performance Status Rating Scale, measures only a single item—functional status. The scale consists of five different levels graded from 0 to 4. A grade of 0 implies "normal activity," whereas a grade of 4 implies "inability to get out of bed." The Karnofsky scale and the ECOG scale have been used primarily to determine patient eligibility for enrollment in a particular study and to predict prognosis.

Other Scales. Recently validated cancer QOL measures include the Quality of Life Index (QL-Index),[72] the Functional Living Index–Cancer (FLIC),[32] the FACT scale,[35] and the EORTC Questionnaire.[24, 49]

The QL-Index was designed to be completed by the physician. The QL-Index comprises five categories of descriptive statements concerning activity, daily living, health, support, and outlook. Each category is scored as 0, 1, or 2, and the scores are summed for an unweighted value meant to represent QOL. The QL-Index has been criticized for a lack of specificity concerning cancer site and treatment and for the exclusion of QOL dimensions and has been praised for its brevity. Physicians can complete the questionnaire in less than a minute.

The FLIC is a patient-administered 22-item questionnaire originally validated on 837 cancer patients over a 3-year period (Table 37–4). Four principal areas of functional importance are defined: (1) vocational/activity,

(2) affect/ psychological state, (3) social interaction, and (4) somatic sensation. Each question is scored from 1 to 7 on a hybrid scale. An overall score is derived by summing scores on all questions without weighting individual QOL dimensions.

The FACT scale is a patient-administered 28-item general cancer QOL measure that can be supplemented with site and treatment modules. The initial validation process for the FACT scale involved 845 patients with cancer and 15 oncology specialists. In addition to a total score, subscores can be generated for physical, functional, social, and emotional well-being and for the patient's relationship with the physician. The FACT scale also allows patients to assign personal value to each QOL area. Cella is presently investigating a head and neck module to supplement the core FACT scale.[35]

The EORTC Study Group validated the first version of its core QOL questionnaire (QLQ-C36) in 537 lung cancer patients. Following this study, the core questionnaire was revised to a 30-item core instrument—the QLQ-C30. The QLQ-C30 consists of six function scales—physical functioning (5 items), role functioning (2 items), cognitive functioning (2 items), emotional functioning (4 items), social functioning (2 items), and global QOL (2 items)—and three symptom scales (pain, fatigue, and emesis). Individual items assessed include sleep disturbance, constipation, diarrhea, appetite loss, dyspnea, and financial impact of the illness. The QLQ-C30 is patient-administered and can be completed in a relatively short time (generally less than 11 minutes).

Head and Neck–Specific Questionnaires

Many head and neck QOL questionnaires have been developed for use across the broad spectrum of head and neck cancers: List's Performance Status Scale for Head and Neck Cancer Patients,[73] the EORTC Core QOL Questionnaire With a Head and Neck Module,[24] the University of Washington (UW) QOL Questionnaire,[23, 74, 75] Cella's FACT Scale With a Head and Neck Module,[35] and the University of Michigan Head and Neck Specific QOL Instrument[76] are among these.

List's Performance Status Scale for Head and Neck Cancer Patients. List's Performance Status Scale is a clinician-rated tool for measuring the unique disabilities of head and neck cancer patients in the areas of eating and speaking (Table 37–5). Patients receive a functional rating score in three subscales—eating in public, understandability of speech, and normalcy of diet. In each subscale, a list of items is arranged in a hierarchy, with normal function and total incapacitation receiving scores of 100 and 0, respectively. Reliability and validity were demonstrated in 181 patients with cancer of the head and neck, representing a range of diagnoses such as cancer of the oral cavity, pharynx, larynx, and other head and neck sites. Furthermore, when these patients were divided into four groups based on the extent

TABLE 37–5 List's Performance Status Scale for Head and Neck Cancer Patients

Eating in public
100 No restriction of place, food, or companion (eats out at any opportunity)
 75 No restriction of place, but restricts diet when in public (eats anywhere, but may limit intake to less "messy" foods, e.g., liquids)
 50 Eats only in presence of selected persons in selected places
 25 Eats only at home in presence of selected persons
  0 Always eats alone
Understandability of speech
100 Always understandable
 75 Understandable most of the time; occasional repetition necessary
 50 Usually understandable; face-to-face contact necessary
 25 Difficult to understand
  0 Never understandable; may use written communication
Normalcy of diet
100 Full diet (no restriction)
 90 Peanuts
 80 All meat
 70 Carrots, celery
 60 Dry bread and crackers
 50 Soft, chewable foods (e.g., macaroni, canned/soft fruits, cooked vegetables, fish, hamburger, small pieces of meat)
 40 Soft foods requiring no chewing (e.g., mashed potatoes, apple sauce, pudding)
 30 Pureed foods (in blender)
 20 Warm liquids
 10 Cold liquids
  0 Nonoral feeding (tube feeding)

From List MA, Ritter-Sterr C, Lansky SB: A performance status scale for head and neck cancer patients. Cancer 66:564–569, 1990.

of their surgery (wide local excision, partial laryngectomy, total laryngectomy, and flap reconstruction), significant group differences were found in all three performance subscales.

EORTC Core QOL Questionnaire With a Head and Neck Module. A disease-specific module for cancer of the head and neck to supplement the QLQ-C30 has recently been validated.[24] The module consists of 21 items measuring disease-related symptoms and treatment-related adverse effects. These items include questions concerning problems with tasting, swallowing, talking, producing saliva and mucus, and breathing through the nose. The module was completed by 126 patients. Thirty-three percent of patients had cancer in the oral cavity, 13% in the pharynx, 19% in the larynx, 18% in the skin, and the remaining 18% in the salivary glands, paranasal sinuses, thyroid gland, or cervical lymph nodes without a known primary. The EORTC QLQ-C30 with a head and neck module was found to discriminate between groups of patients before, during, and after treatment with radiation, and between acute, subacute, and late disease– and treatment-related symptoms and toxicity. For example, problems with soreness in the mouth, swallowing, and salivation/mucus production were worst halfway through the radiation course, while change in taste was greatest immediately after treatment completion. The questionnaire's high acceptance and compliance rates among patients add to its utility as a practical QOL instrument.

Before the publication of the EORTC head and neck module, Jones and associates developed a head and neck QOL questionnaire based on the EORTC core questionnaire to which a specific head and neck module had been added.[77] In the questionnaire, 14 questions specific to cancer of the head and neck were scored on an interval from 0 to 3. Responses to each question ranged from "not at all" to "very much." In Jones' study, 48 patients who had undergone surgical treatment for cancer of the head and neck completed the questionnaire (a response rate of 98%). For analysis, the patients were divided into five groups: laryngectomy (15), craniofacial procedure (11), pharyngolaryngoesophagectomy (5), "other operation" (4 patients who underwent a hemiglossectomy, 3 tonsillectomy, and 2 thyroidectomy), and patients with clinical recurrence. In each group, different problem areas were identified. Laryngectomy patients reported speech difficulties and hyposmia. Craniofacial patients described visual problems, headaches, and a diminished sense of taste and smell. Pharyngolaryngoesophagectomy patients described eating- and speech-related problems. Patients with recurrence reported problems with speech, self-consciousness, smell, taste, and eating. In Jones' opinion, the results indicate that additional studies should use the EORTC questionnaire to increase the clinician's understanding of functional problems, which in turn would aid rehabilitation efforts.

UW QOL Questionnaire. The UW QOL questionnaire was designed to be specific for head and neck patients.[23] It is patient-administered and generally can be completed in less than 5 minutes. The scale comprises 10 categories, each of which describes important daily living dysfunctions or limitations about which patients complain, that result from cancer of the head and neck or its treatment effects. Each of the nine categories includes several options that allow the patient to describe his or her own current functional status.

The highest level, or "normal" function, is assigned 100 points, whereas the lowest level, or greatest dysfunction, is scored 0 points. Each category contributes equally to the final score of the questionnaire of 1000 points. This questionnaire was administered to 75 head and neck cancer patients on three separate occasions: (1) several days preoperatively, (2) immediately postoperatively, (3) and 3 months postoperatively. Patients were grouped according to their clinical stage (T1, T2, T3, or T4). The questionnaire was found to be sensitive enough to detect not only the expected large differences in QOL for T3- and T4-stage cancer patients after treatment, but also the more subtle changes that may occur in T1- and T2-stage patients.

The UW QOL instrument was further assessed for internal consistency with the use of data collected from 550 patients. Based on this analysis, the domains have been modified to eliminate "employment" and "dryness," and a global QOL inquiry has been added. The internal consistency of the UW QOL-R (revised) scale is high (Cronbach's alpha = .85).[74]

Recently, Rogers and colleagues analyzed the addition of two questions regarding mood and anxiety. Their results indicate that the addition of these two questions has strengthened the UW QOL instrument by providing previously absent probes in the psychosocial realm.[75]

◼ QUALITY OF LIFE ASSESSMENT IN HEAD AND NECK CANCER

Two types of QOL studies have been done in cancer of the head and neck—those that report assessment strategies and QOL instruments and those that document QOL in specific patient populations. The purpose of QOL research in head and neck cancer has been threefold: (1) to use QOL as an outcome measure of treatment, (2) to assess the rehabilitation needs of patients, and (3) to determine the pretreatment QOL of patients so that QOL can be used as a predictor of prognosis. Site-specific and treatment-specific QOL questions account for the majority of QOL research in head and neck cancer. Particularly in cases where different treatments have nearly equivalent cure rates but different functional problems, questions of QOL have been raised to guide the selection of treatment. This particularly applies to treatment decisions for patients with cancer of the larynx.[65, 78-85]

The survival of patients with advanced cancer of the glottis treated with primary surgery is often reported as being the same as that for patients treated with radiotherapy or radiochemotherapy. Surgical treatment for cancer of the glottis can include removal of the entire larynx and loss of laryngeal speech, whereas radiotherapy preserves voice. The perception of a better post-treatment QOL, even in situations where radiotherapy has a less likely chance of cure, may lead patients to choose radiotherapy instead of surgery.

Harwood's comparison of post-treatment QOL between patients treated with radiotherapy and those treated with surgery illustrates the importance of using a QOL measurement for treatment selection for patients with cancer of the larynx.[79] In his series of 129 patients (113 patients treated with radiotherapy and 16 treated with surgery) who were rated in every parameter of voice (volume, pitch, ability to communicate, rate of speech) except for dryness of the throat, successfully irradiated patients had better ratings than did surgical patients. Moreover, less than 50% of laryngectomy patients were working after treatment had been completed, whereas more than 80% of the irradiated patients were working. The treatment groups of this series were comparable by stage. In the group of successfully irradiated patients, there were 89 T1 or T2 tumors and 24 T3 or T4 tumors. The initial stages of the surgery patients included 9 T1 or T2 tumors and 7 T3 or T4 tumors. One T1 and two T2 patients received a partial laryngectomy, whereas the other 13 surgical patients received a total laryngectomy. Functional rating scores were not stratified by partial or total laryngectomy, but the successfully irradiated T3 and T4 patients (the irradiated subgroup with the expected worse function) still maintained higher functional rating scores than did the entire surgery group.

More recently, Terrell and coworkers have analyzed the survivors from the Veterans Administration Laryngeal Cancer Study. Using a cross-sectional technique, they have demonstrated that the group treated with chemoradiation had a better QOL ($P < .05$) than those who had undergone laryngectomy.[86]

Other QOL studies have pointed out the overall impact of combined therapy, indicating that combined-modality treatment is a predictor for increased severity of symptoms and poor function after treatment completion.[2, 87]

Radiation is often chosen as the primary treatment not only for advanced laryngeal cancer but also for many other stage III and IV head and neck cancers. Recognizing the need to measure radiation-induced QOL changes so that treatment toxicities could be compared, Browman and associates developed and validated the Head and Neck Radiotherapy Questionnaire (HNRQ).[22] The HNRQ is interviewer-administered and consists of 22 questions that deal with radiation symptoms related to the following six domains: oral cavity, throat, skin, digestive function, energy level, and psychosocial status. Each question includes seven possible response options listed according to the degree of impairment with a Likert scale.

In a prospective, randomized, double-blind study of concurrent 5-FU and radiotherapy in the treatment of advanced head and neck cancer, the HNRQ was able to measure acute morbidity due to radiotherapy and to discriminate between patients receiving 5-FU and those receiving placebo. A total of 175 patients with cancer of the oral cavity, oropharynx, hypopharynx, or larynx receiving a 6.5-week course of radiotherapy were randomly assigned to receive concomitant fluorouracil or saline placebo. The HNRQ was administered weekly for the 6.5 weeks of treatment and for 4 weeks after treatment. The mean HNRQ and its domain scores showed significant declines during treatment, with a nadir in the placebo group near the end of treatment (week 7) and subsequent improvement over the next 3 to 4 weeks. The differences in mean HNRQ and all domain scores between placebo and fluorouracil groups were also highly significant.

Harrison and associates used List's Performance Status Scale to assess the functional outcome of patients with base of tongue cancer who had been treated with radiotherapy and/or surgery. In his series of 30 patients with squamous cancer of the base of the tongue, patients treated with external beam irradiation plus brachytherapy maintained an excellent QOL.[88] The mean scores were 83% for eating in public (indicating virtually no restrictions on where to eat), 93% for understandability of speech (virtual normal speech), and 75% for normalcy of diet (some restrictions on certain types of foods). Performance scores were also separated by T stage (8 patients had T1 tumors; 13 had T2 tumors; 8 had T3 tumors; and 1 had T4 tumor). Functional outcome did not deteriorate with advancing disease, but the relatively small number of patients prevented statistical confirmation of an association between performance status and T stage.

In a separate study by Harrison and associates, when 30 patients (21 with T1 or T2 tumors; 9 with T3 or T4 tumors) with squamous cell cancer of the base of the tongue treated with primary radiation were compared with 10 patients (5 with T1 or T2 tumors; 5 with T3 or T4 tumors) treated with primary surgery, patients treated with radiotherapy had consistently better performance scores.[89] All the patients treated with primary surgery had resection of tumor at the base of the tongue, neck dissection, and postoperative radiotherapy. The authors did not indicate either the extent of the surgery (whether patients required laryngectomy [total or partial], mandibulotomy, or hemimandibulectomy) or the type of repair. Because primary radiotherapy and surgery have similar local control and survival rates, the authors stated that these results suggest that radiotherapy ought to be the preferred treatment for T1 or T3 lesions and that surgery may not be needed for all T4 lesions.

Before any modality, either surgical or radiotherapeutic, becomes the accepted primary treatment for a particular type of cancer of the head and neck, the long-term effects of that modality on QOL should be known. The results of Larson's retrospective study of 148 patients with cancer of the oral cavity or oropharynx (39 T1 tumors, 69 T2 tumors, 17 T3 tumors, and 3 T4 tumors) treated only with radiotherapy and free of disease for at least 5 years (median of 119 months) support this particular need.[90] The study reported a 56.3% overall incidence of soft tissue ulceration, osteonecrosis, or spontaneous fracture. Osteonecrosis had occurred within 2 years of radiotherapy in 42% of patients with radiation-induced osteonecrosis (44 patients), within 3 years in 56% of patients, and within 5 years in 82% of patients. Of the 44 patients with osteonecrosis, 18 required subsequent partial or hemimandibulectomy. The incidence of lesser complications, such as pain, dryness, induration, atrophy, or trismus, was not reported but was likely higher. The findings of this study exemplify the high incidence and clinical significance of the late morbidity of radiotherapy for early-stage cancer. When choosing treatment, the physician must be aware of information concerning both the short- and long-term morbidity associated with a particular treatment. Additional QOL studies may provide additional information.

Deleyiannis and coinvestigators administered the UW QOL questionnaire to a group of 13 patients undergoing combined surgery and postoperative radiotherapy versus primary radiotherapy for advanced curable oropharyngeal cancer. Treatment (whether primary radiotherapy [n = 7] or combined surgery and postoperative radiotherapy [n = 6]) was significantly associated with a worsening of QOL. This was particularly true in the QOL domains of chewing and swallowing. Patients who underwent surgery appeared more likely to suffer from disfigurement and from a worsening of speech but had greater pain relief than did patients who received primary radiotherapy.[91]

Numerous investigators have conducted trials using induction chemotherapy plus radiotherapy in patients with locally advanced head and neck cancer.[84, 92–94] Induction chemotherapy has not been shown to improve survival rates, but it may play an important role in preserving laryngeal function. Consequently, investigators are interested in identifying the chemotherapy regimens that have the highest complete response rate, highest rate of organ preservation, longest survival, and lowest toxicity. Because toxicity directly impacts on QOL, the effects of chemotherapy on QOL have been assessed in a number of domains. Previous studies have measured physical well-being, mood, pain, nausea and vomiting, and appetite.[22, 95] Hematologic effects, such as neutropenia and thrombocytopenia, and nonhematologic effects, such as acute hepatic failure and renal failure, have also been measured.[93, 94] A standard QOL questionnaire (such as Browman's HNRQ) for chemotherapy trials in cancer of the head and neck can facilitate comparisons of toxicity across different studies and drug regimens.

A common purpose of QOL measurement is to assess the rehabilitation needs and the rehabilitative outcome of reconstructive surgery. Perhaps the most extensive use of functional parameters in rehabilitative analysis has been for patients with oral or oropharyngeal cancer.[96–98] Teichgraeber and associates in 1985[97] compared three groups of patients with oral or oropharyngeal cancer who had received radiation alone (20 patients), surgery alone (20 patients), or combined therapy (11 patients). The sites of primary tumors were anterior tongue (26 patients), base of the tongue (9 patients), floor of the mouth (6 patients), retromolar-anterior faucial pillar (RMT-AFP) (4 patients), alveolar ridge (4 patients), and buccal mucosa (2 patients). Patients were assessed in the following domains: speech intelligibility, articulation, tongue mobility, swallowing, employment status, activity level, pain level, weight, salivary flow, status of mandible and teeth, and taste. Overall, patients with RMT-AFP, base of the tongue, and anterior tongue cancers had the best speech scores, whereas patients with buccal mucosa, alveolar ridge, and floor of the mouth cancers had the worst scores. Radiotherapy patients had the best speech and swallowing function, and those treated with combined therapy had the worst function. When oral reconstruction techniques were compared, those patients with intraoral skin grafts had the best speech results. Patients with tongue flap reconstruction had better speech results than those treated with primary closure, but the primary closure patients had the best deglutition scores. The uneven distribution of the oral lesions by site and the limited number of patients necessitate that the results of this study be reassessed in a larger prospective study.

In 1987, McConnel, Teichgraeber, and Adler used a protocol similar to Teichgraeber's 1985 protocol to compare three types of oral cavity reconstruction: skin grafts, hemitongue flaps, and myocutaneous flaps.[98] Speech and swallowing were studied in 15 surgical patients with T2 or T3 tongue and/or floor of the mouth lesions. Functions evaluated included speech intelligibility, articulation, tongue mobility, diadochokinesis, and oral phase swallowing. This study demonstrated that tongue mobility was the most significant variable in determining postoperative speech results and that patients with split-thickness skin grafts had the best speech and swallowing function.

Komisar published the first studies of the functional results of mandibular reconstruction for patients who had undergone composite resection of oropharyngeal cancer.[99, 100] In his 1990 series, seven patients underwent reconstruction with a metal plate and a free bone graft taken from the iliac crest. One patient underwent reconstruction with only a metal plate. In the reconstructed group, two patients also received myocutaneous flaps. In the group of eight patients who did not undergo mandibular reconstruction, seven received myocutaneous flaps for oral closure. The functions of deglutition, mastication, and cosmesis were compared between patients with and without reconstruction. There was no significant difference in deglutition. Mastication was worse and cosmesis was improved among the patients with reconstruction. Patients with reconstruction also had a greater number of hospitalizations secondary to complications from the reconstructive procedure. Kosimar concluded that aggressive surgical reconstruction of the mandible for lateral defects does little to improve the QOL of patients with oral pharyngeal cancer.

In 1991, Urken and colleagues demonstrated the functional advantages of free-tissue transfer in oromandibular reconstruction.[101] Using a number of tests to assess overall well-being, cosmesis, deglutition, oral competence, speech, length of hospitalization, masticatory function, and dental rehabilitation, Urken compared 10 patients who underwent one-stage oromandibular reconstruction using the iliac crest–internal oblique free flap and dental rehabilitation with osseointegrated implants versus 10 patients with similar soft tissue and bone defects who underwent no bony reconstruction of the mandible. In the group of patients with nonreconstructed mandibles, three required a pectoralis major flap for oral cavity reconstruction. One patient had reconstruction with a hemitongue flap. The defect in the remaining six patients was closed primarily. In almost all functional and psychosocial categories, patients who had undergone reconstruction had higher scores. The average length of hospitalization for patients with reconstruction (20.1 days) was not significantly higher than the length of hospitalization (19.7 days) for patients who had not undergone reconstruction. In addition, patients with mandibular reconstruction achieved a functional level closer to that of their pre-disease state and were able to resume employment and social activities more frequently than patients who had not undergone reconstruction.

Urken's study represents the type of critical analysis of post-treatment function that is necessary for the evaluation of surgical therapy. Without such analysis, treatment decisions are based on the surgeon's preference. However, this study did not address pretreatment status and the possible confounding factor that the group of patients who had reconstruction might have had a pretreatment functional status significantly better than that of patients who did not undergo reconstruction. Patients with relatively low pretreatment functional status might not be good surgical candidates for microvascular free-flap reconstruction and would be expected to have a lower postoperative functional status based solely on their pretreatment status.

One indication that the group of patients who had undergone reconstruction might have been a subgroup with a particularly high level of pretreatment functioning and low operative risk is the decreased incidence of complications among these patients compared with the total series of patients who underwent reconstruction with microvascular free flaps at the same institution. In the series of 200 patients who received microvascular free flaps (from which 120 received vascularized bone–containing free flaps for mandibular and midface reconstruction), major complications (including death, severe neurologic dysfunction, and 31 reoperations for ischemia of the flap, infection, or donor site problems) occurred in 18% of patients, and minor complications that did not require surgical intervention (i.e., hardware exposure, seroma) occurred in 9.5% of patients. Five and 13 patients experienced, respectively, postoperative delirium tremens and pneumonia.[102] Alternatively, in Urken's subgroup of 10 patients who had undergone mandibular reconstruction, no major or minor complications were reported. One patient had a prolonged hospitalization due to alcohol withdrawal, and three patients underwent removal of their fixation plate at 9 to 12 months because of sinus tracts secondary to loose screws. A prospective, randomized study with pretreatment QOL evaluation could address questions concerning the confounding influence of pretreatment QOL.

To address specific areas relevant to head and neck cancer surgery, a subset of domains can be used, as in the studies by Kuntz and coworkers[103] and Terrell and associates,[61] who analyzed shoulder function after various forms of neck dissection. Both studies documented a significant negative impact from the classic radical neck dissection when compared with accessory nerve preservation. Similarly, Brown and colleagues used the speech and swallowing domains of the UW QOL to assess outcomes of two different forms of palatal reconstruction after resection for cancer. They were able to document better outcomes when a pharyngeal flap was used to supplement radial forearm flap reconstruction.[104]

◼ QUALITY OF LIFE AS A SCREENING MECHANISM

One of the most appropriate and altruistic targets for the head and neck QOL movement will be to make the transition from analysis to action. Now that the areas of greatest negative impact on QOL have been highlighted, it is entirely reasonable to expect that we should focus on methods to eliminate or treat them. Our goal should be to *improve* the health and QOL of our head and neck cancer patients as a result of the therapeutic encounter.

Pursuing this line of thought, a number of groups have analyzed patients with head and neck cancer, have demonstrated high levels of anxiety, depression,[105, 106] and alcoholism[107] in these patients, and have studied the impact these disorders have on treatment compliance[108, 109] and disability.[2, 107]

Because it is the patient who ultimately bears the consequences of treatment, treatment decisions should be based on patient (not physician) attitudes toward quality as well as quantity of life. Patients should have all the information about the consequences of treatment available to them before receiving treatment and should actively participate with their physicians in medical decision making concerning their care. Patients may choose to preserve their QOL at the risk of having decreased survival times. For example, in one study of attitudes toward the quantity and quality of life, approximately 20% of the volunteers interviewed chose radiotherapy instead of surgery for a stage T3 carcinoma of the larynx so that they could maintain their voices, even though radiotherapy is associated with a lower survival rate.[78] Because the volunteers who were interviewed did not have cancer, the results of this study should be interpreted with caution. Clinicians are aware of the devastation wrought by locoregional recurrence, but patients have no way to perceive the risk or reality of that situation when choosing initial therapy. Recurrence could change patients' attitudes toward quantity and quality of life. For example, patients who had initially chosen a less radical treatment for the purpose of preserving their pretreatment QOL might find that the decline in QOL caused by recurrence and subsequent treatment is worse than the QOL decline expected by a more radical initial therapy. Perhaps a study of how attitude toward QOL changes in patients with recurrence, and how this change if anticipated by patients may affect initial treatment selection, is warranted.

◖ THE FUTURE

The infrequent use of QOL assessment in earlier head and neck clinical trials was founded on the belief that QOL was unmeasurable and undefinable. Clinicians have traditionally searched for "hard data," that is, variables that could be accurately and repeatedly measured and expressed in numbers.[110, 111] Consequently, the results of treatment have been expressed in terms of such variables as survival, tumor response rates, and tumor size. Data concerning a patient's functional status, distress, pain, ability to work, and other qualities of life were often considered to be too "soft" to merit scientific attention and thus were excluded from scientific analysis of diagnosis and treatment. These exclusions denied the importance of the aspects of life perhaps most meaningful to the patient and diverted attention from the clinician's obligation to provide comfort and relief, not just cure.

The challenge was that the "soft" data of QOL research needed to be "hardened" and made intellectually respectable. Reliability and responsiveness are the crucial criteria for acceptance of information as hard data. Recent head and neck cancer QOL measures, in particular the UW QOL questionnaire and Browman's HNRQ, have demonstrated not only reliability but also responsiveness. Moreover, QOL data have been used to critically analyze reconstructive techniques and to influence treatment selection in clinical trials in which two different treatments led to similar survival rates but a significant discrepancy in QOL. Thus, the present and future challenge of head and neck cancer research is to work toward the routine inclusion of QOL outcome measures in clinical trials. QOL might

prove to be the most sensitive and powerful measure of treatment efficacy.

Improving Study Design

Because of the lack of a universally accepted definition of QOL and the existence of a number of QOL instruments, investigators who wish to conduct QOL studies must clearly indicate what they mean by QOL and must identify the particular QOL domains that are to be measured. One appraisal of the quality of QOL measurements in the medical literature found that in a sample of 75 articles with the term "quality of life" in their titles, only 15% conceptually defined QOL and only 47% identified the target domains. Moreover, no article distinguished overall QOL from health-related QOL.[33] The results of this study highlight the need for investigators to more clearly differentiate between disease-specific health status, general health status, health-related QOL, and overall QOL.

Schwartz and associates reviewed 445 abstracts discussing "quality of life" or "health status" in head and neck cancer patients. Sixty-one articles were scrutinized, with the finding that 40 different QOL instruments were used and only 18% of studies were hypothesis-driven.[112] The authors set the stage for future investigation in head and neck QOL by stating, "Despite these barriers, the importance of using QOL outcomes in evaluating head and neck cancer treatment has grown because it shows promise as a means of deciding between treatments when no survival advantage is afforded by one modality over another. However, if the results of QOL studies are not made meaningful to clinicians, the potential of these measures will not be realized. Therefore, we make the following recommendations. Studies using instruments to measure QOL outcomes and to compare groups should be precise in their identification of what construct is to be measured, for example, health-related quality of life (HrQOL), functional status, or depression. Comparator groups should be identified a priori and a testable hypothesis should be presented. Finally, the clinical importance of reported differences must be interpreted using familiar anchors or minimally important differences until the instruments are more widely used and their scores understood."[11]

The medical care system in the United States is currently reassessing managed care. In a managed care system, medical services are often ranked in order of importance based on a cost-effectiveness analysis and the perceived health benefit gained from the treatment. A cost-effectiveness analysis dictates a priority list based on a calculated cost-to-benefit ratio. Increasingly, physicians are asked to demonstrate the benefit of a treatment in terms of QOL with the purpose of justifying financial reimbursement. For example, the Oregon Health Services Commission prioritized its list of health care services on the basis of net expected health "benefits."[113] "Benefits" were generally restricted to include the final outcomes of longevity plus QOL. Intermediate outcomes, such as tumor shrinkage, were not considered for the priority ranking. Consequently, in cancer of the head and neck where treatment may not significantly prolong life but may either improve or reduce a patient's QOL, investigators must learn to use QOL measures to quantify the effects of treatment and thus justify the need for and the selection of treatment. Patient satisfaction with medical care will also undoubtedly increase as patients realize that their QOL is one of their physicians' primary concerns.

Refining QOL Research

At the beginning of the 21st century, we can state that QOL research in general, and specifically head and neck cancer QOL research, has a solid methodological basis. It is time to deal with the next set of challenges, many of which have been well defined by Morton.[114]

The NIH-sponsored conference on "Measuring and Reporting Quality of Life in Head and Neck Cancer" (McLean, Virginia, 2002) was assembled in large part to achieve consensus on existing QOL measures, outline current challenges, and highlight areas for further research. In particular, it is important that we work toward the following goals:

1. Identify a small set of accepted instruments.
2. Collaborate in data accumulation to reduce the impact of heterogeneous sites, stages, and forms of treatment.
3. Use QOL as a therapeutic tool to identify those patients in need of early intervention and treatment for conditions such as depression, anxiety, and alcoholism.
4. Increase the emphasis on well-designed hypothesis-driven studies.
5. Broaden societal and third party payer awareness that head and neck cancer patients are uniquely affected by their illness and its treatment. In general, they require more intensive support when compared with patients with common cancers.
6. Clarify the meaning of numeric representation of QOL. How does the score from a head and neck cancer–specific QOL instrument describe a patient's QOL experience?

REFERENCES

1. Weymuller EA Jr: Moratorium on multi-institutional head and neck cancer trials. Head Neck 16:529–530, 1994.
2. Terrell JR, Nanavati K, Esclamado RM, et al: Health impact of head and neck cancer. Otolaryngol Head Neck Surg 120:852–859, 1999.
3. Gritz ER, Carmack CL, deMoor C, et al: First year after head and neck cancer: Quality of life. J Clin Oncol 17:352–360, 1999.
4. Coniglio JU, Netterville JL: Guidelines for patient management. In Bailey BJ (ed): Head and Neck Surgery—Otolaryngology. Philadelphia, JB Lippincott, 1993, p 1022.
5. Burns L, Chase D, Goodwin WJ: Treatment of patients with stage IV cancer: Do the ends justify the means? Otolaryngol Head Neck Surg 97:8–14, 1987.
6. Gamba A, Romano M, Grosso IM, et al: Psychosocial adjustment of patients surgically treated for head and neck cancer. Head Neck 14:218–223, 1992.
7. Fletcher AE: Measurement of quality of life in clinical trials of therapy. Recent Results Cancer Res 111:216–230, 1988.
8. Moinpour CM, Feigl P, Metch B, et al: Quality of life end points in cancer clinical trials: Review and recommendations. J Natl Cancer Inst 81:485–495, 1989.
9. Gotay CC, Korn EL, McCabe MS, et al: Quality-of-life assessment in cancer treatment protocols: Research issues in protocol development. J Natl Cancer Inst 84:575–579, 1992.
10. Poon MA, O'Connell MJ, Moertel CG, et al: Biochemical modulation of fluorouracil: Evidence of significant improvement of survival and quality of life in patients with advanced colorectal Cancer. J Clin Oncol 7:1407–1418, 1989.
11. Kornblith AB, Anderson J, Cella DF, et al: Quality of life assessment of Hodgkin's disease survivors: A model for cooperative clinical trials. Oncology 4:93–101, 1990.
12. Walczak JR, Brady M: Comparison of quality of life (QOL) in ovarian cancer patients participating in a national cooperative troup phase III randomized trial. Proc Am Soc Clin Oncol 10:A1185, 1991.
13. Ganz PA, Lee JJ, Siau J: Quality of life assessment: An independent prognostic variable for survival in lung cancer. Cancer 67:3131–3135, 1991.
14. Stewart AL, Greenfield S, Hays RD, et al: Functional status and well-being of patients with chronic conditions. Results from the Medical Outcomes Study. JAMA 262:907–913, 1989.
15. Tarlov AR, Ware JE, Greenfield S, et al: The Medical Outcomes Study: An application of methods for monitoring the results of medical care. JAMA 262:925–930, 1989.
16. Office of Disease Prevention, Office of Medical Applications of Research, National Cancer Institute: Workshop on quality of life research in cancer clinical trials. Presented at the NCI Annual Conference, July 16–17, 1990, Bethesda, Maryland.
17. Office of Science Policy and Legislation, National Institutes of Health: Workshop on quality of life assessment: Practice, problems, and promise. Presented at the NIH Annual Conference, October 15–17, 1990, Bethesda, Maryland.
18. Drettner B, Ahlbom A: Quality of life and state of health for patients with cancer in the head and neck. Acta Otolaryngol 96:307–314, 1983.
19. Gotay CC, Moore TD: Assessing quality of life in head and neck cancer. Qual Life Res 1:5–17, 1992.
20. Ringash J, Bezjak A: A structured review of quality of life instruments for head and neck cancer patients. Head Neck 23:201–213, 2001.
21. Long SA, D'Antonio LL, Robinson EB, et al: Factors related to quality of life and functional status in 50 patients with head and neck cancer. Laryngoscope 106:1084–1088, 1996.
22. Browman GP, Levine MN, Hodson DI, et al: The head and neck radiotherapy questionnaire: A morbidity/quality-of-life instrument for clinical trials of radiation therapy in locally advanced head and neck cancer. J Clin Oncol 11:863–872, 1993.
23. Hassan SJ, Weymuller EA: Assessment of quality of life in head and neck cancer patients. Head Neck 15:485–496, 1993.
24. Bjordal K, Kaasa S: Psychometric validation of the EORTC core quality of life questionnaire, 30-item version and a diagnosis-specific module for head and neck cancer patients. Acta Oncol 31:311–321, 1992.
25. Ferrans CE, Powers MJ: Psychometric assessment of the quality of life index. Res Nurs Health 15:29–38, 1992.
26. Cella DF, Tulsky DS: Quality of life in cancer: Definition, purpose, and method of measurement. Cancer Invest 11:327–336, 1993.
27. Cella DF, Cherin EA: Quality of life during and after cancer treatment. Compr Ther 14:69–75, 1988.
28. Ferrans CE, Powers MJ: Quality of life index: Development and psychometric properties. ANS Adv Nurs Sci 8:15–24, 1985.
29. Calman KC: Quality of life in cancer patients—an hypothesis. J Med Ethics 10:124–127, 1984.
30. Aaronson NK, Bullinger M, Ahmedzai S: A modular approach to quality-of-life assessment in cancer clinical trials. Rec Results Cancer Res 111:231–248, 1987.
31. Aaronson NK: Quality of life assessment in clinical trials: Methodologic issues. Control Clin Trials 10:195S–208S, 1989.
32. Schipper H, Clinch J, McMurray A, et al: Measuring the quality of life of cancer patients: The Functional Living Index—Cancer: Development and validation. J Clin Oncol 2:472–483, 1984.
33. Gill TM, Feinstein AR: A critical appraisal of the quality of quality-of-life measurements. JAMA 272:619–626, 1994.
34. Piccirillo JF: Development and validation of the head and tumor outcome measure (HTOM). Information about importance scales and the HTOM was communicated by personal correspondence.
35. Cella DF, Tulsky DS, Gray G, et al: The functional assessment of cancer therapy scale: Development and validation of the general measure. J Clin Oncol 11:570–579, 1993.
36. Patrick DL, Deyo RA: Generic and disease-specific measures in assessing health status and quality of life. Med Care 27:S217–232, 1989.
37. Bergner M, Bobbitt RA, Carter WB, et al: The Sickness Impact Profile: Development and final revision of a health status measure. Med Care 19:787–805, 1981.

38. Bush JW: General health policy model/quality of well-being (QWB) scale. In Wenger NK, Mattson ME, Furber CD, et al (eds): Assessment of Quality of Life in Clinical Trials of Cardiovascular Therapies. New York, Lejack Publishing, 1984.

39. Ware JE, Sherbourne CD: The MOS 36-Item Short-Form Health Survey (SF-36). I. Conceptual framework and item selection. Med Care 30:473–483, 1992.

40. Deyo RA, Inui TS, Leninger J, et al: Physical and psychosocial function in rheumatoid arthritis. Arch Intern Med 142:879–892, 1982.

41. Bergman B, Sullivan M, Sorenson S: Quality of life during chemotherapy for small cell lung cancer. II. A longitudinal study of the EORTC core quality of life questionnaire and comparison with the Sickness Impact Profile. Acta Oncol 31:19–28, 1992.

42. Hart LG, Evans RW: The functional status of ESRD patients as measured by the Sickness Impact Profile. J Chron Dis 40:S117–S136, 1987.

43. Augustinsson LE, Sullivan L, Sullivan M: Physical, psychologic, and social function in chronic pain patients after epidural spinal electrical stimulation. Spine 11:111–119, 1986.

44. Schrier AC, Dekker FW, Kaptein AA, et al: Quality of life in elderly patients with chronic nonspecific lung disease seen in family practice. Chest 98:894–899, 1990.

45. Feinstein AR: The pre-therapeutic classification of comorbidity in chronic disease. J Chron Dis 23:455–468, 1970.

46. Piccirillo JF, Wells CK, Sasaki CT, et al: New clinical severity staging system for cancer of the larynx: Five year survival rates. Ann Otol Rhinol Laryngol 103:83–92, 1994.

47. Karnofsky DA, Burchenal JH: Clinical evaluation of chemotherapeutic agents in cancer. In McLeod CM (ed): Evaluation of Chemotherapeutic Agents. New York, Columbia University Press, 1949.

48. Criteria Committee of the New York Heart Association: Diseases of the heart and blood vessels: Nomenclature and criteria for diagnosis. Boston, Little, Brown, 1964.

49. Sprangers MAG, Cull A, Bjordal K, et al: The European Organization for Research and Treatment of Cancer approach to quality of life assessment: Guidelines for developing questionnaire modules. Qual Life Res 2:287–295, 1993.

50. Osoba D: Lessons learned from measuring health-related quality of life in oncology. J Clin Oncol 12:608–616, 1994.

51. Weymuller EA Jr, Yueh B, Deleyiannis FWB, et al: Quality of life in patients with head and neck cancer. Arch Otolaryngol Head Neck Surg 126:329–335, 2000.

52. Spilker B: Quality of life trials. In Guide to Clinical Trials. New York, Raven Press, 1991, p 377.

53. Spilker B: Definitions and conceptual issues. In Quality of Life Assessments in Clinical Trials. New York, Raven Press, 1990, p 11.

54. Spilker B: Quality of life trials. In Guide to Clinical Trials. New York, Raven Press, 1991, p 371.

55. Spilker B: Functional disability scales. In Quality of Life Assessments in Clinical Trials. New York, Raven Press, 1990, p 115.

56. Spilker B: Interpreting quality of life data. In Guide to Clinical Trials. New York, Raven Press, 1991, p 729.

57. Hutchinson TA, Boyd NF, Feinstein AR: Scientific problems in clinical scales as demonstrated by the Karnofsky Index of Performance Status. J Chron Dis 32:661–666, 1979.

58. Schag CC, Heinrich RL, Ganz PA: Karnofsky Performance Status revisited: Reliability, validity and guidelines. J Clin Oncol 2:187–193, 1984.

59. Anderson JP, Bush JW, Berry CC: Classifying function for health outcome and quality-of-life evaluation: Self versus interviewer modes. Med Care 24:454–470, 1986.

60. Spilker B: Definitions and conceptual issues. In Quality of Life Assessments in Clinical Trials. New York, Raven Press, 1990, p 20.

61. Terrell JE, Welsh DE, Bradford CR, et al: Pain, quality of life, and spinal accessory nerve status after neck dissection. Laryngoscope 110:620–626, 2000.

62. Rogers SN, Hannah L, Lowe D, et al: Quality of life 5–10 years after primary surgery for oral and oro-pharyngeal cancer. J Craniomaxillofac Surg 27:187–191, 1999.

63. Ganz PA, Haskell CM, Figlin RA, et al: Estimating the quality of life in a clinical trial of patients with metastatic lung cancer using the Karnofsky Performance Status and the Functional Living Index—Cancer. Cancer 61:849–856, 1988.

64. Spilker B: Chronic rheumatic disease. In Quality of Life Assessments in Clinical Trials. New York, Raven Press, 1990, p 451.

65. Deleyiannis FW-B, Weymuller EA Jr, Coltrera MD, et al: Quality of life after laryngectomy: Are functional disabilities important? Head Neck 21:319–324, 1999.

66. Nunnally JC: Psychometric theory. New York, McGraw-Hill, 1978.

67. Selby PJ, Chapman JAW, Etazadi-Amoli J, et al: The development of a method for assessing the quality of life of cancer patients. Br J Cancer 50:13–22, 1984.

68. Kramer MS, Feinstein AR: Clinical biostatistics: LIV. The biostatistics of concordance. Clin Pharmacol Ther 29:111–123, 1981.

69. Landis RJ, Koch GG: The measurement of observer agreement for categorical data. Biometrics 33:159–174, 1977.

70. Zubrod CG, Schneiderman M, Frei E, et al: Appraisal of methods for the study of chemotherapy of cancer in man: Comparative therapeutic trial of nitrogen mustards and triethylene thiophosphoramide. J Chron Dis 11:7–33, 1960.

71. American Joint Committee (AJC) on Cancer: Manual for Staging of Cancer, 4th ed. Philadelphia, Lippincott, 1992.

72. Spitzer WO, Dobson AJ, Hall J, et al: Measuring the quality of life of cancer patients: A concise QL index for use by physicians. J Chron Dis 34:585–597, 1981.

73. List MA, Ritter-Sterr C, Lansky SB: A performance status scale for head and neck cancer patients. Cancer 66:564–569, 1990.

74. Weymuller EA Jr, Alsarraf R, Yueh B, et al: Analysis of the performance characteristics of the UW QOL and modification of the instrument. Arch Otolaryngol Head Neck Surg 127:489–493, 2001.

75. Rogers SN, Gwanne S, Lowe D, et al: The addition of mood and anxiety domains to the University of Washington quality of life scale (UW-QOL R). Head Neck (in press).

76. Terrell JE, Nanavati KA, Esclamado RM, et al: Head and neck cancer—specific quality of life instrument validation. Arch Otolaryngol Head Neck Surg 123:1125–1132, 1997.

77. Jones E, Lund VJ, Howard DJ, et al: Quality of life of patients treated surgically for head and neck cancer. J Laryngol Otol 106:238–242, 1992.

78. McNeil BJ, Weichselbaum R, Pauker SG: Speech and survival tradeoffs between quality and quantity of life in laryngeal cancer. N Engl J Med 305:982–987, 1981.

79. Harwood AR, Rawlinson E: The quality of life of patients following treatment for laryngeal cancer. Int J Radiat Oncol Biol Phys 9:335–338, 1983.

80. Llewellyn-Thomas HA, Sutherland HJ, Hogg SA, et al: Linear analogue self-assessment of voice quality in laryngeal cancer. J Chron Dis 37:917–924, 1984.

81. Karim ABMF, Kralendonk JH, Njo KH, et al: Radiation therapy for advanced (T3T4N0-N3M0) laryngeal carcinoma: The need for a change of strategy: A radiotherapeutic viewpoint. Int J Radiat Oncol Biol Phys 13:1625–1633, 1987.

82. Weiss MH: Head and neck cancer and the quality of life (Editorial). Otolaryngol Head Neck Surg 108:311–312, 1993.

83. Ackerstaff AH, Hilgers FJM, Aaronson NK, et al: Improvements in respiratory and psychosocial functioning following total laryngectomy by the use of a heat and moisture exchanger. Ann Otol Rhinol Laryngol 102:878–883, 1993.

84. The Department of Veterans Affairs Laryngeal Cancer Study Group: Induction chemotherapy plus radiation in patients with advanced laryngeal cancer. N Engl J Med 324:1685–1690, 1991.

85. Rockley TR, Robin PE, Powell J, et al: Primary treatment of cancer of the larynx. J Laryngol Otol 105:459–462, 1991.

86. Terrell JE, Fisher SG, Wolf GT: Long-term quality of life after treatment of laryngeal cancer. Arch Otolaryngol Head Neck Surg 124:964–971, 1998.

87. deGraeff A, deLeeuw JRJ, Ros WJG, et al: Pretreatment factors predicting quality of life after treatment for head and neck cancer. Head Neck 22:398–407, 2000.

88. Harrison LB, Zelefsky MJ, Sessions RB, et al: Base-of-tongue cancer treated with external beam irradiation plus brachytherapy: Oncologic and functional outcome. Radiology 184:267–270, 1992.

89. Harrison LB, Zelefsky MJ, Armstrong JG, et al: Quality of life after treatment for squamous cell cancer of the base of tongue—A comparison of primary radiation therapy versus primary surgery. Presented at the 33rd Annual Meeting of The American Society of Therapeutic Radiology and Oncology, New Orleans, 1993.

90. Larson DL, Lindberg RD, Lane E, et al: Major complications of radiotherapy in cancer of the oral cavity and oropharynx: A 10 year retrospective study. Am J Surg 146:531–536, 1983.

91. Deleyiannis FW-B, Weymuller EA Jr, Coltrera MD: Quality of life of disease-free survivors of advanced (stage III or IV) oropharyngeal cancer. Head Neck 19:466–473, 1997.
92. Forastiere AA: Cisplatin and radiotherapy in the management of locally advanced head and neck cancer. Int J Radiat Oncol Biol Phys 27:465–470, 1993.
93. Shirinian MH, Weber RS, Lippman SM, et al: Laryngeal preservation by induction chemotherapy plus radiotherapy in locally advanced head and neck cancer: The M.D. Anderson Cancer Center experience. Head Neck 16:39–44, 1994.
94. Urba SG, Forastiere AA, Wolf GT, et al: Intensive induction chemotherapy and radiation for organ preservation in patients with advanced resectable head and neck carcinoma. J Clin Oncol 12:946–953, 1994.
95. Coates AC, Gebski V, Stat M, et al: Improving the quality of life during chemotherapy for advanced breast cancer: A comparison of intermittent and continuous treatment strategies. N Engl J Med 317:1490–1495, 1987.
96. Velanovich V: Choice of treatment for stage I floor-of-mouth cancer: A decision analysis. Arch Otolaryngol Head Neck Surg 116:951–956, 1990.
97. Teichgraeber J, Bowman J, Goepfert H: New test series for the functional evaluation of oral cavity cancer. Head Neck Surg 8:9–20, 1985.
98. McConnel FMS, Teichgraeber JF, Alder RK: A comparison of three methods of oral reconstruction. Arch Otolaryngol Head Neck Surg 113:496–500, 1987.
99. Komisar A, Warman S, Danziger E: A critical analysis of immediate and delayed mandibular reconstruction using A-O plates. Arch Otolaryngol Head Neck Surg 115:830–833, 1989.
100. Komisar A: The functional result of mandibular reconstruction. Laryngoscope 100:364–374, 1990.
101. Urken ML, Buchbinder D, Weinberg H, et al: Functional evaluation following microvascular oromandibular reconstruction of the oral cancer patient: A comparative study of reconstructed and nonreconstructed patients. Laryngoscope 101:935–950, 1991.
102. Urken ML, Weinberg H, Buchbinder D, et al: Microvascular free flaps in head and neck reconstruction. Report of 200 cases and review of complications. Arch Otolaryngol Head Neck Surg 120:633–640, 1994.
103. Kuntz AL, Weymuller EA Jr: The impact of neck dissection on quality of life. Laryngoscope 109:1334–1338, 1999.
104. Brown JS, Zuydam AC, Jones DC, et al: Functional outcome in soft palate reconstruction using a radial forearm free flap in conjunction with a superiorly based pharyngeal flap. Head Neck 19:524–534, 1997.
105. Hammerlid E, Persson LO, Sullivan M, et al: Quality-of-life effects of psychosocial intervention in patients with head and neck cancer. Otolaryngol Head Neck Surg 120:507–516, 1999.
106. D'Antonio LL, Long SA, Zimmerman GJ, et al: Relationship between quality of life and depression in patients with head and neck cancer. Laryngoscope 108:806–811, 1998.
107. Deleyiannis FW-B, Thomas DB, Vaughan TL, et al: Alcoholism: Independent predictor of survival in patients with head and neck cancer. J Natl Cancer Inst 88:542–549, 1996.
108. McDonough EM, Boyd JH, Varvares MA, et al: Relationship between psychological status and compliance in a sample of patients treated for cancer of the head and neck. Head Neck 18:269–276, 1996.
109. Bjordal K, Ahlner-Elmqvist M, Hammerlid E, et al: A prospective study of quality of life in head and neck cancer patients. Part II: Longitudinal data. Laryngoscope (in press).
110. Schipper H, Levitt M: Measuring quality of life: Risks and benefits. Cancer Treat Rep 69:1115–1123, 1985.
111. Feinstein AR: An additional basic science for clinical medicine: I. The constraining fundamental paradigms. Ann Intern Med 99:393–397, 1983.
112. Schwartz S, Patrick DL, Yueh B: Quality-of-life outcomes in the evaluation of head and neck cancer treatments. Arch Otolaryngol Head Neck Surg 127:673–678, 2001.
113. Hadorn DC: Setting health care priorities in Oregon: Cost-effectiveness meets the rule of rescue. JAMA 265:2218–2225, 1991.
114. Morton RP: Quality of life: Current status and future directions. In Shah JP, Patel SG (eds): Head and Neck Cancer, vol IV. Lewiston, NY, BC Decker, 2001, pp 119–125.

Name: _____

Date: _____

University of Washington Quality of Life Questionnaire (UW-QOL)

This questionnaire asks about your health and quality of life **over the past seven days**. Please answer all of the questions by checking one box for each question.

1. **Pain**. (Check one box: ☑)
   - ☐ I have no pain.
   - ☐ There is mild pain not needing medication.
   - ☐ I have moderate pain—requires regular medication (codeine or nonnarcotic).
   - ☐ I have severe pain controlled only by narcotics.
   - ☐ I have severe pain, not controlled by medication.

2. **Appearance**. (Check one box: ☑)
   - ☐ There is no change in my appearance.
   - ☐ The change in my appearance is minor.
   - ☐ My appearance bothers me but I remain active.
   - ☐ I feel significantly disfigured and limit my activities due to my appearance.
   - ☐ I cannot be with people due to my appearance.

3. **Activity**. (Check one box: ☑)
   - ☐ I am as active as I have ever been.
   - ☐ There are times when I can't keep up my old pace, but not often.
   - ☐ I am often tired and have slowed down my activities although I still get out.
   - ☐ I don't go out because I don't have the strength.
   - ☐ I am usually in bed or chair and don't leave home.

4. **Recreation**. (Check one box: ☑)
   - ☐ There are no limitations to recreation at home or away from home.
   - ☐ There are a few things I can't do but I still get out and enjoy life.
   - ☐ There are many times when I wish I could get out more, but I'm not up to it.
   - ☐ There are severe limitations to what I can do, mostly I stay at home and watch TV.
   - ☐ I can't do anything enjoyable.

5. **Swallowing**. (Check one box: ☑)
   - ☐ I can swallow as well as ever.
   - ☐ I cannot swallow certain solid foods.
   - ☐ I can only swallow liquid food.
   - ☐ I cannot swallow because it "goes down the wrong way" and chokes me.

6. **Chewing**. (Check one box: ☑)
   - ☐ I can chew as well as ever.
   - ☐ I can eat soft solids but cannot chew some foods.
   - ☐ I cannot even chew soft solids.

7. **Speech**. (Check one box: ☑)
   - ☐ My speech is the same as always.
   - ☐ I have difficulty saying some words but I can be understood over the phone.
   - ☐ Only my family and friends can understand me.
   - ☐ I cannot be understood.

8. **Shoulder**. (Check one box: ☑)
   - ☐ I have no problem with my shoulder.
   - ☐ My shoulder is stiff but it has not affected my activity or strength.
   - ☐ Pain or weakness in my shoulder has caused me to change my work.
   - ☐ I cannot work due to problems with my shoulder.

9. **Taste**. (Check one box: ☑)
   - ☐ I can taste food normally.
   - ☐ I can taste most foods normally.
   - ☐ I can taste some foods.
   - ☐ I cannot taste any foods.

10. **Saliva**. (Check one box: ☑)
    ☐ My saliva is of normal consistency.
    ☐ I have less saliva than normal, but it is enough.
    ☐ I have too little saliva.
    ☐ I have no saliva.

11. **Mood**. (Check one box: ☑)
    ☐ My mood is excellent and unaffected by my cancer.
    ☐ My mood is generally good and only occasionally affected by my cancer.
    ☐ I am neither in a good mood nor depressed about my cancer.
    ☐ I am somewhat depressed about my cancer.
    ☐ I am extremely depressed about my cancer.

12. **Anxiety**. (Check one box: ☑)
    ☐ I am not anxious about my cancer.
    ☐ I am a little anxious about my cancer.
    ☐ I am anxious about my cancer.
    ☐ I am very anxious about my cancer.

Which issues have been the most important to you <u>during the past 7 days?</u>
Check ☑ up to 3 boxes.
☐ Pain	☐ Swallowing	☐ Taste
☐ Appearance	☐ Chewing	☐ Saliva
☐ Activity	☐ Speech	☐ Mood
☐ Recreation	☐ Shoulder	☐ Anxiety

GENERAL QUESTIONS

Compared to the month before you developed cancer, how would you rate your health-related quality of life? (check one box: ☑)
☐ Much better
☐ Somewhat better
☐ About the same
☐ Somewhat worse
☐ Much worse

In general, would you say your **health-related quality of life** <u>during the past 7 days</u> has been: (check one box: ☑)
☐ Outstanding
☐ Very good
☐ Good
☐ Fair
☐ Poor
☐ Very poor

Overall quality of life includes not only physical and mental health, but also many other factors, such as family, friends, spirituality, or personal leisure activities that are important to your enjoyment of life. Considering everything in your life that contributes to your personal well-being, rate your **overall quality of life** <u>during the past 7 days.</u> (check one box: ☑)
☐ Outstanding
☐ Very good
☐ Good
☐ Fair
☐ Poor
☐ Very poor

Please describe any other issues (medical or nonmedical) that are important to your quality of life and have not been adequately addressed by our questions (you may attach additional sheets if needed).

Index

Note: Page numbers followed by the letter f refer to figures; page numbers followed by the letter t refer to tables.